contents in brief

THIRD EDITION

MATERNITY
NURSING

Care of the Childbearing Family

Laurie N. Sherwen, PhD, RN, FAAN
Professor and Dean
School of Nursing
The College of New Jersey
Ewing, New Jersey

Mary Ann Scoloveno, EdD, PNP, RN
Associate Professor
Rutgers, The State University of New Jersey
College of Nursing
Newark, New Jersey

Carol Toussie Weingarten, PhD, RN
Associate Professor
College of Nursing
Villanova University
Villanova, Pennsylvania

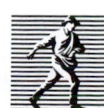

APPLETON & LANGE
Stamford, Connecticut

www.appletonlange.com

99 00 01 02 03/ 10 9 8 7 6 5 4 3 2 1

Prentice Hall International (UK) Limited, *London*
Prentice Hall of Australia Pty. Limited, *Sydney*
Prentice Hall Canada, Inc., *Toronto*
Prentice Hall Hispanoamericana, S.A., *Mexico*
Prentice Hall of India Private Limited, *New Delhi*
Prentice Hall of Japan, Inc., *Tokyo*
Simon & Schuster Asia Pte. Ltd., *Singapore*
Editora Prentice Hall do Brasil Ltda., *Rio de Janeiro*
Prentice Hall, *Upper Saddle River, New Jersey*

Library of Congress Cataloging-in-Publication Data
Sherwen, Laurie Nehls, 1947–
    Maternity nursing : care of the childbearing family / Laurie N.
Sherwen, Mary Ann Scoloveno, Carol Toussie Weingarten. — 3rd ed.
        p.   cm.
    Rev. ed. of: Nursing care of the childbearing family / Laurie N.
Sherwen, Mary Ann Scoloveno, Carol Toussie Weingarten. 2nd ed.
© 1995.
    Includes bibliographical references and index.
    ISBN 0-8385-7083-6 (case : alk. paper)
    1. Maternity nursing.   2. Family nursing.   I. Scoloveno, Mary
Ann.   II. Toussie Weingarten, Carol, 1949– .   III. Sherwen, Laurie
Nehls, 1947– . Nursing care of the childbearing family.   IV. Title.
    [DNLM: 1. Maternal–Child Nursing.   2. Obstetrical Nursing.
3. Patient Care Planning nurses' instruction.   4. Pediatric Nursing.
5. Perinatology nurses' instruction.   6. Pregnancy nurses'
instruction.   WY 157.3S554m 1999]
RG951.S473   1999
610.73'678—dc21
DNLM/DLC
for Library of Congress   98-31091

Editor-in-Chief, Nursing: Sally J. Barhydt
Acquisitions Editor: Nancy Anselment
Development Editor: Janet Foltin
Production Service: York Production Services
Associate Art Manager: Maggie Belis Darrow
Designer: Mary Skudlarek
Illustrators: Barbara Cousins; Network Graphics
Cover photo: See page 1019

PRINTED IN THE UNITED STATES OF AMERICA

ISBN 0-8385-7083-6
90000
9 780838 570838

To my mother and father, Marjory and William Nehls, and to
Nancy, Bill, and David, my sister and brothers . . .
I thoroughly enjoyed growing up in our family,
To my students, faculty, and colleagues . . .
for all that you have taught me about being a leader,
And, of course, to my husband and friend, Doug . . .
who never loses faith in me and what I can accomplish.

Laurie Nehls Sherwen

To my husband Red . . .
after all these years,
To my children, Bobby, Maria, Michael, and his girlfriend Maria . . .
for their unending love and support,
To my mother and in memory of my father . . .
who taught me the meaning of love,
To my old friends Jane and Judy . . .
who always make me feel special
(when we grow old, we will wear purple),
And a special tribute to my joy, Alex . . .
who makes it wonderful to move up a generation.

Mary Ann Scoloveno

To Michael . . .
my husband and soul-mate for all time,
To "Mamacita," Gladys Toussie Markuson . . .
my mother, first role model, and inspiration,
To Jeanne Toussie Jacobwitz . . .
sister, pal, and colleague throughout our lives,
To Benita Goldin Ross . . .
who is like a sister to me,
And to Sandra Myers Gomberg, Evelyn Krosnick, Jacqueline Smith Mileto,
Monique Raphel High Pesta, and Pamela DeShields Young . . .
whose friendship means more than words can express.

Carol Toussie Weingarten

To nursing students, Robert L. Scoloveno, Jr., and Robin M. Weingarten . . .
with great joy we have watched you grow and choose to follow your own careers in nursing.
To you and to all nursing students, our love and hopes for the future of our profession.

Laurie Nehls Sherwen
Mary Ann Scoloveno
Carol Toussie Weingarten

contents

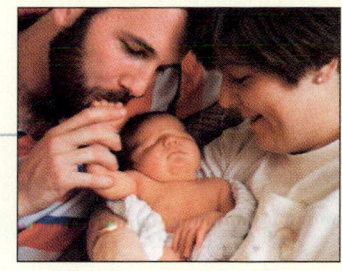

PART ONE
THE CHILDBEARING FAMILY

PART TWO
PREPARING FOR PREGNANCY AND BIRTH

PART THREE
PREGNANCY

PART FOUR
BIRTH

PART FIVE
THE POSTPARTUM PERIOD

contributors

Donna M. Barry, RN, MSN, NPC
Instructor
School of Nursing
Muhlenberg Regional Medical Center
Plainfield, New Jersey
Chapter 19

Barbara L. Cannella, RNC, MS, CNS
Instructor
College of Nursing
Rutgers, The State University of New Jersey
Newark, New Jersey
Chapters 20 and 24

Marcia Cauley Costello, PhD, RD
Assistant Professor
College of Nursing
Villanova University
Villanova, Pennsylvania
Chapters 14 and 31

Sandra L. Gomberg, MSN, RN
Chief Operating Officer
Temple University Children's Medical Center
Philadelphia, Pennsylvania
Chapter 34

Claire E. Lindberg, PhD, RN, CNSc, NPC
Assistant Professor
College of Nursing
Seton Hall University
South Orange, New Jersey
          and
Nurse Practitioner
Health and Wellness Center
Montclair State University
Upper Montclair, New Jersey
Chapter 7

Linda G. McClellan, RNC, MSN
Educator for Women's and Infants' Care
Allegheny University Hospital–City Avenue
Philadelphia, Pennsylvania
High-Risk Newborn Consultant

Carol Millan, RNC, MS
Instructor
School of Nursing
Muhlenberg Regional Medical Center
Plainfield, New Jersey
Chapter 19

Karen H. Morin, DSN, RN
Professor
School of Nursing
Widener University
Chester, Pennsylvania
Chapter 8

Patricia A. Mynaugh, PhD, RN
Associate Professor
College of Nursing
Villanova University
Villanova, Pennsylvania
Chapter 23

Geraldine O'Hare, MSN, CRNP
Certified Registered Nurse Practitioner
The Children's Hospital of Philadelphia
Primary Care Center at Cobbs Creek
Philadelphia, Pennsylvania
Chapter 30

Ellen Shuzman, PhD, RNC, MSN
Director of Education and Development
Perinatal Clinical Specialist
St. Peter's Medical Center
New Brunswick, New Jersey
Chapter 28

▶ Contributors to the Second Edition

Mary Ann Best, PhD, RN

Kathleen D. Black, RNC, MSN

Denise H. Braun, MSN, RN, FACCE

Wendy C. Budin, MSN, RNC

Pamela S. Chally, PhD, MN, RN

Nancy Collis-Mele, RNC, MSN

Susan K. Fabry, MS, PNP, CS, RN

Judy Custer Garbinski, MNEd, RN

Renee Helm Gosselin, MSN, RN

Cynthia B. Hughes, EdD, RNC, PNP

Barbara S. Kiernan, MSN, PNP, CS, RN

Donna G. Knauth, MS, RNC

Charlotte Koehler, MN, CCE, IBCLC

Joanne MacKenzie, MScN, RN

Cathy Kahn Recht, MS, RN

Caryle G. Wolahan, EdD, RN, FAAN

reviewers and consultants

Elizabeth W. Black, MSN, RN, CNS
Assistant Professor, Nursing
Gwynedd-Mercy College
Gwynedd Valley, Pennsylvania

Barbara L. Cannella, RNC, MS, CNS
Instructor
College of Nursing
Rutgers, The State University of New Jersey
Newark, New Jersey

Donna Costello-Nickitas, PhD, RN
Associate Professor
Hunter-Bellevue School of Nursing
Hunter College–City University of New York
New York, New York

Geri Diemer, PhD, RN
Clinical Professor
School of Nursing
University of Wisconsin–Madison
Madison, Wisconsin

Rosemarie F. DiLandro, MS, RNC, NP
Women's Health Nurse Practitioner
Planned Parenthood of Suffolk County, Inc.
Smithtown, New York

David E. Jacobwitz, MD, FACOG
Morristown OB-GYN Associates, PA
Morristown, New Jersey

Jeanne Toussie Jacobwitz, CNM, MSN, MPH
Formerly Director, Nurse Midwifery Services
Robert Wood Johnson University Hospital
New Brunswick, New Jersey

Susan Jay, PhD, RN
Director of Neonatal Nurse Practitioner Program
School of Nursing
East Carolina University
Greenville, North Carolina

Amy Levi, CNM, PhD(cand.)
Director, Claire Lintilhac Nurse Midwifery Service
Fletcher Allen Health Care
Burlington, Vermont

Ruth Marcott, PhD, RN
Associate Professor
School of Nursing
University of Texas
Galveston, Texas

Linda G. McClellan, RNC, MSN
Educator for Women's and Infants' Care
Allegheny University Hospital–City Avenue
Philadelphia, Pennsylvania

Alice Obrig, MS, MPH, EdD
Assistant Professor
School of Nursing
Fairfield University
Fairfield, Connecticut

Linda C. Pugh, PhD, RNC
Director of Professional Education Programs and
    Associate Professor
School of Nursing
Johns Hopkins University
Baltimore, Maryland

Sheila Rock, MSN, RN
Course Coordinator Emeritus
College of Nursing
University of Illinois at Chicago
Chicago, Illinois

Karen D. Springer, MS, CNM
Assistant Professor
The University of Texas School of Nursing
Galveston, Texas

Michael S. Weingarten, MD, MBA, FACS
Chief, Division of Vascular Surgery
Crozer-Chester Medical Center
Upland, Pennsylvania
          and
Clinical Associate Professor of Surgery
School of Medicine
University of Pennsylvania
Philadelphia, Pennsylvania

preface

In caring for the childbearing family, nurses share in life's most profound and poignant moments. *Maternity Nursing: Care of the Childbearing Family*, third edition, provides a foundation for nursing students and for nurses caring for families during the reproductive years. The book focuses on the family and spans topics ranging from women's health issues to childbearing and care of the newborn and infant in both low- and high-risk situations. The family-centered approach to the content, the scope of each chapter, the color illustrations and photographs, and accompanying pedagogy are designed to promote excellence in clinical practice. Clinical reasoning and critical thinking are emphasized, as diagnostic, ethical, and therapeutic decision making are integrated throughout the book. This textbook is also designed to foster awareness and application of research related to parent–newborn health, to stimulate consideration of ethical issues relating to childbearing, and to promote appreciation for culturally sensitive nursing care based on the unique needs of each family.

Scientific advances continue to influence obstetric and neonatal technology; however, technology provides tools to use judiciously. Although technologic advances are discussed throughout the textbook, nurses are challenged to consider their risks, as well as benefits, and to use technology thoughtfully and appropriately.

Care of the childbearing family is too complex for any one discipline. For this reason, an interdisciplinary focus and collaborative aspects of care are integrated throughout the textbook, along with unique nursing implications. Effective health care requires collaboration among nurses, other health care providers, family members, and members of the broader community.

▶ Organization Around Wellness, Risk, and Alternative Care Settings

Childbearing is a low-risk experience for most families, although some families are regarded as high risk due to real or potential problems. Many health care providers specialize in wellness care during childbearing, and some specialize in high-risk care. Students as well as practitioners need easy access to information on both low- and high-risk conditions. In addition, families are cared for in many environments, including hospitals or birthing centers, ambulatory care clinics, and homes. Consequently, the third edition of *Maternity Nursing: Care of the Childbearing Family* provides an integrated perspective on the current nature of childbearing. This book focuses on wellness and the healthy aspects of childbearing, high-risk conditions related to childbearing, and community-based as well as hospital-based care during childbearing. Five broad themes are developed within the book: The Childbearing Family (trends and issues); Preparing for Pregnancy and Birth; Pregnancy; Birth; and The Postpartum Period (which includes the newborn period). Chapters in each part include low- and high-risk considerations and settings for childbearing.

Chapters 1 through 4 outline the current status of parent–newborn health care; perinatal health and high-risk health care; clinical reasoning; and family and pregnancy-related theories. Chapters 5 through 7 discuss issues related to preconceptional health, such as human sexuality, human reproduction, and women's health. An understanding of these areas is vital to the care of the childbearing family. In addition, specific issues that women currently face as they strive for healthy outcomes for themselves and their families are highlighted throughout the book.

Chapters 8 and 9 concern issues involved in planning a family and the educational preparation a family needs throughout the childbearing cycle. Chapters 10 through 12 address high-risk aspects of pregnancy and birth with discussions of reproductive risks, age-related concerns during pregnancy, and psychosocial concerns of high-risk childbearing families.

Discussion of the pregnancy experience begins with an overview of the growth and development of the embryo and fetus (Chapter 13) and details the important role of nutrition during childbearing (Chapter 14). Pregnancy entails continual change; however, early, middle, and late pregnancy have specific characteristics. Traditionally, pregnancy is described by trimester. From our years in clinical nursing education, we have found that students consistently have difficulty caring for clients during different trimesters when content is presented only as pregnancy. To deliver optimal nursing care in any one trimester, students must understand the pregnant woman and her family at that particular time. Therefore, we have again, as in our first and second editions, taken a holistic, although more streamlined, trimester approach in Chapters 15 through 19. In this edition, however, chapters about care of the low-risk pregnant woman and family during each trimester are now followed by chapters about care of the high-risk client so that students may understand the continuum of health and illness as it relates to specific phases of pregnancy. These chapters have been extensively revised and reorganized to avoid repetition and to focus specifically on the unique aspects of assessment and care required during each trimester. Chapter 20 concludes this part with a discussion about community-based nursing during pregnancy.

Chapters 21 through 27 discuss the intrapartum period and continue the nursing process format with specific chapters focusing on physiologic and psychologic changes, assessment, and nursing care during this phase of the childbearing cycle. Both low- and high-risk aspects of the intrapartum period are explored. Chapters 21, 22, and 24 present care of the low-risk intrapartum client. Chapter 23 concerns managing pain during childbirth, an issue relevant to both low- and high-risk women. The care of the family at risk during birth is the focus of Chapter 25, and the cesarean birth experience is discussed in Chapter 26. Finally, Chapter 27, new to this edition, examines birthing in community-based settings.

Chapters 28 through 33 deal with both low- and high-risk aspects of care of the postpartum woman and newborn. Postpartum and newborn nutrition is discussed in Chapter 31 and, in Chapter 33, specific attention is given to the low-birth-weight infant, a major health care issue in the United States. Chapter 34, a new chapter that concludes the book, examines community-based nursing during the postpartum and newborn periods.

► Learning Aids

The chapters in this new edition have been carefully developed and updated to promote learning and review of information. Each chapter begins with a vignette that explores an issue discussed in the chapter. (Please note that the names of the people in the photos that appear with the vignettes have been changed to protect their privacy.) Key terms are in boldfaced type throughout the text. Chapter Highlights aid review of important points discussed in each chapter. Critical Thinking Questions at the ends of the chapters encourage students to apply the information learned from the chapters to the vignettes at the beginning of the chapters. Current references focus on practice and research resources. A glossary of key terms appears at the end of the book.

Other features are incorporated to enhance learning:

- Five chapters present the ideas and beliefs of different cultural groups relating to health care practices and approaches to childbearing: African-American (Chapter 15); East Asian, with particular focus on the Japanese-American family (Chapter 17); Chicano (Chapter 18); Puerto Rican (Chapter 22); and American Indian (Chapter 28).
- Color photographs and illustrations have been designed to illustrate specific teaching points and to portray the human aspects of nursing care.
- Numerous tables and boxes summarize and highlight key points within the chapters.
- Women's Health features highlight issues that are of special importance to women, such as social trends, sexuality, health problems, violence against women, substance abuse, family planning, infertility, and genetic counseling.
- Research Abstracts are presented as clinically focused discussions of relevant nursing research studies that consist of succinct descriptions of the actual studies and sections entitled Application to Practice that help students apply the results of the research to the concepts presented in the chapters. Research is integrated throughout the book; the abstracts reinforce the importance of nursing research in parent–newborn nursing.

- Nursing Alerts highlight life-threatening and/or extremely important information about specific maternal and fetal/newborn conditions.
- Ethical Decision Making features examine the ethical implications of specific issues related to childbearing through statement of the issues and questions posed to students for their consideration.
- Client Teaching features present strategies that nurses can use to educate clients about various aspects of pregnancy, labor and delivery, and the postpartum and newborn periods.
- Commonly Asked Questions provide examples of questions that clients may ask about specific aspects of childbearing
- Critical Thinking in Care Planning features incorporate case studies and plans of care that are presented in terms of assessment, nursing diagnosis, expected client and family outcomes, nursing action/intervention with rationales, and evaluation.
- Three appendices that concern the transfer of drugs into human milk, standard laboratory values for childbearing women, and selected maternal–child health Internet sites are also included in the book.
- The comprehensive Index facilitates locating specific information in the book.

► Teaching–Learning Package

Several educational ancillaries enhance the scope of this textbook.

- A *Clinical Companion*, prepared by Mary Ann Scoloveno, EdD, PNP, RN, and packaged with the textbook, explores additional issues in the areas of women's health and community-based maternity nursing care and reinforces essential concepts relating to assessment and management of the childbearing family during pregnancy, labor and delivery, and the postpartum and newborn periods.

- An *Instructor's Manual*, written by Helen Van Hoozer, MA, supplements the text chapter-by-chapter and includes chapter synopses; key terms and phrases; learning outcomes; activities; available resources such as video series, CD-ROM, computer-assisted instruction, and written materials; "Quizits" to test and extend students' knowledge of chapter content and promote achievement of the learning outcomes; questions for research; and supplemental materials for use with the activities. The *Instructor's Manual* also includes the printed version of the *Computerized Testbank.*
- An updated *Computerized Testbank,* prepared by Barbara Cannella, RNC, MS, CNS, in an IBM format with NCLEX-type questions that tests learners' knowledge of essential chapter content.
- A *Review and Study Guide,* prepared by Elaine Zimbler, MA, RN, presents case studies, key terms, key concepts, and questions relating to the case studies for each chapter in the textbook. More than 100 NCLEX-type questions are included at the end of the guide to help students prepare for the NCLEX-RN.
- A set of four-color acetate *Transparencies,* selected from the textbook's illustrations, may be used for classroom instruction.

As practicing nurses, researchers, and educators, we are committed to family-centered care for all childbearing families. We believe that nurses have a crucial role in ensuring that compassionate, expert care be delivered to clients regardless of their risk or socioeconomic status. Today, as the health care delivery system is undergoing major change, the need has never been greater for nurses with creative solutions to health care dilemmas.

Laurie Nehls Sherwen
Mary Ann Scoloveno
Carol Toussie Weingarten

acknowledgments

During our preparation of the third edition of *Maternity Nursing: Care of the Childbearing Family,* some very special people generously shared their talents and time with us. Denise Braun, MS, RN, FACCE; Linda Carmen Copel, PhD, RN; Marcia Cauley Costello, PhD, RD; Christine Danser, MS, CNM; Ninetta Dickerson, RN, IBLC, MSN-NNP; David E. Jacobwitz, MD, FACOG; Jeanne Toussie Jacobwitz, CNM, MSN, MPH; Linda G. McClellan, RNC, MSN; Vincent C. Mileto, MD, FACOG; Donna Faust Patterson, PhD, RN, CRNP; Mary Anne Ritchie, PhD, RN; Michael E. Ross, MD, MBA; Hester M. Sonder, MD, FACOG; Alice Zal, DO; and H. Michael Zal, DO, FACN, always made time to answer our questions, no matter how basic or complex. We greatly appreciate the reference consultation so competently given by Louise Green, MLS, and Jacqueline H. Mirabile, MS in LS.

As practicing nurses, we have often been impressed with the creativity, competence, and compassion of colleagues. Our book has given us the chance to record some of these dimensions of care through original color photographs of staff in action in wellness and acute care settings. The photo opportunities for this book would not have been possible without help from Barbara Cannella, RNC, MS, CNS; Amy Levi, CNM, PhD(cand.); Denise Roy, MSN, CNM; Ellen Shuzman, PhD, RNC, MSN; and the staffs of St. Peter's Medical Center in New Brunswick, New Jersey, the West Philadelphia Community Center in Philadelphia, Pennsylvania, and The Birth Center in Bryn Mawr, Pennsylvania. Many of the wonderful photographs of nurses, families, and newborns were taken by photographer George D. Dodson, with additional photos provided by Mary Ann Scoloveno and Carol Toussie Weingarten. The descriptive and informative color illustrations were executed by Barbara Cousins and Network Graphics.

We are also grateful to the many clients who allowed us to share in the joy or, at times, the sorrow of their childbearing experiences. Their commitment to helping others by sharing their own situations was inspiring.

Writing the third edition of this major core textbook presented unique challenges, especially as we endeavored to restructure and tailor the book to meet the needs of nurses and nursing students at the start of the millenium. We are fortunate to have family and friends whose love and support have remained with us through the years of our work. We are especially grateful to Cassandra Barnett, MS, PNP; Nina Chianese, MS, RN; Nancy and Ian Clelland; Donald and Geysah DePalma; John and Rose DePalma; Michael and Kathleen DiChiara; Catherine Hill; Lauren and Marin Jacobwitz; Arthur Krosnick, MD; John Lewy, MD; Noreen Mahon, PhD, RN; Marty and Gladys (Toussie) Markuson; Georgia and William Nehls, Jr.; Lisa and David Nehls; Marjory and William Nehls; Maryann Rose, RN; Barry and Dena Ross; David A. Ross; Mitchell Ross, MD; Heather Sinclair Ross; Eileen Scarinici, MS, FNP; Dolores Scoloveno; Grace Sherwen; Patricia Sherwen; and Theresa M. Valiga, EdD, RN. We thank Maria and Robert Scoloveno, Jr. for preparing Appendix C.

Special thanks go to the excellent and committed staff at Appleton & Lange. They have become like a second family to us, particularly through the demands of this third edition. As with our second edition, Editor-in-Chief Sally Barhydt provided support, vision, and expert advice throughout the project. Maggie Darrow's expertise with the illustration program make this edition of the book exceptional. We especially acknowledge Janet Foltin, our developmental editor, for her competence, compassion, and collegiality. The quality of the book is a tribute to Janet's hard work. Words cannot express how deeply we respect and admire Janet.

Our students and colleagues at The College of New Jersey, Rutgers, The State University of New Jersey, and Villanova University continue to inspire us and provided invaluable insight as we worked on this edition. We also appreciate the many readers who have shared their thoughts with us through the years and who use our book in their work with childbearing families.

The three of us have known each other and worked on various projects together for over 20 years and have shared the growth and development of our own children and pets. What began as dreams of three young nurses has blossomed into lifelong friendship and professional collaboration. We know that among our readers will be classmates or colleagues who share hopes of publication and dare to see themselves as authors for the next generation. To you we offer our example, our encouragement, and the work of ourselves and our colleagues from which you will chart the future nursing care of the childbearing family.

Laurie Nehls Sherwen
Mary Ann Scoloveno
Carol Toussie Weingarten

guide to
key features

CHAPTER HIGHLIGHTS

Set of bulleted statements that highlight the essential topics presented in the chapter.

CHAPTER VIGNETTE AND CRITICAL THINKING QUESTIONS

Each chapter opens with a vignette related to the specific chapter content. At the end of the chapter, the student is asked to revisit the opening vignette in context with the concepts discussed in the chapter, and respond to critical thinking questions.

Chapter Highlights

- Educational preparation is a necessary part of prenatal care and involves the family.

- Nearly all pregnant clients who receive prenatal care have access to some type of educational program. Educational programs need to be accessible, affordable, culturally sensitive, well timed, and tailored to the learning needs of clients.

- Education for childbearing ideally should begin before conception so that lifestyle changes can be made and the couple can be helped to achieve maximum wellness.

- Education for childbearing may span the childbearing year or be done at individual prenatal visits or in one day.

- Educational preparation of the childbearing family focuses on the physiologic and psychologic needs of the family and addresses issues such as relaxation/stress reduction, self-care practices, and exercise.

- Prepared childbirth methods include psychophysical preparation, psychoprophylaxis, the LeBoyer method, the Bradley method, and hypnosis.

- Clients have several choices for childbirth attendants; e.g., physicians, certified nurse-midwives, certified midwives, and lay midwives.

- Choices for delivery settings include hospitals, free-standing birth centers, and the client's home. Most American women deliver in a hospital.

After reading the vignette at the beginning of this chapter, use what you have learned to answer these questions.

1. If you were the nurse supervising the Denglers' childbirth education class, how would you respond to Tamika's lack of confidence in her ability to concentrate on her breathing patterns?

2. What other questions might Tamika and Rashid have about preparation for labor and delivery?

3. Despite Tamika's worry about mastering breathing techniques, what benefits do you think this couple will receive from participating in a childbirth preparation program?

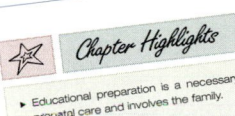

Critical Thinking Questions

Tamika and Rashid Dengler, who are 36 weeks pregnant, are attending a childbirth education class. As part of class activities, they are practicing patterned breathing for use in labor and delivery. Rashid helps Tamika to lie on the floor on her side; he kneels behind her and supports her back with a pillow. Tamika focuses her attention on her favorite bracelet, a gift from Rashid, and begins the breathing pattern. Rashid breathes with her. Tamika suddenly realizes she forgot to make two important phone calls. She abruptly stops the exercise. Rashid also stops and asks, "What happened?" Tamika sighs and states, "I don't know how I can concentrate on breathing when I have a million other thoughts running through my mind. Will I be able to do this when I really am in labor?" ■

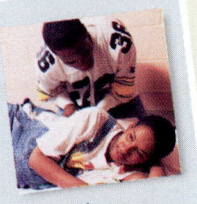

9

Educational Preparation for Childbirth

DRUG GUIDE
Helpful information on common drugs used in maternity care is highlighted.

▶ DRUG GUIDE: HEPARIN

ACTIONS/INDICATIONS

Inhibits thrombus and clot formation through the inactivation of thrombin and the potentiation of antithrombin III. Indicated for prophylaxis and treatment of various thromboembolic disorders, venous thrombosis, pulmonary embolism. Also treatment of atrial fibrillation with embolization, diagnosis and treatment of disseminated intravascular coagulation, and treatment of peripheral arterial embolism.

DOSAGE

Administered by IV infusion, intermittent IV injection, or deep SC injection for full-dose therapy and deep SC injection for low-dose therapy. *Full-dose therapy: IV infusion:* Initial bolus dose of 5000 U by direct IV, then 20,000 to 40,000 U in 1000 mL isotonic sodium chloride solution over 24 hours. *Intermittent IV injection:* Initial dose of 10,000 U followed by 5000 to 10,000 U every 4 to 6 hours. *Deep SC:* Initial dose of 10,000 to 20,000 U IV, usually preceded by bolus dose of 5000 U IV, then 8000 to 10,000 U every 8 hours or 15,000 to 20,000 U every 12 hours. Follow PTT (partial thromboplastin time) for adjustment of doses in all regimens. *Low-dose therapy:* 5000 U SC every 8 to 12 hours. *Disseminated intravascular coagulation:* 50 to 100 U/kg by IV infusion or IV injection every 4 hours. If no improvement after 4 to 8 hours, heparin therapy should be discontinued.

CONTRAINDICATIONS AND PRECAUTIONS

Hypersensitivity to pig or beef proteins. Use with caution in cases in which the risk of hemorrhage is increased, such as dissecting aneurysm; ulcerative GI lesions; diverticulitis; hemorrhagic blood dyscrasias; menstruation; ovulation; threatened abortion; subacute bacterial endocarditis; increased capillary permeability; arterial sclerosis; severe hypertension; renal, hepatic, or biliary disease; eye, brain, or

spinal cord surgery; continuous tube drainage from any orifice; and spinal tap or spinal anesthesia.

ADVERSE REACTIONS

Most common: minor bleeding. *Less common:* CV—major hemorrhage; hematologic—thrombocytopenia, localized or disseminated thromboses (white clot syndrome); GI—elevated liver enzymes; local reactions—with deep SC injection, local irritation, erythema, mild pain, hematoma, ulceration, or cutaneous and subcutaneous necrosis; other—hypersensitivity reactions, osteoporosis, and spontaneous fractures in clients receiving ≧10,000 U/day for 3 or more months.

DRUG INTERACTIONS

- Aspirin, nonsteroidal anti-inflammatory agents, dipyridamole: Inhibit platelet function and may increase risk of hemorrhage.
- Streptokinase, urokinase: May increase risk of bleeding.
- Dihydroergotamine: May potentiate antithrombogenic effects of heparin.
- IV nitroglycerin: May antagonize anticoagulant effect of heparin.
- Probenecid: Enhances the duration and intensity of effects produced by heparin.

NURSING IMPLICATIONS

- Assess blood coagulation studies. If not within therapeutic range, contact physician.
- Assess for signs of bleeding (e.g., epistaxis, blood in urine, ecchymosis).
- Observe needle sites for hematoma, swelling, heat, redness, and pain.
- Teach client and her partner the signs of hemorrhage and the rationale for the treatment.

vent subacute bacterial endocarditis at time of delivery in women with prosthetic heart valves or grafts. When the cervix is fully dilated and the fetus is engaged, prompt forceps delivery is indicated unless an easy, spontaneous vaginal delivery is imminent (Cunningham et al., 1997). Epidural anesthesia is preferred because it generally offers greater hemodynamic stability. However, hypotension is potentially lethal in the pregnant cardiac client, and great care must be taken to avoid it. Blood loss should be minimized. Fundal massage and intravenous oxytocin are suggested. Oxytocin should be administered slowly to avoid hypotension. Early ambulation reduces the increased risk for deep-vein thrombosis and thromboembolism in the postpartum period.

Although pregnancy in class III and IV heart disease is contraindicated, women markedly compromised may become pregnant and wish to continue the pregnancy. Management of these clients includes bedrest throughout the pregnancy. Hospitalization is usually required. The focus of care for women in cardiac failure (class IV) is medical rather than obstetric. Delivery for any woman in frank failure carries with it a high mortality rate.

▶ Nursing Diagnoses

Examples of nursing diagnoses for the client with heart disease are:

NURSING ALERT
Highlight life-threatening or extremely important information about specific maternal and fetal / newborn conditions.

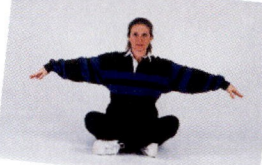

! Nursing Alert

A pregnant woman may acquire toxoplasmosis (an infection caused by the protozoan *Toxoplasma gondii*) through contact with infected cat feces or by eating raw or undercooked infected meat. To decrease or prevent infection, a pregnant woman should: avoid contact with the cat's litter box; have someone else clean the litter box (*T. gondii* mature within 24 hours of leaving the cat's body); wash hands well after contact with the cat; wear gloves for gardening and wash hands well (neighborhood cats often have access to home garden areas and *T. gondii* can survive actively in soil after feces decompose); and eat only well-cooked meat. Screening for toxoplasmosis antibodies may be done before pregnancy or at the first prenatal visit. Women should promptly report any flu-like symptoms to their health care providers.

flicts related to sexual desire during a culturally "taboo" period, lack interest, or be embarrassed regarding the pregnant shape (see Chapter 5).

Desire for physical closeness and expression of sexuality are normal and may be encouraged for the low-risk, healthy couple. To provide client teaching, the nurse needs to assess the couple's attitude toward sexuality, their cultural backgrounds, and their fears and concerns. Sexuality encompasses more than intercourse. Kissing, touching, and cuddling are also sexual expressions.

Bathing/Swimming. Bathing, swimming, and showering are allowed throughout pregnancy. Tub baths and swimming should be avoided after rupture of the membranes because of the possibility of infection. Women should avoid or be very careful taking tub baths late in pregnancy because their center of gravity has shifted, making them vulnerable to falls.

Exposure to very high temperatures, as in saunas or hot tubs, should be avoided because of the possible harmful effects on the fetus related to increased maternal body temperature.

Personal Hygiene. Daily showering controls odors related to sweating and normal vaginal secretions. Douching is not recommended for the pregnant woman.

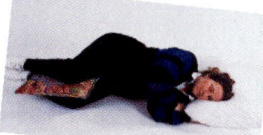

FIGURE 9–2. Resting position for a pregnant woman: lying on the left side with a pillow supporting the upper legs.

♀ Women's Health

Sexual intercourse between a pregnant woman and her partner is usually contraindicated in situations in which the woman has either uterine bleeding, rupture of the membranes, or strong uterine contractions after orgasm and in cases in which the woman has a history of premature labor or premature rupture of the membranes.

WOMEN'S HEALTH
Issues of special importance to women are highlighted and integrated throughout the text where most appropriate.

 ### Critical Thinking in Care Planning

Care of an Infant Experiencing Feeding Problems

Amy Hirschburg and her son Jason, 6 months old, visit the clinic for a six-month checkup. Amy reports that Jason has been very irritable lately and has not been sleeping through the night. She also reports that she has been "watering down" the formula lately to "make it last." Her husband Stephen has recently lost his new job as a city bus driver and

they have had difficulty in paying their bills and having enough money to buy food for the family. Jason's weight is 13.5 pounds and his height is 24.5 inches. This places him in the 10th percentile for weight and the 15th percentile for height. Income screening reveals that the family is eligible for WIC.

▶ Assessment

- 6-month-old male infant experiencing growth failure
- Weight: 13.5 lbs (10th percentile)
- Height: 24.5 in. (15th percentile)
- Mother reports "watering down" infant formula to "make it last"
- Mother reports lack of money for food or formula purchases
- Family is income eligible for WIC

Nursing Diagnosis

Altered nutrition, less than body requirements, related to infant's inadequate formula intake

Expected Client/Family Outcomes	Nursing Action/Intervention	Evaluation
By the end of the visit, the client will: • Identify how improper feeding can lead to infant growth failure.	Explain importance of preparing infant formula according to package directions. *Rationale:* Growth failure is due to insufficient kcal and nutrient intake.	Client provides return demonstration on correct preparation of formula and describes the effects of feeding diluted formula.
• Make appointment for enrollment in WIC.	Contact local WIC program for client referral. *Rationale:* Referral to WIC provides a means of obtaining necessary food in order to prevent further weight loss in infant.	Client reports that she has contacted WIC and is receiving benefits.
• Receive WIC vouchers for infant formula, infant cereal, and infant juice.	Review how WIC foods/formula can be integrated into meal plan. *Rationale:* Enrollment in WIC provides sufficient formula and infant food.	
• Work with the nurse in developing a healthy menu plan for the infant.	Develop a healthy meal schedule for infant. *Rationale:* Client and family benefits from a specific plan to follow.	Client describes menu plan and family's adherence to it.

CRITICAL THINKING IN CARE PLANNING
A case study is presented and a plan of care is developed based on that study. This allows the student to apply the nursing process to the childbearing experience.

► Chronic Hypertension

Hypertensive cardiovascular disease is marked by the formation of fatty deposits within the arterial walls. This increases vascular resistance to the flow of blood and increases the work of the heart. Tissue perfusion throughout the body is diminished as a result, and over a period of years all organs will be adversely affected. Hypertensive cardiovascular disease is a continued elevation of blood pressure of 140/90 or higher before pregnancy or before the 20th week of gestation in the absence of trophoblastic disease.

Many factors are associated with the development of hypertensive cardiovascular disease. Major factors include family history of hypertension, race (increased prevalence among African-Americans), a sedentary lifestyle, use of tobacco, excessive use of alcohol, obesity, a diet high in cholesterol and triglycerides, a stressful lifestyle and inappropriate means of coping, and a history of PIH. The client with chronic hypertension may have an underlying predisposing condition such as renal disease.

It is difficult to distinguish chronic hypertension from PIH, particularly in a woman who has not received early prenatal care. Because blood pressure may normally decrease in the first and second trimesters, blood pressure measurements for the woman with chronic hypertension may appear normal. Typically, as pregnancy progresses the blood pressure returns to its hypertensive state.

Nursing and Collaborative Assessment

Chronic hypertensive disease, in contrast to preeclampsia, is suggested by the observation of hemorrhages and exudates in the optic fundi; plasma creatinine concentrations greater than 1 mg/dL; plasma urea nitrogen concentrations greater than 20 mg/dL; and the presence of other predisposing chronic diseases such as diabetes, connective tissue disease, or renal disease.

Complications of chronic hypertension in pregnant women include abruptio placentae, intrauterine growth retardation, and superimposed preeclampsia.

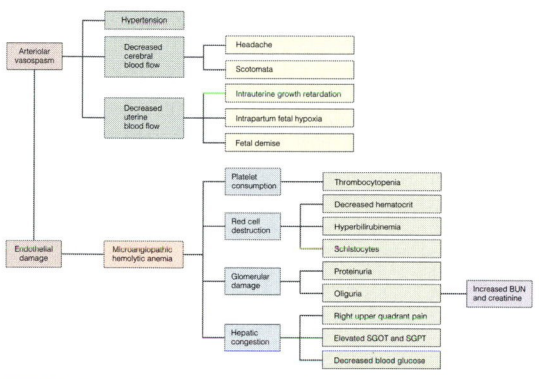

FIGURE 19–3. Physiologic alterations occurring in the HELLP syndrome. BUN: blood urea nitrogen; SGOT: serum glutamic-oxaloacetic transaminase; SGPT: serum glutamic-pyruvic transaminase. *(Reproduced, with permission, from Whittaker, A.A. et al. (1986). Hemolysis, elevated liver enzymes, and low platelet count syndrome. Nursing care of the critically ill obstetric patient. Heart and Lung 15:402–408.)*

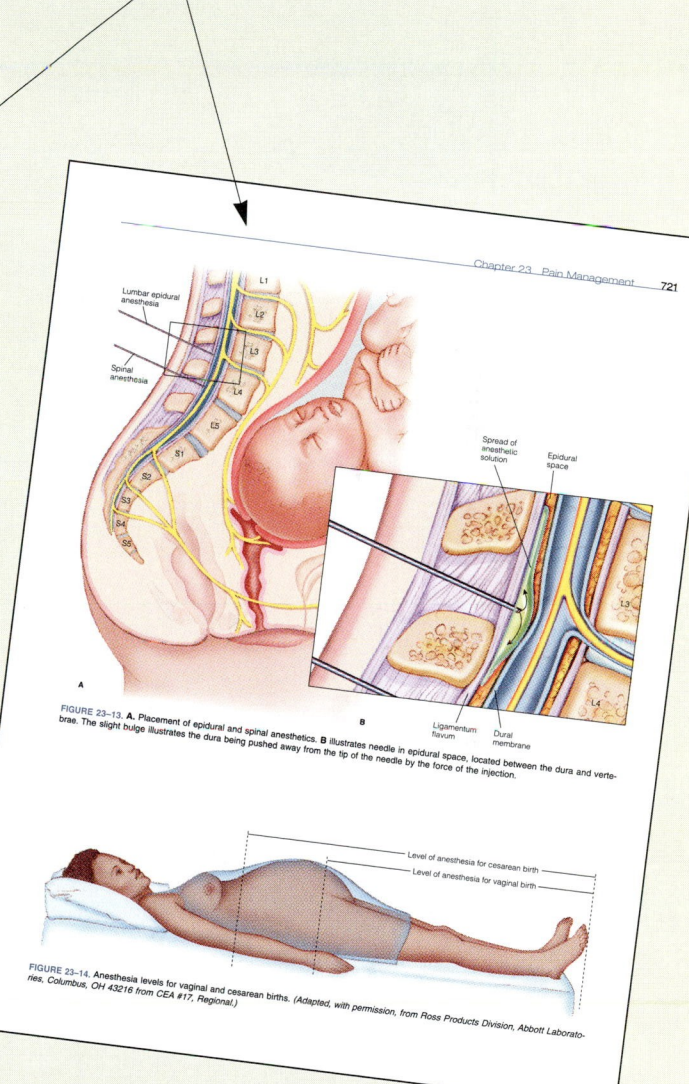

FIGURE 23–13. **A.** Placement of epidural and spinal anesthetics. **B** illustrates needle in epidural space, located between the dura and vertebrae. The slight bulge illustrates the dura being pushed away from the tip of the needle by the force of the injection.

FIGURE 23–14. Anesthesia levels for vaginal and cesarean births. *(Adapted, with permission, from Ross Products Division, Abbott Laboratories, Columbus, OH 43216 from CEA #17, Regional.)*

 Commonly Asked Questions

Menstruation

What is a normal menstrual period?

A normal menstrual period represents the shedding of the lining of the uterus. Menstrual flow includes blood, some endometrial tissue, white blood cells, and mucus.

How long should menstrual periods last?

There is considerable variation among the length of menstrual periods among women. Menstrual periods can last from 2 to 8 days.

How often does menstruation occur?

Although the menstrual cycle has traditionally been described as being about 28 days long, cycles vary greatly among women. Menstrual cycles also vary within the same woman by about 5 to 10 days. Menstruation reflects complex physical, psychologic, and environmental interactions, such factors as extreme weight loss, vigorous physical activity, and emotional stress can affect menstrual patterns.

How much blood is lost?

About 30 to 100 mL of blood is lost during menstruation. The amount of flow depends on factors like the thickness of the endometrium and certain medications.

Are clots abnormal?

Because of the presence of fibrinolysin, which breaks down clots, menstrual flow does not tend to clot. Clots may represent heavy bleeding related to a variety of pathologic causes. Clots also occur, however, in normal, healthy women. A study of hemoglobin or hematocrit should be routine at gynecologic visits and can indicate whether excessive bleeding is taking place during menstruation.

How much iron do women lose during menstruation?

Women can lose about 0.5 to 1 mg of iron daily in menstrual flow.

Should exercise be restricted during menstruation?

There is no reason why a woman cannot continue with her usual pattern of activities. Indeed, such exercises as brisk walking and tennis may promote feelings of well-being and reduce menstrual discomforts.

Should vaginal sprays or douches be used to prevent menstrual odor?

No. Despite vigorous advertising campaigns, vaginal sprays or douches should not be used by the healthy woman; these preparations can cause such problems as rashes, itching, and burning. Showering, bathing, or external cleansing with water or water and gentle soap, as well as regular changing of pads or tampons, is sufficient. Normal menstrual flow has a mild "fleshy" odor. Foul-smelling discharge could indicate abnormal conditions such as infection and should be reported to the health care provider without delay.

Can a woman get pregnant during her period?

Although the menstrual phase is the least fertile time during a woman's cycle, pregnancy could, in theory, occur. The graafian follicle begins to mature in the ovary while menstruation is taking place in the uterus. Considering that sperm can live up to 6 days, unprotected intercourse could possibly result in pregnancy.

Is it all right for a woman to have intercourse during menstruation?

The healthy woman does not have to refrain from intercourse on the basis of menstruation alone. Religious, cultural, or other personal beliefs do, however, affect sexual behavior during menstruation. Women need to be informed about the risk of pregnancy with unprotected intercourse at any time during the menstrual cycle. Although contact with vaginal secretions is an important source of transmission of certain diseases, menstruation can bring the male into direct contact with his partner's blood. This may be a concern for some couples.

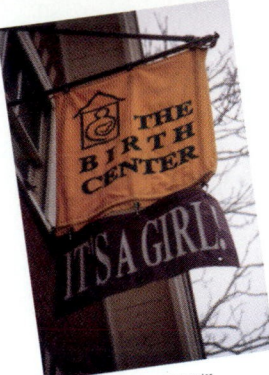

Home birth is defended as a safe alternative to hospital birth in certain medically and obstetrically low-risk populations when a skilled birth attendant is present and a modern hospital system is available to provide backup if needed (Olsen, 1997). Opponents of home birth feel that childbearing is unpredictable and that birth at home presents an unnecessary risk to mother and infant. Opponents also claim that decreases in perinatal morbidity and mortality may be the result of the shift to hospital deliveries and the use of technologies that have been developed over the last 50 years. Supporters of home birth state that most complications can be predicted and that major obstetric difficulties are rare.

A planned home birth is the most controversial of birth alternatives. The nature of obstetric problems and the lack of credible research demonstrating the safety of home birth indicate that this controversy is likely to continue. Nevertheless, some clients do choose home birth, and nurses working with childbearing families need to be aware of this.

In many states, lay midwives, rather than physicians or CNMs, attend home births. Physicians and CNMs may hesitate to attend scheduled home births

FIGURE 9–8. Birth center.

believe that attentive screening, client cooperation, and care delivered by CNMs with appropriate physician backup make the centers a safe option, and transfer rates are usually low.

A challenge is presented to hospital-based nurses who work with clients transferred from birth centers. The nurses must first evaluate their own feelings about out-of-hospital births. During a transfer, they welcome the transferred client, her support person, and the nurse-midwife; all should work together to ensure a positive birth experience. The collaborative effort is facilitated by previous planning. Nurses who work on hospital units that are backups for a birth center should meet with birth center staff to devise collaborative strategies for transfers.

Home Births. Among the reasons women may have a home birth are inability to reach a hospital (geography), desire for a family-centered birth experience away from a hospital, and unplanned delivery at home. Accurate data on the safety of home birth are lacking, as are figures for the actual number of home births.

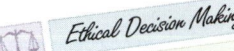

Ethical Decision Making

Nurse Sheila Moran, who specializes in care of high-risk obstetric patients, is on duty when Sunnie Bart is brought to the hospital for emergency cesarean delivery. Sunnie, suspicious of hospitals, planned to deliver her first baby at home where she was attended by her husband Stephan. Neither Sunnie nor Stephan had prior experience with childbirth. After 12 hours of difficult labor without progress, Stephan called for help, and Sunnie was brought by ambulance to the hospital, where fetal distress was identified.

1. What do this couple's actions indicate about their values and attitudes toward the health care system?
2. What conflicts might the nurse expect the couple to experience?
3. How might the nurse be expected to feel about this couple and their situation?
4. What strategies might the nurse use to ensure this couple receives high-quality care?

ETHICAL DECISION MAKING
Ethical implications of issues related to childbearing are discussed and questions are posed for consideration.

CLIENT TEACHING
Guidelines/strategies that nurses can use to educate clients and their families about various aspects of pregnancy, childbirth, and the postpartum and newborn periods.

▶ TREATMENT OPTIONS FOR PRIMARY DYSMENORRHEA

NONPHARMACOLOGIC TREATMENT
- heat (warm baths, showers, heating pad)
- back or abdominal massage
- mild exercise
- relaxation
- imagery

PHARMACOLOGIC TREATMENT
- NSAIDs
- combination oral contraceptives

may institute the measures without consulting a health care provider. Nurses can suggest alternative therapies to augment the woman's own ideas and provide reassurance as well as education about dysmenorrhea.

Client Teaching

Primary Dysmenorrhea

The nurse can suggest the following actions to help a client manage the discomfort related to primary dysmenorrhea:

- Take 400 mg of ibuprofen every 6 hours beginning one week before the start of your menses
- Continue to take the ibuprofen for 48–72 hours after your menses begin
- Take the ibuprofen with food to avoid stomach upset
- Apply warmth to your lower abdomen and back with either a hot bath or shower or a heating pad or warm pack
- To make a warm pack, put a warm, moist face towel in a Ziploc bag, wrap it in a pillowcase, and place it against the area of pain
- When using a heating pad or warm pack, test the temperature with your hand or wrist before applying it to your skin
- Do not sleep with a heating pad or warm pack as it may cause burns
- Drink warm tea or other warm drinks
- Walk at a moderate pace for 15 minutes to half an hour when you experience discomfort

Treatment of secondary dysmenorrhea is based on treating the underlying cause if one can be identified. The woman with secondary dysmenorrhea may undergo additional diagnostic testing which may be stressful and uncomfortable. Testing may include pelvic ultrasounds and surgical diagnostic modalities such as laparoscopy and hysteroscopy (see Chapter 10 for discussion of laparoscopy). Hysteroscopy involves inserting an instrument into the uterine cavity to look for intrauterine polyps or fibroids which may be a source of pain and increased bleeding (Klotz, 1995). Women undergoing diagnosis and treatment of secondary dysmenorrhea need additional support and education from their nurses as well as physical care prior to, during, and after any surgical or other invasive procedures.

Two common causes of secondary dysmenorrhea are endometriosis (see Chapter 10 for discussion of endometriosis) and leiomyomas. Leiomyomas are benign fibroid tumors of the smooth muscle of the uterus, which depend on estrogen for their growth. They can be located within the uterine wall (intramural) or in the cervix or broad ligament (intraligamentous), grow towards the surface of the uterus (subserous), or protrude into the uterine cavity (submucous). While many women with leiomyomas have no symptoms, they are a frequent cause of secondary dysmenorrhea. Common symptoms caused by leiomyomas are pelvic pressure, urinary frequency, pelvic bloating and congestion, dyspareunia, and heavy menstrual bleeding (Forrest, 1994). Leiomyomas are the most common reason, aside from cancer, for hysterectomy (surgical removal of the uterus) (Wilcox, Koonin, Pokras, Strauss, Xia, & Peterson, 1994). Leiomyomas can be treated with methyl prednisone acetate, which decreases bleeding and suppresses tumor growth, or with gonadotropin-releasing hormone agonists (GnRH-a) such as Leuprorelin and Nafarelin, which suppress tumor growth and shrink existing tumors. An alternative procedure to hysterectomy is myomectomy, where only the fibroid and a small amount of surrounding uterine tissue is removed.

Research Abstract

Implications of Bedrest for the High-Risk Pregnant Woman

A focused qualitative study was designed to investigate the experiences of 24 high-risk pregnant women on prolonged bedrest. The 24 women involved were confined to bedrest at home or in the hospital, from 7 to 50 days. The majority of participants were white, married, well-educated women who had planned this pregnancy. The age range was from 18 to 36 years. Ten were primiparas, and 14 were multigravida. Diagnoses were varied as follows: placenta previa (n = 7), premature rupture of membranes (n = 4), pregnancy-induced hypertension (n = 5), and preterm labor (n = 8). Twelve were in a hospital on bedrest, 3 were at home, and 9 had been in bedrest in both places.

The methodology involved diary keeping by the subject, field notes, and an interview. The focus was on the emotional and psychologic aspects of bedrest.

The researchers used a stress process model to classify data. Themes of stressors fall into three categories: situational, environmental, and family. Some situational themes were assumption of the sick role, uncertainty as to the fetus' well-being, and lack of control. Environmental stressors included feeling like a prisoner, "missing out," and "feeling bored." Family stressors were concerns

about children and role reversal. Stress manifested itself in women's emotional reactions, such as guilt, anger, depression, and loneliness. Socially, stress manifested as altered relationships with others. The physical side effects of stress and prolonged bedrest included altered wake and sleep cycles, digestive changes, muscle wasting, weakness, and fatigue.

Mediators for stress included tangible physical or emotional support by family, friends, and health care providers. Answering questions was seen as the most significant contribution of the nurse. Expression of a sense of caring by the nurse was also highly important. Many women found that educating themselves about their high-risk condition was helpful.

Application to Practice

This focused study provides qualitative data about the stressors experienced by the high-risk antepartum client confined to bedrest, and what nursing can do to help the client cope with this situation.

Source: Gupton, A., Heaman, M., & Ashcroft, T. (1997). Bedrest from the perspective of the high-risk pregnant woman. Journal of Obstetric, Gynecologic, and Neonatal Nursing, 26(4) 423–430.

RESEARCH ABSTRACT
Relevant nursing research studies are summarized to help students apply the results of the research to the concepts in the chapters.

Fibrinogen is converted to fibrin, causing a state of hypofibrinogenemia (depletion of fibrinogen). Platelets and fibrin are consumed by the formation of large numbers of microemboli, which are tiny clots, throughout the vascular bed. Clots are lysed (or dissolved), resulting in increased levels of fibrin split products. Fibrin split products have anticoagulant properties. The increase in fibrin split products, decrease in number of platelets, and reduction of fibrinogen combine to result in generalized hemorrhage. The woman may bleed extensively, for example, from venipuncture sites, and she may demonstrate petechiae and oozing from mucous membranes and gums. Hematomas may develop. The disseminated microemboli can cause ischemia of vital organs, resulting in any number of organic dysfunctions.

Collaborative Assessment
Women at risk for DIC are assessed for signs and symptoms of generalized bleeding and screened periodically for its development. Table 19–11 summarizes blood tests which are commonly used to assess for DIC. In areas where laboratory analysis is readily available, clotting time and bleeding time tests have been widely replaced by the determination of the prothrombin time, partial thromboplastin time, platelet count, and measurement of products of fibrin degradation (fibrin split products).

Collaborative Management
The objectives of treatment include prompt identification of DIC, elimination of the causative factor,

I

The Childbearing Family

Tamara Hunter, RN, BSN, has been a staff nurse within the maternity unit of a community hospital for the last two years. Her care of families during both the labor and delivery and postpartum experiences has given her a great amount of satisfaction. She is especially interested in the period between the birth of the newborn and the discharge of the family from the hospital.

Tamara met with a colleague who is a masters-prepared neonatal nurse practitioner who specializes in the care of the high-risk newborn at the health care facility at which she is employed. Tamara explores this and other areas of specialization through journal articles and conversations with other maternity nurses and considers the possibility of obtaining an MSN as an advanced practice nurse, a pediatric nurse practitioner focusing on the healthy newborn. Although she is excited about this opportunity, she is also a little apprehensive about it, mainly because she is concerned that concentration on the care of the newborn will affect her commitment to the childbearing family as a whole. ∎

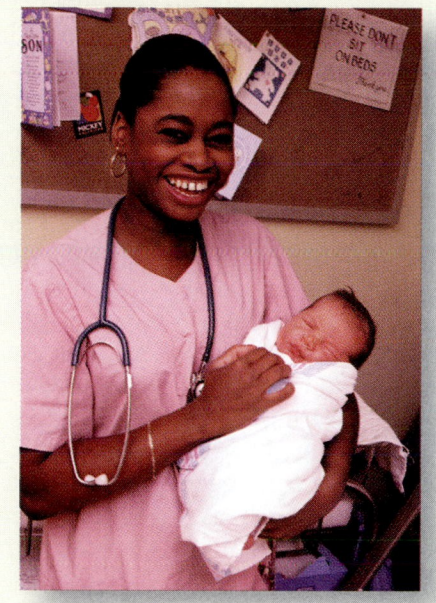

1
——————

Trends and Issues in Care of the Childbearing Family

Technologic innovations enable health care providers to ensure the survival of many low-birth-weight infants and many sick infants who would have died 10 years ago. Although health care providers can do much for many people in our society, many more live with impairments or do not live because barriers restrict their access to care.

Morbidity and mortality associated with childbearing have improved dramatically in the past 50 years in the United States, but this country continues to lag far behind other industrialized nations in overall infant mortality statistics. Adequate prenatal care is seen as essential in improving pregnancy outcomes for both mother and neonate.

This chapter explores both historical and contemporary trends relating to the care of childbearing families. The influence of factors such as managed care, roles of advanced practice nurses, and case management in childbearing care is discussed as well as future trends in the delivery of this care.

The challenge to nurses and other health care professionals in the 21st century will be to improve access to care for all individuals in our society, and in particular to ensure appropriate prenatal care to childbearing women. With continued movement into managed care arrangements, care delivery to pregnant women, children, and families must balance cost with quality. Through education, practice, and research, nurses can and must play an important role in helping to achieve these health care objectives.

► HISTORICAL TRENDS

The provision of care to childbearing families has evolved over the course of many centuries. The evolution of this care can be identified through the changing terms used to describe the provider and recipient of care. The earliest term used to refer to providers of care to childbearing women was **midwife.** This term was derived from *mid,* meaning "with," and *wif,* meaning "wife" or "woman." It was used as early as the Middle Ages, around 1303. Noble women were responsible for the delivery of infants for the serfs on their estates. Hence, they served as the midwives during the Middle Ages.

The branch of medicine that dealt with the practice of assisting in childbirth was known as **midwifery** until the latter part of the 19th century in the United States and Great Britain. At that time, the term *obstetrics* was introduced. The word is derived from the Latin *obstetrix,* meaning "midwife," and is also related to the Latin *obstare,* meaning "to stand by or in front of."

Obstetrics is currently defined as that branch of medicine that deals with the phenomena and management of pregnancy, labor, and the postpartum in low- and high-risk circumstances. Midwifery is still the term used to delineate the practice of a nurse who is responsible for management of childbearing women and neonates within a health care system that provides for collaborative management and referral (American College of Nurse-Midwives, 1993).

An important phase in the provision of care to childbearing families occurred after World War II, when the focus of care shifted from the provider of care to the recipient. **Maternity care** was the term used to denote a broader focus to health care, involving psychosocial and cultural aspects of the woman as well as physiologic aspects.

Today, the focus of practice has expanded to include the childbearing family as a whole, as well as the woman. Health care providers recognize that when one member of the family system is affected by pregnancy and birth, all other members are also affected and the family structure changes.

The evolution of concepts, definitions, and terms related to care of the childbearing family demonstrates a broadening perspective. The focus has shifted from the provider to the woman as recipient of care and finally to the entire family unit as recipient of care. The evolving concept also demonstrates the importance of nurses as an integral part of the health care team.

An example of family-centered care can be seen in modern childbirth centers. The family is encouraged to plan for the birth experience, and to use the center as an environment which will bring the family closer together by the birth. Nurses are integral to the process in this environment as both the providers of care, such as the certified nurse-midwife, who delivers the newborn and manages not only the pregnancy, but also the postpartum and newborn periods, and as childbirth center staff nurses during the prenatal, labor and delivery, and postpartum/newborn periods. Certified nurse-midwives and professional registered nurses participate as part of the birth team, collaborating with parents, siblings, and extended family members during the entire childbearing experience. Chapter 9 explores in greater depth the childbearing experience in a childbirth center.

► CONTEMPORARY ISSUES AND TRENDS

Among the most notable trends in care of the childbearing family has been the improvement in maternal and infant outcomes that has occurred worldwide over the past half century. In contrast to this trend, however, the ranking of the United States relative to other industrialized nations has actually worsened in recent decades. This has led many health care providers and policy makers in the United States to question aspects of the current health care delivery system for mothers and infants. A review of current U.S. vital statistics illustrates both of these trends.

▶ Current Vital Statistics

Maternal, neonatal, and infant mortality rates have decreased dramatically over the past 35 to 41 years (March of Dimes Birth Defects Foundation, 1997). Table 1–1 summarizes these rates. Data on which vital statistics are based are collected periodically. Analysis of these statistics is time consuming; thus, statistics for a year may not be reported until several years later. The National Center for Health Statistics, part of the U.S. Department of Health and Human Services, is a resource for current statistics. Other organizations, such as the March of Dimes, often compile the statistics in a more usable form.

These vital statistics serve as a sort of "report card" concerning delivery of health care to mothers, newborns, and infants. They point to improvements in health care of these groups, and also to the areas that still need improvement. For example, statistics still demonstrate a great disparity between infant mortality rates of white and black infants. As integral members of the health care delivery team for childbearing families, nurses are responsible for developing solutions to problems producing negative statistics.

Definitions

Definitions of vital statistics related to the childbearing cycle are necessary to ensure both a standard method for reporting births and maternal and infant mortality and morbidity rates across the United States and an understanding of the meaning of reports of vital statistics (see the box entitled Vital Statistics: Definitions).

Statistics related to these definitions are reported by the government for the categories of "white" and "black" mothers and infants. Thus, the term *black* rather than *African-American* is used to describe mothers and infants in the following discussion and tables.

Infant Mortality

The infant mortality rate is often cited as the gauge of the health of a nation. The lowest infant mortality rate ever recorded in the United States (8.0 infant deaths per 1000 live births) was recorded in the year 1994. Among white infants, the rate was 6.6, down from 7.6 in 1990. The rate for black infants, however, was 15.8 in 1994 compared with 18.0 in 1990. Although rates for both black and white infants continue to decline at approximately the same rate per year, the rate for black infants continues to remain more than twice as high as the rate for white infants (March of Dimes, 1997; Taylor, Katz, & Moos, 1995). Figure 1–1 illustrates the declining rates and the difference between black and white infant deaths. Clearly, segments of the U.S. population have health needs that still go unmet.

▶ TABLE 1–1

Maternal, Neonatal, and Infant Mortality Statistics for the United States, 1960–1994

	1960	1970	1980	1990	1992	1994
Maternal Mortality						
(Maternal deaths per 100,000 live births from complications of pregnancy, childbirth, and the puerperium)						
Total	37.1	21.5	9.2	8.2	7.8	8.3
White	26.0	14.4	6.7	5.4	5.0	6.2
Black	103.6	59.8	21.5	22.4	20.8	18.5
Neonatal Mortality						
(Infant deaths per 1000 live births before 28 days old, exclusive of fetal deaths [20 weeks of gestation to delivery])						
Total	18.7	15.1	8.5	5.8	5.4	5.1
White	17.2	13.8	7.5	4.8	4.3	2.6
Black	27.8	22.8	14.1	11.6	10.8	10.2
Infant Mortality						
(Infant deaths from birth to 1 year of age per 1000 live births)						
Total	26.0	20.0	12.6	9.2	8.5	8.0
White	22.9	17.8	11.0	7.6	6.9	6.6
Black	44.3	32.6	21.4	18.0	16.8	15.8

Source: March of Dimes Birth Defects Foundation, 1997.

▶ VITAL STATISTICS: DEFINITIONS

BIRTH RATE

Annual number of live births per 1000 population

LIVE BIRTH

An infant who, at birth, demonstrates signs of life such as breathing, heartbeat, and voluntary muscle movements

STILLBIRTH

An infant past the point of viability who is born dead

ABORTUS

A fetus or embryo removed or expelled from the uterus at 20 weeks or earlier, or weighing less than 500 g, or measuring less than 25 cm

NEONATAL MORTALITY RATE

Number of infant deaths occurring in the first 28 days of life per 1000 live births

PERINATAL MORTALITY RATE

Number of stillbirths plus number of neonatal deaths per 1000 live births

INFANT MORTALITY RATE

Number of deaths of infants under 12 months of age per 1000 live births

MATERNAL MORTALITY RATE

Number of maternal deaths resulting from the reproductive process per 100,000 live births

DIRECT MATERNAL DEATH

Death of the mother resulting from reproductive complications of pregnancy, labor, postpartum, or interventions; for example, maternal death from hemorrhage as a result of cervical lacerations of labor

INDIRECT MATERNAL DEATH

Death of a mother not directly related to the childbearing cycle but resulting from a previously existing disease or a disease not related to reproduction that developed during the childbearing cycle and was aggravated by the pregnancy; for example, maternal death from mitral valve disease during childbearing

Maternal Mortality

In 1994, 328 women were reported to have died in the United States from complications of pregnancy, childbirth, and the postpartum. The maternal mortality rate was 8.3 deaths per 100,000 live births in 1994. This rate is 66% higher than the objective sought for the year 2000—5% per 100,000 live births. Similar to the statistics for black and white infant deaths, black women were over three times more likely to die of complications related to pregnancy than were white women (March of Dimes, 1997).

International Infant Mortality Rates

In 1993, the United States ranked 25th among industrialized nations in infant mortality rate, behind such countries as Singapore, Ireland, and Italy. Japan ranked first with the lowest infant mortality rate (4.4) (March of Dimes, 1997). Table 1–2 compares ranking for selected countries for 1993. Despite a continued decline in the infant mortality rate, the United States is losing ground in comparison with other industrialized countries. In 1991, the United States ranked 22nd among industrialized countries in infant mortality rate, only to have slipped 3 ranks in 3 years.

Some possible reasons exist for the discrepancy between the United States and other developed countries. Other countries do a better job of ensuring infant survival than the United States by:

1. Having readily available, easily understood provider systems for prenatal care
2. Removing economic barriers to access to prenatal care
3. Linking prenatal care to comprehensive social and financial benefits that support the optimal health and well-being of mothers and infants

The United States leads the world in spending on health. Measures of health care use and health status do not provide evidence that the United States has a superior health care system for its large expenditure levels. Such insights may have relevance for policy development in the United States.

▶ Access to Prenatal Care

It has long been understood that one of the primary factors related to infant mortality in the United States is the increase in delivery of low-birth-weight infants.

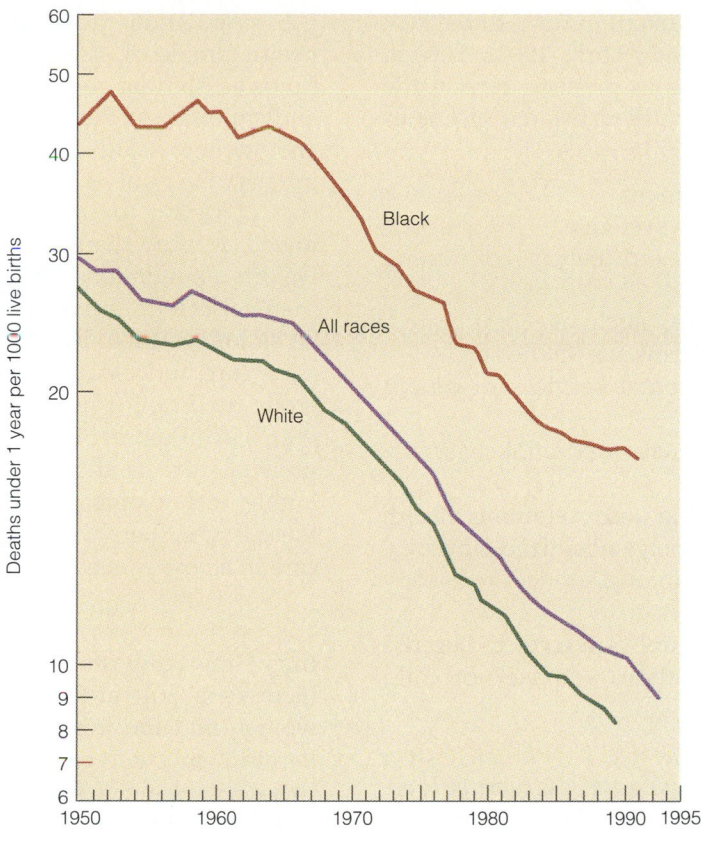

FIGURE 1–1. Infant mortality rates by race: United States 1950–1992. *(Adapted from Kochanek, K., & Hudson, B. (1995). Advance report of final mortality statistics.* Monthly Vital Statistics Report, 43*(suppl 6), 11.*

▶ **TABLE 1-2**

International Comparisons of Infant Mortality Rates, 1993*

Rank	Country	Rate	Rank	Country	Rate
1	Japan	4.4	20	Spain	7.2
2	Finland	4.4	21	New Zealand	7.2
3	Singapore	4.7	22	Israel	7.8
4	Hong Kong	4.8	23	Belgium	8.2
5	Sweden	4.8	24	Greece	8.3
6	Norway	5.1	25	**United States**	**8.4**
7	Denmark	5.4	26	Czech Republic	8.5
8	Switzerland	5.6	27	Cuba	9.4
9	Germany	5.8	28	Portugal	9.6
10	Ireland	6.0	29	Kuwait	12.3
11	Australia	6.1	30	Hungary	12.5
12	England and Wales	6.2	31	Chile	13.1
13	Netherlands	6.3	32	Poland	13.4
14	Canada	6.3	33	Puerto Rico	13.4
15	Austria	6.5	34	Costa Rica	13.8
16	Scotland	6.5	35	Bulgaria	15.5
17	France	6.8	36	Russian Federation	20.3
18	Northern Ireland	7.1	37	Romania	23.3
19	Italy	7.2			

*Includes countries that reported infant mortality rates to the World Health Organization
Rates are per 1,000 live births
Note: Rankings are based on more than 1 decimal place
Source: March of Dimes Birth Defects Foundation, 1997.

Low birth weight has been linked, in turn, to the lack of prenatal care (Martin, 1997; York, 1993). Several barriers to a woman's access to prenatal care in the United States have been identified (March of Dimes Birth Defects Foundation, 1997).

• Limited financial resources
• Uncoordinated service systems
• Individual behaviors and beliefs concerning health care
• Bureaucratic obstacles, such as complicated, lengthy application forms for Medicaid
• Unavailability of maternal services in certain parts of the country
• Underfunded and overcrowded publicly supervised clinics
• Difficulty in recruiting and retaining health care providers in publicly subsidized clinics
• Lack of coordination among services for needy individuals
• Inaccessibility to prenatal care services because of transportation, location, and lack of child care facilities

The Committee on Perinatal Health (COPH), in its document entitled *Toward Improving the Outcome of Pregnancy: The 90s and Beyond* (Committee on Perinatal Health, 1995), has issued several recommendations that address access to care, including the provision for ambulatory prenatal care and infant care and the improvement of the availability of perinatal providers.

Strategies to achieve these recommendations include broadening health insurance coverage for childbearing women and infants, improving coordination and funding of public programs, simplifying bureaucratic procedures, increasing the number of maternal care providers, establishing a national council on children and health, and raising public awareness throughout the country.

▶ Issues in the Delivery of Care

Contemporary issues that affect the care delivered to the childbearing family may be divided into four major areas: economic, social, legislative and legal, and technologic. In addition, managed care is an issue that transcends all these areas. Although these areas and issues are discussed briefly below, because of their importance, the issues identified are elaborated on throughout the text.

Economic Issues

Shifting demographics and an increased emphasis on costly technologic interventions have created a crisis in the health care system today (Hadley, 1996). As the U.S. population grows older and experiences more health problems, the focus of health programs and funds is shifting more on the elderly than mothers and children. At the same time, technologic advances are helping health care providers to keep preterm infants alive, but at great cost to society. The lifetime cost of caring for a low-birth-weight infant is estimated at more than $500,000 (March of Dimes Birth Defects Foundation, 1997). Paradoxically, the cost of prenatal care that may prevent low birth weight can be as low as $400. In addition, the influence of managed care and cost containment has the potential to erode funding for maternal and newborn health programs even more. Surely, society must recognize that prenatal care is more cost effective than intensive, highly technologic care of sick infants. Because of these issues, there will be a continuing need to deliver care in a cost-effective manner.

Social Issues

Infant mortality statistics do not reflect the current increase in drug and other substance use by pregnant women and the number of infants born exposed to harmful substances. Punitive actions taken against pregnant substance abusers do little to encourage early and consistent prenatal care among these women.

Legislative and Legal Issues

Managed care arrangements, discussed below, have attempted to limit the hospital stay after a normal birth to a maximum of 24 hours, by refusing to pay for more time in the hospital for mother and normal newborn. In many states, consumers have rallied against managed care companies, and secured legislation against such forced discharges. Such trends fos-

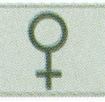

Women's Health

The problem of substance abuse by pregnant women is aggravated by the close relationship between women and infants infected with human immunodeficiency virus (HIV) and the use of drugs. Both HIV infection and drug use occur frequently in urban, minority, low-income women—those already at risk for adverse pregnancy outcomes. There is a great demand and need for services for these individuals, a goal that cannot be met by current funding levels for health care.

tered by practices of managed care companies will likely continue (Ferguson & Engelhard, 1997).

In addition, malpractice continues to be an issue having an impact on maternal and infant care. Issues of malpractice for providers of care to childbearing families affect not only the nature of care delivered but also the recruitment and retention of health care professionals in this specialty. Increases in malpractice premiums among physicians, certified nurse-midwives, and advanced practice nurses in maternity have curtailed services to recipients of public programs who are at high risk for problems.

Malpractice issues have not only created a shortage of providers for the childbearing family, but have also increased tension among members of the inter-disciplinary team, including consumers. This tension is worsened as competition among providers increases because of managed care arrangements. Certified nurse-midwives (CNMs) and nurse practitioners (NPs) provide a high quality, cost-effective alternative to physician care, and are often seen as providers of choice under these arrangements.

Technologic Issues

Technology today is a double-edged sword. On one hand, technologic advances have greatly improved the outcome of pregnancy for high-risk pregnant women and have facilitated survival of infants who would have died 10 years ago. On the other hand, increased technology has contributed to the burdensome cost of neonatal and maternal care and the rate of cesarean deliveries.

Computer systems are also technologies whose use has increased significantly in the care of childbearing families (Fig. 1–2). Although they have been very beneficial in coordinating data bases and in transferring information between sites around the country, they do have a potential to dehumanize care. For example, when computers are placed at the mother's bedside, nurses may spend a large part of the mother's stay in the unit inputting data into the computer instead of interacting with the mother.

Managed Care

Within the past 10 years, managed care has perhaps been the major influence on health and nursing care delivery, including care during childbearing. Managed care can broadly be defined as health insurance plans that combine three elements: delivery of health care services, financing of those services, and controlling the use of the services. Most managed care plans also have a specific network of health care providers (i.e., physicians, NPs, physical therapists, etc.) who are available to care for individuals enrolled in the plan. Providers and provider organizations (e.g., a

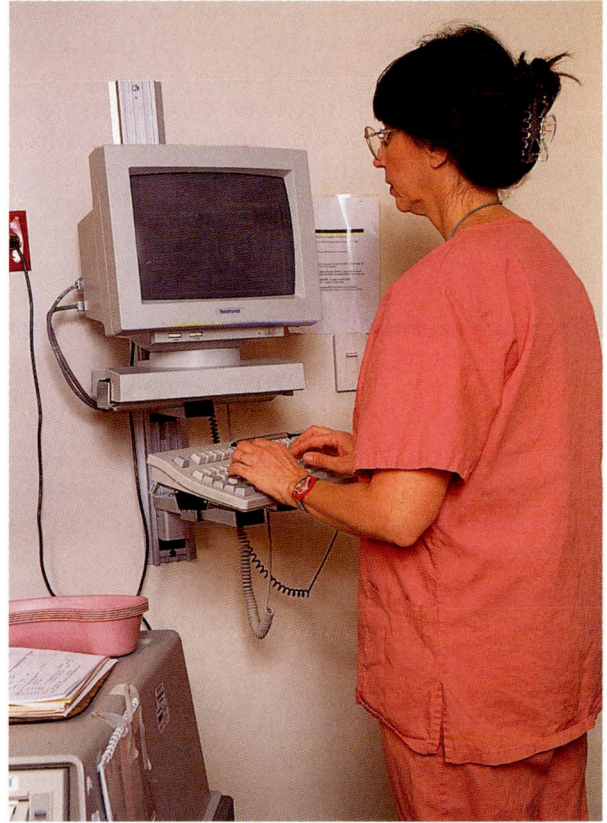

FIGURE 1–2. The computer can be a useful tool in helping the nurse record assessment findings about the client during childbirth.

hospital or nurse-managed clinic) are paid a specific fee for each client covered by the plan in advance of any health care being offered. Thus, the less costly the care provided per client, the more money left for the provider. Usually the plan imposes some restrictions on the provider the client is able to choose, often in the form of surcharges or refusal of coverage for use of providers who are not within the health maintenance organization's (HMO's) provider network. As of 1995, 20% of the population in the United States was receiving health insurance under managed care arrangements, including 23% of Medicaid beneficiaries and 9% of Medicare beneficiaries. Enrollment in managed care arrangements is rapidly enlarging as private and public employers and federal and state entitlement programs change their insurance carriers from fee-for-service models to managed care models (Weisman, 1996). Managed care has been seen as the answer to cost escalation in health care (Bendell, 1997). Most managed care companies (which include HMOs, insurance companies, and other institutions) contract with providers and facilities to provide care for individuals insured under their plan and then negotiate fixed reimbursement rates for services provided by the providers and facilities.

The philosophy of managed care organizations, in general, includes health promotion and disease prevention, with the aim of avoiding serious disease and more costly treatment services. However, as managed care has developed a larger share of the health insurance market, managed care organizations have been able to negotiate contracts with providers and health care facilities which provide less money per client served to those who provide health care services. Providers have had to take on larger case loads of clients to meet expenses of running their operations and make a reasonable profit. Managed care has been criticized for creating a climate in which providers have very little time and few resources with which to provide care for many individuals. The financing arrangements within managed care often provide financial disincentives for providers to give adequate services to their clients (Weisman, 1996), since the less money spent on the client, the more money left for the provider or provider organization.

Specifically, providers may no longer be able to perform a wide battery of expensive tests or perform costly procedures, even when they believe they are justified. The managed care company simply will not pay for such tests or procedures. An example of a breakdown in provision of necessary services due to managed care financing is the issue of mastectomy clients being discharged 48 hours or less after surgery, because managed care companies refuse to provide reimbursement for longer stays. In many states, government has stepped in and legislated longer and more appropriate hospital stays, allowing women in this situation more opportunity for nursing care to prevent complications or more education concerning care of self.

Managed care, in and of itself, is not inherently "bad care." Nor is fee-for-service care, which focuses on pathology and disease, inherently "good care." Potentially, managed care's focus on health promotion and illness prevention may provide an excellent modality for maintenance of optimum well-being of the population. However, the current focus of managed care on economics and cost containment has the potential for a negative impact on the health of the population, including childbearing families. The ideal situation, which nurses and nursing organizations such as the American Nurses Association (ANA) advocate, provides a balance between the two models: a focus on health and high-quality, cost-effective care (Ferguson & Engelhard, 1997).

► Trends in Nursing Care

Trends in nursing care of the childbearing family are reflected in nursing practice, nursing education, and nursing research.

Nursing Practice

Trends in nursing practice include the development of standards of care by the profession; increase in specialization, certification, and practice parameters of advanced practice nurses; movement of nursing care into the community-based nursing environment; consumer involvement in childbearing care; the role of nurse practitioners in care of childbearing families; the use of unlicensed assistive personnel to deliver care; and case management.

Standards. The profession of nursing has an obligation to the public to deliver high-quality nursing care. In an effort to meet this obligation, nursing standards have been developed by several nursing organizations, among them the ANA and the Association of Women's Health, Obstetric, and Neonatal Nursing (AWHONN). The standards for maternity nursing practice apply to homes, alternate birthing centers, hospitals, and ambulatory care settings. They identify health, demographic, environmental, and psychosocial parameters.

Because standards reflect current knowledge in the field, they are dynamic and subject to change; however, they always represent levels of practice agreed on by leaders in the profession or specialty.

Increased Specialization, Certification, and Practice Parameters of Advanced Practice Nurses. The increased complexity of care given to childbearing families has led to more specialization of maternity nurses; for example, a maternity nurse may specialize solely in the care of the well neonate. In addition, advanced practice nurses, including both clinical nurse specialists and NPs, are gaining in-depth knowledge through advanced degrees and seeking recognition and credibility through certification mechanisms. Both AWHONN and ANA offer a variety of certifications in maternal–newborn nursing. Finally, NPs are delivering primary care to healthy pregnant women and their families.

Community-Based Nursing and Home Health Care. The practice setting for nurses who care for childbearing families is shifting from acute care institutions to the home and community. The changing economic climate of health care and managed care arrangements will necessitate that more maternity clients be discharged within 24 hours of birth, which will require a shift to community-based care (McGregor, 1996). Even high-risk maternity and neonatal clients are being cared for at home. Technologies that were formerly available only in the hospital are now in the home as well. Nurses who practice in the community have had to refocus their practice to incorporate skills that were once needed only in hospitals. In addition, discharge of clients into community, home, and ambulatory care settings, has increased the importance of the case manager role, a role nurses are readily assuming (see discussion below). (See Chapters 20, 27, and 34 for a discussion of community-based maternity and neonatal care.)

Consumer Involvement in Childbearing Care.
Consumer involvement has affected delivery of care to childbearing families. By speaking their needs and desires, consumers have created several changes: preparation of clients for involvement in childbirth; the vaginal birth after cesarean (VBAC); movement away from circumcision of newborns; alternative childbirth settings; and family-centered maternity care. These consumer-fostered trends are discussed throughout the text.

Family-centered maternity care deserves particular mention here. This concept of care, perhaps more than any other philosophy that has affected the health care industry, has had a major impact on how nurses deliver care to childbearing families. In family-centered maternity care, emphasis is placed not only on the delivery of safe, quality care to the mother and neonate, but also on care that fosters family unity. The concept of family-centered maternity care comprises several components:

1. Childbirth preparation for both partners (and for siblings as well)
2. Involvement of the father in the entire birthing process
3. Choice of birthing environment when possible (all hospitals should have a birthing room as an alternative to traditional labor and delivery suites)
4. Sibling visitation
5. Early discharge programs for mothers and infants
6. Strategies to foster family members' attachment to the newborn
7. Parental leave options for both parents

These components are discussed in detail elsewhere in the text. In addition, nursing management for families throughout the childbearing cycle is based on a family-centered care philosophy.

Nurse Practitioners.
Increasingly, especially in the managed care environment, NPs are being recognized as alternative providers to family medicine physicians for primary health care delivery (Sinclair, 1997). NPs are in collaborative practice with physicians, may practice independently, or work in a variety of health care agencies or HMOs. NPs practice under their own professional license as a nurse, and are thus able to practice autonomously in their areas of expertise. The NPs likely to be most involved with childbearing families are pediatric nurse practitioners (PNPs), family nurse practitioners (FNPs), women's health nurse practitioners (WHNPs), neonatal nurse practitioners (NNPs), or perinatal nurse practitioners. NPs are master's-prepared with rigorous preparation in assessment, diagnosis, and treatment of minor illnesses. All NPs engaged in practice must be certified by a practitioner credentialing agency, such as the American Nurses Credentialing Center, which sets practice standards.

Practitioner training emphasizes advanced assessment through the client history and physical exam, and diagnosis and treatment of minor health problems. In most states, the NP can prescribe medications and order diagnostic tests. Practitioner training also stresses educating and promoting health for the client and family. In addition, NP training prepares the practitioner for one of the key responsibilities of the primary provider in a managed care setting: screening and referring clients to specialists. NPs can provide high-quality services to families by acting as advocates, by influencing health policy, and by strengthening behaviors that keep the client and family healthy. Research has consistently documented the high levels of care delivered by NPs and client satisfaction in receiving this care. A major source of satisfaction is the manner in which NPs incorporate the client and family in decision making concerning care (Sherwen, 1997).

Unlicensed Assistive Personnel.
The current emphasis of managed care on cost containment has produced some highly negative situations in hospitals and other health care agencies. Traditionally, registered nurses represented about two thirds of the hospital workforce, making salaries for nurses one of the biggest items in the budget (Simpson, 1997). Forced by lowered reimbursement provided by managed care companies, hospitals and other health care facilities have found ways to decrease their budget (Huston, 1996). Decreasing salaries for personnel who provide client care has become one way to cut the budget. "Downsizing" registered nurses and replacing them with unlicensed assistive personnel

(UAP) is one way to accomplish this decrease in salaries. UAP are health care workers who have no defined body of knowledge or educational preparation upon which to base their practice. UAP are also uncredentialed and there is no state or federal regulatory body to validate their competence (AWHONN, 1997). Since they command a lower salary than RNs, UAP are being hired by hospitals and health care facilities, provided with some training in skills and tasks such as intravenous catheter insertion and obtaining ECG recordings, and charged with providing client care.

Although unlicensed personnel in the form of orderlies and nursing assistants have long been a part of staffing on nursing units, they were generally trained in a nursing model to provide assistance to, rather than replace, RNs. In a survey by AWHONN, half of the nurses polled indicated that up to 10% of the RN positions in their clinical settings are being replaced with UAP positions (Simpson, 1997). Finally, nurses are responsible for the practice of UAP on their units and must delegate tasks to them without knowing how they were trained or what skills they have obtained. This practice increases the nurse's liability risk and may put his or her license in jeopardy.

Nurses, nursing organizations, and physicians have all voiced concern about these changes in the so-called "skill mix" of the personnel providing client care and fear that this trend will have adverse effects on client outcomes. However, to date there is insufficient data to support or disprove this belief. AWHONN, as well as other nursing organizations, has issued a statement concerning UAP and the care of women and infants (AWHONN, 1997). It cautions that UAP can assist, but not replace RNs. While UAP can perform repetitive tasks which are clearly defined and for which they have been trained, they cannot perform the essential nursing processes of assessment, diagnosis of a problem, planning client care, implementation of that care, and evaluation of the client outcomes.

Nurses have responded to the potential threat to client safety due to the use of UAP through organized action to inform consumers about the differences in training and abilities between RNs and UAP. An example of this is the recent campaign by the New York State Nurses Association, which educated consumers about the differences between RNs and other personnel. Nurses in maternity and women's health care can contribute to consumer awareness of this issue by ensuring that clients know that they are receiving care by an RN. This can be done by introducing oneself as a registered nurse and by wearing a name tag that clearly states the wearer's name and the title Registered Nurse.

Case Management. "Case management" is a term and role used frequently in managed care arrangements, and in a variety of integrated or partially integrated care delivery systems. An "integrated" health care delivery system is one in which a broad range of services and health care agencies are managed under one business system. For example, an integrated health care system may include a home health agency, community hospital, ambulatory care clinic, acute care hospital, nursing home, and hospice. While the concept of case management can be applied to many role functions in managed care, it is only fully operational in a highly integrated system of care. The ideal function of a case manager is to guide a client through the multitude of health resources, from outpatient, primary care services, through acute services, through rehabilitation and back to the community, and finally, through death, in a smooth, "seamless" manner. However, many nurses and other health care professionals are working as case managers in partially integrated systems. Further, the nature of the case management function also varies. In contrast to the ideal of providing "holistic" health-related care for a client as the level of care alters with the health status, some case managers primarily function as "utilization reviewers" or "monitors," ensuring that health care resources are not wasted. Indeed, case management as a role has often been associated, inappropriately, with the more negative side of managed care arrangements. However, the role has great potential, when carried out in its full sense, to ensure a high-quality health care experience for clients. Nurses, with their orientation to care for the total human being, are ideal professionals to function as case managers.

Specific tools or techniques are often used by case managers to measure outcomes of care. These tools have also found their way into general practice of several disciplines. In fact, some are seen as multidisciplinary tools, which several professionals will follow, each contributing to a part of the total plan. The tools of case management are critical/clinical paths, protocols/algorithms, and risk assessment/outcome measurement instruments. Critical/clinical paths and protocols/algorithms are designed to "standardize" routine care between professional providers, and risk assessment/outcome measurement instruments are used to determine if specific interventions actually result in the desired client outcome. Because critical/clinical paths are written by representatives of the disciplines involved in the care of pregnant women and their families, they provide a framework for gaining consensus among the team members about the care requirements for childbearing families. This greatly enhances consistency and reduces nonclientrelated and nonessential variability in care from one family to another (Bower, 1997).

Nursing Education

Many nursing leaders have become concerned with the manner in which schools of nursing educate future nurses to practice with childbearing families. It has been suggested that health care professionals, including nurses, should be prepared to provide culturally relevant, sensitive care that incorporates health education and counseling. Further, they must provide cost-effective care in new environments in community-based ambulatory care settings and in homes. For the nurse to successfully implement the components of care for childbearing families, nursing education must reflect appropriate curricular content.

On the graduate level, programs are available for nurses to gain in-depth knowledge in specialized areas of advanced maternal–newborn nursing. Some of these areas include specialty practice in perinatal nursing, neonatal nursing, and home health care of childbearing families. In addition, nurse practitioners practice in the areas of neonatal, pediatric, family, and women's health practice as primary care providers. Also, many nurses are being prepared in master's programs or post-master's certificate programs as case managers.

At both the undergraduate and graduate levels, the economics of health care and technical equipment used in maternity care settings must be understood by the nurse. The educational process must include coverage of advanced technology, so nurses are comfortable with these advances and can explain use of such technology to their clients. Use of informatics and computer technology is also essential in maternity care.

Nursing Research

Nursing research concerned with the childbearing family attempts to explain variables concerned with the childbearing experience and to shed light on problems relating to clinical practice. Thus, research in this area tends to focus on current priorities in delivery of health care to childbearing families.

Nursing research that answers some of the questions related to childbearing is both quantitative and qualitative. Quantitative research is rigorously designed and controlled to develop and test theories by focusing on the relationships among variables identified as important to care of childbearing families and individuals. Qualitative research focuses on describing phenomena and evolving theories of importance to nursing and uses more naturalistic, less controlled research methods. Both types of research are necessary

to expand our understanding of the childbearing family. Chapters in this text contain Research Abstracts that describe and comment on both quantitative and qualitative studies concerned with childbearing.

Priorities for federal and private funding of nursing research in the area of childbearing often parallel major national concerns. For example, at this time, a high research priority identified by the National Institute for Nursing Research at the National Institutes of Health (NIH) is research dealing with low-birth-weight infants and outcomes of care delivery. Similarly, one of the highest priorities for the nation's health is lowering infant mortality and morbidity rates.

Nursing research on childbearing families will expand the knowledge base for practice. Nurses need to incorporate research findings into their practice.

▶ Future Trends in Delivery of Care to Childbearing Families

Several authors have attempted to identify a probable (and a preferable) future for health care and nursing (Cox, 1997; Korniewicz & Palmer, 1997). The following trends in health care are likely to continue well into the future, and will have an impact on the care delivered to childbearing families:

1. The health care industry will continue to be dominated by cost-containment strategies
2. Access to high-technology, expensive forms of care will be limited
3. Hospitals and other health agencies will continue to merge, downsize, and form large health systems covering large geographic areas
4. Nurses, as well as physicians, will provide primary care to clients in a variety of managed care arrangements
5. Community- and home-based care will become a predominant mode of care delivery
6. Professional organizations, such as AWHONN and ANA, will become more and more involved in the political arena

Within this volatile environment, improvement of the outcome of pregnancy must become a national priority. It is essential for the United States to develop a care system that ensures optimal health for childbearing families. In 1990, the COPH was convened to define strategies for improving the outcome of pregnancy. They developed and published, in 1995, key recommendations essential for improving the outcome of pregnancy. Those recommendations that

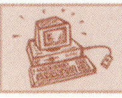

Research Abstract

Students' Perception of Nursing as a Career

To increase the number of nurses who are culturally sensitive to inner-city populations, a wide variety of ethnically and racially diverse students must choose nursing as a career. However, ethnic minorities comprise just slightly more than 7% of registered nurses in the United States. If colleges are to recruit culturally diverse nursing students, they must first know how high school students perceive nursing. The purpose of this cross-sectional descriptive survey was to (1) Explore the perception of urban high school students concerning nursing as a career; (2) Examine the congruence between students' "ideal" careers and nursing; and (3) Explore the perceptions of nursing held by students in ethnic and racial groups.

A large, racially diverse urban high school in New England was the site of the study. A questionnaire consisting of 17 Likert-like items to measure attitudes toward an ideal career and 17 similar items to measure perceptions of nursing as a career was administered to all 451 junior students attending school that day. Two hundred and ninety-one students (65%) responded; 276 surveys were usable. The sample represented 116 (42%) males and 160 (58%) females between 15 and 17 years old. Ninety-six (35%) were White, 96 (35%) African-American, 49 (18%) Latino, 20 (7%) Asian, and 15 (5%) "other." Ninety-six percent of the sample said they planned to go to college.

Construct validity was examined using factor analysis which yielded four factors on the ideal career dimension and four on the nursing career dimension. The ideal career factors were knowledge, power, activity, and security. The nursing career dimensions were activity, power, evaluation, and knowledge.

Students perceived nurses as caring people who work with their hands, work very hard, and are very busy. They were least likely to see nurses as leading others, making decisions, having power, and making a lot of money. Female students, as opposed to male, also perceived nurses as being less caring than they wished to be. T-tests revealed that there were significant differences ($p = <.01$) on every item. In each case, students perceived nursing as not meeting the requirement they wanted in an ideal career. When ethnic and racial groups were compared concerning differences in their perceptions of nursing, no significant differences among the groups were found. All ethnic and racial groups were unlikely to see nurses as leaders who could make decisions for themselves, were very powerful, and made a lot of money. Additionally, post hoc tests also revealed that the Asian females were least likely to view nurses in a positive light.

The strong lack of congruence between the students' ideal career and nursing does not bode well for the students' consideration of nursing as a career. The authors recommend that nurse educators gear recruitment strategies to ethnic and racial minorities, correct inaccurate perceptions, highlight traits in nursing that are valued by each ethnic group, and develop mentoring opportunities.

Application to Practice

This study provides useful information concerning reasons why young people currently choose not to go into nursing as a career. This trend is of great concern, as health care becomes more complex, and the nursing workforce ages and moves towards retirement. Nursing leaders have been unable to promote a more positive image of nursing in the general public, and nurse educators, especially in baccalaureate programs, have not been able to develop effective recruitment strategies aimed at college-bound high school students of all racial and ethnic groups. If nursing is to survive as a profession, recruitment of young people into baccalaureate programs will need to become a priority.

Source: Reiskin, H., & Haussler, S.C. (1994). Multicultural students' perception of nursing as a career. Image: Journal of Nursing Scholarship, 26(1), 61–64.

define trends in delivery of care for childbearing families include (Committee on Perinatal Health, 1995):

- A focus on health promotion and health education. This focus should begin long before conception, and in fact, should begin in elementary school.
- A focus on reproductive awareness. New strategies to reach each man and woman of childbearing age concerning reproductive health should be incorporated into the practice of all health providers.
- A focus on preconception and interconception care. Risk reduction should be emphasized and family planning counseling and services should be routinely available to all individuals. Annual preconception or interconception visits, as well as prepregnancy planning visits, should become standards of care.
- Ambulatory prenatal care. Early risk assessment, followed by appropriate care, consultation, or referral, must be a universal and ongoing component of prenatal care. Families should be directed to the appropriate care delivery agencies (e.g., medical center for high-risk pregnancy; childbirth center for low-risk pregnancy).

- Inpatient perinatal care. Women should be able to deliver in the appropriate environment, as above.
- Infant care. Perinatal services must extend through the first year of life, with access to pediatric care and a regular source of care for all infants. Early intervention services should be structured to include appropriate care for infants.
- Access to perinatal providers. Strategies need to be developed to improve access of childbearing families to appropriate providers, including perinatologists, neonatologists, midwives, PNPs, and so on.

Because of the potential consequences of these recommendations to childbearing families, nurses who practice with this population will need to understand both societal and health care trends and their implications for health care delivery. In addition, nurses will need to assume active roles in policy decisions to ensure that adequate resources are allocated to mothers, infants, and their families. Nurses can be instrumental in advocating health-related prenatal care as well as care for high-risk childbearing families.

Chapter Highlights

- While increased knowledge and improvements in technology over the past 50 years have greatly improved the outcomes for mothers and infants in the United States, infant mortality statistics reveal that many women and children do not benefit from these improvements.

- The discrepancy in rates of mortality between black and white infants and mothers is a clear indication that the system of care for childbearing families is failing.

- An important priority for the nation is to reduce the infant mortality rate.

- Contemporary economic, social, legislative and legal, technologic, and health care delivery trends provide a context for viewing the nature of care delivered to childbearing families.

- By understanding current issues and trends, nurses are better able to formulate and implement strategies that contribute to the well-being and care of childbearing families.

- Nursing practice, education, and research will continue to change in response to the evolving needs of the childbearing population.

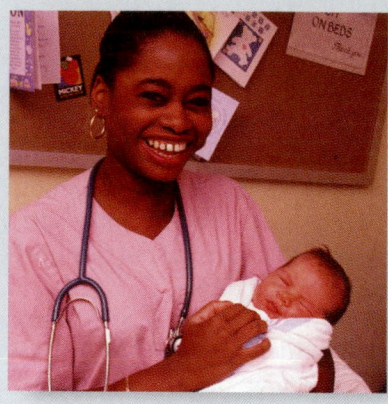

After reading the vignette at the beginning of this chapter, use what you have learned to answer these questions:

1. What actions can Tamara Hunter employ to ensure that her preparation as a pediatric nurse practitioner (PNP) focusing on well-newborn care will enhance her relationships with the families with whom she interacts?

2. What benefits are gained by increased specialization in maternity nursing in terms of improvements in maternal and infant outcomes?

3. Are there any drawbacks to specializing in one area of maternity nursing in relation to the quality of care delivered?

Critical Thinking Questions

► References

American College of Nurse-Midwives. (1993). *Educating nurse-midwives: A strategy for achieving affordable, high-quality maternity care.* Washington, DC: Author.

Association of Women's Health, Obstetrics, and Neonatal Nursing. (1997). *The role of unlicensed assistive personnel in the nursing care of women and newborns. Position statement.* Washington, DC: Author.

Bendell, A. (1997). Health care in the 1990s: Changes in health care delivery models for survival. *Journal of Obstetric, Gynecologic, and Neonatal Nursing, 26*(2), 212–216.

Bower, K. (1997). Case management and clinical paths: Strategies to support the perinatal experience. *Journal of Obstetric, Gynecologic, and Neonatal Nursing, 26*(3), 329–333.

Committee on Perinatal Health. (1995). *Toward improving the outcome of pregnancy: The 90s and beyond.* White Plains, NY: March of Dimes Birth Defects Foundation.

Cox, R. (1997). Family health care delivery for the 21st century. *Journal of Obstetric, Gynecologic, and Neonatal Nursing, 26*(1), 109–118.

Ferguson, S., & Engelhard, C. (1997). Short stay: The art of legislative quality and economy. *AWHONN Lifelines, 1*(1), 17–23.

Hadley, E. (1996). Nursing in the political and economic marketplace: Challenges for the 21st century. *Nursing Outlook, 44*(1), 6–10.

Huston, C. (1996). Unlicensed assistive personnel: A solution to dwindling health care resources or the precursor to the apocalypse of registered nursing? *Nursing Outlook, 44*(2), 67–73.

Korniewicz, D., & Palmer, M. (1997). The preferable future for nursing. *Nursing Outlook, 45*(3), 108–113.

March of Dimes Birth Defects Foundation. (1997). *StatBook: Statistics for monitoring maternal and infant health.* White Plains, NY: Author.

Martin, G. (1997). Real managed care (from Kubler-Ross to better outcomes). *Journal of Perinatology, 17*(2), 93–94.

McGregor, L. (1996). Short, shorter, shortest: Continuing to improve the hospital stay for mothers and newborns. *MCN, American Journal of Maternal-Child Nursing, 21*(4), 191–196.

Reiskin, H., & Haussler, S.C. (1994). Multicultural students' perception of nursing as a career. *Image: Journal of Nursing Scholarship, 26*(1), 61–64.

Sherwen, L. (1997). Nurses: Primary care professionals. *Exceptional Parent, 27*(3), 42–43.

Simpson, K. (1997). Unlicensed assistive personnel: What nurses need to know. *AWHONN Lifelines, 1*, 26–31.

Sinclair, B. (1997). Advanced practice nurses in integrated health care systems. *Journal of Obstetric, Gynecologic, and Neonatal Nursing, 26*(2), 217–223.

Taylor, G., Katz, V., & Moos, M.K. (1995). Racial disparity in pregnancy outcomes: Analysis of black and white teenage pregnancies. *Journal of Perinatology, 15*(6), 480–483.

Weisman, C. (1996). Introduction: Proceedings of women's health and managed care: Balancing cost, access and quality. *Women's Health Issues, 6*, 1–4.

York, R. (1993). Maternal factors that influence inadequate prenatal care. *Public Health Nurse, 10*(4), 241–244.

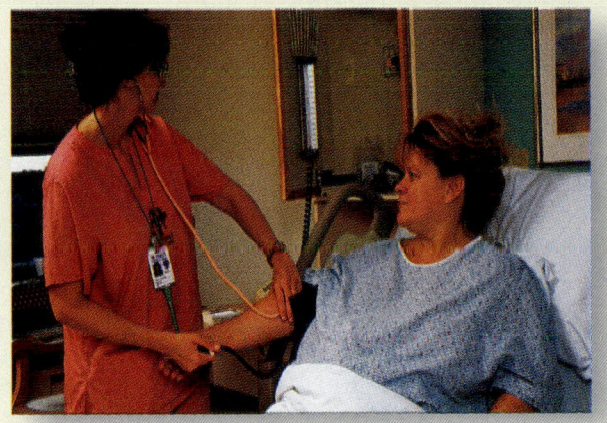

Cathleen Harris is admitted to the labor and delivery unit in the first stage of labor, with her cervix dilated at 2 cm. This is Cathleen's and her husband Bill's second pregnancy.

Margaret Kiely, RN, is monitoring Cathleen's progress in labor. On admission, Cathleen's vital signs are T = 37.4°C (99.3°F); P = 90 beats/minute; R = 15 respirations/minute; BP = 110/70. The fetal heart rate is 140 beats/minute. As Cathleen begins the fourth hour of the active phase of labor, the nurse notes an increase in her blood pressure to 130/98, with an increase in the fetal heart rate to 154 beats/minute. Contractions are occurring every 3 minutes and each lasts approximately 60 seconds.

The nurse informs Cathleen and Bill about these changes and tells them that she will need to contact Cathleen's obstetrician, Dr. Aizawa, and the perinatalogist and neonatologist on call within the unit. Cathleen grasps Bill's hand and asks: "Is it really necessary to have all these doctors here? Why can't just you and Dr. Aizawa help us and our baby?" ■

2

The Perinatal Experience

The perinatal period spans the developmental stages of fetal and neonatal life. The concept of the perinatal period is important, because many of the stresses and hazards that affect the fetus have either a direct or an indirect effect in the neonatal period. Moreover, jeopardy to life is greater during this period than at any subsequent time in the person's life cycle. Of the deaths occurring in the first year of life, about two thirds occur in the first 28 days. If fetal loss is added to this statistic, then the perinatal period is the greatest threat to life for a given time interval (March of Dimes Birth Defects Foundation, 1997).

This chapter provides an overview of the perinatal perspective, including factors influencing care of low-risk and high-risk childbearing families. A framework of perinatal nursing is presented, describing the components of care for the low-risk and high-risk client. Perinatal care is, by nature, collaborative. Thus, the framework for perinatal nursing presented in this chapter emphasizes collaborative care, but structures this care in a manner that parallels the steps of the nursing process. A model for interdisciplinary team development is also presented, with an emphasis on the need for role flexibility, mutual cooperation, and communication in achieving truly collaborative interdisciplinary care.

Several historical trends in perinatal care, most importantly regionalization or perinatal services and transport to clinical facilities offering different levels of specialized care, have contributed to a decline in perinatal mortality over the past 40 years. However, the advent of managed care has forced a reconceptualization of regionalization (Joffe & Black, 1997). Whatever systems of care are in place, the perinatal nurse will play an important role in achieving improved birth weight and access to care for members of lower socioeconomic groups, who are particularly at risk for poor perinatal outcome.

Regardless of whether nurses practice with healthy or compromised childbearing clients and neonates, identification of risk status is an inherent part of the nursing process. Thus, all maternity nurses will need to maintain the perinatal perspective.

▶ PHILOSOPHY OF PERINATAL CARE

Although nothing is inherent in the term "perinatal care" to indicate that it concerns high-risk or low-risk mothers, fetuses, and neonates, in practice the concept deals with identifying risk factors on a continuum from low to high risk. What does it mean to classify a mother, fetus, or neonate as high or low risk and to include that person in a system of perinatal care delivery? Nurses and other health care professionals assess and screen mothers, fetuses, and neonates throughout pregnancy and the neonatal period. The physiologic and psychologic strengths of the family are determined, as well as possible vulnerabilities and problems. In other words, they determine the risk status of a woman and family, be it low or high.

Within this broad perspective, probable and definite risk factors are identified as early in the pregnancy as possible. For example, adolescents or women over age 35 may be identified as being at risk for problems in the perinatal period. In addition, some women enter the childbearing cycle with a condition such as diabetes, which might profoundly affect the course of the pregnancy for both mother and fetus. Similarly, some neonates are born with inherent problems, such as prematurity, which may produce a poor reproductive outcome for mother and neonate in certain circumstances and may affect their subsequent development and well-being. These families would be considered high risk; however, problems can be prevented or treated if childbearing families are assessed early and risk factors identified.

Timely intervention, made possible by careful monitoring of high-risk mothers, fetuses, and neonates, helps to optimize reproductive outcome for all involved. The goals of high-risk and low-risk maternity care are identical: optimum well-being for mother, neonate, and family. Identification of the risk status of the childbearing family alerts the health care team to problems that may emerge during the course of the pregnancy or the neonatal period. Interventions can thus be begun in the most timely fashion to prevent or minimize a poor reproductive outcome (Dujardin, Clarysse, Criel, DeBrouwere, & Wangata, 1995).

▶ DEFINITION OF TERMS

Although authorities agree that the perinatal period spans fetal and neonatal life, there is disagreement as to when this period begins. Some authorities say that the perinatal period begins as early as conception; others say it begins as late as 28 weeks of gestation. The confusion rests on the lack of knowledge of when the fetus can reasonably survive outside of the uterus, that is, the **point of viability.** The estimate that is given as the lowest point of viability is 20 weeks of gestation, with some states using 24 or 28 weeks as the point of viability for statistical purposes. For clarity, 20 weeks of gestation will be used here as the point of viability. Thus, the **perinatal period** is defined as the period from 20 weeks of gestation through the 28th day of neonatal life for purposes of reporting outcomes of low-risk and high-risk pregnancies.

Perinatal nursing is broader by definition than those definitions used for statistical purposes. Because risk status should be identified early in the pregnancy or even in the preconception period, and because the nurse cares for the childbearing family throughout the span of gestation and the neonatal period, **perinatal nursing** is defined as the practice of professional nursing in response to the needs of the high-risk or low-risk family throughout the prenatal, intrapartum, postpartum, and neonatal periods. **High-risk perinatal nursing** is the practice of nursing of childbearing families who have an increased probability of either psychosocial or physical illness, disability, or death, that is, the nursing care of childbearing families assessed to have a high-risk status.

Other terms relevant to perinatal care are defined in Chapter 1 and in Table 2–1.

▶ CONCEPTUAL FRAMEWORK FOR PERINATAL NURSING

Perinatal nurses structure their care delivery for families in various states of risk using the nursing process. In addition, they must tailor their care to complement care delivered by other members of the interdisciplinary team. Figure 2–1 provides a framework that identifies the components that form the basis for perinatal nursing. These components parallel the steps of the nursing process. They are nursing assessment of reproductive and developmental health, the decision-making process and nursing diagnoses, collaborative planning and intervention, and evaluation and revision of outcome criteria.

Several factors are associated with the expertise of perinatal nurses. These include their educational preparation, personal and professional experience, and the attitudes, beliefs, and values that make up their personal philosophies regarding perinatal care.

▶ Nursing Assessment of Reproductive and Developmental Health

As a member of the health care team, the perinatal nurse systematically assesses the expectant parents, fetus, neonate, family, and environment. The expectant parents are assessed for physiologic, sensory, motor, language, cognitive, educational, self-help, and emotional/behavioral factors. Physiologic parameters are assessed in the fetus. Assessment of the neonate includes the same factors assessed in the expectant parents, with the added dimension of neonatal temperament. The family is assessed for structure and dynamics. Assessment of the environment includes assessments of the home, community, work, and school environments (Fig. 2–2). The cultural affiliation of the family is also assessed.

Assessment of these parameters provides the nurse with the data base from which decisions and

---

▶ TABLE 2–1

Definitions Relevant to Perinatal Nursing

Term	Definition
Stillbirth rate	Number of stillborn infants per 1000 population
Neonatal period	First 28 days of life; the period of greatest mortality in childhood, with the highest risk occurring in the first 24 hours of life
Neonatal death	Death of an infant before 29 days of life
Perinatology	Specialty of obstetric medicine devoted to care of the high-risk mother and fetus
Neonatology	Specialty of pediatric medicine devoted to care of the high-risk neonate; if the infant remains hospitalized for several months after birth, the neonatologist often provides care for that infant beyond the age of 28 days
High-risk pregnancy	Pregnancy in which the woman has an increased chance of developing a psychosocial or physical illness or dying; or a pregnancy in which the fetus has an increased chance of developing an illness or dying; or both
High-risk neonate	Infant who has an increased possibility of developing a psychosocial or physical illness or disability or of dying at birth or in the near future
High-risk postpartum client	Woman who has, during the first 6 weeks after delivery, an increased chance of developing a psychosocial or physical illness or dying as a result of the childbearing process

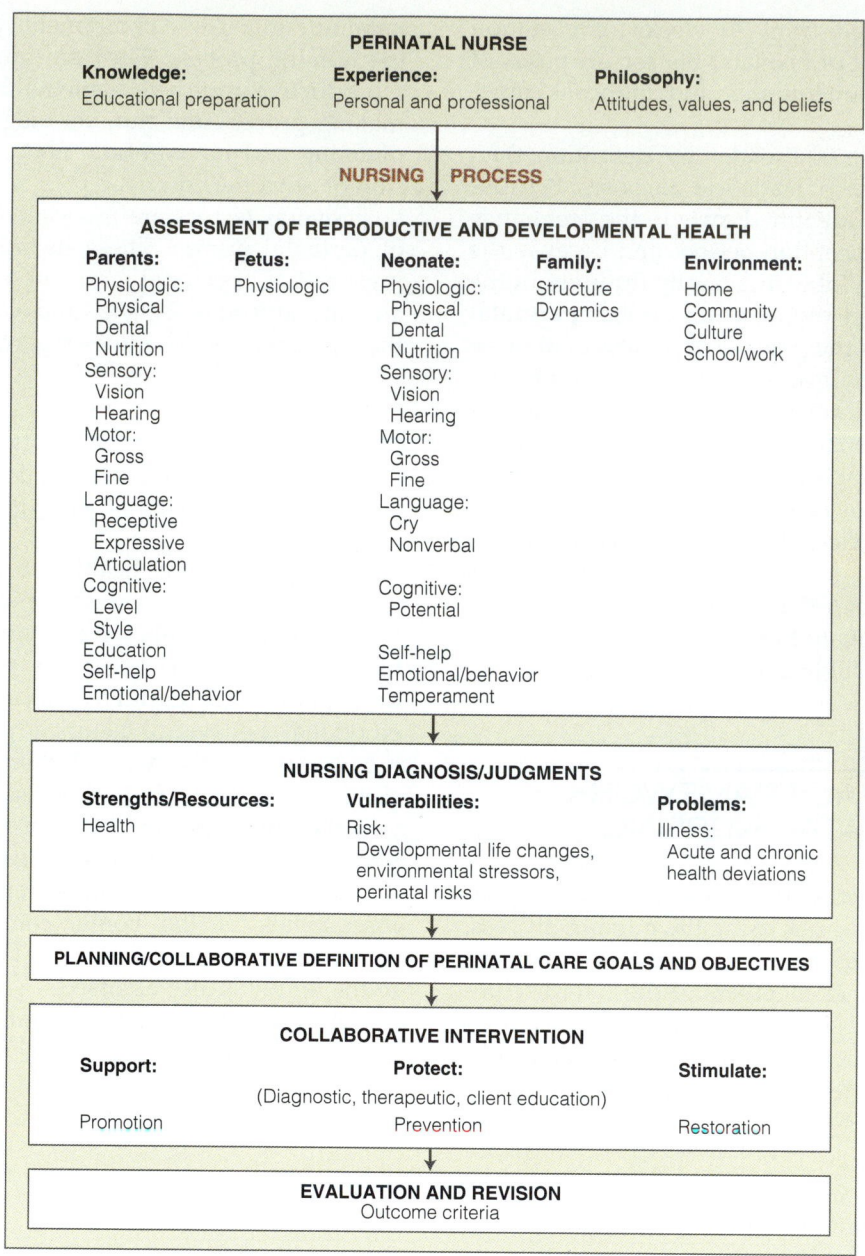

FIGURE 2–1. Conceptual framework for perinatal nursing.

nursing diagnoses are made relative to the health status of the perinatal family. Assessment concepts significant to both reproductive and developmental parameters of the childbearing family are also included (Vecchi, Vasquez, Radin, & Johnson, 1996).

▶ The Decision-Making Process and Nursing Diagnoses

The framework for nursing assessment, as well as nursing decisions, is a health–risk–illness continuum.

Assessment about health provides the basis for decisions about client/family strengths and resources. Assessment related to risk provides the basis for decisions about vulnerabilities. Assessment related to illness provides the basis for decisions about both acute and chronic health deviations or problems.

Data collected during the initial assessment and on subsequent visits are used to develop nursing diagnoses and direct the collaborative development of goals and objectives on which the plan of care (including diagnostic, therapeutic, and client education interventions) is formulated.

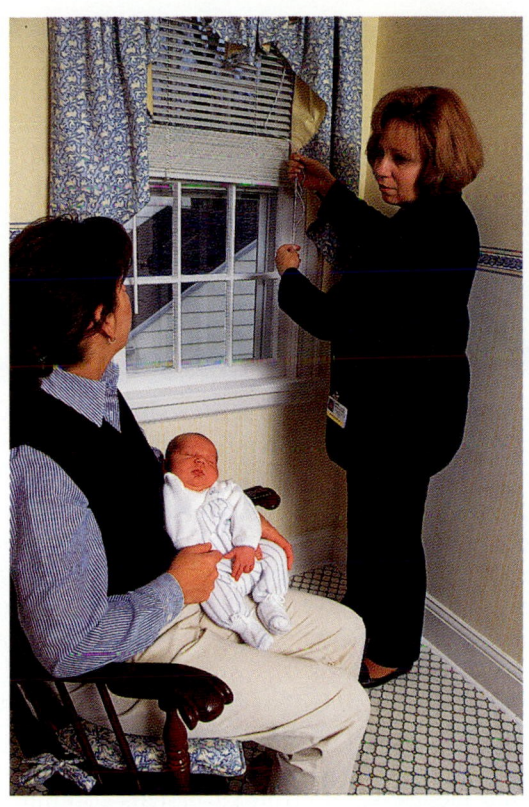

A

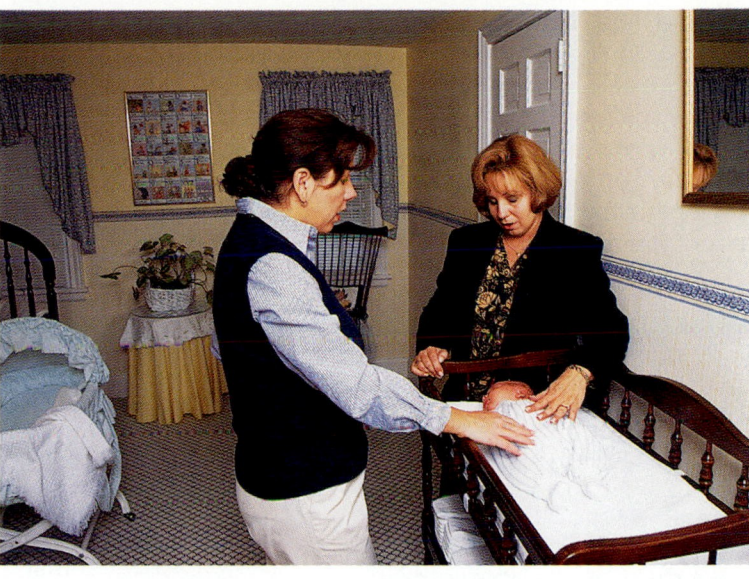

B

FIGURE 2–2. An important role for the nurse on a perinatal/neonatal interdisciplinary team is assessment of the home environment and review of safety measures with the family. **A.** Keeping cords of blinds away from young children. **B.** Maintaining a firm hold on the newborn while on the changing table.

▶ Planning and Collaborative Goal Setting

Nursing assessment and diagnoses concerning the family are pooled with data gathered by other professionals on the interdisciplinary team. Nursing and other data form the basis of collaborative goals for the family and will direct the management plan and interventions developed by the team, which also includes the family. Goal planning is accomplished through team discussion and sharing of discipline-specific perceptions (Fig. 2–3); the process of negotiation will determine the plan and the coordinated, collaborative interventions of team members. Plans and goals of interdisciplinary teams are often represented in critical pathways, algorithms, clinical paths, or predictive pathways.

▶ Collaborative Intervention

Collaborative intervention is an important dimension of the framework for perinatal nursing outlined in Figure 2–1. The nurse collaborates with other members of an interdisciplinary team to promote health, prevent complications, and restore the client to a level of health care that will promote well-being for the childbearing family.

Decisions about health care for the client and the family require the integration of information from a variety of sources. Although the health–illness continuum is used within this framework, nurses must recognize that perinatal families have dynamic and changing health states. Thus, the high-risk client may

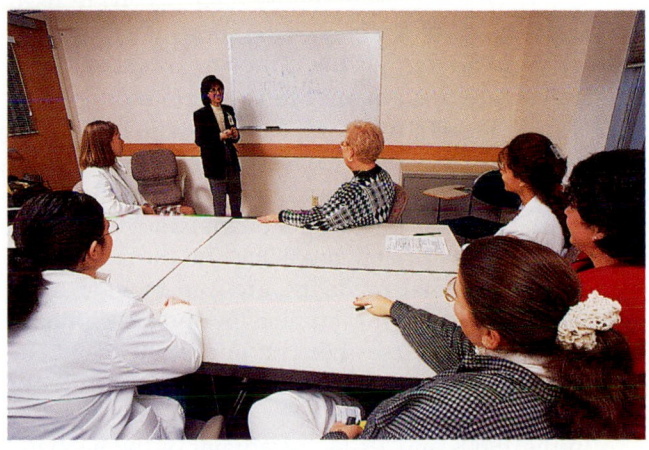

FIGURE 2–3. Interdisciplinary health care team meeting.

become a low-risk client with comprehensive interventions. Similarly the adolescent mother may be considered at risk because of age, but healthy self-care practices may produce a good reproductive outcome for mother and neonate. Strengths and resources exist at the same time as problems and vulnerabilities. Care for the perinatal family should therefore include three types of intervention:

1. *Health promotion.* Activities that support and enhance existing strengths and resources
2. *Health protection* (illness prevention). Activities that protect the family from stressors
3. *Restoration.* Activities that stimulate the family's ability to adapt

▶ Evaluation and Revision of Outcome Criteria

The final phase of the framework of perinatal nursing includes care and revisions based on these evaluations. Because the nursing process is cyclic, the nurse reassesses the perinatal family on an ongoing basis.

▶ HISTORICAL FACTORS AND TRENDS IN PERINATAL CARE

It has been known for some time that certain situations in the prenatal, intrapartum, postpartum, and neonatal periods can have an adverse effect on maternal and fetal/neonatal outcome. It was not, however, until the 1950s that health care providers began to focus on the relationship between specific factors and their outcomes. A study in 1951 identified cerebral palsy as being linked to high-risk factors during the childbearing cycle (Luke, 1993). By the 1950s, a number of states developed maternal mortality committees. These committees gathered data that were used to direct activities designed to reduce maternal mortality. The decade of the 1950s thus became the age of neonatal awareness among health care providers.

During the 1960s and 1970s, further investigation contributed to the knowledge of risk factors associated with morbidity and mortality. The 1960s has been termed the decade of fetal medicine, and the 1970s, the decade of perinatal medicine. In the 1980s, the concept of perinatal medicine grew to include management of childbearing families by interdisciplinary teams, on which nurses became important members. This trend has continued into the 1990s (Institute for Family-Centered Care, 1996).

In the 1960s and 1970s the advent of the neonatal intensive care unit (NICU) and improved technologi-

cal advances contributed greatly to the sharp reduction in the infant mortality rates. This reduction was primarily due to improved survival in low-birth-weight infants, primarily premature infants. These low-birth-weight infants accounted for 57% of all infant deaths; the majority of these deaths occurring within the first 30 days of life (March of Dimes Birth Defects Foundation, 1997).

▶ Regionalization

The progress that has been made in reducing mortality was to a great extent due to regionalization of perinatal care. In the mid-1960s, leaders in the delivery of perinatal care at a national level, including obstetricians, neonatologists, and pediatricians, recognized that a change was necessary in the way perinatal health services were delivered to improve the reproductive and developmental outcomes for families at risk.

Technical developments, the creation of the NICU, and its subsequent reduction in infant mortality prompted the formation of a national Committee on Perinatal Health (COPH) in 1976. This committee was made up of members of the joint committee on perinatal health of the American Medical Association, the American College of Obstetricians and Gynecologists (ACOG), the American Academy of Family Physicians, and the American Academy of Pediatrics. Their report, *Toward Improving the Outcome of Pregnancy* (TIOP I), outlined a regionalized system for organizing and maximizing resources with an emphasis on inpatient perinatal services (COPH, 1977; Evans & Friedland, 1995; March of Dimes Birth Defects Foundation, 1997). The new way of organizing services was called **regionalization.** As described in the report, regionalization refers to "the development, within a geographical area, of a coordinated cooperative system of maternal and perinatal health care in which, by mutual agreements between hospitals and physicians and based upon population needs, the degree of complexity of maternal and perinatal care each hospital is capable of providing is identified so as to accomplish the following objectives: quality care to all pregnant women and newborns, maximal utilization of highly trained perinatal personnel and intensive care facilities, and assurance of reasonable cost effectiveness" (COPH, 1977).

The basic premise of regionalization should be a single standard of care for all perinatal clients. Any mother and her fetus/neonate/infant should have equal access to whatever aspect of perinatal care they need. To provide the best care in a cost-effective manner, all perinatal care institutions in a given region were organized so that appropriate levels of perinatal care were available to a perinatal client at different facilities within a geographic area. Thus, through transporting childbearing women or neonates of different risk status to an appropriate facility within that geographic area, each family would receive appropriate care in a cost-efficient, high-quality manner.

The concept of regionalized perinatal care described in TIOP I was an excellent one; however, the system of perinatal care was still inadequate. Many women in the United States, especially those who are living in poverty and African-American, are still without perinatal health services of reasonable quality. Regionalization, as originally proposed, failed to provide universal *prenatal care* and to identify and manage high-risk pregnancies in a successful manner.

In addition, recent changes in the financing of health care delivery may have contributed to the eroding of the regional health care system. Increased competition for clients, more uninsured clients, and managed care have all affected the system, resulting in hospitals and health care providers operating outside of the system. An example of this is a blurring among services offered at traditionally high-risk and low-risk facilities. For example, a community hospital may hire a neonatologist and keep low-birth-weight infants in its own NICU rather than transport the infant to a large academic health center where the infant would have received care in a traditional regionalized system. It became apparent that new systems of perinatal care had to be developed to meet the needs of pregnant women and neonates in the changing health care environment.

Regionalization in the Changing Health Care System

Over the course of the past 10 years, the expansion and development of regionalized perinatal care has faltered. This was largely because of clinical and financial issues created by institutional and individual competition for clients, which overshadowed the original intent of this system of care (Pollack, 1996). In addition, by the mid-1980s the United States was experiencing a slowdown in the reduction in infant mortality noted in the early years of regionalization. While transport to institutions where specialists and technology were available had a great effect on infant mortality, it became evident that other factors needed to be considered in a system of perinatal care.

In 1976, TIOP I proposed a model system for regionalized perinatal care and defined three levels of inpatient hospital care based on the level of technology and maternal–fetal specialists available at the facilities. If a pregnant woman or neonate was at too high risk to be cared for at one level, they were to be

transferred to the next level where more sophisticated high-risk care was available. Due to the factors already mentioned however, it was clear that further improvement in the outcome of pregnancy required emphasis on preparation for successful childbearing, full access to perinatal care, and new regionalized perinatal care structures (COPH, 1995).

In 1990, the COPH was reconstituted to respond to a changing environment and to make further recommendations for the regionalization of perinatal care in the 1990s and beyond. Ten underlying assumptions served as a framework for their deliberations (COPH, 1995):

1. Perinatal care includes services along a continuum beginning before conception and extending through the first year of infant life.
2. The perinatal care system should be designed to improve pregnancy outcome for the total population and to ensure optimal health for every woman and infant. Additional effort is required to realize these goals for medically or socially high-risk women.
3. A system approach to delivery of perinatal care, with structures and mechanisms for accountability, is needed to ensure that appropriate care is accessible to all.
4. The organization and structure of perinatal care must be responsive to individual needs. Significant and continuing improvements in outcome depend on providing medically appropriate and culturally competent care to each family.
5. Structures should be flexible at the state and local level. No one model can be applied across the nation, and community-level involvement is essential to success.
6. Perinatal care providers include a mix of public and private, health and nonhealth, and ambulatory and inpatient practitioners and facilities that must be coordinated to meet the needs of women and infants.
7. Preventive services are the most effective way to improve pregnancy outcome. This includes health promotion and health education, as well as family planning and prepregnancy risk-reduction efforts.
8. Effective technology must be applied to perinatal problems. Proven therapeutic interventions should be continued because they save lives and reduce disabilities.
9. Data and research are needed to assess the effectiveness of current efforts and to develop new knowledge that can be used to improve the outcome of pregnancy.

10. Financing adequate to support the perinatal care system is required. Key elements include personal health care coverage for women and infants, adequate payment for providers, and support for structural elements of the system.

The COPH, made up of a wide variety of consumers and health professionals, including nurses, issued its report; *Toward Improving the Outcome of Pregnancy: The 90s and Beyond* (TIOP II). Like TIOP I, the report focuses primarily on the organization and structure of perinatal services. However, TIOP II includes a broader continuum of perinatal care than TIOP I, ranging from health education, preconception, and prenatal care to birth services and care through the first year of life. TIOP II also calls for better integration of services across the broad continuum of necessary services, as well as more emphasis on prevention, risk identification, and data collection and evaluation (Evans and Friedland, 1995).

Regionalization mainly focuses on the relationships between providers in a system of care. TIOP I defined three levels of care, to be delivered in hospitals, based on responsibility, services, and technology. For example, a Level I institution, such as a community hospital with minimum technology and no maternal–fetal medical specialist on staff, delivered low-risk women and neonates; a Level II institution, with a moderate amount of sophisticated technology and high-risk maternal–fetal personnel such as perinatologists, neonatologists, and perinatal nurse practitioners, delivered women and neonates at moderate risk; and a Level III institution, with high levels of technology and many maternal–fetal medical and nursing specialists on staff delivered women and neonates at the highest risk. TIOP II expanded the emphasis on provider relationships between levels of risk care by recommending that individual providers be organized into networks, and that states or substate regions develop boards with the responsibility of coordinating services. Further, TIOP II recommended that the three levels of care be modified, enhanced, and promoted to include basic, speciality, and subspecialty care. These levels of care could be continued for inpatient care and initiated for ambulatory prenatal care as well. The three new levels of care delivery to mothers and neonates are:

- Basic providers (including family physicians, certified nurse-midwives, general practitioners, nurse practitioners and obstetricians);
- Specialty care providers (including obstetricians and experienced family physicians); and
- Subspecialty care providers (including maternal–fetal medicine specialists and geneticists).

The three levels of hospital care continue in recommendations made by COPH, although TIOP II drops the designation of Level I, II, and III and substitutes the terms basic, specialty, and subspecialty care. In addition, TIOP II acknowledges that the three levels of inpatient care can be co-located within one hospital or facility—a major change from TIOP I.

TIOP II includes recommendations that perinatal regions should be clarified to avoid duplication or fragmentation of services. The COPH also recommends that geopolitical boundaries for regions be established across the country. Structural reforms and ongoing accountability of care of a total population depend on having well-defined perinatal regions (Evans & Friedland, 1995).

Accountability would be achieved through state and regional perinatal boards, which would serve as planning and coordinating bodies for the state. In each region, the perinatal boards would facilitate the formation of perinatal care networks. They would also provide links to other state agencies, address activities such as planning, monitoring access to care, collecting data, and providing education to providers. In general, the boards' roles would be to monitor affordable, available, and appropriate care for all women and infants (Evans & Friedland, 1995). Figure 2–4 depicts the proposed structure for perinatal care in states and regions.

While TIOP II proposes many important changes in the structure of the system of perinatal care, these changes face many barriers to implement; for example, a lack of funding and staff expertise, lack of defined regional boundaries, weak collaboration among agencies and providers, and poor coordination of research efforts and data collection. Perinatal boards at the state or substate regional level may also have varying levels of authority, and hence, varying ability to enforce or regulate networks. There is evidence, however, that some states or regions are already developing structures or models that include some of the tenets of TIOP II. For example, Pollack (1996) analyzed perinatal services in six metropolitan regions. An alternative to traditional regionalization based on a reorganization of existing perinatal services into a coordinated system was defined that appropriately used and selectively developed the resources of community hospitals with moderate-risk nurseries (those formerly designated as Level II nurseries) operating under closely monitored definitive guidelines for care. A group of private practice neonatologists functioned in cooperation and as equal partners with an established university facility (formerly designated as a Level III facility) and staff. This model was found to provide safe, efficient, and cost-effective care.

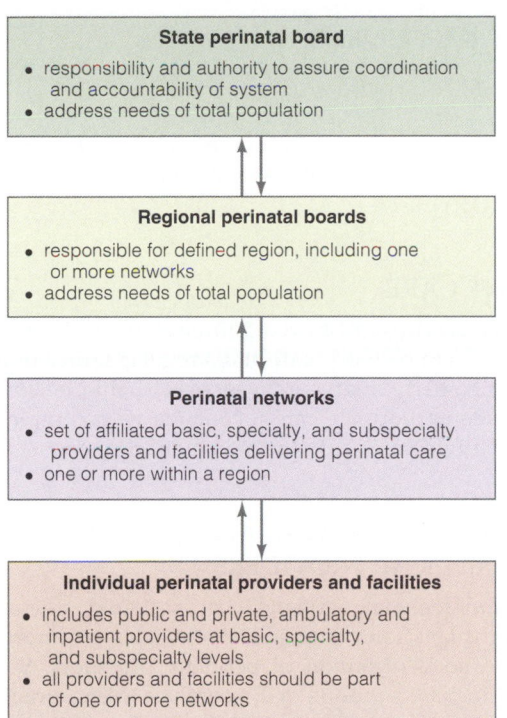

FIGURE 2–4. Proposed structure for perinatal care in states and regions. *(Reproduced, with permission, from Committee on Perinatal Health (COPH). (1995).* Toward improving the outcome of pregnancy: The 90s and beyond. *White Plains, NY: March of Dimes Birth Defects Foundation.)*

A second model described in the literature (Rowley, 1995) restructured perinatal care in order to reduce the disparity in infant mortality rates between African-American and Caucasian infants. The author describes a model that assumes that prenatal care will reduce risks and enhance protective factors by

the appropriate use of two prevention strategies: the high-risk prevention strategy and the population-based prevention strategy. The high-risk prevention strategy is associated with clinical care. It consists of establishing a perinatal network for screening and assessment of a woman's risk for a specific poor pregnancy outcome and the provision of appropriate medical and social interventions for those found to be at high risk. The population-based prevention strategy is based on the principle that moderate and achievable change by the population covered by the network as a whole might greatly reduce mortality. The goal of the strategy is to shift the entire distribution of exposure to prenatal care in a favorable direction. This strategy is seen as possibly effective for low-risk African-American women without major risk factors (Rowley, 1995). Other examples exist as well. New state and regional initiatives focus on coordinating resources and care in an effort to improve care of women and infants, as well as efficiently use resources. TIOP II's newly defined recommendations have the potential to continue the positive effects produced by TIOP I. See box on page 26 entitled Key COPH Recommendations Essential for Improving the Outcome of Pregnancy for a summary of TIOP II recommendations.

▶ Transport

Within a geographic area, if the perinatal client requires a level of care different from what the closest hospital or clinical facility can offer, the client is transported to another facility with more appropriate resources (Fig. 2–5). If the caregivers predict that the neonate will require neonatal intensive care, every

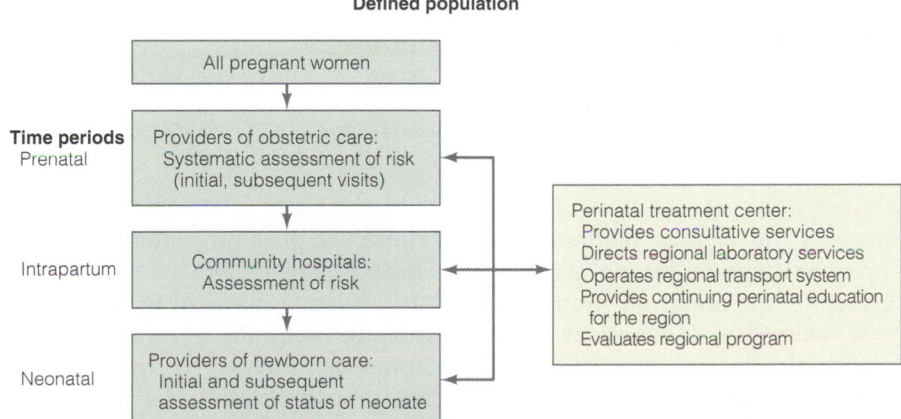

FIGURE 2–5. Conceptual model of a regional perinatal system within a defined geographic area. *(Reproduced, with permission, from Merkatz, I., & Johnson, K. (1976). Regionalization of perinatal care for the United States.* Clinical Perinatology, *3, 272.)*

► KEY COPH RECOMMENDATIONS ESSENTIAL FOR IMPROVING THE OUTCOME OF PREGNANCY

HEALTH PROMOTION AND HEALTH EDUCATION

In collaboration with families and health professionals, every school (K–12) should develop and implement a plan for comprehensive school health education that includes age-appropriate reproductive health information.

REPRODUCTIVE AWARENESS

New strategies to reach each man and woman of childbearing age with reproductive awareness messages should be implemented. All health providers should employ reproductive health screening to reduce risks.

STRUCTURE AND ACCOUNTABILITY

Perinatal regions should be well defined to ensure accountability for care of a total population. State and regional perinatal boards should be established with the authority and responsibility for ensuring, providing, or coordinating nonclinical activities such as planning, monitoring access, data collection, and provider education.

PRECONCEPTION AND INTERCONCEPTION CARE

Risk reduction should be emphasized and family planning counseling and services routinely available. Preconception or interconception visits annually, as well as a prepregnancy planning visit, should become standard components of care.

AMBULATORY PRENATAL CARE

Early risk assessment, followed by appropriate care, consultation, or referral, must be a universal and ongoing component of prenatal care; medical and social services may be needed.

INPATIENT PERINATAL CARE

Three levels of perinatal care defined in the 1970s should be modified, enhanced, and promoted. Three types of facilities should be recognized: basic, specialty, and subspecialty perinatal centers, with all facilities integrated into networks of care.

INFANT CARE

Perinatal services must extend through the first year of life, with access to pediatric care and a regular source of care for all infants. Early intervention services should be structured to include appropriate care for infants with complex problems and integrated into the regionalized system.

IMPROVING THE AVAILABILITY OF PERINATAL PROVIDERS

State and regional perinatal boards should assesss need, develop plans, and implement strategies to improve the supply and distribution of perinatal providers. Strategies should include supports and incentives to encourage qualified providers to deliver perinatal care.

DATA, DOCUMENTATION, AND EVALUATION

Every state should have a perinatal data program to facilitate accountability and to provide information for monitoring the system and perinatal outcome, including population-based and clinical data.

FINANCING PERINATAL CARE

Any health care reform plan should include a benefit package that meets the unique needs of pregnant women and infants, and a process for updating the benefit package to add effective new interventions. Financing mechanisms should be determined for nonclinical services and used to support perinatal system structures.

Source: Committee on Perinatal Health, 1995.

---

effort is made to transport the woman before delivery. Transfer of the pregnant woman to another perinatal center is referred to as **maternal transport;** transfer of a neonate is referred to as **neonatal transport.** Maternal or antepartal transport in comparison with neonatal or postnatal transport is associated with decreased neonatal mortality and shorter hospital stays. Therefore early recognition of high-risk fetal conditions and maternal transfer is preferred. However, advanced labor or high-risk intrapartum condi-

tion may prohibit maternal transport (McCormick & Richardson, 1995).

When a nurse practitioner, nurse-midwife, obstetrician, or family practice physician determines that transport is required, the appropriate facility in that geographic location is called and advised that a transport is needed. When the receiving facility ascertains that transport is indicated and when a bed is available for the mother and neonate, the transport is arranged. Prior to transport, the "sending" agency must stabi-

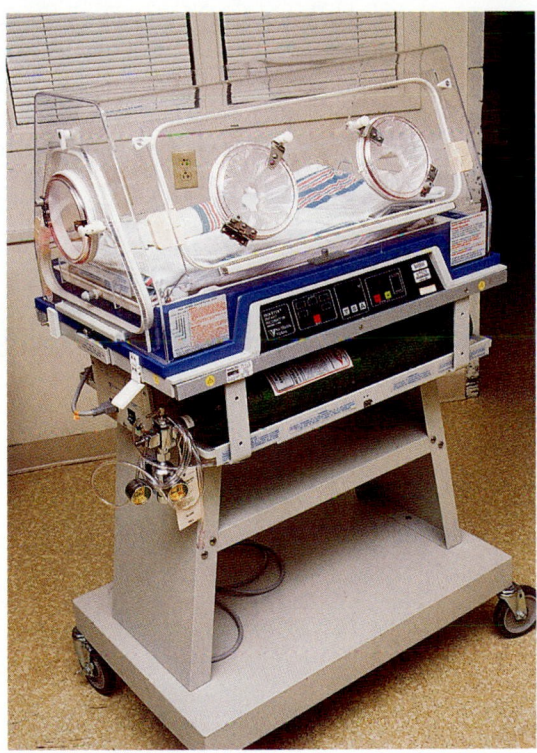

FIGURE 2–6. Perinatal transport vehicle.

lize and support the perinatal family to reduce the possibility that an emergency will develop in the transport vehicle.

The transport vehicle is usually a privately owned ambulance, ambulance helicopter, or fixed-wing aircraft that is under contract for transport purposes. The transport team may be a group of nurses, a group of paramedics especially trained for perinatal emergencies, an obstetric resident, or a respiratory therapist and nurse. Most of the supplies and equipment available in the intensive care unit are carried in the transport vehicle (Fig. 2–6).

Before departing from the facility of origin, the transport team assesses the client, provides treatment as needed, instructs the client and family about the transport procedure and the location of the receiving agency, and then proceeds with the transport. If the individual to be transported is the neonate, parents are provided an opportunity to see the neonate prior to transport.

On arrival at the receiving agency, the client and family are assisted in their adaptation to the emergency situation and transfer. If the client's condition warrants a transfer back to the original agency, a transfer is then made back to the sending hospital or other appropriate facility. This is a method of providing risk-appropriate care in a cost-effective manner as

close geographically to the client's home as possible. Thus, the transport "road" is a two-way street.

▶ Barriers and Access to Prenatal Care

Low birth weight in infants is one of the most devastating high-risk problems during the perinatal period. It is also believed to be one of the primary factors related to infant mortality in the United States today. Low birth weight has been linked directly to lack of prenatal care (Wirtschafter, 1995). One of the primary concerns, then, of nurses and other health care professionals involved in perinatal care must be to improve access to prenatal care, thus helping to reduce low birth weight and decrease infant mortality. Equal access to prenatal care is a prerequisite for successful systems of perinatal care. Reduction of barriers to quality prenatal care for all pregnant women must be a national priority.

Two broad issues are related to access to prenatal care. They are nonfinancial barriers to care and components of prenatal care effective in reducing low birth weight.

Nonfinancial Barriers to Prenatal Care

Three categories of nonfinancial barriers to prenatal care exist: (1) public policy/system barriers (inconvenient locations and hours of service, inadequate support and use of nurse-midwives, maldistribution of providers, lack of transportation, and multiple eligibility requirements for benefits); (2) provider barriers (negative behavior characteristics, inadequate education regarding psychosocial and cultural aspects of care, and communication problems between providers); and (3) client barriers (lack of knowledge about the importance of prenatal care, fear of the system and health care providers, denial and ambivalence about pregnancy, and lack of incentives to seek care). These areas must be addressed through greater public awareness and action in order to improve access to care for low-risk and high-risk women of all socioeconomic levels (Evans & Friedland, 1995).

Many programs exist across the country which attempt to reduce barriers to prenatal care. For example, programs may utilize a "one-stop shopping" model. Such a program would allow women to enroll in Medicaid and WIC programs where they receive prenatal care. Another example of a program would be one which employs an outreach worker to drive a van through the city and transport pregnant women who have not yet entered prenatal care to an appropriate prenatal care provider or clinic. There are many other examples of programs currently in operation, often due to the initiative of nurses, which are in action throughout the country.

Components of Prenatal Care

Seven categories of prenatal care have been identified as most effective in reducing the incidence of low birth weight: (1) initial and ongoing risk assessment, (2) individualized care based on case management, (3) nutritional counseling, (4) education to reduce or eliminate unhealthy habits, (5) stress reduction, (6) social support services, and (7) health education.

Prenatal care should be individually tailored to each woman's needs, degree of risk present, and mutually determined goals. Low-risk mothers require only selected categories of components and a minimal number of visits; women at high risk require almost all of the components and frequent visits.

▶ Concept of Risk

In order to employ the primary strategy of early risk identification and the provision of appropriate care,

---

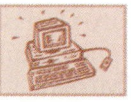

Research Abstract

Association Between Abuse During Pregnancy and Low Birth Weight

Physical abuse during pregnancy is seen as a risk to the health of both mother and infant. The purpose of this study was to examine the link between abuse during pregnancy and both risk factors for and joint relationship with low birth weight (defined by the Institute of Medicine [IOM]).

A sample of 1,203 pregnant women was drawn from two public prenatal clinics. The ethnic composition was African-American (n = 414), Hispanic (n = 412), and White (n = 377). The majority of women were between 20 and 29 years; 30% were teenagers. Women were urban residents and most had incomes below the poverty level. Each woman was entered into the study at the first prenatal visit.

Instruments used were the Abuse Assessment Screen (AAS), the Conflict Tactics Scale (CTS), the Index of Spouse Abuse (ISA), and the Danger Assessment Scale (DAS). All instruments had acceptable reliability and validity. In addition, 5 clusters of IOM-defined risk factors associated with low birth weight (LBW) were used to conduct a blind evaluation of each woman's medical record following delivery.

In this sample, abuse during pregnancy affected one in six women. As an aggregate and for each ethnic group, women abused during pregnancy delivered a higher percentage of LBW infants than nonabused women (p < .025). White women, followed by Hispanic women, experienced the most and severest episodes of abuse. For all ethnic groups, the perpetrator was almost always someone the woman knew intimately. Women abused during pregnancy were at risk for being less than 17 years of age, unmarried, having less than a 15-pound weight gain, less than 24-month interpregnancy interval, infections, anemia, smoking, and alcohol/drug use.

The investigators conclude that abuse during pregnancy is a significant risk factor for LBW infants, comparable to the commonly recognized risk factors cited above. The findings document a connection between abuse during pregnancy, IOM risk factors, and increased risk of lower infant birth weight.

Application to Practice

As the investigators suggest, all pregnant women should be assessed for abuse, regardless of when they initiate their first prenatal visit. If abuse is identified, it is essential to initiate intervention strategies designed to counteract this situation and other associated risk factors for LBW. Further, abused pregnant women need to be offered education, advocacy, and community referral information.

Source: McFarlane, J., Parker, B., & Soeken, K. (1996). Abuse during pregnancy: Association with maternal health and infant birth weight. Nursing Research, 45(1); 37–42.

risk assessment should be early and ongoing. Identification of perinatal clients at risk ideally begins before pregnancy or at the first prenatal visit and continues throughout the perinatal period. Risk factors are defined as characteristics that indicate a higher probability of adverse outcomes and help guide the actions of the woman, her social support network, and the providers. Once the nurse-midwife, nurse practitioner, obstetrician, perinatologist, or perinatal team identifies the woman or fetus at risk, collaborative management by the team is initiated.

Many factors may influence the maternal–fetal status and the status of the neonate. Chapters 15, 17, and 18, which provide a detailed description of assessment during pregnancy, identify these factors. Generally, there are three categories of risk factors:

1. *Medical.* Known medical complications, such as diabetes, may occur before or during pregnancy. Genetic factors posing a risk to the fetus, such as Tay-Sachs disease, fit into this category. Also included are lifestyle factors such as smoking that add an increased risk to the pregnancy.
2. *Obstetric or reproductive.* Past pregnancy conditions can suggest risk to the current pregnancy. An example is previous preterm labor and delivery.
3. *Psychosocial.* Socioeconomic status, social support systems, and psychological adaptation to pregnancy may affect the pregnancy, the treatment, and client compliance. This category—which includes the factors that are perhaps the most difficult to change and are the most often ignored—is a vital part of a holistic risk assessment.

Medical, reproductive, and psychosocial risks may be viewed on a continuum, as depicted in Table 2–2.

To ensure an appropriate level of care delivery, perinatal care should be based on a standardized antenatal risk assessment tool as part of the ongoing prenatal record. ACOG's antepartum record has been recommended by the COPH (March of Dimes Birth Defects Foundation, 1997) for standardized use in an effort to improve communication among providers of care for clients throughout the perinatal period, both inpatient and outpatient (Fig. 2–7). Some guidelines for referral to the appropriate provider or perinatal care center are given in Figures 2–8 and 2–9 and in Table 2–3.

▶ **TABLE 2-2**

Medical, Reproductive, and Psychosocial Risk Continuum and Nursing Actions

Type of Risk	Health	At Risk	Illness
Medical	Assess client for change in at-risk/ill status. Educate client about pregnancy and medical condition, available resources. Educate client about health maintenance in pregnancy, reportable signs and symptoms of illness.	Assess client for risk and treat/monitor. Educate client about risk status, management, outcomes, and resources.	Assess client for change in status. Educate client about illness. Assist client to optimal level of health.
Reproductive	Assess client for change in at-risk/ill status. Educate client about childbirth, self-care, infant care and management, nutrition, and resources.	Assess client for risk and treat/monitor. Educate client about risk status, management, outcomes, and resources.	Assess client for change in status. Educate client about illness, possible deviations from normal.
Psychosocial	Assess mother/family for developmental tasks, psychological adaptation to pregnancy. Assess client support systems. Assess client socioeconomic status, adequacy of home environment, access to food of adequate nutritional value, available transportation to health care.	Assess mother/family for developmental, situational crisis. Educate mother/family about resources, support groups, classes, financial aid, WIC.	Assess mother/family for change in status. Educate mother/family about disability, rehabilitation, and financial aid. Refer to social service as necessary.

ACOG Antepartum record

Date _____

Name _____
        Last   First   Middle

ID # _____ Hospital of delivery_____

Newborn's physician _____ Referred by _____ Final EDD_____

Birth date Age Race Marital status	Address
Mo Day Yr S M W D SEP	
Occupation Education	Zip: Phone: (H) (O)
☐ Homemaker (Last grade completed)	Insurance carrier/Medicaid #
☐ Outside work	
☐ Student Type of work	

Emergency contact:	Relationship:	Phone:

Total preg	Full term	Premature	Abortions induced	Abortions spontaneous	Ectopics	Multiple births	Living

Menstrual history

LMP ☐ Definite ☐ Approximate (month known) Menses monthly ☐ Yes ☐ No   Frequency: Q _____ Days   Menarche _____ (Age onset)

      ☐ Unknown ☐ Normal amount/duration Prior menses _____ Date   On BCPs at concept. ☐ Yes ☐ No   hCG + ___ / ___ / ___

Past pregnancies (Last six)

Date Mo/Yr	GA weeks	Length of labor	Birth weight	Type delivery	Anes.	Place of delivery	Perinatal mortality Yes/No	Treatment preterm labor Yes/No	Comments/complications

Past medical history

	O Neg + Pos	Detail positive remarks Include date and treatment		O Neg + Pos	Detail positive remarks Include date and treatment
1. Diabetes			16. Rh sensitized		
2. Hypertension			17. Tuberculosis		
3. Heart disease			18. Asthma		
4. Rheumatic fever			19. Allergies (drugs)		
5. Mitral valve prolapse			20. GYN surgery		
6. Kidney disease/UTI					
7. Neurologic/epilepsy					
8. Psychiatric			21. Operations/hospitalizations (year and reason)		
9. Hepatitis/liver disease					
10. Varicosities/phlebitis					
11. Thyroid dysfunction			22. Anesthetic complications		
12. Major accidents			23. History of abnormal PAP		
13. History of blood transfus.			24. Uterine anomaly		

	Amt/Day Prepreg	Amt/Day Preg	# Yrs use			
				25. Infertility		
				26. In utero DES exposure		
14. Tobacco				27. Street drugs		
15. Alcohol				28. Other		

Comments: _____

_____

_____

_____

_____

(Cont.)

FIGURE 2–7. Standard antenatal risk assessment tool. *(From ACOG Antepartum Record. Copyright 1989. Revised April 1992. The American College of Obstetricians and Gynecologists, 409 12th Street, SW, Washington, DC 20024-2188.)*

Genetics screening

Includes patient, baby's father, or anyone in either family with:

	Yes	No		Yes	No
1. Patient's age ≥ 35 years			10. Huntington chorea		
2. Thalassemia (Italian, Greek, Mediterranean, or Oriental background): MCV< 80			11. Mental retardation		
			If yes, was person tested for fragile X?		
3. Neural tube defect (meningomyelocele, open spine, or anencephaly)			12. Other inherited genetic or chromosomal disorder		
			13. Patient or baby's father had a child with birth defects not listed above		
4. Down syndrome			14. ≥ 3 first-trimester spontaneous abortions, or a stillbirth		
5. Tay-Sachs (eg, Jewish background)					
6. Sickle cell disease or trait			15. Medications or street drugs since last menstrual period		
7. Hemophilia					
8. Muscular dystrophy			If yes, agent(s):		
9. Cystic fibrosis			16. Other significant family history (see comments)		

Comments: _____

_____

_____

_____

_____

_____

Infection history	Yes	No		Yes	No
1. High risk AIDS			4. Patient or partner have history of genital herpes		
2. High risk hepatitis B			5. Rash or viral illness since last menstrual period		
3. Live with someone with TB or exposed to TB			6. History of STD, GC, chlamydia, HPV, syphilis		
			7. Other (see comments)		

Comments: _____

_____

_____

_____

_____ **Interviewer's signature** _____

Initial physical examination

Date ___ / ___ / ___   Prepregnancy weight _____   Height _____   BP _____

	Normal	Abnormal				
1. HEENT	☐ Normal	☐ Abnormal	12. Vulva	☐ Normal	☐ Condyloma	☐ Lesions
2. Fundi	☐ Normal	☐ Abnormal	13. Vagina	☐ Normal	☐ Inflammation	☐ Discharge
3. Teeth	☐ Normal	☐ Abnormal	14. Cervix	☐ Normal	☐ Inflammation	☐ Lesions
4. Thyroid	☐ Normal	☐ Abnormal	15. Uterus	☐ Normal	☐ Abnormal	☐ Fibroids
5. Breasts	☐ Normal	☐ Abnormal	16. Adnexa	☐ Normal	☐ Mass	
6. Lungs	☐ Normal	☐ Abnormal	17. Rectum	☐ Normal	☐ Abnormal	
7. Heart	☐ Normal	☐ Abnormal	18. Diagonal conjugate	☐ Reached	☐ No	_____ CM
8. Abdomen	☐ Normal	☐ Abnormal	19. Spines	☐ Average	☐ Prominent	☐ Blunt
9. Extremities	☐ Normal	☐ Abnormal	20. Sacrum	☐ Concave	☐ Straight	☐ Anterior
10. Skin	☐ Normal	☐ Abnormal	21. Arch	☐ Normal	☐ Wide	☐ Narrow
11. Lymph nodes	☐ Normal	☐ Abnormal	22. Gynecoid pelvic type	☐ Yes	☐ No	

Comments (Number and explain abnormals): _____

_____

_____

_____

_____

_____ **Exam by** _____

(Cont.)

FIGURE 2–7. *Continued*

ACOG Antepartum record

Name _____
           Last   First   Middle

| Drug allergy: |
| Anesthesia consult planned ☐ Yes ☐ No |

Problems/plans	**Medication list:**	Start date	Stop date
1.	1.		
2.	2.		
3.	3.		
4.	4.		

EDD confirmation	**18–20-week EDD update:**
Initial EDD:	Quickening ___ / ___ / ___ + 22 wks = ___ / ___ / ___
LMP ___ / ___ / ___ = EDD ___ / ___ / ___	Fundal ht. at umbil. ___ / ___ / ___ + 20 wks = ___ / ___ / ___
Initial exam ___ / ___ / ___ = ___wks = EDD ___ / ___ / ___	FHT w/fetoscope ___ / ___ / ___ + 20 wks = ___ / ___ / ___
Ultrasound ___ / ___ / ___ = ___wks = EDD ___ / ___ / ___	Ultrasound ___ / ___ / ___ + ___wks = ___ / ___ / ___
Initial EDD ___ / ___ / ___ Initialed by _____	Final EDD ___ / ___ / ___ Initialed by _____

32–34-week EDD–uterine size concordance (± 4 or more CM suggests the need for ultrasound evaluation)

Visit date (year _____)													
Weeks gest. (best est.)													
Fundal height (CM)													
Presentation													
FHR present: F = fetoscope D = doptone													
Fetal movement: + = present O = absent													
Prematurity: signs/symptoms:* + = present O = absent													
Cervix exam (Dil./Eff./Sta.)													
Blood pressure: Initial													
Blood pressure: Repeat													
Edema + = present O = absent													
Weight (prepreg: _____)													
Cumulative weight gain													
Urine (glucose/ albumin/ketones)													
Next appointment													
Provider (initials)													
Test reminders	8–18 weeks CVS/AMNIO/MSAFP			24–28 weeks glucose screen/RhIg									

Comments: _____

_____

_____

_____

_____

_____

_____

*For example: vaginal bleeding, discharge, cramps, contractions, pelvic pressure.   (Cont.)

FIGURE 2–7. *Continued*

Laboratory and Education

Initial labs	Date	Result	Reviewed
Blood type	/ /	A B AB O	
Rh type	/ /		
Antibody screen	/ /		
HCT/HGB	/ /	_____ % _____ g/dl	
Pap smear	/ /	Normal / Abnormal / _____	
Rubella	/ /		
VDRL	/ /		
GC	/ /		
Urine culture/screen	/ /		
HBsAg	/ /		

Comments/additional lab

8–18-week labs (when indicated)	Date	Result
Ultrasound	/ /	
MSAFP	/ /	_____ MOM
Amnio/CVS	/ /	
Karyotype	/ /	46, XX or 46, XY / other ____
Alpha-fetoprotein	/ /	Normal ____ Abnormal ____

24–28-week labs (when indicated)	Date	Result
HCT/HGB	/ /	_____ % _____ g/dl
Diabetes screen	/ /	1 HR _____
GTT (if screen abnormal)	/ /	_____ FBS _____ 1 HR _____ 2 HR _____ 3 HR
Rh antibody screen	/ /	
RhIG given (28 wks)	/ /	Signature _____

32–36-week labs (when indicated)	Date	Result
Ultrasound	/ /	
VDRL	/ /	
GC	/ /	
HCT/HGB	/ /	_____ % _____ g/dl

Optional lab (high-risk groups)	Date	Result
HIV	/ /	
HGB electrophoresis	/ /	AA AS SS AC SC AF ↑A$_2$
Chlamydia	/ /	
Other	/ /	

Plans/Education (counseled ☐)

☐ Anesthesia plans _____

☐ Toxoplasmosis precautions (cats/raw meat) _____

☐ Childbirth classes _____

☐ Physical activity _____

☐ Premature labor signs _____

☐ Nutrition counseling _____

☐ Breast or bottle feeding _____

☐ Newborn car seat _____

☐ Postpartum birth control _____

☐ Environmental/work hazards _____

☐ Tubal sterilization _____

☐ VBAC counseling _____

☐ Circumcision _____

☐ Travel _____

Requests _____

Tubal sterilization

Consent signed   ___ / ___ / ___   Date ___   Initials _____

FIGURE 2–7. *Continued*

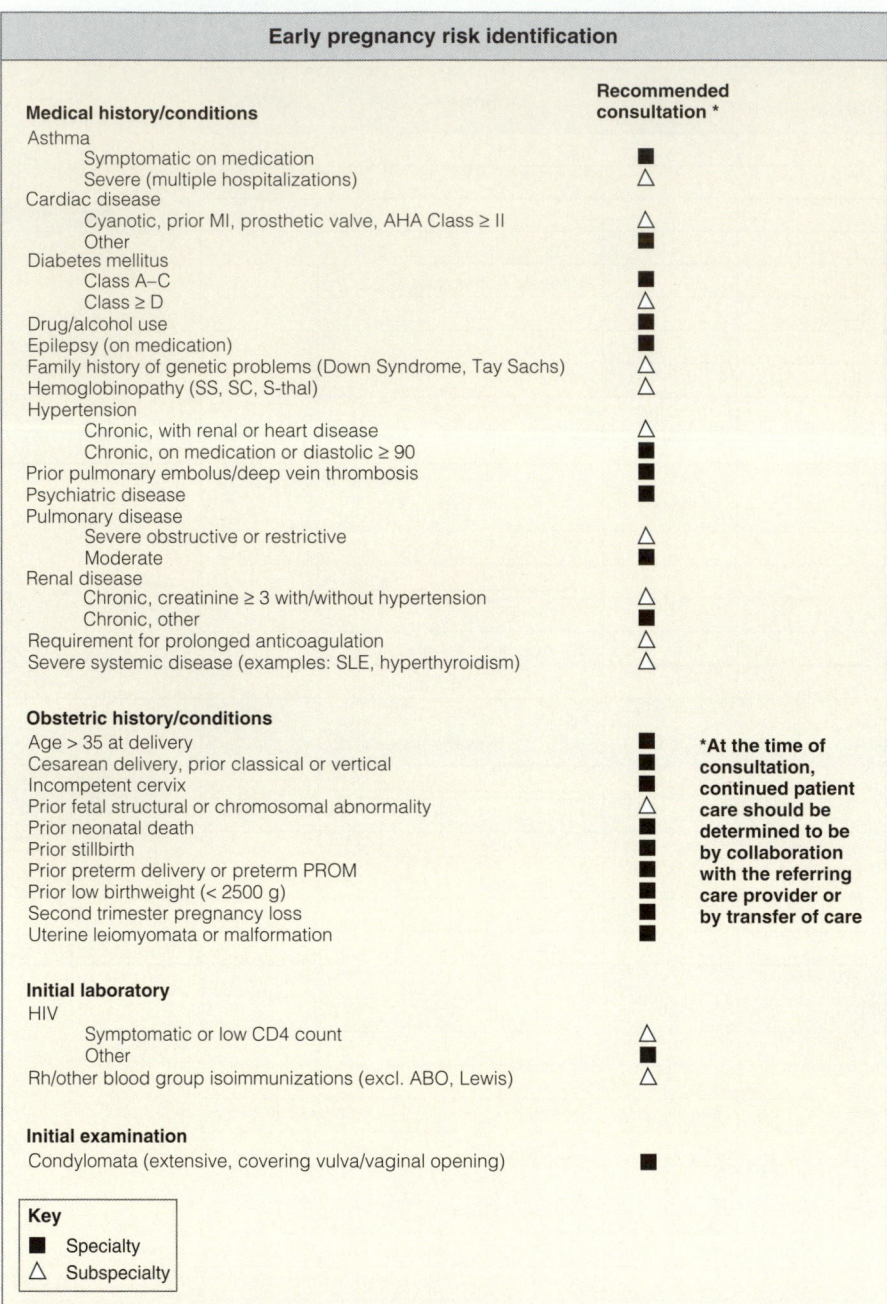

FIGURE 2–8. Early pregnancy risk identification. *(Reproduced, with permission, from Committee on Perinatal Health, 1995.)*

▶ CAREGIVERS IN PERINATAL CARE

The practice of having a single health care provider attend to the needs of the perinatal client has all but disappeared from today's health care system. Obstetricians rely on consultation from pediatricians, and appropriate therapeutic decisions cannot be made without information from the nurse at the bedside. Perinatal clients with complications require the coordinated, sophisticated interaction of allied health care professionals and a large group of multidisciplinary specialists, as well as physicians and nurses, to ensure quality care.

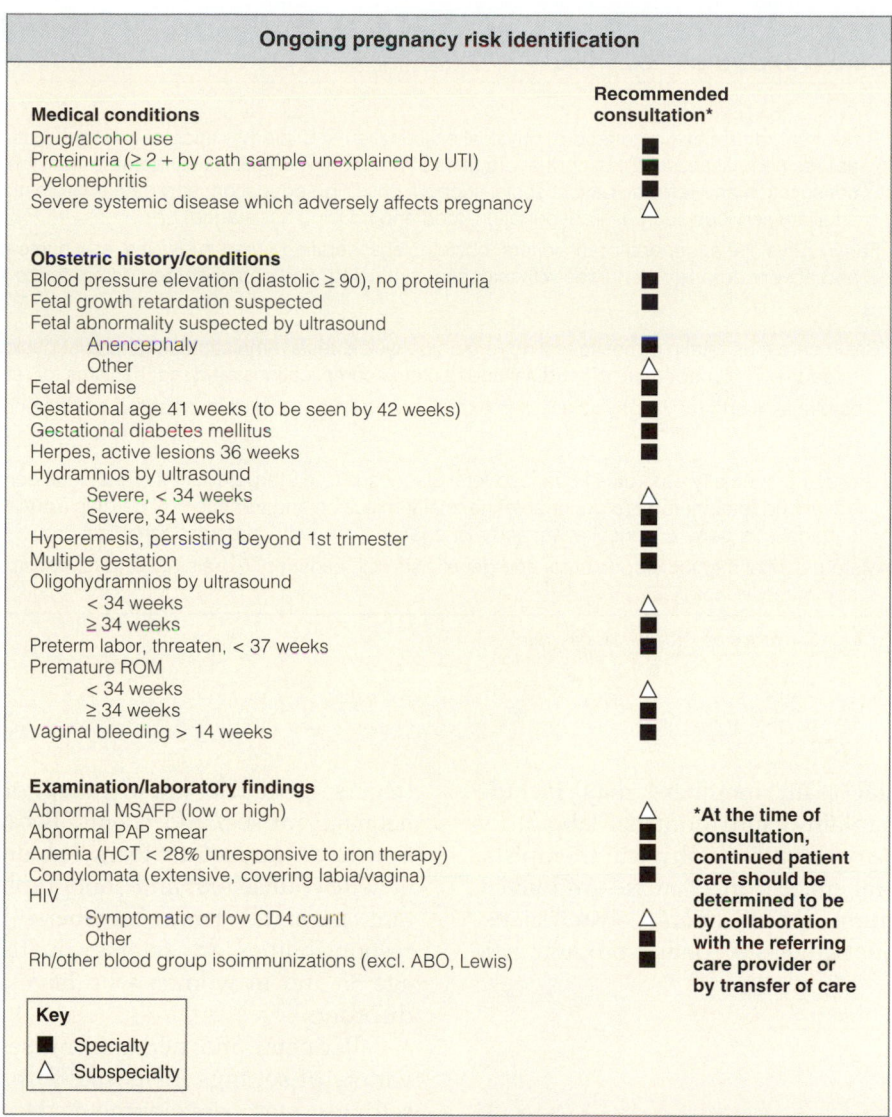

FIGURE 2–9. Ongoing pregnancy risk identification. *(Reproduced, with permission, from Committee on Perinatal Health, 1995.)*

▶ Collaboration as a Basis for Perinatal Care

Collaboration means working with other individuals or groups of individuals to achieve a goal. In perinatal settings, collaboration is multidisciplinary, interdisciplinary, and intradisciplinary; it includes the family; and it is a team effort to provide the highest quality of perinatal health care.

In collaborative management, the role of a given team member depends on that person's expertise and relationship with the client and family. A factor that never changes is the need for all team members to value one another's contributions and to work together as a team to achieve the best possible outcome. The continued reduction of infant mortality and morbidity will not occur through further development of technology alone. In the future emphasis must be placed on the development of approaches to prevent high-risk births, principally prenatal care. This will require additional nursing resources as well as the efforts of the entire perinatal team.

▶ The Interdisciplinary Team

An interdisciplinary approach to the provision of perinatal care is no different than the team approach required for the delivery of any other type of health

▶ **TABLE 2-3**

Ambulatory Prenatal Care Providers and Expertise

Basic Prenatal Care

Capabilities   Risk-oriented prenatal care record, physical examination and interpretation of findings, routine laboratory assessment, assessment of normal progress of pregnancy, ongoing risk identification, mechanisms for consultation and referral, psychosocial support, childbirth education, and care coordination (including referral for ancillary services such as transportation, food and housing assistance)

Provider Types   Family physicians, general practitioners, obstetricians, certified nurse-midwives, and nurse practitioners and advanced practice nurses with experience, training, and demonstrated competence

Specialty Care

Capabilities   Basic care plus fetal diagnostic testing (e.g., biophysical tests, amniotic fluid analysis, basic ultrasound); expertise in management of medical and obstetric complications; and mechanisms for referral and consultation

Provider Types   Obstetricians and family physicians with experience, training, and demonstrated competence

Subspecialty Care

Capabilities   Basic and specialty care plus advanced fetal diagnoses (e.g., targeted ultrasound, fetal echocardiology); advanced fetal therapy (e.g., intrauterine fetal transfusion and treatment of cardiac arrhythmias); medical, surgical and genetic consultation; and management of severe maternal complications

Provider Types   Maternal–fetal medicine specialists and geneticists with experience, training, and demonstrated competence

Reproduced, with permission, from Committee on Perinatal Health, 1995.

care today. Perinatal team members may include social workers, chaplains, nutritionists, laboratory technicians, respiratory therapists, physical therapists, transport team members, certified nurse–midwives, women's health nurse practitioners, obstetricians, perinatologists, neonatologists, neonatal nurse practi-tioners, pediatric nurse practitioners, perinatal and neonatal nurses, and clients. Because genetic evalua-tion is an important team responsibility, geneticists, genetic counselors, and sonographers are also impor-tant perinatal team members. Examples of their responsibilities are fetal evaluation in women over age 35 and in women who have a history of genetic disorders.

Perinatal and neonatal nurses provide care in a variety of settings including outpatient and inpatient settings, staff development departments, perinatal outreach programs, and maternal and neonatal trans-port teams. As in any nursing situation, roles and tasks vary from time to time. For example, the nurse in the NICU may have primary responsibility for care of the neonate. On the other hand, clinical nurse spe-cialists may have the responsibility of coordinating care for the neonate, mother, and family in high-risk situations.

 *Ethical Decision Making*

A pregnant woman can expose her fetus to significant risk by the choices she makes for her individual lifestyle. As a nurse caring for this client, consider the following questions:

1. Because a fetus is totally dependent on the mother for protection, do you think society reserves a right to dictate healthy maternal behaviors?

2. Since smoking can be as harmful as illegal drugs to the fetus, should it be prohibited in pregnancy?

3. Would such bans deter pregnant women with unhealthy lifestyles from seeking prena-tal care?

▶ Model for Interdisciplinary Care

Each clinical facility or system of care will develop a model for development of an interdisciplinary team. In any viable model for interdisciplinary care, the responsibility for assessment, decision making, deliv-ery of service, and evaluation is shared by the differ-ent disciplines constituting the team. The philosophy supporting the model must be one of providing service to clients through a shared commitment to group goals, achieved through interdisciplinary team planning (Lasker, 1997). Several factors have the potential to influence the development of interdisciplinary teams and their effectiveness: philosophy, professionalism, territoriality, communication and influence, role identity, and team development.

Philosophy

Commitment of the team members to collaboratively determine priorities is essential to the development of an effective team. The client and family are seen as essential team members. A commitment must be made to the client and family needs rather than to a professional's ego.

Professionalism

The behavior acquired by the team members during their disciplinary educational program affects how each member will function within the interdisciplinary team. Nurses have traditionally functioned under the direction of the physician. As a member of the interdisciplinary team the nurse must assert autonomy and exhibit expertise in professional nursing in a manner that complements but does not threaten either the physician or other professionals. This issue is particularly difficult for a nurse practitioner whose role function may, indeed, overlap with some role functions of a physician. Often nurses experience conflicts related to authority and territoriality that have developed through their socialization during the nursing educational program and practice.

Nurses who are just beginning their practice often experience significant frustration. They have the ability to provide competent care to childbearing families, but probably need a period of 6 months to a year and continuing education to function efficiently on a high-risk interdisciplinary team.

Territoriality

All members of the interdisciplinary team rely on basic knowledge from the physical, natural, behavioral, nursing, and medical sciences and from the humanities. Although nursing focuses on the whole person and the family, other professions may have more precisely defined territory. Within the interdisciplinary team conflict emerges where there is an overlap into others' territory. Boundaries must be negotiated between team members, and it takes time for norms to be established within the group. Problems often develop in settings where there are frequent personnel changes. The overall effectiveness of the team is dependent on the capabilities of the individual members to collaborate, cooperate, communicate, and interact as an interdependent group of individuals.

Communication and Influence

Influence may be defined as any interpersonal interaction with psychologic effects. Each member of the team must acquire influence. Nurses, at different levels of preparation, develop influence through precise suggestions and demonstration of expertise in their roles.

Role Identity

Effective team members are able to give and take and perform a variety of roles within the team dependent on what is needed to meet client needs. Specifically, the nurse must (1) define the nursing role, (2) recognize the overlap between the disciplines, (3) learn what other disciplines can do and be aware of the territoriality issues and boundaries, and (4) develop influence and share in the distribution of power.

The components of the nursing role may be difficult to specify. Different settings and client populations demand different nursing activities. However, there are specific nursing responsibilities common to all perinatal care settings:

1. *Promotion and maintenance of health.* Identification of the particular needs of the perinatal client that interfere with functioning (problems, acute or chronic health deviations), as well as vulnerabilities (aspects of health promotion relative to potential health problems).
2. *Facilitation of growth and development.* Anticipatory guidance, childbirth education, labor support.
3. *Supportive counseling.* Providing or referring the family for genetic, grief, or supportive counseling.
4. *Teaching.* Teaching self-care skills, strategies to promote development and minimize risk.

Other responsibilities emerge based on the family and situational needs, the level of preparation and expertise of the nurse, and the other professionals represented on the team.

Team Development

Development and administration of this complex team are best accomplished through on-the-job, simultaneous teaching of all the specialized team members, as a collective group. The new graduate of a nursing program, or any professional program for that matter, requires at least a 6-month orientation before he or she can become an integral member of

▶ **TABLE 2–4**

A Model for Orientation of the Perinatal Interdisciplinary Team

Site	Provide program in actual setting in which care is to be provided.
Planning	Involve all team members in program planning.
	Involve learners in the definition of learning needs.
Implementation	Involve all team members in the teaching of the program.
	Involve the learners in the conduct of the program when possible.
Evaluation	Use both learner-focused and client-focused outcome criteria to evaluate the impact of the program.
	Involve all team members in the evaluation of the program.

the team. Some professionals require even more time. For example, neonatologists must complete a minimum of a 1-year "hands-on" clinical fellowship training program following a pediatric residency before being able to function as a capable team member. Table 2–4 provides a model describing the components of such an orientation program.

Even in a community hospital, perinatal care relies on an interdisciplinary philosophy. The team may contain fewer specialists, but nursing, medicine, and other support disciplines are still represented. The need for on-site training is as essential in the community-based nursery as it is in a university-based medical center (a subspecialty care provider).

Team members must be able to relate what they learn to the specific resources of their unit. Thus, the majority of the activities directed at developing a perinatal interdisciplinary team should occur in the setting in which care is to be provided.

The educational program must also be directed toward the same interdisciplinary group that will be involved with providing care in the clinical setting. Thus, specialists in obstetric and pediatric medicine as well as nurses from both of these practice areas must be included in the program.

The orientation program will be most effective when it is provided by other members of an interdisciplinary team. Team members integrate content more readily when there is another specialist in their discipline to relate to on the faculty. Appropriate orientation into the role of interdisciplinary team member therefore requires the efforts of all of the members of the perinatal team.

Critical Thinking in Care Planning

Care Plan for Maternal Transport for Preterm Delivery

Karen Blake is a 16-year-old high school student who is now 29 weeks pregnant. Karen lives with her mother, Ms. Blake, who works as a secretary to support her single-parent family. Ms. Blake's insurance pays for Karen's medical care, but will not provide for the infant's care.

At 29 weeks of gestation, Karen is admitted to a basic perinatal hospital with frequency, urgency, dysuria, and uterine contractions. Shortly after Karen is admitted to the labor and delivery unit, her membranes rupture spontaneously. Karen's obstetrician performs a vaginal examination and determines that Karen's cervix is 80% effaced and 3 cm dilated. Her contractions are mild to moderate in strength, 4 minutes apart, and 40 seconds in duration. Karen's obstetrician advises Karen and her mother that delivery of the 29-week infant is imminent and that arrangements will be made for Karen to be transported to a subspecialty perinatal center.

Karen and her mother begin to cry when they realize they will have to leave their trusted obstetrician and move to a strange and distant hospital.

The Blakes are reassured that they can maintain telephone contact with their family obstetrician. In addition, the perinatal nurse in the basic perinatal hospital gives Ms. Blake a map of the route to the subspecialty perinatal center as well as a diagram of the hospital. She also informs Ms. Blake about state money available to help pay for the infant's hospital expenses. Karen's obstetrician then arranges for Karen's transport to the subspecialty perinatal center by the hospital transport team. When the team arrives, they estimate that the 45-minute trip to the center can probably be made before delivery of Karen's infant. They review with Ms. Blake instructions on how to reach the new hospital and then proceed with the transport.

▶ Assessment

- Client transported to subspecialty perinatal center
- Client and family receiving care from unfamiliar members of interdisciplinary team

- Client and her mother cry when they leave their trusted obstetrician
- Client's mother states: "How will we pay for the baby's hospital bill?"

Nursing Diagnosis

Anxiety, related to transport to unfamiliar birth setting.

Expected Client/Family Outcomes	Nursing Action/Intervention	Evaluation
Client and her mother will use hospital resources with relative ease.	Orient client and her family to agency, including neonatal intensive care unit. *Rationale:* Lack of familiarity with subspecialty perinatal facility will increase client/family anxiety.	Client is oriented to environment. Client's mother visits cafeteria.
Client and her mother will maintain contact with familiar obstetrician and nurse at basic perinatal agency.	Arrange phone call with basic perinatal center team. Encourage client and her mother to express feelings. Facilitate the presence of client's mother with client at subspecialty perinatal facility.	Client's mother talks with team at basic perinatal agency. She is present with client at subspecialty perinatal facility.

(continued)

Critical Thinking in Care Planning *continued*

Expected Client/Family Outcomes	Nursing Action/Intervention	Evaluation
	Rationale: Client/family need to maintain relationship with familiar caregivers at basic perinatal agency who have been identified as a support. Social support helps to alleviate anxiety.	

Nursing Diagnosis

Anxiety, related to anticipated high cost of neonatal care.

Expected Client/Family Outcomes	Nursing Action/Intervention	Evaluation
Client's mother will talk with social worker about financial aid.	Arrange for a social worker to meet with family and discuss financial needs. *Rationale:* Social worker is appropriate member of interdisciplinary team to arrange financial assistance via state funding.	Client's mother talks with social worker and states: "She thinks we can get state money."

Chapter Highlights

► Perinatal nursing is the practice of professional nursing in a variety of settings in which families seek assistance in maintaining health, preventing health problems, or restoring health throughout the prenatal, intrapartum, postpartum, and neonatal periods.

► The framework for perinatal nursing parallels the steps of the nursing process and includes assessment of reproductive and developmental health, decision-making process and nursing diagnoses, planning and collaborative goal setting, collaborative intervention, and evaluation and revision of outcome criteria.

► The Committee on Perinatal Health (COPH) and other organizations and individuals have proposed national initiatives and models of care designed to resolve problems associated with perinatal care.

► Systems of care designed to deliver perinatal services across the country, such as regionaliza-tion, are plagued with many problems in providing services, especially to medically underserved populations.

► The COPH, in its 1995 report entitled *Toward Improving the Outcome of Pregnancy: The 90s and Beyond,* recommended that individual perinatal providers be organized into networks supervised by state regional perinatal boards and that the levels of care be reorganized to include basic, specialty, and subspecialty care.

► Significant improvements in providing perinatal care can occur by increasing access to prenatal care for low- and high-risk pregnant women and neonates, developing better means of identification of high-risk pregnancies, and increasing availability of intensive perinatal services for families who need them.

► Perinatal nursing occurs within the context of an interdisciplinary health care team.

Chapter Highlights continued

▶ Perinatal nurses have a major role in management of families in need of perinatal services and in the political solutions needed to resolve problems associated with perinatal care.

▶ Perinatal nursing actions involve teaching, promotion and maintenance of health, facilitation of growth and development, provision of support, counseling, assessment of risk, and management of complex sophisticated technology.

After reading the vignette at the beginning of this chapter, use what you have learned to answer these questions:

1. What are the factors in this situation that compel Margaret Kiely to draw on the expertise of other members of the interdisciplinary health care team?

2. What approach should the nurse use in explaining the role of the interdisciplinary health care team with Cathleen and Bill Harris so as to allay their concerns about this aspect of care?

3. In what ways can the nurse most effectively fulfill her role as a member of the interdisciplinary health care team in this situation?

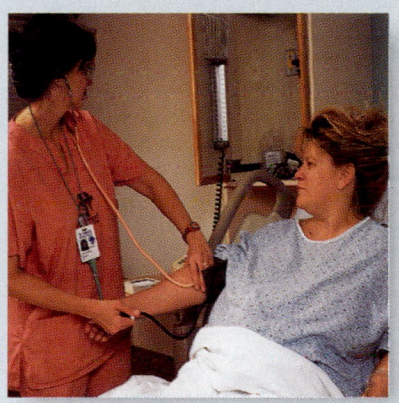

Critical Thinking Questions

▶ References

Committee on Perinatal Health (COPH). (1977). *Toward improving the outcome of pregnancy: Recommendations for the regional development of maternal and perinatal health services.* White Plains, NY: March of Dimes Birth Defects Foundation.

Dujardin, B., Clarysse, G., Criel, B., DeBrouwere, V., & Wangata, N. (1995). The strategy of risk approach in antenatal care: Evaluation of the referral compliance. *Social Science Medicine, 40*(1), 529–535.

Evans, A., & Friedland, R. (1995). Background on TIOP: Recommendations through the lens of managed care. In F. Katz & A. Lane (Eds.), *Perinatal care in the changing health system* (pp. III-3-III-11). Washington, DC: National Academy of Social Insurance.

Institute for Family-Centered Care. (1996). Family-centered care and managed care: Are they compatible? *Advances in Family-Centered Care, 3*(1), 1–30.

Joffe, M.S., & Black, K.D. (1997). *The healthy start initiative: A community-driven approach to infant mortality reduction—Vol V. Collaboration with managed care organizations.* Arlington, VA: National Center for Education in Maternal and Child Health.

Lasker, R.D. (1997). *Medicine and public health: The power of collaboration.* New York: New York Academy of Medicine.

Luke, B. (1993). The changing pattern of infant mortality in the U.S.: The role of prenatal factors and their obstetrical complications. *International Journal of Gynecology and Obstetrics, 40,* 199–212.

March of Dimes Birth Defects Foundation. (1997). *Statbook: Statistics for monitoring maternal and infant health.* White Plains, NY: Author.

McCormick, M., & Richardson, D. (1995). Access to neonatal intensive care. *The Future of Children, 5*(1), 162–175.

McFarlane, J., Parker, B., & Soeken, K. (1996). Abuse during pregnancy: Association with maternal health and infant birth weight. *Nursing Research 45*(1), 37–42.

Pollack, L. (1996). An effective model for reorganization of perinatal services in a metropolitan area: A descriptive analysis and historical perspective. *Journal of Perinatology, 16*(1), 3–8.

Rowley, D. (1995). Framing the debate: Can prenatal care help to reduce black-white disparity in infant mortality? *Journal of the American Medical Women's Association; 50*(5), 187–193.

Vecchi, C.J., Vasquez, L., Radin, T., & Johnson, P. (1996). Neonatal individualized predictive pathway (NIPP): Discharge planning tool for parents. *Neonatal Network, 15*(4), 7–13.

Wirtschafter, D. (1995). Perinatal services in the era of managed care: A Kaiser Permanente physician's perspective. *Journal of Perinatology, 15*(5), 414–417.

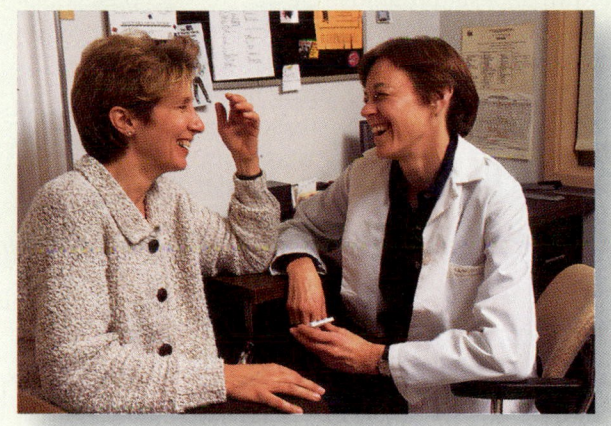

Jeanne Goodwin is 8 weeks pregnant with her third child. During her second prenatal visit, Ann Salzman, RN, CNM, updates Jeanne's health history and conducts the physical examination. Among the findings are: resting pulse rate: 86 beats/minute; respirations: 17 respirations/minute; BP: 115/70; uterus: pear-shaped, approximately doubled in size; and presence of Chadwick's sign (mucous membranes of the vulva, vagina, and cervix are bluish).

After the physical examination, the nurse discusses the findings with Jeanne and proceeds to update the plan of care based on the wellness diagnosis of asset in the health of the mother related to normal physical changes in the first trimester. When the nurse informs Jeanne that she is experiencing a high level of wellness, Jeanne is visibly surprised and states: "I don't feel particularly well, especially in the morning when I get out of bed and am immediately sick to my stomach." ∎

3

Clinical Reasoning and the Childbearing Family

The complexity of clinical practice requires that students learn how to deliver nursing care to clients based on theoretical knowledge and skills relevant to clinical practice situations. To plan and manage care for childbearing families, nurses use a clinical reasoning process that incorporates critical thinking skills.

This chapter describes the clinical reasoning process, including the types of nursing decisions involved in the process. The relationship of clinical reasoning to critical thinking and to the nursing process is also discussed.

▶ THE CLINICAL REASONING PROCESS

Clinical reasoning is a decision-making process used by nurses when caring for clients in a variety of clinical settings. Nursing decisions include diagnostic, ethical, and therapeutic judgments that are made in collaboration with the client. These judgments are made in complex clinical situations where the nurse identifies client response patterns to health and illness and recognizes alternative explanations for clinical circumstances. The clinical reasoning process includes all the cognitive skills implied in client assessment and management of care and also involves the whole process of critical thinking.

▶ Critical Thinking and Clinical Reasoning

Critical thinking is an inherent cognitive activity in the clinical reasoning process and is an approach to inquiry in which nurses examine clinical and professional issues and search for effective answers (Saucier, 1995). The box entitled Characteristics of Critical Thinking summarizes the elements of critical thinking.

People use critical thinking in many different types of situations in which there are no problems to solve. (Miller & Babcock, 1996). Therefore, although critical thinking and clinical reasoning are closely related, they are not identical. For example, the method used to conduct a scientific experiment in a microbiology class, or the deliberations used to buy a piece of clothing, also incorporate critical thinking.

▶ Decision Making in Clinical Reasoning

Clinical reasoning is used by nurses who care for childbearing families to assess the health patterns and environmental dimensions that may affect the individual's and family's health; to analyze overall health and actual or potential health problems; to plan, implement, and evaluate therapeutic interventions; and to resolve ethical dilemmas.

Diagnostic Decision Making

Diagnostic decision making, a component of clinical reasoning, is a process of collaboration among the nurse, the client, and members of the interdisciplinary team, resulting in a nursing diagnosis. The process includes collecting information, interpreting the information, clustering the information, and naming the cluster.

Nurses collect information when they observe the client and obtain the client's health history. Because of their clinical knowledge, nurses know which observations are important, what questions to ask, and how to interpret the information. They cluster the information by grouping the defining signs and symptoms into a diagnostic category (Dexter et al., 1997). A list of nursing diagnosis categories has been developed and approved by the North American Nursing Diagnosis Association (NANDA). Each of the nursing diagnosis categories has four components: (1) label, (2) definition, (3) etiologic or related factors, (4) defining characteristics. Nurses choose the appropriate nursing diagnosis label by matching the cluster of information they have identified with the definitions and defining characteristics of the NANDA labels (Carroll-Johnson & Paquette, 1994; NANDA, 1996). Table 3–1 provides an example of a NANDA-approved diagnosis that may be applicable to a childbearing family.

▶ CHARACTERISTICS OF CRITICAL THINKING

- Purposeful and goal directed
- Conceptual
- Rational and objective (conclusions are reached on the basis of evidence)

- Analytical (supported by a knowledge base and enhanced by skill in application)
- Autonomous and creative
- Essential to problem solving and decision making

▶ **TABLE 3–1**

Example of a NANDA-Approved Nursing Diagnosis

Label	Breastfeeding, effective
Definition	State in which a mother–infant dyad/family exhibits adequate proficiency and satisfaction with the breastfeeding process
Related factors	Basic breastfeeding knowledge; normal breast structure; normal infant oral structure; support sources; maternal confidence
Defining characteristics	
Major	Mother able to position infant at breast to promote a successful latch-on response; infant content after feeding; regular and sustained infant sucking at breast; appropriate infant weight for age
Minor	Signs and/or symptoms of letdown reflex; eagerness of infant to nurse, maternal verbalization of satisfaction with breastfeeding process

Source: North American Nursing Diagnosis Association, 1996.

There is some concern among nurses that most of the NANDA diagnostic labels describe health problems. Some diagnostic labels that do reflect health include: Health-Seeking Behaviors; Family Coping: Potential for Enhanced; Effective Breastfeeding; and Anticipatory Grieving (Carroll-Johnson & Paquette, 1994). The limited number of NANDA labels reflecting wellness can be problematic for the nurse caring for childbearing families who are essentially healthy clients. NANDA does, however, recognize the importance of a wellness diagnosis which is a clinical judgment about a client in transition from a specific level of wellness to a higher level of wellness.

Wellness diagnoses are stated in a somewhat different manner than problem diagnoses. Specifically, the NANDA labels are stated in positive terms by using such qualifiers as "effective," "positive," and "enhanced." For example, if a cluster of infor-

mation demonstrates that a healthy parent–child relationship exists, the nursing diagnosis may be stated as "effective parenting." Others call wellness diagnoses strength diagnoses. In other words, the nursing diagnosis is made after careful assessment of client strengths (e.g., effective family communication pattern).

Diagnostic Decision Making Using Patterns. Some nurses state wellness as well as illness diagnoses in terms of, and after assessment of, client patterns. **Patterns** are defined as sequences of behavior over time, rather than isolated instances. Gordon (1987) has identified a typology of 11 functional health patterns that can be used during diagnostic decision making (Table 3–2).

NANDA also identifies patterns, called **human response patterns,** that reflect the pattern and organi-

▶ **TABLE 3–2**

Gordon's Typology of Functional Health Patterns

Pattern	Description
Health perception and health management	Client's perception of health and well-being and how health is managed
Nutritional and metabolic	Food and fluid consumption relative to metabolic need and pattern indicators of local nutrient supply
Elimination	Excretory function (bowel, bladder, skin)
Activity or exercise	Exercise, activity leisure, and recreation
Cognitive and perceptual	Sensory status and cognitive level
Sleep and rest	Sleep, rest, and relaxation
Self-perception and self-concept	Self-concept and perceptions of self (e.g., body comfort, body image, feeling state)
Role relationship	Role engagements and relationships
Sexuality and reproductive	Satisfaction/dissatisfaction with sexuality; reproductive history
Coping and stress tolerance	General coping mechanisms and effectiveness in terms of stress tolerance
Value and belief	Values, beliefs, or goals that guide choices or decisions

Source: Gordon, 1987.

▶ **TABLE 3-3**

Human Response Patterns as Described by NANDA

Choosing	Selection among alternatives
Communicating	Transmission of information or feelings
Exchanging	Mutual act of giving and receiving
Feeling	Sensation, apprehension, subjective awareness
Knowing	Acquisition of factual information, principles, and actions through observation, inquiry, or information
Moving	Activity; changing position; excretion; action
Perceiving	Development of awareness through the senses
Relating	Establishment of affiliations or connections
Valuing	Concern; assignment of worth, usefulness, or importance

zation of individuals as they interact with the environment. Table 3–3 defines the NANDA human response patterns that can be used by the nurse during diagnostic decision making.

Wellness-oriented diagnoses may also be organized by functional health patterns. An example of such a diagnosis is "adequate sexual functioning associated with adaptation to changes associated with childbearing as evidenced by report of satisfactory sexual relationship." The organizing functional health pattern in the example is the sexuality and reproductive pattern. Each of the wellness nursing diagnoses is defined and described in terms of health status, contributing factors, and defining characteristics.

No matter what system is used for assessment and diagnosis labeling, diagnostic decision making always involves collecting data, clustering the data, and naming the cluster. It is an important part of the clinical reasoning process used by the nurse.

Ethical Decision Making

Ethics is the branch of philosophy that examines what our behavior ought to be in relation to ourselves, other human beings, and the environment. It includes the study of theories, principles, and values that are used to explore beliefs and behaviors. **Ethical deci-sion making** is a problem-solving process with specific emphasis on the careful examination of alternatives and thoughtful justification of the choice of actions required. All actions must be justified on the basis of ethical principles. Table 3–4 defines ethical principles that are relevant to nursing practice.

Ethical decision making comprises the following steps (Aiken & Catalano, 1994):

1. Perceiving the problem or dilemma
2. Determining and obtaining relevant factual information (collecting data, analyzing data related to the ethical dilemma)
3. Aiming at conceptual clarity—explaining adequately what is being talked about (What does it mean to have the "right to life"?); stating the dilemma (the critically ill newborn's right to death with dignity versus the nurse's obligation to preserve life and do no harm)
4. Considering the choices of actions
   a. By listing the possible courses of action without considering the consequences
   b. By constructing and evaluating arguments by identifying alternatives from the list of choices with an ethical reason for each
   c. By anticipating objections; evaluating arguments using ethical principles

▶ **TABLE 3-4**

Ethical Principles

	Principle	Definition
	Respect	Recognition of the dignity of each person
	Autonomy	Recognition of an individual's ability to make his or her choices
	Nonmaleficence	Duty to do no harm
	Beneficence	Duty to do good
	Confidentiality	Protection of the individual's right to privacy
	Fidelity	Duty to keep promises
	Veracity	Truthfulness
	Justice	Obligation to be fair to everyone

5. Making the decision; acting on the choices
6. Reflecting on the outcome

The ethical decision-making process, by its nature, creates differences of opinion. Sound, ethical decision making requires collaboration among the client, family, nurse, and other members of the health care team.

Therapeutic Decision Making

Therapeutic decision making is a component of clinical reasoning used by nurses when they plan and implement nursing care. It is a problem-solving process in which the nurse takes the following actions:

1. Collects information through assessment
2. Establishes data-based nursing diagnoses
3. Plans with the client by setting goals, prioritizing the goals, and formulating intervention strategies
4. Implements the plan of care
5. Evaluates the plan through outcome criteria

The therapeutic decision-making process focuses on planning, implementing, and evaluating care. To plan effectively, nurses need to assess the client and formulate nursing diagnoses; they use the diagnostic decision-making process when making therapeutic judgments. Therapeutic decision making is one of the cornerstones that underlies the nursing process. Other disciplines that deliver therapeutic services also adapt therapeutic decision making in determining their discipline-specific interventions.

▶ THE NURSING PROCESS

Clinical reasoning leading to diagnostic, ethical, and therapeutic judgments can be achieved through the nursing process, which includes assessment, nursing diagnosis, planning, implementation, and evaluation.

The **nursing process** is the "action component" of theory-based nursing practice and is the systematic method of delivering nursing care. The nursing process provides a way of communicating to others on the health care team the holistic needs of the client (Gross, 1994).

The nursing process can be viewed as a unit consisting of phases. Each phase is dependent on the phases that precede and follow it and in actual practice cannot be separated from them. The nursing process is cyclic and the phases overlap; however, for purposes of analysis, each phase of the nursing process is discussed separately.

▶ Preprocess Goals

The following goals need to be achieved before the nursing process begins:

- Establishment of trust between client and nurse
- Definition of the nurse's and client's respective roles in the nursing care situation
- Establishment of client comfort in the chosen role
- Establishment of a positive environment to pursue the nursing process

▶ Assessment

Assessment, the first phase of the nursing process, is the collection of data to determine a client's present and past health and functional status and to evaluate the client's coping patterns and responses to therapeutic interventions. Assessment data are obtained by interview, physical examination, observation, review of records and reports, and collaboration with colleagues.

▶ Nursing Diagnosis

The nurse formulates the nursing diagnosis through the diagnostic decision-making process (Carpenito, 1993). A **nursing diagnosis** is a nursing judgment or conclusion referring to a potential or actual problem or strength of a client that falls within the scope of nursing intervention. As was previously noted, formulating nursing diagnoses related to healthy childbearing families can be somewhat problematic. Insufficient emphasis may be placed on planning nursing care to enhance wellness and strengths of the family. An example of a wellness-oriented diagnosis for the childbearing family is "joy related to the birth of a healthy baby."

This textbook gives examples of wellness (or strength)-oriented diagnoses, as well as examples of problem-oriented nursing diagnoses. Both wellness- and problem-oriented nursing diagnoses are included under the features entitled Critical Thinking in Care Planning throughout the text.

▶ Planning

In the third phase of the nursing process, **planning,** goals are set and prioritized, and methods are designed to resolve problems, reach goals, and assist the client to achieve a higher level of wellness. Planning involves a deliberate approach to setting well-

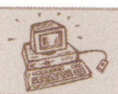

Research Abstract

Assessment of Low-Birth-Weight Infants for Cerebral Palsy

The increase in the prevalence of cerebral palsy (CP) is related in part to increased survival of low-birth-weight (LBW) infants. The purpose of this study was to evaluate the accuracy of screening neurological assessment by a trained nurse examiner in the identification of neurological abnormality consistent with the diagnosis of CP and to assess the use of goniometric measurement as a component of the nurse's screening assessment. Goniometry is the objective measurement of joint motion and mobility, and is used to determine the existence of neuromuscular disability and evaluate response to therapeutic intervention.

A total of 1,105 newborns weighing 500 to 2,000 g at birth, all live births and transported-in infants treated at one institution, were enrolled in a prospective study. Extensive data were collected on each mother–infant pair at birth, and each infant was prospectively screened by ultrasound examination for the presence of brain lesions. Nine hundred and one were alive and available for follow-up examination at age 2. Motor status was quantitatively assessed by a nurse who was specially trained in the use of the goniometer and in the measurement and evaluation of muscle tone and reflex in both healthy and impaired children. Evaluations were assessed for interrater reliability at three intervals.

Children were categorized by the nurse after the screening examination into 5 groups: definitely normal, probably normal, uncertain, probably abnormal, and definitely abnormal. Any child classified as other than definitely normal was referred to one of 4 consulting child neurologists for evaluation. Medical charts of children not examined were reviewed for evidence of CP.

When compared with either a neurologist's definitive diagnosis or chart abstraction evidence of CP, the nurse's referral, after examination including the goniometric assessment, was an excellent screen. The sensitivity of the nurse's evaluation, that is, the ability to identify those children at risk of

CP, was high. Of the 116 children with a diagnosis of CP from a neurologist's examination or medical record review, 113 (97.4%) were classified by the nurse as neurologically abnormal. Of the 183 children referred by the nurse for definitive neurological evaluation, 113 had evidence of CP resulting in a positive predictive value of the nurse's screening examination of 61.7%. Of the 534 children not referred, 531 were free of CP, resulting in a negative predictive value of 99.4%. Thus the nurse's ability to rule out children without CP was also high. The investigators concluded that the sensitivity of abnormal goniometry, or its ability to correctly identify those children with CP, was relatively high (sensitivity = 85.5%). The specificity of goniometry, or its ability to identify those children without CP, was fair (431 of 519 children without CP had normal goniometric measurements for a specificity of 83%). The results of this study indicate that goniometric measurement, as an adjunct to the nurse's global neurological assessment, provides quantitative information that can support the clinical suspicion of tonal abnormality. However, its low specificity renders it a poor choice as a screening tool when used in isolation.

Application to Practice

This study points out the importance of nurse-conducted screening activities for the ongoing health care of LBW infants. Nurses are most often the professionals who see children on an ongoing basis for well-child care. With assistance of screening tools, the nurse can accurately identify children who have, and who do not have, CP. This study also points out the limitations of screening instruments, no matter how sophisticated, when used in isolation of a highly trained practitioner who can think critically.

Source: Pinto-Martin, J.A., Torre, C., & Zhao, H. (1997). Nurse screening of low-birth-weight infants for cerebral palsy using goniometry. Nursing Research, 46 (5); 284–287.

defined goals, validating data obtained by assessing the client's problem, establishing priorities, and making decisions about interventions to solve the problems. The nurse and client need to determine both long-term goals and short-term, immediate goals. These goals provide the blueprint for the remaining phases of the nursing process and are the basis for determining the best way to achieve goals.

▶ Implementation

The fourth phase—the action phase—of the nursing process, **implementation,** comprises the start and completion of the actions necessary to accomplish the previously defined goals. The nurse may carry out the actions alone or may coordinate the therapeutic actions of others.

Independent nursing interventions are those actions that fall under the scope of a nurse practice act and that the nurse performs independently. Interdependent nursing interventions are those therapeutic actions that the nurse performs in collaboration with other health care professionals, such as physicians, physical therapists, and nutritionists. Health care of childbearing families is a highly complex endeavor, requiring the combined efforts of nurses and other health care professionals.

▶ Evaluation

Evaluation, the last phase, is the review of changes experienced by the client as a result of the nurse's actions. The nurse must compare preset goals, also called **outcome criteria,** with the actual attainment or progress toward attainment of the goals in practice. Data on whether goals are reached provide feedback by which the original planning for the client may be altered or revised. Perhaps the goals were inappropriate or the actions and methods designed to reach them were inadequate. The evaluation component of the nursing process allows for needed revisions in the plan of care. The process is cyclic: evaluation leads back to further assessment.

▶ CLINICAL REASONING AND THE CHILDBEARING FAMILY

Clinical reasoning, and use of the nursing process, are essential in delivering care to childbearing families. As demonstrated in the Critical Thinking in Care Planning features throughout the text, the nurse uses these processes to plan and implement effective care strategies for the childbearing woman, her family, and the newborn throughout the entire childbearing cycle. The nursing process, based in trust, defines the professional relationship that the nurse establishes with the family. Clinical reasoning, critical thinking, and diagnostic and ethical decision making enables the nurse to engage in the nursing process to ensure a positive outcome of the childbearing cycle for the family.

Chapter Highlights

▶ Clinical reasoning, used by nurses when they care for clients, is a decision-making process that includes diagnostic, ethical, and therapeutic judgments.

▶ Critical thinking is the basis for clinical reasoning, and is a way in which nurses examine clinical and professional issues and search for effective answers.

▶ Diagnostic decision making is an important part of clinical reasoning and involves collecting, interpreting, and clustering information, and finally, naming the cluster.

▶ Wellness diagnoses are particularly important in the care of childbearing families, since childbearing is often a "healthy" state.

▶ Ethical decision making, also part of clinical reasoning, is a problem-solving process that emphasizes examination of alternatives and justification of choices of action on the basis of ethical principles.

▶ Therapeutic decision making, which includes diagnostic decision making, is used by nurses to plan and implement nursing care.

(continued)

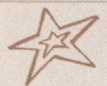

Chapter Highlights continued

▶ The nursing process includes assessment, nursing diagnosis, planning, implementation, and evaluation.

▶ Critical thinking is essential to and provides the basis for the nursing process.

After reading the vignette at the beginning of this chapter, use what you have learned to answer these questions.

1. If you were the nurse responsible for planning and coordinating Jeanne Goodwin's care, how would you explain the significance of the wellness diagnosis in enhancing her and her family's strength during the childbearing experience?

2. What priorities and goals would you establish to help Jeanne maintain and enhance her level of wellness for the remainder of her pregnancy?

3. Which aspects of the clinical reasoning process do you think are relevant in the management of Jeanne's prenatal care?

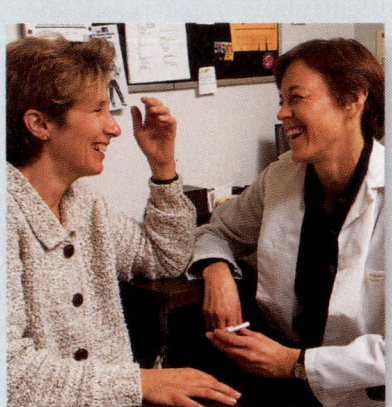

Critical Thinking Questions

▶ References

Aiken, T.D., & Catalano, J.T. (1994). *Legal, ethical, and political issues in nursing.* Philadelphia: F.A. Davis.

Carpenito, L.J. (1993). *Nursing diagnosis: Application to clinical practice* (5th ed.). Philadelphia: J.B. Lippincott.

Carroll-Johnson, R.M., & Paquette, M. (1994). *Classification of nursing diagnoses: Proceedings of the Tenth Conference.* Philadelphia: J.B. Lippincott.

Dexter, P., Applegate, M., Backer, J., Claytor, K., Keffer, J., Norton, B., & Ross, B. (1997). A proposed framework for teaching and evaluating critical thinking in nursing. *Journal of Professional Nursing, 13*(3), 160–167.

Gordon, M. (1987). *Nursing diagnosis: Process and application* (2nd ed.). New York: McGraw-Hill.

Gross, J.W. (1994). Learning nursing process: a group project. *Nursing Outlook, 42*(6), 279–283.

Miller, M.A., & Babcock, D.E. (1996). *Critical thinking applied to nursing.* St. Louis, MO: Mosby.

North American Nursing Diagnosis Association. (1996). *Nursing diagnoses: Definitions and classifications.* Philadelphia: Author.

Pinto-Martin, J.A., Torre, C., & Zhao, H. (1997). Nurse screening of low-birth-weight infants for cerebral palsy using goniometry. *Nursing Research, 46*(5), 284–287.

Saucier, B.L. (1995). Critical thinking skills of baccalaureate nursing students. *Journal of Professional Nursing, 11*(6), 351–357.

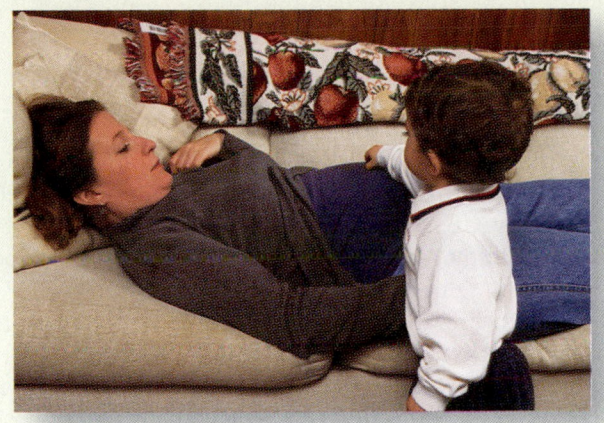

Melissa Hamilton, who is in her 20th week of pregnancy with her second child, arrives home with her 3-year-old son, Kevin. The day has been spent attending her scheduled prenatal visit and meeting with a real estate agent about putting their two-bedroom house up for sale. Tired, Melissa lies down on the sofa. Kevin comes to her, smiles, and puts his hand over her stomach.

Melissa wonders how Kevin will respond to his baby sister after her birth. She and her husband Sean have told him about the baby and he seems happy about having a new playmate, but still demands much of Melissa's attention. Melissa and Sean are also unsure about selling their house. Although they need a larger home, Melissa does not want to lose the friendships they have developed among their neighbors. During her prenatal visit earlier in the day, Melissa had considered talking to Linda Doherty, RN, about her concerns with the changes that the new baby would bring for her and her family, but wondered if the nurse would be able to help her cope with these stressful events. ■

4

Theories for Understanding the Childbearing Family

The conceptual models that nurses use in working with the childbearing family are abstract and describe only general approaches to the study of childbearing. Theories, or specific statements, are needed to describe, explain, or predict phenomena related to pregnancy and childbearing. Specific theories are guidelines for the nurse delivering care to mothers, infants, and families in the real world.

Many theories proposed by disciplines other than nursing relate to the pregnancy cycle and other aspects of life and further define the phenomenon of childbearing. These theories, which are discussed in some depth in this chapter, are frequently used by nurses to form the basis or rationale for nursing practice with childbearing families, infants, and mothers. The theories discussed include: family theory, crisis theory, bonding or attachment theory, separation–individuation theory, and transcultural care theory.

Many of these theories were not developed specifically for understanding childbearing families. Nurse investigators and others, however, have developed theories that are relevant to childbearing families through research with pregnant women, some of which are related to the psychosocial aspects of childbearing. These theories are also discussed in this chapter.

▶ FAMILY STRUCTURE AND FUNCTION

The family unit is probably one of the most vital considerations of the maternity nurse. Regardless of its form, the family is the basic unit of our society and, as such, is the social institution that has the greatest effect on individuals and how they develop. It has been called the "primary group," because of its importance in the life of an individual.

Family is defined as a small social system made up of individuals related to each other by reason of strong reciprocal ties and constituting a permanent household (or cluster of households) that persists over years (Gelles, 1995). Members usually enter through birth, adoption, or marriage and leave only by death. Even divorce or abandonment cannot totally remove a person from his or her family, although such events dramatically alter the nature of the relationships within the family system.

In the United States, the stereotype of a family is that of two parents and their children, with grandparents who do not reside in the same household. The concept of family, however, has expanded over time to include groups of unrelated people, as well as blood relatives, living and caring for each other.

Because of the diverse nature of the makeup of families, different terms are used to describe the types of families found in our society. Table 4–1 describes some family types that have relevance to childbearing.

The family unit occupies a vital position between the individual and society and has two functions, or roles (Gelles, 1995). These functions are (1) to meet the needs of the individuals who form the family unit and (2) to meet the needs of the society of which it is a part. These functions for society and the individual can only be met by the family unit.

▶ TABLE 4–1

Types of Families

Type	Description
Nuclear	Consists of two parents and their children, usually associated with an extended family network not living in the same household. Two subtypes of nuclear families are family of origin (the group into which a person is born) and family of procreation (the group into which people enter as adults and in which they usually appear in the position of husband or wife, mother or father).
Extended	Any family or individual who has a relationship with a nuclear family and to whom the nuclear family looks for consultation and support. Extended family members may be relatives (e.g., grandparents) or collateral relationships (e.g., friends).
Single-parent	Consists of one parent raising children as a result of separation, divorce, death, or being unmarried. Although many single-parent families are headed by women, they may also be headed by men.
Binuclear	Consists of two parents who have terminated the spousal relationship, live in two separate households, and cooperate in the responsibilities of parenting. They have usually been awarded joint custody of the children by the courts.
Reconstituted (stepfamily)	Consists of remarried adults with children from the husband's and/or the wife's previous marriage. This family may be considered *blended* if children result from the present marriage.
Same-sex	Consists of two adults of the same sex with or without children.
Communal	Group of unrelated adults and children dedicated to a common purpose.

The function of the family as it relates to the individual is important during the phase of childbearing. The family provides for survival and ensures development of the newborn, infant, and dependent child. For adults, it meets affectional, socioeconomic, and sexual needs. For all members, it serves as a buffer between the individual and society. Thus, family theory, of all theories relating to childbearing, deserves attention as a basis for understanding client behaviors during pregnancy, birth, and the postpartum period.

Childbearing and rearing are two primary tasks the family fulfills for society. The family unit provides a stable, recognized, legitimate unit for bringing new members into a society and for socializing those members so that they can function in society.

▶ THE FAMILY DEVELOPMENTAL CYCLE

The family system, as an integrated entity, may grow and develop in a sequential fashion, similar to how an individual person develops. Childbearing is one of the most important stages of the family cycle since it entails a major reorganization of family structure and function. Such major reorganization of a system may produce a developmental crisis. (See the section entitled "Crisis Theory" later in this chapter.) This section discusses the childbearing family in the developmental crisis of reorganizing to incorporate a new member and the special developmental challenges faced by economically disadvantaged families.

▶ A Dynamic System

The life cycle of the family is a dynamic process that has three phases: beginning, middle, and end. During the beginning phase, the major theme of family function and of the developmental tasks is establishment. The middle phase theme is expansion, extension, maintenance, and continuation. The end phase theme and tasks are related to transition, contraction, and completions (Gelles, 1995). Each of these phases can be identified; the success of achieving developmental tasks can be assessed; and diagnoses concerned with family needs, strengths, and weaknesses can be formulated.

▶ Family Developmental Tasks

Family developmental tasks are specific to a given stage of development in the family life cycle. They are directed toward maintenance and continuation of family well-being at a particular period during the life cycle. In a classic work, family developmental tasks are described by Duvall (1977) as the growth responsibilities a family must accomplish at its stage of development to (1) satisfy its biologic requirements, (2) meet cultural demands, and (3) satisfy its own aspirations and values. Tasks shift with each stage of the family life cycle.

Like an individual, a family can succeed or fail in meeting tasks or growth responsibilities that arise at various stages in the life cycle. Family success in mastering tasks leads to success in mastering subsequent tasks in new developmental stages. Failure, however, leads to later difficulty and disapproval from society.

Family developmental tasks arise when the needs of one or more family members come together with the expectations of society in terms of family performance. Internal (subsystem) tension and pressure combine with societal expectations (input) to produce a need for family system change. The need for change (which can be viewed as a developmental crisis for the family) creates new tasks, which must be mastered by the family to resolve the crisis, restore homeostasis, and become ready for the next stages of development.

Duvall and others have identified critical stages in the family life cycle when the family must solve specific developmental tasks. Duvall's focus is primarily on childrearing. Thus, critical events that require the family to accomplish developmental stages are such family-related phenomena as getting married, giving birth, launching young adults, and adjusting to the "empty nest." Stress on the family system is inevitable during the various stages of growth, and this stress encourages family solution of developmental tasks. Unpredictable events, however, such as birth of a child with disabilities, untimely death of a member, or natural disasters, may complicate the picture. Thus, family systems, as well as individual systems, may have situational crises as well as normal developmental crises where family developmental tasks are expected and predictable.

▶ Duvall's Eight-Stage Family Life Cycle

Duvall identifies eight stages of family development (see box entitled Eight Stages of Family Development). Other theoreticians have elaborated on this scheme, but it remains the predominant mode of viewing the life cycle.

► EIGHT STAGES OF FAMILY DEVELOPMENT

Stage 1   Beginning: married couple without children
Stage 2   Childbearing: oldest child under 30 months
Stage 3   Preschool: oldest child 30 months to 6 years
Stage 4   School-age: oldest child 6 to 13 years
Stage 5   Teenage: oldest child 13 to 20 years

Stage 6   Launching: period between when the oldest child leaves home and the youngest child leaves
Stage 7   Middle: "empty nest" until retirement
Stage 8   Aging: retirement to death of both spouses

Developmental Tasks of the Beginning Family

While there are eight stages to the family developmental cycle, due to the focus on childbearing in this book, only the two stages that deal with childbearing are described in detail. During the establishment phase of marriage, the basic family system tasks (dependent on the couple's social status, ethnic and racial group, and family background) are:

1. Finding, furnishing, and maintaining a first home
2. Establishing mutually satisfactory means of support
3. Allocating responsibilities
4. Establishing mutually acceptable personal, emotional, and sexual roles
5. Interacting with in-laws, relatives, and community
6. Planning for children (including using contraceptives, deciding to have children, and dealing with pregnancy)
7. Maintaining couple motivation and morale

Developmental Tasks of Childbearing

The childbearing stage of the family life cycle begins with the birth of the first child and continues until the firstborn is in preschool. During this stage, husband and wife must make the difficult transition to parenthood, a process that is the focus of later chapters in this book. Tasks for the childbearing family include:

1. Arranging space (territory) for a child
2. Financing childbearing and childrearing
3. Assuming mutual responsibility for child care and nurturing
4. Facilitating role learning of family members (i.e., assuming the maternal and paternal roles)
5. Adjusting to changed communication patterns in the family to accommodate a newborn and young child
6. Planning for subsequent children
7. Realigning intergenerational patterns (i.e., establishing grandparent–grandchild subsystems)

8. Maintaining family members' motivation and morale
9. Establishing family rituals and routines

► The Life Cycle of Economically Disadvantaged Families

Living in poverty does not make a family dysfunctional; many families do fulfill the developmental needs of members despite poverty. Poverty, however, is still a very powerful negative force on a family, especially as many economically disadvantaged families in the United States are also made up of minority individuals (McAdoo, 1993, 1997). Some major stressors on these families have been described:

1. Ongoing intrusion of a variety of agencies and officials in the family's daily life
2. Discriminatory societal attitudes, especially if the family is not of the dominant cultural group
3. Constant bombardment with complex, extreme, and unrelenting situations over which the family has little control
4. Great interdependence of family members financially and emotionally (Survival for one member often depends on survival of other members.)
5. Continual stress and change (The family is at a great disadvantage in dealing with normal developmental stressors over time.)

It is important for the nurse to recognize that families often do learn a variety of creative responses to deal with an impoverished and hostile environment. Not everything the family does is maladaptive; behaviors must be assessed in the context of the family's specific situation. However, several observations are relevant to families of various ethnic groups who live in poverty. Some identifiable patterns are evident:

1. The life cycle is disturbed by many unpredictable life events and stresses (situational crises).

2. The family has few resources available to cope with crises.
3. Life cycle stages are shortened, with blurred transitions between stages.
4. Families living in poverty are often headed by women and are often extended family structures.

Developmental Stages

The phrase *shortened life cycle stages* means that families living in poverty often have less calendar time to complete developmental stages. Moreover, at each stage with its "normal" maturational crises, several unpredictable situational crises often occur. Members of economically disadvantaged families are frequently prevented from solving the developmental tasks of each stage. Consequently, it becomes more difficult to meet the tasks of subsequent stages. The three developmental stages of poor families are described below.

Stage 1: Adolescence or Unattached Young Adulthood.
During this stage, the young person faces three tasks.

1. *Establishing the self as a person.* Children either are pushed out of the home early or are seen as an important source of support for the family. Peer groups, for example, gangs, often attain major importance in the young person's life.
2. *Attempting to find work.* This is often difficult for poor minority youths. The "underground" economy has great appeal.
3. *Developing intimate heterosexual peer relationships.* Much sexual experimentation occurs among young people. Girls may see pregnancy and motherhood as their only chance at having an identity; boys, because there are few economic opportunities, often become transients in heterosexual relationships.

Stage 2: The Family with Children.
Three tasks are accomplished by families living in poverty during this stage.

1. *Forming a marital system.* This is difficult because of chronic stress and conflicts over use of time and money.
2. *Taking on parental roles.* Young parents often identify with single peers and avoid the parental role. If the mother accepts Aid to Families with Dependent Children (often called "welfare"), the father is often pushed into the role of "peripheral male."
3. *Realigning relations with the extended family.* Because extended family boundaries may be

more flexible among low-income ethnic groups, a young parent(s) may be easily accepted into the extended family hierarchy.

Stage 3: The Family in Later Life.
The task of this stage, becoming a grandparent and turning over the reins to the next generation, is difficult for the elderly living in poverty. Generally, there is no "empty nest" and older family members must still contribute to make financial ends meet. These individuals are often grandparents by midlife and may find themselves rearing a young parent and his or her child as "siblings." Further, with expansion of the drug culture and human immunodeficiency virus (HIV) infection, grandparents are more and more finding themselves as the persons responsible for rearing their grandchild as biologic parents become unable to do so (Dowdell & Sherwen, 1998). For example, the woman in African-American families is often described as someone who cannot move out of the child care role.

The life cycle described above may be more relevant for some groups of economically disadvantaged families than others. Culture and whether the family lives in a rural or urban environment affects to some extent how poverty shapes the family life cycle. Yet it is most likely that the life cycle is shortened in some manner for all families living in poverty. This, as well as the necessity to deal with continual situational crises, makes achievement of developmental tasks difficult for family members.

▶ OVERVIEW OF THE CHILDBEARING FAMILY

Childbearing is a developmental challenge for the family system. Within the system, a variety of changes in structure, function, and existing subsystems occur. Pregnancy and the perinatal period initiate such reorganization. Indeed, many changes must be completed before the infant's birth. The chapters in this book focus in depth on changes that occur in the family system and its members during pregnancy and childbirth. This section is an overview of some of these changes.

▶ Changes in Family Patterns

For the family unit as a whole, and for the expectant woman and man as individuals, childbearing represents both a developmental crisis and a developmental opportunity for maturation and growth. The family and its members will change in irreversible ways. As a

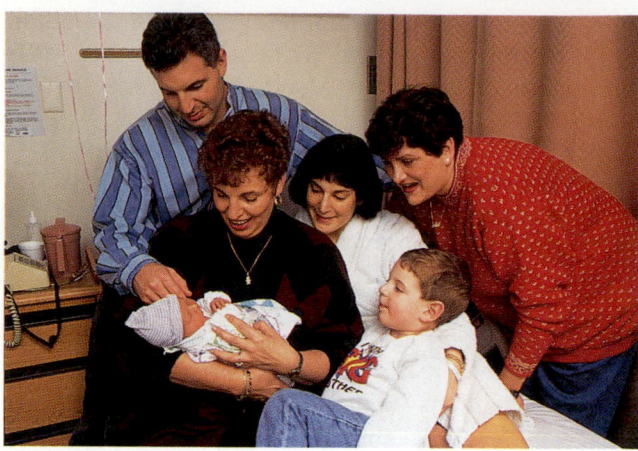

FIGURE 4–1. Pregnancy and the birth of a child result in significant changes both within the family unit and between the family and the rest of society.

result, they may experience internal family stress. Prior to birth of an infant, the man and woman may function as relatively independent individuals. After pregnancy, however, the couple participates in the creation and shaping of a new human being who will, to some

extent, reflect each of them and their relationship. Thus, during childbearing, the expectant woman and man experience major and important shifts in themselves, in their relationship with each other and with others outside the nuclear family, and in the patterns of their family as a whole (Fig. 4–1).

Changes that occur in the psychologic makeup of the expectant woman are now fairly well recognized, and changes that occur in the expectant man are a current focus of interest. Little emphasis, however, has been placed on the couple as a unit and the changes that inevitably occur in their patterns of interaction or in the family as a whole. Table 4–2 outlines some of the changes that may occur in the family system during the childbearing cycle.

▶ Environmental Effects on the Family System

The family system in rearing and socializing children receives input from many other systems in its environment, such as the health care and school systems. Many institutions and systems have a stake in how the family rears its children; the family has an oblig-

---

▶ TABLE 4-2

Family Changes During the Childbearing Cycle

Family Component	Change During Childbearing
Structure	First pregnancy involves shift from stable dyad to a volatile triangle. Subsequent pregnancies involve development of several complex, shifting triangular structures. Family members must occasionally cope with being the "isolate" in a triangle. Stress and tension may increase.
	Additional subsystems must be established: mother–child; father–child; sibling; grandparent–grandchild
Power	Patterns often alter; egalitarian power patterns often become more "traditional," with father as decision maker. Fetus and newborn may become very powerful in family system, producing major changes in parents' behavior and family patterns.
Boundaries	Mother's boundary incorporates another human within, the embryo–fetus. Becomes a "protective" container for fetus, progressively closing in and focusing her attention inward.
	Father's boundary must expand to give support and become empathetic with mother.
	Family boundary must become highly permeable to selected input, for example, health care and education.
Affect or feelings	Stress arising from structural change may alter feeling tone in family system. Danger signs are perception of hidden anger and hostility; pervasive depression; and apathy, unresponsiveness, or "flat" emotion.
Intergenerational patterns and roles	Parents' parents must "move up" a generation to become grandparents.
	Each member of the family system (both nuclear and extended) must assume new roles— whether it is a first or subsequent pregnancy.
Communication patterns	Family members must learn to communicate as a triangle. One member needs to learn to be a temporary outsider or "isolate" left out of communications, because only two people can communicate at one time.
Cultural background and rituals	Family members from different cultural backgrounds may have different values concerning pregnancy and childbearing, may perceive new roles differently, and may have different practices and rituals for this event. Differences can produce family conflict and stress.

ation to develop individuals who fit into society, a culture, and an extended family. Input from the environment can produce family stress and tension or can be supportive. Society's expectations of parental roles and functions may conflict with family expectations. For example, some schools see the educational system as a proper source for sex education for children. Many parents see their children's sex education as a task belonging to them in their parental role. Conversely, a family nurse practitioner may reinforce a parent's role as caretaker of a premature infant.

▶ Changing Roles of Women

The changes in the status of women have had an impact on the family. Women today are more educated than their mothers were and are seeking to define their new social roles. It has been reported that by 1991, 53% of women with children returned to the work force in the first year of their infant's life (Carnegie Task Force, 1994). This fact may be disturbing to some; however, research indicates that women who are employed function, in general, as well as women who are not employed in such areas as household activities, infant care, social and community activities, and self-care activities (Mercer, 1995). Research also shows that family functioning and child development are not affected when a woman returns to work after delivering a preterm infant. Indeed, maternal employment may have a beneficial effect on child development and family functioning (Arendell, 1997).

▶ NURSING INTERVENTIONS

The structural change and accompanying stress of childbearing produce a developmental crisis (or challenge) for the family. This crisis requires the family to master several developmental tasks to attain a higher level of growth and complexity. New coping strategies must evolve for the family to master these tasks. It is thus not surprising that a model for nursing interventions with the childbearing family comes from crisis theory. Table 4–3 provides a framework for nursing interventions during the precrisis, crisis, and postcrisis phases.

The nursing interventions outlined in Table 4–3 for the family in crisis are, necessarily, broad and general. The nurse needs to assess each pregnant woman and her family and adapt such interventions to the family's unique needs and attributes. Later chapters give more insight into specific forms of intervention, which are dependent on unique aspects and needs of the childbearing family.

▶ TABLE 4–3

Nursing Interventions for the Three Phases of Crisis

Goal of Nursing Intervention
To assist the family to capitalize on the growth potential inherent in the crisis.

Level	Nursing Interventions
Precrisis: Predictable risks and development events in the life cycle (childbearing)	Provide anticipatory guidance; discuss changes in family structure concerned with adding a new member. Assess risk factors, potential family strengths and weaknesses, past coping and problem solving, resources. Implement health teaching. Implement health promotion or maintenance strategies.
Crisis: Coping strategies not sufficient to deal with changes in family structure and problems in development (pregnancy, birth, the newborn)	Clarify the problem(s). Assist the family in gaining an understanding of the situation. Accept the family. Use appropriate interpersonal and institutional resources. Assist the family to express feelings. Assist the family to explore alternative means of problem solving. Assist the family to use new resources and strategies.
Postcrisis: Crisis has been resolved, leading to a higher, the same, or lower level of family function	Support the family in its new strategies of resolution. Emphasize growth potential in solutions. Attempt to reverse or lessen effects of maladaptation through appropriate rehabilitative effort or therapy.

Research Abstract

Development and Validation of Research Instruments for Use in Maternity Nursing

The Perception of Birth Scale (POBS) was developed in 1979 by Marut and Mercer to measure women's perceptions of their childbirth experiences—either vaginal or unplanned cesarean deliveries. While reliability and validity data have been obtained on the instrument over the years, a complete factor analysis on the instrument was necessary. The purpose of this study was to conduct an exploratory factor analysis to determine the underlying subscale structure of the POBS psychometrically.

The sample for the study was drawn from a larger study of adaptation to cesarean birth. The sample included 345 women; 100 had unplanned cesarean deliveries, and 245 had vaginal deliveries. All delivered healthy full-term infants and none of the women were classified as high-risk. Most women (89%) were primiparas.

A final sample size of 320 cases were used for the factor analysis. Twenty-five of the original 29 POBS items produced five factors. Factor 1 was labeled Delivery Experience; Factor 2, Labor Experience; Factor 3, Delivery Outcome; Factor 4, Partner Participation; and Factor 5, Awareness. Items in each factor were internally consistent, and the factors were shown not to overlap (that is, they demonstrated low correlations with each other).

The investigators concluded that the factor analysis yielded a 25-item instrument consisting of 5 factors or subscales. The ability of the POBS to capture a wide range of women's perceptions of the birth experience and the internal consistency reliabilities of each factor or subscale indicated that the instrument could be used for research purposes. However, further development of the POBS is still necessary. Three subscales have few items (Delivery Outcome, Partner Participation, and Awareness) and lower reliability. Additional items need to be developed to improve the performance of these subscales. In addition, four of the original scale items were dropped from the final version, either because they did not meet the appropriate threshold (a correlation called a loading criteria) that allowed them to be included in any one of the 5 factors or because they loaded almost equally on more than one factor (items cannot be part of more than one subscale). Unfortunately, two of the unusable items dealt with the mother's worry about the baby, which is an intuitive dimension of perception of the birth experience. The investigators therefore also recommended that further research include rewording the two items dealing with concern about the baby.

Application to Practice

This study clearly points out the amount of development necessary to construct a truly valid and reliable instrument. Nursing research in parent–child nursing, and other areas, has been at a disadvantage because of the lack of such instruments to measure nursing phenomena. Nurses still use many questionable instruments and often develop their own instruments for a study. More psychometric studies, such as the one described here, are necessary to allow nurse researchers to collect data that can serve as the basis for development of nursing interventions.

Source: Fawcett, J., Knauth, D. (1996). The factor structure of the perception of birth scale. Nursing Research, 45(2); 83–86.

▶ THEORIES FOR UNDERSTANDING THE CHILDBEARING FAMILY

▶ Crisis Theory

Crisis is defined as the impact of an event that challenges the assumed state of an individual and forces that individual to change his or her view of, or readapt to, the world, to himself or herself, or to both (Caplan, 1964). Life events likely to induce a crisis have two broad criteria: (1) they are of basic importance to the individual or family, and (2) they cannot be solved by means of previous problem-solving mechanisms. Pregnancy, birth, and role transitions are examples of such events. During the period of disequilibrium early in the crisis situation, people are more willing to accept help and are more open to change. Therefore, crisis theory has commonly been used as a theoretical base, or framework, for nursing interventions. A crisis framework is useful for assessing individuals as well as for analyzing the family system.

There are two types of crises: **situational** (or **accidental**) and **developmental** (or **maturational**). A situational crisis is an unexpected, stressful external event that may or may not coincide with a developmental crisis. (See Chapter 12 for a description of a situational crisis: a high-risk pregnancy.) A developmental crisis, with which this chapter is concerned, is somewhat different. It is viewed as "normal," because most persons and families experience such crises routinely in the process of growth and development. These crises are generally viewed as periods of marked physical, psychologic, and social change that are characterized by disturbances in life's pattern. During these periods, biopsychosocial stimuli poses certain tasks that must be faced and mastered by the person or family with a reasonable degree of effectiveness if the next maturational stage is to yield its full potential for further growth and development.

An extensive body of literature concerning transition to parenthood in normal families comes from the field of family sociology. It suggests that couples must master family tasks if they are to move successfully to the next stage of development and that most parents experience crises in the first year of adjusting to the birth of a first baby.

The concept of developmental tasks specific to childbearing can apply both to the individual and to the family as a whole. Numerous research studies have investigated the question of whether transition to parenthood represents a crisis in terms of psychologic upheaval for the individual and for the family. The predominant view is that for a minority of families, perhaps 20%, a true crisis occurs. For the majority of families, however, parenthood would more accurately be considered a transition period, or developmental event, that does not provoke a major life crisis, although it may provoke a series of minicrises.

During each developmental phase, the person or family is subject to unique stresses different from those of previous phases and to developmental tasks specific to that phase. Accompanying the phases may be high levels of anxiety, because the individual or family may experience major changes in functions and behaviors. With appropriate support from others, however, the person or family is likely to meet the challenges posed by growth and development. Thus, developmental crises are viewed as normal, providing

opportunity for a new sense of self-mastery for an individual or family who successfully completes the developmental tasks posed by the transitions.

A single developmental situation such as childbirth can produce different reactions in families, ranging from equilibrium to complete disorganization. There is evidence to support that characteristics of the family itself and the stressor event interact to determine the extent of a crisis situation. These characteristics include

- The nature of the stressor (That is, is it expected and desired, as in the birth of a planned-for child, or is it unexpected and feared, such as a high-risk pregnancy?)
- The number of crisis events facing the family at the same time (e.g., the birth of a first child coupled with loss of a parent's job or death of an extended family member)
- The way the family defines and gives meaning to the crisis event (That is, is the event seen as a challenge, where everyone has the opportunity to grow, or is it seen as forcing unwanted change on the family?)
- The internal resources a family has for dealing with crisis (such as strengths of individual members, affection between members, flexible role patterns in the family)
- The external resources a family has for dealing with crisis (such as social support networks— extended family, parent groups, friend networks)
- The ability of the family to change and adapt to the crisis event through development of short- and long-term coping strategies

When a crisis is handled well by the person or family, it results in a higher, more complex level of functioning through the development of new coping strategies. When a crisis is handled poorly, however, it can lead to a decline in the level of functioning and possibly major disorganization.

▶ Bonding and Attachment Theories

Considerable confusion surrounds the similar theories of bonding and attachment: how they relate, their differences, and the importance of the two theories during childbearing. These two theories are discussed together because they relate closely and are often used interchangeably.

Bonding Theory

Bonding theory has received a large amount of attention from the mass media, and many parents are familiar with the term. A bond is defined as "a unique relationship between two people that is specific and endures over time (Klaus & Kennel, 1982). The term **bonding** is used most often to refer to a rapid process, occurring immediately after birth, that reflects mother-to-infant attachment (not the infant's attachment to the mother) (Mercer, 1995). This process of establishing a bond between mother and newborn is seen as being facilitated by physical and skin-to-skin contact between mother and newborn (Fig. 4–2). Infant suckling, visual contact between mother and infant, and the mother's fondling of the infant are involved. Similar behaviors on the part of the father and infant are said to result in a bond as well.

Two major factors said to influence bond formation between parent and infant are (1) parental background and (2) care practices (i.e., at the location of the birthing) (see box entitled Factors Influencing Bonding).

Because health care personnel cannot really hope to change parental background to improve bonding, much of the focus of nursing intervention is on the birthing period. A major component of bonding theory is the concept of a sensitive period for the mother (and to some extent the father) immediately following

birth. During this **maternal-sensitive period** (Klaus & Kennel, 1982), which occurs in the first few hours and days following the infant's birth, complex interactions between mother and child occur and help to establish a bond between them.

During the maternal-sensitive period, which coincides with the time following birth often spent in the hospital by most mothers and infants, the mother is particularly sensitive and open to forming a bond with her infant. Bond formation involves many interrelated processes, which are actually reciprocal interactions between mother and infant (i.e., both mother and infant contribute to bond formation through their actions, such as mutual gazing). The behaviors indicating bonding are discussed in more detail in Chapter 28.

Bonding and Separation

One of the major outgrowths of bonding theory was the belief that separation of the mother and infant immediately after birth might interfere with the bonding process. Much concern with separation emerged from studies of sick or premature infants who were separated from their mothers because they required special care in intensive care nurseries. Some of these infants were subsequently abused by parents. It was feared that separation of sick infants from their mothers interrupted bonding and thus negatively affected the emerging parent–child relationship.

The notion that any separation of normal infants and their mothers immediately postpartum may hurt the future mother–infant relationship was an easy theoretic step. The media presented sensationalized concepts of bonding to susceptible parents, who came to believe that unless they bonded immediately to their newborn, their relationship to their child would be ruined forever. Parents who were separated from their newborn after birth were upset and concerned and even felt guilty.

Problems with Bonding Theory

As often happens when a theory gains such popularity, critics emerged and attempted to point out flaws in the ideal of bonding. The critics argued two basic points. First, formation of a relationship (i.e., parent–infant relationship) evolves out of many experiences rather than one specific "event," such as the immediate postpartum period in the hospital. This criticism points to the complexity of human behavior and the numerous factors that shape the person.

Second, several investigators have challenged the idea that there is a sensitive period in humans. They believe that the theory that concerns animal attachment to offspring does not apply to humans, who are infinitely more complex than animals.

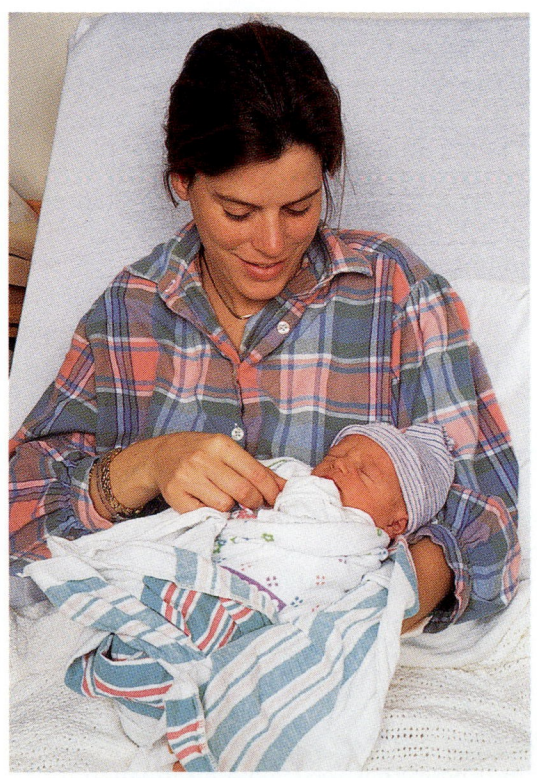

FIGURE 4–2. Bonding between a mother and her newborn.

► FACTORS INFLUENCING BONDING

PARENTAL BACKGROUND

- Care parents received from their parents
- Genetic and other inborn endowments
- Culture
- Relationships in the family
- Experiences with previous pregnancies

CARE PRACTICES

- Interventions of caregivers during and after the birthing process
- Institutional practices concerning birth (behavior of physicians, nurses, and other hospital personnel)
- Care and support parents receive during labor and delivery
- Course of events during the first days of the postpartum period and newborn life (especially the amount of separation of mother and infant)
- Rules of the health care facility

Regardless of the justification of these criticisms, another factor should be considered in attempting to arrive at a more flexible concept of bonding for the nurse and other professionals working with childbearing families. A danger in the idea that early separation can lead to permanent damage to the mother–infant relationship is the unhappiness and guilt it can cause to those parents who are aware of this theory and who are separated from their infants. They may come to believe that serious damage has been done to the present and future relationship and nothing they can do afterward can "fix" it. Other parents who cannot be present at a birth, for example, adoptive parents, may be discouraged in their efforts to relate to their adoptive children from the start. In addition, professionals may begin to treat all parents the same way. If a mother chooses not to be with her infant, she may be seen as a candidate for a parenting disorder, with little consideration given to other factors that might be present (e.g., fatigue). One way to look more flexibly at bonding is to consider it in relation to the process of attachment.

Attachment Theory

The **attachment relationship** theory, developed in the late 1960s by Bowlby (1969) and Ainsworth (1969), proposes that the affectional tie between mother, father, and infant develops out of response patterns that ensure that infants will be cared for during their years of dependency. This relationship is said to develop over the first year of life, with the quality of attachment between mother and infant at 1 year relating to later social and cognitive development of the child. Early attachment behaviors coming from the infant are specific to humans and are elicited by any human adult (Fig. 4–3). As the infant grows and develops, the responses become increasingly complex and directed to particular others in the infant's environment. The nature of the relation is mutual—affection grows in *both* the mother (or father) and the infant, over time. Secure attachment between mother and infant is the basis for trust, which allows the infant to function eventually as an independent individual apart from parents.

Bonding may set the stage, in a positive direction, for the developing patterns of interactions between mother and infant during the first year and help ensure the attainment of secure attachment between

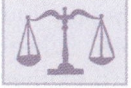 *Ethical Decision Making*

"Bonding" is a theoretical concept that has been highly popularized in both the professional and popular media. Bonding is, however, a difficult concept to measure scientifically. To date, no reliable and valid measurement instrument has been developed to quantify this phenomenon. Yet nurses continue to rate maternal–infant bonding using a variety of instruments and checklists of dubious value. Two issues are involved:

1. Should nurses make judgments about and interventions concerning bonding (and the future parent–child relationship that bonding is said to affect) based on unvalidated assessment tools?

2. Conversely, should the nurse not assess the process and risk missing a truly disturbed (or potentially disturbed) maternal–infant interaction?

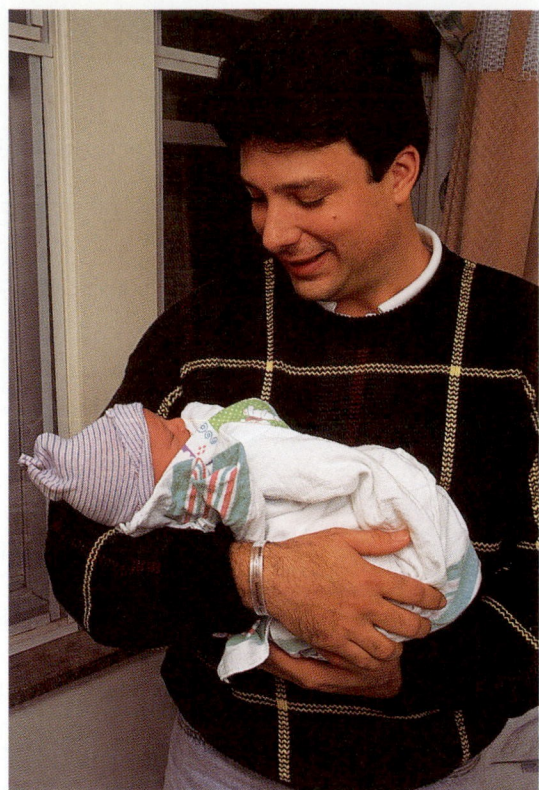

FIGURE 4–3. A father eliciting attachment behaviors from his newborn.

both mother and infant at 1 year and after. Separation during this time, however, does not prevent subsequent positive patterns of interaction between mother and infant and the development of affectional ties over the first year of the infant's life.

Nurses working with the childbearing family have opportunities to assess parent–infant interaction, interpret the meaning of infants' behaviors to parents, and promote positive parenting behaviors. Not only should nurses critically evaluate instruments used to measure parent–infant interaction, but they should also consider other factors that impact on attachment, such as cultural beliefs and practices, styles of parenting, patterns of interactions, and illness. It has been suggested that nurses move "beyond bonding" and view childbearing as a major transition in the life of a family. Nurses can be more effective by using this time when parents' interest in learning is heightened to determine what the parents want to know and help them meet their needs.

▶ Separation–Individuation Theory

Bonding and attachment are only half of the process necessary for the evolution of a positive mother–child–family relationship. A complementary process must occur—separation or, more accurately, separation–individuation. As noted in the previous discussion of theories of bonding and attachment, separation has acquired a somewhat negative connotation. Many believe that separation of the mother and infant interferes with bonding and the evolving mother–child relationship; however, the lack of separation–individuation experience can also be detrimental to the evolution of a healthy mother–child relationship.

The term *separation* is defined as the infant's psychologic development track of differentiation, distancing, boundary formation, and disengagement from the mother. *Individuation* refers to the infant's development of psychologic autonomy, that is, the development of his or her own unique personality characteristics. **Separation–individuation** is the process by which the infant separates psychologically from the mother to become an autonomous individual. The theory of separation–individuation was first developed by Mahler, who spoke of the process as the psychologic birth of the human infant (Mahler, Pine, & Bergman, 1975).

Separation–individuation is a sort of psychologic "hatching" from the maternal–infant common boundary. The mother and infant are said to occupy the same "field" during pregnancy, having a common boundary. This state is said to continue for a time after birth. The theoretic focus of separation–individuation theory is the means by which the infant separates from the symbiotic unity with the mother and becomes an autonomous, independent individual.

Nursing Alert

Nursing assessment of the parent–infant interaction must be conducted carefully and sensitively so that both the family's concerns about this relationship and the nurse's role in caring for them are acknowledged. A hasty judgment on the nurse's part about the quality of the attachment relationship that is based either on questionable evaluation instruments or limited observation time with the family can cause distress and uncertainty within the family unit and perhaps affect the relationship between the nurse and the family.

Both attachment and separation can be viewed as potentially helpful and harmful phases of the developmental process. Both must be present in interrelations between mother, infant, and other family members for normal growth and development to occur; problems seem to arise when there is too much attachment or separation. The responsibility of the nurse and others working with parents and children may be not so much ensuring that bonding occurs for all time, but instead assessing the progressive change in proportions of attachment and separation– individuation at various phases of the life cycle. (See Chapter 17 for a discussion about the effect of the separation–individuation pattern on the siblings' experience during the second trimester of pregnancy.)

► Transcultural Care Theory

Transcultural nursing is nursing care that recognizes and respects the way in which different cultures perceive, know, and practice health care. The idea of transcultural nursing and transcultural care was proposed by Leininger in the mid-1960s. She has since developed the idea into a theory of nursing that she calls *transcultural care diversity and universality* (Leininger, 1985). This theory of care is highly relevant to nursing, "because it gets to the heart and nature of nursing, and [it] . . . has the greatest potential to explain nursing phenomena and actions" (Leininger, 1985).

Leininger's theory states that different cultures perceive, know, and practice care in different ways. Yet there are some commonalities about care among all cultures in the world. Identifying the differences and similarities among cultures can provide a basis for nursing knowledge that can be used to guide nursing care decisions and actions to benefit clients.

The nursing profession, as the profession most interested in providing holistic care to individuals, must be knowledgeable about and skilled in values, beliefs, and health–illness practices of different cultures. Lack of this knowledge and skill results in a gap in provision of competent nursing care. Because cultural factors are one major force that influence the quality of health and nursing care given to people, omission of cultural factors is a major obstacle to providing care (Baker, 1996). See box entitled Concepts in Transcultural Nursing for a description of the concepts that are important in the understanding of transcultural nursing care.

Health Care Systems
Two other related aspects of transcultural nursing and care concern the professional health care system and the folk health care system and the differences between the two. These two systems of health care

► CONCEPTS IN TRANSCULTURAL NURSING

ETHNOCENTRISM
Assumption that one's own beliefs and ways of doing things are the best or superior. Example: Given the belief that strict asepsis is essential to the well-being of mother and infant, some nurses may consider other cultures' birth practices that do not occur in sterile environments as "barbaric."

CULTURAL IMPOSITION
Imposition of one's own values, beliefs, and practices on the client, family, or community in the belief that one's own lifeways are "best" and from ignorance of others' cultural practices. Example: Some nurses place great value on father participation in the birth process, which ignores cultural variation in perception of appropriate masculine roles.

CULTURAL EXCLUSION
Conscious or unconscious avoidance or omission of cultural values and practices because they are seen as inferior, incompetent, or too difficult. Individuals whose cultural practices differ from those of the dominant culture are excluded or not treated as individuals and, in turn, feel left out and demeaned. Example: Inability of a health care professional to acknowledge a client's need to avoid exposure to cold air due to her belief that such exposure can harm her baby.

CULTURAL ACCOMMODATION
Process in which the needs of clients are met appropriately, cultural practices are respected, and clients' lifeways are recognized. Example: Use of folk health practices in addition to professional health ideas in the delivery of care.

Source: Simkin, 1996.

currently exist in the United States, as well as in other cultures (and countries). It is vital that nurses understand the two systems to promote cultural accommodation and provide therapeutic, culturally sensitive care.

The **professional health care system** consists of people who have received a formal professional education and have assumed health care roles serving clients. These individuals include nurses, physicians, social workers, pharmacists, and physical and occupational therapists. In the United States, formal education is based on Western ideologies of health care.

In contrast, the **folk** (local, indigenous) **health care system** consists of people who are not formally educated but have assumed service roles to help people in their own community on the basis of local beliefs and practices. These folk health caregivers are prepared through informal experiential methods and reflect local cultural health beliefs and practices. Folk practices develop through daily life experiences in each culture and are related to the group's social structure. They are generally known and recognized by members of the particular community or cultural group.

Most individuals in the professional health care system fail to recognize the folk health care system, or if they are aware of it, they usually belittle it as "non-scientific," "superstition," "quackery," and so on. Until health care professionals recognize and respect the folk system along with the professional system, conflicts with clients from different cultures and gaps in health care services will result. The two systems are complementary and, together, can provide optimum health services to people.

Clashes between the professional health care system and professional caregivers and the client's cultural beliefs and folk health care system often result in great stress for the client and perhaps even the client's ignoring the prescription for care offered by the professional health care system. Flexibility, understanding, respect, and incorporation of the client's culture and cultural practices facilitate acceptance of the professional and his or her health ideas by the client and reduce client stress.

Developing Cultural Awareness

How can a nurse develop the ability to give culturally appropriate health care to clients from different cultures? The primary way is through the education system. Transcultural nursing is a specialty area in nursing, just as is maternal–infant nursing. Transcultural care concepts should, however, be considered in all phases of the nursing curriculum and in continuing education.

Several strategies can help one develop cultural awareness:

1. The student may explore his or her own cultural background.
2. The student may then learn about a different culture by reading literature, attending seminars, enrolling in formal courses, and so forth.
3. The student may conduct a small-scale cultural profile of a community and attend cultural events in a community.
4. The student may direct study to learning cultural norms of the people met in nursing practice.

Of course, major anthropologic and ethnographic study is necessary before one can gain a true understanding of cultural groups. Many individuals actually live and participate in a culture to gain an understanding of that group. The enormous variety of cultural groups makes it impossible for the nurse to be a universal expert. It is, however, vital that nurses recognize culture as one of the most important considerations in care delivery. If care practices suggested to the pregnant woman of a particular cultural group conflict with her beliefs and values, they will not be carried out, no matter how good they are.

Finally, the student must realize that nursing itself is a culture. When viewed from a different perspective, nursing practices might seem barbaric or inappropriate. The student needs to keep an open, flexible mind concerning health care and other culturally based beliefs, as well as remain aware of culture as a major factor in a person's beliefs and practices about health and other behaviors.

► THEORIES CONCERNING PSYCHOSOCIAL ASPECTS OF CHILDBEARING

The theories discussed in this section differ from those in the previous section in a very important way. Theories discussed in the first section were not necessarily developed from research or observations on pregnant women, newborns, or families. Although they are useful in explaining phenomena that occur in childbearing families, they also explain phenomena in other situations that have nothing to do with pregnancy.

The theories to be discussed in this section were developed specifically from research and observations on childbearing families. Thus, they relate specifically to pregnancy and help flesh out the picture of individuals and families experiencing pregnancy. Concepts introduced in these theories, such as role development or fantasy during pregnancy, are elaborated on in future chapters discussing psychosocial changes during each trimester. The specific theoretic concepts to be explored here include psychosocial changes in the mother during pregnancy (including the experience of becoming a mother, maternal role assumption, role conflict and attainment of the maternal role, establishment of a relationship with the fetus, and fantasies during pregnancy), psychosocial changes in the father during pregnancy (including paternal role assumption and paternal pregnancy experiences, especially paternal style and the couvade syndrome), experiences of siblings during pregnancy, and experiences of grandparents during pregnancy.

▶ Psychosocial Changes in the Mother: An Overview

Pregnancy and becoming a parent represent major changes in the life of a woman. It has been theorized that pregnancy represents a period of transition between two completely different lifestyles or ways of viewing oneself in the world: from woman-without-a-child to woman-and-child (Lederman, 1996). This transition involves psychologic incorporation of this new image of woman-and-child into the woman's self-concept. Although this change in view of self is most dramatic with a first child, it occurs with additional births as well. The relationship a mother establishes with her child is uniquely different with each pregnancy and is independent of any relationship with a previous child. That is why, for example, a woman who has a stillborn child cannot replace that child or that relationship with another child.

The psychosocial change women experience may be described as a shift in their self-image, beliefs, values, priorities, behavior patterns, relationships with others, and problem-solving (coping) skills. Various factors have been proposed as influencing the psychologic dynamics accompanying pregnancy. These include the woman's characteristic coping mechanisms, stage of pregnancy, her current life stresses, her stage in the life cycle, the symbolic meaning of the pregnancy to her, and her relationship within her family. In other words, psychologically during the course of the pregnancy, the woman evolves a new perceptual framework by which to interpret her world. The psychologic inclusion of the infant into the woman's view of herself as woman-and-child is interdependent with and symmetrically parallel to the biologic development of the fetus and the pregnancy. This chapter

and subsequent others examine the changes occurring in each trimester as the woman adapts and accommodates to the process of having a child and becoming a mother.

Becoming a Mother

Acceptance of Pregnancy. Accepting the pregnancy is one of the first changes a woman must make for a successful transition in lifestyle. This acceptance refers to a woman's adaptive responses to all of the changes inherent in prenatal growth and development (Lederman, 1996). A woman who cannot accept the pregnancy will find it very difficult to accept the changes necessitated by pregnancy, childbirth, and interaction with the newborn.

In general, low acceptance of pregnancy has been associated with unplanned pregnancy, greater conflicts and fears, many physical discomforts during pregnancy, and depression. Acceptance of pregnancy, on the other hand, has been linked to feelings of happiness and enjoyment of the pregnancy, little physical discomfort, moderate mood swings, and relatively little reported ambivalence during the first trimester. Complete acceptance of pregnancy is rare, however. Some ambivalence was felt to be "normal." Most ambivalence concerned two areas: financial security and changed lifestyle (including the motherhood–career conflict) (Lederman, 1996).

Particular areas need to be assessed concerning a woman's acceptance of pregnancy:

1. Extent to which the pregnancy was planned and wanted by the woman and her partner
2. Amount of time the woman is happy versus depressed during the pregnancy (this may have different meanings depending on the woman's trimester of pregnancy)
3. Amount of reported discomfort during pregnancy and the woman's response to the discomfort
4. Extent to which the woman accepts or rejects changes in her body
5. Amount of ambivalence or experienced conflict concerning the pregnancy expressed by the woman near term

Self-Image and Body Image During Pregnancy. Other aspects of the psychologic change a woman undergoes during pregnancy are self-image and body image. Evolution of a new view of the self is an essential component of the new, altered sense of self as mother-and-child. Self-image and body image will be different, depending on the woman's trimester of pregnancy. There are three interdependent spheres of self that influence the psychologic transition to role of mother: the ideal self, the self-image, and the body image (Mercer, 1995).

The ideal self is composed of all the attributes, qualities, and images a person would like to have and hopes to include in the self. For the pregnant woman, the ideal self represents her image of the "ideal mother" she would like to become.

Self-image refers to the more reality-oriented, active self. It is the self that interacts with the real world, here and now. It incorporates both the ideal self and the body image, holding the desirable aspects of the ideal self as a standard of behavior to be attained. This "self" of the expectant mother will evaluate how successfully or unsuccessfully she will be at attaining maternal behaviors.

Body image during pregnancy has to do with a woman's perception of her size, how she moves, and her own physical beauty or ugliness. One vital component of body image that plays a role during pregnancy is body boundary. **Body boundary** during pregnancy becomes an important protector of the fetus; it literally keeps the fetus inside the woman's protective container of a body.

As the pregnancy cycle progresses, the woman's perception of the body boundary increases over and above the actual physical size of the pregnant body and the actual weight gain.

Role Assumption and Maternal Adaptation

Attainment of the maternal role has been studied by many nurse researchers and clinicians. Reva Rubin, Ramona Mercer, and Regina Lederman are prominent nurses who have described the process of maternal role attainment and adaptation. Assuming and adapting to the role of "mother" are parts of a long-term process. The psychologic changes a woman undergoes during pregnancy that enable her to assume the maternal role actually build on a lifelong process of informal socialization of learning a feminine identity.

Feminine Identity. Feminine identity has been defined as a woman's definition of herself and of the outside world (Mercer, 1995). Feminine identity begins as early as there is a sense of self, around 2 years of age. A little girl may develop an identity of what it means to be female by playing with dolls, wearing ruffled dresses, and interacting with people who expect her to act like a "little lady." A girl may also develop a feminine identity by engaging in "gender-free" activities and playing with toys not deemed specific for girls or boys. She may also develop her identity by associating with and playing with little boys.

The feminine identity undergoes development at various phases of a woman's life—during the preschool period, school-age period, puberty, adolescence, childbirth, and menopause. It is especially affected by periods in the life cycle in which there is marked physical, physiologic, and psychologic change, such as puberty, pregnancy, and menopause. During the massive changes that occur during pregnancy, many factors affect the evolution of feminine identity into a sense of being a mother.

Many of a woman's personality traits (e.g., her temperament, belief system, or level of assertiveness) determine how well she adapts to the maternal role. The expectant woman's perception of and relationship with her own mother are seen as key in the process of adapting to the maternal role. Furthermore, the extent of stress (including marital disharmony) affects the woman's attainment of the maternal role and identity.

Maternal Identity. Maternal identity is an internalization of the maternal role. Identity formation occurs anew with each pregnancy. There is no carryover or transference of a maternal identity from one child to the next. Formal anticipatory socialization for the role of mother begins during pregnancy as the woman progresses through the psychologic incorporation of the infant into her self-system and self-concept. However, the complete formation of a maternal identity awaits the birth of the infant and identification of the child in reality (Mercer, 1995).

Maternal Role Attainment. Maternal role attainment, that is, acquisition of the mothering role, is described as a process that begins prenatally and ends with formation of a maternal identity during the infant's first year. For first-time mothers, it is a process in which the mother achieves competence in the role and integrates the mothering behaviors into her established role set, so that she is comfortable with her identity as a mother (Mercer, 1995).

The goal of identification with a motherhood role for primigravidas is for the mother to refocus her thinking away from the single self and toward the mother–infant unit. Identification of the motherhood role involves two important factors: the woman's motivation to assume that role and the extent of her preparation for a motherhood role. Furthermore, identification of the role is closely related to the woman's relationship with her own mother (Lederman, 1996).

Identification with a Motherhood Role in Multigravid Women. Identification with a motherhood role is different for multigravid and primagravid women. Even though multigravid women have already made the transition to the role of woman-with-child, they have to again form a maternal identity as mother to this infant (Lederman, 1996). In particular, women often worry about the changes another child will require in their lives. They are also often concerned with how their children will accept a sibling.

In general, past experience with motherhood is an asset to most multigravid women during the process of identification with a motherhood role. Prior experience provides the mother with knowledge about what to expect in her role as mother of an infant and also gives her some degree of confidence regarding the nature of the tasks to be performed. Nonetheless, she must still prepare herself emotionally, physically, financially, and in other ways for the challenges that will undoubtedly occur as the result of being the mother of more than one child.

Regardless of how many children a woman has, she still thinks about her own mother with respect to her pregnancy and expanding motherhood role, but to a lesser extent than do primigravid women. The standard for a multigravid woman is her own previous mothering experience.

Role Conflict and Attainment of the Maternal Role

Assumption of a role does not always proceed smoothly. For several reasons, a person may not "fit" a particular role. These situations are commonly labeled role conflicts, and they evolve continually for individuals who must function in a complex social structure. Role conflicts may develop in several ways. For example, there may be major discrepancies between the anticipated role and the experienced role. Large shifts from familiar to unfamiliar roles or to roles that have conflicting but desired goals may also produce role conflict. Furthermore, inadequate preparation for the role or vague and ambiguous role definitions may also produce role conflict in the individual (Mercer, 1995).

Another potential source of role conflict stems from an individual's membership in multiple groups. It is likely that at least one role necessary for social interactions in one group will be incompatible with a role necessary for interactions in a second group. The necessity to give up or alter one or both roles may produce conflict for the individual.

Several potential situations that may directly produce conflict in a woman attempting to move into the maternal role are inability to achieve the "good mother" role, lack of knowledge and preparation for the maternal role, and career conflicts.

Inability to Achieve the "Good Mother" Role. Role conflict increases if a mother believes she

cannot imitate the "good mother" of her childhood or has unrealistic expectations of the behaviors she will perform as the "good mother." If perceptions of her own mother are unrealistic and idealistic, a woman may fear her perceived inability or be unable to emulate the desired behaviors. She then sees herself as functioning in the role of the "bad mother."

Lack of Knowledge and Preparation for the Maternal Role. Despite efforts in some school systems to make adolescents aware of issues related to parenting, most young people lack preparation. In the "modern" nuclear family, guidelines for parenting are confusing and role models less apparent than in some other family types. Stressors include the lack of guidelines for successful parenting; the abruptness of the transition to parenthood at the birth of a child; the need to redesign old roles rapidly and adapt to new ones; the pressure to reassess goals, values, and priorities associated with new roles; and the desire to determine alternative means of gratification from the new roles (Arendell, 1997).

This source of conflict may be lessened by childbirth preparation during pregnancy and by family living courses in high school. This problem in role assumption, however, will probably continue as society becomes more complex and mobile and the role of parent becomes more vague.

Career Conflicts. One major source of conflict in attaining the maternal role is career conflicts. A career is often seen as a source of self-respect, self-confidence, and independence for a woman (Lederman, 1996). The crucial question is whether a woman can successfully integrate career and family roles.

Women's Health

The enactment of the Family and Medical Leave Act of 1993 may offer the new mother a way to handle the conflict she experiences in integrating her maternal and career roles. This legislation allows workers with companies of 50 or more employees to take up to 12 weeks of unpaid leave from their jobs following the birth or adoption of a child or to care for seriously ill family members. During this leave, health insurance benefits are maintained and employees are able to return to either their former positions or to comparable ones in the company.

Establishing a Relationship with the Fetus

During the course of pregnancy, and the transition to a new lifestyle and the maternal role, a mother needs to establish a relationship with the infant-to-be (the fetus). This relationship with the fetus is thought to be the first stage in establishing a relationship with the newborn and then the child. Many clinicians have sought ways to strengthen maternal attachment or "bonding" to the fetus in utero (Mercer, 1995).

The fetus (unless the woman has ultrasound) is only a reality, however, during the second trimester, when fetal movements can be felt. The abstract child is then transformed into the "real" child.

Fantasy During Pregnancy: An Overview

Fantasy is an important factor in assumption of the maternal role and transition into the lifestyle of woman-and-child. Fantasies during pregnancy allow a woman to have a "dress rehearsal" for labor and delivery and "mothering" of an infant. Realistic fantasies of potential problems that might occur during pregnancy and labor and delivery can help the woman prepare herself to cope with these problems or complications, should they occur. Finally, especially during the third trimester, fantasies may give the nurse clues to concerns the woman may have about pregnancy, birth, and mothering (Mercer, 1995).

▶ Psychosocial Changes in the Father: An Overview

With the advent of family-centered maternity care, nurses find themselves caring for the whole family, not just the maternal–infant dyad. Suddenly, what the father and siblings feel and do is important, and this knowledge is necessary for delivery of nursing care to the childbearing family unit. Knowledge concerning fathering and the father's experience during pregnancy and childbirth still lags well behind knowledge concerning the mother; however, a beginning in understanding fathering has been made.

Fathers, as well as mothers, must make a major lifestyle change during the childbearing cycle (Hawkins & Dollahite, 1997). The man must gain a new perceptual framework, that of man-and-child, to be able to father his infant. The changes a father must undergo to make the necessary lifestyle shift can, at present, be grouped into two categories: (1) changes concerned with development of the role of father and (2) changes in the man's experiences that occur during his partner's pregnancy.

Development of the Father Role

The role of father can be seen to develop in three interdependent ways:

1. Through personal and environmental factors that occur during the man's course of development
2. Through participation in the childbearing cycle
3. Through interactions with the newborn infant

Developmental Factors. Generally in the course of growing up in a family, a young boy identifies with both his mother and father. Thus, to some extent, his adult personality and attitudes retain some nurturing (mothering) aspects as well as the more traditional and heavily emphasized, instrumental (fathering) aspects (Dollahite, Hawkins, & Brotherson, 1997). In many men, then, there is a desire to "create life" like their mothers and to nurture.

Other developmental factors associated with the father role have been identified. These include the man's childhood experience with his own father, marital satisfaction, and experience with infants.

Participation in the Childbearing Cycle. A father's active participation and involvement in pregnancy, labor, and delivery strengthen his perception of himself in the father role. This involvement also assists his partner in seeing him as a father. Participation in the childbearing cycle also seems to have an influence on the evolving father–infant relationship and on paternal attachment.

Father–Infant Interactions and the Father Role. The father's interaction with his newborn infant promotes bond formation between father and infant and solidifies the father role (Palkovitz, 1997). Fathers have been shown to be able to nurture a newborn as efficiently as mothers and to function as competent infant caregivers.

The Father's Psychosocial Experiences During Pregnancy

The Couvade. *Couvade* is an anthropologic term designating a set of rituals or behaviors in certain cultures that regulate paternal actions during childbirth. It is derived from the French verb *couver*, which means "to brood" or "to hatch." In the cultural groups in which couvade is practiced, a man is assisted, by performing certain rituals, to assume the role of father and to gain acknowledgment of this major transition from his partner and his society.

Interestingly enough, some men in the predominant Western cultures go through what has been called the **couvade syndrome** (Gerson, 1997)—bodily symptoms experienced by a father during the course of his partner's pregnancy. Symptoms include gastrointestinal disorders, nausea and vomiting, increased or decreased appetite, backache, toothache, syncope, fatigue, leg cramps, and weight gain.

Couvade phenomena have had several interpretations. Most commonly, they are believed to be an expression of the father-to-be's involvement in the pregnancy and identification with his partner. Theoretically, the more the father-to-be identifies with the mother-to-be and is involved in the pregnancy, the more he experiences the couvade symptoms.

Stages of the Pregnancy Experience for Men. Although much is still unknown about the progression of the pregnancy experience for an expectant father, researchers have identified six stages through which men involved in the pregnancy (those who are responsive to the pregnancy and their feelings about it) pass (Palkovitz, 1997).

1. Getting ready period (when the couple attempts to create a pregnancy)
2. Stage of conception (when conception is medically confirmed)
3. End of the first trimester
4. Midpregnancy
5. Stage of turning toward father and fathering (between 15 and 25 weeks of pregnancy)
6. End of pregnancy (26 weeks to end of pregnancy)

The father-to-be's concerns in each of these stages are discussed in Chapters 15, 17, and 18.

Paternal Fantasies During Pregnancy. Expectant fathers also experience fantasies about the course of the pregnancy and the infant-to-be during pregnancy. It may be that fantasy performs a similar function during pregnancy for the expectant man as it does for the expectant woman. Like those of the expectant mother, an expectant father's fantasies become more vivid toward the end of pregnancy, although some might be present in the first two trimesters as well. In general, however, men seem to be more reluctant to admit to having fantasies (both day- and night dreams) during pregnancy than are their partners.

Styles of Paternal Involvement in Pregnancy. Some fathers are "attuned" to their pregnancy experiences and some are not. Fathers who are attuned are able to describe their inner experiences concerning the pregnancy (Gerson, 1997). A now classic theory (May, 1980) explains, in part, the phenomenon of an expectant father's involvement (or noninvolvement) in his partner's pregnancy. A man's involvement can be seen on a continuum between two opposing dimensions: detachment and involvement (Fig. 4–4). The varying levels of detachment and

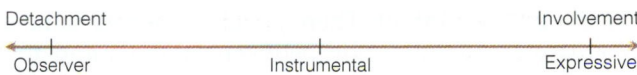

FIGURE 4–4. Continuum between paternal detachment and involvement in pregnancy.

involvement characterize three styles of paternal pregnancy involvement.

- *Observer style.* The man reports certain emotional distance from the pregnancy and sees himself largely as a bystander. This style is the most detached of the three, involves little decision making in the pregnancy, and can be associated with either a happy or an unhappy affective state.
- *Expressive style.* The man reports a highly emotional response to pregnancy and sees himself as a full partner in it. Fathers adopting this style often have a high incidence of pregnancy symptoms. These fathers also expect to actively parent their children.
- *Instrumental style.* The man emphasizes tasks to be accomplished and sees himself largely as a caretaker or manager of the pregnancy. These fathers downplay the emotional impact of the pregnancy and pride themselves in carrying out traditional functions central to their role as husband and father. They "take care of business," often making appointments for their partners, keeping partners on diets, and making major purchases and decisions concerning the infant. This style represents the midpoint on the detachment–involvement continuum.

▶ The Sibling's Experience: An Overview

Very little is known about how children in a family adapt to pregnancy and a new infant. Even more baffling is the manner in which a first-born child moves into the new role of brother or sister with the birth of a new infant. It has been estimated that some 80% of children in the United States grow up with siblings. Furthermore, the patterns of sibling interactions seem to be established during infancy of the later-born child and continue throughout childhood. These interactions may influence the nature of later relationships between the siblings and may even have an influence on the personality development of each child. Thus it is an area of concern for the nurse delivering family-centered care.

The relationships between parents and children in a family also may alter during pregnancy and after birth of a new infant. There generally seems to be an increase in confrontation between mothers and first-born children and a decrease in maternal availability to the first-born child. Even during pregnancy, the anticipation of the expected birth may affect the parent–child relationship and parental availability to the first-born child.

There are also many changes in sibling behavior with birth of a new infant. Withdrawal and antagonism, especially in relation to the new baby, are common. This phenomenon is well known as *sibling rivalry*. Current child preparation programs offered by health care facilities during pregnancy and sibling visitation, sibling bonding, or sibling presence at the birth are all seen as ways to improve relationships and promote attachment between older children and the new infant. There is, however, little documentation as yet to indicate that these programs actually do improve behaviors of older children. This requires extensive nursing research.

There is indication that some factors that cannot be altered may play a role in an older child's adaptation to a new baby. The child's age may be a factor, as children younger than 5 are more likely to become upset by a sibling's birth. In addition, the child's existing personality and the nature and stability of the parent–child relationship may be the most important factors in sibling adjustment. Nurses have a major role in helping the family develop an individualized strategy to support and prepare a child for the mother's pregnancy, labor and delivery, and introduction of the new sibling. They may also need to support the family throughout the older child's course of adjustment to a new sibling.

▶ The Grandparents' Experience: An Overview

To date, there has been very little research on the psychosocial aspects of becoming a grandparent or the role of grandparents in families. With the changes in family structure in recent years as well as the current social and economic climate, however, grandparents (grandmothers in particular) are assuming the role of primary care provider or are sharing the role with the parent or parents (Kornhaber, 1996). Although grandparents often form vital support structures for parents after the birth of an infant, in some families, grandparents may produce many conflicts for the childbearing family. Subsequent chapters discuss the scant information that exists about the role grandparents play in the childbearing family.

Critical Thinking in Care Planning

Care of the Family Experiencing a Developmental Crisis

Sara Scott, age 21, met Mike Phillips, age 22, at a friend's party and they began dating. After a 3-month romance, they decided to get married. Mike's salary as a sports equipment salesman and Sara's salary as a receptionist for an insurance company would allow them to maintain Mike's studio apartment.

For the first 2 months after their wedding, Sara and Mike had an active social life. In the third month, Sara missed her menstrual period. A home pregnancy test indicated that she was pregnant. Both Sara and Mike were surprised but pleased.

Sara's parents began to pressure the couple to move into the four-room upstairs apartment in their house in the suburbs. Mr. and Mrs. Scott reasoned that the couple could save money and have more room for the baby, and Sara could get prenatal care from Mrs. Scott's obstetrician-gynecologist. Mike was not in favor of the move because he felt uncomfortable living so close to Sara's parents and would have to commute to work.

For the first month of Sara's pregnancy the couple continued to live in their city apartment. Sara was bothered with "morning sickness" and numerous other discomforts of pregnancy and received prenatal care from a public hospital's clinic to save money. Their social life ceased, and Mr. and Mrs. Scott constantly voiced their disapproval of the situation. Finally, Mike reluctantly agreed to move to the Scott's upstairs apartment. Sara resigned from her job at the insurance company because she did not feel well enough to commute to her job. With only one salary, Mike and Sara became dependent on financial support from Mr. and Mrs. Scott. They lived rent-free, and Sara's parents agreed to pay for her prenatal care and the delivery at their local hospital.

As the pregnancy progressed, Mike and Sara found that they had little to talk about and almost no interests in common. Sara spent her days with her mother. Mike found Sara's expanding body unattractive. Commuting to work was tiring, and he began to stay after work to socialize with his friends. Mike began to be more and more concerned with his ability to support a wife and baby on his salary. When he went home, he and Sara fought and he knew that Mr. and Mrs. Scott thought he was "no good."

▶ Assessment

- Have not established tasks of early family: living arrangements, finances, roles, interactions with extended family, planning a family, maintaining motivation and morale.
- Difficulty in transition from dyad to triangle during pregnancy.
- Has turned over power to extended family.
- No long-term nuclear family goals established.

- Husband is withdrawing from nuclear family and extended family intruding into boundaries.
- Hostility, anger, unresolved conflict.
- Spouses have not assumed adult family roles.
- Dysfunctional communication.

Nursing Diagnosis

Ineffective family coping: Compromised related to inability of family to meet developmental tasks of childbearing family because of poor resolution of earlier tasks.

(continued)

Critical Thinking in Care Planning *continued*

Expected Client/Family Outcomes	Nursing Action/Intervention	Evaluation
The nuclear family will regain a stable, workable, positive structure and function.	Crisis Intervention strategies: Help nuclear family understand crisis. Assist nuclear family to express feelings openly. Assist nuclear family to explore other means of problem solving and coping. *Rationale:* The family unit develops as does each individual. Family development occurs in stages, each with tasks that must be mastered. Families experience developmental crises. Thus, crisis intervention strategies are appropriate here.	The nuclear family reorganizes structure and function in a positive manner.
The nuclear family will successfully master the developmental tasks of early family (thus providing a strong base for mastering the next stage's tasks)		The nuclear family accomplishes necessary developmental tasks.

Chapter Highlights

▶ The family is a network of relationships that meets the needs of both the individuals who form the family unit and of the society of which it is a part.

▶ The family undergoes stages of development similar to that experienced by the individual, where several developmental tasks, among them childbearing, must be accomplished.

▶ Childbearing leads to a variety of changes in the family system, among them shifts in patterns concerned with power, boundaries, feelings, communication, and cultural rituals; environmen-

tal influences that can lead to either stress or growth; and the evolving roles of women.

▶ Pregnancy and birth may be seen as a potential crisis situation for families with all the inherent challenges and opportunities for family growth.

▶ Bonding, attachment, and separation–individuation theories describe how family members develop necessary affectional ties to each other and, in addition, function as separate, autonomous individuals.

Chapter Highlights *continued*

▶ Culture is a vital aspect of each individual's makeup, and nursing care delivered must be culturally relevant and sensitive.

▶ Other theoretical concepts related to childbearing include psychosocial changes that occur in the mother, father, siblings, and grandparents during pregnancy and childbirth.

After reading the vignette at the beginning of this chapter, use what you have learned to answer these questions:

1. Which concepts or principles within family developmental or crisis theory can Linda Doherty, RN, use in helping Melissa and Sean Hamilton cope with the changes that are occurring within their growing family?

2. What challenges does Melissa Hamilton face in the psychologic integration of her infant into both her view of herself and her family's life?

3. How can the nurse promote Melissa Hamilton's identification with her role as mother for both Kevin and her new baby?

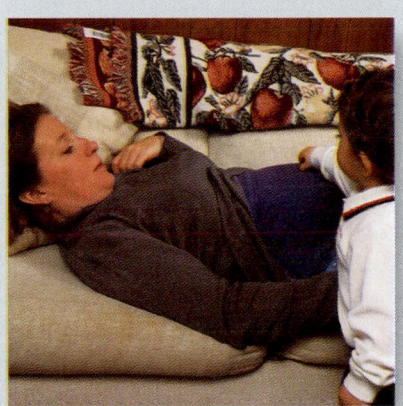

Critical Thinking Questions

▶ References

Arendell, T. (1997). *Contemporary parenting.* Thousand Oaks, CA: Sage.

Ainsworth, M. (1969). Object relations, dependency, and attachment: A theoretical review of the infant–mother relationship. *Child Development, 40;* 969–1025.

Baker, C. (1997). Cultural relativism and cultural diversity: Implications for nursing practice. *Advances in Nursing Science, 20*(1); 3–11.

Bowlby, J. (1969). *Attachment and loss.* New York: Basic Books.

Caplan, G. (1964). *Principles of preventive psychiatry.* New York: Basic Books.

Carnegie Task Force. (1994). Starting points: Meeting the needs of our youngest children. New York: Carnegie Corporation of New York.

Dollahite, D.C., Hawkins, A.J., & Brotherson, S.E. (1997). Fatherwork: a conceptual ethic of fathering as generative work. In A.J. Hawkins and D.C. Dollahite (Eds.), *Generative fathering.* (pp. 17–35). Thousand Oaks, CA: Sage.

Dowdell, E.B., & Sherwen, L.N. (1998). Grandmothers who raise grandchildren. *Journal of Gerontological Nursing, 24*(5), 8–13.

Duvall, E. (1977). *Marriage and family development* (5th ed.). Philadelphia: JB Lippincott.

Fawcett, J., & Knauth, D. (1996). The factor structure of the perception of birth scale. *Nursing Research, 45*(2), 83–86.

Gelles, R.J. (1995). *Contemporary families.* Thousand Oaks, CA: Sage.

Gerson, K. (1997). An institutional perspective on generative fathering: creating social supports for parenting equality. In A.J. Hawkins and D.C. Dollahite (Eds.), *Generative fathering* (pp. 36–51). Thousand Oaks, CA: Sage.

Hawkins, A.J., & Dollahite, D.C. (1997). *Generative fathering.* Thousand Oaks, CA: Sage.

Klaus, M., & Kennel, J. (1982). *Parent-infant bonding* (2nd ed.). St. Louis: CV Mosby.

Kornhaber, A. (1996). *Contemporary grandparenting*. Thousand Oaks, CA: Sage.

Lederman, R.P. (1996). *Psychosocial adaptation in pregnancy* (2nd ed.). New York: Springer.

Leininger, M. (1985). Transcultural care diversity and universality: A theory of nursing. *Nursing and Health Care, 6,* 209–212.

Mahler, M., Pine, R., & Bergman, A. (1975). *The psychological birth of the human infant*. New York: Basic Books.

May, K.A. (1980). A typology of detachment/involvement styles adopted during pregnancy by first-time fathers. *Western Journal of Nursing Research, 2,* 445–453.

McAdoo, H.P. (1997). *Black families*. Thousand Oaks, CA: Sage.

McAdoo, H.P. (1993). *Family ethnicity*. Thousand Oaks, CA: Sage.

Mercer, R.T. (1995). *Becoming a mother*. New York: Springer.

Palkovitz, R. (1997). Reconstructing "involvement": Expanding conceptualizations of men's caring in contemporary families. In A.J. Hawkins and D.C. Dollahite (Eds.), *Generative fathering* (pp. 200–216). Thousand Oaks, CA: Sage.

Simkin, P. (1996). The experience of maternity in a woman's life. *Journal of Obstetric, Gynecologic, and Neonatal Nursing, 25*(3), 247–252.

Ben and Nina Huang have been married for 6 years. Ben owns his own accounting business and Nina is a music teacher in the local high school. They live in a two-bedroom apartment that is centrally located to both their jobs. For relaxation, Ben and Nina enjoy going out to dinner, seeing friends, and taking weekend trips and vacations.

Recently, Ben and Nina have been discussing their plans for starting a family, a desire that both of them share. Nina is anxious to make an appointment with the nurse practitioner at the women's health clinic for a full physical examination and wants Ben to accompany her so that they can discuss discontinuation of their family planning method with the nurse. Although Ben is excited about the prospect of becoming a father, he is concerned that his emotional and sexual relationship with Nina will change as a result of their desire to conceive a child. Ben wants to talk to Nina about these feelings, but is reluctant to bring the subject up out of fear that Nina would doubt his commitment to their future. ▪

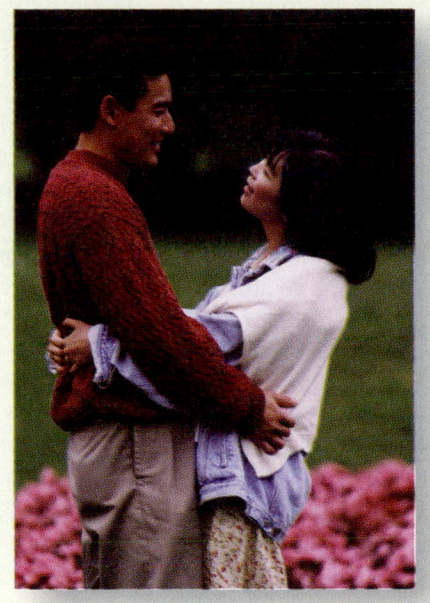

5

Human Sexuality

Sexuality has been defined as the part of life that has to do with being male or female. Sexuality in an individual evolves and matures as an interactional process in a biologic environment influenced by family members, friends, church, culture, and social and school factors.

Issues related to sexuality are at the forefront of health concerns today. Unplanned pregnancy, particularly in adolescents, is an important and serious concern. Furthermore, sexually transmitted diseases (STDs), among them the life-threatening human immunodeficiency virus (HIV) infection, have stimulated parents, health professionals, and educators to support the spread of information about protective behaviors related to sexuality. The increased awareness of sexual abuse of children has led to aggressive measures to ensure protective sexual education of children.

This chapter explores sexuality in terms of its biologic and developmental components and its cultural and behavioral expression throughout the life span. Sexuality during the childbearing phase of family life is highlighted as one life cycle phase. Nursing implications for the human sexuality process are woven throughout the narrative.

► SEXUAL SELF-CONCEPT

How individuals perceive themselves in terms of gender, masculinity or femininity, and their adoption of effective sex-role behaviors has an effect on their relationships with peers, adults, and members of the opposite sex; on play and work choices; and on their developmental expression of human sexuality. This interrelationship of biology, psychology, sociology, and culture is basic to the individual's sexual self-concept.

Gender is a biologic concept that refers simply to an individual's sex, male or female. Children's idea of their gender is usually fixed by 3 years of age. Biologic differences between males and females include (as discussed in Chapter 6) primarily chromosomal and anatomic differences and physiologic differences in the endocrine and genitourinary systems.

Nonbiologic concepts also are important for an understanding of sexuality. **Masculinity** and **femininity** are culturally prescribed, reinforced characteristics of the sexes that are independent of gender. **Sex-role behaviors** are behaviors commonly assigned to men and women; these are more likely to change in response to situational demands. Sex-role attributes are elements of culturally accepted characteristics of masculinity and femininity that are more sta-

ble over time. Thus, biologic gender, ideas of masculinity and femininity, and appropriate sex-role behaviors all affect one's developing sexuality (Wilson, 1995).

Theories about sex-role development and sex-role behaviors have varied. Freud's theory of biologic determinism suggested that sexuality is instinctively patterned; he based his sexual development theories primarily on the male. Social learning theory postulated that sex-role behaviors are learned the way other behaviors are learned—through reward, punishment, and observation of behaviors that are in agreement with family, social, and cultural groups. A third model, the cognitive developmental model, portrayed the child as actively structuring his or her own experience. The child, from the age of $1\frac{1}{2}$ to 3, categorizes himself or herself as a male or female and then, in the light of this definition, begins the process of "cognitive rehearsal" in which the appropriate sex roles are acted out.

► Sex-Role Behaviors

Regardless of how children learn sex-role behaviors, it is clear that development of sex-role behaviors begins in infancy. Classic studies by John Money of individuals with physical abnormalities of the genital tract supports this view (Money & Ehrhardt, 1972). Money found that the psychologic aspects of sexuality are independent of the biologic aspects; that is, a sexually ambiguous individual at birth, if labeled a female and socialized as a female, will comfortably take on the psychologic identity of a female.

In an early but authoritative review of sex-role research, Maccoby and Jacklin (1974) examined differences between boys and girls. They concluded that intelligence was equal between the sexes; however, there were fairly well-established differences between the sexes in the areas of verbal skills (girls), visuospatial ability (boys), mathematical ability (boys), and aggressiveness (boys). Other studies disagree with these conclusions, which support biologically based differences in cognition and sex-role behavior (Meyer-Bahlburg, 1995). Fausto-Sterling (1985) contends that although there may be a biologic origin for such differences, the actual differences are very small. Furthermore, there are differences among individuals within each sex that, in certain instances, would be as great as the differences between the sexes. Fausto-Sterling concludes that definitive statements about biologically based sex-role differences cannot be made until research methods improve.

▶ Femininity, Masculinity, and Androgyny

Femininity and masculinity are concepts that take on meaning in the context of the sociocultural environment of the individual. As any child grows up in a community, he or she receives messages about what masculinity and femininity mean.

Traditionally, the role of female in the United States has been to be popular, desirable, marriageable, and able and willing to bear children. More recently, feminists have aimed to incorporate the characteristics of activity, assertiveness, and achievement as part of the feminine perception. Although our sense of identity is tied early and closely to a perception of being male or female, the concepts of femaleness and maleness are not as value laden as we think. For example, women have many strengths that are necessary for a society to meet human needs. Society has not, however, been willing to identify these characteristics as strengths and therefore to benefit from women's skills.

Other characteristics that have traditionally been viewed as feminine include being affectionate, nurturant, yielding, and understanding, all of which are expressive behaviors. Characteristics that have traditionally been viewed as masculine include being aggressive, independent, analytic, and competitive.

Individuals who incorporate both feminine and masculine characteristics are termed **androgynous.** Androgynous individuals may possess greater behavioral flexibility, which may be related to increased mental health and personal competence. It is also believed that males and females with a masculine sex-role orientation may have higher self-esteem.

▶ Cultural Factors

An understanding of sexuality today requires a look across cultures. Cross-cultural studies have supported the existence of sex differences in the areas of aggressiveness and dominance (Whiting & Whiting, 1975). The expression of sexual behaviors and the characteristics of masculinity and femininity differ across cultures. Thus, although most cultures believe in sex-role stereotypes, these stereotypes differ among cultures. Not all cultures expect women to be passive, dependent, and gentle. In some cultures sexual expression differs; for example, sexual stimulation has been used as a pacifier for newborns and as an aid in weaning older infants. In other cultures, children play at intercourse during childhood; and real intercourse may begin as early as the age of 8 or 10.

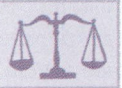 *Ethical Decision Making*

The influence of cultural attitudes on sexual self-concept is powerful and leads the nurse to consider several controversial questions such as:

1. Is sex education the responsibility of the parents, the school, or both?
2. Should sexual abstinence be stressed and family planning information deemphasized until adolescents are older?
3. Should abstinence be taught and birth control information provided to adolescents?
4. Should condoms be distributed to teenagers in school?

The American cultural attitude toward sexuality has been described as paradoxical. Parents and adults have been described as protective or prohibitive concerning sexual behavior. They discourage the expression of sexual behaviors such as masturbation and sex play by children and adolescents. Yet society has excited youth with media images of youthful sensuality and sexuality. Recently, popular musicians have been criticized by African-American women for linking violence and sex as a positive image. Superficial communications, which glamorize sexual behavior but lack meaningful information, have been linked to the high adolescent pregnancy rate in the United States. Adults in our society have also been reluctant to take on the role of sex educators. Our culture has been contrasted with European cultures, which have encouraged more open communication and expression of sexuality and hence more responsible sexual behavior (Schlegel, 1995).

▶ SEXUAL RESPONSE CYCLE

The sexual response cycle is the physiologic manifestation of the interplay of sexual interest, culture, and psychology. This cycle has been studied and reported in detail largely as a result of the pioneering work of Masters and Johnson (1966, 1970). It can be initiated by an individual alone as in masturbation or through a relationship with another person.

Masters and Johnson (1966, 1970; Masters, Johnson, & Kolodny, 1986) emphasized that the entire human body, including the nervous system, is involved in sexual arousal. Two particular responses are important during the sexual response cycle, myotonia and vasocongestion.

Myotonia, or muscle tension, increases throughout the body during sexual stimulation and is controlled by the peripheral nervous system (PNS). During sexual arousal, there are links between the sense organs (input) of the PNS, the central nervous system, and the output branches, the somatic and autonomic branches. The facial, abdominal, pelvic, back, leg, and arm muscles, which are controlled by the somatic branch of the PNS, all show increased activity and tension during the sexual response cycle.

In the circulatory system, **vasocongestion,** or blood pooling, increases the size of many parts of the body. One type of vasocongestion occurs in erectile tissue, where the blood fills specially constructed spaces in the nipples, clitoris, and penis. The shaft of the penis is made up of spaces and cavities like a sponge. The blood vessels leading into the tissue dilate, permitting an increased inflow of blood, thereby filling the spaces in the erectile tissue with blood. The fibrous tissue surrounding the erectile tissue limits the expansion, and the pressure causes the penis to maintain a rigid structure.

A second type of vasocongestion occurs when existing blood vessels engorge with blood; this results in the increased size of breasts and labia and the color changes noted in the labia minora, for example, during sexual arousal. Vaginal lubrication is a by-product of vasocongestion. As the vaginal capillaries increase in size, the fluid pressures are altered in the walls of the vagina, and increased fluid passes into the vagina. Each capillary is surrounded by smooth muscle; when the smooth muscles are stimulated by the sympathetic branch of the autonomic nervous system they contract and the vessel shrinks. When sympathetic stimulation *decreases,* as during sexual arousal, the blood pressure in the vessels causes them to expand because of the relaxed smooth muscle. The expansion of many vessels at one time causes vasocongestion in nonerectile tissue.

Different organ systems are innervated by the sympathetic and parasympathetic branches of the PNS. Although most organs are dominated by one or the other branch, the sex organs receive messages from both branches. In females, vasocongestion and orgasm appear to be under sympathetic control. Orgasm is a genital reflex consisting of contractions of certain genital muscles controlled by spinal neural centers. On the other hand, penile erection is primarily a parasympathetic response, and ejaculation is a sympathetic response.

In addition to Masters and Johnson's model of the sexual response cycle, discussed in depth here, Kinsey et al. (1948, 1953) and Kaplan (1979) also described models of the sexual response cycle. Table 5–1 contrasts these models. Basically, the models differ in the inclusion or omission of a phase. All the models have an excitement (or buildup) phase and an orgasm phase, but although each researcher observed the process of resolution or the return of the body to prestimulation levels, Kaplan (1979) did not label this as a separate phase, thus minimizing its importance.

Four similar phases of the sexual response cycle have been described for both males and females by Masters and Johnson (Masters & Johnson, 1966; Masters, Johnson, & Kolodny, 1982, Masters, Johnson, & Kolodny, 1986): excitement, plateau, orgasm, and resolution. The same sexual response cycle is begun regardless of the type of sexual stimulation, be it masturbatory, mechanical, coital, or fantasy, although the response varies in intensity and duration. Masters and Johnson also make the point that the phases are not always clearly separated from one another. There is a consistent pattern of progression, but sometimes the excitement phase is rapid and leads quickly to orgasm, and other times the excitement phase builds up over hours (Masters, Johnson, & Kolodny, 1986). Masters and Johnson reported the most intense orgasmic response from masturbation.

Kaplan's (1979) modification of the human sexual response cycle included principally the addition of the desire phase and the concept that each phase is governed by a separate neurophysiologic system. Sexual desire, or sexual appetite, is promoted by the hormone testosterone, in both sexes, and by two neurotransmitters, serotonin and dopamine. These are important in mediating sexual desire. External stim-

▶ **TABLE 5–1**

Theoretical Models of the Sexual Response Cycle

Theorist	Year		Phases			
Kinsey	1948, 1953	—	Buildup	—	Orgasm	Aftereffects
Masters and Johnson	1966	—	Excitement	Plateau	Orgasm	Resolution
Kaplan	1979	Desire	Excitement	—	Orgasm	—

uli, such as an emotional bond to another person; sensory cues, such as erotic media; or smells may act as stimuli to sexual desire.

Tables 5–2 and 5–3 depict the physiologic sexual response of females and males according to Masters and Johnson's phases in the sexual response cycle. These tables describe the particular responses noted in the various organ systems.

Subjectively, the orgasmic phase is the peak pleasurable experience in both sexes. Women have the potential for multiple orgasms and may experience the second or third orgasm as the most pleasurable. In men, the orgasm with the largest ejaculate is experienced as the most pleasurable and this is usually the first orgasm. The orgasms of women have been described as twice as long as men's and of greater intensity. Individual variations, of course, do result in differences from these generalizations. The vasocongestion of the female is generalized to the entire pelvic area, in contrast to the male's more localized congestion, and the total blood volume removed by muscle contraction is greater in the female.

Another unique feature of the female sexual response is that the uterine contractions in women during orgasm show the same recorded pattern as the first stage of labor; they differ only in amplitude.

▶ **TABLE 5-2**

Physiologic Sexual Response: Women

Excitement	
Vagina	Vaginal lubrication occurs
	Inner two thirds of vagina lengthen and distend, change to dark purple color
	Outer third of vagina fills with blood
Labia	Labia minora enlarge, become more deeply colored
	Labia majora flatten and thin, move away from midline
Uterus	Uterus elevates, pulling on vagina and making a tent or open area at inner third of vagina
Breasts	Breasts increase in size
	Nipples become erect
Cardiovascular/respiratory	Heart rate slows early, then increases in rate
	Blood pressure elevates as phase progresses
	Breathing may increase in rate
Skin	Sex flush (measleslike rash on chest or upper abdomen)
Plateau	
Vagina	Vaginal opening decreases by one third
Labia	Labia minora turn from pink to bright red in nulliparous women and from red to deep wine in multiparous women
Clitoris	Retracts from unstimulated position to inaccessible place under clitoral hood
Skin	Sex flush spreads to all areas of breasts, chest, and abdomen
Orgasm	
Vagina	Contractions begin in outer third of vagina at 0.8-second intervals and recur from 3 to 15 times; time between contractions lengthens and strength of contractions decreases
Uterus	Contracts, similar to labor
Rectum	Rectal contractions linked in time with vaginal contractions
Muscular	Release of muscular spasm, some loss of voluntary control, with spasms and contractions of many muscle groups
Cardiovascular/respiratory	Heart rate two times normal
	Blood pressure increases by one third
	Breathing rate three times normal
Resolution	
Breasts	Loss of nipple erection, slower loss of breast volume
	Sex flush and swelling around nipples disappear
Skin	Film of perspiration covers body
Vagina	Congestion in outer third of vagina disappears
	Congestion in vaginal walls disappears in 15 minutes or longer
Labia	Labia majora return to unstimulated size
	Labia minora return to prestimulation color in 15 seconds, return to prestimulation size more slowly
Clitoris	Within 5 to 10 seconds clitoris returns to normal position, loss of vasocongestion slower
Uterus	Uterus descends to unstimulated position
Cardiovascular/respiratory	Blood pressure, breathing, and heart rate return to prestimulation condition
Urinary	Urge to urinate, particularly in nulliparous women

Reproduced, with permission of the Masters and Johnson Institute, St. Louis, Missouri, from Masters, W.H., & Johnson, V.E. (1966). Human sexual response. Boston: Little, Brown.

► **TABLE 5-3**

Physiologic Sexual Response: Men

Excitement	
Penis	Erection caused by blood engorgement, increases in size
Scrotum/testes	Scrotal skin tenses, becomes congested and thick
	Testes rise higher in scrotum, increase in size as much as 50%
Breasts	Nipple erection and swelling
Muscular	Increasing spasm of long muscles of legs and arms and abdominal muscles
Rectum	Some voluntary contractions late in phase
Cardiovascular/respiratory	Heart rate slows initially, then quickens
	Breathing may increase late in phase
Plateau	
Skin	Sex flush occurs (not as frequent as in women) over chest, neck, and face
Muscular	Increased muscular tension of face, neck, abdomen, and limbs
Penis	Glans penis enlarges
Testes	Increase from 50 to 100% in size
	Elevation of testes fully accomplished
Cardiovascular	Blood pressure elevates as phase progresses
Orgasm	
Penis	Penile muscle contraction and urethral contractions result in actual ejaculation of the seminal fluid out of the penis
Testes	Contractions of testes, prostate gland, and seminal vesicles as they collect sperm and seminal fluid and expel them into the entrance of the urethra
Muscular	Release of muscular spasm, some loss of voluntary control with spasms and contractions of many muscle groups
Rectum	Contractions linked to genital contractions
Cardiovascular/respiratory	Heart rate, blood pressure, and breathing increase, generally higher than in women
Resolution	
Penis	After ejaculation 1/2 erection is lost quickly; second stage is slower
Scrotum/testes	Scrotal wall reverts to uncongested state
	Testes descend rapidly in most men, loss of swelling
Skin	Skin flush disappears
	Perspiration usually confined to palms and soles of feet, but sometimes widespread
Breasts	Nipple erection lost
Muscular	Loss of muscle tension over a 5-minute period
Cardiovascular/respiratory	Heart rate, blood pressure, and breathing return to prestimulation state

Reproduced, with permission of the Masters and Johnson Institute, St. Louis, Missouri, from Masters, W.H., & Johnson, V.E. (1966). Human sexual response. Boston: Little, Brown.

Women with hysterectomies also experience intense orgasms. The sexual arousal of women occurs more readily during the luteal phase or the last 14 days of the menstrual cycle. This is a result of increased pelvic congestion, increased vaginal fluid, and subsequent increased "interest."

Women's Health

The experience of orgasm among women is variable. Orgasmic response is influenced by several factors, such as woman's health status, emotional feelings, sexual desire, and external stimuli.

Masters and Johnson (1966) interpreted sexual functioning as an interaction between the biophysic and psychosocial systems. These systems could reinforce or inhibit each other. In an individual who has acquired positive attitudes and values about gender, sex role, and characteristics of masculinity and femininity and has a positive image as a sexual being, the biologic and sexual response cycle will be enhanced.

Certain cultural characteristics of femininity and masculinity may inhibit or enhance the biophysic response cycle. Feminine characteristics of affection and affiliation may enhance the sexual relationship, whereas passivity and submissiveness may contribute to denial and suppression of individual sex needs. Similarly, a masculine identity of assertiveness and activity may contribute to healthy acknowledgment and pursuit of a sexual relationship, but competitiveness and independence may inhibit the affectionate relationship underlying the sexual relationship.

▶ SEXUALITY OVER THE LIFE SPAN

The individual's experience and understanding of sexuality over the life span change as a function of cognitive, psychosocial, cultural, and physiologic maturation. Masters' and Johnson's (1966) important documentation and research on the human sexual response point out that the physiologic experience of sexual arousal and consummation shows little variation over the life span. The physiologic phenomena, however, are only one component of human sexuality. Other components, such as the behavioral, social, and psychologic expressions of sexuality in the developing individual from infancy through adulthood, do vary over the life span (Lancaster, 1994). Central to the concept of sexual development is the awareness of sexuality blossoming over time and being affected by and changing as a result of developmental life cycles and situational occurrences. The act of first intercourse, then, is not an end but an incident occurring at some point during the sexual process. The sexual unfolding stage begins in adolescence for most individuals but is not limited to these chronologic years. Some individuals may deal with the challenges of sexual unfolding at a much later age.

▶ Infancy

Sexuality is a characteristic of *all* children and evidence of the functioning of the human sexual response cycle is demonstrated in infancy when an infant boy has an erection and an infant girl has signs of fluid in her vagina. When the infant discovers his or her genital organs through touch, he or she is initiating the sexual response cycle. The behaviors associated with unfolding sexuality include looking at and touching the genitalia in the first year of life. These early experiences of touching accompany the feeling of pleasure associated with the genitalia.

▶ Toddler Through School-Age Period

Gesell and others (1974) have summarized the usual stages of sexual awareness and sex play in the young child as follows:

- 2½-year-olds: show interest in urination and the different postures girls and boys assume as well as their genital differences
- 3-year-olds: verbalize interest in gender differences
- 4-year-olds: play games of "show" and continue verbal play and names related to elimination and other people's bathrooms
- 5-year-olds: display modesty and engage in less bathroom play
- 6-year-olds: participate in mild sex play ("hospital"), exhibitionism, and bathroom talk
- 7-year-olds: express less interest in gender differences and bathroom talk
- 8-year-olds: display a high interest in sex and engage in peeping, smutty jokes, and whispering
- 9-year-olds: express interest in the details of their own organs and may begin sex swearing and reciting sex poems
- 10-year-olds: like smutty jokes
- 11- and 12-year-olds: interest in sex may peak

Within each of these stages, periods of intense interest in sex are interwoven with periods of less interest. Many children progress through these stages exhibiting a wide range of individual variations. Gesell and colleagues (1974) describe "twosomes" occurring at 6, 7, and 8, followed by an interest in the opposite sex that is expressed as a movement away, a dislike of "jerkos" and "nerds." Exploratory behaviors resulting in pleasure in the preschool and older child include mutual touching between boys and girls, simulated sexual games, and repetitive self-stimulation of genitalia, or masturbation. The response of peers, siblings, parents, or other adults to this behavior affects the development of a child's sexual awareness.

In the psychoanalytic view of childhood sexuality, the parents are the primary love objects of a child's sexual hugs and longings. Continuing maturity demands that the child give up these desires and replace parents with love objects outside the family. This perspective of sexuality is accompanied by childhood behaviors that depict the child as being close first to mother, then to the opposite-sex parent, and then to peers. The child may display intrusiveness and jealousy of the marital relationship at certain stages. The child may also talk of marrying the parent of the opposite sex and physical embraces of the loved parent may imitate more adult sexual embraces.

▶ Adolescence

During adolescence the individual experiences dramatic physiologic, cognitive, psychologic, social, and sexual development. At the onset of puberty, the hormonal changes and subsequent physical changes will have an effect on an individual's self-image (Wilson, 1995), self-esteem, and social relationships with same-

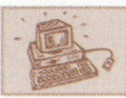

Research Abstract

Influence of Personal and Family Beliefs on Adolescent Parenting

In literature, adolescent parenting is almost universally seen as a non-normative life event that results in negative long-term consequences for mother and child. This view, however, distorts the real world circumstances of many low-income and working class teenagers. It also overlooks how mothering is a rite of passage to adulthood for many low-income teens and may lead to positive feelings about the self. A longitudinal interpretive study was undertaken to explore how young mothers define and redefine the self over time and to discover the turning points and transitions in young mothers' notions of the self and their visions of the future. The goal of the study was to describe patterns in young mothers' narratives of self and their visions of the future, and how they vary in the context of personal and family history. The basis of the study was the concept of phenomenology of everyday practices and the notion of a socially embedded identity formed through dialogue.

The current narrative describes a follow-up study, the "second phase" in a longitudinal, qualitative research project. Thirteen of 16 original young mothers enrolled in the study, and 11 of 18 family members and 3 male partners participated in this phase of the research. Families were African-American or non-Latina White and reflected diverse household structures and socioeconomic backgrounds. The mean age of mothers was 15.6 years when they gave birth to their first-born child; at the time of this study, their mean age was 19.4. Five of the mothers had given birth to an additional child, 5 were married, 8 had high school or equivalent diplomas, and 5 had obtained vocational training. Data consisted of detailed narratives obtained during three visits. In a separate visit, grandparents described changes in their lives. Interviews were taped, transcribed verbatim, and analyzed following a hermeneutic approach. This approach involves a systematic process that unfolds as the researcher's understanding of human actions and situations gains depth from multiple readings and analysis.

For this sample, mothering was not described as a negative event that jeopardized future plans but, rather, created a sense of responsibility and supplied a social identity that was familiar and consistent with family and cultural meanings of becoming a woman. The teenagers began to experience a future by reorganizing their lives around the identity of mothering as they struggled to develop a responsive self. Those teens who had access to continued schooling, day care for their children, and family support experienced a relatively smooth transition to motherhood. However, teens having conflicted, coercive relationships or families whose lives were surrounded by danger or extreme poverty found being a mother burdensome and precarious.

The investigators concluded that young mothers' views of the self and the future were not ordered by ideal norms of the life course. Instead, their views were ordered by meanings and practices inherent in their families and communities.

Application to Practice

The above study provides evidence that challenges current thinking about adolescent pregnancy. Nurses caring for pregnant teens from diverse racial, cultural and socioeconomic backgrounds need to be aware of cultural beliefs related to pregnancy. Families may provide an environment for the teen and her child that fosters the young mother's sense of self and ability to move forward in a positive direction.

Source: Smith-Battle, L., & Leonard, V. W. (1998). Adolescent mothers four years later: Narratives of the self and visions of the future. Advances in Nursing Science, 20*(3), 36–49.*

sex and opposite-sex peers (see Chapter 6 for discussion of puberty).

Kriepe (1983) views adolescent sexual expression as dependent on four dynamic forces: (1) acceptance of physical maturation, (2) attainment of adult thinking skills, (3) achievement of independence, and (4) achievement of an adult identity. Physically mature adolescents may not be emotionally mature, and early sexual development is not necessarily accompanied by early achievement of independence or attainment of adult thinking skills (Kriepe, 1983). See Chapter 11 for discussion of the factors influencing sexual activity in adolescents.

The adolescent years are an incredibly needy period in terms of sexuality. Adolescents are immature in knowledge, impulse control, relationships, self-esteem, and identity, but have strong feelings of sexuality. This combination requires guidance and maturity from parents and other adults. Furthermore, for sexually active teenagers, the multiple partners experienced during adolescence, anxiety about performance, and societal taboos against open sexual expression cause teenagers to participate in "fast sex in awkward places." A lack of adequate information can lead to a high-risk climate for STDs, impotence or premature ejaculation in men, or early pregnancy or orgasmic dysfunction in women.

▶ Adulthood

During the childrearing phase, couples must adapt their needs for marital intimacy and privacy to the changes of pregnancy, lactation, and the needs of their children. Frequently it is the parents' private time that is diminished and sacrificed, to the disadvantage of their sexual relationship. Sexuality becomes a family process as parents recognize their children's developing sexuality and create a family environment in which they can grow and flourish.

The end of the reproductive years—voluntarily through tubal ligation or vasectomy or through menopause—signifies sexuality as distinct from the procreative period. This stage may be welcomed by adults as a period of freedom from early childrearing cares or may be associated with a feeling of loss and aging (Edwards & Booth, 1994).

Masters and Johnson (1966), in their study of middle-aged and elderly men and women, established several important points, the major one being that people of all ages respond sexually past menopause. There is no definitive age of cessation of sexuality; however, several changes do occur in the sexual response cycle as an individual ages. In the older woman, sex flush occurs less frequently, labia

majora do not move away from the midline, labia minora lose the response of enlargement, vaginal lubrication occurs at a slower rate, the vagina's ability to increase in width and depth decreases, and the subjective experience of orgasm diminishes.

In the older man, the amount of time necessary to attain an erection is lengthened, but the erection is maintained for longer periods. The loss of erection is more rapid and the force of ejaculation and the intensity of contractions is reduced. The scrotum has reduced vasocongestion. There is less elevation of the testes and the increase in the size of the testes is not evident.

▶ SEXUAL HISTORY

Taking a sexual history is a skill that the nurse develops with experience. Acquiring the ability to gather the most relevant information in a timely manner in the context of a warm, open, trusting relationship is indeed a valued achievement. Taking a sexual history incorporates all the skills necessary for taking a nursing history along with additional sensitivity. In our culture, for the most part, sexual information is private; there is an unwillingness to share and trust this information to others. Our sexual self-esteem is closely related to some of our core self-concepts: male, female, masculinity, femininity. The sharing of problems and conflicts in this area should be valued and treated as confidential. The individual's need for self-worth must be respected.

If a sexual problem is suspected or identified, a more thorough sexual history is warranted for the purpose of identifying a long-term or situational problem. Focusing on the client as a whole individual aids the nurse in deciding if external stress, such as financial worries, may be spilling over to affect the sexual relationship or if the primary problem resides in the sexual relationship itself. More appropriate consultation or referral can be made with this complete information. Effective communication between nurse and client about sexual matters is achieved by the health care professional's awareness of her or his own self on the sexual continuum, comfort with his or her unfolding or maturing sexuality, and the ability to learn to communicate with others in this area.

Specific strategies that nurses can use when taking a sexual history include the following:

- Assume everyone does everything
- Give positive feedback to the individual
- Follow the lead of the client, that is, listen carefully to the client's messages about what concerns her or him

- Avoid using ambiguous expressions like "making love" for vaginal intercourse and be familiar with and use when appropriate the special vocabularies of cultural or economic groups like "prick" (for penis) or "cunt" (for vagina).
- Be aware of particular sexual customs and norms that predominate in specific groups
- Use eye-to-eye contact
- Validate the client's responses by clarifying and restating the question or response
- Avoid statements such as "everyone does that"

Depending on the setting, checklists and standard forms can aid in sexual history taking. The box entitled Sexual History Components summarizes the types of information that may be included on these tools. The baseline data gathered from standard forms can open doors for more deeply probing questions. A Planned Parenthood agency will have such a form; a postpartum unit may need to add sexuality as an assessment or educational area to the history form.

Important general categories for a nurse to assess during the sexual history include any change in the individual's experience of sexuality. If these changes are the result of the biologic health of the individual's genitourinary tract, the nurse needs to assess the structures involved, taking into account the variations that result from developmental differences.

▶ SEXUALITY AND THE CHILDBEARING COUPLE

▶ Pregnancy

Much of the knowledge about the sexual response cycle during pregnancy again comes from the early work of Masters and Johnson (1966). Later researchers have supplemented this work. Findings are not always consistent and, although researchers report on group findings, it is clear that individual variations and responses to sexuality need to be respected throughout the pregnancy cycle. Table 5–4 summarizes alterations in the sexual response cycle that may occur during pregnancy.

Certain physiologic changes related to the breast tissue and pelvic viscera affect the sexual response cycle in pregnant women. Enlargement of glandular tissue and increased vascularity of the breasts often lead to breast tenderness in early pregnancy. This can decrease a woman's interest in having her breasts stimulated during foreplay. Breast tenderness tends to decrease in the second and third trimesters. Increased pelvic vascularity occurring during pregnancy can lead to changes in sexual interest and increased orgasmic experiences, as well as such signs of uterine irritability as abdominal cramping, aching, and low backache.

▶ SEXUAL HISTORY COMPONENTS

GENERAL PHYSICAL, DEVELOPMENTAL, AND LIFESTYLE FACTORS:

Past history of systemic illness, e.g., diabetes
History of STDs, e.g., vaginitis
Progression of physical sexual maturity (e.g., onset of menarche, regularity of menses)
Past history of contraceptives, abortions, fetal or newborn losses
Current review of symptoms
Nutrition, drugs, and alcohol use
Past history of abuse

PSYCHOSOCIAL FACTORS:

Progression through and accomplishment of age-appropriate psychosocial tasks
Body image, satisfaction with physical appearance
Self-concept, self-evaluations about gender, femininity or masculinity, etc.
Past parent–child relationship, attitudes and values conveyed toward sex
Quality of current intimate relationships

PAST SEXUAL ACTIVITY:

Age of first intercourse
Frequency
Types of sexual contact
Partners, number, ages, sex
Problems, satisfaction, and orgasmic competency
History of sexual abuse

CURRENT SEXUALITY RELATED TO CHILDBEARING:

Attitudes, myths, or knowledge related to sexuality and childbearing
Change in frequency
Change in sexual interest
Techniques of intercourse
Satisfaction and problems
Spouse agreements or differences

▶ **TABLE 5-4**

Changes in Sexual Response Cycle During Pregnancy

Excitement	
Labia	Increased engorgement of labia majora
	Labia minora two to three times unstimulated size
Vagina	Increased vaginal lubrication
Breasts	Increased enlargement and congestion of breast tissue
Plateau	Increased pelvic congestion
Orgasm	Increased orgasmic intensity, duration, and frequency
Resolution	Sustained pelvic congestion and, therefore, possibly sustained sexual tension

In general, the increased vascularity of the entire pelvis with resulting vasocongestion promotes coital orgasm in the pregnant woman. For this reason women who have not achieved orgasm prior to conception may well experience orgasm for the first time during pregnancy. The increased volume of the pelvic venous bed during pregnancy enhances the capacity for sexual tension and improves orgasmic intensity, frequency, and pleasure. Increased orgasmic competency during pregnancy may also be related to improved relaxation related to sexuality and affirmation of womanliness.

In addition to the general changes in the sexual response cycle already described, other researchers have looked at factors affecting sexual interest during pregnancy. Sexual drive and interest are not altered by pregnancy. Other factors influencing the pregnant couple can, however, result in increased or decreased interest in sexuality. General factors affecting sexual activity during pregnancy, other than the pregnancy itself, include age of the mother, length of the marriage, quality of the marital relationship, and the pre-existing sexual relationship. Sexual frequency during pregnancy seems to be increased in younger mothers and younger marriages.

Research has established that sexual desire in pregnant women can be expressed in one of three ways: (1) women in whom sexual activity and desire remain constant throughout pregnancy; (2) women in whom sexual activity declines steadily over the pregnancy; and (3) women in whom sexual activity declines in the first and third trimesters but increases during the second trimester. Both men and women perceived declines in sexual activity as negative for the relationship.

Factors in early pregnancy other than breast tenderness that can inhibit sexual interest are the symptoms of early pregnancy—fatigue, nausea, and vomiting. On the other hand, satisfaction stemming from the knowledge that the couple has been able to con-

ceive, freedom from having to use contraceptives, and increasing pelvic congestion may contribute to a woman's or couple's increased interest in sexuality. The woman or couple who will be experiencing sexuality for its own sake may find this stressful; others may experience it as joyous.

During the second trimester, Masters and Johnson (1966) reported a marked increase in eroticism and effectiveness of sexual performance. In fact, sexual performance can surpass that in the nonpregnant state. Many of the "nuisance" symptoms of the first trimester have disappeared. The pregnant woman's body has changed. These changes may be perceived either as very attractive and sensual or as unappealing to the pregnant woman and her spouse, affecting sexual interest accordingly.

During the third trimester Masters and Johnson (1966) reported a decrease in sexual interest. A variety of reasons have been put forth to explain this change. During the third trimester women report more physical complaints, such as pelvic tension and backaches. Discomfort with increased body weight and body shape and difficulty in finding comfortable sexual positions are also cited as decreasing sexual activity. Medical advice or medical contraindication is another factor in the decrease in sexual activity during the third trimester. Marital partners also are concerned about the safety of the fetus and frequently choose to decrease sexual activity during the last trimester.

The identified changes discussed in the woman's sexual patterns may be similar with the man's changes (the man may also experience decreased sexual interest in the last trimester) or dissimilar (the man or woman may have sustained interest in sex throughout the pregnancy). These disruptions require adaptation by the sexual couple.

Two specific issues underlie couples' general concern for fetal safety and influence their decision to persist or abstain from intercourse: (1) precipitation of premature labor and (2) introduction of infection or air embolism into the uterine cavity. Although hypotheses have suggested a relationship among prostaglandins, semen, increased oxytocin level, and uterine contractions (see Chapter 21), clinical evidence connecting orgasm to the onset of premature labor is lacking. Neither clinical nor research evidence upholds a relationship between premature labor and intercourse late in pregnancy for normal women without a high-risk history. A relationship may exist between these factors for women with a known history of premature onset of labor.

Oral–genital sexual activity has been associated with air embolism late in pregnancy. For this reason, blowing into the vaginal area during late pregnancy is not advised.

▶ Childbirth

Oxytocin, a hormone produced by the pituitary gland, initiates uterine contractions, triggers milk letdown for breastfeeding mothers, and is found in the bloodstream during vaginal dilation. This hormone appears to link the three experiences of birth, lactation, and orgasm and may account in part for the sensual or erotic feelings experienced by some women when giving birth or breastfeeding. Orgasms have been reported by some women during the second stage of labor as a result of increased vasocongestion when the clitoris is engorged and the woman is bearing down. Not all women perceive the delivery or breastfeeding experience with this degree of sensuality and the health care professional must be sensitive to the range of normal experiences for individual women.

▶ Postpartum Period

Because sexuality is not simply a function of biologic or physiologic changes, the postpartum period reflects the contradictions and complexities of the childbearing period. Physiologically, pelvic vasocongestion and hence enhanced sexuality have lifted with delivery of the infant. Perineal irritation or pain secondary to tears, episiotomy repairs, or rectal hemorrhoids may occur during this period. In addition, fatigue, anxiety, vaginal discharge, and breast soreness may result in decreased sexual interest. Furthermore, negative feelings about body image, lack of privacy, and appropriate timing for marital intimacy may also contribute to a woman's diminished sense of sexuality in the postpartum period.

On the other hand, breastfeeding mothers continue to experience enlargement and engorgement of the breasts, which in some women has resulted in a feeling of enhanced sexual stimulation to the plateau or orgasmic level. Physiologically, the nipple becomes erect and lengthens during breastfeeding, a reaction that also occurs during sexual arousal. Oxytocin is released as the infant suckles on the breast and, as a result, uterine muscle fibers contract rhythmically as in sexual arousal. An enhanced sense of femininity or womanliness as a result of the birthing experience and breastfeeding may also contribute to a positive interest in sexuality.

Labor and breastfeeding both have physiologic similarities to the orgasmic experience, and some women have subjectively noted and described this response. The association of breastfeeding and sexuality has been accepted by some women and enjoyed, whereas other women have felt anxious and guilty. Conversely, body contact and fatigue secondary to the breastfeeding experience may result in diminished sexual interest and drive and temporary loss of the breast as an erogenous zone. Sexual excitement may stimulate the milk letdown reflex, which may also alter the woman's or couple's sexual enjoyment.

Research indicates that sexual intimacy returns to prepregnancy levels by 12 weeks postpartum (Tulman, Fawcett, Grablewiski, & Silverman, 1990), although in some couples, an interest in and desire for sex comes even earlier. Other researchers report fatigue, anxiety, and preoccupation with the infant as factors that affect the marital relationship negatively for up to a year. Levels of estrogen drop after delivery, causing decreased lubrication and a tighter, more sensitive vagina. Until ovulation occurs, both breastfeeding and nonbreastfeeding mothers can be considered to be "estrogen starved." Vulvar and vaginal tissues may be more sensitive or sore during intercourse or genital manipulation. Monilial infections may flare during the postpartum period, causing uncomfortable sex.

Obstetric tears or a torn or stretched perineal body may inhibit sexual satisfaction or delay this process further in other couples. If an episiotomy was performed after delivery, intercourse can be resumed in 2 weeks. Positive aspects of episiotomy repair may include heightened sensitivity over the repair area or a tighter vagina. Extremely stretched tissues or poorly repaired tears or episiotomies, however, may lead to changes in vaginal muscles or the size of the vaginal orifice, thus altering the tone of the vagina. This may change the man's or the woman's sensation of the penis in the vagina and alter the sexual response cycle. Postpartum (Kegel) exercises may be encouraged to increase and maintain perineal and vaginal tone. It is important to note that a loose vagina occurring after a precipitous delivery, closely spaced pregnancies, or large babies is balanced by the vasocongestion that occurs during sexual stimulation. The vasocongestion, which is often increased after childbirth, makes the vagina very snug.

Lochia (the spongy layer of the decidua that is discarded as vaginal discharge during the first few days after delivery) may continue up to 6 weeks after delivery. Intercourse may be resumed during the alba, or whitish, phase. Its normal odor or presence, though, may be a barrier against sexual activity for some couples over a longer period. Open communications between partners and a health provider are important to identify any sexual alterations as a result of the pregnancy or postpartum process.

The literature has often emphasized a woman's sexual responsiveness during the childbearing year. In fact, a woman's comfort with her own sexuality may be related to her ease in adaptation to the parenthood role. Furthermore, high estrogen and progesterone levels during pregnancy may increase the vascular bed in the pelvis, contributing to long-range improvements in sexual arousal and potential for orgasm.

Fathers may be particularly unprepared for a sustained interruption of sexual relations in the postpartum period. Fathers' sense of well-being has been found to be most closely related to their perception of the quality of the marital relationship. The quality of sexual functioning is an important aspect of marital satisfaction and is an important component of the male's concept of self. Alterations in sexuality for fathers may more directly affect their self-concept and marital functioning. Nurses need to be aware that childbearing may affect sexual responsiveness of the marital partners differently and that men, in particular, may need assistance in adapting to the inevitability of change in their sexual partners.

▶ Nursing Implications: Sexuality and Childbearing

Nurses who care for the childbearing couple must obtain a complete database, including a detailed sexual history. Ideally, the history taking should include both partners. If the father cannot be physically present at some point for interviewing, careful attention should be given to obtaining information about his perspective. For example, the interviewer might ask, "Did your partner want this pregnancy?" "Does your partner have any feelings about sex possibly hurting the baby?" A complete database provides knowledge of common needs of childbearing couples as well as specific problem identification.

Sexuality is often considered a secret and taboo subject. Sexual attitudes and values are formed over a lifetime, and these attitudes must be considered and respected. All couples can benefit from simple factual information about factors affecting sexuality during pregnancy and the postpartum period, safe sexual practices during childbearing, and common problems and concerns (e.g., comfortable sexual positions).

As in other aspects of intimate relationships, the couple's ability to communicate openly, identify and voice concerns, be open to new information, be flexible, and adapt to new ways of problem solving are all strengths that enhance sexual functioning. These aspects of a relationship, particularly in young marriages, may need reinforcement or development. A sexual relationship between partners that already includes a variety of methods of stimulating each other, use of different positions for intercourse, and orgasmic competence is different from one in which partners are just beginning to explore their sexual

selves and only achieve satisfaction infrequently. Sensitivity to these relationship differences and the ability to communicate information in a nonjudgmental manner are critical to the success of sexual education and counseling.

The nurse can provide simple, factual information. For example, (1) grooming and hygiene may need to be modified during pregnancy to enhance the sexual self; (2) increased vaginal discharge, heat sensitivity, nausea, and vomiting may contribute to a need for increased baths, mouth care, and deodorant; and (3) attractive feminine clothes can highlight a woman's increased voluptuousness and yet accommodate the pregnant or nursing mother's body shape (many women with small breasts enjoy their breast development during this period).

Timing for intimacy may have to be reevaluated during the childbearing cycle as fatigue, gastrointestinal disturbances, or demands from the new infant or siblings may make previous rituals of sexual intimacy inappropriate. The late-night sexual contact may now be a time when the woman experiences great fatigue or complains of sore nipples because of frequent nursings. Anticipation by the couple about changing time and relationship demands can help them to think about the need to set up time for themselves as a couple alone and schedule child care.

The techniques of intercourse may change for pregnant couples as pregnancy progresses. Manual

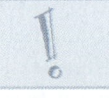

Nursing Alert

The nurse should communicate that penile–vaginal intercourse can be considered safe for pregnant couples except in the following situations:

- History of repeated early miscarriage
- History of uterine abnormalities or cervical incompetence (if cervical banding has taken place, couples may have intercourse)
- History of premature onset of labor (women should avoid orgasm but not necessarily intercourse)
- History of premature rupture of the membranes because of the risk of introduction of bacterial infection
- Unexplained vaginal bleeding
- Unexplained abdominal pain

fondling and mouth stimulation may be suggested as alternatives to penile–vaginal intercourse. The side-by-side, rear-entry, or female-superior positions may be suggested as alternatives to the male upright (missionary) position. Deep penetration may be uncomfortable during periods of pelvic vasocongestion, and these alternate positions may control the rate and depth of penetration. Rear entry when the woman is in the knee–chest position will also aid in shifting pelvic contents upward. This avoids direct pressure on the abdomen and frees the hands for manual stimulation.

Touching, caressing, and holding are important alternatives if orgasm and intercourse are contraindicated. The nurse may suggest back rubs, full-body massage, sensual stroking, hugging, and use of vibrators as important forms of sexual communication. The nurse should encourage the couple to communicate about changing erogenous zones during the childbearing cycle (e.g., nipple soreness, episiotomy scar sensitivity).

▶ SEXUALLY TRANSMITTED DISEASES

More than 50 diseases and syndromes are currently classified as STDs. **Sexually transmitted diseases** constitute a category of diseases transmitted through sexual intercourse and intimate sexual contact with the genitals, mouth, or rectum. This does not mean that sexual intercourse is the exclusive mode of transmission. Some STDs (HIV infection, syphilis, gonorrhea) may be transmitted perinatally from the mother to the fetus; other STDs, such as moniliasis, may result from changes in host factors, such as diabetes; still others (HIV, hepatitis B) occur as a result of blood-to-blood contact from such means as shared contaminated needles. Nevertheless, they all share the definition of STDs in that a principal means of transmission is sexual contact.

Several factors in today's society have contributed to the magnitude of STDs:

- *The large number of persons in the population at high risk (young adults).*
- *Changing sexual behaviors.* Sexual intercourse occurs earlier among women aged 15 to 19 years. The number of single adults has increased because of postponement of marriage, divorce, or widowhood, resulting in an increased multiplicity of sexual partners.
- *A higher proportion of infections with multiple modes of transmission that is being transmitted sexually.* Examples are hepatitis A and B, HIV, and group B streptococcus.

- *Increasing incidences of diseases associated with sex-for-drugs prostitution.*
- *Diversion of local STD control efforts to combat the threat of HIV infection.*

STDs are important health concerns for several reasons other then the discomfort of the acute symptoms of the disease. The effects of untreated STDs can lead to pelvic inflammatory disease (PID) in women or other types of irreversible organ damage. This damage to the genital area leads to scarring and adhesions within the reproductive tract, ultimately contributing to infertility, ectopic pregnancies, reproductive loss, and neoplasms. In addition, the risk of a mother contracting STDs is increased during pregnancy. Finally, HIV infection, an internationally acknowledged STD with exceedingly high mortality rates at present, has alerted everyone to the life-threatening consequences of STDs and the financial and human cost to society in general.

Some of the common STDs discussed briefly here are summarized in Table 5–5. In the 1960s and 1970s the two major "venereal diseases," as they were then called, were syphilis and gonorrhea, and the three minor diseases were chancroid, lymphogranuloma venereum, and granuloma inguinale. There has been a rise in the incidence of these three formerly minor diseases, although the incidence is far less than for the major STDs. The greatly expanded list in the 1990s includes more than 20 organisms that spread disease person to person during sexual contact including *Chlamydia trachomatis,* herpes simplex virus type 2, cytomegalovirus, hepatitis virus, *Candida albicans, Trichomonas vaginalis,* enteric bacteria, ectoparasites, and HIV.

Women are alerted to the possibility of infectious disease in the reproductive tract principally by the symptoms of discharge, pain, and itching. Not all STDs result in clear symptoms, thus making diagnosis and treatment difficult for both the client and the health care practitioner.

▶ Perinatal Transmission

Certain STDs pose significant and potentially life-threatening health risks to both the mother and the fetus. **Perinatal transmission,** or infection from the mother to the fetus, involves several possible routes, as follows:

- Transplacental transmission occurs when the infected maternal blood results in placentitis, which then spreads to the fetus (cytomegalovirus and syphilis are thought to be transmitted from the mother to the fetus in this way)

Summary of the Principal Sexually Transmitted Diseases

Disease and Etiologic Agents	Typical Clinical Presentation	Presumptive Diagnosis (warrants full treatment and follow-up)	Therapy	Complications and Sequelae
Nongonococcal Urethritis (NGU)				
Chlamydia trachomatis: Other sexually transmitted agents can cause NGU and include *Ureoplasma urealyticum, Trichomonas vaginalis, Candida albicans,* and herpes simplex virus.	Men usually have dysuria, frequency, and mucoid to purulent urethral discharge. Some men have asymptomatic infections. Steady female sexual partners of men with chlamydial NGU are likely to have chlamydia.	Men with typical clinical symptoms are presumed to have NGU when their gonorrhea tests are negative and they have either WBCs[a] on Gram's stain of urethral discharge or sexual exposure to an agent known to cause NGU. Asymptomatic men with negative gonorrhea tests are also presumed to have NGU if they have at least 4 WBCs per oil immersion field on an intraurethral smear.	Azithromycin 1 g PO in single dose; or doxycycline 100 mg PO, 2 times daily for 7 days. *Treatment during pregnancy:* Erythromycin base 500 mg PO, 4 times daily for 7 days; or amoxicillin 500 mg PO, 3 times daily for 7 days.	Urethral strictures, prostatitis, epididymitis. Chlamydial NGU may be transmitted to female sexual partners, resulting in mucopurulent endocervicitis, PID, and other adverse outcomes (see below).
Mucopurulent Cervicitis (MPC)				
Chlamydia trachomatis is the principal pathogen, although *Neisseria gonorrhoeae,* herpes simplex virus, *Candida albicans,* and *Trichomonas vaginalis* can also produce cervicitis (see relevant panels).	The client may be symptomatic or asymptomatic, and a yellow mucopurulent endocervical exudate may be present. Cervical ectopy appears to correlate with cervical infection with this agent.	The presence of yellow mucopurulent endocervical exudate or the finding of this exudate on a white cotton-tipped swab of endocervical secretions suggests infection with *C. trachomatis.* In women without visible exudate, the presence of 10 or more polymorphonuclear leukocytes per 1000× field on a Gram-stained specimen of endocervical mucus (without contamination by vaginal cells) also allows a presumptive diagnosis.	If *N. gonorrhoeae* is not found, treatment should be given as noted above for NGU. *Treatment during pregnancy:* Erythromycin base 500 mg PO, 4 times daily for 7 days; or amoxicillin 500 mg PO 3 times daily for 7 days.	Ascending infections may lead to symptomatic or asymptomatic endometritis, salpingitis, ectopic pregnancy, and subsequent infertility. Ascending infection during pregnancy may lead to adverse obstetric outcomes, conjunctivitis, or pneumonia in the infant, and puerperal infection.
Gonorrhea				
Neisseria gonorrhoeae, a gram-negative diplococcus.	When symptomatic, men usually have dysuria, frequency, and purulent urethral discharge. Women may have mucopurulent endocervical exudate, abnormal menses, or dysuria, or may be asymptomatic. Anorectal and pharyngeal infections are common. These may be symptomatic or asymptomatic.	Microscopic identification of typical Gram-negative intracellular diplococci on smear of urethral exudate (men) or endocervical material (women). Cervical specimens that are Gram-stain-tested should also be cultured for *N. gonorrhoeae.* *Or* Growth on selective medium demonstrating typical colonial morphology, positive oxidase reaction, and typical Gram's stain morphology.	A wide range of antimicrobial therapy is available. For example, for uncomplicated urethral, endocervical, or rectal infection, ceftriaxone 125 mg IM in single dose; or cefixime 400 mg PO in single dose; or ciprofloxacin 500 mg PO in single dose; or ofloxacin 400 mg PO in single dose and azithromycin 1 g PO in single dose; or doxycycline 100 mg PO, 2 times daily for 7 days. For uncomplicated infection of the pharynx,	PID,[a] ectopic pregnancy, infertility. Men are at risk for epididymitis, sterility, urethral stricture, and infertility. Newborns are at risk for ophthalmia neonatorum, sepsis, arthritis, meningitis, rhinitis, vaginitis, urethritis, and inflammation at sites of fetal monitoring. All infected, untreated persons are at risk for disseminated gonococcal infection (includes septicemia, arthritis, dermatitis, meningitis, and endocarditis).

(continued)

Summary of the Principal Sexually Transmitted Diseases

Disease and Etiologic Agents	Typical Clinical Presentation	Presumptive Diagnosis (warrants full treatment and follow-up)	Therapy	Complications and Sequelae
			ceftriaxone 125 mg IM in single dose; or ciprofloxacin 500 mg PO in single dose; or ofloxacin 400 mg PO in single dose and azithromycin 1 g PO in single dose; or doxy-cycline 100 mg PO, 2 times daily for 7 days. *Treatment during pregnancy:* ceftriaxone 125 mg IM in single dose; or cefixime 400 mg PO in single dose. For women unable to tolerate ceftriaxone or cefixime, spectino-mycin 2 g IM in single dose. For treatment of presumptive *C. trachomatis* infection, erythromycin base 500 mg PO, 4 times daily for 7 days or amoxicillin 500 mg PO, 3 times daily for 7 days.	
Human Papillomavirus (HPV) DNA virus of papovavirus family.	Soft pink to white raised lesions, usually painless, with multiple fingerlike projections. Malodorous vaginal discharge, pain and burning with urination, and pruritus may occur.	Presence of one or more lesions on the external genitalia, perineum, or anus. For subclinical lesions, colposcopy with directed biopsy.	Podofilox 0.5% solution (applied with cotton swab) or gel (applied with finger) to warts 2 times daily for 3 days, followed by 4 days of no therapy; or imiquimod 5% cream applied with finger to warts at bedtime 3 times weekly for as long as 16 weeks; or cryotherapy with liquid nitrogen or cryoprobe; or podophyllin resin 10 to 25% in compound tincture of benzoin applied to each wart and allowed to air dry; or trichloroacetic acid or bichloroacetic acid 80 to 90% applied only to warts and allowed to dry; or surgical removal by tangential scissor excision, tangential shave excision, curettage, or electrosurgery; or intralesional interferon; or laser surgery.	*Females:* may be associated with carcinoma of the cervix, vagina, vulva, and anus. Males: may be associated with carcinoma of the penis and anus. Neonates: laryngeal papillomatosis.

Summary of the Principal Sexually Transmitted Diseases

Disease and Etiologic Agents	Typical Clinical Presentation	Presumptive Diagnosis (warrants full treatment and follow-up)	Therapy	Complications and Sequelae
			Treatment during pregnancy: cryotherapy with liquid nitrogen or cryoprobe or surgery.	
Herpes Genitalis Herpes simplex virus (HSV) types 1 and 2, DNA viruses that cannot be distinguished clinically.	Single or multiple vesicles appear anywhere on the genitalia. Vesicles spontaneously rupture to form shallow ulcers, which may be very painful. They resolve spontaneously without scarring. The first occurrence is termed *primary infection* (mean duration 12 days). Subsequent, usually milder, occurrences are termed *recurrent infections* (mean duration 4.5 days). The interval between clinical episodes is termed *latency.* Viral shedding occurs intermittently during latency.	When typical genital lesions are present or a pattern of recurrence has developed, herpes infection is likely. A presumptive diagnosis is further supported by direct identification of multinucleated giant cells with intranuclear inclusions in a clinical specimen prepared by Papanicolaou or other histochemical stain; by typical HSV morphology by electron microscopy; or by detection of HSV antigens by monoclonal or polyclonal antibody detection systems. (*Note:* Antibody detection systems may detect biologically inactive viral particles. Primary HSV infection is presumed if any initially negative serologic titer becomes significantly detectable in convalescent serum.)	*First clinical episode:* To reduce the signs and symptoms, use acyclovir 400 mg PO 3 times daily for 7 to 10 days; or acyclovir 200 mg PO 5 times daily for 7 to 10 days; or famciclovir 250 mg PO 3 times daily for 7 to 10 days; or valacyclovir 1 g PO 2 times daily for 7 to 10 days. For clients who have severe symptoms or complications that necessitate hospitalization, an alternative regimen is acyclovir 5 to 10 mg/kg body weight IV every 8 hours for 5–7 days. *Recurrent genital herpes:* for episodic recurrent infection, acyclovir 400 mg PO 3 times daily for 5 days; or acyclovir 200 mg PO 5 times daily for 5 days; or acyclovir 800 mg PO 2 times daily for 5 days; or famciclovir 125 mg PO 2 times daily for 5 days; or valacyclovir 500 mg PO 2 times daily for 5 days. For daily suppressive therapy, acyclovir 400 mg PO 2 times daily; or famciclovir 250 mg PO 2 times daily; or valacyclovir 250 mg PO 2 times daily; or valacyclovir 500 mg PO once/day; or valacyclovir 1,000 mg PO once/day. *Treatment during pregnancy:* Systemic acyclovir should be avoided in pregnant women without life-threatening (disseminated) infection.	*Males and females:* Neuralgia, meningitis, ascending myelitis, urethral strictures, and lymphatic suppuration may occur. *Females:* Fetal wastage may be increased. *Neonates:* Virus from an active genital infection may be transmitted during vaginal delivery, causing neonatal herpes infection. Neonatal herpes ranges in severity from clinically inapparent infections to local infections of the eyes, skin, or mucous membranes, to severe disseminated infection that may involve the central nervous system. The infection has a high case fatality rate and many survivors have ocular or neurologic sequelae.

(continued)

Summary of the Principal Sexually Transmitted Diseases

Disease and Etiologic Agents	Typical Clinical Presentation	Presumptive Diagnosis (warrants full treatment and follow-up)	Therapy	Complications and Sequelae
Cytomegalovirus (CMV) Infection				
Herpes virus.	Primary infection is largely asymptomatic, but clients may experience myalgia, chills, and malaise. Lymphadenopathy and hepatosplenomegaly may be present.	Antibody tests; positive CMV-specific IgM test and fourfold rise in IgG antibody titer.	No treatment currently exists.	*Neonates:* Congenital CMV infections: mental retardation, microencephaly, intracranial calcification, chorioretinitis, hearing loss, cerebral palsy, hepatosplenomegaly, thrombocytopenia, hepatitis with jaundice, and/or anemia.
Syphilis				
Treponema pallidum spirochete with regular spirals and characteristic motility.	*Primary:* The classic chancre is located at the site of exposure. All genital lesions should be suspected to be syphilitic. *Secondary:* Clients may have a highly variable skin rash, mucous patches, condylomata lata, lymphadenopathy, or other signs. *Latent:* Clients are without clinical signs. *Tertiary:* Dependent on whether client has neurosyphilis or cardiovascular syphilis.	*Primary:* Clients have typical lesion(s) and positive serologic test for syphilis (STS) or their present titer is at least fourfold greater than the last, or there has been syphilis exposure within 90 days of lesion onset. *Secondary:* Clients have the typical clinical presentation and a strongly reactive STS. *Latent:* Clients have serologic evidence of untreated syphilis without clinical signs. *Tertiary:* Various combinations of STS results, abnormalities of cerebrospinal fluid (CSF) cell count, or reactive VDRL-CSF with or without clinical manifestations.	*Primary and secondary, or early, syphilis:* Benzathine penicillin G 2.4 million units IM in one dose. For nonpregnant, penicillin-allergic clients, doxycycline 100 mg PO 2 times daily for 2 weeks or tetracycline 500 mg PO 4 times daily for 2 weeks. *Syphilis of indeterminate length, or of more than 1-year duration, or late latent syphilis:* Benzathine penicillin G 7.2 million units total; 2.4 million units IM, weekly for 3 consecutive weeks. *Tertiary syphilis:* Benzathine penicillin G 7.2 million units total; 2.4 million units IM, weekly for 3 consecutive weeks. *Treatment during pregnancy:* Penicillin regimen appropriate for stage of syphilis (see above). For pregnant women with penicillin allergies, desensitization is required followed by treatment with penicillin.	Both late syphilis and congenital syphilis are preventable with prompt diagnosis and treatment of early syphilis. Sequelae of late syphilis include neurosyphilis (general paresis, tabes dorsalis, and focal neurologic signs), cardiovascular syphilis (thoracic aortic aneurysm, aortic insufficiency), and localized gumma formation. Sequelae of congenital syphilis include premature birth, intrauterine growth retardation, hepatosplenomegaly, CNS involvement, and ocular lesions.
Vaginitis				
Trichomonas vaginalis, a motile protozoan with an undulating membrane and four flagella.	Presentations vary from no signs or symptoms to erythema, edema, and pruritus of the external genitalia. Excessive and malodorous discharge is a common finding.	There are no presumptive criteria for this diagnosis.	Metronidazole 2 g PO in single dose *Treatment during pregnancy:* Metronidazole 2 g PO in single dose *after* 1st trimester.	Secondary excoriations. Recurrent infections are common.

Summary of the Principal Sexually Transmitted Diseases

Disease and Etiologic Agents	Typical Clinical Presentation	Presumptive Diagnosis (warrants full treatment and follow-up)	Therapy	Complications and Sequelae
Fungal vaginitis Predominantly *Candida albicans,* dimorphic fungi, which grow as oval budding yeast cells and as chains of cells (hyphae).	Females may experience dysuria, pruritus, and cheesy-white, curdlike discharge. Male sexual partners may develop urethritis, balanitis, or cutaneous lesions on penis.	Presumptive criteria are the typical symptoms of vaginitis or vulvitis, microscopic identification of yeast (budding cells or hyphae) in Gram's stain, or culture that shows positive result for a yeast species.	Miconazole 2% cream 5 g intravaginally for 7 days; or miconazole 200 mg vaginal suppository, 1 suppository for 3 days; or miconazole 100 mg vaginal suppository, 1 suppository for 7 days; clotrimazole 1% cream 5 g intravaginally for 7–14 days; or clotrimazole 100 mg vaginal tablet, 2 tablets for 3 days; or clotrimazole 500 mg vaginal tablet, 1 tablet in single application; or terconazole 0.4% cream 5 g intravaginally for 7 days; or terconazole 0.8% cream 5 g intravaginally for 3 days; or terconazole 80 mg vaginal suppository, 1 suppository for 3 days; or fluconazole 150 mg PO, 1 tablet in single dose; or butoconazole 2% cream 5 g intravaginally for 3 days; or tioconazole 6.5% ointment 5 g intravaginally in single application. *Treatment during pregnancy:* miconazole, clotrimazole, or terconazole (see above), 7 days of therapy recommended.	Fungal vaginitis in pregnancy increases the risk of neonatal oral thrush.
Bacterial vaginosis Predominantly *Gardnerella vaginalis.*		Presumptive criteria include three of the following: • a homogeneous gray or white, adherent discharge; • vaginal pH greater than 4.5; • release of a fishy-smelling amine mixed with 10% KOH; • presence of "clue cells."	Metronidazole 500 mg PO, 2 times daily for 7 days; or clindamycin cream 2%, 1 full applicator (5 g) intravaginally at bedtime for 7 days; or metronidazole gel 0.75%, 1 full applicator (5 g) intravaginally 2 times daily for 5 days; or metronidazole 2 g PO in single dose; or clindamycin 300 mg PO 2 times daily for 7 days.	May be associated with infectious complications of pregnancy, such as chorioamnionitis and puerperal infection and preterm labor and with polymicrotract infections in nonpregnant women, such as endometritis, salpingitis, and PID.

(continued)

Summary of the Principal Sexually Transmitted Diseases

Disease and Etiologic Agents	Typical Clinical Presentation	Presumptive Diagnosis (warrants full treatment and follow-up)	Therapy	Complications and Sequelae
			Treatment during pregnancy: for high-risk pregnant women (those who have previously delivered a premature infant) who are asymptomatic: metronidazole 250 mg PO 3 times daily for 7 days; for low-risk pregnant women (those who previously have not had a premature delivery) who are symptomatic: metronidazole 250 mg PO 3 times daily for 7 days.	
Human Immunodeficiency Virus (HIV) Infection				
Also referred to as acquired immunodeficiency syndrome (AIDS) in its terminal phases, lymphadenopathy-associated virus, and AIDS-related retrovirus. (All are agreed to be the same virus, which contains RNA and is in the retrovirus family.)	Symptoms range from minimal to full clinical syndrome of HIV infections. Clients with full clinical syndrome of HIV infection often give a history of nonspecific symptoms for months prior to diagnosis. These symptoms may include easy fatigue, poor appetite, weight loss, lymphadenopathy, diarrhea, fever, and night sweats. Other symptoms specific to opportunistic diseases occur in clients with HIV infection, such as purple to bluish skin lesions associated with Kaposi's sarcoma (KS) or shortness of breath and nonproductive cough resulting from *Pneumocystis carinii* pneumonia (PCP). Symptoms for infants include failure to thrive, lymphadenopathy, hepatosplenomegaly, encephalopathy, PCP, lymphocytic interstitial pneumonia (LIP), recurrent bacterial infection, recurrent diarrhea, and kidney and heart failure.	Presumptive diagnosis of HIV infection is usually made on clinical evidence, supported by serologic tests for antibodies to HIV. Once an individual is infected, current research suggests the individual remains infected indefinitely and may transmit the infection to others. As yet unidentified factors may influence which infected individuals develop HIV disease and which particular opportunistic illness may occur.	To date, no treatment has been identified to eradicate the virus or reverse the immunologic dysfunction associated with HIV infection. Standard therapy consists of treating opportunistic diseases aggressively as they occur. Zidovudine (AZT, ZDV) suppresses HIV replication and is FDA approved for adults and children. It may slow progress of the disease. Newer drugs, such as indinavir and delavirdine, are being successfully used for treatment in combination with ZDV. ZDV treatment should be offered to all HIV-infected pregnant women after the first trimester.	The outcome in clients with HIV infection is not completely understood. AIDS eventually develops in almost all HIV-infected persons. In one study of HIV-infected adults, AIDS developed in 87% within 17 years after infection.

[a]WBCs, white blood cells; PID, pelvic inflammatory disease

Source: U.S. Centers for Disease Control and Prevention, 1998; Youngkin & Davis, 1998.

- Transmembranous transmission results when cervical infection or endometrial infection spreads to the membranes and hence to the fetus
- Vertical transmission: occurs as a result of exposure to infected cervical or vaginal secretions at the time of delivery (herpes simplex virus type 2 is predominantly transmitted this way)
- Breast milk transmission occurs when breast milk is the reservoir for the organism (some cases of HIV infection in infants have been attributed to this route)

▶ Chlamydia trachomatis Infection

In the United States, *Chlamydia trachomatis* infection is one of the most frequently contracted STDs and occurs frequently among sexually active adolescents and young adults.

Four million new infections are reported annually (American Social Health Association, 1994). Chlamydiae are small intracellular parasites with two nucleic acids; they infect the mucosa and are susceptible to antibiotics. In women, the principal signs of infection are vaginal discharge and pruritus, although an infection may be asymptomatic. Clinically these symptoms are not distinctive and cannot be differentiated from those of gonorrhea. In fact, chlamydiae are frequently found in mixed infections, such as with *Neisseria gonorrhoeae, Candida albicans,* or *Trichomonas vaginalis.* Chlamydia infection can be diagnosed by isolation and growth of the organism after culture or through serologic tests. The usual drug of choice in *nonpregnant* women is azithromycin or doxycycline (U.S. Centers for Disease Control and Prevention, 1998). For pregnant women erythromycin base or amoxicillin are the drugs indicated (U.S. Centers for Disease Control and Prevention, 1998). See Chapter 19 for further discussion of *C. trachomatis* infection during pregnancy.

▶ Gonorrhea

Gonorrhea is the second most frequently occurring STD in listings of annual new infections by the Centers for Disease Control and Prevention (CDC). It is also identified as a serious infectious disease in terms of its sequelae: PID or pelvic abscess, ectopic pregnancy, and infertility. Gonorrhea has also been associated with chorioamnionitis, premature labor, premature rupture of membranes, and postpartum endometritis. Gonorrhea is caused by *Neisseria gonorrhoeae,* a gramnegative diplococcus, and can be diagnosed by his-

tory, by microscopic examination, and by culture of the organism. Cultures can be taken from the endocervical canal, rectal area, and pharyngeal area.

Most clients who contract gonorrhea are single and under 25. Women with decreased levels of estrogen are at greater risk of developing gonorrheal vulvovaginitis; thus, women who are premenstrual, in the postpartum period, or are postmenopausal are at higher risk. The initial site is the lower reproductive tract; if untreated, the organisms ascend to produce upper reproductive tract illness. Irritation, discharge (yellow and purulent), and painful, frequent urination are symptoms, but it is estimated that at least 50% of women with gonorrhea are asymptomatic. Symptoms, if present, usually occur 2 to 5 days after exposure.

Because of the increase in infections caused by penicillin-resistant organisms and the high rates of coinfection with chlamydia, current CDC guidelines include presumptive treatment of chlamydia infection. The medication regime is ceftriaxone, cefixime, ciprofloxacin, ofloxacin and azithromycin, or doxycycline for nonpregnant women. Ceftriaxone or cefixime can be used for pregnant women.

▶ Human Papillomavirus

Human papillomavirus (HPV) is a slow-growing DNA virus of the papovavirus family. More than 60 types of HPV have been identified; at least 20 have been associated with genital infection. Condyloma acuminata, or genital warts, are a frequent manifestation of HPV and are the most commonly diagnosed viral STD. The true scope of HPV is not known because asymptomatic and subclinical infections are more prevalent than genital warts. HPV infections are classified as clinical, subclinical, or latent (Youngkin & Davis, 1998).

Genital warts and warts on the cervix and in the vagina, urethra, and anus are most frequently caused by HPV types 6 and 11 (U.S. Centers for Disease Control and Prevention, 1998). Certain types of HPV (most notably 16 and 18) have been linked to carcinoma of the cervix, vagina, vulva, anus, and penis. HPV can be diagnosed by physical examination and colposcopy and biopsy for subclinical lesions, dysplasia, and malignancy (Youngkin & Davis, 1998). Genital warts are soft pink to white raised tumors with multiple fingerlike projections resembling cauliflower. Genital warts can proliferate and become friable during pregnancy (U.S. Centers for Disease Control and Prevention, 1998).

Treatment of genital warts should be guided by client preference, available resources, and the experience of the health care provider (U.S. Centers for Disease Control and Prevention, 1998). Available regimens for the nonpregnant woman are therapies administered either by the client (podofilox and imiquimod) or by the health care provider (cryotherapy, podophyllin resin, trichloroacetic acid, bichloroacetic acid, interferon, and surgery) (U.S. Centers for Disease Control and Prevention, 1998). Cryotherapy or surgery can be used for pregnant clients.

▶ Herpes Simplex Virus Type 2 Infection

Genital herpes, caused by herpes simplex virus type 2 (HSV-2), has been diagnosed in at least 45 million people in the U.S. (U.S. Centers for Disease Control and Prevention, 1998). The highest incidence of HSV-2 infection is in adolescent women. The initial infection usually occurs 3 to 7 days after exposure to the virus. The primary infection (the initial illness after exposure) can include such diverse symptoms as fever, headache, malaise, chills, anorexia, and painful urination. The typical lesions of HSV-2 are found on the labia, perineum, vulva, vagina, and bladder and are initially heralded by burning and numbness. This sensation is followed by vesicles, which rupture and result in shallow, painful ulcers. These initial lesions can last 3 to 6 weeks. The first episode of this chronic illness is generally more severe and longer lasting than recurrences. Treatment of the first episode for nonpregnant women consists of either acyclovir, valacyclovir, or famciclovir. The safety of acyclovir and valacyclovir in pregnant women has not been established (U.S. Centers for Disease Control and Prevention, 1998). After the initial episode, the HSV-2 virus is thought to lie dormant in sensory nerve ganglia and thus can recur throughout the lifetime. Identified triggers for recurrence include menstruation, fever, stress, and infectious illness. Recurrent herpes is characterized by typical HSV lesions at the site of viral entry that are fewer, less painful, and resolve more rapidly than primary herpes lesions (Youngkin & Davis, 1998). Treatment of recurrent episodes consists of either acyclovir, famciclovir, or valacyclovir. In addition, daily suppressive therapy with acyclovir, famciclovir, or valacyclovir can reduce the number of recurrences among clients who have frequent recurrences (U.S. Centers for Disease Control and Prevention, 1998). There is no known cure for HSV-2.

During pregnancy, both mother and fetus are at increased risk of HSV-2 infection. The transmission rate of primary HSV-2 in pregnant women may be as high as 50%, whereas neonatal transmission of HSV-2 is estimated to be only 3 to 5%. See Chapter 19 for additional discussion of HSV-2 infection during pregnancy.

Because of the painful and recurring nature of the disease, and the risk to the mother and fetus during pregnancy, a great deal of publicity about this disease was generated during the early and mid-1980s. Anxiety and stress about the symptoms and sequelae of this STD require a great deal of psychosocial support from a caring, sensitive nurse. More positively, for many women who pay attention to lifestyle factors and maintain a healthy therapeutic regimen, many of the symptoms of HSV-2 can be controlled during recurrences.

▶ Cytomegalovirus Infection

Cytomegalovirus (CMV) is transmitted through various routes including both sexual contact and perinatal transmission. It is a herpes virus and is found in saliva, respiratory secretions, breast milk, cervical secretions, and semen. Many children secrete CMV in their urine. One million new cases are identified annually according to the CDC (American Social Health Association, 1994). Further, 55% of young adults have CMV antibodies in their blood.

In adults, CMV is thought to pattern itself after HSV-2 in that it probably lies dormant in host tissue indefinitely and is reactivated periodically and particularly during pregnancy. For adults, even the primary infection is largely asymptomatic. Certain blood and liver function tests mirror mononucleosis infection in the adult, but there is a lack of throat, tonsil, or lymph symptomatology. No treatment currently exists for CMV.

Transmission of the infection to the fetus may result in defects in every organ system and subsequent central nervous system dysfunction. Fetuses at greatest risk are those whose mothers have a primary infection with CMV. Chapters 13 and 19 discusses effects of CMV on the pregnancy and fetus.

▶ Syphilis

In 1990, more than 50,000 cases of syphilis were reported in the U.S. (Youngkin & Davis, 1998). Although increases in syphilis infection have occurred in all cultural and ethnic groups, the greatest increases are among *young* women and heterosexual men in inner-city African-American and Latino populations.

The *Treponema pallidum* spirochete is transmitted by sexual contact, blood transfusion, or accidental inoculation to the adult and transplacentally to the fetus. In the adult, depending on the type of sexual contact experienced, the painless ulcer or chancre (the initial sign of syphilis) may be found on the lip, tongue, nipple, fingers, anus, or genital area 10 to 90 days after exposure. Many syphilitic ulcers are atypical, so all genital lesions should be considered suspicious.

Six weeks after the primary chancre the secondary stage occurs and frequently includes a generalized rash, For the first 2 to 4 years after initial exposure there may be recurrences. During this time, the so-called early latency period, the individual is infectious to other individuals and to the fetus. The tertiary phase follows the latency period and is characterized by conditions relating to neurosyphilis, cardiovascular syphilis, or other expressions of the disease (for example, meningeal irritation and aortic diastolic murmur). The later stages present a much lowered risk of communicability. Syphilis is diagnosed through screening blood tests, such as the Venereal Disease Research Laboratories (VDRL) test, or rapid plasma reagin (RPR) test, followed by a confirmatory fluorescent treponemal antibody absorbed (FTA-ABS) test and *T. pallidum* immobilization (TPI) (see Chapter 15 for discussion of screening tests for syphilis during the first trimester). Syphilis is treated most effectively with benzothine penicillin G; however, doxycycline, tetracycline, or erythromycin may be used for individuals with penicillin allergies. Clients who experience allergic reactions to penicillin, including pregnant women with syphilis in any stage and clients with neurosyphilis, should be desensitized and treated with penicillin (U.S. Centers for Disease Control and Prevention, 1998). Untreated congenital syphilis in the infant results in high mortality rates and in multiple-body-system pathology.

The Jarisch-Herxheimer reaction is an acute febrile reaction often accompanied by headache, myalgia, and other symptoms that may occur after any therapy for syphilis. It may precipitate labor or cause fetal distress in pregnant patients. It is treated symptomatically (U.S. Centers for Disease Control and Prevention, 1998).

▶ Vaginitis

Several types of vaginitis are included as STDs. They are those caused by *Trichomonas vaginalis, Gardnerella vaginalis,* and *Candida albicans* (which causes vulvovaginitis). Trichomoniasis occurs in approximately 3 million women annually (Moulton & Montgomery, 1995) and is responsible for one-fourth of vulvovaginitis complaints (American College of Obstetricians and Gynecologists, 1996). *Trichomonas* infection is caused by a unicellular protozoan and results in

vaginal discharge in 30% of women. The vaginal discharge has been described as profuse, frothy, and malodorous. Small hemorrhages give the cervix the classic "strawberry" appearance. Pruritus and dysuria may also be symptoms of infection with this organism, which frequently resides in the vagina, the urethra, the bladder, and Skene's glands. As many as 60% of women who have gonorrhea are also found to have trichomoniasis. Women presenting with symptoms of either infection should be evaluated for both. The usual diagnosis of *T. vaginalis* infection is made by microscopic examination of a saline wet mount in which motile trichomonads are seen. The recommended treatment is 2 g (in a single dose) of metronidazole. This is *not* recommended during the first trimester of pregnancy. Alternative iodine preparations also pose a risk to the fetus because excessive absorption of iodine may result in suppression of the fetal thyroid.

Candidiasis actually results from an overgrowth of organisms constituting 25% of a woman's normal vaginal flora. *C. albicans,* a saprophytic fungus, causes 90% of yeast infections. An estimated 75% of women will have at least one episode of candidiasis (U.S. Centers for Disease Control and Prevention, 1998). It frequently coexists with trichomoniasis. Symptoms in some women include intense pruritus and a cheesy-white, curdlike discharge. Many women do not have this discharge. Often, but not always, the vagina will be bright red with white plaques. The overgrowth of *Candida* is attributed to changes in host factors. Frequent triggers, which alter host resistance and thus result in infection, include pregnancy, diabetes, use of broad-spectrum antibiotics, and HIV infection. Diagnosis of candidal infection is by Gram's stain or by wet-mount examination under the microscope. The treatment of choice is local vaginal therapy, particularly miconazole, clotrimazole, terconazole, fluconazole, butoconazole, and tioconazole. During pregnancy, treatment with miconazole, clotrimazole, and terconazole is recommended.

Bacterial vaginosis results from overgrowth of the organism *Gardnerella vaginalis* (formerly called *Hemophilis vaginalis*). Although bacterial vaginosis is associated with having multiple sex partners, it is unclear whether it results from acquisition of a sexually transmitted pathogen (U.S. Centers for Disease Control and Prevention, 1998). This infection is typically identified by its fishy foul odor and yellow-gray vaginal discharge. The vaginal wall appears normal. It is diagnosed by the presence of "clue cells" under the microscope, a pH greater than 4.5, and a fishy odor. Clue cells are vaginal epithelial cells to which Gram-negative organisms are attached. The most effective treatment is metronidazole and clindamycin.

► Human Immunodeficiency Virus Infection

An in-depth discussion of infection with HIV is inappropriate in this chapter; however, it is a life-threatening STD affecting the mother, infant, family, and society. The three principal routes of transmission of HIV are (1) sexual contact with infected body fluids; (2) contact with infected blood or blood products via transfusion, organ transplants, shared needles, or accidental needle stick injury; and (3) transmission from an infected woman to her infant prenatally, at birth, or during breastfeeding (Youngkin & Davis, 1998). Infection with HIV causes HIV disease, the terminal phase of which is acquired immunodeficiency syndrome (AIDS). Although antiretroviral therapies, which include nucleoside reverse transcriptase inhibitors (NRTI) such as zidovudine (also called AZT or ZDV), protease inhibitors (PI) such as indinavir (also called Crixivan), and non-nucleoside reverse transcriptase inhibitors (NNRTI) such as delavirdine (also called Rescriptor) (Elion, 1997) have been shown to benefit people with HIV, there is still no known cure. As with the epidemiology of other STDs, a high-risk group for infection with HIV is the inner-city, disadvantaged minority population, primarily African-American and Latino. Intravenous drug use, homosexuality, and heterosexual contact with an intravenous drug user or bisexual partner are critical lifestyle factors contributing to the increased likelihood of HIV infection.

To be considered HIV positive, an individual must test positive for the HIV antibody three times, twice with the ELISA screening test and once with the more specific, and expensive, Western blot test or immunofluorescence assay (IFA). A positive result means that an individual is considered infected for life and can transmit the virus to others, even if he or she has no symptoms. If the individual tests negative, there is still the possibility that he or she will convert to an antibody-positive status. The interval between when a person is exposed to the virus and develops antibodies may be as long as 6 months. The interval between infection and development of AIDS can range from a few months to 10 years.

There is growing evidence that HIV is becoming a truly heterosexually transmitted disease, although links to the drug culture and gay community continue to exist. As of 1995, about 20 million people were infected with HIV; 36% were women (Stine, 1996). Heterosexual transmission from an intravenous-drug-using male partner to a nonusing sexual partner occurs in about 40% of cases. Transmission can occur after only one at-risk sexual encounter or after repeated contact over several years. An increased risk of infection is likely in conditions in which blood is present or tissue is damaged, such as cervicitis, vaginitis, and menstruation.

A large percentage (52%) of women with HIV infection are intravenous drug users themselves. Because women using intravenous drugs may have limited social or economic resources, prostitution may be a means of support for the drug habit and family, thus contributing to the double risk of infection from contaminated needles or heterosexual transmission.

For the childbearing family, fetal infection can be the result of transmission from a mother who was infected through her own intravenous drug use or through heterosexual contact with an intravenous drug user or bisexual partner. It is estimated that three quarters of HIV-infected children were infected through perinatal transmission. Perinatal transmission is as of yet poorly understood. Three typical models are suggested: transplacental passage, vertical transmission (contact with maternal blood or vaginal secretions during labor and delivery), and postpartum ingestion of breast milk (Whipple, 1992).

The frequency of perinatal transmission when the mother is HIV positive, and has not been treated with zidovudine during pregnancy, is currently considered to be approximately 15 to 25% (U.S. Centers for Disease Control and Prevention, 1998). Both symptomatic and asymptomatic infected mothers can transmit HIV to their infants. HIV can be transmitted in more than one pregnancy, and each infant is at risk of developing HIV infection. See Chapter 19 for additional information on HIV infection during pregnancy.

For nurses, information regarding HIV infection and other STDs cannot be separated from the emotional response evoked by individuals concerned about HIV or AIDS. Even considering whether to be tested creates a crisis in a person's life—a crisis that is worsened if the results are positive and by no means ended if the results are negative.

Many of the individuals confronted by HIV infection have already experienced social isolation and rejection because of a different lifestyle, poverty, drug use, or minority status. Their social, economic, and educational resources are limited. This is the background with which they face another crisis. Denial, anger, fear, somatization, sexual dysfunction, depression, and thoughts of suicide are a range of anticipated emotional responses to the possibility of HIV infection. Mothers who give birth to children infected with HIV experience guilt and grief. A complex assessment and management plan for this illness provided either at an on-site setting or through referral is a challenge for all health care professionals and warrants in-depth attention.

Education regarding means of transmission remains the most important public health strategy for controlling the spread of HIV. Educational efforts

Ethical Decision Making

The AIDS epidemic has raised many ethical and moral issues, especially in the area of sexuality and reproduction. As a nurse caring for clients who must deal with this crisis, consider the following questions:

1. Should all pregnant women be tested for the HIV antibody? (Currently, such testing is voluntary.)
2. What responsibility do health care providers have to inform partners of clients who test positive for HIV?
3. Who should be informed if an individual tests positive for the HIV antibody?
4. Should health care providers be required to care for clients who test positive for the HIV antibody or have HIV infection?

should be targeted particularly at groups with high-risk behaviors for whom the message should be simple, direct, clear, and culturally specific. It has been suggested that if women of childbearing age who are at high risk for HIV infection would avoid pregnancy, there would eventually be no new cases of pediatric HIV; however, advising these women not to become pregnant is controversial and may reflect the caregiver's bias. HIV is associated with high-risk behaviors, not with specific groups or individuals.

It is recommended that all pregnant women should be offered HIV testing because of the ability of current treatments to reduce the likelihood of perinatal transmission (U.S. Centers for Disease Control and Prevention, 1998). In particular, recent findings indicating that treatment with zidovudine during pregnancy can reduce mother-to-infant transmission rates to 8% if administered to women during the later stage of pregnancy and during labor and to infants for the first 6 weeks of life, make identification of infected pregnant women vital (U.S. Centers for Disease Control and Prevention, 1998). Because of the delay in seroconversion and also the possibility of new exposure to an HIV-infected individual, some authorities suggest that testing should be repeated in the third trimester of pregnancy.

Specialized education, counseling, and intervention programs should be aimed at substance abusers, who are estimated to account for a substantially rising proportion of new cases of HIV infection. This popu-

lation poses a significant risk to childbearing women and their children in terms of the spread of HIV.

▶ Health Education and Sexually Transmitted Diseases

STDs have been identified as one of 15 health priority areas for national prevention and control. The important priorities are (1) to reduce the incidence of gonorrhea, syphilis, and gonococcal PID; (2) to provide accurate and timely education about STDs to every junior and senior high school student; and (3) to train health care providers so that 95% will be capable of diagnosing and treating all currently recognized STDs (American Medical Association, 1992).

Some of the key activities identified by a World Health Organization/Pan American Health Organization Scientific Group related to this issue include (1) health education, (2) disease detection (Fig. 5–1), (3) appropriate treatment, (4) partner tracing and client counseling, (5) clinical service evaluation, (6) training, and (7) research.

Though nurses should be involved in all of these activities, it is clear from past experience that one professional or one strategy alone will not solve the problem of HIV infection, STDs, or drug abuse. Instead, multifaceted, multimedia, and multidisciplinary approaches have the greatest hope for success.

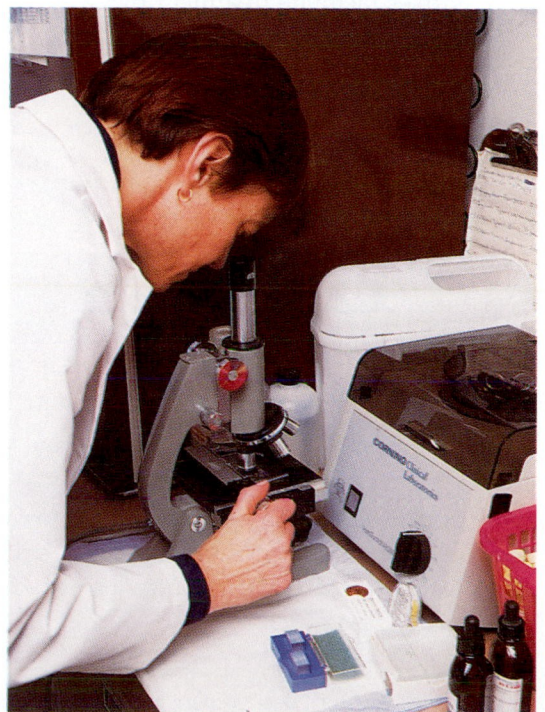

FIGURE 5–1. The detection of sexually transmitted infections through microscopic examination of cultures is an important responsibility for the nurse in her role as health educator.

Health education is a broad mandate to be implemented at the health promotion and at the primary, secondary, or tertiary level of prevention. Health education includes providing information about STDs, the mode of transmission, and healthy protective behaviors aimed at reducing the incidence of such diseases. Health education strategies need to be creative and developmentally, culturally, educationally, and linguistically appropriate and can include:

- Posters
- Brochures
- Telephone audiotapes
- Ads in school newspapers
- Films
- Classes led by peer educators
- Classes using a variety of techniques such as role playing, group discussions, one-to-one teaching contacts, and essay assignments in which drugs or AIDS is the topic

Education is aimed at multiple target populations and should be appropriate for low-risk groups, high-risk groups, and parents or spouses of those in high- or low-risk groups. In particular, educational strategies must be devised to reach adolescents, who because of their developmental stage are seen as the "next wave" of the HIV epidemic.

Professional nurses, through careful history taking, symptom analysis, observation and recording of physical findings, and referral contribute to disease detection. Nurses facilitate treatment by:

- Educating clients
- Monitoring clients' cooperation with the medical regimen

- Addressing supportive measures that will enhance treatment (such as fluid intake and hygiene practices)
- Fostering healthy lifestyle behaviors
- Investigating treatment cooperation issues
- Modifying regimens accordingly
- Evaluating new approaches that promote treatment cooperation and ensure the practice of safe sex

Contacting and treatment of sexual partners are important adjuncts to treatment. The nurse focuses on the responses of the client to treatment as well as on monitoring the response of the client's support system or family to the detection and treatment regimen. Pregnancy poses a particular health risk to the mother because of increased susceptibility to disease and contraindications to certain drug therapies. STDs also present a substantial health risk to the fetus. Active anticipatory education and counseling related to this life cycle phase are warranted.

Furthermore, the nurse has a responsibility to influence policy making through such community roles as parent, politically involved voter and lobbyist, PTA member, community organization member, and Girl Scout or Boy Scout leader. The problem of HIV infections or STDs or drug abuse will not be solved by a superlative 20-minute presentation by a nurse but by widespread distribution of information and acknowledgment by all of society that this is a problem our adult members and children must address. Certainly nursing, together with other groups and individuals, has a key role to play in this endeavor.

Chapter Highlights

▶ Sexuality is an integral aspect of human functioning across the life span.

▶ Concepts such as masculinity, femininity, androgyny, biologic gender, sex-role behaviors, and cultural factors are important in an understanding of sexuality.

▶ The four phases of the sexual response cycle for both males and females are excitement, plateau,

orgasm, and resolution and are accompanied by specific physiologic responses in various organ systems.

▶ The individual's experience and understanding of sexuality over the life span change as a function of cognitive, psychosocial, cultural, and physiologic maturation.

▶ The primary purpose of taking a sexual history is to identify a long-term or situational problem

Chapter Highlights continued

with either an individual's or couple's sexual functioning.

► Physiologic and psychosocial changes during pregnancy, childbirth, and the postpartum period can have a significant impact on both sexual desire and sexual response of childbearing couples.

► Societal and cultural changes over the past two decades have led to an increasing incidence of STDs, such as *Chlamydia trachomatis* infection, gonorrhea, human papillomavirus infection, herpes simplex virus type 2 infection, cytomegalovirus infection, syphilis, vaginitis, and HIV.

► Nursing responsibilities related to health education and STDs include counseling clients concerning sexual expression and safe sex practices, planning consumer programs directed toward prevention of STDs, and determining policies on the institutional, local, and national levels related to sexuality.

After reading the vignette at the beginning of this chapter, use what you have learned to answer these questions:

1. What types of approaches can the nurse practitioner take in counseling Ben and Nina Huang about the aspects of childbearing on their sexual relationship?

2. What aspects of Ben and Nina Huang's sexual history would help the nurse practitioner in developing effective interventions to help the couple understand and resolve their concerns about their sexual relationship and childbearing?

3. In what ways would physiologic, psychosocial, or cultural factors play a part in how this coup;le views their sexuality and childbearing?

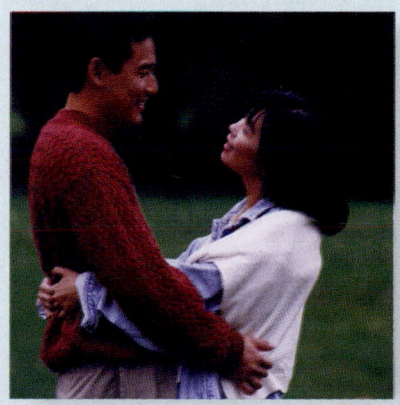

Critical Thinking Questions

► References

American College of Obstetricians and Gynecologists. (1996). Vaginitis. *ACOG Technical Bulletin, 221*, 1–9.

American Medical Association. (1992). Culturally competent health care for adolescents: A guide for primary care providers. Chicago: Department of Adolescent Health, AMA.

American Social Health Association. (1994). *STD (VD): Questions, answers.* Research Triangle Park, NC: Author.

Edwards, J.N., & Booth, A. (1994). Sexuality, marriage, and well-being: The middle years. In A.S. Rossi (Ed.), *Sexuality across the life course* (pp. 233–260). Chicago: The University of Chicago Press.

Elion, R. (1997). *Do you know your options? An updated guide to anti-retroviral therapies.* Washington, DC: National Association of People with AIDS.

Fausto-Sterling, A. (1985). *Myths of gender.* New York: Basic Books.

Gesell, A., Ilg, F.L., Ames, L.B., & Rodell, J.L. (1974). *Infant and child in the culture of today: The guidance of development in home and nursery school*. New York: Harper & Row.

Kaplan, H. (1979). *Disorders of sexual desire*. New York: Brunner/Mazel.

Kinsey, A.C., Pomeroy, W.B., & Martin, C.E. (1948). *Sexual behavior in the human male*. Philadelphia: W.B. Saunders.

Kinsey, A.C., et al. (1953). *Sexual behavior in the human female*. Philadelphia: W.B. Saunders.

Kriepe, R.E. (1983). Prevention of adolescent pregnancy: A developmental approach. In E.R. McAnarney (Ed.), *Premature adolescent pregnancy and parenthood* (pp. 37–59). New York: Grune & Stratton.

Lancaster, J.B. (1994). Human sexuality, life histories, and evolutionary ecology. In A.S. Rossi (Ed.), *Sexuality across the life course* (pp. 39–62). Chicago: The University of Chicago Press.

Maccoby, E., & Jacklin, C. (1974). *The psychology of sex differences*. Stanford, CA: Stanford University Press.

Masters, W.H., & Johnson, V.E. (1966). *Human sexual response*. Boston: Little, Brown.

Masters, W.H., & Johnson, V.E. (1970). *Human sexual inadequacy*. Boston: Little, Brown.

Masters, W.H., Johnson, V.E., & Kolodny, R.C. (1982). *Human sexuality*. Boston: Little, Brown.

Masters, W.H., Johnson, V.E., & Kolodny, R.C. (1986). *Masters and Johnson on sex and human loving*. Boston: Little, Brown.

Meyer-Bahlburg, H.F.L. (1995). Psychoneuroendocrinology and sexual pleasure: The sexual aspect of sexual orientation. In P.R. Abramson & S.D. Pinkerton (Eds.), *Sexual nature, sexual culture* (pp. 135–153). Chicago: The University of Chicago Press.

Money, J., & Ehrhardt, A.A. (1972). *Man & woman, boy & girl: The differentiation and dimorphism of gender identity from conception to maturity*. Baltimore: Johns Hopkins University Press.

Moulton, A.W., & Montgomery, K.M. (1995). Approach to the patient with a vaginal discharge. In A.H. Goroll, L.A. May, & A.G. Mulley (eds.), *Primary care medicine: Office evaluation and management of the adult patient* (3rd ed.). Philadelphia: J.B. Lippincott.

Schlegel, A. (1995). The cultural management of adolescent sexuality. In P.R. Abramson & S.D. Pinkerton (Eds.), *Sexual nature, sexual culture* (pp. 177–194). Chicago: The University of Chicago Press.

Smith-Battle, L., & Leonard, V.W. (1998). Adolescent mothers four years later: Narratives of the self and visions of the future. *Advances in Nursing Science, 20*(3), 36–49.

Stine, G.J. (1996). *Acquired immune deficiency syndrome: Biological, medical, social, and legal issues* (2nd ed.). Englewood Cliffs, NJ: Prentice-Hall.

Tulman, L., Fawcett, J., Grablewiski, L., & Siverman, L. (1990). Changes in functional status after childbirth. *Nursing Research, 39,* 70–75.

U.S. Centers for Disease Control and Prevention. (1998). 1998 guidelines for treatment of sexually transmitted diseases. *Morbidity and Mortality Weekly Report, 47*(RR-1), 1–111.

Whipple, G. (1992). Women and AIDS: Sexuality issues. *Nursing Outlook, 40,* 56–63.

Whiting, B.B., & Whiting, I.W.N. (1975). *Children of six cultures*. Cambridge, MA: Harvard University Press.

Wilson, J.D. (1995). Sex hormones and sexual behavior. In P.R. Abramson & S.D. Pinkerton (Eds.), *Sexual nature, sexual culture* (pp. 121–134). Chicago: The University of Chicago Press.

Youngkin, E.Q., & Davis, M.S. (1998). *Women's health: A primary care clinical guide* (2nd ed.). Stamford, CT: Appleton & Lange.

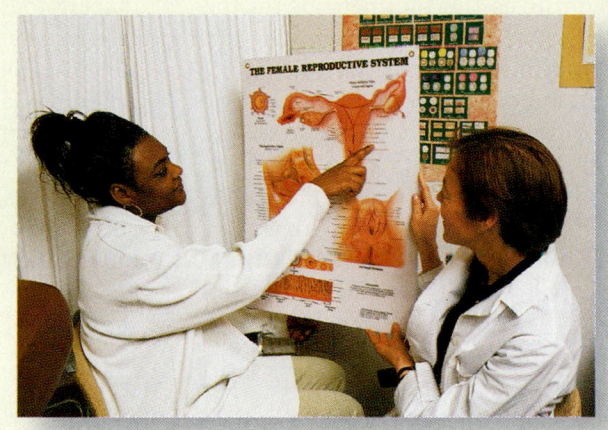

Shaila Jackson, a 23-year-old nulliparous woman, is attending a well-woman health examination at a local women's health center. While reviewing Shaila's health history, Ann Salzman, CNM, MSN, notices that Shaila is looking intently at a chart showing the female reproductive system. She smiles and asks, "Do you have any questions that you would like to ask me before we start your physical examination?"

Shaila glances quickly at the nurse-midwife and then lowers her eyes. She replies, "I recently read in a magazine that women should examine their genital area every month. But, I'm not sure how to do that and I don't completely understand the drawings." The nurse-midwife says, "Let's look at these diagrams and I'll explain each structure and its function. Feel free to ask questions as we talk. If you'd like, you can use a hand mirror to watch while I evaluate your reproductive organs." Shaila replies, "I'm interested in learning how everything works, but I'm not sure if I'll feel comfortable examining myself. Is it really necessary?" ∎

6

Human Reproduction

At no other time in the life cycle of a human being is the interplay of genetics and environment so apparent as when the sperm fertilizes the ovum to begin the development of a unique individual. Growth and development of the resulting individual will be influenced by the transmission of genetic material and by the presence of a healthy uterine environment. The ovum and sperm each carry to the union a half-share of genetic information so that the united cell receives the full amount of genetic information required for directing the growth and development of the new individual. Both the male and female reproductive systems are designed to ensure the successful union of the sperm and the ovum.

This chapter describes the genetic aspects of human reproduction, puberty, the anatomy of the male and female reproductive systems, and the processes of spermatogenesis and oogenesis. The chapter concludes with a description of the phases of the menstrual cycle, including the ovarian and endometrial cycles. A thorough knowledge of this content is required by the nurse who cares for the woman and her partner prior to and during pregnancy.

▶ GENETIC ASPECTS OF HUMAN REPRODUCTION

Each human being has unique hereditary characteristics that are the result of contributions of genetic material by the ovum and sperm at conception. Hereditary characteristics are determined by genes that appear in pairs (alleles) on the chromosomes within the human cell nucleus. It is estimated that there are between 30,000 and 50,000 gene pairs in each human cell nucleus.

Genes are the basic units of inheritance and are composed of deoxyribonucleic acid (DNA). A double-stranded molecule in the shape of a coiled ladder, DNA is present in the nucleus of each human cell. The genes in each cell nucleus are tightly intertwined in the DNA of the chromosomes. The functions of DNA include replication during cell division, coding for the production of structural proteins and enzymes, and regulation of the rate of synthesis of these proteins and enzymes.

Chromosomes are the threadlike structures within the nucleus of the cell that carry the genes. They are formed by the winding of DNA molecules around protein molecules like thread around a spool. Genes are arranged linearly along the chromosomes, with each gene having a particular location (locus). A gene locus on one chromosome has a matching gene locus on its paired chromosome.

The human cell has 23 pairs of chromosomes (46 total) in its nucleus, half donated by the mother and half by the father. Twenty-two pairs ($n = 44$) of chromosomes are identical in males and females; they are called **autosomes.** The remaining two chromosomes, called sex chromosomes, are alike in the female (XX) and different in the male (XY). To view the chromosomes in terms of number and structure, a photomicrograph is obtained of the chromosomes and each chromosome is arranged in numerical order in a **karyotype** (Fig. 6–1). (See Chapter 10 for further discussion about the use of karyotypes in genetic counseling.)

▶ Cell Division

Human cells divide by mitosis or meiosis. **Mitosis** occurs when a parent cell having 46 chromosomes forms two daughter cells, each having 46 chromosomes identical to the parent cell. Mitosis is the process by which body cells are duplicated for growth in the developing fetus and child and damaged or dead cells are replaced in the adult. **Meiosis** is the process of reduction division, during which the parent cell with 46 paired chromosomes forms four daughter cells (called gametes), each with 23 unpaired chromosomes. In other words, the total number of chromosomes in an ovum or sperm is reduced by half, so that when the gametes unite during fertilization, the resulting one-celled human organism contains the necessary 46 chromosomes. Meiosis occurs in ovum and sperm cell formation.

Before cells divide, DNA replication must occur. The double strand of DNA must unwind and separate. The individual strands then serve as a model for a new double strand of DNA to be formed (Fig. 6–2). The result is two new strands of DNA that are genetically identical to the original DNA strands. If the DNA strand is not replicated exactly, genetic mutations can occur during cell division, causing a permanent change in the genetic material (see Chapter 10 for a discussion about numerical chromosomal abnormalities).

Mitosis

Mitotic division has five stages: interphase, prophase, metaphase, anaphase, and telophase (Fig. 6–3).

Interphase I, the stage before cell division occurs, is sometimes called the "resting stage" of cell division. During this phase, no chromosomal activity can be observed under the microscope (Fig. 6–3A); however, it is thought that the strands of DNA are not actually "resting" during this stage and that DNA replication actually occurs near the end of interphase.

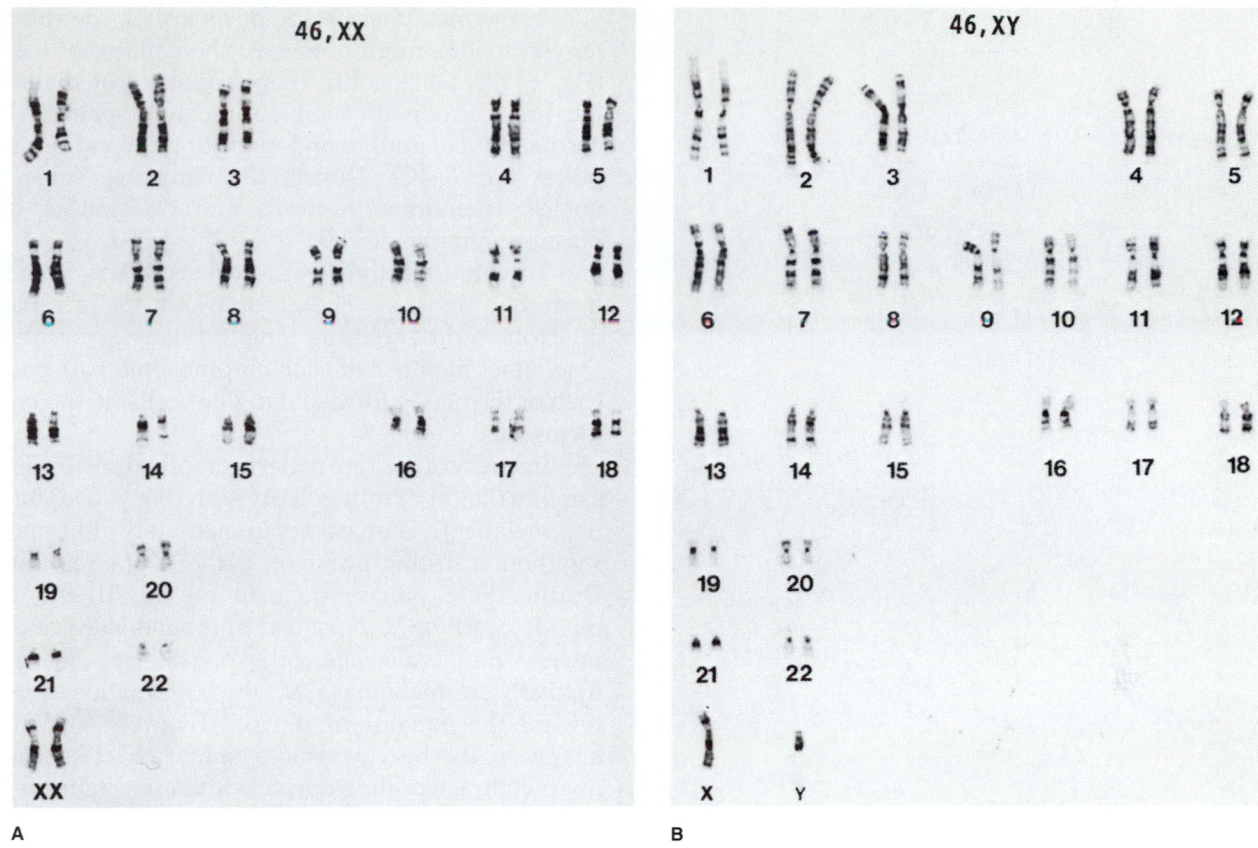

FIGURE 6–1. Normal chromosomes at metaphase. **A.** Female karyotype. **B.** Male karyotype.

Protein synthesis, which is required before a cell can begin mitosis and actually divide, is also thought to occur during interphase. During protein synthesis, one strand of DNA serves as the model for the formation of messenger ribonucleic acid (mRNA). This process, called transcription, takes place in the nucleus of the cell. The transcribed mRNA transports the DNA code for individual genes. Once formed, mRNA travels from the cell nucleus to the cytoplasm, where translation occurs. During translation, amino acids are brought into place in an ordered sequence to form a polypeptide chain resulting in the final gene product. If the message of the DNA is not transcribed and translated exactly, the result may be an altered gene product (e.g., a structural protein or enzyme) that does not adequately carry out its function.

During prophase, cell division begins (Fig. 6–3B). The chromosomes begin to coil and condense and develop a definite shape, appearing as two duplicated longitudinal halves called chromatids. The two chromatids are held together in a constricted area called the centromere. If the centromere is located in the center, the chromosome appears X-shaped; if it is located

at one end of the chromosome, the chromosome has a wishbone or Y-shaped appearance.

During prophase, two centrioles (cytoplasmic structures) can be seen at one side of the nucleus. By the end of prophase, the centrioles begin moving apart and are separated by spindle fibers made up of protein. The nuclear membrane disappears during this phase.

During early metaphase, the centrioles are pulled to opposite poles of the cell (Fig. 6–3C). The chromatid pairs move back and forth within the spindle fibers as they are tugged toward first one pole and then the other. Finally, they line up along the equator of the cell (middle of the cell), marking the end of metaphase.

At the beginning of anaphase, the centromeres separate simultaneously in all the chromatid pairs. The spindle fibers contract and draw the chromatids of each pair apart toward the centrioles at the opposite poles of the cell (Fig. 6–3D). Each chromatid then becomes a separate chromosome.

During early telophase (also called interphase II), the chromosomes have reached the opposite poles. The spindle fibers disperse and the cytoplasm divides. The

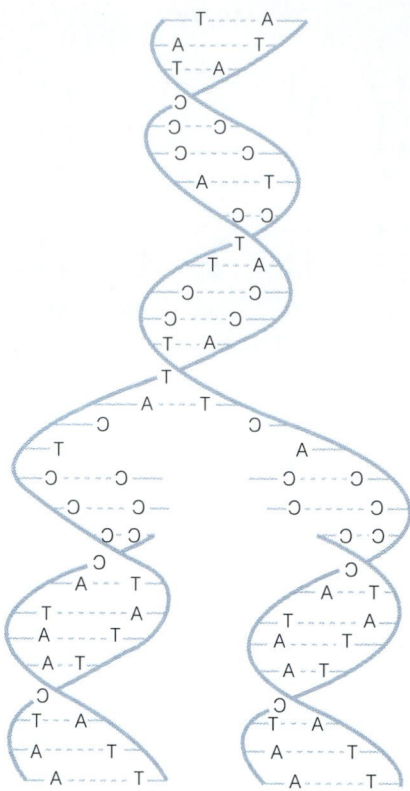

FIGURE 6–2. DNA replication resulting in two strands of DNA identical to the parent DNA.

nuclear membrane re-forms, separating each newly formed nucleus from the cytoplasm. The sister chromatids unwind and uncoil and are no longer visible under the microscope. At the end of telophase, the parent cell is divided into two daughter cells that are genetically identical to the original cell (Fig. 6–3E). The two cells are exactly alike in genetic material and each has 46 chromosomes. The cells then reenter interphase I.

Meiosis

Meiosis consists of two successive cell divisions, resulting in the formation of four daughter cells, each with a haploid (or halved) number of chromosomes (23).

During the first cell division (meiosis I), the chromosomes coil and condense (Fig. 6–4). They have already duplicated and formed four sister chromatids. During prophase I, there is a close association of the four sister chromatids of the paired chromosomes. In fact, the chromatids physically exchange genetic material, accounting for the wide variation of traits among individuals who are children of the same parents. During this stage, the nuclear membrane disappears, the centriole duplicates, and the centriole pairs each migrate toward opposite poles of the cell (Fig. 6–4A).

In the metaphase stage of meiosis I, the four sister chromatids migrate toward the equator of the cell (Fig. 6–4B). During the anaphase stage of meiosis I, the first meiotic division occurs, with paired sister chromatids separating and migrating toward opposite poles (Fig. 6–4C). During the telophase stage, the nuclear membrane re-forms and division of cytoplasm occurs (Fig. 6–4D).

The first cell division in meiosis differs from that in mitotic division. The chromosome pairs separate intact instead of splitting longitudinally as in mitosis. One intact member of each chromosome pair goes to each of the newly formed daughter cells by the end of meiosis I.

In meiosis II, the pattern of cell division is the same as that in mitotic cell division (Fig. 6–5). The second meiotic division occurs immediately after meiosis I without a resting phase or further DNA replication. During the prophase stage of meiosis II, the chromatids continue to be coiled and condensed and the nuclear membrane again disappears (see Fig. 6–3B, mitosis). In metaphase II, the chromatids migrate toward the equator of the cell (Fig. 6–5A). During anaphase II, the centromere splits and the spindle fibers contract, pulling the individual sister chromatids toward opposite poles of the cell (Fig. 6–5B). At telophase II, the cytoplasm again divides. The result of the meiotic division is four daughter cells, each with 23 chromosomes (Fig. 6–5C), or half as many chromo-

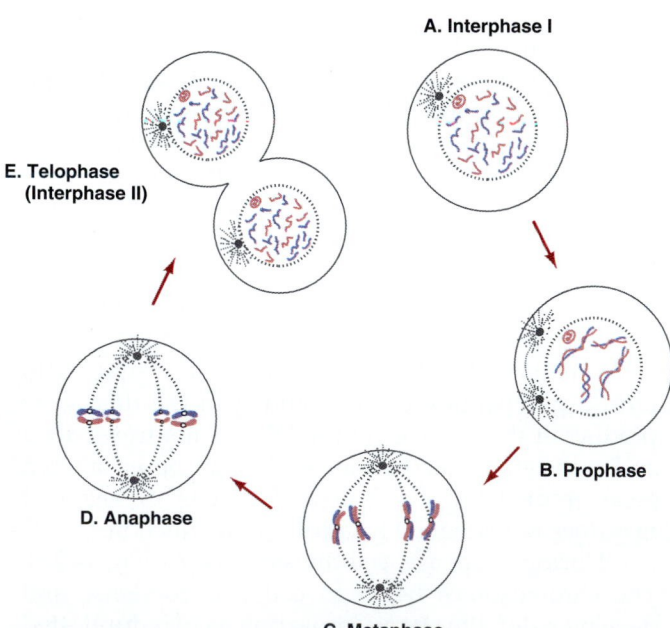

FIGURE 6–3. Mitosis. *(Adapted, with permission, from Hay, W.W., Groothuis, J.R., Hayward, A.R., & Levin, M.J. (1997). Current pediatric diagnosis and treatment (13th ed.). Stamford, CT: Appleton & Lange, p. 886.)*

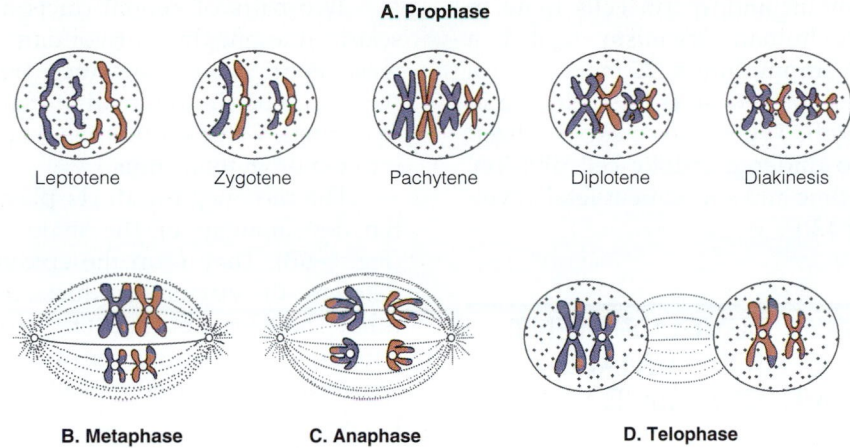

FIGURE 6–4. First meiotic division (meiosis I). *(Reproduced, with permission, from Stenchever, M.A. (1973). Human cytogenics: A workbook in reproductive biology. Cleveland, OH: The Press of Case Western Reserve University.)*

somes as the original cell. One of these 23 chromosomes is a sex chromosome. If the parent cell is an ovum, each of the four resulting daughter cells will contain one X sex chromosome; but if the parent cell is a sperm, two of the daughter cells will contain X chromosomes and two will contain Y chromosomes.

► Gametogenesis

Gametogenesis is the process by which the sperm and ovum are produced. During gametogenesis, mei-

otic cell division occurs, resulting in a haploid number of chromosomes (23) in the daughter cells, or gametes. Sperm cell formation is referred to as spermatogenesis and ovum cell formation as oogenesis. (These processes are described later in the chapter.)

► Fertilization

Fertilization occurs when a sperm penetrates the outer layer of the ovum, setting off a chain of events that results in the development of a human embryo.

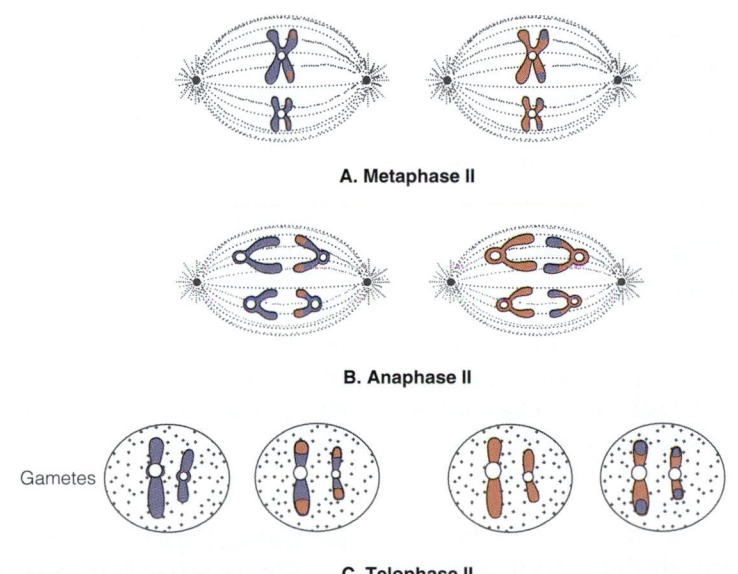

FIGURE 6–5. Second meiotic division (meiosis II). *(Reproduced, with permission, from Stenchever, M.A. (1973). Human cytogenics: A workbook in reproductive biology. Cleveland, OH: The Press of Case Western Reserve University.)*

At fertilization, the ovum and sperm cells unite to form a single-celled human organism (called a zygote), containing 46 chromosomes (22 pairs of autosomes and 1 pair of sex chromosomes [XX resulting in a female, XY in a male]). The single-celled, fertilized zygote then begins to undergo mitotic cell division, which initiates embryonic and subsequent fetal development. (See Chapter 13.)

► EMBRYOLOGIC DEVELOPMENT OF THE MALE AND FEMALE REPRODUCTIVE SYSTEMS

The male and female reproductive systems begin development during the embryonic period (the period beginning the third week after fertilization and continuing to approximately the eighth week). The structure and function of the reproductive organs in both sexes follow an organized and complex pattern of development.

The sex of the embryo is determined at fertilization by the genetic makeup of the sperm that fertilizes the ovum. If an X-bearing sperm unites with an X-bearing ovum, the resulting sex chromosome complex will be XX and the genetic sex of the embryo, female. If a Y-bearing sperm unites with an X-bearing ovum, the sex chromosome complex will be XY and the genetic sex, male.

Although the genetic sex of the embryo is determined at fertilization, the reproductive organs initially begin to develop in the same way in both sexes. In fact, there is no difference in the appearance of the reproductive organs of males or females until about the seventh week of gestation. This period in which the female and the male internal reproductive organs and external genitalia are similar is referred to as the indifferent or undifferentiated stage of development.

► Development of the Internal Reproductive Systems

The immature gonads are first seen during the fifth week of embryologic development when thickened epithelial cells form gonadal ridges. Fingerlike epithelial cords soon grow from the gonadal ridge of each gonad. Each indifferent gonad now consists of an outer cortex and an inner medulla. In embryos with an XX sex chromosome complex, the cortex differentiates into an ovary, and the medulla regresses. In embryos with an XY sex chromosome complex, the medulla differentiates into a testis and the cortex regresses.

Two pairs of genital ducts also develop in both sexes, mesonephric (wolffian duct) and paramesonephric (müllerian duct) (Fig. 6–6A). The ducts come together in the median plane in both sexes and fuse into a Y-shaped uterovaginal canal, which opens into the urogenital sinus.

The mesonephric ducts play an essential role in the development of the male reproductive system (Fig. 6–6B). They form the epididymides, the ductus deferens, the ejaculatory ducts, and the efferent ductules. The lateral portion of the duct forms the seminal vesicle. The remainder of the male genital system consists of the urethra, which gives rise to the prostate gland.

In female embryos, the mesonephric ducts regress and the paramesonephric ducts develop into the female reproductive tract. The unfused portions of paramesonephric ducts develop into the uterine tubes. The fused portions form the uterovaginal primordium, which develops into the epithelium and glands of the uterus and the fibromuscular vaginal wall. Fusion of the paramesonephric ducts brings together two peritoneal folds, forming right and left broad ligaments (Fig. 6–6C).

In genetic males, primitive sperm (called spermatogonia) are formed during fetal life. Beginning during puberty, formation of spermatogonia again occurs; these primitive sperm cells continue to form and mature into spermatozoa throughout the male's fertile years.

In genetic females, primitive ova (called oogonia) are formed during fetal life. Through mitosis, thousands of oogonia are formed. Because no oogonia are formed postnatally, females are born with the primary oocytes (about 400,000) that they will have throughout their reproductive years.

The fetal testes produce two hormones: a nonsteroidal inducer substance and androgens. The inducer substance stimulates the development of the mesonephric ducts into the male genital tract. It also suppresses the development of the müllerian glands. Unlike the testes, which produce hormones to stimulate male development, the ovaries are not needed to stimulate primary sexual female development. It is most likely the absence of testicular hormone that stimulates primary sexual development in the female.

► Development of the External Reproductive Systems

Development of the external genitalia in males and females also begins with an undifferentiated stage for

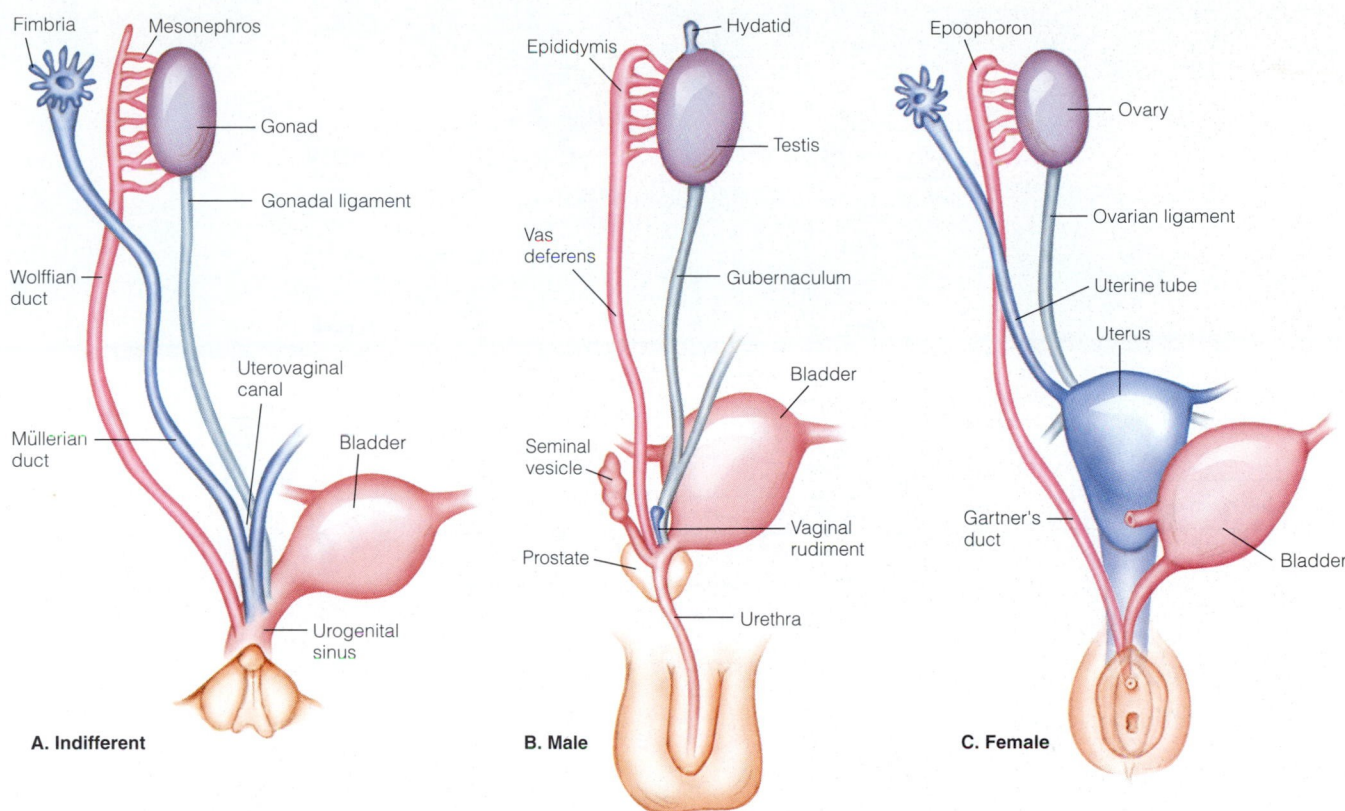

Fimbria

Mesonephros

Gonad

Gonadal ligament

Wolffian duct

Uterovaginal canal

Müllerian duct

Bladder

Urogenital sinus

A. Indifferent

Epididymis

Hydatid

Testis

Vas deferens

Gubernaculum

Bladder

Seminal vesicle

Prostate

Vaginal rudiment

Urethra

B. Male

Epoophoron

Ovary

Ovarian ligament

Uterine tube

Uterus

Gartner's duct

Bladder

C. Female

FIGURE 6–6. Development of the internal reproductive structures. *(After Corning, H.K., & Wilkins, L. Redrawn and reproduced, with permission, from Withaus, R.H. (1974). Textbook of endocrinology (5th ed.). Philadelphia: W.B. Saunders.)*

about the first 7 weeks (Fig. 6–7). A genital tubercle develops in both sexes in the fourth week. On either side of a cloacal membrane, labioscrotal swellings and urethral folds develop. The genital tubercle becomes longer and is called a phallus.

By the tenth week of development, the male testes secrete fetal androgen (testosterone) hormone. Under the influence of testosterone, the anterior part of the genital tubercle develops into the penis. The urethral folds fuse together to form the spongy urethra; the external opening of the urethra moves to the glans penis and an opening is evident at the tip of the penis. The labioscrotal swellings grow larger, fuse, and develop into the scrotum (Fig. 6–7).

In the absence of fetal testosterone, the female clitoris is formed from the genital tubercle. In the female, the urethral folds do not fuse, giving rise to the labia minora. The labioscrotal swellings become the labia majora. Two openings, the urethral and vaginal openings, are formed between the labia minora (Fig. 6–7).

▶ PUBERTY

Puberty is defined as the developmental phase in males and females that results in physical maturity and the capacity to reproduce. The changes that occur are hormonally mediated and take place over several years. The rate at which individuals physically mature is highly variable, but the sequence of events is very predictable. Secondary sex characteristics, those that distinguish the sexes, are used to identify the pattern of events. The sequence of events for females includes (Tanner, 1962, 1978):

- Appearance of breast buds
- Appearance of pubic hair (about 16% develop pubic hair prior to breast enlargement)
- Change in vaginal secretions
- linear growth acceleration
- Appearance of axillary hair
- Ovulation

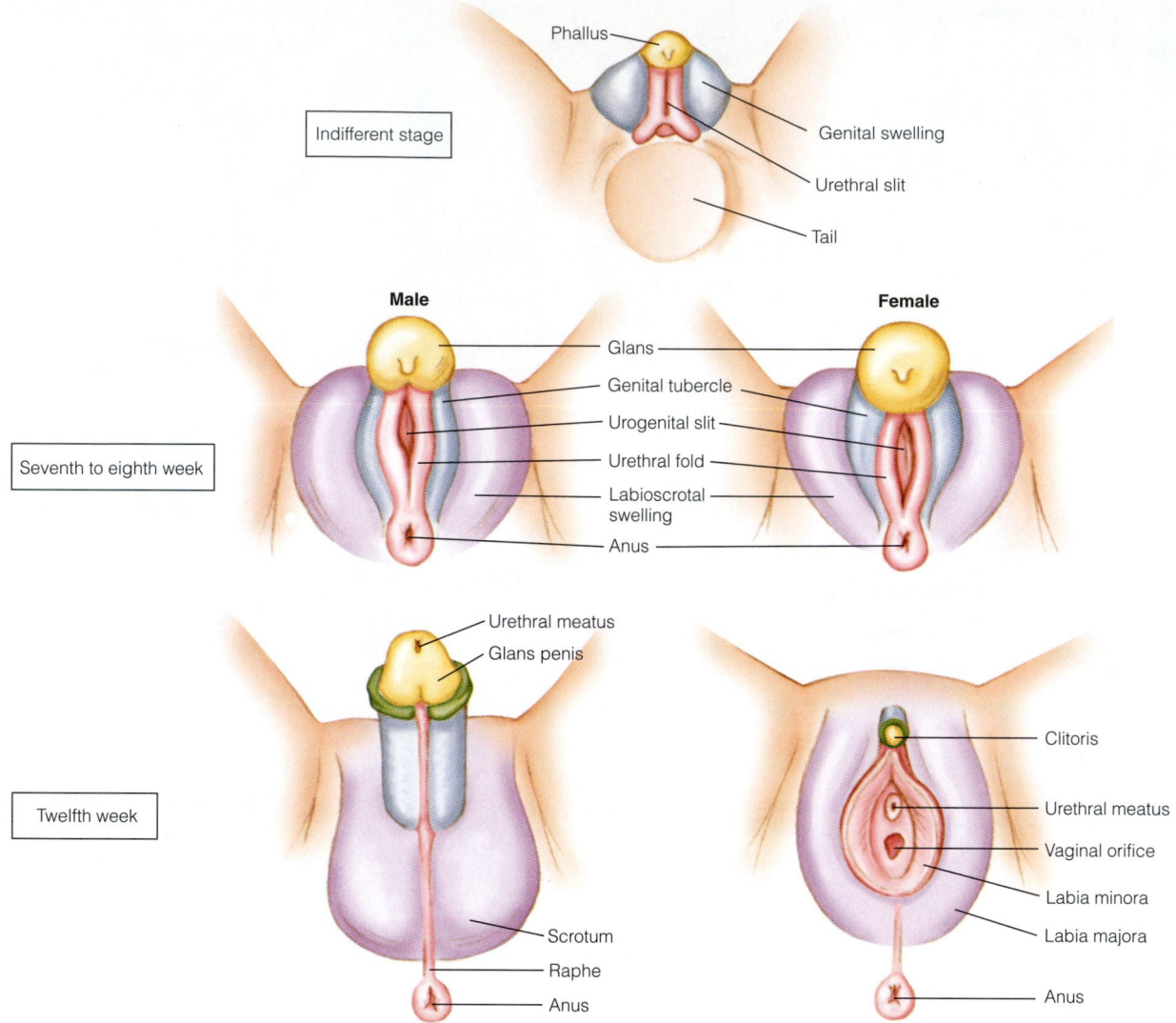

FIGURE 6–7. Development of the external reproductive structures. *(Reproduced, with permission, from Ganong, W.F. (1995). Review of medical physiology (17th ed.). Norwalk, CT: Appleton & Lange, p. 384.)*

For boys, the sequence of events includes (Tanner, 1962, 1978):

- Testicular enlargement
- Appearance of pubic hair
- Increased growth of the penis
- First ejaculation
- Peak height growth
- Axillary hair
- Beginning facial hair
- Voice deepening

Tanner (1962) divides the period of puberty into five stages based on secondary sex characteristics. The secondary sex characteristics assessed in boys include the size of the male genitals and the development of pubic hair. For girls, pubertal development is assessed by the size of the breasts and the development of pubic hair.

▶ Stages in Pubertal Development in Boys

The stages of pubertal development in boys are (Copeland, 1986; Tanner, 1962):

1. Size of genitals:
   - Stage 1: childhood size of the penis, testes, and scrotum
   - Stage 2: enlargement of the testes and scrotum
   - Stage 3: enlargement of the penis
   - Stage 4: further growth of the testes, scrotum, and penis

- Stage 5: male genitals are adult in size and shape
2. Development of pubic hair:
   - Stage 1: no pubic hair
   - Stage 2: sparse growth of slightly pigmented hair at the base of the penis
   - Stage 3: dark coarse hair sparsely spread over the junction of the pubis
   - Stage 4: pubic hair that is adult in type
   - Stage 5: pubic hair is adult in type and quantity, extending to the thighs

The adolescent growth spurt in boys occurs on the average between the ages of 12 and 16 years, coinciding with Tanner's stages 3 and 4. Ejaculation of semen usually occurs before the growth spurt, whereas the androgen-induced enlargement of the larynx (which stimulates voice changes) corresponds to the growth spurt (Tanner, 1962; Copeland, et al., 1986). Axillary hair appears during stage 4, and facial hair develops slightly after the appearance of axillary hair.

▶ Stages in Pubertal Development in Girls

Breasts and pubic hair are used as assessment parameters for pubertal development in females. The stages of pubertal development in girls are (Copeland, 1986; Tanner, 1962):

1. Development of breasts:
   - Stage 1: preadolescent phase (papillae only)
   - Stage 2: breast bud stage (mound of breast and papilla is formed, with areolar enlargement)
   - Stage 3: enlargement of the breasts and areola continue, without separation of their contours
   - Stage 4: nipple and areola form a secondary mound above the level of the breasts
   - Stage 5: adult stage: areolar recession and appearance of mature breasts

The breasts do not develop symmetrically, as one is usually slightly larger than the other.

2. Development of pubic hair:
   - Stage 1: no pubic hair
   - Stage 2: sparse growth of long, slightly dark fine hair
   - Stage 3: hair becomes darker and curlier and spreads over the symphysis
   - Stage 4: texture and curliness of hair is similar to that of an adult but has not spread to the thighs

- Stage 5: hair is adult in quality and quantity and growth is spread to inner aspect of thighs and abdomen

The female pubertal growth spurt begins earlier than in boys, usually between the ages of 9 and 13 years. Female growth begins to accelerate in stage 2 and reaches a peak in stage 3. Voice changes also occur in girls but are not as pronounced as those in boys. Axillary hair appears, on average, 2 years after the onset of pubic hair development. The first menstrual period occurs during stage 4 of female breast development and follows the growth spurt (Marshall & Tanner, 1969; Tanner, 1962). In stage 5, ovulation occurs.

▶ Hormonal Influences on Puberty

The changes at puberty are influenced by hormones secreted by the anterior pituitary gland. These hormones are called gonadotropins and include follicle-stimulating hormone (FSH) and luteinizing hormone (LH), also referred to as interstitial cell-stimulating hormone (ICSH) in the male.

During puberty, the hypothalamus secretes gonadotropin-releasing factor (GnRF), which stimulates the anterior pituitary gland to release the gonadotropins FSH and LH. Follicle-stimulating hormone provokes the growth of ova in the ovary and of sperm-producing cells in the male testis. The cells in the ovary and testis in turn produce female and male sex hormones (estrogen in the female and testosterone in the male). These sex hormones are responsible for the development of the secondary sex characteristics.

The regulatory mechanisms for the onset of puberty are not fully understood. The hormones produced by the anterior pituitary gland are thought to be controlled through a feedback mechanism by the hypothalamus. One theory suggests that prior to puberty, immature ovaries and testes secrete small amounts of hormones. The hypothalamus, being sensitive to the inhibiting effect of these small quantities of hormones, does not stimulate the anterior pituitary gland to produce gonadotropins. At puberty, the hypothalamus becomes less sensitive to the feedback and begins stimulating the pituitary gland to secrete the gonadotropins in increasing amounts until a new equilibrium is reached in late adolescence, when maturation occurs.

When puberty is complete, the estrogen-dominated females have wider hips, a broader skeleton, and more fat distribution, particularly in the breasts, hips, and thighs, than their male counterparts. Testosterone-dominated males have larger skeletons, greater muscle mass, and broader shoulders than females.

► THE MALE REPRODUCTIVE SYSTEM

The mature male reproductive system consists of internal and external genital organs. The external organs are the penis and the scrotum; the internal organs are the testes, epididymides, ductus deferens (vas deferens), ejaculatory ducts, and urethra. Accessory glands of the male reproductive system include the seminal vesicles, the prostate gland, and the bulbourethral glands (Cowper's glands) (Fig. 6–8).

► External Genital Organs

Penis

The **penis** functions in both the reproductive and urinary systems. It is called the male organ of copulation because it deposits sperm in the female vagina during sexual intercourse. The penis also conducts urine from the body through the urethral meatus, which is located at the tip of the penis.

The penis consists of a body, or the shaft, and a cone-shaped end, or glans. The shaft contains three cylindrical masses of erectile tissue, two dorsal corpora cavernosa and one ventral corpus spongiosum.

These bodies are surrounded by the tunica albuginea, a layer of dense fibrous connective tissue that helps control the distension of the erectile tissue.

The corpus spongiosum contains the urethra and becomes enlarged at the distal end of the penis to form the glans penis. The penis is covered by loose skin. The skin covering the glans penis is called the foreskin, or prepuce. Surgical removal of the foreskin is referred to as **circumcision.**

Blood is supplied to the penis mainly through the internal and external pudendal arteries and veins. The penis is innervated by sympathetic and parasympathetic nerve fibers. (See Chapter 5 for a discussion of the changes that occur in this organ during sexual arousal.)

Scrotum

The **scrotum** is a pouchlike structure, divided in the middle by a septum (raphe), forming two scrotal sacs. Each scrotal sac contains one testis, one epididymis, and parts of the spermatic cords. The left scrotal sac is usually longer than the right because the left spermatic cord is longer.

The scrotum is made up of fascia and smooth muscle, together called the tunica dartos. When exposed to cold, the dartos muscle and cremaster

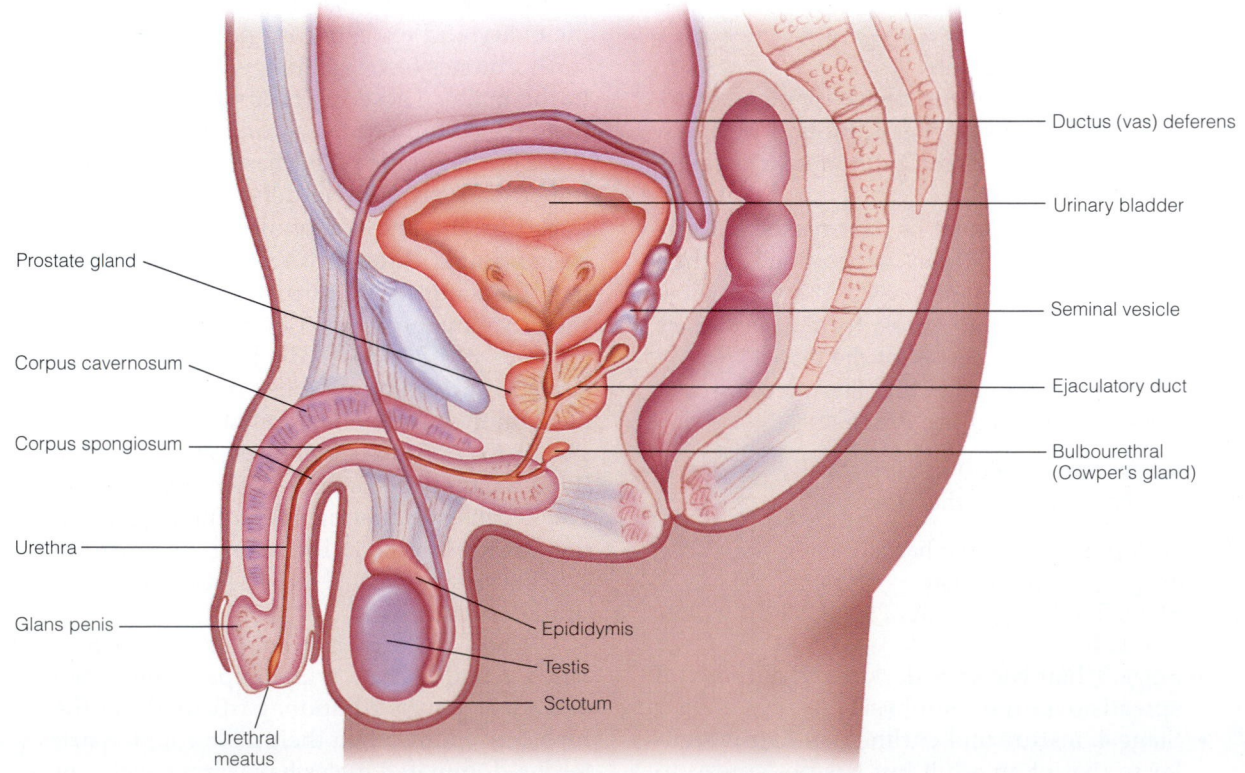

FIGURE 6–8. Male reproductive organs.

Prostate gland
Corpus cavernosum
Corpus spongiosum
Urethra
Glans penis
Urethral meatus
Epididymis
Testis
Sctotum
Ductus (vas) deferens
Urinary bladder
Seminal vesicle
Ejaculatory duct
Bulbourethral (Cowper's gland)

muscle of the spermatic cords contract, causing the scrotum to appear wrinkled. This mechanism draws the scrotum closer to the body for warmth.

Scrotal temperature is 2°C lower than internal body temperature and is the ideal temperature for spermatogenesis, which occurs in the testes. If, during development, the testes do not descend into the scrotum, the temperature of the body will inhibit spermatogenesis.

▶ Internal Genital Organs

Testes

The **testes** are two oval-shaped organs located in the scrotum. Each testis is approximately 4 to 5 cm long, 2 to 3 cm in diameter, and 10 g in weight. A single testis is located in each of the scrotal sacs. The testes are suspended on each side by **spermatic cords.** The spermatic cords, which begin slightly above the inguinal canal, pass through the canal into the scrotum.

The testes are surrounded by a membrane called the tunica vaginalis and by the tunica albuginea. The tunica albuginea projects inside each testis and forms septa, which divide the testis into about 250 lobules. Each lobule contains one to three convoluted (coiled and folded) tubules referred to as the **seminiferous tubules.**

The seminiferous tubules come together to form thin-walled spaces, the rete testis, which in turn form efferent ducts, which go through the tunica albuginea and empty into the epididymis.

The seminiferous tubules contain two types of cells: Sertoli cells and interstitial cells of Leydig. Sertoli cells provide nutrients and enzymes to the immature spermatocytes during the maturation process. The interstitial cells of Leydig produce testosterone, the main male sex hormone.

Spermatogenesis. **Spermatogenesis** is the process by which spermatogonia, the fetal sperm cells, are transformed into mature sperm. The spermatogonia remain inactive in the seminiferous tubules of the testes until they begin to increase in number at puberty. Mitotic divisions allow the spermatogonia to grow and transform into primary spermatocytes, the largest sperm cells in the tubules.

The primary spermatocytes undergo the first meiotic division, forming two secondary spermatocytes about half the size of the primary spermatocytes. The secondary spermatocytes undergo a second meiotic division, forming four haploid spermatids having 23 chromosomes each; the spermatids are about half the size of the secondary spermatocytes. The spermatids attach to the Sertoli cells and are transformed into four mature sperm cells, or spermatozoa, after several weeks in the epididymis.

A mature sperm consists of a head, neck, middle piece, and tail (Fig. 6–9). The head forms the bulk of the sperm and consists of the nucleus, which is covered by a membrane called the **acrosome.** The acrosome contains enzymes that assist in the penetration of the ovum by the sperm (see Chapter 13). The neck of the sperm contains centrioles, which carry the chromosomal material of the sperm. The middle piece of the sperm contains mitochondria, arranged in a coil, which provide the sperm with energy. The tail, or flagellum, is long and moves the sperm through the female reproductive tract.

Spermatogenesis is hormonally mediated in the male. During puberty, the hypothalamus secretes releasing hormones, which stimulate the anterior pituitary gland to secrete FSH and ICSH.

FSH stimulates the production of sperm by the seminiferous tubules; ICSH stimulates the interstitial cells of Leydig to secrete testosterone. When the testosterone levels in the blood are elevated during sperm production, a substance called inhibin is released from the Sertoli cells. This substance inhibits the release of FSH by the anterior pituitary gland. Also, the elevated testosterone levels inhibit the release of ICSH so that the interstitial cells of Leydig

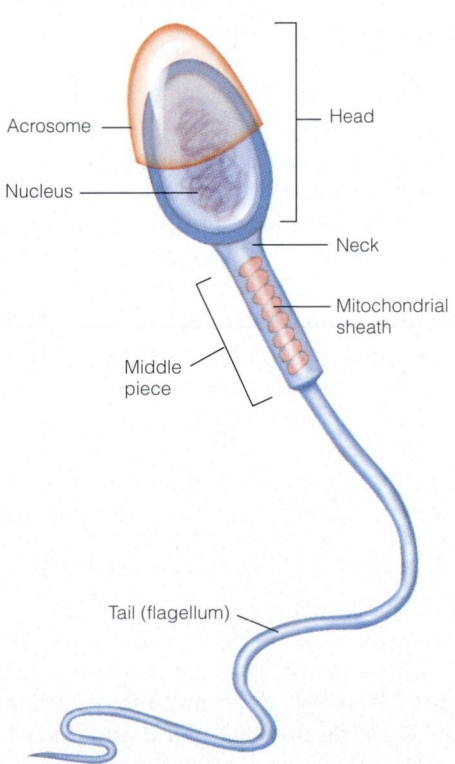

FIGURE 6–9. Structure of the sperm.

do not produce testosterone. As the blood levels of testosterone drop, the inhibitory effects of inhibin and testosterone on FSH and ICSH are lost; FSH again stimulates the seminiferous tubules to produce sperm and ICSH stimulates the production of testosterone.

Testosterone and other male hormones secreted by the testes, as well as steroids secreted by the adrenal cortex, are called androgens. Testosterone, the most prevalent and potent of the testicular hormones, stimulates the development of the secondary sex characteristics in the male and is needed for the production of mature sperm and seminal fluid. It is produced throughout the life of a man, although secretions of testosterone begin diminishing after the age of 40.

Epididymis

The **epididymis** is a duct consisting of a coiled tubule that is located above and behind each testis. If stretched the tubule would measure about 20 ft (6 m) in length. Each epididymis extends from the efferent duct at the top of each testis to the ductus deferens. The purpose of the epididymis is to store sperm received from the seminiferous tubules. When the sperm enter the epididymis, they are immotile. After 2 to 3 weeks in the epididymis, the sperm become relatively motile and their maturation is completed. The wall of the epididymis consists of smooth muscle, which contracts during ejaculation, pushing the sperm into the ductus deferens.

Ductus Deferens (Vas Deferens)

The **ductus deferens** (vas deferens) is continuous with the duct of the epididymis and is approximately 18 in. (46 cm) long. It is made up of layers of smooth muscle. A ductus deferens arises from the posterior wall of each testis and joins the spermatic cord. After joining with the spermatic cord, each ductus deferens passes through the inguinal canal, enters the pelvic cavity, and passes downward to the posterior wall of the urinary bladder. Before reaching the entrance to the bladder, the ductus deferens enlarges. The enlargement, called the ampulla, is a place where sperm can be stored. Each ampulla joins with a duct from the seminal vesicle and becomes known as the ejaculatory duct.

Ejaculatory Ducts

The **ejaculatory duct** is continuous with the ductus deferens and is formed by the union of the seminal vesicle and the ductus deferens. The ejaculatory ducts extend through the prostate gland and end at the prostatic urethra. Each duct ejects sperm received from one of the testes into the prostatic urethra.

Urethra

The **urethra,** the passageway for both sperm and urine in the male, extends from the neck of the bladder to the glans penis. It is surrounded by the prostate gland and consists of three sections: prostatic urethra, membranous urethra, and cavernous urethra.

The prostatic urethra extends from the bladder through the prostate gland, where the ejaculatory ducts join it to the membranous urethra. The membranous urethra extends from the prostastic urethra through the urogenital diaphragm, the floor of the pelvic cavity, where it forms the urethral sphincter. The membranous urethra becomes the cavernous urethra, which is made up of spongy erectile tissue and extends through the penis. The reproductive purpose of the urethra is to eject semen (the fluid containing spermatozoa) outside the body.

▶ Accessory Glands

The **accessory glands** of the male reproductive system consist of the seminal vesicles, the prostate gland, and the bulbourethral glands (Cowper's glands). The male accessory glands secrete materials into the semen. The purpose of these secretions is to provide nutrients to the sperm and to increase the fluid in which the sperm are transported.

Seminal Vesicles

The **seminal vesicles** are two pouchlike structures that join the end of each ductus deferens to become the ejaculatory ducts. The seminal vesicles secrete a viscous fluid that contains fructose, fibrinogen, proteins, and prostaglandins. During ejaculation, the fructose provides energy to the sperm, increasing the motility and fertilizing ability of the sperm. Fibrinogen, a plasma protein, adds to the viscosity of the seminal fluid. Proteins provide nutrients to the sperm. Prostaglandins may assist the movement of the sperm to the female fallopian tubes by stimulating uterine contractions.

Prostate Gland

The **prostate gland,** a single gland located beneath the bladder, surrounds the base of the urethra and adds to the semen by secreting a milky fluid. The fluid assists in the motility of the sperm and contributes to the alkalinity of the semen because it contains bicarbonate ions. Prostatic secretions also contain small amounts of lipids, enzymes, and citric acid.

The prostate gland has several lobes, measures approximately 4 cm in diameter, and is made up of both glandular and muscular tissue. When the muscular tissue contracts, the milky fluid is secreted into the urethra.

Bulbourethral Glands

The **bulbourethral glands (Cowper's glands)** are located in the urogenital diaphragm on either side of the membranous urethra. These glands secrete a lubricating substance that coats the surface of the urethra. This fluid is alkaline and assists in neutralizing the acidic environment of the male urethra and female vagina. This increases the viability of sperm, which need an alkaline environment for survival.

▶ Semen

Semen, or seminal fluid, is ejaculated with the sperm from an erect penis. It consists of the secretions of the accessory glands and the epididymis. Each ejaculate contains 2 to 6 mL of fluid with a pH of 7.35 to 7.50. The alkalinity of the fluid buffers the sperm from the acidity of the vaginal secretions. Each milliliter of semen contains about 50 to 150 million sperm. In addition to other substances, the seminal fluid contains the enzyme hyaluronidase, which helps the sperm penetrate the ovum.

▶ Transport of Spermatozoa

After the spermatids are formed, they are pushed into the epididymis, which stores the sperm and contributes secretions to the seminal fluid. The sperm begin to move in the epididymis. Through muscular contraction, the sperm are transported from the epididymis to the ductus deferens. When the ductus deferens contracts, the sperm are transported to the duct of the seminal vesicle. The seminal vesicle adds nutrients to the seminal fluid and joins the ejaculatory duct. The ejaculatory duct transports the sperm through the prostate gland to the prostatic urethra, where the sperm exit the body through the penis at the external urethral opening (see Fig. 6–8).

There is no cyclic nature to the production and transport of sperm. Sperm are viable in the male reproductive tract for several weeks. When mature sperm are ejaculated, they live for 48 to 72 hours in the female reproductive tract. Sperm that are not ejaculated dissolve and are reabsorbed.

▶ THE FEMALE REPRODUCTIVE SYSTEM

The female reproductive system consists of external and internal genital organs. The external organs are called the **vulva** or pudendum and include the mons veneris (mons pubis), labia majora, labia minora, clitoris, vaginal vestibule, urethral meatus, introitus and hymen, opening of Skene's glands and Bartholin's glands, and perineum. The internal organs include the ovaries, fallopian tubes (oviducts), uterus, and vagina (Figs. 6–10 and 6–11). The structures of the female reproductive tract are needed for copulation, fertilization, implantation of the fertilized ovum, and development and birth of the fetus.

▶ External Genital Organs

Mons Veneris (Mons Pubis)

The **mons veneris** (mons pubis) is a fatty pad that covers the anterior portion of the symphysis pubis (Fig. 6–10). After puberty, the female mons veneris is covered by curly hair distributed in a triangular pattern. The base of the triangle is formed at the upper margin of the symphysis pubis. The apex of the triangle of hair growth is found over the labia majora. This triangular distribution of hair is referred to as the escutcheon and may differ in women of varying ethnic backgrounds. The mons veneris acts as a cushion for the pelvic bones.

Labia Majora

The **labia majora,** two lateral folds of adipose tissue covered by skin and hair, extend posteriorly from the mons veneris to the anterior border of the perineum, where they merge to form the posterior commissure. The labia majora are approximately 7 to 8 cm long, 2 to 3 cm wide, and 1 to 1.5 cm thick.

The labia majora are covered with stratified squamous epithelium that is richly supplied with sebaceous glands. Beneath the skin is a layer of thin, poorly developed muscle, called the tunica dartos labialis, and a mass of adipose tissue. In nulliparous women, the inner surface of the labia majora looks like a mucous membrane, whereas in multiparous women, it appears more skinlike. After repeated childbearing, the labia majora are less prominent and with menopause they begin to atrophy (Cunningham et al., 1997).

Blood is supplied to the labia majora from the internal and external pudendal arteries. The labia majora have extensive venous drainage. The veins communicate with the dorsal vein of the clitoris, the veins of the labia minora, and the perineal veins. This extensive plexus of veins can result in varicosities during pregnancy and can contribute to hematoma formation during labor and delivery (Cunningham et al., 1997).

The labia majora also have an extensive lymphatic system both under the skin and deeper within the subcutaneous tissue. Innervation is also extensive,

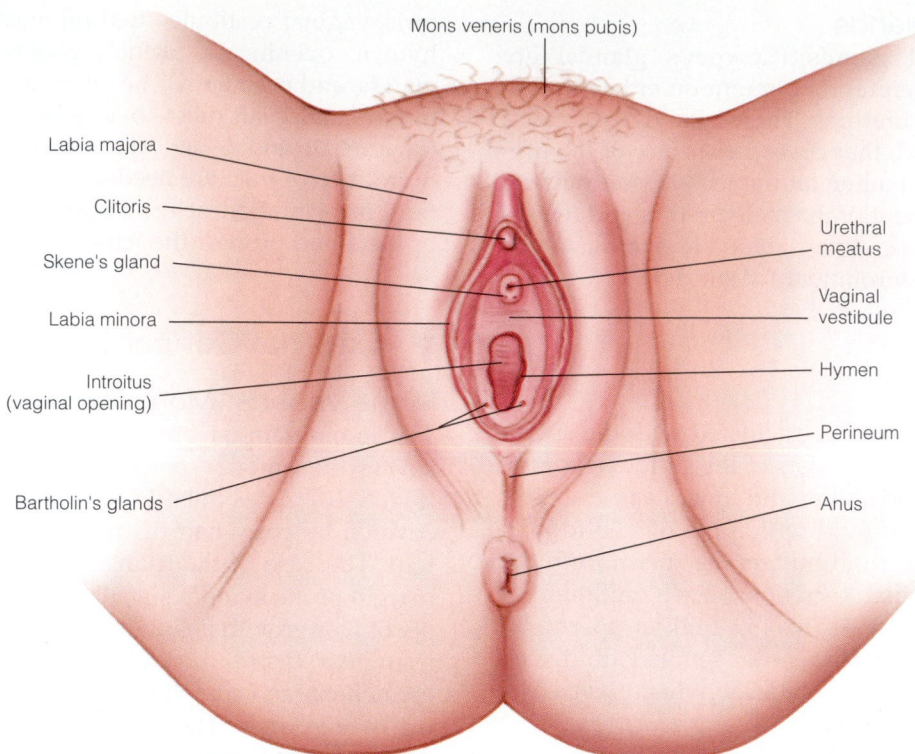

FIGURE 6–10. External female reproductive organs (adult parous woman). (*Reproduced, with permission, from DeCherney, A.H., & Pernoll, M.L. (1994).* Current obstetric and gynecologic diagnosis and treatment *(8th ed.). Norwalk, CT: Appleton & Lange, p.16.)*

involving the anterior hypogastric nerves, which supply the superior portion of the labia majora, and the posterior iliac nerves, which innervate the gluteal area. The nerve supply makes the labia majora sensitive to painful stimuli, pressure, and temperature.

Labia Minora

The **labia minora,** two thin, pink folds of tissue located on the inner surface of the labia majora, extend dorsally on either side of the vaginal orifice and are not covered with hair. The labia minora are covered with stratified squamous epithelial cells, which are continuous with the mucous membrane of the vagina. The tissues of the labia minora unite to form two thin plates of skin: the lower plate forms the frenulum of the clitoris, and the upper plate forms the prepuce of the clitoris. Inferiorly, the labia minora extend toward the perineum and fuse to form the fourchette. The fourchette, the posterior ring of the vaginal introitus (opening), is easily visible in nulliparous women. In multiparous women, the labia minora usually appear as if they are part of the labia majora (Cunningham et al., 1997).

The interior folds of the labia minora consist of erectile tissue containing many blood vessels. The main arteries supplying the labia minora come from the superficial perineal artery and from the rete of the labia majora. Venous drainage is by way of the perineal and vaginal veins. The labia minora are supplied by many nerve endings, making them very sensitive to stimuli such as touch.

Clitoris

The **clitoris** is a small structure found posterior to the mons veneris. It is similar to the penis in the male because it is made up of erectile tissue that is highly sensitive to sexual arousal. The clitoris has a richer nerve supply than the male penis, being innervated primarily through the terminal branch of the pudendal nerve.

The clitoris consists of a glans, a corpus (body), and two crura. The glans contains spindle-shaped cells, which are highly sensitive to stimuli. It is covered by the prepuce, a hoodlike structure formed by the labia minora. The body is made up of two corpora cavernosa, similar to the corpus spongiosum in the male penis. The crura extend laterally and are attached to the inferior rami of the pubis to form the central body of the clitoris.

The pudendal artery supplies blood to the clitoris. The nerve supply is mainly found within the prepuce. The clitoris is one of the principal erogenous

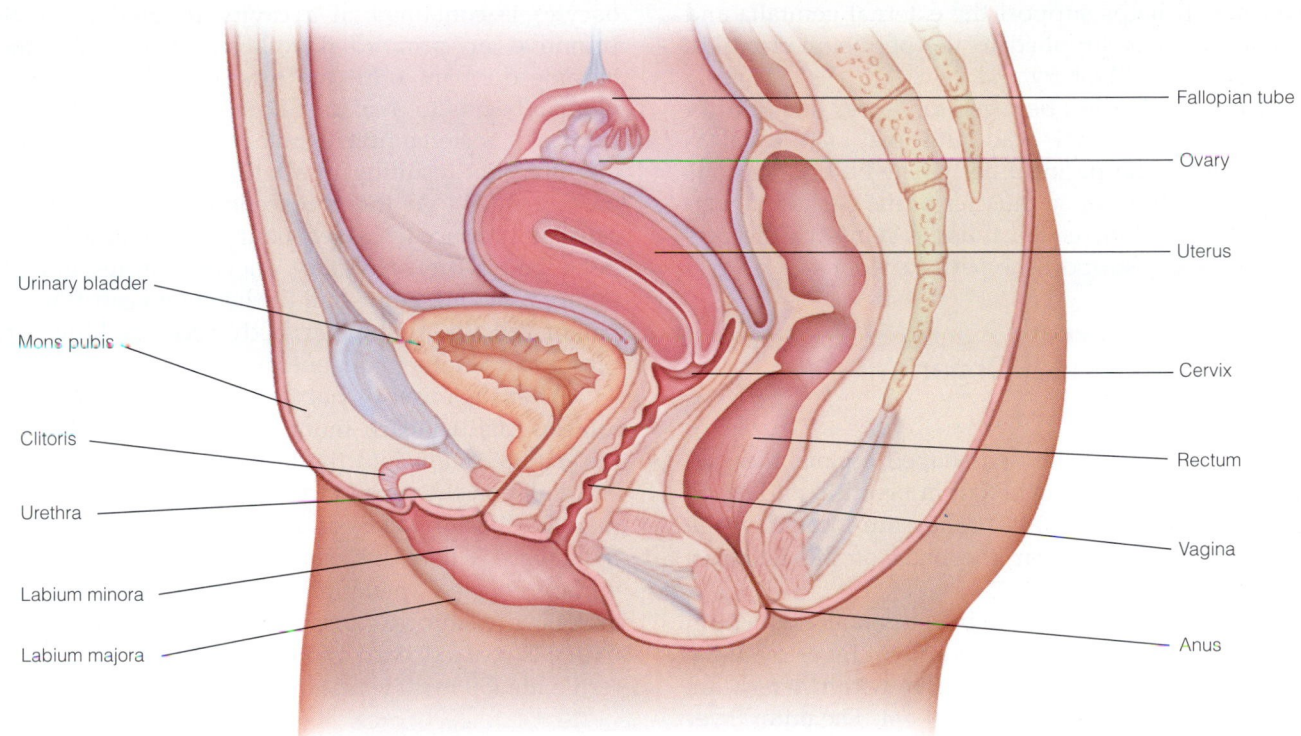

FIGURE 6–11. Internal female reproductive organs.

organs of women; it rarely exceeds 2 cm in length even in a state of erection (Cunningham et al., 1997).

Vaginal Vestibule

The vaginal vestibule is an almond-shaped area extending from the clitoris to the fourchette. The urethral meatus (the opening of the urethra), the introitus (the opening of the vagina) and hymen, and the openings of the ducts of Bartholin's and Skene's glands are found in the vestibule.

Urethral Meatus. The **urethral meatus** is in the middle of the vestibule, 1 to 1.5 cm below the clitoris. It is located above the vaginal opening and appears slitlike and puckered.

The **paraurethral glands (Skene's glands)** usually open on either side of the urethra. The openings are small, each measuring about 0.5 mm in diameter. Skene's glands secrete a lubricating substance into the vaginal vestibule.

Introitus and Hymen. The **introitus** is located in the lower portion of the vestibule and differs in size and shape among women. The introitus may be partially covered by a thin, connective tissue membrane called the **hymen.** The hymen may be ruptured through sexual intercourse, physical activity, or use of tampons. The idea that virginity can be established by an intact hymen is false, although some cultures may still adhere to this belief. Once the hymen is ruptured, hymenal tags called hymenal caruncles (carunculae myrtiformes) remain.

Bartholin's glands open on either side of the introitus at approximately 5 and 7 o'clock above the bulbocavernous muscles of the vagina. They are a pair of glands measuring 0.5 to 1 cm in diameter. The ducts are 1.5 to 2.0 cm long and transport a secretion originating in the glands.

The glands lubricate the introitus with a clear, viscous secretion, particularly at the time of sexual arousal.

Perineum

The **perineum** is the area between the vagina and the anus. It is made up of connective tissue, muscles, fascia, and adipose tissue. The pelvic diaphragm and the urogenital diaphragm support the perineum. The pelvic diaphragm consists of the levator ani and coccygeus muscles, which support the pelvic structures. Between the levator muscles pass the vagina, urethra, and rectum. The urogenital diaphragm, which is found below the pelvic diaphragm, consists of deep transverse perineal muscles, the sphincter of the membranous urethra, and internal and external fascial coverings. It helps support the external genitalia and vagina. Blood is supplied to the perineum from the internal pudendal artery and vein.

The area that lies between the lower one third of the posterior vaginal wall and the anal canal is referred to as the perineal body. The bulbocavernous muscles, the transverse muscles of the perineum, and the external sphincter ani muscles reinforce the perineal body and support the perineal floor.

▶ Internal Genital Organs

Ovaries

The **ovaries** are two almond-shaped organs, measuring 2 to 5 cm in length, 1.5 cm in breadth, and 0.6 to 1.5 cm in width (Fig. 6–11). They are located in the upper pelvic cavity near the ends of the fallopian tubes.

Each ovary is covered by germinal epithelium and consists of an outer cortex and an inner medulla. The cortex contains epithelial cells, within which are ova in various stages of development. The outer layer of the cortex is made up of the tunica albuginea. The medulla consists of loose connective tissue, numerous arteries and veins, some smooth muscle fibers, nerves, and lymphatic vessels.

The ovaries are supported by uteroovarian ligaments, mesovarium, and infundibulopelvic ligament. The uteroovarian ligaments are made up of connective tissue and muscle fibers. They extend from the uterine cornua (part of the uterus where the fallopian tubes open) to the lower pole of the ovary, anchoring the ovary to the uterus.

The mesovarium is a short tissue, consisting of two layers of peritoneum, which connect the ovary to the posterior portion of the broad ligament. The mesovarium contains branches of the ovarian and uterine arteries.

The infundibulopelvic ligament is the suspensory ligament of the ovary. It consists of a fold of peritoneum arising from the upper, outer pole of the broad ligament and extending to the pelvic wall. The infundibulopelvic ligament supports and suspends the ovary. It attaches to the mesovarium and contains the ovarian artery, veins, and nerves, which branch off into the mesovarium.

The functions of the ovary are development and expulsion of ova and secretion of the female hormones, estrogen and progesterone. The process by which the mature ova are formed is called oogenesis.

Oogenesis. In the female, ovum formation is called **oogenesis.** Primitive oogonia enlarge to form primary oocytes before birth. Each of the primary oocytes is contained in a cavity referred to as the primitive or primordial follicle. These cells then become dormant until the time of puberty, when a woman begins to ovulate. Shortly before ovulation, a primary oocyte completes meiosis I, or the first meiotic division, resulting in a haploid number of chromosomes (23). At the completion of meiosis I, two cells are produced, the secondary oocyte and the first polar body. The secondary oocyte matures into the ovum, receiving almost all of the cytoplasm from the parent cell; the first polar body receives little cytoplasm and begins to degenerate.

After the onset of puberty, one of the primordial follicles matures each month and ruptures, releasing the mature ovum into the fallopian tube (ovulation). At ovulation the secondary oocyte begins the second meiotic division (meiosis II) but progresses only to metaphase, where division is arrested. When the secondary oocyte is penetrated by a sperm, the second meiotic division is completed. Usually one mature ovum is formed each month throughout a female's fertile life (30 to 40 years).

Fallopian Tubes (Oviducts)

Two **fallopian tubes,** also referred to as **oviducts** and uterine tubes, extend laterally from the uterine cornua to the ovaries. Each measures approximately 8 to 14 cm in length and is divided into four areas: (1) interstitial portion, (2) isthmus, (3) ampulla, and (4) infundibulum. The interstitial portion is found within the uterine musculature and extends upward and outward from the uterine cavity. The isthmus is the narrow, straight portion of the tube that adjoins the uterus. The isthmus passes into the wider, more tortuous portion called the ampulla. The ampulla ends in the funnel-shaped infundibulum, which is covered with projections called **fimbriae.** The fimbriated end of the tube opens into the peritoneal cavity. The longest of the fimbriae, the fimbria ovarica, forms a shallow gutter that reaches the ovary.

The wall of the tube is made up of four tissue layers, as described below:

- Serous (or peritoneal): completely covers the tube except for a small portion at the lower border.
- Subserous: contains the blood and nerve supply to the tube.
- Muscular: arranged in an inner, circular and an outer, longitudinal shape, which is more prominent at the uterine end of the tube. The musculature of the tube is responsible for the continuous rhythmic tubal contractions, which become more intense at the time of ovulation.

- Mucous: contains ciliated epithelial cells, which are found most abundantly at the fimbriated end of the tube. At the time of ovulation, the cilia at the fimbriated end of the tube assist in directing the ovum into the tube; the cilia in the rest of the tube propel the ovum toward the uterus.

Blood is supplied to the fallopian tubes by the ovarian and uterine arteries. The nerves that supply the tubes are derived from the parasympathetic and sympathetic nervous systems.

Fertilization occurs in the distal third of the fallopian tube, and the fertilized ovum is transported through the tube to the uterus (see Chapter 13). The environment in the tube assists in the nourishment of the fertilized ovum before it reaches the protection of the uterus.

Uterus

The **uterus** is a pear-shaped, muscular organ, which in the nonpregnant woman is situated between the urinary bladder and the rectum. It varies in size and shape according to age and number of pregnancies. In the prepubertal girl, the uterus measures from 2.5 to 3.5 cm. Before the first pregnancy, the uterus of the adult woman measures approximately 5.5 to 8 cm and weighs from 50 to 60 g. In women who have been pregnant the uterus measures 9 to 10 cm in length and weighs about 80 g.

Blood is supplied to the uterus by the uterine and ovarian arteries. The uterine artery, the terminal branch of the hypogastric arteries, is the principal source of blood to the uterus. The ovarian artery, a branch of the aorta, divides into small branches as it extends to the ovary. The main stem of the ovarian artery anastomoses to the ovarian branch of the uterine artery (Fig. 6–12). Both the uterine and ovarian arteries enter the uterus via the broad ligament. Blood from the uterus and vagina is returned through a venous plexus, the uterovaginal plexus, which is located in the uterine muscle. The uterovaginal plexus joins the uterine vein and empties into the hypogastric vein.

The nerve supply for the uterus is derived from the sympathetic and parasympathetic nervous systems. The sympathetic nervous system causes muscular contraction, whereas the parasympathetic nervous system inhibits uterine muscular contraction.

The uterus has the ability to increase to 500 times its capacity during pregnancy. It provides a safe, nourishing environment for the fertilized ovum to grow and develop. During labor, the muscular contractions of the uterus help the descent and expulsion of the products of conception.

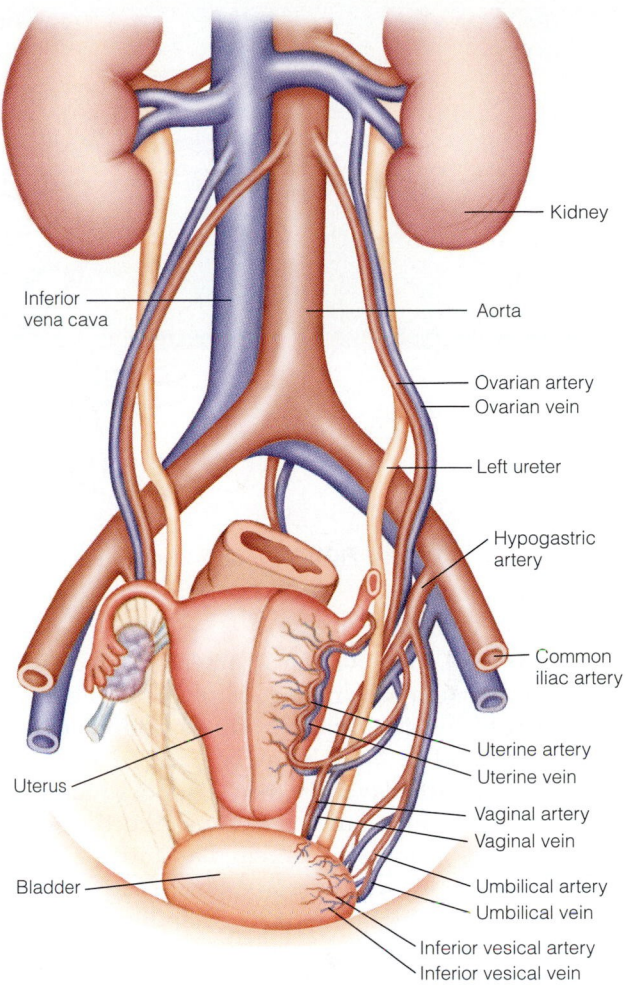

FIGURE 6–12. Blood supply to the internal female reproductive organs.

The uterus is divided into two major parts, the corpus, or upper two thirds, and the cervix, or lower third. The upper portion of the corpus, extending above the attachment of the fallopian tubes, is called the fundus.

Corpus. The **corpus,** or body, of the uterus is made up of three layers: the perimetrium, or outer serous layer; the myometrium, or muscular middle layer; and the endometrium, or innermost layer.

The **perimetrium** is formed by peritoneum, extending from the anterior wall of the uterus to the surface of the bladder. It also covers the surface of the superior vaginal fornix and forms the anterior wall of the pouch of Douglas. At the lateral margins of the uterus, the peritoneum forms broad ligaments.

The **myometrium** is continuous with the muscular layer of the fallopian tubes and the vagina. The smooth muscle fibers of this layer extend into the

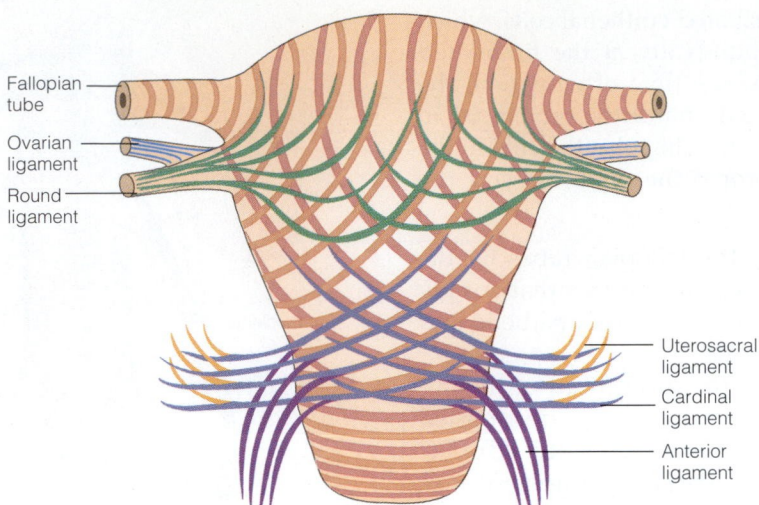

Fallopian
tube

Ovarian
ligament

Round
ligament

Uterosacral
ligament

Cardinal
ligament

Anterior
ligament

FIGURE 6–13. Schematic arrangement of directions of muscles of the myometrium.

round, cardinal, and ovarian ligaments. Three layers of muscles make up the myometrium. The outer layer is composed of longitudinal fibers found mostly around the fundus; these help expel the fetus during labor. The middle layer is made up of interlacing muscle fibers, which run in various directions. The inner layer is composed of circular muscle fibers, which hypertrophy, forming a sphincter at the internal os of the cervix (Fig. 6–13). The bundles of smooth muscle of the myometrium are united by connective tissue.

The **endometrium** is made up of a single layer of ciliated columnar epithelium, glands, and stroma. The thickness of the endometrial lining depends on the stage of the menstrual cycle, and ranges from 0.5 to 5 mm.

Late in the menstrual cycle, under the influence of estrogen and progesterone, the endometrial layer is composed of two layers: the surface layer, or zona functionalis, and deep layer, or zona basalis. The zona functionalis is expelled during menstruation, whereas the zona basalis remains.

The glands extend through the whole surface of the endometrium. They secrete a thin alkaline fluid that keeps the uterus moist, assists in the transport of sperm, and nourishes the fertilized ovum before its implantation in the uterus.

The endometrial lining also has coiled or spiral arteries, which respond to hormonal influence during the menstrual cycle and pregnancy. During pregnancy, these arteries contribute to the blood supply of the placenta (see Chapter 13).

Isthmus. The **isthmus** of the uterus is located between the corpus and the cervix. It measures 5 to 7

mm and is significant during pregnancy because it is necessary to the formation of the lower uterine segment (see Chapter 15).

Cervix. The lowest portion of the uterus, or the neck, is called the **cervix.** The cervix is 2 to 3 cm long. The **internal os** of the cervix divides the uterine cavity (corpus) and the cervical canal. The **external os** of the cervix opens into the vagina.

The muscular wall of the cervix is not as thick as that of the corpus of the uterus. It is composed mainly of collagenous and elastic tissue, which gives the cervix the ability to stretch during the labor and delivery process.

The cervical canal is also lined with columnar ciliated epithelium, containing mucus-secreting glands. The cervical mucosa provides an alkaline environment for the sperm during ovulation and lubrication for the vaginal canal.

The cervix is divided into a vaginal portion and a supravaginal portion. The lower area of the vaginal portion of the cervix is referred to as the portico vaginalis, or ectocervix. At the lower extremity of the ectocervix is the external cervical os. On speculum examination, the external os varies in appearance. Before childbirth it is regular and spherical in appearance; after childbirth it appears like a transverse slit that divides the external os into anterior and posterior lips (Fig. 6–14).

The ectocervix is lined with squamous stratified epithelium, which is continuous with the squamous epithelium of the vagina. The point at which the squamous epithelium and the columnar epithelium meet is called the **squamocolumnar junction.** The location of the squamocolumnar junction differs according to

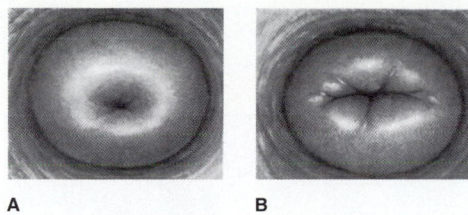

FIGURE 6–14. Appearance of the external os. **A.** Before childbirth. **B.** After childbirth. *(Reproduced, with permission, from Cunningham et al. (1997). Williams obstetrics (20th ed.). Stamford, CT: Appleton & Lange, p. 47.)*

age and number of deliveries. In women who have given birth one or more times, the squamous epithelium may extend up the cervical canal, lining up to one half of the canal. The lips of the cervix in a woman who has given birth may also appear everted (ectropion).

The supravaginal segment of the cervix is covered with peritoneum on its posterior surface. It is surrounded by the pubocervical, uterosacral, and transverse cervical ligaments, which provide stability to the uterus.

Ligaments of the Uterus. The uterus is supported in the pelvic cavity by ligaments, which include the broad, round, and uterosacral or sacrouterine ligaments (Figs. 6–13 and 6–15).

The **broad ligaments** extend on either side of the uterus to the pelvic floor, dividing the pelvic cavity into anterior and posterior compartments. Each broad ligament consists of folds of peritoneum, continuous with those of the abdominal peritoneum. The folds of peritoneum are divided into upper and lower borders and form the following structures:

- Upper border: broad ligaments enfold the fallopian tubes (which are attached to the broad ligament at the mesosalpinx) and the ovarian and round ligaments and form the infundibulopelvic (or suspensory) ligament.
- Lower border: broad ligaments form the cardinal and anterior ligaments (consisting of dense connective tissue) that are joined to the supravaginal portion of the cervix and contain the uterine vessels and lower portion of the ureter.

The two **round ligaments** are found on either side of the fundus. They are continuous with the ovar-

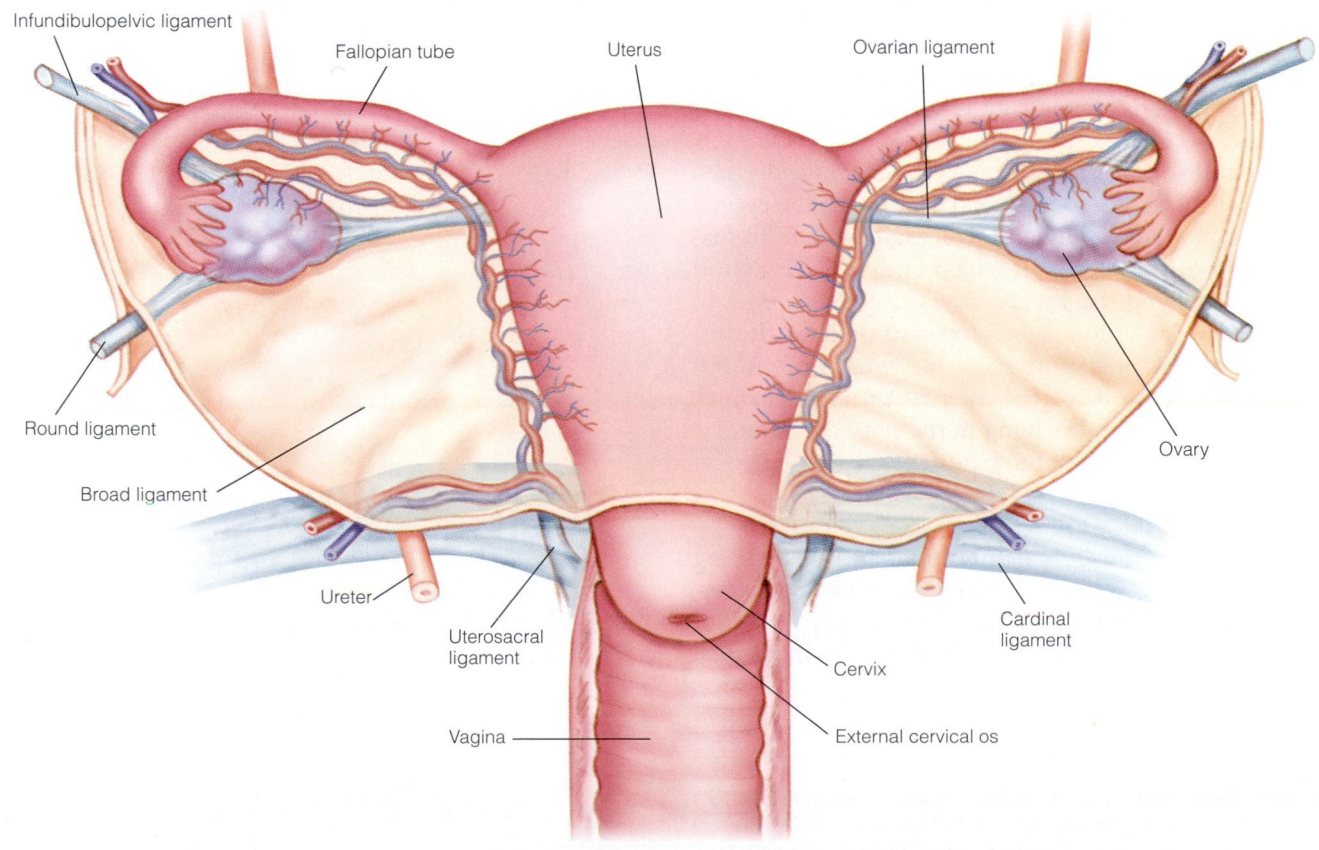

FIGURE 6–15. Ligaments of the uterus.

ian ligaments and run through the folds of peritoneum of the broad ligament. The round ligaments extend through the inguinal canal to the labia majora, attaching the uterus to the external genitalia. These ligaments consist of smooth muscle cells, connective tissue, blood vessels, and nerves. The round ligaments provide support to the uterus, especially during pregnancy when they enlarge considerably.

The two **uterosacral** (sacrouterine) **ligaments** extend from the supravaginal portion of the cervix to the sacrum. They insert on the lateral borders of the first and second sacral vertebrae. The uterosacral ligaments are covered with peritoneum and consist of connective tissue and some smooth muscle, blood vessels, and nerves. They serve to support the corpus and cervix, keeping the uterus in the anterior position.

Uterine Positions. The uterine position is not fixed within the pelvic cavity. The position may vary according to posture or gravity. If the nonpregnant woman is in an upright position, the body of the uterus is almost horizontal, flexed anteriorly, with the fundus resting on the bladder. The cervix is back toward the sacrum, with the external os at about the level of the ischial spines.

Displacement of the uterus may occur, causing a variation in the position of the organ. Women with variations in the position of the uterus may complain of symptoms such as back pain and dysmenorrhea. Examples of variations of uterine placement include retroflexion, retrocession, anteflexion, and retroversion (Fig. 6–16).

Retroflexion of the uterus is the term used when the corpus of the uterus bends back toward the cervix, resulting in a sharp angle. **Retrocession** refers to displacement of the uterus in which both the cervix and the corpus bend backward toward the sacrum. In **anteflexion,** the uterus bends forward on itself. **Retroversion** of the uterus may occur with or without retroflexion. A retroverted uterus turns backward, with the uterine fundus lying in the pouch of Douglas instead of anteriorly on the bladder.

Vagina

The **vagina** is a musculomembranous tube, extending from the uterus to the vulva and measuring an average 10 cm in length. It is located between the bladder and rectum. Anteriorly, the vagina comes in contact

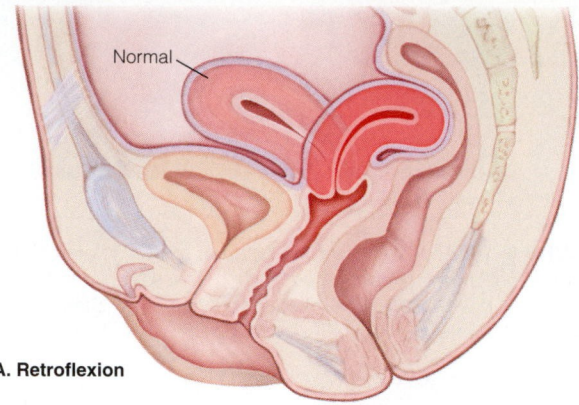

A. Retroflexion

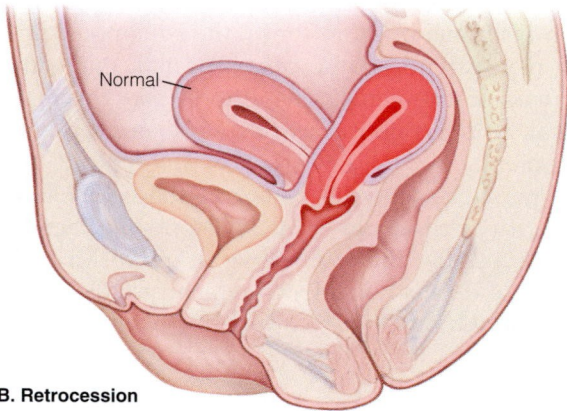

B. Retrocession

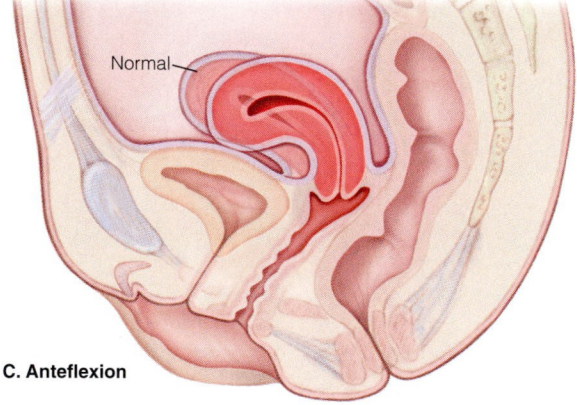

C. Anteflexion

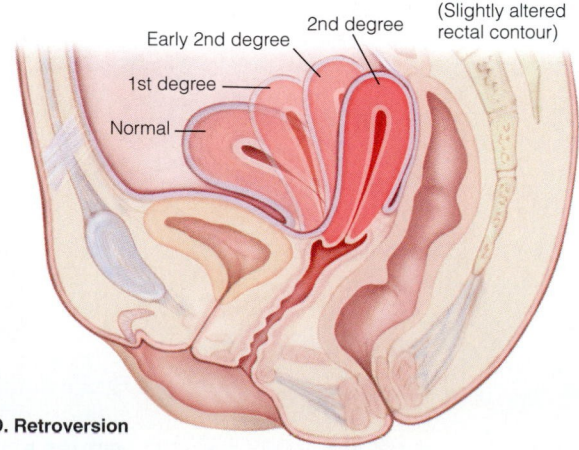

D. Retroversion

FIGURE 6–16. Variations in uterine position. *(Reproduced, with permission, from DeCherney, A.H., & Pernoll, M.L. (1994). Current obstetric and gynecologic diagnosis and treatment (8th ed.). Norwalk, CT: Appleton & Lange, p.16.)*

with the bladder and urethra. The connective tissue separating the vagina from the bladder and urethra is called the vesicovaginal septum. Posteriorly, between the lower portion of the vagina and rectum, the connective tissue separating the vagina from the rectum is called the rectovaginal septum.

The vaginal canal has many elastic folds or rugae in its muscular walls, allowing the canal to expand during intercourse and childbirth. Mucous membranes line the vaginal canal, and the hymen may partially cover the introitus. The mucosa of the vagina is made up of stratified squamous epithelium.

The lower portion of the cervix projects into the upper 1 to 2 cm of the vagina. A blind vault or recess surrounds this area, which is divided into anterior, posterior, and two lateral fornices. The posterior fornix is deeper than the anterior and lateral fornices because the vagina is attached higher on the posterior wall of the cervix than on the lateral or anterior walls. The anterior wall of the vagina measures 6 to 8 cm in length; the posterior wall measures 7 to 10 cm in length.

The environment of the vaginal canal is acidic and responds to hormonal levels throughout the menstrual cycle. When stimulated by estrogen, the vaginal mucosa metabolizes glycogen. Glycogen metabolism is promoted by lactobacilli, normal bacterial inhabitants of the vagina. As a result of glycogen metabolism, lactic acid is produced, causing the pH of the vagina to become acidic, ranging from 4.0 to 5.0 in an adult woman in the reproductive years. The acidic environment minimizes the possibility of vaginal infection.

The vagina receives its blood supply from branches of the uterine, inferior vesicle, and internal pudendal arteries. The network of veins follows the path of the arteries. Blood from the vagina is returned through the uterovaginal venous plexus, which empties into the hypogastric veins.

The vagina functions as the female organ of copulation and the passage for menstrual flow. It also forms part of the birth canal and is capable of significant distension and expansion during labor and delivery.

▶ Musculoskeletal Supports for the Genitalia

The female reproductive organs are supported by the bony pelvis. In addition, fibromuscular structures support the external and internal genital organs.

Bony Pelvis

The **bony pelvis** consists of four bones that are joined together by ligaments. The four bones include the paired innominate bones, the sacrum, and the coccyx. Each innominate (hip) bone is composed of the fusion of the ilium, the ischium, and the pubis. Anteriorly, the paired innominate bones are joined at the symphysis pubis and posteriorly they are joined to the sacrum, forming the sacroiliac joints.

The sacrum is a heavy bone that is formed by the union of five sacral vertebrae. The superior border of the sacrum is prominent because the sacrum is directed downward and backward. The sacral prominence is referred to as the sacral promontory, an important landmark when assessing the size of the female pelvis. The coccyx is loosely articulated with the lower border of the sacrum, making the coccyx movable. In some women the coccyx may be fused to the sacrum.

The pelvis is divided into two parts, the false pelvis and the true pelvis. The line that marks the false pelvis from the true pelvis is called the iliopectineal line, which is part of the linea terminalis. Above the iliopectineal line is the false pelvis, which is bounded posteriorly by the lumbar vertebrae, anteriorly by the abdominal wall, and laterally by the iliac fossae. The false pelvis has little significance in maternity care.

Below the iliopectineal line lies the true pelvis, which is significant in maternity care. The true pelvis may be divided into the pelvic inlet, midpelvis, and pelvic outlet, the dimensions of which are important to the passage of the fetus during labor and delivery. (See Chapter 15 for a complete discussion of the true pelvis.)

The true pelvis is classified according to its shape using the Caldwell–Moloy classification system. The pure types of pelvic shapes include gynecoid, android, anthropoid, and platypelloid (Fig. 6–17).

The **gynecoid pelvis** has a slightly oval inlet, with the anteroposterior diameter of the inlet being slightly less than the transverse diameter (Fig. 6–17A). The sides of the posterior segment of the pelvis are spacious and well rounded. The ischial spines are not prominent and the pubic arch is wide. The sacrum is somewhat hollow and the sacrosciatic notch is well rounded. This type of pelvis is also called the **female pelvis.** Its structure facilitates the passage of the fetus during labor and delivery. This type of pelvis is found in 50 to 55% of women.

The **android pelvis,** also known as the **male pelvis,** has a heart-shaped outline (Fig. 6–17B). This type of pelvis has a wedge-shaped inlet because the sides of the posterior segment tend to form a wedge at the juncture with the anterior segment. The anterior pelvis and the subpubic arch are narrow and the ischial spines are prominent. The sacrum inclines forward in the pelvis with little or no curvature, and the sacrosciatic notch is narrow. Women with android pelves (about 20%) usually need cesarean deliveries.

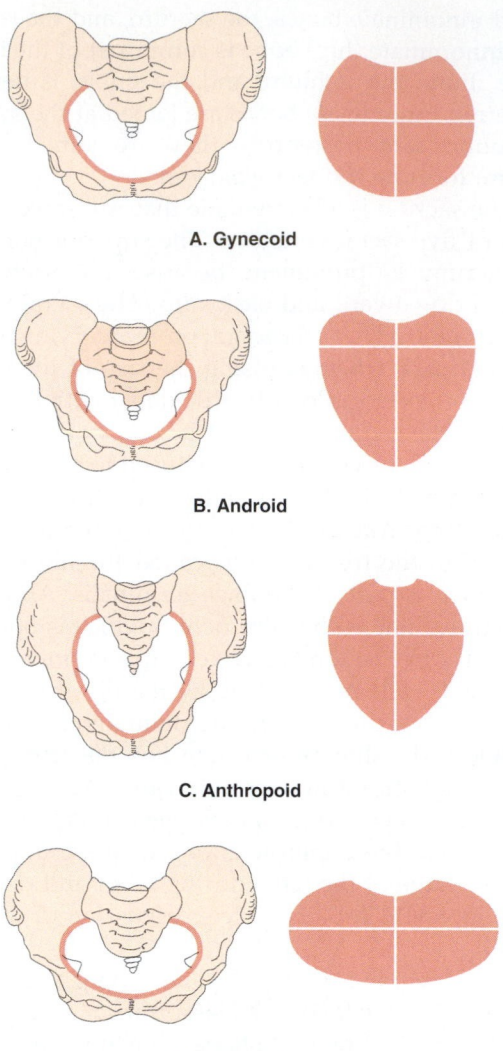

A. Gynecoid

B. Android

C. Anthropoid

D. Platypelloid

FIGURE 6–17. Variations of female pelves. Lines in diagrams at right (after Steele) show the greatest diameters of the pelves at left. *(Reproduced, with permission, from Benson, R.C. (1983). Handbook of obstetrics and gynecology (8th ed.). Los Altos, CA: Lange Medical Books.)*

The **anthropoid pelvis** (Fig. 6–17C) is oval in shape, with the largest diameter of the inlet running antero-posteriorly. The anterior and posterior segments are narrow and pointed and the walls are straight. The side walls converge and the sacrum is straight, making this type of pelvis deep. The interspinous diameter and the subpubic arch are wide and the ischial spines are prominent. The anthropoid pelvis is more common in non-Caucasian than in Caucasian women, making up about one fourth of the pure variety of pelves in Caucasian women and nearly one half of those in non-Caucasian women (Cunningham et al., 1997).

The **platypelloid pelvis** has a flattened gynecoid shape (Fig. 6–17D). The inlet is oval with a wide

transverse diameter and a short anteroposterior diameter. The posterior segment is flat and the angle of the anterior pelvis is wide. The interspinous diameter is also wide. In this type of pelvis, the sacrum is well curved and rotated backward, making the sacrum short, the pelvis shallow, and the sacrosciatic notch narrow. The platypelloid pelvis is rare in comparison with other pure pelvic varieties and is found in less than 3% of women.

Women's pelves may be one of the four pure types described above or may be of an intermediate or mixed type. When describing the intermediate pelvis, the posterior segment is described first and the anterior segment next (e.g., android–anthropoid) (Pernoll, 1991).

Pelvic Muscles

The pelvic structures are supported by the muscles of the pelvic floor, which insert at various points around the bony pelvis (Fig. 6–18). The pelvic floor consists of the muscular pelvic diaphragm, which separates the pelvic cavity from the perineal space. The levator ani muscles and the coccygeus muscle make up the pelvic diaphragm. Each of the levator ani muscles is, in turn, composed of pubococcygeus and iliococcygeus muscles. The pubococcygeus muscle is the most specialized of the muscles of the pelvic floor, expanding to allow delivery of the newborn and contracting to support the pelvic structures. The iliococcygeus muscles join the pubococcygeus muscle proper and insert into the lateral margins of the coccyx. These muscles act like a musculofascial layer.

The ischiococcygeus or coccygeus muscles occupy most of the posterior portion of the pelvic floor. They originate from the ischial spines and insert into the coccyx and the fifth sacral vertebra. These muscles supplement the levator ani muscles in supporting the pelvic contents. The obdurator internus muscles form the lateral walls of the pelvis.

The perineum lies below the pelvic diaphragm, bounded superiorly by the levator ani muscles and the coccygei. The central portion of the perineum, called the perineal body, is formed by the anal sphincter, two levator ani muscles, the superficial and deep transverse perineal muscles, and the bulbocavernosus muscles. These muscles reinforce the perineum and support the perineal floor.

Collectively the muscles of the pelvic floor are referred to as the circumvaginal muscles. Childbearing may weaken the tone of pelvic floor muscles, causing problems later in life, such as lack of urinary control. Research has demonstrated that exercise of these muscles before and during pregnancy improves the strength and tone of the circumvaginal muscles (see Chapters 9 and 28).

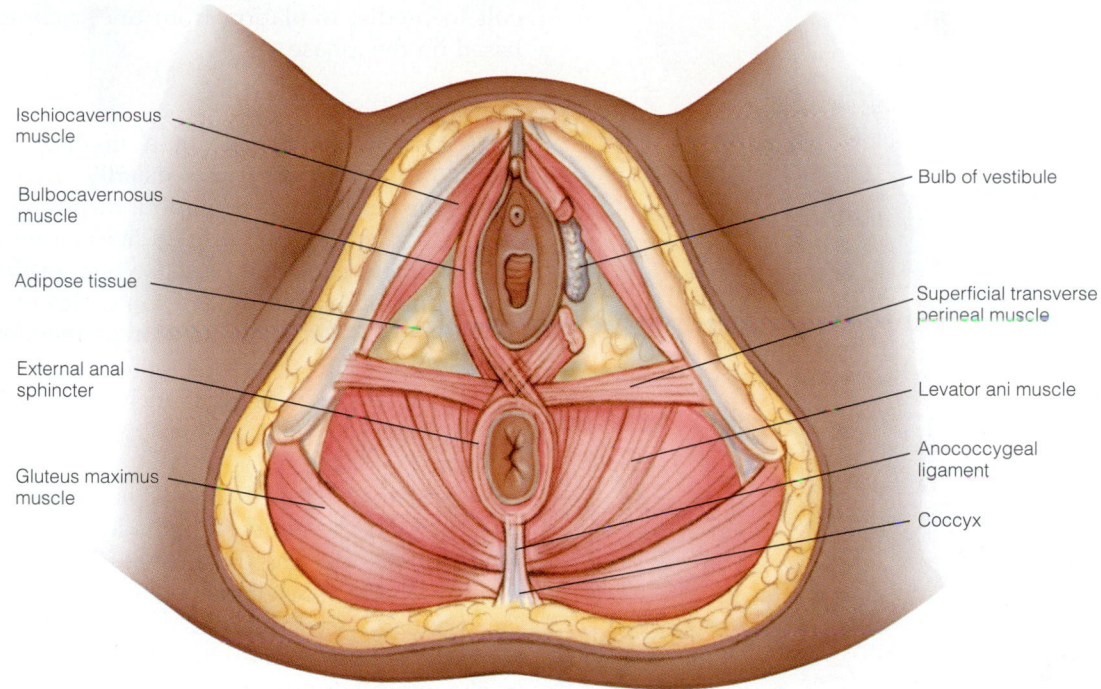

FIGURE 6–18. Pelvic musculature (inferior view). *(Reproduced, with permission, from DeCherney, A.H., & Pernoll, M.L. (1994). Current obstetric and gynecologic diagnosis and treatment (8th ed.). Norwalk, CT: Appleton & Lange, p.16.)*

► Mammary Glands (Breasts)

The **mammary glands** or breasts are considered accessory glands of the female reproductive system because of their role in lactation. The breasts, which are modified sebaceous glands, are located over the pectoral muscles on either side of the anterior wall of the chest.

Externally, each breast is covered with skin and has an areola and a nipple (Fig. 6–19). The **areola** is pigmented and contains modified sebaceous glands referred to as **Montgomery's glands.** Montgomery's glands make the surface of the areola rough. In the center of the areola is the nipple, which consists of erectile tissue. Milk ducts drain milk into the nipple during lactation.

Internally, each breast is divided into 15 to 20 lobes. Each lobe is further divided into lobules consisting of glandular tissue within adipose tissue. The size of the breasts is determined by the amount of adipose tissue they contain and has no relationship to the ability to lactate. The lobules contain acinic cells, which are composed of connective tissue and capillaries. The milk is secreted from the acinic cells into the mammary ducts. The mammary ducts dilate as they reach the nipple to form ampullae, where the milk is stored. They narrow as they approach the nipple and

are known as **lactiferous ducts.** The lactiferous ducts transport the milk from the ampullae to the nipple.

Blood is supplied to the breasts by the intercostal and internal mammary arteries. Blood from the mammary glands is returned through the mammary veins.

► THE MENSTRUAL CYCLE

The **menstrual cycle** occurs cyclically in the sexually mature female throughout the reproductive years. It comprises two interrelated cycles, the ovarian and the endometrial, which occur continuously and influence the ability of a woman to reproduce. The menstrual cycle begins with the first day of menstruation and ends with the onset of menses the following month. The length of the cycle may vary from about 24 to 35 days, averaging 28 days. The duration of the menstrual flow is variable, lasting anywhere from 2 to 8 days.

► Ovarian Cycle

The **ovarian cycle** may be divided into four parts for descriptive purposes: follicular phase, ovulation, luteal phase, and premenstrual phase.

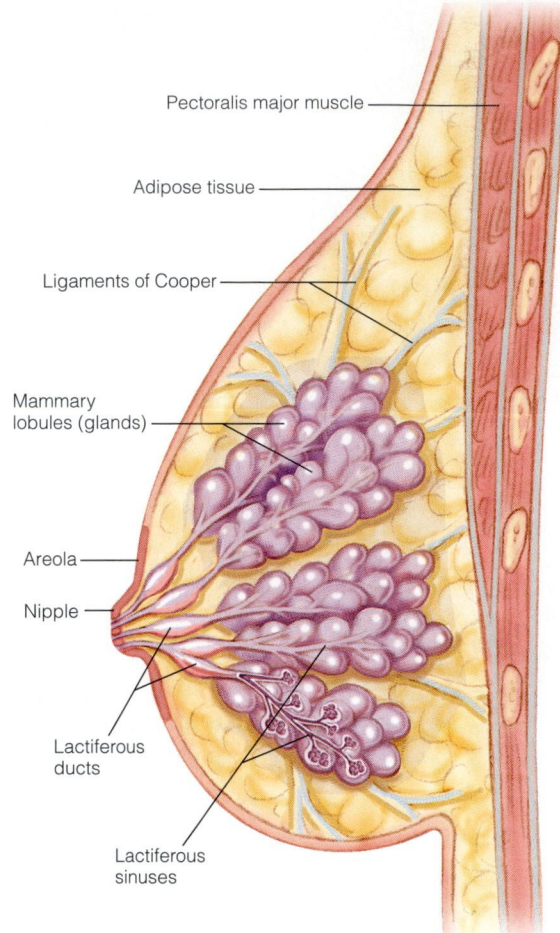

Pectoralis major muscle

Adipose tissue

Ligaments of Cooper

Mammary
lobules (glands)

Areola

Nipple

Lactiferous
ducts

Lactiferous
sinuses

FIGURE 6–19. Anatomy of the mammary gland and supportive structures.

Follicular Phase

The follicular phase begins about the third to the fifth day of the cycle; there is great variability in its length. During this phase, FSH secreted by the anterior pituitary gland stimulates a number of primitive or primordial follicles to develop. Each of the follicles contains an immature ovum. A proliferation of cells occurs within the follicles, stimulated by FSH, with follicular fluid developing between the cells. The hormone estrogen is secreted by all of the developing follicles, but secretion is greatest in the dominant follicle that will reach maturity. As the estrogen secretion increases, it triggers a negative feedback mechanism in the hypothalamus and anterior pituitary gland, inhibiting the secretion of FSH. When the ovum in the dominant follicle reaches maturity, the follicle ruptures and the ovum is expelled during ovulation. Only the dominant follicle matures to this point; the other follicles are pushed aside and degenerate. The length of the follicular phase varies so that it is diffi-

cult to predict ovulation from one cycle to the next based on this phase.

Ovulation

Ovulation is the release of a mature, unfertilized ovum from the ovary and usually occurs 14 days before the next menstrual period. If sperm are present, fertilization will occur 24 to 48 hours after ovulation. Because there is a brief period when fertilization can occur, it is important to have some idea of the timing of ovulation when planning a pregnancy. Women can be taught the subjective signs that sometimes accompany ovulation. These signs include ovulatory cervical muccorrhea and ovulatory pain called mittelschmerz.

Ovulatory cervical muccorrhea occurs for 1 to 3 days around the time of ovulation. Women can be taught to be alert to the increased slippery vaginal discharge, which resembles the uncooked white of an egg. Ovulatory cervical muccorrhea is "runny" in consistency, and a woman will have a slippery sensation as she wipes her vulva after urination.

A second sign of ovulation, ovulatory pain or **mittelschmerz,** occurs in approximately 25% of women. The pain occurs at the time of ovulation in either lower quadrant, although it is more frequent in the lower right quadrant. Ovulatory pain may also alternate regularly from one side to the other in successive cycles. The pain is located over the ovarian region (suprapubic) and is frequently accompanied by pressure and ache in the rectum and a feeling of gaseous distension. The pain lasts from 1 to 3 days, with the peak of the discomfort at the estimated time of ovulation.

Objective signs of ovulation include changes in basal body temperature, spinnbarkeit, and the fern pattern of the cervical mucus. See Chapter 10 for a discussion about basal body temperature analysis.

Spinnbarkeit, or elasticity of the ovulatory cervical mucus, is a helpful guide in predicting the day of ovulation. Activity of the endocervical glands is maximal at the time of ovulation because of the increase in secretion of estrogen by the ovary. Within 2 to 3 days before ovulation, there is a dramatic change in the cervical mucus, from no elasticity to an ability to stretch an average of 10 to 20 cm. There is a rapid decrease in this ability after ovulation (Fig. 6–20). Spinnbarkeit is also a sign that the viscosity of the cervical mucus is such as to enhance mobilization of the sperm through the mucus.

Another objective sign of ovulation is the absence of **ferning,** the fernlike pattern of the cervical mucus under microscopic examination. About the time of ovulation, ferning reaches its maximum profusion because of the high estrogen levels. After ovulation,

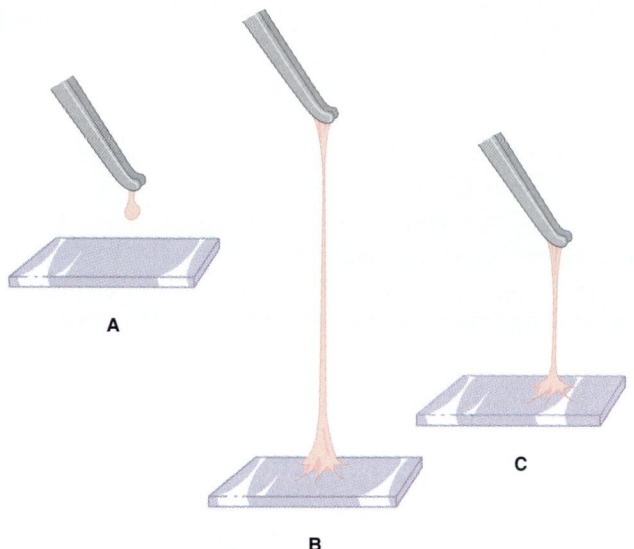

FIGURE 6–20. Determining elasticity of cervical mucus (spinnbarkeit) to predict day of ovulation. **A.** Three days before ovulation. **B.** Day of ovulation. **C.** Day after ovulation.

the cervical mucus no longer manifests this pattern because progesterone is present. The degree of fern pattern is usually directly related to the degree of muccorrhea and spinnbarkeit.

Luteal Phase

After ovulation, the cells in the ruptured follicle increase in size and fill with a yellow material called lutein. The follicle is now called the corpus luteum, or yellow body. Luteinizing hormone is secreted by the anterior pituitary gland and stimulates the corpus luteum to secrete progesterone. During the luteal phase, both estrogen and progesterone are secreted by the follicle. If fertilization does not occur, the corpus luteum reaches full development in 8 to 10 days and begins retrogressing. Concentrations of LH become low and the production of estrogen and progesterone declines rapidly. The decline in circulating estrogen and progesterone triggers a positive feedback mechanism to the hypothalamus, which stimulates the anterior pituitary gland to begin secreting FSH in preparation for a new cycle.

Premenstrual Phase

The premenstrual phase occurs 2 to 3 days before menstruation. The corpus luteum retrogresses, with a concomitant decline in estrogen and progesterone levels. These changes in hormone levels are followed by shedding of the endometrial lining (zona functionalis) during menstruation.

▶ Endometrial Cycle

In all stages of the ovarian cycle the endometrium of the uterus demonstrates changes in response to hormone levels. The **endometrial cycle,** sometimes referred to as the **uterine cycle,** includes changes in the uterus that are stimulated by hormones during the ovarian cycle. The endometrial cycle may be divided into three phases: proliferative, secretory, and menstrual. It is significant to note that there is individual variation in the activity of the ovary and the effect on the uterus. The changes in the ovarian and uterine cycles are not coincident in time. In other words, the follicular phase of the ovarian cycle is not absolutely parallel to the proliferative phase of the endometrial cycle. The changes are continuous throughout the cycle and the phases are artificial, used for descriptive purposes only.

Proliferative Phase

In the early part of the proliferative phase of the endometrial cycle, immediately after menstruation, the endometrium is very thin and the endometrial glands are narrow. Under the influence of estrogen secreted by the ovary, the cells of the endometrium multiply by mitosis and the endometrium thickens. As the proliferative phase progresses, the endometrium becomes even thicker as a result of glandular hyperplasia and growth of the stroma. The stroma becomes edematous as a result of stimulation of estrogen and increases in ions, water, and amino acids. During this phase, the endometrium proliferates from approximately 0.5 to 5 mm in height and increases approximately eightfold in thickness. This proliferation of cells serves to prepare the uterus for implantation of the fertilized ovum. The proliferative phase of the endometrial cycle varies in length among women. For example, a 28-day menstrual cycle has a shorter proliferative phase than a 32-day cycle. Unlike the proliferative phase, the secretory or postovulatory phase of the cycle is fairly consistent so that it can be predicted that ovulation will occur about 14 days prior to menstruation.

Secretory Phase

After ovulation, under the influence of estrogen supplemented by progesterone secreted by the ovary, the endometrial glands become increasingly tortuous. There is increased edema of the stroma and dense coiling of the spiral vessels. The endometrium during the secretory phase is succulent and rich in glycogen, preparing for implantation of the fertilized ovum and growth of the embryo. The endometrial changes that occur during this phase are precise and must be mediated by progesterone, which is secreted by the ovary

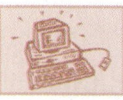

Research Abstract

Evaluation of Therapeutic Response Patterns in the Woman Experiencing Premenstrual Syndrome

Since symptoms and symptom change vary within an individual over time, it is important to describe individual symptom patterns in order to understand a client's experience of symptoms and treatment. Premenstrual syndrome (PMS) is a disorder which involves multiple symptoms and behaviors occurring along or about the menstrual cycle. Since PMS is cyclic, both pattern and time are important in evaluation of symptoms and treatment effect. Little is known about the pattern of perimenstrual symptom clusters across the menstrual cycle phase or across multiple cycles. Further, since it is the individual woman who suffers symptoms, an evaluation strategy which provides insight into individual patterns of responses and the effects of treatments is of vital importance clinically. The purpose of this interrupted time-series study was to determine the effectiveness of a multiple component nursing intervention aimed at relieving the symptom severity and distress associated with PMS and to describe the occurrence of individual patterns of symptoms and symptom pattern change.

In a time-series design, each woman is considered as one experiment and serves as her own control. Data on the woman, taken at one time, are compared with data on the same woman taken at a later point in time. Internal validity of the design is maintained by using multiple measures and establishing a stable baseline of behaviors prior to introducing the treatment. In this study, daily and weekly measures were collected across seven complete menstrual cycles in five women meeting restrictive sampling criteria. The baseline phase included three complete menstrual cycles followed by a seven-week intervention phase and a post-intervention phase of three menstrual cycles. Women included in the study had PMS, were between 32 and 41 years (mean = 37), had a regular menstrual cycle, no major health problems, were on no medications or hormones, and had no existing psychiatric illness. In addition to PMS, all women met the criteria for perimenstrual negative affect (PNA), which include such affective states as anger, depression and anxiety, among others.

PNA symptom perception and evaluation (the dependent variable) was measured by a self-report symptom checklist, The Menstrual Symptom Severity List, a highly reliable and valid method which incorporates symptoms selected from the most commonly used menstrual symptom rating scales. Each woman completed this checklist as part of a Daily Health Diary. The experimental treatment used in this study was a system of non-pharmacologic strategies involving self-monitoring, personal choice, self-regulation, and self/environmental modifications, administered within a group format of peer support and professional guidance. After data were collected on a baseline phase of three menstrual cycles, data were collected as each woman began the experimental treatment phase (one to two menstrual cycles), followed by data collection on three post-treatment menstrual cycles.

The data analysis consisted of two phases: a within-individual time-series analysis or pretreatment baseline behavior of 90 daily data points, and an "interrupted" (that is, the treatment "interrupted" the baseline behavior) time-series analysis of treatment effect of 120 daily data points. A statistic, called the auto-correlation function, which compares a woman's own data with itself, was used to identify significant patterns of symptoms and treatment effects.

Three symptom severity patterns emerged from the baseline data analysis: a "classic" PMS pattern, a premenstrual magnification pattern, and a social week pattern (which bore no relationship to the menstrual cycle at all). Related to the therapeutic treatment, patterns of therapeutic response emerged from the time-series analysis of post-treatment data compared with baseline symptom severity patterns: a "normalized" response pattern where symptom severity declined to a mild cyclic process and an "unstable" response pattern that remained reactive.

The investigator concluded that the use of auto-correlation analysis allows the clinician to

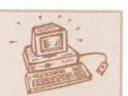

Research Abstract *continued*

reveal underlying symptom patterns that would go unnoticed with traditional summary statistics. Results from this study provide a clinically relevant framework for evaluating therapeutic response patterns in the individual woman experiencing PMS.

Application to Practice

This complex study points to limitation of traditional experimental designs, which capture data at only one point in time. For most clinical situations, it is a pattern of symptoms, and effects of treatments, that is relevant in therapeutic interventions. This form of research clearly extended the knowledge of nursing therapeutics by evaluating the therapeutic effect of a treatment with an emphasis on the individual over time.

Source: Taylor, D.L. (1994). Evaluating therapeutic change in symptom severity at the level of the individual woman experiencing severe PMS. Image, *26(1); 25–32.*

during the luteal phase of the ovarian cycle. If a biopsy of the endometrium is done during this phase and demonstrates changes in the endometrium consistent with the secretory phase, it can be said that ovulation has taken place. The secretory phase of the menstrual cycle lasts about 14 days. About 2 or 3 days before menstruation, in response to the decline in levels of estrogen and progesterone, there is a reduction in endometrial tissue fluid, a decrease in blood flow, and disintegration of the stromal cells.

Menstrual Phase

The cellular debris, blood, and mucus that are found with degeneration of the endometrium are discharged through the cervix to the vagina and out of the body via the introitus. Other materials in the menstrual flow include prostaglandins, a unique class of tissue hormones, which have a role in the initiation of menstruation and possibly contribute to the menstrual discomfort that some women experience (Cunningham, et al., 1997). The menstrual phase lasts from about the first to the fifth day of the menstrual cycle. Toward the end of this phase FSH, secreted by the anterior pituitary gland, stimulates the secretion of estrogen by the ovarian follicles and the endometrial lining is reconstructed in a new cycle.

▶ Hormonal Activity During the Menstrual Cycle

The menstrual cycle is hormonally mediated through the activity of the hypothalamus, anterior pituitary gland, and ovaries. When stimulated by the hypothalamus, the anterior pituitary gland produces gonadotropin. One of these hormones, FSH, stimulates the growth and development of the graafian follicle. The follicle secretes estrogen, which stimulates proliferation of the endometrial lining of the uterus. When ovulation occurs, the anterior pituitary gland secretes LH, which stimulates development of the corpus luteum. The corpus luteum secretes progesterone, which further develops the lining of the uterus in preparation for the fertilized ovum. In the absence of pregnancy, the corpus luteum degenerates, decreasing the levels of estrogen and progesterone and causing the uterus to shed its lining during menstruation. The decline in estrogen and progesterone triggers a positive feedback to the hypothalamus, which stimulates the anterior pituitary gland to secrete FSH once again. Summaries of the hormones of the ovarian cycle and the action of the pituitary gonadotropins are found in Table 6–1.

▶ **TABLE 6-1**

Milestones in the Correlation of Ovarian and Endometrial (Menstrual) Cycles

				Phase			
	Menstrual 1–5 Days	Early Follicular 6–8 Days	Advanced Follicular 9–13 Days	Ovulation 14 Days	Early Luteal 15–19 Days	Advanced Luteal 20–25 Days	Premenstrual 26–28 Days
Ovary	Corpus albicans forms from corpus luteum of preceding cycle. Follicular recruitment proceeds.	Follicles mature and the chosen or dominant follicle develops.		Ovulation occurs, and granulosa cells in the ruptured follicle are luteinized.	Vascularization of granulosa lutein cells occurs, and corpus luteum forms. Follicular atresia begins.	Corpus luteum matures and follicular atresia continues.	Corpus luteum regresses, and follicular recruitment is initiated for the next cycle.
Estrogen	Low level is derived principally from extraglandularly produced estrone. Little estradiol-17β is secreted by the ovary.		Estradiol-17β secretion, principally by granulosa cells of the dominant follicle, increases strikingly, maximal rates being attained just prior to the LH surge.	Immediately after, or coincident with, ovulation, there is an abrupt, indeed, precipitous decline in estradiol-17β secretion.	There is a gradual and progressive postovulatory rise in estradiol-17β secretion by the corpus luteum.	Maximal rates of postovulatory estradiol-17β secretion are attained. Luteal-phase estradiol-17β secretion rates, however, are not nearly as great as those observed in the immediate preovulatory phase.	Estradiol-17β secretion declines precipitously and, as during menstruation, the principal estrogen produced is estrone, which is formed in extraglandular sites.
Progesterone	Secretion is low. There is little secretion of progesterone by the adrenal cortex, and the corpus luteum of the preceding ovarian cycle has regressed.		During the follicular phase of the ovarian cycle, progesterone levels remain low. This is because human granulosa cells cannot synthesize cholesterol, the obligate precursor of progesterone, but are dependent on LDL cholesterol that can be obtained from the blood only after vascularization of the granulosa cells after ovulation.	Progesterone secretion increases steadily as a consequence of the availability of LDL and LH action to effect cholesterol side-chain cleavage.	Progesterone secretion remains high until the end of the advanced luteal phase.		Progesterone secretion declines precipitously.

Milestones in the Correlation of Ovarian and Endometrial (Menstrual) Cycles

				Phase			
	Menstrual 1–5 Days	Early Follicular 6–8 Days	Advanced Follicular 9–13 Days	Ovulation 14 Days	Early Luteal 15–19 Days	Advanced Luteal 20–25 Days	Premenstrual 26–28 Days
Endometrium	Menstrual desquamation and early reorganization of endometrial glandular epithelium occur.	Glandular epithelium proliferates as a result of many mitoses.	There is pseudo-stratification of nuclei—no secretion, early stromal changes.	Subnuclear vacuoles that are rich in glycogen appear.	Vacuoles migrate to the luminal surface. Mitosis ceases. The endometrial glands become very tortuous.	Vacuoles have been secreted and decidualization commences. Stromal edema and enlargement of stromal cells are prominent.	Stromal cells are disrupted and disintegrate. Leukocyte infiltration and interstitial hemorrhage occur.
Pituitary Secretion							
FSH	The FSH levels that had become modestly increased coincident with the decline in steroid secretion by the regressing corpus luteum of the preceding cycle now decline.		FSH secretion is at all times pulsatile in nature but during the proliferative phase of the ovarian cycle, prior to the LH surge at midcycle, FSH levels remain low.	A significant surge in FSH secretion, albeit less prominent than that of LH, heralds the commencement of the ovulatory process.	After the midcycle gonadotropin surge, FSH levels fall abruptly to levels similar to those found during the preovulatory phase of the cycle.		As steroid secretion by the regressing corpus luteum diminishes, there is a modest but significant increase in FSH.
LH	Levels of LH are low and reasonably constant until just prior to ovulation.			Coincident with, or just after, the striking increase in estradiol-17β secretion by the dominant follicle, there is a striking increase in LH secretion—the LH "surge."	Levels of LH are low and reasonably constant until just prior to ovulation.		

LH, luteinizing hormone; LDL, low-density lipoprotein; FSH, follicle-stimulating hormone.

Adapted, with permission, from Cunningham, F.G. et al. (1997). Williams obstetrics (20th ed.). Stamford, CT: Appleton & Lange, p. 82.

Chapter Highlights

▶ Human reproduction is dependent on the transmission of genetic material via the ovum and sperm at conception, with each of these specialized cells contributing half of the chromosomes containing the hereditary characteristics for the new individual.

▶ Mitosis occurs as a result of replicative division in which a cell having 46 chromosomes divides to form two identical daughter cells, each having 46 chromosomes.

▶ Meiosis is a process of reduction division in which the number of chromosomes in a cell is reduced by half.

▶ The male reproductive system is made up of external (penis and scrotum), internal (testes, epididymides, ductus deferens, ejaculatory ducts, and urethra), and accessory organs (seminal vesicles, prostate gland, and bulbourethral glands).

▶ The female reproductive system consists of external (mons veneris, labia major, labia minora, clitoris, vestibule, and perineum) and internal (ovaries, fallopian tubes, uterus, and vagina) organs.

▶ The menstrual cycle consists of the ovarian and endometrial cycles.

After reading the vignette at the beginning of the chapter, use what you have learned to answer these questions.

1. What benefits will Shaila Jackson gain in understanding the structure and function of her reproductive system?

2. In educating Shaila Jackson about the organs of the female reproductive system, what factors (e.g., psychosocial, cultural) should Ann Salzman, CNM, MSN, consider?

3. What other methods can Ann Salzman use to enhance and clarify the teaching she is providing to Shaila Jackson?

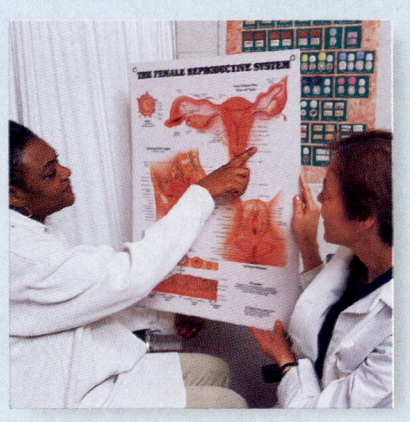

Critical Thinking Questions

▶ References

Copeland, K.C. (1986). Variations in normal sexual development. *Pediatric Review, 8*(2), 47–55.

Cunningham, F.G. et al. (1997). *Williams obstetrics* (20th ed.) (p. 47). Stamford, CT: Appleton & Lange.

DeCherney, A.H., & Pernoll, M.L. (1994). *Current obstetric and gynecologic diagnosis and treatment* (8th ed.) (p. 16). Norwalk, CT: Appleton & Lange.

Ganong, W.F. (1995). *Review of medical physiology* (17th ed.) (p. 384). Norwalk, CT: Appleton & Lange.

Marshall, W.A., & Tanner, J.M. (1969). Variations in pattern of pubertal changes in girls. *Archives of Disease in Childhood, 44,* 291.

Tanner, J.M. (1962). *Growth at adolescence* (2nd ed.). Oxford, England: Blackwell Scientific.

Tanner, J.M. (1978). *Into man: Physical growth from conception to maturity.* Cambridge, MA: Harvard University Press.

Taylor, D.L. (1994). Evaluating therapeutic change in symptom severity at the level of the individual woman experiencing severe PMS. *Image, 26*(1), 25–32.

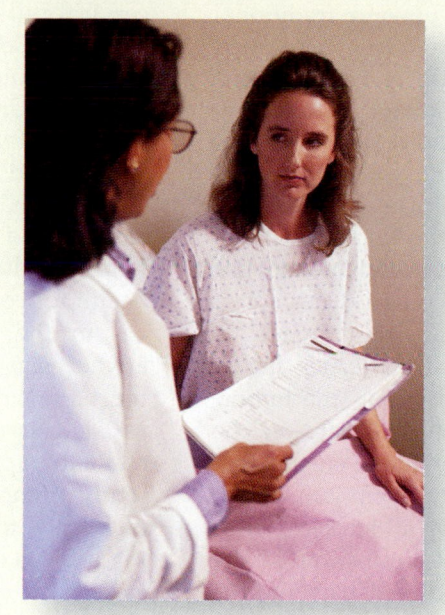

Patricia Ingham, RN, is helping 25-year-old Christine Larson to prepare for a gynecologic examination as part of her periodic health visit. As the nurse describes the assessments that the nurse practitioner will conduct during the examination, she notes that Christine appears nervous and fearful when the nurse refers to the Papinicolaou (Pap) smear that will be obtained as part of the routine screening procedures. The nurse then remembers from Christine's health history that she had contracted human papillomavirus (HPV) two years ago and had been successfully treated for this infection.

Patricia Ingham touches Christine's hand gently and asks, "Are you afraid about the results of the Pap smear, given your history of HPV?" Christine swallows hard and, looking at the nurse, replies, "When I was diagnosed with HPV, the doctor told me that I may be at risk of developing cervical cancer. Although the Pap smear was normal last year, I'm terrified that the next test will be abnormal. Is there anything I can do that will help me overcome this fear?" ∎

7

Issues in Women's Health

Women are unique and different from men in their health care needs. New models for the provision of women's health care, which go beyond traditional gynecologic and obstetric care, are being developed and put into practice. Nursing care of women must include attention to both the physiologic and psychologic needs of this population. Issues such as socioeconomic status, sexual orientation, violence against women, and substance use and abuse are as important to a woman's health as are the management of discomforts related to menstruation and menopause and screening for breast and gynecological cancers.

This chapter describes the current trends in women's health care and the critical issues facing women's health nurses. It also discusses the importance of the woman's periodic health visit and the strategies that nurses can implement to ensure that this encounter with the health care system will lead to the adoption of healthy lifestyles by all female clients. The chapter concludes with an examination of the concerns women have in regard to menstruation, the climacteric and menopause, breast cancer and breast diseases, and gynecological cancers. The nurse is a vital participant in caring for and supporting women as they face the various challenges within their lives.

▶ TRENDS AND ISSUES IN WOMEN'S HEALTH AND HEALTH CARE

Health has been defined in many ways. In 1946 the World Health Organization defined health in a holistic manner as including physical, mental, and social well-being (World Health Organization, 1979). Although this concept of health has long been accepted by health care professionals, until recently women's health care has been guided by a philosophy that focused primarily on issues related to the reproductive system such as contraception, fertility, and menstruation.

From the 1800s through the middle of the 20th century, women's health care was provided primarily by male physicians for two reasons: one, legislation gave physicians exclusive control over health care and, two, women were excluded from the profession through exclusion from medical schools. As late as 1980 paternalistic and condescending attitudes towards women were being instilled in medical students and residents during their training (Geary, 1995).

Under the influence of the women's health movement of the 1960s and 1970s, women began to demand respect for and take control of their bodies.

Self-help groups such as the Boston Women's Health Book Collective were formed. Feminists advocated cervical self-exam and early pregnancy terminations at home (Geary, 1995). Women's and feminist groups opened clinics to provide female-centered health care services. Groups such as the National Women's Health Network, the National Black Women's Health Project, and the National Latina Health Organization were formed during this time to monitor public policy as it related to women's health, act as advocates for women's health, and provide information about health to women.

In the last 30 years, there have been many advances in women's health, but most were related to reproductive health including fetal monitoring, assisted reproductive technologies, hormone replacement therapies, and advances in contraception. Currently attention is being directed toward primary care of women that involves a more holistic view, including a focus on life span issues, including chronic diseases such as hypertension, cardiac disease, and psychosocial influences on health. More female health care practitioners, including nurse practitioners and physicians, are available today, and these practitioners have helped bring a more woman-centered approach to medicine and health care.

Nurses have long been advocates for women's issues in health care. Changes related to maternal involvement in pediatric care, paternal involvement in birthing, and a return to more natural and less medically oriented birth options were initiated by nurses, most of whom were women themselves and many of whom were mothers who understood these issues both personally and professionally. Nurses continue to advocate for better health care for women.

In our current society, women have fewer pregnancies and spend relatively little of their adult life in childbearing. In addition, women can expect to live over a third of their lives after menopause, that is, after their reproductive functions have ceased. This trend points to the need for health care providers to plan primary care for women from a life span perspective that includes reproductive health care but also looks beyond it. To deliver optimal care to women the nurse needs to consider the whole woman, including physical, psychologic, and emotional aspects.

Medical care for women has also been criticized as being based on a male model of health and illness. Nonreproductive illnesses such as heart disease have been studied primarily in men, with treatments being developed based on these studies and then applied to women. The inappropriateness of this model is illustrated by statistics that show that women's health is indeed different from men's. Women of all ages tend to suffer from acute health conditions (lasting no more than 3 months) 20–30% more than do men (Verbrugge, 1992), conditions that include injuries, infections, and digestive disturbances. Women are also more likely than men to suffer from nonfatal chronic conditions such as anemia, thyroid conditions, arthritis, migraine headaches, and heart rhythm disorders. Both short-term and long-term disabilities are also more common among women. According to Verbrugge (1992), women's activities are restricted due to disorders or illnesses about 25% more days per year compared to men. Women also have higher rates of long-term disabilities including limitations of mobility, strength, and endurance. However, although females may suffer more illness and disability in life, they have the advantage over males in terms of survival and longevity. In the United States, females have a life expectancy that is about 7 years longer than their male counterparts and are less likely to die at any given age (Phillips, Sexton, & Blackman, 1997). Men also have higher rates of mortality from all the leading causes of death including cardiac diseases, cancer, accidents, and stroke (Verbrugge, 1992). Differences in health between women and men are a function of social and cultural influences as well as biological differences.

▶ Sociocultural Influences on Women's Health

Family Structure and Multiple Roles

The women's movement, which began in the late 19th and early 20th centuries and gained momentum and renewed focus during the 1960s and 1970s, has had significant effects on the position of women and the roles they assume within our society. Changes in the family structure have also occurred and include increased numbers of single parent families, usually headed by women. A higher percentage of women have entered the workforce and their salaries are often integral to their families' financial stability. Although women now shoulder all or part of the family's economic burden, they are still responsible for the majority of household and family care tasks (Quimby, 1994). Mothers still assume the major burden of child care, including arranging for day care, sick care, and social activities. Women are thus placed in the stressful position of trying to succeed in their jobs and careers while continuing to invest significant time and energy in household duties and child care.

In addition to being the major child care providers within the family unit, more than 50% of women become responsible for one or more aging parents, just as they themselves reach middle age

(Quimby, 1994). While assuming the burden of caring for elderly parents or other relatives, women may also be working and taking care of minor children, often adolescents (Acheson, 1997). Collins (1994) has called women the "safety net" for our health care system since women provide the majority of unpaid health care to the elderly. Many of these caregivers are themselves elderly and the impact of this responsibility on their own health can be significant.

Poverty

Women are more likely than men to be poor and to lack health insurance (Acheson, 1997). Two thirds of all adults living below the poverty level are women and 35% of the poor in America live in households headed by women. About a third of women who head households work outside of the home but many are on public assistance or depend on the income of other family members. Many of these women have low educational levels and 4 out of 5 receive no financial support from the fathers of their children (Woods, 1995). Women are more likely to be employed in low-paying jobs such as retail sales, food service, and service industries. Women are also more likely than men to be unemployed, work part-time, or in jobs where health insurance is not provided. In all age groups, women earn only 70% of what men earn.

Poverty is associated with poor physical and mental health (Quimby, 1994). Sexually transmitted diseases (STDs), including acquired immunodeficiency syndrome (AIDS), complications of pregnancy, childbirth, substance abuse, and addiction are all among the health problems which are more common among low-income women.

One third of homeless individuals are women and more than two thirds of homeless families are headed by single women. Homelessness is also associated with serious health problems such as violence, substance abuse, chronic disease, and inadequate nutritional intake.

Low-income and homeless women not only have poorer health, but also have restricted access to health care due to such factors as lack of health insurance, lack of providers in their neighborhoods, and lack of transportation. Women who work for low hourly wages often cannot take time off from their jobs to wait long hours in crowded clinics to get health care.

Longevity

Longer life spans for people in general and for women in particular are accompanied by an increased incidence of disease and disability. Chronic illnesses such as cancer, arthritis, cardiovascular disease, hypertension, and osteoporosis are among the health problems of elderly females. Urinary incontinence is common among elderly women and may be due to poor muscle tone, urinary tract infections, or medications. Coupled with decreases in mobility, urinary incontinence can lead to social isolation and depression.

Another problem affecting the health of elderly women is polypharmacy. Multiple prescriptions sometimes from different providers can lead to changes in both mental status, such as delirium and depression, and physical status, including insomnia, impairment of motor functions, and orthostatic hypotension, all of which can lead to falls. In spite of the increased risk of side effects among this group, health care providers prescribe tranquillizers to elderly women over twice as often as they prescribe them to elderly men (Horton, 1995).

Even as life spans have increased, families have become scattered over longer distances, so the elderly often live far from their children, grandchildren, and other relatives. Smaller families also mean fewer relatives available to provide physical assistance and emotional support to elderly women. More than half of women who live to the age of 85 enter nursing homes (Collins, 1994) and 75% of nursing home residents are women (Woods, 1995).

Poverty also disproportionately affects elderly women, who account for 72% of the aged poor in America (Woods, 1995). Many elderly women are forced to use their savings and sell off their assets to meet expenses when their husbands are ill, leaving them with little to live on after their husbands die. Widows may also lose their insurance coverage when their mates die, thus, many elderly women do not have private health insurance and rely on Medicare, the federally financed insurance program for the elderly. Medicare does not pay for long-term nursing home care; the elderly who need these services must spend down their savings to qualify for Medicaid, which provides benefits for the poor.

Elderly women living in the community may lack transportation to stores to purchase food and other necessities and may have difficulty acccessing health care due to lack of transportation or to physical disability.

Lesbian and Bisexual Women

A **lesbian** is a woman whose primary erotic attractions and affectional desires are for women (Denenberg, 1994; Downey, 1995). A **bisexual** is a person who has erotic attractions for and may have had sexual experiences with individuals of both sexes. The majority (77%) of women who consider themselves lesbians have had sexual experiences with men at varying times during their lives for various reasons (Downey, 1995). About 3–5% of women in the United States identify themselves as lesbians; however, the number may be higher. Lesbian women do not always disclose their sexual orientation to health care providers, primarily because of fear of rejection, ridicule, discrimination, and breach of confidence. These same fears can lead lesbian women to forego needed care so as to avoid interactions with personnel in the health care system.

Lesbian women have many of the same health care needs as heterosexual women and some additional concerns. Although STDs are less likely to be acquired during sex between two women, many lesbian women have also had sex with men and are at risk for acquiring these diseases from men. Lesbian women also suffer from gynecologic problems such as endometriosis, fibroids, vaginosis, cervical cancer, and breast cancer and are in need of pelvic and breast examinations, mammograms, and Papanicolaou (Pap) smears. As with all women, screening should be based on assessment of individual risk. Lesbian women have high rates of alcoholism, illicit drug use, and nicotine use, which may be related to the stress of being a member of a minority community or to the fact that the gay social scene traditionally revolves around gay bars and parties (Downey, 1995). The National Lesbian Health Care Survey reported high incidences of physical abuse during childhood or adulthood (37% of lesbians), rape and other sexual attack (32%), and sexual abuse by a family member while growing up (19%) among lesbians (Bradford, Ryan, & Rothblum, 1994). The need for mental health services is high among this population. Half of the women in this survey had received counseling for depression and over three fourths had received some form of mental health services. Over half of the lesbians surveyed had thought about committing suicide and 18% had attempted it (Bradford, Ryan, & Rothblum, 1994).

Health Care System

Two major issues confront women's health nurses in the health care system today: the evolution of managed care as the primary means of third-party reimbursement, and the dilution of nursing care through the use of unlicensed assistive personnel (UAPs) in inpatient, outpatient, and long-term care facilities.

Managed care can offer access to comprehensive primary care services to women through providing a complete package of services, improving prevention and screening services, reducing out of pocket health care costs, and decreasing the need for unnecessary procedures. However, at this time it is unsure if managed care will realize this potential, especially as large numbers of low-income women are enrolled in managed care through Medicare and Medicaid. These women have a wide range of health and social problems, including inadequate nutrition, drug and alcohol addiction, and high rates of STDs, conditions which the managed care model did not originally take into consideration.

The Commonwealth Fund Survey of Women's Health (Collins & Simon, 1996) found that although managed care companies provided reimbursement for a wide range of preventive services including mammograms, Pap smears, and contraceptive services, barriers existed which prevented women from receiving adequate preventive care, such as:

- Cost
- Lack of coverage for the service
- Inability to get an appointment with the provider of the service
- Lack of counseling by the managed care physician
- Inadequate amount of time spent with the physician
- Poor client–physician communication
- Existence of requirements for staying within the provider network
- Need for referrals from the primary care provider for visits to specialists and for diagnostic tests and treatments

Ironically, managed care has provided more opportunities for employment for nurse practitioners as physicians and health care facilities seek ways to provide quality care within the lower reimbursement levels.

The use of UAPs to deliver client care is controversial since it touches on issues related to professionalism, cost containment, and quality assurance (see Chapter 1 for discussion about UAPs). This development will continue to have a significant impact on the delivery of women's health services.

Policy and Research Issues

In the early 20th century the first laws related to women's health began to appear and were intended to protect women as the weaker sex and for the sake of their children. Most of these regulations related to women in the workforce, such as laws to regulate the maximum number of hours women could work per week. Other laws related to women's reproductive functions. As early as 1859 states began to enact laws that placed abortion under the control of physicians by limiting the procedure to cases in which a physician deemed it necessary to save the woman's life (Geary, 1995). In the early 1900s laws allowed for surgical sterilization without the woman's consent in cases where the woman was judged to be retarded or mentally ill. Many poor and non-white women were

sterilized under these regulations (Ladd-Taylor, 1992). As late as the 1970s many doctors followed a formula developed by the American College of Obstetricians and Gynecologists to determine which women could have a tubal ligation. The formula required that the woman's age multiplied by the number of living children she had equal at least 120 before she was "eligible" for sterilization. In most cases the woman's husband was required to consent to the tubal ligation before it could be performed (Geary, 1995).

By the 1970s women's rights activists began to protest the current policies regarding surgical sterilization and abortion. In 1974 the Department of Health, Education and Welfare issued the first guidelines for sterilization which required that the woman herself give informed consent and required a waiting period between consent and surgery. In 1973 the historic Supreme Court Decision in the case of *Roe v. Wade* led to legalized abortion in the United States, although there were and continue to be barriers in terms of access to this service.

In 1965 Medicaid regulations provided health care to women and children through government funding. The Women, Infants, and Children (WIC) program was established as part of these regulations and provides pregnant women, infants, and young children with nutritional supplements in an effort to decrease infant and child mortality.

Throughout the late 20th century women's rights activitists, including many nurses, have continued to advocate for changes in women's health policies at the government level. For many years, medical care for women in nonreproductive matters such as cancer and cardiac disease had to rely on research carried out almost exclusively on male subjects. One reason that was frequently given for not including women in clinical research trials was that women might be pregnant and the treatments being tested might harm a fetus. In 1983 the United States Public Health Service convened the Task Force on Women's Health Issues that recommended increased emphasis be placed on women's health research, including research on improved methods of contraception for both men and women. In 1986 the National Institutes of Health (NIH) issued a policy requiring inclusion of minority and female subjects in relevant clinical research studies. The Office of Research on Women's Health (ORWH) of NIH was formed in 1990 to monitor implementation of these policies. At the same time, increased funding for women's health research was allocated. The Women's Health Initiative, a 14-year, $625 million study, was established by the NIH to examine the effects of hormone replacement therapy, diet, and exercise on coronary heart disease, breast and colon cancer, and osteoporosis. The ORWH has also supported important studies on women's reproductive health, urologic disorders, autoimmune disorders, occupational health, and disability issues. Other recent government initiatives in women's health include the appropriation of $50 million for Pap smears and mammograms for low-income women. The Agency for Health Care Policy and Research also has an Office of Women's Health which is dedicated to improving disease prevention and screening efforts as well as to determining the most effective interventions for various disorders.

▶ Critical Issues Facing Women's Health Nurses

Violence Against Women

Violence against women occurs within all ethnic and socioeconomic groups and is thought to be related to societal issues of dominance and control over women and children. Women can be victims of violence during many developmental periods (including childhood, adolescence, adulthood, and the later years) and in various types of relationships.

Studies have shown that as many as 17% of all adult women were sexually abused by a family member during childhood (Campbell & Landenburger, 1995). The U.S. Preventive Services Task Force (1996) reports that the incidence of child sexual abuse may be as high as 450,000 cases per year in the United States. While discussion of abuse during childhood is beyond the scope of this book, it is important for nurses to remember that women who were abused during childhood may suffer the repercussions of that abuse throughout their adult lives. Adult manifestations of child sexual and physical abuse may manifest themselves in women as low self-esteem, social isolation, guilt, substance use and abuse, sexual disorders, depression, and post-traumatic stress disorder. Physical consequences of sexual abuse in childhood include damage to reproductive organs and STDs that can lead to chronic pelvic pain and infertility. Women who were sexually abused as children may have increased fear, discomfort or pain during gynecological examinations and procedures, or childbirth. These women need additional emotional support from nurses during routine gynecological procedures and during labor and delivery.

Domestic violence includes physical, sexual, and psychologic abuse by a spouse or domestic partner. The true incidence of domestic violence is unknown, primarily due to underreporting by its victims. It has been estimated that about half of the women who are abused fail to report these violent acts to the police (Horton, 1995). Underreporting may be due to fear of reprisals by the perpetrator, shame, economic depen-

dence on the abuser, or a feeling that the abuse is minor or that it will not happen again. Women also do not report violence, including rape, for fear that the police will be ineffective or insensitive towards them (Horton, 1995). Despite the bias caused by underreporting, statistics on abuse of women are alarming. It is estimated that nearly 1,000,000 women are victims of assault, rape, or robbery each year by their male partners (U.S. Preventive Services Task Force, 1996). Battering and physical abuse may account for 22–35% of emergency room visits made by women each year (Horton, 1995). In addition, 8–17% of women report being battered during pregnancy (Horton, 1995). Teenage women may also be battered by persons with whom they have a dating or sexual relationship. Homicide is often a result of domestic violence. Women who are murdered are usually killed by a spouse, boyfriend, or other family member, and victims of domestic violence are four times more likely to be murdered (Bailey, Kellermann, Somes, Banton, Rivara, & Rushforth, 1997).

Abuse of the elderly by family members and other caretakers at home and in long-term care facilities includes physical and psychologic abuse, withholding of food, clothing and medical care, financial exploitation, and forced social isolation. It is estimated that 4–10% of the elderly are victims of physical or psychologic abuse (Horton, 1995; U.S. Preventive Services Task Force, 1996). Data have indicated that the majority of elderly women who are abused (86%) are subjected to this treatment at the hands of a relative, with 40% of these women being the victims of spousal abuse (Suggs, 1995). Abuse of elderly women by spouses may be part of a pattern of domestic violence that has characterized the marriage for many years. As women live longer and are more often economically and socially dependent on others, they are more frequently the victims of elder abuse.

Lenore Walker (1979), a psychotherapist who studied battered women, described the lives of battered women in her Cycle Theory of Violence. This theory helps to explain why women remain in relationships where they are abused and sometimes eventually murdered. It describes three phases in the cycle of battering that vary in timing and intensity within and between couples (see box entitled Cycle Theory of Violence).

Violence against women is typically underrecognized by the health care profession. This is illustrated by the fact that only about 5% of women who have been abused are identified as victims of domestic violence in the medical record. Nurses have a moral obligation to intervene to stop the cycle of violence. The first step in intervention is identification of women who are abused. Women who are victims of

▶ CYCLE THEORY OF VIOLENCE

- Tension-Building Stage. Minor battering or abusive incidents occur, including verbal abuse, slapping, or throwing objects. The woman tries to pacify the abuser by nurturing him and being compliant with his wishes. She may also accept blame for his actions or rationalize his actions as being caused by outside factors such as stress at the workplace. Alternatively, she may try to avoid conflict by staying out of his way. However she reacts, these minor battering episodes will continue to escalate despite her efforts to defuse the tension building within the batterer.

- Acute Battering Incident. Tension continues to grow and the compensatory mechanisms of the woman become ineffective. The result is an uncontrolled release of rage from the batterer and is expressed in a major incident of abuse. This occurrence is usually short lived but very violent and often includes both verbal and sexual abuse, such as forced intercourse or sodomy, in addition to physical battering. There is nothing the woman can say or do to prevent the battering. If police are called, it is usually during this phase. The woman may hide or run from the house to avoid even more severe injury. More commonly, women endure the abuse and then isolate themselves for several hours or days as if in a state of post-traumatic shock. Delays in seeking care for injuries caused during the abuse often occur because of the tendency to become depressed, listless, and helpless after this incident.

- Loving Kindness and Contrite Loving Behavior. Sometimes called the Honeymoon Phase, it is characterized by kindness, loving behavior, and contrition on the part of the batterer and immediately follows violent abuse. The woman is showered with attention and gifts as the batterer tries to make up for his abusive behavior. If she is hospitalized because of the abuse, he may refuse to leave her and will look after her every need. The batterer is convinced and may manage to convince others that he is truly sorry and will never again engage in such violence again. However long this phase lasts, it will eventually end, and the tension-building phase will begin again, signaling a repeat of the cycle.

Source: Walker, 1979.

abuse may not tell anyone unless they are asked directly. Clinical signs of violence include chronic pain such as abdominal or pelvic pain or headache, other vague physical complaints, and multiple injuries, especially in the central part of the body, including the head, chest, abdomen, and genitalia.

Women who are beaten or abused may overuse alcohol or illicit or prescription drugs as a way to self-medicate their physical and psychic pain. Another clinical outcome of physical or psychologic abuse is depression.

The nurse can use the following guidelines to provide intervention to an abused woman:

- Create a safe environment for discussing the abuse
- Assure the client of confidentiality
- Inform the woman that she will not be abandoned if she is unwilling or unable to leave the abuse relationship
- Question the woman alone
- Ask direct questions such as: "Have you been hit, slapped, kicked, or injured by someone?" or "Have you been forced to have sex by anyone?"
- Take notice of the presence of new and old injuries during the physical examination and describe them in the chart

- Describe (in the client's words) how the injuries were obtained
- Record the time and date of the assault, the name of the suspected assailant, and the relationship of the suspected assailant to the client
- Advise the client that she is not at fault in the abuse and that she has the right to be safe
- Refer the client to a social worker for assistance in locating a safe place such as a shelter and obtaining an order of protection against the abuser
- Help the client who is not ready to leave the relationship to develop an escape plan when violence recurs (such as having a bag packed with items such as clothing and medications for herself and her children and hiding it where the abuser will not find it)
- Provide the client with the address of a shelter for battered women or with telephone numbers of appropriate referral agencies
- Report abuse of minors or elderly people to the appropriate state authorities

Rape is forced sexual intercourse. It is estimated that 133,000 women are victims of rape or attempted rape each year (Horton, 1995). Only 44% of rapes are committed by people who are strangers to the victims. Fifty-five percent of the women who are raped know

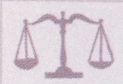

Ethical Decision Making

Many nurses feel unsure of how to therapeutically intervene with a woman who is a victim of domestic violence. There are many issues related to care of a woman who is in an abusive relationship and many nurses feel powerless when confronted with such a client. A common situation is one in which a woman presents to the health care system with injuries or other signs that suggest that she has suffered physical, emotional, or sexual abuse, but she does not admit to the abuse. Alternately, she may admit to the abuse but refuse to leave the abuser and may even defend the abuser's actions. This situation raises the following questions:

1. Should all women be asked about present or past abuse?
2. If the woman appears with signs of abuse should she be confronted with the nurse's suspicions?
3. Should nurses and other health care workers be expected to continue to provide care to women who are abused but refuse to leave the relationship?
4. How far should the nurse go to protect the client from the abuser?
5. Should the nurse support continuation of the relationship or should she condemn the abuser and the relationship?

their assailant. Rape can occur within marriage and is often part of a battering relationship. Most states recognize forced sexual intercourse within marriage as rape. Date or acquaintance rape is rape by someone whom the victim knows or with whom she may even have a social or dating relationship.

Women who have been raped are often bought to the emergency room where they are examined and their injuries are treated. Forensic evidence such as scrapings from under fingernails, pubic hair combings, and fluid from the vagina is collected during the examination and saved for future court proceedings. These women, who are experiencing severe crisis, may feel doubly assaulted if the examination and evidence collection are not handled in a professional and

sensitive way. Nurses can provide emotional support to these women in much the same way as they can to women who are victims of physical abuse by assuring the victim that the assault was a criminal act and that she was in no way at fault and by recording statements by the victim and descriptions of the assault and of the injuries sustained.

Substance Abuse

The terms "substance use," "abuse," and "addiction" can be applied to alcohol, legal and illegal drugs, and nicotine. Women may use substances for recreational purposes or in a compulsive manner. Recreational use refers to occasional modest use of a substance for pleasure. Compulsive use is the frequent use of a drug in spite of the fact that there may be adverse medical or social consequences. Addiction is preceeded by compulsive use and is defined as chronic, compulsive substance use (Flagler, Hughes, & Kovalesky, 1997). The state of craving or needing a drug, either physiologically or psychologically, is called dependence.

Substance use and abuse can lead to adverse physical, emotional, social, and legal consequences. Substance abuse among women is related to high levels of stress, physical, sexual, and psychologic abuse, depression, post-traumatic stress syndrome, and other mental disorders. Women who are addicted to substances often report having few or no supportive persons in their lives. Another consequence of substance abuse is increased risk of exposure to STDs, including human immunodeficiency virus (HIV) and hepatitis, through sharing needles with other drug users and engaging in unsafe sexual behavior such as unprotected sex or sex with multiple partners or with partners who are at risk for STDs in exchange for drugs.

Alcohol. Although women are less likely than men to report drinking alcoholic beverages, 40–51% of all women are reported to use alcohol and 2% consume more than 5 drinks a day (Horton, 1995). Many women start drinking during adolescence and 30% report binge drinking which is defined for women as more than 3 drinks at a time (Horton, 1995). There are racial and ethnic differences in alcohol use and abuse among women. Asian, African-American, and Hispanic women are more likely than Caucasian and Native American women to abstain completely from alcohol. High incidences of alcohol use and abuse have been reported among Native American and Alaskan Native women. These women suffer from increased morbidity and mortality as a result of this use (Jessup, 1997).

The consequences of alcohol use among women include liver disease, anemia, malnutrition, hypertension, obesity, gynecological disorders, miscarriage, and birth defects. Women are known to be more susceptible to the physiologic action of alcohol due to decreased body water content and to decreased activity of gastric alcohol dehydrogenase, an enzyme which metabolizes alcohol in the digestive system before it can enter the bloodstream. These factors lead to decreased tolerance of alcohol by women, increased intoxication after ingesting a comparable amount of oxygen, and increased damage to the body with prolonged or intense use. High rates of drinking problems and alcoholism in the families of female alcoholics also point to a genetic predisposition (Jessup, 1997).

Controlled Substances. Drug use includes illicit and prescription drugs that are taken for nonprescribed uses. Categories of drugs that can be abused include central nervous system depressants such as barbiturates, tranquillizers, hallucinogens, antidepressants, narcotics, and opiates and stimulants including amphetamines (Flagler, Hughes, & Kovalesky, 1997). Government surveys show that approximately 35% of white women, 24% of Hispanic women, and 27% of African-American women between the ages of 12 and 35 admitted to having used illegal drugs and 10%, 9%, and 12%, respectively, were recent or current users (Substance Use and Mental Health Services Administration, 1994). It is common for women who use substances to engage in polydrug use, that is, use of more than one drug or substance. Adverse health consequences of drug use are varied and depend on the drug or the amount used. Severe effects include acute cardiovascular disease such as stroke or myocardial infarction from using cocaine; hepatitis, HIV infection, AIDS, bacterial endocarditis and pulmonary embolism from using injection drugs such as heroin or cocaine; and respiratory complications from chronic marijuana use (U.S. Preventive Services Task Force, 1996). The legal and social consequences of illegal drug use include incarceration, homicide, suicide, motor vehicle accidents, and disruption of families and communities (U.S. Preventive Services Task Force, 1996).

The U.S. Preventive Services Task Force (1996) recommends including questions about alcohol and drug use (legal and illicit) when conducting complete and episodic client histories, especially in high-risk groups. Nurses are ideal health providers to assess women for drug use because of their communication skills, which enable them to establish a trusting and helping relationship. Alcohol and drug use assessment should always be approached in a nonjudgmental manner and confidentiality must be maintained. Nurses should assess the types of substances used, the frequency of consumption of each substance, and

quantities consumed. It is helpful to know the circumstances in which use takes place, i.e., only at parties, on weekends versus every day before and after school.

Traditional drug and alcohol treatment programs were originally developed for men who could be sent to a residential treatment center for up to a month for intensive therapy that was paid for by their company's health insurance policy. Follow-up programs often involved multiple meetings at nights or on weekends. Until the late 1980s, alcohol and drug rehabilitation did not address the specific needs of women. At that time the problem of perinatal substance abuse received government attention and a few demonstration projects that addressed the needs of pregnant substance abusers were started. The majority of treatment programs still do not address the needs of women who are responsible for the care of their children. Women are often afraid to enter inpatient treatment programs for fear they may lose their children to the foster care system and be unable to reunite their families when they are discharged.

Nurses need to be aware of the types of treatment programs available in their communities that might meet the needs of women who have child care responsibilities. Programs based on the twelve step model, which relies on peer support and meetings located in the community, are often more practical for women with children. Other treatments such as disulfiram, methadone maintenance, antidepressants, supportive therapy, acupuncture, or biofeedback can support recovery programs in some instances (Kearney, 1997). Women who are in drug or alcohol recovery need support and encouragement from nurses. A multidisciplinary case management approach to providing rehabilitation services, job training, and child care to facilitate re-entry into community life are most beneficial in assisting women to maintain recovery.

Smoking. Nicotine is an addictive substance that is available legally in the form of cigarettes, cigars, and smoking and chewing tobacco. Most women who use nicotine smoke it in the form of cigarettes. Currently about 1 of every 4 women in the United States smokes cigarettes, with the highest rates in the 25–44 age group (28%) (Horton, 1995). Historically, more men have smoked than women, but this gap is closing and the numbers are approximately equal, with women making up approximately half of the 46 million adults who smoke in this country (Scheibneir, 1997). While the number of women who smoke has declined by 21% since 1965, the number of women who are heavy smokers (>25 cigarettes/day) has increased from 13% to 23% (Horton, 1995). This trend is of concern because many of the adverse physiologic effects of smoking appear to be somewhat dose-related. The profile of women who are likely to smoke includes women who are separated or divorced, less educated women, and women from lower socioeconomic groups. Native American women are more likely to smoke than Caucasians, African Americans, or Hispanics. Hispanics and Asian American women are least likely to smoke although the rates of smokers among the women in these groups increase with length of time since immigration to the United States (Horton, 1995). African-American women are less likely to initiate and maintain successful smoking cessation than Caucasian women once they have started to smoke (Scheibneir, 1997).

It is estimated that more than 140,000 deaths of women in the United States each year are smoking related (Horton, 1995). Lung cancer, which is known to be strongly linked to cigarette smoking, is now the leading cause of cancer deaths in women, exceeding even breast cancer. Cigarette smoking is related to increased risk for many other serious health conditions including cancers of the mouth, esophagus, kidney, bladder, and cervix, chronic lung disease, cardiovascular diseases, and osteoporosis. In addition, cigarettes increase the risk for heart attack and stroke among women who take oral contraceptives (Horton, 1995).

Nurses should question all women about use of nicotine at each health visit. Information should be obtained about type of tobacco ingested or inhaled and amount. Studies have shown that health care providers including nurses can be effective in assisting clients to stop smoking. The National Heart, Lung, and Blood Institute (1993b) recommends that nurses follow the four-step process described here in helping their clients, including women, to stop smoking:

- *Ask* smokers about their smoking habits at each visit
- *Advise* smokers about the effects that smoking has on their health and the benefits of smoking cessation
- Negotiate a *"quit date"* with the smoker
- *Follow up* by telephone and at each visit to see if clients have been successful at quitting

Client-centered materials on smoking cessation are available from many groups, including the National Heart, Lung, and Blood Institute of the U.S. Department of Health and Human Services and the American Cancer Society. Many smoking cessation techniques and aids are available including individual and group interventions, nicotine patches, and nicotine gum. The antidepressant bupropion has recently been approved as a nonnicotine aid to smoking cessa-

tion. A complete discussion of smoking cessation techniques is beyond the scope of this book.

Sexually Transmitted Diseases

Sexually transmitted diseases affect women throughout their life span. Consequences of STDs in women include pelvic inflammatory disease, miscarriages, ectopic pregnancies, infertility, and even death. In women, many STDs are asymptomatic for at least part of their natural history. During this asymptomatic period the infection can cause damage to internal organs and in some cases be transmitted to others, including the fetus during pregnancy. STDs are more readily transmissible from men to women than from women to men due to anatomic and physiologic factors. Male and female condoms are the only devices on the market that reliably protect against these diseases. However, neither of these devices can be used without the knowledge of the male partner. Societal and cultural values have favored males as the decision makers in sexual matters, making it difficult for some women to initiate use of a device that could protect her against infection. Sexually transmitted diseases will remain major causes of morbidity and mortality among women until reliable, safe, and effective female-controlled methods of protection are developed. See Chapters 5 and 19 for further discussion of STDs.

Mental and Emotional Disorders

Depression occurs more than twice as often among women than men with prevalence rates among women of 20–25% as compared with 7–12% among men (Cole, Christensen, Raju, & Feldman, 1997). There are several recognized forms of depression, including chronic depression, minor depression, bipolar disorder, and major depression. Major depression is the most common severe mental illness found in women and major depressive episodes are also more common among women (4.5–9%) than among men (2.3–3.2%) (Cole, Christensen, Raju, & Feldman, 1997; Horton, 1995).

The prevalence rate of depression in women is highest between the ages of 25 and 44 (Horton, 1995). Among adolescents, females have consistently higher rates of depression than males. Among the elderly, 50–60% of women have mild depression and 1–3% have major depression (Horton, 1995). Risk factors for depression in women include young age, low income, lower educational level, unemployment, high-stress job, lack of social support, lack of perceived control over life, lack of a sense of personal accomplishment, and lack of a sense of independence (Horton, 1995). Contrary to public belief, menopause is not a risk factor for depression, nor does it cause depression. Depression in midlife women may be related to life transitions such as changes in family structure and the need to care for elderly parents. Increased rates of depression in elderly women may be related to such life events as loss of a spouse, social isolation, failing physical health, and economic changes.

Depression may co-exist with physical illness, other mental/emotional disorders including substance abuse, and with stressful life events. Symptoms of depression include the following:

- Depressed mood
- Anhedonia (loss of pleasure in living)
- Physical symptoms (insomnia, excessive fatigue, changes in appetite, agitation)
- Psychologic symptoms (trouble concentrating, difficulty making decisions, hopelessness, decreased self-esteem)

Either depressed mood or anhedonia must be present along with five other symptoms for a diagnosis of depression to be made. Nurses should be alert to signs of depression in their female patients. Depression can be treated with a combination of counseling, psychotherapy, and medication.

Suicide

Although males commit suicide at 4 to 7 times the rate of females, suicide is a leading cause of death among females ages 5 to 44. Among 15 to 24-year-old women, suicide is the third leading cause of death. At least part of the difference in suicide rates between the genders is the tendency of females to use less lethal methods than males. Females are therefore less likely to succeed in their suicide attempts. Depression is a major risk factor for suicide; therefore, all depressed clients should be assessed for suicide risk. When a client shows signs of depression, nurses should directly ask about suicide.

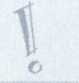 *Nursing Alert*

Clients who are at high risk for committing suicide can be identified by the following characteristics: expression of hopelessness with their lives; intention to commit suicide; and development of a specific plan that involves a lethal method such as a gun or hanging, which is available to them. Prompt intervention is necessary if these conditions occur (Cole, Christensen, Raju, & Feldman, 1997).

Eating Disorders

Anorexia nervosa and bulimia nervosa are eating disorders that occur almost exclusively among females. **Anorexia nervosa** is characterized by extreme weight loss greater than 15% of ideal body weight related to inadequate intake of nutrients. Ninety to ninety-five percent of cases of anorexia nervosa are among young females and 9% of women with anorexia nervosa die, either from consequences of malnutrition or from suicide (Horton, 1995). Anorexia is more common among dancers, competitive athletes, gymnasts, skaters, and fitness buffs. Although there may be a biological predisposition to eating disorders, anorexia nervosa is thought to be due to a combination of personality and sociocultural factors including obsessive-compulsiveness, disturbed body image, the idealization of thinness, an irrational fear of obesity, and a desire to develop the ideal body for a certain sport. A characteristic of anorexia nervosa is the denial of illness even while weight loss and other physical changes threaten a client's health and life.

Anorexia nervosa may begin slowly or suddenly. The anorexic develops an obsessive preoccupation with food, dieting, and weight along with excessive compulsion for exercise. Physical signs of anorexia nervosa include rapid and extreme weight loss, amenorrhea, loss of hair, development of lanugo, hypothermia, decreased heart rate, and decreased blood pressure. Admission to the hospital may be needed to correct dehydration, electrolyte imbalances, and abnormalities in liver and cardiac function. Sometimes tube feeding is required until behavioral interventions and psychotherapy can begin to correct the underlying psychiatric and emotional disorders and the individual can begin to develop more normal eating patterns. For many individuals, anorexia nervosa persists throughout the life span characterized by exacerbations and remissions.

Bulimia nervosa is characterized by binge eating followed by purging by self-induced vomiting. It is a distinct eating disorder from anorexia nervosa, although sometimes women have both disorders either at the same time or at different times. While anorexia nervosa often begins in early adolescence, bulimia nervosa more often begins between the ages of 17 and 25 (Horton, 1995). This disorder is also more common in women than in men, with 10 times as many women diagnosed with the disorder.

Clients experiencing bulimia nervosa are usually obsessed with their body shape or size. Compulsive exercising or dieting are sometimes seen as the bulimic woman tries to compensate for the calories she has taken in. During an episode of binging the woman may consume as many as 15,000 calories within a 1–2 hour time period. Binge eating is generally a secretive behavior and individuals report a feeling of being out of control. Some bulimic clients will also take laxatives and diuretics to aid in the purging process. Feelings of guilt, shame, depression, and anxiety are also associated with bulimic episodes.

Physical signs of bulimia nervosa include gum disease, tooth decay, esophagitis, gastritis, menstrual disturbances, cardiac arrhythmias, dehydration, and electrolyte imbalances. Some women develop swollen salivary glands, which gives them a round faced appearance.

Bulimia nervosa is usually treated on an outpatient basis with behavioral therapy and sometimes with antidepressants. Occasionally, women with bulimia nervosa may also have to be hospitalized due to medical complications but this is not as common as in anorexics. Bulimics as well as anorexics often do not complete the recommended course of therapy and this can become a lifelong disorder as well.

▶ NURSING CARE OF WOMEN

▶ The Woman's Periodic Health Visit

Goals and Principles

The periodic health visit provides an opportunity for the nurse to focus on the goals of primary prevention, secondary prevention, and health promotion. Primary prevention involves specific actions that prevent disease (U.S. Preventive Services Task Force, 1996) such as providing rubella immunization to the nonpregnant woman and teaching women to use condoms to avoid infection with STDs. Secondary prevention aims to detect diseases as soon as possible after onset in order to provide treatment that cures the disease, or slows progression of the disease and limits disability (U.S. Preventive Services Task Force, 1996). One example of secondary prevention is using the Pap smear to detect precancerous and cancerous changes in cervical cells and provide early treatment. Cervical cancer has a nearly 100% cure rate if detected early. Screening for high blood pressure and high cholesterol are also examples of secondary prevention.

Approximately 50% of all deaths in the United States are related to risky behaviors such as smoking, alcohol and illicit drug use, poor dietary intake, and sedentary lifestyle (U.S. Preventive Services Task Force, 1996). Health promotion refers to activities that aim to prevent death and disease by increasing public awareness of health-related lifestyle factors and by promoting healthy behaviors. Health promotion for the healthy woman might include teaching about diet and exercise to reduce her risks for cardiovascular disease.

Traditionally disease prevention and health promotion for women were limited to reproductive issues. The current trend towards holism in women's health care necessitates a perspective that includes consideration of women's social and psychologic needs as well as attention to all body systems. Although many women visit a gynecologist for their yearly breast and pelvic exam, there is an emerging trend towards a system wherein the woman receives gynecologic preventive care and screening within the context of her general health care. Nurses have important roles in providing primary care to women including assessment of health risks and health conditions, screening, and designing interventions to promote wellness and decrease the impact of illness. In addition nurses provide education aimed at health promotion and illness prevention, give support during wellness care, and ensure appropriate referrals.

Nurses function on a variety of levels in providing health services to women. Registered nurses have a major role in assessment, intervention, and health education. Advanced practice nurses such as clinical nurse specialists (CNSs), nurse practitioners (NPs), and certified nurse midwives (CNMs) provide comprehensive health assessments including complete physical examinations. State laws vary regarding advanced practice nurses but in many states, NPs, CNS, and CNMs may also order lab tests and prescribe medications including birth control pills and devices. A team approach that involves all members of the health and wellness team and that focuses on accomplishing client and family-centered goals is most effective.

Timing of the periodic health visit has been the subject of much controversy. Current recommendations tailor the timing of the periodic health examination to the health needs of each individual woman, although there are specific recommendations made by various authorities for the time intervals between certain screening and interventions. Although the periodic health visit is often initiated by the client, nurses are often in a position to recommend that a woman obtain this care on a regular basis and should assist the woman in formulation of a comprehensive program of health screening and activities directed at maintaining wellness.

Strategies

In an outpatient setting the nurse is frequently responsible for greeting the woman and initiating the health care process. Welcoming each client in a friendly, respectful manner encourages the open communication that is crucial to obtaining accurate information about the woman's physical, emotional, and psychosocial status. After greeting the client and introducing herself, the nurse should provide basic anticipatory guidance about the visit including:

1. A brief explanation of what can be expected to occur during the visit. The client should be made aware that a history will be taken, a physical examination will be performed, and specific screening procedures will be conducted.
2. Names and credentials of the personnel who will interview or examine her. For example, the nurse could tell the client that her examination will be performed by Ms. D. Smith, a nurse practitioner.
3. Explanation of other services that may be performed during the visit such as health education, social work, or referrals to other needed agencies.
4. Discussion of the time requirements for providing comprehensive wellness assessment. The client should be advised how long she can expect to spend in the health care facility for her initial visit and if she will have to set aside additional time for screening tests such as mammography. It is also helpful to provide clients with estimates of time requirements when they schedule their appointments.

Several strategies can be employed to ensure that the client receives optimum care during her wellness evaluation. These include the following:

1. Ensure that sufficient time is set aside for evaluation. The client's initial evaluation can require up to an hour and a half but subsequent visits may require less time. Make sure that time is provided for the client to ask questions and voice her concerns.
2. Provide the client with privacy for all aspects of the visit including the history, examinations, procedures, and individual education sessions. No client should be expected to discuss her health and concerns within earshot of other clients, family members, or staff members who are not involved in her care. Clients may withhold important information such as information on physical or sexual abuse or substance use, if they feel that family members or strangers may be able to hear. Likewise, confidentiality must be maintained by providers, with information shared between providers only as necessary for the provision of optimum care. Information about a client should never be discussed in public places such as hallways, elevators, or the employee cafeteria.
3. Approach the client with a nonjudgmental, interested professional attitude. The ability to ask questions in a nondirective and nonthreatening manner, combined with good listening and observation skills, facilitates assessment while increasing client comfort. When taking a health history, nurses should keep in mind that not all women are heterosexual and should avoid language that conveys this assumption. For example, in collecting demographic data, the nurse can ask: "What is your partner's name?" rather than "What is your husband's name?" Sexual assessment should include a question about sexual orientation such as "Are you sexually active with men, with women, or with both men and women?"
4. Conduct client assessment in a collaborative manner to decrease repetition, increase efficiency, and improve communication. Advance discussion of roles and responsibilities between nurses and other providers of care can lead to development of an effective approach to client assessment and care. Multidisciplinary care conferences allow providers to share necessary information and develop a comprehensive plan of care.
5. Provide anticipatory guidance about the examination techniques and their purposes, offer emotional support during the examination, and teach relaxation techniques to use during the examination. These interventions foster a therapeutic working relationship with the client while helping her through the examination and procedures.

Assessment

Comprehensive assessment includes compiling a client data base that includes both subjective and objective data. The history provides subjective data, that is, information reported by the client and/or possibly by family members or caretakers. The physical examination and laboratory tests provide objective data. Laboratory data is composed of the results of the analysis of various specimens which may be obtained before (e.g., urine sample), during (e.g., cervical and vaginal specimens), and after (e.g., blood samples) the physical examination. Comprehensive assessment is necessary to provide high-quality wellness care and is a standard to which nurses may be legally held.

The complete health history includes a thorough report of the client's current and past health and is usually obtained prior to the physical examination (Fig. 7–1). Table 7–1 outlines the relevant information sought for a well woman's health history. Information provided by the history directs health care providers during the physical examination and identifies areas that require a specific focus. This information is also used to identify the woman's perception of her

▶ **TABLE 7-1**

Guidelines for Health History of a Well Woman

Background

Name, address

Birthplace, date of birth

Religion; racial background; languages spoken, primary language

Education, particular learning difficulties

Current employment

Financial status (client's perception of whether income is adequate)

Health insurance

Alternative health care, past and present (e.g., herbalists)

Overall satisfaction with lifestyle

Marital status: if appropriate, partner's name, occupation, address, health; client identification of problems such as drug abuse; client evaluation of relationship (including incidents or fear of abuse)

Children: ages, addresses, health status; child care; perceived parenting problems

Significant other background: similar to partner information

Cultural beliefs related to wellness, prevention, diet, reproduction, treatment, healers

Reasons for visit; concerns; goals for visit

Present state of health

  Client's perception of usual health status and of being at risk for health problem

  Allergies

  Medications; special health requirements

Past health history

  Previous wellness visits; illnesses (hospitalization, surgery, childhood illnesses)

  Accidents, injuries; immunizations (type, date); medications

Family history

  Acute or chronic illnesses, particularly client's parents, grandparents, siblings; congenital problems

  Deaths (dates and reasons)

  Attitudes and practices related to wellness

Overview of Body Systems

General

Feelings of wellness; fatigue, chills, fever, weakness, hot flashes, night sweats, unexplained feelings of illness

Integument

Skin: general appearance, rashes, lesions, moles and any changes in their appearance

Hair: change in hair growth or loss; chemical treatments

Nails of hands and feet: change in color, shape, condition

Head, Eyes, Ears, Nose, Throat (HEENT)

Head: headaches (location, duration, frequency, treatments, perception of cause); dizziness; loss of consciousness; injury

Eyes: vision problems (specify), eyeglasses or contact lenses, infections, tearing, pain, surgery or injury, date of last eye exam, family history of eye disease

Ears: tinnitus, discharge, pain, history of infection, hearing impairment, vertigo, hearing aid, date of last hearing exam

Nose and sinuses: nasal discharge; bleeding (frequency, amount, client's perception of cause); sinus problems, frequency of colds; loss of smell; nasal obstruction; drug use (snorting); smoking; treatments (prescribed or self-treatment); nasal surgery

Mouth: hygiene; knowledge and regularity of oral hygiene practices; prosthetics (dentures, braces); lesions on lips or in mouth (frequency, severity); excessive salivation; condition of teeth; difficulty speaking; change in taste of foods; sore or

bleeding gums; discolored mucosa or teeth; last dental exam; regularity of evaluations

Throat: difficulty swallowing, soreness, irritation, infections, hoarseness, coughing, treatment (prescribed or self-directed)

Neck: Swelling, soreness, stiffness, lumps, thyroid problems

Cardiovascular

Chest pain, palpitations, claudication, varicosities, edema, shortness of breath; number of pillows used for sleeping; mottling of skin; hypertension; history of heart murmur, rheumatic fever, congenital heart problems; cardiac disease; smoking; exercise patterns; exercise tolerance

Respiratory

Shortness of breath; difficult or painful breathing; cyanosis; cough (productive, nature of secretions, blood); allergies, wheezing, history of respiratory infections (type, treatments); night sweats; history of emphysema, asthma, tuberculosis, bronchitis; date and results of chest x-rays; tuberculin tests; smoking habits; respiratory medication

Gastrointestinal

Appetite; difficulty swallowing; bowel patterns and changes (diarrhea, constipation, hemorrhoids, rectal bleeding, frank blood in stool or tarry stools); jaundice; history of ulcers; nausea, vomiting, gallbladder disease, hepatitis; anorexic or bulemic behaviors; use of antacids, laxatives, or other drugs; history of enteric infections or parasites (dates, treatment, outcome)

Urinary

Frequency; color change; polyuria; urgency; pain, burning, itching; pyuria, hematuria, nocturia; foul odor; hesitancy, incontinence, leakage; history of urinary tract infection or trauma (dates, treatment); use of diuretics or other drugs

Reproductive

Breasts: Pain, lumps, lesions, nipple discharge, history of breast disease (types and dates of treatment), understanding of breast self-examination, regularity of self-examinations, client's perceptions of own risks for breast disease

Menstruation: date last menstrual period began; age at menarche; length of cycles, duration of menses, regularity; menorrhagia, metorrhagia, dysmenorrhea; premenstrual symptoms; treatments for menstrual problems

Family planning: Birth control (attitude toward practice; methods used now and in past; level of understanding of methods; satisfaction with methods; problems)

Obstetrics: Current possibility of pregnancy; previous pregnancies (planned, unplanned), outcomes; dates and types of deliveries; infants' birth weight and status, obstetric or neonatal complications and treatments; infertility problems and treatments

Gynecology: Vaginal discharge (nature, amount, duration, odor); itching, burning, lesions; past vaginal infections (type, dates, treatments); problems of infectious (e.g., STDs) or noninfectious origin (e.g., endometriosis, fibroids, infertility, miscarriage or pregnancy loss, surgery), including dates and treatments; date of last Pap test; understanding and practice of genital self-examination

Sexual history: Frequency of sexual relations; sexual orientation; satisfaction with the sexual relationship; client's perception of problems or concerns related to own sexuality or sexual relationship; understanding of risk for STDs; history of risky sexual behaviors including multiple partners, risky partners, and unprotected intercourse

▶   **TABLE 7-1 (continued)**

Guidelines for Health History of A Well Woman

Musculoskeletal

Pain, stiffness, limited movement; history of injury or disease; redness, swelling, deformed joints or skeleton (e.g., scoliosis); vigorous activity (regular practice or recent undertaking)

Neurologic

Seizures (type, onset, treatment, level of control); tremors; problems with balance or speech; weakness or paralysis (transient or permanent); problems with gait; paresthesias; loss of consciousness; loss of memory; mood swings, depression, anxiety, or other mental symptoms; drug use and effects

Hematopoietic

Anemia (type, treatment); sickle-cell (trait or disease); bleeding or other blood disorders, including frequent unexplained bruising; transfusions (dates, reasons, reactions); family history of hemophilia

Lymphatic

Pain, tenderness, swelling, infection of any nodes

Endocrine

Change in glove or shoe size; hirsutism; excessive sweating or thirst; polyuria; polyphasia; goiter; other endocrine problems and treatments; heat or cold intolerance; unexplained weight change

Lifestyle

Nutrition

Access to adequate food; location of meals; food preparation (self or others); typical daily or weekly diet; vitamin and mineral supplements; preferred foods; snacking patterns; fluids (type, amount, including alcoholic beverages); food allergies (type of reaction); dietary supplements (type, amount, duration); recent weight gain or loss; salt, caffeine intake; ingestion of nonfood items; client's perception of weight; weight control practices; satisfaction with current nutritional status and weight; weight fluctuations, use of diet aids

Smoking

Nonsmoker, current smoker (how long, amount smoked, brand); understanding of effects of smoking; desire to quit, attempts; history of smoking-related illnesses; smokers in home and work environment

Drug Use

Present or past use (prescription or recreational, type, and route of administration); history of intravenous drug use; history of sharing needles or other drug equipment; treatment programs (date and effects of treatment); illnesses related to drug use (cellulitis, hepatitis, HIV seroconversion, HIV infection)

Alcohol

Current intake (amount, type, frequency); previous or current history of alcohol treatment; alcohol-related illnesses (physical, mental, social)

Occupations

Present or past jobs (includes work for monetary or nonmonetary pay and work of housewives); job satisfaction; description of the physical work environment, including size of work area, ventilation, noise levels, safety measures, exposure to chemical or other potentially hazardous conditions (e.g., asbestos, benzene, oils), stress (means of relieving stress, support from others, occupational transitions, and client's reactions), exposure to heat or cold, protective devices available and used; client's perceptions of specific present or past occupational hazards

Exposure to Infectious Diseases

Known exposure at home, work, or during travel; contact with animals or animal excrement, especially cat feces

Sleep, Rest, Exercise and Activity Patterns

Amount and pattern of sleep and rest; amount and type of exercise; regularity and level of exercise; client's reaction to exercise and perception of own activities

Stress Patterns

Client's perception of acute or chronic stress; reactions to stress and ways of coping; effectiveness of coping strategies; individuals who help client deal with stress

Safety

History of trauma; history of current or past mental or physical abuse

Interpersonal Relationships

Support system; resource people; degree of social isolation

physical, psychosocial, and educational needs and her strengths and supports and to develop a plan of care. The comprehensive history should be obtained at the woman's first visit to a provider and updated at subsequent visits.

At all visits the nurse should give special attention to gynecologic, sexual, and reproductive concerns including reproductive history, menstrual history, contraceptive use, prevention of STDs, and sexual history. This provides data for interventions related specifically to female sexuality and reproduction. Any nurse who works with female clients should be confident in his or her abilities to do a comprehensive sexual assessment. See Chapter 5 for information on how to take a sexual history.

Subjective information is best obtained from the client in an area where privacy can be assured. In some instances, such as when the client is mentally handicapped or cannot speak the same language as the nurse, a third party must be present to provide information or to translate questions and answers. If language translation is necessary it is important to obtain a translator who speaks both languages well, understands confidentiality issues, and is trained in medical terminology. Use of family members as translators is sometimes necessary but is not ideal as this raises issues of privacy, confidentiality, and accuracy.

Comprehensive physical assessment of the client may be done by an NP or other qualified health care provider. The registered nurse participates in this

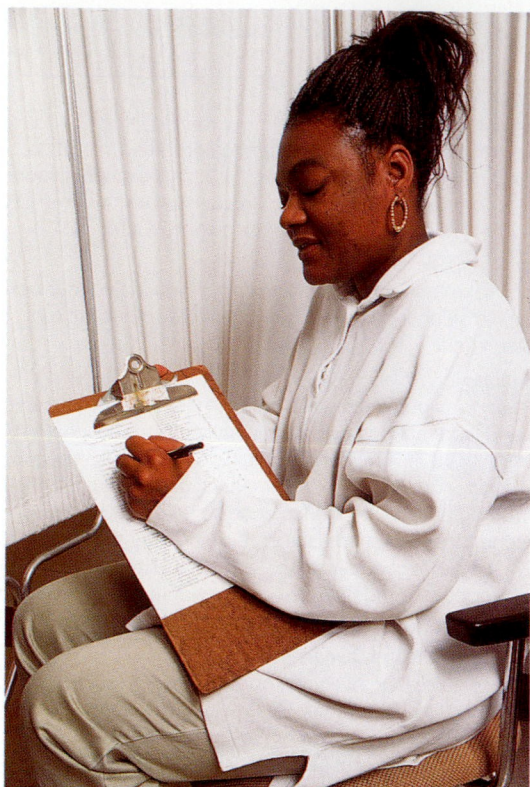

FIGURE 7–1. An essential part of the assessment process is having the client complete a well woman history.

process by providing emotional and physical support to the client, obtaining data such as vital signs, and assisting the examiner. The client should be given a gown to change into and a drape or sheet should be arranged to provide maximum privacy while exposing only the part of the body being examined. The nurse assists the woman on and off the examining table as necessary to ensure safety and helps in positioning her for maximum comfort during the examination. Table 7–2 provides an outline for the comprehensive general physical examination of the female client. Breast and gynecological examinations may be performed by the primary care practitioner or the client may be referred to a gynecologic specialist for these services. If a gynecological examination is to be performed during the same visit as the comprehensive general physical examination, a female staff member should remain in the room to protect both the client and examiner from misunderstandings, misconduct, or charges of misconduct. Information specific to the gynecological examination is provided below.

Health Promotion and Screening

The U.S. Preventive Services Task Force (1996) has compiled guidelines for health interventions aimed at

▶ **TABLE 7-2**

Sample Outline for a Well Woman Physical Examination

Name

Age

Height

Weight

Vital signs
  Temperature
  Pulse
  Respirations
  Blood pressure (both arms; sitting, standing, supine)

General Impression

Neurologic Status
  Mental status; motor function; reflexes

Integument
  Skin color, texture, lesions (breaks, bruising, rashes, sores, pigmented areas, moles or warts, infected areas); hair (skin or hair parasites); nails (fingernails, toenails)

HEENT
  Head: Size, lesions, lumps, scaling, parasites; facial symmetry; edema
  Eyes: Alignment; lids; lacrimal apparatus; conjunctiva; cornea; sclera; irises; pupils; lenses; ophthalmoscopic; presence of infection; pupils equal round and reactive to light and accommodation (PERRLA)
  Ears: Hearing; external ear; otoscopic (ear canals, tympanic membranes)
  Nose and sinuses: Nasal septum; mucosa; presence of inflammation, discharge, lesions, polyps; pain or tenderness
  Oral cavity: Condition of mouth; lesions or bleeding of lips, gums, tongue, or oral cavity; condition of teeth (obvious decay, missing teeth; oral appliances), condition of tongue, pharynx, tonsils; pain or soreness
  Neck: Masses, edema, tenderness; position of trachea; nonpalpable thyroid, lymph nodes

Chest:
  Character and rate of respirations; symmetry of chest expansion; lungs clear; masses or tenderness; presence of infections

Breast
See Table 7–5

Cardiac and Peripheral Vascular
  Presence, rate, and regularity of cardiac and peripheral pulses; no carotid bruits; no heart murmurs; color and temperature of extremities; any evidence of varicosities or phlebitis; any evidence of needle tracks, shunts, or other vascular invasions

Abdomen
  Symmetry; muscle tone; presence of masses; tenderness; scars; bowel sounds; aortic size; nonpalpable and nontender spleen, kidneys; no liver enlargement or tenderness; presence of hernias; no lymph node enlargement or tenderness

Genitalia and Anal Area
See Table 7–5

Musculoskeletal
  Neck: pain, condition of temporomandibular joint
  Back: posture, pain or tenderness, deformity or curvature
  Extremities: symmetry of arms and legs; pain in joints, muscles, redness, swelling; restricted movement

Concluding Impression

preventing premature death and disability. The guidelines include age-based recommendations for screening tests, counseling interventions, immunizations, and chemoprophylactic regimens. Recommendations are based on screening and interventions which have been shown to affect the leading causes of morbidity and mortality for each age group. Table 7–3 lists the leading causes of death among women identified by the U.S. Preventive Services Task Force for each of the age groups from adolescence through older adulthood. Table 7–4 summarizes the recommendations for interventions to be performed during the periodic health visit. Frequency of intervention is provided where a specific frequency is recommended. These recommendations are aimed at the general population of individuals, that is, those who are free from symptoms of the disease or target condition. Additional interventions are recommended for individuals at high risk for other conditions affecting their health, well-being, or life span.

Timing of the periodic health visit should be individualized depending upon the client's age and risk profile. Health promotion screening and interventions should not be confined to the periodic health visit. Many individuals do not use the health care system on a routine basis for preventive health services due to barriers of cost, time, and accessibility. For these individuals it is crucial to initiate health promotion and disease prevention interventions during each encounter.

The education nurses receive in health promotion, health education, and risk assessment make them ideal professionals to carry out the recommendation of the U.S. Preventive Services Task Force. Nurses have traditionally been acutely concerned with health promotion and screening, especially in their roles as public health nurses. Nurses also participate in health promotion and screening on other levels such as in the outpatient setting and in schools.

Gynecological and Breast Examination

The gynecologic examination includes examination of the breast and related structures, external genitalia, vagina, cervix, uterus and adnexa, and rectum. In some settings the gynecologic health history and gynecologic examination are performed separately from other health assessments and screening. In other settings it is possible to address other health needs along with the gynecological examination and thus provide more holistic care. The nurse working in a setting that provides only gynecologic care should be alert to indications of health problems in other body systems and to clients' concerns about nongynecological health matters and be prepared to assist clients in obtaining appropriate care for those concerns. Even in a strictly gynecological setting, the minimal assessment should include assessment of vital signs, height, weight, heart, lungs, and abdomen in addition to assessment of the breasts and external and internal genital organs.

Immediately prior to the gynecological examination the nurse should provide the woman with the opportunity to empty her bladder. A full bladder increases the woman's discomfort during the pelvic examination and may decrease accuracy of the physical findings. At this time, the nurse may also ask the woman to collect any necessary urine specimens. Table 7–5 illustrates the components of the physical examination of the breasts and internal and external genitalia.

To decrease risk of infection and increase the client's confidence in her care, the nurse should always wash hands before and after the examination using proper handwashing technique. Universal precautions should be observed during this examination as during all client contacts. Nails should be kept short and jewelry should not be worn on the hands to

▶ **TABLE 7–3**

Leading Causes of Death Among Women by Age Group

Age Group	Cause of Death
11–24	Accidents Homicide Suicide Cancer
25–34	Accidents Cancer Homicide Suicide
35–44	Cancer Heart disease Accidents Suicide
45–54	Cancer Heart disease Cerebrovascular disease Accidents
55–64	Cancer Heart disease Cerebrovascular disease Lung disease
65–84	Heart disease Cancer Cerebrovascular disease Lung disease
> 85	Heart disease Cerebrovascular disease Cancer Lung disease

Source: Woods, 1995.

▶ **TABLE 7-4**

Interventions for Women Recommended by U.S. Preventive Services Task Force (USPSTF) for Periodic Health Exam

Intervention	Age Group	Frequency	Notes
Screening			
Height and weight	≥ 11		
Blood pressure	≥ 11	≥ every 2 years if last reading < 140/85; every year if last systolic reading < 140 and last diastolic 85–95	At each client visit[a]
Papanicolaou (Pap) test	≥ 11	≤ every 3 years for all sexually active women who have a cervix	First Pap smear at age 18 or earlier if sexually active and then every year until 3 consecutive normal Paps. After 3 consecutive normal Paps, physician discretion is recommended.[b]
Chlamydia screen	< 20	If sexually active	Frequency given by USPSTF is "during routine gyn exams"
Rubella serology or vaccination history	> 12	At first clinical visit	All nonimmune, nonpregnant women should be counseled appropriately and offered vaccination. Nonimmune pregnant women should be counseled and offered vaccination immediately postpartum.
Assess for problem drinking	≥ 11		Screening can be done through careful history-taking or use of standardized questionnaires
Total blood cholesterol	45–65	≥ every 5 years	≥ every 5 years age ≥ 20[c]
• Fecal occult blood • Sigmoidoscopy	≥ 50	Annually (fecal occult blood testing)	Annually ≥ 40 (fecal occult blood testing)[b]
Mammogram +/– clinical breast exam	50–69	Every 1–2 years	Ages 40–49 (yearly)[b] Ages 40–49 (based on risk)[d]
Vision screening	≥ 65		
Hearing screening	≥ 65		
Counseling			
Injury prevention			
• Lap/shoulder belts	≥ 11		
• Bicycle/motorcycle/ATV helmets	≥ 11		
• Smoke detectors	≥ 11		
• Safe storage/removal of firearms	≥ 11		
• Hot water heater < 120–130 degrees F	> 65 > 65		
• CPR training household members	> 65		
Substance use			
• Avoid tobacco use and smoking cessation	11 ≥ 65		Frequent assessment of tobacco use and frequent repetition of messages about avoidance of smoking and smoking cessation are recommended.
• Underage drinking	11–21		
• Illicit drug use	11–25		
• Avoid alcohol and drugs while driving, swimming, boating, etc.	≥ 11		Include questions about drug use when taking history
Sexual behavior			
• STD prevention	≥ 11		Counseling should be tailored to individual risk behavior after careful assessment of such behavior.
• Contraception	Age 11 to end of childbearing years		
Diet and exercise			
• Balanced diet/ limit fat and cholesterol	≥ 11		
• Adequate calcium	≥ 11		
• Regular physical activity	≥ 11		

▶   **TABLE 7–4 (continued)**

Interventions for Women Recommended by U.S. Preventive Services Task Force (USPSTF) for Periodic Health Exam

Intervention	Age Group	Frequency	Notes
Dental health			
• Regular dental visits	≥ 11		
• Brush/floss daily	≥ 11		
Immunizations			
• Tetanus-diphtheria booster	≥ 11	• Booster at 11–16 years and then every 10 years	
• Hepatitis B	11–24	• If not previously immunized	
• MMR	11–12		
• Rubella	> 12	• If not immune	
• Pneumococcal	> 65	• Routine revaccination not recommended	
• Influenza	> 65	• Annually	
Chemoprophylaxis			
• Multivitamin with folic acid daily	Childbearing years		
• Hormone replacement	Peri- and post-menopausal		

Note: *Interventions are for the general population and should be modified based on specific individual and population risks.

[a]JNC V, 1993.
[b]American Cancer Society, 1997.
[c]National Heart, Lung, and Blood Institute, 1993a.
[d]National Institutes of Health, 1997.

Source: U.S. Preventive Services Task Force, 1996.

decrease both the risk of injury to the client and the chance that examination gloves will tear during the examination. Since clients may be allergic to materials such as latex or iodine which may be used in routine examinations, the nurse should question them about allergies prior to the examination. After specimens are obtained gloves can be lubricated with a water soluble lubricant to increase comfort during the bimanual examination.

During the gynecological examination, specimens are often collected from the cervix or vaginal walls for assessment of disorders such as cervical cancer and for testing for STDs and vaginal infections. For these tests, proper sampling technique is important.

Client Participation in the Gynecological and Breast Examination. Many women regard the gynecologic examination with negative feelings such as dread, embarrassment, fear, and anxiety. This is probably related to cultural norms that designate the breasts and genitals as private areas not to be seen or touched by another person except within a sexual relationship. The examination itself is physically invasive and can be uncomfortable. Vaginal and perineal infections, lacerations, unhealed episiotomies, and post-menopausal changes in the vaginal wall are conditions that can cause pain during a gynecological examination. Another source of emotional and physical discomfort can be the lithotomy position, which is usually used for the external and internal genital examination. Clients may also fear that abnormalities may be found, especially if they know that they may be at risk for STDs or cancer. Women may fear that health care professionals will pass judgment on their behavior or will breach confidentiality related to the findings of their examination and screening tests. In addition, women who have been subject to sexual abuse may view the physical examination as traumatic and a further loss of personal control (Chalfen, 1993).

Certain techniques can increase the woman's emotional and physical comfort during the examination. The gynecological examination can be used as a tool for education and empowerment of the female client. This approach involves giving the woman the opportunity to participate in the examination and through that participation to learn about her anatomy and physiology, breast self examination (BSE), and vulvar self-examination. The examination also provides an atmosphere that encourages the woman to discuss issues related to reproduction and sexuality, makes her feel more in control of the examination process, and makes the examination less threatening. The following strategies can be implemented to make

► **TABLE 7-5**

Components of Clinical Breast and Gynecologic Physical Examination

I. Breast Examination

Focus

- Breasts   Size, symmetry, dimpling, lesions, scars, masses, thickening, tenderness, inflammation, implants
- Nipples   Everted or inverted, discharge, crusting, scars
- Lymph nodes   Size, condition, tenderness

| Inspection | Palpation | | Client Education |
	Positioning	Technique	
Client Sitting: Inspect breasts first with client's arms at her side, then with her arms overhead, and finally with her hands firmly on hips and elbows forward (chest muscle flexion).	**Client Sitting:** Axillary, subscapular, pectoral, clavicular, and lateral lymph nodes are palpated (see Fig. 7–2 for location of lymph nodes in the breast). **Client Lying Down:** The breast is flattened, which facilitates lump detection. *Supine:* Woman lies on her back on the examining table. A small folded towel or wedge is positioned under her shoulder on the side being examined, which distributes breast tissue more evenly. The woman places her hand behind her head. *On her side:* Woman lies on the hip opposite the breast being examined and rotates her shoulders so that they are flat against the examining table. Her hand on the side to be examined is placed against her forehead. This positioning flattens breast tissue for examination.	**To Identify Lumps:** Examiner palpates with the pads of the middle three fingers (fingertips are not used). Light, medium, and firm pressure is applied throughout the breast to detect abnormalities. Palpation should be done in a systematic way to ensure complete coverage of the breast tissue. The examiner can use a pattern such as parallel lines, concentric circles or the wedge (see Fig. 7–4 on page 166). The entire breast, from the clavicle to the inframammary ridge and from midsternal to posterior axillary line should be palpated. Palpate well into the axilla. Palpate the areola. Palpate each nipple gently.	Breast self-examination is taught and client's mastery of the technique and understanding of its importance are evaluated. Teaching may be done by staff nurse, nurse practitioner, or physician.

II. Genitalia Examination

Positioning	Inspection	Palpation	Client Education
Lithotomy: To promote comfort, head and shoulders are elevated to semisitting position; stirrups are adjusted to comfortable length for woman's height to prevent excessive hip abduction; client's hands are placed at her sides (not overhead) to avoid tightening of abdominal muscles; relaxation techniques, such as deep breathing, may be practiced. **Speculum:** Speculum should be neither too hot nor too cold. It may be lubricated with small amount of warm water; however, water is used sparingly to avoid interference with specimen results.	**External** • Hair distribution • Color and condition of vulva and perineum • Lesions, rashes, masses, swelling, varicosities, parasites, discharge • Bruising, lacerations, scars • Needle track marks in groin or elsewhere • Unnatural odor **Internal** (with speculum in place): *Specimens* may be obtained from the vagina and cervix.	**Internal** (following removal of speculum and application of lubricant to glove) *Uterus:* Size, shape, masses, tenderness *Adnexa:* Masses, tenderness	Client may watch examination using a mirror held near her knees or vulva. Self-examination of the vulva may be taught using this method of inspection. Client technique is evaluated.

► **TABLE 7–5 (continued)**

Components of Clinical Breast and Gynecologic Physical Examination

II. Genitalia Examination (cont.)

Positioning	Inspection	Palpation	Client Education
	Vagina • Condition and color of mucosa • Lacerations, lesions, discharge, cystocele or rectocele, muscle tone, unnatural odor, bruising *Cervix* • Color and condition • Erosions, cysts, lesions, discharge from os, trauma, string from intrauterine device		

III. Rectal Examination

Positioning	External Inspection	Internal Palpation
Lithotomy	Inflammation, hemorrhoids, signs of trauma	(Using well-lubricated glove) Hemorrhoids, masses in rectum or adnexa (palpated through rectovaginal wall), sphincter tone, bleeding, pain

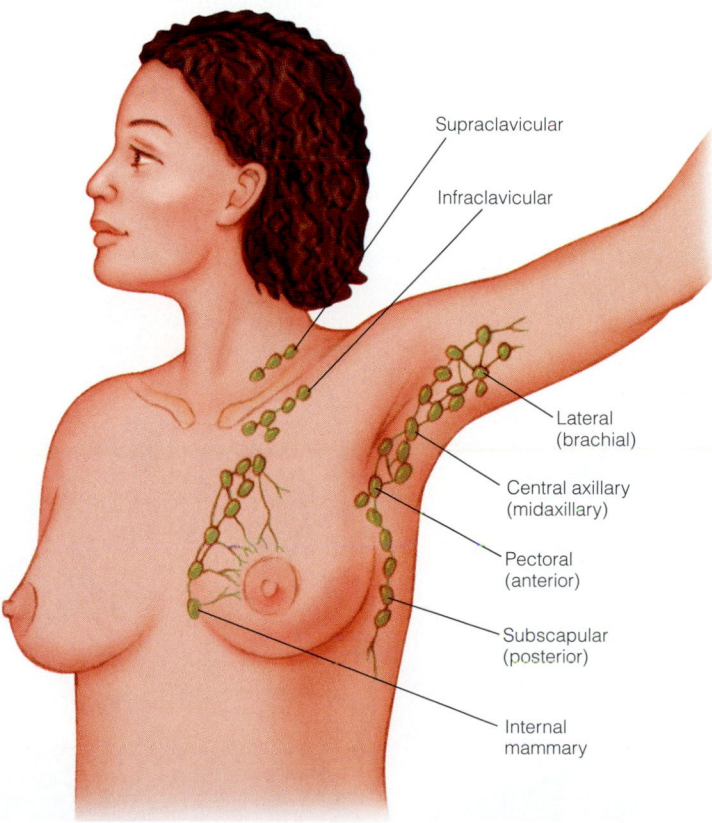

FIGURE 7–2. Location of the subscapular, central axillary, anterior pectoral, supraclavicular, and infraclavicular nodes in the female breast.

the examination an educational and empowering experience:

1. Promote the client's comfort and privacy by ensuring that the door to the examination room remains closed while she is undressed and that she is covered as much as possible during the examination by a gown and/or drapes. Set the stirrups at a comfortable angle to avoid painful abduction of her hips and cover them with padding to reduce contact with the cold metal surface (Fig. 7–3). Keeping the room at a comfortable temperature also increases her comfort and helps her relax.

2. Adjust the examination table and the drapes so that the woman's head is elevated and she can see the face of the person examining her. That person should be sure to make eye contact with the client at intervals during the examination, to proceed slowly and carefully and to inform the woman about the process of the examination as it is being done.

3. Offer the woman a mirror and show her how to position it during the internal and external genital examinations so she can view the procedures. This approach helps the nurse and examiner to explain reproductive anatomy and physiology as well as procedures to the woman. Many women have never viewed their genitalia and are grateful to be given the chance to do this and to learn what each structure is and what it is for. Be sure to allow time for her to ask questions as the exam proceeds.

4. Help the woman to relax during the examination and during any uncomfortable procedures by encouraging muscle relaxation and slow relaxed breathing.

▶ Menstruation and Menstrual Disorders

Menstruation

Menstruation, the shedding of the uterine lining at the end of the menstrual cycle, is a normal cyclic physiologic event during the reproductive years. Historically and in some cultures today the process is surrounded by myth, secrecy, and even ceremony. As people from many different cultures continue to immigrate to the United States nurses will encounter women with many different beliefs surrounding menstruation. Taboos related to menstruation are still seen today in language which refers to menstruation as "the curse," "my friend," or "my period." Because some women are reluctant to discuss menstruation and menstrual difficulties, the nurse must incorporate assessment of the menstrual cycle and menstrual discomforts at every visit.

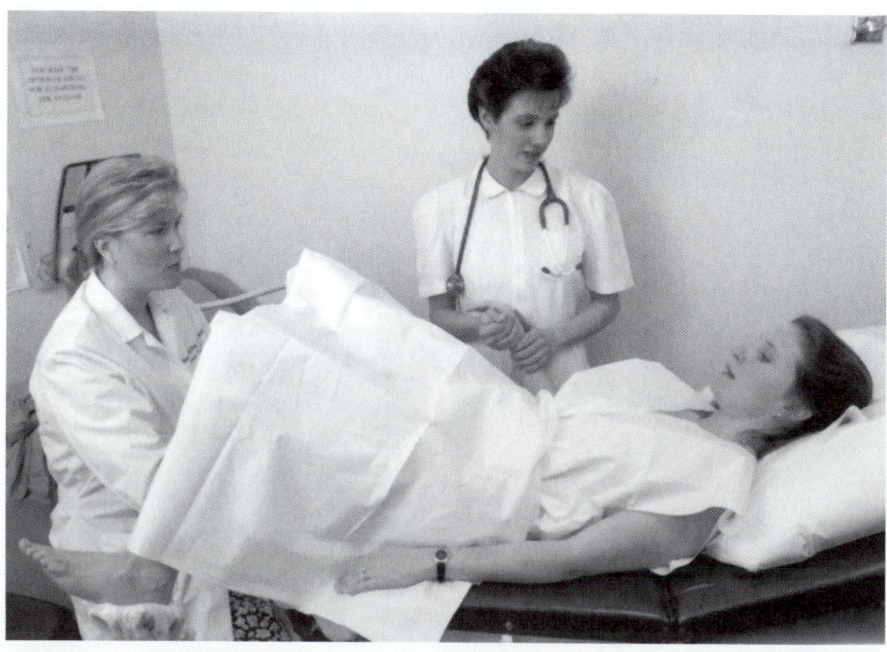

FIGURE 7–3. The client is placed in the lithotomy position during regular gynecologic examinations. Her feet are in stirrups, arms rest comfortably at her sides, and her head is slightly elevated.

Puberty refers to the period during which the endocrine and gametogenic functions of the ovaries develop. Puberty lasts from 1 to 8 years with an average length of 4 years. During puberty the female gains 20–25% of her final adult height and 50% of her adult ideal body weight (Becker, 1995). Secondary sexual characteristics, including breasts and pubic hair, also develop during puberty. One milestone in puberty is **menarche,** the first menstrual period, which can take place in girls as young as 9 or as old as 16. The average age of menarche in the United States is 12.7 years (Brown & Corbett, 1995).

Nursing care of the menstruating girl and woman includes education about physiologic and psychologic aspects of menstruation. School nurses play a large part in educating girls about menstruation before menarche. Some girls may be upset or frightened by the onset of their first menstrual period or need assistance in managing the flow.

Menstrual hygiene is an important topic for nurses to discuss with menstruating women and girls. Commercially produced alternatives for absorbing menstrual flow include sanitary pads and tampons. Sanitary pads are produced in a variety of sizes, thicknesses, and absorbencies and may be attached to the undergarments with adhesive strips or held on by a special belt. They should be changed frequently to prevent buildup of bacteria that can cause odor and increase the woman's risk for urinary tract infection. Pads containing deodorants are also marketed but are not recommended as the deodorant products can cause irritation. Daily showering and perineal cleansing should be sufficient to control menstrual odors. Women should be advised that cleaning out the vagina after menstruation using commercial or homemade douches is unnecessary and may lead to irritation or infection.

Tampons are inserted into the vagina to absorb menstrual flow. Many women find that tampons are a hygienic and comfortable alternative to pads. Tampons can be worn by most menstruating women and girls and do not cause tearing of an intact hymen. Women may need education about how to insert a tampon, especially if they are not familiar with their own anatomy. Tampons are also produced in a variety of sizes and absorbencies. Manufacturers of tampons are required to conform to standard labeling of their products as junior, regular, super, or super plus absorbency. Use of super absorbent tampons has been associated with a rare infection called **toxic shock syndrome** (TSS). TSS is an acute illness caused by a toxin produced by a strain of *Staphylococcus aureus* bacterium. It is characterized by hypotension, high fever, and a rash which is followed by peeling of the skin, especially on the palms and soles. Multiple organ systems can become involved. Although TSS is rare (1/100,000 menstruating women), it is fatal in 2–4% of cases (American Academy of Pediatrics, 1997; Creehan, 1995). To prevent TSS, women should be instructed to change tampons frequently and to use the least absorbent tampon needed to control the menstrual flow. Women with a history of TSS should be advised not to use tampons (American Academy of Pediatrics, 1997).

Premenstrual Syndrome

Premenstrual syndrome (PMS) refers to a variety of physical, emotional, and behavioral symptoms that can occur during the luteal phase of the menstrual cycle (after midcycle and decreasing or disappearing at the start of or shortly after the start of menstruation). Although symptoms vary from woman to woman, each woman tends to have a consistent pattern of symptoms that are cyclical. Women who complain of PMS often begin to have symptoms during adolescence or young adulthood. Symptoms typically worsen as the woman ages, and stop at menopause (Gise, 1995). PMS occurs in women all around the world, although the specific manifestations may vary from culture to culture. As many as 95% of all women report that they have at least one premenstrual symptom (Gise, 1995).

The cause of PMS is still unknown although there is evidence that it is related to the hormones estrogen and progesterone. Abnormal levels of serotonin, a neurotransmitter, may also be a factor. Risk factors for PMS include a personal or family history of mood disorders, anxiety disorders, or substance abuse and a family history of a mother, sister, or daughter with PMS. Women who have been sexually abused also are more likely to suffer from PMS (Gise, 1995).

Over 150 symptoms have been described as occurring with PMS but most women report only a few to several symptoms or discomforts (see the box entitled Common Symptoms of Premenstrual Syndrome). Controversy has long existed over whether PMS is an endocrine disorder, a psychiatric disorder, or a set of physiologic changes caused by normal hormonal cycling.

Four types of premenstrual syndromes have been described (Gise, 1995):

1. Premenstrual symptoms or changes occur in women who have one or more mild to moderate symptoms which do not interfere with daily functioning. As many as 95% of all women fall into this category. Most of these women do not seek care for their symptoms.

2. Premenstrual syndrome occurs in women who have two more symptoms which they feel are

Commonly Asked Questions

Menstruation

What is a normal menstrual period?

A normal menstrual period represents the shedding of the lining of the uterus. Menstrual flow includes blood, some endometrial tissue, white blood cells, and mucus.

How long should menstrual periods last?

There is considerable variation among the length of menstrual periods among women. Menstrual periods can last from 2 to 8 days.

How often does menstruation occur?

Although the menstrual cycle has traditionally been described as being about 28 days long, cycles vary greatly among women. Menstrual cycles also vary within the same woman by about 5 to 10 days. Menstruation reflects complex physical, psychologic, and environmental interactions; such factors as extreme weight loss, vigorous physical activity, and emotional stress can affect menstrual patterns.

How much blood is lost?

About 30 to 100 mL of blood is lost during menstruation. The amount of flow depends on factors like the thickness of the endometrium and certain medications.

Are clots abnormal?

Because of the presence of fibrinolysin, which breaks down clots, menstrual flow does not tend to clot. Clots may represent heavy bleeding related to a variety of pathologic causes. Clots also occur, however, in normal, healthy women. A study of hemoglobin or hematocrit should be routine at gynecologic visits and can indicate whether excessive bleeding is taking place during menstruation.

How much iron do women lose during menstruation?

Women can lose about 0.5 to 1 mg of iron daily in menstrual flow.

Should exercise be restricted during menstruation?

There is no reason why a woman cannot continue with her usual pattern of activities. Indeed, such exercises as brisk walking and tennis may promote feelings of well-being and reduce menstrual discomforts.

Should vaginal sprays or douches be used to prevent menstrual odor?

No. Despite vigorous advertising campaigns, vaginal sprays or douches should not be used by the healthy woman; these preparations can cause such problems as rashes, itching, and burning. Showering, bathing, or external cleansing with water or water and gentle soap, as well as regular changing of pads or tampons, is sufficient. Normal menstrual flow has a mild "fleshy" odor. Foul-smelling discharge could indicate abnormal conditions such as infection and should be reported to the health care provider without delay.

Can a woman get pregnant during her period?

Although the menstrual phase is the least fertile time during a woman's cycle, pregnancy could, in theory, occur. The graafian follicle begins to mature in the ovary while menstruation is taking place in the uterus. Considering that sperm can live up to 6 days, unprotected intercourse could possibly result in pregnancy.

Is it all right for a woman to have intercourse during menstruation?

The healthy woman does not have to refrain from intercourse on the basis of menstruation alone. Religious, cultural, or other personal beliefs do, however, affect sexual behavior during menstruation. Women need to be informed about the risk of pregnancy with unprotected intercourse at any time during the menstrual cycle. Although contact with vaginal secretions is an important source of transmission of certain diseases, menstruation can bring the male into direct contact with his partner's blood. This may be a concern for some couples.

► COMMON SYMPTOMS OF PREMENSTRUAL SYNDROME

EMOTIONAL

Emotional lability (sudden sadness or tearfulness), anxiety, irritability, anger, hostility, loneliness

COGNITIVE/BEHAVIORAL

Difficulty concentrating, forgetfulness, impaired judgment, social withdrawal, interpersonal conflict, changes in sexual desire, insomnia, bouts of substance abuse, decreased productivity and efficiency

BREASTS

Tenderness and pain

SKIN

Acne, recurrence of herpes and other skin disorders

GASTROINTESTINAL

Abdominal bloating, food cravings, appetite changes, diarrhea, constipation

OTHER

Vasomotor instability (hot flushes), palpitations, dizziness, headache, fatigue, edema, weight gain

Ginsburg, 1995; Plouffe, Rausch, Khrein, & Stewart, 1994.

problematic but do not interfere with their daily activities. Although they may discuss their symptoms with their health care providers, they usually do not need interventions other than over-the-counter medications. About one third of women have premenstrual syndrome.

3. Premenstrual disorder occurs in women who have at least one emotional/mood related symptom such as depression or anxiety and four or more other symptoms. The American Psychiatric Association identifies this category as Premenstrual Dysphoric Disorder (PMDD) which is classified as a depressive or mood disorder (American Psychiatric Association, 1994). Women with this level of PMS constitute a small minority of women (<4%).

4. Premenstrual exacerbation occurs in women who have physical or mental disorders which worsen during the luteal phase of the menstrual cycle. Examples include mood disorders, anxiety disorders, personality disorders, migraine headaches, asthma, endometriosis, and seizures. Premenstrual exacerbations are different from other premenstrual syndromes in that they do not completely resolve at any phase of the menstrual cycle.

It is not possible to diagnose PMS through history and physical examination alone although these can help rule out other disorders. Diagnosis of any of the PMS disorders requires that the woman keep a daily symptoms diary for at least two months and submit that diary to her health care provider for review. In this diary she records her symptoms on each day, their severity, and the presence or absence of menstrual flow. PMS is diagnosed based on a pattern of symptoms with a sharp drop in number and severity of symptoms in the week after menstruation. If there is not at least one symptom-free week each month the woman may have premenstrual exacerbation rather than one of the other premenstrual syndromes. Keeping a symptom diary is complex and time consuming and the woman will need education from the nurse about how to complete the symptom diary. There is no specific diagnostic test which is helpful in identifying PMS but some tests may be helpful in diagnosing other commonly coexisting conditions such as hypothyroidism and anemia (Plouffe, Rausch, Khrein, & Stewart, 1994).

Treatment of PMS is aimed at relieving the woman's specific symptoms. For example, a woman who is bothered by breast tenderness might be given a prescription for bromocriptine and a woman who is troubled by edema might be advised to restrict her salt intake or might be given a prescription for a mild diuretic. Many women do not need to be treated with medications but find that their PMS is manageable with a routine of exercise and dietary modification such as decreasing salt intake to minimize water retention. See box entitled Treatment Options for Women with Premenstrual Syndrome.

Education and support for the woman and her family are major roles for nurses in the treatment of PMS. Women with PMS are often led to feel that they are "crazy" or unstable because their behavior varies with their menstrual cycle. Nurses can provide support by advising women and their families of the biological basis for PMS and by assisting them with diagnosis

► TREATMENT OPTIONS FOR WOMEN WITH PREMENSTRUAL SYNDROME

NONPHARMACOLOGIC TREATMENT

- Education and supportive therapy
- Stress reduction techniques
- Dietary modification
- Vitamins and/or minerals
- Exercise

PHARMACOLOGIC TREATMENT

- Bulk-forming agents
- Diuretics
- (NSAIDs) Non-steroidal anti-inflammatory drugs
- Bromocriptine
- Hormonal agents
- Antidepressants
- Antianxiety agents

and treatment. Advising women and their families on techniques to cope with the stress caused by living with PMS is another important aspect of nursing care.

Dysmenorrhea

Dysmenorrhea is pain during menstruation and is a common complaint of female clients. Primary dysmenorrhea is related to normal increases in prostaglandin levels during menstruation and is not considered to be related to a disease or pathologic process. As many as 75% of women experience primary dysmenorrhea (Klotz, 1995). Secondary dysmenorrhea is pain during menstruation which is related to a disease process. The nurse needs to realize that both types of dysmenorrhea represent real physical conditions experienced by women from all backgrounds and socioeconomic groups and are not related to psychological states. Pain is a subjective and personal experience. A woman's experience of menstrual discomforts and her expression of those discomforts may be affected by her cultural and psychosocial background.

Primary dysmenorrhea usually begins in adolescence with the onset of ovulatory menstrual cycles and is most common among women in their teens and twenties. Women using intrauterine devices for contraception usually have increased primary dysmenorrhea. The incidence of primary dysmenorrhea decreases with age. The pain associated with primary dysmenorrhea usually occurs during the first day or two of the menstrual period and is described as crampy in nature. It is usually located in the suprapubic area, lower back, and inner thighs and may be accompanied by nausea and vomiting. Exercise and oral contraceptives can decrease the pain of primary dysmenorrhea. While most women with this type of dysmenorrhea are able to carry out their normal activities, some women suffer from pain that is disabling and interferes with their ability to function during a few days of their menstrual cycles.

Secondary dysmenorrhea tends to occur in women older than 25 and increases with age (Klotz, 1995). Causes of secondary dysmenorrhea include endometriosis, pelvic inflammatory disease, fibroid tumors, and cervical and uterine abnormalities. Women with secondary dysmenorrhea often complain of pain that may begin before menstruation and increases in intensity over time. Onset, location, and duration of symptoms depend on the underlying disease process. Associated symptoms also depend on the pathologic cause and may include dyspareunia (pain with intercourse), rectal pressure and pain with defecation, prolonged menstrual periods, heavy bleeding, and shortened menstrual cycles.

Assessment of the woman with dysmenorrhea includes a careful history and physical examination performed to establish whether the pain is related to a pathologic condition. The woman's answers to the following questions about her pain can help determine whether she has primary or secondary dysmenorrhea.

- What is the pain like?
- How severe is the pain?
- Where is the pain located?
- Has the pain interfered with or prevented usual activities and how?
- When does the pain start?
- How long does the pain last?
- Are there any other symptoms present?
- What makes the pain worse? Better?
- How long have you had this type of pain?
- Has the pain increased, decreased, or stayed the same over time?
- What have you tried to relieve the pain? Has it helped?

Primary dysmenorrhea can be relieved by nonpharmacologic therapies alone or by a combination of nonpharmacologic and pharmacologic therapies (see box entitled Treatment Options for Primary Dysmenorrhea). Many women with primary dysmenorrhea

▶ TREATMENT OPTIONS FOR PRIMARY DYSMENORRHEA

NONPHARMACOLOGIC TREATMENT

- Heat (warm baths, showers, heating pad)
- Back or abdominal massage
- Mild exercise
- Relaxation
- Imagery

PHARMACOLOGIC TREATMENT

- NSAIDs
- Combination oral contraceptives

---

may institute the measures without consulting a health care provider. Nurses can suggest alternative therapies to augment the woman's own ideas and provide reassurance as well as education about dysmenorrhea.

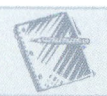

Client Teaching

Primary Dysmenorrhea

The nurse can suggest the following actions to help a client manage the discomfort related to primary dysmenorrhea:

- Take 400 mg of ibuprofen every 6 hours beginning one week before the start of your menses
- Continue to take the ibuprofen for 48–72 hours after your menses begin
- Take the ibuprofen with food to avoid stomach upset
- Apply warmth to your lower abdomen and back with either a hot bath or shower or a heating pad or warm pack
- To make a warm pack, put a warm, moist face towel in a Ziploc bag, wrap it in a pillowcase, and place it against the area of pain
- When using a heating pad or warm pack, test the temperature with your hand or wrist before applying it to your skin
- Do not sleep with a heating pad or warm pack as it may cause burns
- Drink warm tea or other warm drinks
- Walk at a moderate pace for 15 minutes to half an hour when you experience discomfort

Treatment of secondary dysmenorrhea is based on treating the underlying cause if one can be identified. The woman with secondary dysmenorrhea may undergo additional diagnostic testing which may be stressful and uncomfortable. Testing may include pelvic ultrasounds and surgical diagnostic modalities such as laparoscopy and hysteroscopy (see Chapter 10 for discussion of laparoscopy). Hysteroscopy involves inserting an instrument into the uterine cavity to look for intrauterine polyps or fibroids which may be a source of pain and increased bleeding (Klotz, 1995). Women undergoing diagnosis and treatment of secondary dysmenorrhea need additional support and education from their nurses as well as physical care prior to, during, and after any surgical or other invasive procedures.

Two common causes of secondary dysmenorrhea are endometriosis (see Chapter 10 for discussion of endometriosis) and leiomyomas. Leiomyomas are benign fibroid tumors of the smooth muscle of the uterus, which depend on estrogen for their growth. They can be located within the uterine wall (intramural) or in the cervix or broad ligament (intraligamentous), grow towards the surface of the uterus (subserous), or protrude into the uterine cavity (submucous). While many women with leiomyomas have no symptoms, they are a frequent cause of secondary dysmenorrhea. Common symptoms caused by leiomyomas are pelvic pressure, urinary frequency, pelvic bloating and congestion, dyspareunia, and heavy menstrual bleeding (Forrest, 1994). Leiomyomas are the most common reason, aside from cancer, for hysterectomy (surgical removal of the uterus) (Wilcox, Koonin, Pokras, Strauss, Xia, & Peterson, 1994). Leiomyomas can be treated with methyl prednisone acetate, which decreases bleeding and suppresses tumor growth, or with gonadotropin-releasing hormone agonists (GnRH-a) such as Leuprorelin and Nafarelin, which suppress tumor growth and shrink existing tumors. An alternative procedure to hysterectomy is myomectomy, where only the fibroid and a small amount of surrounding uterine tissue is removed.

Amenorrhea

Amenorrhea refers to the absence of menses. Primary amenorrhea refers to failure to menstruate by age 16, whether or not there is normal development of secondary sexual characteristics or to failure to menstruate by age 14 and lack of development of secondary sexual characteristics by that time. Causes of primary amenorrhea include genetic disorders, endocrine disorders, and anatomic abnormalities. Secondary amenorrhea refers to absence of menses for 6 months after normal menstruation has been established. The primary physiologic causes of secondary amenorrhea include the normal events of pregnancy, lactation, and menopause. Secondary amenorrhea can also be caused by disorders of the hypothalamic-pituitary-ovarian axis, endocrine disorders such as hypothyroidism, pituitary tumors, marked weight loss, eating disorders, medications including oral and injectable contraceptives, contraceptive implants and phenytoin (Dilantin), and uterine or cervical scarring from such sources as radiation or surgery. Excessive exercise and situational stress are also common causes of secondary amenorrhea.

Assessment of amenorrhea includes a thorough history and complete physical and gynecological examination. The review of systems should focus on symptoms related to hormonal changes such as hair loss, skin changes, intolerance to heat and cold, hot flashes, increased nervousness, or fatigue. The nurse should be sure to explore lifestyle and situational factors, most notably unprotected intercourse, intense physical training, and increased stress. Laboratory testing should begin with a pregnancy test and can include measurements of serum levels of thyroid hormones, pituitary hormones, follicle stimulating hormone, estrogen, and progesterone. Other tests might include pelvic ultrasound and computerized axial tomography scans. Treatment of primary and secondary amenorrhea depends upon the cause. Emotional support and education are two important roles for the nurse in the diagnosis and treatment of primary and secondary amenorrhea.

▶ The Climacteric and Menopause

Ovarian function decreases as part of the normal aging process eventually resulting in cessation of the menstrual cycle. **Menopause** refers to the permanent cessation of ovarian function and is defined retrospectively after there have been no menstrual periods for twelve consecutive months. The average age of menopause in the United States is 50 (The Contraceptive Report, 1995). Menopause can also be brought on at any age by surgical removal of the ovaries or by destruction of the ovaries by chemicals or radiation. The 5–10 year period of gradual decrease in ovarian hormone production prior to the menopause is called the **climacteric. Perimenopause** refers to the period of time which includes the climacteric menopause, and the first few years after menopause. The changes which occur during the perimenopause represent a normal physiological transition in a woman's life. A woman can now expect to live about a third of her life after she has reached menopause.

Women are born with a large number of oocytes which are surrounded by primordial follicles (See Chapter 6). The number of follicles decreases as the woman ages due to both ovulation and follicular degeneration. As a result, both ovulatory function and the production of the ovarian hormones estrogen and progesterone decrease. This process eventually disrupts the negative feedback loop which, during an ovulatory menstrual cycle, inhibits production of follicle-stimulating hormone (FSH) and luteinizing hormone (LH). FSH and LH rise markedly at menopause. The serum level of FSH is sometimes used to provide a definitive measurement of a woman's menopausal status. FHS > 40 mIU/ml on 2 occasions one week apart is considered to be diagnostic of menopause (Garner, 1994).

During the climacteric, as ovarian function decreases and levels of circulating estrogen drop, a number of physiologic and structural changes occurs. The menstrual cycle becomes increasingly unpredictable as ovulatory cycles decrease. It is not uncommon for menstrual flow to be heavier and longer and for the cycles to be longer. Some women will have scantier bleeding, or shorter and less frequent menses. Bleeding or spotting between menses also is common. Although some cycles are anovulatory, it is impossible to predict when the final ovulatory cycle will occur so women who wish to avoid pregnancy should still use contraception until they have definitely passed menopause. Irregular menstrual bleeding is a distressing aspect of the climacteric for many women and may lead to embarrassment and inconvenience. Repeated episodes of heavy bleeding sometimes lead to anemia and may require medical or surgical treatment (Garner, 1994; LeBoeuf & Carter, 1996).

Vasomotor Instability

The most common and classic symptom of the perimenopausal period is vasomotor instability, commonly known as the "hot flash" or "hot flush." Hot flashes, which vary in frequency and intensity, are reported by 85 to 88% of perimenopausal women to some degree (Garner, 1994; LeBoeuf & Carter, 1996). It is not unusual for women to mention the discomfort they are experiencing from these hot flashes during a routine physical or gynecological examination.

Hot flashes are related to variations in the level of circulating estrogen. Although the exact cause of hot flashes is unknown, a surge in LH followed by a rapid increase in the core body temperature has been noted (LeBoeuf & Garner, 1996). The rise in body temperature leads to perspiration, which is sometimes profuse. The hot flash can last anywhere from a few seconds to a few minutes. Vasomotor instability usually starts a few years prior to menopause and lasts for one to as long as five years (Garner, 1994). It is often worse at night and may awaken the woman repeatedly from sleep. Disruption of normal sleep patterns can lead to fatigue, mood changes, difficulty concentrating, and emotional lability. Women also report embarrassment and distress from hot flashes and sweating that may occur in public.

Breast and Urogenital Changes

Glandular tissue in the breast is gradually replaced with adipose and connective tissue causing the breasts to become smaller and less firm. The tissue of the vulva, vagina, and uterus also undergo atrophic changes. Pubic hair thins, the labia minora and majora become smaller, the vagina becomes shorter and narrower, and the uterus decreases in size.

Changes in the vaginal epithelium lead to an increase in the vaginal pH, which makes the woman more susceptible to vaginal infections. The thick folds in the vaginal walls, known as rugae, flatten, making the vaginal walls smooth. Thinning of the vaginal walls, decreased blood flow to the vagina, and decreased ability to produce lubrication during sexual stimulation may cause discomfort during intercourse.

Loss of pelvic floor muscle tone can lead to prolapse of the uterus, bladder (cystocele), and/or rectum (rectocele), especially in women who have had many vaginal deliveries or difficult vaginal deliveries. Women with poor pelvic muscle tone may develop stress incontinence, which is leakage of urine with increased pelvic pressure such as that caused by coughing, sneezing, or laughing (Newman & Burns, 1997). Loss of muscle tone in the bladder and urethra may lead to incomplete bladder emptying, increased urinary frequency, and urinary incontinence (Krissovich & Safran, 1997). These physiologic changes lead to an increased incidence of urinary tract infections in middle-aged and older women.

Osteoporosis

Bone mass begins to decrease after age 35 and the rate of loss accelerates as estrogen levels drop after menopause. Post-menopausal women are at increased risk for **osteoporosis,** a disease in which deterioration

of the microarchitecture of the bone leads to a decrease in bone mass. When bone mass decreases sufficiently, bones become fragile and are more likely to break. Osteoporosis leads to 1.5 million fractures each year in the United States (National Osteoporosis Foundation, 1997) and 80% of the 25 million Americans who have osteoporosis are women (National Osteoporosis Foundation, 1995).

Common sites of fractures due to osteoporosis are the vertebrae and the hips. Vertebral fractures cause loss of height and stooped posture. Hip fractures lead to increased rates of hospitalization, need for long-term care, assistance in activities of daily living, prolonged disability, and, sometimes, death (National Osteoporosis Foundation, 1997).

Although age-related loss of bone mass occurs in all individuals certain factors are associated with increased risk of developing osteoporosis, as follows:

- Female
- Caucasian or Asian race
- Small-boned and thin stature
- Early menopause
- Smoking
- Alcohol use
- Sedentary lifestyle
- Family history of osteoporosis

Adequate calcium intake throughout the lifetime can decrease a woman's risk of postmenopausal osteoporosis as can adequate weight-bearing exercise and avoidance of nicotine and excessive alcohol intake. Estrogen replacement therapy after menopause also helps prevent osteoporosis by decreasing the rate of bone loss. Adequate calcium intake is of critical importance in the postmenopausal period. Postmenopausal women should consume 1,000 mg of calcium/day if they are on estrogen replacement therapy and 1,500 mg/day if they do not take estrogen.

Diagnosis of osteoporosis prior to fractures allows for treatment and preventive measures designed to prevent falls and avoid fractures and is primarily performed through measurement of bone density. Bone densitometry measures bone mineral density in key parts of the skeletal system including spine, hip, forearm, or in the whole body. During a bone density scan, the client lies flat on a table and the scanner passes over her body. The test is painless and the amount of radiation exposure is lower than that of a standard chest X-ray. During the scan, a computer calculates the woman's bone density relative to the bone density expected in healthy young women and a deviation score is calculated. Women whose bone density is more than 2.5 standard deviations below normal are said to have osteoporosis (Kessenich, 1997). Osteopenia, which precedes osteoporosis, is defined as bone mass density of more than 1 standard deviation but less than 2.5 standard deviations below normal. Individuals who are found to have osteopenia can be counseled to modify their diet, take calcium supplements, increase their weight-bearing exercise and further monitor their bone density as preventive measures against development of osteoporosis.

Estrogen replacement therapy or medications which slow bone loss such as calcitonin or bisphosphonates may be prescribed for postmenopausal women who have osteoporosis or osteopenia. Nurses need to educate women on osteoporosis prevention and treatment. For women who have osteoporosis, fall prevention is especially important to reduce the risk of fractures and resultant disability.

Cardiovascular Disease

Lower estrogen levels in postmenopausal women lead to increased risk for cardiovascular disease. Heart disease is the number one cause of death among women aged 65 and older. Levels of high-density lipoproteins, which have a protective effect against cardiovascular disease, decrease after menopause. Low-density lipoproteins and total cholesterol, which are each associated with higher risk of cardiovascular disease, increase. The incidence of hypertension also increases in postmenopausal women. Forty-one percent of women aged 45–64 and 47% of women older than 64 have hypertension (Horton, 1995). Cigarette smoking, obesity, sedentary lifestyle, and diabetes are additional risk factors for cardiovascular disease among women. Postmenopausal estrogen replacement therapy reduces the level of low-density lipoproteins, increases high-density lipoproteins, and reduces the risk for cardiovascular disease among women (Horton, 1995; Moore & Noonan, 1996).

Hormone Replacement Therapy

Many of the adverse physiologic effects of menopause can be reduced by replacing endogenous estrogen with exogenous estrogen. Estrogen replacement therapy has been shown to decrease cardiac risk, decrease risk of osteoporosis, relieve symptoms of urogenital atrophy, and decrease or eliminate the discomforts associated with vasomotor instability. Estrogen replacement therapy, however, has been shown to increase a woman's risk for hyperplasia of the lining of the uterus, leading to increased rates of endometrial cancer (Gambrell, 1997; Moore & Noonan, 1996). For women who have an intact uterus, various combinations of estrogen and progesterone are prescribed. These combination routines, shown in Table 7–6, are known as hormone replacement therapy (HRT) and provide the benefits of estrogen replacement without the increased risk of endometrial cancer.

Estrogen is available in various forms including oral, vaginal creams, and transdermal patches. The newest form is an estrogen-saturated ring that is inserted intravaginally. Vaginal estrogen creams are very effective in reducing the discomforts associated with urogenital atrophy but they are generally prepared in an oil base. Women should be advised that simultaneous use of estrogen vaginal cream and latex condoms may increase the risk of condom breakage.

The dose of estrogen that has been shown to prevent osteoporosis and cardiovascular disease is 0.625 of conjugated estrogen or the equivalent of any other form of estrogen. Progesterone is most commonly administered in oral form. Occasionally, when menopausal discomforts are not controlled by estrogen, an androgen is added to the routine. Side effects of HRT include vaginal bleeding, breast tenderness, headache, bloating, nausea, and mood changes. There is controversy over whether HRT increases the risk of

▶ **TABLE 7–6**

Hormone Replacement Therapy Regimens

Hormone	Hormone Regimen (30 day cycles)	Notes
Continuous Estrogen	**Estrogen** every day of the month	Recommended only for women who have had hysterectomies
Cyclic Combined	**Estrogen** and **Progesterone** together on days 1–25	Withdrawal bleeding occurs during days 26–28
Continuous Combined	**Estrogen** and **Progesterone** together every day of the month	No withdrawal bleeding after the first 12 months. Usually irregular bleeding first 6–12 months
Cyclic	**Estrogen** on days 1–25 **Progesterone** on days 13–25	Withdrawal bleeding during days 25–30
Continuous Estrogen with Intermittent Progesterone	**Estrogen** every day of the month **Progesterone** for 12 days (usually days 1–12)	Withdrawal bleeding during days 13–17

Source: Gambrell, 1997; Moore & Noonan, 1996.

breast cancer (Gambrell, 1997; Moore & Noonan, 1996). Hormone replacement therapy is contraindicated in women with a history of estrogen-dependent cancers, pregnancy, abnormal vaginal bleeding, liver disease, and thromboembolic disease.

Nursing Care of Perimenopausal Women

Nurses can play a major role in the health care of women during their middle and older years by providing education and emotional support. Table 7–7 lists some nonpharmacological interventions that nurses can suggest for women coping with perimenopausal discomforts.

Many women are unaware of the uses, benefits, and risks of HRT and are unable to make an informed decision about its use. Nurses can provide both education and guidance about HRT based on an assessment of the individual women's health risks. Many women will choose not to take HRT. Women who do choose this therapy need education as to proper dosing and side effects of their hormone regimen. Women who are on HRT should be advised to continue their monthly BSEs, have a yearly mammogram, and continue to have routine Pap smears. Additional testing, including endometrial biopsy or ultrasounds, may be ordered in some cases. All women in midlife and after benefit from counseling about the value of healthy lifestyle habits including adequate physical exercise, stress reduction, low fat diet, adequate calcium, weight reduction if obese, and avoidance of smoking, illicit drug use, and excessive alcohol use. Positive health practices such as these will help all women to decrease risks for heart disease and osteoporosis.

▶ Breast Care and Breast Diseases

Screening for Breast Disease

Changes within the breast can lead to benign or malignant conditions. Women's health nurses must be knowledgeable about breast assessment, and be prepared to provide appropriate education, counseling, support, and referrals should abnormalities be detected by the woman herself or by health care providers.

One important health promotion activity is teaching the techniques and principles of BSE and periodically reinforcing those principles. While all women need periodic clinical breast examinations performed by a nurse or physician, monthly BSE is recommended as an additional inexpensive method of

---

▶ **TABLE 7–7**

Nonpharmacologic Interventions for Perimenopausal Discomforts

Discomfort	Intervention
Vasomotor flushes	Wear layered clothing Drink cool beverages Obtain adequate ventilation Use a fan Avoid ingestion of caffeine, spicy foods, and alcoholic beverages
Vaginal dryness/discomfort during intercourse	Continue sexual activities Increase length of foreplay to allow time for vagina to lubricate Use water soluble lubricants during intercourse Use long-acting vaginal moisturizers
Insomnia	Drink warm milk or chamomile tea at bedtime Avoid caffeinated foods and beverages in the evening Avoid daytime naps Get adequate physical exercise
Urinary symptoms	Perform Kegel exercises Empty bladder frequently Consume adequate fluids Avoid foods and fluids that cause diuresis such as tea, coffee, watermelon Use pessary for pelvic organ prolapse Use absorbent pads
Irritability, nervousness, feeling "down"	Perform relaxation exercises Get adequate physical exercise Use positive imagery Interact with available social supports Plan diversionary activities

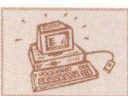

Research Abstract

Factors Influencing Depression Among Midlife Women

The purpose of this study was to examine the relationship of certain factors to depressed mood among midlife women. Factors hypothesized to contribute to depressed mood among midlife women included menopausal changes, vasomotor symptoms, stressful life context, socialization for midlife, and health status. To participate in the study, women had to be 35–55 years old, have had a menstrual period within the last year, have an intact uterus and at least one ovary, be nonpregnant and nonlactating, and be able to speak and read English. The final sample was 337 women ranging in age from 35 to 55 years old. Most of the women (80%) were European-American, with African-American and Asian women each accounting for 8% of the total sample. The mean educational level of the women was 15 years of schooling.

Based on the evidence found through their review of prior studies, the authors hypothesized that women undergoing menopausal changes will experience more vasomotor symptoms and that vasomotor symptoms will be related to higher levels of depressed mood. Women with positive socialization towards midlife will experience a less stressful life context during the menopause and will have fewer vasomotor symptoms and therefore indirectly, less depressed mood. Women with good health will have less depressed mood. Women with good health were expected to have less stress, less severe vasomotor symptoms, and less depression.

Menopausal changes were assessed by asking women to report whether or not they had changes in their menstrual cycle in the last 6 months including changes in the length or regularity of the cycle. The Washington Women's Health Diary was used to assess vasomotor symptoms. Socialization towards midlife was measured with a scale that measured attitudes towards aging and with a scale that measured attitudes towards menopause. Health status was measured by a series of questions that asked women to self-rate their health, compare their health with other women their age, and to indicate whether they had any chronic illnesses. Stressful life context was measured with a stressful life events scale and depressed mood was measured with the Center for Epidemiologic Studies Depression Scale and the SCL-90 Depression Scale.

Fourteen percent of the participants had experienced changes in the length of their menstrual cycle and 18% experienced increased cycle irregularity within the last 6 months. Seventeen percent reported hot flashes and sweats. Socialization towards midlife was positive among the participants. Women reported a mean of 10 negative life events in the past year, with a range of 0 to 83. The median rating of health among these women was 4 = "very good." They also rated their health as about the same as others their age and reported a median of 2 chronic illnesses. Results showed that menopausal changes and vasomotor symptoms had no significant effects on depressed mood. Stressful life context was the strongest predictor of depressed mood and poor health also predicted depressed mood among these midlife women. Health status also predicted stress. Socialization for midlife predicted stress and vasomotor symptoms and stress predicted vasomotor symptoms. Negative socialization resulted in increased stress and increased vasomotor symptoms. The authors concluded that menopausal events, including menopausal cycle changes and vasomotor symptoms, do not affect depressed mood in midlife women, but that depressed mood is affected by stress and poor health.

Application to Practice

It is often taught, and many people believe, that menopause causes psychological symptoms including depression and that depression is an inevitable aspect of midlife for women. This study clarifies some of the factors that may be related to depression in midlife women. Women who present with depressed mood in midlife should not be advised that this is related to menopausal changes or symptoms. Clinicians need to look for other causes of depression besides menopause in midlife women. Women with depressed mood should be assessed for stressful life context and

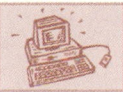

Research Abstract continued

acute or chronic health problems. The relationship among negative socialization for midlife, increased life stress, and increased vasomotor symptoms points out that women should be presented with a positive picture of menopause and midlife. Nurses should advise women that midlife can be a healthy and positive time of life and emphasize ways to manage symptoms and physical changes. Depression in midlife women should be taken seriously by health care professionals and not minimized or ignored as "just part of menopause." Interventions for depression should include interventions aimed at decreasing life stress and health problems.

Source: Woods, N.F., Mitchell, E.S. (1997). Pathways to depressed mood for midlife women: Observations from the Seattle women's health study. Research in Nursing and Health, 20; 119–129.

screening for breast cancer since it has the potential to aid in discovery of cancer at an early and more curable stage. In addition, the majority of breast masses are detected by the woman herself. See box entitled American Cancer Society Recommendations for Breast Self-Examination and Clinical Breast Examination for recommended intervals for periodic clinical breast examination and BSE. Figure 7–4 describes essential elements of BSE. The clinical breast examination is described in Table 7–5.

Successful BSE is a self-care practice that incorporates knowledge of the appropriate timing and techniques, a positive and willing attitude, and performance skills. Teaching strategies for BSE include use of pamphlets, films, slide-tape programs, lectures, and one-on-one teaching. Hands-on one-on-one teaching with return demonstration has been shown to be a more effective teaching method for BSE than passive methods such as pamphlets or videotapes. The opportunity to practice BSE on a model and receive corrective feedback from an instructor is a crucial element in the development of women's skill in BSE. The degree of skill acquired can be assessed through return demonstration.

BSE should be taught as a self-care practice, beginning in adolescence. Monthly BSE allows the woman to develop familiarity with the normal contours and texture of her breasts. Women should examine their breasts after their menstrual period (day 4, 5, 6, or 7 of the menstrual cycle) when the breasts are less tender and not swollen. Postmenopausal or pregnant women should choose a day in the month, such as the first, and do BSE on that day of each month. Some women resist routine BSE due to fear of cancer or cultural proscriptions against touching or handling their breasts. The nurse should allow time for discussion of feelings and fears during teaching sessions and emphasis should be placed on the positive health benefits of BSE. Women should be advised to contact their health provider without delay if they discover or suspect any abnormality in their breasts. A woman's significant other can be taught breast examination techniques in cases where the woman is unable to perform BSE independently.

▶ AMERICAN CANCER SOCIETY RECOMMENDATIONS FOR BREAST SELF-EXAMINATION AND CLINICAL BREAST EXAMINATION

≥ 20 YEARS OLD

Breast self-examination every month

20–39

Clinical breast examination every three years

≥ 40 YEARS OLD

Clinical breast examination every year

WHY DO THE BREAST SELF-EXAM?

There are many good reasons for doing a breast self-exam each month. One reason is that it is easy to do and the more you do it, the better you will get at it. When you get to know how your breasts normally feel, you will quickly be able to feel any change, and early detection is the key to successful treatment.

REMEMBER: A breast self-exam could save your breast – and save your life. Most breast lumps are found by women themselves, but in fact, most lumps in the breast are not cancer. Be safe, be sure.

WHEN TO DO BREAST SELF-EXAM

The best time to do breast self-exam is right after your period, when breasts are not tender or swollen. If you do not have regular periods or sometimes skip a month, do it on the same day every month.

HOW TO DO BREAST SELF-EXAM

1. Lie down and put a pillow under your right shoulder. Place your right arm behind your head.

2. Use the finger pads of your three middle fingers on your left hand to feel for lumps or thickening. Your finger pads are the top third of each finger.

3. Press firmly enough to know how your breast feels. If you're not sure how hard to press, ask your health care provider. Or try to copy the way your health care provider uses the finger pads during a breast exam. Learn what your breast feels like most of the time. A firm ridge in the lower curve of each breast is normal.

4. Move around the breast in a set way. You can choose either the circle (A), the up and down line (B), or the wedge (C). Do it the same way every time. It will help you to make sure that you've gone over the entire breast area, and to remember how your breast feels.

5. Now examine your left breast using right hand finger pads.

6. If you find any changes, see your doctor right away.

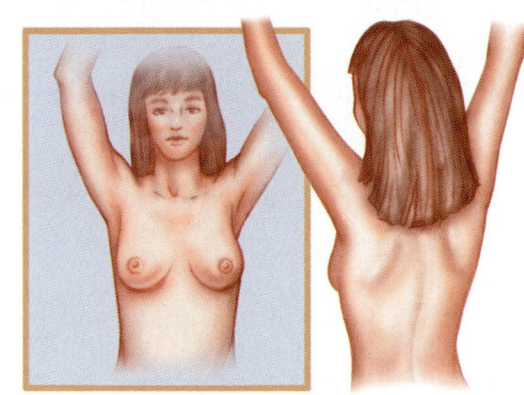

FOR ADDED SAFETY

You should also check your breasts while standing in front of a mirror right after you do your breast self-exam each month. See if there are any changes in the way your breasts look: dimpling of the skin, changes in the nipple, or redness or swelling.

You might also want to do a breast self-exam while you're in the shower. Your soapy hands will glide over the wet skin making it easy to check how your breasts feel.

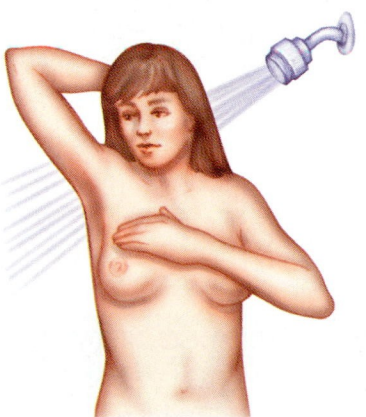

FIGURE 7–4. Breast self-examination. *(Reproduced, with permission, from the American Cancer Society, 1997.)*

An experienced clinician can detect a breast mass as small as 1 cm by palpation. By the time a mass has reached that size it has probably been present for at least two years. At this stage, 20–30% of cancerous tumors have already begun to metastasize to the lungs or other areas of the body. **Mammography,** or X-ray imaging of the breasts, can detect breast masses that are too small to be palpated by even an experienced clinician (Fig. 7–5). Mammography may help increase length of survival after a diagnosis of breast cancer due to earlier detection. Clinical trials among women aged 50–60 have shown that regular screening mammograms can reduce breast cancer mortality by one third in this age group (National Institutes of Health, 1997). Results of research related to younger women, mammography, and breast cancer survival are less clear and various recommendations have been proposed for women younger than 50, including screening mammogram every year and screening based on individual risks (see Table 7–4). Diagnostic mammograms can also be used to aid in diagnosis of breast lumps that have been discovered through BSE or clinical breast examination. As mammograms use very low dose radiation, the risk of yearly mammogram screening is negligible.

Because the breasts must be compressed between two surfaces to get a good image, women can experience discomfort during a mammogram and some may experience pain or minor bruising for a few days afterwards. For women who are premenopausal, it is more comfortable to schedule their mammogram just after their menses when the breasts are less tender. All women should be advised not to use powder or deodorant on or near their breasts on the day of their

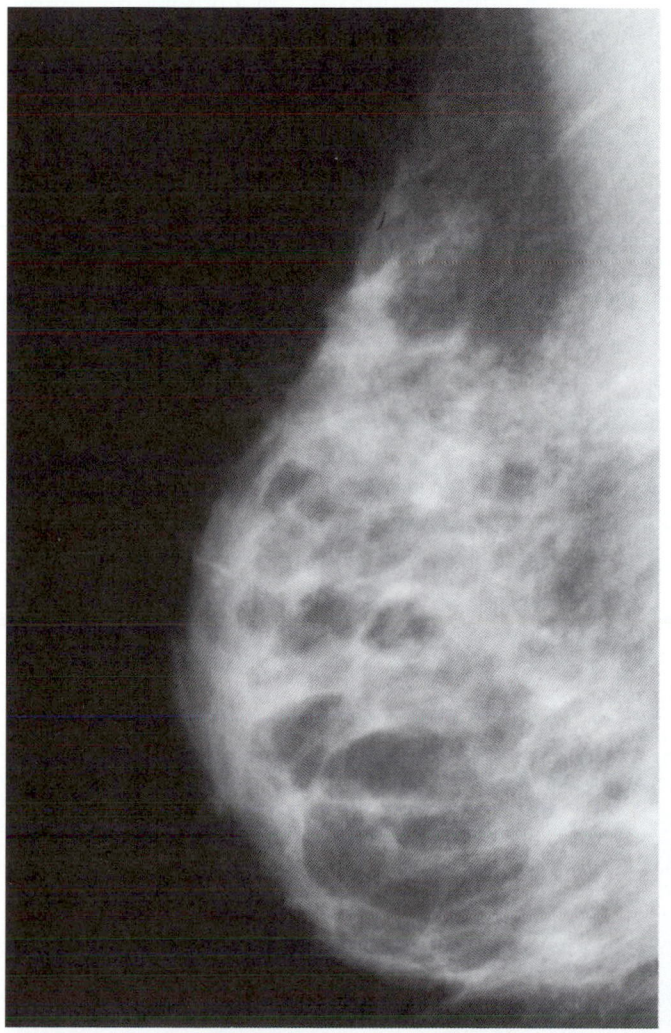

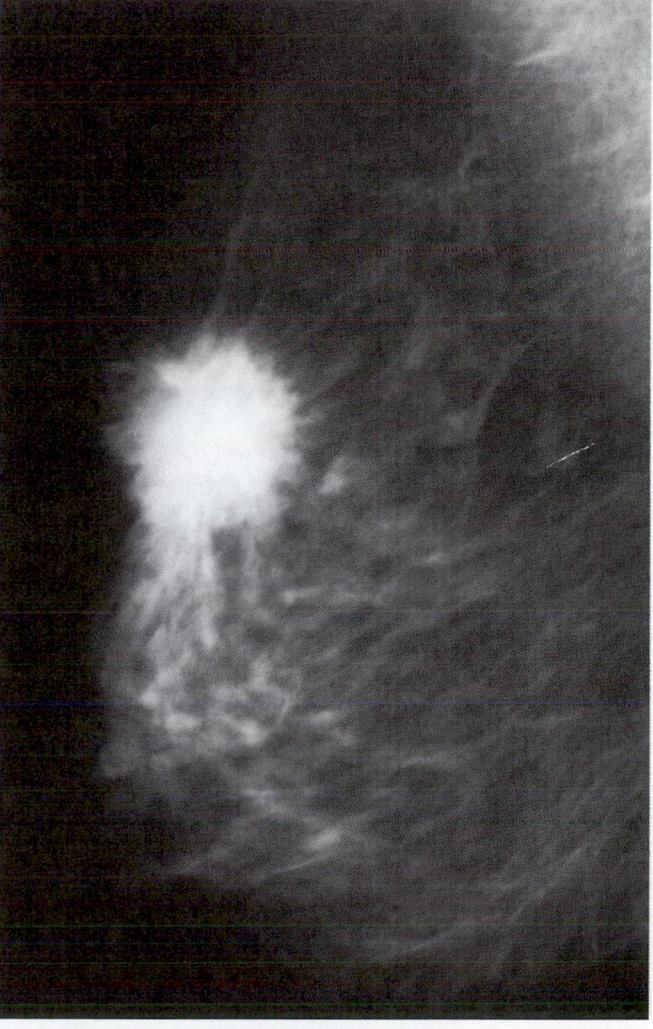

A   B

FIGURE 7–5. Mammography. **A.** Normal mammogram. **B.** Abnormal mammogram.

mammogram as these substances can lead to false positive results.

Some women may react to the idea of mammography with fear and anxiety. They may be fearful that a cancer will be discovered, or they may have heard other women discuss the discomforts they have experienced during the procedure. Some women may avoid mammography because it involves having someone handle their breasts, an action associated with sexual relationships or with prior sexual abuse. Nurses should be sensitive to these issues and provide support and guidance to women who need mammograms as well as education about the procedure and its potential for decreasing their risks of dying from breast cancer. Mammograms and other forms of breast screening, including education about BSE, are sometimes performed in special centers designated for such purposes alone. These centers usually offer a calm, relaxed, and woman-centered atmosphere, which may increase a woman's comfort and sense of safety during breast screening procedures (Fig. 7–6). In these centers, the radiologist may be available to read the mammogram while the woman waits, sparing her the anxiety of waiting days or weeks for her results.

Benign Breast Diseases

The female breast undergoes changes from puberty to menopause due to the effects of estrogen and progesterone. Estrogen stimulation during puberty causes proliferation of the vascular, glandular, fatty and, connective tissues. Menopausal changes in the breast have been described earlier in this chapter. There are also changes in the breast due to the cyclic hormonal changes of the menstrual cycle.

Hormonal stimulation of the breast tissue may also result in benign (noncancerous) breast disease. Benign breast disease, including fibrosis of the tissue, cyst formation, or abnormal proliferation (growth) of cells, is extremely common and may result directly from hormonal effects on the breast tissue or from abnormal responses to hormonal stimulation.

Fibrocystic breast changes, formerly called fibrocystic breast disease, include thickening of the breast tissue, formation of cysts, hyperplasia of the epithelium of the ducts, and duct ectasia. Symptoms usually include breast tenderness or pain (mastodynia), which is most often bilateral. The pain is cyclic, beginning one to two weeks prior to menstruation and resolving during the menstrual period. Some women report pain in their breasts all throughout their menstrual cycle. Clinically, the breasts are nodular or lumpy. There may be dominant masses, some of which may arise and regress quickly. Nipple discharge may be present in some cases. Treatment depends on the age of the woman and the type of changes present. Although fibrocystic changes are not cancerous, some women who have these benign tumors are at increased risk for breast cancer in the future. This is especially true for women who also have a positive family history of breast cancer.

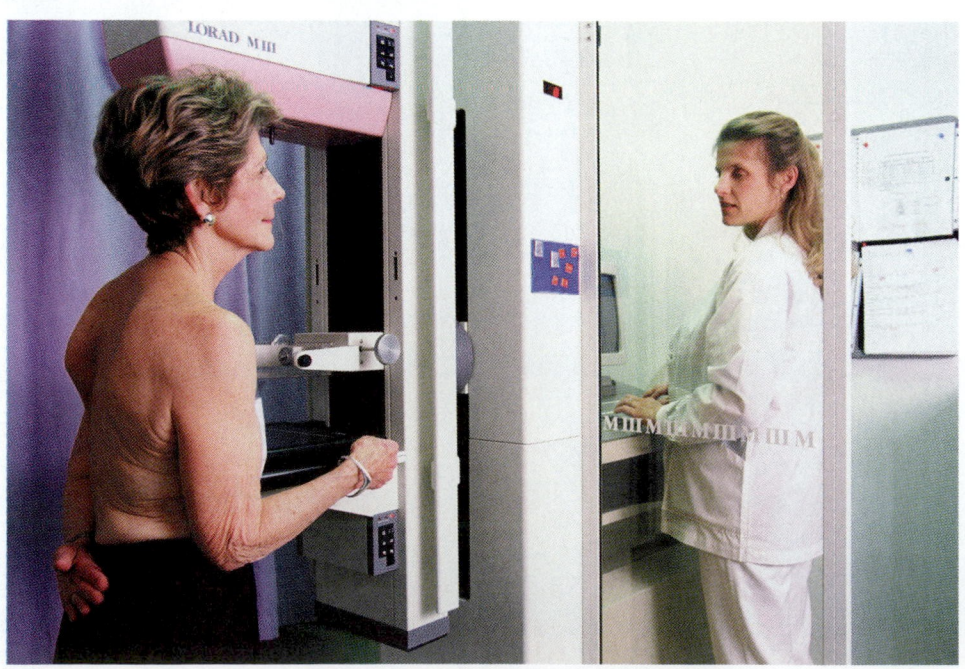

FIGURE 7–6. A client undergoing a mammography.

Fibroadenomas are fibrocystic changes which result in small solid benign tumors, usually between 1 and 2 cm in size. Fibroadenomas are felt as small, painless, round, firm, discrete masses which are moveable. They are often described as feeling like a "pea" or a "marble." Most often fibroadenomas are single but sometimes they are found in both breasts. The most common site is the upper outer quadrant of the breast. They begin to develop between the ages of 15 and 25 (Miller, 1995), but may not be palpable until they have been developing for some years. If the woman is less than 25 years old when the fibroadenoma is discovered, the surgeon may decide to leave it alone as the possibility of malignancy in a tumor of this sort is very low in this age group. In women older than 25, biopsy to rule out breast cancer is advised (Miller, 1995). Biopsy may be done using a fine needle which is inserted into the mass to remove cells for analysis, or by surgical excision of the mass and subsequent analysis of the cells.

Cysts may also form, commonly in both breasts. Cysts are fluid-filled sacs of varying sizes ranging from one to many centimeters in diameter. Unlike fibroadenomas, multiple cysts are likely to be present and both breasts are usually involved. Cysts are most common in women between ages 30 and 50 but do not commonly occur after menopause. Cysts may arise quickly, sometimes seemingly overnight. Cysts which are close to the surface of the breast often feel soft or compressible because of the fluid inside. Cysts deep in the breast often feel like hard, smooth lumps or masses. Aspiration using local anesthesia is the usual treatment of choice. After numbing the skin a long needle is inserted into the cyst and the fluid is removed, causing the cyst to collapse. The fluid may be sent for laboratory analysis. Any cyst that does not disappear after aspiration, reoccurs, produces bloody fluid when aspirated, or is suspicious for cancer when the fluid is analyzed in the lab, should be removed and biopsied.

Duct ectasia is a condition that includes dilatation of the major mammary ducts under the nipple, resulting in inflammation and bloody nipple discharge. This condition tends to occur during perimenopause and is a common cause of nipple discharge in women in their fifties (Branch, 1994). Women may present with a mass under the nipple or in the areola, which may cause the nipple to retract. A sticky, greenish, brownish, cream-colored, or bloody discharge from the nipple is usually present. Nipple discharge without palpable mass may be present in less advanced cases, although there is usually redness and swelling around the areola and the area is tender to palpation. Axillary lymphadenopathy may be present on the affected side in advanced cases.

Intraductal papillomas are another form of benign breast disease that can cause nipple discharge. In this case a tumor in the mammary duct, which is usually too small to palpate, causes discharge of serous or slightly bloody fluid from the nipple of the affected breast. Usually there is only one tumor, affecting only one mammary duct. Occasionally the tumor may grow large enough to be felt by the woman or her clinician. This type of tumor is also most common in the perimenopausal period.

Diagnosis of nipple discharge and associated conditions includes laboratory analysis of the discharge which may include tests for occult blood and a Pap smear. Mammograms are also commonly obtained. Treatment is usually surgical removal of the associated tumor and its affected duct in a procedure called a wedge resection. The tissue removed is sent to the lab for biopsy to rule out cancer.

Supporting the Woman Undergoing Diagnosis of Breast Disease

Although most breast lumps and most cases of nipple discharge are not malignant, many women respond to such a finding with fear and anxiety, most of which is related to fear of cancer. Several nursing care strategies may be used to assist the woman who needs further diagnosis and treatment.

Case management is a systematic process of identifying, mobilizing, facilitating, and monitoring appropriate use of health care resources (Benoit, 1996). While one aim of case management is control of costs by eliminating inappropriate use of resources, from a nursing point of view, case management can enable the client to obtain the most appropriate care in a timely manner. This involves making referrals to the appropriate specialists and facilities for diagnosis and treatment and assisting the woman to obtain timely appointments with those providers. The nurse may direct the woman to community-based financial and social services. Women may also need direction and assistance in navigating the health insurance system. For a woman with a breast mass, timely, appropriate care decreases anxiety and distress associated with waiting for final diagnosis and treatment and may even increase her chances of survival if the mass is malignant. Nurses are the ideal health professionals to provide case management services to women with breast masses because nurses understand the implications of diagnosis and treatment, are informed about treatment options and providers, and understand the psychologic implications of having breast disease of any kind.

When a breast mass is identified in a primary care setting, prompt referral for mammography and other diagnostic services is important. Results of such testing should be obtained as quickly as possible and communicated to the client. Setting up an appointment for follow-up enables the health care provider to discuss results, treatment options, and referrals with the woman in person. Face to face meetings also allow for assessment of the woman's reaction to her diagnosis. Women sometimes become distraught after learning that they have a breast mass or after learning that a mass is malignant or requires further treatment. The nurse can provide the woman with a private place and a supportive environment until she is calm enough to leave the facility. If necessary someone identified by the woman as a supportive person can be called to escort the woman home. Enlisting assistance of psychological support personnel may be appropriate in some instances.

Anticipatory guidance for further testing and treatment that follow a finding of any abnormality in the breast is helpful. The nurse should provide information on what tests or procedures are necessary and how those tests can be arranged. Most women appreciate information about how the tests are performed and what information is obtained through each test. Discussing sensations that are experienced during a given test or procedure and how any discomforts can be managed is also helpful. This type of information should be provided when the woman is calm and receptive. Providing printed information in the woman's own language enables her to review what she has been told at her leisure. Follow-up phone calls to women to ensure their understanding of information provided are also a way to provide additional support during the diagnostic period.

Emotional support is another important nursing intervention for the woman with a breast mass. Prior to definitive diagnosis through biopsy, the nurse should never reassure the client that the mass is probably benign. The nurse can more appropriately demonstrate support by remaining with the client, encouraging her to express her feelings, and by providing concrete assistance as already discussed. Providing the client with a phone number she may call for further help or to talk to a supportive person is another assistance that nurses can provide.

Breast Cancer

Breast cancer is the most common cancer among women. Over 43,500 women died from breast cancer in the United States in 1993 (American Cancer Society, 1997) making breast cancer second only to lung cancer as a cancer-related cause of death. The American Cancer Society estimated that in 1997, 180,200 new cases of breast cancer would be identified among women living in the United States (American Cancer Society, 1997).

Five-year survival rates for both African-American and Caucasian women have increased steadily since 1960, from 63 to 85% for Caucasian women and from 46 to 70% for African Americans (American Cancer Society, 1997). Increased survival rates may in part be due to earlier detection through breast examination and mammography. The highest incidence of breast cancer occurs among Caucasians (116/100,000), Hawaiians (106/100,000), and African Americans (95/100,000). African-American women have the highest death rates from breast cancer (31/100,000), followed by Caucasian (28/100,000) and Hawaiian women (25/100,000) (National Cancer Institute, 1997a). Decreased access to health care and lower screening rates may be related to decreased survival rates among African Americans.

While the overall incidence of breast cancer among women is about 110 cases for every 100,000 women (American Cancer Society, 1997), risk increases with age. A woman's risk for breast cancer by age 30 is only 1 in 2,525. By age 50, however, it is 1 in 50 and by age 80 a woman's risk for breast cancer increases to 1 in 10 (National Cancer Institute, 1997).

The cause of breast cancer is unknown although it is thought to be a combination of genetic, hormonal, nutritional, and environmental factors. Several risk factors for breast cancer have been identified in addition to female gender and age, as follows (Couzi & Davidson, 1997):

- History of breast cancer in one breast
- First degree relative (mother, sister, or daughter) with breast cancer
- Atypical hyperplasia found on prior biopsy
- Nulliparous state
- First child later than age 30
- First menstrual period prior to age 12
- Menopause after age 55
- Defects in certain genes (BRCA1 and BRCA2)

Lesions suspicious of breast cancer may be identified through physical examination and/or through mammography or ultrasound. On physical examination, breast cancer presents as a fixed mass with poorly defined borders. Usually the mass is unilateral but cancer may affect both breasts simultaneously. Cancerous breast lumps may or may not be painful. There may be dimpling of the skin over the mass or nipple retraction. A clear, yellow, or bloody discharge may be present, usually from only one nipple. In advanced breast cancer palpable lymph nodes may be present in the axilla, supraclavicular, or infraclavicular areas. Definitive diagnosis is through biopsy.

Breast cancers are most likely to originate in the epithelial lining of the mammary ducts. This type of carcinoma accounts for 70–80% of all breast cancers

(National Cancer Institute, 1997b). Less frequently cancer may arise in the epithelial lining of the lobules. Paget's disease, which accounts for about 1–4% of all breast cancers (Branch, 1994), is a cancer of the nipple, often associated with a ductal carcinoma under the nipple. Inflammatory cancer of the breast, which accounts for about 1% of all breast cancer (Branch, 1994), manifests as a swollen breast with diffuse red or brawny induration of the skin of the breast ("peau d'orange" skin). Inflammatory breast cancer is a rapidly spreading cancer that carries a poor prognosis for survival.

Breast cancer is classified into five stages based on size of the tumor, presence of and extent of lymph node involvement, and presence of metastasis (tumor spread) to distant sites. Table 7–8 illustrates breast cancer staging. Distant sites include lymph nodes in the supraclavicular area, as well as to other organs such as the liver or lungs. "In situ" breast cancer refers to cancer confined to the epithelium of a mammary duct or lobule. This type of cancer usually presents as microcalcifications found on mammography. If in situ carcinoma is undetected and untreated it has a high probability of developing into invasive breast cancer, that is, of spreading throughout the ductal system and developing into higher grade tumors (Kuter, 1995).

Survival after breast cancer depends on early diagnosis and treatment. Treatment of breast cancer is based on the stage of the disease, the general health and age of the client, whether the client is pre- or post-menopausal, and whether the tumor is estrogen or progesterone dependent. Treatment modalities include:

- Total mastectomy (removal of the breast)
- Lumpectomy (removal of the lump and surrounding tissue)
- Radiation therapy
- Chemotherapy
- Hormonal therapy

Lymph nodes are often removed for biopsy to determine if there has been disease spread or as a measure to contain spread of the disease. Therapies that conserve the breast, including lumpectomy and lumpectomy followed by radiation therapy, have been shown to be equivalent to mastectomy in terms of survival and recurrence for clients with cancers discovered at Stage II or lower (Strozzo, 1998) and are less physically disfiguring and emotionally devastating. Tamoxifen, a nonsteroidal antiestrogen, is an example of a hormonal treatment for estrogen dependent breast cancer types. Tamoxifen competes with estrogen at receptor sites throughout the body including those cancerous cells dependent upon estrogen for growth and survival. Tamoxifen is used for treatment of both early and advanced estrogen dependent breast cancer, often in combination with other modalities such as surgery or radiation therapy.

Breast reconstruction lessens physical disfigurement and improves body image in a woman who has undergone mastectomy. Prior to or in the absence of reconstruction, the nurse should advise the woman about breast prostheses and clothing that will improve her self-image.

Nursing care of the woman with breast cancer includes anticipatory guidance and education about breast cancer, its prognosis, and treatment. Nurses are also involved in care of the woman in the immediate postsurgical hospitalization, during prolonged chemotherapy or radiation treatment, and throughout the rehabilitation phase. Postsurgical care includes management of fluid and electrolyte balance, infection surveillance, teaching of self-care skills, and emotional and psychological support. Nurses also teach the woman to perform exercises to assist in rehabilitation of the chest and arm muscles after surgery.

▶ **TABLE 7-8**

Breast Cancer Staging

	Stages				
	0	I	II	III	IV
Tumor size	in situ (no identifiable tumor mass)	< 2 cm	< 5 cm	any size with extension to chest wall or skin	any size with or without extension to chest wall or skin
Lymph node involvement	none	none	none or movable axillary nodes on ipsilateral side	movable or fixed nodes on ipsilateral side, or internal mammary nodes on ipsilateral side	any movable or fixed nodes
Metastasis	none	none	none	none	present

Source: National Cancer Institute, 1997b.

Referral to community-based care for continued assistance with rehabilitation is appropriate. Reach to Recovery is a self-help group that provides emotional support and counseling for women who have had breast cancer surgery. Breast self-examination should be strongly encouraged in women who have survived breast cancer due to the risk of recurrence in the same or the other breast.

▶ Gynecological Cancers

The three most common sites of gynecological cancers are the cervix, the lining of the uterus (endometrium), and the ovary. These three types of cancer have been projected to account for over 76,000 new cases of cancer in 1997.

Cervical Cancer

Over 14,000 of the 76,000 new cases of cancer will be diagnosed as invasive cervical cancer. Rates of invasive cervical cancer have declined steadily since 1973 primarily due to screening with the Pap smear. Death rates from cervical cancer declined by 48% from 1971 to 1993, because early detection allowed for treatment of the cancer before it reached the invasive stage (American Cancer Society, 1997). Ninety-one percent of women diagnosed with invasive cervical cancer when it is still localized to the cervix are alive 5 years after diagnosis. African-American women are twice as likely to die from cervical cancer than Caucasian women.

Cervical cancer is most strongly linked to infection with the human papillomavirus (HPV). There are over 60 known strains of HPV. Strains 31, 33, 35, 51, 52, 16, 18, 45, and 56 are most closely associated with cervical cancer while strains 6, 11, 42, 43, and 44 are associated with cancer but to a lesser extent (American College Health Association, 1997; Carson, 1997; Muntz, 1995). Although cervical cancer is found in women in all socioeconomic groups, it is more common in women of low socioeconomic status. Other risk factors for cervical cancer include (American Cancer Society, 1997; Carson, 1997):

- Early age at first intercourse
- Infection with other STDs
- Multiple sexual partners
- Sex with men who have had multiple partners
- Poor nutrition, including deficiencies of vitamins A and C
- Compromised immune system such as found in women with HIV/AIDS
- Alcohol consumption
- Cigarette smoking

Cervical cancer is most often asymptomatic, although some women with cervical changes may have abnormal vaginal discharge, bleeding, or spotting in earlier stages. In late stages cervical cancer may cause pain and symptoms characteristic of spread to other organs. Women who were exposed to diethylstilbestrol (DES) in utero are at high risk for both cervical and vaginal cancer. DES was given to many pregnant women to prevent miscarriage between 1940 and 1971 resulting in prenatal exposure of millions of women alive today.

Many cases of cervical cancer can be prevented through educating women about its causes and providing them with information on safer sexual practices. Women should also be encouraged to change other behaviors such as smoking and alcohol use, which lead to increased risk for cervical cancer.

Cervical screening with the Pap smear is an inexpensive and relatively accurate method of screening for cervical cancer and for precancerous changes. A woman should have her first Pap smear when she becomes sexually active or at age 18, whichever is sooner. Table 7–4 presents guidelines for routine cervical cancer screening. The Pap smear is not foolproof however. About 1 in every 100 Pap smears results in a false negative (interpreted as negative when in reality a cancerous or precancerous condition is present), due to errors in collecting, preserving, or interpreting the sample.

Pap smears have traditionally been collected by scraping a wooden spatula across the cervix and smearing the cells obtained in a thin layer on a glass slide. To reach cells in the endocervix a thin cytobrush or a "broom" is used; those cells should also be thinly applied to the slide, either next to or on top of the cells obtained with the spatula. The cells should be applied to the slide as soon as they are collected and the slide should be sprayed with the appropriate fixative *immediately* after the cells are applied. Failure to apply the fixative before the cells dry from contact with the air causes unsatisfactory or uninterpretable smears. Other causes of unsatisfactory Pap smears include vaginitis or cervical infections, menstruation or other vaginal bleeding, use of douches, spermicides, and vaginal creams within two days prior to the Pap smear, and lubricant placed on the speculum prior to insertion (American College Health Association, 1997; Muntz, 1995). Unsatisfactory smears need to be repeated using the proper technique. After collection and fixation, the slides must be properly labeled and transported to the laboratory for interpretation.

Pap smears are usually done during a periodic health visit, family planning, or routine gynecological checkup. Women should be advised not to douche, have intercourse, or use intravaginal medications, tampons, or contraceptives for 48 hours prior to their scheduled appointment if a Pap smear is to be done. The test should be rescheduled if these conditions are not met or if the woman is menstruating, has other vaginal bleeding, or has a vaginal infection.

Newer methods of collecting and interpreting Pap smears promise to improve accuracy. The FDA has recently approved a new method of specimen transport which eliminates the need to apply the cells to a slide. In this new method of collection, the cells on the spatula are stirred into a preservative liquid in a specimen container and the cytobrush is sent to the lab in the same container. The specimen is then centrifuged to separate out the cervical cells, which are then spread thinly on the slide. This method separates cellular debris from the sample, making it easier to interpret. New automated screening devices have also been approved by the FDA for certain limited uses. These devices should reduce the number of false negative readings but significantly increase the costs of screening.

Interpretation of the Pap smear is done by a qualified cytopathologist who examines the cells under a high-power microscope and determines the presence and degree of cell pathology. Changes suspicious for precancerous conditions are called dysplasia. Dysplastic cells show evidence of abnormal growth patterns such as abnormal appearing nuclei that are greatly enlarged, leading to a high nucleus: cytoplasm ratio. Dysplasia can be mild, moderate, or severe, and the degree of dysplasia correlates with the degree of change in the cell structure.

If there are no identified cell abnormalities, the Pap smear is reported as normal. If there are abnormal cells present, they are classified according to a standard classification system. The Bethesda System, a commonly used system for classifying cervical cell cytology, was developed by an expert panel convened by the National Cancer Institute. The Bethesda System classifies cervical cell dysplasia as follows:

- Atypical Squamous Cells of Undetermined Significance (ASCUS) refers to changes in the squamous cells of the cervix which are not dysplastic changes.
- Low-Grade Squamous Intraepithelial Lesion (LSIL) includes cellular changes characteristic of infection with HPV (koilocytotic or condylomatous atypia) or of mild dysplasia.
- High-Grade Squamous Intraepithelial Lesion (HSIL) refers to moderately to severely dysplastic cells. HSIL also includes carcinoma in situ, which refers to the presence of abnormal cells throughout the entire thickness of the epithelial cell layer. Intraepithelial lesions (LSIL

or HSIL) do not extend beyond the surface layer of cells on the cervix.
- Atypical Glandular Cells of Undetermined Significance (AGUS) refers to the presence of a different type of cell, which may be present on the cervix in an atypical form. These cells may originate in the endocervix or in the endometrium of the uterus.

The Bethesda System also requires that the final report include a statement on the adequacy of the specimen received in the lab. The report also describes other types of cellular changes, such as those caused by the organisms responsible for vaginitis, the virus herpes simplex, or bacteria such as coccobacilli.

Another commonly used classification system for cervical changes relies on assigning a numerical category based on the number of dysplastic cells found on the surface of the cervix. This system refers to dysplastic changes as Cervical Intraepithelial Neoplasia (CIN) and is as follows:

- CIN 1: mild dysplasia equivalent to LSIL
- CIN 2: moderate dysplasia
- CIN 3: severe dysplasia or carcinoma in situ

CIN 2 and CIN 3 are both considered HSIL in the Bethesda System.

The Pap smear is not considered diagnostic of cancer; it must be followed by other tests before making a definitive diagnosis. Further testing and treatment is based on the Bethesda classification and the knowledge that many low-grade cervical lesions do not progress to cancer. If a Pap smear shows ASCUS with inflammatory changes caused by infection, the infection should be treated if possible and the Pap smear repeated 3 months after completion of treatment. If a Pap smear shows ASCUS and the woman is in a low-risk category for cervical cancer, the clinician may elect to wait and repeat the test in 3–4 months. Women who are at higher risk for cervical cancer, such as those with a history of prior abnormal Pap smears and those infected with HIV, should be referred for further diagnostic biopsies, as should women with LSIL, HSIL, or CIN 1–3.

Colposcopy is another screening technique for cervical cancer and uses stereoscopic magnification to visualize the vulva, vagina, and cervix. The clinician looks for changes in the surface of these organs such as changes in vasculature, color, and surface pattern. Endocervical curettage, which is removal of cells from the endocervical canal, should be performed at the same time. Cone biopsy is another method of removing cervical cells for further diagnosis, which involves removal of a cone-shaped wedge of tissue from the cervix, which is then sent to the lab for examination of the tissue. If biopsy confirms LSIL or HSIL or invasive cancer, further treatment is necessary.

Cervical cancer is staged according to amount of local spread and presence or absence of metastasis to other pelvic organs and distant metastasis (see box entitled Stages of Cervical Cancer). Abnormal cells confined to the cervix are removed using cryotherapy, or excised using either laser or LEEP (loop electrosurgical excision procedure). Lesions found on the vagina or vulva during colposcopy or during a routine gynecological examination can be treated with liquid nitrogen or various chemotherapeutic agents such as imiquimod cream, tricholoracetic acid, or 5-Fluorouracil cream. Hysterectomy, radiation therapy, or more radical surgical techniques are sometimes necessary when the cancer has spread beyond the cervix.

Following local therapies such as cryotherapy or LEEP, the nurse should make sure that the woman receives instructions for postsurgical self-care. While these will vary for different treatment modalities, they commonly include restrictions on vaginal intercourse, use of tampons or douches until the surgical site has healed, and instructions for cleansing and drying the external genitalia. Women will appreciate anticipatory guidance about vaginal bleeding. Possible postsurgical discharge can be copious. An appointment for a postsurgical check will be necessary. It is important that clients understand the need for continued surveillance for recurrent cancer with Pap smears every 3–6 months (Muntz, 1995). As with treatment for any disease that may be sexually transmitted, women treated for cervical cancer should be advised on safer sexual practices.

An abnormal Pap smear can be very stressful: It carries with it overtones of uncertainty over causes and outcomes that may include malignancy and death. Women with abnormal Pap smears almost always have to undergo some form of treatment, repeat testing, or further diagnostic procedures. The association of abnormal Pap smears with HPV infection raises the possibly stigmatizing issue of sexual transmission. Nurses can decrease the psychological impact of an abnormal Pap smear by contacting the woman personally with her results and providing accurate information on the level of abnormality found and the type of follow up necessary.

Endometrial Cancer

Endometrial cancer is cancer of the uterine lining and is the most common type of cancer affecting the uterine corpus. Incidence of endometrial cancer is about 21/100,000 women. About 35,000 new cases of endometrial cancer were expected in 1997 (American Cancer Society, 1997). The five-year survival rate for endometrial cancer is 95% if the cancer is discovered in an early stage but only 66% if it has begun to spread (American Cancer Society, 1997). Endometrial cancer is unusual in women under 40 years of age.

Risk factors for endometrial cancer are:

- Estrogen, including use of estrogen without progesterone for postmenopausal HRT
- Early age at menarche
- Late age menopause
- Obesity
- Nulliparity or low parity
- History of failure to ovulate
- History of tamoxifen therapy

Factors associated with decreased risk of endometrial cancer are use of oral contraceptives and pregnancies.

▶ STAGES OF CERVICAL CANCER

0

In situ—non-invasive, intraepithelial

I

Invasive, confined to cervix

II

Spread to vaginal wall but confined to upper two-thirds of vagina

III

Includes lower one-third of vagina and/or extension to pelvic sidewall

May be fixed to bony structures of pelvis

IV

Extension beyond reproductive organs to other pelvic organs such as bladder or rectum and/or distant metastatic spread

Source: Robboy, Duggan, & Kurman, 1994.

There is no routine screening test for endometrial cancer, which usually presents as abnormal uterine bleeding or spotting. The Pap smear does not screen for endometrial cancer as it only collects cells from the outside of the cervix. Annual pelvic examinations are recommended for women over 40 (American Cancer Society, 1997). They should be questioned about bleeding between menstrual periods, heavy or irregular menstrual periods, and periods of amenorrhea followed by bleeding or spotting. A woman who has undergone menopause who has unexpected vaginal bleeding or spotting warrants a diagnostic workup for endometrial cancer. Pain and other systemic symptoms usually are not present unless the cancer is advanced and has spread to other organ systems.

If endometrial cancer is suspected, an endometrial biopsy or dilatation and curettage (D&C) can be performed to collect cells from the lining of the uterus to be analyzed by a pathologist. The thickness of the uterine lining can be measured with ultrasound and is sometimes recommended instead of endometrial biopsy or D&C. If a diagnosis of endometrial cancer is made, hysterectomy is the most likely treatment, often followed by radiation or chemotherapy.

Ovarian Cancer

Ovarian cancer is often referred to as a "silent" cancer, because it lacks definitive signs or symptoms in its early stages. Ovarian cancer accounts for 4% of all cancers in women and will lead to over 14,000 deaths in 1997 (American Cancer Society, 1997). Ovarian cancer is often not diagnosed until it has grown and spread, and this leads to a low overall five-year survival rate of 46%.

Risk factors for ovarian cancer are:

- Age (peaking in the 70s)
- Nulliparity
- Family history of ovarian cancer
- Presence of defects or mutations in the BRCA1 and BRCA2 genes

Pregnancy and oral contraceptives appear to be protective against ovarian cancer.

There is no routine screening test for ovarian cancer but the American Cancer Society recommends an annual pelvic examination along with careful assessment by history for all women over 40 years of age (American Cancer Society, 1997).

The most common symptom of ovarian cancer is enlargement of the abdomen but this is often mistaken by the woman as weight gain or muscle weakness. Vaginal bleeding is a rare symptom. Women may also complain of vague abdominal discomforts such as increased distension and gas, or of pelvic pressure. Women over 40 with these symptoms and discomforts should be evaluated for ovarian cancer. Diagnostic modalities include pelvic examination, ultrasound, and blood tests for CA 125, a tumor marker.

Treatment of ovarian cancer begins with surgery. One or both ovaries may be removed and often the fallopian tubes and uterus are removed as well. Further surgery may be indicated depending on degree of tumor growth and spread. Radiation and/or chemotherapy often follow surgery. In advanced cases, palliative measures such as nutritional support and management of pain and other symptoms help optimize the quality of life.

Nursing care of women with gynecological cancers involves management of the woman in the hospital setting before and after surgery as well as in the outpatient setting. Women who have had debilitating cancer surgery or treatments often become candidates for community-based care services provided by or directed by nurses. Chemotherapy, management of its side effects, and palliative therapy is often provided by nurses who administer treatments and coordinate care for these clients.

Critical Thinking in Care Planning

Care of a Woman with Osteoporosis Risk

Janet Wu, 53 years old, comes to the health center for a well woman periodic health visit. Ms. Wu is an Asian American with a small, thin build. Her height is 5'1" and her weight is 92 lbs. Ms. Wu does not smoke or drink alcoholic beverages. Her lifestyle is essentially sedentary. She works as a computer programmer in a large university and drives to work every day. She sits at her keyboard for about 10 hours each day and watches television or does light housework at night. She has not menstruated in three years, having achieved a normal menopause at age 50. Ms. Wu's bone density scan shows slightly lowered bone density in both hips and in her spine, leading to a diagnosis of early osteopenia. There is no evidence of new or old fractures. Ms. Wu is lactose intolerant. After discussion with her nurse practitioner and her nurse, Ms. Wu decides not to take hormone replacement therapy. Her next visit is scheduled for 1 month.

▶ Assessment

- Client states she does not know what is "wrong with her bones."
- Client does not drink milk or consume dairy products and has a low intake of leafy green vegetables.
- Client does not currently take calcium supplements.
- Client has sedentary job and no established exercise pattern.
- Bone density scan shows lowered bone density.

Nursing Diagnosis

Knowledge deficit related to osteopenia and osteoporosis.

Expected Client/Family Outcomes	Nursing Action/Intervention	Evaluation
Client is able to identify the basic pathology of osteoporosis and discuss its causes and prevention.	Teach client the pathology of osteoporosis and the contributing factors that can lead to decreased bone mass. *Rationale:* Client is more likely to adopt lifestyle changes necessary to halt progress of the disease if she understands the reasons for the recommendations.	When asked, the client is able to state the causes of osteoporosis, its manifestations, and preventive measures.

Nursing Diagnosis

Altered nutrition, less than body requirements related to calcium intake

Client will increase calcium intake to at least 1500 mg daily.	Advise client to increase her intake of nondairy foods that contain calcium including such foods as salmon, turnips and collard greens, spinach, and cooked dried beans. Advise client to take 1500 mg/day of calcium supplement, preferably as calcium carbonate. *Rationale:* Increased calcium in diet and in the form of supplements decreases bone loss and replaces lost bone.	Client increases intake of calcium in form of diet and supplements as demonstrated by 24-hour diet recall and assessment of use of supplements at next visit.

Critical Thinking in Care Planning continued

Expected Client/Family Outcomes	Nursing Action/Intervention	Evaluation
Client will obtain an adequate intake of vitamin D.	Advise client to consume foods such as egg yolks, which contain vitamin D, and to go out into the sun as much as possible. Advise client to take a multivitamin with vitamin D or calcium supplements that contain vitamin D. *Rationale:* Vitamin D is required for the absorption and reabsorption of calcium from the intestine and kidney.	Client reports increased exposure to sunlight and adequate intake of vitamin D as demonstrated by 24-hour recall. Bone density scan in 1 year shows increased or stable bone density.

Nursing Diagnosis

Risk for trauma from falls related to decreased bone density

Client will adopt a program of both weight bearing and aerobic exercise at least 4 times/week for 30–60 minutes.	Advise client of the relationship between bone loss and sedentary lifestyle. Assist client to plan appropriate exercise routine and schedule. *Rationale:* Weight-bearing exercises such as jogging, brisk walking, and weight training build bone density.	Client reports establishment of adequate exercise program by next visit. Bone density scan in 1 year shows increased or stable bone density.
Client will alter home environment to decrease safety hazards and will adopt safer practices outside of the home.	Advise client to remove scatter rugs, keep stairwells well lighted, and remove debris from floors. Sidewalks should be kept clear of ice and snow. Advise client to wear proper footwear and safety gear in and out of the home, especially during exercise. *Rationale:* Adoption of safety measures inside and outside of the home will decrease the risk of falls that may result in fractures due to osteoporosis.	At next visit, client will report that she has altered her home environment to decrease fall risk and has adopted use of safe footwear and equipment. Client will remain free of fractures.

Chapter Highlights

▶ Factors influencing women's health in the United States today include family structure and multiple roles, poverty, longevity, sexual orientation, components of the health care system, and policy and research issues.

▶ Violence, substance use and abuse, smoking, sexually transmitted diseases, mental and emotional disorders, suicide, and eating disorders are critical issues currently facing women and their health care providers.

▶ The woman's periodic health visit gives nurses the opportunity to focus on the goals of primary and secondary prevention and health promotion for the client.

▶ Nursing care of the well woman includes education about the physiologic and psychologic aspects of menstruation.

▶ Health-related issues for women during the menopause and postmenopause include vasomotor instability, urogenital atrophy, osteoporosis, and cardiovascular disease, which can be managed through a combination of methods such as diet, exercise, and the use of hormone replacement therapy.

▶ Breast self-examination, clinical breast examination, and mammography are important methods for screening women for breast cancer.

▶ Nursing strategies that can be used to support women undergoing diagnosis of breast cancer include making referrals to appropriate specialists and facilities for diagnosis and treatment; directing clients to community-based, financial, and social services; ensuring prompt referral for mammography and other diagnostic services; setting up face-to-face appointments to discuss results, treatment, and referrals; providing anticipatory guidance for further testing and treatment; and demonstrating support for clients by encouraging them to express their feelings and by providing assistance as needed.

▶ Nursing care of the woman with breast cancer includes anticipatory guidance and education about breast cancer, its prognosis, and treatment.

▶ The three most common sites of gynecological cancers are the cervix, the endometrium, and the ovary.

▶ The Pap smear is an inexpensive and effective method of screening for cervical cancer and enables early detection and care of this disorder.

▶ Annual pelvic examinations for women over 40 are recommended as screening methods for endometrial and ovarian cancer.

▶ Nursing care of clients with gynecological cancers involves management in both outpatient and acute care settings and referral of clients to appropriate community-based services.

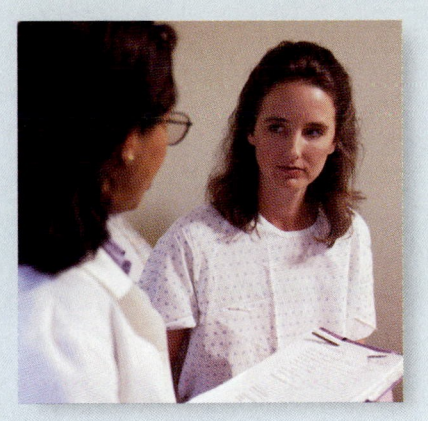

After reading the vignette at the beginning of this chapter, use what you have learned to answer these questions.

1. As part of her role in supporting Christine Larson during the gynecologic examination, what nursing strategies can Patricia Ingham, RN, use to help this client regard this situation as an opportunity to enhance her health?

2. Why is it important for the nurse to address Christine Larson's anxiety about screening procedures such as the Pap smear before the gynecologic examination is begun?

3. What other aspects, besides physiologic, may affect Christine Larson's response to and participation in the periodic health visit?

Critical Thinking Questions

► References

Acheson, L. (1997). Women in the United States health care system. In J. Λ. Rosenfeld (ed.), *Women's health in primary care* (pp. 9–18). Baltimore: Williams & Wilkins.

American Academy of Pediatrics. (1997). Staphylococcal toxic shock syndrome. In G. Peter (ed.), *1997 Red book: Report of the Committee on Infectious Diseases* (24th ed.) (pp. 481–482). Elk Grove Village, IL: Author.

American Cancer Society. (1997). *Cancer facts and figures—1997.* Atlanta, GA: Author.

American College Health Association Task Force on HPV and Other STDs. (1997). Genital human papillomavirus disease: Diagnosis, managment and prevention. Baltimore: Author.

American Psychiatric Association. (1994). *Diagnostic and statistical manual of mental disorders* (4th ed.). Washington, DC: Author.

Bailey, J., Kellermann, A., Somes, G., Banton, J., Rivara, F., & Rushforth, N. (1997). Risk factors for violent death of women in the home. *Archives of Internal Medicine, 157,* 777–782.

Becker, J. (1995). Adolescent medicine. In D. Lemcke, J. Patiison, L. Marshall, & D. Cowley (eds.), *Primary Care of Women* (pp. 15–24). Norwalk, CT: Appleton & Lange.

Benoit, C. (1996). Case management and the advanced practice nurse. In J. Hickey, R. Ouimette, & S. Venegoni (eds.), *Advanced practice nursing: Changing roles and clinical applications* (pp. 107–125). Philadelphia: J. B. Lippincott.

Bradford, J., Ryan, C., & Rothblum, E. (1994). National lesbian health care survey: Implications for mental health care. *Journal of Consulting and Clinical Psychology, 62,* 228–242.

Branch, L.G. (1994). Breast health. In E. Youngkin & M. Davis (eds.), *Women's health: A primary care clinical guide* (pp. 281–308). Norwalk, CT: Appleton & Lange.

Campbell, J., & Landenburger, K. (1995). Violence against women. In C.I. Fogel & N.F. Woods (eds.), *Women's health care: A comprehensive handbook* (pp. 407–425). Thousand Oaks, CA: Sage.

Carson, S. (1997). Human papillomatous virus infection update: Impact on women's health. *The Nurse Practitioner, 22,* 24–30, 35–37.

Chalfen, M. (1993). Obstetric-gynecologic care and survivors of childhood sexual abuse. In L.C. Andrist (ed.), *AWHONN's clinical issues in perinatal and women's health nursing: Women's issues in women's health care nursing* (pp. 191–195). Washington, DC: Association of Women's Health, Obstetric, and Neonatal Nurses.

Cole, S., Christensen, J., Raju, M., & Feldman, M. (1997). Depression. In M. Feldman & J. Christensen (eds.), *Behavioral medicine in primary care: A practical guide* (pp. 177–192). Stamford, CT: Appleton & Lange.

Collins, J. (1994). Women and the healthcare system. In E. Youngkin & M. Davis (eds.), *Women's health: A primary care clinical guide* (pp. 3–15). Norwalk, CT: Appleton & Lange.

Collins, K., & Simon, L. (1996). Women's health and managed care: Promises and challenges. *Women's Health Issues, 6,* 39–44.

Couzi, R., & Davidson, N. (1997). Breast cancer and prevention. In J. Rosenfeld (ed.), *Women's health in primary care* (pp. 683–702). Baltimore, MD: Williams & Wilkins.

Creehan, P. (1995). Toxic shock syndrome: An opportunity for nursing intervention. *Journal of Obstetric, Gynecologic, and Neonatal Nursing, 24,* 557–561.

Denenberg, R. (1994). *Report on lesbian health.* Washington, DC: National Gay and Lesbian Task Force Policy Institute.

Downey, J. (1995). Health care for lesbians. In D. Lemcke, J. Pattison, L. Marshall, & D. Cowley (eds.), *Primary care of women* (pp. 42–46). Norwalk, CT: Appleton & Lange.

Flagler, S., Hughes, T., & Kovalesky, A. (1997). Toward an understanding of addiction. *Journal of Obstetric, Gynecologic, and Neonatal Nursing, 26,* 441–448.

Forrest, D. (1994). Common gynecologic pelvic disorders. In E. Youngkin & M. Davis (eds.), *Women's health: A primary care clinical guide* (pp. 241–280). Norwalk, CT: Appleton & Lange.

Gambrell, R. (1997). *Hormone replacement therapy* (5th ed.). Durant, OK: Emis Medical.

Garner, C. (1994). The climacteric, menopause, and the process of aging. In E. Youngkin & M. Davis (eds.), *Women's health: A primary care clinical guide* (pp. 309–343). Norwalk, CT: Appleton & Lange.

Geary, M. (1995). An analysis of the women's health movement and its impact on the delivery of health care in the United States. *The Nurse Practitioner, 20,* 24–35.

Ginsburg, K. (1995). Some practical approaches to treating PMS. *Contemporary OB/GYN, May,* 24–48.

Gise, L.H. (1995). Premenstrual syndromes. In D. Lemcke, J. Pattison, L. Marshall, & D. Cowley (eds.), *Primary care of women* (pp. 410–420). Norwalk, CT: Appleton & Lange.

Horton, J. (1995). *The women's health data book: A profile of women's health in the United States* (2nd ed.). Washington DC: Elsevier Science.

Jessup, M. (1997). Addiction in women: Prevalence, profiles and meaning. *Journal of Obstetric, Gynecologic, and Neonatal Nursing, 26,* 449–458.

JNC V. (1993). The fifth report of the Joint National Committee on Detection, Evaluation & Treatment of High Blood Pressure (JNC V). *Archives of Internal Medicine, 153,* 154–183.

Kearney, M. (1997). Drug treatment for women: Traditional models and new directions. *Journal of Obstetric, Gynecologic, and Neonatal Nursing, 26,* 459–468.

Kessenich, C. (1997). Obtaining a diagnosis of postmenopausal osteoporosis. *Lippincott's Primary Care Practice, 1,* 474–484.

Klotz, M. (1995). Dysmenorrhea, endometriosis and pelvic pain. In D. Lemcke, J. Pattison, L. Marshall, & D. Cowley (eds.), *Primary care of women* (pp. 420–432). Norwalk, CT: Appleton & Lange.

Krissovich, M., & Safran, R. (1997). Urinary incontinence in adults. *Lippincott's Primary Care Practice, 1,* 361–381.

Kuter, I. (1995). Breast cancer. In D. Lemcke, J. Pattison, L. Marshall, & D. Cowley (eds.), *Primary care of women* (pp. 188–205). Norwalk, CT: Appleton & Lange.

Ladd-Taylor, M. (1992). Women's health and public policy. In R.D. Apple (ed.), *Women, health and medicine in America: A historical handbook* (pp. 383–402). New Brunswick, NJ: Rutgers University Press.

LeBoeuf, F., & Carter, S. (1996). Discomforts of the perimenopause. *Journal of Obstetric, Gynecologic, and Neonatal Nursing, 25,* 173–180.

Miller, J. (1995). Benign breast disorders. In D. Lemcke, J. Pattison, L. Marshall, & D. Cowley (eds.), *Primary care of women* (pp. 206–213). Norwalk, CT: Appleton & Lange.

Moore, A., & Noonan, M. (1996). A nurse's guide to hormone replacement therapy. *Journal of Obstetric, Gynecologic, and Neonatal Nursing, 25,* 24–31.

Muntz, H. (1995). Cervical cancer screening and management of the abnormal Papanicolaou smear. In D. Lemcke, J. Pattison, L. Marshall, & D. Cowley (eds.), *Primary care of women* (pp. 467–476). Norwalk, CT: Appleton & Lange.

National Cancer Institute. (1997a). Breast cancer and mammography statistics. [On-line]. Available: http://rex.nci.nih.gov/MAMMOG-WEB/STATS-CHARTS.html.

National Cancer Institute. (1997b). Breast cancer [On-line]. Available: http://cancernet.nci.nih.gov/clinpdq/soa/Breast-cancer-physician.html#3.

National Heart, Lung, and Blood Institute (1993a). Detection, Evaluation & Treatment of High Blood Cholesterol in Adults (NIH Publication No. 93-3096). Washington, DC: U.S. Government Printing Office.

National Heart, Lung and Blood Institute. (1993b). Nurses: Help your patients stop smoking (NIH Publication No. 92-2962). Washington, DC: U.S. Government Printing Office.

National Institutes of Health. (1997). *Consensus development statement: Breast cancer screening for women Ages 40–49.* [On-line]. Available: http://odp.od.nih.gov/consensus/statements/cdc/.

National Osteoporosis Foundation. (1995). *Position paper: Current perspectives on diagnosis, prevention and treatment of osteoporosis.* Washington, DC: Author.

National Osteoporosis Foundation. (1997). Important disease facts. [On-line]. Available: http://www.nof.org/.

Newman, D., & Burns, P. (1997). New approaches for managing stress incontinence in women. *Lippincott's Primary Care Practice, 1,* 382–387.

Phillips, J., Sexton, M., & Blackman, J. (1997). Demographic overview of women across the lifespan. In K.M. Allen & J.M. Phillips (eds.), *Women's health across the lifespan: A comprehensive perspective* (pp. 17–35). Philadelphia: J. B. Lippincott.

Plouffe, L., Rausch, J., Khrein, I., & Stewart, K. (1994). Premenstrual syndrome: Update on diagnosis and management. *The Female Patient, 19,* 53–60.

Quimby, C. (1994). Women and the family of the future. *Journal of Obstetric, Gynecologic, and Neonatal Nursing, 23,* 113–122.

Robboy, S., Duggan, M., & Kurman, R. (1994). The female reproductive system. In E. Rubin & J. Farber (eds.), *Pathology* (2nd ed.) (pp. 909–971). Philadelphia: J. B. Lippincott.

Scheibneir, M. (1997). In harm's way: Childbearing women and nicotine. *Journal of Obstetric, Gynecologic, and Neonatal Nursing, 26,* 477–484.

Strozzo, M. (1998). An overview of stage I and stage II breast cancer for the primary care provider. *Lippincott's Primary Care Practice, 2,* 160–169.

Substance Use and Mental Health Services Administration. (1994). *National household survey on drug abuse: Population estimates 1993.* (SMA Publication No. 94-3017). Washington, DC: Author.

Suggs, N. (1995). Domestic violence. In D. Lemcke, J. Pattison, L. Marshall, & D. Cowley (eds.), *Primary care of women* (pp. 112–123). Norwalk, CT: Appleton & Lange.

The Contraceptive Report. (1995). *Weighing the risks and benefits of hormone replacement therapy after menopause.* Houston, TX: Baylor College of Medicine.

U.S. Preventive Services Task Force. (1996). *Guide to clinical preventive services* (2nd ed.). Baltimore: Williams & Wilkins.

Verbrugge, L. (1992). Pathways of health and death. In R.D. Apple (ed.), *Women, health and medicine in America: A historical handbook* (pp. 41–79). New Brunswick, NJ: Rutgers University Press.

Walker, L. (1979). *The battered woman.* New York: Harper & Row.

Wilcox, L., Koonin, L., Pokras, R., Strauss, L., Xia, A., & Peterson, H. (1994). Hysterectomy in the United States, 1988–1990. *Obstetrics and Gynecology, 83,* 549–555.

Woods, N.F. (1995). Women and their health. In C.I. Fogel & N.F. Woods (eds.), *Women's health care: A comprehensive handbook* (pp. 1–22). Thousand Oaks, CA: Sage.

Woods, N.F., & Mitchell, E.S. (1997). Pathways to depressed mood for midlife women: Observations from the Seattle women's health study. *Research in Nursing and Health, 20,* 119–129.

World Health Organization. (1979). Constitution of the World Health Organization. In T.L. Beauchamp & J.F. Childress (eds.), *Principles of biomedical ethics* (pp. 284–285). New York: Oxford University Press.

II

Preparing for Pregnancy and Birth

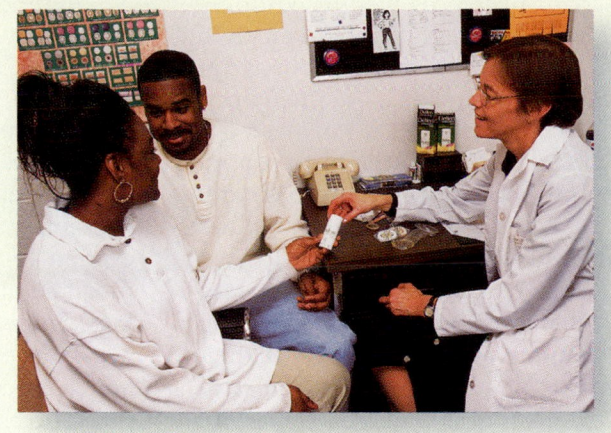

Scott and Shaila Jackson are meeting with Ann Salzman, CNM, MSN, for a contraceptive counseling session at a local health center. Shaila tells the nurse-midwife that she and her husband are considering changing their method of contraception. Shaila has used a diaphragm successfully for the past two years, but they would like to change to a method that "requires less planning." Both Shaila and Scott want to delay childbearing for "at least 3 more years."

During their discussion about available contraceptive methods, Shaila expresses interest in the use and benefits of the pill or other long-acting female contraceptives. The nurse-midwife notices, however, that Scott does not express a preference for any method and keeps glancing at Shaila, as if trying to catch her attention. The nurse-midwife asks, "Scott, what is your opinion about these methods?" Scott looks nervously at Shaila and replies, "I know that Shaila and I agreed to talk about using something other than the diaphragm, but I'm not sure if I like any of these methods better. Don't these other methods have side effects?" ∎

8

Family Planning

Conception control is not a new concept. Attempts at control date back at least 5000 years. Poisonous, deadly, often ineffective substances were used orally by both men and women and vaginally by women to prevent or terminate pregnancy. Most couples have at some time sought freedom from the risk of pregnancy. Not until the late 1800s and early 1900s, however, did women themselves become active in the birth control movement, and not until the 1960s were birth control methods openly discussed with women in health care settings (Finch & Green, 1963).

Today, several factors encourage the trend toward smaller families and planning childbearing: changing lifestyles, economics, improved contraceptive technology, and better methods of communicating information about contraceptive technologies as a part of health care services.

The terms *birth control, contraception,* and *family planning* have been used interchangeably. Family planning is the broadest concepts and includes assessing the genetic, physical, psychosocial, cultural, and religious concerns of individuals or couples considering reproduction. It also involves seeking solutions to infertility, controlling when a pregnancy occurs, and voluntarily interrupting pregnancy. Birth control and contraception generally refer to the methods employed to avoid or space pregnancies. This chapter discusses reproductive decision making, risk assessment in the reproducing couple, contraceptive counseling, pregnancy prevention methods, and pregnancy termination.

▶ REPRODUCTIVE DECISION MAKING

It used to be so simple: women and men married and engaged in sexual intercourse, which usually resulted in pregnancy (Cushner, 1986). Human reproduction was characterized primarily by one feature—chance. Today, however, human reproduction is quite different. The primary characteristic at this time is not chance, but choice. Today couples may choose to become parents without choosing to marry or they may choose to be sexually active and avoid unintended pregnancies or births (Hatcher et al., 1994).

Despite the reproductive options available today, most women can still be expected to have a child eventually. Data continue to show that most women in the United States will probably have two children in their lifetime and that their childbearing will be compressed into an ever-narrowing span of time. Thus there is strong evidence that family size in the United

States is becoming increasingly limited to no, one, or two children.

Reproductive decisions today are based on complex value systems in which alternatives are considered, each having its own risks, benefits, and uncertainties (Hatcher et al., 1994). The desire to reproduce, intelligence, educational background, career goals, financial considerations, and ethical, moral, and religious beliefs are all factors considered in reproductive decision making. Many women who practice contraception continue to regard the possibility of getting pregnant and having a baby with some positive feelings. Some women also associate contraception with negative feelings. Thus many women have to maintain a balance of conflicting emotions that on any given occasion may determine the use or nonuse of their contraceptive method (Miller, 1986). At any one time, the motivation to avoid conception may be weighed against the perceived risk of conception occurring. Other factors that may influence a woman's use or nonuse of a contraceptive method are the attitudes of her partner or even of extended community members, such as close friends and other family members.

The innate desire for children may be predetermined by cultural and personal influences and may be fixed in early childhood. It is determined by both individual experience in the family and by more widespread cultural influences of society and the individual's specific ethnic or religious group. The desire for children may vary with time, place, socioeconomics, race, and religious beliefs (Westhoff, 1996b).

Financial considerations are becoming increasingly significant in today's reproductive decision making. The cost of raising a single child in an affluent society is considered prohibitive by some. Raising two or three children is more than many are willing to undertake financially.

▶ Reproductive Decision Making for At-Risk Couples

When a couple has an increased risk of having a child with a birth defect or genetic disorder, that risk will influence their reproductive decision making. Subjective interpretation of risk and past experience with a problem are two factors that highly influence such a couple's reproductive decision making.

Subjective interpretation of risk by a couple is influenced by many factors. The same objective risk may mean different things to different people and in fact may mean different things to the same person at different times in his or her life (Westhoff, 1996b).

What one person considers a high risk may be a low or acceptable risk to another.

One factor that may influence risk perception is past experience with the "odds." Many couples believe that a 1% risk of having a child with Down syndrome is low. But a 20-year-old couple's risk of having a child with Down syndrome is approximately 1 in 2000; if they happen to be the 1 in 2000 that has already had one affected child, the couple's risk is higher than it was before their first affected child was born, because having one Down child increases the chance of having a second affected child.

A second factor that may influence risk interpretation is the nature and severity of the disorder for which the family is at risk. A 5% risk of having a child who will survive many years with severe mental retardation may have much more significance for a couple than a 25% risk of having a child who will die shortly after birth.

Past experience with a disorder may also have a big impact on the couple's subjective interpretation of risk. If a woman herself was born with a cleft lip and palate, how she felt about her own birth defect while growing up may directly influence how she perceives her 3% risk of having a similarly affected child.

A nurse's interpretation of risk may influence a couple's reproductive decision making. How risk figures are expressed may influence a couple's reproductive choices. A risk may be presented as a 1 in 4 risk, a 25% risk, or a 3 to 1 chance against having an affected child. When presenting risk figures to families it may be helpful to present both absolute and relative risk figures. In communicating to a couple that their risk of having a child with a birth defect is 1%, it should be remembered that the same couple's risk may be 100 times greater than the general population risk; thus it may be important for them to hear this risk figure in more than one way. It is also important for the nurse to inform the couple that their specific risk must be added to the 3% general population risk that any reproducing couple faces of having a child with a birth defect.

A decision regarding reproductive behavior must not be unduly influenced by the health care provider. Nurses need to be supportive, nonjudgmental, and nondirective in the counseling they provide. Nurses are responsible for ensuring that the information a couple receives is factually correct and presented in a sensitive manner. It is also important to allow adequate time for questions and discussion when a couple receives this information. Follow-up supportive counseling should be offered to the family as well. Nurses can help couples sort through the information available to them and support them in the reproductive decisions they make.

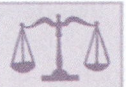

Ethical Decision Making

A controversial area in health care is the control of reproduction, including fertility. The innate desire for children exists in most individuals, regardless of cultural, ethnic, or personal lifestyle factors. Consider the following issues as they relate to reproductive decision making for various populations:

1. What rights and options for reproduction are available to homosexuals?
2. For individuals with HIV infection?
3. For individuals who are likely to pass on severe genetic problems to their children?
4. For individuals who are mentally retarded?

▶ ASSESSMENT OF RISK IN THE REPRODUCING COUPLE

A pregnancy at risk is one in which there is an increased chance of morbidity or mortality for the mother, fetus, or infant. A pregnancy is also considered high-risk when a pregnancy is unplanned or undesired or the individual or couple is unable to adequately care for the child economically, socially, or psychologically (Sherwen & Miele, 1986).

▶ Provider Responsibilities

Identifying families at risk and communicating the risk to them are responsibilities of the health care provider. Health care providers have been held liable for not identifying families at risk. Courts have recognized wrongful conception claims of parents who seek damages after the birth of a healthy but unplanned child born as a result of a failed sterilization or abortion or the improper filling of a birth control prescription (Donovan, 1984). Thus there is legal precedent that health care providers have responsibility to ensure access to competent and comprehensive family planning services. Furthermore, the advent of the Human Genome Project makes the use of genetic counseling more compelling (Kopala, 1997). Health care providers also have the responsibility to assess common risk factors and to provide correct information about reproductive risks that are identified. Nurses must be able to provide specific, accurate, and understandable information to clients so that they may make informed reproductive decisions. Nurses should not attempt to influence reproductive decisions according to their own values or desires. The information regarding reproductive alternatives should be provided in an environment that is as value free as possible.

▶ Approaches to Risk Assessment

A number of approaches are useful in identifying individuals or couples at risk. These include obtaining a thorough family history, assessing psychosocial factors, identifying racial and ethnic background, and parental age, and discussing maternal health history, past reproductive history, and, when applicable, a history of the present pregnancy.

Family Health History

A thorough family history may give clues to risk status. Specific questions about individual family members should be asked regarding the health status of all first-degree (parent, child, and siblings) and second-degree (half-siblings, grandparent, aunt, uncle, niece) relatives. Of concern would be the identification of a history of multiple miscarriages, stillbirths, children who are born with birth defects or who have died at a young age, any pathologic condition that occurred more than once in a family, or any known genetic disorders. If the family history reveals that this pregnancy is the result of a consanguineous mating (intercourse between individuals related by blood), the risk of having a child with a genetic disorder may be increased.

Psychosocial Factors

Low level of education, low socioeconomic status, associated poor nutrition and limited access to prenatal care increase a couple's risk of having a low-birth-weight child. Occupation is often related to socioeconomic status. The highest incidence of perinatal loss, in families in which the father is present, occurs when the father is in semiskilled labor or a manual occupa-

tion. The lowest loss rate occurs when the father is a professional or a farmer. The highest incidence of perinatal loss, however, occurs in families in which the father is absent.

Racial and Ethnic Background

It is also important to identify both racial and ethnic background, because perinatal risk is increased in specific groups (see Chapters 16 and 19). In addition, some genetic disorders are associated with specific ethnic groups. These are listed in Table 8–1.

Parental Age

Advancing maternal age is associated with an increasing risk of having children with chromosomal abnormalities (see discussion in Chapter 10). Recent studies, however, suggest that there is a small but increasing risk for single-gene abnormalities associated with advancing paternal age. Maternal age less than 17 is a risk factor associated with low birth weight. An adolescent father may often provide a poor or absent support system for the mother or the child.

Maternal Health History

Women who have low weight for height or chronic hypertension are at risk of having low-birth-weight children (Carmichael & Abrams, 1997; Creasy & Resnick, 1994). Maternal metabolic disorders such as juvenile-onset insulin-dependent diabetes increase two- to three-fold a woman's risk of having a child with a birth defect. Genetic disorders such as maternal myotonic dystrophy or maternal phenylketonuria (PKU) can result in the birth of an infant with significant health or learning problems.

In addition to collecting information about preexisting disorders or conditions, it is also important to assess the lifestyle and environmental hazards to which women are exposed that pose significant risks to their fetuses and infants. These hazards include smoking; use of alcohol, prescription drugs, recreational drugs, and caffeine; and contact with radiation and environmental chemicals. See Chapter 13 for a discussion of fetal teratogens.

▶ **TABLE 8–1**

Genetic Disorders Associated with Specific Racial and Ethnic Groups

Genetic Disorder	Racial or Ethnic Group	Carrier Frequency	Incidence
Cystic fibrosis	Caucasians	1 in 20	1 in 600
Tay-Sachs disease	Ashkenazi Jews	1 in 25	1 in 2500
Sickle cell anemia	African Americans	1 in 10	1 in 400
Thalassemia	Mediterraneans	1 in 25	1 in 2500

Reproductive History

An individual or couple's reproductive history should be reviewed, including information about reproduction with other partners. Of specific concern is the identification of recurrent fetal wastage and of previous children who were born preterm, or with low birth weight, stillborn, or malformed, or who have since died.

History of the Present Pregnancy

An interval between pregnancies of less than 6 months increases a woman's risk of having a low-birth-weight infant. Poor nutrition and weight gain are other crucial risk factors that have been identified, along with multiple gestation, preeclampsia, eclampsia, oligohydramnios or polyhydramnios, and bleeding during pregnancy (Cunningham et al., 1997).

Assessment of exposure to potential teratogens during pregnancy is important. (See Chapters 13 and 19 for discussions of the effect of specific infections on the mother and fetus.) Other health problems, such as maternal obesity, are associated with an increased risk for neural tube defects and possibly other central nervous system abnormalities (Morin, 1998; Tinkle & Sterling, 1997).

▶ Diagnostic Decision Making and the Nursing Process

Many nursing diagnoses may be derived from data obtained during the assessment. Table 8–2 gives some examples of nursing diagnoses for the couple who is at reproductive risk. Figure 8–1 depicts the nursing process for this couple.

▶ GENETIC EVALUATION AND COUNSELING

An individual or couple who is identified as having an increased reproductive risk should be referred for genetic evaluation and counseling and, if necessary, prenatal diagnosis and high-risk, obstetric care. Genetic counseling refers to the problem-solving process concerning the occurrence or risk of genetic disorders in the family. Genetic counseling has the following goals:

- To provide the family with a better understanding of the medical facts, prognosis, management, inheritance, risk of recurrence, and alternatives for dealing with the risk
- To make the family aware of the educational, health care, and reproductive options available
- To help the family make the best possible adjustment to the disorder's presence or to its risk

The genetic counseling process has evolved over time, and though it may have started as a service to produce primarily reproductive information and options, most genetic counseling services today provide diagnostic consultation and confirmatory testing. These services also use a case-management approach for providing information, support, and follow-up to families and to individuals affected with genetic disorders.

▶ TABLE 8–2

Examples of Nursing Diagnoses for Couple at Reproductive Risk

Nursing Diagnosis	Contributing Factors
Risk for reproductive anxiety	Related to: • Family history of birth defects or genetic disorders • Ashkenazi Jewish background • Advancing maternal age • Maternal diabetes • Maternal drug or alcohol use • Viral illness or high fever during pregnancy
Body image disturbance	Related to: • One member of the couple identified to be a "carrier" of a genetic disorder (e.g., female identified as carrier of gene for Duchenne muscular dystrophy or male identified as carrier of gene for Huntington's disease) • One member of the couple identified to be infertile (e.g., female with 45, X or 46, XY or male with 47, XXY)
Anticipatory grieving	Related to: • Couple identified to be at risk of having child with birth defect or genetic disorder • Previous pregnancy losses including miscarriage, pregnancy termination, stillbirth, or liveborn child who has since died

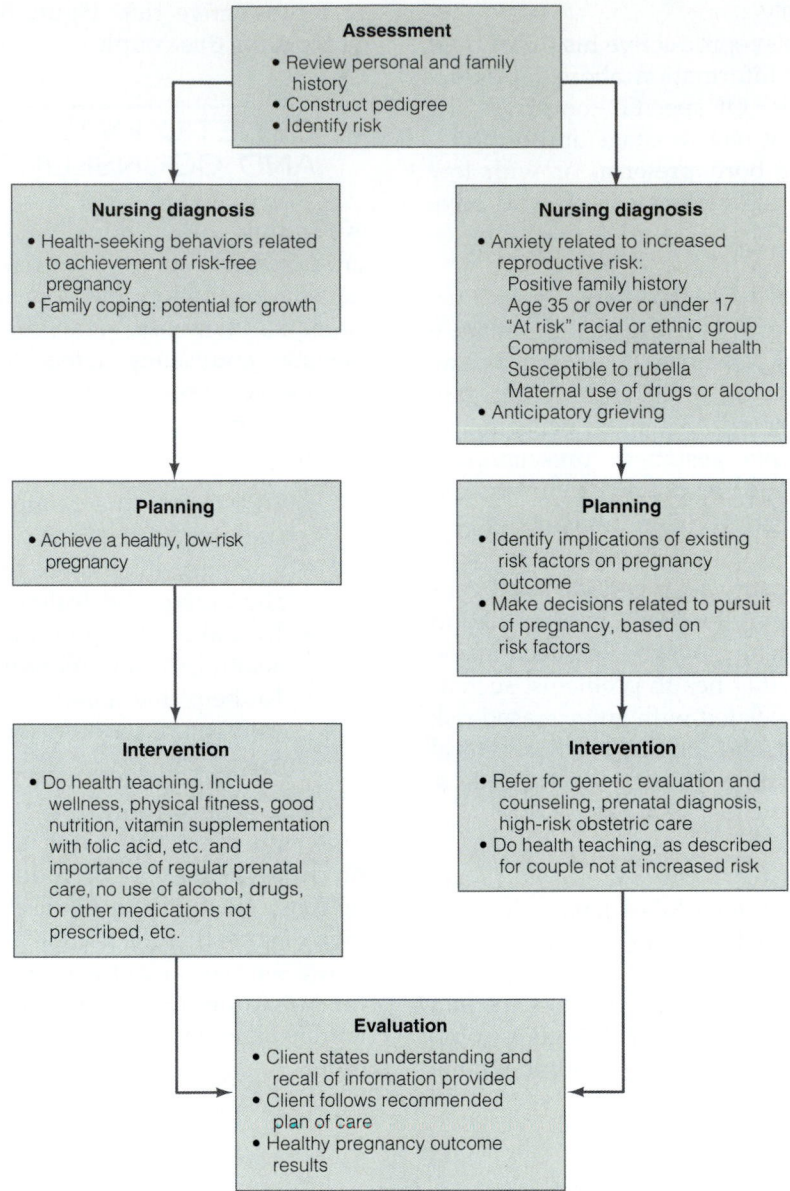

FIGURE 8–1. The nursing process. Assessment of a family planning pregnancy, with subsequent nursing diagnoses, planning, interventions, and evaluation.

If an individual or couple is believed to be at risk before or during pregnancy, a referral should be made for genetic evaluation and counseling. The genetic specialist reviews the family and other history, pertinent records, and the health care provider's evaluation, and constructs an in-depth pedigree. Risk factors identified are carefully considered.

The individual or couple is then scheduled for a genetic counseling visit. If indicated, diagnostic tests, such as chromosome analysis, are carried out (see Chapter 10). If a specific diagnosis can be confirmed,

informative and supportive counseling is provided in the clinic. A plan is made for follow-up counseling, and if necessary, referrals for prenatal diagnostic testing or high-risk obstetric care are done.

▶ PRENATAL DIAGNOSIS

Several methods of prenatal screening and diagnosis have been developed. Some of the more common include maternal serum alpha-fetoprotein (MSAFP) monitoring, amniocentesis, chorionic villus sampling, cordocentesis, ultrasonography, magnetic resonance imaging (MRI), and roentgenograms (x-rays). Many birth defects or genetic disorders may be diagnosed prenatally using more than one of these methods. In addition, several methods are often used to more carefully describe or monitor the birth defect or genetic disorder identified in the fetus.

Chapters 15, 17, and 18 describe in greater depth the assessment techniques used during each trimester. Table 8–3 summarizes the defects that may be identified by prenatal diagnostic screening. The outcome of prenatal diagnostic evaluation is usually reassuring, and the couple is informed that the disorder being investigated is not present in the expected child. For some couples an abnormality is identified. They must decide whether to continue or terminate their pregnancy. Pregnancy termination when a birth defect is identified is discussed later in this chapter.

▶ CONTRACEPTIVE COUNSELING

The motives for contraceptive use are unique, and the choice of method and its meaning to the couple are highly individual. According to Cunningham and associates (1997, p. 1339), "in no other branch of medicine are social, religious and political forces more obvious than in family planning." Thus the full range of contraceptive alternatives must be discussed with a client, so that a fully informed and satisfactory choice can be made. Individual differences must be respected by the nurse.

Maternity and community-based nurses have an important role in the care of a client seeking information about planning a family or avoiding pregnancy. The nurse must ensure that information, guidance, and methods are available to all clients. If the nurse feels unqualified or uncomfortable giving such information, she or he should tell the client and provide an appropriate referral.

Every nurse who provides information about contraception or assists individuals or couples to plan their families should be aware of available methods of contraception and their advantages and disadvantages. The individual or couple's contraceptive choice may vary throughout the life span depending on many factors (Hatcher et al., 1994):

- Self-image
- Personal values
- Sexual activity
- Age
- Religious beliefs
- Family traditions
- Cultural practices
- Expense
- Availability of bathroom facilities
- Frequency of intercourse
- Number of children
- Acceptable risk of pregnancy
- Illness or physical problems
- Level of comfort with the body and its functions

Thus, the nurse should pay attention to physical and financial barriers that are identified, as well as past success with methods used when discussing pregnancy prevention methods (Stewart, 1996).

An important point to remember when assisting clients to select a suitable contraceptive method is that choice may involve the _couple's_ decision. Unlike most health measures, pregnancy prevention ideally

---

▶ **TABLE 8-3**

Fetal Abnormalities That May Be Identified by Prenatal Diagnostic Screening

Fetal Abnormalities	Prenatal Diagnostic Screening Test					
	Amniocentesis	_CVS[a]_	_Cordocentesis_	_Ultrasonography_	_MRI[a]_	_X-Ray_
Chromosomal abnormalities	+[b]	+	+	−	−	−
Neural tube defects	+	−	−	+	±	±
Biochemical defects	+	+	+	−	−	−
Molecular defects	+	+	+	−	−	−
Skeletal anomalies	−	−	−	+	+	±
Soft tissue anomalies	−	−	−	+	+	−
Prenatal infections	+	−	+	−	−	−
Hemolytic disease	+	−	+	−	−	−

[a]CVS, chorionic villus sampling; MRI, magnetic resonance imaging.
[b]+, method can be used; −, method not useful; ±, method may be useful, but is usually not used for this purpose.

involves the participation of both male and female partners. Optimally, nurses should encourage the man's participation and provide an opportunity for him to share in the selection of the method and, ultimately, in the responsibility for fertility control. Recent data indicate that men do perceive they have equal responsibility (Grady, Tanfer, Billy, & Lincoln-Hanson, 1996). In some ethnic/cultural groups, if a woman chooses a method of contraception that her partner disapproves of, the couple will most likely not use the method.

Planning a family deals with the client's sexuality; therefore, a private setting should always be provided for the counseling session. The client's feelings about family plans should be explored in a nonjudgmental way. All contraceptive methods should be discussed and summarized to allow an informed decision to be made by the client(s). There is no single "best method" of contraception, only the method that works best for the individual client or couple.

▶ Informed Consent

The issue of informed consent is particularly important in the area of contraceptive counseling. Healthy clients may request information about contraceptive methods, often without specific health indications. The nurse helps the client to have enough information about the proposed method to make a sound decision. Sufficient information is provided by discussing the available methods and their risks, benefits, and effectiveness.

Risks
Every contraceptive method has risks, although lack of contraception and resulting pregnancy poses greater risks (Cunningham et al., 1997). Risks may be associated with the method itself or the risk of pregnancy as a result of contraceptive failure or misuse. The nurse must discuss how often the method is associated with mortality and morbidity and such problems as hospitalization, hysterectomy, infection, loss of fertility, pain, or nuisance side effects. It should be noted that the maternal mortality associated with pregnancy is far greater than mortality associated with any commonly used contraceptive.

A method may also have what might be termed "inconvenience risks," such as making sexual intercourse less pleasant. Partner dissatisfaction or embarrassment associated with the method may also occur.

Finally, the risk of pregnancy, should a method fail, must be discussed, including how often a preg-

nancy occurs (Table 8–4), what the dangers of pregnancy are to this woman, and what major life disruptions would occur with pregnancy.

Benefits
Therapeutic effects are associated with many of the methods of contraception; for example, condoms may reduce the risk of sexually transmitted diseases (STDs) and oral contraceptives regulate and lighten menstruation. The nurse should explain these benefits, as well as the contraceptive benefits to the client. The therapeutic benefits may influence an individual or couple's decision regarding which method of birth control to choose.

Effectiveness
The primary concern of clients seeking contraception is most likely the effectiveness of a method. When counseling clients about effectiveness, nurses must be familiar with two types of effectiveness rates: theoretical and use. The theoretical effectiveness rate is the method's effectiveness in preventing pregnancy under ideal conditions (when it is completely understood and used correctly at all times). This is the method's maximum rate of effectiveness. If pregnancy occurs, it is due to a failure of the method itself, not how the method is being used. The use effectiveness rate takes into consideration the method's effectiveness with actual use. Not surprisingly, some people use the method correctly and others use it carelessly or incorrectly. Use effectiveness rates are lower because of human error.

▶ Cost

An individual or couple must be informed about what their ongoing expenses will be in using a contraceptive method. If cost imposes a hardship for the individual or couple, alternative contraception or a means of obtaining the desired method less expensively should be offered.

▶ Literacy

Parker and colleagues (1996) addressed the relation between contraceptive use and literacy. Although no studies were found, several relevant points are made from their review of the literature. Reading level of many commercially prepared client instructions was at an average grade reading level of 10.3 while those prepared by health care professionals were at a 8.7 grade reading level. It is quite possible that informa-

▶ **TABLE 8-4**

First-Year Perfect Use and Typical Failure Rates of Pregnancy Prevention Methods

Method	Perfect Use (%)	Typical Failure Rates (%)
Male sterilization (vasectomy)	0.1	0.15
Female sterilization (tubal ligation)	0.4	0.4
Progestin implants		
Norplant	0.09	0.09
Injectable progestogen		
Depo-Provera	0.3	0.3
Intrauterine device		
Progestasert	1.5	2.0
ParaGard or Copper T380A	0.6	0.8
Oral contraceptive agents		
Combined	0.1	—
Progestogen only	0.5	—
Condom		
Male	3	12
Female	5	21
Diaphragm (with spermicidal agent)	6	18
Cervical cap (with spermicidal agent)		
Nulliparas	9	18
Multiparas	20	36
Coitus interruptus	4	19
Periodic abstinence		
Postovulation	1	—
Symptothermal	2	—
Ovulation	3	—
Calendar	9	—
Spermicidal agents (foams, jellies, creams, vaginal suppositories)	6	21
Chance	85	85

Adapted, with permission, from Hatcher R.A. et al. (1994). Contraceptive technology (16th Rev. ed.). New York: Irvington.

tion clients receive about contraception is beyond their reading, and thus, their comprehension level.

▶ Contraceptive Counseling with Teenagers

The number of sexually active teenagers has increased substantially over the past two decades. Concomitantly, the age at which teenagers report their first experience with sexual intercourse has declined. In 1981, pregnancy occurred in 1.4% of 14-year-old girls. This percentage continues to rise throughout the teen years, with 10% of 19-year-olds becoming pregnant (Moore, Adler, & Kegeles, 1996). At least 85% of pregnancies occurring in the teen years are unintended (Grimes, 1995). The reasons cited for this high unintended pregnancy rate include poor education in areas of family living, sexuality, and contraception, not only by the schools but also by the family and church, and the lack of access to both contraceptive information and contraceptive methods. In addition, there seems to be a "double standard" regarding sexuality that is ever present in a teenager's daily life. Sex is portrayed in books and magazines and on television and radio as something wonderful and desirable. Very early, however, many teens have received the message regarding the taboos associated with sex outside of marriage. See Chapters 5 and 11 for additional discussion of teenage sexuality.

The legal rights of minors to obtain contraceptive services without parental consent is an area of concern to all health professionals involved in providing family planning services. The laws related to minors' rights to contraception vary from state to state. In 1977, the U.S. Supreme Court ruled that minors have a right to contraceptives. To date, there have been no rulings on the rights of minors to prescriptive contraceptives. Nurses must remain informed regarding the current legal statutes in the state in which they practice. Providing adequate information is one way to increase most effective contraceptive use. When a couple or an individual has weighed the benefits and risks of the methods available, made a choice based on which methods best meet their needs, and fully understands how to use the method, the likelihood of discontinuation and misuse is substantially reduced. The following sections discuss currently available methods to prevent pregnancy.

► PREGNANCY PREVENTION METHODS

Various approaches can be adopted to organize information about the many pregnancy prevention methods. Frequently, contraceptive choices are categorized according to method of action. The approach adopted in this text, however, is to discuss pregnancy prevention methods in descending order of effectiveness (see Table 8–4).

► Sterilization

Effectiveness and Action

Both male (**vasectomy**) and female (**bilateral tubal ligation**) sterilization (also known as voluntary surgical contraception or USC) are extremely efficient in preventing pregnancy.

The typical failure rate after a vasectomy is 0.15%; after a tubal ligation the typical failure rate is 0.4%. Consequently, for individuals who no longer wish to have children, sterilization is an effective, safe

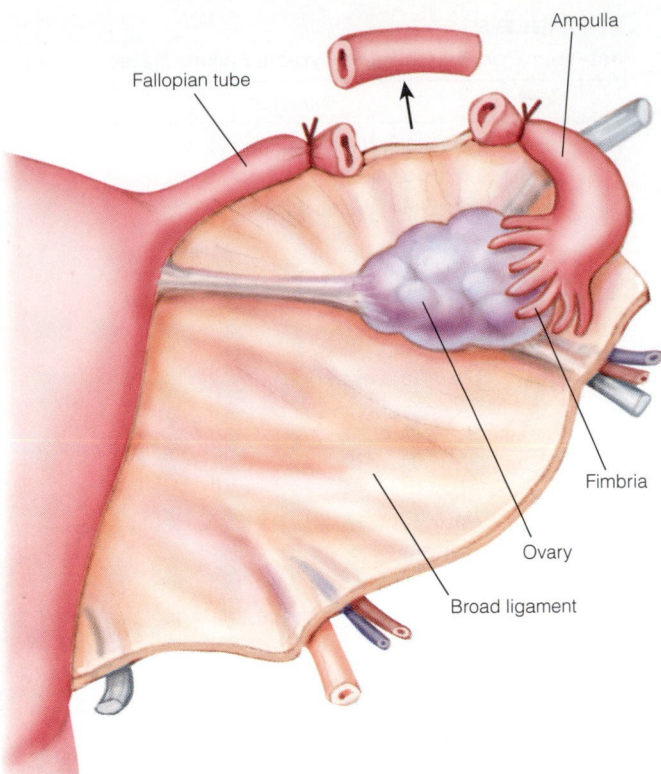

FIGURE 8–3. One method to achieve sterilization is tubal ligation. The fallopian tubes are excised following ligation.

choice (Hatcher et al., 1994). In fact, by 1988, sterilization was the contraceptive method of choice among married and formerly married women (Peterson et al., 1996). Although tubal ligation is very effective, recent data (Peterson et al., 1996) indicate that the failure rate is greater than usually reported. Futhermore, ethnicity and risk may be related in analyzing effectiveness rates, with more black women likely to experience a sterlization failure than white women. Thus, ethnicity may serve as an indicator for other risk factors that remain to be assessed.

Sterilization is accomplished by creating an artificial obstruction in either the vas deferens (vasectomy) or the fallopian tubes (bilateral tubal ligation). Vasectomy is a relatively simple procedure during which both vasa are isolated, cut, and tied (Fig. 8–2). Vasectomy can also be performed using a "no-scapel" technique (Hatcher et al., 1994). A puncture, rather than a scapel incision, is made in the scrotum and the vas deferens are reached through that puncture hole. This method is reported to have fewer complications than the scapel method. Coagulation may also be used to create the obstruction in the vas. Given the nature of the procedure, a vasectomy can be performed in an appropriately equipped and staffed physician's office

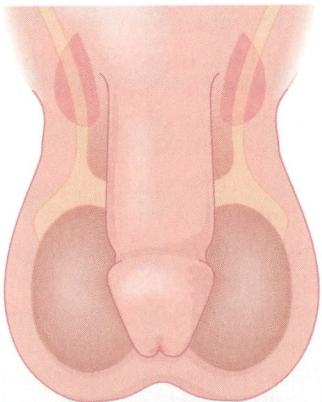

FIGURE 8–2. Vasectomy procedure. Interruption of both ductus (vas) deferens.

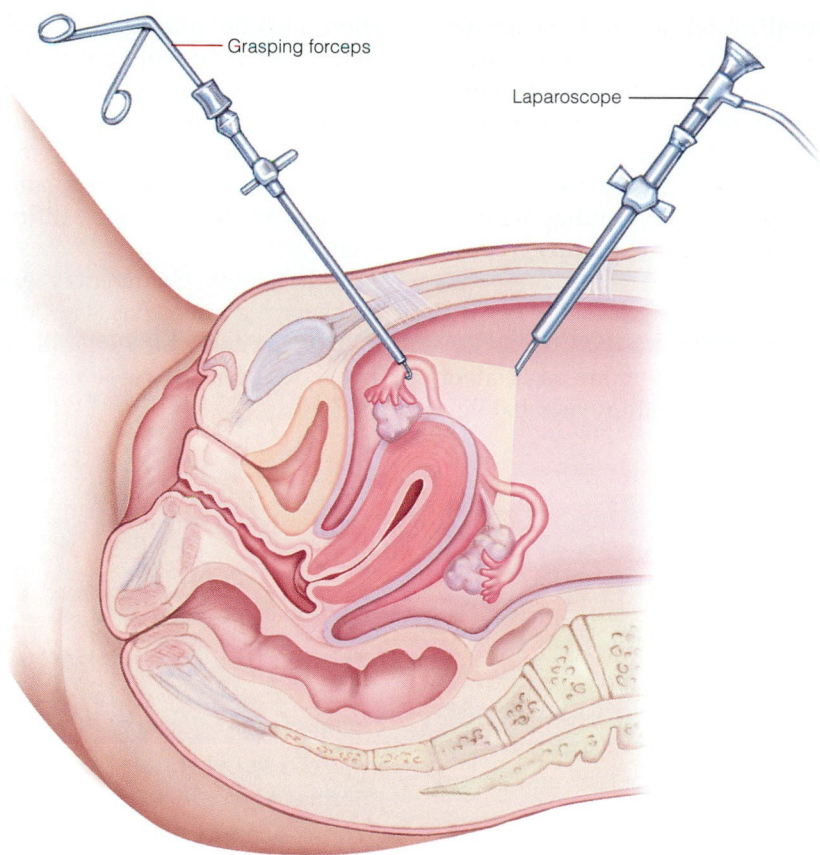

Grasping forceps

Laparoscope

FIGURE 8–4. Laparoscopy. The laparoscope is used to visualize tubal sterilization accomplished through minilaparotomy incision at level of pubic hair line. *(Redrawn, with permission, from Hatcher, R.A. et al. (1994).* Contraceptive technology *(16th Rev. ed.). New York: Irvington.)*

under either local or spinal anesthesia (Hatcher et al., 1994). Consequently, the client may go home as early as 15 to 30 minutes after the procedure has been completed (if local anesthesia is used) (Hatcher et al., 1994). Sterility is achieved after a vasectomy when a minimum of 15 ejaculations have been produced. To ensure sterility, the client can have his semen evaluated under a microscope for sperm count after 15 ejaculations have occurred.

A vaginal or abdominal route may be taken for access to the fallopian tubes. The tubes are obstructed by means of rings, bands, ligation (Fig. 8–3), or coagulation (Hatcher et al., 1994). Unless ovulation occurred within 48 hours before the surgical procedure, sterility is immediate.

Minilaparotomy and laparoscopy (Fig. 8–4) are two methods frequently used for tubal sterilization. Of the two methods, the former is the easier. A feature of both procedures is that they can be performed under local anesthesia; consequently, these procedures are frequently done on an outpatient basis.

Although in the past a hysterectomy was performed for sterilization, because of cost, required recovery time, and physical and emotional impact, it is no longer justified as a means of pregnancy prevention.

Informed Consent

Because of the nature and permanency of the procedure, an informed consent should be obtained. The general irreversibility of the procedure should be stressed, the procedure simply but accurately explained, and risks and benefits clearly described by the physician in terms that are easily understood by the client. An additional consent may be required for the type of anesthesia to be employed. Currently, spousal consent is not required.

Benefits

All methods of sterilization are considered permanent and consequently are extremely effective overall. In addition, when compared with other pregnancy prevention options, sterilization is an inexpensive procedure—the financial outlay occurs once rather than on a monthly or more frequent basis. Another benefit is the singular nature of the sterilization procedure, which frees the client from having to make repeated contraceptive decisions. Lastly, sterilization provides a pregnancy prevention option that is independent of coitus, a desirable attribute for any contraceptive method.

Risks and Contraindications

As with any operative procedure, there are associated risks. Complications related to vasectomy or tubal lig-ation include infection, bowel perforation, hemorrhage, and incisional pain as well as potential complications associated with the type of anesthesia. For instance, an individual is more susceptible to pulmonary complications after the use of general anesthesia. The type of surgery and the methods used in the sterilization procedure influence the complications seen.

Vasectomy clients may experience epididymitis and sperm granulomas. The former, treated with scrotal support and heat, generally resolves within 7 days. The latter typically resolves on its own (Hatcher et al., 1994).

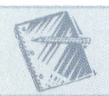 *Client Teaching*

Sterilization

Client teaching instructions relating to sterilization procedures are grouped into general postprocedure considerations and specific guidelines related to either a vasectomy or tubal ligation.

General Considerations:

- Rest for about two days before resuming normal activities.
- Avoid strenuous activity for about 1 week to prevent undue pressure to the excision area.
- Know the early danger signs associated with sterilization:
  - Bleeding from the incision site
  - Excessive pain
  - Dizziness with fainting
  - Temperature greater than 100.4°F
- Resume sexual intercourse between 3 and 7 days after the procedure. Call a health care professional if you experience discomfort once sexual activity is resumed.
- Take a mild analgesic, such as codeine or aspirin, for incision pain. Observe appropriate interval times for these medications to avoid oversedation or undersedation.

Teaching for a Client Experiencing a Vasectomy:

- Purchase and wear a good scrotal support continuously for the first 2 days. Apply an ice pack to the scrotum for at least 4 hours immediately after the procedure to lessen discomfort (Hatcher et al., 1994).
- Take a sponge bath, not a shower or tub bath, for the first 48 hours after the procedure. To promote comfort, take sitz baths for 48 hours after the procedure.
- Use another pregnancy prevention method for 4 to 6 weeks after the procedure since sterility is not achieved immediately.

Teaching for a Client Experiencing a Tubal Ligation:

- Sponge bathe for the first 48 hours after the procedure (Hatcher et al., 1994). Pat rather than rub the incision dry.
- Wear loose undergarments to avoid irritating the incision.
- If you were using other contraceptive methods before the procedure, no other preventive methods need to be taken after the procedure. However, if you were not using other methods, you need to use other pregnancy prevention measures after the procedure if intercourse has occurred within the 48 hours before the procedure or occurs within the first few days of the procedure.

Recent studies implicate vasectomy with an increased incidence of prostate cancer (Giovannucci, Ascherio, et al., 1993; Giovannucci, Tosteson, et al., 1993). The risk appears highest in those men who have had a vasectomy for more than 20 years. In another study, however, age at which the vasectomy was performed was found to be a more significant risk factor than length since vasectomy (Hayes et al., 1993). Given that the etiology of prostate cancer is poorly understood, the specific reason for the increased incidence of prostate cancer remains unclear.

Women undergoing sterilization occasionally experience a change in menstrual patterns. This is thought to be due to the change in pregnancy prevention method rather than to the procedure itself: frequently, an intrauterine device is removed or an oral contraceptive is stopped shortly before the procedure. Consequently, increased menstrual flow could be attributed to these factors rather than to the sterilization procedure itself. One study indicated that up to 5 years may elapse before these changes are evident (Wilcox, Martinez-Schnell, Peterson, Ware, & Hughes, 1992). Sterilization does *not* protect against STDs.

Occasionally, both men and women may wish to reverse the sterilization procedure. For either sex, reversal success is dependent on the initial surgical procedure (Hatcher et al., 1994); that is, such factors as the amount of tube (vas or fallopian) removed and the use of coagulation as the ligation method influence the success of the reversal procedure. Although sperm will be found in the ejaculate of 81 to 98% of men undergoing a vasectomy reversal procedure, members of both sexes should consider sterilization permanent (Hatcher et al., 1994).

Teaching

Information about the sterilization procedure is given to the client before the procedure and again before the client goes home.

► Progestin Implants (Norplant System)

Effectiveness and Action

The Norplant system, which provides levonorgestrel, is a very effective pregnancy prevention method with a less than 1% annual failure rate. The cumulative pregnancy rate is 3.7% for the 5-year period (Hatcher et al., 1994). Because the pregnancy rate increases significantly after 5 years, this system requires replacement (Kaunitz & Jordan, 1997). An attractive feature of the implants is the resulting lower serum level of levonorgestrel in comparison to oral agents. This effect is accomplished by means of the continuous delivery system of the six Silastic tubes (Fig. 8–5). Norplant's contraceptive action, effective within 24 hours of insertion, is thought to be similar to that of the progestin-only pill. The cervical mucus thickens,

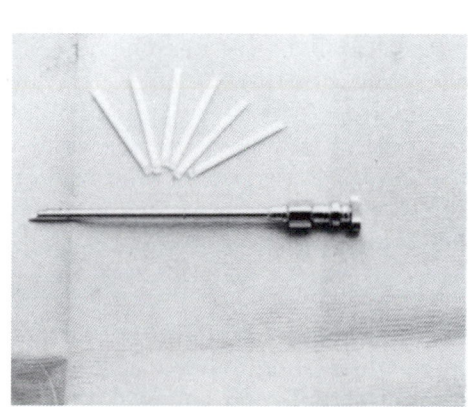

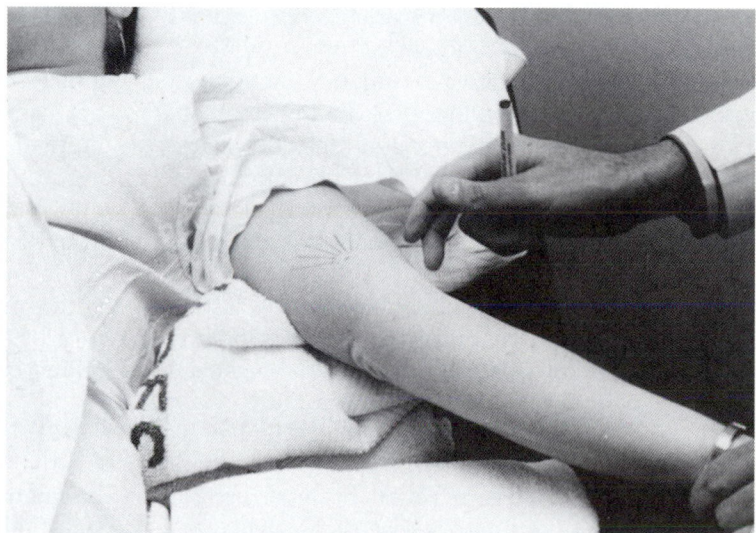

A   **B**

FIGURE 8–5. Norplant System (levonorgestrel implants), a reversible, 5-year-progestin-only contraceptive. **A.** Silastic tubes. **B.** Outline of insertion on the medial aspect of the arm. *(Reproduced, with permission, from Lemcke, D.P., Pattison, J., Marshall, L.A., & Crowley, D.S. (1995).* Primary care of women. *Norwalk, CT: Appleton & Lange, p. 489.)*

which interferes with sperm access, the endometrial surface changes, and the luteinizing hormone (LH) surge needed for ovulation is inhibited (Kaunitz & Jordan, 1997). The pregnancy prevention effectiveness is influenced by weight, with those weighing more than 70 kg having a greater chance of becoming pregnant. However, amount of risk is associated with type of implant. Hard capsules have a 5-year failure rate of 9.3% while soft capsules have a failure rate of 2.4% (Hatcher et al., 1994).

Informed Consent

As with any form of pregnancy prevention, the client should be well informed about the benefits, risks, and side effects of Norplant. In addition, the insertion of the implants is a minor surgical procedure. Therefore, the health care provider should obtain written informed consent in which the effects of the implants are explained prior to the procedure. Having the client retain a copy helps reinforce the information.

The Norplant system has become a target for personal injury lawyers who contend that the silicone content of the tubes has caused disease; to date, no cause and effect relationship has been proven by scientific research (Cunningham et al., 1997). However, lawsuits and perception of problems have been decreasing use of this method. Given the class action suits filed in 1994 (Kalmuss, Davidson, Cushman, Heartwell, & Rutling, 1996; Klitsch, 1995), informed consent becomes even more critical in terms of potential problems with removal.

Benefits

One of the most attractive characteristics of Norplant is its reversibility. A one-time procedure provides a continuous, safe, and effective pregnancy prevention method independent of intercourse (Hatcher et al., 1994). Because Norplant is estrogen free, the client should not experience such side effects as nausea and breakthrough bleeding. Unlike oral contraceptives, Norplant produces no daily hormone surge (Hatcher et al., 1994).

Several noncontraceptive benefits may be associated with the use of Norplant implants. These include "scanty menses or no menses; decreased menstrual cramps and pain; and suppressed ovulatory pain (mittelschmerz)" (Hatcher et al., 1994, p. 292). The risk of endometrial and ovarian cancer is also decreased. Women with implants seem to be at less risk for developing pelvic inflammatory disease as well.

Risks and Contraindications

Menstrual changes, particularly during the first year, are very common (Hatcher et al., 1994). In fact, alter-

Women's Health

Due to the estrogen-free composition of Norplant, these implants are an option for those clients for whom estrogen-containing pregnancy prevention methods are contraindicated (for example, clients with a history of thrombophlebitis or thromboembolic disorder, cerebrovascular accident, or coronary artery disease).

ations in menstruation are experienced by approximately 75% of users during the first year (Kalmuss et al., 1996). These changes vary in nature, ranging from the absence of menses to bleeding that is irregular and extended. Headache is reported to be the second most common side effect and a frequent reason offered for discontinuing the implants (Kalmuss et al., 1996). These side effects may disappear as the hormonal (levonorgestrel) level reaches its maintenance level. Weight gain has also been associated with Norplant. In addition, increased incidences of bilateral breast tenderness and acne have been reported in Norplant users. Norplant users are not at increased risk of ectopic pregnancy. Women who have a history of heart attacks, are predisposed to developing subacute bacterial endocarditis, suffer from migraines, or who, because of personal or religious beliefs, do not tolerate irregular bleeding are not considered to be good candidates for Norplant. Women who have had a pulmonary embolus, are taking antiseizure medications such as phenytoin, have unexplained uterine bleeding, or are pregnant are also discouraged from choosing Norplant implants (Hatcher et al., 1994). Lastly, Norplant should be used with great caution in those women who have a history of allergies or whose acne became worse when taking combined pills.

Teaching

Clients considering Norplant as their method of pregnancy prevention should have a clear understanding of the insertion and removal process. In addition, ensuring that clients receive intensive education about possible side effects, particularly menstrual cycle changes, can contribute to client satisfaction with the method (Hatcher et al., 1994). Clients should be instructed to keep the insertion area clean and dry for several days after the procedure. Furthermore, they should report any of the following to their health care provider: signs of infection at the site (pus, pain); severe headaches that are repetitive, any migraine headaches, or blurred vision; delayed menstrual periods, abdominal pain, or heavy vaginal bleeding.

Clients should be made aware that health care providers need special education for insertion and removal of the implants. This specialized knowledge may limit client accessibility, particularly in more remote areas. The client should give this fact consideration in the event that educated personnel may not be available for either insertion or removal.

Insertion does involve a small incision. Some clients may be concerned that they will experience pain during the procedure. Hatcher and colleagues (1994) offer several suggestions to assist with the removal of the capsules. These include using more (6–8 mL vs 3 mL) of local anesthetic, creating a larger incision (1 cm vs 4 mm), and positioning the client for comfort. This information should be shared with prospective clients.

Clients should be made aware that the implants must be replaced in 5 years, as effectiveness decreases after this time. They should be informed that the implants do *not* provide protection against most STDs. Consequently, clients at risk should be counseled to use barrier methods as well.

▶ Injectable Progestogen (Depo-Provera, Noristerat)

Effectiveness and Action

Both medroxyprogesterone acetate (Depo-Provera), sometimes called depomedroxyprogesterone (DMPA), and norethindrone exanthane (Noristerat, or NET) are highly effective pregnancy prevention agents, with typical failure rates of 0.3 and 0.4%, respectively. Both are long-acting progestins administered intramuscularly. Because DMPA was approved as a pregnancy prevention option in June 1992, a more detailed discussion of that drug follows. The most effective time to administer DMPA is within 5 days of beginning menses (Kaunitz & Jordan, 1997). The appropriate dose is 150 mg, given every 3 months (Hatcher et al., 1994; Kaunitz & Jordan, 1997). DMPA's ultimate result is suppression of graafian follicle development. Because of the prolonged effect of DMPA, women have a "grace period" of about 2 weeks should they be late for another injection (Hatcher et al., 1994; Kaunitz & Jordan, 1997).

Informed Consent

A client's choice of a pregnancy prevention method should always be based on the most comprehensive information available for all options. Consequently, the health care provider should make every effort to ensure that the client is aware of the benefits, side effects, and contraindications for DMPA. One way to involve the client in the exchange of information is via a written informed consent. Such a strategy provides the client with the opportunity to reflect on the choice and to identify any concerns. Giving the client a copy of the informed consent provides a concrete reference point for both client and provider.

Benefits

DMPA's efficacy is well recognized, especially for those women for whom other methods are not acceptable (Westfall, Main & Barnard, 1996). Like Norplant, DMPA is another option not associated with sexual intercourse, thereby enhancing a woman's flexibility and increasing her privacy (Hatcher et al., 1994). The discomforts associated with menstruation may be decreased or alleviated resulting from alterations in the menstrual flow. Amenorrhea has been reported in more than half of the women who use it for 1 year. Because menstrual flow is decreased, anemia may be lessened. The risk of endometrial cancer is significantly lowered in DMPA users. Both seizure frequency and incidence of sickle-cell anemia crisis are reported decreased in those women who are amenorrheic (Archer et al., 1997).

Risks and Contraindications

Amenorrhea, desirable by some clients, may be considered such a serious side effect that other clients will discontinue DMPA. Sangi-Haghpeykar and colleagues (1996) report bleeding patterns as one of the major reasons to discontinue the drug, a finding supported by Westfall, Main, and Barnard (1996). If this should be the case, a client may wish to use NET, as less amenorrhea is associated with it. A client could also experience abdominal bloating, headaches, dizziness, weight gain (1–3 kg), and, possibly, mood changes. Although fertility may take up to a year to return, studies indicate that DMPA does not lead to long-term infertility (Hatcher et al., 1994). Breast cancer risks are similar to those associated with oral contraceptive use. Data indicate that women who become estrogen deficient consequent to DMPA may suffer from osteoporosis. However, when the drug is discontinued, bone density increases (Archer et al., 1997). Nonetheless, caution should be exercised.

Teaching

As DMPA does *not* protect against the AIDS virus, clients should be instructed to continue use of other barrier methods. In addition, clients need to use another method for 2 weeks after receiving the injection. A schedule of return visits that takes into account client needs as well as the 3-month time limit can be established at the time of the first injection. Clients should receive extensive instruction regarding the changes in menstrual pattern. Clients should also be encouraged to seek medical advice when concerned about the changes. Other suggestions for seeking medical help include the occurrence of headaches, depression, heavy bleeding, or weight gain (Hatcher et al., 1994).

▶ Intrauterine Devices

Effectiveness and Action

Of the methods currently used to prevent pregnancy, the intrauterine device (IUD) ranks fifth in effectiveness (see Table 8–4). Progestasert users have an expected pregnancy rate of 2.0%, and the rate for ParaGard T380A users is 0.8%. One factor influencing these rates is age: the older the client, the lower the expected pregnancy rate.

Intrauterine devices (small metal or plastic forms that are placed in the uterus to prevent implantation of a fertilized ovum) are thought to exert their pregnancy-preventive action in one of two ways: movement of the ovum through the fallopian tubes is accelerated and sperm migration is impeded (Hatcher et al., 1994).

Two IUDs are currently available: Progestasert and ParaGard, Model T380A, or CuT 380A (Pasquale, 1996) (see Fig. 8–6). Progestasert releases progesterone into the uterine cavity from a storage area on the device. The increased levels of progesterone alter the uterine environment. Should fertilization occur, implantation is prevented. Because the Progestasert device has a monofilamented tail, the incidence of infection is decreased. Progestasert needs to be replaced after 1 year: this is a positive attribute because an opportunity is provided for the health care provider to reassess the client and to perform an annual breast examination and Pap smear.

The other IUD currently available is the ParaGard, or CuT 380A or Model T380A. This IUD is the more effective device to date, with "a first year efficacy rate greater than 99 percent" (Westhoff, 1996b, p. S22). This T-shaped device has copper wire wrapped around its stem and copper collars on its horizontal arms. It, too, has a monofilamented tail. The exact mechanism of action is not currently known. It is, however, thought

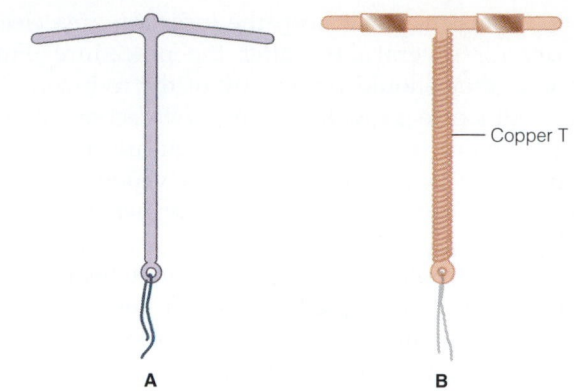

FIGURE 8–6. Intrauterine devices. **A.** Progestasert. **B.** ParaGard, Model T380A, or CuT 380A. *(Adapted, with permission, from DeCherney, A.H., & Pernoll, M.L. (1994). Current obstetric & gynecological diagnosis & treatment (8th ed.). Norwalk, CT: Appleton & Lange, p. 679.)*

that copper inhibits migration of sperm, thus preventing fertilization (Westhoff, 1996). Unlike Progestasert, ParaGard can remain in place for 10 years before being replaced. Good preventive health habits should be fostered in clients with this IUD. These habits include continuing to have an annual cervical cytology screening and breast examinations.

Informed Consent

The IUD, particularly the Dalkon shield, received much negative publicity during the 1980s. Many women who used this device developed serious pelvic infections. The Dalkon shield was implicated in 10 to 15 deaths. The design of the Dalkon shield enhanced bacterial entry into the uterus. Its tail consisted of hundreds of fibers encased in a sheath. The fibers were thereby isolated from the cervical mucus, which destroys bacteria, and organisms had direct access to the uterus and fallopian tubes. As a result of litigation, production of the Dalkon shield and three other devices was discontinued (Westhoff, 1996a). The FDA, however, never withdrew its approval for use of the IUD.

Current manufacturers are very aware of the legal history of the IUD. Progestasert manufacturers have brochures available that explain in detail the mechanisms of action and the effectiveness of their product. Side effects, risk factors, and warning signs are also described (Westhoff, 1996a). Both physician and client are encouraged to sign it. Each section is to be initialed by the client (Westhoff, 1996a).

ParaGard manufacturers have developed a similar pamphlet. The client's initials are required after each major section of the document (12 in all). In addition, both client's and physician's signatures are required at the end of the document. Information within the document is comprehensive.

Benefits

The major benefit of the IUD is that compliance is not an issue. In fact the highest continuation rates for a pregnancy prevention method are associated with IUD users (Pasquale, 1996; Westhoff, 1996a). Use of an IUD also appears to decrease a woman's risk for endometrial and cervical cancer (Rosenblatt et al., 1996; Westhoff, 1996a). Furthermore, copper IUDs seem to offer a better protection against endometrial cancer (Rosenblatt et al., 1996). Candidates for the IUD are those women who are in a monogamous relationship, have had at least one child, and are free of any pelvic inflammatory disease (Pasquale, 1996).

Risks and Contraindications

The incidence of pelvic inflammatory disease increases when the IUD is used, particularly within the initial 4-month period following insertion (Burkman, 1996; Pasquale, 1996). Pelvic inflammatory disease that occurs after this time is associated with sexually transmitted pathogens (Burkman, 1996). Consequently, careful aseptic technique should be used to decrease the introduction of bacteria during insertion of the IUD (Burkman, 1996). The risk of pelvic inflammatory disease is increased in nulliparous women, in those having multiple sexual partners, and in those having frequent intercourse (Westhoff, 1996). The incidence of tubal infertility among nulliparous women has been suggested to be approximately twice that of nonusers. No change in fertility rates, however, has been reported in the literature (Pasquale, 1996).

Uterine perforation has been associated with the IUD. This risk is rare, with an occurrence of 1 in 1000 to 1 in 5000 insertions (Pasquale, 1996). Its occurrence is confirmed by ultrasound or x-ray.

One of the more common problems is a tendency for increased uterine cramping. This discomfort is influenced by the shape and size of the IUD as well as the obstetric history and physical status of the uterus. Increased bleeding is also associated with an IUD in place. Alterations in bleeding may be manifested by increased amount of bleeding, increased number of menstrual days, and intermittent spotting. This increased blood loss may also result in a decrease in hematocrit, overtly demonstrated by weakness and pallor (Hatcher et al., 1994). Spontaneous expulsion of the IUD occurs in 5 to 6% of users within the first year. Symptoms range from cramping

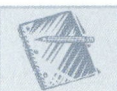

Client Teaching

Use of an Intrauterine Device

The following instructions should be discussed with the client before use of an IUD:

- Learn how your IUD works and what side effects may occur. Read the package insert before using the IUD.
- You should be able to feel the IUD string in your vagina after the device is inserted. First, however, before it is inserted, feel the back of your vagina to familiarize yourself with the area; this preparation will make it easier for you to find the IUD string after the IUD has been inserted.
- You need to check the string frequently during the first few months after IUD insertion. During that period, take special care to check the string before having sexual intercourse.
- Use a second contraceptive method during the first few months after the IUD is inserted.
- Check the string's placement after each of your periods.
- If unusual cramping occurs during your period, check the string's placement.
- The IUD may be expelled without your being aware of it. Because this tends to occur during menses, make it a habit to check tampons or pads for evidence that the device was expelled.
- Know the danger signs associated with IUD use:
  - Abnormal spotting, bleeding or discharge (discharge could signal infection)
  - Abdominal pain or pain during intercourse
  - Fever, chills, or generally not feeling well
  - String missing or shorter or longer than usual
  - A late period (could signal pregnancy)

to actually feeling the device in the vagina (Hatcher et al., 1994).

Contraindications to the use of the IUD as a pregnancy prevention option include suspected or known pregnancy, presence of an acute pelvic infection or a history of pelvic inflammatory disease, presence of uterine anomalies, and suspected or known malignancies. Women who have a history of pelvic inflammatory disease, who have multiple sexual partners, who have never had a child, and who are younger than 25 should be offered another pregnancy prevention option rather than the IUD (Pasquale, 1996).

Should pregnancy occur with an IUD in place and removal does not occur, there is a 50% chance of spontaneously aborting the fetus. The risk is lower if the device is removed. The risk of ectopic pregnancy is increased 6 to 10 times when Progestasert is used (Hatcher et al., 1994).

Teaching

Clients choosing IUDs as their pregnancy prevention method need to be informed about the associated risks and about how to check for the continued presence of the IUD. Furthermore, clients need to be comfortable touching their genitalia, as assessment of IUD placement is their responsibility. Nutritional habits should be assessed and plans identified to increase daily iron intake. It may be necessary to review basic nutritional information with the client. Should iron be prescribed, methods of counteracting some of the side effects should be addressed. Clients also must understand that an IUD does not protect against STDs.

▶ Oral Contraception

Combined Oral Contraceptive Agents

Effectiveness and Action. **Oral contraceptive** pills are among the most effective methods of reversible pregnancy prevention (Potter, Oakley, deLeon-Wong, & Canamar, 1996). Combined oral contraceptive agents have a lowest expected failure rate of 0.1%, comparable to that of male sterilization. Typical failure rate, however, is 3% and is attributed to high rate of discontinuation by users for nonmedical reasons (Hatcher et al., 1994). In other words, pregnancy may result because an individual stopped taking the oral contraceptive because of inconvenience or expense, not because it was not exerting its pregnancy prevention action.

Combined oral contraceptive agents are preparations containing both an estrogen and a progestin. These hormonal preparations exert their pregnancy preventive effects by:

1. Suppressing hormonal reproduction in the hypothalamus and the anterior pituitary, resulting in the inhibition of ovulation (Hatcher et al., 1994)

2. Altering the endometrial surface so that it is unfavorable for implantation
3. Altering peristalsis and secretions within the fallopian tubes, thereby interfering with sperm, ovum, and gamete movement
4. Accelerating the degeneration of the corpus luteum, removing the source of needed hormones for the continuation of pregnancy
5. Changing the consistency of cervical mucus, creating a hostile environment

Many preparations are currently available in the United States: the difference among products is in the amounts of estrogen and progestin. The pills are available in either 21-day or 28-day packages. Because risks associated with oral contraceptive agents increase as hormonal concentrations increase the amount of estrogen in most preparations is 35 μg or less (Baird & Glasier, 1993).

Efforts continue to be directed toward the development of oral contraceptives pills that have low amounts of estrogen and progestogen. Currently there are two new progestin preparations available in the United States (desogesterol and norgestimate), although another (gestodene) is available in Europe. One of the new preparations, composed of 150 μg of desogestrel (a new progestin) and 20 g of ethinyl estradiol (estrogen), is reported to be very effective in preventing pregnancy (Reifsnider, 1997). These newer preparations are called the "third generation" of contraceptive pills because they contain lower doses of both estrogen (<30 μg) and progestogen. Second generation pills contained less than 50 μg of ethinyl estradiol. First generation pills contained more than 50 μg of ethinyl estradiol. Thromboembolic events have been reported to be more frequent in women using the third generation pills (Spitzer et al., 1996), although Suissa and colleagues (1997) did not find this when pills were prescribed to first-time pill users, even when the progestin was desogestrel, which has been reported to have the highest incidence of thromboembolic events (Reifsnider, 1997). Schwartz and associates (1997) obtained similar findings and stated "reduction in the estrogen content of oral contraceptives has greatly enhanced the cerebrovascular safety of these commonly prescribed medications" (p. 602). Interestingly, third-generation pill users are not at increased risk of myocardial infarction when they were compared to second-generation pill users (Lewis et al., 1996, 1997). Thus, health care providers need to carefully screen clients in terms of risk and consider using a preparation containing norgestimate, which has the lowest rate of thromboembolic events associated with it (Reifsnider, 1997). Examples of third-generation oral contraceptives include Desogen, Ortho-Cept, and Ortho-Cyclen (Gallagher & Fuller, 1997).

Informed Consent. Figure 8–7 presents one institution's efforts to provide comprehensive information to clients and to document that they received the information. Having a client sign the consent form reinforces the seriousness of the decision.

The client choosing an oral contraceptive should know the early signs of potential problems. The health care provider is encouraged to assess the client's level of understanding of the written and

---

ORAL CONTRACEPTIVE CONSENT FORM

I agree that I am receiving birth control Pills of my own free will. Pills are the method of family planning which I have chosen from all the methods that have been explained to me. The advantages and disadvantages of the other methods of birth control have been explained to me.

BENEFITS: I am aware that oral contraceptives are *not* guaranteed to be 100% effective. It is my understanding that combined birth control Pills can be 99% effective if I take them exactly according to instructions. I understand that progestin-only Pills (Minipills) are slightly less effective even if I follow the instructions. I understand that some women experience the following *benefits* from using birth control Pills:

- Decreased menstrual cramps
- Decreased menstrual bleeding
- More regular menstrual bleeding
- Decreased pain at the same time of ovulation
- Less risk of acute gonococcal pelvic inflammatory disease (gonorrhea infection in the tubes)
- Improvement in acne
- Less risk of cancer of the uterus or ovary
- Less risk of benign breast tumors and/or ovarian cysts

RISKS: I have been told to watch out for the following danger signals and return to the clinic or make contact with my clinician at once if I develop one of these problems. These could be warnings of serious or even life-threatening illness.

EARLY DANGER SIGNS

caution

A ■ Abdominal pain (severe)
C ■ Chest pain (severe), cough, shortness of breath
H ■ Headache (severe), dizziness, weakness, or numbness
E ■ Eye problems (vision loss or blurring), speech problems
S ■ Severe leg pain (calf or thigh)

See your clinician if you have any of these problems, or if you develop depression, yellow jaundice or a breast lump.

I am aware that while using oral contraceptives, I could have the following side effects, many of which can be temporary:

Major problems		*Minor problems*	
•	Blood clot of the leg or the lung	•	Nausea
•	Stroke or heart attack	•	Spotting between periods
•	Gallbladder disease	•	Less menstrual bleeding
•	One type of liver tumor	•	Breast tenderness
•	Death	•	Weight gain
		•	Headache
		•	Depression
		•	High blood pressure
		•	Splotchy darkening of the skin on my face
		•	Worsening of acne
		•	Infections in the vagina

I have been told that most of the serious problems in Pill users happen to women over 30 who are heavy smokers (15 or more cigarettes a day).

STOPPING PILLS: I have been told that I may stop using the Pills *at any time*. I have been told I should use another means of birth control until I have had three regular periods before attempting to become pregnant. I have also been informed that if my periods were very irregular, very heavy, and/or very painful before taking Pills, they may return to this pattern when I stop taking Pills.

INSTRUCTIONS for the use of birth control Pills have been given to me in writing and I have been given a patient package insert for my specific brand of Pill.

QUESTIONS: I have been given the chance to ask questions about all forms of birth control and about the Pill in particular. My questions have been answered to my satisfaction.

_____
Signature

FIGURE 8–7. Informed consent form for oral contraceptive counseling. *(Reproduced, with permission, from Hatcher, R.A. et al. (1988). Contraceptive technology, 1988–1989, (14th ed.). New York: Irvington.)*

verbal information presented. Appropriate changes in the level of instruction should be made to ensure a client's understanding of the results of her decision.

Benefits. Many noncontraceptive benefits are associated with oral contraceptives. Women experience a decrease in amount and length of menstrual flow, a lessening of menstrual cramps, and a greater regularity of menstrual cycles. Because of the decrease in menstrual flow, pill users are less susceptible to iron-deficiency anemia (Hatcher et al., 1994). Although the mechanisms are not fully known, oral contraceptives do offer the user protection against pelvic inflammatory disease (Hatcher et al., 1994). No evidence, however, has been found to indicate that there is the same protection against HIV. In addition, evidence indicates that chlamydial growth is enhanced by oral contraceptives. A client who is exposed to multiple sexual partners should be encouraged to use a second method that more effectively prevents infection, such as a condom with spermicide or diaphragm.

There is evidence that oral contraceptives exert a protective action against both endometrial and ovarian cancers (Hatcher et al., 1994). Recent data, however, indicate that women who use oral contraceptives are at increased risk for the development of adenomatous cervical carcinomas (Thomas et al., 1996). However, a cause-effect relationship is hard to prove. Women who choose oral contraceptives alone do not have any benefits of barrier or spermicidal protection from the human papillomavirus. They may also have cytologic screening more often for cervical cancer, thus leading to greater detection (Cunningham et al., 1997).

Other conditions that appear to benefit from oral contraceptive administration include endometriosis and fibrocystic breast disease. Both are diminished. Oral contraceptives also affect bone density in a manner similar to estrogen replacement thereby preventing osteoporosis (Hatcher et al., 1994).

Risks and Contraindications. Oral contraceptives have been associated with an increased incidence of cardiovascular complications, specifically stroke, hypertension, clot formation, and heart attack (Hatcher et al., 1994). Current literature, however, implicates the concentration of hormones in combination oral contraceptive agents; that is, the risk is lower for medium- and low-fixed-dose preparations (Schwartz et al., 1997). Furthermore, according to Hatcher and colleagues (1994), the occurrence of cardiovascular risks has been demonstrated in a select group of women:

- Women who smoke, are overweight, and do not exercise
- Women who are older than 50
- Women who have other health problems such as hypertension, diabetes, and heart or vascular disease
- Women who have a family history of diabetes or a heart attack in a person under the age of 50, particularly heart attack in a female family member.
- Women who have an elevated cholesterol level or a high LDL/HDL cholesterol ratio

On the other hand, recent studies indicate that healthy, nonsmoking women over 35 are at no greater risk of serious cardiovascular disease when taking oral contraceptive preparations containing less than 50 µg of estrogen (Hatcher et al., 1994). Although oral contraceptive pills alter lipid metabolism, the major cardiovascular risks are associated not with atherosclerosis but with thrombus formation (Spitzer et al., 1996). Counseling with regard to signs and symptoms of clot formation is important.

Oral contraceptives exert both negative and positive effects on lipid metabolism, a noteworthy characteristic given our society's preoccupation with cholesterol levels and efforts to lower them. Estrogenic effects are that HDL and HDL_2 increase, LDL decreases, and triglycerides increase (Baird & Glasier, 1993). Opposite effects are true for progestin; that is, they tend to decrease HDL and HDL_2, increase LDL, and decrease triglycerides (Baird & Glasier, 1993). Third-generation pills tend to increase HDL and triglycerides and may offer some protective cardiovascular benefits (Crook, 1997). Consequently, a lipoprotein profile consisting of total cholesterol, HDL-cholesterol, and total triglycerides may be obtained before beginning either oral contraceptives or hormone replacement therapy.

The association between oral contraceptive use and breast cancer has been under investigation for many years; it is unclear whether oral contraceptives are related to its development (Cunningham et al., 1997). Currently, for women who presently take combined oral contraceptives or who stopped taking them within the past 10 years, data indicate that these women are at a small increased relative risk of having breast cancer diagnosed (Collaborative Group on Hormonal Factors in Breast Cancer, 1996). There does not appear to be an increased risk for those women who stopped taking combined oral contraceptives more than 10 years ago. Furthermore, women who used oral contraceptives and are diagnosed with breast cancer have cancers that are not as clinically advanced as the cancers in those women

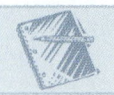

Client Teaching

Combined Oral Contraceptives

The following instructions should be discussed with the client before use of combined oral contraceptives:

- The oral contraceptive may be initiated in different ways; therefore, follow the instruction given by your health care provider.
- Take the oral contraceptive at a similar time each day, thereby establishing a pattern of administration.
- Read the package insert before you begin taking the oral contraceptive.
- If you experience bleeding between periods, it may be alleviated by taking the oral contraceptive at the same time every day.
- Some drugs, such as phenytoin (Dilantin), interfere with the protection afforded by the oral contraceptive. You may need to use a second method along with the pill.
- Check your pill package each day as a way to avoid overlooking a "missed" dose.
- When you miss taking a pill, take it as soon as you remember. Similarly, if you miss two pills, take them as soon as you realize the omission, then take two pills the following day.
- If you miss one or two pills, use an additional contraceptive method for the next 7 days.
- Be very familiar with an alternative form of contraception.
- Know the early danger signs associated with oral contraceptive use:
  - Severe calf or thigh pain
  - Abdominal pain
  - Chest pain, cough, or shortness of breath
  - Severe headache, dizziness, weakness, or numbness
  - Loss of vision or blurring
  - Speech problems

does not seem to influence risk. The possibility that race plays a role in risk status has been noted with older African-American and other non-white women demonstrating a potentially stronger response to the effects of contraceptives (Brinton et al., 1997). However, long-term results of studies of the newer low-dose oral contraceptives are not yet available; the high overall incidence of breast cancer (1 in 9 women) also makes finding a small increased risk difficult (Cunningham et al., 1997).

The relationship between oral contraceptives and liver cancer remains unclear (Hatcher et al., 1994; Waetjen & Grimes, 1996). Women who used contraceptives with more than 50 μg of estrogen do, however, have a slight risk of liver disease (Hannaford, Kay, Vessey, Painter, & Mant, 1997). Conflicting data exist regarding the relationship between oral contraceptives and skin cancer.

Minor risks associated with oral contraceptives include the development of oily skin or acne, absence of menses, midcycle spotting or breakthrough bleeding, breast discomfort or fullness, and possibly depression. Women may also experience persistent nausea, morning sickness, or a weight gain.

Contraindications to combined oral contraceptives vary. Table 8–5 lists precautions in the use of this contraceptive method.

Teaching. Teaching about benefits and risks should be reinforced; the fact that no protection is provided against HIV should be stressed. Information about the pill's action should be reinforced and the method of taking the pill clearly explained (21-day versus 28-day preparations). Measures should be taught that facilitate adherence to the regimen, for example, taking the pill before going to bed or on rising.

Progestogen-Only Contraceptive Agent

Effectiveness and Action. The progestins found in the progestin-only pill (**minipill**) are the same as those found in combined oral contraceptives, except that they are present in smaller doses. Minipills contain 0.5 mg or less of a progestin used daily (Cunningham et al., 1997). They are an effective pregnancy prevention option with a lowest expected failure rate of 0.5%. Progestin-only pills exert their effect by altering the endometrial surface of the uterus as well as the consistency of cervical mucus.

The minipill is an alternative hormonal agent for those women who have a history of mild hypertension or headaches or who have experienced some of the less pleasant effects of combined oral contraceptive pills (morning sickness, persistent nausea, weight gain).

who did not take contraceptives. Age at which contraceptive use began may influence risk of breast cancer: beginning use before age 20 is associated with a higher risk than is beginning use at a later age. Type of estrogen or progestogen preparation

▶ **TABLE 8–5**

Precautions in the Provision of Combined Oral Contraceptives

Refrain from providing combined oral contraceptives for women with the following diagnoses:

Precautions	Rationale/Discussion
Thrombophlebitis or thromboembolic disorder or a history thereof	Estrogens promote blood clotting, therefore, women with other risk factors for excess blood clotting are at risk for future blood clotting problems with oral contraceptives. However, thromboembolic events related to known trauma or an intravenous needle are not necessarily a reason to avoid use of pills.
Cerebrovascular accident or a history thereof	Estrogens promote blood clotting. Women with other risk factors for excess blood clotting are at risk for future blood clotting problems with oral contraceptives.
Coronary artery or ischemic heart disease or a history thereof	Women with angina, heart attacks, or congestive heart failure may have valvular heart disease, coronary artery disease, kidney failure, or other serious disease. These women are at high risk for fatal complications during pregnancy and should strongly consider voluntary surgical contraception, or a reliable progestin-only method like Norplant or injectables. If these are not acceptable, the risks associated with low-dose oral contraceptives are almost certainly lower than the risks associated with pregnancy.
Known or strongly suspected breast cancer or a history of breast cancer	In theory, the hormones in oral contraceptives might cause some lumps to grow. Some clinicians and some clinical protocols suggest that women found to have a breast mass should not be provided combined oral contraceptives until cancer of the breast has been ruled out. Other clinicians are comfortable prescribing pills while the cause of the breast mass is being evaluated. Lumps which are suspicious should be evaluated.
Known or strongly suspected estrogen-dependent neoplasia or a history thereof	It is generally accepted that exogenous estrogens should not be provided to women with cancer of the reproductive organs. Estrogens may stimulate the growth of some cancers of the reproductive organs.
Pregnancy or pregnancy quite strongly suspected	Pregnancy would not be strongly suspected in a woman who had taken her last cycle of pills on schedule and has gone through 21 active pills and her 7 placebo pills without bleeding. In this instance the next package of pills should be started on schedule.
	Current data do NOT show that hormonal contraceptives taken during pregnancy cause any significant risk of birth defects because the doses are so low. However, since exposing the fetus to any medication could in theory cause birth defects, hormonal contraceptives should not be given to pregnant women. Ideally, women who have missed pills should be tested for pregnancy before continuing their cycles.
Benign hepatic adenoma or liver cancer or a history thereof	Progestins and estrogens affect the general functioning of the liver and should not be used during acute hepatitis. Use of oral contraceptives is associated with a higher risk of a rare benign liver tumor (hepatocellular adenoma). However, recent studies in the developing world by WHO found no evidence that combined oral contraceptives use causes liver cancer.
Markedly impaired liver function at present time	Progestins and estrogens affect the general functioning of the liver and should not be used during acute hepatitis. Some clinicians suggest that combined pills should not be used in clients with hepatitis until liver function tests have returned to normal.

▶   **TABLE 8-5** *(continued)*

Precautions in the Provision of Combined Oral Contraceptives

Exercise caution if combined oral contraceptives are used or considered in the following situations and carefullly monitor for adverse effects:

Precautions	Rationale/Discussion
Over 35 years old and currently a heavy smoker (15 or more cigarettes a day)	Cigarette smoking is the most important risk factor for vascular disease in women. Women over age 35 who smoke are at increased risk of heart attack, stroke, and other blood clotting problems. The mechanisms of this increased risk are not proven, but both estrogen and smoking increase the body's tendency to form blood clots. All smokers should be warned of this risk and all women should be advised to stop smoking.
Migraine headaches that start after initiation of oral contraceptives	Migraine headaches have been associated with an increased risk of stroke; however, some women report an improvement in their headaches with oral contraceptives.
Hypertension with resting diastolic blood pressure of 90 or greater or a resting systolic blood pressure of 140 or greater on three separate visits, or an accurate diastolic measurement of 110 or more on a single visit	A woman under 35 who is otherwise healthy and whose blood pressure is controlled by medication can elect to use oral contraception. For women who are over 35, the progestins and estrogens in combined oral contraceptives can slightly increase blood pressure. Women who have high blood pressure are already at increased risk for heart problems; using oral contraceptives can increase this risk.
Diabetes mellitus	Women with diabetes are at increased risk of heart disease and stroke, particularly if the woman smokes. Estrogens and progestins may slightly decrease glucose tolerance but this is unlikely to happen with low-dose oral contraceptives. Women with uncontrolled diabetes are also at high risk for poor pregnancy outcome, and need a very reliable contraceptive.
Elective major surgery or major surgery requiring immobilization planned in next 4 weeks	With the current low-dose pills, the problems associated with pill use and elective surgery have decreased.
Undiagnosed abnormal vaginal/uterine bleeding	Although oral contraceptives are often used to manage heavy bleeding, clinicians should be sure that the cause of the bleeding is known before prescribing oral contraceptives. The causes of irregular bleeding include: intrauterine and ectopic pregnancy, breast feeding, pelvic inflammatory disease, cancer of the reproductive tract, early or premenopause, hypo- or hyperthyroidism, and other gynecological problems.
Sickle cell disease or sickle C disease	Clients with sickle cell trait can use oral contraception. Progestins stabilize the red blood cell membrane. The risk of thrombosis in women with sickle cell disease or sickle C diseases is theoretical (and medical-legal).
Lactation	Estrogen very slightly decreases the quality and the quantity of breast milk, while progestins are galactogens, promoting breast milk production. Breastfeeding alone is an adequate contraceptive when the mother is still amenorrhic and not substituting other foods or liquids for breastfeeding meals. Thus, oral contraceptive use is only indicated when breastfeeding is no longer adequate, and when other methods are unacceptable. Some experts advise against combined pills entirely when other alternatives such as the minipill are available. If estrogen-containing contraceptives are the only available option, breastfeeding should be well established (at least 6 weeks' postpartum) before low-dose estrogen-containing pills are introduced.
Gestational diabetes	Low-dose formulations do not produce a diabetic glucose tolerance response in women with previous gestational diabetes, and there is no evidence that oral contraception increases the incidence of overt diabetes mellitus. It is believed that women with previous gestational diabetes can use oral contraception with annual assessment of the fasting glucose level.

(continued)

► **TABLE 8-5** *(continued)*

Precautions in the Provision of Combined Oral Contraceptives

Exercise caution if combined oral contraceptives are used or considered in the following situations and carefully monitor for adverse effects:

Precautions	Rationale/Discussion
Active gallbladder disease	Oral contraceptives may accelerate the development of gallbladder disease in women already susceptible to it. The mechanism is unclear, but it probably relates to effects of the pill on cholesterol metabolism.
Congenital hyperbilirubinemia (Gilbert's disease)	Women with this condition can be started on oral contraceptives but monitored carefully for jaundice hyperbilirubinema.
Over 50 years of age	Women over 50 are at increased risk for heart and cerebrovascular disease. Estrogens promote blood clotting. Women with other risk factors for blood clotting, particularly women age 35 or older, are at risk for future blood clotting problems with oral contraceptives. Women over 50 should consider using lower-dose estrogen replacement therapy.
Completion of term pregnancy within the past 10–14 days	When a woman starts oral contraceptives during the third postpartum week, she safely avoids the hypercoaguable state that occurs immediately after delivery (10–14 days).
Cardiac or renal disease or history thereof	These women are at high risk for fatal complications during pregnancy and should strongly consider voluntary surgical contraception, or a reliable progestin-only method like Norplant or injectables. If these are not acceptable, the risks associated with low-dose oral contraceptives are almost certainly lower than the risks associated with pregnancy.
Conditions likely to make it very difficult for a woman to take oral contraceptives consistently and correctly	Mental retardation, major psychiatric illness, alcoholism, or other chemical abuse, and/or a history of repeatedly taking oral contraception or other medications incorrectly, make compliance with taking oral contraceptives difficult.
Family history of hyperlipidemia	Hyperlipidemia increases a woman's risk for atherosclerotic heart disease.
Family history of death of a parent or sibling due to myocardial infarction before age 50	Myocardial infarction in a mother or sister is especially significant and indicates a need for lipid evaluation.

Source: Reproduced, with permission, from Hatcher, R.A. et al. (1994). Contraceptive technology (16th Rev. ed.). New York: Irvington.

Informed Consent. As with combined oral contraceptives, the client needs to be aware of the benefits and risks associated with progestin-only pills. After a thorough explanation, a consent form should be signed (see Fig. 8–7).

Benefits. Dysmenorrhea is lessened, but not to the extent achieved by use of combined oral contraceptives. Although two possible major benefits of combined oral contraceptives—protection against both endometrial cancer and pelvic inflammatory disease—are influenced by progestins, no data are currently available to suggest that similar protection exists when progestin-only contraceptive pills are taken (Hatcher et al., 1994). Both headaches and hypertension occur less frequently.

Progestin-only preparations do not affect lactation. Thus, they are an excellent pregnancy prevention option for a breastfeeding mother (Hatcher et al., 1994).

Recently, pills containing only norgestrel or levonorgestrel are recommended for women considering contraceptive implants. After 4–6 months of using this medication without problems, trying the implants is considered reasonable (Cunningham et al., 1997).

Risks and Contraindications. Irregular bleeding is more common with this form of contraceptive pill. The same absolute contraindications that apply to combined oral contraceptives are applicable to the progestin-only preparation (see Table 8–5). Should pregnancy occur, the likelihood of an ectopic pregnancy is greater when the minipill is taken.

Teaching. The information required about progestin-only pills is similar to that needed by clients using combined oral contraceptives. Often a woman who is starting oral contraceptive use is given a 3-month supply of pills. This procedure encourages the client to return to the health care facility to receive her additional prescription. In this manner health care providers can assess the client's possible side effects, level of knowledge, and use patterns of the oral contraceptive method.

▶ Condoms

Female Condom

The **female condom** (Fig. 8–8) is a polyurethane sheath with a flexible polyurethane ring at each end. The ring at the open edge remains outside the vagina and covers the labia. The ring at the closed end of the sheath fits under the symphysis like a diaphragm. In vitro tests have shown the condom impermeable to HIV, cytomegalovirus, and hepatitis B virus. The Reality female condom was approved by the FDA in May 1993 and is sold over the counter. It can be used only once. This fact, plus its cost, approximately $2.50/condom, are the main disadvantages (Reifsnider, 1997). The female condom has reported use–effectiveness rates of 79%. The method effectiveness rate increases to 95% when used for a year (Gollub, Stein, & el-Sadr, 1995). These investigators found that women liked the female condom because they felt protected, "they like the sensation (soft, natural, nondrying) of the device" (p. 156), and that they felt in control of their own protection, because they did not have to negotiate with their partner for protection. Past experience with male condoms, a woman's own attitudes about using male condoms, and her perception of her partner's fidelity can influence a woman's use of the female condom (Gil, 1995). Although not frequent, women have reported that they have had problems inserting the female condom, problems with the inner ring, and problems with keeping the condom in place during intercourse (Gollub, Stein, & el-Sadr, 1995).

Male Condom (without Spermicides)

Effectiveness and Action. The **male condom** (Fig. 8–9) is the most reversible form of male pregnancy prevention options, with the exception of coitus interruptus (Hatcher et al., 1994). Made of either latex rubber (basic or thin) or skin (processed collagen tissue) and placed over the erect penis, the condom is a barrier to the transmission of semen into the vagina. Condom production must adhere to stringent FDA standards (Hatcher et al., 1994).

Although the lowest expected failure rate is 2%, typical failure rate for the condom is 12%. Efficacy of this method appears to be inversely influ-

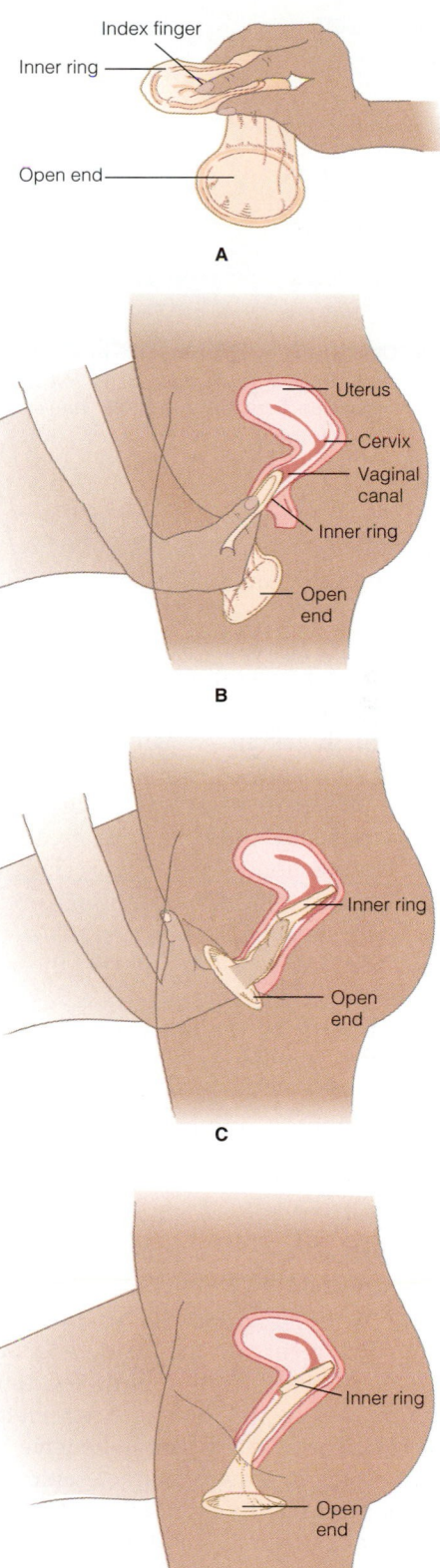

FIGURE 8–8. Reality female condom. Insertion and positioning. **A.** Inner ring is squeezed for insertion. **B.** Sheath is inserted similar to a tampon. **C.** Inner ring is pushed up as far as it can go with index finger. **D.** Reality condom in place. *(Courtesy of The Female Health Company.)*

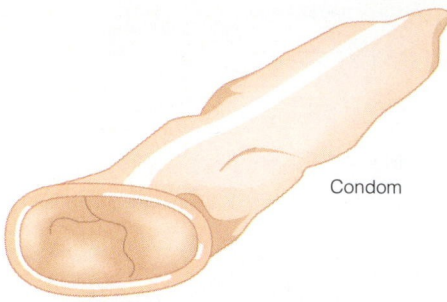

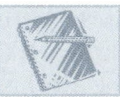
Condom

FIGURE 8–9. Unrolled male condom with reservoir tip. *(Reproduced, with permission, from Lichtman, R., & Papera, S. (1990). Gynecology: Well-woman care.* Norwalk, CT: Appleton & Lange, p. 80.)

reluctant to use it. Use of a thinner condom that is lubricated and textured may, however, enhance sensitivity.

Foreplay is interrupted during application of the condom, making condom use objectionable. Encouraging partner participation in the application of the condom may contribute to a more mutually positive experience. Finally, men in certain ethnic or cultural groups may reject the use of condoms. Generally, other options should be suggested for these couples.

enced by age: the younger the user, the higher the failure rate.

Benefits. A major benefit is the protection the condom affords in decreasing the chance of STDs and HIV (Anderson, Brackbill, & Mosher, 1996; Santelli, Davis, Celentano, Crump, & Burwell, 1995). Furthermore, it has been suggested that use of nonoxynol-9 with the condom may provide even greater, though not absolute, protection against HIV (Hatcher et al., 1994). Latex rather than skin condoms provide the best protection against STDs. However, such products may provide an effective alternative for those individuals who are latex sensitive.

Another benefit is the increased level of male participation in pregnancy prevention. Condoms may be the couple's primary preventive method or their backup method. Condom use can enhance sexual intimacy by involving both partners in its application.

Although length and width remain relatively constant, the client has a variety of options when choosing a condom. Condoms can be smooth or ribbed. They may be lubricated or not lubricated, have spermicidal agents on the inside and outside of the sheath, and be tapered. Some condoms have sperm reservoirs at the tip, others do not. Hatcher and colleagues (1994) present a comprehensive guide to condoms that considers these characteristics.

Condoms are readily accessible. They may be purchased over the counter in any pharmacy at very little cost. Furthermore, the client has a choice of quantity to purchase. The client may purchase one or many condoms.

Risks and Contraindications. Glans sensitivity is reduced by the condom. This fact makes many men

Client Teaching

Use of a Male Condom

The following instructions should be discussed with the client before use of a condom:

- Use a condom every time you have sexual intercourse.
- Put the condom on before the penis enters the vagina.
- To apply the condom, roll it over the erect penis to the base of the penis.
- Ensure that sufficient excess condom (about one-half inch) remains at the tip to collect semen.
- Spermicidal latex condoms or spermicidal foam offers additional protection against infection.
- For lubrication, use contraceptive foam, water, or K-Y jelly; do **not** use petroleum jelly, such as Vaseline.
- Your partner may help to apply the condom, as it can be a pleasurable experience for both of you.
- If possible, use another form of pregnancy prevention with the condom.
- When the penis is withdrawn from the vagina, hold the rim (top edge) of the condom to prevent semen from spilling.
- Check the condom for tears before throwing it away.
- Use a condom only once.

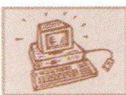

Research Abstract

Condom Use Among Divorced and Separated Women

This study investigated STD risk reducing behaviors, specifically condom use, using the Interaction Model of Client Health Behavior (IMCHB) in a convenience sample of 254 white, middle class, mostly educated women who ranged from 20 to 49 years. Data were collected via questionnaires distributed by a variety of professionals to clients known to be separated or divorced. Use of a condom was very low: 41% had not used condoms since their change in marital status, 38% used condoms some of the time, while 21% used condoms on a regular basis. Furthermore, condom use was more frequent in women who reported they used "barrier, withdrawal, rhythm, or no method of contraception" (p. 111) [fertile group], possibly because they were older, had fewer children, and reported using condoms more frequently with their former spouse. Non-fertile women were those who "were temporarily or permanently incapable of pregnancy (oral contraception, tubal ligation, hysterectomy, menopause)" (p. 111). In the fertile subgroup condom use was supported by: positive feelings towards condoms on the part of the woman and her partner, her past experience with condoms with her spouse, and the woman's perception of partner support. Condom use in the non-fertile group was enhanced by: length of the most recent relationship, number of children at home, partner's receptivity to condoms, and the woman's perception of her competence in using a condom. When findings were examined relative to the IMCHB and group [fertile versus non-fertile] membership, the following was evident: All women were involved in risky behavior and the model helps identify a group of variables that contribute to understanding this health behavior.

Application to Practice

Two findings are particularly applicable to intervention by nurses: the participants' perceived competence in terms of assuring condom use and their feelings towards condoms. Nurses can help women assess their sexual behavior in terms of risk and develop responsibility for their behavior. Thus, nurses can discuss assertive strategies useful in conveying the woman's decision to use condoms. Nurses can encourage partners to participate in contraceptive decisions by attending health care visits, developing written materials to share with a partner, and supporting the expectation that responsibility for decreasing risky sexual behavior is a critical activity for both partners. Nurses can also incorporate explicit, yet simple instructions about the use of condoms during interactions with women. Repeat demonstration may be helpful to ascertain a woman's degree of comfort with a condom.

Source: Marion, L.C., & Cox, C.L. (1996). Condom use and fertility among divorced and separated women. Nursing Research, 45, 110–115.

Teaching. The client should be well informed about the benefits of condom use. The client should also be made aware of the characteristics that are perceived as less attractive. It is imperative that the client understand how the condom is applied.

Until recently, little was known about male preferences and perceptions in relation to condom use. Grady and colleagues (1993), using a national sample of 3210 men, determined that men often use a condom because usage demonstrates caring and concerned qualities. Among the men studied was the perception that using condoms implied that either the man or his partner had AIDS. The proportion of the sample indicating fear that the condom would break far exceeded the actual breakage rates.

Although not frequent, condoms do break. In fact, in a sample of young men (17–22 years of age), Lindberg, Sonenstein, Ku, and Levine (1997) report that almost one quarter of the sample had experienced breakage of at least one condom during the prior 12 months. Factors influencing success with condoms included past experience with condoms and "recent sex education" (p. 128). Success rates improve when condoms are used by experienced, motivated individuals (Rosenberg & Waugh, 1997).

Women who are at risk for contracting STDs need to be supported in their efforts to have their partners use condoms even when these women are using another method of pregnancy prevention. Findings indicate that women whose attitudes towards safer sex are positive, who have been able to refuse sex when their partner does not wear a condom, and who believe in the condom's ability to protect against STDs will incorporate condoms into their pregnancy prevention actions (Santelli, Davis, Celentano, Crump, & Burwell, 1995). Furthermore, in one study (Anderson, Brackbill, & Mosher, 1996), never-married women who were younger, earned more money, had not been sexually active for long, and who had not chosen a permanent method of pregnancy prevention or were taking oral contraceptives, were more likely to use condoms.

Partner relationship also influences use of condoms (Santelli, Kouzis, Hoover, Polaczek, Burwell, & Celentano, 1996). These investigators suggest that "efforts to increase women's skills at negotiating sexual relationships could also increase their ability to use condoms with male partners or to refuse unwanted sexual advances" (p. 107). These comments are supported by Detzer and colleagues (1995) who determined that women perceived several barriers to use of condoms, including partner's perception.

Findings from these studies can be incorporated into the health care provider's approach to condom use. Assessing and addressing client concerns may enhance client use of an inexpensive method of pregnancy prevention.

▶ Diaphragm (with Spermicidal Agents)

Effectiveness and Action

Similar to the condom, the **diaphragm** is a physical barrier between cervix and sperm. As is evident from Table 8–4, although the lowest expected failure rate is 6%, the typical failure rate for diaphragm users is 18%, three times that of the IUD and 1.5 times that of the condom. Among barrier methods, however, the diaphragm is most effective in preventing pregnancy. Pregnancy occurs in 4 to 8% of women using a diaphragm and in 10 to 13% using a cervical cap (Trussell, Strickler, & Vaughan, 1993). Effectiveness is also influenced by user characteristics; women using the diaphragm who have intercourse three or more times a week and are younger than 30 are at greatest risk for experiencing accidental pregnancy (Hatcher et al., 1994).

The most common style of diaphragm has a flexible rim and a rubber cup that is shaped like a dome (Fig. 8–10). The dome is the portion that covers the cervix. For additional pregnancy prevention action, spermicidal jelly can be placed in the dome and around the rim of the diaphragm (Fig. 8–11). Because diaphragms need to be fitted on an individual basis, a variety of sizes are available. The largest rim size that fits the client comfortably is selected. The diaphragm should stay in place 6 to 8 hours after intercourse to achieve maximum pregnancy prevention action. The diaphragm should be removed within 24 hours to avoid risk of toxic shock syndrome (TSS) (Hatcher et al., 1994).

Benefits

The diaphragm (and spermicidal agent) may provide some protection against such STDs as gonorrhea. The diaphragm's protective action against HIV or chlamydia is not known and a client should not select the diaphragm because of the unfounded belief that she will have good protection against STDs. The incidence of cervical neoplasia has been reported to decrease with diaphragm use. The reduction is thought to be caused by the decreased transmission of human papillomavirus (HPV) (Hatcher et al., 1994; Tagg, 1995).

The diaphragm offers a high degree of protection without the influence of exogenous hormones. In addition, women wear it only when it is needed. Many women prefer a method that helps them retain control.

Risks and Contraindications

Women who use the diaphragm are at an increased risk for the development of urinary tract infections (UTIs) (Tagg, 1995). Reasons for this increased risk include possible urethral obstruction, alteration in normal vaginal flora as a consequence of diaphragm use, questionable postcoital voiding habits, and possibly the bactericidal effects of spermicidal jelly (Tagg, 1995).

Women may develop an allergy to either the rubber used in the construction of the diaphragm or the spermicidal agent used in its application. In addition,

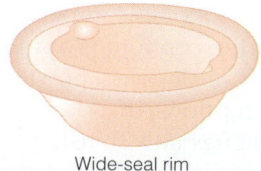

Wide-seal rim

FIGURE 8–10. Diaphragm: note the wide-seal rim and rubber cup. *(Redrawn, with permission, from Hatcher, R.A. et al. (1988). Contraceptive technology, 1988–1989 (14th ed.). New York: Irvington.)*

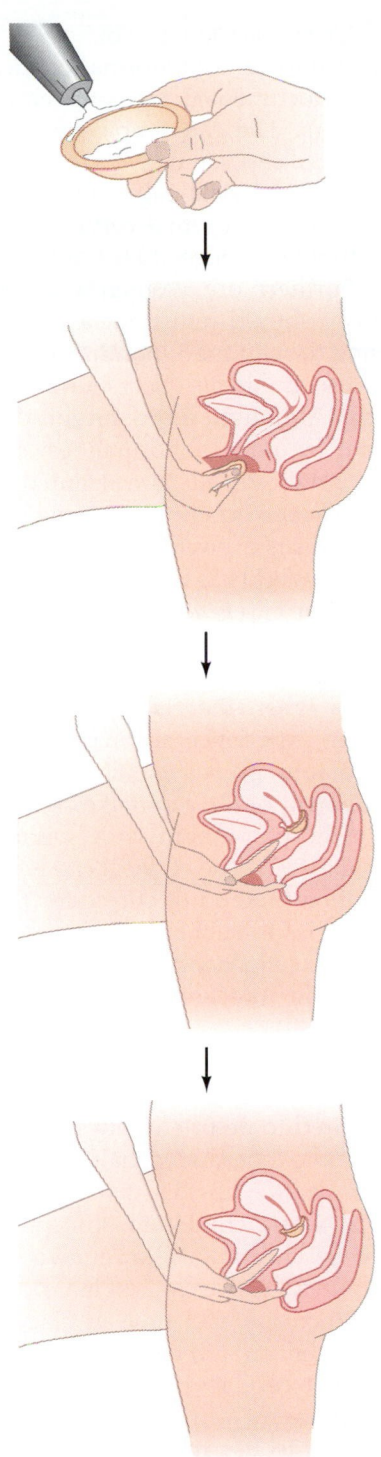

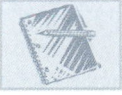

FIGURE 8–11. Application of spermicide and placement of diaphragm.

both partners can develop an irritation as a result of the spermicidal agent.

The risk of the development of TSS as a result of diaphragm use is under study, with conflicting results being demonstrated. Nonetheless, the health care provider should provide explicit directions that decrease the likelihood that TSS will occur. Minor risks include the development of a foul-smelling vaginal discharge, pelvic discomfort, and possible vaginal trauma as a result of prolonged wear or diaphragm rim pressure (Hatcher et al., 1994).

A disadvantage is that intercourse must be planned with this method of pregnancy prevention. Couples may find that use of the diaphragm interferes with spontaneity of intercourse and may not use it, thereby increasing the chance of conception. Some clients find the spermicidal cream or gel "messy." Indeed, women may need to wear a light "minipad" or panty shield the next day.

Women who have had a history of UTIs or TSS, are allergic to rubber, have abnormal vaginal anatomy, or cannot learn the proper method of inserting the diaphragm should consider another form of pregnancy prevention.

Teaching

The client needs to have a good understanding of her body and be comfortable with it. She also needs to be motivated to prevent pregnancy and plan intercourse (Beckman & Harvey, 1996). She needs to know how to insert the diaphragm (see Fig. 8–11), what discomforts may occur, and the signs and symptoms of TSS. Care

Client Teaching

Use of a Diaphragm

The following instructions should be discussed with the client before use of a diaphragm:

- Use the diaphragm with a spermicidal agent every time you have sexual intercourse.
- Apply more spermicide each time you have intercourse.
- Leave the diaphragm in 6 to 8 hours after intercourse.
- Remove your diaphragm at least once during a 24-hour period to decrease the risk of TSS.
- Know the signs of TSS:
  - (High) fever
  - Diarrhea and vomiting
  - Faintness, weakness
  - Muscle aches, sore throat
  - Rash resembling sunburn

of the diaphragm should also be explained: it is washed with mild soap and water, placed in a case after it is dry, kept away from heat, and inspected regularly for damage.

▶ Cervical Cap (with Spermicidal Agents)

Effectiveness and Action

As Table 8–4 indicates, the effectiveness of the cervical cap (with spermicidal agent) is comparable to that of the diaphragm, with a typical failure rate of 18% in nulliparous women. In parous women, the failure rate doubles (Hatcher et al., 1994). Effectiveness of the cervical cap as a pregnancy prevention method is dependent on consistency of use (Beckman & Harvey, 1996).

The **cervical cap** acts to prevent pregnancy in the same manner as the diaphragm. Because the rubber cap is fitted over the cervix, it serves as a physical barrier between sperm and cervix (Fig. 8–12). The cap can be compared to a thimble, with the portion that would cover the finger being the portion inserted over the cervix.

The Prentif Cavity Rim cervical cap, which was approved by the FDA for national use in May 1988, is the only cap available for contraceptive use in the United States (see the section entitled Future Trends in Pregnancy Prevention for discussion of new products). As with the diaphragm, the cervical cap must be fitted for the individual; it is available in four sizes.

Benefits

The cervical cap is an option for diaphragm users who are unable to continue using that method because of recurrent urinary infections associated with diaphragm use. The cervical cap is also an alternative for women who are unable to use oral contraceptives.

The cervical cap is less restrictive than the diaphragm in that it can be worn for up to 48 hours and does not require as much spermicide as the diaphragm. In addition, if the user inserts the cervical cap several hours prior to coitus, she does not need to reapply spermicide before coitus or with repeated intercourse.

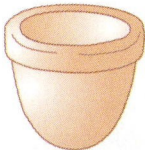

FIGURE 8–12. Prentif Cavity Rim cervical cap. (*Redrawn, with permission, from Hatcher, R.A. et al. (1988).* Contraceptive technology, 1988–1989 *(14th ed.). New York: Irvington.*)

Risks and Contraindications

Conversion of normal to abnormal cervical cytology tests has been documented for both cervical cap and diaphragm users. The rates, however, are different: 4% for the cervical cap versus 1.7% for the diaphragm. Consequently, the cervical cap should be prescribed only for women with normal cervical cytology tests and those without evidence of HPV infection (Hatcher et al., 1994). Furthermore, women who choose to use the cervical cap should return for a cervical cytology test after using the cap for 3 months. An annual cervical cytology test should also be included in the client's plan of care. Although more recent data indicate fewer cervical cytology abnormalities, conscientious surveillance of these results is warranted.

Allergic reaction to either the rubber cap or the spermicidal agent is a possibility, as with diaphragm use. Another possibility is the occurrence of TSS, particularly when the cap is worn for extended periods.

Other risks include unpleasant vaginal odor, difficulty inserting and removing the cap, and discomfort or trauma when the cervical cap is used. Cap users, however, experience fewer urinary side effects (UTIs) than diaphragm users (Hatcher et al., 1994). User misplacement of the cap makes it a less effective method than the diaphragm with spermicide (Cunningham, et al., 1997). The cervical cap is not the pregnancy prevention method of choice for those women who have allergies to rubber or spermicide; a history of TSS, cervical cell changes (dysplasias), or UTIs; vaginal or pelvic infections; or a history of HPV (Hatcher et al., 1994).

Teaching

The time required to be fitted with the cervical cap is between a half to one and a half hours. The client needs to be aware of this to make appropriate arrangements (work, child care, transportation). The client should be encouraged to remove the cap after 48 hours of use, as cap wear, vaginal odor, and incidence of TSS increase with time in place (Hatcher et al., 1994). The client should be instructed in the proper care of the cap (see Client Teaching feature entitled "Use of a Diaphragm"). In addition, the client should be instructed *not* to use the cap if there are signs of infection or if she is menstruating (Clinical Dialogue, 1993).

▶ Coitus Interruptus

Effectiveness and Action

Coitus interruptus is withdrawal of the penis from the vagina during intercourse, and ejaculation outside of the woman. Theoretically, with coitus interruptus, sperm do not come in contact with the cervix, preventing pregnancy. Penile withdrawal has a typical failure rate of 19%, comparable to diaphragm and cervical cap failure rates. This method of pregnancy prevention is used by few couples in this country. However, "it is one of the most widely used temporary methods worldwide" (Rogow & Horowitz, 1995).

Benefits

Coitus interruptus requires neither device nor chemical. No cost is involved. This method of pregnancy prevention may enhance a couple's communication, and they may explore other means of sexual satisfaction.

Risks and Contraindications

Many couples consider withdrawal as very effective in preventing pregnancy in that ejaculation occurs outside the woman's body; however, this method requires excellent self-control. Consequently, in the excitement of impending orgasm, the male partner may not be able to exert sufficient control to withdraw prior to ejaculation (nor may the female partner wish him to do so).

The incidence of conception is related to the number of orgasms. Multiple orgasms occurring over a short period increase sperm concentration in preejaculation fluid. Therefore, even if the male partner withdraws prior to ejaculation, the female partner may be exposed to a sufficient number of sperm to result in conception.

The sex act is interrupted at a crucial moment with this method. Consequently, a factor to consider is that the sexual pleasure of both partners may be diminished when coitus interruptus is used.

Teaching

To use this method most effectively, the man should urinate and then wipe off the tip of the penis before insertion, thereby decreasing the chance of unknowingly introducing sperm into the vagina (Hatcher et al., 1994). Risks should be emphasized and alternative contraceptive methods discussed. The couple may wish to use a spermicide should ejaculation occur while the penis is in the vagina. If coitus interruptus is the method adopted, the couple's decision should be reinforced, given that some method is better than no method.

Furthermore, the health care provider should make every effort to provide information about alternative methods of achieving orgasm, especially when the possibility of decreased sexual pleasure is very real. Mutual masturbation is one example of an alternative method. In addition the health care provider will need to keep in mind the religious and cultural beliefs of the couple, as these factors can influence the reception of the information given (Rogow & Horowitz, 1995).

▶ Periodic Abstinence (Natural Family Planning)

Effectiveness and Action

Four methods of periodic abstinence, also called natural family planning, are identified in Table 8–4. Lowest expected failure rates range from 1 to 9%. The typical failure rate for all methods is 20%. Effectiveness is based on the accurate definition of the fertile period to be avoided (Trent & Clark, 1997). Although methods of assessment vary, all periodic abstinence options are based on not having intercourse when the female partner is considered to be fertile. All methods require extensive instruction for maximum effectiveness.

Using the **postovulation method,** the couple may have intercourse only after the occurrence of ovulation has been determined. Sufficient time, generally at least 3 days, should elapse between ovulation and intercourse. For example, if a woman's normal cycle is 30 days, ovulation (see discussion of calendar method) may occur on day 16 of the cycle. The couple abstains from the time of menstruation until three days after ovulation, for a total of 19 days of abstinence. Consequently, in this example the couple has 11 "safe" days during a 30-day cycle in which to have intercourse. This method is hypothesized to be the most effective of the abstinence methods.

The **symptothermal method** combines the assessment of body symptoms with temperature readings. Basal body temperature (BBT) is taken and documented on a daily basis, as are cervical mucus changes. In addition, women employing this method observe for such other signs and symptoms as spotting, breast tenderness, and midcycle pain (mittelschmerz). Cervical palpation is sometimes employed with the symptothermal method. By using her middle finger, a woman can assess the consistency of the cervix; the cervix becomes softer, and more open during ovulation (Trent & Clark, 1997).

Both the thermal method and the cervical mucus method are forms of the **ovulation method,** which is dictated by the average length of cycle. The *thermal method* assesses changes in the BBT. Using an expanded-scale thermometer, the woman takes her temperature (usually oral) every morning on awakening, before undertaking any activity. To facilitate this, she can shake down the thermometer before going to bed the previous night. Temperature readings are then recorded and inspected for an elevation (see Fig. 10–8). When the temperature remains elevated for 3 days, ovulation is thought to have occurred (Trent & Clark, 1997). Intercourse is then considered safe and can occur after this time. When used in conjunction with other methods, the thermal method helps predict ovulation. Hatcher and colleagues (1994) provide very comprehensive instructions on this method.

The *cervical mucus method* assesses changes in cervical mucus as a result of hormonal fluctuations associated with the normal menstrual cycle (Trent & Clark, 1997). As ovulation approaches or occurs, the characteristics of cervical mucus change. It becomes more abundant and stretchy, thin, clear, and slippery. Table 8–6 summarizes cervical mucus changes during the menstrual cycle. Some users of this method rely on bodily sensations of lubrication, moisture, and stickiness rather than the actual characteristics. The symptothermal method is often used to enhance the ovulation method.

The **calendar method** provides the individual or couple with opportunity to determine when intercourse should be avoided because of the presence of an ovum. This method identifies the couple's fertile period and is based on three assumptions: "(1) ovulation occurs on day 14 (plus or minus 2 days) before the onset of the next menses; (2) sperm remain viable for 2 to 3 days; and (3) the ovum survives 24 hours." (Hatcher et al., 1994, p. 332).

To enhance its predictive abilities, and before using this method, the client must maintain a menstrual calendar documenting the length of her menstrual cycle for an 8-month period. The period of abstinence can be determined once the pattern of the cycle is apparent; the earliest fertile day is then calculated by subtracting 20 days from the length of the shortest cycle. Subtracting 10 days from the woman's longest cycle identifies the woman's latest fertile day. Because truly regular cycles are experienced by few women, and because an abnormal cycle is not unusual over a single year, this method is now gener-

ally supplemented by more reliable assessment methods (Trent & Clark, 1997).

An alternative to periodic abstinence, with well-defined assessment measures, is **total abstinence** (complete avoidance of intercourse). This form of pregnancy prevention is acceptable and should be recognized and accepted by health care professionals. Other forms of expressing the individual's sexuality should be explored when total abstinence is chosen.

Benefits

Periodic abstinence is a pregnancy prevention method for those for whom other methods are unacceptable. For example, the Billings Ovulation Method has been well received and followed in India (Indian Council of Medical Research Task Force on Natural Family Planning, 1996). Abstinence may be preferable for physical, ethical, or religious reasons. Moreover, periodic abstinence methods increase a woman's understanding of her body and a couple's awareness of their fertility. Communication between partners is fostered by use of such a pregnancy prevention method.

Disadvantages

Periodic abstinence methods have several disadvantages. For example, meticulous record keeping is required. In addition, using a method necessitates that it be followed daily. Consequently, motivation must remain high for both partners. Extensive training, over several months, is required to enhance effectiveness. Sexual spontaneity may be stifled. Because mothers who are breastfeeding may be unable to determine safe, or infertile, periods, this method is not recommended for them. In addition, this method does not provide protection from STDs.

No absolute contraindications have been determined. Irregular menstrual cycles and temperature charts, however, may impede periodic abstinence methods in preventing pregnancy.

▶ **TABLE 8–6**

Cyclic Characteristics of the Cervix and Cervical Mucus

Time of Cycle	Amount	Viscosity	Appearance	Spinnbarkeit	Ferning	Cervix
Postmenstruation	Moderate	Thick	Cloudy	None	None	Firm, closed
Nearing ovulation	Increasing	Somewhat thick to thin	Mixed/cloudy and clear	Moderate	Moderate	Firm, closed
Ovulation	Maximum	Very thin and slippery	Clear	Maximum 2–3 or more inches	Well developed	Soft, open
Postovulation (about 3 days)	Decreasing	Thin	Mixed cloudy and clear	Minimal or none	Minimal or none	Firm, closed
Nearing menstruation	Minimal	Thick	Cloudy	None	None	Firm, closed

Reproduced, with permission, from Hatcher, R.A. et al. (1988). Contraceptive technology, 1988–1989 (14th ed.). New York: Irvington. Adapted from Health Education Bulletin, July 1979, by the National Clearinghouse for Family Planning Information DHEW, Bureau of Community Health Services.

Teaching

Couples who choose periodic abstinence require extensive education to be able to accurately document and assess their efforts. If a combination of methods is used, all components must be addressed. Hatcher and colleagues (1994) present a comprehensive discussion of needed instruction. Couples who wish to use natural family planning methods (NFP) as their means of pregnancy prevention need support and guidance. There are several international NFP organizations that can direct couples to specially prepared individuals who can assist and instruct them in NFP methods.

In addition, Moreno and colleagues (1997) present an alternative method that is based on the relation between peak salivary electrical resistance (SR) and an increase in vaginal resistance. Called the CUE™ method, it appears to be as effective in defining a woman's fertile period as is the ovulation method.

► Spermicidal Agents

Spermicidal agents include foams, jellies, film, and suppositories.

Effectiveness and Action

As Table 8–4 indicates, the lowest expected failure rate of spermicidal agents is 6%; typical failure rate is 21%, and may be as high as 50% (Hatcher et al., 1994). Spermicides are readily accessible in pharmacies. Combination of spermicidal agents with a second method, such as a condom or diaphragm, enhances their effectiveness.

Spermicidal agents consist of an inert substance that holds the spermicidal chemical in place. The spermicidal chemical is usually nonoxynol-9, the same chemical used in certain condoms (see section entitled "Male Condom"). Pregnancy is prevented by means of active destruction of sperm by the chemical.

Another over-the-counter product is a spermicidal film called Vaginal Contraceptive Film (VCF). Measuring only 2 × 2 in., this translucent paper-thin square dissolves into a cohesive gel when inserted into the vagina. It is achieved within 15 minutes and inserted at least 5 minutes before intercourse. Effectiveness is maintained for up to 1 hour after insertion (Hatcher et al., 1994). If used correctly with a condom, VCF is 100% effective.

Benefits

Because a variety of spermicidal agents are manufactured, the client has considerable flexibility in choosing the form most suitable to his or her needs. Many are individually packaged, adding greater user

appeal. Significant protection against chlamydia and gonorrhea is gained by using spermicidal agents.

Risks and Contraindications

Occasionally an allergic response may occur, or suppositories may not melt or foam when placed in the vagina. An unpleasant taste may be noted by couples having oral–genital sex. The possibility that spermicidal agents may have teratogenic effects has been studied. Results do not support any association (Cunningham et al., 1997); however, controversy continues.

Teaching

Clients need to be informed about proper insertion techniques and signs and symptoms of an allergic response. Insertion times should be clearly understood. Table 8–7 presents a review of the various spermicides and their method of action.

► Ineffective Methods

Despite the wide variety of contraceptive methods available, some individuals still practice methods that are ineffective in preventing conception. Douching is an example.

Douching, or cleansing of the vagina to rid it of sperm, has been used to prevent conception for centuries. Such agents as citrus, herbs, cola, and lye have been used with poor or even lethal results. The use effectiveness rate of douching is less than 60%. When vaginal spermicides are used, it is especially important not to douche for at least 6 hours after intercourse because the spermicide will be rendered ineffective.

► New Trends in Pregnancy Prevention

Lactational Amenorrhea Method

Historically, in the United States, breastfeeding has been considered to be a unreliable method of pregnancy prevention. However, recent data (Hatcher et al., 1994; Hight-Laukaran et al., 1997; Labbok, et al., 1997; Ramos, Kennedy & Visness, 1996) indicate that women can use the lactational amenorrhea method as an introductory or interim postpartum method. When a mother meets the following criteria she has less than a 2% chance of becoming pregnant: the woman must be amenorrheic, be fully or almost fully breastfeeding, and less than 6 months postpartum. Breastfeeding is further defined to include:

(a) breastfeeding frequency must be a pattern comparable to at least 10 short or 6 long breastfeeds

► **TABLE 8-7**

Spermicides

Representative Products (Brand Names)	Spermicidal Agent	Action	Comments
Film: Vaginal Contra-ceptive Film (VCF)	Nonoxynol-9	Contraceptive protection begins 15 minutes after insertion; remains effective no more than 1 hour	Small, thin sheets

Foam:
  Delfen, Emko, Koromex Emko
  Because, Emko Prefil
	Nonoxynol-9
	Nonoxynol-9
		Contraceptive protection is immediate; remains effective for at least 1 hour	Aerosol container
			Small container

Jellies and Creams: Conceptrol, Delfen, Koromex Jel, Ortho Gynol II, Ramses	Nonoxynol-9	Contraceptive protection is immediate. When used alone, remains effective at least 1 hour; when used with diaphragm or cap, remains effective at least 6–8 hours	Reuseable applicator
Koromex Cream, Ortho Gynol Concep-trol Jel, Milex Shur Sheal Jel	Octoxynol Nonoxynol-9		Reuseable applicator Single-use packets
Suppositories and Tablets: Encare, Intercept, Koromex Inserts, Prevent, Semicid	Nonoxynol-9	Contraceptive protection begins 10–15 minutes after insertion; remains effective no more than 1 hour	

Adapted, with permission, from Hatcher, R.A. et al. (1994). Contraceptive technology (16th Rev. ed.). New York: Irvington.

within 24 h; (b) supplemental feedings of no more than 1 ounce (30 ml) per week of supplement in month 1, nor more than 2 ounces (60 ml) in month 2, 3 ounces in month 3, etc.; (c) no replacement of breastfeeds with other feeds, and no more than 10% of feeds or food can be other than direct breastfeeding; and (d) breastfeeding must be maintained with both day and night feeding and no long intervals between feeds (Labbok et al., 1997, p. 329.)

Long intervals were defined as either one episode of greater than 10 hours between feeds or frequent episodes of greater than 6 hours between feeds. This method of pregnancy prevention is very supportive of breastfeeding mothers. An alternative method must, however, be used should any of the three criteria no longer be present. Although this method has been well received in less-developed countries where many more women breastfeed, its use in the United States may be limited by the need to adhere to breastfeeding exclusively during the first six months postpartum. Nonetheless, breastfeeding women should be informed about this option.

Emergency Contraception

Emergency contraception "refers to specific contraceptive methods that can be used as emergency mea-sures to prevent pregnancy after unprotected intercourse" (von Hertzen & Van Look, 1996, p. 52). It is considered a backup method of pregnancy prevention. Previously, emergency contraception was often called the "morning after pill." However, use of the term "emergency" conveys the idea that one can obtain treatment immediately rather than waiting until the morning (Ellertson, 1996) and is, in fact, a 24-hour a day option. This method can also be used sporadically or irregularly, rather than on an ongoing basis (Ellertson, 1996).

This form of contraception has been viewed as a form of abortion by some individuals. However, understanding its mode of action helps dispel this misconception (Grimes, 1997). Although not clearly understood, ovulation is blocked by the combination of estrogen-progestin present in the emergency pills (Glasier, 1997). Thus, pregnancy is prevented. As implantation initiates a pregnancy, this drug cannot be considered an abortifacient (Grimes, 1997). Furthermore, this regimen "cannot disrupt an established pregnancy" (Grimes, 1997, p. 1078).

Recently, a specific regimen, the Yuzpe regimen (estrogen plus progestin), was approved by the FDA for use as a contraceptive (Grimes, 1997). This regimen involves ingesting two doses of pills: one pill contains 100 mcg of ethinyl estradiol (estrogen component) and one pill contains 1.0 mg of norgestrel (progestin component). The first dose "is taken within 72 hours of unprotected intercourse and the second is taken 12 hours later" (Trussell, Ellertson, & Stewart, 1996 p. 58). Thus the total amount of each drug ingested is 200 mcg ethinyl estradiol and 2.0 mg of norgestrel. It is reported to have about a 75% effectiveness rate (Chez & Chapin, 1997; Lindberg, 1997; Trussell, Ellertson, & Stewart, 1996).

There are several common side effects of this dose of combination pregnancy prevention pills, most notably nausea and vomiting (Lindberg, 1997). Should vomiting occur within an hour of taking the pills, the dose may be repeated. Vomiting can be lessened if the woman ingests food or takes an antiemetic prior to taking the pills (Chez & Chapin, 1997; Lindberg, 1997). Other than these side effects, this method is considered safe (Chez & Chapin, 1997; Davies, 1997).

Additional methods of emergency contraception include administering high doses of estrogen over a five day period, as is currently done in the Netherlands (Glasier, 1997), and inserting a copper IUD. An attractive feature associated with using an IUD is that it introduces a consistent method of pregnancy prevention (Lindberg, 1997).

The need for emergency contraception presents an excellent opportunity to discuss alternative pregnancy prevention methods that are more effective. Every effort should be made to help the woman choose one of the methods discussed in this chapter before she leaves the office, clinic, or emergency room. In addition, emergency contraception should be discussed whenever pregnancy prevention methods are discussed. Data indicate that neither users nor health care professionals are familiar with emergency contraception methods (Delbanco, Mauldon, & Smith, 1997; Gold, Schein, & Coupey, 1997; Harper & Ellertson, 1995). Table 8–8 presents information about the type of pills available as well as the education that should accompany their administration.

▶ **TABLE 8-8**

Emergency Contraceptive Pills

Brand	Pills per Dose	Ethinyl-Estradiol per Dose (μg)	Levonorgestrel per Dose (mg)*
Ovral	2 white pills**	100	0.50
Alesse	5 pink pills**	100	0.50
Nordette	4 light-orange pills**	120	0.60
Levlen	4 light-orange pills**	120	0.60
Lo/Ovral	4 white pills**	120	0.60
Triphasil	4 yellow pills**	120	0.50
Tri-Levlin	4 yellow pills**	120	0.50

*The progestin in Ovral, Lo/Ovral and Ovrette is norgestrel, which contains two isomers, only one of which (levonorgestrel) is bioactive. The amount of norgestrel in each dose is twice the amount of levonorgestrel.

**The treatment schedule is one dose within 72 hours after unprotected intercourse and another dose 12 hours later.

Instructions

1. Take the first dose when possible, no later than 72 hours after unprotected sex. One hour before taking the pills, take the anti-nausea medication suggested by your clinician. Eat a snack or drink a glass of milk to reduce the risk of nausea.

2. Take the second dose 12 hours after the first dose. Remember to eat a snack and take the anti-nausea medication, if suggested, 1 hour prior to this dose.

   About one-third of users experience mild, temporary nausea that should subside within a day. If you vomit within an hour after taking a dose, call your clinician. You may need to repeat a dose.

   Watch for pill danger signals over the next week. See your clinician as soon as possible if you experience any of the following:
   - Severe calf or thigh pain
   - Chest pain, cough or shortness of breath
   - Severe headaches, dizziness, weakness or numbness
   - Blurred vision, vision loss or trouble speaking
   - Severe abdominal pain
   - Yellowing of the eyes

3. Your next period should begin within 3 to 4 weeks. If it does not begin, or the flow is significantly less than normal, see your clinician for a pregnancy test. If you think you are pregnant, check with your clinician as soon as possible.

4. Get started as soon as you possibly can with a method of birth control you can use every time you have sex. Emergency contraceptive pills are meant for one-time, emergency protection.

5. Protect yourself from AIDS, other sexual infections and pregnancy. Use condoms every time you have sex if you think you might be at risk. Emergency contraceptive pills don't protect against sexually transmitted infections.

Reproduced, with permission, from Trussell, J., Koenig, J., Ellerton, C., & Stewart, F. Preventing unintended pregnancy: The cost-effectiveness of three methods of emergency contraception. American Journal of Public Health 87: 932–937; Hatcher, R.A. et al. (1994). Contraceptive technology (16th Rev. ed.). New York: Irvington.

Commonly Asked Questions

What should I do if the condom my partner or I am using breaks?

You should see your health care provider as soon as possible after you have noticed that breakage has occurred. There is a regimen presently in use that is about 75% effective in preventing pregnancy after intercourse. However, it is important that you receive this medication within 72 hours. This is a topic to discuss with your health care provider before this occurs so that you know what to do.

I am breastfeeding. What pregnancy prevention methods are available for my use?

There are several methods that you can use. Those that contain progestin only do not adversely affect breast milk. Examples of these include: Norplant, Depo-Provera, the Progestasert IUD, and progestin-only contraceptive pills. A new method is called the Lactational Amenorrhea Method. This method is considered an interim method of pregnancy prevention and requires total or almost total breastfeeding. That means that supplemental feedings are not used. One advantage to this method is that you can get breastfeeding well established before you use an alternative method such as an IUD.

I have heard that there is a low-dose oral contraceptive pill on the market. What does that mean?

Low-dose oral contraceptive pills have less than 50 μg of an estrogen preparation. The most recent preparations tend to have less than 30 μg. This means that there are fewer side effects and complications.

I am thinking about using an IUD. What can you tell me about them?

IUDs are very effective in preventing pregnancy. However, there are several things to consider about IUDs. If you have many sexual partners, the IUD is not the pregnancy prevention method for you, as the risk of infection increases as the number of partners increases. You also need to be comfortable with your body, as having an IUD in place requires that you check for its placement. Lastly, it is generally used with women who have had at least one child.

▶ Future Trends in Pregnancy Prevention

Although many pregnancy prevention methods are available, many individuals still have unmet needs (Document, 1996). Thus, work continues on refining current methods as well as developing new methods that allow for greater client freedom. Biodegradable capsules, such as Capronor (administered through a tube), Annuelle (fused pellets), or injectable microspheres function similarly to Norplant. An alternate version of Norplant, Norplant-2, is also being investigated (Reifsnider, 1997). This system only has two, rather than six, rods. Similarly, a two-rod levonorgestrel containing implant, LNG ROD, has been studied, with positive results (Sivin, Lahteenmaki, et al., 1997; Sivin, Viegas, et al., 1997). Another implant, Implanon, is undergoing preliminary studies, as are two progestins: nesterone (ST-1435) and nomegestrol. Both of these have reported pregnancy rates of less than 1% (Reifsnider, 1997). Monthly injectables, such as norethisterone enanthate and estraial valerate (Mesigyna), and depot medroxyprogesterone acetate and estradial cypionate (Cyclofem), that consist of estrogen and progestin or only progestin, such as levonorgestrel butanoate, are either available or are being tested in other countries. Cyclofem will marketed as Cyclo-Provera in this country (Klitsch, 1995). Bohamondes and colleagues (1996) report a favorable assessment of the Unijet® as a method of administering Cyclofem. This system prevents reuse of needles, a significant factor in less well-developed countries.

Work continues on refining vaginal rings. A vaginal ring consists of "a soft, silastic device that lies transversely across the upper vagina and measures 50–55 mm in diameter" (Reifsnider, 1997, p. 92). Both progestin-estrogen and progestin-only rings are being evaluated. The latter appear to exert less of a pregnancy prevention action. A new preparation of vaginal film containing benzalkonium chloride rather than nonoxynol-9 is currently under investigation (Mauck, Baker, Barr, Abercrombie, & Archer, 1997; Mauck, Baker, Barr, Johanson, & Archer, 1997). This preparation is being investigated because "it may cause less irritation to mucosal tissues, it may cost less to manufacture, and its lower hygroscopicity should make it more stable in warm, humid climates of developing countries and less likely to stick to the fingers" (Mauck, Baker, Barr, Johanson, & Archer, 1997, p. 97). A transdermal progestin cream is also being developed that may be particularly useful with breastfeeding mothers (Reifsnider, 1997). A new vaginal sponge is also being investigated (Klitsch, 1995).

Other pregnancy prevention methods under investigation include both gonadotropin releasing hormone (GnRH) agonists and antagonists. Developmental work on a birth control vaccine continues as well.

Several new IUDs have been developed. Four are copper based: the FlexiGard, the Multiload 375, the Nova T, and the UCDcu (Reifsnider, 1997). The only hormone-releasing IUD, the Levenova/Mirena IUD, contains levonorgestrel that is "released at a rate of 20 µg per day and prevents pregnancy for at least 5 years" (Reifsnider, 1997, p. 93). Two new cervical caps have been developed. The Femcap, which may be useful for those women who cannot be fitted with the Prentif Cavity Rim cap, has a cap and a brim, and can be used with oil-based lubricants. This cap will probably be available by the year 2000 (Hatcher et al., 1994). Another cap, Lea's Shield, enhances cervical fit. It is not currently available but is in clinical trials (Klitsch, 1995).

The preceding discussion has presented potential alternatives for women; however, research efforts have also been directed toward the development of _male_ pregnancy prevention methods. Weekly injections of testosterone enanthate have been effective in decreasing the sperm count in men (Klitsch, 1995; Reifsnider, 1997). However, whether this method would be well received is questionable (Ringheim, 1995). A dual-implant system is also being considered (Klitsch, 1995), as are the GnRH agonists and antagonists. Calcium channel blockers, such as mifepristone and nifidepine, have been noted to have pregnancy prevention actions. However, their use is still experimental. Gossypol, found in cottonseed, is presently being tested in China at half its original dosage. It appears to be very effective, with no associated side effects (Reifsnider, 1997).

As is evident, the future holds many alternatives for individuals and couples seeking to prevent pregnancy. Certainly, as many choices as possible should be made available to meet individual and couple needs. With the increased number of options is the responsibility of the health care professional to provide comprehensive and complete information on which the client can make a knowledgeable choice.

▶ PREGNANCY TERMINATION

Approximately half of all pregnancies are unintended; however, many women decide to continue their pregnancy. The decision-making process regarding whether to continue or terminate a pregnancy begins when a woman first suspects she is pregnant. The process may be brief or may require weeks or even months. During this time a woman should have an opportunity to discuss openly with a nurse or other health care professional whether she wishes to continue her pregnancy. The discussion should include a review of the woman's situation, age, marital status, family stability, socioeconomic status, personal goals and values, religious beliefs, and many other psychosocial factors. A pregnancy risk assessment should be carried out so that a woman may weigh identified risk factors and reproductive options.

Elective (voluntary) **abortion** is the "interruption of pregnancy before viability at the request of the woman, but not for reasons of impaired maternal health or fetal disease" (Cunningham et al., 1997, p. 594). Women have terminated undesired pregnancies for many generations, whether their culture approved or disapproved. Accurate statistics regarding pregnancy termination are difficult to determine, especially in countries where the procedure is not legal. An estimated one elective abortion occurs for every 3 live births in the United States (Cunningham et al., 1997).

Despite the slight decline in the pregnancy termination rate, the majority of U.S. adults continue to approve of legal pregnancy termination. One classic study showed that 90% of the adults in the United States approved of legal termination if a woman's health was endangered by the pregnancy; 83% approved if the woman became pregnant as a result of rape; 83% approved if there was a strong chance that the fetus had a serious birth defect; 52% approved if the family could not afford the child; 48% approved if the woman was not married and did not wish to marry; 47% approved if a woman was married but did not desire the child; and 41% percent approved for "any reason" (Granberg & Granberg, 1980). However, given the change in political climate, one must question whether similar findings would be obtained today.

▶ Legal Status of Pregnancy Termination in the United States

On January 22, 1973, the U.S. Supreme Court announced a decision in two landmark cases (_Roe v._

Wade and *Doe v. Bolton*) related to pregnancy termination. A summary of the decision follows (Hatcher et al., 1994).

1. The decision to have an abortion rests with the pregnant woman and her health care provider during the first trimester.
2. During the second trimester, the state may intercede through regulation of the abortion procedure in ways that are "reasonably related to her health" (Hatcher et al., 1994, p. 474). State intercession is predicated on concern for the woman's health.
3. The state may choose to regulate and even prohibit abortion when a pregnancy has progressed to the point of fetal viability. These restrictions are based on the state's "interest in the potentiality of human life" (Hatcher et al., 1994, p. 474); however, an abortion may be performed if medical judgment indicates that the woman's health or life is jeopardized by not having an abortion.

On July 1, 1976, the Supreme Court held that the state cannot impose the requirement of consent by a third party on a woman's right to abortion. This "veto" power cannot be exercised by a spouse or a parent (Supreme Court). Despite strong antitermination sentiments in some populations, the Supreme Court repeatedly upheld a woman's right to pregnancy termination, until July 3, 1989. At that time, the Supreme Court, in *Webster v. Reproductive Health Services,* upheld a Missouri law that in effect gave individual states a much greater ability to restrict pregnancy termination. In this ruling, a law banning use of state facilities and prohibiting state employees from performing abortions was upheld. Furthermore, a provision requiring physicians to perform tests to determine whether a 20-week-old fetus could survive outside the uterus was also upheld on the grounds that such testing furthered the state's interest in protecting potential human life. Although the Supreme Court decision stopped short of reversing *Roe v. Wade,* other test cases pending in the Supreme Court might result in its overthrow. Health care professionals must remain aware of the possible impact of the July 3, 1989, Supreme Court ruling on current and future contraceptive technology. As individual states make decisions concerning the beginnings of life and their responsibility in that area, certain contraceptive methods (for instance, the morning-after pill) also may be called into question.

Since 1977 Congress and state legislatures have imposed many restrictions related to federal and state funding of pregnancy terminations. Although the fed-

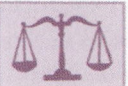

Ethical Decision Making

The two major cases concerning pregnancy termination, *Roe v. Wade* in 1973 and *Webster v. Reproductive Health Services* in 1989, have established the foundation for federal and state involvement in this area. As a nurse working with clients who may want to explore this option, the consideration of the following issues may be useful in clarifying your opinions about pregnancy termination:

1. Do you see a conflict between a woman's right to terminate a pregnancy and the ability of individual states to intervene in that decision?
2. How would you weigh the interests of the parties in this matter so that equal consideration is given to each and decisions are made to achieve satisfactory outcomes for all involved?

eral government (as of 1981) provides funding for terminations only in the case of a threat of death to the mother should she carry the pregnancy, some states have chosen to provide funding for these services for welfare-eligible clients.

The availability of legal pregnancy terminations has dramatically decreased the maternal mortality and morbidity previously associated with illegal, criminal terminations (Henshaw, 1986). Prior to legalization, terminations were responsible for the majority of maternal deaths in urban areas, with estimates of 800 to 5000 maternal deaths per year (Henshaw, 1986).

▶ Psychosocial Factors Affecting Pregnancy Termination

In most societies, a high value is placed on women in their role as mothers, and powerful systems of reinforcement operate to make motherhood central to women's lives. A decision to terminate a pregnancy is rarely made without some conflict of emotions because of the complex values associated with womanhood and motherhood. Even if the child is unwanted, the woman may on some levels desire to remain pregnant as a symbol of potency, vitality, or reconnection with inner wishes and desires. Though some unintended pregnancies can be completely accidental and the result of a contraceptive method failure, many result from contraceptive misuse or nonuse. An "accidental" pregnancy sometimes is a mechanism used to affect relations with important people in a woman's life, such as a husband, lover, or parents. Women also become pregnant as a result of rape or an abusive relationship.

Some teenagers become pregnant to demonstrate their sexuality and maturity and to bolster their self-concept. An infant may be desired, in some instances, as someone to love them. The use of contraceptive methods may be avoided because it represents planning regarding sexual activity, which they feel is taboo. On finding she is pregnant, a teenager may decide that she cannot face the responsibilities of caring for and raising a child and thus elects abortion.

A woman may become pregnant to force a lover into marriage or save a troubled marriage or other relationship. She may then find that the pregnancy did not produce the desired result and elect to terminate the pregnancy.

Poor physical or mental health can result in pregnancy termination. A woman to whom pregnancy poses a risk to her physical or mental health may choose termination.

Termination may be chosen if a pregnancy is untimely. Finishing an education, reaching a personal or professional goal, recent marriage, recent childbirth, and reduced income are reasons why some women elect a pregnancy termination.

Sociocultural factors can also play an important role in a decision to seek pregnancy termination. If termination is illegal, a woman may risk minimal prosecution to terminate her pregnancy. If social values condemn terminations, she faces disapproval by peers, family members, and members of her community. When pregnancy terminations are legal and societal values are more accepting, deciding to have a termination may be less traumatic.

Although at this time the United States places no legal restrictions on early pregnancy terminations and few requirements on later ones, this does not mean that every woman who desires to terminate a pregnancy has equal access. The ability to obtain a termination is greatly influenced by such factors as the availability and accessibility of facilities providing these services, methods of financing health care services, and personal and economic resources.

For women without health insurance or adequate means to pay for a termination, the lack of facilities providing this service can be a problem. In the United States, termination of pregnancy is, like all health care, usually an option dependent on adequate income and availability.

The situation for poor women has become particularly difficult in the last several years. Since the enactment of the Hyde Amendment, which restricted federal funds for pregnancy termination, funding has dropped for Medicaid patients. Many states have even chosen not to fund the terminations the federal government left to state control. The Supreme Court ruling, which resulted in the closing of publicly subsidized facilities in Missouri, will exacerbate this situation as other states follow suit.

The impact of this decrease in publicly funded pregnancy terminations is felt in many ways. Women with no or low income who are intent on having a termination often delay their procedure while seeking the necessary funds. This leads to an increase in the complication rate because the pregnancy termination takes place at a later gestational age. It often also results in the need for a more costly procedure for a second-trimester abortion. Women with low income who are able to raise the money for their own terminations may do so at the expense of their rent or utility bills, food, clothing, or by fraudulent use of relatives' insurance policies. Extreme desperation may lead to self-induced abortion or even suicide.

▶ Counseling Regarding Pregnancy Termination

The nurse is often a key professional in providing counseling to women considering pregnancy termination. The need to make responsible decisions about an unwanted or problem pregnancy may become apparent in a prenatal or family planning clinic or in another health care setting. The nurse may begin initial discussion and assistance in beginning to solve problems with women or couples facing an unintended pregnancy.

Many women need to think beyond their initial reaction to the unintended pregnancy. They need to be encouraged to consider all options, such as placing the baby for adoption, that are available to them. It is important for the nurse to encourage the woman to make the decision herself, even though she may feel confused and ambivalent, because of pressure from her partner, other family members, or peers. Regret and emotional sequelae may be minimized when the choice is not perceived as being forced by others. Exploring alternatives helps to realistically clarify the situation. In thinking through each choice she should explore not only present feelings and relationships, but also future circumstances, goals, and needs.

The nurse or counselor should also explain the abortion procedure required for the client's stage of gestation, how it is done, its discomforts, safety, risks, duration, cost, and follow-up care instructions. Written information summarizing this discussion should be provided to the client to ensure informed choice or consent.

Many psychosocial factors are weighed in the decision to continue or terminate a pregnancy. If a woman is involved in a stable relationship she may wish to include her partner in the decision-making process. It is important, however, for the woman's desires to be respected in this regard.

As prenatal diagnostic techniques have become more sophisticated and accessible, more women are choosing to determine if the child they are carrying has a birth defect or genetic disorder. The decision to terminate a pregnancy because of an abnormality in the fetus presents additional psychosocial factors that complicate the woman or couple's decision-making process and thus is dealt with later in this chapter.

▶ Termination Procedures

Pregnancy terminations may be carried out during the first trimester (during the first 13 weeks after the beginning of the last menstrual period) or the second trimester (from 14 to 24 weeks of gestation). If a woman suspects she may be pregnant but no positive diagnosis has been made, a menstrual extraction or a vacuum aspiration of uterine contents can be carried out before the woman's first missed period.

First-Trimester Pregnancy Terminations

Mifepristone (RU-486). With FDA approval granted, this drug became available for use in 1997. It exerts its abortive action by "softening and breaking down the endometrial lining" (Mackenzie & Yeo, 1997, p. 86). This drug is highly effective in terminating pregnancy before 8 weeks of gestation when given in conjunction with misoprostol, a prostaglandin analogue. A woman desiring this method receives 600 mg of mifepristone that is ingested while in the presence of the health care provider. The woman remains in the office or clinic for a 30-minute observation period to assess her response to the medication. Should she tolerate the medication well, she is permitted to resume her scheduled activities. In addition, she is scheduled for a follow-up appointment in 36–48 hours to receive the 40 μg of misoprostol. When this dose is given, she is required to remain at the health care facility for

about 4 hours, during which time the products of conception should be expelled (Mackenzie & Yeo, 1997). The majority (60%) of women undergoing medical abortion will expel the products of conception within this time while the remaining women will abort at home. In order to assure that the abortion is complete, the woman is scheduled for a return visit in 7–10 days, during which she will have a pelvic examination (Mackenzie & Yeo, 1997). Should the abortion be incomplete, the woman is scheduled for surgical intervention.

Women seem to be fairly receptive to this form of abortion (Harvey, Beckman, Castle, & Coyteaux, 1995). Although interviewed before this method became available, about one third of the participants indicated that they would use this method. Reasons cited for choosing this method included: produces fewer complications, does not require anesthesia, can be used early in pregnancy, and seems to be more natural. Four disadvantages were identified: the need for numerous visits, the possibility that expulsion will be painful, the perception that this method may be perceived as being too easy, and the discomfort with a new method (Harvey, Beckman, Castle, & Coyteaux, 1995).

Menstrual Extraction. **Menstrual extraction** may be performed if a client's menstrual period is less than 2 weeks late. Some clients choose not to confirm the presence of the pregnancy to avoid the ethical dilemma of continuing or terminating the pregnancy.

Menstrual extraction is performed by inserting a sterile plastic cannula into the endometrial cavity. Suction is then applied with a large syringe to withdraw the uterine contents. This procedure is performed on an outpatient basis, requires neither anesthesia nor cervical dilation, and takes only a few minutes to complete. It is also low in cost.

Vacuum Aspiration. Pregnancies that are less than 12 to 13 weeks of gestation may be terminated by **vacuum aspiration** using a cannula and suction. The cervix must be dilated; the amount of dilation required is determined by the gestation of the pregnancy. After cervical dilation, the cannula is introduced into the uterus and a small suction pump is used to remove the products of conception. The procedure takes less than 10 minutes to complete and is usually performed under local anesthesia to the cervix and on an outpatient basis. The client is allowed to go home within 1 to 4 hours of the procedure.

Dilation and Curettage. **Dilation and curettage** (D&C) is similar to vacuum aspiration except that the uterine walls are scraped with a curet instead of by suction.

Second-Trimester Pregnancy Terminations

Dilation and Evacuation. A **dilation and evacuation** (D&E) is very similar to a D&C. It can be used for pregnancy termination between 13 and 24 weeks of gestation. With a D&E, the cervix requires substantially more dilation, because the products of conception are much larger. Local anesthesia is used for this procedure and the woman is usually allowed to go home on the same day as the procedure.

Prostaglandin Instillation. **Prostaglandin instillation** may be used to terminate a pregnancy around 15 weeks of gestation. Prostaglandin can be inserted vaginally as a suppository into the cul-de-sac or administered intraabdominally into the amniotic sac. It is used to induce uterine contractions. After instillation of prostaglandin, uterine contractions usually begin within a few hours. Uterine contractions continue until the fetus is delivered. Hospitalization is required for this method and the woman should be observed for nausea, vomiting, cervical lacerations, and tissue reactions. The major disadvantage to the use of this method late in pregnancy is the possibility that a live fetus may be delivered.

Saline Induction. **Saline termination** may be used after 16 weeks of gestation. An amniocentesis is performed to remove some of the amniotic fluid. After the amniotic fluid is removed, a hypertonic saline solution is introduced into the amniotic sac. Uterine contractions usually begin within 12 to 24 hours. The labor may last 10 to 24 hours. The woman needs to be hospitalized and must be treated similarly to other women in labor. Sometimes, prostaglandin instillation and saline induction are used in combination for pregnancy termination.

Hysterotomy. **Hysterotomy** is removal of the products of conception through an incision in the uterine and abdominal walls. It is rarely used for pregnancy termination. It may be the method chosen when other termination methods are contraindicated or used when a woman desires a sterilization procedure at the same time.

▶ Risk Factors and Complications

The risks associated with pregnancy terminations since terminations have become legal are minimal.

The complications that have been observed are less likely if:

- The pregnancy is terminated early.
- The client is healthy.
- The clinician performing the procedure is well trained and experienced.
- The uterus is not severely anteverted or retroverted.
- The client understands the warning signs for post-termination complications.
- Prompt follow-up care is immediately accessible.
- Careful examination of the products of conception is carried out to ensure complete termination and to rule out the possibility of a molar or ectopic pregnancy.
- Rh immune globulin is given to Rh-negative women.
- The client does not have infection such as gonorrhea or chlamydia.
- The client is not ambivalent about having the termination or believes she can cope with the ambivalent feelings she may be experiencing.
- Local anesthesia is used rather than regional or general anesthesia and *Laminaria digitata* is used to soften the cervix (Hatcher et al., 1994).

The five most common posttermination physical problems observed include bleeding, infection, retained products of conception or uterine blood clots, continuing pregnancy, and cervical or uterine trauma (Hatcher et al., 1994). Clients should be instructed verbally and given written instructions to contact the clinic or physician if any of the following physical signs occur: fever and chills, foul-smelling discharge, heavy bleeding, severe abdominal pain, and nausea and vomiting. They should be informed to avoid intercourse, use of tampons, and douching for approximately 2 weeks to reduce the risk of introducing bacteria that may cause infection. A discussion should take place regarding plans for further reproduction. If a woman desires a contraceptive method, she should be provided with this method and instructed on its use. She should also be instructed to call if she is experiencing emotional difficulties.

The woman who has terminated a pregnancy early for psychosocial indications should be informed that a grief reaction is common among women who have terminated pregnancies. In usual situations, women should be evaluated 2 weeks after termination for both physical and emotional adjustment to the procedure. At that time a decision about further follow-up evaluation or counseling may be made.

► Termination of Pregnancy for a Birth Defect or Genetic Indication

Terminating a pregnancy for a birth defect or a genetic indication is an area that has only been recently studied. Grief after such a termination is significant and can be long-lasting.

In one study 13 women who had previously terminated their pregnancies in a 2½-year period were interviewed (Thomson, 1985). Two of the 13 women continued to express a significant grief reaction after their termination. They had experienced major physical changes such as weight loss, the need for medication to sleep, and a change in behavior, particularly exhaustion. They expressed a significant amount of anger and guilt about their termination.

Four women continued to express a moderate grief reaction. They had difficulty maintaining their activity level and continued to feel quite angry about their loss.

Two women continued to express a mild grief reaction after their termination. They became tearful during the interview and expressed significant sadness about their loss.

Five of the 13 women interviewed appeared to have a well-resolved grief process. They expressed sadness about their loss but did not feel anger or guilt about their termination experience.

These differences in grief resolution were compared with the length of time since the termination. No major differences were observed in the women who terminated their pregnancies during the year prior to the interview compared with the women who had terminated 1 to 2 years before and those who had terminated more than 2 years before the interview.

The one factor identified that might be associated with women's resolution of their grief was birth or adoption of other children into the family after the termination.

Of the eight women who were having difficulty coping, four were planning no further children because of their increased age, their risk, or their past experience. Two of the eight women were facing a significant risk of recurrence (25%) and had not yet decided about future children. Another two of the eight women were planning pregnancies "at some time in the future."

Many factors may complicate the grief process following termination of pregnancy because of a birth defect or genetic disorder:

1. The individual or couple may have chosen to keep the news of the pregnancy private until the results of the prenatal diagnostic testing were known. The pregnancy may have been kept a secret so that if an abnormality was identified and the pregnancy was terminated, fewer people would need an explanation. This means, however, that fewer people could provide support.

2. Some women have not yet resolved their ambivalent feelings about the pregnancy. The pregnancy may have been untimed or undesired, but the decision to undergo prenatal diagnostic testing shows intent to continue the pregnancy.

3. An individual or couple who receives abnormal prenatal diagnostic results has little time for anticipatory grief. The couple may be given information about the abnormality present in the fetus one day, and termination of pregnancy may occur the next.

4. A termination of pregnancy late in the second trimester causes substantial physical pain. Cramping and blood loss occur, along with emotional anguish, all of which magnify a woman's vulnerability.

5. Guilt is a feeling expressed by almost all couples who have a child with a birth defect or genetic disorder. Most individuals or couples believe that it must be something they did or did not do to cause their child to have this problem. Thus, the guilt may add to the already complicated grief process.

6. Couples who terminate their pregnancy may not have an opportunity to see or hold their lost baby. They can only fantasize about how their baby might have looked and what he or she would have become. Usually no funeral or memorial service is held. The baby is not given a name. There may be no birth or death certificate. Nothing of the pregnancy remains. The couple has experienced a significant loss and yet it is not acknowledged by many friends, family members, or most of society.

7. Many women who have had prenatal diagnostic tests are nearing the end of their reproductive life. They may have other children who are young adults and leaving home and they may be at an age where they are beginning to be concerned about menopause. These factors too can complicate the grief process.

8. Caregivers, friends, and family may have difficulty recognizing or acknowledging that the loss of this pregnancy is significant. Many health care providers have trouble understanding why a woman would be so upset about her pregnancy termination when this is the course of action she has chosen. It is diffi-

cult for health care providers to understand that in this situation, a couple is forced to choose between two difficult alternatives, to terminate the pregnancy or to continue the pregnancy and have a child with a birth defect or genetic disorder.

Because significant grief is associated with a pregnancy termination for a birth defect or genetic indication, it is important that these families receive ongoing follow-up care after this event.

Whenever possible a couple terminating a pregnancy for a genetic indication should be seen at the time of their termination by a health care provider equipped to provide support and follow-up counseling. At the time of the termination, supportive grief counseling should be initiated. The significance of the loss should be acknowledged and the couple should be encouraged to express their sadness. A plan should be made for follow-up counseling.

Two to six weeks after the loss, the woman should have a postpregnancy evaluation. The results of any evaluation done on the fetus should be discussed with the couple. Their level of grief and the support systems available to them should be assessed. A discussion should also take place regarding future reproductive plans and methods of contraception if the couple desires.

Four to six months after the loss, a second visit with the couple should take place. This will occur at about the time of the estimated due date. It is a date that the couple will have on their minds, perhaps for many years. Again, the couple's level of grief and the support systems available should be assessed. Further discussion regarding reproduction should take place.

Depending on how the couple is coping, a third visit may be scheduled 6 to 12 months after the due date. By then the couple's grief should be fairly well resolved. They should be looking toward the future rather than back at their loss. If a delayed or distorted grief reaction is identified at this time or at any time during this process, a referral for more in-depth psychologic counseling is considered.

Pregnancy termination for a birth defect or a genetic disorder can have a tremendous impact on a couple. Support and intervention are needed to help the couple in this time of crisis. Figure 8–13 diagrams the nursing process as it relates to a client who has had a pregnancy terminated.

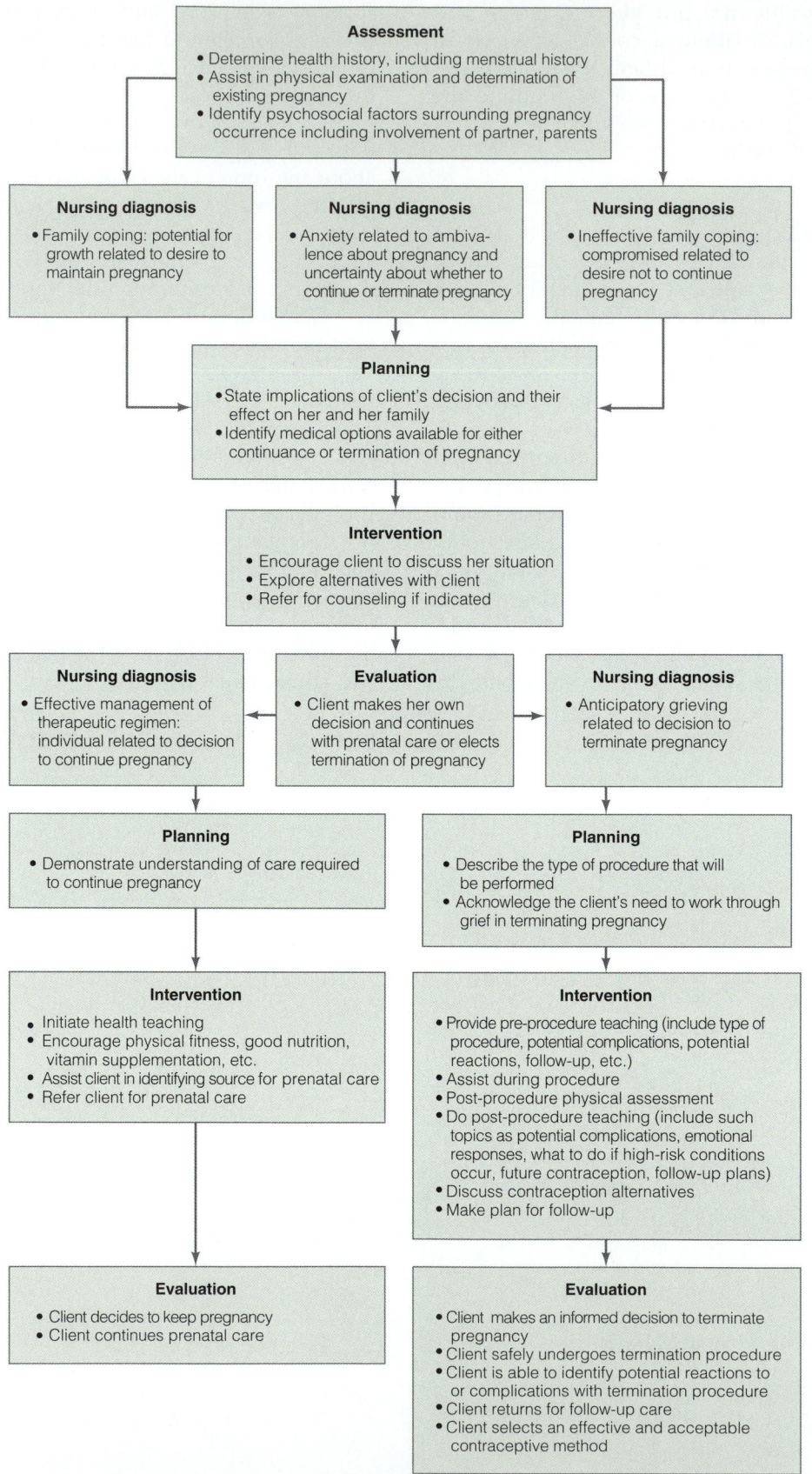

FIGURE 8–13. The nursing process as it relates to a woman who has had a pregnancy terminated.

Critical Thinking in Care Planning

Care of the Couple During Contraceptive Decision Making

Alice and Joe Paul have just delivered their fifth baby, a healthy 9-pound girl. Mother, father, and siblings are attaching well to the new baby.

Alice and Joe have been married for 6 years. Their other children are ages 5, 3, 2, and 1 years. When the nurse assesses the couple for discharge planning, Alice confides in her that although she is very happy with this baby, she hopes it will be her last. She states, "We just can't afford any more children and it's so hard to take care of so many little ones."

Alice and Joe also confide that their religious beliefs prevent use of the pill, barrier methods, or sterilization. They have been using the rhythm and coitus interruptus methods, which have not been effective, as their last three children were unplanned. After reviewing with the couple the various methods of contraception, the couple decides to use the symptothermal method to control their fertility.

▶ Assessment

- Couple indicates that they would like to use a more effective contraceptive method:
  - Have five children ages 5, 3, 2, 1, and newborn
  - State that last three were unplanned

- State that they have used "rhythm and coitus interruptus" unsuccessfully
- Have religious beliefs that preclude use of certain contraceptives
- Couple states that they would like to use the symptothermal method.

Nursing Diagnosis

Ineffective family coping: Compromised related to needed family planning

Expected Client/Family Outcomes	Nursing Action/Intervention	Evaluation
The couple will agree on a method that is compatible with their needs and beliefs before discharge.	Discuss advantages and disadvantages of available contraceptive methods.	Couple identifies a method for planning their family at the end of the discharge planning session.
The couple will relate reduced anxiety in use of the chosen method at the 6-week visit. Concerns about limiting the family size will not interfere with attachment behaviors in the immediate puerperium.	Support the couple in choosing a contraceptive method that is compatible with their religious and cultural beliefs and family needs and lifestyles. Discuss past contraceptive history with couple and identify why they feel it was not effective. *Rationale:* Discussing contraceptives in a nonjudgmental manner alleviates anxiety and motivates clients to use method properly. Anxiety can interfere with attachment behaviors; alleviation of anxiety fosters family attachment. Considering the culture and religious beliefs fosters comfort with use of contraception.	At the 6-week visit, couple relates confidence in using chosen method. At the 6-week visit, family relates and demonstrates appropriate attachment behaviors.

(continued)

Critical Thinking in Care Planning *continued*

Nursing Diagnosis

Knowledge deficit, related to selected family planning method.

Expected Client/Family Outcomes	Nursing Action/Intervention	Evaluation
On discharge, the couple will discuss effectiveness, use, and advantages and disadvantages of chosen method.	Demonstrate use of the basal thermometer, use of the chart, and methods of interpretation to couple. *Rationale:* Knowledge about usage and effectiveness of contraceptive method fosters proper and effective use.	Couple is able to discuss the effectiveness, procedure, and evaluation criteria for chosen method.
During the 6-week postpartum visit, the couple will demonstrate effective use of chosen contraceptive method.	Teach changes in cervical mucus in relation to ovulation (spinnbarkeit). Teach couple about subjective signs of ovulation such as mittelschmerz. Teach couple procedures for taking basal temperature and evaluating the temperature in relation to menstrual cycle. *Rationale:* Demonstration reinforces learning.	During 6-week visit, couple demonstrates use of the basal temperature and interprets chart that they have kept. The couple describes the objective and subjective signs of ovulation.
	Refer couple to classes on natural family planning. *Rationale:* Referral to support groups enhances learning.	The couple informs the nurse at the 6-week visit that they have attended a natural family planning support group.

Chapter Highlights

▶ Nurses have an important role in assisting individuals with family planning and act as teachers, counselors, and support and resource people for couples making contraceptive choices.

▶ The approaches that are used to identify individuals or couples at reproductive risk include obtaining a family history, assessing psychosocial factors, identifying racial and ethnic background and parental age, and discussing maternal health history, past reproductive history, and history of the present pregnancy.

▶ Genetic counseling is a problem-solving process that examines the occurrence or risk of genetic disorders in the family and involves prenatal diagnosis and, if necessary, high-risk obstetric care.

▶ A major component of contraceptive counseling is informed consent that is based on discussion of the available methods and their risks, benefits, and effectiveness.

▶ A variety of contraceptive methods are available and include, from the most effective to the least

Chapter Highlights continued

effective, sterilization, progestin implants, injectable progestogen, intrauterine devices, oral contraceptive agents, condoms, diaphragms, cervical caps, coitus interruptus, periodic abstinence, and spermicidal agents.

▶ Now trends in pregnancy prevention include the lactational amenorrhea method and emergency contraception.

▶ Pregnancy termination requires complex decision making and support of the client throughout the process.

After reading the vignette at the beginning of this chapter, use what you have hearned to answer these questions.

1. How can Ann Salzman, CNM, MSN, advocate for Scott and for Shaila Jackson in their reproductive decision making?

2. What information about available contraceptive methods should the nurse-midwife provide to help Scott and Shaila Jackson select a method that is most appropriate for them and their lifestyles?

3. How would the nurse-midwife help this couple to identify a contraceptive method that would be best for them?

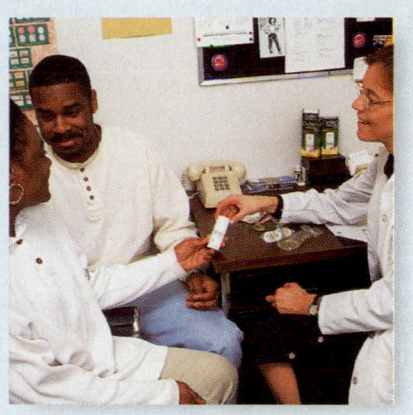

Critical Thinking Questions

▶ References

Anderson, J.E., Brackbill, R., & Mosher, W.D. (1996). Condom use for disease prevention among unmarried U.S. women. *Family Planning Perspectives, 28,* 25–28, 39.

Archer, B., Irwin, D., Jensen K., Johnson, M.E., & Rosie, J. (1997). Depot medroxyprogesterone. Management of side-effects commonly associated with its contraceptive use. *Journal of Nurse-Midwifery, 42,* 104–111.

Baird, D.T., & Glasier, A.F. (1993). Hormonal contraception. *The New England Journal of Medicine, 328,* 1543–1549.

Beckman, L.J., & Harvey, S.M. (1996). Factors affecting the consistent use of barrier methods of contraception. *Obstetrics and Gynecology, 88,* 65S–71S.

Bohamondes, L., Marchi, N.M., Cristofoletti, M. de L., Nakagava, H.M., Pellini, E., Araujo, F., & Rubin, J. (1996). Uniject® as a delivery system for the once-a-month injectable contraceptive Cyclofem® in Brazil. *Contraception, 53,* 115–119.

Brinton, L.A., Gammon, M.D., Malone, K.E., Schoenberg, J.B., Daling, J.R., & Coates, R.J. (1997). Modification of oral contraceptive relationships on breast cancer risk by selected factors among younger women. *Contraception, 55,* 197–203.

Burkman, R.T. (1996). Intrauterine devices and pelvic inflammatory disease: Evolving perspective on the data. *Obstetrical and Gynecological Survey, 51,* S35–S41.

Carmichael, S.L., & Abrams, S. (1997). A critical review of the relationship between gestational weight gain and preterm delivery. *Obstetrics and Gynecology, 89,* 865–873.

Chez, R.A., & Chapin, J. (1997). Emergency contraception. The pill's little-known secret goes public. *Lifelines, 1*(5), 28–31.

Clinical dialogue. (1993). Fitting the cervical cap. *Contemporary Obstetrics/Gynecology, 38,* 99–104.

Collaborative Group on Hormonal Factors in Breast Cancer. (1996). Breast cancer and hormonal contraceptives: Further results. *Contraception, 54,* 1S–25S.

Creasy, R.K., & Resnik, R. (1994). *Maternal-fetal medicine. Principles and practices* (3rd ed.). Philadelphia: J. B. Lippincott.

Crook, D., on behalf of the UK Desogen Study Group. (1997). Multicenter study of endocrine function and plasma lipids and lipoproteins in women using oral contraceptives containing desogestrel progestin. *Contraception, 55,* 219–224.

Cunningham, F.G., MacDonald, P.C., Gant, N.F., Leveno, K.J., Gilstrap, L.C., Hankins, G.D.V., & Clark, S.L. (1997). *Williams Obstetrics (20 ed.).* Stamford, CT: Appleton & Lange.

Cushner, I.M. (1986). Reproductive technologies: New choices, new hopes, new dilemmas. *Family Planning Perspectives, 18,* 129–132.

Davies, J.E. (1997). A second chance at preventing pregnancy. *ADVANCE for Nurse Practitioners, 5* (11), 43–47.

Delbanco, S.F., Mauldon, J., & Smith, M.D. (1997). Little knowledge and limited practice: Emergency contraceptive pills, the public, and the obstetrician-gynecologist. *Obstetrics and Gynecology, 89,* 1006–1011.

Detzer, M.J., Wendt, S.J., Solomon, L.J., Dorsch, E., Geller, B.M., Friedman, J., Hauser, H., Flynn, B.S., & Dorwaldt, A.L. (1995). Barriers to condom use among women attending planned parenthood clinics. *Women and Health, 23* (1), 91–102.

Document. (1996). Contraceptive research and development: Looking to the future. *Family Planning Perspectives, 28,* 272–274.

Donovan, P. (1984). Wrongful birth and wrongful conception: The legal and moral issues. *Family Planning Perspectives, 16,* 64–69.

Ellertson, C. (1996). History and efficacy of emergency contraception: Beyond coca-cola. *Family Planning Perspectives, 28,* 44–48.

Finch, B.E., & Green, H. (1963). *Contraception through the ages.* Springfield, IL: Charles C Thomas.

Gallagher, R., & Fuller, C.A. (1997). A new generation of oral contraceptives. *ADVANCE for Nurse Practitioners, 5*(11), 39–81.

Gil, V.E. (1995). The new female condom: Attitudes and opinions of low income Puerto Rican women at risk for HIV/AIDS. *Qualitative Health Research, 5,* 178–203.

Giovannucci, E., Ascherio, A., Rimm, E.B., Colditz, G.A., Stampfer, M.J., & Willett, W.C. (1993). A prospective study of vasectomy and prostate cancer in U.S. men. *Journal of the American Medical Association, 269,* 873–877.

Giovannucci, E., Tosteson, T.D., Speizer, F.E., Ascherio, A., Vessey, M.P., & Colditz, G.A. (1993). A retrospective study of vasectomy and prostate cancer in U.S. men. *Journal of the American Medical Association, 269,* 878–882.

Glasier, A. Emergency postcoital contraception. (1997). *The New England Journal of Medicine, 337,* 1058–1064.

Gold, M.A., Schein, A., & Coupey, S.M. (1997). Emergency contraception: A national survey of adolescent health experts. *Family Planning Perspectives, 29,* 15–19, 24.

Gollub, E.L., Stein, Z., & el-Sadr, W. (1995). Short-term acceptability of the female condom among staff and patients at a New York City hospital. *Family Planning Perspectives, 27,* 155–158.

Grady, W.R., Klepinger, D.H., Billy, J.O., & Taufer, K. (1993). Condom characteristics: The perceptions and preferences of men in the United States. *Family Planning Perspectives, 25,* 67–73.

Grady, W.R., Tanfer, K., Billy, J.O., & Lincoln-Hanson, J. (1996). Men's perceptions of their roles and responsibilities regarding sex, contraception and childbearing. *Family Planning Perspectives, 28,* 221–226.

Granberg, D., & Granberg, B. (1980). Abortion attitudes 1965–1980: Trends and determinants. *Family Planning Perspectives, 12,* 250–261.

Grimes, D. (ed.). (1995). Contraception and adolescents: Highlights from the NASPAG Conference. *The Contraception Report: Contraception and Adolescents, VI* (3), 4–7, 10–11, 14.

Grimes, D.A. (1997). Emergency contraception: Expanding opportunities for primary prevention. *The New England Journal of Medicine, 337,* 1078–1079.

Hannaford, P.C., Kay, C.R., Vessey, M.P., Painter, R., & Mant, J. (1997). Combined oral contraceptives and liver disease. *Contraception, 55,* 145–151.

Harper, S., & Ellertson, C. (1995). Knowledge and perceptions of emergency contraceptive pills among a college-age population: A qualitative approach. *Family Planning Perspectives, 27,* 149–154.

Harvey, S.M., Beckman, L.J., Castle, M.A., & Coyteaux, F. (1995). Knowledge and perceptions of medical abortion among potential users. *Family Planning Perspectives, 27,* 203–207.

Hatcher, R.A., Trussell, J., Stewart, F., Stewart, G.K., Kowal, D., Guest, F., Cates, W. Jr., & Poindexter, M.S. (1994). *Contraceptive technology* (16th Rev. ed.). New York: Irvington.

Hayes, R.B., Pottern, L.M., Greenberg, R., Schoenberg, J., Swanson, G.M., Liff, J., Schwartz, A.G., Brown, L.M., & Hoover, R.N. (1993). Vasectomy and prostate cancer in U.S. blacks and whites. *American Journal of Epidemiology, 137,* 263–269.

Henshaw, S. (1986). Trends in abortions 1982–1984. *Family Planning Perspectives, 18,* 34.

Hight-Laukaran, V., Labbok, M.H., Peterson, A.E., Fletcher, V., von Hertzen, H., & Van Look, P.F.A. (1997). Multicenter study of the Lactational Amenorrhea Method (LAM): II. Acceptability, utility, and policy implications. *Contraception, 55,* 337–346.

Indian Council of Medical Research Task Force on Natural Family Planning. (1996). Field trial of Billings Ovulation Method of natural family planning. *Contraception, 53,* 69–74.

Kalmuss, D., Davidson, A.R., Cushman, L. E., Heartwell, S., & Rutlin, M. (1996). Determinants of early implant discontinuation among low-income women. *Family Planning Perspectives, 28,* 256–260.

Kaunitz, A.M., & Jordan, C.W. (1997). Two long-acting hormonal contraceptive options. *Contemporary OB/GYN, February,* 27–38, 43–48, 50–51.

Klitsch, M. (1995). Still waiting for the contraceptive revolution. *Family Planning Perspectives, 27,* 246–253.

Kopala, B. (1997). The Human Genome Project: Issues and ethics. *MCN, the American Journal of Maternal/Child Nursing, 32,* 9–15.

Labbok, M.H., Hight-Laukaran, V., Peterson, A.E., Fletcher, V., von Hertzen, H., & Van Look, P.F.A. (1997). Multicenter study of the Lactational Amenorrhea Method (LAM): I. Efficacy, duration, and implications for clinical application. *Contraception, 55,* 327–336.

Lewis, M.A., Heinemann, L.A.J., Spitzer, W.O., MacRae, K.D., & Bruppacher, R, for the Transnational Research Group on Oral Contraceptives and the Health of Young Women. (1997). The use of oral contraceptives and the occurrence of acute myocardial infarction in young women. *Contraception, 56,* 129–140.

Lewis, M.A., Spitzer, W.O., Heinemann, L.A.J., MacRae, K.D., Bruppacher, R., & Thorogood, M; on behalf of the Transnational Research Group on Oral Contraceptives and the Health of Young Women. (1996). Third generation oral contraceptives and risk of myocardial infaction: An international case-control study. *British Medical Journal, 312,* 88–90.

Lindberg, C.E. (1997). Emergency contraception: The nurse's role in providing postcoital options. *Journal of Obstetric, Gynecologic, and Neonatal Nursing, 26,* 145–152.

Lindberg, L.D., Sonenstein, F.L., Ku, L., & Levine, G. (1997). Young men's experience with condom breakage. *Family Planning Perspectives, 29,* 128–131, 140.

Mackenzie, S.J., & Yeo, S. (1997). Pregnancy interruption using mifepristone (RU 486). A new choice for women in the USA. *Journal of Nurse-Midwifery, 42,* 86–90.

Marion, L.C., & Cox, C.L. (1996). Condom use and fertility among divorced and separated women. *Nursing Research, 45,* 110–115.

Mauck, C.K., Baker, J.M., Barr, S. P., Abercrombie, T.J., & Archer, D.F. (1997). A phase 1 comparative study of contraceptive vaginal films containing benzalkonium chloride and nonoxynol-9. Postcoital testing and colposcopy. *Contraception, 56,* 89–96.

Mauck, C.K., Baker, J.M., Barr, S.P., Johanson, W.M., & Archer, D.F. (1997). A phase-1 comparative study of three contraceptive vaginal films containing nonoxynol-9. Postcoital testing and colposcopy. *Contraception, 56,* 97–102.

Miller, W.B. (1986). Why some women fail to use their contraceptive method: A psychological investigation. *Family Planning Perspectives, 18,* 27–32.

Moore, P.J., Adler, N.E., & Kegeles, S.M. (1996). Adolescents and the contraceptive pill: Impact of beliefs on intention and use. *Obstetrics and Gynecology, 88,* 48S–56S.

Moreno, J.E., Khan-Dawood, F.S., & Goldzieher, J.W. (1997). Natural family planning: Suitability of the CUE™ method for defining the time of ovulation. *Contraception, 55,* 233–237.

Morin, K.H. (1998). Perinatal outcomes of obese women: A critical review of the literature. *Journal of Obstetric, Gynecologic, and Neonatal Nursing, 27,* 431–440.

Parker, R.M., Williams, M.V., Baker, D.W., & Nurss, J.R. (1996). Literacy and contraception: Exploring the link. *Obstetrics and Gynecology, 88,* 72S–77S.

Pasquale, S. (1996). Clinical experience with today's IUD. *Obstetrical and Gynecological Survey, 51,* S25–S29.

Peterson, H.B., Xia, Z., Hughes, J.M., Wilcox, L.S., Tylor, L.R., Trussell, J., for the U. S. Collaborative Review of Sterilization Working Group. (1996). The risk of pregnancy after tubal sterilization: Findings from the U. S. Collaborative Review of Sterilization. *American Journal of Obstetrics and Gynecology, 174,* 1161–1170.

Potter, L., Oakley, D., de Leon-Wong, E., & Cañamar, R. (1996). Measuring compliance among oral contraceptive users. *Family Planning Perspectives, 28,* 154–158.

Ramos, R., Kennedy, K.I., & Visness, C.M. (1996). Effectiveness of lactational amenorrhea in prevention of pregnancy in Manila, Philippines: Non-comparative prospective trial. *British Medical Journal, 313,* 909–912.

Reifsnider, E. (1997). On the horizon: New options for contraception. *Journal of Obstetric, Gynecologic, and Neonatal Nursing, 26,* 91–100.

Ringheim, K. (1995). Evidence for the acceptibility of an injectable hormonal method for men. *Family Planning Perspectives, 27,* 123–128.

Rogow, D., & Horowitz, S. (1995). Withdrawal: A review of the literature and an agenda for research. *Studies in Family Planning, 26,* 140–153.

Rosenberg, M.J., & Waugh, M.S. (1997). Latex condom breakage and slippage in a controlled clinical trial. *Contraception, 56,* 17–21.

Rosenblatt, K.A., Thomas, D.B., & The WHO Collaborative Study of Neoplasia and Steriod Contraceptives. (1996). Intrauterine devices and endometrial cancer. *Contraception, 54,* 329–332.

Sangi-Haghpeykar, H., Poindexter, A.N., Bateman, L., & Ditmore, J.R. (1996). Experience of injectable contraceptive users in an urban setting. *Obstetrics and Gynecology, 88,* 227–233.

Santelli, J.S., Davis, M., Celentano, D.D., Crump, A.D., & Burwell, L.G. (1995). Combined use of condoms with other contraceptive methods among inner-city Baltimore women. *Family Planning Perspectives, 27,* 74–78.

Santelli, J.S., Kouzis, A.C., Hoover, D.R., Polacsek, M., Burwell, L.G., & Celentano, D.D. (1996). Stage of behavior change for condom use: The influence of partner type, relationship and pregnancy factors. *Family Planning Perspectives, 28,* 101–107.

Schwartz, S.M., Siscovick, D.S., Longstreth, W.T., Psaty, B.M., Beverly, K., Raghunathan, T.E., Lin, D., & Koepsell, T.D. (1997). Use of low-dose oral contraceptives and stroke in young women. *Annals of Internal Medicine, 127,* 596–603.

Sherwen, L.N., & Miele, N. (1986). Assessing and identifying the high-risk pregnancy: A holistic approach. *Topics in Clinical Nursing, 8,* 33–34.

Sivin, I., Lahteenmaki, P., Ranta, S., Darney, P., Klaisle, C., Wan, L., Mishell, D.R., Lacarra, M., Viegas, O.A.C., Bilhareus, P., Koetsawang, S., Piya-Anant, M., Diaz, S., Pavez, M., Alvarez, F., Brache, V., LaGuardia, K., Nash, H., & Stern, J. (1997). Levonorgestrel concentrations during use of levonorgestrel rod (LNG ROD) implants. *Contraception, 55,* 81–85.

Sivin, I., Viegas, O., Campodonico, I., Diaz, S., Pavez, M., Wan, L., Koetsawang, S., Kiriwat, O., Piya-Anant, M., Holma, P., el din Abdalla, K., & Stern, J. (1997). Clinical performance of a new two-rod levonorgestrel contraceptive implant; A three-year randomized study with Norplant® implants as controls. *Contraception, 55,* 73–80.

Spitzer, W.O., Lewis, M.A., Heinemann, A.J., Thorogood, M., & MacRae, K.D., on behalf of the Transnational Research Group on Oral Contraceptives and the Health of Young Women. (1996). Third generation oral contraceptives and risk of venous thromboembolic disorders: An international case-control study. *British Medical Journal, 312,* 83–88.

Stewart, F.H. (1996). Contraception in the United States: Overview and priorities for improvement. *Obstetrical and Gynecological Survey, 51*(12), S4–S7.

Suissa, S., Blais, L., Spitzer, W.O., Cusson, J., Lewis, M., & Heinemann, L. (1997). First-time use of newer oral contraceptives and the risk of venous thromboembolism. *Contraception, 56,* 141–146.

Tagg, P.I. (1995). The diaphragm: Barrier contraception has a new social role. *Nurse Practitioner, 20* (12), 36–42.

Thomas, D.B., Ray, R.M., & the World Health Organization Collaborative Study of Neoplasia and Steriod Contraceptives. (1996). Oral contraceptives and invasive adenocarcinoma and adenosquamous carcinomas of the uterine cervix. *American Journal of Epidemiology, 144,* 218–289.

Thomson, E. (1985). Early pregnancy loss. *March of Dimes/Birth Defects Foundation, Original Article Series, Strategies for Genetic Counselling, 23,* 37–44.

Tinkle, M.B., & Sterling, B.S. (1997). Neural tube defects: A primary prevention role for nurses. *Journal of Obstetric, Gynecologic, and Neonatal Nursing, 26,* 503–512.

Trent, A.J., & Clark, K. (1997). What nurses should know about natural family planning. *Journal of Obstetric, Gynecologic, and Neonatal Nursing, 26,* 643–648.

Trussell, J., Strickler, J., & Vaughan, B. (1993). Contraceptive efficacy of the diaphragm, the sponge, and the cervical cap. *Family Planning Perspectives, 25,* 100–105.

Trussell, J., Ellertson, C., & Stewart, F. (1996). The effectiveness of the Yuzpe regimen of emergency contraception. *Family Planning Perspectives, 28,* 58–64, 87.

von Hertzen, H., & Van Look, P.F.A. (1996). Research on new methods of emergency contraception. *Family Planning Perspectives, 28,* 52–57, 88.

Waetjen, L.E., & Grimes, D.A. (1996). Oral contraceptives and primary liver cancer: Temporal trends in three countries. *Obstetrics and Gynecology, 88,* 945–949.

Westfall, J.M., Main, D.S., & Barnard, L. (1996). Continuation rates among injectable contraceptive users. *Family Planning Perspectives, 28,* 275–277.

Westhoff, C.L. (1996a). Current assessment of the use of intrauterine devices. *Journal of Nurse-Midwifery, 41,* 218–223.

Westhoff, C.L. (1996b). The IUD in evolution. *Obstetrical and Gynecological Survey, 51,* S20–S24.

Wilcox, L.S., Martinez-Schnell, B., Peterson, H.B., Ware, J.H., & Hughes, J.M. (1992). Menstrual function after tubal sterilization. *American Journal of Epidemiology, 135,* 1368–1381.

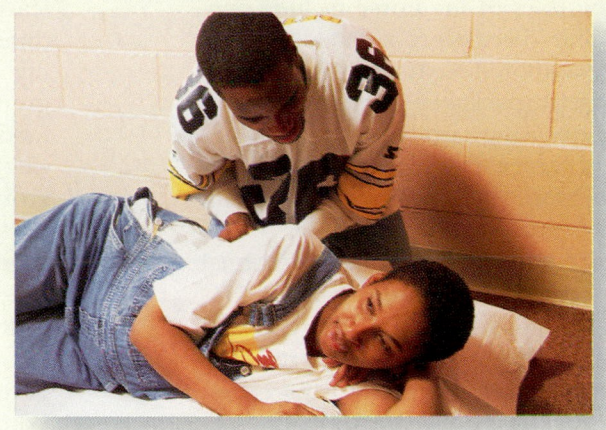

Tamika and Rashid Dengler, who are 36 weeks pregnant, are attending a childbirth education class. As part of class activities, they are practicing patterned breathing for use in labor and delivery. Rashid helps Tamika to lie on the floor on her side; he kneels behind her and supports her back with a pillow. Tamika focuses her attention on her favorite bracelet, a gift from Rashid, and begins the breathing pattern. Rashid breathes with her. Tamika suddenly realizes she forgot to make two important phone calls. She abruptly stops the exercise. Rashid also stops and asks, "What happened?" Tamika sighs and states, "I don't know how I can concentrate on breathing when I have a million other thoughts running through my mind. Will I be able to do this when I really am in labor?" ∎

9

Educational Preparation for Childbirth

The opportunity for client teaching arises in nearly every setting in which nurses interact with pregnant families. The teaching roles of the nurse include one-to-one explanation and discussion, client education classes, and nurse-authored pamphlets, articles, books, and audiovisual packages directed toward education of the childbearing family. These roles are equally important; however, the scope and focus of the roles are not the same and, therefore, different objectives and strategies are required.

All clients require and benefit from educational preparation for childbearing and early parenting. Differences in cultural and educational background among clients challenge the nurse to present material that is acceptable and understandable to the client. This chapter discusses appropriate educational preparation that includes teaching related to physical and psychosocial changes of childbearing, childbirth alternatives, and ways in which the client and her family can best be prepared for advancing pregnancy, labor, delivery, and the newborn.

► TEACHING AND LEARNING CONSIDERATIONS DURING CHILDBEARING

Much has been written about how people learn. The process, of course, requires information (cognitive domain), but also involves the learner's attitude and readiness to learn (affective domain) and the learner's ability to perform whatever skills are necessary (psychomotor domain) (Bloom, 1982). For example, if a couple wants to use a certain method of childbirth preparation, they must be given information about childbirth and the techniques necessary for the method. In addition, they must be motivated to seek out the teaching sessions and attend them. If their knowledge base is incomplete, if they do not care to learn about the method, or if they do not master the techniques, they cannot be expected to have a positive birth experience using their chosen approach. If the nurse presents information on a level the couple cannot understand, if classes are held at times incompatible with the couple's work schedules, or if opportunity for supervised practice is not provided during the classes, the nurse, rather than the clients, establishes an ineffective teaching–learning situation.

Whether providing on-the-spot teaching in a labor room or planning a series of childbirth classes, the nurse must consider several factors:

1. Who are the learners? What are their demographic characteristics, especially with regard to their cultural backgrounds and socioeco-nomic and educational levels? Although it may be assumed that people are capable of learning, teaching strategies differ greatly for different learners. For example, diet counseling for women from financially poor backgrounds needs to focus on low-cost nutritious foods, whereas price might not even be a consideration for women from wealthy backgrounds. The client's cultural background must also be considered when devising appropriate teaching strategies. The box entitled Teaching Strategies for Clients from Diverse Cultures presents teaching strategies appropriate for clients from various cultural backgrounds.

2. What is the purpose and length of the teaching–learning situation? Is the nurse providing anticipatory guidance for one clinic visit? Is the nurse assuming a major ongoing responsibility for assisting couples to prepare for childbirth through a series of classes? Definition of the purpose and length of the teaching–learning situation is essential to the planning of any content.

3. In what setting will the teaching–learning situation take place? Will the nurse be interacting with the client in an examination room, a labor and delivery suite, a postpartum room, a birth center, or a classroom? Will more than one client or client–family be present, as in a prepared childbirth class? Assessment of the setting is crucial to the development of effective strategies.

4. What does the nurse expect the learners to be able to do after attending the teaching sessions? Will they be able to state in their own words reasons to avoid over-the-counter medications? Will they be able to demonstrate relaxation and control techniques as taught in prepared childbirth classes? Whether teaching takes place in a clinic or classroom, the nurse needs to specify in advance behavioral objectives for each client. These objectives need to be stated in terms of readily observable or measurable client behaviors. Such expressions as "clients will *know,* will *feel,* will *understand,*" need to be avoided, as these are not possible to evaluate as stated. Clients could, however, demonstrate knowledge by defining "false labor" or by performing a certain breathing technique appropriately.

In a classic project, Bloom and colleagues developed a taxonomy of educational objectives. (1982; Krathwohl et al., 1982) This taxonomy provided a means for classifying educational goals from the simplest to the most complex learning behaviors. It dealt with three major domains of learning: cognitive, affective, and psychomotor. The cognitive domain focused on the recall or identification of knowledge and on the development of intellectual abilities and skills. The affective domain dealt with objectives describing interest, attitudes, and values and the evolution of appreciations and adequate adjustment. The psychomotor domain focused on the development of manipulative or motor skills (Bloom, 1982). Developed as a means to facilitate communication, the taxonomy allowed an individual in a teaching role not only to identify what behaviors or goals were expected of the learners but also to state those goals in an appropriate fashion.

5. What is to be taught? How much content can realistically be presented? What content *must* be presented by the nurse? What material can be presented through teaching aids, such as written literature and audiovisual presentations in a clinic or class? The nurse must realize that "everything" cannot be taught at once or by one person. For example, it is more important for a woman contemplating pregnancy to be taught about the potential hazards of drugs and alcohol than it is for her to be taught about infant care. Client assessment helps the nurse tailor an educational program to meet the unique learning needs of the family. Information is prioritized so that the most important concepts are adequately presented. These decisions evolve from consideration of where the client is in the childbearing cycle, the extent of the nurse's teaching role, where the teaching will take place, and the amount of time available for teaching. One *ineffective* strategy is to present large amounts of detailed information in a short period. In addition, nurses should note the amount of time available for nurse–client interaction and follow a presentation schedule. Teaching plans give the nurse an agenda to ensure that a standard of information is provided to all clients.

6. What content will be presented by other health professionals? Although teaching is a major nursing role, it is not solely the domain of nursing. Nurses often refer clients to childbirth education programs that are taught in part by other health care professionals. Nurses caring for a childbearing family should identify topics that they will present and topics that will be presented by other health care profession-

als, for example, fellow nurses, nurse-midwives, physicians, and nutritionists. Through collaboration, teaching is less likely to be duplicated, time is used more effectively, and the expertise of each professional is more likely to be employed. The nurse has the responsibility to find out what is being taught and to make certain that other health care professionals working with the childbearing family know what information will be covered by the nurse. Collaborative teaching plans and instruction guides, listing teaching content, the individuals who will cover the content, the dates and special comments are ways to implement an interdisciplinary approach. Nurses must also assess their own feelings regarding their teaching roles and identify behaviors that they use to deal with the discomfort they have in teaching–learning situations.

7. Which strategies will be most effective in helping clients achieve objectives? Which methods will present the material most clearly? To determine these answers, a nurse must be creative. Strategies that work effectively with one client or group of clients may not be as helpful with others. For example, if a woman cannot read, visual presentations and discussions are considered. Although teaching aids such as films, models, and games can help learning, they should not replace nurse–client discussion.

8. Which methods of evaluation are appropriate for the clients and for the teaching–learning situation? Although paper-and-pencil tests are common in school, they may not be the best choice in clinical settings. Return demonstrations or a client's presenting information in her own words are more suitable. Evaluation should always directly relate to the objectives. For example, if one objective of a class on infant bathing specifies that the mother will independently bathe her infant according to the procedure shown in the class, the evaluation should assess whether mothers who attended the class did indeed bathe their infants in the prescribed manner.

9. What questions will aid in evaluation or provide additional information needed by the nurse for client assessment? The ability to ask effective questions is an art that can be developed by the nurse with careful thought, consultation, and practice. The nurse should not rely on questions that require culturally conditioned "yes" or "no" answers or that assume

▶ TEACHING STRATEGIES FOR CLIENTS FROM DIVERSE CULTURES

Respect the client's traditions and ideas. Know your limits. Be kind. Share your knowledge.

Understand belief systems surrounding pregnancy, labor and birth, and postpartum/infant care for the client population. Listen to the client's questions. Clients will tell you their values, customs, and priorities through their questions.

Plan a teaching strategy:

- Teach the smallest amount needed to do the job. List only a few words at a time.
- Make your points as vividly as you can. Use simple language. Illustrate. Use active voice. Use headings.
- Have clients restate and demonstrate the information. Have clients share in a group and translate information into real-life situations.
- Review repeatedly. Skip records and calendars; different cultures have different time orientations.

The plan must be "by the people, for the people."

ENVIRONMENT

- Make your environment acceptable to your population.
- Make the location a place in which clients can find sameness with themselves.
- Provide clients with positive role models: posters, artwork from community members or organizations, enlargements of 35-mm photographs of members of the community.

ONE-ON-ONE COUNSELING

- Keep a file of commonly asked questions; use many illustrations, not many words.
- Create a flip chart with illustrations of common cultural beliefs and expected health care practices.
- Make up flash cards with common procedures in clients' language, including illustrations.
- Set up a language bank. Have accessible bilingual staff, client education materials in clients' language, list of common phrases for clinical area, on-site community college language course.

GROUP EDUCATION

- Encourage group discussion.
- Avoid questions that require "yes" or "no" answers.

- Encourage discussion of cultural approaches.
- Role-play what to do in various situations, and have the learners provide the cues.
- Set up link on the community level for referral for health care.

VIDEOS

- Interact with your audiovisual.
- The more you interact, the more your audience will interact.
- Turn off the video, show certain sections, and talk over parts.
- In previewing films, choose those not longer than 10 minutes. Look for people from the culture in the film. Note use of street or professional language. Determine accuracy of information and target audience.

WRITTEN MATERIALS

- Present written materials in a culturally acceptable manner.
- Use advance organizers. Put first things first. Summarize and review.
- Use active voice and conversational style. Use short words and sentences. Keep concept density low. Use words consistently.
- Avoid stylized pictures. Avoid cartoons, which can be confusing. Use simple pictures, drawings, or diagrams. Include all anatomic parts; this makes it easier for clients to locate body parts and also provokes less fear.
- Develop written materials in languages used by clients. To avoid inaccurate or insulting translations, have translations done only by individuals who know the language and subject well.
- Some people cannot read; however, clients can learn effectively despite their inability to read or write. Alternative strategies should be used in this situation. Any printed material should rely on a pictorial presentation.

Courtesy of Christina Ippolito Moore, RN, MS.

---

that the client has a great deal of obstetric information (see box entitled Examples of Effective and Ineffective Questions for Use with the Childbearing Family). Teaching effectively does not require that the nurse discuss each piece of content. Alternative strategies, for example, videos shown in clinic waiting rooms or at the bedside on the postpartum unit, can provide information and allow more nurse–client time for teaching other important topics. Client education materials have been developed by private and nonprofit groups for the childbearing family. The cost of appropriate audiovisual packages can be included in

▶ EXAMPLES OF EFFECTIVE AND INEFFECTIVE QUESTIONS FOR USE WITH THE CHILDBEARING FAMILY

EFFECTIVE QUESTIONS

What brings you to the clinic today?

What has been making you feel uncomfortable since your last visit?

What worries or concerns do you have about this pregnancy, labor and delivery, your new baby, and so forth?

What have you liked about the prepared childbirth series?

What did you find not to your liking about the prepared childbirth series? What things would make the classes more helpful to future expectant parents?

Can you describe the diet you have been following since your last visit? In what ways have you found the prescribed prenatal diet to be easy to follow (or difficult to follow)?

Show me how you do the psychoprophylactic breathing exercises.

INEFFECTIVE QUESTIONS

How are you?

Do you have any questions?

Are you following the diet instructions you received at your last visit?

Is everything okay?

Do you know how to do the breathing exercises for labor and delivery?

Do you like the prepared childbirth classes?

---

unit and program budgets. Nurses can also author these types of packages and seek grants for financial support in their development. A less expensive method is to collaborate on the production of health promotion programs with faculty and students in the nursing program at a local university. Frequently, students receive course credit for working on such projects. In addition, nursing faculty who want to remain clinically involved may find that collaborative projects to produce educational materials for the childbearing family are a way to meet this personal objective. Such collaborative projects between nursing faculty and nurses in clinical practice also strengthen relationships between nursing education and nursing service.

10. What factors related to the physical needs and convenience of childbearing clients need to be considered in teaching–learning situations? For example, classes planned for third-trimester clients need to incorporate opportunities for breaks, movement, and change of position, as pregnant women have difficulty sitting for long periods. Classes should be scheduled so that couples can easily attend.

An extensive literature exists on the topics of teaching and learning. Table 9–1 lists categories of learning objectives with examples of their application to childbearing clients. Broad consideration of teaching–learning theory and its application to nursing is, however, beyond the scope of this textbook.

▶ PREPARATION OF THE EXPECTANT PARENTS

▶ Educational Preparation Classes During Different Phases of Childbearing

Although procreation is a normal cultural expectation, it is not easy. The physical and emotional changes of childbearing, often accompanied by alterations in lifestyle, can produce situational and developmental crises for the childbearing family (see Chapter 4). Educational preparation can allay fears and involve clients in selecting lifestyle behaviors that promote obstetric health and make them aware of risk factors during childbearing. Ideally, prenatal education should begin prior to pregnancy; formalized classes should start early in pregnancy and extend across the childbearing year, that is, from conception to 3 months after delivery (Biasella, 1993). This gives the family time to absorb information, to understand the processes of childbearing and beginning parenthood, and to make informed choices about their childbearing experience. Table 9–2 presents a content outline for prenatal education.

Preconception

Factors that extend from earliest childhood have an impact on general health and on parenting perceptions and practices throughout the adult years. Such elements include the individual's lifestyle, state of health, own experiences with parents or parenting fig-

▶ **TABLE 9-1**

Selected Categories of Learning Objectives

Category	Example of Objective ("The pregnant couple will . . .")
Cognitive	
Knowledge	
Define	Define terms specific to pregnancy.
Identify	Identify the components of a healthy pregnancy diet.
Comprehension	
Interpret	Interpret experienced physiologic changes during pregnancy.
Translate	Translate health practices to self-care during pregnancy.
Application	
Apply	Apply exercises learned during childbirth classes to a 15-minute practice session.
Affective	
Valuing	
Accept	Accept responsibility for developing a birth plan.
Commit	Commit to health care practices during pregnancy.
Psychomotor	
Skill Acquisition	
Acquire	Acquire skills in caring for a newborn.
Physical Ability	
Endure	Endure labor and delivery with the help of learned breathing techniques.

ures, cultural heritage, religious background, personal attitude, current support and situation, schooling, and exposure to media portrayals of families and parents.

A primary nursing goal during this period is non-judgmental assessment of the client, including her informal and formal preparation for parenthood. The nurse should realize that not all of life's prepregnancy experiences are desirable or positive. For example, a woman whose family depends heavily on her income may realistically be worried about the amount of time she can manage away from work or the quality of child care that she can afford.

During the preconceptional phase, clients expecting to get pregnant may become interested in learning about or selecting obstetric caregivers and care settings. Education dealing with obstetric choices is therefore important.

Despite years of schooling, many American children receive little information about childbearing and parenting. Nurses can participate in preconceptional education as consultants, speakers, and teachers in schools, community and religious organizations, and in wellness care settings. They can author, produce, and consult on media projects dealing with childbearing and they can counsel clients in clinical settings. Topics related to preconceptional preparation for childbearing might include physical and mental health, the importance of early prenatal care, safety, risk factors (including alcohol and other drugs), and strategies for selecting obstetric caregivers and obstetric facilities.

First Trimester

Early-pregnancy education for a family during the first trimester may be sponsored by individuals or groups, such as childbirth education associations, clinics, physicians, certified nurse-midwives, and obstetric nurses. In addition, the media reach large viewing, listening, and reading audiences. Some early pregnancy educational programs exist; however, most prenatal teaching is done during the third trimester to prepare clients for the "big event" of childbirth.

The first trimester is when men and women choose obstetric caregivers and settings and seek early obstetric care; they begin a relationship with health care providers that will continue at least through the postpartum period. Although some women have prior contact through gynecologic care visits or previous obstetric experiences, others make contact for the first time. It may be difficult for clients to obtain information about alternative obstetric settings; however, client education through the media or by groups that do not have a vested interest in a particular agency may help present the range of obstetric choices available to the family. Nurses also need to evaluate the extent to which their teaching presents obstetric options objectively.

The major purposes of first-trimester prenatal education are to explain the changes taking place within the woman's body, identify changes within the family system, assist clients to identify normal reactions to being newly pregnant, and offer information that may help pregnant clients to identify risk factors

▶ **TABLE 9-2**

Outline for Prenatal Education

At the earliest contact between client and nurse, a teaching plan is developed. This reflects the unique learning needs of each client and incorporates information that health care providers identify as essential for all pregnant women to know and information that clients identify as learning priorities. The outline is reviewed with the client and updated whenever necessary. Client referral to individuals or organizations sponsoring childbirth education can also be appropriate for meeting overall learning objectives.

Preconception

How pregnancy occurs (menstrual cycle)

Lifestyle factors with potential impact on becoming pregnant and on early pregnancy: drugs such as alcohol, nutritional status, general health, occupational and environmental considerations

Alternatives in childbirth settings and in obstetric caregivers

Pregnancy tests

Myths about conception and pregnancy

First Trimester

Feelings about pregnancy, ambivalence, developmental tasks of early pregnancy, age-related issues

Family reactions to pregnancy, first-trimester emotional responses of expectant fathers

Early-pregnancy physical changes

Sexuality during the first trimester

Lifestyle factors with potential impact on early pregnancy: drugs such as alcohol, nutrition (including prescribed vitamin and iron supplements), general health, exercise, rest, occupational and environmental considerations

Warning signs of early pregnancy

Fear of miscarriage (suggested presentation as a topic in a group setting)

First-trimester diagnostic tests for maternal/fetal well-being (as appropriate)

Client expectations for pregnancy and childbirth

Options available to client within the selected prenatal and delivery setting, tour of birthing facility

Anticipatory guidance regarding what to expect at prenatal visits

Sibling concerns, telling other children about pregnancy

Resources within the caregiving agency or private practice and within the community (including relevant literature)

Second Trimester

Feelings about pregnancy, acceptance of pregnancy, developmental tasks of midpregnancy, age-related issues

Family responses to progressing pregnancy, second-trimester responses of expectant fathers

Fetal growth and development

Midtrimester physical changes, relief of discomforts associated with enlarging fetus and physical changes

Sexuality during the second trimester

Lifestyle factors with potential impact on midpregnancy: drugs such as alcohol, smoking, nutrition (including prescribed vitamin and iron supplements), general health, exercise, body mechanics, rest, occupational and environmental considerations, stress

Changes in activities of daily living related to midpregnancy

Warning signs of midpregnancy

Diagnostic tests for assessment of maternal/fetal well-being (as necessary)

Client's expectations for pregnancy and birth

Client's fears and anxieties related to second trimester

Sibling concerns

Client expectations for pregnancy and childbirth, confirmation of registration for third-trimester prenatal classes

Third Trimester

Feelings about pregnancy, developmental tasks of third trimester

Preparation for labor, delivery, and parenting (Content may be given by health care providers during prenatal visits or can be offered in greater depth during a series of prepared childbirth classes)

Client expectations for labor and birth, progress of prepared childbirth classes

Family reactions to advanced pregnancy; third-trimester emotional responses of expectant fathers; sibling preparation

Late-pregnancy physical changes, management of discomforts related to late pregnancy

Sexuality during the third trimester

Lifestyle factors with potential impact on late pregnancy: drugs such as alcohol, nutrition (including prescribed vitamin and iron supplements), smoking, general health, exercise, body mechanics, rest, occupational and environmental considerations

Signs of labor, "true" labor versus "false" labor, physiology of labor and delivery, passenger, passage, powers, and psyche in labor

Positioning in labor

Techniques useful during labor and delivery

Analgesia and anesthesia during labor and delivery, medications used during labor and delivery; nonpharmacologic strategies for pain management (breathing strategies, relaxation techniques, massage, etc.)

Technology and childbirth, assessment of fetal maturity, potential for induction or augmentation of labor, potential use of electronic fetal monitoring, intravenous infusions, and so on

Variations in labor

The high-risk experience: potential for operative obstetrics (e.g., forceps, episiotomy, cesarean childbirth); potential for transfer from birthing center, home, or birthing room because of obstetric complications; potential for family-centered birth despite operative obstetrics

Warning signs of late pregnancy, signs and symptoms of premature labor

Review of birth plan, anticipatory guidance regarding what can be expected within the selected labor and delivery setting

Discussion of fears and concerns related to late pregnancy, labor and delivery, or postpartum

Role-play and activities for problem solving during parturition.

Tour of labor and delivery setting

Preparations for client's stay in hospital or birth center, preparations for a home birth

Preparations for other family members during client's birthing experience and immediate recovery (e.g., child care for siblings)

Preparations for the newborn, selection of a pediatric caregiver (may include a prenatal introductory meeting)

Infant nutrition, preparation for breastfeeding or bottle feeding

Early parenting

What to expect from caregivers and the health care system during labor, delivery, and postpartum

Anticipatory guidance for postpartum (includes physical and emotional changes, family changes, and strategies for coping)

Resources available during third trimester and postpartum

and to make lifestyle changes that can promote good health for themselves and their unborn baby.

Early prenatal education may also reduce the confusion and anxiety that precedes late pregnancy (when classes were most often offered). In addition, it may challenge women to learn more about pregnancy, childbirth, and parenting.

Formats for prenatal education range from a single class only for pregnant women to a series of classes for women and their support persons. Probably no "best" format can be recommended for all first-trimester teaching settings.

Success of first-trimester programs depends largely on the commitment of the nurse and the sponsoring agency. Commitment extends beyond words to the provision of adequate funds, space, time, and personnel to make such a program possible. In designing first-trimester classes, the nurse must assess current literature, the client population, factors that motivate clients to attend sessions, and the resources available in his or her own setting. Networking with nurse colleagues who have been involved in first-trimester prenatal education is also suggested.

A teaching plan is used for each class and is based on assessment of the pregnant family's learning needs. The plan has several functions:

- To identify learning objectives in terms of client behaviors
- To specify content that needs to be presented to help the woman and her family during childbearing and early parenthood
- To designate criteria to be used to evaluate client achievement of learning goals

The plan follows the steps of the nursing process. It is reviewed for each prenatal visit, and attainment of learning objectives is marked as pregnancy progresses. It is not appropriate to wait until the postpartum period to evaluate all objectives stated in the teaching plan.

Second Trimester

Discussion of midpregnancy educational programs is rare in the literature. Formal midpregnancy classes are not widely available. Those in existence tend to focus on exercise during pregnancy and are taught by individuals with interest in physical fitness. For couples seeking prenatal care through hospital or private physician-based practices, educational preparation evolves mainly from office and clinic visit encounters with individual health care providers. A more comprehensive education is often provided by nurse-midwives. A strong philosophic emphasis on collaboration between client and caregiver is a highlight of midwifery services, and client teaching is a major midwifery priority throughout the childbearing year.

Couples in midpregnancy may attend early-pregnancy classes. As discussed earlier, these classes may be designed for clients who are new to a prenatal care service, whether they initially come during the first, second, or third trimester. Assessment of class members allows the nurse to identify the particular learning needs of the group and to direct course content accordingly. Table 9–2 presents a suggested outline of content relevant to midpregnancy.

Third Trimester

Third-trimester classes tend to focus on physical, emotional, and lifestyle factors associated with the last part of pregnancy and on preparation for the labor and birth experience. In response to criticisms that third-trimester classes did not provide adequate preparation for beginning parenthood, many now include content relevant to concerns of the early postpartum and newborn periods. Some series include classes after participants have delivered.

Originally, many third-trimester pregnancy classes focused on a particular method of childbirth; most educational preparation was therefore devoted to mastering a certain technique. Drawbacks of this approach included a sense of failure on the part of couples who were unable to follow the method exactly or who did not experience a low-risk vaginal delivery and a sense of anger about delivery in a setting where medical or nursing staff were unsupportive of the selected method. Although each method has had enthusiastic supporters, no single method has been proven "best" for all couples. Another criticism of the classes is the limitation of content to pregnancy, labor, and delivery. Today, third-trimester education, which has become available to most clients, tends to be varied. It focuses less on a particular method than on approaches that blend aspects of various methods.

Childbirth Educators

Currently, anyone with an interest in childbirth preparation can call herself or himself a childbirth educator. No local, state, or national board regulates who teaches or what is taught. Certain major organizations, such as the American Society for Psychoprophylaxis in Obstetrics (ASPO) and the International Childbirth Education Association (ICEA), offer programs that can lead to certification in this specialty. They also specify standards for childbirth preparation classes and sponsor educational programs on childbirth-related topics. Membership in the organization does not, however, signify that an individual has advanced training in childbirth education.

Nurses need to know about the childbirth education programs offered in their geographic areas and about the backgrounds of the people offering those programs. In addition, evaluation of clients' satisfaction with the classes and their levels of preparation for labor and delivery and the postpartum can provide additional clues to the quality of programs. Nurses who provide childbirth education need to accept their own responsibility to remain current in this specialty by attending appropriate conferences, by joining childbirth education groups, by completing continuing education courses, and by reviewing relevant literature. Nurses should not assume that their own personal or clinical experiences, although necessary and important, provide them with all they need to know about childbirth education.

Current trends have brought many changes in childbirth education (Zwelling, 1996). Prenatal education is considered standard practice instead of a radical concept. Although greater outreach is needed, education has been extended to such hard-to-reach groups as low-income and minority populations that previously would not have had access to such teaching. More options exist for nonpharmacologic pain management. The scope of education has been expanded to include such topics as preconception, early pregnancy, cesarean education, breastfeeding, and newborn care (Biasella, 1993; Zwelling, 1996). The nature of educational programs has become more eclectic in order to reflect clients' needs. The term "parent education" more accurately describes current programs than the traditional term, "childbirth education."

Many educational programs are sponsored by hospital systems. This sponsorship has several advantages. A wider population can be serviced; clients may attend classes in the same facility in which they will deliver; and continuity of care can be fostered when some of the childbirth educators work on the childbearing units, have thorough knowledge of the facility, and may actually care for the family. Negative aspects of this trend include: use by hospitals of such classes as marketing vehicles; lack of attention to ensuring that classes are staffed by individuals who can provide high quality education; lack of encouragement for staff to seek childbirth educator certification; limitation of information about childbirth options to what is provided at a certain facility; and potentially greater acceptance of technologic interventions and less emphasis on nonpharmacologic alternatives in childbearing (Zwelling, 1996).

▶ Information for Prenatal Clients

Education throughout pregnancy focuses on the physiologic and psychosocial needs of the family. Informa-

tion for clients that is specific to a particular trimester of pregnancy is usually introduced prior to that stage. In addition, much content has relevance for more than one trimester.

Relaxation/Stress Reduction

Pregnant couples can learn to reduce stress by active relaxation. Relaxation can be taught as a coping strategy to deal with the changes encountered during pregnancy, as well as labor and delivery. Clark (1986) identifies several stress management interventions, including breathing awareness, relaxation sigh, imagery, breathing and imagery, biofeedback, progressive relaxation, self-hypnosis, thought stopping, and coping skills training.

Self-Care Practices

Education about self-care focuses on information the couple may need to use in coping with activities of daily living.

Posture and Movement. The pregnant woman is taught proper body mechanics as early in pregnancy as possible. Thus, as her center of gravity shifts because of the enlarging uterus, she will be able to move more safely and easily. When standing, the woman should keep her shoulders, back, hips, knees, and feet in a straight line. She is taught to use her legs rather than her back muscles when stooping or lifting. The pregnant woman is also encouraged to sit with her legs crossed (tailor sitting). This strengthens the inner thigh muscles (Fig. 9–1). The recommended position when resting is lying on the left side in a lateral Sims' position, with pillows supporting the upper legs (Fig. 9–2).

Clothing. In general, loose-fitting skirts and pants that stretch are most appropriate for pregnancy. Maternity clothing can be fashionable as well as comfortable and need not be costly or new. Many women share maternity clothing.

Maternity girdles are usually not necessary unless the abdomen is large and pendulous. Maternity pantyhose often can provide better fit and more support than regular pantyhose in a larger size. Constricting items such as garters and tight waist bands may interfere with venous return and should be avoided.

The pregnant woman should also avoid high-heeled shoes, as they may cause back discomfort and affect balance. Maternity bras may be used to support the breasts and promote comfort. Cotton-crotch underpants or panty shields should also be worn, as they absorb moisture.

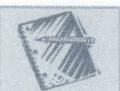

Client Teaching

Stress Management Interventions

To reduce stress related to the childbearing experience, the nurse can teach the pregnant woman the following interventions:

- **Breathing awareness**   Concentrate on inhaling and exhaling while lying on a blanket on the floor with your legs straight and slightly apart, arms at your side away from your body, your palms up, and your eyes closed. (Due to such concerns as supine hypotension women in advanced pregnancy should avoid lying flat on their backs.)

- **Relaxation sigh**   Sigh deeply on exhalation while standing or sitting.

- **Imagery**   Imagine yourself in a safe and pleasant place when you feel stressed.

- **Breathing and imagery**   Begin by using imagery. When you inhale, picture energy rushing into your lungs. When you exhale, picture the energy flowing to all parts of your body.

- **Biofeedback**   Identify tensions in various parts of your body and then let go of these tensions.

- **Progressive relaxation**   Tighten and relax muscle groups, beginning with your hand and moving down to your foot. Check for relaxation in each muscle group before moving on to the next muscle group. Practice imagery while you are relaxing these muscles.

- **Self-hypnosis**   Learn this technique from a person who is knowledgeable in it. A wakeful state of deep relaxation can be achieved by use of positive statements.

- **Thought stopping**   Interrupt unwanted thoughts with the command "stop" and follow it by reassuring and accepting self-statements.

- **Coping skills training**   Achieve relaxation by saying the following stress/coping statements to yourself:
  1. There's nothing to worry about.
  2. I'm going to be all right.
  3. I can get help if I need it.
  4. Take it step by step.
  5. I did well!
  6. Situations don't have to overwhelm me anymore.
  7. I can do this.

Lifestyle/Habits. The childbearing couple is taught positive health care practices. Teaching focuses on reinforcing a client's health, promoting lifestyle practices, and addressing high-risk behaviors identified by the client's history. Rationales for changing behaviors such as smoking and drinking alcohol are explained. The couple is also taught about potentially harmful environmental factors.

Employment. Most pregnant women should be able to work as long as they feel comfortable; however, physical or psychologic risks for pregnancy must be considered. In certain circumstances, women may not be able to continue with their usual work during pregnancy.

Sexuality. Sexual desires and behaviors may change during pregnancy. The nurse needs to be aware of clients' individual responses to sexuality throughout the childbearing cycle. Women and their partners may normally fear hurting the fetus, experience conflict over fetal "presence" during lovemaking, have con-

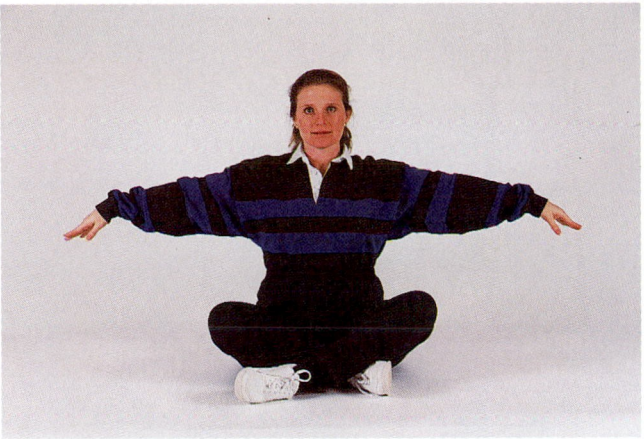

FIGURE 9–1. Tailor sitting.

flicts related to sexual desire during a culturally "taboo" period, lack interest, or be embarrassed regarding the pregnant shape (see Chapter 5).

Desire for physical closeness and expression of sexuality are normal and may be encouraged for the low-risk, healthy couple. To provide client teaching, the nurse needs to assess the couple's attitude toward sexuality, their cultural backgrounds, and their fears and concerns. Sexuality encompasses more than intercourse. Kissing, touching, and cuddling are also sexual expressions.

Bathing/Swimming. Bathing, swimming, and showering are allowed throughout pregnancy. Tub baths and swimming should be avoided after rupture of the membranes because of the possibility of infection. Women should avoid or be very careful taking tub baths late in pregnancy because their center of gravity has shifted, making them vulnerable to falls.

Nursing Alert

A pregnant woman may acquire toxoplasmosis (an infection caused by the protozoan *Toxoplasma gondii*) through contact with infected cat feces or by eating raw or undercooked infected meat. To decrease or prevent infection, a pregnant woman should: avoid contact with the cat's litter box; have someone else clean the litter box (*T. gondii* mature within 24 hours of leaving the cat's body); wash hands well after contact with the cat; wear gloves for gardening and wash hands well (neighborhood cats often have access to home garden areas and *T. gondii* can survive actively in soil after feces decompose); and eat only well-cooked meat. Screening for toxoplasmosis antibodies may be done before pregnancy or at the first prenatal visit. Women should promptly report any flu-like symptoms to their health care providers.

Exposure to very high temperatures, as in saunas or hot tubs, should be avoided because of the possible harmful effects on the fetus related to increased maternal body temperature.

Personal Hygiene. Daily showering controls odors related to sweating and normal vaginal secretions. Douching is not recommended for the pregnant woman.

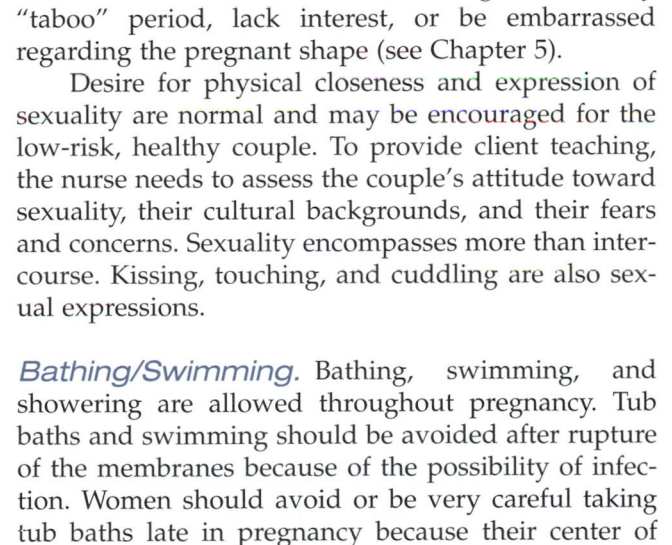

FIGURE 9–2. Resting position for a pregnant woman: lying on the left side with a pillow supporting the upper legs.

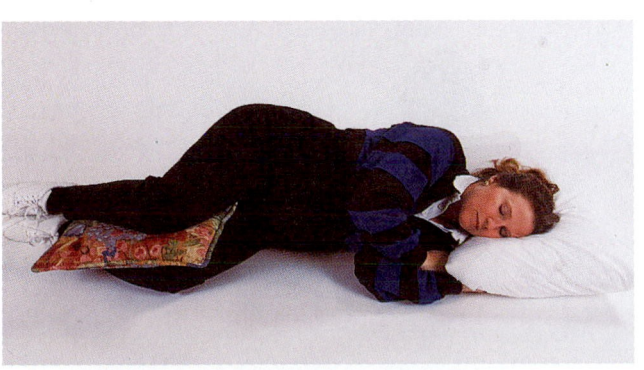

Women's Health

Sexual intercourse between a pregnant woman and her partner is usually contraindicated in situations in which the woman has either uterine bleeding, rupture of the membranes, or strong uterine contractions after orgasm and in cases in which the woman has a history of premature labor or premature rupture of the membranes.

Travel. Long-distance travel by train or plane is not contraindicated during pregnancy; however, travel to regions of the world where health care is not available or where the incidence of disease is high is not recommended during pregnancy. Pregnant women need to protect themselves and their fetuses from physical trauma during travel. Seat belts, including lap and shoulder straps, should be worn when traveling in a car. Automobile accidents may result in fetal loss or placental separation.

Exercise

Regular exercise is a means of promoting health. Benefits of physical exercise during pregnancy include toning and strengthening of maternal muscles and the cardiovascular system, promotion of physical stamina, release of tension, an overall sense of well-being, and preparation for labor and delivery. Various prenatal exercises are recommended to strengthen muscle tone in preparation for delivery and the postpartum period.

Kegel Exercises. Kegel exercises, also called pelvic floor exercises, are done to strengthen the pubococcygeal muscle. This muscle provides support for the bladder, urethra, vagina, uterus, and rectum. Kegel exercises increase vaginal tone and elasticity in preparation for labor and delivery. Increased tone may also influence sexual pleasure during pregnancy and after birth of the baby. The pubococcygeal muscle may be identified by voluntarily stopping a stream of urine. The pressure sensation is caused by contraction of this muscle (Lichtman & Papera, 1990). Many different techniques are used to teach Kegel exercises. For example, the exercise can be done slowly, contracting the muscle up to 10 seconds. The exercise can also be done with rapid squeezing and releasing (flutter exercises) (Lichtman & Papera, 1990). The client can perform Kegel exercises anywhere; the exercises do not need to be limited. The increased tone of the pubococcygeal muscle is beneficial during pregnancy and afterward.

Pelvic Tilt. Pelvic tilt exercises help relieve backache and also strengthen the abdominal muscles. The client tucks the buttocks; this flattens the lower back. The pelvis tilts slightly upward. She then relaxes the back muscles, which allows the hips to return to the natural position. It is basically a rocking movement. Pelvic tilt exercises can be done in three different positions (Department of Health Services, 1987): (1) The client stands against a wall and presses her lower back against the wall. (2) The client positions herself on her hands and knees, arching her lower back and then relaxing to a flat back (Fig. 9–3). (3) The client lies on

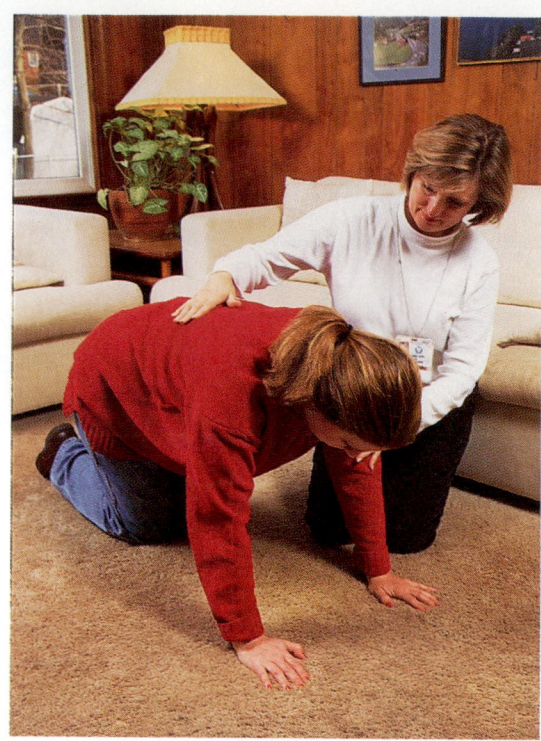

FIGURE 9–3. Pelvic tilt exercises: the client has positioned herself on her hands and knees, arches her lower back, and then relaxes it to a flat position.

the floor on her back and bends her knees; she presses her lower back flat against the floor and then relaxes (Fig. 9–4).

Leg Raises. A pregnant woman may lie on her back with her knees bent and feet flat on the floor. She

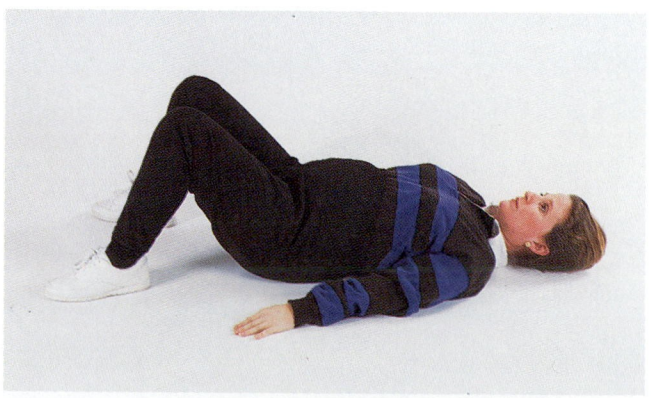

FIGURE 9–4. Pelvic tilt exercises: the client lies on the floor on her back, bends her knees, and presses her back flat against the floor.

is shown how to straighten one leg by lifting the foot into the air and holding it momentarily off the floor. Leg raises strengthen abdominal muscles (Fig. 9–5).

Concerns About Sports and Exercise. Many types of prenatal exercise classes have been organized. A nurse must be familiar with them before referring a client. Moderate exercise during pregnancy has many benefits, but exercise may also provoke concerns. Fetal hyperthermia may result from increased production of heat during maternal exercise; however, in a temperate climate without extreme heat or humidity, the body usually dissipates heat efficiently. Vigorous exercise may also cause fetal hypoxia; the increased oxygen demands of peripheral maternal muscles may draw blood from the uterus, thereby providing less blood to the fetus.

Maternal safety may also be threatened by exercise. Throughout the first trimester, the mother's ability to perform sports or exercise is not affected substantially. During the second and third trimesters, however, as the uterus expands and hormones alter the musculoskeletal system, changes occur in her center of gravity, balance, and gait. In addition, her joints and ligaments weaken, predisposing them to tearing. She becomes at risk for injury, especially in sports that require speed, precision, and balance.

Various opinions exist about what and how much exercise is safe. Generally, the healthy pregnant woman can engage in exercise that does not result in excess physical strain. The nurse needs to identify what specific plans the client has for activities and to assess the woman's interpretation of mild, moderate, and heavy exercise. For the nurse to provide advice, the client's unique physical condition and responses to exercise must be evaluated. Good common sense is also helpful.

A pregnant woman should be advised to contact her health care provider if she develops these warning signs during exercise:

- Persistent pain or tenderness, especially chest, back, pubic, or hip pain; a ripping sensation followed by pain
- Onset of uterine contractions
- Headache, "lightheadedness"
- Vaginal bleeding
- Leakage of fluid from the vagina
- Nausea and vomiting (not the usual morning sickness)
- Difficult breathing
- Palpitations
- Increase, decrease, or cessation of fetal movements
- Heart rate greater than 130 beats per minute
- Dyspnea

► CHOICES IN CHILDBIRTH

Current options for childbearing families have evolved during years of professional and lay groups' working with and against each other. Nurses need to realize that no educational program or delivery alternative is unconditionally accepted for the childbearing family. Nevertheless, the heterogeneous nature of the American population requires that educational preparation on the safe choices in childbearing be available to enable clients to make informed choices.

► Development of Current Delivery Alternatives

Before the 20th century, nearly all births in the United States occurred out of the hospital. Women planned to deliver at home, where they would be assisted by a woman experienced in childbirth, a midwife, or a physician. Limited transportation, few hospitals, and the level of hospital technology did not make hospital birth a desirable choice for many families. Hospitals were regarded as places for the sick, feeble, and dying, not for women undergoing a normal process. This trend persisted into this century (Weingarten & Jacobwitz, 1987).

Changes in patterns of obstetric care and childbirth accompanied social and technologic changes in the early 20th century. For example, it is estimated that midwives performed 38% of all deliveries in New York City in 1913 (Mattson & Smith, 1993). In the

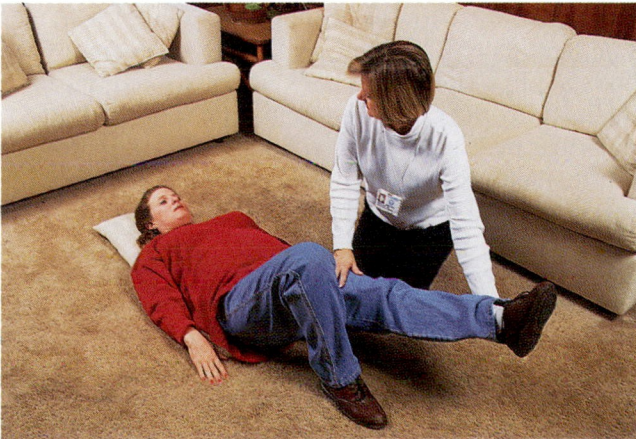

FIGURE 9–5. To strengthen abdominal muscles, a pregnant woman may be taught to alternately raise one leg then the other from a bent position straight up off the floor.

following years, however, midwife-attended births decreased. By 1935, midwifery came to be centered mainly among families living in poverty and among African-Americans in the rural South. This change may have occurred because educational programs for midwives were lacking and fewer women aspired to become midwives. Over time, the United States came to have no well-educated group skilled in home births.

The rate of hospital births increased from 39.6% in 1935 to 99% of all births in the United States in 1979 (Devitt, 1977; Zwelling, 1996). Pregnancy and birth began to be viewed as pathologic phenomena that required technologic intervention. Some of these practices, for example, the use of forceps, were thought a greater hazard to client health if used in a home rather than hospital. Thus, physicians' support of in-hospital deliveries was strengthened.

The movement within medicine to organize obstetrics as a specialty reinforced the abnormal aspects of birth (Varney, 1997). Obstetric analgesia and anesthesia promoted the thought among women that childbirth in a hospital was safer and less painful.

Restrictive isolation policies also developed early in this century with concern for the high rate of morbidity and mortality of hospitalized children with infectious disease. Visitors were thought to introduce disease. Thus evolved the practice of separating parents from their hospitalized child, whether the infant was ill or in a well baby nursery (Klaus, Kennel, & Klaus, 1996).

Not until the late 1960s did major changes begin to take place in obstetric practice. The women's movement had a great impact. Opposition was directed toward a woman's lack of control over her body, rigidity of hospital policies, separation of women from their support persons during childbirth, and definition of childbirth as high-risk pathology even for healthy women. As the case was presented for pregnancy as a normal life event, attention was drawn to educational preparation for childbirth and the right of women to make choices concerning their birth experiences.

By the late 1960s and early 1970s, in response to consumer demand, nurse-midwifery programs in the United States began to grow again, and nurse-midwives became more widely available. They were a choice of childbirth attendant for healthy, low-risk women. Nurse-midwives strove to ensure a satisfying, family-centered birth experience for their clients. Their background in nursing, advanced training in obstetrics, and success on a national certifying examination for the American College of Nurse-Midwives (ACNM) established a professionally educated group

of birth attendants whose philosophy evolved from commitment to childbirth as a manifestation of health.

► Methods of Preparing for Childbirth

A number of prepared childbirth methods have been developed to help childbearing clients cope with childbirth. These methods include: psychophysical preparation, psychoprophylaxis, the Leboyer method, the Bradley method, and hypnosis.

Childbirth educators also may offer eclectic approaches that incorporate aspects of different methods. Despite the variation in childbirth methods, all involve a combination of physical and psychologic techniques. Each method requires prenatal education that includes discussions of what labor and delivery are like, a support person attending the laboring woman, and the woman's relaxing of specific muscles, breathing in a controlled manner, and using her muscles effectively in delivery.

Psychophysical Preparation: Grantly Dick-Read

Grantly Dick-Read, a British physician, pioneered the development of childbirth preparation methods. Dick-Read derived his belief in the emotional beauty of childbirth by designing a process of prenatal and intrapartum education and exercise. He questioned why young people were not routinely educated for childbearing. Dick-Read felt this lack of education contributed to high levels of anxiety for pregnant women. He believed that, with a prescribed educational program, women could be assisted to decrease their fear and, therefore, muscular tension in childbirth (Dick-Read, 1944). Through studied relaxation methods, women could learn to control specific muscle groups and prevent or inhibit a spiral of fear, tension, and pain. According to Dick-Read, many of the body's physiologic reactions were related in their intensity to the body's muscle tone. For Dick-Read, muscular relaxation reduced the muscle tone throughout the body to a minimum. The primary goal of his work was childbirth without fear.

Dick-Read believed that lessons in relaxation could be given during the earliest stages of pregnancy. During the late 1940s when Dick-Read's book became available in the United States, his approach was thought radical and revolutionary. Although his techniques were never completely developed as a method, a modified Dick-Read approach was.

Psychophysical preparation focused on a woman's ability to work along with the forces of labor by relaxing and breathing more rapidly and more deeply as the intensity of contractions increased. In prenatal class discussions group members could raise topics related to their own learning needs; breathing and relaxation techniques were presented as aids for breaking the fear–tension–pain spiral. The breathing technique for the Dick-Read method is primarily abdominal, with the depth and rapidity of breathing increasing as uterine contractions increase during the first stage. During the second stage of labor, a mother pants to prevent pushing and holds her breath to aid pushing. Toward the end of labor, if the abdominal breathing is not enough rapid chest breathing may be done.

Dick-Read was the first to use the term **natural childbirth,** a method of childbirth in which neither analgesics nor anesthetics are used. It caught on readily and eventually was applied to any method of preparation and education for labor that prevents or decreases the need for pain-relieving medication.

Psychoprophylaxis: Lamaze Technique

Psychoprophylaxis is the training of mind and body to select an appropriate reaction to stressful stimuli (Chabon, 1966). The psychoprophylactic method is based on principles first developed in the former Soviet Union and used widely there and in China. It was introduced in France in 1951 by the French physician Ferdinand Lamaze. Originally it was called the Pavlov method, because it was based on the stimulus–response, conditioned reflex theory of the Russian physiologist Pavlov. Psychoprophylaxis was popularized in the United States by Marjorie Karmel, whose book *Thank You, Dr. Lamaze* (1959) joyously describes the satisfaction the author experienced using this technique during her delivery in Paris. Her work made a landmark contribution to the changing of obstetric practice and was instrumental in raising support for establishment of the American Society for Psychoprophylaxis in Obstetrics (ASPO), a childbirth education organization.

The main focus of the psychoprophylactic technique (the **Lamaze technique**) was to alter the perception of pain in childbirth through the use of the mind. Women would attend prenatal classes to learn activities and breathing patterns that would allow them to control their experience of pain during uterine contractions. By maintaining a high level of alertness and conscious activity during labor and delivery and by using conditioned responses, a woman could control her muscles and alter her perception of pain. The techniques were best used with the active support of the woman's partner and members of the attending health care team. According to Chabon (1966), "the

greater this support, the more successful the exercise techniques." Prenatal classes, especially those beginning prior to the third trimester, could also promote communication between parents-to-be, helping them to work more effectively together during labor.

The psychoprophylactic technique taught prenatally is very structured and evolves from conditioning, concentration, and discipline. The exercises and relaxation and breathing patterns of psychoprophylaxis are tools that a couple can use to deal with the stress of childbirth. The pain reduction techniques may diminish distress associated with labor by helping the woman to remain in control.

The first breathing pattern in the Lamaze method is called slow-paced breathing. It begins with a deep cleansing breath and involves a focal point or focus of attention, effleurage (light touch massage of the abdomen), and slow-paced breathing (about 6 to 10 breaths per minute). It ends with a deep cleansing breath. The support person or practitioner may breathe with the woman to help her focus her attention, may perform massage, and may check for relaxation.

For stronger contractions, modified paced breathing is used. The woman begins to breathe slowly through her nose or mouth; breathing becomes faster as the contraction reaches its peak and slows as the contraction ends. A cleansing breath is then taken.

For very strong contractions, modified paced breathing is accompanied by increased concentration. The modified paced breathing is, at its maximum, twice the normal breathing rate or about one breath every 2 seconds (about 30 breaths per minute maximum). The woman is taught that the faster the breathing is the more shallow it must be, and the slower it is the deeper. This ensures the proper exchange of oxygen and carbon dioxide and prevents hyperventilation.

Childbirth without Violence: The LeBoyer Method

In 1975, Frederick LeBoyer introduced a delivery technique that was intended to improve the newborn's birth experience. LeBoyer's method included dimming the lights in the delivery room, placing the baby on the mother's warm abdomen, waiting up to 6 minutes before cutting the umbilical cord while the mother gently massaged the baby, and submerging the baby in warm water after the cord is cut. This delivery technique was believed to lessen the so-called "birth trauma" that concerned some psychotherapists, although no scientific evidence indicates that the LeBoyer method of birth helps an individual in future psychosocial development. Many parents, however, report a positive birthing experience.

The Bradley Method

The hallmark of the Bradley method is that the husband or partner of the mother is the primary labor coach; the method is also referred to as *husband-coached childbirth.* The physiologic components of the Bradley method are breath control, abdominal breathing, and general body relaxation that is in harmony with the body, labor, and contractions. The major breathing technique is slow abdominal relaxed breathing, which may become more rapid as the contractions intensify. The Bradley method focuses on breath control while the mother is in a comfortable position, which can be individualized for each woman. Deep mental relaxation is simultaneously pursued.

Hypnosis

Hypnosis is another effective approach to pain control in labor. The technique requires a great deal of time, training, and intensity.

Effectiveness

Prenatal education classes are now considered part of standard obstetric practice. How effective are they? The answer to this often-asked question depends on how the term "effective" is used. For example, preparation that affords a couple the opportunity to learn about and discuss pregnancy, labor, and delivery can be effective in establishing a partnership between clients and health care providers. In addition, educational preparation that focuses on a shared delivery experience between the client and her support person can effectively foster communication between family members. Antenatal classes for women and their partners who want the classes have been identified as one of the forms of care likely to be beneficial (Enkin, Keirse, Renfrew, & Neilson, 1995). In a recent study, Hart and Foster (1997) found that couples who attended childbirth education classes reported a sense of control during labor and delivery; they found a relationship between subjects' perceived control and overall evaluation of their childbirth experiences. Research does not clearly support claims that prepared childbirth techniques alone ensure healthier babies or that fewer labor and delivery complications occur.

Support for prepared childbirth has ranged from passionate endorsement to the more pragmatic view that knowledge is better than ignorance. Researchers have had difficulty in isolating specific outcomes, but that does not lessen the importance of educational preparation for childbirth and parenting. Childbirth education is a complex topic, presented in many different ways in different settings. Researchers face difficult tasks in identifying its specific and subtle benefits and effects, especially when research is based on objectives deemed appropriate to health professionals rather than to clients (Enkin et al., 1990; Shearer, 1996).

Disadvantages

A possible disadvantage of prepared childbirth classes is the sense of failure that may be experienced by women and their partners if they are unable to follow through with the program as it was taught. Receiving anesthesia or analgesia could also be a source of disappointment. Advocates of the Bradley method are so strongly opposed to analgesia and anesthesia that teachers must maintain a high rate of medication-free deliveries among their students to remain certified by the American Academy of Husband-Coached Childbirth (AAHCC). This could be a burden on the childbearing couple.

At times, couples undertake prepared childbirth education with unrealistic expectations of easy, pain-free deliveries. Such hopes can lead to a sense of failure and negative feelings if the delivery experience is very different.

Women who have unplanned cesarean deliveries are at risk for a situational crisis related to the operative birth and may grieve the loss of the expected low-risk birth experience. To help address this problem, cesarean birth classes are often available and nurses and other health care providers do try to ensure a positive birth experience for couples who experience cesarean deliveries.

Currently, many childbirth educators attempt to present labor and delivery realistically and strive to help clients feel good about themselves whatever the delivery outcome. Nurses need to identify and address client expectations at the beginning of the educational program. Alternative birth plans may also help reduce disappointment should a high-risk condition arise. Support partners should be specifically included in classes and planning, as women may have a difficult time if they feel that their family members think they have failed.

Prepared Childbirth and Technology

Technologic advances in obstetrics provide aids to care for childbearing women. One example of such obstetric tools is the electronic fetal monitor. Occasionally, technology may control childbirth and be used as an excuse to prevent a family-centered birth experience. Nurses need to share appropriate information with clients about technical equipment and procedures and to provide them with opportunities to discuss questions they may have. In addition, nurses

Research Abstract

Couples' Attitudes toward Childbirth Participation: Relationship to Evaluation of Labor and Delivery

This descriptive, correlational survey used a pretest-posttest design to investigate the relationship between couples' prenatal attitudes toward childbirth participation and perceptions of their labor and delivery experiences. The researchers administered the Prenatal Attitude toward Childbirth Participation Scale, along with a personal data form, to 119 couples before and after their 6-week childbirth education classes at a tertiary care hospital. The Labor Delivery Evaluation Scale, the Labor Agency Scale, and the Delivery Agency Scale were given to the couples in the hospital after delivery. Of the group, 73 couples completed the postdelivery questionnaires before discharge. Results supported the hypothesis that the couples and the mothers and fathers individually would have a greater sense of control in labor and delivery after completing the classes. Couples who had normal vaginal deliveries perceived more control during labor and delivery than couples who had vacuum assisted or cesarean births; they also evaluated their childbirth experiences more positively than those with assisted or cesarean births.

Application to Practice

This study indicates certain benefits of childbirth education classes. The study suggests that health care providers and prenatal educators should focus on couples' chances to exercise control during childbirth and on recognizing the need to release control to the health care team during emergency situations. These findings support previous studies and clinical observations, indicating that women who require obstetric interventions perceive their birth experiences as less satisfying than those who have normal vaginal deliveries. Nurses and other health care providers can use these results as a challenge to find ways in which high-risk situations can be more positive for couples. By focusing on couples, the study also provides information useful to prenatal educators, who need to focus their content on the needs of both partners. As the authors themselves point out, study results should be considered in light of such limitations as a small, homogeneous sample size, a small (n = 36) group of uncomplicated deliveries, and the absence of a control group of couples who did not attend the childbirth education series. The study also highlights the importance of using appropriate research instruments, sensitive enough to identify variables being studied.

Source: Hart, M.A., & Foster, S.N. (1997). Couples' attitudes toward childbirth participation: Relationship to evaluation of labor and delivery. Journal of Perinatal and Neonatal Nursing, 11(1), 10–20.

should use strategies that allow clients to use both methods for prepared childbirth and necessary technology.

▶ Choice of Childbirth Attendant and Setting

A woman giving birth may be cared for by one of several types of attendants. Settings for delivery include hospitals, free-standing birth centers, and homes. Choice is available, too, in birthing equipment. Special birthing beds and chairs are designed to accommodate individual differences and position preference (Fig. 9–6).

Childbirth Attendants

Physicians. Physicians are the largest group of professionals performing deliveries in the United States. Educational preparation includes graduation from medical or osteopathic school, at least one year of postmedical school clinical training, and national and state licensure. Although deliveries can legally be performed by any physician, most are done by obstetricians, who have completed several years of postgraduate training in obstetrics. Many are also certified by the American College of Obstetricians and Gynecologists.

Certified Nurse-Midwives. **Certified nurse-midwives** (CNMs) are registered nurses who have

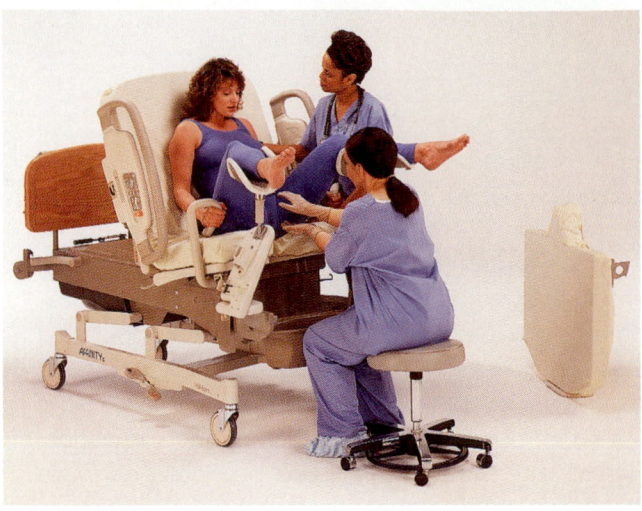

FIGURE 9–6. Birthing beds are designed to accommodate the needs or wishes of a particular client. Before a birth, a nurse should instruct the woman about how the bed will be used. *(Courtesy of Hill-Rom, Batesville, IN.)*

completed postgraduate training in nurse-midwifery. These educational programs focus on maternal/newborn health and normal deliveries. The certification examination is sponsored by the American College of Nurse-Midwives (ACNM). As of January, 1997, nearly 7000 nurse-midwives had been certified by the ACNM and ACNM Certification Council, Inc. (ACNM, 1997). CNMs are licensed by the state where they practice; states determine restrictions on the scope and location of practice.

Certified Midwives. Certified midwives are not nurses. These individuals have graduated from a special program for non-nurses that meets criteria specified by the ACNM. These programs either require a baccalaureate degree for admission or grant no less than a baccalaureate degree. Upon successful completion of the midwifery program, the graduate is able to take the national certification examination to become a Certified Midwife (ACNM, 1997).

Lay Midwives. **Lay midwife** is a general term used to describe an individual who attends births, but who is not a nurse-midwife or physician. Specific educational standards are not established. Some may have had sufficient training and experience to care aptly for childbearing families; others may only be interested in the birth process and have little formal training. Some states require licensure; however, most do not. Lay midwives rarely have hospital or licensed birth center privileges; they attend clients most often in homes.

Childbirth Setting

In making decisions about where and with whom to deliver, family members must interact. They must be well informed about facilities in their geographic area, know the implications for their family and baby, and they should be able to identify their goals for their birth experience (see Table 9–2). Despite the availability of options, most families choose to deliver in hospitals.

A family's past experiences and attitudes, level of risk, and socioeconomic background are other factors that influence their choice. Personal feelings of alienation, lack of control, desire to participate in decision making, and frustration with inflexible hospital policies are among the reasons that clients seek an alternate birth experience. The family's ability to pay for services influences their selection of a delivery alternative. For example, a family that does not have obstetric insurance may simply seek care from the cheapest source or opt for no prenatal care. In other situations, couples may be reimbursed by their insurance company only if delivery is in a hospital.

Table 9–3 summarizes the advantages and disadvantages of three types of birth experience. The hospital setting and obstetrician-attended birth are the primary recommendations for the high-risk client. Alternatives are restricted to low-risk clients.

Hospitals. Hospital facilities may provide only low-risk services for healthy mothers and infants; some hospitals can handle specific high-risk conditions. Others can provide technology and staff expertise for those at highest risk. Hospitals may also offer a variety of options. Those that provide high-risk care may also offer family-centered care in which CNMs attend births.

Women who have moderate to high-risk complications include those with severe diabetes, cardiac or thyroid disorders, or premature labor, or those who have a fetus diagnosed with such abnormalities as Rh disease, hydrocephaly, and certain genetic disorders. They should have access to a hospital with a perinatologist and neonatologist and a neonatal intensive care unit (NICU). For financial and staffing reasons, high-risk care tends to be concentrated in regional centers (see Chapter 2).

Many women today labor, deliver, and recover in a **hospital birthing room** (Fig. 9–7). In that setting, the client is not transferred from a labor room to a delivery room, unless the mother or fetus is in distress. Women may be moved to the postpartum unit after a recovery and bonding period; however, in some hospitals, women remain in the same room until discharge. A support person and occasionally other rela-

▶ **TABLE 9-3**

Advantages and Disadvantages of Different Birth Settings

Type	Advantages	Disadvantages
Hospital	Security, availability of emergency equipment Potential use of birthing room Availability of professional staff Availability of latest technology For multiparous women, some quiet time alone Contact with other new mothers Insurance coverage of birth expenses Availability of analgesia and anesthesia, if necessary	Impersonal and routine care Potential rigid rules Restrictive visiting policies Increased risk of unnecessary interventions Use of unnecessary medications Hospital limitation of options (e.g., ambulation) Separation from other children at home Separation from other family members
Birth center	Continuity of care Homelike setting Opportunity for couple to participate actively in care Wellness orientation Less expensive Extensive information on childbirth readily available Discharge within 24 hours Early and extended contact with newborn Ability to have any significant others present	Possibility of transfer to another facility Appropriate only for low-risk women (may be "risked out" at any time) Limited accessibility Possibility of needing emergency care Possibility that insurance may not cover delivery Possibility that regional anesthetics may not be available Sense of failure if client needs to be transferred to acute care facility
Home	Emotionally satisfying for all family members Familiar environment Opportunity for family members to participate actively in birth Wellness orientation Least expensive birth option Early and extended contact with newborn	Possibility that emergency interventions may be needed Difficulty in finding qualified birth attendants Difficulty in accessing transportation to acute-care setting if needed Possibility that insurance may not cover home birth Unavailability of analgesia and anesthesia Appropriate only for low-risk women

tives or friends may remain with the client. Sibling attendance is uncommon. In establishing birthing rooms, hospitals have attempted to create a family-centered, homelike birth experience. This represents attempts to make institutional goals more congruent with a family's emotional needs as well as with consumer and professional desires. Birthing rooms in hospitals have continued to develop in response to

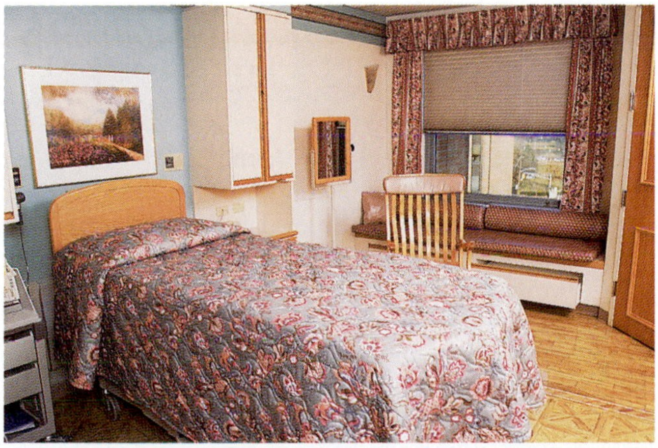

FIGURE 9–7. Hospital birthing room.

consumer demand for a beautiful, homelike environment and in response to competition among hospitals for clients.

Some hospitals have strict criteria concerning who may use a birthing room; some permit only women at lowest risk. To clarify such limitations, prenatal education classes should identify for couples who is allowed to use a birthing room or, indeed, if such a room is established at an institution. Other hospitals have more lenient criteria and routinely permit women who expect to deliver vaginally to use the birthing room, even if they are not at lowest risk. Clients need to know that backup facilities are readily available in a hospital birthing room.

Free-Standing Birth Centers. **Birth centers** provide homelike birthing experiences outside a hospital (free-standing) (Fig. 9–8). They offer a compromise between hospital and home births. Birth centers are usually licensed by the state in which they are located. They provide some emergency care on the premises and transportation to a backup hospital, should the need arise.

Birth centers are based on the belief that childbirth for most women is a normal life event; thus, safe, satisfying, health-oriented, family-focused births

Commonly Asked Questions

What delivery settings are currently available?

Hospitals (traditional hospitals, hospitals including birth centers or birthing rooms), free-standing birth centers and homes.

What is a free-standing birth center?

Free-standing birth centers provide care for child-bearing families; the centers often offer well-woman care to women who are not pregnant. The term "free standing" refers to their location outside a hospital.

Is delivery in a free-standing birth center safe?

Years of experience and several studies have demonstrated that delivery in a licensed free-standing birth center is a safe alternative for healthy, low-risk families.

Can healthy women who choose to deliver in a hospital still be cared for by certified nurse-midwives?

Yes. Many, but not all hospitals currently have CNMs on their staffs. CNMs may be employed by the hospital, may be in joint practice with physician groups, or may have their own private practices and deliver their clients at the hospital.

What are hospital birthing rooms?

In trying to normalize and make birth experiences more family centered (and also to attract childbearing clients), many hospitals have constructed labor and delivery areas that mimic homelike environ-ments. These rooms can be beautiful and cozy, with obstetric equipment concealed behind cabinets, such comfortable furniture as rocking chairs, and private bathrooms that include showers and whirlpool tubs. Women can labor, deliver, and recover in these rooms. In some hospitals, women can continue to have use of the rooms during their postpartum course.

A local hospital is advertising beautiful new birthing rooms. Will this ensure a family-centered birth experience?

Not necessarily. While lovely surroundings are desirable, the attitude and approach of the birth attendants are more important aspects in ensuring a family-centered birth experience.

My husband and I are looking forward to sharing our baby's birth. If I should unexpectedly need a cesarean delivery, can we remain together?

Not necessarily. Hospitals vary widely in their policies. Be sure to discuss this with your midwife or obstetrician during a prenatal visit so that you are clear about the policies in the facility you select. Many hospitals have prenatal cesarean classes for couples who want to remain together. However, in some hospitals, support people may be denied the chance to share delivery simply because they have not been to classes. In certain high-risk circumstances, the obstetrician may request that no family member be in a cesarean room, regardless of his having taken classes.

---

can take place away from an acute care hospital, in a more homelike setting. Staff usually encourage a client to include whomever she wishes in the birth event. Prenatal care is given at the center, and the family has many opportunities to get to know the birth center and its staff. The birth center may be owned by physicians, CNMs, lay groups, or any combination thereof. Licensed birth centers have physicians available for consultation whenever appropriate.

Only women who are healthy and have no history of contraindicating medical, obstetric, or psychiatric problems may qualify for care in a birth center.

No client can be assured that the birth will take place at the center, because a high-risk condition may develop during pregnancy or labor and necessitate transfer to an acute care hospital. In such situations, the CNM may deal with the client's potential frustration, anger, and sense of failure by remaining with her and her partner as a support person during transport and throughout the hospital delivery.

Questions are often asked about the safety of birth centers, especially because transfers for complications involve delay. Collaborative planning between the facilities is essential. Advocates of the centers

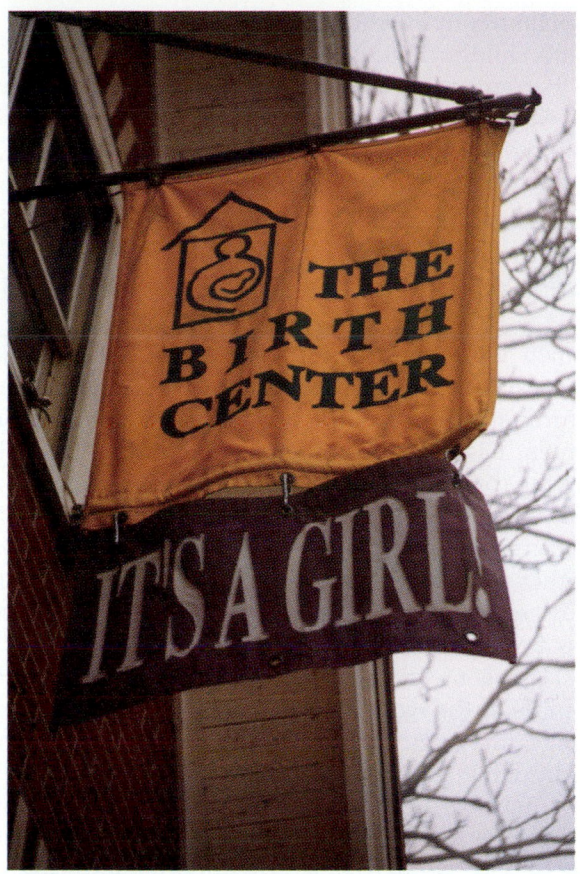

FIGURE 9–8. Birth center.

Home birth is defended as a safe alternative to hospital birth in certain medically and obstetrically low-risk populations when a skilled birth attendant is present and a modern hospital system is available to provide backup if needed (Olsen, 1997). Opponents of home birth feel that childbearing is unpredictable and that birth at home presents an unnecessary risk to mother and infant. Opponents also claim that decreases in perinatal morbidity and mortality may be the result of the shift to hospital deliveries and the use of technologies that have been developed over the last 50 years. Supporters of home birth state that most complications can be predicted and that major obstetric difficulties are rare.

A planned home birth is the most controversial of birth alternatives. The nature of obstetric problems and the lack of credible research demonstrating the safety of home birth indicate that this controversy is likely to continue. Nevertheless, some clients do choose home birth, and nurses working with childbearing families need to be aware of this.

In many states, lay midwives, rather than physicians or CNMs, attend home births. Physicians and CNMs may hesitate to attend scheduled home births

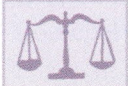 *Ethical Decision Making*

Nurse Sheila Moran, who specializes in care of high-risk obstetric patients, is on duty when Sunnie Bart is brought to the hospital for emergency cesarean delivery. Sunnie, suspicious of hospitals, planned to deliver her first baby at home where she was attended by her husband Stephan. Neither Sunnie nor Stephan had prior experience with childbirth. After 12 hours of difficult labor without progress, Stephan called for help, and Sunnie was brought by ambulance to the hospital, where fetal distress was identified.

1. What do this couple's actions indicate about their values and attitudes toward the health care system?
2. What conflicts might the nurse expect the couple to experience?
3. How might the nurse be expected to feel about this couple and their situation?
4. What strategies might the nurse use to ensure this couple receives high-quality care?

believe that attentive screening, client cooperation, and care delivered by CNMs with appropriate physician backup make the centers a safe option, and transfer rates are usually low.

A challenge is presented to hospital-based nurses who work with clients transferred from birth centers. The nurses must first evaluate their own feelings about out-of-hospital births. During a transfer, they welcome the transferred client, her support person, and the nurse-midwife; all should work together to ensure a positive birth experience. The collaborative effort is facilitated by previous planning. Nurses who work on hospital units that are backups for a birth center should meet with birth center staff to devise collaborative strategies for transfers.

Home Births. Among the reasons women may have a home birth are inability to reach a hospital (geography), desire for a family-centered birth experience away from a hospital, and unplanned delivery at home. Accurate data on the safety of home birth are lacking, as are figures for the actual number of home births.

where hospitals or licensed birth centers are readily accessible. Beyond the issue of the safety of home birth itself is the issue of defense in a malpractice suit. Fear of litigation and difficulty in defending one's actions in an unlicensed and unsupported setting are deterrents to the most well-intentioned obstetric professional.

▶ A SINGLE CLASS FOR CHILDBIRTH EDUCATION

Historically, a series of childbirth classes were conducted one evening a week for 6 to 8 weeks and each class lasted 2 or 2½ hours. This method was believed the most effective because participants had time to practice breathing and relaxation techniques outside the class and then reinforce those techniques during the next session. The classes also fostered friendships and support among group members. Today, many expectant women have busy schedules with full-time or part-time careers. Most partners are also employed, and often the mother and partner have conflicting work schedules. To meet the changing needs of expectant couples, many locations have developed a "one-day childbirth" class, which basically includes essential information about childbirth but without the week-by-week repetition and practice. A brief assessment form, completed when the client signs up for the class, can provide information about the specific needs and learning styles of the class participants (Bridgewater & Wiman, 1998). Reading material and handouts may be mailed to participants before the class meets so that they may learn about basic concepts before attending. This increases flexibility and eliminates the problems of missing a series of classes because of conflicts or time constraints. Although an abbreviated format is not the ideal learning situation, the class does provide needed information to the

expectant couple who might otherwise be unable to attend childbirth classes. Nurses need to be aware of the barriers to educational opportunities for clients and work within their time limitations to provide the best possible learning experience.

▶ CHILDBIRTH CLASSES FOR PHYSICALLY DISABLED WOMEN

Women with physical disabilities feel the same joy and excitement, apprehension and ambivalence regarding their pregnancy and birth as do able-bodied women. Disabilities should not be seen as obstacles denying prenatal education (Rogers & Matsumura, 1991). With some modifications, women with disabilities can usually participate in classes in the same way as other women. Any limitations of a disability should be discussed with the woman and her partner before class begins; if needed, appropriate modifications to the class content and process should be made. For example, if the woman has a spinal cord injury, some changes may be necessary in teaching relaxation and conditioning exercises. Also, signs of the onset of labor may be different for the woman with a spinal cord injury. It may be helpful to instruct the woman how to observe the shape of her abdomen during the last weeks of pregnancy or teach her how to palpate contractions with her fingertips. Women who are visually impaired benefit greatly from handouts printed with enlarged type, and this can usually be accomplished easily with a computer. Women who are blind benefit from listening to videos, tapes, and CDs on labor and birth. Educators recognize that each person has unique and individual needs. The goals of childbirth classes apply to all: to educate women on the process of labor and birth and empower them to make informed decisions for themselves and their babies.

Critical Thinking in Care Planning

Care of the Family Preparing for Childbirth

Sabrina and Bart Matthews are expecting their third child. Sabrina, 34 years old, is 28 weeks pregnant. Since her first child was born 10 years ago, Sabrina has been a homemaker. Bart is a lineman for the telephone company. Their children, Coleen (10) and George (6), are in good health and attend public school. The couple states that the whole family is looking forward to the new baby, and they would like some information to read at home.

At her routine prenatal appointment, Sabrina says to the nurse: "I would really like to try the Lamaze method and have Bart with me. We didn't take classes with the other two kids, because Bart never wanted to. He now would like to see the baby born." Sabrina delivered her previous babies with an epidural block. They were normal spontaneous vaginal deliveries.

▶ Assessment

- 28-week pregnant multiparous woman
- No childbirth preparation classes with previous births
- Delivered previous pregnancies with epidural block
- Two previous normal spontaneous deliveries

- States "I would really like to try the Lamaze method and have Bart (husband) with me."
- Two siblings, a girl, age 10 and a boy, age 6

Nursing Diagnosis

Family coping: Potential for growth, related to childbirth preparation

Expected Client/Family Outcomes	Nursing Action/Intervention	Evaluation
By the end of the visit, the client will be able to identify childbirth preparation classes and sibling preparation classes available in the area.	Discuss differences in types of childbirth preparation (e.g., Lamaze, Bradley). Provide client with a list of dates, places, instructors, and goals of Lamaze classes and sibling classes. *Rationale:* Childbirth preparation should fit the family's needs and lifestyle.	When asked, client identifies potential childbirth preparation classes she and her husband might attend.
During the third trimester, the couple will attend a series of childbirth preparation classes (Lamaze).	Assess client's understanding of Lamaze childbirth preparation and knowledge of labor and delivery. *Rationale:* Learning begins with the individual's level of knowledge regarding the subject matter.	When questioned, couple relates that they are attending a childbirth preparation class.
During the third trimester, the siblings will attend a sibling preparation class.	Give client supplemental reading materials related to Lamaze preparation and sibling preparation. *Rationale:* Supplemental reading materials help to reinforce concepts and clear up misunderstandings.	When questioned, client relates that her children are attending a sibling preparation class.
	Discuss client's perceptions of previous deliveries and how they previously prepared their daughter for their son's birth. *Rationale:* Previous experiences identify knowledge deficits, misconceptions, and also strengths.	Client discusses perceptions of previous deliveries.

(continued)

Critical Thinking in Care Planning continued

Nursing Diagnosis

Knowledge deficit (husband), related to participation in childbirth preparation and labor and delivery.

Expected Client/Family Outcomes	Nursing Action/Intervention	Evaluation
By the end of this visit, couple will identify goals and contents of Lamaze preparation.	See earlier interventions. *Rationale:* See earlier rationale.	See earlier evaluation.
The next prenatal visit will be scheduled during the birth center's evening hours so that husband can attend.	Encourage client to bring husband to prenatal visits. *Rationale:* Including the supporting other in health care encourages active participation and informed decision making.	Husband attends next prenatal visit with client and asks questions.
		Husband discusses pros and cons of attending classes and birthing; couple makes decision.
	Schedule visits at a time convenient to husband. *Rationale:* Prenatal care should be accessible and available at times congruent with family members' needs.	
	Discuss husband's feelings about attending classes and birthing and perceptions of wife's previous labors and deliveries. *Rationale:* Considering the clients' feelings and perceptions helps formulate a trusting relationship.	Couple decides whether husband will coach or if an alternative is more desirable.
By the end of the third trimester, if husband agrees to participate, he will be prepared in the role of support person, or agree to attend labor and delivery, with an alternative person being coach.	Provide husband with information and supplemental reading materials regarding childbirth preparation. *Rationale:* Supplemental reading reinforces learning.	
	Discuss the role of support person with husband and alternatives available. *Rationale:* Information regarding role and alternate strategies for participation allows for informed decision making.	

Chapter Highlights

▶ Educational preparation is a necessary part of prenatal care and involves the family.

▶ Nearly all pregnant clients who receive prenatal care have access to some type of educational program. Educational programs need to be accessible, affordable, culturally sensitive, well timed, and tailored to the learning needs of clients.

▶ Education for childbearing ideally should begin before conception so that lifestyle changes can be made and the couple can be helped to achieve maximum wellness.

▶ Education for childbearing may span the childbearing year or be done at individual prenatal visits or in one day.

▶ Educational preparation of the childbearing family focuses on the physiologic and psychologic needs of the family and addresses issues such as relaxation/stress reduction, self-care practices, and exercise.

▶ Prepared childbirth methods include psychophysical preparation, psychoprophylaxis, the LeBoyer method, the Bradley method, and hypnosis.

▶ Clients have several choices for childbirth attendants; e.g., physicians, certified nurse-midwives, certified midwives, and lay midwives.

▶ Choices for delivery settings include hospitals, free-standing birth centers, and the client's home. Most American women deliver in a hospital.

After reading the vignette at the beginning of this chapter, use what you have learned to answer these questions.

1. If you were the nurse supervising the Denglers' childbirth education class, how would you respond to Tamika's lack of confidence in her ability to concentrate on her breathing patterns?

2. What other questions might Tamika and Rashid have about preparation for labor and delivery?

3. Despite Tamika's worry about mastering breathing techniques, what benefits do you think this couple will receive from participating in a childbirth preparation program?

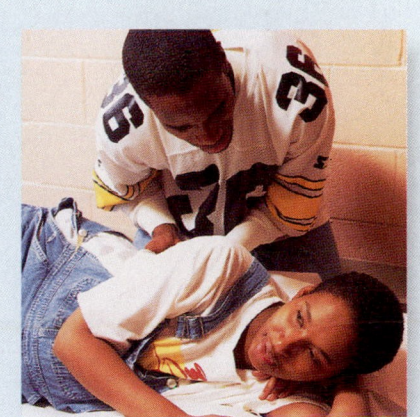

Critical Thinking Questions

► References

American College of Nurse-Midwives, Division of Accreditation (1997). Education programs accredited by the ACNM Division of Accreditation [booklet]. Washington, DC: Author.

Biasella, S. (1993). A comprehensive perinatal education program. *AWHONN'S Clinical Issues in Perinatal Nursing, 4*, 5–19.

Bloom, B. (Ed.). (1982). *Taxonomy of educational objectives: Cognitive domain* (25th ed.). New York: Longman.

Bridgwater, N. (1998). Childbirth education options: Exploring one day classes. *AWHONN's Lifelines, 2*(2), 49–52.

California Department of Health Services. (1987). *Natural remedies for pregnancy discomforts.* Sacramento, CA: Coalition for the Medical Rights of Women and Educational Programs Associates.

Chabon, I. (1966). *Awake and aware.* New York: Delacorte Press.

Clark, C.C. (1986). *Wellness nursing: Concepts, theory, research and practice.* New York: Springer.

Devitt, N. (1977). The transition from home to hospital birth in the United States. *Birth and the Family, 4*, 47–58.

Dick-Read, G. (1944). *Childbirth without fear.* New York: Harper & Brothers.

Enkin, M.W., Keirse, M.J., Renfrew, M.J., & Neilson, J.P. (1995). Effective care in pregnancy and childbirth: A synopsis. *Birth, 22*(2), 101–110.

Hart, M.A., & Foster, S.N. (1997). Couples' attitudes toward childbirth participation: Relationship to evaluation of labor and delivery. *Journal of Perinatal and Neonatal Nursing, 11*(1), 10–20.

Karmel, M. (1959). *Thank you, Dr. Lamaze.* New York: Dolphin Books.

Klaus, M.K., Kennel, J., & Klaus, P.H. (1996). *Bonding: Building the foundations of secure attachment and independence.* Reading, MA: Merloyd Lawrence.

Krathwohl, D.R., et al. (1982). *Taxonomy of educational objectives: Affective domain* (13th ed.). New York: London.

Lichtman, R., & Papera, S. (1990). *Gynecology: Well woman care.* Norwalk, CT: Appleton & Lange.

Mattson, S., & Smith, J. (Eds.). (1993). Preparation for childbirth. In L.M. Mullaly (Ed.), *Core curriculum for maternal-newborn nursing.* (pp. 126–144). Philadelphia: W.B. Saunders.

Olsen, O. (1997). Meta-analysis of the safety of home birth. *Birth, 24*(1), 4–13.

Rogers, J., & Matsumura, M. (1991). *Mother to be: A guide to pregnancy and birth for women with disabilities.* New York: Demos.

Shearer, E.L. (1995). Commentary: Many factors affect the outcome of prenatal classes. *Birth, 22*(1), 27–28.

Varney, H. (1997). *Varney's midwifery* (3rd ed.). Sudbury, MA: Jones and Bartlett.

Weingarten, C.T., & Jacobwitz, J.T. (1987). Alternatives in childbearing: Choices and challenges. In L.N. Sherwen (Ed.), *Psychosocial dimensions of the pregnant family* (pp. 193–218). New York: Springer.

Zwelling, E. (1996). Childbirth education in the 1990s and beyond. *Journal of Obstetric, Gynecologic, and Neonatal Nursing, 25*, 425–432.

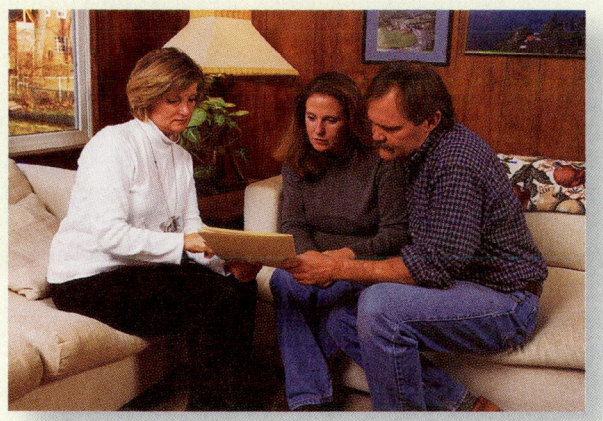

Stephen and Andrea Nolan, ages 34 and 32, respectively, are expecting their first child. Andrea is 10 weeks pregnant. As part of their prenatal care, the couple has been advised to participate in an assessment to evaluate the risk of passing a genetic disorder to their baby. Pamela Fields, RN, MSN, meets with Stephen and Andrea and describes the nature of the information that she will be collecting from them in order to conduct the risk assessment. The nurse begins to question the couple about their own and their families' health histories and explains the use of a genogram as a tool to identify family members who are or could be at risk for a genetic disorder.

In response to the nurse's questions, Stephen states that his sister Elizabeth, who died at age 10, suffered from cystic fibrosis. As the nurse makes note of this fact, Andrea, who looks visibly concerned, asks: "What can you tell us about the chances of our passing this disease to our baby?" Stephen reaches out and grasps Andrea's hand tightly. "We want to be prepared," he states, "for whatever happens." ∎

10

Families with Reproductive Risks

The process of human reproduction usually results in the birth of healthy infants. In some instances, however, problems can occur, creating major life crises for the family. Examples are genetic abnormalities of the infant and the family stress of infertility. In each case, family members experience a loss. Families who give birth to a child with a genetic abnormality grieve for the loss of the perfect child; families facing infertility grieve over the loss of the children they never had.

Genetic problems include autosomal chromosomal abnormalities, which are those abnormalities involving the first 22 pairs of chromosomes, and sex chromosomal abnormalities, which are abnormalities involving the pair of sex chromosomes. Genetic problems can be further classified according to the pattern of inheritance: single-gene inheritance or multifactorial inheritance. **Single-gene (Mendelian) inheritance** is the pattern of inheritance in which the presence of one gene can cause the expression of a trait. The **multifactorial (non-Mendelian) pattern of inheritance** is a result of the interaction of genetic and environmental influences. This mode of inheritance causes the largest number of birth defects in humans.

Other problems of human reproduction center on **infertility** (diminished or absent ability to conceive or produce a viable offspring). Infertility can be specific to problems of the female or male partner, to a combination of female and male problems, or to unexplained causes.

Families experiencing reproductive problems, such as genetic abnormalities and infertility, are often on an intense emotional roller coaster ride. The happiness that is supposed to accompany pregnancy leads to the despair surrounding the couple's inability to produce a perfect child. Nurses need to identify the emotional as well as physiologic needs of these couples. Empathetic nursing care helps the family reach a healthy resolution to the crises.

▶ GENETIC AND STRUCTURAL CHROMOSOMAL ABNORMALITIES

Genetic disorders represent the major causes of congenital malformations in children. Chromosomal abnormalities represent 20–25% of congenital malformations. They are also identified in about 50% of early spontaneous abortions (Cunningham et al., 1997).

Normal human body cells have a complement of 46 chromosomes: 22 pairs of autosomes and 1 pair of sex chromosomes. The gene complement of the individual is referred to as the **genotype;** the characteris-

tics or appearance of the individual as a result of the genotype and environmental factors is called the **phenotype.** Individuals with genetic abnormalities usually have characteristic genotypes as well as phenotypes.

Chromosomal abnormalities that occur in the first 22 pairs of chromosomes are called autosomal chromosomal abnormalities. Abnormalities may also occur in the pair of sex chromosomes: these are called sex chromosomal abnormalities. Chromosomal abnormalities may be further classified into numerical chromosomal abnormalities, resulting in an individual who has too many or too few chromosomes, and structural chromosomal abnormalities, resulting in an individual who usually has the complement of 46 chromosomes, but a piece of a chromosome may be missing or an extra piece of chromosomal material may be attached. In either case the individual has too many or too few genes, resulting in abnormalities in both growth and development.

▶ Numerical Chromosomal Abnormalities

Numerical chromosomal abnormalities are usually a result of **nondisjunction,** an error in cell division in which the paired chromosomes fail to separate at anaphase. This error may occur during mitotic cell division or during the first or second meiotic divisions (Moore, 1993). (For a detailed discussion of cell division, see Chapter 6.) Numerical chromosomal abnormalities may occur in either the autosomes or the sex chromosomes. When a chromosome is missing so that the human body cells contain one less than the normal complement of 46 chromosomes, the numerical abnormality is called a **monosomy.** When human body cells have three chromosomes along a pair rather than the normal two, the abnormality is called a **trisomy.**

Numerical Autosomal Abnormalities

Numerical autosomal abnormalities involve the first 22 pairs of chromosomes, or autosomes. A monosomy of the autosomes is very rare in living persons because this abnormality is usually not compatible with life.

Trisomies of the autosomes are the result of nondisjunction in the ovum or sperm in which either germ cell has 24 instead of 23 chromosomes. When fertilization occurs, the new individual has a complement of 47 chromosomes instead of the normal 46 chromosomes. The most common numerical autosomal abnormality is **Down syndrome** or **trisomy 21,** in which there are three number 21 chromosomes

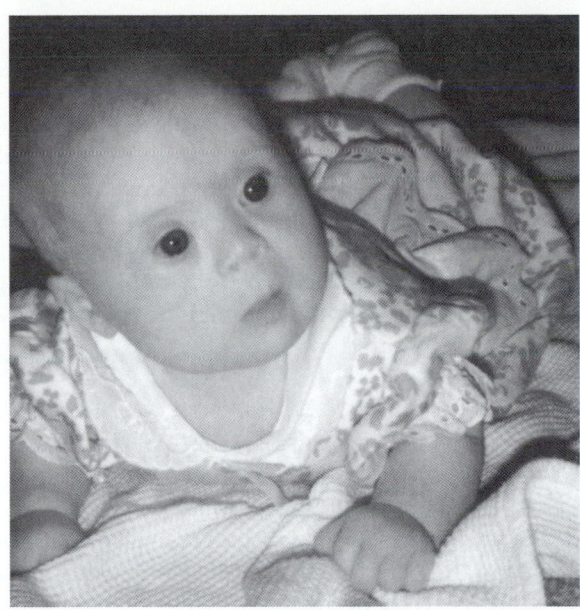

FIGURE 10–1. An infant with Down syndrome as a result of trisomy 21. Among the clinical manifestations are almond-shaped eyes and low-bridged nose. Often the infant's tongue protrudes.

instead of two. Children with this syndrome have phenotypes that distinguish them from other members of the same family (Fig. 10–1). Other examples of trisomies of the autosomes include trisomy 18 (Edwards' syndrome) and trisomy 13 (Patau's syndrome).

These autosomal trisomies are less common than trisomy 21, and children with these conditions usually die during infancy (Table 10–1). Autosomal trisomies occur with increasing frequency as maternal age increases and are usually due to nondisjunction in oogenesis. This is particularly true of trisomy 21, which is found in 1 in 1550 births in mothers under the age of 25, but in about 1 in 25 births in mothers over the age of 45.

Numerical Abnormalities of the Sex Chromosomes

Numerical abnormalities of the sex chromosomes are relatively common and may result in monosomies and trisomies (Rudolph, Hoffman, & Rudolph, 1996). In the vast majority of cases, these abnormalities do not produce the severe handicaps that are present with autosomal numerical abnormalities. The reason for this stems from the unique characteristics of the X chromosome.

During early divisions of the fertilized ovum, only one X chromosome is biologically active; the others are inactivated. The number of inactivated X chromosomes is one less than the total number of X chromosomes found in the nucleus of the cell. The inactivated X chromosome is one of the last chromosomes to replicate its DNA. The **Barr body** or sex chromatin body is thought to represent this genetically inactive, late-replicating X chromosome.

▶ **TABLE 10–1**

Examples of Numerical Chromosomal Abnormalities

Chromosomal Disorder	Average Incidence	Characteristics
Autosomal Disorders		
Trisomy 21 (Down syndrome)	1:700	Mental retardation; flat occiput; upper slant to palpebral fissures; protruding tongue; broad, short hands with simian creases; possible congenital heart defects
Trisomy 18 (Edwards' syndrome)	1:5000	Mental retardation; low-set malformed ears; prominent occiput; congenital heart defects; failure to thrive; usually death in infancy
Trisomy 13 (Patau's syndrome)	1:7000	Mental retardation; bilateral cleft lip and palate; polydactyly; malformed ears; death early in infancy
Sex Chromosome Disorders		
Turner's syndrome (45 total chromosomes, X sex chromosomes)	1:2500	Female; short stature; webbed neck; negative sex chromatin test; absence of sexual maturation at puberty; amenorrhea; broad chest with widely spaced nipples; sterile
Klinefelter's syndrome (47 chromosomes, XXY sex chromosomes)	1:1000	Male; tall, long legs in relation to trunk; mental deficiency of varying degree; small testes; absence of sperm or oligospermia; 80% are sex chromatin positive
Triple X syndrome (47 chromosomes, XXX sex chromosomes)	1:1000	Female; normal in appearance; two sex chromatin bodies; may be mentally retarded; fertile
XYY syndrome (47 chromosomes, XYY sex chromosomes)	1:1000	Male; tall, long head; may display antisocial behavior; normal appearance and sexual development
Fragile X syndrome	1:1250	Male: mild to severe mental retardation Female: may not be affected

Normal female body cells have one active and one inactivated X chromosome; thus, females are sex chromatin positive. The normal male body cells have one active and no inactivated X chromosomes; thus, males are sex chromatin negative. Whenever an increased number of X chromosomes exist, all but one of the X chromosomes replicate late; and when one of the two X chromosomes has a structural abnormality, it often replicates late. X chromosome abnormalities (in number or structure) are more compatible with life and cause less profound effects than those of the autosomes because the genetic material that causes the abnormality is found in the inactive, late-replicating X chromosome.

Most monosomies of the sex chromosomes result in death of the embryo. It is estimated that 20% of early spontaneous abortions are the result of sex chromosome monosomies (Cunningham et al., 1997). **Turner's syndrome,** a genetic abnormality affecting females, is an example of a monosomy of the sex chromosomes in which the child survives. This syndrome occurs when nondisjunction during spermatogenesis results in the absence of the paternal X chromosome. Female children with Turner's syndrome have 45 chromosomes: 44 autosomes, and 1 X chromosome.

Trisomies of the sex chromosomes may also be found; however, the characteristic physical features of these abnormalities usually do not appear until adolescence (see Table 10–1). Sex chromatin patterns are used to detect some of the trisomies of the sex chromosomes. For example, when their cells are examined microscopically, females who have an XXX sex chromosome complement will have two masses of sex chromatin; males who have an XXY sex chromosome complement will usually have one mass of sex chromatin (Moore, 1993).

▶ Mosaicism

Mosaicism is a genetic mutation that results in an unequal number of chromosomes in the cells. Mosaic individuals thus have cells with varying genetic constitutions or genotypes; some of the body cells have one number of chromosomes (e.g., 47 or 45), and others have another number of chromosomes (e.g., 46). Most individuals who are diagnosed as mosaic have a mixture of normal cells with 46 chromosomes and trisomic cells with 47 chromosomes. The usual cause of mosaicism is nondisjunction during early cell division of the fertilized ovum. Mosaic individuals may display handicaps such as mental deficiencies, but these handicaps are usually less serious than those of persons with trisomies or monosomies.

▶ Structural Chromosomal Abnormalities

Abnormalities in the structure of the chromosomes usually occur when a piece of a chromosome breaks and is missing or transfers from one chromosome to another chromosome. Most of these abnormalities are caused by environmental factors such as exposure to radiation and drugs. The type of abnormality that develops depends on what happens to the pieces of chromosomes that are broken.

Translocation

Translocation is the transfer of a piece of one chromosome to a nonhomologous chromosome (one that is not part of the transferring chromosome's matched pair). Such transfers can occur between any two chromosomes in the genotype during the process of meiosis or mitosis. (DeCherney & Pernoll, 1994). If two chromosomes undergo breaks and exchange pieces, the individual will have no missing or extra chromosomes and is said to be a **balanced translocation carrier.** The balanced translocation carrier may produce germ cells (ovum or sperm) with the abnormal translocation chromosome, causing his or her offspring to have an abnormal extra chromosome. For example, a woman with a balanced translocation between chromosome number 21 and chromosome number 14 or 15 may produce offspring with Down syndrome. The syndrome in this case is caused by a translocation trisomy instead of an autosomal trisomy; the fertilized ovum has two normal number 21 chromosomes (one from the mother and one from the father), and an extra piece of number 21 chromosome attached to chromosome 14 or 15. Offspring that are affected with this syndrome have an extra chromosome even though their body cell chromosome count is 46. Three to four percent of individuals with Down syndrome have translocation trisomies. These are not related to increasing maternal age. Either mother or father can be a carrier of the translocation, with a 1 in 5 chance of an offspring being affected if the mother is a carrier and a 1 in 20 chance if the father is a carrier.

Deletion

Deletions occur when a chromosome breaks and a portion of the chromosome is lost. An example of a chromosomal structural abnormality caused by a deletion is the **cri du chat (cat's cry) syndrome.** In this syndrome, there is a deletion of the short arm of the number 5 chromosome. Infants with this syndrome display a characteristic weak, high-pitched, catlike cry. They also have small heads (microcephaly), severe mental retardation, failure to thrive, and congenital heart disease.

Structural Abnormalities of the Sex Chromosomes

The most common structural abnormality of the sex chromosomes is the **isochromosome.** This abnormality is caused by an injury to the X chromosome during meiosis, resulting in loss of the short arm of one X chromosome. The cell in this abnormality divides transversely instead of longitudinally. After the arm breaks, rehealing occurs, forming the isochromosome, both arms of which originate from the chromatids of a single arm of the original chromosome. Individuals with this abnormality, therefore, lack the genes that are normally found on the other arm of the chromosome (Rudolph et al., 1996). Individuals affected by this abnormality are usually short in stature and display some of the same characteristics as those who have Turner's syndrome.

▶ Patterns of Inheritance and Abnormalities

Inheritance may be classified as single-gene (Mendelian) inheritance or multifactorial (non-Mendelian) inheritance. The genes found along the chromosomes determine the structure and function of the proteins and enzymes of the human body. These genes determine eye color, hair color, blood and tissue type, and existence of a genetic disorder such as phenylketonuria (PKU), cystic fibrosis, or sickle cell anemia.

Single-Gene Inheritance

Genes, like the chromosomes, come in pairs, half received from the mother and half received from the father. The gene that is expressed by the individual is referred to as **dominant;** the gene that is present but not expressed by the individual is called **recessive.** Individuals who have one dominant gene and one recessive gene for a trait are **heterozygous** for that trait. Conversely, individuals who have identical genes in a pair are **homozygous** for that trait. A recessive trait may be expressed by the individual if there is no dominant gene on either chromosome of the pair. There are four types of single-gene patterns of inheritance: autosomal dominant, autosomal recessive, X-linked dominant, and X-linked recessive.

Autosomal Dominant Disorders. Autosomal dominant disorders are caused by a single altered gene along one of the autosomes. The disease trait is a heterozygous trait in which one gene in the pair is normal and the other gene in the pair is abnormal. The single altered gene is dominant, thus causing the individual to express the abnormal trait. These disorders may occur as the result of a new mutation

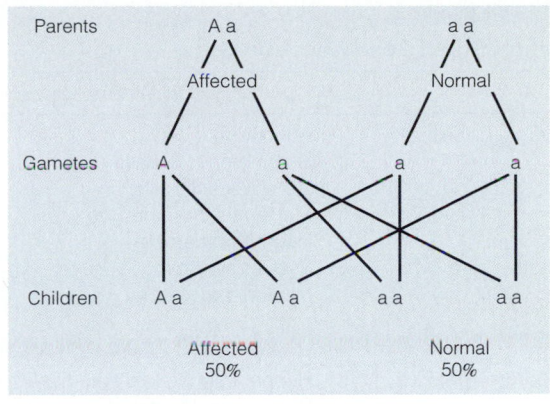

FIGURE 10–2. Diagram illustrating autosomal dominant inheritance. *(Reproduced, with permission, from Blackman, J. (1990). Medical aspects of developmental disabilities in children birth to three (2nd ed.). Rockville, MD: Aspen Publishers, pp. 152–153.)*

(change in genetic material) in an individual ovum or sperm cell, or they may be inherited from one parent or the other who is affected by the disorder. An individual who has an autosomal dominant disorder has a 50% risk of passing the gene to each of his or her offspring. In other words, each offspring of an affected parent has a 1 in 2 chance of demonstrating the disorder. If the parent does not transmit the abnormal gene to the offspring, the child will be normal and his or her offspring will be normal. Males and females are equally likely to be affected because the gene does not involve the sex chromosomes. Figure 10–2 illustrates the pattern of autosomal dominant inheritance; Table 10–2 lists some common autosomal dominant disorders.

Autosomal Recessive Disorders. Autosomal recessive disorders are expressed in an individual when both members of an autosomal gene pair are altered. Although both parents carry the recessive altered genes, they are not affected by the disorder because they are heterozygous for the trait and the altered gene does not express itself. When two individuals carrying the same recessive altered gene reproduce, however, they may both pass the altered gene to their offspring, who will then have no normal gene to carry out the necessary function. Both parents are called carriers of the autosomal recessive disorder, and they have a 25% risk of passing the disorder to each of their offspring. That is, each offspring has a 1 in 4 chance of demonstrating the disorder. Moreover, each offspring has a 1 in 2 (50%) chance of being a carrier of the recessive trait even though the offspring is normal and does not express the disorder; each child also has a 1 in 4 (25%) chance of not having the disease and not being a carrier.

► **TABLE 10–2**

Common Single Gene Abnormalities

	Dominant Disorders	Recessive Disorders
Autosomal disorders	Achondroplasia Huntington's disease Tuberous sclerosis Marfan's syndrome Neurofibromatosis Stickler syndrome Myotonic dystrophy	Cystic fibrosis Galactosemia Glycogen storage disease Hurler's syndrome Limb-girdle muscular dystrophy Maple syrup urine disease Phenylketonuria Sickle cell anemia Tay–Sachs disease
X-linked disorders	Hypophosphatemia (vitamin D-resistant rickets) Cervico-oculo-acoustic syndrome	Duchenne muscular and Becker muscular dystrophies Hemophilia A Hemophilia B Hunter's syndrome Color blindness Lesch–Nyhan syndrome Glucose-6-phosphate dehydrogenase deficiency

Because parents must pass the same altered gene for expression of the disorder to occur in their children, parents who are closely related (consanguineous matings) are more likely to produce offspring with the recessive disorder than parents who are unrelated. Again, males and females are equally likely to be affected, because the genes are not present in the sex chromosomes. Moreover, specific populations may have a higher frequency of recessive disorders than other populations. For example, sickle cell anemia is found more frequently in black populations than in white populations. Figure 10–3 illustrates the pattern of autosomal recessive inheritance; Table 10–2 lists examples of these disorders.

X-Linked Dominant Disorders.

X-linked dominant disorders are extremely rare in humans. They are the result of an alteration in a gene located along an X chromosome. Because females have two X chromosomes, these disorders occur twice as often in females as in males. X-linked dominant disorders are passed from an affected male to all of his daughters, because the daughters receive the father's altered X chromosome. None of his sons are affected, because they receive their father's Y chromosome.

A female with an X-linked dominant disorder has a 50% chance of passing the altered genes to her daughters and sons. Each child of a female with the X-linked dominant disorder will then have a 1 in 2 chance of expressing the disorder. Figure 10–4 illustrates the pattern of X-linked dominant inheritance; Table 10–2 lists X-linked dominant disorders.

X-Linked Recessive Disorders.

X-linked recessive disorders are much more common than X-linked dominant disorders. They occur more frequently in males than in females, because males have a single X chromosome and the single X chromosome carries the altered gene. When males receive a "single dose" of the altered gene, therefore, they express the disorder. Females, on the other hand, have two X chromosomes, one that carries the abnormal gene for the trait and one with a normal gene to carry out the function of the trait. Females must have the gene present in a "double dose" or in both X chromosomes to be affected. On rare occasions, however, females show some characteristics of the disorder because the X chromosome carrying the normal trait is randomly inactivated, allowing the abnormal trait to express itself.

A female who is a carrier of a gene that causes an X-linked recessive disorder has a 50% risk of passing

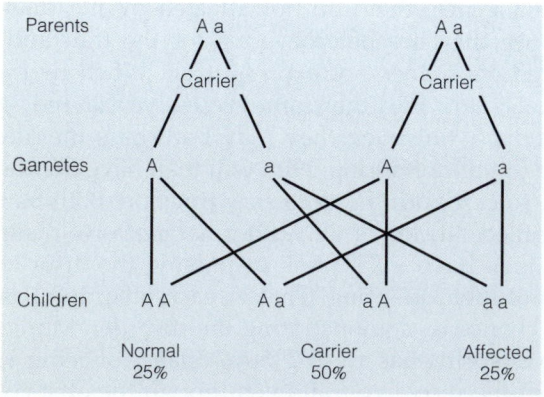

FIGURE 10–3. Diagram illustrating autosomal recessive inheritance (*Reproduced, with permission, from Blackman, J. (1990). Medical aspects of developmental disabilities in children birth to three (2nd ed.). Rockville, MD: Aspen Publishers, pp. 152–153.*)

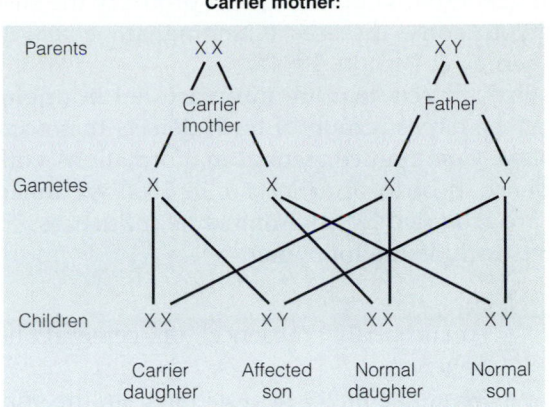

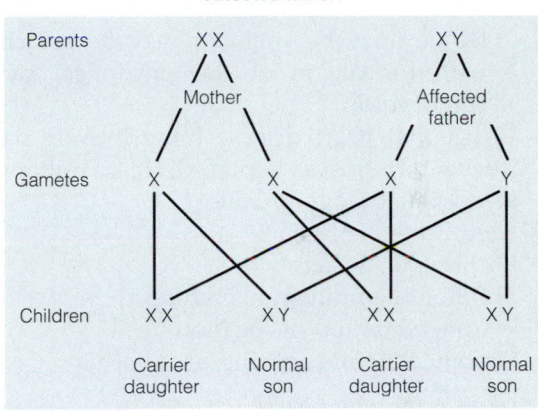

FIGURE 10–4. Diagram illustrating X-linked dominant inheritance. *(Reproduced, with permission, from Blackman, J. (1990). Medical aspects of developmental disabilities in children birth to three (2nd ed.). Rockville, MD: Aspen Publishers, pp. 152–153.)*

FIGURE 10–5. Diagram illustrating X-linked recessive inheritance. *(Reproduced, with permission, from Blackman, J. (1990). Medical aspects of developmental disabilities in children birth to three (2nd ed.). Rockville, MD: Aspen Publishers, pp. 152–153.)*

the abnormal gene to her sons. Each son will have a 1 in 2 chance of demonstrating the disorder. The female carrier also has a 50% chance of passing the altered gene to her daughters, who will then have a 1 in 2 chance of becoming carriers of the altered gene. The son who is affected by the X-linked disorder has a 100% chance of passing the variant X to his daughters because the affected father has only one X to pass on. Fathers cannot transmit the altered gene to their sons because they transmit the Y instead of the X chromosome to their sons. Figure 10–5 illustrates the pattern of X-linked recessive inheritance; Table 10–2 lists some common X-linked recessive disorders.

Fragile X Syndrome

Fragile X syndrome is a relatively newly recognized condition. It is the most common cause of mental retardation known, occurring in about 1 per 1200 males and 1 per 2500 females (American College of Obstetricians and Gynecologists, 1995). In this condition there is a break in the X chromosome caused by a

mutation in the Fragile X Mental Retardation 1 gene (FMRI). Males who have this syndrome are typically affected because they have only one X chromosome. Females, on the other hand, are usually normal because they have two X chromosomes; the abnormal gene on one X chromosome is compensated for by the normal gene on the other X chromosome. Heterozygous females have a 50% chance of passing the abnormal gene to their children. Males who carry the fragile X gene will pass the abnormal gene to all of their daughters. Many affected families have two or more children with fragile X syndrome (Jackson & Vessey, 1996).

▶ Multifactorial Inheritance and Abnormalities

Many human characteristics are determined by multifactorial inheritance, accounting for the wide variation seen among normal humans in such areas as size, intelligence, blood pressure, and probably the susceptibility to some diseases (Cunningham et al., 1997; DeCherney & Pernoll, 1994).

Birth defects that are multifactorial in origin are by far the largest group of birth defects that occur in humans. Common congenital malformations with an incidence at birth of at least 1 in 1000 are inherited and are modified by environmental influences. These defects include the following:

- Neural tube defects
  - Anencephaly (absence of cerebral hemispheres)
  - Myelomeningocele (opening in the lumbosacral vertebrae through which the meningeal sac and spinal cord protrude)
  - Spina bifida (opening in the lumbosacral vertebrae; may be slight or may be associated with protrusion of the meningeal sac or spinal cord)
- Congenital heart disease (may include patent ductus arteriosus, septal defects, pulmonary stenosis, tetralogy of Fallot)
- Cleft lip or cleft palate
- Orthopedic defects
  - Talipes equinovarus (clubfoot)
  - Congenital hip dislocation
- Umbilical hernia and inguinal hernia

Multifactorial birth defects have a polygenic component in which the cumulative effect of many genes produces the expression of the disorder. Many theories have been proposed regarding the mechanisms of multifactorial inheritance. None of these theories, however, has been readily accepted by all scientists and clinicians.

Some facts are known. For example, multifactorial disorders tend to cluster in families and are found more frequently among relatives than in the general population. Unlike the risk of single-gene disorders, which remains the same with each pregnancy, the risk of multifactorial disorders increases when more than one member of the family has the disorder. For example, the risk for the single-gene disorder sickle cell anemia is 25% (1 in 4) for each pregnancy if both parents carry the recessive gene for the trait, regardless of the number of children in the family who have the disorder. In contrast, a family who has a child with the multifactorial birth defect spina bifida has a greatly increased risk of having a subsequent child with the disorder (from 1 in 2000 before the birth of the first affected child to 1 in 40 after the birth of the affected child). Moreover, the more severe the defect, the more likely the risk of recurrence in subsequent siblings. For example, the risk of recurrence is greater for future siblings of a child with bilateral cleft lip

(5.6%) as opposed to one with a unilateral cleft lip (2.6%).

Multifactorial birth defects also vary among races, so that there may be a higher incidence of certain defects among persons of one particular race than in persons of other races (Rudolph et al., 1996). For example, umbilical hernias are found more frequently in black infants than in white infants. Sex also plays a role in multifactorial inheritance. Certain conditions, like pyloric stenosis, occur more frequently in males than in females.

Environmental factors also contribute to multifactorial birth defects. Seasonal variations, exposure to toxic chemicals, radiation, and certain altitudes seem to contribute to these defects. There also seem to be variations in occurrence from place to place in the world. Interestingly, not all of these defects appear to be environmentally induced, because the frequency of such abnormalities in identical twins, termed *concordance*, is four to eight times greater than in nonidentical twins and other siblings (DeCherney & Pernoll, 1994).

Overall, multifactorial defects are identified in about 1% of newborns. In most cases, a simple pattern of inheritance cannot be demonstrated, and risk rates are difficult to estimate. In general, the risk of significant malformation in any pregnancy is approximately 1 to 2%. The risk of a second malformed child is about 5%, with the risk increasing with subsequent malformed children (Cunningham et al., 1997). Even with the difficulty in providing accurate risk rates for multifactorial birth defects, the risk for these defects is still much lower than for single-gene defects (Rudolph et al., 1996).

▶ CARE OF THE FAMILY AT RISK FOR GENETIC DISORDERS

▶ Nursing and Collaborative Assessment

Nursing and collaborative assessment for potential or actual genetic disorders focuses on counseling and support of the family. A comprehensive family history and genogram provide the nurse with information about the family pedigree. This information includes health and illness data as well as information about psychosocial factors, racial and ethnic background, parental age, maternal health history, reproductive history, and history of present pregnancy, when applicable (see Chapter 8). The child who is born with a suspected or actual genetic abnormality is given a complete physical examination to determine the extent of the disability caused by the defect.

To determine risk status for genetic abnormalities, the constitution of the chromosomes in number and structure is assessed by obtaining a photomicrograph of the chromosomes and arranging them in numerical order. This arrangement, called the **karyotype,** is used by the geneticist and other members of the health care team to assess alterations in chromosome number and structure and risk of abnormalities to present or future offspring. The karyotypic assessment of individuals is done by analysis of 20 to 50 chromosome spreads for chromosome number. Several spreads are required to determine whether the cells have different chromosome counts (e.g., mosaicism). Photographs are taken of representative chromosome spreads and karyotypes are constructed. Banding techniques also are used to determine numerical counts of chromosomes. In this technique, the cells are stained at metaphase to determine the banding patterns of each chromosome. It is thus possible to identify every chromosome in the karyotype and clearly identify translocations and trisomies. Sex chromatin (Barr body) analysis also may be done to determine the number of X chromosomes present in the cells. The number of X chromosomes is the number of Barr bodies plus one.

▶ Nursing and Collaborative Management

Risk determination for genetic disorders or birth defects allows the couple to become involved in reproductive decision making (see Chapter 8). Nurses, in collaboration with other health care team members,

Commonly Asked Questions

What is the purpose of seeing a genetic counselor?

A genetic counselor helps you to understand the way heredity and environmental factors contribute to disorders. The counselor also helps you to identify the risks of recurrence of a disorder in your family and the options available to you for dealing with the risk. Genetic counselors give you the information so that you can make an informed decision about your options.

When the genetic counselor told us that the probability of having a child with sickle cell anemia was 25%, did that mean that if we have four children, only one of the children will have the disease?

No. Sickle-cell anemia is a recessive disorder. This means that if both you and your partner carry the gene for sickle cell anemia, you are carriers of the disease. With each pregnancy, you have a 1 in 4 or 25% chance of having a child with the disease, a 2 in 4 or 50% chance of having a child who will carry the trait for the disease, and a 1 in 4 or 25% chance that the child will neither have the disease nor carry the trait for the disease.

Why is it only probable that my male children will develop hemophilia if I carry the gene for hemophilia? I have no signs of the disease and I am a female.

Hemophilia is called an X-linked disease. Females have two X chromosomes; males have one X chromosome and one Y chromosome. If the X chromosome that the male receives from his mother has the abnormal gene for hemophilia, the male child will exhibit the disease because he only has the abnormal X chromosome. With females, even if they receive the abnormal X chromosome, the normal X chromosome usually takes over the function. Female children who have the abnormal X chromosome can pass this chromosome on to their male children who will develop hemophilia.

Will genetic testing be able to tell us about all the possible congenital health problems that our child may have?

No. There are congenital health problems that will not be identified through genetic testing. Genetic testing identifies those problems that are coded in the chromosomes and genes. We now know of more than 5,000 single-gene disorders. There are probably more that we have not identified. Examples of congenital health problems that cannot be identified through genetic testing include congenital rubella syndrome and other infections.

support the couple through the decision-making process. If the woman is pregnant, several antenatal tests can be done to assess for genetic disorders (see Chapters 15, 17, 18). The nurse needs to provide the couple with factual information about the tests and the risks and benefits of the testing procedures. Emotional support for the couple and other family members is important because of the anxiety-producing nature of the testing procedures and the possibility of actual genetic problems.

Faced with the risk of having a child with a genetic abnormality, the couple will need to engage in reproductive decision making regarding the present pregnancy, if applicable, or future pregnancies. For example, a couple who is presented with the risks of having a child with Down syndrome may decide that they will take the risk and that if, through antenatal testing, the fetus is found to have Down syndrome, they will carry the pregnancy to term and care for the child. The nurse should never attempt to influence a couple with regard to their present or future child-bearing decisions. Rather, the couple should be supported through the decision-making process in a nonjudgmental manner. The nurse assists the couple by providing them with information; however, the decision must be made by the couple.

If a child is born with a genetic disorder, the family will need a great deal of emotional support from the nurse and other members of the health care team. The family must be allowed to grieve for the loss of the "perfect" child that they had imagined during the pregnancy. The family also needs information regarding support services for follow-up care of the child, such as developmental centers and foundations that are specifically dedicated to the child's disorder. The nurse can help to promote family coping by coordinating the services of a variety of resources for families who are confronted with children who have genetic disorders or who are at risk for genetic disorders.

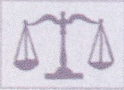 ## Ethical Decision Making

Advances in human genetics are rapidly occurring. By the year 2005 it is anticipated that the entire human genome (the complete gene complement of a human) will be mapped and all 70,000–100,000 genes will be identified (Jones, 1996). There is a possibility that any individual can be screened genetically for medical as well as social problems. The Human Genome Project generates important ethical questions about the type of genetic information that should be generated and the genetic manipulations that should be allowed (Murray & Livny, 1995).

1. Who should be screened genetically?
2. What genetic information should be disseminated and who should control the release of this information?
3. What ethical problems are posed for individuals, employers, and insurance companies related to genetic screening?
4. How will genetic information change health care?
5. How will genetic information change individual lives?

▶ INFERTILITY

Infertility represents a major life crisis to more than 15% of couples of childbearing age in the United States. About 5 million couples are infertile. At least one of six couples experiences the stress of infertility in their lifetime, with some indication that the incidence is on the rise (Whiteford & Gonzalez, 1995; Zinaman & Uhler, 1996).

The increased incidence of infertility may be related to the postponement of childbearing until after the optimum age of fertility (i.e., ages 24 to 30), the increased prevalence of sexually transmitted diseases (STDs), especially gonorrhea and chlamydia, and the side effects associated with some contraceptive methods. Environmental hazards and stress also are thought to contribute to the problem. It has been estimated that smoking more than one pack of cigarettes per day, for example, decreases the chance of pregnancy by more than 20% (Benson & Pernoll, 1994). Further, the higher incidence of infertility may reflect the fact that more people are currently seeking help for this problem.

Infertility is generally defined as the inability to conceive after 1 year of regular sexual intercourse without contraception. **Primary infertility** is defined as the inability to conceive with no previous history of pregnancy. **Secondary infertility** is the inability to conceive after one or more successful pregnancies. **Sterility** is absolute inability to conceive. **Fecundity** is the ability to participate in the production of a child.

Fecundability is the chance of becoming pregnant per month of exposure. Young, healthy couples having frequent intercourse have a 28% chance of pregnancy per month.

The criterion of 1 year in the definition is based on statistics for a normal population of couples who are not using contraception; these statistics show that approximately 50% of all sexually active couples conceive in the first three months and 85% conceive in 1 year (Ransom & McNeeley, 1997).

Probable causes for infertility are found in 85 to 90% of couples after careful evaluation. Factors related to the female partner account for 40 to 50% of infertility problems; factors related to the male partner account for an additional 30%; and a combination of factors related to both male and female partners account for another 20 to 30%. Approximately 50% of those couples who seek treatment conceive. Pregnancy occurs in 15 to 20% of infertile couples even without treatment (Benson & Pernoll, 1994).

▶ Problems Related to the Female Partner

It is assumed that the prerequisites for fertility in the female are the ability to produce a normal ovum capable of fertilization in the fallopian tube and a healthy endometrium, in which the fertilized ovum implants and which is capable of nourishing the embryo fetus. Problems with fertility associated with the female partner can be grouped with respect to the pelvic factor, the ovulatory factor, and the cervical factor.

The Pelvic Factor

The pelvic factor contributes to female infertility by creating problems with fertilization or implantation of the fertilized ovum in the uterus. The pelvic factor includes infection of the pelvic organs, endometriosis, and structural disorders.

Infections. Infections of the vagina, cervix, fallopian tubes, and endometrium may contribute to infertility. Infections can interfere with the viability of the sperm by making the environment of the cervix and vagina hostile to sperm. Infections of the endometrial lining of the uterus may contribute to difficulty in implantation and survival of the fertilized ovum. Because of the increased incidence of pelvic inflammatory disease, partly as a result of the rising incidence of STDs, infections of the fallopian tubes are becoming more common. Adhesions and scar tissue in the tubes interfere with fertilization and transportation of the fertilized ovum to the uterus. Infections

may also interfere with the healthy functioning of the ovaries.

Endometriosis. **Endometriosis,** a condition in which endometrial tissue grows outside the uterine cavity, may also contribute to female infertility. Endometriosis, an important health problem of women, is estimated to be present in 10 to 15% of women in the reproductive years. The prevalence of this condition increases to 30% among infertile women (Chin, 1997). It is thought that endometriosis has a polygenic or multifactorial etiology because women relate a family history of the disease (Lemcke, Pattison, Marshall, & Cowley, 1995)

Endometriosis is diagnosed when functional endometrium or tissue resembling the uterine lining is found implanted outside the uterus. Although endometriosis may be found in other areas of the body, it is found most frequently on the ovaries and in the cul-de-sac, particularly on the uterosacral ligaments, the rectosigmoid, the posterior cervix, and on the peritoneum of the broad ligaments (Fig. 10–6) (Chin, 1997).

Women with endometriosis have a progressive disease that may cause pelvic pain as well as infertility. Women often report that the pain begins one to two days prior to their menses and lasts throughout their flow (Lemcke et al., 1995).

Pain, however, is not a consistent symptom and is not always proportional to the extent of the endometriosis. Asymptomatic endometriosis is found in women with infertility (Lemcke et al., 1995).

The relationship between endometriosis and infertility has been extensively investigated. Moderate and severe endometriosis is related to pelvic adhesions. Implants involving the ovaries, the most common site of endometriosis, may impair ovulation, and implants involving the fallopian tubes may interfere with transportation of the fertilized ovum through the tube. Adhesions in the cul-de-sac caused by endometriosis may lead to a noncongenitally retroverted uterus. Moreover, endometrial implants may secrete prostaglandins that possibly interfere with ovulation and tubal function. Mild endometriosis as well as advanced disease can cause infertility, although the mechanism by which this occurs is unknown (Benson & Pernoll, 1994).

Structural Disorders. Structural disorders associated with female infertility include malformation of the uterus and fibroid tumors. Malformation of the uterus is congenital. A **bicornuate** or **septate uterus** may be completely or partially y-shaped. A complete septum may extend to the external os, creating a double uterus with two separate uterine cavities, or the septum may be partial and not extend to the internal or external os (Fig. 10–7). Uterine fibroid tumors may also impede implantation of the fertilized ovum in the endometrium.

The Ovulatory Factor

The ovulatory factor contributing to female infertility includes problems related to ovulation and hormonal

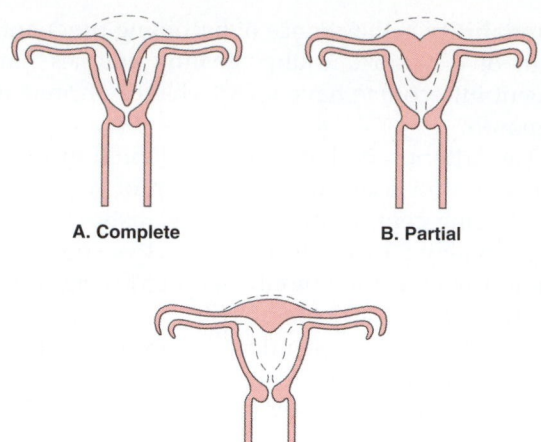

A. Complete   **B. Partial**

C. Arcuate

FIGURE 10–7. Septate uteri. *(Reproduced, with permission, from Cunningham, F.G., MacDonald, P.C., Gant, N.F., Leveno, K.J., Gilstrap, L.C., Hankins, G.D.V., & Clark, S.L. (1997).* Williams obstetrics *(20th ed.). Stamford, CT: Appleton & Lange, p. 642.)*

activity. Hormone activity is important to ovulation and the development of a healthy endometrium capable of nourishing the fertilized ovum. Problems arising from dysfunction of the pituitary, thyroid, or adrenal glands or the ovaries may impede these processes. Anovulation (failure of the ovaries to produce or release ova) may be related to increased levels of prolactin, secreted by the anterior pituitary gland. It is thought that prolactin may cause anovulation by blocking the action of gonadotropins on the ovaries (DeCherney & Pernoll, 1994). Significant increases in prolactin may indicate the presence of a pituitary adenoma, a prolactin-secreting tumor, causing ovulatory failure and amenorrhea. Secretion of elevated levels of steroid hormones by the adrenal glands may also affect ovulation because the increased androgen production blocks the action of the female hormones estrogen and progesterone.

Estrogen and progesterone secretion by the ovary may also be inadequate. If the secretion of estrogens is inadequate during the follicular phase of the menstrual cycle, the woman may not ovulate. If, on the other hand, progesterone production during the luteal phase is inadequate, the woman may ovulate but abort the fetus. Luteal-phase inadequacy is characterized by a defective endometrial response caused by insufficient progesterone output (Ransom & McNeeley, 1997).

The Cervical Factor

The cervical factor contributing to female infertility includes disturbances in the cervical environment that affect the survival and motility of the sperm. The cervical mucus should normally change under the influ-

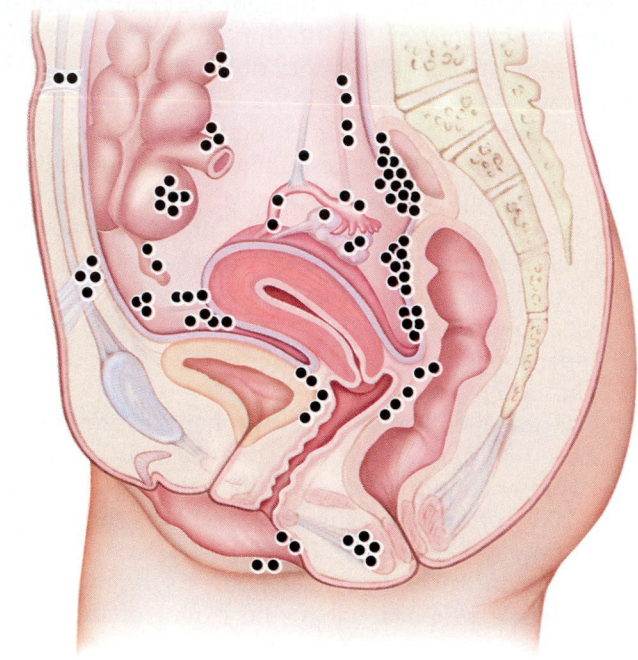

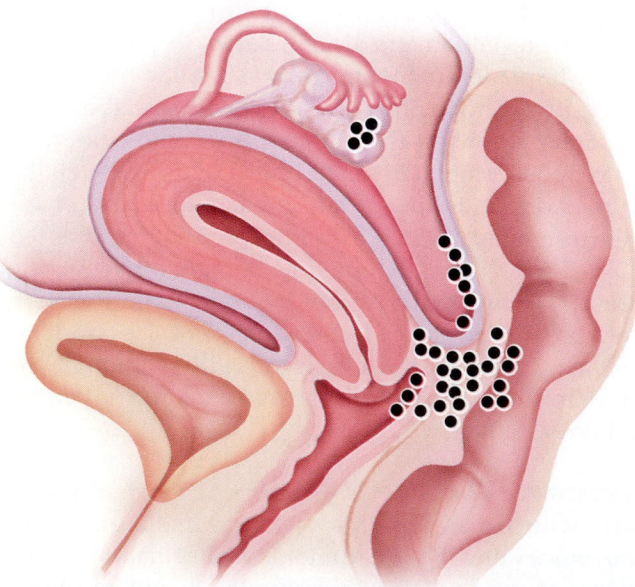

FIGURE 10–6. Common sites for endometriosis. *(Reproduced, with permission, from Way, L.W. (Ed.). (1994).* Current surgical diagnosis and treatment *(10th ed.). Norwalk, CT: Appleton & Lange, p. 985.)*

ence of estrogen and luteinizing hormone at the time of ovulation. If the production of these hormones is low or if cervicitis (inflammation of the cervix) is present, sperm may be impeded or destroyed by a hostile cervical mucus (De Cherney & Pernoll, 1994).

▶ Problems Related to the Male Partner

It is assumed that the prerequisites for fertility in the male include production of sufficient numbers of mature sperm that are motile and are able to be transported through the male reproductive tract. Problems related to male factor infertility may thus be grouped into problems in sperm production, motility, and transport.

Sperm Production Problems

The average number of sperm deposited in the vagina is 70 million per milliliter of semen, with a semen volume of 2 to 6 mL. A sperm count of 20 million or below in 2 to 6 mL of semen is suggestive of inadequate sperm production. Inadequate sperm production may be caused by infections, mechanical problems, or environmental influences.

Infections. Infections of the reproductive organs that affect sperm production include gonorrhea and chlamydia. Testicular inflammation (orchitis) caused by mumps in adulthood may also be associated with low sperm production. A high fever in the male, causing prolonged elevation of temperature in the scrotum, will also affect the quantity and quality of sperm ejaculated.

Mechanical Problems. Mechanical factors related to low sperm production include a varicocele, a varicose vein in a spermatic cord, and cryptorchism (undescended testicles). Both impede spermatogenesis by causing the sperm to be at a temperature higher than that needed for spermatogenesis.

Environmental Influences

Environmental influences on sperm production include exposure to radiation and industrial chemicals, which may injure the testicles. Excessive smoking and alcohol intake may also lower sperm production by decreasing testosterone levels. Intake of certain drugs such as some antihypertensive agents and marijuana may also cause hypospermatogenesis. Moreover, in utero exposure to diethylstilbestrol (DES) has been linked to inadequate sperm production (Benson & Pernoll, 1994). Finally, malnutrition, stress, and the use of hot tubs may also be related to inadequate production of sperm.

Sperm Motility Problems

Problems in sperm production are interrelated with problems in sperm motility. Sperm motility is due to flagellar action and is necessary for the maintenance and transport of sperm. Greater than 60% of the sperm per ejaculate should be motile for effective fertility. Factors that may affect the motility of sperm include decreased levels of testosterone, which may lower the level of seminal plasma needed for motility and transport, infection, and prostate disease.

Sperm Transport Problems

Problems that affect the ability of the male to transport sperm through his reproductive tract and deposit them in the female may also occur. The male reproductive tract may be obstructed by scar tissue formation as a result of infections. An injury to the vas deferens will also impede the transport of the sperm.

The adequacy of deposition of sperm in the female is dependent on the ability of the male to ejaculate. Problems with ejaculation may be the result of **impotence** (the inability to achieve an erection), **premature ejaculation** (untimely ejaculation), or **retrograde ejaculation,** a condition in which the sperm flow backward into the bladder instead of out of the penis. Retrograde ejaculation may be caused by diabetes mellitus, surgical trauma, or neurologic damage. Hypospadias, a congenital abnormality in which the male urethra opens on the shaft of the penis instead of the glans, may also cause problems in ejaculating sperm high in the vagina.

▶ Combined Problems

Combined problems, those that are attributed to both partners, include problems with sexual technique and sexual timing, as well as with immunologic responses to sperm.

Sexual Technique and Timing

Certain positions during sexual intercourse favor transport of the sperm to the cervical opening (e.g., woman on her back with knees flexed). Also, to enhance the delivery of sperm to the cervical opening, the woman can remain on her back with her knees flexed for 10 to 15 minutes after intercourse.

Another problem that can be categorized as a combined problem is the couple's lack of knowledge regarding the timing of intercourse during the fertile period and the life span of the sperm and ovum. Fertility is favored when the frequency of intercourse is every 36–48 hours from 3 to 4 days before until 2 days after ovulation. Couples can be reassured that they can have intercourse on consecutive days and as frequently as they wish in the periovulatory period. Normal sperm can fertilize ova for 24 to 48 hours after ejaculation. However, the ovum can be fertilized for only about 6 to 12 hours after ovulation (Lemcke et al., 1995).

Immunologic Factors

Another theory of the etiology of infertility focuses on immunologic factors involving the female or male partner. For example, some women develop antibodies against their partners' sperm, with the result that healthy sperm do not survive the hostile cervical environment. The male partner also may have an autoimmune response to his own sperm. In this condition, the male makes antibodies against and destroys his otherwise healthy sperm. Antibodies to sperm may be found in the blood as well as in genital secretions.

▶ Unexplained Infertility

Although the etiology of infertility can be explained in 85 to 90% of infertile couples, at times, even after careful investigation, the cause of infertility remains unexplained. Unexplained infertility is more common when the female partner is in her late 30s or early 40s (Lemcke et al., 1995). Because many of these couples will achieve a pregnancy without treatment, causation of and treatment for unexplained infertility remain unproven.

▶ CARE OF THE INFERTILE COUPLE

Infertility represents a life crisis to couples. Couples describe feelings of social isolation and alternating feelings of hope and disappointment. They also perceive a loss of control of their lives (Imeson & McMurray, 1996). Infertility investigation and treatment may be threatening and uncomfortable for the couple, but because infertility is central to their lives, they actively seek such investigations and treatment in an effort to solve the problem. Nurses can assist infertile couples to make treatment decisions, to focus on successful aspects of their lives, and to move on with their lives despite treatment outcomes (Olshansky, 1996).

Nurses and other members of the health care team should begin the infertility investigation in a supportive atmosphere for the couple. The goals of the initial steps of the workup include performing a health assessment of the couple, determining possible etiologies, providing correct advice and support, and facilitating referrals. From the beginning, the nurse should also be aware of any religious limitations that the couple may perceive about infertility treatment (Fryday, 1995).

▶ Nursing and Collaborative Assessment

Health History

Both partners should be seen early in the investigation so that a complete history of each partner can be obtained and assistance can be provided in creating an atmosphere in which the partners can support each other. A detailed history includes present and past health status and family, social, sexual, and reproductive data. At the outset, the couple should be asked if the infertility is primary or secondary in nature and the length of time they have been attempting a pregnancy. The health history includes data regarding childhood illnesses, immunizations, allergies, hospitalizations and serious illnesses, accidents and injuries, medications, and habits. Social data include information related to family relationships and support systems, as well as ethnic and religious affiliations. Occupational, educational, and financial status are important parts of the social data base. The couple's patterns of health care and of daily living are also considered in this portion of the history. A review of systems provides the nurse with significant data regarding the health of the partners in general and the problem of infertility specifically.

The sexual history includes pertinent data related to the couple's sexual practices and perceptions of their sexuality. This part of the history can be threatening to an infertile couple, who may view having children as an important aspect of their sexuality. The history should be approached in a supportive and nonthreatening manner so that the couple feel comfortable in discussing such sexual functions as frequency of intercourse and techniques used during intercourse.

The reproductive history also may provoke anxiety in the couple because it focuses attention on possible perceived inadequacies. A history of pregnancies, abortions, live births, and stillbirths, as well as any surgical interventions, such as tubal ligation and vasectomy, is elicited.

For the woman, a detailed menstrual history includes onset, duration, frequency, regularity, and problems of menstruation, as well as a history of premenstrual symptoms and dysmenorrhea. Questions are asked that are relevant to the pelvic, ovulatory, and cervical factors. A history of infections of the pelvic organs, including pelvic inflammatory disease, vaginitis, and cervicitis, may be significant to the problem of infertility. Additional important problems include a history of endometriosis and disorders of the pituitary, thyroid, or adrenal glands, which may indicate problems in hormonal activity. Any history of structural disorders such as congenital malformation of the uterus and fibroid tumors also is significant. In addition, a contraceptive history is taken and any information regarding systemic or chronic illness or past surgeries is recorded.

With respect to the male factor, significant findings in the health history include infections of the reproductive organs, orchitis (inflammation of the testes), mumps in adulthood, and prostatitis (inflammation of the prostate). Any history of factors that may cause prolonged elevation of temperature in the scrotum should also be assessed. These factors may include high fevers, exposure to heat from the environment, wearing of tight underclothes, excessive exercise, and use of hot tubs. A history of surgery, such as herniorrhaphy or vasectomy reversal surgery, may also be significant. The male may also have had a problem with varicocele or hydrocele (fluid in the scrotum) in the past, as well as endocrine disorders involving the pituitary and thyroid glands.

Certain findings in the history may be significant for both male and female partners. These include environmental factors such as exposure to radiation or toxic substances (e.g., lead). The use of drugs such as alcohol and marijuana should also be assessed as should use of medications that may affect sexual functioning (e.g., some antihypertensive drugs).

Both partners are also asked about a history of STDs and their mothers' use of DES. Occupational data that may provide information regarding work-related stress and occupational hazards is also obtained. The couple are asked questions about the frequency of coitus, premature ejaculation, and use of lubricants that may be spermicidal.

The complete health history is an important assessment tool for the nurse and other members of the health care team. It provides information regarding general health, as well as relevant data specific to the problem of infertility. It also enables the nurse to determine the way the couple defines the problem, how they have coped with problems in the past, and who is identified as their support network. The infertility study is tedious and sometimes fraught with disappointment. It also assumes that the couple will take part in the testing and intervention procedures. It is during the initial health history that the nurse can provide a supportive atmosphere for the couple and information to the couple regarding the workup.

Physical Examination

The next step in the infertility investigation is a complete physical examination. Included in the examination is a pelvic examination for the female. The structure of the vagina is carefully assessed, as are the shape and size of the cervix, uterus, and ovaries. Signs of pelvic inflammatory disease or palpable tubal or ovarian masses should be noted. An enlarged uterus may indicate the presence of fibroid tumors, which may prevent implantation of the fertilized ovum. The cervix is also assessed to determine if production of clear, copious, acellular mucus is evident. Cervical and vaginal specimens are taken to determine the possibility of infection.

As part of the complete assessment of the male, an examination of the male genitalia is performed. The structure, size, and shape of the penis, scrotum, testes, and prostate are assessed, and the scrotum is palpated for varicocele. Any abnormal discharge from the penis also is assessed.

The physical examination also affords the nurse or other health care practitioner an opportunity to assess secondary sex characteristics of the partners. Absent or minimal secondary sex characteristics may indicate reproductive immaturity and endocrine problems. During the physical examination, the nurse has an opportunity to educate the partners regarding anatomy and physiology and reproductive function. An assessment of each partner's feelings also may be made at this time. The nurse acts as the couple's advocate throughout the infertility investigation (McCullorn, 1996).

Diagnostic Tests

Diagnostic testing during the infertility assessment focuses on adequacy of ova and sperm production and possible impediments to fertilization. The most frequently conducted tests first evaluate male factor infertility and the ovulatory factor in the female: semen analysis, sperm penetration assay, postcoital test, basal body temperature analysis, and endometrial biopsy. The evaluation of cervical factor infertility is determined through physical examination and properly timed postcoital examination. The hysterosalpingogram and laparoscopy evaluate the pelvic factor. Other tests that may be performed include thyroid function tests, complete blood count, and urinalysis.

Semen Analysis. The semen analysis provides information regarding the number, structure, and motility of sperm. It also determines the volume and viscosity of the semen and the presence of infection or agglutination of the sperm. The male partner is instructed to abstain from ejaculation for 48 to 72 hours prior to the collection of the specimen. The specimen may be obtained through masturbation, coitus interruptus, or use of a special condom called a seminal pouch. Regular condoms should be avoided as they contain spermicides. The semen analysis is repeated several times at greater than 74 day intervals to allow further spermatogenesis to occur (Ransom & McNeeley, 1997). In general, a sperm count below 20 million in 2 mL of semen with less than 60% motility 2 hours after ejaculation is suggestive of an infertility problem.

The semen analysis should be done early in the infertility investigation. It provides needed information and is noninvasive.

Sperm Penetration Assay.

The sperm penetration assay (SPA) tests the functional capacity of sperm to penetrate and fertilize the ovum. It is based on the ability of human sperm to penetrate zona-free hamster eggs in the laboratory. There is a correlation between the ability of ejaculated sperm to penetrate zona-free hamster eggs and their ability to fertilize human ova. There is also a significant relationship between the ability of the sperm to penetrate the zona-free hamster eggs and sperm count, motility, and structure. Mean penetration rates for hamster ova are shown to be significantly higher in males with proven fertility than in those who are categorized as infertile. These infertile men may not be identified routinely through semen analysis because semen analysis gives no information relative to the ability of the sperm to penetrate the ovum.

Postcoital Test.

The initial interaction of the sperm and the female genital tract can also be assessed. The **postcoital (or Sims-Huhner) test** is performed late in the follicular phase of the menstrual cycle. The purpose of this test is to determine the clarity and consistency of the cervical mucus and the viability and motility of the sperm in the cervical environment. The couple is instructed to have intercourse within 8 hours of the examination, after abstaining from intercourse for 48 hours.

The optimal time for performing the test is 1 to 2 days prior to expected ovulation, when the cervical mucus normally undergoes characteristic changes consistent with peak estrogen secretion by the ovary. The presence of sodium chloride precipitation in the cervical mucus at this time results in a ferning pattern when the mucus is viewed under a microscope. Vaginal ultrasound can provide immediate feedback regarding the timing of the test by determining the presence or absence of a dominant follicle. The presence of sperm and sperm motility also are assessed (DeCherney & Pernoll, 1994).

If the results of the postcoital test reveal cervical mucus that is cloudy and cellular, a less than optimum environment for sperm survival, or few viable and motile sperm, the test should be repeated. The test is usually repeated within the same menstrual cycle or during the next menstrual cycle.

Basal Body Temperature Analysis.

The purpose of the basal body temperature (BBT) chart is to determine if ovulation has occurred. The woman is instructed to take her temperature on awakening each morning. In the first half of the menstrual cycle, prior to ovulation, the BBT is usually below 98°F (36.7°C). Just prior to ovulation, when estrogen level has reached a peak, a drop in the BBT occurs. Following ovulation, there is a rise in BBT of 0.5 to 1°F (0.3 to 0.6°C). The temperature continues to remain higher until the premenstrual phase of the cycle, with a decline in progesterone. The woman should chart the BBT on a graph for three consecutive cycles, noting the onset of menses, illness, or other factors that might interfere with the readings. She should also indicate times when intercourse has occurred. Figure 10–8A is a graph of an anovulatory cycle; Figure 10–8B is an ovulatory chart.

Basal body temperature charting is a relatively simple procedure. Like semen analysis, however, it can be anxiety-laden, reminding the partners that a problem exists and placing a burden on the couple to schedule sexual intercourse.

Endometrial Biopsy.

The endometrial biopsy is performed during the luteal phase of the menstrual cycle to determine if ovulation has occurred and to provide information related to the condition of the endometrium. The test is done 5 to 7 days prior to the onset of menses. A sample of endometrial tissue is taken with a curette after the cervix is gently dilated. The endometrium at this time should be secretory in nature because of the influence of progesterone after ovulation. A proliferative endometrium indicates that ovulation has not taken place or that a luteal-phase deficiency may be present. Progesterone assays may be done to complement the endometrial biopsy. A plasma progesterone level greater than 5 ng/mL and a urinary pregnanediol level of at least 2 mg per 24 hours are indicative of ovulation.

Hysterosalpingogram.

The **hysterosalpingogram** usually follows the previously mentioned tests and is used to evaluate the pelvic factor. This test is done in the early proliferative phase of the cycle to avoid interfering with ovulation or an early pregnancy. A radiopaque dye is instilled into the uterus and fallopian tubes to determine their patency. Through fluoroscopy and x-ray techniques the tubes are visualized. When the tubes are patent, the

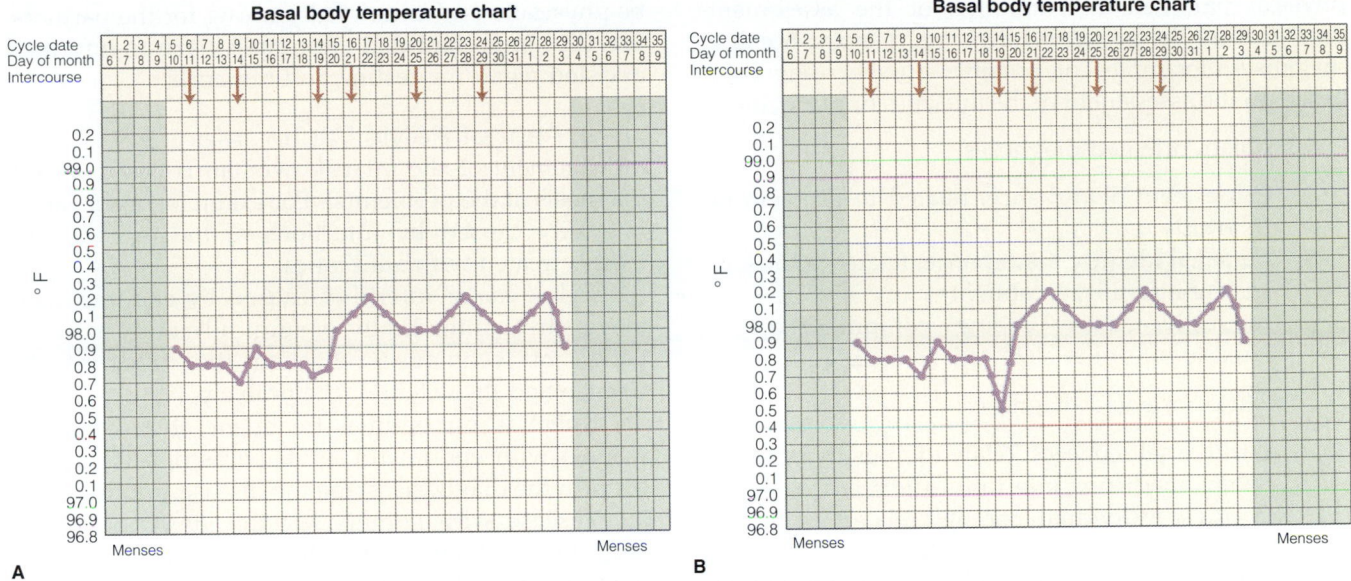

FIGURE 10–8. Basal body temperature chart. **A.** Anovulatory cycle. **B.** Ovulatory cycle.

radiopaque substance enters the peritoneal cavity. If the tubes are not patent, the substance does not enter the cavity and the diagnosis of tubal occlusion is made.

The hysterosalpingogram may be therapeutic as well as diagnostic in that previously occluded tubes may be opened through insertion of the dye. Other tests for tubal patency, such as the laparoscopy, are therefore performed at least 6 months after the hysterosalpingogram to allow conception to occur. Hysterosalpingograms may be performed without anesthesia and on an outpatient basis (Soules & Mack, 1995).

Laparoscopy. A **laparoscopy** is a procedure performed in the early follicular phase of the menstrual cycle that allows direct visualization of the pelvic organs. The woman may be given general, regional, or local anesthesia. An instrument called a laparoscope is inserted, usually at the level of the umbilicus. The peritoneal cavity is distended with carbon dioxide so that the pelvic structures can easily be visualized and assessments can be made for tubal patency and such pelvic pathology as endometriosis, cysts, and pelvic inflammatory disease. Some minor postoperative discomforts are associated with insertion of the laparoscope and distension of the peritoneal cavity with carbon dioxide. The woman can, however, be assured that normal activity can be resumed 1 to 2 days after the procedure.

Other Tests

Other tests may be ordered when specific problems are suspected. These include hormonal assays and immunologic tests. Luteinizing hormone, estrogen, and progesterone assays are sometimes performed.

The detection of sperm antibodies is the basis for immunology testing in the infertility workup. Screening tests for antisperm antibodies in either partner can be done for autoantibodies in the male or serum antibodies in the female (Benson & Pernoll, 1994).

Immunologic testing is often done when infertility is unexplained. Its role has become more useful as the impact of immunologic reactions on infertility has become more apparent.

▶ Nursing Role in Care of the Infertile Couple

The nursing role in the care of the infertile couple is varied. In collaboration with other health care team members, nurses act as counselors and advocates for the infertile couple.

▶ Nursing Diagnoses

Nurses begin the initial assessment through history taking and physical examination of both partners. The assessment data includes psychosocial as well as physical parameters. Evaluation of the assessment data enables the nurse to formulate relevant nursing diagnoses. Examples of possible nursing diagnoses based on the assessment of the infertile couple include:

Problem-oriented diagnoses:

- Self-esteem disturbance, related to problem of infertility
- Personal identity disturbance, related to unsuccessful infertility treatment
- Ineffective family coping: compromised, related to infertility study of the couple

Wellness-oriented diagnoses:

- Positive self-concept, related to positive coping behaviors during infertility study
- Positive individual coping, related to social support of the infertile couple
- Effective coping, related to positive family adaptation throughout infertility study of the couple

► Nursing and Collaborative Management

The nurse plans and implements care with the couple. Management of the infertile couple is dependent on the etiology of the problem and the goals of the couple. The nursing role includes providing the couple with anticipatory guidance about testing and possible treatments. As an advocate, the nurse ensures that both partners understand the risks, as well as the benefits, of the various treatments. Success rates associated with the treatments should be given so that a clear understanding of the possibility of pregnancy is achieved. The nurse also provides unbiased support to the couple throughout the decision-making process.

Infertility assessment and treatments can be tedious, time consuming, and costly. They may also be physically and emotionally taxing for the partners. It is thus important that the couple make an informed decision regarding testing and therapies.

Treatment of Pelvic Factor Infertility

Management of the infertile woman is based on the diagnosis of the problem(s). For example, pelvic factor infertility caused by infections of the reproductive tract is treated with antibiotics.

Pelvic factor infertility caused by endometriosis may be treated medically, or surgically, or by a combination of techniques reflecting the needs of the woman and the extent of the problem.

There is no optimal treatment of the infertile woman with endometriosis. Laparoscopy is used to confirm the diagnosis, stage the disease, and treat visible disease with surgery, electrocautery, or a CO_2 laser beam (Ransom & McNeeley, 1997). Medical treatment for endometriosis includes drugs that suppress ovulation and menstruation in an effort to heal the endometrial lesions of endometriosis. The drugs that may be used include gonadotropin-releasing hormone (GnRH) agonists, danazol, progestins, and oral contraceptives (see Table 10–3).

Infertility associated with the fallopian tubes may be caused by infections, adhesions, or endometriosis. As stated previously, tubal blockage is sometimes resolved by a hysterosalpingogram, which may clear the tubes of remnants of mucus.

Structural defects related to the uterus may also be treated with surgical intervention. Myomectomies, removal of uterine fibroid tumors, and reconstructive surgery for congenital malformation of the uterus have been performed to enhance fertility.

Treatment of Ovulatory Factor Infertility

Treatment of ovulatory factor infertility is based on the etiology. For example, treatment for thyroid disease may include replacement therapy for hypothyroidism, and medications, radioiodine, or surgery for hyperthyroidism.

► TABLE 10-3

Drugs Used to Treat Endometriosis

Drug[a]	Route	Side Effects
GnRh agonists	IM Intranasal IM abdominal implant	Hot flashes, insomnia, vaginal dryness, headache
Danazol (synthetic androgen)	PO	Weight gain, voice changes, hot flashes, decreased breast size, vaginitis
Progestins	PO IM	Breakthrough bleeding, weight gain, bloating, mood swings
Continuous non-cyclic oral contraceptives	PO	Breast tenderness, nausea, breakthrough bleeding

[a]These medications inhibit FSH, LH, ovulation and menstruation and may be given for 3–6 months.

Problems related to ovulation or the follicular and luteal phases of the menstrual cycle also may be treated pharmacologically. In anovulatory women, clomiphene citrate (Clomid) may be given to induce ovulation (see Drug Guide: Clomiphene Citrate (Clomid)).

Another agent used to stimulate follicular growth is human menopausal gonadotropin (hMG). This drug is a purified preparation of FSH and LH extracted from the urine of postmenopausal women. The drug stimulates ovarian follicular growth and maturation directly. To induce ovulation, human chorionic gonadotropin (hCG) must be given after the administration of hMG and when the assessment of the woman indicates that sufficient follicular maturation has occurred, coinciding with the LH surge. Follicular maturity is measured by estrogen levels, ultrasound scans, and the quality and quantity of cervical mucus. Estrogen levels may be obtained by determining plasma estradiol levels and obtaining a 24-hour urine sample for urinary excretion of estrogen. Appearance and volume of the cervical mucus, spinnbarkeit, the elasticity of the ovulatory cervical mucus, and ferning patterns also help to identify the LH surge, as do over-the-counter ovulation predictor kits. Side effects of hCG therapy include ovarian enlargement and ovarian hyperstimulation syndrome. The incidence of multiple fetuses following this type of therapy is 20 to 40%. Like other forms of treatment for infertility, therapy is expensive and requires commitment on the part of the couple and health care provider so that the timing of the tests needed to detect the LH surge and the timing of intercourse can be optimal. It is imperative, as with any type of therapy, that the couple make an educated choice as to the acceptance or rejection of treatment.

Infertility associated with luteal-phase inadequacy may be caused by increased prolactin secretion by the anterior pituitary gland (hyperprolactinemia). Elevated levels of prolactin inhibit FSH and LH secretion and their actions on the ovary so that ovulation does not occur. Bromocriptine mesylate (Parlodel) may be prescribed to inhibit prolactin secretion by the anterior pituitary gland (see Drug Guide: Bromocriptine Mesylate (Parlodel)).

Luteal-phase inadequacy is also treated with clomiphene citrate during the follicular phase of the cycle. The medication improves follicle growth, enhances follicular estrogen production, and prepares the endometrium for luteal development. Some authorities suggest that progesterone supplementation is also needed to improve pregnancy outcome.

▶ DRUG GUIDE: CLOMIPHENE CITRATE (CLOMID)

ACTIONS/INDICATIONS

Acts as an estrogen receptor blocker in the hypothalamus, resulting in increased rates of secretion of FSH and LH, resulting in ovarian stimulation of the graafian follicle and ovulation. It is indicated in anovulatory women with normal liver function and normal endogenous estrogen levels. It is ineffective in women with primary pituitary or ovarian failure.

DOSAGE

Administered orally only. The starting dose is 50 mg once daily for 5 days at any time if there is no recent uterine bleeding or on the fifth day of the cycle if uterine bleeding occurs. If ovulation does not occur, 100 mg once daily for 5 days can be tried during the next cycle. If ovulation does not occur after second treatment, the second treatment is repeated during the next cycle. Therapy should not generally extend beyond 3 to 4 cycles.

ADVERSE REACTIONS

CNS: dizziness, visual disturbances, insomnia, depression. *GI:* bloating, nausea, vomiting. *Reproductive:* ovarian hyperstimulation, heavier menses, multiple gestation (twins most common), breast discomfort. *Fetal:* birth defects.

DRUG INTERACTIONS

Danazol may inhibit response to clomiphene.

NURSING IMPLICATIONS

1. Teach woman to begin taking medication on fifth day of cycle and to take the drug at the same time each day.
2. Reinforce teaching about drug and potential risks and benefits.
3. Teach woman to report symptoms of hot flashes, nausea, vomiting, headache, visual symptoms.
4. Instruct woman to stop taking drug if pregnancy is suspected.
5. Alert the couple to the risk of multiple births.
6. Explain the probable duration of the treatment.
7. Teach woman to evaluate ovulation by charting basal body temperatures and using over-the-counter test kits that detect the LH surge.

▶ DRUG GUIDE: BROMOCRIPTINE MESYLATE (PARLODEL)

ACTIONS/INDICATIONS

Used to inhibit prolactin secretion by the anterior pituitary gland with little or no effect on other pituitary hormones. It is indicated for luteal-phase inadequacy caused by hyperprolactinemia in the absence of a pituitary tumor.

DOSAGE

Administered orally. Usual dosage is 5 to 7.5 mg/day with a range of 2.5 mg to 15 mg/day for up to 6 months or until pregnancy occurs.

ADVERSE REACTIONS

CNS: dizziness, fainting, insomnia, headache. *GI:* nausea, vomiting, constipation, diarrhea. *CV:* hypotension.

DRUG INTERACTIONS

Erythromycin causes increased serum bromocriptine levels and toxic effects.

NURSING IMPLICATIONS

1. Teach woman to monitor ovulation.
2. Teach woman to discontinue drug when ovulation is suspected.
3. Teach woman to take drug with food and exactly as prescribed.
4. Blood pressure should be monitored in first few days of therapy.
5. Caution woman about dizziness as well as other side effects.
6. Teach client to discontinue drug when pregnancy is suspected.

However, support of the luteal phase with additional progesterone has been used with variable success (Ransom & McNeeley, 1997).

Pharmacologic therapies for infertility may extend the menstrual cycle, thus delaying the onset of menses. The nurse should prepare the couple for this prospect so that they do not experience false hope that a pregnancy has occurred, compounding their disappointment if it has not.

Treatment of Cervical Factor Infertility

If the cause of infertility is determined to be cervical, estrogen therapy may be used prior to anticipated ovulation for several months. Low-dose estrogen is thought to enhance the quantity and quality of the cervical mucus and make it more receptive to sperm. If low-dose estrogen therapy is ineffective, hMG may be used. When the cervical mucus is altered because of inflammation or infection, some practitioners advocate the use of a tetracycline (doxycycline) for both partners (DeCherney & Pernoll, 1994). Intrauterine insemination of the partner's sperm may be offered to the couple if the cervix is hostile and when antibodies are present (Ransom & McNeeley, 1997).

Treatment of Male Factor Infertility

Treatment of male factor infertility focuses on the adequacy of production, number, motility, and structure of sperm and is based on the ability of the sperm to survive the cervical environment and penetrate the ovum.

If the cause of infertility is oligospermia (few sperm), changes in lifestyle may help to correct it. The man should be advised to avoid prolonged exposure to heat sources, such as hot tubs and restrictive clothing, which may interfere with sperm production and viability. Sources of radiation and chemical hazards should be assessed, as should the use of alcohol, drugs, and tobacco. Clomiphene citrate, gonadotropins, gonadotropin hormone-releasing hormone, and androgen rebound therapies may be used to increase sperm count.

If after treatment the sperm count remains low, artificial insemination of the woman with her husband's sperm (AIH) may be considered. Because sperm occur in highest concentration and are most motile in the first few drops of semen, the ejaculate is split and the first fraction saved. This may be done several times, and the resulting first-fraction-split ejaculates are combined and inseminated into the female partner. The use of split ejaculates enhances cervical mucus penetrability and sperm characteristics when the semen volume is high and the sperm count is low (Benson & Pernoll, 1994).

If insemination using the male partner's sperm is ineffective, or azoospermia (no sperm) or severe oligospermia is present, artificial donor insemination (ADI) may be presented to the couple as an option. A newer technique, intracytoplasmic sperm injection (ICSI), where sperm is injected directly into the ovum, has been successful when the male partner is severely oligozoospermic.

Problems related to ejaculation may be caused by impotency, especially during the infertility study itself when the man is under pressure to perform. A supportive, nonjudgmental atmosphere is needed for the couple, along with reassurance that this may be a transient problem. Sexual counseling also may be required.

If a varicocele is diagnosed, surgery to ligate the spermatic vein is sometimes performed. Varicocele ligation has demonstrated improvement in sperm parameters in up to two thirds of infertile men; however, postoperative pregnancy rates have not been different between the treated and untreated (Benson & Pernoll, 1994).

Treatment of male factor infertility is varied, and the benefits of therapies aimed at improving sperm production, motility, viability, and structure are inconclusive. Ideally, management is directed to specific causation, as nonspecific therapies have produced disappointing results.

Treatment of Combined Problems

When infertility results from a combined problem, such as faulty sexual technique or lack of knowledge related to timing of sexual relations, sexual counseling is warranted. The need for counseling also should be assessed throughout the infertility workup because the procedures and the perception of the couple of the need to perform may interfere with sexual functioning.

If the combined problem is immunologic, treatment aimed at reducing sperm antibodies is sometimes implemented. Sperm autoimmunity in men may be treated by immunosuppression with steroids. The man's semen and serum, as well as the woman's cervical mucus, are monitored for antibody titers to evaluate the effectiveness of the therapy. If it is found that the woman has antibodies to her partner's sperm, condom therapy is usually recommended. The couple is instructed to use condoms during intercourse for 6 months; this reduces exposure to sperm and may decrease the female partner's sensitivity. Sperm antibody titers are retested after the therapy and the couple is encouraged to attempt conception.

Treatment of Unexplained Infertility

When investigations fail to reveal a cause for infertility, treatment may then be based on possible causes. Because of the high spontaneous pregnancy rate in unexplained infertility, however, the effectiveness of the various treatments is difficult to assess. Treatments have included correction of anatomic problems and the use of hormonal manipulation during the follicular and luteal phases of the cycle. Treatment for immunologic factors also has been attempted to decrease sperm antibodies, with few conclusive results. It is difficult to assess whether treatments aimed at improving cervical mucus or the use of antibiotics for infections have more than a placebo

effect. The choice of no treatment and the hope for spontaneous pregnancy may be a better option than treatment that has not been proven.

The treatment of infertility is most effective when a causative factor is identified. Diagnosis and treatment of ovulatory disorders have demonstrated relatively good results, and tubal infertility may be treated effectively with microsurgery. Treatment of male infertility is, however, often ineffective and largely empirical. Although new techniques have been developed in the treatment of infertility, any treatment should be based on the decision of the couple themselves after they have received a full, unbiased appraisal of their problem and the probability of successful management.

Assisted Reproductive Technology

Assisted reproductive technology (ART) has been called "the brave new world of baby making." The procedures require a substantial investment of monetary and personal resources. The procedures can cost $6000 to $10,000 per cycle.

In vitro fertilization–embryo transfer (IVF-ET) is a technique used in the management of infertile couples that encompasses removal of a mature ovum from a woman's ovary, fertilization of the ovum with a sperm in a petri dish, and reimplantation of the embryo into the woman's uterine cavity. In vitro fertilization is often referred to as test tube fertilization in the popular press. Criteria for selection for IVF–ET include a normal semen sample and ovarian accessibility at laparoscopy.

To encourage the development of numerous ova, all IVF–ET programs use the technique of superovulation. The following drugs are used to induce superovulation: (1) clomiphene citrate alone; (2) hMG alone; (3) a combination of clomiphene citrate and hMG; (4) pure human FSH alone or in combination with hMG and clomiphene citrate; or (5) luteinizing hormone-releasing hormone. The maturity of the follicles is usually monitored, by performing ultrasound and by measuring serum estradiol and LH levels. Human chorionic gonadotropin is given to mature the oocytes. When the largest follicle reaches a diameter of approximately 20 mm, the mature ova are recovered through follicular aspiration during laparoscopy. The extracted ova are placed in a simple culture medium, and sperm in a concentrated suspension are added (50,000 of the most active sperm per oocyte). Following fertilization, the zygote is allowed to develop to the four- to eight-cell stage, about 48 to 72 hours after insemination, when the embryo is transferred to the uterine cavity of the mother. Often several embryos are transferred to increase the chances of pregnancy. Some of the fertilized ova are sometimes frozen to be used in additional cycles if pregnancy is not sustained. The success rate of in vitro fertilization (pregnancy and delivery of a healthy newborn) is reported to be approximately 20%.

Ovum Transfer. Ovum transfer was developed for infertile women as an alternative to IVF–ET. It involves insemination of a donor female at the time of ovulation with semen from the husband of an infertile woman. Three to four days after insemination, the embryo is transferred to the uterus of the infertile woman, who carries the pregnancy. Genetically the donor is the mother.

Gamete Intrafallopian Transfer. Another reproductive technologic procedure used in the treatment of infertility is **gamete intrafallopian transfer** (GIFT). Developed in 1984, GIFT involves the direct transfer of preovulatory oocytes and washed sperm into the fallopian tubes after aspiration of the ovarian follicles at laparoscopy. The technique attempts to mimic the early physiologic processes that lead to pregnancy in the human by placing both male and female gametes at the normal site of fertilization. As in in vitro fertilization, mature oocytes are aspirated from the female client after she has been treated with hormones to promote superovulation and hCG to mature the ova. These ova are evaluated and then loaded into a catheter for transfer. The catheter is also loaded with a preparation containing 100,000 sperm. The sperm and ova may be separated by an air bubble in the catheter. The catheter tip is guided approximately 1.5 cm into the fimbriated end of the fallopian tube and the contents of the catheter are gently discharged, permitting natural fertilization and cleavage (Fig. 10–9).

The GIFT procedure can be used only with women who have at least one intact, functional fallopian tube, because after fertilization occurs, the zygote must be able to travel through the tube to the uterus for implantation. The woman must also have one accessible ovary on which to perform the follicular aspiration. The success rate for GIFT is reported as between 25 and 50%.

An advantage of GIFT over IVF–ET is that the entire procedure is performed during the laparoscopy, thereby eliminating the 2-day laboratory incubation period and subsequent introduction of the embryo into the uterine cavity required postlaparoscopy in IVF–ET. Moreover, techniques have recently been described whereby ova are obtained transvaginally instead of during laparoscopy although with less success (Lemcke et al., 1995). The ova and sperm are then transferred into the fallopian tubes transcervically under ultrasound guidance. A disadvantage of the GIFT procedure is the speed with which laboratory

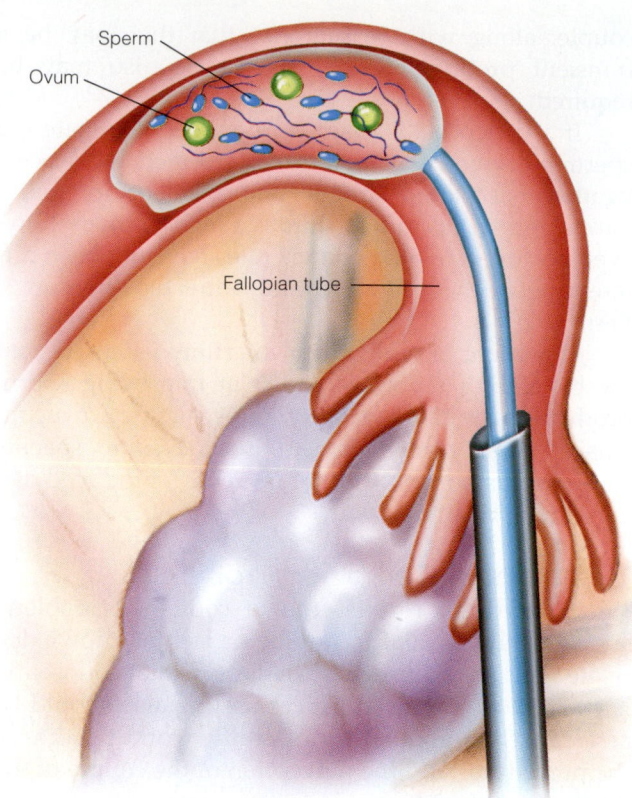

FIGURE 10–9. Gamete intrafallopian transfer (GIFT). Insertion of a catheter containing sperm and ova into the fimbriated end of the fallopian tube.

personnel must work while the client is under anesthesia. Further, GIFT is more expensive than IVF–ET.

Zygote Intrafallopian Transfer. **Zygote intrafallopian transfer** (ZIFT) is a combination of IVF and GIFT in which the ova are fertilized in the laboratory and then transported to the fallopian tube for development and transport to the uterus. There is conflicting evidence about the differences in results between GIFT, ZIFT, and IVF–ET. Until recently, most authors reported higher implantation and pregnancy rates with GIFT and ZIFT compared with IVF–ET. The rates are now considered comparable by some authorities.

Assisted Hatching. Assisted hatching (AZH) is a fairly new ART. This technique presumes that there will be a problem with the embryo breaking out or "hatching" from the zona pellucida of the fertilized ovum when the embryo is transferred to the uterus. Assisted hatching occurs when an enzyme is injected into a small portion of the zona to dissolve the zona pellucida while the embryo is held in place. The hope is that the embryo will "hatch" out of the ovum and implant into the uterus.

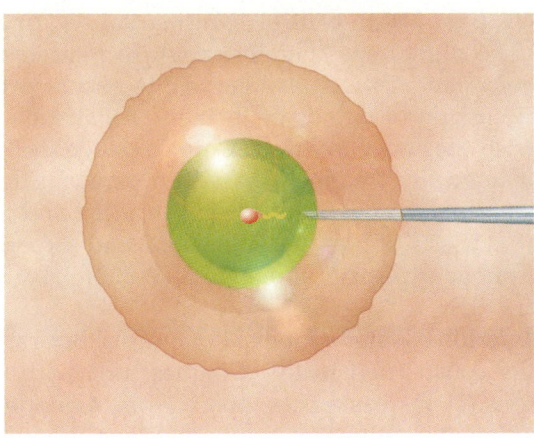

FIGURE 10–10. Intracytoplasmic Sperm Injection (ICSI). The ovum is held steady by a flat-nosed pipette and is fertilized with sperm contained in a micro-needle.

Intracytoplasmic Sperm Injection. With ICSI, a single sperm is placed into the cytoplasm of the ovum. This technique has allowed couples with sperm counts too low for IVF to reconsider the option (Lemcke et al., 1995). With ICSI, the ova are retrieved in the same way that they are retrieved for IVF or GIFT. However, the ova are then fertilized in the laboratory by direct injection of a single sperm into each ovum (see Figure 10–10). Forty-eight hours later the resulting embryos are transferred into the uterus. Some embryos may be frozen for later attempts at pregnancy. For infertile couples with male-factor problems, ICSI is a major advance in achieving fertility (Gvakharia, Greer, Lipshultz, & Lamb, 1995).

Implantation of Frozen Ova. Until recently frozen ova could not be fertilized by sperm because frozen ova were considered too fragile. This new technology protects the ova with a chemical solution before the ova are frozen. The solution mimics the follicle, the protective capsule around the ova in the

Nursing Alert

Success rates for pregnancies using ARTs do not necessarily mean delivery of a baby at term; rather, they may mean clinical pregnancy rates. A clinical pregnancy is a pregnancy that has developed to the stage where a gestational sac can be visualized on ultrasound.

ovary. After thawing, each ovum is injected with a single sperm and then fertilized ova are transferred into the uterus.

▶ Psychologic Aspects of Infertility

Infertility is a major life crisis for many couples. Menning has described a predictable sequence (surprise, denial, grief, isolation) in the couple's response to infertility. This includes surprise, stemming from the couple's assumption that they are fertile and the fact that typically they have practiced birth control to await the right time to have children. Denial of the problem also is common and acts as a protective mechanism for the couple. It should, however, be short term so that the couple may gain realistic awareness and acceptance of the problem (Menning, 1988).

Grief is the most common response to infertility. Even when the diagnosis is tentative, the couple will experience a period of grief for the children they never had. In fact, the couple with an inconclusive diagnosis of infertility may have profound cyclic feelings of hope and despair, high stress, and chronic sorrow (Hainsworth, Eakes, & Burke, 1994; Imeson & McMurray, 1996; Schoener & Krysa, 1996).

Isolation is another common response, and may be a result of lack of social support. Well-meaning friends who suggest solutions to the problem, such as "relax and you'll get pregnant," may instead cause the couple to isolate themselves further from support systems. This isolation delays the grief process and places strains on the marital relationship and friendships (Hirsch & Hirsch, 1995). It has been documented that infertile individuals feel greater dissatisfaction with themselves and their marriage than couples who are not infertile, and women experience greater stress over time and have greater emotional investment than males (Halman, Andrews, & Abbey, 1994).

Common behaviors observed in infertile couples may have different meanings (Sandelowski, 1994). Physical inability to have a child may be perceived as personal inadequacy and social failure. The infertile couple often feel helpless. Having made the decision to have children, the couple may perceive that their options have been taken away. They may respond with anger toward family members or health care providers who delve into intimate details of their lives. The perception that testing and sexual relations must be programmed also may cause anger, directed at those who place them in uncomfortable situations. Old marital conflicts may be reawakened and the couple may feel they are losing control of their life plans.

Guilt is also a common feeling among infertile couples and may stem from a prior history of premar-

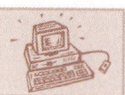

Research Abstract

Psychosocial Effects of Infertility

This study explored the psychosocial effects of infertility and the role of support for couples over time. It was hypothesized that infertile individuals experience decreased social support and contentment, lower levels of marital and sexual satisfaction, and lower self-esteem over time. It was further hypothesized that those infertile persons with higher levels of social support would be less affected.

Ninety-four subjects were recruited through a national newsletter for an infertility support group. Of the subjects who entered the study, 41% completed it. The results indicated that perceived support as well as contentment and self-esteem increased, rather than decreased, over time. Social support was positively related to contentment, marital satisfaction, sexual satisfaction, and sex-role identity.

Application to Practice

Nurses can play an important role in helping couples cope with the stress of infertility over time. Nursing strategies should focus on the social support needed by the couple. Infertile couples often experience cycles of hope and despair that can accompany the infertility treatment. These couples require empathetic nurses who act as advocates and counselors for infertile individuals.

Source: Hirsch, A.M., & Hirsch, S.M. (1995). The long-term psychosocial effects of infertility. Journal of Obstetric, Gynecologic, and Neonatal Nursing, 24*(6), 517–522.*

ital sex, use of birth control, extramarital sex, or abortion. The nurse may therefore wish to interview the partners alone, as well as together, to ensure privacy for discussion of details of their lives that each does not wish the other to know. Couples make decisions about infertility treatment based on personal beliefs, their partners' beliefs, physician advice, and emotional stress. Couples feel alienated and experience pain, public exposure, and stigma (Whiteford & Gonzalez, 1995).

Infertility is not a medical diagnosis, but rather a socially constructed reality. Couples cope with infertility by (1) increasing the space from reminders of infertility, (2) instituting measures for regaining control, (3) acting to increase self-esteem, (4) looking for hidden meaning, (5) giving in to feelings, and (6) sharing the burden with others. Many couples report feelings of isolation that are increased by the inappropriate responses of others (Imeson & McMurray, 1996). The longer the couple remains infertile, the less likely they are to feel in control of their lives. To regain control, both partners must work through the grief process to reach a sense of resolution. Nurses and other health care team members often can provide the support necessary for the couple to resolve the crisis of infertility in a positive manner. In addition, the couple may be referred to RESOLVE, the support organization founded in 1973 by Barbara Eck Menning, a nurse. This organization disseminates educational information and also provides needed referral services for infertile couples.

As various treatments for infertility are pursued and found unsuccessful, the couple is faced with several choices. They may discontinue further treatment, with the possibility of remaining childless. Adoption may be another option that the couple will pursue; however, it is important that the couple resolve their loss of biologic parenting so that parenting of an adopted child can be a positive experience. The options of artificial insemination, by the partner or a donor, and other assisted reproductive technology procedures may also be suggested to the couple. It is imperative that the nurse understand the couple's feelings regarding these technologies. Sometimes the zeal of health care professionals for new procedures leads them to ignore the couple's reasons for finding such procedures unacceptable. It is important that the couple be supported through their infertility investigation and treatment. Regardless of whether couples choose to continue or terminate the treatment, their wishes should be respected by the health care staff.

Critical Thinking in Care Planning

Care of the Infertile Couple

John and Rosemary Long, 32 and 30 years respectively, have been attempting a pregnancy for 2 years. The couple comes to the health center for evaluation of their infertility. John is found to have an extremely low sperm count with low motility. John is treated with clomiphene citrate and his sperm count does not improve. Options are discussed with the couple, including artificial insemination with donor sperm and intracytoplasmic sperm injection (ICSI) with in vitro fertilization (IVF).

► Assessment

- Client states: "We don't understand how ICSI and IVF work."
- Couple states: "We shouldn't have used birth control for so long. Do you think we made ourselves infertile?"

Nursing Diagnosis

Knowledge deficit, related to treatments for infertility.

Expected Client/Family Outcomes	Nursing Action/Intervention	Evaluation
By the end of the visit, the couple will: • Describe the treatment modalities. • Identify the risks and benefits of each treatment. By the next visit, the couple will make an informed decision as to subsequent treatment.	Teach clients procedure used for insemination using donor's sperm: • Highly concentrated sperm suspension is used. • Donor is screened for HIV, other diseases, or genetic problems. • Insemination into the cervix occurs at the time of ovulation. • Success rate greater than 30% is reported. Teach clients the ICSI procedure: • The ova are retrieved just as if you are undergoing IVF. • Each egg is fertilized in the laboratory by direct injection of a single sperm into each ovum. • Two days later, the resulting embryos are placed into the uterus. • Extra embryos are frozen for later attempts at pregnancy. • The fertilization rate per ovum using ICSI is about 70%. • The pregnancy rate per cycle attempt is about 40%. *Rationale:* Infertility treatment requires decision making on the part of the couple. Realistic decision making requires knowledge of alternatives, risks, and benefits.	When asked, clients: • Discuss each of the treatment alternatives and procedures involved. • List risks and benefits associated with each treatment. • Discuss the chances of success or failure of each treatment. Clients make a knowledgable decision about treatment or decision not to pursue treatment.

(continued)

Critical Thinking in Care Planning continued

Nursing Diagnosis

Self-esteem disturbance, related to guilt about possibly contributing to infertility.

Expected Client/Family Outcomes	Nursing Action/Intervention	Evaluation
By the end of the first visit, the couple will: • Identify their feelings related to their infertility • Focus on making decisions about treatments.	Listen and offer support in a nonjudgmental manner. Acknowledge the clients' feelings of hope and despair. Answer questions concerning infertility and their feelings of causation. *Rationale:* Guilt is a salient feature of infertility. Infertility represents the loss of the fantasized child. Give unbiased support to couple through their decision-making processes. Give couple realistic explanations about their condition. Refer to RESOLVE. *Rationale:* Supporting the couple in a nonjudgmental manner fosters resolution of grief. Support organizations such as RESOLVE assist the couple to cope with the infertility and work through their grief.	Couple relates their feelings freely to nurse. Couple realistically relates their infertility problem. Couple discusses their future plans concerning infertility.

Chapter Highlights

▶ Genetic disorders include disorders of the auto-somes and disorders of the pair of sex chromosomes.

▶ Chromosomal abnormalities may be classified as numerical chromosomal abnormalities or structural abnormalities.

▶ In single-gene inheritance, the gene that expresses itself is referred to as dominant; the gene that is present but does not express itself is called recessive.

▶ Multifactorial disorders occur as a result of the interaction of genes and environmental influences.

▶ Infertility may be a result of problems of the female partner, including pelvic, ovulatory, and cervical factors.

▶ Male factor infertility is related to sperm production, motility, and transport.

▶ Treatment of infertility is based on the etiology of the problem and may be medical, surgical, or both.

▶ Assisted reproductive technology includes newer techniques in infertility treatment.

▶ Genetic disorders and infertility are major life crises for the family.

▶ Nurses can provide the needed support to help families through the crises of genetic disorders and infertility.

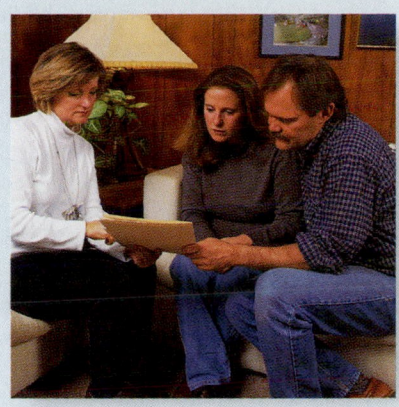

After reading the vignette at the beginning of this chapter, use what you have learned to answer these questions.

1. Based on the information obtained through the risk assessment, how would you as the nurse providing genetic counseling to Stephen and Andrea Nolan, explain the risk of their child expressing the gene for cystic fibrosis?

2. With the knowledge of a family history of a genetic disorder such as cystic fibrosis, what type of support and information would the Nolans need from the nurse in order to cope with this situation?

3. What do you see as the benefits of the genetic counseling process? Do you think that participation in this process has any drawbacks for the childbearing family?

Critical Thinking Questions

▶ References

American College of Obstetricians and Gynecologists; Committee on Genetics (1995). Fragile X syndrome. Committee opinion no. 161. Washington, DC: Author.

Benson, R.C., & Pernoll, M.L. (1994). *Handbook of obstetrics and gynecology* (9th ed.). New York: McGraw-Hill.

Chin, H.G. (1997). *On call obstetrics and gynecology.* Philadelphia: W.B. Saunders.

Cunningham, F.G., MacDonald, P.C., Gant, N.F., Leveno, K.J., Gilstrap, L.C., Hankins, G.D.V., & Clark, S.L. (1997). *Williams obstetrics* (20th ed.). Stamford, CT: Appleton & Lange.

DeCherney, A.H., & Pernoll, M.L. (1994). *Current obstetric and gynecologic diagnosis and treatment* (8th ed.). Norwalk, CT: Appleton & Lange.

Fryday, M. (1995). Treating infertility in Roman Catholics. *Nursing Standard, 10*(5), 31–34.

Gvakharia, M., Greer, J.A., Lipshultz, L.I., & Lamb, D.J. (1995). Treating male-factor infertility with ICSI. *Contemporary Urology, 7*(9), 58–59, 61–63, 67.

Hainsworth, M.A., Eakes, G.G., & Burke, M.L. (1994). Coping with chronic sorrow. *Issues in Mental Health Nursing, 15*(1), 59–66.

Hirsch, A.M., & Hirsch, S.M. (1995). The long-term psychosocial effects of infertility. *Journal of Obstetric, Gynecologic, and Neonatal Nursing, 24*(6), 517–522.

Halman, L.J., Andrews, F.M., & Abbey, A. (1994). Gender differences and perceptions about childbearing among infertile couples. *Journal of Obstetric, Gynecologic, and Neonatal Nursing, 23*(7), 593–600.

Imeson, M., & McMurray, A. (1996). Couples' experiences of infertility: A phenomenological study. *Journal of Advanced Nursing, 24*(5), 1014–1022.

Jackson, P.L., & Vessey, J.A. (1996). *Primary care of a child with a chronic condition* (2nd ed.). St. Louis: Mosby.

Jones, S.L. (1996). Genetics: changing health care in the 21st century. *Journal of Obstetric, Gynecologic, and Neonatal Nursing, 25*(9), 777–783.

Lemcke, D.P., Pattison, J., Marshall, L.A., & Cowley, D.S. (1995). *Primary care of women.* Norwalk, CT: Appleton & Lange.

Menning, B.E. (1988). *Infertility: A guide for the childless couple* (2nd ed.). Englewood Cliffs, NJ: Prentice-Hall.

McCullorn, M.I. (1996). The nurse as patient advocate and counselor . . . infertility nurse. *Infertility and Reproductive Medicine Clinics of North America, 7*(3), 483–493.

Moore, K.L. (1993). *The developing human: Clinically oriented embryology* (4th ed.). Philadelphia: W.B. Saunders.

Murray, T.H., & Livny, E. (1995). The human genome project: ethical and social implications. *Bulletin of the Medical Library Association, 83*(1), 14–21.

Olshansky, E.F. (1996). A counseling approach with persons experiencing infertility: Implications for advanced practice nursing. *Advanced Practice Quarterly, 2*(3), 42–47.

Ransom, S.B., & McNeeley, S.G. (1997). *Gynecology for the primary care provider.* Philadelphia: W.B. Saunders.

Rudolph, A.M., Hoffman, J.I.E., & Rudolph, C.D. (1996). *Rudolph's pediatrics* (20th ed.). Stamford CT: Appleton & Lange.

Sandelowski, M. (1994). On infertility. *Journal of Obstetric, Gynecologic, and Neonatal Nursing, 23*(9), 749–752.

Schoener, C.J., & Krysa, L.W. (1996). The comfort and discomfort of infertility. *Journal of Obstetric & Neonatal Nursing, 25*(2), 167–172.

Soules, M.R., & Mack, L.A. (1995). Imaging of the reproductive tract in infertile women: Hysterosalpingography, ultrasonography, and magnetic resonance imaging. In W.R. Keye, R.J. Chang, R.W. Rebar, M.R. Soules (eds.), *Infertility evaluation and treatment.* Philadelphia: W.B. Saunders.

Whiteford, L.M., & Gonzalez, L. (1995). Stigma: The hidden burden of infertility. *Social Science and Medicine, 40*(1), 27–36.

Zinaman, M.J., & Uhler, M.L. (1996). Clinical and laboratory assessment of male infertility. *Physician Assistant, 20*(3), 101–102, 105–108, 110.

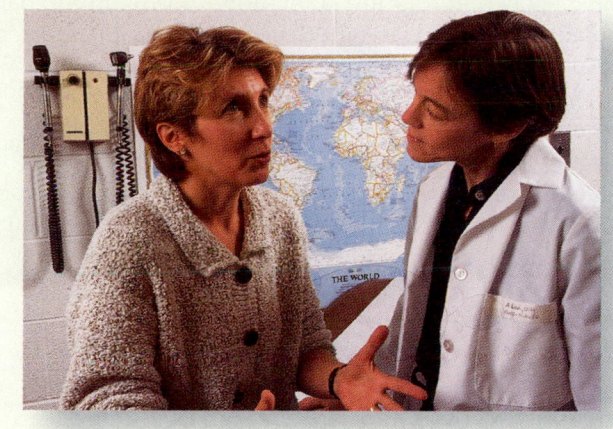

Jeanne Goodwin, age 36, is 8 weeks' pregnant with her third child. Her two older children, 8-year-old Lisa and 6-year-old Daniel, are from Jeanne's first marriage. Jeanne and her second husband, Anthony, also have another son, Christopher, age 10, from Anthony's first marriage. Jeanne and Anthony have been married for two years.

During her prenatal visit, Jeanne confides in Ann Salzman, CNM, MSN, that although she and Anthony are happy and excited about sharing a child together, they are concerned about the older children's relationship with the newest member of the family. Jeanne says, "The children just now seem to be getting used to living together. I'm worried that they think that Anthony and I will love the baby more than we love them. What can we do to help them feel that they are as important to us as the baby is?" ■

11

Age-Related Considerations for Pregnancy

Childbearing at the extremes of reproductive life is becoming more common. Adolescents and women over 35 have unique needs that require alterations in the care traditionally provided to childbearing women in their 20s. Although women in both groups do have uncomplicated pregnancies and deliver robust infants, adolescents and older mothers are considered at high risk for a variety of age-related physical and psychosocial conditions.

Adolescence is a time of transition between childhood and adulthood. The teenager struggles for independence and development of an adult identity. For most adolescents, pregnancy is an unplanned, unwanted event that adds to the complexity and difficulty of the teen years. The adolescent is faced with many choices that greatly affect her future. Working with the adolescent and her significant others, the nurse, in collaboration with other health care providers, can do much to promote healthy outcomes.

The woman over 35 may view pregnancy as a planned, desired event; some women may have become pregnant as a result of interventions using reproductive technology. Others may be surprised and shocked at the idea of pregnancy at their stage of life. Concerns of the older pregnant woman include managing health problems related to the aging process and a higher risk of having a baby with genetic abnormalities.

This chapter discusses adolescent growth and development, adolescent sexual development, effects of early childbearing on adolescents, costs and risk factors of adolescent pregnancy, and nursing care of the pregnant adolescent. It also examines the advantages and disadvantages of delayed childbearing, pregnancy outcome and mature women, and nursing management of the mature pregnant woman and family.

▶ ADOLESCENT PREGNANCY

Sexual activity among American teenagers has increased greatly over the last three decades (Grimes, 1995a). By the age of 18 about 56% of females and 73% of males have had intercourse. The rate of teen births increased greatly from 50.6 per 1000 women in 1984 to 62.1 in 1991. Since then there has been a steady decline in teen pregnancy rates and birth rates to 54.7 per 1000 women in 1996. However, despite what statistical trends seem to indicate, between 1984 and 1996 there was an overall increase in the rate of live births to teenagers (USDHHS, 1997; March of Dimes Birth Defects Foundation, 1997). Teen pregnancy, as well as risks of sexually transmitted disease (STDs), continue to be problems (Grimes, 1995b).

In the United States, adolescent pregnancy is common in all social, economic, and racial groups (Cunningham et al., 1997). Approximately 85% of teenage pregnancies are unintended, compared with a rate of 55% of total unintended U.S. pregnancies (Grimes, 1995a). One third of adolescent mothers will have a second or third child while still teenagers (Bragg, 1997). Only about 40% of teenagers seek contraceptive services within a year of becoming sexually active; about half of unintended pregnancies occur in the first six months after sexual activity is begun. Although the likelihood of intercourse and the use of contraceptives increase with age, early start of intercourse among young teenagers (age 13–14) does not happen frequently; young teenagers who have had intercourse may have been forced to do so (Grimes, 1995a; U.S. Centers for Disease Control and Prevention, 1995). This highlights the importance of screening for abuse for all pregnant clients.

Only a small number of pregnant teens are married. However, nearly all teens keep their babies (Bragg, 1997; Thompson, Powell, Patterson, & Ellerbee, 1995). An unintended, out-of-wedlock pregnancy is a life-changing event with long-term implications for the teens involved, their families and society.

The United States has one of the highest teen pregnancy rates and abortion rates among industrialized nations. Almost 1 million American teens become pregnant each year. The American teen pregnancy rate of 11% exceeds the rate of 5% in other Western countries (Esparza & Esperat, 1996). Studies have not identified American teenagers as more sexually active than teenagers in Western Europe. However, their consistent use of effective contraception is lower (Grimes, 1995a).

Adolescent pregnancy brings potentially high-risk physical and psychosocial situations. Comprehensive health care is therefore needed early in pregnancy. Principles of adolescent growth and development must be understood by the nurse and incorporated into an ongoing nursing care plan.

▶ Adolescent Growth and Development

Adolescence spans the growth period between childhood and adulthood. The number of years required for completion of this period varies, because each youth progresses through this period at a unique pace. The onset of adolescence, puberty, is a time of rapid physical, psychologic, and social development that leads to maturity. Adolescence often brings years of confusion, years in which the individual wavers between accepting the responsibilities of adulthood and fleeing to the security of childhood.

As hormonal influences become apparent, the adolescent may feel that he or she is locked into a stranger's body that changes daily in appearance and function. Fluctuating emotions result, complicating the youth's struggle with such issues as identity development, value formation, and decision making. The manner in which adolescents confront these issues, along with their genetic potential and life experiences, determine the complexity of this period for the youth and the family. Adolescence must be completed before the status of adult can be attained.

Developmental Tasks of Adolescence

Adolescence can be subdivided into three stages: early adolescence (which begins with puberty and consists of ages 10 to 13); middle adolescence (ages 14 to 16); and late adolescence (ages 17 to 21) (Crockett & Petersen, 1993; USDHHS, 1991). Age ranges are assigned to each stage, but these are arbitrary, as each adolescent progresses through these stages at a different rate. The nurse must therefore assess each adolescent's developmental stage in planning appropriate care (Drake, 1996).

Adolescence brings the transition from childhood to adulthood. Under normal circumstances, cognitive growth continues, and the adolescent learns to understand the effects of his or her behavior. As the teen years pass, the egocentric world of the early adolescent evolves into the sociocentric world of the adult. The impulsive behavior of the early adolescent gives way to understanding of complex abstract concepts and ability to control impulsive behavior. As the adolescent matures into adulthood, he or she better defines a personal identity and prepares to assume an independent functional role in society (Crockett & Petersen, 1993). Table 11–1 summarizes biopsychosocial development during adolescence.

▶ Adolescent Sexual Development

Factors Influencing Sexual Activity

Blending a sexual identity into an emerging adult personality is one of the greatest challenges facing the adolescent. Several factors may influence adolescents to become sexually active:

- Early onset of physical maturity
- Influence of media; sexuality portrayed as desirable in many media sources (TV, films, magazines, videos)
- Hormonal changes

- Desire for reassurance that they are sexually "normal" and "grown up"
- Rebellion from family
- Peer pressure
- Desire to belong to a group or to feel that someone could be attracted to them
- Feelings of being invulnerable
- Less social stigma of an unmarried and uncommitted sexual relationship
- Lack of community and parental support and supervision

Sexual feelings become stronger during adolescence, as teenagers mature physically. In addition, adolescents today live in a world where sexuality is used to imply maturity and the adult status that adolescents are so eagerly seeking. Sexual overtones are everywhere, and adolescents may be confused by conflicting messages. The media portray the sophisticated adult as one who uses sexual expressions effectively; yet when adolescents attempt to imitate this behavior they are reminded of their young age and told to ignore the signals being sent by their maturing bodies. Adolescents on television are often portrayed as having no notion of protection, consequences, or social responsibility to their partners or to themselves. On television and in films, sexuality is presented to teens as a casual and carefree activity, despite the reality of human immunodeficiency virus (HIV) infection and other STDs.

Adolescents today tend to become sexually mature at an earlier age. The age of puberty has been decreasing about 1 to 3 months each decade over the last 175 years in the United States with puberty occurring between the ages of 8 and 13 in girls and 9 and 14 in boys (Ganong, 1994). The average age of menarche is 12.7 years (see Chapter 7). Although adolescent females may be anovulatory for the first 1 to 3 years after menstruation starts, this is not an absolute, and many girls do conceive during this period.

All adolescents, even those prepared for the physiologic changes, have many questions about their sexual "normalcy" and may become preoccupied with these concerns. As the adolescent's sexual feelings become stronger, he or she must develop ways to release sexual tension. Hormonal changes and the resulting urges encourage sexual experimentation (Brooks-Gunn & Paikoff, 1993). Masturbation, leading to orgasm, remains the primary means of sexual expression for the majority of boys and for many girls during adolescence.

As the adolescent's need for independence from the family increases, rebellion against parents and their values and beliefs frequently results. For many adolescents, engaging in a sexual relationship outside

▶ **TABLE 11–1**

Biopsychosocial Development During Adolescence

Stages	Characteristics	Developmental Tasks
Early adolescence (age 10–13 yrs)	Onset of puberty, becomes concerned with developing body	Adolescent has major questions concerning normalcy of physical maturation; often concerned about the stages of sexual development and how his or her process relates to peers of same gender.
		Occasional masturbation.
	Begins to expand social radius beyond family and concentrate on relationships with peers	Can begin to encourage some external responsibilities alone in consultation with parents, i.e., visit with health care provider, contacts with school counselors.
	Cognition is usually concrete	Concrete thinking requires dealing with most health situations in a simple, explicit manner using visual as well as verbal cues.
Middle adolescence (age 14–16 yrs)	Pubertal development usually complete and sexual drives emerge	Explores ability to attract opposites. Sexual behavior and experimentation (same and opposite sex) begin.
		Masturbation increases.
	Peer group sets behavioral standards, although family values usually persist	Peer group will often have an effect on compliance; peers rather than parents may offer key support for such activities as visits to health care providers.
	Conflicts over independence	Increased assumption of independent action, together with continued need for parental support and guidance; able to discuss and negotiate changes in rules.
		Ambivalence on part of adolescent in discussion and negotiation.
	Cognition begins to be abstract	Begins to consider full range of possibilities with poor ability to integrate into real life because ego identity not fully formed and cognitive growth not complete.
Late adolescence (age 17–21 yrs)	Physical maturation complete. Body image and gender role definition is secured.	The adolescent begins to feel comfortable with relationships and decisions regarding sexuality and preference. Movement to individual relationships becomes more important than peer group.
	Relationships are no longer narcissistic; there is a process of giving and sharing.	Adolescent more open to specific questioning regarding behavior.
	Idealistic	Idealism may lead to conflicts with family.
	Emancipation is nearly secured	With emancipation, the young person begins to more fully recognize the consequences of his actions.
	Cognitive development is complete	Most are capable of understanding a full range of options for health issues.
	Functional role begins to be defined	Often interested in significant discussion of life goals because this is the primary function of this stage.

Adapted, with permission, from Rudolph, A.M. (1996). Rudolph's pediatrics (20th ed.). Norwalk, CT: Appleton & Lange, p. 39.

of marriage may be one way of demonstrating independence. Some adolescent males view fathering a child as a way to enhance their masculinity (Marsiglio, 1993).

Adolescents may be pressured into becoming sexually active by their partners. Peer pressure also influences sexual activity (Fig. 11–1). Adolescents, especially males, brag about their sexual conquests. An adolescent may not want to carry the stigma of being the only virgin in the group. As inexperienced adolescents listen to tales of sexual adventures, they have no way of knowing that many stories are invented to impress the listener; thus teens may become sexually active, not from sexual desire, but from the need to belong to the group.

The increase in sexual activity among adolescents has also been attributed to societal and cultural changes in the United States. One of the most significant changes is the increasing number of single-parent families in the country. Many parents also work outside the home. Adolescents frequently assume duties that were held by adults in the family,

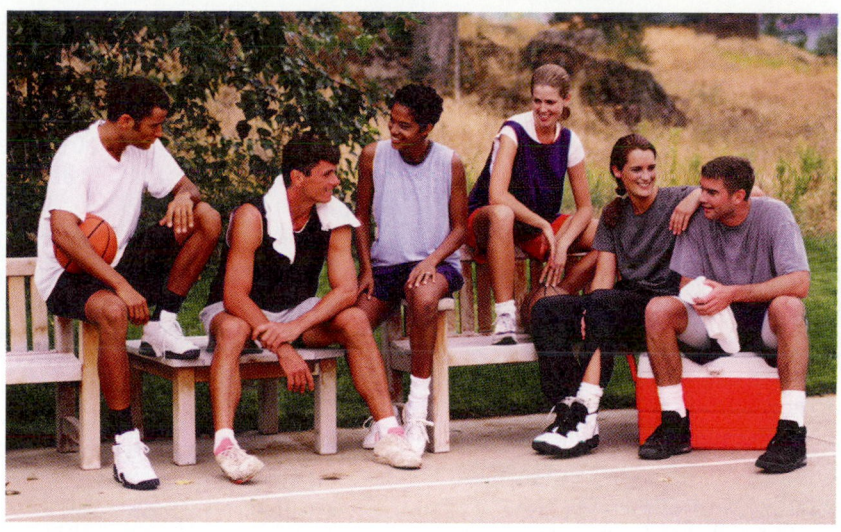

FIGURE 11–1. Peer pressure can have an impact on an adolescent's behaviors.

thus increasing their feelings of maturity. Since the 1980s, adolescents have spent less and less time with adults (Perry et al., 1993). Many adolescents spend long periods in unsupervised situations at home while parents are out, which increases the opportunity for sexual activity.

The media has an enormous impact on teenagers at a time when they are struggling to form their own identities. As noted by Seplow and Storm (1997), watching TV consumes about 40% of all the hours Americans are not committed to working, eating, sleeping, or doing chores. The average teenager spends about 21 hours per week watching television (Bragg, 1997). Television and other media have become the core of culture. When TV was first developed, families together would watch programs, which were directed toward general audiences. With current trends, many households have more than one television set. Family members no longer view programs together (Seplow & Storm, 1997), and parents and teens often do not discuss the messages conveyed in these programs. Many programs watched by teenagers deal heavily with sex, violence, and dysfunctional relationships. The media presents teens with images of self-worth based on sexuality and adulthood as characterized by drinking, spending money, and being sexually active, often without consequences or loving relationships (Bragg, 1997).

Sex Education for Adolescents

Some adolescents are not able to communicate with their parents about sexual topics. The responsibility for discussing information and values about sexuality is frequently left to the schools or religious institutions. Incorporation of sex education into the curriculum can increase knowledge about reproduction and pregnancy risk (Brooks-Gunn & Paikoff, 1993). Research results, however, are mixed concerning outcomes of sex education for adolescents, as it is difficult to assess to what degree school-based programs postpone or prevent adolescent sexual activity and pregnancy. Creative educational methods and strategies need to be devised to better reach adolescents with an appropriate message concerning responsible sexual behavior (U.S. Centers for Disease Control and Prevention, 1993). Unfortunately, many teenagers continue to have unprotected sexual intercourse and therefore remain at risk for unintended pregnancy and disease (Grimes, 1995b).

In addition to the traditional sex education classes, several school districts across the country have opened clinics located on the school grounds. These clinics provide primary health services for the school population, and may also provide sexual counseling services (Kirby et al., 1993). Some institutions actually dispense contraceptive devices.

These clinics have many advantages. Students are able to receive the services they need in familiar surroundings. The services are convenient and confidential. Peers use the clinic so the adolescent feels "safe" seeking information. In addition, because adolescents are the only population served, staff working in the clinic are well informed about adolescent growth and development.

▶ Alternatives Available to the Pregnant Adolescent

When an adolescent girl becomes pregnant, she can get married and have the child, have an abortion, place the infant for foster care or adoption, rear the child alone, or allow her parents or other family members to rear the child. Prior to the 1960s, the majority of adolescents either married or placed the infant for adoption after a "hush-hush" pregnancy. The legitimacy of the birth and the reputation of the adolescent and her family were of primary concern.

The 1960s marked the beginning of a sexual and cultural revolution that changed society's norms. Today teen idols such as actresses and rock stars openly discuss the advantages of single parenthood. Adolescents may follow their example, not considering that these famous women have resources far beyond the adolescent's resources, or that stardom does not necessarily mean emotional health.

Some adolescents choose to marry after pregnancy is confirmed, although this option is becoming less common. Two factors appear to influence whether or not a couple decides to marry: age and cultural expectations. The older a young woman is when she conceives, the more likely she is to marry. Socioeconomic status and culture also influence whether a couple marries or not; Caucasians marry more often than African-Americans (Kahn & Anderson, 1992).

The adolescent's search for independence is often stifled by an early marriage, as financial concerns may force the young couple to live with family members. Although this arrangement provides tangible support for the couple, such as room, board, and perhaps infant care, it may prevent the young couple from developing an independent, mature marital relation-

ship. The adolescents may continue to rely on parents or other adults to make their decisions or may be forced to accept outside opinions because of their continuing dependent status. Different cultural groups, however, perceive this arrangement in a more positive manner. Some families easily incorporate the young couple.

Even if the couple decides to set up a separate household, financial difficulties and problems stemming from emotional immaturity are common. The principal effects of early childbearing on adolescents include:

- Decrease in satisfactory job opportunities
- Increase in high school dropouts
- Delayed independence from parents
- Increased divorce rates
- Larger family size
- Increased reliance on public assistance or other financial difficulties

Adolescent marriages are more likely to end in divorce than adult marriages.

Many adolescents terminate their pregnancies by abortion. An accurate number of teenage abortions is difficult to estimate since several states do not collect data on the age of women obtaining abortions.

Abortion is not an easy decision for most young women. Adolescents are aware of conflicting religious and moral views about abortion and are affected by these ideas. Many adolescents do not know where to seek services or lack a means of transportation to the facilities. Others do not have the money or resources needed for an abortion. Still others do not accept the pregnancy until the fetus becomes active and physical changes are undeniable. Some may enter emergency rooms in labor and claim they did not know they were pregnant.

Placing the infant for adoption is an alternative that fewer younger women are selecting. As cultural taboos against out-of-wedlock births have faded, more adolescents are choosing to raise the child alone or with the help of family members.

Various organizations can assist the adolescent who elects to place her baby for adoption. Both state-licensed and religious-affiliated adoption agencies exist throughout the United States. Private adoptions are also becoming more common. In this situation an attorney is usually the intermediary between the couple, seeking an infant to adopt, and the young mother. The couple usually pays the mother's medical expenses and often supplements her living expenses during her pregnancy. Although this adoption option is becoming more common, it is important that the laws of each state be known, so that the adoption is not jeopardized.

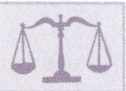 *Ethical Decision Making*

As a nurse providing care for adolescents, you will encounter many controversial issues that relate to the rights of adolescents and to adolescent parenting, such as:

1. Should parents be held legally responsible for the sexual activities of their teenagers?
2. Who should inform parents of a teenager's pregnancy?
3. Should parental consent be required for a teenager under 18 to have an abortion?

The adolescent who does place her infant for adoption has made a very difficult decision and requires tremendous support from the health care team and her family members. The adolescent may desire to see and spend time with her newborn before discharge. This is normal. Many mothers who place their infants for adoption state that they use this time to say goodbye to their child.

Currently, about 95% of teens keep their babies. The adolescent who decides to keep the infant needs a great deal of guidance, education, and support to make the transition to parenthood and then to parent successfully. Although some pregnant adolescents come from families and backgrounds that well meet economic and emotional needs, many pregnant adolescents come from socially, economically, or emotionally high-risk families that have complex needs that predate pregnancy. The presence of an infant can further complicate difficult situations. Indeed, many cases of child abuse involve teen mothers (Bragg, 1997).

In some settings the grandmother takes on the mothering role. The adolescent mother may shift between being grateful for her mother's or grandmother's help and feeling resentful for her intrusion. This can lead to conflict and confusion in the family. In some cultural groups, however, the adolescent mother and her infant are easily incorporated into the extended family.

▶ Effects of Early Childbearing on Adolescents

The Adolescent Mother

Effects of early childbearing on the adolescent mother include developmental, educational, and economic factors. The impact of these factors is also affected by the adolescent's personal and family situation prior to the pregnancy.

For the pregnant teenager, the developmental tasks of adolescence are complicated by the developmental tasks of pregnancy (Drake, 1996). For example, in normal developmental circumstances, nonpregnant adolescents are concerned with their changing body images. Reflecting the influence of the media and the slender "ideal" propagated in U.S. society, the nonpregnant adolescent girl may be dissatisfied with the increase in size and weight that occurs during the teen years. Pregnancy compounds these feelings, as the adolescent experiences physical prenatal changes that she may perceive as unattractive.

Pregnancy is a crisis for most adolescents. As physiologic changes reduce the adolescent's feeling of self-control, fear of the unknown may intensify her emotions, and she may act indifferent or "tough" to mask her terror.

Parents of adolescents who become pregnant respond in many ways to this news. Feelings of shock, anger, disappointment, betrayal, and shame may be experienced from confirmation of their daughter's sexual activity as well as from the pregnancy. Parents frequently ask, "Where did we go wrong?" Some parents may force the adolescent from the home and believe "she is too disruptive" and "she has made her bed, now she can lie in it." Believing their daughter was taken advantage of, others blame the father of the baby and try to prevent any contact between him and their daughter. After an initial "shock," many parents come to accept and support their daughters. Reactions to pregnancy reflect such factors as religious and cultural background, whether the parent or other family member had a baby out of wedlock, whether the adolescent was previously pregnant, the nature of usual family dynamics, and the presence of preexisting family problems.

Despite laws that forbid schools to expel pregnant girls, many do drop out of school and do not return. Even bringing an infant or young child to a school-based day-care program can be overwhelming for a teenager. Subsequently, lack of formal education limits the economic and social opportunities of the young mother (Grimes, 1993; Podgurski, 1993; Roye & Balk, 1997). An estimated one in three adolescents who give birth will become pregnant again within 2 years, thus further limiting opportunities (Grimes, 1993). Early parenthood also delays the adolescent's transition to emotional, financial, and social independence. Although some pregnant teenagers marry, many do not, and the baby usually then resides with the mother and/or her family. As noted in *Healthy People 2000: National Health Promotion and Disease Prevention Objectives* (USDHHS, 1991), female-headed families tend to be poorer than two-parent families, as they do not have a second wage earner, women tend to earn lower wages than men, and because teenage mothers frequently lack education and job skills. Roye and Balk (1997) described a special program for pregnant teenagers and their mothers. In addition to promoting communication and positive relationships, the program's results indicated higher self-esteem and lower school dropout rates among those who participated.

Currently, teenage pregnancy in the United States does not carry the same widespread social stigma that it once did, when an unmarried pregnant girl was considered "ruined." Among some peer groups, pregnancy may be viewed as confirmation of the girl's womanliness.

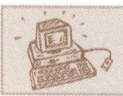

Research Abstract

Caring for Pregnant Teens and Their Mothers

This article described results of a program that included inner city pregnant teenagers and their mothers or significant mothering person. Begun in 1993, the program recruited 154 pregnant teens. A group of teens who refused to participate or who were cared for before the program started was also used so that results could be compared for teens whose mothers participated with teens whose mothers did not. Study participants filled out questionnaires before starting the program and, again, several years later, when open-ended questions were also asked of the teens and the grandmothers. The program was scheduled to coincide with the teen's prenatal visits. A social worker first met for two one-hour sessions with the grandmother; the teen joined them for the third session; and the social worker met alone with the grandmother for the fourth session. The social worker met with the teen and grandmother at the time of the infant's first and second well-baby visits; additional sessions were an offered option. The pregnant teenager's program meanwhile included every other week visits until the third trimester when weekly visits began, classes taught by a pediatric nurse practitioner or certified nurse-midwife, and, after delivery, monthly visits during the first year, every 2 months during the second year, and visits every 3–6 months until the infant turned 3 or the mother turned 19. When the babies were between 2 and 5 years old, the group was contacted again; 65 mothers and 15 grandmothers were available for follow-up by telephone or mail. Results indicated that important goals of the program were met. The teens whose mothers participated in the program were less likely to have dropped out of school, had a lower incidence of repeat pregnancy and higher self-esteem than those whose mothers did not participate in the program. Furthermore, grandmothers reported the program helped them cope with their feelings, helped improve their relationships with their daughters and the communication between them, and helped the entire family.

Application to Practice

This study documented the effectiveness of a program that focused on grandmothers as well as their pregnant teenage daughters. Adolescent pregnancy is a socially high-risk situation and a crisis for many families. The authors not only based their program on interventions for pregnant teens, but devised a program that had a goal of fostering mother–daughter relationships during a turbulent time. Programs such as this are time consuming and, in the current climate of managed care, are difficult to carry out. However, as the authors point out, decreasing repeat pregnancy, bolstering self-esteem in a high-risk population, preventing school dropout, and fostering family relationships result in economic as well as social benefits. This study provides an example of how a high-risk group was targeted, how a special program was implemented, and how results were identified.

Source: Roye, C.F., & Balk, S.J. (1997). Caring for pregnant teens and their mothers, too. MCN, American Journal of Maternal Child Nursing, 22(3), 153–157.

The Adolescent Father

Sexual activity continues to rise for adolescent boys, as well as for adolescent girls. Traditionally, boys tended to become sexually active at younger ages than girls. Despite sexual activity, most adolescent boys do not intend for pregnancy to occur. The onset of sexual activity by an adolescent male is influenced by such factors as his degree of independence from the family, whether he or a close family member was born out of wedlock, cultural background, attitude of the peer group, and susceptibility to the effects of the media.

Pregnancy superimposes the challenges of fatherhood upon the developmental tasks of adolescence. However, the teenage father is unlikely to be better able to assume the responsibilities of pregnancy and parenthood than the teenage mother. Like the adolescent mother, the adolescent father may be faced with negative responses of family (including the girl's family) members. He may also experience a sense of crisis and such feelings as anger, depression, and isolation. Some adolescent fathers, particularly those from lower socioeconomic and educational backgrounds, view impregnating a woman as enhancing their masculinity; these individuals also tend to have greater likelihood of not using measures to prevent a subsequent pregnancy (Marsiglio, 1993).

Although adolescent pregnancy does result from casual sex, many adolescent males are involved in a "meaningful" relationship with their partner. They usually have similar socioeconomic backgrounds, common educational achievement, and are within 3 to 4 years of each other in age.

Research indicates that the quality of the relationship with the baby's father is important for a young mother. For example, in a study of 36 adolescent mothers and their infants, Diehl (1997) found that paternal involvement and support were associated with more positive mother–infant interactions. Even within a subgroup of teen mothers with low self-esteem, involvement with the baby's father was associated with more positive mother–infant interactions.

There is a lack of information about the long-term involvement of adolescent fathers with their infants. Actual involvement reflects such factors as the desire of the adolescent father to be involved with his child, the nature of the relationship between the adolescent father and mother, whether or not the couple marries, acceptance of the adolescent father by the young mother's significant others, and other social factors that encourage or discourage paternal involvement. Other influences often affect the father's involvement with the adolescent mother and their baby. For example, government regulations concerning payment of public assistance and Aid to Families with Dependent Children may force the father to live elsewhere. In some places, if a male admits to fathering a child born to a mother less than 16 years of age, he can be charged with rape.

Nurses working with pregnant adolescents should recognize that the amount of a father's participation in the pregnancy may be determined by the wishes of the mother and by the relationship of the couple. Some fathers may desire to marry the mother; others deny responsibility for the pregnancy; still others do not wish to marry the mother, but want to participate in the pregnancy and the rearing of the child.

Some adolescent mothers, because of pregnancy resulting from casual sex, incest, or rape, do not wish to name the father of the baby or do not want contact between the father and the baby. Health care

Women's Health

Early childbearing can have serious psychosocial implications. Examples include decreased verbal and nonverbal interactions between mother and infant, lack of confidence about ability to be capable parents, maladaptive parenting responses, and inconsistent care given to infants and children by adolescent parents.

providers should intervene to assist the girl if sexual abuse is suspected.

When the couple desires, the father can be encouraged to attend prenatal visits and classes, serve as the labor coach, and assume partial responsibility for child care. His participation can strengthen the relationship with his unborn child and may enhance the father's desire to remain a part of his child's life. The father's support may also promote maternal–fetal attachment.

The Older Father

Adolescent girls may become pregnant by older male partners, rather than by an adolescent male. While some such relationships are strong, as Bragg (1997) notes, the difference in age may indicate a power imbalance within the couple, which in turn might provide a situation for "less than voluntary" sexual behavior.

▶ Costs and Risks of Adolescent Pregnancy

Adolescent pregnancy is accompanied by high personal and social costs. Personal costs, such as inhibition of educational and other opportunities, have been presented. However, society is also deprived of potential contributions from its members and challenged to meet the needs of people who are in economic hardship. It is hard to separate effects of adolescence, poverty, lack of prenatal care, and high-risk behaviors on pregnancy outcome. These risk factors tend to occur together and add to the costs of adolescent pregnancy. In a study of attachment behaviors of pregnant adolescents (Bloom, 1995), only 6 (12%) of 47 low-income pregnant teenagers had completely uncomplicated pregnancies. Such complications as gestational diabetes, STDs, cervical dysplasia, anemia, intrauterine growth retardation, and preterm labor

▶ RISK FACTORS RELATED TO ADOLESCENT PREGNANCY

- Socioeconomic factors
- Inadequate or no prenatal care
- Use of tobacco, alcohol, and other substances
- Sexually transmitted diseases
- Lack of social support
- Poor nutritional status
- High stress

- History of abuse
- Higher risk of maternal death for young teens (13–15 years) than for women 20–24 years (Bragg, 1997)
- Problems for the infant, including higher rates of illness, injury, and death for infants of mothers younger than 17 years than for infants of older women (Bragg, 1997)

affected the rest of the group. See box entitled Risk Factors Related to Adolescent Pregnancy.

▶ Adolescent Pregnancy and Maltreatment

Adolescents may be considered at risk for physical or mental maltreatment. According to the Council on Scientific Affairs of the American Medical Association (1993), adolescents experience maltreatment at rates equal to or greater than rates of abuse for younger children. Nevertheless, adolescents are more often viewed as being responsible for the maltreatment and are less likely to be reported to child protective services than are younger children. Premature sexual activity and unintended pregnancy are risk behaviors associated with maltreatment (Council on Scientific Affairs, 1993; Grimes, 1995a). Research supports the widespread incidence of maltreatment of pregnant adolescents. Unlike pregnant adolescents who had not been abused, the sexually victimized adolescents began intercourse earlier and were more likely to be involved with alcohol and other drugs, to have exchanged sex for money, and to report that their own children had been abused or taken from them by Child Protective Services. Parker and associates (1993) found that 182 (26%) of their sample of 691 pregnant teenagers and adult women had been victims of physical or sexual abuse within the past year. A higher percentage of teens (31.6%) than adults (23.6%) reported abuse during the past year; more teens (21.7%) than adult women (15.9%) experienced abuse during the pregnancy.

Research limitations and the underreporting of maltreatment during adolescence make identification of the incidence of abuse difficult. However, nurses need to realize that pregnancy during adolescence often reflects high-risk behavior and can be both a cause and reflection or turmoil between the teenager and significant others. Maltreatment is widespread;

assessment and appropriate intervention should be part of prenatal care.

▶ Nursing and Collaborative Assessment

As for any pregnant woman, assessment combines history, physical examination, and laboratory testing. The history is updated at each subsequent visit; physical examination and laboratory testing continue to be performed according to protocols for particular gesta-

Nursing Alert

As part of screening for abuse of the pregnant adolescent:

- Prepare in advance; make certain you know what to do in your setting when an abused pregnant adolescent is identified; be aware of referrals, resources, etc.
- Interview the adolescent in private
- Ask the adolescent whether she has been harmed or if she feels unsafe. This is also part of the regular prenatal care interview.
- Make certain that a physical examination identifies any injuries; document all evidence of injury, as well as the client's explanation of how the injury occurred
- Discuss a plan for the adolescent's safety
- Provide appropriate education about violence and abuse
- As indicated, follow local/state guidelines for reporting physical/sexual abuse of a minor

tional periods. In taking a history, the nurse must realize that the teenager is dealing both with the changes of adolescence and of pregnancy. Special attention needs to be devoted to the adolescent's response to being pregnant, developmental level, educational background, learning needs, economic level, and support systems. Physical and laboratory assessment of the pregnant adolescent is similar to prenatal assessment for the older pregnant woman. Although teenagers, particularly young teenagers, may be at higher risk for such conditions as poor nutritional status, preeclampsia, and preterm labor, all pregnant women should be assessed for these conditions. High-risk lifestyle factors indicate need to assess for such conditions as STDs, substance abuse, and maltreatment.

▶ Nursing Diagnoses

Evaluation of assessment data enables the nurse to develop relevant nursing diagnoses. Examples of possible nursing diagnoses that are based on assessment of the pregnant adolescent include:

Problem-oriented diagnoses:

- Personal identity disturbance, related to premature childbearing and maternal role demands
- Altered nutrition (less than body requirements), related to adolescent dietary patterns
- Social isolation from peers, related to impending motherhood and feeling different from peers

Wellness-oriented diagnoses:

- Progressive individual coping, related to social support during pregnancy
- Enhanced self-esteem, related to paternal involvement in pregnancy

▶ Nursing and Collaborative Management

A comprehensive plan that addresses the physical and psychosocial needs of the pregnant adolescent should be developed (see Critical Thinking in Care Planning later in the chapter). Management strategies for the pregnant adolescent focus on beginning care as early as possible during pregnancy and promoting ongoing care throughout pregnancy. In ideal circumstances, sexually active teens would be receiving regular gynecologic care prior to pregnancy; in reality, many teenagers do not. Indeed, adolescents often need to overcome barriers in order to receive care (see box entitled Examples of Barriers to Care for Pregnant Adolescents) (Hogan, 1993; Millstein, 1993).

Educating the public about the importance and location of prenatal care helps spread the word to adolescents. Articles in the print media and public service announcements during radio and television programs, popular with teenagers, are important for prenatal public health promotion. Volunteer endorsement of prenatal care by celebrities who serve as role models to teens also is helpful.

Prenatal care that is accessible in location and available in after school, evening, and weekend sessions prevents having to choose between attending school or obtaining prenatal care. In-school educational and service programs for pregnant teens can also foster continuation in school while making care accessible (Warrick, Christianson, Walruff, & Cook, 1993). School-based classes can also focus on building self-esteem to help teens dealing with problematic behaviors of others such as smoking (Winkelstein, 1995). In addition, consolidating services so that teens are able to be scheduled for comprehensive care at each session and in one location can conserve time and minimize stress for the adolescent and help

---

▶ EXAMPLES OF BARRIERS TO CARE FOR PREGNANT ADOLESCENTS

- Lack of financial support. Lack of knowledge about programs such as Medicaid to help pay for prenatal care.
- Lack of accessible sites for prenatal care.
- Problematic hours for private or clinic health care provider (lack of after school, evening, or weekend sessions).
- Lack of information about the importance of early prenatal care.
- Fear of the examination.
- Fear of lack of confidentiality on the part of health care providers.

- Fear of punitive attitudes on behalf of health care providers.
- Problems with the prenatal care delivery system—e.g., long waits, ever-changing staff, lack of sensitivity of staff to the special needs of adolescents.
- Lack of support from significant others. Lack of "someone to turn to" or fear of informing significant others.
- Denial of the pregnancy. Hopes that the pregnancy is not "real."

ensure that the adolescent appears not only for her examinations, but also for prescribed tests and interventions. School-based programs also allow the childbirth educator the chance to be visible to students and to influence attitudes about sexuality and pregnancy within the student population (Podgurski, 1993). Some pregnant teens also have problems related to substance use. Indeed, over the past decades, teen use of alcohol and other drugs has increased (Bragg, 1997).

Providing prenatal care for adolescents requires time, patience, and understanding by all levels of staff and at every contact with the adolescent. Staff need to be educated in the care of adolescents and to recognize and complement adolescent mothers' positive efforts; such strategies help to support self-confidence and an atmosphere conducive to sharing feelings and asking questions (Fleming, Munton, Clarke, & Strauss, 1993). Staff also need to be sensitive to client cultural backgrounds and to consider such factors as acculturation as well as ethnic background when planning and providing care (Reynoso, Felice, & Shragg, 1993).

Ideally, the same staff would care for an adolescent at each of her visits. Many ambulatory care settings, however, do not have consistent medical coverage; resident and attending physicians may rotate through prenatal care settings, and the teenager may be examined by a different individual at each visit. Nurses are the health care providers who are most likely to interact with the adolescent on an ongoing basis. Nurses can also do much to orient new physicians to the special needs of adolescents and to expected standards of care.

Management begins with the adolescent's initial contact with the health care system. Many teenagers are afraid to telephone for an appointment. A rude or uncaring receptionist can discourage the teenager from coming for prenatal care. The adolescent's first interaction with health care providers will greatly influence her carrying out the health care plan. Most adolescents do not come to their first visits alone and may be accompanied by their mothers, boyfriends, or significant others. In some cases of abuse, such as incest, the adolescent may be accompanied by the individual who has abused her. The health history often includes sensitive material that the adolescent may not have shared with significant others. For this reason and to encourage the teenager to express her thoughts freely, the adolescent is interviewed privately. As with any client, responses are confidential.

If an adolescent senses that the nurse is rushed or that the adolescent is just another "case," the atmosphere needed to build trust and rapport will not exist. Continuity of staff needs to be provided to establish and maintain trusting relationships. The nurse must understand the normal growth and development of adolescents, as well as the problems that accompany teenage pregnancy (see box entitled Strategies for Helping Teen Parents).

Adolescents need to be presented with available options in a nonjudgmental manner. Support services should be offered for whatever decision the adolescent makes, and may include referrals for abortion services, adoption agencies, and social services. In accordance with the views of certain religious organizations, prenatal clinics that they sponsor may not refer a client directly for abortion services. Community nursing agencies, parent education programs, and alternative educational or residential education programs may be suggested.

▶ STRATEGIES FOR HELPING TEEN PARENTS

- Talk to the teens. Ask such questions as, "How can I make this time easier for you? What do you need from me?"
- Use simple, easy to understand language. Be sure to include both the young mother and the father.
- Explain all procedures and what to expect.
- Encourage the father to participate in a way that is comfortable for him. Examples include giving the mother juice and labor coaching.
- Make sure teen parents are aware that holding hands, back rubs, and other types of helpful touch are encouraged in the hospital or birth center and can be a great source of support and comfort.
- Find out the teens' situations. Refer teens to postpartum and parenting support groups for teens. Get to know the

people to whom you are referring the teens, if possible. This fosters continuity of care and helps to personalize care if you know what and whom you are talking about.
- Identify community resources teens can turn to for counseling, crisis intervention, and other types of support. Make sure these are available in your practice area and that there are pamphlets for staff to give out as appropriate.
- Discuss strategies for personalizing care to meet the unique needs of teens at unit staff meetings. Arrange for in-service speakers or conferences to help staff develop skill in working with pregnant teenagers.

Source: Mills, 1997.

As with any client, the adolescent needs to be included in her plan of care. Procedures must be explained beforehand. Recognizing that many adolescents fear physical examination, the nurse should provide anticipatory guidance, promote privacy and comfort during examination, and ensure that either the nurse or a supportive staff member is with the adolescent during the examination.

Educational Preparation

Through one-to-one sessions and through parent education classes, nurses serve as teachers for pregnant adolescents. The adolescent's knowledge of childbearing should be assessed. The adolescent may have many misconceptions about childbearing, promoted by relatives, friends, and popular media. The pregnant adolescent should be encouraged to take part in childbirth and parenting education programs and ideally should be referred to classes specifically for teenagers. These classes not only cover pregnancy, fetal growth and development, labor and delivery, and early parenting, but also address concerns unique to teenagers. Such topics as substance abuse, STDs, and maltreatment should also be part of educational programs. The nurse should encourage the adolescent to bring a support person, who may also serve as labor coach. Nurses have served in this capacity in situations where the adolescent has no one else. Teens identified as having problems with alcohol or other drugs ideally should be referred for counseling and programs specifically designed for adolescents. Problems associated with substance-abusing pregnant teens extend beyond pregnancy and need long-term strategies (Bragg, 1997).

Parenting content is part of educational preparation for pregnant adolescents; some parenting programs may begin in the prenatal period and continue after the birth of the baby. Small group classes allow pregnant adolescents to share experiences and express feelings about pregnancy and parenting. Many adolescents have not had much experience with the raising of small children; their perceptions of parenting are based on media images such as television commercials, where the infant is cute and well behaved. In teen parenting groups, nurses can serve as resources and facilitators to help dispel myths and promote parenting skills. Such creative strategies as having adolescents draw self-portraits afford opportunities for them to share feelings about self, family, and the infant, and for the nurse to provide support, encouragement, and education.

Health care providers should begin to discuss future methods of planning a family with pregnant adolescents before the first infant is born. An assessment should be made of the adolescent's future goals and her lifestyle. By discussing this information before delivery, the adolescent is assisted in considering her future and in making her own plans regarding future childbearing.

▶ DELAYED CHILDBEARING

Women who give birth after age 35 are referred to as **mature gravidas** or mature clients. Thirty-five is actually an arbitrary selection, based on the need to give some classification structure to aging and childbearing. There is no magic reason why 35 should be so identified; some experts have suggested use of a sliding scale instead (Cunningham et al., 1997).

Later motherhood is not a new trend. Such factors as lack of available, effective contraceptives; social approval of large families; and high childhood mortality were historically related to women having children as long as they were able to have children. However, choosing to postpone having children until the midthirties or later and a larger number of pregnant women in their later reproductive years reflect changes in patterns of childbearing (Stark, 1997).

Normal biologic pregnancy does not occur after menopause. However, reproductive technology has made pregnancy resulting from implantation of fertilized human donor ova into a human female possible for women who would not be able to become pregnant due to changes from the aging process (Check, Nowroozi, Baruea, Shaw, & Saver, 1993). Although such births are rare, childbearing by women who more commonly are in the grandparent age group raises many ethical, financial, and medical issues.

▶ Factors Influencing Delayed Childbearing

Women give many reasons for delaying childbearing and childrearing. A major influence has been the increase in job opportunities and careers for women. A young woman's dreams are no longer solely oriented to thoughts of finding a husband and having children. Today, young women are entering diverse careers, many of which were closed to women of previous generations. Many young women enter the work force or the university setting seeking skills for a career, not merely a job. Hard work and advanced degrees offer previously unavailable opportunities for the young woman of today.

The years from 20 to 30 are often critical in establishing oneself in a profession. The option of taking time out to search for a partner or start a family may not be available to the woman who wants to advance in a career. Once a woman is successful in her field, the decision to change her status by adding the mothering role may require much thought and introspection. Some couples delay parenting for financial reasons.

Late and repeat marriages also are given as reasons for delaying motherhood (Kitzinger, 1995). As more and more youths elect to attend college and as educational expenses increase, the attraction of early marriages has diminished. When young adults do marry as students, they are often forced to hold down jobs as well as fulfill their educational responsibilities.

As social bans on divorce have been lifted, the number of repeat marriages has increased. Many women take some time out after a divorce to determine the qualities that they are seeking in a partner and a relationship. These couples may need time to establish their identity as a couple and often further delay childbearing for several years.

Improved contraceptive methods have allowed the postponement of childbearing. Infertility has also been a factor delaying childbearing.

▶ Advantages of Delayed Childbearing

The decision to have a child after the age of 35 is one that is seldom made without thought. Although women describe being aware of the ticking of the biologic clock, the determining factor is usually not based on physiology alone. Most women who decide to become parents consider the options carefully, weighing the pros and cons.

Many women reach this period in their development having accomplished their professional goals and having become ready to realize the personal goal of parenthood. Although they are successful in their chosen careers, many state that they are left with the feeling that something is missing from their lives. They have a sense of being unfulfilled, and believe that having a child will fill this void. These feelings are quite different from those of the immature adolescent who may be searching for someone to love her. The older mother tends to be more emotionally mature, to be involved in a stable marriage, and to have greater financial and family resources to help with childbearing than the younger woman (O'Reilly-Green & Cohen, 1993). She also benefits from varied adult life experiences.

If the mature client desires to combine her career with motherhood, her employer may be more likely to make concessions to keep a valuable employee. She may receive special benefits as incentives to continue working. These may include more flexible working hours, on-site child care, and additional vacation benefits. Because of her financial status, she may also be able to have household help that younger women cannot afford, which eases the strain of combining working and parenting. Women may also head their own businesses. Arrangements for childbearing and childcare, although not necessarily easy, are then usually within their control.

▶ Disadvantages of Delayed Childbearing

Disadvantages can be associated with delayed parenting. Childbearing and childrearing require alterations in well-established life patterns, which can be stressful and not wholly pleasant to change (Stark, 1997). Rearing small children at an older age can be emotionally and physically draining. Career pressures, as well as difficulties in obtaining adequate rest, exercise, and nutrition while on the job, can add stress to a pregnancy.

Having a second or subsequent family brings unique challenges. The mother and/or her partner is starting over again. Previous spouses and children may not welcome the pregnancy. Children seek a sense of stability and belonging; parents need to be sensitive to their children's feelings of being "discarded" in favor of a new family or "not really belonging" because their parents are no longer together and someone else has arrived. Parents are faced with the tasks of maintaining and building bonds with children from their previous relationships and integrating the newborn into their families. Many parents are able to blend children from previous and present relationships into loving and successful families, but others experience conflict and must contend with emotional and behavioral difficulties.

Although delayed childbearing is becoming increasingly "in fashion," older parents tend to have

 Women's Health

A mature client and her partner may feel uncomfortable in childbirth education classes with much younger participants. The childbirth educator can help the couple become part of the group and should address their concerns. Classes may also be held for groups of mature gravidas.

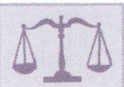

Ethical Decision Making

Reproductive technology has now made it possible for postmenopausal women to carry an implanted pregnancy to term and to become mothers in their 50s and 60s. This situation raises such questions as:

1. Should women in their senior years become mothers?
2. Should health care providers agree to facilitate their becoming mothers?
3. Who should pay the high cost related to reproductive manipulation?
4. Men do become fathers during their senior years. Is denying women the chance to become mothers at the same ages as men "right" or "fair?"

difficulty finding peers with young families. Most people in their 40s have completed their families and frequently have grown children. Peers tend to be involved with their school-age, teenage, or young adult children and may no longer be interested in concerns related to infant care. The mature mother also may have difficulty relating to the woman in her 20s, who is at a very different point in life.

Older mothers may not be able to count on help from their own parents, who may be elderly and have health care concerns of their own. As one mother observed, "I was taking my son to the babysitter's and my 84-year-old father to adult day care."

▶ Pregnancy Outcome and the Mature Woman

Pregnancy at an advanced maternal age, particularly after age 40, is associated with increased complications (see box entitled Health Problems and Risks Associated with Pregnancy Over 35). Traditionally, older pregnant clients are considered high risk, although many are healthy. Conflicting results in the research literature and limitations of studies make identification of complications related to age alone difficult; it is also hard to specify at which age complications actually occur. However, medical or chronic problems such as heart disease and cancer can emerge or intensify as women age. These conditions can have adverse effects on pregnancy; unfortunately, delayed childbearing and the presence of young children do not ensure longevity or protect against disease. Nevertheless, despite a higher incidence of pregnancy

▶ HEALTH PROBLEMS AND RISKS ASSOCIATED WITH PREGNANCY OVER 35

MATERNAL COMPLICATIONS

- Diminished fertility, as part of the aging process.
- Medical complications of chronic illnesses, which intensify with duration of the illness.
- Higher incidence of hypertension. Higher perinatal mortality in older hypertensive women.
- Increased incidence in gestational diabetes and overt complications of diabetes.
- Increased number of hospitalizations related to cardiovascular, neurologic, connective-tissue, renal, and pulmonary disorders, which increase in incidence and severity due to maternal age.
- Increased rate of cesarean deliveries due to such factors as prolonged labor, increased hypertensive disorders, and more fetal monitoring.
- Increased incidence of ectopic pregnancy.
- Increased risk of maternal mortality (estimated to be nearly four times the risk for women aged 20 to 24), related to the medical and obstetrical problems that may complicate pregnancy in older women.

- Increased incidence of placenta previa, across levels of parity.
- Increased incidence of twins and triplets.
- Psychologic stress, related to such factors as being categorized as high risk, undergoing prenatal testing, and fearing that time is running out.

FETAL AND NEONATAL COMPLICATIONS

- Increase in chromosomal abnormalities.
- Increased risk of spontaneous abortion.
- Increased risk of preterm delivery and fetal growth retardation.
- Increased incidence of low birth weight (perhaps related to the increased incidence of hypertensive and vascular complications).
- Higher incidence of macrosomic infants, perhaps related to such factors as maternal obesity, multiparity, diabetes.

Sources: Adashek, Peaceman, Lopez-Zeno, Minogue, & Socol, 1993; Check, et al., 1993; Cunningham, et al., 1997; Edge & Laros, 1993; Langer & Langer, 1993; O'Reilly-Green & Cohen, 1993; Williams & Mittendorf, 1993.

complications, neonatal outcome is usually good. Pregnancy for the mature woman is regarded as safe, especially if she is healthy (Cunningham et al., 1997).

► Nursing and Collaborative Assessment

Assessment for the mature client is essentially the same as for a younger pregnant woman; however, assessment is tailored toward the unique circumstances of delayed childbearing. The health history focuses on gathering data related to a couple in their middle years of adulthood. Topics that provide important information for developing a care plan include previous and current health concerns, obstetric history, family situation, use of reproductive technologies to become pregnant, multiple roles, and psychologic responses to pregnancy on the part of the client and her significant others.

Because the mature client is considered at risk, a variety of screening tests are recommended that would not be routinely ordered for younger women. Such tests include chorionic villus biopsy or amniocentesis and ultrasound scanning. Women who would never elect abortion also may choose genetic screening. Normal results may allay anxiety; knowing in advance about the birth of a baby with an abnormal genetic condition gives the client and her family time to receive support and to prepare for the birth of the infant with special needs.

Other assessment tools relate to identification of specific or psychosocial problems, for example, the existence of hypertension or diabetes, or pregnancy occurring in a family with children from a previous relationship that ended bitterly.

► Nursing Diagnoses

Evaluation of assessment data enables the nurse to develop relevant nursing diagnoses. Examples of possible nursing diagnoses that are based on assessment of the mature pregnant client include:

Problem-oriented diagnoses:

- Parental role conflict, related to incompatibility between parent and career roles
- Anxiety, related to testing for genetic abnormalities
- Fear, related to higher risk of cesarean delivery

Wellness-oriented diagnoses:

- Potential asset in parenting, related to maturity and planned pregnancy

► Nursing and Collaborative Management

Management for the healthy, mature pregnant woman with no existing health problems is similar to management of the younger client. However, anticipatory guidance and support need to be provided in regard to the additional screening recommended for these women. Common beliefs and misconceptions about complications exist, and the older client may fear the development of complications. Prenatal testing and the concerns of health care providers who consider testing necessary are sources of psychologic stress for many, even when the results are negative.

Management for the client with existing or emergent problems focuses on the nature of the problem. For example, establishing good diabetic control even before pregnancy is attempted has been related to a decrease in congenital anomalies and stillbirth, which are recognized complications of diabetes (Edge & Laros, 1993).

Many mature women carefully plan their pregnancies; some are pregnant with the assistance of reproductive technology. They may worry about not having a "perfect, normal" baby or fear losing a child with little time to conceive another (Kitzinger, 1995). Adding the complex role of parenting may not be as easy as expected, especially for well-educated clients who are successful in other areas of life. Interventions that anticipate such feelings and provide guidance and support are needed.

Not all older clients are happy to be pregnant. Indeed, some may have thought they were "going through menopause." The client and her partner may react with disbelief, as the thought of childbearing at this stage in life may be shocking. These couples need nonjudgmental support as they consider reproductive options and ways of integrating childbearing and childrearing into their lives.

Health care providers need to be able to refer mature clients to appropriate learning resources. Books, videotapes, and reprints of articles in the popular press help meet learning needs. Childbirth education programs, specifically for the older woman, allow for interaction among mature clients in small group settings and foster the development of peer support networks.

Critical Thinking in Care Planning

Care of the Pregnant Adolescent

Melinda, age 15, arrives at the clinic with amenorrhea of 3 months. Her boyfriend, age 16, is with her. When talking with the nurse both refuse to make eye contact and instead look at the floor. They occasionally hold hands and glance at each other briefly. Melinda bites on her fingernails and plays with her long hair.

When questioned, Melinda states that she and her boyfriend have been sexually active for 6 months about twice a week. Withdrawal has been the only form of birth control used. She denies any alcohol, tobacco, or drug use, and reports that she has been trying to diet for the last 2 months. She states that she is afraid that she is pregnant and begins to cry. She has not told her parents about her fears. A physical examination shows changes consistent with a 12-week pregnancy, and her pregnancy test is positive.

► Assessment

- Age 15 years; 5'8", 125 lbs.
- Amenorrhea 3 months
- Positive pregnancy test
- Increased uterine size
- Unplanned pregnancy
- Client states that she would like to keep pregnancy
- Client slumps when she walks, and wears baggy clothes

- Client states that she does not want a "big belly," that she feels ugly, and that she is trying to diet
- Client states that she has been dieting so that the pregnancy would not show; she has lost 3 pounds in the last month
- Client cries when talking about telling her parents that she is pregnant and states that she is afraid to tell her parents
- Client states that she knows very little about pregnancy and childbirth

Nursing Diagnosis

Body image disturbance, related to physical changes of advancing pregnancy.

Expected Client/Family Outcomes	Nursing Action/Intervention	Evaluation
Client will demonstrate acceptance of her changing body image as evidenced by: • Speaking positively about her changing body. • Gaining adequate weight each month.	Encourage client to attend teen pregnancy support groups so that she can share her feelings. *Rationale:* Adolescents believe in the imaginary audience. If they feel unattractive, they are certain that everyone agrees with their assessment. Peer support is very important to adolescents. Teen pregnancy groups can discuss problems and feelings regarding pregnancy.	Client no longer tries to hide her pregnancy. Client talks positively about her pregnant body. Client attends teen pregnancy support group. Client gains appropriate weight each month.

(continued)

Critical Thinking in Care Planning *continued*

Nursing Diagnosis

Altered nutrition, less than body requirements.

Expected Client/Family Outcomes	Nursing Action/Intervention	Evaluation
Client will consume an adequate amount of essential nutrients and calories as evidenced by: • Weight gain of approximately 25–35 pounds. • No acetone in the urine. • Food diary reflecting appropriate intake.	Assess pattern of weight changes at each visit. Check urine at each visit. Take a diet history at the first prenatal visit, and encourage client to keep a food diary. Explain why client needs various nutrients, stressing their importance to her health as well as to fetal growth. Help client and her mother plan meals that are nutritious and acceptable. *Rationale:* Adolescents have specific food likes and dislikes and eat trendy foods. Many of their favorite foods, such as pizza and hamburgers, do contain essential nutrients, and can be supplemented to ensure sufficient intake of the needed nutrients.	Client gains weight appropriately and does not have acetone in the urine. Client's food diary reflects adequate prenatal nutrition.
Reports of taking multivitamin supplements each day, as prescribed.	Confirm that client has vitamin/mineral supplement. Teach client how to take her vitamin/mineral supplements. *Rationale:* Vitamin/mineral supplements help meet nutritional needs during pregnancy.	Client reports that she is taking her multivitamin supplements daily.

Nursing Diagnosis

Altered family processes, related to premature pregnancy.

Client's parents will demonstrate acceptance of the pregnancy as evidenced by: • Supporting client's decision to have the baby. • Allowing client to remain at home during her pregnancy. • Providing emotional support. • Attending prenatal visits.	Support client's decision to tell her parents about the pregnancy. Allow client to role-play possible parental responses. *Rationale:* Parents of pregnant adolescents frequently react with anger and express disappointment that the pregnancy occurred. Pregnancy is a crisis situation, regardless of a woman's age, and requires physical and emotional support. Role playing allows the client the opportunity to rehearse possible responses to her parents' reactions. Counsel parents about expected changes of pregnancy and the danger signals. Encourage family counseling if parents are unable to accept the pregnancy. If available, refer to a teen/grandparent program. *Rationale:* Counseling can foster communication among family members and help resolve problems.	Client continues to live at home. Client's parent comes to prenatal visits with her, offering support. Client's parents help her make plans for the infant to be included in the family.

Critical Thinking in Care Planning continued

Nursing Diagnosis

Knowledge deficit, related to physical and psychosocial changes of pregnancy and fetal growth development.

Expected Client/Family Outcomes	Nursing Action/Intervention	Evaluation
Client will demonstrate knowledge of pregnancy as evidenced by: • Making and keeping prenatal appointments. • Following the plan of care developed with the health care team. • Reporting any danger signals to the health care team promptly. • Stating in her own words changes of pregnancy and fetal growth and development. • Attending teen prenatal education program.	Determine client's present knowledge about pregnancy and childbirth; build on this knowledge base in terms that client can understand, at each visit, by providing information about the physical, social, and psychologic changes of pregnancy, and fetal growth and development. *Rationale:* Adolescents are self-centered and "now" oriented, and health teaching should focus on the adolescent and her current expectations. Explaining why changes are occurring and what to expect next enhances the acceptance of these changes. Answer client's questions. Discuss danger signals and appropriate responses. *Rationale:* Talking about growth and development of the fetus makes the pregnancy more real, and encourages prenatal attachment. Explain why vital signs, urine, and weight gain are monitored. *Rationale:* Explaining why procedures are carried out will help client understand the importance of prenatal visits. Encourage client to participate in prenatal and childbirth classes, especially one designed for adolescents, if available. *Rationale:* Attending classes with peers provides client with peer support and gives her the chance to share her fears and concerns with others her age who are also pregnant.	Client makes and keeps clinic appointments. Client follows the plan of care developed with the health team. Client reports any warning signs that occur. Client describes in her own words expected changes of pregnancy and fetal growth and development. Client attends prenatal and childbirth classes regularly.

Nursing Diagnosis

Alteration in adolescent development, related to premature pregnancy.

Client will demonstrate acceptance of the pregnancy as evidenced by: • Making an informed decision about the continuation of the pregnancy. • Seeking and participating in comprehensive antepartum care.	Provide factual information about alternatives available. *Rationale:* Adolescents seldom have factual information about options like adoption. They have heard "scare stories," but have no realistic expectations of alternatives. Refer client to appropriate agencies for support of her decision. *Rationale:* Pregnant adolescents need to be referred to a social worker for help with social, financial, and educational concerns, if they elect to continue the pregnancy.	Client makes an informed decision about continuation of her pregnancy based on her future goals and aspirations. Client is able to discuss options available to her, and to consider the pros and cons of each. Client reports that she has initiated contact with appropriate referral agencies.

Chapter Highlights

▶ Over the years, social and cultural values have changed. Women under 20 and over 35 routinely bear children.

▶ Pregnancy can be complicated by age extremes.

▶ Socioeconomic and cultural factors, family and peer support, and early and comprehensive health care affect an adolescent's well-being.

▶ Adolescent pregnancies usually do not result from careful planning.

▶ The nurse can influence the course of the adolescent's pregnancy by providing education, support, and a guide to resources.

▶ Delayed childbearing has advantages and disadvantages. Advantages include maturity, financial stability, planning for the child, and the opportunity to have established a career. Disadvantages relate to stresses of childrearing at an older age, lack of assistance from aging parents, and preexisting health problems that evolve with the aging process.

▶ Plans of care must be designed to meet the specialized needs of both pregnant adolescents and mature pregnant clients.

After reading the vignette at the beginning of this chapter, use what you have learned to answer these questions:

1. In conducting an assessment of Jeanne Goodwin, what data would help Ann Salzman, CNM, MSN, respond to the client's concerns about the effect of the baby's arrival on the family situation?

2. What types of nursing interventions would promote the integration of the child into the family?

3. In terms of coping with the stressors involved in blending children from previous and current relationships into one family, what are the advantages and disadvantages of being "older" or "mature" parents in this situation?

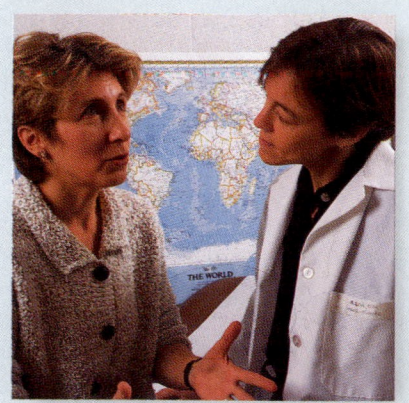

Critical Thinking Questions

▶ References

Adashek, J.A., Peaceman, A.M., Lopez-Zeno, J.A., Minogue, J.P., & Socol, M.L. (1993). Factors contributing to the increased cesarean birth rate in older parturient women. *American Journal of Obstetrics and Gynecology, 169,* 936–940.

Bloom, K.C. (1995). The development of attachment behaviors in pregnant adolescents. *Nursing Research, 44,* 284–289.

Bragg, E.J. (1997). Pregnant adolescents with addictions. *Journal of Obstetric, Gynecologic, and Neonatal Nursing, 26*(5), 577–584.

Brooks-Gunn, J., & Paikoff, R.L. (1993). Sex is a gamble, kissing is a game: Adolescent sexuality and health promotion. In S.G. Millstein, A.C. Petersen, & E.O. Nightingale (Eds.), *Promoting the health of adolescents: New directions for the twenty-first century* (pp. 180–208). New York: Oxford University Press.

Check, J.H., Nowroozi, K., Barnea, E.R., Shaw, K.J., & Sauer, M.V. (1993). Successful delivery after age 50: A report of two cases as a result of oocyte donation. *Obstetrics and Gynecology, 81,* 835–836.

Council on Scientific Affairs, American Medical Association. (1993). Adolescents as victims of family violence. *Journal of the American Medical Association, 270,* 1850–1856.

Crockett, I.J., & Petersen, A.C. (1993). Adolescent development: Health risks and opportunities for health promotion. In S.G. Millstein, A.C. Petersen, & E.O. Nightingale (Eds.), *Promoting the health of adolescents: New directions for the twenty-first century* (pp. 13–17). New York: Oxford University Press.

Cunningham, F.G., MacDonald, P.C., Gant, N.F., Leveno, K.J., Gilstrap, L.C., Hankins, G.D.V., & Clark, S.L. (1997). *Williams obstetrics* (20th ed.). Stamford, CT: Appleton & Lange.

Diehl, K. (1997). Adolescent mothers: What produces positive mother–infant interaction. *MCN, American Journal of Maternal Child Nursing, 22*(2), 89–95.

Drake, P. (1996). Addressing developmental needs of pregnant adolescents. *Journal of Obstetric, Gynecologic, and Neonatal Nursing, 25*(6), 518–524.

Edge, V., & Laros, R.K., Jr. (1993). Pregnancy outcome in nulliparous women aged 35 or older. *American Journal of Obstetrics and Gynecology, 168,* 1881–1885.

Esparza, D.V., & Esperat, M.C.R. (1996). The effects of childhood sexual abuse on minority adolescent mothers. *Journal of Obstetric, Gynecologic, and Neonatal Nursing, 25*(4), 321–330.

Fleming, B.W., Munton, M.T., Clarke, B.A., & Strauss, S.S. (1993). Assessing and promoting positive parenting in adolescent mothers. *MCN, American Journal of Maternal Child Nursing, 18,* 32–37.

Ganong, W.F. (1994). Physiology of reproduction. In A.H. DeCherney & M.L. Pernoll (Eds.), *Current obstetric and gynecologic diagnosis and treatment* (8th ed.) (pp. 124–145). Norwalk, CT: Appleton & Lange.

Grimes, D.A. (Ed.). (1993). Contraceptive services in school-based clinics: The Baltimore experience. *The Contraception Report, 4,* 4–6.

Grimes, D.A. (Ed.). (1995a). Contraception and adolescents: Highlights from the NASPAG Conference. *The Contraception Report: Contraception and Adolescents, VI*(3), 4–7, 10–11, 14.

Grimes, D.A. (Ed.). (1995b). Trends in sexual behavior among high school students in the United States: The Youth Risk Behavior Survey. *The Contraception Report: Contraception and Adolescents, VI*(3), 12–14.

Hogan, I.G. (1993). Teenagers' perceptions of barriers to prenatal care. *Southern Medical Journal, 86,* 737–741.

Kahn, J.R., & Anderson, K.E. (1992). Intergenerational patterns of teenage fertility. *Demography, 29,* 39.

Kirby, D., Resnick, M.D., Downes, B., Kocher, T., Gunderson, P., Potthoff, S., Zelterman, D., & Blum, R.W. (1993). The effects of school-based health clinics in St. Paul on school-wide birthrates. *Family Planning Perspectives, 25,* 12–16.

Kitzinger, S. (1995). *Birth over thirty-five.* In P. Simkin (Ed.) New York: Penguin Books.

Langer, O., & Langer, N. (1993). Diabetes in women older than 40 years of age: Social and medical aspects. *Obstetrics and Gynecology Clinics of North America, 20,* 299–311.

March of Dimes Birth Defects Foundation. (1997). StatBook: Statistics for monitoring maternal and infant health. Washington, DC: Author.

Marsiglio, W. (1993). Adolescent males' orientation toward paternity and contraception. *Family Planning Perspectives, 25,* 22–31.

Mills, C.B. (1997). Taking time to care: Making ways to help teen parents. *AWHONN Lifelines, 1*(5), 72.

Millstein, S.G. (1993). A view of health from the adolescent's perspective. In S.G. Millstein, A.C. Petersen, & E.O. Nightingale (Eds.), *Promoting the health of adolescents: New directions for the twenty-first century* (pp. 97–118). New York: Oxford University Press.

O'Reilly-Green, C., & Cohen, W.R. (1993). Pregnancy in women aged 40 and older. *Obstetrics and Gynecology Clinics of North America, 20,* 313–331.

Parker, B., McFarlane, J., Soeken, K., Torres, S., & Campbell, D. (1993). Physical and emotional abuse in pregnancy: A comparison of adult and teenage women. *Nursing Research, 42,* 173–178.

Perry, C.L. et al. (1993). The social world of adolescents. Family, peers, schools and the community. In S.G. Millstein, A.C. Petersen, & E.O. Nightingale (Eds.), *Promoting the health of adolescents: New directions for the twenty-first century* (pp. 73–96). New York: Oxford University Press.

Podgurski, M.J. (1993). School-based adolescent pregnancy classes. *Clinical Issues in Perinatal and Women's Health Nursing, 4,* 80–91.

Reynoso, T.C., Felice, M.E., & Shragg, G.P. (1993). Does American acculturation affect outcome of Mexican-American teenage pregnancy? *Journal of Adolescent Health, 14*(4), 257–261.

Roye, C.F., & Balk, S.J. (1997). Caring for pregnant teens and their mothers, too. *MCN, American Journal of Maternal Child Nursing 22*(3), 153–157.

Seplow, S., & Storm, J. (1997). How TV redefined our lives. *The Philadelphia Inquirer,* A1, A16–A17.

Stark, M.A. (1997). Psychosocial adjustment during pregnancy: The experience of mature gravidas. *Journal of Obstetric, Gynecologic, and Neonatal Nursing, 26,* 206–211.

Thompson, P.J., Powell, M.J., Patterson, R.J., & Ellerbee, S.M. (1995). Adolescent parenting: Outcomes and maternal perceptions. *Journal of Obstetric, Gynecologic, and Neonatal Nursing, 24*(8), 713–718.

U.S. Centers for Disease Control and Prevention. (1993). Teenage pregnancy and birth rates—United States, 1990. *Morbidity and Mortality Weekly Report, 42,* 733–737.

U.S. Centers for Disease Control and Prevention. (1995). Adolescent health: State of the nation—Pregnancy, sexually transmitted diseases and related risk behaviors among U.S. adolescents (DHHS Publication No. (CDC) 099-4630). Atlanta: U.S. Department of Health and Human Services, Public Health Service.

U.S. Department of Health and Human Services, Public Health Service. (1991). *Healthy people 2000: National health promotion and disease prevention objectives, full report with commentary* (DHHS Publication No. (PHS) 91-50212). Washington, DC: U.S. Government Printing Office.

U.S. Department of Health and Human Services. (1997). *Vital statis-*

tics report shows significant gain in health [On-line]. Available: http://www.dhhs.gov/

Warrick, L., Christianson, J.B., Walruff, J., & Cook, P.C. (1993). Educational outcomes in teenage pregnancy and parenting programs: Results from a demonstration. *Family Planning Perspectives, 25,* 148–155.

Williams, M.A., & Mittendorf, R. (1993). Increasing maternal age as a determinant of placentia previa. More important than increasing parity? *Journal of Reproductive Medicine, 38,* 425–428.

Winklestein, M.L. (1995). Teaching pregnant adolescents to cope with environmental smoke. *MCN, American Journal of Maternal Child Nursing 20*(1), 38–42.

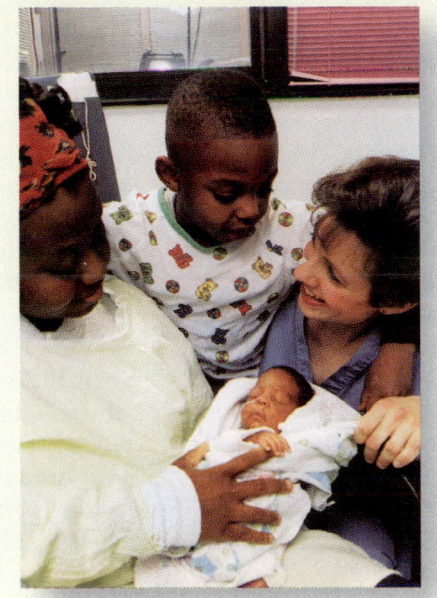

Grant Reed, born at 33 weeks of gestation, is admitted to the neonatal intensive care unit (NICU) in a regional medical center. Due to his premature status and need for aggressive nutritional management, Grant is placed on tube feedings. For the first three days, Grant's parents, Audra and William Reed, visit the NICU to be with their son and to participate in his care.

On the fourth day of Grant's stay in the NICU, Audra arrives at the medical center with her older son Jesse, age 5. Elizabeth Thompson, RN, greets them at the door of the NICU. Audra introduces Jesse to the nurse and states, "I've explained to Jesse what he will see and hear when he's in the NICU and he seems ready to visit with his new brother. I'm worried, though, that Jesse may be frightened when he sees Grant's feeding tube. Do you have any suggestions about how I can help Jesse handle this situation?" ■

12

Psychosocial Concerns of the High-Risk Childbearing Family

High-risk childbearing families are those whose physical, emotional, or social situations threaten their health, well-being, and development during the childbearing year. Every high-risk condition has broad and complex psychologic implications. Meeting the psychosocial needs of high-risk childbearing families requires strategies evolving from an understanding of crisis, grief, and mourning. Although high-risk conditions can have far-reaching negative psychologic effects on the childbearing family, they can also have positive, growth-producing outcomes. A unified, consistent, and interdisciplinary approach among multiple health care providers promotes adaptation to childbearing and parenthood for high-risk clients. By providing education, culturally sensitive support, and appropriate referrals, nurses can help clients and their families understand and cope with high-risk conditions.

Every nurse working with childbearing families will encounter clients who become high risk, even in such wellness settings as birth centers. Nurses therefore need to be prepared to deal with high-risk situations, if only on a temporary basis prior to a client's transfer.

This chapter discusses the concept of high risk and the psychosocial concerns experienced by families during high-risk pregnancy and the intrapartum period. It also explores the role of the nurse in caring for families of a high-risk newborn and nursing strategies to help families cope with perinatal death.

▶ THE CONCEPT OF HIGH RISK

High-risk clients are those whose physical, emotional, or social situations present some threat to their health, well-being, or development. In its broadest sense, the concept of high risk extends throughout the childbearing year from preconception through the postpartum and neonatal period. Some high-risk conditions, such as diabetes, chronic substance abuse, or a turbulent marriage, may have existed before conception. Others, such as the onset of premature labor, stillbirth, or the birth of an infant needing neonatal intensive care, may occur suddenly or without known cause. Many such high-risk conditions as cesarean delivery and the birth of a very premature infant have implications that extend beyond the childbearing year. Clients may be high risk for one or more reasons.

▶ The High-Risk Client and High-Risk Family

Any high-risk condition affects the entire family. In every high-risk situation, the ability of individuals to function appropriately within the context of their family or everyday activities is threatened in some way. Childbearing and early parenthood involve stress and role transition in the best of circumstances; however, high-risk parenting adds pressure and requires different, complex role changes. In addition, such situations as the loss of an infant or the need for neonatal special care affect both parents and family members simultaneously. The support system available to each partner can be jeopardized, as both parents and family members are grieving. Any high-risk situation should therefore immediately classify the family, and not simply the client, as high risk. Parents need information about their baby's condition, treatment, and prognosis when the need for special care is identified and the baby is admitted to the neonatal intensive care unit (NICU) (Heuer, 1993).

Through contact with clients in prenatal, intrapartum, postpartum, and neonatal settings, nurses are able to aid in high-risk identification, assessment, interventions, and follow-up. Working with high-risk clients requires the ability to blend scientific and technologic expertise with compassion and skill in interpersonal relationships. Nurses need to be aware of how the client's cultural background may affect adaptation to high-risk status or behaviors in crisis and grief. For example, a client may be greatly distressed but may not openly cry because of cultural emphases on self-discipline and control. Clients from certain Asian cultures may not initiate questions for fear of insulting the health care provider. In addition, nurses are challenged to help clients develop confidence in their own abilities to cope and to assist the high-risk family to develop joy and skill in beginning parenthood. Implementation of quality care also involves a collaborative approach that includes other health care professionals, such as physicians, social workers, and pastoral care representatives.

▶ THEORETICAL BASES OF HIGH-RISK CARE

▶ Crisis

Crisis theory presents a general model that readily applies to clients across the life span and in just about every type of clinical setting. Crisis is a state of upset or disequilibrium in which a person struggles with a situation that he or she perceives to be temporarily beyond personal ability to comprehend or to control (Caplan, 1982). A crisis forces a person to readapt his or her view of self, of the environment, or both. A shift between realistic and unrealistic expectations produces stress and anxiety that can become severe enough to prevent functioning in the usual manner. A sense of crisis can persist for days or weeks until the person is able to work out ways of dealing with the current predicament and of adapting to possible future life changes.

During the course of a lifetime, nearly everyone can expect to encounter several crises. Some may be developmental or maturational crises, that is, broad life changes that occur during growth and development, such as the transition to parenthood (see Chapter 4 for discussion of developmental crises). Others may be situational crises, that is, crises occurring in relation to particular and unexpected circumstances, such as having an infant admitted to a NICU. Situational crises may or may not occur along with developmental crises.

Not every new life event is accompanied by a crisis. The term *crisis* refers to a state or to an individual's *reaction* to a potentially threatening event and not to the specific event itself. Crisis is therefore a manifestation of a person's unique perception (see Chapter 4 for a discussion of the characteristics of an individual's or family's perception of a crisis that determine the degree to which crisis is experienced).

Crisis resolution, for situational as well as developmental crises, may move in a healthy direction, with the client and family learning new adaptive responses and actually evolving toward a higher level of functioning; however, a crisis that is poorly resolved or dealt with in a maladaptive manner can become prolonged or result in a lower level of functional ability for the client and family. The potential threats presented by a crisis are accompanied by opportunities for the client and her family to grow, develop new life patterns, and become better able to deal with future problems.

► Loss, Grief, and Mourning

Feelings of loss emerge when a person perceives that something of value has gone or been taken away. Grief comprises the emotional and physical responses to loss. Mourning is the process of grieving and working through grief. Grief-producing situations in parent–neonate nursing range from inability to have a vaginal delivery to dealing with a stillbirth or the birth of an infant with a severe congenital anomaly. As with feelings of crisis, the nature of grief depends on the individual's unique perception. Perception, in turn, evolves from many complex factors, for example, the client's cultural and religious background, presence of other family members, support (or lack of support) from significant others, previous life experi-

ences, and physical status. Both crisis and grief are accompanied by emotional upheaval; indeed, grief may follow crisis, especially situational crises. The box entitled Nursing Strategies for Childbearing Clients Experiencing Crisis and Grief summarizes interventions that nurses can use to help these clients.

Much has been written on the topic of loss and grief, especially with reference to death and dying and birth of an abnormal infant. Researchers and clinicians have identified a predictable emotional pattern of grieving responses among adults (Kubler-Ross, 1969; Lindemann, 1944). Variation in the number of stages or phases defining the grieving process exists among theorists; however, the emotional processes they describe are similar. In working with high-risk families, the nurse needs to understand crisis, grief, and mourning and to be prepared to deal with clients' psychologic and psychosomatic reactions. Seven facets of grief and mourning are described below.

Shock and Disbelief
During this stage the client reacts to the news of the high-risk condition, which is interpreted as a loss. The client may be stunned and unable to concentrate or to make decisions, but may appear outwardly calm. Health care providers may mistakenly interpret this reaction as the client's handling the situation without difficulty. Somatic symptoms, such as light-headedness, sweating, palpitations, and gastrointestinal discomforts, may accompany shock and disbelief. Clients may also try to avoid or to deny the high-risk condition and its impact. "It can't be true" and "This can't be happening to me" are common statements.

Anger
Many clients express anger, which may be directed against staff, other family members, or themselves. In addition, they may express anger by blaming themselves or others (e.g., "Why me?"), quarreling or fighting with other family members, or finding fault with nursing and medical care.

Bargaining
When a high-risk condition exists that is perceived as a loss, clients may seek to bargain in the hope that if they do not behave in a certain way all will be well. For example, they may promise to attend religious services, be a "better" person, or donate to charities. Through bargaining, clients try to attain some control over a difficult situation.

► NURSING STRATEGIES FOR CHILDBEARING CLIENTS EXPERIENCING CRISIS AND GRIEF

Anticipate the potential for crisis and grief. For example, clients who receive news of a high-risk condition, particularly a condition requiring a change in lifestyle or having long-term implications, may be expected to experience crisis.

Assess the event itself and its implications for the client's health and well-being.

Assess the client's and family's responses in light of their religious and cultural backgrounds.

Provide an atmosphere of privacy and confidentiality to encourage the client to express feelings.

Allow adequate time to discuss the high-risk condition and the family's feelings. Listen carefully, but do not make unrealistic promises, such as "Everything will turn out fine." Having another nurse temporarily "cover" other clients can allow the staff nurse the uninterrupted opportunity to talk with a client in crisis.

Help clients identify physical, emotional, and behavioral responses related to crisis and grief. Reassure clients when responses are normal. Promptly enlist the assistance of mental health and security resources if clients'

responses pose a threat to the health or safety of themselves or others.

Ensure that the client receives support in coping with crisis and grief. Assist the client in identifying sources of support within her own network of family and friends. Offer to speak with significant others if the client so desires. Provide the client with referrals, for example, for appropriate support groups, for telephone "hot line" assistance, for relevant counseling, or for appropriate financial aid services. Make certain that a plan for follow-up of the client experiencing crisis and grief is implemented—for example, telephone contact at regular intervals or home visits if appropriate.

Communicate with other health care providers directly involved in the family's care so that a consistent and supportive approach may be implemented.

Provide a mechanism to deal with tension on the part of health care providers, such as interdisciplinary staff conferences, so that staff members can discuss their own feelings related to working with clients in crisis and grief.

Developing Awareness of the Loss and Acute Mourning

When a person becomes acutely aware of a loss, feelings of helplessness, hopelessness, depression, and guilt may emerge. The individual may be unable to sleep, yet feel exhausted; somatic symptoms such as shortness of breath, lack of muscular power, and intense subjective distress may be experienced; these feelings may recur in waves. From her study of mothers who lost a child through death, Wong (1980) observed that the phase of developing awareness evolves into a period of yearning and pining for the dead child. During this time mothers often become irritable as they evaluate the relationship they had with the child. They also experience feelings of anger, guilt, and bitterness at everyone, including themselves.

Guilt

"Why didn't I take better care of myself during my pregnancy?" "Why did I continue to clean house by myself?" "Why didn't I come to see my baby more often in the special care nursery?" "Why wasn't I kinder to my wife when she was pregnant?" These are examples of feelings that may be experienced, although not verbalized, by clients. In cultures that view death or illness as punishment for sin, guilt

becomes an especially difficult burden. Many high-risk conditions, such as the development of preeclampsia, are beyond parental control; however, others, such as substance abuse, do harm the fetus and compromise the health of the newborn. A major challenge is to assist clients in acknowledging that being at risk or having an infant at risk does not mean they are "bad" or "undeserving" of good health or health care. Clients need to understand conditions over which they had no control and to receive anticipatory counseling about guilt feelings. Staff may become angry with clients whose behaviors, such as drug abuse or sexual promiscuity, injured the fetus or newborn; however, little is gained by moralistic scolding. Health care providers need to focus first on their own feelings of working with these parents so they can develop therapeutic plans of care that focus on current and future goals. Feelings of guilt make clients vulnerable to comments of staff and family members. Dealing directly with the potential for guilt is a goal that is helped by collaboration among nurses, physicians, social workers, and chaplains involved in client care.

Estrangement

In a study of grieving families, Wong (1980) noted that communication between husband and wife

Nursing Alert

The following behaviors may be indications of severe depression in a woman who has experienced either a high-risk condition, birth of an abnormal infant, or death of an infant and should be noted so that appropriate actions can be taken:

- Increase or decrease in weight (more than 15% of total body weight)
- Inability to perform daily living activities such as self-care practices and care of older siblings
- Thoughts about suicide with or without a plan to take action on these thoughts
- Acute desire for solitude

tended to lessen after the death of a child, because each partner tried to avoid hurting the other with talk of their loss. This fear of upsetting each other extended to relationships with other children. A "detachment" process seemed to occur within the family and could be manifested either by emotional distancing or by absence from the home.

Acceptance of the Loss

During this phase the person begins to be less preoccupied with memories of the loss and is able to think more realistically about the event (Lindemann, 1944). The client is able to resume normal activities and develop new interests. Time, thought, and sufficient mourning need to take place before the client can arrive at this stage. Health care providers should not confuse the calm outward appearance the client may display in reaction to a recent loss with acceptance of the loss.

▶ PREPREGNANCY CONCERNS OF THE POTENTIALLY HIGH-RISK COUPLE

Certain physical conditions place a couple at risk for poor pregnancy outcome or threaten maternal well-being. These conditions can be as varied as heart disease, diabetes, collagen diseases, and habitual spontaneous abortions. For the couple, the desire to have a

child is accompanied by fears about what pregnancy would entail, whether the health of the mother would be jeopardized, and whether the birth of a healthy infant would be possible. Previous high-risk obstetric history, neonatal intensive care experience, or loss of a pregnancy or infant can also have strong emotional impact on the couple.

Nurses have important roles in education and support of couples contemplating a high-risk pregnancy. Nurses can help in identifying the risks pregnancy poses to mother and fetus. Nurses can discuss the nature of the high-risk care that will be required and help clients in identifying life pattern changes that will evolve with the high-risk pregnancy. Nurses can help correct misconceptions, provide emotional support, and also serve as sources of referral for couples in need of in-depth counseling.

For certain clients, such as those with severe heart disease or those who are infected with the human immunodeficiency virus (HIV), pregnancy at any time is not advised. Clients need to be given that information and emotional support thereafter.

Ultimately, the decision to become pregnant or not to become pregnant is made by the client or the couple. The nurse has important roles in providing information that will help clients make their own decisions about pregnancy and in making certain that clients' fears and concerns are adequately addressed.

A normal human reaction is to want to reassure couples that high-risk technology and staff can help them have a healthy infant. Health care expertise can assist many couples, yet some high-risk clients will not be able to have a pregnancy or the birth of a healthy child. Health care providers therefore need to use a hopeful, yet realistic approach when counseling the high-risk client and family.

Successful outcome of a high-risk pregnancy often depends on a close working relationship among the client, nurses, and other health care professionals. A haphazard or uncoordinated approach on the part of various health care professionals can add to the client's stress and prevent the establishment of a trusting relationship. Nurses therefore need to collaborate with other members of the interdisciplinary team in developing an organized approach to the high-risk client.

▶ PSYCHOSOCIAL CONCERNS DURING HIGH-RISK PREGNANCY

Nearly every high-risk situation has the potential to become an emotionally unhealthy situation or a situation in which a family develops new and effective ways of coping. Concepts of crisis, grief, and mourning must be tailored to specific client situations. The nurse needs to realize that high-risk conditions are accompanied to some degree by special emotional needs on the part of clients and families. The nurse must be prepared to anticipate problems, undertake interim crisis intervention, collaborate with other health care professionals, and make appropriate referrals.

▶ Maternal Tasks During High-Risk Pregnancy

An individual evolves through different developmental stages during the life process. Successful achievement of expected life tasks at various stages leads to further emotional maturation and ability to deal successfully with future tasks. Developmental theory applies well to pregnancy, because a woman normally faces certain stages or tasks during transition to the motherhood role. These maternal tasks, according to Rubin (1984), are safe passage for the woman herself and her fetus, acceptance by others, binding-in to the child, and giving of oneself.

More research is needed to document comparative similarities and differences between high-risk and low-risk pregnant clients in their ability to meet developmental tasks of pregnancy. In a high-risk pregnancy, a mother's uncertainty over her health and that of the fetus and anxiety related to pregnancy outcome can hamper her ability to feel she has mastered the task of safe passage. Feelings of guilt or rejection over the high-risk condition can prevent a woman from feeling accepted by significant others. Abused women, already feeling rejected and fearing for their safety, are at great risk.

Maternal–fetal attachment is a task accomplished by both high-risk and low-risk women. However, the high-risk mother, who may fear the loss of the fetus or newborn or who is very ill, may avoid the task of binding-in to the fetus. A woman may also become "desperate" to produce a child and anxiously wait for any indication of fetal life. The high-risk mother must often make greater changes in lifestyle than the healthy pregnant woman; especially when bedrest or hospitalization is required. The high-risk mother who has a normal infant and returns to good health may take pride in her "sacrifices"; the mother who suffers a perinatal loss may feel that her efforts have produced nothing but sorrow.

The great variation among etiology, course, and outcomes that constitute maternal–fetal risk makes identification of a model for developmental tasks during high-risk pregnancy difficult. The ability of the high-risk client to meet tasks of pregnancy depends on the reason for high-risk status and the quality of support she receives to help her meet the tasks of pregnancy. Nursing interventions regarding maternal tasks during high-risk pregnancy evolve from assessment of unique high-risk client needs in relation to normal developmental tasks of pregnancy. This topic continues to warrant further research.

▶ Threats to Self-Image

High-risk pregnancy poses several threats to a client's self-image. Three of these sources are the client herself, the client's significant others, and health care providers.

Pregnancy is a womanly process. Many cultures, including traditional U.S. society, define success of a marriage in terms of ability to produce healthy offspring. In being considered high-risk, a woman may feel that she is in some way lacking in a basic feminine ability to reproduce. Her concept of herself and her own worth may be compromised, especially if she comes from a background that places high value on reproduction.

High-risk pregnancy often means that the client must look to others for advice and assistance, which may foster an uncomfortable sense of dependency. When hospitalization is required, the client is removed from the home environment. Away from her everyday roles in familiar surroundings, she may experience additional changes in self-image. As one client stated, "Suddenly I felt as if I had lost control of my body and could no longer do anything right. I was going to fail at the one thing all grown up women are supposed to be able to do."

Pregnancy is a time of emotional vulnerability, even for a low-risk client. The importance of social support, especially support from the infant's father, on a woman's transition to parenthood is well known. The high-risk client has potentially greater needs for approval and support because of the problem or problems that may jeopardize her well-being. When hospitalization is necessary, strategies that promote self-confidence and feelings of being loved and valued assume additional importance. For example, the nurse can reinforce the positive aspects of the client's participation in her own care during hospitalization.

At times, a turbulent family background can be the source of risk as well as a major threat to self-image. When high-risk social situations are identified, providing immediate emotional support and referral to social service or mental health specialists can help clients through difficult psychosocial situations.

Women's Health

A high-risk pregnant woman may be blamed for her condition by significant others. In some cases, anger and blame may contribute to verbal or physical abuse of the high-risk pregnant woman.

As previously noted, anger and blame can be direct or indirect manifestations of crisis and grief. Frequently, these emotions are expressed within the high-risk family, regardless of the reasons for high-risk status.

Nurses and other health care providers can have a major effect on client self-image and willingness to continue with care. At times a client's lifestyle is responsible for a high-risk condition. Examples include substance abuse and sexually transmitted diseases. The client may face threats to self-image because of disapproval from health care professionals. Strategies such as staff meetings, focusing on such topics as reactions to working with clients with high-risk behaviors and use of clinical consultants, can be helpful in dealing with the high-risk situation and in promoting client self-image. Prejudicial remarks directed toward clients because of their high-risk status are always to be considered inappropriate and unprofessional.

Health care providers direct much effort toward promoting, maintaining, and restoring the health of the physically ill client and fetus. The "high tech" approach can have a negative effect on a client's self-image, if the emotional aspects of high-risk care are not considered.

▶ Psychologic Impact of Prenatal Diagnosis

Clients at risk for fetal abnormalities that can be identified through diagnostic techniques, such as chorionic villus sampling or amniocentesis, may refuse to accept the pregnancy until normal test results are known. Clients who might consider abortion of an abnormal fetus and clients who fear the possibility of raising an abnormal child may experience anxiety and guilt.

The opportunity to prepare emotionally for the birth of an abnormal infant may also be accompanied by acute crisis and by a long period of prenatal distress. This could be problematic in situations in which the extent of the abnormality is uncertain. The box entitled Nursing Strategies for Families Preparing for the Birth of an Abnormal Infant summarizes nursing actions to help clients cope with this situation.

▶ Implications of High-Risk Pregnancy

For many previously healthy women, high-risk status is a condition that occurs only with pregnancy. For example, women who become severely preeclamptic might have enjoyed active healthy lives prior to their pregnancies. High-risk status has many implications

▶ NURSING STRATEGIES FOR FAMILIES PREPARING FOR THE BIRTH OF AN ABNORMAL INFANT

Accept the family's decision to have an abnormal child; avoid imposing one's personal values or opinions.

Identify the potential for crisis related to birth of an abnormal infant, even in the best of circumstances.

Make certain that a consistent collaborative approach is used among all health care providers. When possible, minimize the number of different health care providers who work with the client, so that an emotionally supportive relationship can be established between the client and caregivers and the client is not continuously interacting with strangers.

Make certain that the client is well educated about the potential status of the infant.

Assist clients in identifying ways in which they will inform others about the infant.

Help clients identify ways they will cope with the infant.

Provide referrals to counseling and to support groups, such as parents of children with Down syndrome.

Make certain that preparations are made prenatally, if the infant's condition requires specialized equipment and services.

Discuss realistically the positive aspects of the expected infant.

Assist the parents to have the best delivery and early parenting experience possible.

for childbearing. Maternal or fetal outcome may be uncertain. More frequent and intensive assessment is needed during pregnancy. Extended hospitalization is possible. In addition, clients may have to give up the chance to select birth options. (Although secondary to physical well-being, this can compound feelings of loss and disappointment during childbearing.) In some cases, clients and their families must be transferred to high-risk hospital centers that are far from their homes. Hotel, meal, telephone, and transportation costs for family members may add to financial burdens; other children may greatly miss their mother's presence in the home. High-risk pregnancies can always be expected to test a family's resources and to require health care supportive interventions.

Psychologic reactions to a high-risk pregnancy are also affected by the level of the client's physical wellness. In certain high-risk conditions, such as severe preeclampsia, hyperemesis gravidarum, or HIV disease the client may be ill. In multiple gestation, the client may be uncomfortable at all times, especially as pregnancy progresses. Feelings of anguish and anxiety can further compromise physical well-being. Nurses need to plan care that integrates assessment of physical well-being with strategies for emotional support.

▶ Pregnancy After Previous Pregnancy Loss or Death of a Child

Even when physically normal during a subsequent pregnancy, clients who have lost a pregnancy or a child must be considered at risk for increased anxiety and for potential alterations in prenatal attachment. Indeed, during a subsequent pregnancy, couples may simultaneously grieve their prior loss and yet attempt to create bonds of attachment to the developing fetus.

Maternity nurses frequently care for pregnant couples who have experienced prior loss of a pregnancy or a child. Nurses need to anticipate that parents might experience residual or rekindled feelings of grief and loss, no matter how healthy or desired the current pregnancy.

Offering pregnant clients opportunity and encouragement to verbalize feelings about previous loss should be part of any nursing care plan dealing with this subject; however, this topic is often difficult and uncomfortable for health care providers. They may focus on the current pregnancy and give the impression that it is somehow inappropriate to recall painful past experiences. Although the nurse may find it easier to say "but you are now having a healthy pregnancy" and "your bad experience is in the past,"

this approach carries little therapeutic value. As the first level of care planning, nurses need to evaluate their own feelings about this subject and to seek consultation with colleagues whenever necessary.

▶ Prenatal Hospitalization

Prenatal hospitalization is needed when a client is ill enough or potentially ill enough to warrant close and continuous professional attention that cannot be provided in the home setting. Conditions resulting in prenatal hospitalization include severe preeclampsia, uncontrolled diabetes, premature labor, various infections, and fetal surgery. Hospitalization may be for a few days or for several months. All clients hospitalized prenatally are considered to be at high risk.

Prenatal hospitalization plucks the client from a lifestyle routine and superimposes the specter of illness on the transition to parenthood. Several stressors are associated with hospitalization:

- Separation from family members; loneliness and concern over household maintenance. In a study of hospitalized pregnant women, Maloni and associates (1993) found separation from family to be the greatest hospital stressor, despite liberal visiting policies.
- Alteration in family patterns, resulting from need of other family members to maintain the household without the client present; potential for anger and blame directed toward the client by the client herself or family members.
- Worry about other children and the impact of separation from their mother; concern over child care, especially when family members cannot stay in the client's home and the spouse has to work.
- Realization that hospitalization means the client is at very high risk.
- Need to conform to a hospital routine.
- Need to undergo uncomfortable procedures, such as fetal monitoring or frequent blood studies.
- Difficulty resting, related to round-the-clock interruptions.
- Concern over health care bills that may not be completely covered by third-party reimbursement; lack of insurance to cover even basic costs; stress of bills related to hospitalization, such as telephone, television, and child care costs.
- Fear of loss of a job, school, or work opportunity related to premature and prolonged hospitalization.

▶ Problems Associated with Bedrest and with Hospitalization

Bedrest traditionally has been prescribed for women with complications of pregnancy. However, research has not documented great benefits of bedrest in improving pregnancy outcome. In addition, pregnant women on bedrest may experience such negative physiologic changes as muscle weakness and difficulty achieving appropriate weight gain, and psychosocial stress related to the degree of activity restriction (Maloni, 1993; Schroeder, 1998). Research indicates that pregnant women can experience bedrest-induced physiologic deconditioning that persists into the postpartum period and that may not be quickly resolved (Maloni, 1993; Schroeder, 1998). Symptoms of deconditioning include shortness of breath on exertion, muscle soreness, difficulty with mobility, and delayed resumption of activities of daily living.

Bedrest in pregnancy carries high economic, emotional, and physical costs. Loss of work or wages, need for help with household management or child care, and loss of opportunities due to leaving the workforce are among hardships that add to the client's stress and anxiety. However, not all women view bedrest or restricted activity negatively. Some may be glad for the chance to rest; others may feel that bedrest and restricted activity offer a way to raise their chances of having a successful pregnancy (Schroeder, 1998). Anticipatory guidance can help clients understand the experience of bedrest or restricted activity.

In prescribing activity levels, health care providers need to evaluate the client's unique situation and include her in such important decision making. As Schroeder (1998) notes, until clinical research can demonstrate bedrest's effectiveness, it should not be routinely prescribed for clients with such conditions as preterm labor or twin gestation.

Few hospitals have enough high-risk pregnant clients who need inpatient care to justify individual prenatal hospitalization units. Prenatal clients are therefore often hospitalized on postpartum units. Most units are still composed of semiprivate rooms. Private rooms are much more expensive and are covered by insurance only when "medically" justified. Unfortunately, promotion of mental health is usually not considered by insurance companies to be reason enough for a pregnant client to be assigned to a private room. Although attempts may be made by staff to keep prenatal clients together, prenatal clients frequently share rooms with postpartum mothers. Given that the routine low-risk postpartum hospital stay is 1 to 3 days, it is possible that a pregnant client may have more than 20 different roommates during her stay. Some prenatal clients may welcome the chance to room with someone who is well and who has had a healthy infant. Other clients, however, may feel additional stress and upset about their own inability to be healthy or to go home. The presence of an infant in the room and hospital restrictions on visitors when infants are with their mothers may add to these feelings. Nurses therefore need to discuss reactions with the hospitalized pregnant client and, when possible, to work with members of the admitting department to make room arrangements that promote mental health.

The hospitalized pregnant client requires special psychosocial nursing strategies that extend beyond physical care expertise (see box entitled Nursing Strategies for the Hospitalized High-Risk Pregnant Client). The client may include staff among her significant others and build strong working relationships with certain staff members due to her hospitalization during the emotionally vulnerable transition to parenthood. Staffing patterns that foster continuity of care by certain staff members can help to establish a sense of trust. Conversely, an ever-changing stream of unfamiliar faces can contribute to client stress and despair. In some obstetric units, nursing staff care for clients in labor and delivery and postpartum settings. Nurses who have cared for the prenatal client during her hospitalization may therefore work with her during her labor and delivery. As one client reported, "After 6 weeks in the hospital, I was frightened about how the baby would actually be. But I had so much faith in the nurses and doctors caring for me that I knew I wouldn't be abandoned. Whatever happened, I felt they would help me have courage."

▶ The High-Risk Client on Bedrest or Partial Bedrest at Home

Women may be prescribed bedrest or partial bedrest at home. Home care has many psychosocial advantages. For example, the client remains in her own home and does not have to be separated from her family, a very difficult situation when the client has other children. The client, rather than a hospital's staff, has control over schedules and visits from significant others. Financial costs are much lower.

Although the client may welcome the opportunity to be self-reliant, she may nevertheless be anxious about successful management of her condition away from the constant surveillance that hospitalization provides. This can be a problem, especially when bedrest is first begun and if the client lacks self-confidence. Clients may find that family members have difficulty accepting their activity restric-

► NURSING STRATEGIES FOR THE HOSPITALIZED HIGH-RISK PREGNANT CLIENT

Make certain the client and family are informed about her condition, treatment plan, and progress.

Provide time to talk with the client about herself, her fears, and her expectations. Identify ways in which hospitalization does and does not agree with the client's expectations for her pregnancy. Identify the client's and the family's reactions to hospitalization. Assist the client and family in designing ways in which the family can manage at home during the woman's hospitalization.

Reinforce the positive aspects of the client's participation in her own care through hospitalization.

Encourage the client to help in the design of her care schedule, whenever possible.

Encourage the client to wear her own clothes if she so desires, and to have mementos of home brought to the hospital, especially if hospitalization will be prolonged.

Adapt hospital routines whenever possible to allow for a more "normal" lifestyle, despite hospitalization.

Collaborate with members of the interdisciplinary team to provide special services for the client.

Promote emotional, as well as physical, comfort measures. Help clients cope with boredom. Encourage visits from hospital personnel, such as volunteers and the librarian, when appropriate. Have television connected; seek charitable sponsorship if clients cannot pay for television. When possible, participate in the roommate selection process; at times, hospitalized antenatal clients may receive much support from each other.

Identify the importance of spiritual needs during high-risk prenatal hospitalization. If the client desires, refer her to the hospital chaplain, encourage visits from members of the client's spiritual community, and make certain she can attend religious services in hospital if she is physically able. Make certain that religious dietary practices, such as a kosher diet, can be maintained.

Be flexible with regard to visiting hours and visitors, including client's other children, to allow her to be with significant others.

Make certain that the client and family are able to receive childbirth preparation within the hospital setting, for example, through hospital or individual teaching sessions and videotapes shown on a hospital video player.

Develop plan for ongoing emotional support after discharge with client.

---

tions and expect the woman to be able to carry on "as usual," because she is home. Some clients spend weeks or months in bed or on restricted activity as pregnancy progresses. Like hospitalized clients, they face potential physical, emotional, and economic problems. Boredom and lack of activities or companionship during working hours for family members makes pregnancy seem endless and the woman feel isolated (Fig. 12–1). The client on bedrest at home is usually deprived of the educational and social benefits of childbirth preparation classes. See box entitled Strategies for Care of the High-Risk Pregnant Woman at Home on Bedrest or Restricted Activity.

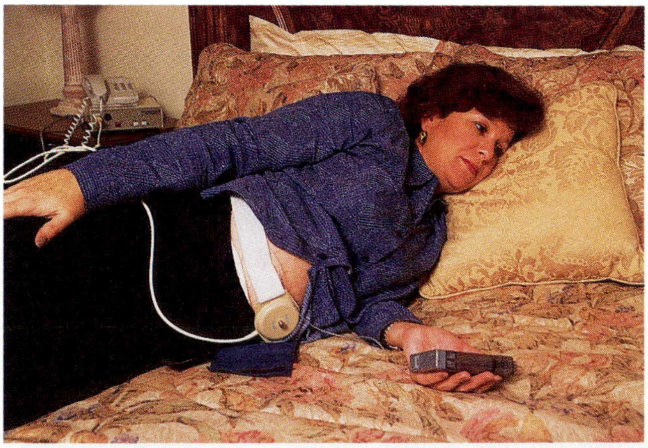

FIGURE 12–1. Prescribed bedrest or partial bedrest at home can result in both advantages and problems for the high-risk client.

► Childbirth Education for the High-Risk Pregnant Client

Lack of access to childbirth education programs is a problem for the high-risk client who is hospitalized or at home on bedrest. In addition to missing content related to labor and delivery, clients and their families lose the often exciting and enjoyable experience of attending a childbirth education program together. Traditionally, teaching for these clients has been done on a one-to-one basis that has focused on high-risk issues and has done little to promote a family-centered delivery experience.

Childbirth classes for hospitalized, high-risk clients and families may be held in the hospital setting. Ideally, the classes would be taught by a certified childbirth educator, experienced in the special needs of high-risk clients. In addition to information needed

▶ STRATEGIES FOR CARE OF THE HIGH-RISK PREGNANT WOMAN
AT HOME ON BEDREST OR RESTRICTED ACTIVITY

Avoid "routine" use of bedrest; make certain that bedrest is only ordered if necessary.

Telephone the client periodically; set a time for a telephone appointment. Make certain to call at the time selected.

Make certain the client knows whom to call in case of emergencies.

Include the client in decision making about level of bedrest/activity restriction. Make certain the client understands the level of activity restriction prescribed.

Make certain the client really can manage with this regimen in the home.

Include family in teaching and discuss ways in which help from significant others is needed.

Refer client for home care services. Such services may include home care nursing visits, home monitoring, etc.

Provide anticipatory guidance. Discuss such topics as physical condition, emotional and economic concerns related to activity restriction as well as to the client's pregnancy.

Provide client and family teaching. Include such topics as the client's physical condition, emotional and economic concerns related to the pregnancy and to activity restriction/bedrest at home, and ways to organize the home environment to meet the needs of a woman on bedrest and her family. Childbirth educators may be available to offer teaching sessions in the client's home, but such personal instruction can be expensive.

When possible, use audiovisual and on-line resources as educational aids. Videotapes are a low-cost option, although clients need access to equipment for viewing; providers of care to homebound pregnant women may seek funding for resources to lend to families. On-line resources for pregnant women also exist; for those women with such computer access, they provide varying types of information and support. Such resources include (Schroeder, 1998):

Sidelines: With support chapters in many areas, Sidelines offers a national, non-profit support network for pregnant women on bedrest. A Resource Center bookstore, list of articles, and peer counseling are among its services. http://home.earthlink.net/~sidelines

ParentsPlace: Such parents' resources as Moms on Bed Rest, fact sheets on bedrest, childbirth, etc. and chat rooms are available. http://www.parentsplace.com

Maintain current contact among all health care providers (certified nurse-midwife, obstetrician, office/clinic nurses) who provide client teaching, home monitoring/home care staff. Ideally, collaborate on identification of care needs and division of teaching content to avoid duplication and to ensure that the client receives important information.

---

by all pregnant clients, the classes would focus on content related to high-risk care, such as hospitalization, possible cesarean delivery, coping with separation from family during hospitalization, and making birth as positive an experience as possible.

In settings where childbirth education classes are not available for the hospitalized client and family, one-to-one teaching between the nurse and the family, the use of audiovisual and interactive learning materials, or both can promote learning.

▶ PSYCHOSOCIAL CONCERNS DURING THE INTRAPARTUM PERIOD

A client's perception of her labor and delivery experience has been noted to be an important factor in her transition to motherhood and postpartum adaptation (Lederman, 1996). Inability to have an expected birth experience has been described as a crisis and has been a source of grief for clients and their spouses. The

high-risk intrapartum experience superimposes the challenge of ensuring a safe delivery on the challenge of promoting a family-centered birth experience.

Clients who are at high-risk during the intrapartum period have either been considered at risk during their pregnancies or become high risk during the intrapartum period. Ideally, health care professionals have had opportunities to provide guidance and support in advance of labor and delivery for those clients who were at risk. In these situations, nurses need to orient the client to the high-risk unit and to review teaching relevant to aspects of high-risk intrapartum care. Although a high-risk client may have had extensive prenatal care, nurses in the labor and delivery unit should not simply assume that she and her family are well informed. Assessment of level of knowledge and reaction to the high-risk condition is of primary importance before interventions can be undertaken.

A client with a healthy prenatal history may become high-risk during labor and delivery. Suddenly staff may begin to rush, uncomfortable procedures may be undertaken, and high-risk equipment may be used. In some cases, the client is physically prepared for emergency cesarean delivery. The client may experience a sudden crisis, accompanied by feelings of unreality, fear, and panic. High levels of anxiety can further complicate the intrapartum process.

A major concern during high-risk pregnancy is that the fetus may be born abnormal or nonviable. In many cases, diagnostic fetal tests cannot predict with certainty whether an infant will be born normal; however, birth of the infant is still a future occurrence.

Labor brings the stress of knowing that answers to questions about fetal anomalies and status may soon be apparent. High-risk clients may, therefore, be especially anxious during their stay in labor and delivery units. Although some potential abnormalities turn out to be minor or nonexistent, many present current and future problems. Despite advance preparation, clients experience shock and crisis even in the delivery room. The use of general anesthesia during delivery postpones but does not "spare" the mother grief. The father frequently has to deal with this information by himself until the mother recovers from anesthesia, thus potentially reinforcing a sense of family isolation during crisis.

Some clients, such as severely preeclamptic clients, may feel ill as a result of their high-risk status. In cases where fetal status is potentially in jeopardy, analgesic medications may be restricted. When possible, alternative strategies such as back rubs, assistance with position changes, guided imagery, and attentive labor coaching can promote relaxation and comfort.

Improving outcomes for high-risk clients has sparked the development of advanced obstetric technology. When used judiciously, such technology is able to provide information about maternal and fetal well-being during labor and delivery. Despite the most skillful technical care, the nurse needs to remember that high-risk equipment and procedures are new and frightening for most clients and that sudden transition to high-risk status can be terrifying. The nurse's ability to remain calm, to provide understandable explanations to the client and her family, to collaborate smoothly with other health care providers, and to blend a compassionate approach with technical expertise are essential to effective high-risk care.

The nurse must remember that the father or significant other who accompanies the high-risk client during labor and delivery is also at risk for crisis. The presence of a loving and familiar person can be important to the client. Welcoming the presence of the support person when feasible, including the support person in client teaching, making it possible for couples who planned to share delivery to remain together, and being willing to listen to the fears and concerns of family members can promote psychologic health for the high-risk family during the intrapartum period.

Much has been done to ensure family-centered care for low-risk clients during labor and delivery. Unfortunately, the focus of interventions for the high-risk client is sometimes on pathologic conditions and family-centered care is excluded. Nurses should evaluate current practices and policies regarding the high-risk client and judge whether restrictions are outmoded traditions or truly in the client's best interests.

▶ Birth of a Healthy Infant After a High-Risk Pregnancy

The delivery of a healthy infant after a high-risk pregnancy may create a situational crisis for clients and their families as they try to return to their normal lives. After the stress of being high risk, the client and her family may have difficulty resuming a low-risk lifestyle. For example, clients may be extremely anxious about going home after delivery. They may need reassurance about their own or their infant's health status, and worry whether common variations, such as sleepiness during initial feeding, are signs of pathology.

Nurses can do much to ease transition for a previously at-risk client and her family. Nurses can continue to regard these families as potentially at risk for anxiety related to their childbearing experience. Before discharge, teaching should include feelings related to high-risk status. Postdischarge client follow-up can be conducted either at office or clinic sessions or through home visits or telephone calls at periodic intervals. Clients experiencing acute or prolonged emotional difficulty, related to the high-risk experience, should be referred for counseling.

▶ Birth of an Abnormal Infant

All parents of infants born with abnormalities are considered at psychosocial risk. When parents know about the abnormality prior to childbirth, they have opportunity to receive support and to begin to prepare for their infant; however, many abnormalities are not known until the infant is born. Both situations are accompanied by crisis. Many complex and interrelated factors determine how well parents are able to cope with their infant's abnormality:

- The nature and extent of the abnormality; the degree of mental or physical impairment.
- To what degree, if at all, the abnormality can be corrected through growth and development and medical or surgical means.

- The extent of cosmetic disfigurement.
- The nature and extent of the infant's acute and chronic needs.
- The amount of disruption in the family related to the infant's condition (e.g., need for a parent to stop work, or round-the-clock care required for the infant).
- The nature of specialized care and costs.
- Religious and cultural views about the abnormality.
- Previous experience with individuals with similar abnormalities.
- Support from significant others; their willingness to accept the situation and show love for the parents and the infant.

A consistent, unified team approach helps parents deal with the birth of an infant with an abnormality. Health care providers need to understand that parents may not only grieve for their infant's condition but also for the loss of their fantasized infant and, in some cases, their dreams for the infant. Many of the strategies summarized in the box entitled Nursing Strategies for Families Preparing for the Birth of an Abnormal Infant are also applicable to parents after the birth of an abnormal infant. Individualized support, encouragement, referral to organizations and support groups focusing on children with similar abnormalities, and strategies that reinforce the parents' self-confidence and focus on the positive aspects of the infant help parents to build hope and love during a difficult transition to parenthood.

► PSYCHOLOGIC ASPECTS OF CARING FOR FAMILIES OF A HIGH-RISK NEWBORN

Every infant admitted to a NICU has or is at risk for pathology. Infants in a NICU are observed or treated for life-threatening or disabling conditions. With few exceptions, families of infants in NICUs are considered to be at risk for parenting. Families experience crisis and grief, although these feelings vary. Parental roles have been altered, and parents have lost the opportunity for a healthy, low-risk neonatal experience. Some infants are taken immediately from the delivery room to the NICU. Others are transferred from a low-risk delivery setting to a tertiary-care hospital that has a NICU. Some infants are initially admitted to a well-baby nursery, but later transferred to a NICU, because of the diagnosis of a high-risk condition.

Certainly, nurses working in NICUs need to be skilled in the physical care of the high-risk newborn

and in the psychologic aspects of working with frightened, grieving families; however, all labor-and-delivery nurses, well-baby nursery nurses, and postpartum nurses will at some point work with parents of a high-risk newborn. Mothers of infants in NICUs are cared for on postpartum units. No matter how well prepared a mother is prenatally for the possible birth of a high-risk infant, the reality of having an infant in the NICU is a shock. Nurses must therefore be able to understand the psychologic dimensions of parenting the high-risk infant and be prepared to implement strategies that will help inform and support new parents during such a difficult time in their lives.

► Obstacles to Parenting within the NICU

Several factors related to neonatal intensive care can present obstacles to parenting and have major psychologic impact on the family.

Prevention of Extended Contact
A high-risk delivery experience and the physical status of the infant may prevent the extended contact desirable during and immediately after birth. Such delays can contribute to parental stress (Shields-Poë & Pinelli, 1997). At times the unstable condition of the newborn may require rapid transfer to a NICU for intensive care support. The mother's physical condition may prevent her from seeing her newborn that day or for several days. In cases where the newborn is transferred to another hospital, the mother may not see her newborn until after her own discharge. (Although some hospitals are able to transfer both mother and infant, this is not done in all situations.) When the father accompanies the infant to the NICU, the mother is then left without her main support person.

Reminders of the High-Risk Status of the Newborn
The presence of skilled personnel, use of specialized equipment such as isolettes, nursery rules and procedures such as monitoring of vital signs and laboratory studies can serve as barriers between parents and their infants and are further reminders of the high-risk status of the newborn. Although depending upon the expertise of staff, some parents may feel jealous of the nurses caring for their infant (Lefrak-Okikawa & Lund, 1993). Parents may be terrified at the sight of monitors attached to their infant or by the realization that their infant is in need of such technical support. In addition, parental reactions may include disappointment, grief, horror, self-doubt, and worry over

the infant's normal development. How parents perceive the severity of their baby's illness can also add to their stress (Shields-Poë & Pinelli, 1997).

Lack of Privacy

Lack of privacy within the NICU can have a mixed impact on parenting. The continuously visible presence of skilled personnel may be comforting to parents, especially if the infant is ill or unstable. Yet, the lack of privacy can affect parental reactions and may not satisfy the need for family members to be alone together with the infant, away from the illness atmosphere of the NICU.

Newborn's Appearance and Ability to Interact

The newborn's appearance and ability to interact can be distressing to parents and can have an impact on the developing parent–infant relationship (Wereszczak, Miles, & Holditch-Davis, 1997). The weak, debilitated, premature, or sedated infant differs greatly from the alert, term infant. In addition, a physician's pessimistic view of the infant's chances for a healthy survival could negatively affect the mother's perception of and attachment to her infant (Klaus & Kennell, 1993; Klaus, Kennell, & Klaus, 1995).

Restrictive Visitation Policies

NICUs have restrictive visitation policies that can impede the acquaintance process among family members. Although many NICUs no longer restrict parental visiting, visitation rights are not always extended to other relatives or family friends. Because of concerns over childborne infections, such as chicken pox, sibling visitation in NICUs is often restricted to a "special occasion" within the unit or viewing through the glass windows of a nursery. Ironically, almost any curious nursing or medical student can visit an infant in a NICU, but visitation by family members and their friends may be restricted. Through interviews with nurses in intensive care units, including NICUs, Chesla and Stannard (1997) observed that practices that distanced families from clients contributed to breakdown of nursing care in intensive care units. Such practices included asking families to leave if the client's condition worsened.

▶ Concerns Related to Prematurity and Low Birth Weight

Prematurity refers to birth before the beginning of the 38th week of gestation. Low birth weight refers to all infants weighing less than 2500 g at birth, regardless of the cause and duration of gestation; very low birth weight refers to infants who weigh less than 1500 g at birth. Neonates who weigh less than 500 g at birth often do not survive. Many low-birth-weight infants are also premature. Prematurity and low birth weight remain among the most frequent reasons for NICU stays.

In addition to their acute problems, premature and low-birth-weight infants are at risk for long-term difficulties, such as dependence on respiratory assistance, learning disabilities, and problems with school achievement (Cunningham et al., 1997). Unfortunately, the nature and extent of difficulties, if any, cannot always be predicted. Consequently, parents have additional stress as they "wait and see" how their baby's development evolves and need to continue with health screening and specialized interventions.

As technology and expertise evolve, ethical and other decision-making dilemmas arise about such topics as quality of life, resuscitation of very small and sick infants, costs of care, and how to decide when outcomes are uncertain. These concerns will continue.

Premature birth cuts short the psychologic developmental processes that occur during the third trimester and superimposes a situational crisis on the normal developmental processes of pregnancy and childbirth (Weingarten, Baker, Manning, & Kutzner, 1990). Mothers of premature infants often report "not being ready" for the infant or "still feeling pregnant." Premature birth may also alter the psychologic transition to grandparenthood and therefore add to crisis in the family.

Prematurity recurs in the literature in association with parenting difficulties, ranging from emotional problems of parents and infants to child abuse (Klaus & Kennell, 1993). Although premature birth occurs in all groups of women, the incidence of prematurity is higher among women who are already physically, emotionally, or socioeconomically stressed. It is difficult to conclude from current research that premature birth in itself directly causes parenting problems; however, poor resolution of crisis and grief contributes to the complexity of difficulties surrounding premature birth. Conversely, a supportive environment can foster positive perceptions of the premature infant.

Almost all surviving premature infants are eventually discharged home to their parents. A major nursing challenge is to assist the parents of premature infants to develop joy and skill in beginning parenthood in the context of an intensive care setting. The extended periods premature infants may spend in the NICU and continued postdischarge contacts provide much opportunity for nurses to educate the family about prematurity, to address prematurity-related concerns, and to foster the development of attachment between parents and their premature infants.

In recent years, developmental care, tailored to the unique needs of each infant and family, has been used in NICUs (Brown, Heermann, 1997; Kledzik, Howell, 1996). Originally planned for the preterm infant, this approach to care has been expanded to include high-risk infants and includes strategies that address the infant's environment, promote healthy growth and development, and maximize the quality of parent–infant interactions. (See Chapter 33.)

▶ Intensive Care/Expensive Care

NICU care *is* expensive care. From a financial viewpoint, the daily charge for a stay in a NICU is substantially higher than for care in a well-baby nursery. In addition, infants in a NICU are hospitalized longer than well infants, who may be discharged on the first to third day after birth. Parents of infants in a NICU may not be covered by insurance for all expenses, especially if the infant has a prolonged stay and potential for chronic problems. Even with various public assistance or special care funds, families often must deal with the huge financial stress of bills that can drain their economic resources. Families can also be burdened by costs related to travel, particularly when infants are admitted to regional NICUs far from their homes.

The emotional impact of having an infant in an NICU cannot be measured in dollars. The anxiety that parents experience over the present and future health of their infants can be far reaching. Certain handicapping conditions, such as some types of cerebral palsy or learning disabilities, do not become apparent until the infant grows into childhood. Some parents may continue to harbor concerns, related to their NICU experience, until developmental milestones of childhood are met. As one mother of an infant who had been evaluated in an NICU for potential seizures and then discharged as "normal" stated: "The words 'probably fine' remained in my mind after we took him home from the NICU. Like a dark cloud, they would sometimes float across my mind. It wasn't until 5 years later, as my son 'graduated' from kindergarten, that I could realize he was just as normal as the other kids." For similar reasons, Klaus and colleagues (1995) caution against giving opinions about a baby's future mental impairment, unless health care providers know with absolute certainty the baby is damaged. Citing experience in one of their own settings, they estimated that expert neonatologists made correct predictions of normality or abnormality about half the time.

For some parents, having an infant in a NICU is a social stigma. Some parents feel they are the objects of pity or blame among their significant others, espe-

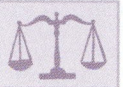

Ethical Decision Making

As the result of infertility interventions, 34-year-old Kate Miller, the mother of a 4-year-old, gives birth to quintuplets at 27 weeks' gestation. All five babies, each weighing less than 1000 grams, are listed as critical in the NICU. Due to their multiple problems, care for each baby is estimated to be over 1 million dollars; if they survive, special needs are expected to continue. With media attention focused on women who have carried larger numbers of fetuses, Kate and her husband Donald have received little publicity. If you were one of the nurses caring for this family, how would you respond to the following issues?

1. What are some of the ethical problems raised by infertility interventions that result in the birth of multiple, low-birth-weight, critically ill newborns?
2. Should potential long-term costs be a factor in choosing and using infertility treatments?
3. Should cost be a factor in deciding whether to continue to treat the babies?

cially if the infant has a condition requiring chronic care. High-risk social behaviors and turbulent home situations are further complicated by a sick infant who requires special and attentive care from already stressed parents.

Nurses must *always* be aware of the broad costs of intensive care. Infants should *never* be admitted for casual reasons or simply because the well-baby nursery staff would feel "safer" if an infant were transferred. One way to minimize the risk of unnecessary NICU admissions is for well-baby nursery nurses to be skilled in assessment and normal variations of the newborn.

▶ NURSING STRATEGIES TO PROMOTE PARENTING WITHIN THE NICU

A multicenter study of families of clients in critical care units, including NICUs, indicated that family members seek assurance that care is being delivered competently, reassurance, access to the client, and accurate information (Dracup, 1993). Nurses can promote parenting of infants in the NICU by:

1. Expecting all parents with an infant in a NICU to face a potential crisis. Realizing that families experience emotional turmoil (Kleiber et al., 1994).
2. Evolving strategies for emotional support from a team approach, including such professionals as physicians, other nurses, social workers, and pastoral care representatives.
3. Discussing with parents the infant's physical condition and reason for stay in the NICU. Has the infant been admitted for observation? Have health problems already been diagnosed? What is the likely prognosis? What current and future plans for the infant have been made?
4. Maintaining a collaborative team approach when providing information to parents. Joint meetings and daily interdisciplinary rounds help staff members provide consistent, supportive care to parents.
5. Anticipating and identifying potential parental reactions to the NICU environment and to the physical condition of the infant. Parents visiting their infants for the first time should be accompanied by a member of the NICU staff who is able to orient them to their infant, to their infant's care routine, and to the NICU. This should also be done if there is a significant change in the infant's condition. Some infants, such as those born very prematurely or those with pronounced congenital anomalies, may look different from the standard of a healthy term infant. Anticipatory guidance must be given to parents prior to their seeing the infant.
6. Promoting the infant's appearance. Infant appearance can have an effect on parental perceptions, and nurses can do much to present infants in the best possible way. Infants need to be kept clean and in a well-organized environment. Whenever feasible, procedures should be undertaken with sensitivity to the parents' feelings. For example, infants' heads should *never* be routinely shaved. One mother described her reaction to her infant's head being shaved. "She was born with a head full of thick hair. When I saw her in the NICU, they had half shaved her head; to me that white scalp looked disfigured. The staff tried to tell me that it was done 'just in case' she needed a scalp vein for an IV, which she never did. It took 9 months for the hair to grow in.

People would stare at her whenever we went out; every time I looked at her I was reminded of the staff's thoughtlessness."
7. Encouraging breastfeeding. Having a baby in the NICU can thwart breastfeeding intentions. Many women, however, can breastfeed successfully. Mothers who do not have conditions that contraindicate breastfeeding (e.g., substance abuse, HIV infection) should be encouraged to breastfeed. Nursing interventions can also include teaching mothers to express and collect milk, assisting mothers with breastfeeding while their babies are in the NICU, providing telephone or home-visit follow-up after discharge or referral to lactation support personnel, and discussing breastfeeding concerns with family members (Meier, Engstrom, Mangurten, Estrada, Zimmerman, & Kopparthi, 1993).
8. Facilitating contact between parents and infant. This can be done in several ways.
   - Discussing with parents the importance of their visits, not only for the infant but also for their own development as parents.
   - Instituting policies, such as unrestricted visiting for parents and for significant others of the parents' choosing. (Parents should not be considered visitors, but integral members of the caregiving team.)
   - Assisting parents to come to visit. (Transportation can be a problem for families who do not have access to cars or who live far from the NICU. Although providing transportation for these families is not within the role of the nurse, relaying this information to social services can possibly help families receive transportation assistance. Hospital auxiliaries or other charitable groups may be willing to contribute either money or services to help these families with transportation.)
   - Providing telephone, e-mail, or letter updates to parents unable to visit. (This is especially important for mothers who are hospitalized elsewhere or for parents who live far from the NICU.)
   - Assisting parents to participate in caring activities such as touching, holding, and feeding the infant if possible (Fig. 12–2).
   - Encouraging parents to bring in pictures of family members for use in the infant's crib as focal points. (Some families may also want to send in tapes to be played for the infant or clothing for the infant to wear.)
9. Providing opportunities for parents to ask questions and encouraging parents to be active

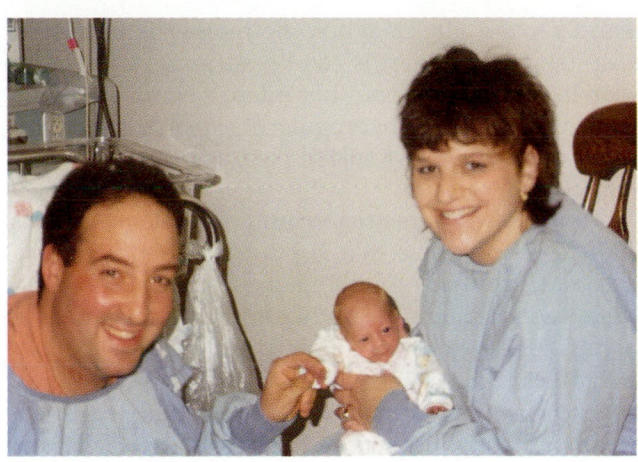

FIGURE 12–2. Family attachment is promoted when parents are encouraged to hold and touch their infant in the NICU.

participants in decisions, related to their infant's care, so they are involved as well as informed (Raines, 1996). Costello and colleagues (1996) reported successful use of individualized parent education binders with updated information about the baby's progress. The binders included such topics as admission information, feeding, parent information, clinical information, and discharge planning. The binders also helped parents to understand and review the baby's status and to communicate with staff.

10. Providing privacy for parents and the infant whenever possible and appropriate. Some units have special "bonding" rooms where parents can be alone with their infants. When this is not possible, the use of removable screens placed around the parents and isolette is helpful.
11. Providing ongoing assessment of development of parenting behaviors and arranging for prompt counseling intervention for parents identified as having difficulty.
12. Encouraging parents to express concerns about siblings and other family members and providing anticipatory guidance about sibling and family responses to the high-risk neonate.
13. Recognizing parents' desires for care that is consistent with their culture and in the best interests of their baby as a member of their family (Raines, 1996).
14. Providing for parental support from other sources, such as support groups for parents of infants in special care. Parents may also receive comfort from being introduced to other

parents who have coped with an infant with a similar condition (Lindsay, 1993). Parents of infants who require surgical repair of congenital anomalies may appreciate seeing photographs of infants who have had successful repair of these types of anomalies.

► Kangaroo Care

Kangaroo care refers to skin-to-skin contact between infant and parents (Drosten-Brooks, 1993; Ludington-Hoe & Golant, 1993; Klaus et al., 1995). Originally used to promote attachment between parents and full-term newborns, kangaroo care is now used successfully with preterm and other ill infants in the NICU. With kangaroo care, the infant, wearing only a diaper, is placed against the bare skin of the parent's chest. The parent then buttons his or her shirt around the infant, so that only the head is visible. Each NICU may have specific criteria for kangaroo care; however, infants who are stable enough to be handled are usually appropriate candidates, even if they require monitoring and ventilatory assistance. A temperature probe remains on the infant's skin to monitor temperature. The warmth of the parent's skin, clothing, and light blankets placed over both can prevent chilling. Coverings can also be adjusted to avoid overheating. With proper precautions, such as good handwashing, infection is not a problem. Benefits of kangaroo care have been reported to include decreased oxygen requirements for the infant, longer quiet sleep periods, shortened hospitalizations, improved parental confidence in caretaking, feelings of closeness to the infant, and increased maternal lactation.

► NURSING STRATEGIES FOR CARE OF PARENTS OF A NEWBORN TRANSFERRED TO A REGIONAL NICU

The preceding discussion applies to almost all parents of infants in NICUs. Parents of a newborn transferred to an NICU from another birthing site have additional, unique needs.

In many states, neonatal intensive care has been concentrated in certain high-risk centers. Theoretically, this allows for the development of specialty units, staffed by health care professionals skilled in the care of critically ill neonates and able to offer the latest in sophisticated technology. Recently, this concept of regionalization has been broadened to include a continuum of care for the prenatal, intrapartum, and postpartum client and family (see Chapter 2 for a discussion about regionalization as an aspect of perinatal care).

Since most childbearing families are not at high risk and do not have infants who require intensive care, birth in wellness-oriented, low-risk childbearing settings is appropriate for them. Indeed, childbearing in a high-risk center may place the healthy client at risk for complications, arising from the often liberal use of obstetric interventions in these facilities. Many hospitals have no need to create high-risk units, because they do not serve a large high-risk population. In addition, a NICU is an enormously expensive unit to maintain; many hospitals cannot afford its upkeep.

Although the regional model of care may decrease neonatal mortality and morbidity, there can be a negative impact on the parents of the transferred infant. The regional center may be a few blocks or a few hundred miles away. In every case, the stress of having an infant who needs a NICU is compounded by maternal–infant separation and the often unexpected reason for transfer. In addition, parents may know the regional center only by reputation; they are compelled to rely on strangers who have not previously been involved in their care.

When the father accompanies the infant on the transport, the mother is left without her significant other. The father is also divided between two hospitals and may feel an additional burden of "having to be strong" for the mother. Concern over being separated from her infant may prompt a mother to make her own health secondary. For example, women who have delivered by cesarean may leave the hospital early and go directly to the NICU, rather than paying attention to their own physical needs for rest and recovery.

In a classic study of parents whose critically ill newborns survived after referral to a regional NICU, Benfield and colleagues (1976) found that most parents experienced grief reactions similar to those whose newborns had died. Parents grieved deeply, regardless of the severity of the infant's illness. The investigators noted that fathers reported dramatic changes in their daily patterns while their wives and infants were in separate hospitals; they also took on a central role in stabilizing the family during this time.

In working with parents of transferred infants, nurses must be aware of the nature of the family's birth experience. Prior to the transfer, the mother should see and touch her infant, whenever possible. Any positive comments about the infant may also be appreciated and remembered by the mother (Klaus et al., 1995; Klaus & Kennell, 1993). On transfer, efforts must be made to orient the family to the facility as well as to the NICU. When the mother is in another hospital, telephone calls can be an important way to keep her informed about her infant's status. Neonatal intensive care units that regularly expect transfers can create areas where exhausted postcesarean or postpartum parents can rest.

Some NICU's restrict visiting to biologic parents. Staff need to realize that supportive friends or relatives are important to the mental health of the father whose wife remains in another hospital. There are few circumstances critical enough to warrant exclusion of a significant other. Frequently, a mother is comforted by knowing that someone she loves and trusts will accompany her husband on her behalf, especially during such a stressful experience. The practice of having a father sit alone with his critically ill infant while a close relative is restricted to an outside waiting room is not therapeutic and should be avoided.

Staff need to realize that transfer of a child to a regional NICU brings other family burdens. Long distances between the NICU and the clients' home and threat of loss of work income may make it difficult for parents to visit. The high costs of hotels and restaurant meals are not covered by health insurance and may deeply affect a family's budget. The needs of siblings and problems associated with finding child care, especially if overnight stays are involved, are additional concerns of parents of the transferred infant. Further, for families living in poverty, such arrangements might not be an option. These social problems deeply affect the emotional well-being of parents of an infant transferred to a NICU and are reasons for referral for social service assistance. In addition, local religious groups may be of assistance through provision of lodging and hospitality to parents of infants in NICUs. Nurses must realize that such problems pertain to parents from all types of social and economic backgrounds.

▶ NURSING STRATEGIES IN CARING FOR SIBLINGS OF A NEWBORN IN THE NICU

In the best of circumstances, the birth of an infant is a stressful event for siblings. When the new infant requires prolonged and intensive parental attention, siblings may feel resentful and anxious. Parents in crisis may seem to place other children "second" in their concern for the sick neonate. The children's lives and schedules may be greatly changed, especially if the parents are gone from the home for long periods, if the siblings are sent to stay with others, or if new arrangements for child care are made. At times, parents may not be able to attend special sibling events, such as school plays, or to host holiday celebrations. Children also worry about their parents' distress. The actual response of the sibling depends on such factors as the child's age, the number of other siblings in the home, the nature of preexisting family relationships, and the amount of change in daily routine related to the infant's hospitalization. The following strategies, which focus on siblings, may be helpful to discuss with parents:

- Siblings should be told about the infant in language they can understand. In addition, parents should tell the siblings what their own feelings are and why. Parents also need to make certain that the child has understood what they are trying to say. The type of explanation should be based on the developmental level of each child. Toddlers, as well as preschool-aged or school-aged children, need information.

- Parents should be encouraged to keep siblings within their own home and not to send them to live with friends or relatives. Although parents may intend to "protect" their children from emotional crisis at home, children may cope better when they remain in their own household. Separating children from their parents may lead to problems. For example, physical and emotional distance created by separation can be extremely disruptive to children and their daily lives. Children may experience more fear from imagining what is wrong with the infant than they would from learning the truth about the situation and coping with it as a family. Children also may believe that their separation from their parents is due either to their behavior or their inability to help their parents during this crisis. When distance and child care problems require that children be sent away, parents need to take care to keep them informed about their own health status and the infant's progress. Parents should be advised to try to maintain usual family routines and standards.

- Parents need to calm siblings' fears that their thoughts or actions caused the infant to be sick or, in cases of perinatal death, to die. Nurses should encourage parents to speak directly to siblings about this topic. Siblings normally have ambivalent feelings about a coming infant. Birth of a high-risk infant or death of the infant may make the siblings feel responsible. In a culture where the media can make anything seem real, sibling guilt feelings need to be addressed.

- Siblings continue to have needs, related to their own developmental level and social network. Parents need to be encouraged to provide special time alone with the siblings to show the sibling he or she is loved and valued.

- Children often have fears about their own health or the health of their parents. Nurses can help parents of a high-risk infant to anticipate these feelings and to reassure the siblings that they are healthy.

- Just as parents may grieve the loss of the fantasized infant, siblings may grieve the loss of the expected brother or sister and may also feel ashamed of the infant's high-risk status. Siblings also may grieve the loss of parental attention.

- Nurses can encourage parents to bring siblings to visit their brother or sister in the NICU, especially if hospitalization is prolonged. Such visits may help siblings to understand more about the infant and to feel a part of the family. (Even in units that do not yet have sibling visitation programs, the sibling may be assisted to view the infant through nursery windows.) Many children handle such visits well; others, however, may be overwhelmed by the NICU and their infant brother or sister. Nurses can advise parents to anticipate a short initial stay with the older child or to bring other adults who can leave the unit if the child becomes overwhelmed.

- Nurses can be instrumental in developing sibling education and visitation programs within the NICU. In this way care can focus on all family members, regardless of their youth. For example, these programs can include: inservice education seminars to help staff to work with parents and siblings within the NICU; developmentally based teaching tools to enhance communication between parents and siblings and to promote family members' participation in the infant's care; sibling visits within the NICU (with appropriate staff screening and supervision).

- During predischarge and postdischarge teaching sessions with parents, nurses need to include the topics of siblings and sibling responses.

- NICU staff should be able to help families identify appropriate children's books and other resources about the NICU and feelings related to a baby in intensive care. Ideally, units would have such resources available for families to use. Funding might be sought from charitable groups or from the hospital's auxiliary.

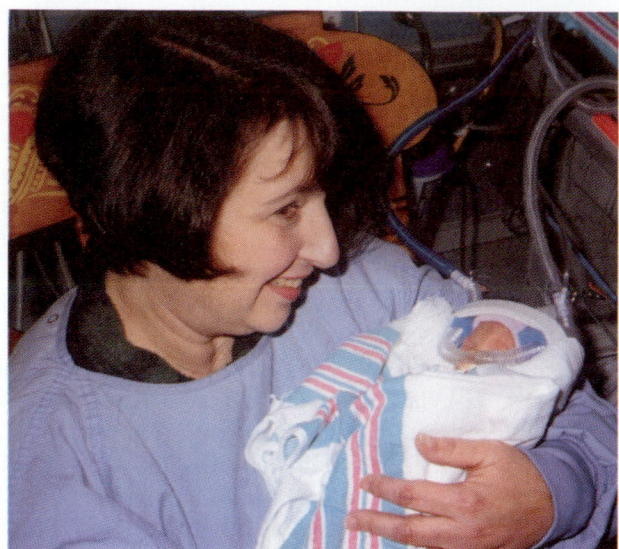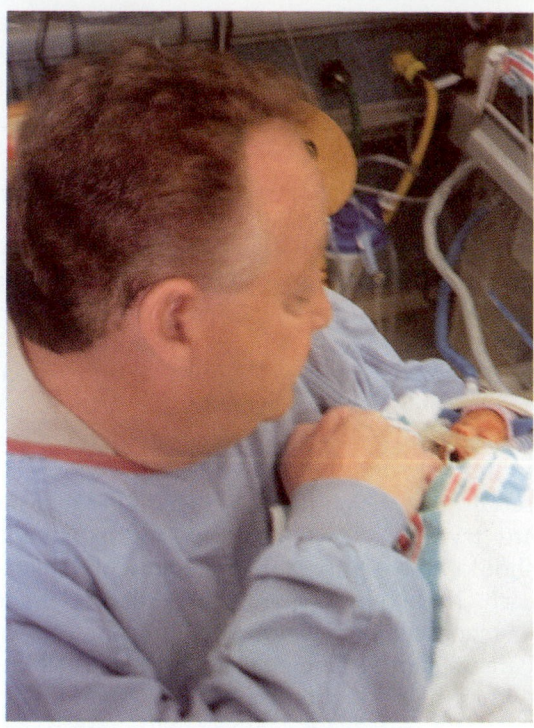

FIGURE 12–3. As part of the nursing care of a newborn in the NICU, grandparents are welcomed into the NICU and are encouraged to interact with their grandchild.

• Nurses can develop or participate in development of learning materials that can promote children's understanding of high-risk infants and NICUs.

tled Nursing Strategies for Care of Grandparents of an Infant in a NICU presents nursing interventions to help grandparents cope with this stressful experience.

▶ NURSING STRATEGIES IN CARING FOR GRANDPARENTS OF A NEWBORN IN THE NICU

Grandparents are often deeply affected by the birth of an infant who requires neonatal intensive care. Concern for the current and future health of the infant is accompanied by feelings of anxiety, worry, and sadness about seeing their own child in distress. Extensive changes have taken place in neonatal intensive care since most grandparents were new parents, and these changes may be overwhelming to grandparents. Nevertheless, grandparents can potentially provide much support to parents (Miles, Carlson, & Funk, 1996); at times, grandparents (especially grandmothers) serve as primary care providers (Fig. 12–3) (Carlson, 1993; McHaffie, 1992). The box enti-

▶ NURSING STRATEGIES RELATED TO DISCHARGE FROM THE NICU

Families look forward to discharge and yet worry about their infant away from the NICU. Families generally come to know and depend upon the expertise of the staff caring for their babies. Although some infants may be discharged needing only routine pediatric follow-up, others will require ongoing specialized care in other inpatient facilities or at home. Despite feelings of relief and happiness about the infant's improved condition, transfer from the NICU can elicit such feelings as fear of the unknown, alienation, helplessness, distrust of a new staff (if a baby goes to a different unit), and concern over not having the technology and personnel of the NICU (Kolotylo, Parker, & Chapman, 1991).

► **NURSING STRATEGIES FOR CARE OF GRANDPARENTS OF AN INFANT IN AN NICU**

Include grandparents or any significant others with the parents' permission, unless these individuals have been designated as primary caretakers for the infant.

Welcome and orient grandparents to the NICU and to the infant.

Encourage grandparents to discuss their concerns.

Encourage grandparent participation in infant care, especially if grandparents will be caretakers after discharge.

Discuss the nature and importance of support needed by the parents of the infant with the grandparents.

Provide specific examples of ways grandparents can help, such as with care of other children.

Dispel myths and misconceptions related to the infant's condition.

Discharge planning begins well in advance of discharge, and may begin as soon as a neonate is admitted to a NICU. Strategies that can help prepare families for discharge include the following:

- Encouraging parental involvement in care of the infant while the baby is in the NICU. Providing support and guidance so that parents can get to know their baby well and develop confidence and independence in caretaking. Klaus and Kennell (1995) have also described the benefits of "nesting," that is, permitting mothers to live in with their infants before discharge. A mother and her infant thereby have an opportunity to share a private room where the mother is the caregiver. Klaus and Kennell believe that nesting is helpful in building confidence and normalizing mothering behavior in the NICU.

- Providing anticipatory guidance about the transfer or discharge, and encouraging the parents to participate in the decision-making process.

- Encouraging parents to express their feelings about discharge from the NICU, and designing care based on their unique needs.

- Ensuring that care evolves from a team approach and that all health care providers are well informed about the current plans for the infant.

- Making certain that the parents or primary care providers are oriented to any new unit, and that they are informed of the time of the actual transfer.

- Making certain that parents or primary care providers have received written as well as verbal information about specialized care or follow-up required after discharge, and making certain that proper arrangements have been made.

- Helping to ease transition through such postdischarge contact as phone calls.

► **NURSING STRATEGIES IN CARING FOR FAMILIES EXPERIENCING PERINATAL DEATH**

► **Nursing Strategies for Care of Parents**

Perinatal death refers to many types of loss related to pregnancy and fertility, including spontaneous abortion, missed abortion, fetal death (formerly called stillbirth), and neonatal death (Association of Women's Health, Obstetric, and Neonatal Nurses, 1998). Perinatal death is an event that can be accompanied by intense feelings of crisis, grief, and loss, especially on the part of the parents.

In the past, perinatal death was treated as a "nonevent," with staff, family, and friends trying to avoid the topic or distract the parents. Parents were given little opportunity to discuss their feelings. Often, well-meaning staff isolated mothers on the postpartum unit or moved them to rooms on another floor; the mothers would then be discharged with plans only for physical follow-up.

Death is a topic that is poorly dealt with or is avoided altogether in U.S. society. Nevertheless, in life's natural order, a person is expected to progress from child to adult and in time to be buried by a member of the younger generation. The parent who experiences a perinatal death has a very different, intense experience. As Kirk (1984) noted, instead of being able to mourn a child she remembers, the mother of a stillborn infant mourns a person she has not known, cannot recall, and yet may not be able to forget. Parents who have other children are faced with the demands of trying to function in the role as they are trying to grieve. Although parents share the common bond of their child's death, mothers and fathers may experience and express their grief differently (Wallerstedt & Higgins, 1996). Parents may also be unaware of their own needs and options when their loss occurs (Primeau & Lamb, 1995).

Fetal loss through miscarriage or termination of pregnancy for genetic reasons can be accompanied by the grief of bereavement; families and health care providers may underestimate the extent of the distress. Zeanah and associates (1993) observed that women who terminated pregnancies for fetal anomalies experienced grief that was as intense as women who had spontaneous perinatal loss.

Parents of an infant who dies after birth have had some opportunity for contact with the "real" infant; however, interactions have frequently taken place within the high-risk hospital environment. Although some infants who die may have had a poor prognosis from birth, others may have progressed well, then died after experiencing an unexpected complication. Parents must deal not only with loss of the fantasy child, but also with the termination of hopes for infant recovery.

In addition to feelings of crisis, grief, and loss, the parents may feel cheated by not being able to have a living child after the pregnancy. According to Parkman (1992), after a normal birth the infant may still be perceived by the mother as part of her bodily or mental self. Death during the perinatal period may then represent loss of a part of the self, just as loss of a body part is perceived. This "injury to the self" may be accompanied by intense feelings of failure, helplessness, and loss of self-esteem as a parent. Anger may be directed toward family members, self, or staff members for not preventing the death. Negative parental reactions may also be intensified when staff are unwilling to address the loss and emotionally "abandon" the client. Such abandonment could take the form of routine postpartum care without discussion of the infant or the pregnancy.

As discussed earlier, maternal attachment to the fetus takes place in high-risk as well as low-risk pregnancies. The infant who experiences fetal death at one time had a very real presence and relationship, especially with the mother.

Nursing strategies for care of parents experiencing a perinatal death require a compassionate, knowledgeable approach. Nurses should realize that grieving parents in crisis may not know about or think of even basic care options. Nursing strategies to assist parents experiencing perinatal loss are discussed below.

Use Knowledgeable, Consistent Approaches and Unhurried Explanations

Most parents have a great need to learn why their infant died. Often, this may be the first question

asked. Staff need to be well informed about the client's individual situation and to have collaborated on a team approach for working with the family. In beginning to resolve grief, parents need to have a trusting relationship with their caregivers. Haphazard, inconsistent responses from health care personnel can add to parental anxiety and distrust. Clients who know in advance that the fetus has died or that their infant is dying should be cared for by the same nurse from admission through delivery, whenever possible.

Staff need to be prepared to answer all questions honestly and directly. When no apparent reason for the infant's death can be identified, staff should share this information. Bilingual interpreters should be sought for any clients who do not speak the same language as health care providers. Staff need to remember that expressions of mourning are influenced by culture.

Information may be presented privately by the physician and reinforced later by the nurse, or presented by a small interdisciplinary group. Members of this group might include the physician, nurse, bereavement social worker, and chaplain. Staff need to select a private setting that will allow for expression of personal feelings and to plan enough time for discussion with the parents. Communication strategies, such as eye contact and touch, are necessary. Staff members may also express their own sadness or empathy with the parents' situation. Klaus and Kennell (1982) described intense, persistent anger toward health care personnel whom parents perceived as being abrupt or as rushing through explanations to obtain autopsy permission. They also noted that parents felt greatly comforted by the nurses or physicians who expressed sadness or empathy with their situation.

Listen

Health care providers often feel compelled to talk when clients experience perinatal death. Families are also helped by health care providers who are able to listen to their feelings or who are simply able to provide what Miles (1993) termed a "silent presence," that is, "the personal use of self, offering an apparently waiting ear and receptive posture so that others may speak." Short comments like "I am so sorry" or "Yes, this is a sad time," can be therapeutic when used in this context.

Avoid Comments That Deny the Existence of the Infant

"You can always have another baby." "Things are better off this way." "You already have children." "You didn't have the chance to really know the baby." Such comments deny the existence of the reason for the client's grief and should be avoided.

Nurses can provide anticipatory guidance about feelings parents and families will experience in relation to perinatal loss. Following perinatal loss, communication among family members may become difficult, as each tries to deal with grief in a personal way. Ideally, both parents should be present during discussion of grieving responses, and this information should be discussed on more than one occasion. Parents can also be encouraged to keep personal journals.

Thoughtfully Select the Environment for Care

The obstetric environment can present additional stresses for the grieving client. Letting the client decide whether to stay on the postpartum unit and making certain that the client experiencing fetal or neonatal death does not have to room with a postpartum mother who has a healthy neonate can strengthen the nurse–client relationship and help clients have some control during a difficult time. Alerting all personnel to the client's condition can help minimize pain related to thoughtless remarks, such as "I'm sorry, I thought you had a baby." In some settings a special symbol, such as a picture of a flower, is placed on the door or chart to alert staff to the special needs of a grieving client.

Encourage Parents to See and Handle the Infant

Frequently, parents conjure monstrous images of what they fear their infant was like. After viewing the infant, however, many feel a sense of relief and peace, even if a congenital anomaly were present. Actually seeing and holding the dead infant may help the couple in the grieving process. Parents should be prepared for the sight of the infant. Simple explanations of what they will see (for example, "the baby is very small and she is pale and still, but otherwise she looks like a baby is expected to look") may be given. Although seeing and holding the dying or dead infant is considered a standard of practice (AWHONN, 1998), parents should make their own decisions and never be forced.

Arrangements should be made for the parents to view or hold the infant in an unhurried, supportive manner. In addition, the infant may be wrapped, garbed, or arranged in a manner that will soften his or her appearance. Parents may or may not wish to be alone with their infant or may wish to see their infant on more than one occasion. Some parents may want other family members to see the infant. Parents also benefit from knowing that the nurse will be nearby, should they not want to continue to be alone with their infant.

Be Respectful

Nurses need to treat the dead fetus or infant with the same respect that would be shown if he or she were alive. This is especially important when a fetus has died, and the mother undergoes labor and delivery. The infant should be presented to the parents in a dignified manner, that is, cleansed, if possible, and wrapped in an infant blanket. Respectful care includes understanding and support for cultural traditions related to grief and death of an infant. For example, some cultural groups, such as Chicanos, may respond demonstratively to death, whereas others, such as certain Native Americans, may express grief in a more quiet manner. Some Southeast Asian families may show grief and depression in the form of somatic complaints, because mental illness is regarded as a disgrace. Supportive, culturally sensitive family-centered nursing care, as well as attention to the way in which the dead infant is presented, can comfort parents during a difficult and vulnerable period.

Help Parents to Make Memories

Parents experiencing a fetal death will have no memories of the infant alive after birth; however, the need to validate that the infant did live persists. Parents should be encouraged to name the infant and to baptize the infant if appropriate to their religion. Nurses and other health care workers can help to create memories by taking a footprint and handprint of the infant or by providing a lock of the infant's hair, the identification band worn by the infant, or the blanket in which the infant was wrapped.

A photograph of the infant contributes to memories. Photographs may be taken while the infant is alive or after death. At times, parents elect not to see the dead infant, but later regret their decision. A photograph, kept by the perinatal staff until requested by the parents, can be a source of comfort and relief. Parents who have seen and held their infants may later treasure any photograph taken.

Facilitate Burial Arrangements and Other Options

Parents have the right to arrange for a private burial for their infant or to have the hospital dispose of the infant's remains. Representatives from the hospital pastoral care program or from the parents' congregation may be asked to conduct a simple service either on the unit or elsewhere. Nurses should know what

Parents' Experience Surrounding the Death of a Newborn Whose Birth Is at the Margin of Viability

In this descriptive study, 8 parents (5 mothers and 3 of their husbands) who had experienced the death of a newborn, weighing less than 500 grams at birth, were interviewed 2 or 3 times in their homes or by telephone between 4 and 15 weeks after their loss. The goal of the study was to describe the parents' own feelings and experiences related to the loss of the baby. Five themes emerged from analysis of the interview data: (1) Realization that the loss was occurring. Most parents did not feel fully prepared for the loss. One couple reported they were given the chance to discuss how much aggressive care they desired for their twins; they were the only couple to say they felt prepared for the death of their babies, even before their birth. Other couples had physicians who tended to discuss newborn survival in terms of gestational age and the possibility of increasing survival if the woman could only stay pregnant longer. (2) Initial response to the loss. Feelings reported included sleep deprivation, adding to exhaustion of labor and delivery, and physical and emotional pain. The mothers reported crying as their first response; fathers felt a loss of control and concern for their wives. (3) Decision making at the time of loss. Decisions had to be made quickly and included: whether to see and hold the newborn while he or she was still alive; whether to hold the baby as he or she died (most of the parents did not want to) or afterward; selecting baptism, infant mementos, burial, autopsy, etc. Parents reported that information, guidance and more time before finalizing decisions were helpful. (4) Components of supportive relationships with others. Acceptance of parents' feelings and behaviors (gentle, appropriate humor, providing a shoulder to cry on, receiving written information on loss, etc. that validated their feelings), being there (being available), and sharing the experience (with another bereaved parent or, in one case, with a nurse) were general characteristics of valued support. Giving information, providing competent care and giving special attention were particular components of support provided specifically by staff. (5) Adjustment at home. Fathers, concerned about their wives and the effects of future pregnancies on them, reported being unable to discuss these worries with their wives. Fathers coped through rigorous physical activity or keeping busy; they felt that the baby's medical problems caused the loss. Mothers reported such intense emotional feelings as emptiness and felt that such situations as being near pregnant women were hard for them. Mothers coped by talking about their loss and by keeping busy; they searched for additional reasons for the newborn's death.

Application to Practice

Newborns with birth weights of 500 g or less have a very poor chance of survival. Experiencing the death of a newborn whose birth is at the margin of viability is very difficult for parents. Findings from this study are similar to observations noted in the literature about perinatal loss and reinforce the importance of support from significant others and from health care providers. Traditionally, the health care literature discusses newborn survival in terms of gestational age. The study highlights the possibility of mothers' inadvertently being made to feel responsible for not being able to maintain their pregnancies longer. The study also notes difficulties surrounding the need for parents to make quick and irreversible decisions about their infant (e.g., whether or not to hold the baby before or as he or she dies, baptism, burial) and differences in bereavement responses between mothers and fathers. The finding that mothers reported intense physical as well as emotional pain highlights the importance of pain interventions for these women. The small sample size limits application of results to other populations and reinforces the need for continuing research. However, the study provides current and in-depth information that is helpful for nurses in planning and implementing care for parents who experience death of a baby born very early and very small.

Source: Kavanaugh, K. (1997). Parents' experience surrounding the death of a newborn whose birth is at the margin of viability. Journal of Obstetric, Gynecologic, and Neonatal Nursing, 26(1); 43–51.

the policies and possibilities are in the facilities where they work (whether cremation is routinely used, common burial with other infants, and so on). The perinatal social worker frequently assists parents in making such arrangements. Burial choices also depend upon the client's cultural and religious background.

A comprehensive checklist for perinatal loss can be developed. Ryan and associates (1991) described the use of a comprehensive checklist to facilitate care after perinatal loss (Fig. 12–4). Use of such a checklist helps to define a standard of care for perinatal loss and helps nurses and health care providers deliver optimum care to clients.

▶ Perinatal Hospice Care

The hospice approach provides supportive and coordinated health care to dying clients within the hospital and in home settings. Originally developed for care of dying adults by Cicely Saunders (1965) in Great Britain during the 1960s, pediatric and neonatal hospice concepts later evolved for care of terminally ill children and infants. Prenatal diagnosis of life-threatening congenital anomalies has extended the concepts of hospice to perinatal care (Calhoun, Hoeldke, Hinson, & Judge, 1997). Through perinatal hospice, health care providers begin support and counseling for grieving families at the time of prenatal diagnosis and continue through delivery and the death of the infant. For example, parents and their significant others are able to see the baby on ultrasound. Depending upon the anomaly, the infant may be born dead, live for a few minutes, or for a longer period. After birth, parents are able to hold, dress, or photograph the infant if they so choose. Comfort measures, such as warmth, cuddling, and feeding of the baby, are offered. An interdisciplinary team of physicians, nurses, social workers, and chaplains works together so the family can experience the high risk pregnancy, birth, and death experience in as positive a manner as possible.

▶ Anticipatory Guidance for Parenting Siblings

Despite perinatal death, clients who have other children are faced with continuing demands of parenthood. Grieving parents also have to deal with children in crisis. In trying to handle competing tasks of parenting children and relinquishing a parenting role, parents may try to distance themselves from their other children. The children may feel excluded as family members or guilty for having caused their parents' grief in some way; at times, they may manifest aberrant attention-getting behaviors. Anticipatory guidance can do much to assist grieving parents in dealing with their other children.

Many of the strategies discussed previously for care of siblings of an infant in an NICU apply to siblings of the infant who dies. As noted, interventions need to be based on understanding of the sibling's developmental level, as well as on such factors as family background. Siblings need to be told simply and directly about the death of the infant. Although they may not verbalize their feelings, children are aware of parental anguish; talking with siblings helps the entire family move through the grieving process. Depending on the age of the sibling, he or she may want to see a picture of the baby, make a special gift, or plant a tree or flowers in memory of the baby (Wallerstedt & Higgins, 1996).

Euphemisms such as "passed away" and "lost" are frequently used for "death." Parents need to take care not to use terms that can confuse or potentially be distressing to children. For example, telling siblings that the infant "went to sleep" or that the "baby was so good that God came for him" will not help a sibling deal effectively with the death, but could contribute to fears about sleep or fears that God will come to take the sibling (Kushner, 1981).

At times parents may feel too upset to answer their children's questions; however, sharing that feeling with the siblings, and reassuring them of their willingness to talk together when they are able, are important.

Finally, attendance of siblings at the infant's funeral is a decision to be made by each family.

▶ Nursing Strategies for Care of Grandparents

Anticipatory guidance about the grieving process needs to be given to grandparents. The parents' desire to hold a dead infant, arrange for a burial, and retain tangible mementos of a fetus who was not born alive may be considered abnormal and "weird" by their significant others. When families are already financially stressed, any money spent for these reasons may be questioned by family members. The old idea that a stillborn is not really an infant may compound parental grief and isolation. Nurses and other health care workers need to assure grandparents and significant others that such behavior related to the fetal death is normal. The couple needs to talk about the loss and should not be told to "just try to forget about it." Grandparents should be encouraged to express their feelings. Many have difficulty dealing with their

Parents' names _____
Address _____
Phone _____
Description of loss: _____

Description of previous loss(es) _____

L.M.P. _____ E.D.C. _____
Weeks of gestation _____
Sex of baby (if known) _____
Religious affiliation _____

	Office Staff	ER Staff	Labor/Delivery	Postpartum	Neonatal ICU	OR Staff	GYN/Post Op	Community Health	Date(s)
Received pregnancy confirmation									
Lab/amnio results	☐	☐	☐			☐			___
Sonogram photo	☐		☐			☐			
Acknowledgment of loss/impaired fertility	☐	☐	☐	☐	☐	☐	☐	☐	___
Bring up the subject									
Refer to the baby/expected child									
Call the baby by name									
Anticipatory guidance about normal grief									
Mother	☐	☐	☐	☐	☐	☐	☐		___
Father	☐	☐	☐	☐	☐	☐	☐		
Family members	☐	☐	☐	☐	☐	☐	☐		
Postloss options given									
To go home/maternity floor/alternate floor	☐	☐	☐						___
Father to remain with mother/private room			☐	☐		☐			
Saw/touched/held baby or products of conception	☐	☐	☐		☐		☐		___
If refused, later offers made									
Family members included in offer	☐	☐	☐		☐		☐		
Received mementos									
Footprints			☐	☐	☐				___
Bracelet			☐	☐	☐				___
Lock of hair			☐	☐	☐				___
Crib card			☐	☐	☐				___
Blanket			☐	☐	☐				___
Tape measure			☐	☐	☐				___
Certificate of life/remembrance	☐	☐	☐			☐	☐	☐	___
Photographs taken									
Given to parents				☐	☐				___
Filed with chart				☐	☐				
Bathed/dressed baby			☐		☐				___
Postdeath options discussed	☐	☐	☐	☐	☐		☐		___
Need/desire for funeral director									
Type/location/timing of service									
Burial/cremation/hospital disposal									
Parent involvement									
Choosing burial outfit/mementos									
Announcements—public/personal									
Religious options									
Baby baptized	☐	☐	☐		☐	☐	☐		___
Clergy notified	☐	☐	☐	☐	☐	☐	☐	☐	
Received information about									
Birth/death certificates	☐	☐		☐	☐		☐	☐	___
Autopsy option discussed	☐	☐	☐	☐	☐		☐		___
Marked chart/room with identifying symbol	☐	☐	☐	☐	☐	☐	☐		___
eg, butterfly, rainbow, rose									
Received literature/suggested readings	☐	☐	☐	☐	☐	☐	☐	☐	___
Hospital admitting office notified	☐	☐							___
SHARE/support group referral made	☐	☐	☐	☐	☐	☐	☐	☐	___

FIGURE 12–4. Comprehensive checklist for perinatal loss. *(Reproduced, with permission, from Ryan, P.F. et al. (1991). Facilitating care after perinatal loss: A comprehensive checklist.* Journal of Obstetric, Gynecologic, & Neonatal Nursing 20, *pp. 385–389.)*

own grief at the loss of the desired infant and with the sight of their own child in emotional pain. Grandparents may benefit from referral to support groups for bereaved families.

► ## Nursing Strategies for Care of Parents Experiencing Death and Survival of Infants of Multiple Gestation

The incidence of multiple gestation (plural births) has risen, especially among older, well-educated Caucasian women, possibly related to the use of fertility drugs. However, twins have been reported to have 5 times the mortality rate of singletons, and triplets have been estimated to have 14 times the mortality rate of singletons (Jewell & Yip, 1995).

Conflicting and complex feelings of joy and grief are experienced when one or more infants in a multiple gestation survives and one or more infants in the same gestation dies. Contrary to myth, parents do not grieve less or simply forget about the loss of one infant in their happiness to have another living infant. Parents faced with the death of an infant from a multiple gestation have special concerns:

- A more acute sense of loss; having "aching arms" despite an infant or infants to hold
- Grief, not only for the lost child, but also for the loss of prestige and attention associated with a multiple birth
- Fears about the health of the surviving infant(s), especially if ill
- Inability to grieve adequately for the dead infant, because of concerns and responsibilities for the living infant(s)
- Potential problems in attachment to the surviving infant(s); concern that their grief will in some way affect the surviving infant(s)
- Worry that the surviving infant(s) will always be a reminder of the dead infant
- Feelings of guilt, failure, or low self-esteem, related to loss of the infant, for example, the perception that the infant's death represented inability to handle multiple children or had some connection to personal thoughts and preferences

The box entitled Nursing Strategies for Parents Experiencing Death and Survival of One or More Infants of a Multiple Gestation summarizes nursing strategies for care of parents experiencing death and survival of one or more infants of a multiple gestation.

► ## NURSING STRATEGIES FOR PARENTS EXPERIENCING DEATH AND SURVIVAL OF ONE OR MORE INFANTS OF A MULTIPLE GESTATION

Anticipate complex feelings of joy and grief, and identify the parents' responses to the loss and survival of the infants.

Ensure that parents are informed about the causes of the infant's death, if known, and about the health status of the surviving infant(s).

Validate the reality, normality, and importance of the parents' feelings. Provide an atmosphere of privacy and enough time for parents to express conflicting feelings, such as concerns over bonding with the surviving infant and comparing the infant who survived with the infant who died. Provide anticipatory guidance about conflicting responses that may normally be experienced on anniversary dates, such as birthdays and holidays.

Encourage parents to verify which infant lived and which died. Assist parents in their progress through the grieving process (e.g., in holding the dead infant and in gathering mementos) although they still have a living infant.

Remind parents of the importance of sharing feelings with each other.

Avoid actions and words that negate or minimize the loss of the infant. Educate parents, their significant others, and health care providers about the negative effects of comments that deny the loss of the infant (e.g., "You're better off with one" or "You should be happy that you do have a baby").

Encourage parents to seek help with child care for the surviving infant without feeling guilty.

Encourage parents to speak freely about the dead infant and also to inform the survivor as he or she gets older. Caution the parents about idealizing the dead infant to the survivor or in ways that would make the survivor feel inadequate.

Refer parents to support groups and to counseling as appropriate.

Reproduced, with permission, from Whitaker, C.M. (1986). Death before birth. *American Journal of Nursing, 86,* 157–158.

► Nursing Strategies for Discharge of Bereaved Parents

Discharge from the hospital can be painful after perinatal death. Although the mother physically goes through postpartum changes, she has no infant to bring home with her or she may bring home only the survivor(s) of her multiple gestation. Parents face mourning rather than the celebration usually accompanying homecoming after childbirth. Nurses can facilitate discharge for parents by providing anticipatory guidance and by asking questions that may help parents cope with their feelings. Nurses can help parents deal with potential questions such as, "How will you tell your friends and neighbors that your baby died?" and "How do you think you will feel when you leave with no baby to take home?" (Estok & Lehman, 1983).

Physical wellness promotes emotional health during grieving. Discharge teaching should include the importance of healthy, healing lifestyle practices such as a well-balanced diet, avoidance of substances such as tobacco, alcohol, and mind-altering drugs, daily exercise, and adequate rest, even if the parents are unable to sleep. The couple should be advised to have a physical examination about 4 months after discharge, because of the potential risk for developing illness during intense grief. Keeping a journal, writing to or about the infant, and reading on grief-related topics may provide comfort. Nurses may also advise couples to postpone major life decisions, if possible, as decision processes can be affected by grief. The importance of sharing feelings with significant others and reaching out for help should be emphasized.

Prior to discharge, clients may be referred to bereavement support groups, available in many communities. These support groups are often organized by parents who have had children in an NICU or who have experienced perinatal death. They may meet regularly and offer a parent-to-parent support network, usually without charge. Support groups frequently work closely with NICU staff; group members may also be available to meet individually with parents within the NICU setting. Some NICUs have developed their own successful perinatal crisis support groups to provide support, information, and other interventions to help clients deal with perinatal loss. These groups may be composed of medical and nursing staff, clergy, social workers, and other parents who have experienced perinatal loss. Such groups may help implement a plan of supportive care for bereaved clients and offer educational programs about perinatal loss to other health care providers and to laypersons.

► Follow-up Nursing Care for Bereaved Parents

Ensuring client follow-up is an essential staff responsibility prior to discharge. Follow-up can take many forms. Telephone calls and home or office visits may take place through social service or through a home or community-based nursing service. In traditional settings, staff nurses usually do not provide postdischarge follow-up care. It is, however, appropriate for staff who have cared for the client during her hospitalization to call to express concern for her postdischarge progress. When available, interdisciplinary grief support teams may begin work with the client at the time of diagnosis or delivery and continue contact after discharge. Their goals may include providing ongoing comfort and support, encouraging grief expression, and promoting the mourning process.

► PSYCHOSOCIAL IMPLICATIONS OF THE DEATH OF A MOTHER

A walk through an old cemetery will often reveal that many young women died in childbirth. Advances in care and technology have greatly decreased the chance of dying during childbearing; today, childbearing women are not expected to die. However, a small number of women do die from such external problems as trauma (e.g., motor vehicle accidents, abuse) and pathologic conditions that pre-date or occur during childbearing (e.g., severe cardiac disease, infections, hemorrhage). At times, emergency cesarean delivery may save the fetus. However, the fetus often dies with the mother; death occurring in the postpartum period leaves a newborn without a mother.

The reasons for a mother's death create unique problems. For example, an HIV-infected infant of a mother who dies of AIDS may not have family able to care for him or her; placement of such an infant can be more difficult than for an uninfected, healthy infant. With appropriate prenatal care, plans for the client and her baby can be made. However, a previously healthy pregnant woman who dies in a car accident or as the result of a pulmonary embolism leaves a family unexpectedly. As one grief-stricken father stated, ". . . I keep waiting to wake from this awful nightmare. How could she be dead? I need to talk to her. All the plans we had for the family, everything . . . is just . . . gone."

Maternal death can result in intense crisis, grief, and mourning for families. When an infant survives, issues related to caretakers emerge. In some cases, lack of social support results in the infant's need for placement through social services. Family members require an organized, caring, team approach. They will need to understand the circumstances of the mother's death and be assisted in making burial arrangements. The father, grandparents, or significant others may need special teaching related to infant care, as well as the opportunity for crisis interventions. The family also should receive information about grief resources in their community and be assisted in making contact. Plans for follow-up, such as telephone calls, should be made.

Staff members may also experience shock, sadness, and grief at the loss of a client. Interdisciplinary staff meetings, including a specialist in grief work, can be helpful as staff struggle to cope with such a tragedy.

▶ SPIRITUAL SUPPORT OF THE HIGH-RISK CHILDBEARING FAMILY

Throughout life, the spiritual dimension of health care can help clients find comfort, strength, meaning, and perseverance to cope with crisis. Spiritual support can be especially important to the high-risk childbearing family. While spirituality may include religion, it is a broader concept that is not confined to specific religions or houses of worship (Miller, 1995; Sumner, 1998). Families do not need to consider themselves "religious" to benefit greatly from spiritual assistance during crisis and mourning.

Many hospitals, especially those with religious affiliations, have pastoral care programs through which chaplains or other pastoral care representatives visit hospitalized clients. Local churches and synagogues may also have individuals available on an "on call" basis (Fig. 12–5). Frequently, these people are skilled in crisis intervention and in dealing with grief and loss. Although representatives from pastoral care routinely meet with clients from their own religion, they can meet with clients regardless of background. As one mother recalled, "We were crying in the back of the unit when the nurse brought the Catholic chaplain to us during rounds. Although we are Jewish, she talked with us privately for over an hour. She was so caring and calm that she helped us to find the spiritual strength to somehow face what we had to. I'd like nurses to know that sorrow is sorrow, not Jewish, Catholic, Protestant or other sorrow."

In providing care that addresses spiritual needs, nurses need to identify the importance of spiritual beliefs and the impact of a client's culture on the

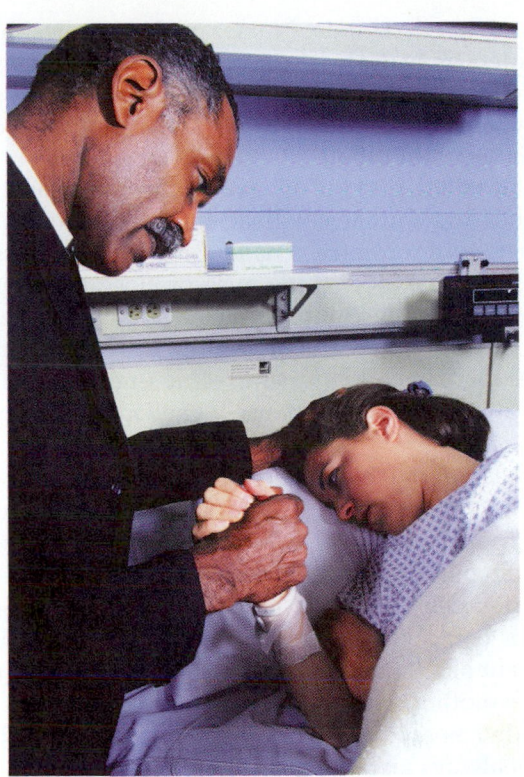

FIGURE 12–5. Spiritual support is often helpful for the high-risk childbearing family.

nature and means of expression of those beliefs. In addition, nurses working with the childbearing family need to know about spiritual resources available at their own hospitals and in their own communities. Whenever possible, nurses should meet their representatives and learn about the services offered. Pastoral care should be regarded as an integral part of the care of the high-risk childbearing family.

At times, clients may request the nurse to pray with them. Joining clients in prayer is appropriate, if the nurse is comfortable with this role (Sumner, 1998); however, nurses should not insist that clients pray or attempt to influence clients with their own religious beliefs.

▶ NURSES' RESPONSES TO CARE OF HIGH-RISK FAMILIES

High-risk conditions bring clients into frequent and extended contact with nurses in clinic, office, hospital, and community-based settings. In situations where primary care is practiced, nurses assume ongoing responsibility for client care planning and delivery. Neonatal special care nurses may work with families for prolonged periods. Nurses and other health care providers may form close professional relationships with clients as they strive together to maintain a pregnancy, ensure a healthy birth, and work toward the discharge of an infant.

As noted previously, every nurse working with childbearing families will at some point come into contact with obstetric crisis. Psychologic stress for staff may be expected, because of close involvement with emotionally draining client situations. Dealing with expected or unexpected high-risk conditions makes parent–child nursing sometimes painful and frustrating, yet also immensely challenging and satisfying.

One of the old-time myths is that health care providers should not become emotionally involved with client situations. By the nature of professional nursing and the amount of time devoted to the care of high-risk clients, nurses *are* involved. Client perception of being cared about is important to the establishment of a therapeutic relationship. As summarized by one mother who gave birth to a healthy infant after extended hospitalization, "My sanity was saved, my spirits always aimed upward, because I was secure in the knowledge that the nurses taking care of me *really do care."*

When a high-risk pregnancy is completed with safe delivery of a healthy and wanted infant, staff members share in the joy and satisfaction. Despite the best and most intensive caring efforts, there are times when adverse maternal, fetal, or neonatal outcomes occur. Severe social problems may result in parents' being unwilling or unable to care for their infant. Situations such as a lost pregnancy, fetal death, or a sick infant who dies after a prolonged intensive care stay are stressful for all staff members who have worked closely with the clients. Further, delivery of care in high-risk situations often generates ethical dilemmas for staff. These difficult conflicting situations produce great stress.

Sometimes the magnitude of a client's hardship does not seem "fair." Staff as well as family members may grieve, experience feelings of helplessness and sorrow, and question whether or not they did all that could be done for the client (Downey, Bengiamin, Heuer, & Juhl, 1995). In addition, staff members may be caught in a variety of ethical dilemmas related to care, as with do not resuscitate orders for a neonate. Over time, "burnout" may occur. Staff may respond by emotionally distancing themselves from co-workers, manifesting a "short temper," starting conflicts with other staff members, or feeling depressed. Frequent staff turnover is another manifestation of stress in high-risk client care settings.

▶ Stress Reduction Strategies for Staff Members Caring for High-Risk Clients

One way to promote excellent high-risk client care is to undertake strategies to help staff emotionally prepare for and deal with these situations. Every unit caring for the childbearing family needs to have staff able to attend to the emotional as well as physical needs of clients, even if the clients are to be transferred to another facility. It is no longer considered revolutionary to acknowledge stress reactions among staff members. Experiencing stress related to client care is not unusual but rather an expected outcome of interactions with other human beings.

Staff planning conferences can explore potential staff reactions and appropriate interventions, should a high-risk condition emerge. In addition, these meetings supply a forum to explore ethical conflicts related to care. These conferences should not be limited to nurses, but should include all personnel working closely with the high-risk client. When a high-risk client has been cared for, unit conferences that focus on staff members' positive and negative feelings about the client and situation can do much to promote feelings of support, sharing, and teamwork among staff. In high-risk units, staff meetings can be a regularly scheduled event, with time provided for discussion of staff feelings. Support from the head nurse or nurse manager and from co-workers, for example, through one-on-one talks among staff members, can be helpful, as can the assignment of two staff members to give direct care to difficult infants, such as those with fatal anomalies. New and inexperienced nurses especially need support (Downey et al., 1995).

Strategies dealing with stressful staff reactions to work with high-risk clients or ethical dilemmas in care delivery include the expertise of mental and spiritual health colleagues and ethics specialists. In some settings, clinical nurse specialists in psychology, psychiatric social workers, psychologists, psychiatrists, or ethicists are available to meet with unit staff members as a group or individually. These individuals may also be available as paid or volunteer consultants to facilities that do not regularly employ such specialists. Nurses can also rely on representatives from pastoral care for help in dealing with feelings about high-risk clients. Some ongoing staff programs are regularly attended by an interdisciplinary group of nurses, physicians, social workers, psychologists, ethicists, and pastoral care representatives.

Adequate staffing, accepting meal periods and short breaks as emotional necessities rather than luxuries, and avoidance of long work stretches or mandated double shifts are stress-relief strategies that are not limited to high-risk situations. Recognition of staff efforts and definition of success in terms of quality care, rather than happy client outcome, are also important. In addition, nurses need to become skilled in recognizing care-related stress and ethical dilemmas among colleagues. Nurses and other health care providers also experience grief over perinatal death, particularly if they have cared for a baby and a family

in NICU. Hammer and colleagues (1992) described rituals of remembrance that staff in their hospital used to deal with such personal feelings as depression, helplessness, and unspoken grief following the death of a child. A particular time was set aside for staff to get together. Sharing feelings, as well as food and a special song ("Let Her Go" by Betsy Rose), helped staff members to gain comfort and strength and to work together effectively.

Critical Thinking in Care Planning

Care of the Parents of a Neonate Transported to a Regional NICU

Mary and Mark Mendez, both 28 years old, experienced a low-risk, uncomplicated pregnancy and planned to deliver at their local community hospital. Mary looked forward to breastfeeding. After 18 hours of labor, however, Mary had an unexpected cesarean delivery for fetal distress. Her membranes had spontaneously ruptured 36 hours prior to delivery.

Baby James, 40 weeks' gestation, had Apgar scores of 8 and 9 and at first appeared well; one day after birth, he was noted to have difficulty maintaining normal body temperature. After a seizure was observed, plans were made for Baby James to be transferred to the neonatal special care nursery at the regional center 20 miles away. His admitting diagnosis was to be "possible sepsis," and intravenous antibiotic therapy was begun. Mary was to remain in the community hospital where she delivered; her husband would accompany the transport team. Although the transfer was to take place during the night, Mary called her mother, sister, and brother-in-law who came immediately to the hospital. Mary and Mark responded to the news of the transfer in a frightened, tearful manner. Mary seemed unable to stop crying and asked her sister to "go in my place for the baby."

▶ Assessment

- Emergency cesarean delivery for fetal distress
- Neonate to be transported to NICU 20 miles away
- Neonate's diagnosis: "possible sepsis"
- Parents visibly upset and tearful

- Parents appear frightened; mother unable to stop crying
- Mother planned to breastfeed; describes disappointment about inability to breastfeed because of neonate's transport to NICU

Nursing Diagnosis

Fear, related to transport of neonate and potential threat to physical well-being of neonate.

Expected Client/Family Outcomes	Nursing Action/Intervention	Evaluation
Prior to transport: • Parents will be able to identify reason for neonate's transfer. • Parents will maintain contact with the neonate. • Supportive family members will be included in transport preparation.	Assess parents' understanding of reason for transport and response to impending transport. Describe the transport and the NICU where neonate will be sent. *Rationale:* Clients may not ask yet still worry about what will happen to neonate and what NICU will be like, especially if they are unable to accompany neonate. Assist mother to nursery; provide opportunity for parents to see and touch neonate. While providing realistic information about neonate, identify positive aspects of neonate's physical status. *Rationale:* Contact with neonate facilitates parent–neonate attachment and helps parents to begin grieving process about high-risk status.	Prior to transport, parents are able to explain in their own words reason for transport. Prior to transport, parents see and hold neonate.

Critical Thinking in Care Planning continued

Expected Client/Family Outcomes	Nursing Action/Intervention	Evaluation
	Provide opportunity for mother's sister and brother-in-law to see and, if possible, touch neonate. *Rationale:* Allowing sister and brother-in-law to see and touch neonate fosters initial family attachment and supportive behavior.	Prior to transport, family members see neonate.
	Encourage a family member to stay with mother while sister-in-law goes with father to NICU. *Rationale:* Support of significant others is needed during periods of crisis.	During transport, a family member stays with mother and sister-in-law accompanies father.

Nursing Diagnosis
Anticipatory grieving, related to separation from neonate and concerns for well-being of neonate.

After transport, mother will be able to express her grief over ill neonate.	Provide privacy for mother. Encourage mother to express feelings; assist her to talk about her concerns and fears; identify her grief reaction as normal. *Rationale:* During vulnerable periods, clients need to be able to express feelings without presence of curious onlookers. The ability to express feelings freely is necessary for healthy crisis resolution.	Mother is provided with privacy. Mother expresses feelings to staff and progresses through grief process.
	Provide phone number of NICU. Encourage mother to call NICU for information about neonate; clarify information received. *Rationale:* Uncertainty can cause additional stress; clarification of information assists client in processing information.	Mother calls NICU and realistically describes information received.

Nursing Diagnosis
Interrupted breastfeeding, related to mother's separation from neonate.

Client will continue with plans to breastfeed by learning use of breast pumps and manual expression of milk.	Encourage mother's breastfeeding plans; teach use of breast pumps and how to manually express milk. Assist mother in bottling, labeling, and storing milk to be brought to neonate in NICU by her family. *Rationale:* Lactation can be established even when neonate is separated from mother. If mother does not begin and maintain lactation, her ability to breastfeed may be compromised. Ability to provide milk for neonate enhances mother's feelings of successful parenting.	Mother is able to use breast pump or manual expression technique to provide breast milk for neonate. Mother continues with plans to breastfeed.

Chapter Highlights

▶ High-risk conditions affect the entire childbearing family and place additional stress on the roles and functions of each family member.

▶ The theoretical bases of high-risk care of the childbearing family include crisis theory and an understanding of loss, grief, and mourning.

▶ Nurses can help couples considering a high-risk pregnancy by identifying the risks the pregnancy poses to mother and fetus, discussing the nature of high-risk care that will be required, explaining the life pattern changes that will occur with the high-risk pregnancy, correcting misconceptions, providing emotional support, and serving as sources of referral.

▶ High-risk pregnancy brings many psychosocial concerns, which include changes in maternal tasks, threats to self-image, problems related to the impact of prenatal diagnosis, and adaptation to the implications of having a pregnancy at high risk.

▶ Clients who have experienced pregnancy loss or the death of a child have special emotional needs.

▶ Prenatal hospitalization adds to the emotional burden for high-risk pregnancy, despite benefits related to physiologic interventions.

▶ Although bedrest has traditionally been prescribed for such conditions as preterm labor, it can also result in physical, emotional, and economic problems for the high-risk client and family.

▶ Childbirth education needs to be tailored to the needs and setting (either hospital or home) of high-risk pregnant women.

▶ The high-risk intrapartum experience superimposes the challenge of ensuring a safe delivery on the challenge of promoting a family-centered birth experience.

▶ Delivery of a healthy infant after a high-risk pregnancy may create a situational crisis for the childbearing family as they try to return to their normal lives.

▶ Clients who give birth to a high-risk infant need a unified, collaborative approach that assists them to maintain their self-esteem, to deal with the loss of their fantasized infant, and to develop a positive relationship with their infant who has special needs.

▶ Every infant admitted to intensive care is considered at risk, although the level of risk depends on the infant's condition.

▶ Nurses need to be aware of obstacles to parenting within the NICU, parents' concerns about prematurity and low birth weight, and the financial and emotional costs of intensive care to the family.

▶ Parents of an infant transferred to a NICU from another birthing site face special problems.

▶ Nursing strategies for families of infants in the NICU must also address the emotional needs of siblings and grandparents.

▶ Discharge of an infant from the NICU can create feelings of both happiness and relief as well as fear and helplessness; nurses need to implement strategies to help families prepare for discharge.

▶ High-risk families may need spiritual support, regardless of whether they previously considered themselves "religious."

▶ Strategies to deal with the emotional impact of high-risk care on staff members should be implemented in NICUs and high-risk settings to prevent stress and potential burnout.

After reading the vignette at the beginning of this chapter, use what you have learned to answer these questions:

1. What strategies can Elizabeth Thompson, RN, suggest to facilitate healthy interaction among Audra Reed and her sons Jesse and Grant?

2. In what ways might a NICU environment present obstacles to parenting?

3. What strengths might the Reeds develop from coping with this high-risk situation?

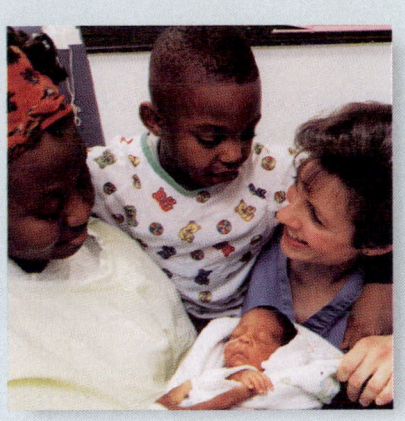

Critical Thinking Questions

▶ REFERENCES

Association of Women's Health, Obstetric, and Neonatal Nurses. (1998). *Standards and guidelines* (5th ed.). Washington, DC: Author.

Benfield, D.G., Leib, S.A., & Reuter, J. (1976). Grief response of parents after referral of the critically ill newborn to a regional center. *New England Journal of Medicine, 294,* 975–978.

Brown, L.D., Heermann J.A. (1997). The effect of developmental care on preterm infant outcome. *Applied Nursing Research, 10,* 190–197.

Calhoun, B.C., Hoeldtke N.J., Hinson R.M., & Judge K.M. (1997). Perinatal hospice: Should all centers have this service? *Neonatal Network,* 16:6, 101–102.

Caplan, G. (1982). Foreword. In M.S. Infante (Ed.), *Crisis theory: A framework for nursing practice* (pp v–vi). Reston, VA: Reston Publishing.

Carlson, G.E. (1993). When grandmothers take care of grandchildren. *MCN, American Journal of Maternal Child Nursing, 18,* 206–207.

Chesla, C.A., & Stannard, D. (1997). Breakdown in the nursing care of families in the ICU. *American Journal of Critical Care,* 6(1), 64–71.

Costello, A., Bracht, M., Van Camp, K., & Carman, L. (1996). Parent information binder: Individualizing education for parents of preterm infants. *Neonatal Network,* 15(5), 43–46.

Cunningham, F.G., MacDonald, P.C., Gant, N.F., Leveno, K.J., Gilstrap, L.C., Hankins, G.D.V., & Clark, S.L. (1997). *Williams Obstetrics* (20th ed.). Stamford, CT: Appleton & Lange.

Downey, V., Bengiamin, M., Heuer, L., & Juhl, N. (1995). Dying babies and associated stress in NICU nurses. *Neonatal Network,* 14(1), 41–46.

Dracup, K. (1993). Helping patients and families cope. *Critical Care Nurse,* 13(Supp.), 4–9.

Drosten-Brooks, F. (1993). Kangaroo care: Skin-to-skin contact in the NICU. *MCN, American Journal of Maternal Child Nursing, 18,* 250–253.

Estok, P., & Lehman, A. (1983). Perinatal death: Grief support for families. *Birth, 10,* 17–25.

Hammer, M., Nichols, D.J., & Armstrong, L. (1992). A ritual of remembrance. *MCN, American Journal of Maternal Child Nursing, 17,* 310–313.

Heuer, L. (1993). Parental stressors in a pediatric intensive care unit. *Pediatric Nursing, 19,* 128–131.

Jewell, S.E., & Yip, R. (1995). Increasing trends in plural births in the United States. *Obstetrics and Gynecology,* 85(2), 229–232.

Kavanaugh, K. (1997). Parents' experience surrounding the death of a newborn whose birth is at the margin of viability. *Journal of Obstetric, Gynecologic, and Neonatal Nursing,* 26(1), 43–51.

Kirk, E.P. (1984). Psychological effects and management of perinatal loss. *American Journal of Obstetrics and Gynecology, 149,* 46–51.

Klaus, M.H., & Kennell, J.H. (1982). Caring for the parents of a stillborn or an infant who dies. In M.H. Klaus & J.H. Kennell (Eds.), *Parent-infant bonding* (pp. 259–292). St. Louis: Mosby.

Klaus, M.H., & Kennell, J.H. (1993). Care of the parents. In M.H. Klaus & A.A. Fanaroff (Eds.), *Care of the high-risk neonate* (4th ed.) (pp. 189–211). Philadelphia: W. B. Saunders.

Klaus, M.H., Kennell, J.H., & Klaus, P.H. (1995). *Bonding: Building the foundations of secure attachment and independence.* Reading, MA: Addison-Wesley.

Kledzik T., & Howell, V. (1996). On becoming an NICU. *Neonatal Network, 15,* 25–33.

Kleiber, C., Halm, M., Titler, M., Montgomery, L.A., Johnson, S.K., Nicholson, A., Craft, M., Buckwalter, K., & Megivern, K. (1994). Emotional responses of family members during a critical care hospitalization. *American Journal of Critical Care, 3,* 70–76.

Kolotylo, C.J., Parker, N.I., & Chapman, J.S. (1991). Mothers' perceptions of their neonates' in-hospital transfers from a neonatal intensive-care unit. *Journal of Obstetric, Gynecologic, and Neonatal Nursing, 20,* 146–153.

Kubler-Ross, E. (1969). *On death and dying.* New York: Macmillan.

Kushner, H.S. (1981). *When bad things happen to good people.* New York: Avon.

Lederman, R. (1996). *Psychosocial adaptation in pregnancy: Assessment of seven dimensions of maternal development* (2nd ed.). New York: Springer.

Lefrak-Okikawa, L., & Lund, C.H. (1993). Nursing practice in the neonatal intensive care unit. In M.H. Klaus & A.A. Fanaroff (Eds.), *Care of the high-risk neonate* (4th ed.) (pp. 212–227). Philadelphia: W.B. Saunders.

Lindemann, E. (1944). Symptomatology and management of acute grief. *American Journal of Psychiatry, 101,* 141–148.

Lindsay, J.K. (1993). Creative caring in the NICU. Parent-to-parent support. *Neonatal Network, 12,* 37–44.

Ludington-Hoe, S.M., & Golant, S. (1993). *Kangaroo care: The best you can do to help your preterm infant.* New York: Bantam.

Maloni, J.A., Chance, B., Zhang, C., Cohen, A.W., Betts, D., & Gange, S.J. (1993). Physical and psychosocial side effects of antepartum hospital bed rest. *Nursing Research, 42,* 197–203.

McHaffie, H.E. (1992). Social support in the neonatal intensive care unit. *Journal of Advanced Nursing, 17,* 279–287.

Meier, P.P., Engstrom, J.L., Mangurten, H.H., Estrada, E., Zimmerman, B., & Kopparthi, R. (1993). Breastfeeding support services in the neonatal intensive-care unit. *Journal of Obstetric, Gynecologic, and Neonatal Nursing, 22,* 338–347.

Miles, A. (1993). Caring for the family left behind. *American Journal of Nursing, 93,* 34–36.

Miles, M.S., Carlson, J., & Funk, S.G. (1996). Sources of support reported by mothers and fathers of infants hospitalized in a neonatal intensive care unit. *Neonatal Network, 15*(3), 45–52.

Miller, M.A. (1995). Culture, spirituality, and Women's health. *Journal of Obstetric, Gynecologic, and Neonatal Nursing, 24:* 3, 257–264.

Parkman, S.E. (1992). Helping families say good-bye. *MCN: American Journal of Maternal Child Nursing, 17,* 14–17.

Primeau, M.R., Lamb, J.M. (1995). When a baby dies: Rights of the baby and parents. *Journal of Obstetric, Gynecologic, and Neonatal Nursing, 24:* 3, 206–210.

Raines, D.A. (1996). Parents' values: A missing link in the neonatal intensive care equation. *Neonatal Network, 15*(3), 7–12.

Rubin, R. (1984). *Maternal identity and the maternal experience.* New York: Springer.

Ryan, P.F., Cote-Arsenault, D., & Sugarman, L.L. (1991). Facilitating care after perinatal loss: A comprehensive checklist. *Journal of Obstetric, Gynecologic, and Neonatal Nursing, 20,* 385–389.

Saunders C. (1965). The last stages of life. *American Journal of Nursing, 65,* 70–75.

Schroeder, C.A. (1998). Bed rest in complicated pregnancy: A critical analysis. *MCN, American Journal of Maternal Child Nursing, 23*(1), 45–49.

Shields-Poë, D., & Pinelli, J. (1997). Variables associated with parental stress in neonatal intensive care units. *Neonatal Network, 16*(1), 29–37.

Sumner, C.H. (1998). Recognizing and responding to spiritual distress. *American Journal of Nursing, 98*(1), 26–30.

Wallerstedt, C., & Higgins, P. (1996). Facilitating perinatal grieving between the mother and the father. *Journal of Obstetric, Gynecologic, and Neonatal Nursing, 25*(5), 389–394.

Weingarten, C.T., Baker, K., Manning, W., & Kutzner, S.K. (1990). Married mothers' perceptions of their premature or term infants and the quality of their relationships with their husbands. *Journal of Obstetric, Gynecologic, and Neonatal Nursing, 19,* 64–73.

Wereszczak, J., Miles, M.S., & Holditch-Davis, D. (1997). Maternal recall of the neonatal intensive care unit. *Neonatal Network, 16*(4), 33–40.

Wong, D.L. (1980). Bereavement: The empty mother syndrome. *MCN, American Journal of Maternal Child Nursing, 5,* 385–389.

Zeanah, C.H., Dailey, J.V., Rosenblatt, M.J., & Saller, D.N., Jr. (1993). Do women grieve after terminating pregnancies because of fetal anomalies? A controlled investigation. *Obstetrics and Gynecology, 82,* 270–275.

III

Pregnancy

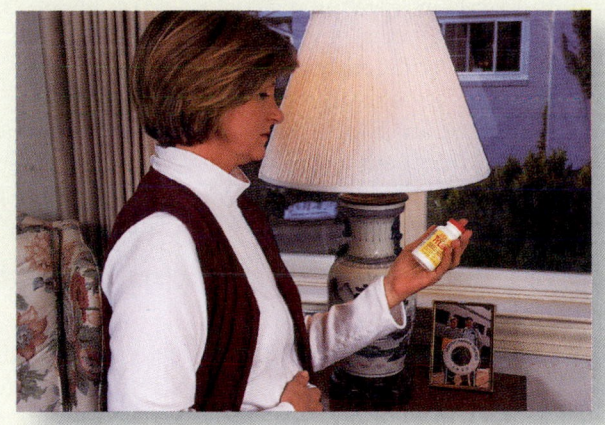

Laura O'Connor, 12 weeks' pregnant, is expecting her third child. While Laura is experiencing a healthy pregnancy, she occasionally has mild headaches, especially after a stressful day with her older children. Today, when talking with her sister-in-law Eileen, Laura closes her eyes briefly and rubs her forehead. When Eileen learns that Laura has been having headaches, she asks, "Why don't you take something to relieve the pain?" Laura responds, "I don't think I should; it might hurt the baby." Eileen says, "I have a friend who took an allergy medication for her sinus headaches when she was pregnant, and the baby was fine. I'm sure if you took it once it wouldn't do any harm."

Later that day, Laura goes to the locked cabinet in which she stores medications and takes out the bottle of acetaminophen. In the directions that are printed on the bottle, she reads that pregnant women are advised to contact a health professional before using the product. Laura thinks to herself, "Do I really need to call the doctor's office about this? It's only a headache." ∎

13

Growth and Development of the Embryo/Fetus

Over the centuries many theories have been put forth to explain fertilization and reproduction. These include the familiar "old wives' tales," some of which had their origins in folk medicine. In modern times, talented researchers have labored diligently to define the molecular events essential to successful reproduction. Their research has resulted in improved pregnancy outcomes, genetic advances, advances in the treatment of infertility, and development of safe and effective birth control methods. Despite the breakthroughs in research contributing to the knowledge of reproductive mechanisms, fertilization and reproduction remain a wondrous process through which a single human egg develops into a 7½-pound infant.

The processes that transform the fertilized human egg into a baby are discussed in this chapter. They include: conception, growth and development during the preembryonic, embryonic, and fetal periods, development of the placenta, and development of twins and multiple births. In addition, effects of the environment on the developing embryo and fetus, including infectious agents, drugs, alcohol, and radiation, are discussed.

The nurse's role during development of the embryo and fetus is one of advocate and counselor. Early in the pregnancy, the mother may not know what to expect; indeed, she may be unaware that she is pregnant and thus unlikely to seek health care. Anticipatory guidance for this period should be provided to women of childbearing age at their regular checkups, in school health classes, in community groups, and through educational materials that are readily available to women of all economic and social groups. This anticipatory guidance should include planning for pregnancy, genetic counseling (if indicated), nutritional counseling, general health counseling, and teaching and counseling regarding embryonic and fetal development. As an advocate, the nurse assists the client in negotiating the health care system during pregnancy, plans for delivery and ongoing care for the mother and her family, coordinates interagency activities, and prepares the family for the new member.

▶ CONCEPTION

The time span during which **conception,** the union of male sperm and female ovum resulting in fertilization, can take place is quite limited in the usual 28-day menstrual cycle. The oocyte, or ovum, is thought to survive only 12 to 24 hours after ovulation. It is now believed that sperm may remain alive in the female reproductive tract up to 72 hours.

Fertilization (the process in which a sperm penetrates the outer layer of the ovum and begins a chain of events resulting in development of the human embryo) usually occurs in the wide lateral portion, or ampulla, of the fallopian tube. Contractility of the fallopian tube is increased as a result of high estrogen levels at the time of ovulation. This heightened contractility serves to move the ovum through the fallopian tube. The high estrogen levels also cause an increase in the amount of cervical mucus, which is less viscous and more easily penetrated by spermatozoa. Spermatozoa move through the cervix, the body of the uterus, and into the fallopian tubes by using their flagella (tails) and by means of uterine contractions. The total critical time span during which fertilization may occur is 24 to 48 hours. This includes the 12 to 24 hours preceding ovulation and the 12 to 24 hours following ovulation; fertilization usually occurs within 24 hours of ovulation. Spermatozoa must remain in the female genital tract 4 to 6 hours before they are capable of fertilizing the ovum.

▶ Prefertilization

The mature ovum is surrounded by two plasma membranes, the zona pellucida and the corona radiata. The zona pellucida is the clear, gelatinous, noncellular layer closest to the cell membrane; its function is not known. The corona radiata is a ring of elongated cells that radiate from the ovum like the gaseous corona around the sun. The zona pellucida and corona radiata are held together by hyaluronic acid, through which the sperm must penetrate to achieve fertilization.

Before a mature sperm can penetrate the corona radiata and zona pellucida, it must undergo **capacitation.** Capacitation is an enzymatic process that results in the removal of plasma protein over the acrosome. The acrosome contains enzymes that are believed to facilitate sperm penetration of the ovum. After capacitation, the acrosome of the sperm undergoes a sequence of events termed the **acrosome reaction.** During this reaction, the acrosome undergoes structural changes: the outer membrane fuses with the overlying cell membrane of the sperm head, and the fused membranes rupture, producing multiple perforations (England, 1996). During the acrosome reaction, the enzymes hyaluronidase and proteinase are secreted by the acrosome. They are released through the perforations in the acrosome of the sperm, and help to dissolve the membranes of the ovum. Progesterone, secreted by the ovum, also seems to stimulate the acrosomal process in the sperm (Fig. 13–1).

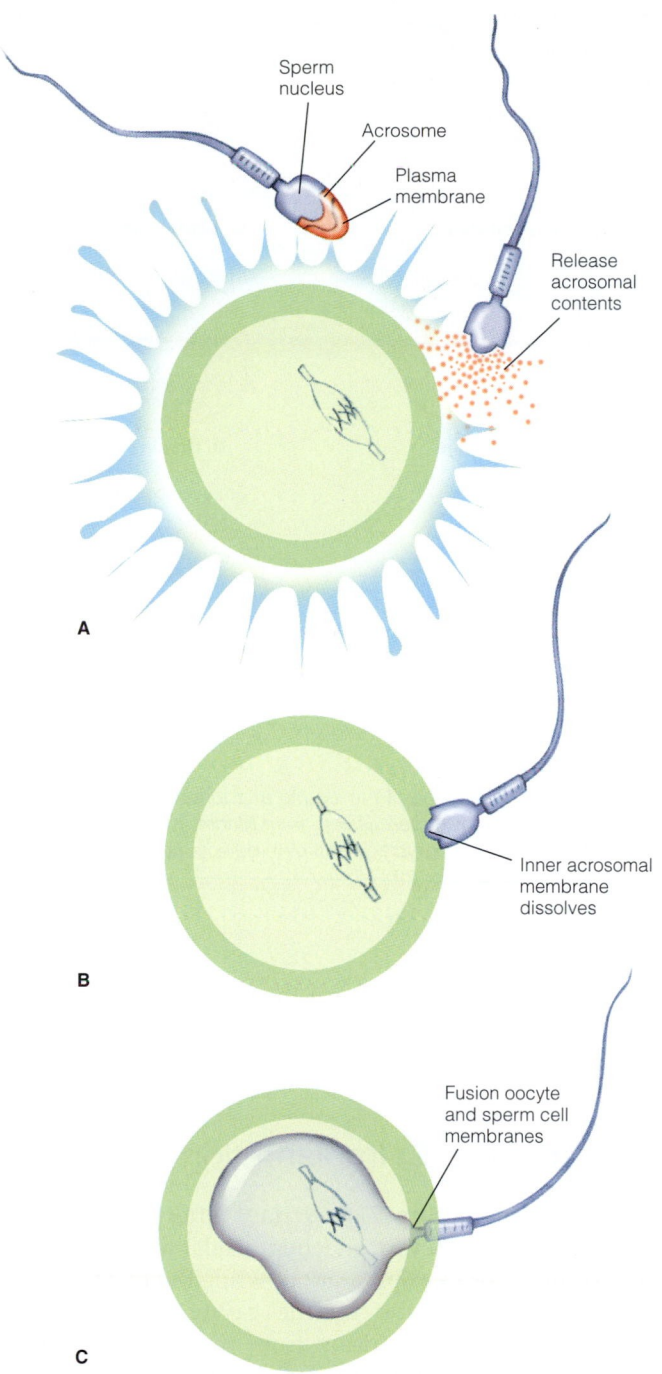

FIGURE 13–1. Acrosome reaction. **A.** Rupturing of the fused membranes of the sperm head and release of hyaluronidase and proteinase through the perforations in the acrosome. **B.** Sperm penetration of the ovum. **C.** Fusion of the sperm and oocyte cell membranes.

▶ Fertilization

As the spermatozoa surround the ovum they deposit minute amounts of hyaluronidase, which break down enough hyaluronic acid in the outer layer to allow one sperm to penetrate the ovum. The head and neck of the sperm enter the ovum and the zona pellucida and the corona radiata fuse. Once the sperm has entered the ovum, the egg responds in three ways: (1) cortical and zona reactions, (2) resumption of the second meiotic division, and (3) metabolic activation (Cunningham et al., 1997).

Cortical and Zona Reactions

The ovum membrane becomes impenetrable to other spermatozoa and the zona pellucida alters its structure and composition, thus preventing more than one sperm from penetrating the ovum.

Resumption of the Second Meiotic Division

It should be recalled that at ovulation the oocyte begins the second meiotic division (meiosis II), but the division is arrested at metaphase (see Chapter 6). The resumption and completion of the second meiotic division occur immediately after entry of one spermatozoa. One of the daughter cells, the second polar body, does not mature. The other daughter cell matures and its nucleus becomes known as the female pronucleus. The female pronucleus contains 22 autosomes and an X sex chromosome.

Metabolic Activation of the Egg

Postfusion activation occurs, including the initial cellular and molecular changes necessary for growth and development associated with early embryogenesis. The activating factor is probably carried by the sperm (Cunningham et al., 1997).

▶ Postfertilization

On penetration of the ovum, the sperm moves forward and lies in close proximity to the female pronucleus. The sperm nucleus enlarges and becomes the male pronucleus, which contains 22 autosomes and an X or Y sex chromosome. The tail of the sperm detaches from the head and degenerates. The male and female pronuclei lose their nuclear membranes, fuse, and randomly intermingle their chromosomes, forming a new one-celled animal, the **zygote** (see Chapter 6).

▶ Factors Important to Fertilization

Fertilization is dependent on three factors: (1) maturation of the ovum and sperm, (2) motility of the sperm or ability of the sperm to reach the ovum, and (3) ability of the sperm to penetrate the zona pellucida and cell membrane of the ovum to achieve active fertilization. The zygote contains a new combination of genetic material that will develop into a new individual, different from anyone else in the world. The zygote will form the embryo and fetus as well as the structures needed to support the fetus during intrauterine life, such as the placenta, the fetal membranes, the amniotic fluid, and the umbilical cord.

▶ PREEMBRYONIC PERIOD

The first 14 days after conception, referred to as the **preembryonic period,** are characterized by rapid cellular multiplication and differentiation, establishment of embryonic membranes, and development of the primary germ layers. At the same time these changes are occurring, the placenta is developing.

▶ Days 1 to 3: Cleavage

Immediately after fertilization, rapid cell division of the zygote begins as the fertilized ovum is transported through the fallopian tube. This early cell division is called **cleavage.** The first cleavage occurs in about 36 hours, with each successive division taking slightly less time, until the process is completed in about 3 days. Although the number of cells in the zygote increases, the size of the developing organism does not increase at this time. Cleavage, which occurs in the fallopian tube, creates smaller cells, known as blastomeres, with each division (Fig. 13–2).

By the third day, a mulberry-like mass of cells (12–16 blastomeres) known as the **morula** has formed. The morula is thought to reach the uterine cavity at about the 12- to 16-cell stage, approximately 60 hours after fertilization.

The morula enters the uterus and is filled with fluid. The fluid within the morula pushes the blastomeres out to the periphery in two layers: the outer layer of cells forms the **trophoblast,** which establishes the nutrient relationship with the uterine endometrium, and the inner layer of cells **(embryoblast),** which differentiates into the embryo. The morula, now known as the **blastocyst,** contains fluid-filled spaces and two layers of cells (Fig. 13–2).

▶ Days 4 to 6: Continued Growth and Differentiation

By the fourth day, the fluid-filled spaces in the blastocyst form one large central space, called the blastocyst cavity. By day 6 the cells of the embryoblast are located at one pole of the blastocyst. These cells eventually form the embryo and amnion. The cells of the

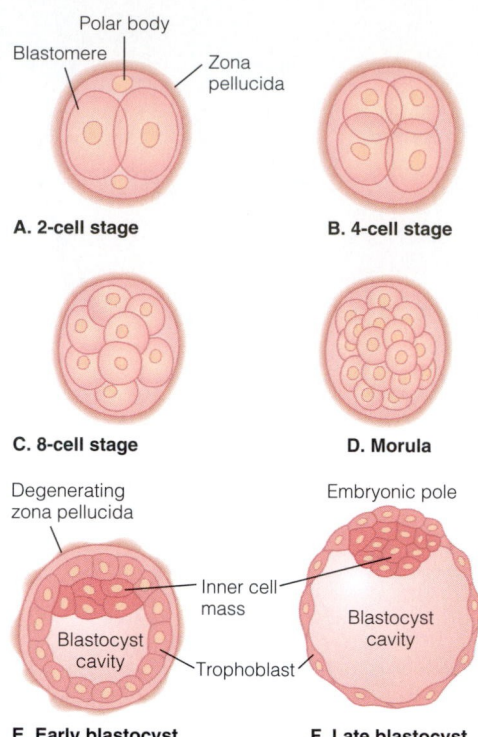

FIGURE 13–2. Cleavage of the zygote and formation of the blastocyst. *(Reproduced, with permission, from Moore, K.L. (1989). Before we are born: Basic embryology and birth defects (3rd ed.). Philadelphia: W.B. Saunders, p. 29.)*

trophoblast flatten and form the epithelial wall of the blastocyst, which eventually develops into the chorion (Figs. 13–2 and 13–3).

▶ Days 7 to 9: Implantation

Implantation occurs 7 to 9 days after fertilization, when the blastocyst attaches itself to the endometrium. Prior to implantation, while the blastocyst is floating freely in the uterine cavity, the fertilized ovum receives its nutrition from the uterine glands, which secrete a mixture of mucopolysaccharides, lipids, and glycogen. Implantation must occur for nourishment to continue.

At the time of implantation, the mucosa of the uterus is in the secretory (progestational) phase of the menstrual cycle. The arteries that supply the layers of the uterus become tortuous, forming a dense capillary bed just beneath the uterine epithelium. The endometrium becomes highly edematous and the uterine mucosa prepares to receive the blastocyst. Implantation often occurs along either the posterior or anterior wall of the body of the uterus. When the trophoblastic layer of cells in the blastocyst contacts the

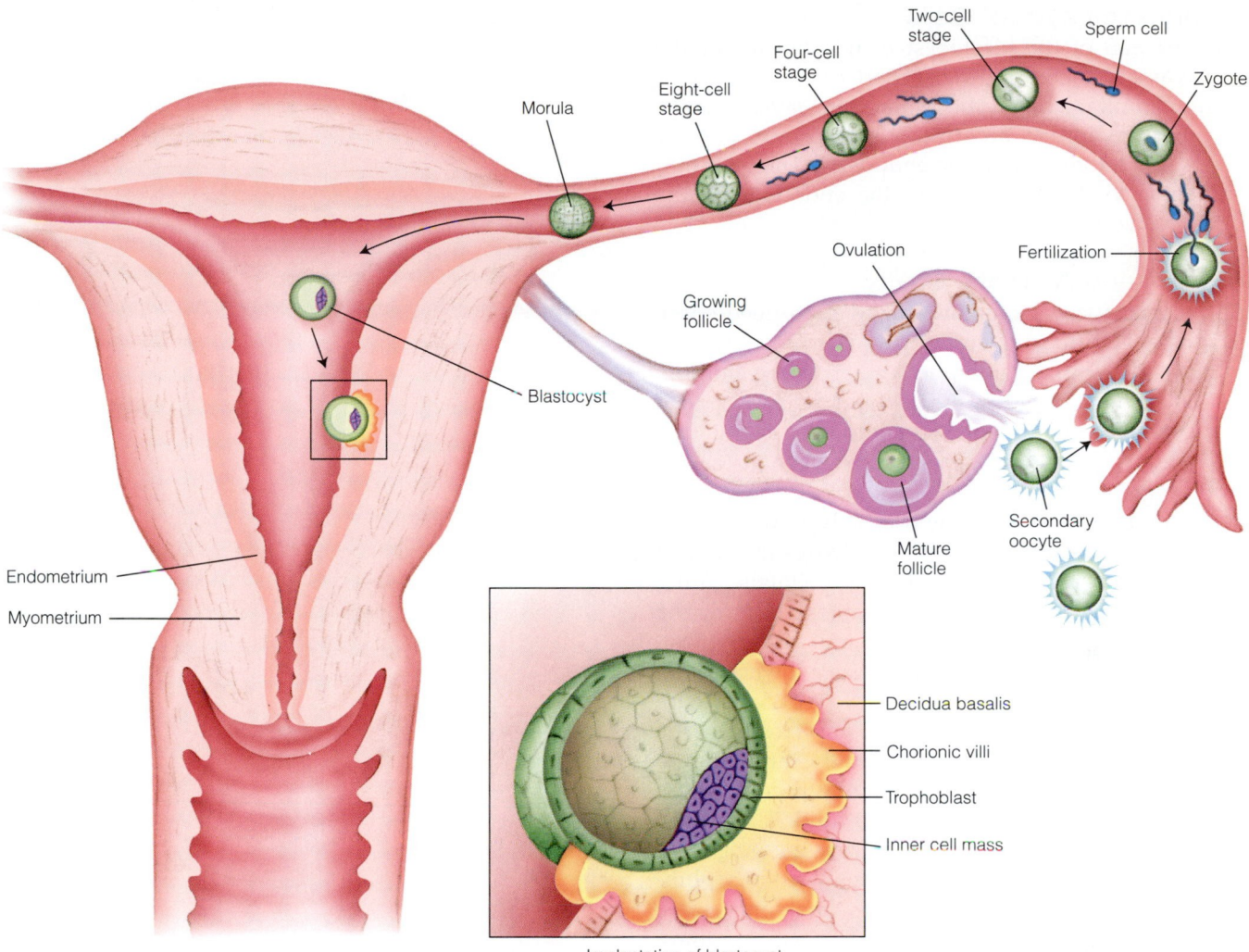

FIGURE 13–3. Sequence of implantation of the blastocyst.

endometrium, the trophoblast differentiates into two layers: the cytotrophoblast, which is composed of cells, and the syncytiotrophoblast, a protoplasmic mass.

Spaces called lacunae appear in the syncytiotrophoblast; these are filled with blood from the ruptured maternal capillaries in the endometrium. The syncytiotrophoblastic lacunae fuse and form lacunar networks; maternal blood flows slowly through these networks and a primitive uteroplacental circulation is established. Oxygenated blood passes into the lacunae from spiral arteries, and deoxygenated blood is removed from them by way of the veins of the uterus.

The blastocyst, now about 1/100th of an inch in diameter, becomes oriented so that the embryonic mass of cells is directed toward the endometrium, which is now known as the **decidua** (see next section). Implantation enables the blastocyst to absorb nutrients

from the glands and blood vessels of the decidua for its subsequent growth and development (see Fig. 13–3).

▶ Week 2: Preplacental Phase

Decidua

The endometrium undergoes changes in response to the action of progesterone to prepare for implantation and nutrition of the fertilized ovum. After implantation, the decidua undergoes several rapid changes. The portion of the decidua directly beneath the site of implantation forms the **decidua basalis** from which the maternal portion of the placenta develops. The portion that overlies the developing ovum and separates it from the rest of the uterine cavity is the **decidua capsularis.** The remaining area of the uterus is lined by the **decidua vera.**

Embryonic Layer of Cells

Implantation of the blastocyst in the decidua of the uterus is completed by the second week of development. Simultaneously, the embryonic layer of cells becomes the **embryonic disc,** which forms two basic layers: the ectoderm and the endoderm. The ectoderm gives rise to the amnion, and the endoderm to the primitive yolk sac.

Amnion and Amniotic Cavity

As the decidua is differentiating, a fluid-filled space develops around the embryo and is lined with a smooth, glistening membrane, known as the **amnion.** As the amnion enlarges, the growing embryo gradually extends into the space, or amniotic cavity, that contains amniotic fluid. The amnion expands as the embryo grows.

Although it is not known exactly how amniotic fluid forms, the volume of fluid increases to between 500 and 1000 mL of clear, slightly yellowish fluid, with a nonfoul characteristic odor, at term. During the first half of pregnancy, the fluid is similar in composition to maternal plasma, except it has a lower protein concentration. Later in pregnancy the fetus contributes to amniotic fluid through urine excretion. The fetus also absorbs amniotic fluid through the gastrointestinal tract by swallowing fluid. As the pregnancy advances, the amniotic fluid is found to contain phospholipids (primarily from the lungs), albumin, urea, uric acid, creatinine, lecithin, sphingomyelin, bilirubin, fat, fructose, inorganic salts, epithelial cells, some leukocytes, various enzymes, **lanugo** (the fine, downy hair that develops on the fetus during the fourth month of gestation), scalp hair, and **vernix caseosa** (a fatty secretion from the fetal sebaceous glands and epidermal cells that coats the skin of the fetus).

The amniotic cavity in which the embryo/fetus is suspended offers protection in several ways. The fluid acts as a cushion, allows for fetal movement, prevents the embryo/fetus from adhering to surrounding tissues, protects the embryo/fetus from infection, and helps to maintain an even temperature for the embryo/fetus.

Yolk Sac

Unlike yolks of other eggs, the **yolk sac** does not provide direct nutrition for the developing embryo/fetus; however, it does have several important functions. It transfers nutrients to the embryo while the uteroplacental circulation is being established and provides blood cells until embryonic/fetal hemopoiesis begins. In addition, cells of the yolk sac become incorporated into embryonic/fetal organs.

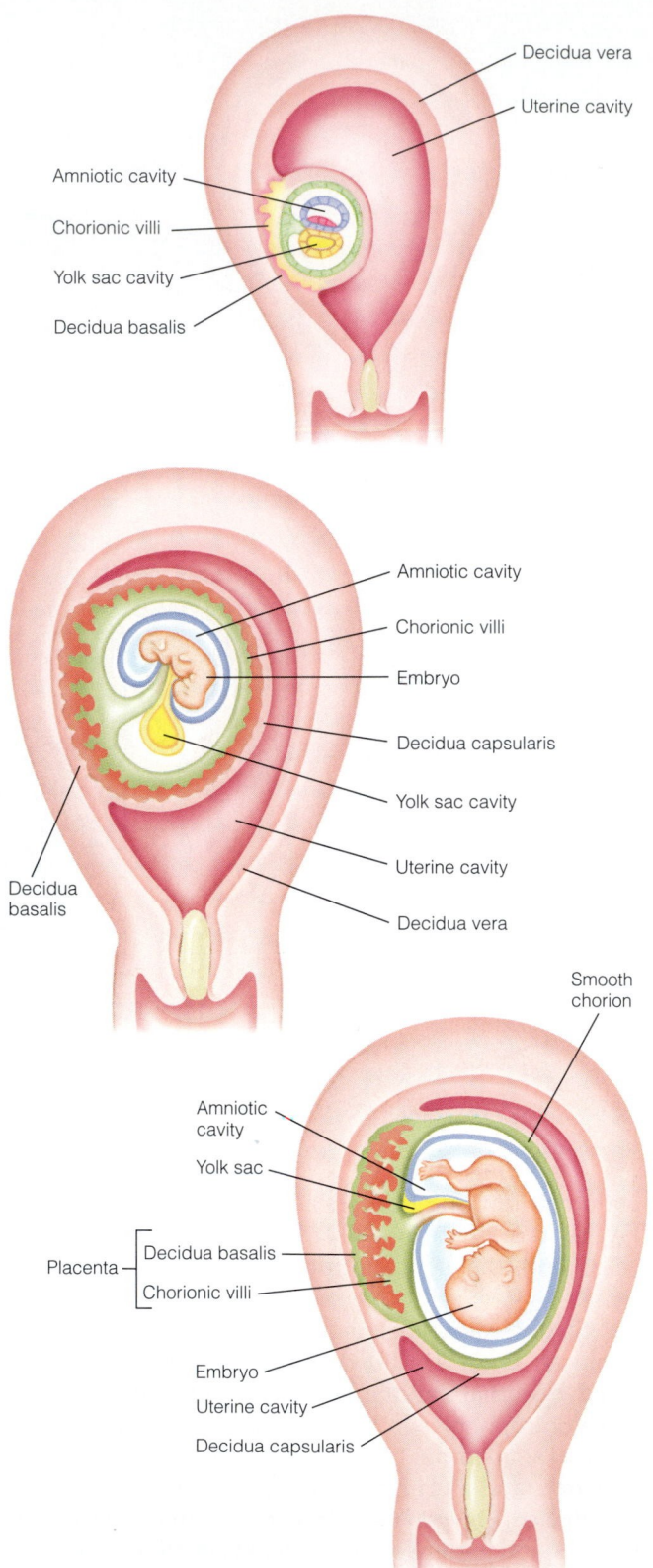

FIGURE 13–4. Sequence of development of the embryo, fetal membranes, and yolk sac during the preplacental phase of development.

▶ **TABLE 13–1**

Body Structures Derived from Primary Germ Layers

Endoderm	Mesoderm	Ectoderm
Epithelium of digestive tract and its glands	Dermis	Epidermis
Epithelium of respiratory tract	Skeleton	All nervous tissue
Epithelium of urinary bladder, gallbladder, and liver	Smooth and cardiac muscles	Hair follicles, nails, and sweat glands
Epithelium of pharynx, auditory tube, tonsils, larynx, trachea, bronchi, and lungs	Connective tissue (cartilage, bone)	Sebaceous glands
	Blood, bone marrow. and lymphoid tissue	Lens, cornea, optic nerve, and internal eye muscles
Primary tissue of liver and pancreas	Endothelium of blood vessels and lymphatics	Internal and external ear
Epithelium of urethra and associated glands, and vagina and associated parts	Fibrous tunic and vascular tunic of eye	Neuroepithelium of sense organs
	Middle ear	Nasal cavity
	Epithelium of kidneys, ureters, adrenal cortex, gonads, and genital ducts	Oral glands and tooth enamel
		Pituitary gland
		Mammary glands

Chorion

The **chorion** is the cellular membrane formed from the trophoblast. The thin, hairlike projections from the chorion are referred to as **chorionic villi.** The villi closest to the uterine wall (chorion frondosum) form the fetal portion of the placenta. The villi farthest from the uterine wall degenerate into a smooth membrane, the chorion laeve. The inner portion of the chorion adheres to the amnion and surrounds the developing fetus and amniotic fluid. The outer portion of the chorion lies against the decidua vera.

Umbilical Cord

The early embryo is connected to the yolk sac by a connecting or body stalk containing two arteries and one vein. During the rapid development of the embryo, the amniotic cavity enlarges and the amnion begins to envelop the body stalk and yolk sac, crowding them together. After the third month, when the amnion has come in contact with the chorion and has obliterated the chorionic cavity, the yolk sac shrinks and is gradually eliminated. The body stalk then lengthens to become the umbilical cord. The vessels in the cord are surrounded by a connective tissue known as **Wharton's jelly.** This tissue is rich in mucopolysaccharides and functions as a protective layer for the blood vessels (Fig. 13–4).

Germ Layers

After implantation, the inner cell mass of the blastocyst begins to differentiate in stages into the three primary germ layers: ectoderm, endoderm, and mesoderm.

At the end of the second week of development, the embryonic disc is bilaminar (two germ layers), consisting of the **ectoderm** (the outermost layer of cells) and the **endoderm** (the innermost layer of cells). At this time a groove, called the **primitive streak,** appears on the ectoderm. A new cell layer is visible on each side of the streak between the ectoderm and the endoderm. The cells migrate into the bottom of the primitive streak and form an intermediate germ layer known as the **mesoderm.** From these germ layers all tissues and organs of the body will develop. Table 13–1 summarizes the structures that are derived from the three germ layers.

▶ PLACENTAL DEVELOPMENT

Thr placenta tends to form and to fix itself in the area of the decidua (decidua basalis) where blood supply is richest. By the fourth month, the placenta has developed two compartments, the fetal portion formed by the chorion frondosum and the maternal portion formed by the decidua basalis. The fetal portion of the placenta is anchored to the maternal portion of the placenta by villi.

As the chorionic villi invade the decidua basalis, a number of wedge-shaped areas are formed; these are known as the placental septa. It is now thought that the placental septa are made up of fetal and maternal tissue. The septa divide the fetal part of the placenta into a number of irregular compartments called cotyledons, consisting of main-stem villi and many branches.

▶ Maternal Placental Structure

During erosion of the decidua basalis by the chorionic villi, blood-filled spaces form and enlarge.

These spaces, originally called lacunae, form a large blood sinus, which is bordered by the chorionic plate on one side and the decidua basalis on the other. The placental septa subdivide the blood sinus into many separate but connecting compartments. Each compartment, in turn, has an intervillous space.

Maternal blood enters the intervillous space through 80 to 100 spiral arteries (endometrial arteries) and is temporarily outside of the maternal circulatory system. The oxygenated blood is propelled toward the chorionic plate (fetal side of the intervillous space). The blood slowly circulates around the surface of the villi, allowing exchange of oxygen and nutrients with the fetal blood. The adequate bathing of the chorionic villi by maternal blood is the most significant factor in ensuring embryo/fetal well-being (England, 1996).

▶ Fetal Placental Structure

The chorionic villi are anchored to the chorionic plate of the trophoblast (fetal portion of placental circulation). Within the chorionic villi of the embryo/fetus are arterial–venous–capillary networks. The arteries, which are the terminal ends of the umbilical arteries, allow deoxygenated blood from the fetus to diffuse into the maternal blood in the intervillous spaces. In addition, oxygen and nutrients from the maternal blood diffuse into the thin-walled fetal veins that eventually converge to form the umbilical vein. The umbilical vein carries oxygenated blood to the fetus (Fig. 13–5).

▶ Placental Membrane

Normally, fetal and maternal blood do not mingle because of the **placental membrane.** This membrane arises solely from fetal tissues composing the chorionic villi. Up to the 20th week of pregnancy, the placental membrane consists of four layers: (1) syncytiotrophoblast, (2) cytotrophoblast, (3) connective tissue core of the villus, (4) endothelium of the fetal capillary.

As pregnancy progresses, some of these layers degenerate, leaving a thin membrane referred to as the **syncytial membrane.** The fetal circulatory network (capillaries, arteries, and veins) lies in close proximity to the syncytial membrane. This thin, intact membrane separates fetal and maternal blood during pregnancy (Fig. 13–6).

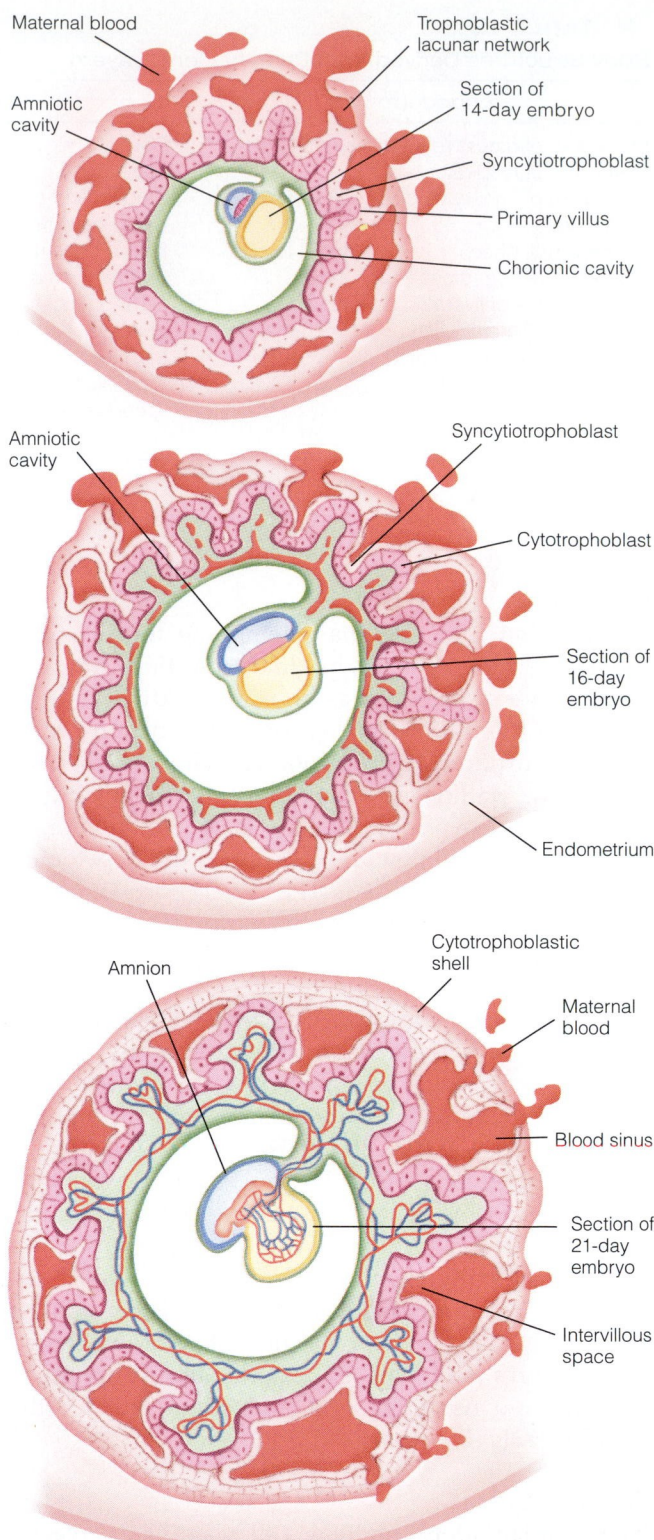

FIGURE 13–5. Longitudinal section of maternal and fetal placental structures.

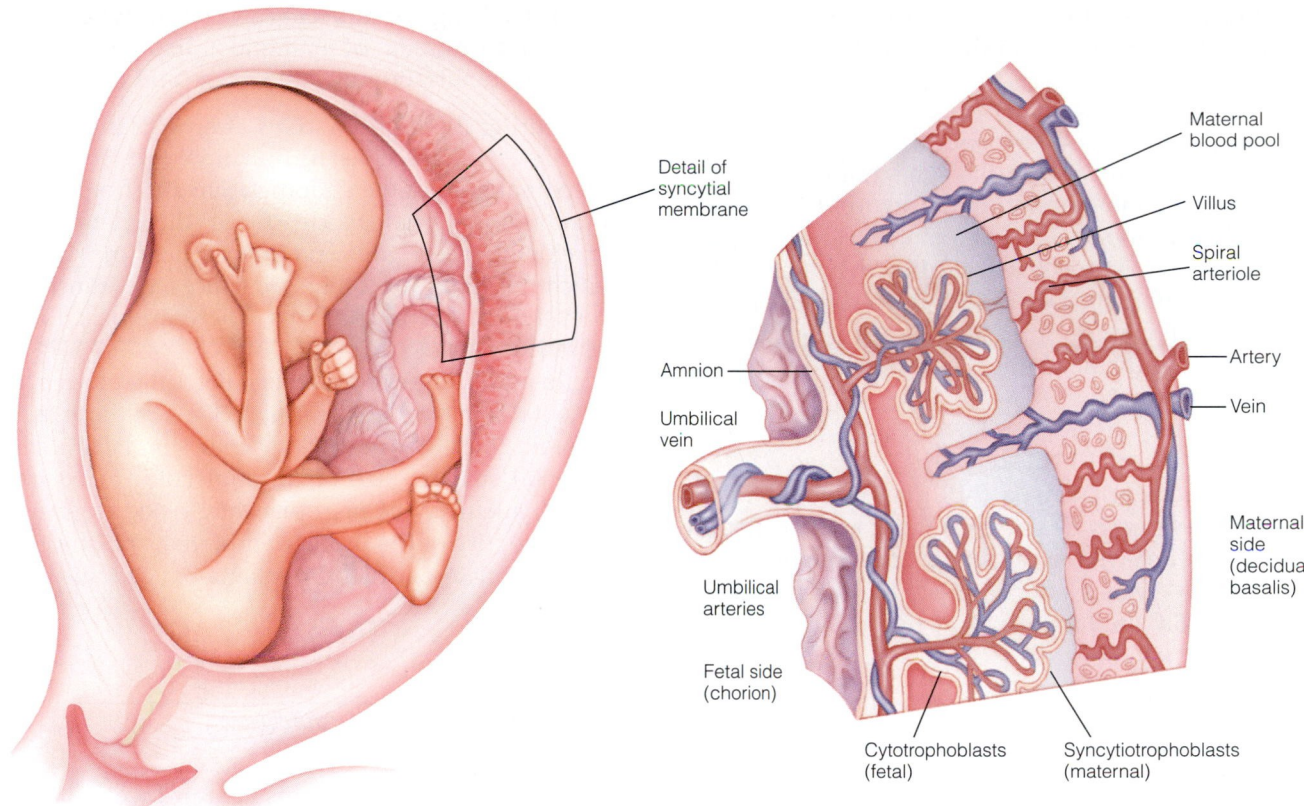

FIGURE 13–6. Vascular arrangement of the placenta, with detail of the syncytial membrane.

► PLACENTAL FUNCTIONS

► Hormone Production

The corpus luteum, which is maintained throughout the entire pregnancy, continues to secrete estrogens and progesterone for about 8 to 10 weeks after fertilization. The placenta also produces four essential hormones: two steroid hormones, estrogen and progesterone, and two protein hormones, human chorionic gonadatropin and human placental lactogen. (See Table 15–2 for a summary of placental hormone functions during pregnancy.)

Estrogen
Throughout pregnancy, the woman is in a hyperestrogenic state. It has been noted that the amount of estrogen produced daily by one woman during pregnancy is equal to that produced by more than 1000 premenopausal women daily (Cunningham et al., 1997). The site of origin of estrogens during most of the pregnancy is the placenta.

Three main forms of estrogen are secreted during pregnancy: estriol, estradiol, and estrone. Estrogen production during pregnancy is dependent on precursors from mother and the fetus. Estriol is the predominant estrogen secreted during pregnancy. The biosynthetic process of estriol formation in the placenta is dependent on steroid secretions from the fetal and maternal adrenals and further processing by the fetal liver. Estradiol and estrone are also formed in the placenta from steroid precursors secreted by the mother and the fetus.

Estrogen is produced as a result of the interplay of the fetus, placenta, and mother. The so-called fetal placental unit is an important regulator of the maternal–fetal environment. The fetus is therefore viewed as an active participant in the healthy progress of the pregnancy (Gumbach, 1996).

Progesterone
Progesterone is also produced in large amounts during pregnancy. After the first few weeks of gestation, little progesterone is produced in the ovary. The

placenta becomes the primary producer of progesterone for the remainder of the pregnancy.

Human Chorionic Gonadotropin

Human chorionic gonadotropin (hCG) is believed to be produced primarily by the syncytiotrophoblast. It is a glycoprotein similar in structure to pituitary luteinizing hormone (LH). Human chorionic gonadotropin appears in the maternal blood by the eighth day after ovulation. Levels of hCG increase steadily, reaching a maximum in 60 to 90 days if fertilization occurs. hCG is the hormone that is detected in current pregnancy tests.

Human Placental Lactogen

Human placental lactogen (hPL) is detectable in the trophoblast as early as the third week after ovulation, and may be detected in the serum of pregnant women as early as 4 weeks after fertilization. This hormone has an action similar to that of human growth hormone.

▶ Transport and Exchange

The main functions of the placenta are

1. Exchange of metabolic and gaseous products between maternal and fetal blood systems
2. Production of hormones
3. Exchange of nutrients and electrolytes
4. Transmission of maternal antibodies
5. Detoxification of some drugs and chemicals.

During the first few days after implantation, the fertilized ovum receives its nutrition directly from the interstitial fluid of the endometrium and from the surrounding maternal tissue. Once the placenta has developed, there are several mechanisms through which nutrients and other substances are transported from the mother to the fetus. These are described in Table 13–2.

In addition, several factors affect the efficiency of placental transport mechanisms. Some of these factors are leakage at the placental barrier site, health of the placental surface, size of the molecules to be transported, adequacy of uteroplacental blood flow, metabolic integrity of the mother and fetus, and the extent to which maternal blood contains oxygen and nutrients.

▶ EMBRYONIC PERIOD

The **embryonic period** begins the third week after fertilization and continues until approximately the eighth week. During this stage, tissues differentiate into essential organs and the main external features develop.

▶ TABLE 13–2

Placental Mechanisms of Transport

Transport Mechanism	Description
Simple diffusion	Movement of substances from an area of higher concentration to an area of lower concentration. Through this mechanism, gases and other simple molecules cross the placenta. Movement depends on the differences in concentration of substances in fetal and maternal plasma, nature of substances, and area of the placenta available for transfer. Some substances transported in this manner are sodium, oxygen, carbon dioxide, and exogenous compounds such as drugs.
Facilitated diffusion	Mechanism whereby the molecule to be transported combines with a protein molecule embedded in the membrane of the placenta. When this molecule is released by the protein molecule into the fetus, the protein molecule is again available to facilitate the diffusion of another molecule across the membrane. This mechanism, which is the primary means of transport of glucose and other sugar molecules, is vital because glucose is the primary energy source of the fetus.
Active transport	Mechanism that operates against a pressure gradient to move a substance from an area of lower pressure to an area of higher pressure. Essential amino acids and water-soluble vitamins are found in higher concentrations in the fetus than in the mother. Through this mechanism, selective amino acids and vitamins are transferred from maternal to fetal blood.
Pinocytosis	Mechanism by which pseudopodial projections from the syncytiotrophoblastic layer engulf small amounts of maternal plasma substances and carry them intact to the fetal circulation. Through this mechanism, complex proteins, some fats, immune bodies, and even some viruses may be transported across the placenta. The mechanism is, however, highly selective; not all maternal antibodies and viruses cross the placental barrier.
Leakage	Transfer of very large materials, such as red blood cells, between mother and fetus through defects or breaks in the placental membrane. This occurs most often at delivery and is responsible for maternal Rh sensitization to fetal red blood cells.

Development of the embryo and fetus follows a cephalocaudal pattern. In other words, the embryo/fetus develops and matures from the head toward the distant extremities. This principle applies to both physical and neurologic development.

► Week 3

During the third week of gestation, the embryonic disc becomes elongated, with a broad cephalic and a narrow caudal end.

► Week 4

By the end of the fourth week, the primitive gut forms and a tubular heart, which develops just outside the body cavity, begins beating, pushing its primitive blood cells through the main blood vessels (Fig. 13–7A). By the 19th to 20th days, the chorionic cavity, which has already begun to form, enlarges; the embryo now is attached to its trophoblastic shell by the body stalk.

Formation of somites (paired, blocklike masses of mesoderm arranged alongside the neural tube of the embryo) occurs during the fourth week. These somites develop into the vertebrae that form the spinal column. Pharyngeal arches and pouches also appear during week 4. The arches form the lower jaw, the hyoid bone, and the cartilage for the larynx. The pouches form the eustachian tube and the cavity of the middle ear, the tonsils, and the parathyroid and thymus glands. The rudiments of the eyes, ears, and nose appear, as do the arm and leg buds.

► Weeks 5 to 8

During the second month of development, the external appearance of the embryo is greatly changed by the enormous size of the head and the formation of limbs, face, ear, nose, eyes, and arm and limb paddles (Fig. 13–7B). The optic cup and lens vesicle of the eye form, nasal pits develop, the heart and circulatory system become more advanced, and the brain differentiates into five areas with ten pairs of cranial nerves. The embryo progresses from a markedly C-shaped body to a structure with a rounded head that is nearly erect and measures approximately 3 cm in length. All major organ systems are formed during the fourth to eighth weeks, hence this is called the period of **organogenesis.** The embryo is most susceptible to factors that interfere with development during this period, with most congenital malformations occurring

at this time (Hanson, 1996). Figure 13–8 is a timetable of human prenatal development from conception to 10 weeks.

► FETAL PERIOD

The period from the end of the eighth week, or the start of the third month, to birth is known as the **fetal period.** This period is characterized by maturation of the tissues and organs and rapid growth of the body. All structures that will be present in the full-term infant are in existence; no new structures will form. Few, if any, malformations arise during this period, although cell death in the central nervous system may be caused by factors toxic to cells and may result in postnatal behavioral disturbances. Growth in length is striking during the third, fourth, and fifth lunar months, whereas increase in weight is most striking during the ninth and tenth lunar months.

In calculating expected delivery dates, most women consider a pregnancy to be 9 months long, starting from their first missed menstrual period. In fact, the average pregnancy is 38 weeks or 266 days in length from the time of conception, or 40 weeks or 280 days from the first day of the last menstrual period. When a woman states that she is 3 months pregnant, she is in fact 12 weeks past her last menstrual period. Thus, most health care providers speak of a pregnancy in terms of lunar or 4-week months. The following discussion uses lunar months and the number of weeks past the last menstrual period to describe the sequence of fetal development. Figure 13–9 illustrates several stages in the development of the fetus.

► Third Lunar Month (Weeks 9–12)

By the end of the 12th week, or third month, the face of the fetus appears more human. Other changes also occur, such as: the ears come to lie close to their definitive position at the sides of the head; centers of ossification appear in most bones; the fingers and toes have differentiated and nail beds form; scattered rudiments of hair appear; and the external genitalia have developed to such a degree that the sex of the fetus can be visually determined. At the end of the third month, reflex activity can be evoked and the fetus is able to make spontaneous movements (Fig. 13–7C). By the end of 12 weeks fetal weight is approximately 45 g and crown–rump length is 87 mm.

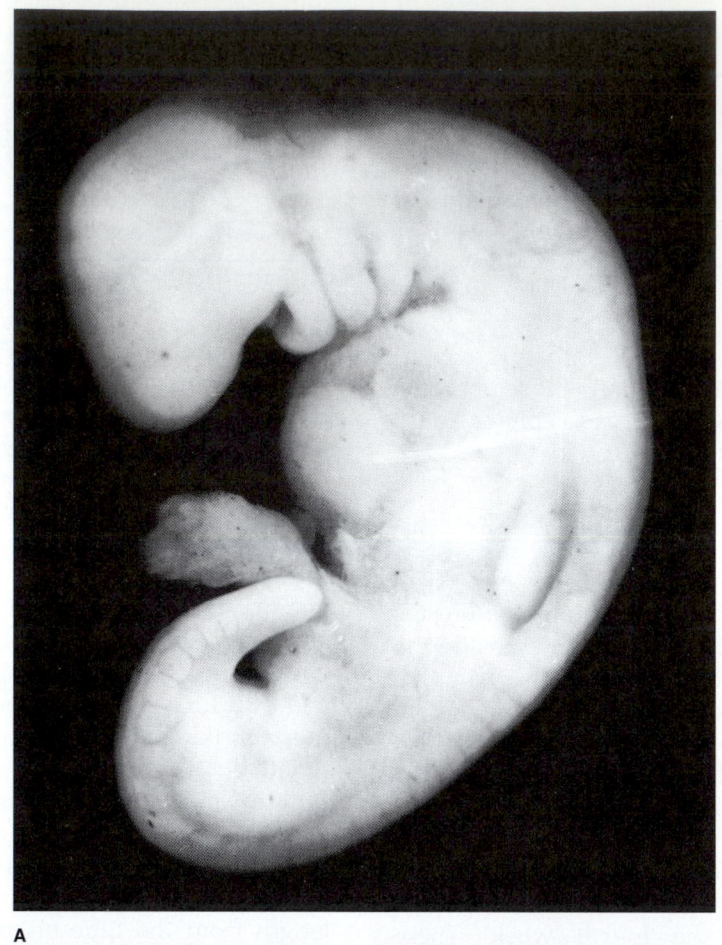

A

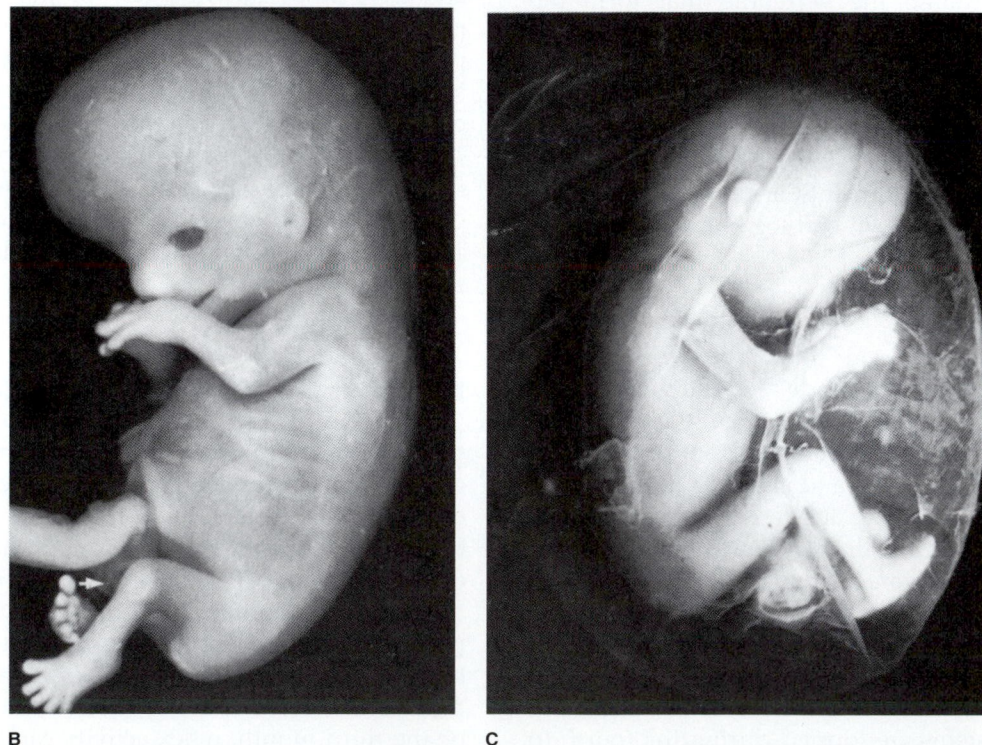

B   C

FIGURE 13–7. Development of the human fetus. **A.** 4 weeks. **B.** 8 weeks. **C.** 12 weeks. *(Reproduced, with permission from Moore, K.L. (1989). Before we are born: Basic embryology and birth defects (3rd ed.). Philadelphia: W.B. Saunders, pp. 65, 69, 100.)*

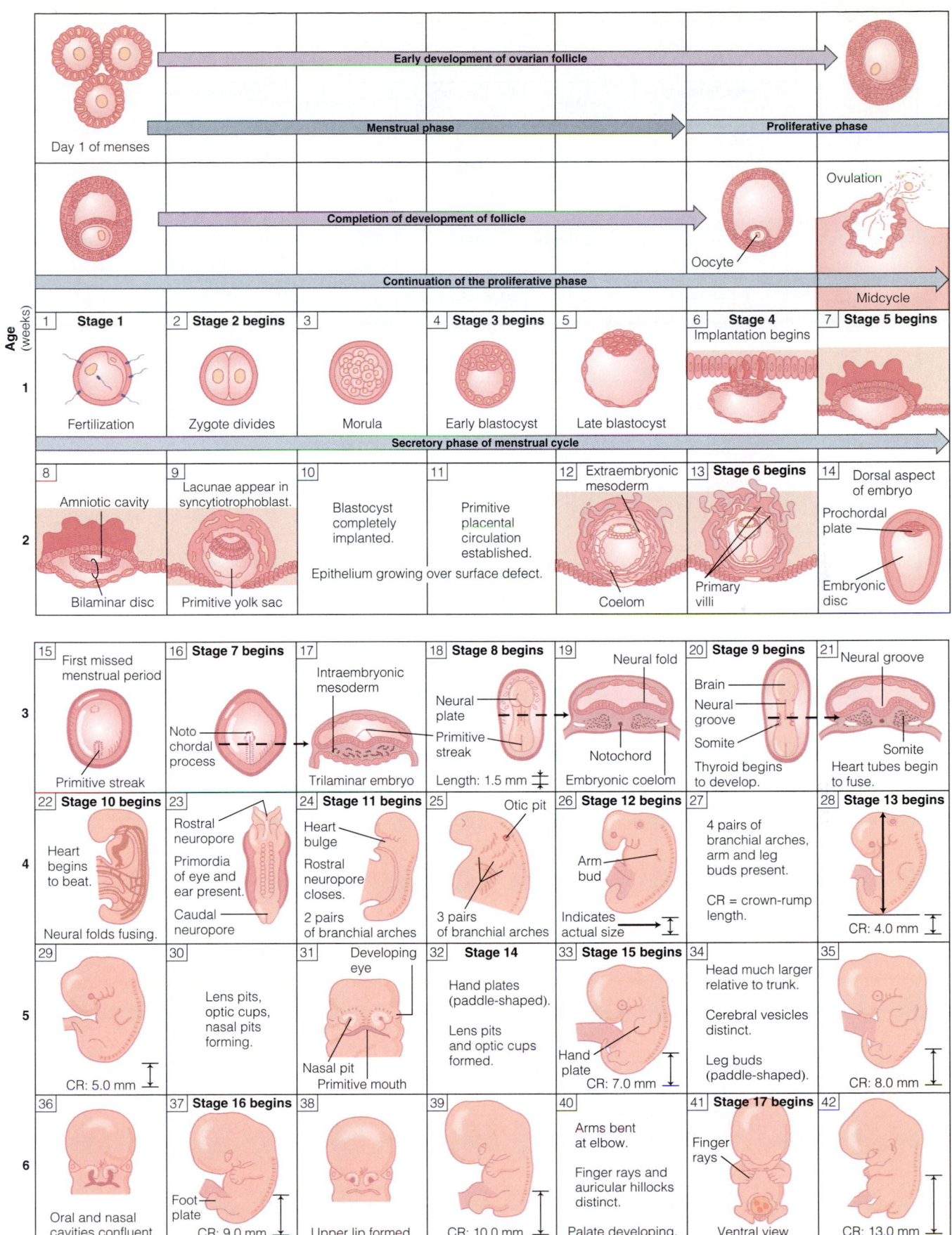

FIGURE 13–8. Human prenatal development, from conception to 10 weeks. *(Reproduced, with permission, from Moore, K.L. (1989). The developing human: Clinically oriented embryology (3rd ed.). Philadelphia: W.B. Saunders, pp. 2–4.)*

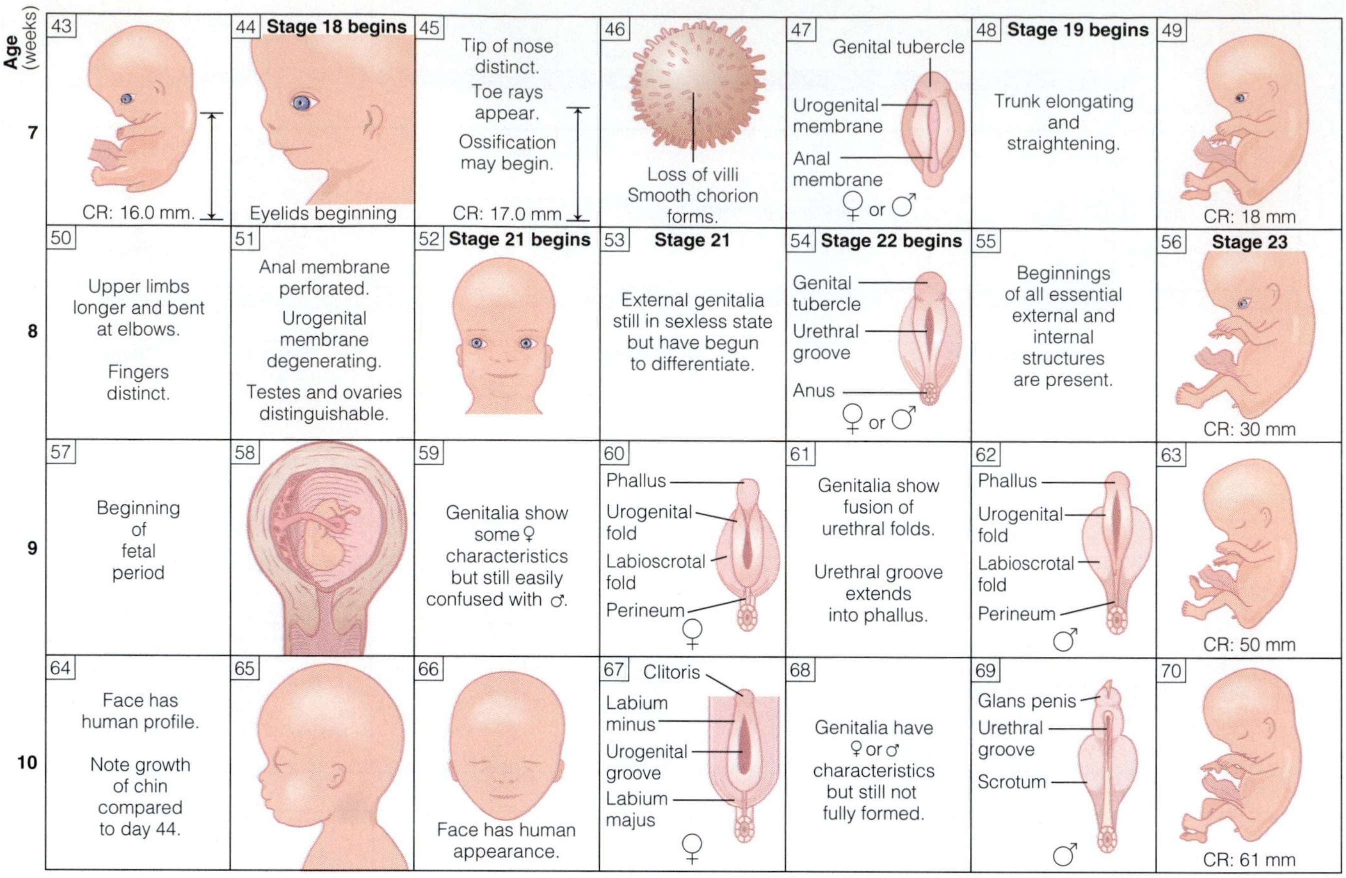

Age (weeks)

7	**43** CR: 16.0 mm.	**44 Stage 18 begins** Eyelids beginning	**45** Tip of nose distinct. Toe rays appear. Ossification may begin. CR: 17.0 mm	**46** Loss of villi Smooth chorion forms.	**47** Genital tubercle Urogenital membrane Anal membrane ♀ or ♂	**48 Stage 19 begins** Trunk elongating and straightening.	**49** CR: 18 mm

| **8** | **50** Upper limbs longer and bent at elbows. Fingers distinct. | **51** Anal membrane perforated. Urogenital membrane degenerating. Testes and ovaries distinguishable. | **52 Stage 21 begins** | **53 Stage 21** External genitalia still in sexless state but have begun to differentiate. | **54 Stage 22 begins** Genital tubercle Urethral groove Anus ♀ or ♂ | **55** Beginnings of all essential external and internal structures are present. | **56 Stage 23** CR: 30 mm |

| **9** | **57** Beginning of fetal period | **58** | **59** Genitalia show some ♀ characteristics but still easily confused with ♂. | **60** Phallus Urogenital fold Labioscrotal fold Perineum ♀ | **61** Genitalia show fusion of urethral folds. Urethral groove extends into phallus. | **62** Phallus Urogenital fold Labioscrotal fold Perineum ♂ | **63** CR: 50 mm |

| **10** | **64** Face has human profile. Note growth of chin compared to day 44. | **65** | **66** Face has human appearance. | **67** Clitoris Labium minus Urogenital groove Labium majus ♀ | **68** Genitalia have ♀ or ♂ characteristics but still not fully formed. | **69** Glans penis Urethral groove Scrotum ♂ | **70** CR: 61 mm |

FIGURE 13–8 (continued). Human prenatal development, from conception to 10 weeks.

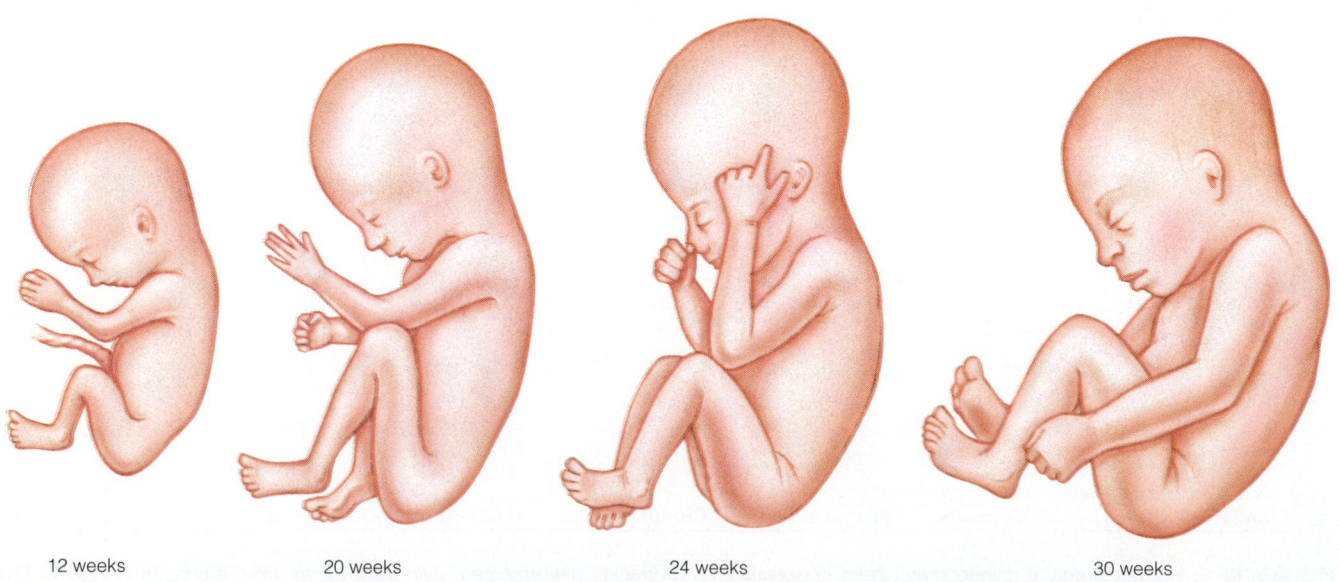

12 weeks   20 weeks   24 weeks   30 weeks

FIGURE 13–9. Human fetal development: 12 weeks, 20 weeks, 24 weeks, and 30 weeks.

▶ Fourth Lunar Month (Weeks 13–16)

During the fourth month the fetus achieves a crown–rump length of approximately 120 mm and, at the end of 16 weeks, weighs about 110 g. Lanugo begins to develop, particularly on the head. The muscles and skeleton are able to hold the fetus more erect. Rudimentary kidneys secrete urine, and the liver and pancreas begin to produce their secretions. The fetus is now quite active.

▶ Fifth Lunar Month (Weeks 17–20)

During the fifth month the fetus increases to a crown–rump length of approximately 200 mm (8 in.) and fetal weight increases to between 435 and 460 g. The lower limbs reach their final relative proportions and the mother begins to feel fetal movements. This sensation is known as **quickening.**

The skin of the fetus becomes coated with vernix caseosa, which protects the fetus' skin from abrasions, chapping, and hardening that would otherwise result from floating in amniotic fluid. **Brown fat** forms during this period. This brown-pigmented tissue, the first adipose tissue deposited in the developing fetus, is found around the adrenals, kidneys, in the neck, between the scapulas, and behind the sternum. Eyebrows, head hair, and nails on both the fingers and toes are visible. By the end of the fifth month, fetal heart tones can be heard with a stethoscope.

▶ Sixth Lunar Month (Weeks 21–24)

The crown–rump length is now approximately 230 mm (9.6 in.). Weight gain during this period is substantial, with the fetus reaching 780 g (1 pound 11 oz). The skin is translucent, pink to red, and wrinkled. The organs are rather well developed and a grasp reflex is present. The alveoli in the lungs are beginning to develop.

▶ Seventh Lunar Month (Weeks 25–28)

The fetus' lungs and pulmonary vasculature develop sufficiently during this period to allow gas exchange to take place. Survival is therefore possible if the infant is born prematurely, although the mortality rate is high. The central nervous system matures dramatically to the stage where it can direct rhythmic breathing movements and control body temperature. The fetus' eyes open and close under neural control. Subcutaneous fat begins to increase.

Infants born at 26 weeks of gestation have a survival rate greater than 45%, if they receive aggressive perinatal care. The survival rate for infants born at 28 weeks, receiving aggressive perinatal care, is greater than 60% (Cunningham et al., 1997).

▶ Eighth Lunar Month (Weeks 29–32)

Subcutaneous fat continues to increase during the eighth month, as does body muscle, bringing the weight of the fetus to approximately 2000 g (4 pounds 6.5 oz) and the crown–rump length to 300 mm (12.5 in.). The lungs are not yet fully developed. The bones, although developed, are still soft and flexible. An infant born during this period has a 70% chance of survival with special care.

▶ Ninth Lunar Month (Weeks 33–36)

The skin of the fetus appears pink and less wrinkled by the ninth month. The fetus is beginning to appear plump and the arms and legs may seem chubby. Lanugo is beginning to disappear, and the nails have grown to reach the fingertips.

The surfactant system of the lungs matures at approximately 36 weeks. **Surfactant,** a phospholipid that maintains alveolar patency and lowers surface tension in the lungs, is evident in increasing quantities. An infant delivered at this time has a 90% chance of survival if he or she receives special care.

▶ Tenth Lunar Month (Weeks 37–40)

The fetus is considered full term at 38 weeks. Very little lanugo remains and the amount of vernix caseosa varies, with the largest deposits in the creases and folds of the skin. The skull has the largest circumference of all parts of the body and is generally positioned downward, which is an important factor in preparing for passage of the infant through the birth canal. The sexual characteristics are pronounced; the testes should be in the scrotum.

At term the fetus weighs about 3000 to 3600 g (6 pounds 10 oz to 7 pounds 15 oz), boys being larger than girls. Boys are also longer than girls, with crown-to-heel length, the commonly used measurement for the newborn, ranging from 48 to 52 cm (19 to 21 in.).

Table 13–3 provides a synopsis of embryonic and fetal development, summarizing the major changes and the development of body and organ systems during various stages of gestation.

▶ **TABLE 13-3**

Summary of Embryonic and Fetal Development

| | First Trimester | | |
| | Embryonic Period | | Fetal Period |
Body System	Lunar Month 1	Lunar Month 2	Lunar Month 3
Integument	Three germ layers are differentiated	Rapid cell differentiation	Nail beds formed, eyelids fused; teeth begin to appear
Cardiovascular	Begins to function; tubular beating; hemopoiesis in yolk sac	Heart and all structures functionally complete: hemopoiesis in liver as yolk sac is incorporated into embryo	Hemopoiesis by liver and spleen
Respiratory	Differentiation of respiratory system and structure; nasal pits, lung buds, trachea, and larynx formed	Formation of three lobes of right lung and two lobes of left lung; bronchi formed with bronchioles dividing	Some respiratory-like movements exhibited
Gastrointestinal	Differentiation of gastrointestinal tract with accessory structure; liver function begins	Urorectal septum formed; oral, nasal cavities, and upper lip formed	Begins to swallow amniotic fluid; bile begins to be secreted by liver; palate and nasal septum fused
Urinary	Urogenital membrane develops into urethral opening; differentiation of kidney		Kidneys begin to function, urine excreted
Reproductive	Sex determined	Urogenital membrane degenerates; testes and ovaries distinguishable; external genitalia begin to differentiate	Gender distinguishable
Musculoskeletal	Rudimentary body parts formed; limb buds present	Muscles developing; extremities, fingers, and toes differentiate; ossification begins; some movement of limbs	Ossification centers present in bones; fetus moves easily
Neurologic	Neural groove formed; brain formed by closure of anterior neural tube; optic cup of eyes formed	Rapid differentiation and cellular growth of central nervous system; cranial nerves developing; lens vesicles appear; ear beginning to form final structure	Grasp and sucking reflexes present; brain and spinal cord developed
Immunologic			Rudimentary immunologic system appears; β lymphocytes appear in liver by 9 weeks

| | Second Trimester (Fetal Period) | | |
Body System	Lunar Month 4	Lunar Month 5	Lunar Month 6
Integument	Downy hair (lanugo) appears on body	Begins to exchange new cells for old in skin; vernix caseosa appears; permanent teeth buds appear	Fingernails present; skin appears red and wrinkled
Cardiovascular	Hemopoiesis by liver, spleen, and bone marrow	Heart sounds heard with stethoscope	
Respiratory			Alveoli forming; surfactant formation begins in alveoli; nares open; fetus displays hiccoughs
Gastrointestinal	Meconium present; gastric and intestinal glands developing		
Urinary	Kidneys assume mature structure		
Reproductive	Uterine development in female; external genitalia well developed		
Musculoskeletal	Rapid skeletal development; joint cavities form; greater spontaneous movement	Quickening (movement felt by mother); skeleton begins to harden	Body straightens; may respond to external sound with movement
Neurologic		Beginning of myelination of spinal cord; sucking reflex present	Alternate periods of sleep and activity; may respond to external sounds; eyes structurally complete; strong grasp reflex
Immunologic	β lymphocytes present in blood and spleen	Detectable level of fetal antibodies	

► **TABLE 13–3** *(continued)*

Summary of Embryonic and Fetal Development

Body System	Third Trimester (Fetal Period)			
	Lunar Month 7	Lunar Month 8	Lunar Month 9	Lunar Month 10
Integument	Eyelids reopen	Begins to store fat; lanugo begins to disappear from face; skin appears less red	Fat deposition continues; lanugo begins to disappear from body; head hair lengthens; earlobes are soft with little cartilage	Lanugo and vernix caseosa both begin to disappear; skin becomes smooth and plump; earlobes are stiff with thick cartilage
Cardiovascular			Increased iron storage by liver	
Respiratory	Respiratory system sufficiently developed so that babies may survive with intensive care; respiratory-like movements apparent		Increased maturity of lungs and surfactant; excellent chance of survival if born; L:S ratio 2:1[a]	
Gastrointestinal		Begins to store fat and minerals		Continues to store fat and minerals
Urinary	Active urine formation			
Reproductive	Testes descend into inguinal canal	One or both testes may descend into scrotal sac		Testes in scrotal sac
Musculoskeletal		Mother may note jerky crying-like movements; minerals stored in bone	Femoral ossification centers formed	Firming of skull and bones; circumference of skull larger than circumference of chest
Neurologic	Central nervous system sufficiently developed so that there is a possibility of survival with intensive care; regulatory activities begin	Fetus can be conditioned to environmental sounds and exhibits good reflex development		All reflexes present
Immunologic				Most IgG is acquired from mother; by term the fetus receives some passive immunity by placental transfer of maternal antibodies

[a]L:S ratio, lecithin:sphingomyelin ratio.

► **Fetal Lung Development**

Fetal lung development is a very complex process affected by the interrelationship of several hormones. Agents that accelerate lung maturation are corticosteroids, thyroid hormones, growth factors, and cyclic adenosine monophosphate (AMP). The role of estrogen and prolactin in lung maturation is not as clear. On the other hand, insulin and hyperglycemia appear to delay lung maturation (Hazinski, 1996).

For the infant to breathe adequately at birth and not to experience respiratory distress syndrome, sufficient quantities of surfactant must be present to allow expansion of the lungs and free exchange of air. Surfactant reduces the surface tension of the alveoli and prevents collapse of the lungs. This reduction in surface tension is necessary for full lung expansion despite the presence of what appears to be adequate respiratory movement.

Movements of the fetal chest have been detected very early in pregnancy. The fetus is capable of respiratory movement from the beginning of the fourth month. By the end of the second trimester, development of air ducts and alveoli, pulmonary vasculature, and muscles of respiration, as well as the coordination of their activities by the respiratory system, reaches a level that allows survival for a short period. The amount of surfactant sufficient to support adequate respiration, however, is not produced until the third trimester, increasing in quantity as the pregnancy progresses (Hazinski, 1996).

► MULTIPLE GESTATION

► Twins

Twins may be either dizygotic (fraternal) or monozygotic (identical). In the United States, the prevalence of twins is 1.08% among Caucasians and 1.36% among African-Americans. Approximately 70% of twin births are dizygotic and 30% monozygotic (England, 1996).

Dizygotic twins originate from two separate zygotes. Because they occur as the result of fertilization of two ova, dizygotic twins are genetically different and may be of the same or different sexes. Dizygotic twins are actually no more alike than other brothers and sisters. They are also delivered more frequently than monozygotic twins. **Monozygotic twins** originate from one zygote. They are therefore genetically identical and of the same sex.

Dizygotic and monozygotic twins also differ with respect to implantation site, placenta, chorion, and amnion. Dizygotic twins have separate implantation sites, placentas, chorions, and amnions, although occasionally their placentas have been known to fuse (Fig. 13–10).

In monozygotic twins, the zygote splits at various stages to form two separate zygotes. The time at which division occurs determines the different structures the twins will share. If division occurs within the first 72 hours of fertilization, the two embryos will be diamniotic and dichorionic, developing two amnions and two chorions. If division occurs between the fourth and eighth days, the embryos will be monochorionic, having separate amniotic sacs covered by a common chorion. If division occurs on about the eighth day, the two embryos will share an amniotic sac (Fig. 13–11).

► Other Multiple Births

Other multiple births—triplets, quadruplets, quintuplets, sextuplets, septuplets, and so forth—may be the result of one zygote (identical), several zygotes (fraternal), or any combination (identical and fraternal). Drugs used to treat infertility may induce multiple births (see Chapter 10).

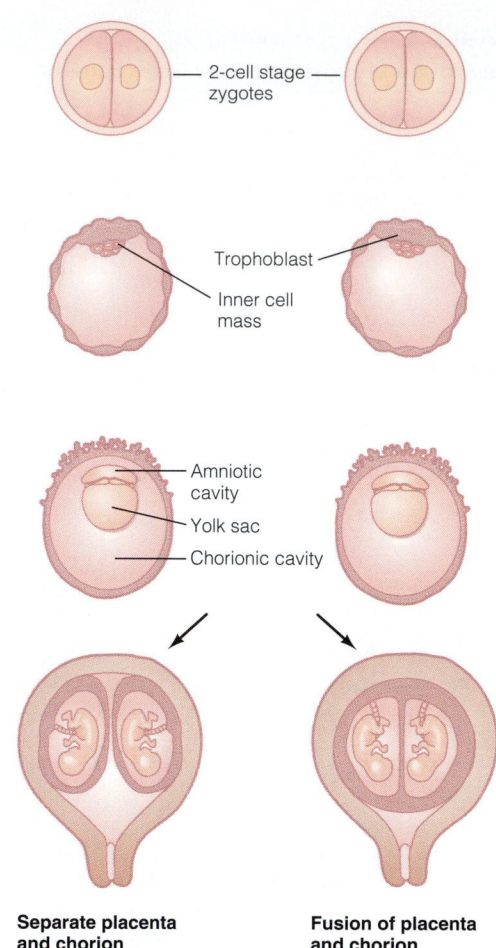

Separate placenta and chorion   **Fusion of placenta and chorion**

FIGURE 13–10. Development of dizygotic twins. *(Reproduced, with permission, from Sadler, T.W. (1990). Langman's medical embryology (6th ed.). Baltimore: Williams & Wilkins, p. 104.)*

► CIRCULATION

► Fetal Circulation

Fetal circulation differs from the circulation that exists in extrauterine life primarily because the fetus secures oxygen and food from maternal blood through the placenta rather than through its own lungs and digestive organs. Fetal circulation is supported by structures such as the umbilical cord, which contains two umbilical arteries and one umbilical vein; the ductus venosus; and the placenta. In addition, the foramen ovale and ductus arteriosus provide detours by which blood bypasses the lungs (Fig. 13–12).

The umbilical vein carries oxygenated, nutrient-bearing blood from the placenta to the fetus. The umbilical vein enters the fetal body through the umbilicus, or umbilical ring, and ascends along the

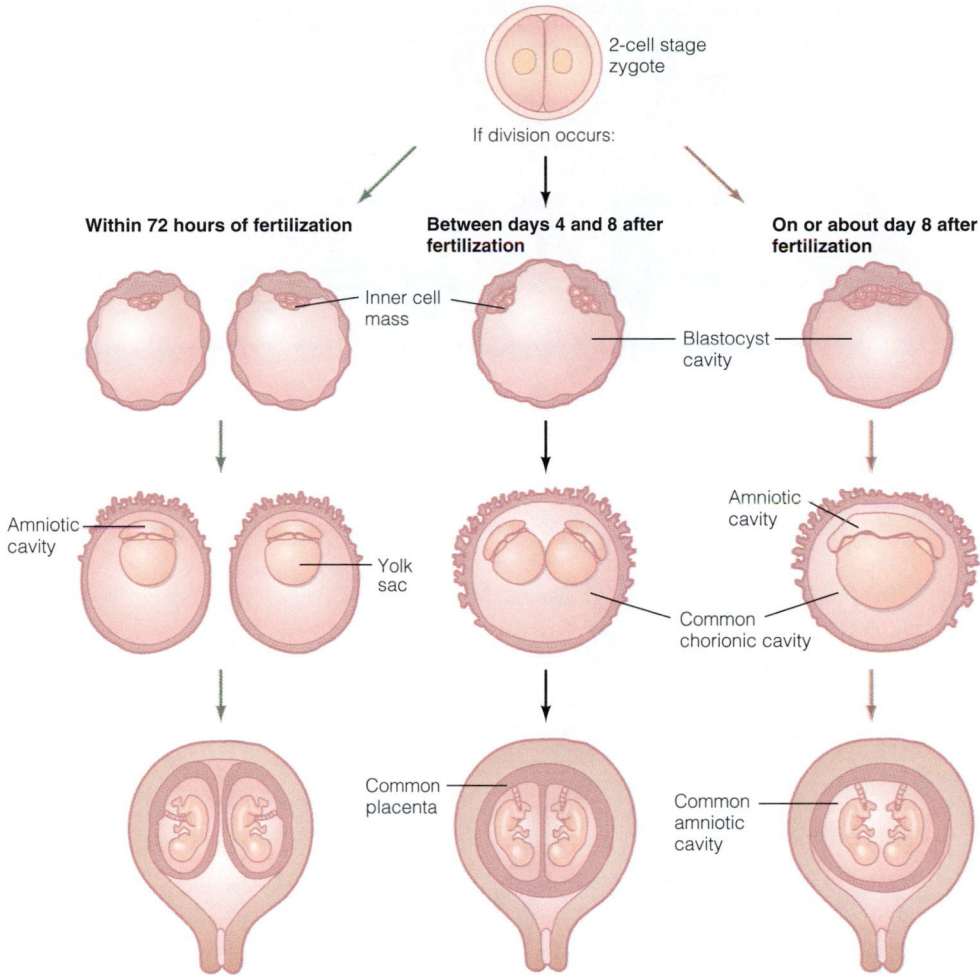

FIGURE 13–11. Possible relationships among fetal membranes in monozygotic twins. *(Reproduced, with permission, from Sadler, T.W. (1990).* Langman's medical embryology *(6th ed.). Baltimore: Williams & Wilkins, p. 105.)*

anterior abdominal wall to the liver, where the vein divides into the portal sinus and the ductus venosus. The portal sinus carries blood to the hepatic veins, located primarily on the left side of the liver. The ductus venosus, or major branch of the umbilical vein, traverses the liver and empties directly into the inferior vena cava.

Highly oxygenated blood from the inferior vena cava mixes with less well oxygenated blood from the veins below the level of the diaphragm and flows into the right atrium of the fetal heart. From the right atrium, the blood passes through the foramen ovale, an opening in the septum between the right and left atria, into the left atrium. Blood then flows into the left ventricle and, finally, is pumped into the aorta. Little or no blood from the superior vena cava, which is less oxygenated, passes through the foramen ovale.

The right ventricle and pulmonary circulation are bypassed; thus, the highly oxygenated blood is pumped directly from the left ventricle and perfuses only two vital organs, the heart and the brain. Blood returning through the superior vena cava empties into the right atrium and passes through the tricuspid valve into the right ventricle. For the most part, this blood is shunted into the descending aorta through the ductus arteriosus. The blood nourishes the trunk and lower extremities. A small amount of blood passes through the lungs, and this provides nourishment only.

The ventricles of the fetal heart work in tandem rather than in series, as a result of the action of the foramen ovale and ductus arteriosus shunts. Cardiac output of the fetal heart is about three times that of an adult at rest and is due partly to the rapid heart rate

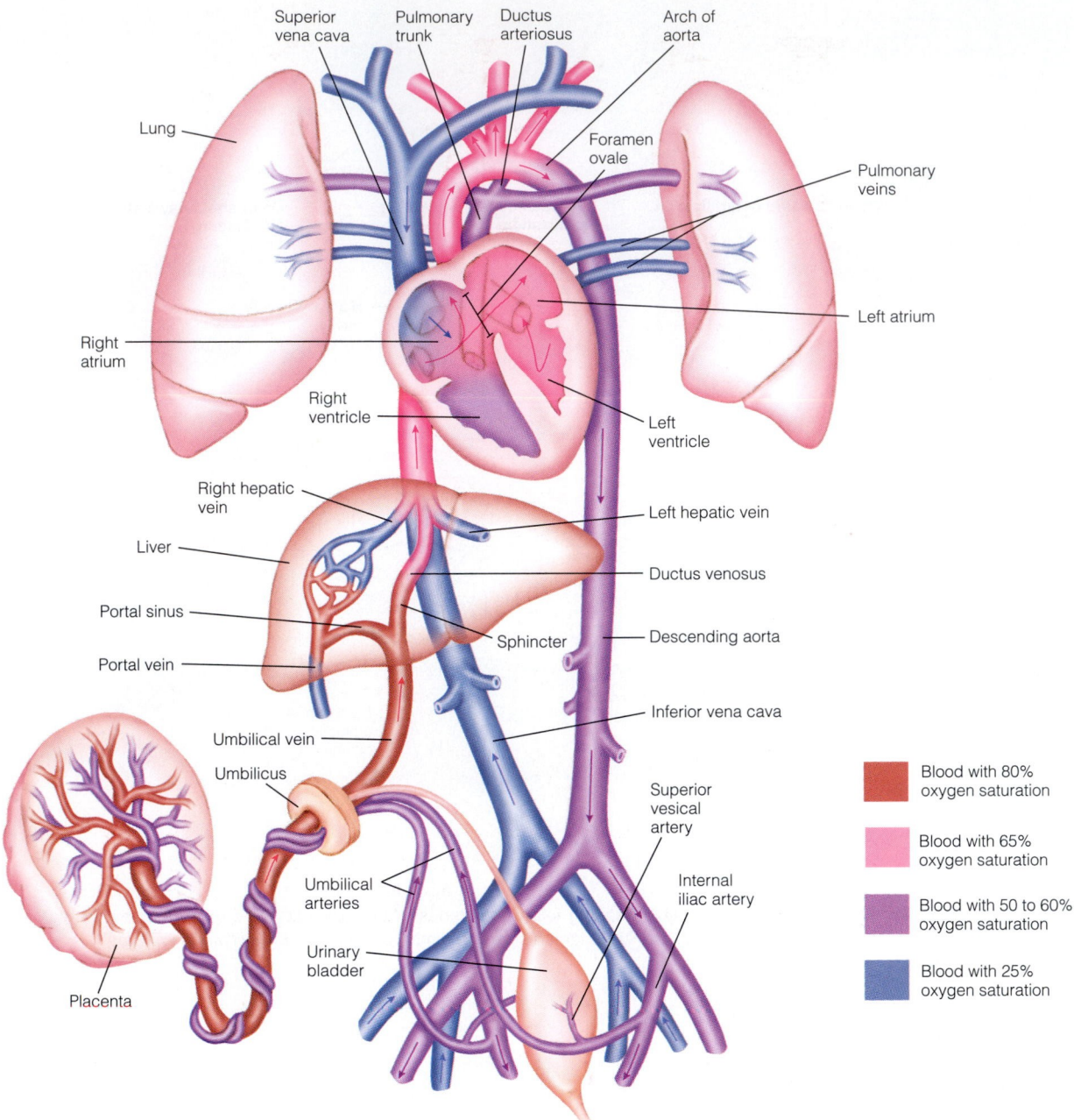

Superior vena cava · Pulmonary trunk · Ductus arteriosus · Arch of aorta

Lung

Foramen ovale

Pulmonary veins

Left atrium

Right atrium

Right ventricle

Left ventricle

Right hepatic vein

Left hepatic vein

Liver

Ductus venosus

Portal sinus

Sphincter

Descending aorta

Portal vein

Inferior vena cava

Umbilical vein

Umbilicus

Superior vesical artery

Internal iliac artery

Umbilical arteries

Urinary bladder

Placenta

Blood with 80% oxygen saturation

Blood with 65% oxygen saturation

Blood with 50 to 60% oxygen saturation

Blood with 25% oxygen saturation

FIGURE 13–12. Fetal circulation.

of the fetus and partly to low peripheral resistance (Hoffman, 1996).

Blood finally returns to the placenta through the two hypogastric arteries, which become the umbilical arteries distally. Carbon dioxide and other waste products are then removed in the placenta, allowing the entire process to be repeated.

At birth the hemodynamics of fetal circulation undergo profound changes. The umbilical vessels, the ductus arteriosus, the foramen ovale, and the ductus venosus normally constrict or collapse with spontaneous or artificial respiration of the infant, or shortly thereafter. As the lungs expand, pulmonary vascular resistance decreases considerably, causing the pressures in the right ventricle and pulmonary arteries to fall. This results in equal pressure in both atria, causing the foramen ovale to close. The umbilical arteries atrophy to become the umbilical ligaments; intraabdominal remnants of the umbilical vein become the round ligament of the liver; and the ductus venosus

► **TABLE 13–4**

Changes in Fetal Circulation After Birth

Structure	Fetal Circulation	Postnatal Change
Umbilical vein	Transports arterial blood to liver and heart	Becomes round ligament of liver
Umbilical arteries	Transports blood to placenta	Become umbilical ligaments
Ductus venosus	Shunts blood to inferior vena cava	Becomes ligamentum venosum
Ductus arteriosus	Shunts blood from pulmonary artery to aorta	Becomes ligamentum arteriosum
Foramen ovale	Connects right and left atria	Closes
Lungs	Contain no air and little blood; are filled with fluid	Fill with air; begin to oxygenate blood
Pulmonary arteries	Transport small amounts of blood to lungs	Transport blood to lungs for oxygenation
Aorta	Receives blood from both ventricles	Receives blood from left ventricle
Inferior vena cava	Transports atrial blood from placenta and venous blood from body	Transports venous blood to right atrium

constricts to form the ligamentum venosum. These changes are outlined in Table 13–4 (see Chapter 30 for an in-depth discussion.)

► **Maternal Placental Circulation**

Fetal circulation is dependent on efficient maternal placental circulation. Maternal blood transports nutrients to the fetus and waste materials from the fetus through the process of diffusion. Maternal arterial blood pressure, intrauterine pressure, pattern of uterine contractions, and factors affecting arteriolar walls are the primary influences on the flow of blood in the placenta.

► **DEVELOPMENTS IN EMBRYOLOGY AND FETOLOGY**

Research in the field of human embryology and fetology is constrained by the ethical, moral, and legal considerations involved in studying and experimenting on humans; however, if advances are to be made in the field of prenatal development, research is necessary. The physiologic risks to the mother and embryo/fetus require that most experimentation and study in this field be performed in the laboratory on animals. Because this type of study can never fully duplicate the actual effects on humans, broad generalizations to humans cannot be made. While federal legislation enacted in 1993 allowed investigators to perform research on fetal tissue from interrupted pregnancies, this practice is still controversial. Such research has, however, major implications for maternal–fetal health and such diseases as Alzheimer's disease. Many people regard this as human experimentation, which raises the issue of the rights of the fetus.

Research in embryology and fetology is proceeding in many areas in an effort to advance medical science and to improve pregnancy outcomes. Among these areas are fetal and maternal nutrition; placental and fetal physiology; physiologic effects of drugs and teratogens on the fetus and placenta; physiologic effects of hormones and enzymes of pregnancy on the fetus and mother; fetal and maternal metabolism; fetal, placental, and maternal circulation; fetal, placental, and maternal pathology; fetal and maternal diseases; fetal immunology; and placental transmission of human immunodeficiency virus (HIV).

The Human Genome Project is another research study that is likely to have a major effect on our knowledge of the development of the embryo and fetus. Identification and mapping of specific genes, including those responsible for genetic alterations of the embryo, may soon allow genes to be routinely manipulated in utero. Cloning, while only accomplished in animals, is most certainly a possibility for humans as well. Many ethical dilemmas are involved with both these possibilities.

Some of the most exciting work is taking place in the area of infertility; for example, techniques such as in vitro fertilization (IVF), in vitro fertilization–embryo transfer (IVF-ET), ovum transfer, gamete intrafallopian transfer, zygote intrafallopian transfer, assisted hatching, intracytoplasmic sperm injection, and implantation of frozen ova (see Chapter 10). Some of these procedures, however, are still generally considered experimental, are very expensive, and are associated with relatively low success rates. More effective techniques are being developed, but with these improvements come new questions regarding the legal, moral, and ethical issues. Complex issues are raised for which no definitive answers are forthcoming.

Continual improvements in the area of prenatal diagnosis through ultrasonography, amniocentesis, chorionic villus sampling (CVS), and percutaneous umbilical cord blood sampling (PUBS) are making these techniques relatively safe, acceptable, and reliable. CVS can be done during the first trimester; however, if used before 9½ weeks it can cause limb reduction defects (Rodeck, 1993). Transvaginal sonography is used for early sonographic evaluation during the first trimester. It gives precise estimates of gestational age by measuring crown–rump length, biparietal diameter, head circumference, and abdominal circumference. PUBS is used to obtain blood samples, primarily for chromosome studies, at about 20 weeks of gestation, after fetal abnormalities have been indicated by prenatal ultrasound (Lasser et al., 1993).

Evaluation of fetal status by means of a biophysical profile is being implemented on a routine basis in an attempt to improve perinatal morbidity and mortality. The biophysical profile is based on multiple discrete variables originating from the fetus. It involves assessing fetal breathing movements, gross fetal body movements, fetal tone, and amniotic fluid volume by dynamic ultrasound imaging, in addition to conducting a nonstress test by Doppler ultrasound (Gebauer & Lowe, 1993).

Embryoscopy, insertion of a minute viewing scope into the mother's abdomen through a needle the size of one used to draw blood, is becoming an invaluable tool in prenatal diagnosis and treatment and fetal surgery. The procedure can be used very early in pregnancy: it has been used as early as 6 weeks, when the embryo is about half an inch long, is shaped like a comma, and has buds for arms and legs.

These methods of prenatal diagnosis have resulted in the further development of intrauterine fetal surgery, which is an option in the treatment of fetuses with such abnormalities as hydrocephalus and hydronephrosis associated with posterior urethral valves. In the future, fetuses with a diaphragmatic hernia and meningomyelocele may be subjects for in utero fetal therapy. The goal of fetal surgery is to provide time for fetal maturity and delivery at or near term by reversing or slowing a destructive process. This type of surgery is highly experimental and risky and may result in fetal death. Nevertheless, fetal surgery is being pioneered in at least 13 centers in five countries (Cunningham et al., 1997). Many ethical, legal, and moral implications will need to be considered as these highly controversial procedures advance.

Research in embryology and fetology is exciting and has considerable potential for improving pregnancy outcomes.

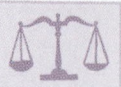

Ethical Decision Making

The potential implications of current and future development in embryology and fetology are both thought provoking and controversial. As a nurse working within the field of reproductive health and acting as an advocate for childbearing families, consider the following questions:

1. Do the benefits of research on fetal tissue from interrupted pregnancies in terms of maternal–fetal health outweigh the ethical implications of human experimentation on a once-developing fetus?
2. To what extent are the assessments and biophysical profiles that can now be carried out to determine fetal status invasive to the mother and child? How should the risks and benefits of these procedures be weighed?
3. Should the use of intrauterine surgery to reverse or slow a fetal abnormality be dependent on the nature and extent of the disorder or should it be implemented in all cases in which the fetus may be susceptible to an adverse outcome after birth?

▶ ENVIRONMENTAL EFFECTS ON THE EMBRYO/FETUS

Several factors contribute to the risks for the mother and fetus throughout pregnancy. Environmental agents may cross the placenta and affect the developing embryo/fetus. Genetic errors may result in functional defects. Approximately 10% of all human malformations are caused by environmental factors, 10% are caused by genetic factors, and the remaining 80% are presumably the result of a complex interplay of several environmental and genetic factors (Hanson, 1996).

The major risk factors with respect to infant mortality are smoking, alcohol abuse, drug use and abuse, occupational hazards, injuries, viruses, and nutritional disorders. These risk factors may also be referred to as teratogens, agents that can cause congenital anomalies in the fetus. It has been determined that any substance given in large enough doses at critical periods of development can be classified as teratogenic.

The embryo is susceptible to a variety of environmental teratogenic influences that are capable of disrupting development. The fetus is also susceptible to teratogens that may result in prematurity, abortion, organ or tissue injury, and possibly malformation.

Three critical periods of development exist: (1) fertilization and implantation, or the first 17 days of gestation; (2) the embryonic period, from day 18 to day 55; and (3) the fetal stage, from day 56 of gestation to delivery. Exposure to teratogens in the first critical period may lead to improper implantation and spontaneous abortion. The embryonic period is the period when the most extensive organ differentiation occurs, the heart in the first 38 days, the arms and legs in the first 49 days, and the teeth in the first 56 days of gestation. Further, differentiation of the palate, external genitalia, and ear occurs in the fetal period. Exposure to teratogens during the embryonic period can cause structural and functional birth defects. During the fetal period, when there is still some organ differentiation, structural defects as well as fetal growth retardation can occur (Fig. 13–13).

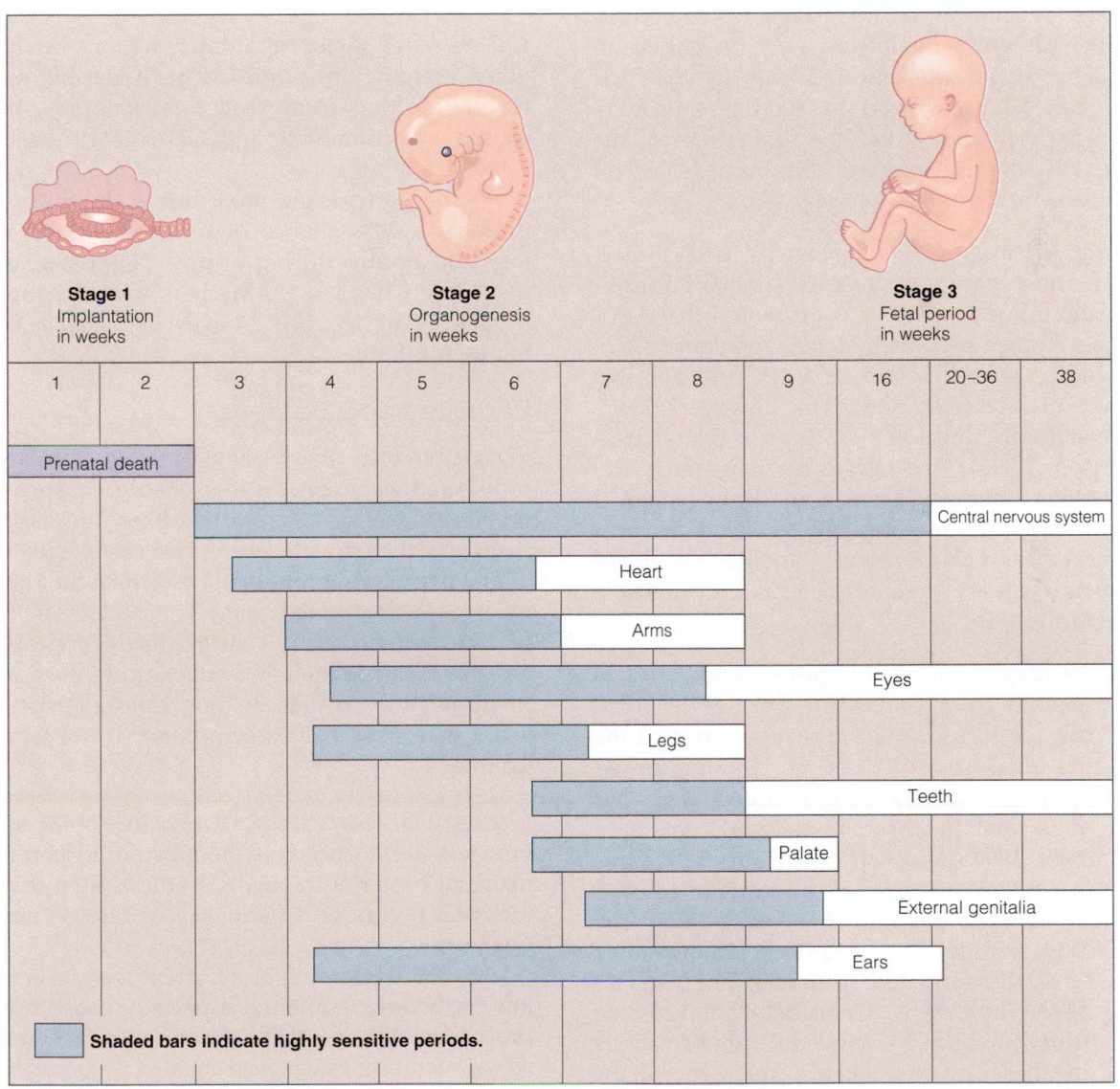

FIGURE 13–13. For the first two weeks after conception, exposure to a teratogen has an all-or-nothing effect. It either disrupts implantation and causes spontaneous abortion or leaves the embryo unharmed. From about the third through the eighth week of pregnancy (when organs form) exposure to a hazardous agent may cause serious structural anomalies. After organ formation and for the remainder of the pregnancy, exposure to fetal toxins will not cause malformation but can interfere with maturation of the central nervous system and retard intrauterine growth or cause cognitive or behavioral abnormalities. *(Reprinted, with permission, from Conover, E. (1994). Guarding against fetal toxins. Registered Nurse, July, 31.)*

Infectious agents known to cause malformations are rubella, cytomegalovirus, herpes simplex virus, HIV, toxoplasma, and group B streptococcus. Environmental and lifestyle factors causing malformations include use of tobacco and drugs, exposure to radiation and chemicals, and occupational hazards.

▶ Infectious Agents

Viruses

Rubella. Rubella infection is preventable through active immunization, yet it continues to be a major cause of birth defects. Several types of malformation may occur, depending on the stage of embryonic development at which the infection occurs. For example, 15–25% of infants infected during the first trimester can be recognized as having congenital rubella in early infancy. After the first trimester, the incidence of severly infected children drops off rapidly (Hanson, 1996) (see Chapter 19).

Cytomegalovirus. Cytomegalovirus (CMV) infection is the most common cause of congenital infections throughout the world. It is estimated that 5–6% of pregnant women become infected, and about 3% of their newborns have evidence of CMV infection. No more than 5% of infected newborns, however, (0.15% overall) eventually develop significant signs of damage (Hanson, 1996). The malformations most frequently seen occur in asymptomatically infected mothers and include microcephaly, cerebral calcifications, blindness and chorioretinitis, and hepatosplenomegaly. Some infants have kernicterus and multiple petechiae of the skin.

Herpes Simplex Virus. Herpes simplex virus is usually transmitted to the infant during the birth process when the virus is shed from the cervix of the lower genital tract. About half of the infants exposed to herpes during delivery become infected. If left untreated it is fatal in approximately 60% of these cases (Martens, 1994), and half of the survivors have untoward neurologic sequelae. Symptoms of the disease develop during the first 3 weeks of life. The infection may manifest as localized inflammatory reactions or as disseminated reactions. The neonate may also be asymptomatic. Occasionally fetuses are infected prior to birth. Congenital abnormalities observed in these infants include microencephaly, microphthalmia, retinal dysplasia, and mental retardation (Hanson, 1996).

Human Immunodeficiency Virus. Perinatal transmission of HIV has been a major concern through-

out the 1980s and early to mid 1990s. While it was concluded fairly early that HIV did not cause birth defects, it was evident that a high percentage of newborns were infected in utero (25–30%). However, with treatment of infected mothers with zidovudine, the incidence of transmission to the fetus is greatly reduced (approximately 8%) (U.S. Centers for Disease Control and Prevention, 1998).

All individuals, regardless of age, and especially those who engage in high-risk behaviors, need to be educated about HIV, its transmission, and ways to reduce the risk of acquiring or transmitting it. Educational programs are an essential component of family planning and prenatal care.

Other Viral Agents. Malformations rarely follow other maternal infections. The hyperthermia (high fever) resulting from viral infections has, however, caused malformations and has recently been implicated as a teratogen.

Varicella (chicken pox) during the first trimester presents a 20% chance of fetal abnormalities if the infection occurs during critical periods of development (see Chapter 19). Mothers with the most common forms of hepatitis B have a 90% chance of infecting their infants.

Parasites and Bacteria

Toxoplasma. Toxoplasmosis results from exposure to infected excretions of household pets such as cats, rabbits, and birds or from handling infected animals that carry the parasite *Toxoplasma gondii.* (See Chapter 9 for a discussion of methods by which the risk of toxoplasmosis can be reduced.) The parasite is transmitted during fetal life, not during the birth process. The most frequent sequela is a subclinical infection that is predominantly ocular. In one third of cases, many years may pass before symptoms are observed (see Chapter 19).

Group B Streptococcus. In some countries, group B streptococcus is the most important cause of neonatal bacterial infection. In the United States, this infection occurs at a frequency of 1 to 30 per 10,000 live births.

Group B beta-hemolytic streptococcus is found in low-birth-weight infants, especially those born after prolonged rupture of the membranes. When the placental membranes are broken, streptococcus can penetrate the protective barrier, grow in the birth canal, and infect the fetus. Women who are susceptible to early rupture of membranes also tend to harbor colonies of streptococcus B. They are also often asymptomatic (see Chapter 19).

▶ Lifestyle and Environmental Hazards

Environmental agents to which a mother is exposed during pregnancy can be categorized into those that the mother chooses as part of her lifestyle, medically prescribed drugs, radiation, environmental chemicals, and occupational hazards.

A woman may choose to use tobacco, recreational drugs, alcohol, and caffeine. Such habits can be changed through counseling; ideally, counseling should occur preconception.

Smoking

Smoking during pregnancy can have adverse effects on fetal growth and development. Studies have shown that smoking during pregnancy is associated with reduced birth weight, reduction in uteroplacental oxygen, and delayed neurologic and intellectual development of children. The adverse effects of smoking are due to the following factors:

- Carbon monoxide, which inactivates fetal and maternal hemoglobin, reducing the amount of oxygen delivered to the fetus
- Nicotine, the vasoconstrictive action of which reduces placental perfusion
- Reduction in maternal appetite, leading to a reduction in caloric intake

In addition to the known risks to the mother, smoking increases the risk of placenta previa, abruptio placentae, premature rupture of the membranes, congenital malformations, respiratory morbidity, spontaneous abortion, bacterial infection, increased risk of sudden infant death syndrome, stillbirth, and infant mortality. Although the substances in cigarette smoke place the fetus at risk in the first trimester of pregnancy, smoking can have harmful effects throughout pregnancy, especially on the developing central nervous system of the fetus. If the mother stops smoking by the 12th week of gestation, the effects on the fetus can be minimized.

Recreational Drugs

The use of "recreational" or illicit drugs by the pregnant woman has caused great concern among investigators and clinicians, because of the documented or potential effects of these drugs on the fetus. Chronic use by the expectant mother of such substances as opium derivatives, barbiturates, and amphetamines can result in intrauterine distress, low birth weight, and drug withdrawal in the newborn. The effects of marijuana on the embryo and fetus are not well documented; however, animal studies have shown that maternal marijuana smoking affects both the male and female reproductive systems. Specifically, delta-9-tetrahydrocannabinol (THC), found in marijuana, may decrease levels of follicle-stimulating hormone, luteinizing hormone, prolactin, and testosterone and may inhibit ovulation and spermatogenesis. Further, THC has been implicated in fetal growth retardation. Chronic users of cocaine and crack during pregnancy have a higher rate of spontaneous abortions, fetal deaths, low-birth-weight and small-for-gestation infants, and infants with depression of interactive behavior and poor organizational response to stimuli, as well as possible learning disabilities. Table 13–5 lists drugs that may be abused and their effects.

The problem of drug use among pregnant women is complex. The majority of these women receive little or no prenatal care and are at greater risk for malnutrition and infections. Further, women who transmit HIV to their fetuses are frequently intravenous drug users or partners of men who are intravenous drug users. The infection is contracted by the mother through contaminated drug paraphernalia or sexual intercourse with an intravenous drug user. The HIV-infected mother may then transmit HIV to her fetus congenitally. These women often do not seek prenatal care until late in pregnancy, sometimes appearing for care when labor has begun. These factors, added to the social and psychologic problems of the mother and the apparent risks to the fetus, require careful health planning by the nurse. The short-term goal may be to reduce the physiologic problems associated with drug use, for the mother and the fetus. Long-term goals include assessment of the medical, social, and psychologic factors that contribute to drug use and management of the addiction through appro-

▶ TABLE 13-5

Selected Drugs of Abuse and Their Possible Effects on the Embryo/Fetus and Neonate

Drug	Effect
Heroin	Intrauterine growth retardation, withdrawal symptoms, respiratory depression, neonatal death
Methadone	Fetal distress, neonatal drug withdrawal
Valium	Possible cleft lip and palate, respiratory depression, hypotonia, hypothermia, low Apgar score
Amphetamines	Possible cleft lip and cleft palate, transposition of the great vessels, learning disabilities
Marijuana	Fetal growth retardation
Cocaine	Spontaneous abortion, fetal death, low birth weight

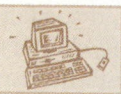

Research Abstract

Implications of Screening for Perinatal Substance Abuse

During the late 1980s and early 1990s the use of drugs by pregnant women gained a great deal of attention. Public concern focused on the effect of drugs on a woman's fetus. This concern led to a variety of legal responses by states. When a legal sanction is linked to findings indicative of maternal prenatal drug use, controversy surrounds whether to test all pregnant mothers and their infants (universal testing) or to test only women who exhibit certain behaviors known to be linked with drug use. Differential hospital policies for testing may lead to problems of selection bias. No data currently exit on the policies and procedures used by hospitals regarding testing a pregnant woman or her neonate. The purpose of this study was to examine hospital perinatal protocols and the criteria used to select pregnant women and neonates for drug testing.

Fifty hospitals that provide maternity care in Cook County, Illinois, were identified through an American Hospital Association listing. Nurse administrators or clinical specialists from 49 of the 50 hospitals responded to a telephone survey which questioned the criteria used to select mothers and infants for testing, the extent to which written informed or oral consent was obtained for drug tests, and the actions taken by hospitals in response to positive drug test results in infants.

The most frequently cited criteria for testing mothers and infants for drug use were verbal admission of drug use, the health provider's suspicion of drug use, a positive diagnosis of HIV or a sexually transmitted disease in the mother, or a combination of these criteria. In addition, failure to obtain written consent from the mother for drug screening occurred in 80% of hospitals when testing was done in newborn units, in 73% of hospitals when testing was done in labor units, and in 53% of hospitals when testing was done in prenatal units. Finally, 94% of hospitals always reported a positive test result to child protection agencies. The discharge of an infant with positive test results was delayed in 65% of newborn units.

This study confirmed the lack of universal drug screening policies in hospitals in a metropolitan area and indicated that the majority of hospitals participating in the survey did not obtain written informed consent from the mother prior to screening. The investigators concluded that universal screening with informed consent for all women, especially as part of routine prenatal care and not connected with criminal sanctions, is seen as useful in identifying drug-abusing mothers who require treatment and in providing early interventions to drug-exposed infants. Further, when sanctions are the consequence of perinatal drug testing, universal drug screening appeared to be a viable option to avoid potential bias and to provide treatment to mothers and neonates.

Application to Practice

This survey provides initial data concerning response of the health care community to perinatal substance abuse. While the conclusion that universal screening of all pregnant women will prevent selection bias when no standard criteria for screening exists is true, the issue is by no means resolved by this approach. This survey clearly indicates that mothers might very well lose custody of their children if positive test results are discovered in their infants. Both universal and selective screening may tend to delay a substance-using pregnant mother's entry into prenatal care for fear that her child will be taken from her. A focus on the underlying causes of substance abuse and ways to help pregnant users, rather than application of punitive actions, is an important consideration for health care providers.

Source: Birchfield, M., Scully, J., & Handler, A. (1995). Perinatal screening for illicit drugs: Policies in hospitals in a large metropolitan area. Journal of Perinatology. *15(3): 208–213.*

priate resources. Nurses should also become involved in planning educational programs for children and adolescents in an effort to prevent drug use at any stage in a person's life, especially pregnancy.

Alcohol

Prenatal damage from maternal alcohol abuse may be one of the most frequent recognizable causes of mental deficiency in the United States. As many as 0.5% of American children may have developmental problems related to maternal alcohol use during pregnancy (Hanson, 1996). Use of alcohol by the expectant mother has been associated with a group of congenital malformations referred to as **fetal alcohol syndrome** (FAS) (see Chapter 32). The severity of the syndrome varies with the amount of alcohol consumed, so that the heavier the drinker, the greater the probability of severe congenital abnormalities. More recent studies, however, have shown that women who drink alcohol in small amounts have a higher incidence of spontaneous abortion. It is now recommended that women consume no alcohol during pregnancy because of the risks to the fetus.

Caffeine

The effect of caffeine in pregnancy is not well documented; there is no scientific evidence to conclude that caffeine is teratogenic. Heavy maternal caffeine consumption may be related to intrauterine growth retardation as a result of reduction of blood flow to the uterus. Nurses should weigh the evidence when counseling pregnant women about caffeine consumption (see Chapter 14).

Medically Prescribed Drugs

Drugs other than those considered "recreational" or illicit also have harmful effects on the developing fetus. Before the thalidomide disaster in the 1960s, it was believed that the placental barrier protected the fetus from drugs taken by the mother. Since that time,

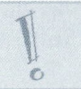

Nursing Alert

Nurses must educate all expectant mothers to exercise caution in relation to any drug they consider using during pregnancy due to potential teratogenic effects on their fetuses (Hanson, 1996).

the placental barrier theory has been discounted and a number of drugs taken by the mother have been associated with birth defects in the offspring.

Thalidomide, a drug once used as an antiemetic during pregnancy, has been proven to cause deformities of the arms, legs, and face in the fetus. The experience with this drug alerted investigators to the need to exercise caution in applying data obtained from animal studies to the human being. No evidence of the teratogenic effects was found when thalidomide was tested on certain animals before its release, yet thalidomide was found to cause malformations in the human fetus. As the effects of thalidomide have been identified only at the expense of thousands of malformed children, it is imperative that malformations related to drug exposure be carefully documented. See box entitled Drugs With Teratogenic Effects in Humans.

Early exposure to high doses of androgenic steroid hormones leads to masculinization of female fetuses. It has also been shown that females exposed in utero to stilbestrol may be at increased risk of developing vaginal cancer 10 or more years after the exposure. Exposure to antineoplastic drugs during pregnancy results in abortion or malformations in 20 to 30% of those fetuses who survive to term.

▶ DRUGS WITH TERATOGENIC EFFECTS IN HUMANS

- Androgens (e.g., testosterone, methyltestosterone, fluoxymesterone, oxandrolone, oxymetholone, ethylestrenol, methandrostenolone, nandrolone, stanozolol)
- Antineoplastic drugs (e.g., methotrexate)
- Coumarin derivatives (warfarin, dicumarol)
- Diethylstilbestrol (DES)
- Ethanol (high, chronic doses)
- Isotretinoin (Accutane)

- Lithium
- Paramethadione (Paradione), trimethadione (Tridione)
- Phenytoin (Dilantin)
- Tetracyclines (demeclocycline, doxycycline, methacycline, minocycline, oxytetracycline, tetracycline)
- Thalidomide (no longer available)
- Valproic acid (Depakene, Depakote)

Tetracyclines have been proven to cause dental staining in offspring because of their strong affinity for osseous and dental tissue.

In addition to the previously mentioned drugs, which have provided strong evidence of teratogenic effects in human populations, many drugs are suspected to be teratogens on the basis of epidemiologic studies, laboratory reports, and case studies. Drugs taken in the first trimester of pregnancy can cause malformations in the embryo/fetus because organogenesis occurs in this period.

The expectant mother should be aware of the known or possible effects of any medications taken during pregnancy. The old adage "better safe than sorry" applies to the use of any substance during pregnancy. Unless the drug is essential to the mother's health (e.g., insulin for diabetic mothers), it should be avoided; if the drug is deemed essential, careful monitoring of the mother and fetus throughout pregnancy is necessary.

Radiation

Exposure to radiation can have teratogenic effects; the nature of the malformation depends on the dose of radiation and the stage of development at which exposure occurred. Organogenesis is the period of development that is most sensitive to radiation. Gross skeletal and central nervous system anomalies are the most common manifestations. Other malformations include ophthalmic defects, impaired motor performance, spina bifida, cleft palate, and defects of the extremities.

Epidemiologic studies have so far indicated that diagnostic ultrasound does not have any measurable

Women's Health

In environments in which pregnant women are exposed to the radiation emitted by video display terminals, the following preventive measures should be followed: minimize the total amount of time in which exposure occurs; shut off equipment when not in use; and sit at least 2 ft from the screen when working in front of these terminals.

or significant biologic effects on the fetus. Additional studies related to microwaves indicate that this form of electromagnetic energy does not have the capacity to produce mutations. It appears from these studies that microwaves and ultrasound do not have sufficient energy to ionize molecules and disrupt DNA. The data on the effects of microwaves and ultrasound are controversial, however, and continued in-depth investigation of these energy sources is needed.

Properly constructed microwave ovens and video display terminals operated under normal conditions appear to emit no or minimal ionizing radiation; they are thus not currently considered a hazard to pregnant women according to some authorities. Others believe that video display terminals may be hazardous to the woman and her fetus. More research needs to be done in this area.

▶ **TABLE 13-6**

Occupational Hazards That May Cause Reproductive Problems or Fetal Congenital Anomalies

Occupation	Hazardous Substance
Textile and garment workers	Cotton and fiber dusts, noise, formaldehyde, dyes, heat, asbestos, solvents, flame retardants
Health personnel	Anesthetic gases, x-rays, alcohol, noise, laboratory chemicals
Electronic assemblers	Lead, tin, antimony, trichloroethylene, methylene chloride, resins
Hairdressers/cosmetologists	Hairspray resins, aerosol propellants, solvents, dyes
Cleaning personnel	Soaps, detergents, heat, enzymes, solvents
Launderers of industrially contaminated clothing	Various industrial chemicals
Photographic processors	Caustics, bromides, iodines, silver nitrate
Plastic workers	Acrylonitrile, formaldehyde, vinyl chloride
Transportation workers	Carbon monoxide, polynuclear aromatics, lead, vibration, microwaves
Painters	Lead, titanium, toluene
Clerks/clerical workers	Trichloroethylene, carbon tetrachloride, formaldehyde, asbestos, cigarette smoke
Printing personnel	Ink mists, methanol, carbon tetrachloride, lead, noise, solvents, trichloroethylene

Reproduced, with permission, from Samuels, M., & Bennett, H.Z. (1983). Well body well earth. *San Francisco: Sierra Club Books.*

Environmental Chemicals

Exposure to environmental chemicals is often beyond the expectant mother's control. One of the most well-documented teratogens in humans is methyl mercury, which has been found in contaminated coastal waters. Pregnant women who ate fish contaminated with this chemical gave birth to children with severe congenital anomalies. Lead, passive smoke, selenium, and a variety of pesticides are also suspected of causing birth defects.

Occupational Hazards

Several occupational hazards have also been identified that may affect male and female reproduction and cause birth defects in the fetus (Table 13–6). Men and women should be made aware of these possible hazards, especially in the reproductive years, to prevent some of their effects on parents and their offspring.

Guiding Principles for Client Education

When one considers the number of teratogens or possible teratogens that may affect parents and their offspring, it is essential to include the possibility of exposure to these agents into the health history and nursing care plan. The box entitled Client Education: Exposure to Teratogens presents the principles that should guide the nurse in teaching expectant parents about known and possible teratogens.

With these principles in mind, the nurse should plan health education programs for couples prior to and during pregnancy so that exposure to teratogens can be prevented.

▶ CLIENT EDUCATION: EXPOSURE TO TERATOGENS

The following principles should be used to educate child-bearing families about known and possible teratogens:

- A teratogen is any agent that can adversely affect the growth and development of the fetus.
- The first trimester is a critical period in the development of the fetus. Exposure to teratogens at this time may cause severe congenital malformations.
- Exposure to teratogens in the second and third trimesters can cause problems related to brain growth, intrauterine growth retardation, and developmental delays in children.

- Neonatal complications such as drug withdrawal have been attributed to maternal drug intake.
- Factors that are not associated with birth defects in animals may be teratogenic in humans.
- Many of the defects caused by teratogens occur before the mother is even aware that she is pregnant, therefore, counseling should be provided prior to pregnancy.
- Informed decision making concerning avoidance of known or suspected teratogens is the responsibility of the client and her family.

Chapter Highlights

▶ After both the sperm and the ova undergo maturation processes, the sperm penetrates the ovum and the ovum responds by cortical and zona reactions, resumption of the second meiotic division, and metabolic activation, all resulting in fertilization of the ovum by the sperm.

▶ The first 14 days of development, known as the preembryonic period, are characterized by rapid growth and development of the fertilized ovum.

▶ By the fourth month, the placenta has developed two compartments, the fetal portion and the maternal portion, and these structures, together with the placental membrane, provide the essentials of life for the growing fetus.

▶ The placenta carries out two important functions during pregnancy: hormone production and transport and exchange of products between the mother and fetus.

▶ During the embryonic period, the third to eighth weeks of development, all major organ systems are formed, which makes this period the time in which the embryo is most susceptible to infectious or environmental agents.

▶ Maturation of the tissues and organs of the fetus occurs during the fetal period, which extends from the third lunar month through the tenth lunar month.

▶ Twins may be either dizygotic (originating from two separate zygotes) or monozygotic (originating from one zygote) and differ with respect to implantation site, placenta, chorion, and amnion.

▶ Fetal circulation is supported by structures such as the umbilical cord, ductus venosus, placenta, foramen ovale, and ductus arteriosus and is dependent on efficient maternal placental circulation.

▶ Developments in embyology and fetology have significant potential for improving pregnancy outcomes.

▶ During the period of embryologic and fetal growth and development, a variety of infectious agents (viruses, parasites, and bacteria), lifestyle hazards (smoking, use of recreational drugs, alcohol, caffeine, and use of medically prescribed drugs), and environmental hazards (radiation, chemicals, and occupational agents) may place the developing human at risk.

▶ The nurse acts as health educator to the family and provides them with information that encourages positive health care behaviors during embryologic and fetal development.

After reading the vignette at the beginning of this chapter, use what you have learned to answer these questions:

1. What educational strategies can be designed to help Laura O'Connor make an informed decision about the use of over-the-counter medications and their potential effects on her fetus?

2. To avoid the use of over-the-counter medications during her pregnancy, what other methods of nonpharmacologic pain relief can be recommended to Laura O'Connor?

3. Given the complex interaction of genetic and environmental factors that may contribute to risks for the mother and fetus, how can the nurse help the client understand these factors and their effects on childbearing?

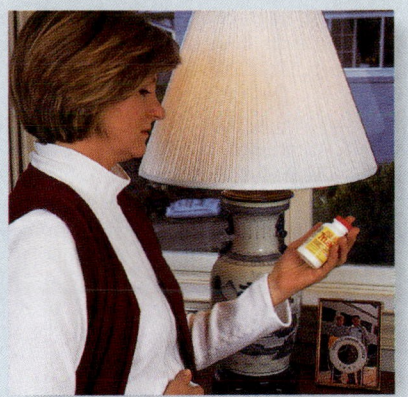

Critical Thinking Questions

▶ References

Birchfield, M., Scully, J., & Handler, A. (1995). Perinatal screening for illicit drugs: Policies in hospitals in a large metropolitan area. *Journal of Perinatology.* 15(3): 208–213.

Cunningham, F.G., MacDonald, P.C., Gant, N.F., Leveno, K.J., Gilstrap, L.C., Hankins, G.D.V., & Clark, S.L. (1997). *Williams Obstetrics* (20th ed.). Stamford, CT: Appleton & Lange.

England, M. (1996). *Life Before Birth* (2nd ed.). New York: Mosby-Wolfe.

Gebauer, L.L., & Lowe, N.K. (1993). The biophysical profile: Antepartal assessment of fetal well-being. *Journal of Obstetric, Gynecologic, and Neonatal Nursing, 2,* 115–124.

Gumbach, M.M. (1996). The endocrine system. In A.M. Rudolph (Ed.), *Rudolph's Pediatrics* (20th ed.) (pp. 1673–1852). Norwalk, CT: Appleton & Lange.

Hanson, J.W. (1996). Teratogenic causes of congenital abnormalities. In A.M. Rudolph (Ed.), *Rudolph's Pediatrics* (20th ed.) (pp. 416–423). Norwalk, CT: Appleton & Lange.

Hazinski, T.A. (1996). The respiratory system. In A.M. Rudolph (Ed.), *Rudolph's Pediatrics* (20th ed.) (pp. 1569–1672). Norwalk, CT: Appleton & Lange.

Hoffman, J.E. (1996). The circulatory system. In A.M. Rudolph (Ed.), *Rudolph's Pediatrics* (20th ed.) (pp. 1409–1568). Norwalk, CT: Appleton & Lange.

Lasser, D.M., et al. (1993). First-trimester fetal biometry using transvaginal sonography. *Ultrasound in Obstetrics and Gynecology, 2,* 104–108.

Martens, K.A. (1994). Sexually transmitted and genital tract infections during pregnancy. *Emergency Medicine Clinics of North America, 12*(1), 91–113.

Morbidity and Mortality Weekly Report. (1998, January 23). *1998 Guidelines for Treatment of Sexually Transmitted Diseases.* Vol 47, No. RR-1. Atlanta, GA: United States Department of Health and Human Services, Centers for Disease Control and Prevention.

Rodeck, C.H. (1993). Prenatal diagnosis: Fetal development after chorionic villus sampling. *Lancet, 1,* 468–469.

U.S. Centers for Disease Control and Prevention. (1998). 1998 guidelines for treatment of sexually transmitted diseases. *Morbidity and Mortality Weekly Report, 47*(RR-1), 1–111.

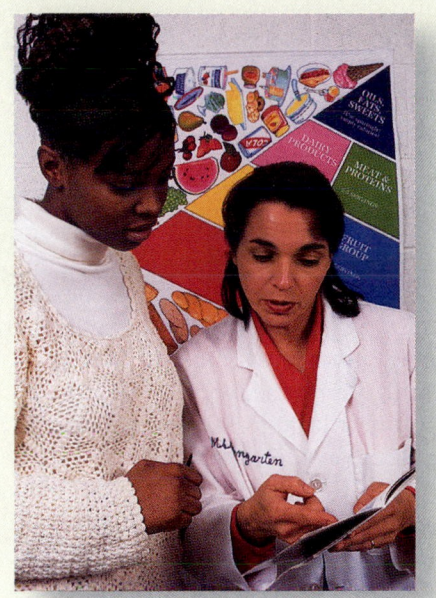

Erika Watson, age 20, is attending her first prenatal visit at a women's health clinic. She is 4 weeks' pregnant with her first child. Her prepregnancy weight was 127 lbs and her height is 5'7". In describing her typical daily intake, Erika states that she usually skips breakfast, has a sandwich or salad for lunch, and either meat or fish and a vegetable for dinner. She states that she knows that this is not a healthy diet and asks for help with nutritional planning.

Before beginning Erika's physical examination, Susan Rosengarten, MSN, NP, reviews the information relating to Erika's nutritional status. The nurse states, "I agree that your diet may not provide you and your baby with all of the necessary nutrients for growth. Let's look at this sample food plan. Tell me which foods you eat and don't eat. Do you see any problems in getting or preparing these foods?" ▪

14

Nutrition During Childbearing

Research in the last several decades has identified the important role of nutrition during pregnancy in influencing maternal and fetal health. The problems related to inadequate maternal nutrition are well recognized by health care professionals. The importance of nutritional health during pregnancy has led to a greater nursing emphasis on obtaining a thorough nutrition assessment, monitoring nutritional status, and promoting nutrition education.

The nurse plays a vital role in conducting the nutrition assessment and acting as a nutrition educator for pregnant women. The frequent contacts nurses have with clients are opportunities to gather information about food practices, lifestyle, and physical changes; to observe clinical signs and symptoms that may reflect nutritional health; to communicate to the client the importance of a healthy diet during pregnancy; and to respond to the client's particular needs or concerns regarding her eating habits.

Nutrition during pregnancy is a complex and diverse subject. This chapter focuses on the specific nutritional requirements of normal healthy pregnant women, as well as those women with special nutritional needs. The collaboration with nutritionists and other members of the interdisciplinary team is also emphasized as a means to ensure comprehensive care of the childbearing woman.

The specific nutritional needs of the postpartum woman, including requirements for breastfeeding, are presented in Chapter 31.

▶ WEIGHT GAIN DURING PREGNANCY

Adequate weight gain during pregnancy is required for maternal health and normal fetal growth and development. The total weight gain should be achieved at a steady rate. Weight gain in the early part of pregnancy promotes maternal tissue accretion (expanded blood volume, energy reserves, uterine growth, placenta). Weight gain in the later stages of pregnancy supports primarily growth of the fetus. Major gains in maternal and fetal organ development and fluid volume do not begin until approximately the 12th week of gestation.

At the end of the first trimester the fetus weighs only 45 g (1.6 oz). After the first trimester, weight gain increases significantly to meet maternal and fetal needs. Only 7 pounds of total weight gained during pregnancy is body fat. The remaining distribution of weight is composed of placental, uterine, fetal, and breast tissue, and blood and other fluid volume. The increased stores of body fat serve primarily as a reserve for energy needed during lactation.

The National Academy of Sciences Institute of Medicine (1990a, 1990b) recommends that pregnant women of normal preconceptional weight gain between 25 to 35 pounds (11.4 to 16 kg) over the course of pregnancy. Weight gain varies among women because of many different factors such as preconceptional weight, age, parity, ethnic origin, socioeconomic status, substance abuse, and level of physical activity. A 10-pound weight range is included in the recommended total weight gain to accommodate these differences. These recommendations were developed to provide guidelines for promoting optimal fetal and maternal health. Low gestational weight gain is associated with a higher risk of delivering growth-retarded infants and higher rates of fetal and infant mortality.

Prepregnancy weight and height measures are used to assess gestational weight gain. For clients whose first visit to the physician is a prenatal checkup, self-reported prepregnancy weight values may be used (although their accuracy is questionable). Weight-to-height ratios are a more valid measure of nutritional status than weight alone as they take into consideration body size. Weight for height can be calculated using **body mass index** (BMI), which is defined as weight (kg)/height (m)^2. Figure 14–1 is a chart used to calculate BMI, and Table 14–1 shows the recommended total weight gain ranges using the BMI.

To monitor weight gain most practitioners use prenatal growth charts as illustrated in Figure 14–2. These charts allow the nurse and client to follow changes in weight gain throughout the pregnancy. The recommended rate of weight gain is shown in Figure 14–2 by the colored lines. The recommended pattern of weight gain for normal body prepregnancy weight for height during the first trimester is 2 to 4 pounds (0.90 to 1.80 kg) and 1 pound (0.45 kg) per

▶ TABLE 14–1

Recommended Total Weight Gain Ranges for Pregnant Women[a] by Prepregnancy Body Mass Index (BMI)[b]

Weight-for-Height Category	Recommended Total Gain	
	kg	lb
Low (BMI < 19.8)	12.5–18	28–40
Normal (BMI 19.8 to 26.0)	11.5–16	25–35
High[c] (BMI > 26.0 to 29.0)	7–11.5	15–25

[a]Young adolescents should strive for gains at the upper end of the recommended range. Short women (< 157 cm, or 62 in.) should strive for gains at the lower end of the range.
[b]BMI is calculated using metric units.
[c]The recommended target weight gain for obese women (BMI > 29.0) is at least 6.0 kg (15 lb).
From National Academy of Sciences Institute of Medicine, 1992.

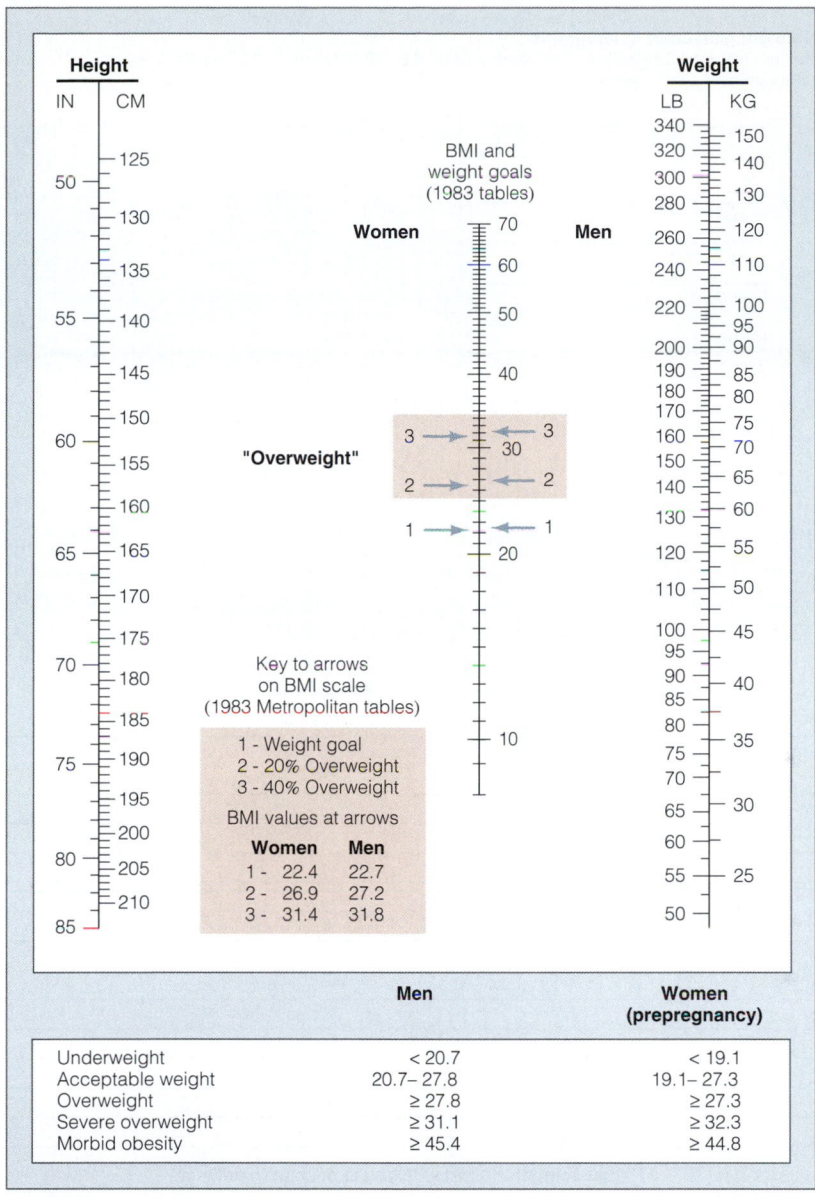

	Men	Women (prepregnancy)
Underweight	< 20.7	< 19.1
Acceptable weight	20.7– 27.8	19.1– 27.3
Overweight	≥ 27.8	≥ 27.3
Severe overweight	≥ 31.1	≥ 32.3
Morbid obesity	≥ 45.4	≥ 44.8

FIGURE 14–1. Nomogram for body mass index (BMI). Weights and heights are without clothing. With clothes, add 5 pounds for men or 3 pounds for women, and 1 in. in height for shoes. Draw a straight line, or place a ruler from your height (left) to your weight (right). At the point where it crosses the BMI line, read your BMI. The accompanying table indicates the BMIs used to define cutoff points. *(Reproduced, with permission, from Burton, B.T., & Roster, W.R. (1985). Health implications of obesity, and NIH Consensus Development Conference. Journal of the American Dietetic Association, 85, 1117–1121.)*

week for the second and third trimesters, for a total of 29 pounds (13.18 kg).

To plot the client's weight on the prenatal growth chart, the nurse must first calculate the client's prepregnancy BMI (see Fig. 14–1). Three separate weight gain recommendations are provided, determined by the categories of obese, high, normal, and low prepregnancy weight. These categories are based on the recognition that the weight gain needs of underweight women are very different from that of obese women. Specific nutritional recommendations for obese and underweight clients are discussed later in this chapter.

If the client's weight gain does not follow the recommended pattern, the first consideration is to doublecheck the measures to determine if there were a measurement or recording error. For normal-weight women whose weight gain is slow in the second or

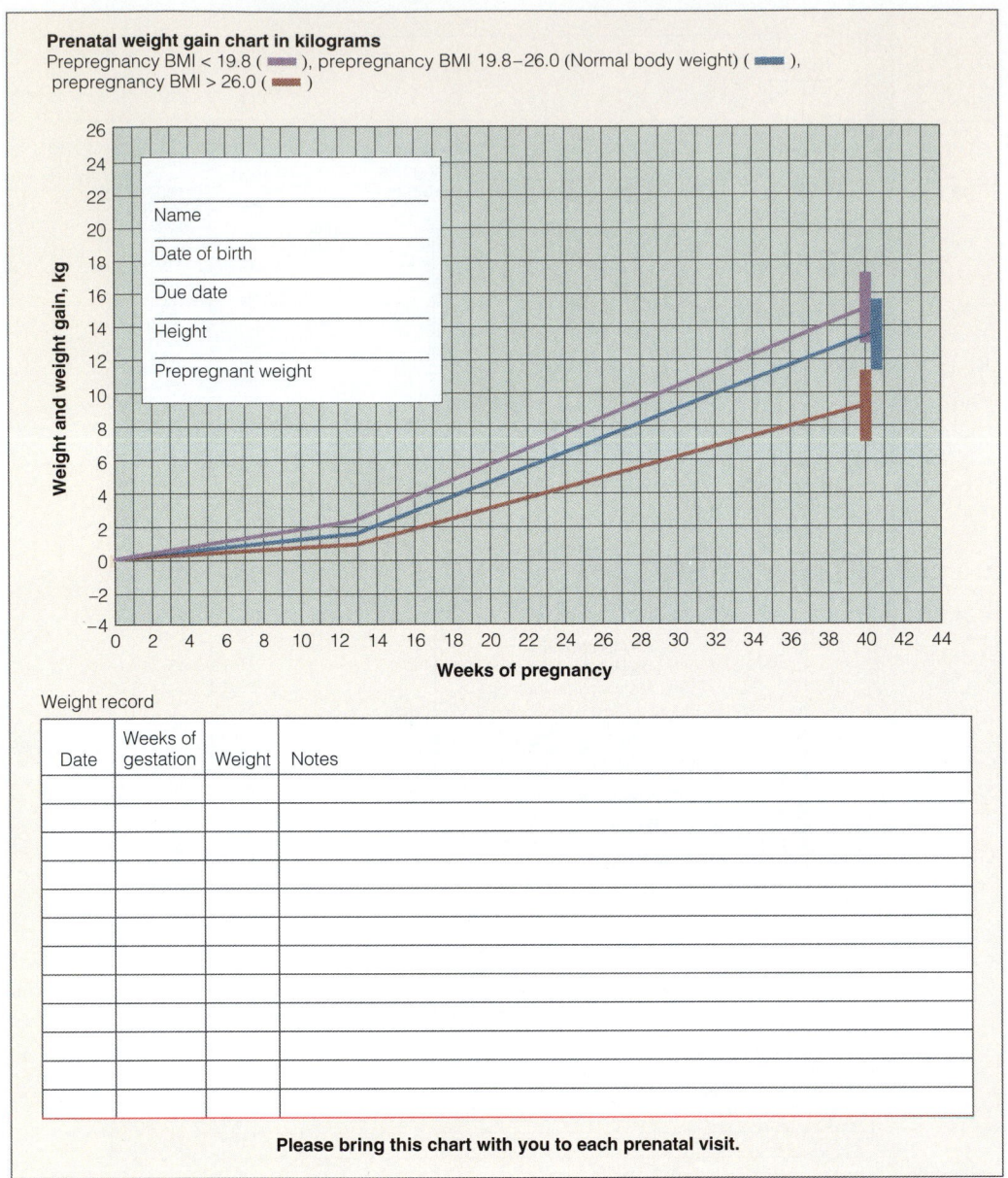

Prenatal weight gain chart in kilograms
Prepregnancy BMI < 19.8 (■■■), prepregnancy BMI 19.8–26.0 (Normal body weight) (■■■),
prepregnancy BMI > 26.0 (■■■)

Name

Date of birth

Due date

Height

Prepregnant weight

Weight and weight gain, kg

Weeks of pregnancy

Weight record

Date	Weeks of gestation	Weight	Notes

Please bring this chart with you to each prenatal visit.

FIGURE 14–2. Prenatal weight gain chart. *(From the National Academy of Sciences Institute of Medicine, Subcommittee on Nutritional Status and Weight Gain During Pregnancy. (1992).* Supplemental materials on nutrition during pregnancy and lactation: An implementation guide. *Washington, DC: National Academy Press.)*

third trimester (gain of less than 2 lb [1 kg] in any one month), the following areas should be explored:

- Does the client complain of such gastrointestinal problems as heartburn, nausea, vomiting, or diarrhea?
- Does the client have a new or preexisting health problem that may interfere with normal food intake?
- Are there any psychosocial problems that may cause a loss in appetite?
- What are the client's attitudes toward weight gain? (For example, is she fearful of gaining excess weight?)

- Does the client have access to sufficient amounts of food?
- Does the client have problems of substance abuse?
- Did the client lose weight since the last visit because of resolution of edema?
- Does the client's kilocalorie expenditure exceed her intake?

In a normal-prepregnancy-weight woman, gain of more than 6.5 pounds (3 kg) in any single month during the second and third trimesters needs further exploration. Excessive weight gain during pregnancy is associated with an increased risk of pregnancy-induced hypertension and a complicated labor. The following questions highlight areas to consider when assessing the causes of rapid weight gain:

- Has the client significantly increased her food intake or significantly decreased her physical activity level?
- Is a multiple gestation possible?
- Are there any signs of edema or gestational diabetes?
- Has the woman stopped smoking recently?

A complete dietary assessment can help to identify factors that may influence alterations in total weight gain. The components of nutrition assessment are discussed later in this chapter.

▶ NUTRIENT REQUIREMENTS

▶ Kilocalories

To achieve the current recommended rate of weight gain, the Food and Nutrition Board of the National Research Council recommends an intake of an additional 300 kcal per day above normal nonpregnant requirements. Total kilocalorie intake should not be below 36 kcal/kg body weight in adult pregnant women. Recommended total kilocalorie intake should be about 2200 kcal per day, or an increase of about 15% above normal requirements. Individual energy

needs, however, reflect basal body requirements, which are dependent on body and muscle size and fat composition, and physical activity level. Therefore, a woman who has a large body mass and exercises regularly may need more than 2400 kcal per day. For the most accurate estimation of energy needs, a thorough nutrition assessment should be conducted.

Because nutrient requirements rise during pregnancy, the extra 300 kcal should come from foods that contribute needed nutrients, such as protein and calcium. The recommended dietary pattern is described in Figure 14–3 and Table 14–2. These are only guidelines to the recommended minimum intake. Individual needs may vary according to the client's specific nutrient requirements and cultural dietary practices (see Evaluation of Cultural Food Practices).

The energy nutrients—protein, carbohydrates, and lipids—are essential in meeting the body's requirements for kilocalories and in performing other vital functions in the body.

▶ Protein

Protein requirements are based on the nutrient needs for synthesis of maternal and fetal tissue and the increase in blood volume that occurs during pregnancy. Approximately one kilogram of protein is stored during pregnancy. More specifically, protein is needed for development of the placenta, enlargement of the uterus, growth of the fetus, formation of the

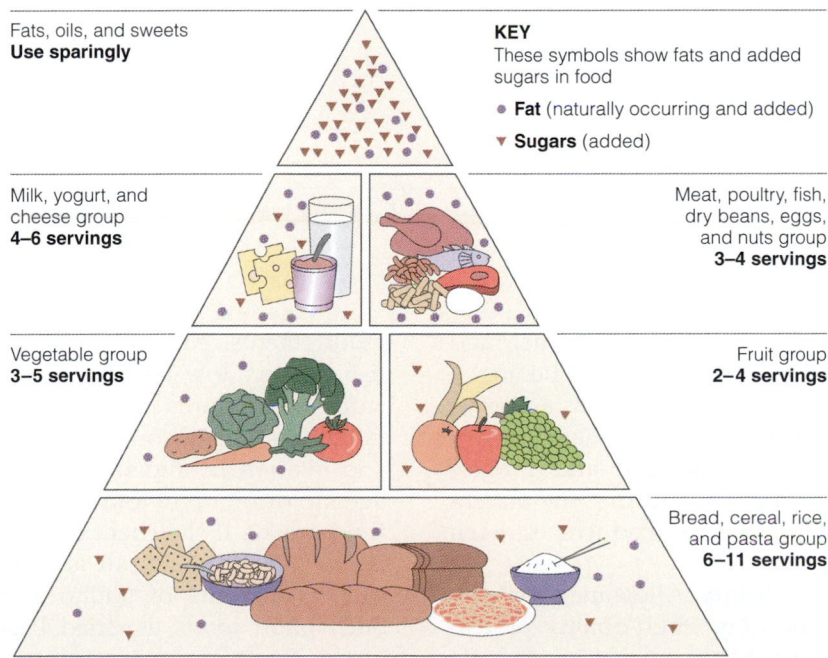

FIGURE 14–3. The Food Guide Pyramid, adapted for pregnant women. *(From the U.S. Department of Agriculture, Washington, DC.)*

► **TABLE 14–2**

Healthy Eating Guide for Pregnant Women

Grain Products	Vegetables	Fruits	Milk and Milk Products	Meat and Protein Foods	Sample Menus
6 to 11 servings a day	**3 to 5 servings a day**	**2 to 4 servings a day**	**4 to 6 servings a day**	**3 to 4 servings a day**	**Breakfast** Orange juice Bran flakes with peaches Muffin or biscuit Milk
• Grain products provide energy, vitamins and minerals. • Fortified breakfast cereals are good sources of folic acid. • Limit pastries, doughnuts, and cookies because they are high in fat.	• Vegetables provide vitamins and minerals. • Leafy green vegetables and beans are good sources of folic acid. • Fresh vegetables are best, but frozen or canned vegetables are acceptable. • Avoid fried vegetables like french fries.	• Fruits provide vitamins and minerals. • Limit fruit drinks with added sugar. Real fruit juice has more of the vitamins you need.	• Calcium builds bones and teeth. • Limit non-dairy milk substitutes. Coffee creamers and condensed milk have low nutritional value. • If lactose-intolerant, purchase specialty products that do not contain milk sugar.	• Protein builds strong muscles and blood. • Liver is a good source of folic acid, but is very high in cholesterol. • Limit high fat and processed meats such as hot dogs, bologna, sausage, spare ribs, corned-beef hash, turkey wings and bacon.	**Lunch** Glass of vegetable juice Egg salad on lettuce Two slices of pumpernickel bread Tomato slices **Dinner** Baked chicken Mixed green salad Baked sweet or white potato Milk Whole wheat roll Apple
Choose these Grain Products 1 slice enriched or whole grain bread 3/4 cup ready-to-eat enriched cereal 1/2 cup oatmeal, grits, or cooked wheat 1 pancake or waffle 1/2 cup spaghetti or noodles 1/2 cup rice, enriched or brown 1 tortilla 1 pita 1 muffin or biscuit 6 soda-type crackers 2 rice cakes	**Choose these Vegetables** 1 cup brussels sprouts 3/4 cup broccoli 1/2 cup spinach 1/2 cup chopped green pepper 1 cup collard greens, kale or cabbage 1/2 cup carrots 1/2 cup squash 1/2 cup eggplant 1/2 cup green beans 1/2 cup sweet peas 1/2 baked potato 1 small sweet potato 1 medium tomato 4–6 medium spears asparagus	**Choose these Fruits** 1 orange 1/2 cup orange or grapefruit juice 3/4 cup cubed watermelon 3/4 cup strawberries 1 small banana 1 apple 1 guava 1 mango 2 tablespoons dried fruit	**Choose these Milk and Milk Products** 1 cup milk: whole, lowfat, skim, powdered, or buttermilk 1 cup yogurt 1 cup cottage cheese 2 1" cubes cheese 1 cup pudding or custard 1-1/2 cups soup made with milk 1 cup ice milk or ice cream	**Choose these Meat and Protein Foods** 2 ounces of beef lamb pork liver chicken turkey fish shellfish 2 eggs 1 cup canned baked beans 1 cup dried peas/beans 1 cup tofu 1 tablespoon peanut butter 1/2 cup nuts	

Reproduced, with permission, from March of Dimes Birth Defects Foundation. (1997). Eating for two: Nutrition during pregnancy. White Plains, NY: Author.

amniotic fluid, increase in maternal tissue, and increased supply of serum proteins such as hemoglobin and albumin. The mother's body builds a reserve of protein during the luteal phase of pregnancy (when the corpus luteum supplies estrogen and progesterone). These stores are later used during the placental phase (i.e., when the placenta produces estrogen and progesterone).

The Recommended Dietary Allowance for protein is 60 g of protein per day. High-quality protein that contains all the essential amino acids in adequate proportions is as important as the total protein

requirements. Animal products such as lean meats, fish, poultry, low-fat dairy foods, and eggs all contain sufficient amounts of the essential amino acids. Low-fat milk is a good source of protein, as well as calcium and vitamin D, and the pregnant woman is encouraged to drink up to four glasses per day as part of her fluid intake. If the client chooses to follow a vegetarian diet that avoids all animal products, she needs proper amounts of amino acids from plant foods. Such plant foods as dried beans, nuts, grains, and seeds, if consumed in appropriate combinations, can supply adequate amounts of protein. To ensure that her protein intake is adequate, a pregnant vegetarian should receive nutritional counseling.

For protein to perform its vital function in promoting the building of tissue, enough calories in the form of carbohydrate and lipids must be available. If kilocalorie intake is inadequate (i.e., inadequate intake of carbohydrates and lipids for energy), protein will not be used for growth and development of new tissue but will instead be used for energy.

► Carbohydrates

The fetus is entirely dependent on the mother for meeting its glucose needs. A fetus requires approximately 30 g of glucose a day, which acts as its primary fuel source. The serum glucose level in the fetus' circulation is about 10 to 20 mg/100 mL lower than that in the maternal circulation. Glucose travels across the placental membrane via facilitated diffusion. Maternal insulin is unavailable to the fetus; therefore, the fetus is dependent on its own supply, which is first produced at 12 weeks of gestation. Glucagon is present in the fetal circulation at 8 weeks of gestation.

As a result of hormonal changes, various alterations in carbohydrate metabolism occur during pregnancy. During the first trimester, the maternal fasting blood glucose level decreases slightly to approximately 75 mg/100 mL of blood because of the increase in glucose supplied to the fetus and the accompanying decrease in insulin production. Glycogen deposits increase in peripheral tissues and hepatic glucose production decreases.

During the second and third trimesters of pregnancy, placental hormones (human placental lactogen, progesterone, estrogen) have a diabetogenic effect (producing a diabetic-like state). Human placental lactogen breaks down adipose tissue and releases glycerol and fatty acids for use as the primary maternal fuel. Estrogen decreases insulin's effectiveness, and cortisol increases the production of glucose by gluconeogenesis. Circulating levels of glucose and maternal amino acids decrease and fatty acids, triglycerides, and ketones increase. There is also maternal peripheral tissue resistance to insulin. During pregnancy, insulin requirements increase up to 70%.

Because of these changes there is a greater risk of starvation ketosis, which is characterized by hypoglycemia, increased nitrogen excretion, raised plasma levels of free fatty acids, and elevated plasma and urinary ketones. This is particularly common in a client who skips meals, especially if she omits breakfast after an overnight fast. Pregnant women should be encouraged to consume three meals a day with nutritious snacks between meals to promote normal blood glucose levels. A minimum intake of 150 g of carbohydrate per day is also advised, but to meet actual kilocalorie requirements during pregnancy, a larger intake of carbohydrate is required. After delivery, insulin requirements return to normal as a result of the excretion of placental anti-insulin hormones.

Carbohydrates should be provided primarily in the form of complex carbohydrates, such as enriched and whole-grain breads and cereals, vegetables, and fruits. Simple carbohydrates or sugars in the diet should be provided mostly from naturally occurring sources, such as fruits and fruit juices. Simple carbohydrates found in such foods as cakes, pies, cookies, candy, and soda should be minimized in the diet, as these foods provide few vitamins and minerals and are high in kilocalories. Total carbohydrate intake should be approximately 50–55% of total kilocalorie intake.

► Lipids

Lipids are required in the diet to provide a concentrated source of energy and essential fatty acids. Maternal fatty acids enter the fetal circulation but are not considered to be a major fuel source for the fetus, as the enzymes required to metabolize fat are present in small amounts. Fatty acids are valuable for the myelinization of nerves and membrane synthesis that occurs in utero; therefore, lipids are essential nutrients for fetal development.

Lipids should be derived from foods high in polyunsaturated and monounsaturated fatty acids, such as vegetable oils. Less emphasis should be placed on foods high in saturated fatty acids such as high-fat red meats, whole milk dairy products, and convenience foods high in fat. The client should choose such foods as lean meats, skinless poultry products, and fish, which are high in protein and low in saturated fat. Total lipid intake should be approximately 30% or less of the total kilocalorie intake. Diets composed of less than 20% of total kilocalories from lipids are not appropriate for pregnant women because they may lack adequate energy.

► Vitamins and Minerals

Vitamins and minerals are essential in the diet to promote the use of energy from protein, carbohydrates, and lipids; to build new tissue; and to act as regulating agents in many metabolic processes in the body. To meet vitamin and mineral requirements, pregnant women, in addition to eating a healthy diet, are often advised to take a multivitamin and multimineral preparation. With the exception of the nutrients iron and folic acid, adequate amounts of vitamins and minerals can be provided in a healthy, well-balanced diet; however, supplements are sometimes recommended as a precautionary measure to ensure adequate vitamin and mineral intake.

Pregnant women should take only those supplements designed for prenatal needs and should avoid any preparation that contains nutrients in higher dosages that may be unsafe. Table 14–3 lists Recommended Dietary Allowances (RDAs) for all vitamins and minerals during pregnancy. Table 14–4 summarizes the physiological functions of vitamins and minerals and common food sources.

Fat-Soluble Vitamins

The fat-soluble vitamins A, D, E, and K are stored in the body; therefore, any excess intake can be extremely toxic. Consuming megadoses of vitamin A during pregnancy has been reported to cause teratogenic effects (Rothman, Moore, Singer, Nguyen, Mannion, & Milunsky, 1995). Vitamin D has also been

shown to be teratogenic when consumed in megadose amounts.

Vitamin A is essential for normal bone development and growth and for growth and maintenance of normal epithelial tissue. Vitamin D is required for normal mineralization of the fetal skeletal system. Vitamin D is a unique nutrient because it is produced in the body by exposure to sunlight of 7-dehydrocholesterol, which is found in the skin. Brief periods of sunlight exposure can provide adequate supplies of the vitamin, which is also supplied by dietary sources such as fish and vitamin-fortified milk.

Protection of the integrity of the cellular membrane and intracellular structures are principal functions of vitamin E. Vitamin K functions in promoting normal blood clot formation, by acting as a cofactor for an enzyme required for the clotting mechanism.

Water-Soluble Vitamins

Vitamin C and the B-complex vitamins—folic acid, niacin (B_3), riboflavin (B_2), thiamine (B_1), vitamin B_6, and vitamin B_{12}—make up the water-soluble vitamins. Although toxic effects from excessive intake of water-soluble vitamins are generally not considered as likely as for the fat-soluble vitamins because excess amounts are excreted in the urine, pregnant women should take vitamin and mineral supplements only as prescribed by their health care provider. Adequate daily intake is essential, however, because the body stores only small amounts of these vitamins.

Vitamin C is required for promoting blood clot and collagen formation. The B-complex vitamins serve chiefly as coenzymes (substances that work along with other enzymes) in the various metabolic pathways of the body. Thiamine functions in carbohydrate metabolism, and riboflavin and niacin in the metabolism of all three energy nutrients.

Folic acid (folacin) needs increase during pregnancy because of the large increase in maternal erythropoiesis and fetal and placental growth. Folic acid is essential for the synthesis of purines and pyrimidines such as DNA and RNA. The relationship between folic acid and birth defects has been studied for more than 40 years. Researchers in the 1960s began to identify a positive relationship between a low folic acid intake and the development of neural tube defects (NTD) (Smithells, et al, 1965). Further investigations supported the original hypothesis by demonstrating that folic acid supplementation during pregnancy prevents the likelihood of the occurrence of a NTD pregnancy in high-risk clients (MRC Vitamin Study Research Group, 1991). In 1992 the U.S. Public Health Service recommended that all women of childbearing age who may become pregnant should take 0.4 mg of folic acid daily (Centers for Disease Control, 1992). As

▶ **TABLE 14–3**

Recommended Dietary Allowances for Reproduction

Nutrient	19–24 y	25–50 y	2nd and 3rd Trimester of Pregnancy
Energy (kcal)	2200	2200	+300
Protein (g)	46	50	60
Vitamin A (RE)[a]	800	800	800
Vitamin C (mg)	60	60	70
Vitamin D (μg)[b]	10	5	10
Vitamin E (mg)[c]	8	8	10
Vitamin K (μg)	60	65	65
Thiamine (mg)	1.1	1.1	1.5
Riboflavin (mg)	1.3	1.3	1.6
Niacin (mg)[d]	15	15	17
Vitamin B_6 (mg)	1.6	1.6	2.2
Vitamin B_{12} (μg)	2.0	2.0	2.2
Folate (μg)	180	180	400
Calcium	1200	800	1200
Phosphorus	150	800	1200
Magnesium	280	280	300
Iron	15	15	30
Iodine	150	150	175
Zinc	12	12	15
Selenium	55	55	65

[a]1 RE (retinol equivalent) = 1 μg or 6 μg β-carotene.
[b]As cholecalciferol. 10 μg cholecalciferol = 400 IU of vitamin D.
[c]α-Tocopherol equivalents. 1 mg d-α = 1 α-TE.
[d]1 NE (niacin equivalent) = 1 mg of niacin or 60 mg of dietary tryptophan.
From National Academy of Sciences, 1989.

Vitamins and Minerals and Their Physiologic Functions During Pregnancy

Nutrient	Physiologic Function	Food Source
Fat-Soluble Vitamins		
Vitamin A	Maintenance of normal epithelial cells, bone growth, and tooth formation	Beef liver, butter, margarine, whole milk, supplemented nonfat milk, dark green leafy vegetables, dark yellow-orange vegetables
Vitamin D	Increased absorption of calcium and phosphorus from maternal gastrointestinal tract, mineralization of fetal bones and teeth	Fortified milk, margarine, fish, liver oils (also supplied via nondietary source through exposure to sunlight)
Vitamin E	Protection of integrity of cellular and intracellular structures, maintenance of red blood cells	Vegetable and seed oils, green leafy vegetables, liver, wheat germ oil
Vitamin K	Promotion of normal blood clot formation by acting as cofactor with enzyme in clotting mechanism	Green leafy vegetables, egg yolk, liver (also produced by microflora of gastrointestinal tract, therefore no established RDA)
Water-Soluble Vitamins		
Vitamin C (ascorbic acid)	Promotion of blood clot and collagen formation, enhancement of absorption of iron, conversion of inactive folic acid to active form	Citrus fruits and juices, green peppers, potatoes, tomatoes, broccoli, cabbage, cantaloupe, strawberries
B-complex vitamins		
Folacin	Synthesis of nucleic acids, production of hemes for hemoglobin, prevention of megaloblastic anemia	Liver, green leafy vegetables, kidney beans, lean beef, whole wheat bread, yeast (vitamin's activity lost with cooking, supplementation of 200–400 µg recommended in latter part of pregnancy)
Niacin (B_3)	Coenzyme in the metabolism of carbohydrates, lipids, proteins	Organ meat, lean meats, poultry, fish, peanuts, vegetables, dry beans, pears
Riboflavin (B_2)	Coenzyme in the metabolism of carbohydrates, lipids, proteins	Milk, eggs, organ meats, veal, beef, cheddar cheese, green leafy vegetables
Thiamine (B_1)	Coenzyme in carbohydrate metabolism	Pork products, organ meats, especially liver, nuts, dried beans, brewer's yeast, wheat germ, whole-grain and enriched breads and cereals
Vitamin B_6 (pyridoxine)	Coenzyme in amino acid metabolism	Meat, poultry, fish, eggs, dairy products, wheat
Vitamin B_{12} (cobalamin)	Maintenance of the myelin sheath of nerve and epithelial cells, maintenance of red and white blood cell formation	Animal proteins, seaweed
Minerals		
Iron	Manufacture of maternal and fetal hemoglobin, increased maternal blood volume (storage of iron compensates for loss of blood during delivery)	Egg yolks, red meats, organ meats, especially liver (Other sources include poultry, fish, dried beans, green leafy vegetables, prunes, but iron in these foods is less efficiently absorbed. Because iron-rich foods may be limited in diet, supplementation with 30–60 mg of ferrous salts is recommended, beginning in the second trimester.)
Calcium and phosphorus	Formation of fetal skeleton and teeth, maternal calcium absorption	*Calcium:* whole milk, nonfat milk, buttermilk, yogurt, hard cheese, green leafy vegetables, sardines, nuts, dried beans *Phosphorus:* nearly all foods, animal proteins, nuts, dried beans, as a food additive in cola drinks and processed foods
Iodine	Synthesis of T_3 and T_4[a]	Iodized salt, saltwater fish, produce grown in iodine-rich soil
Sodium	Normal body metabolism	A variety of fresh and processed foods, especially cured meats, and salty foods such as potato chips, pretzels, salted nuts and popcorn, salted pickles, olives, and relishes
Magnesium	Activation of enzyme systems in energy-producing reactions, synthesis of proteins, nucleic acids, fats	Dark green leafy vegetables, dried beans, nuts, soybeans, whole-grain cereals, milk, meat, seafood
Zinc	Synthesis of DNA and RNA, role in metabolism and maintenance of acid–base balance	Animal proteins, shellfish, especially Atlantic oysters (also found in moderate amounts in eggs, milk, and cheese, and in smaller amounts in legumes, nuts, and whole grains, but zinc from these sources may not be well absorbed)

[a]T3, triiodothyronine; T4, 3,5,3′,5′-tetraiodothyronine (thyroxine).

of 1998 the Food and Drug Administration (FDA) requires that all enriched bread products, enriched flours and corn meals, enriched pasta and rice be fortified with folic acid. Breakfast cereal manufacturers may voluntarily add folic acid to their products (U.S. Food and Drug Administration, 1996).

Vitamin B_{12} (cobalamin) requirements are also related to the development of maternal and fetal tissue. Vitamin B_{12} works together with folic acid to promote the transfer of methyl groups in the synthesis of nucleic acids and purines and pyrimidines.

Vitamin B_6 (pyridoxine) functions as a coenzyme in amino acid metabolism; therefore, as protein requirements increase during pregnancy, B_6 needs are also elevated.

Minerals

Minerals are essential in the diet during pregnancy. Many contribute to cell and tissue formation in the body and work with enzymes to stimulate biochemical reactions. The increase in mineral requirements during pregnancy is based on the normal physiologic changes associated with pregnancy.

Iron. The large increases in iron in maternal blood volume, fetal iron stores, placental iron content, and blood losses during delivery emphasize the need for increased iron requirements during pregnancy. Iron is required to produce hemoglobin, which supplies oxygen to the body's tissues and is also essential in promoting the production of iron-containing enzymes used in oxidation of energy nutrients. Iron stores are formed primarily during the last trimester of pregnancy and provide enough iron to last about 6 months.

Maternal absorption of iron is estimated to be 30% above nonpregnant levels; however, to meet iron needs and prevent iron deficiency anemia, iron supplementation is usually advised during pregnancy. In addition to the RDA of 15 mg, an additional daily supplement of 30 to 60 mg of ferrous salts is recommended beginning about 12 weeks of gestation.

There are conflicting reports regarding the effects of iron deficiency on fetal health. Some studies report an increased incidence of low birth weight and prematurity (Scholl & Hediger, 1994). Possible side effects of iron supplementation, particularly at the higher doses used to treat anemia, include constipation, diarrhea, heartburn, and nausea. Slow-release tablets may help to relieve some of these problems.

Calcium and Phosphorus

Calcium and phosphorus act synergistically to promote fetal skeletal development. Approximately 30 g of calcium is stored in the mother and fetus during pregnancy. The fetus accumulates 25 g of calcium by the time of birth. Most calcium and phosphorus are supplied by the mother to the fetus during the last 4 weeks of pregnancy; however, the mother should consume adequate amounts of calcium and phosphorus throughout pregnancy to build up sufficient stores. Because too much phosphorus may impede calcium absorption, it is recommended that individuals have a one-to-one ratio of calcium to phosphorus in their diet.

To meet increased calcium needs pregnant women need to increase their intakes of dairy products or consider a calcium supplement that provides 600 mg of calcium per day. Women with lactose intolerance should choose low-lactose milk or calcium supplementation, or both, to meet the requirements.

Iodine

Iodine is a vital component of the thyroid hormones, which regulate the body's growth, reproduction, and metabolism. An increase of 25 μg per day is recommended. An iodine deficiency during pregnancy can result in insufficient fetal production of the thyroid hormones, leading to physical and mental retardation.

Sodium

In pregnancy, approximately 950 mEq of sodium is retained. This additional supply of sodium can be found in the fetus (290 mEq), the placenta (57 mEq), the amniotic fluid (100 mEq), the maternal extracellular volume including the uterus (80 mEq), the breasts (35 mEq), the plasma (140 mEq), and edema fluid (240 mEq). Because of the extra requirements for sodium storage in the body, sodium intake should not be restricted during pregnancy. Rigid sodium restriction during pregnancy has been observed to lead to neonatal hyponatremia. Sodium intake should be no less than 2 to 3 g per day. This level can be achieved by the consumption of moderate amounts of sodium in processed foods, with a variety of fresh foods in the diet.

Magnesium

Magnesium functions as a cofactor (a mineral that works with an enzyme) in stimulating the biochemical reactions involved in the metabolism of carbohydrates, lipids, and proteins. Approximately 1 g of magnesium is accumulated by the fetus during pregnancy. The RDA advises an additional 20 mg of magnesium per day. Magnesium deficiency can lead to neuromuscular dysfunction.

Zinc

The mineral zinc is thought to be important for normal growth of tissues. An adequate zinc intake is achieved by a diet high in both proteins and calories.

Women's Health

Engaging in a moderate exercise program during pregnancy provides many benefits to the woman and her baby. For pregnant clients who pursue exercise regimens, the following nutritional considerations should be observed:

- Drink 12 to 24 oz of water before, during, and after exercising to prevent dehydration
- Consume foods that will supply an adequate amount of kilocalories to meet the increased requirements of pregnancy and the demands of physical exercise

▶ Water

Water is frequently overlooked as a nutrient. Its role in promoting a healthy pregnancy is as important as that of vitamins and minerals. Water functions in the processes of digestion, absorption, excretion, and circulation. It acts as the body's solvent and transport medium for nutrients and body substances. Water also assists in maintaining a homeostatic body temperature. Because of the increases in blood and fluid volume, it is recommended that pregnant women drink eight 12-oz glasses of water per day.

▶ SUBSTANCES TO AVOID DURING PREGNANCY

Many clinicians and practitioners believe that certain substances should be avoided during pregnancy. Some of these substances include components of the diet such as caffeine and alcohol as well as the practice of pica. The nurse, when taking a health history, assesses the client's use of these substances. Through teaching and counseling, the nurse provides the pregnant woman and family members with information that allows them to make decisions concerning positive health care practices.

▶ Caffeine

Caffeine is a stimulant present in many beverages (coffee, tea, cola and cocoa beverages), foods (chocolate), and medications. Sources of caffeine are listed in Table 14–5. Questions regarding safe intake of caffeine during pregnancy are focused primarily on its ability

to cross the placenta and enter the fetal circulation. The teratogenicity of caffeine in humans has not been clearly demonstrated. Caffeine consumption has been associated with an increased risk of low-birth-weight infants in some studies (Fenster, Eskenazi, Windham, & Swan, 1991), but other factors may have affected the results (Godel, 1992).

Despite the lack of convincing evidence, the FDA in 1981 issued a warning concerning caffeine use in pregnancy. Until further information is known, pregnant women should avoid excessive daily intake (more than 500 mg) of caffeine during pregnancy. When conducting a nutrition assessment, the nurse should question the client about her caffeine consumption and recommend caffeine-free beverages such as water and fruit juices.

▶ Alcohol

Because of the devastating effects of alcohol on fetal growth and development, total abstinence should be recommended during pregnancy. Even the consumption of a healthy diet cannot prevent the teratogenic effects of ethanol in pregnancy. (See Chapter 32 for further discussion of fetal alcohol syndrome.)

▶ Pica

Pica, the unusual craving for nonfood items, may begin during the first trimester of pregnancy. Sub-

▶ TABLE 14–5
Common Sources of Caffeine

Beverage or Food	Caffeine (mg)[a]
Coffee	
Drip (5 oz)	146
Percolated (5 oz)	110
Instant, regular (5 oz)	53
Decaffeinated (5 oz)	2
Tea	
1-minute brew (5 oz)	9–33
3-minute brew (5 oz)	20–46
5-minute brew (5 oz)	20–50
Canned iced tea (12 oz)	22–36
Cola drinks (12 oz)	
Coca-Cola	65
Pepsi-Cola	43
Tab	50
Cocoa and chocolate	
Cocoa drink (6 oz)	10
Milk chocolate (1 oz)	6
Baking chocolate (1 oz)	35

[a]Strength of brew and length of brewing time influence caffeine content of hot beverages; additionally, caffeine content of domestic teas is less than that of imported black teas.

stances ingested by pregnant women practicing pica include dirt or clay, starch, ice or refrigerator frost, wall plaster, cigarette ashes, coffee grounds, and burnt matches. Clay and starch are the more common substances consumed by women practicing pica. Several theories exist to explain this behavior, which is also observed during other stages of the life cycle, such as childhood. Some theories associate pica with sociocultural beliefs. Other research studies have reported that pregnant women have a craving or "taste" for clay or starch. Potential complications associated with pica include maternal malnutrition as a result of displacement of nutritious foods in the diet, decreased bioavailability of essential nutrients, parasitic infections from contaminated clay, congenital lead poisoning from maternal consumption of wall plaster, and dystocia from fecal impaction as a result of clay ingestion. Case reports of fetal and maternal mortality from practices of pica have also been described (Horner, 1991).

All pregnant clients should be screened for pica during initial assessment. For example, the nurse can ask: "Do you ever eat any nonfood items such as clay, cornstarch, or large amounts of ice?" Because of the high rate of iron deficiency among individuals practicing pica, screening for pica is recommended if a woman is anemic; screening for anemia is recommended if a woman practices pica. Other tests, such as serum lead levels, may be performed according to the hazards related to substances ingested. Clients should be counseled on the dangers associated with potentially harmful pica practices. When a client reports the practice of pica, suggest alternative behaviors, such as choosing a healthy snack when experiencing a craving, or recommend an alternative activity, such as going for a walk.

► NUTRITION SCREENING AND ASSESSMENT

Nutrition services in a perinatal clinic should include specific protocols for nutrition screening and assessment. The development of these procedures should involve the entire perinatal interdisciplinary team: nurse, physician, nutritionist, social worker, and all other personnel involved in the provision of health services.

Nutrition screening and assessment serve several purposes: it allows for early detection and correction of nutrition-related abnormalities or disorders; it establishes baseline data for further evaluation of the client's health status; and it promotes formulation and implementation of plans for intervention. The nursing process in management of nutritional problems includes the following steps:

1. Assessment of nutritional status
2. Formulation of nursing diagnosis
3. Design of a plan for intervention to improve nutritional status
4. Implementation of strategies to meet identified goals and objectives
5. Evaluation of the effectiveness of the plan with appropriate recommendations

► Nursing and Collaborative Assessment

The purpose of the initial nutrition screening is to elicit data about the client's nutritional status. This information is usually obtained during the first prenatal visit, when anthropometric measurements such as

► MATERNAL NUTRITIONAL RISK FACTORS

- Adolescence (less than 3 years postmenarche)
- Human immunodeficiency virus (HIV)
- Three or more pregnancies within 2 years
- History of abortions, pregnancy complications, low-birth-weight infants, or perinatal loss
- Multiple fetuses
- Low socioeconomic status
- Anorexia nervosa, bulimia nervosa, binge disorder
- Restrictive diets (veganism, fad diets)
- Heavy smoking (more than 20 cigarettes per day)
- Excessive alcohol intake (chronic use of more than 5 oz

whiskey per day or its equivalent in beer or wine) or history of binge drinking
- Drug addiction
- Unsupervised use of pharmacological doses of supplements
- Chronic systemic diseases
- Prepregnant weight with a BMI ≥ 26.0
- Anemia
- Inadequate weight gain (less than 1 kg per month)
- Excessive weight gain (3 kg per month) possibly associated with fluid retention

height and body weight are obtained, laboratory studies are conducted, and a physical examination is performed. The data obtained at this screening verify the existence of any nutritional risk factors and help prioritize the mother's health care needs. Maternal risk factors may be present at the onset of pregnancy or may develop during or after pregnancy (see box entitled Maternal Nutritional Risk Factors). Identification of risk factors helps the nurse plan nutrition intervention and refer the appropriate clients to the nutritionist for further assessment of nutritional status.

In many health care settings, registered dietitians are available to conduct the assessment, but in most facilities, the collection of data requires the collaboration of the entire health care team. There are four components of the assessment process: dietary data, anthropometric measurements, biochemical indexes, and physical examination. A diagnosis or plan should not be based on one component alone but should instead evolve from assessment of all four components. Assessment data can be recorded on a separate form for prenatal nutrition history (Fig. 14–4) or can be integrated into the health assessment form, depending on the protocol of the health care facility.

Dietary Data

The nurse may use the health history, 24-hour dietary recall, or food diary to elicit information about a client's diet. The health history provides information about the type of diet being followed, who does the shopping and cooking, and any cultural practices related to diet. Of particular importance are the following:

1. Factors that affect eating patterns, especially nausea, vomiting, constipation, diarrhea, and pica
2. Attitudes toward weight gain
3. Socioecononomic factors relevant to food intake (marital status, family size, education, income, occupation, and activity level)
4. Type of diet being followed (cultural influences on the diet) (see next section entitled "Evaluation of Cultural Food Practices")
5. Practice of food faddism (faddist diets that are inadequate in nutrients)
6. Sources of food (Who purchases the food? Where is it purchased? Is any food produced in the home? Does the family have or need assistance with food purchasing [e.g., food stamps, WIC program]?)

Name: _____ Age: _____ Date: _____
Height: _____ Present weight: _____ Preconceptual weight: _____ BMI: _____
Recent weight loss/gain: _____

Dietary modifications (eg, low sodium): _____
Food allergies/intolerances: _____
Prescribed medications: _____
Vitamin/mineral supplements: _____
Medical history: _____
Obstetric history: _____
Social history: _____
Dental history: _____
Physical activity: _____
Education: _____ Occupation: _____
Marital status: _____ Number in household: _____ Person responsible for food shopping/cooking: _____
Kitchen facilities: stove _____ refrigerator: _____ running water: _____
Unusual/fad dietary habits (eg, pica): _____
Cultural/ethnic food practices: _____
Number of meals/snacks per day: _____
Alcohol intake: _____ Caffeine intake: _____
Federal assistance (eg, Food Stamp Program, WIC): _____
Labs: Hct: _____ Hgb: _____ Others: _____
Clinical data: _____
Nutritional status: high risk: _____ moderate risk: _____ low risk: _____
Major nutritional problems: _____

FIGURE 14–4. Prenatal nutritional assessment tool.

7. Food preparation (How and where is food prepared? Who prepares the food? What cooking and storage facilities are available?)
8. Amounts and types of fluid consumed with and between meals
9. Consumption of substances detrimental to maternal and fetal health (e.g., alcohol)
10. Prescribed medications that interfere with nutrient use by the body
11. Relationship, as viewed by the pregnant client, between food intake and health of the fetus and herself

The 24-hour dietary recall is the method most frequently used to estimate a client's nutrient intake, because it is simple to administer. In this method, the client recalls her food intake of the previous day. The nurse or registered dietition acquires the information during an interview with the client, or the client reports it on a self-assessment form. To improve the reliability of the recall, the interviewer should carefully review that day's intake with the client, with particular attention to items that are frequently omitted, such as condiments, dressings, butter, margarine, gravies, and snacks. Omission of a food group such as milk should prompt the interviewer to ask the client if the item is normally found in her diet. This may be accomplished by using an abbreviated form of a food frequency questionnaire that asks specifically how many times per day, per week, or per month the client consumes a particular food.

Another dietary evaluation method is the food diary. The client keeps a record for at least 4 days (preferably one weekend and two weekdays) listing every food item she consumes. The diary may also provide information related to the client's lifestyle, such as the location and time of meals and with whom the client ate.

With the information acquired with the dietary assessment tools, the nutrient content of the diet can be calculated by hand or by use of a computer program with a nutrient data bank. To evaluate nutrient intake accurately, the diet should be compared with the RDAs for women during pregnancy (see Table 14–3). From these results, dietary interventions can be planned.

Evaluation of Cultural Food Practices. Cultural food practices can influence food consumption during pregnancy in a variety of ways. Beliefs and behaviors that are culturally related can affect the way in which foods are cultivated, distributed, purchased, prepared, served, and consumed, or avoided. A pregnant client's ethnic and geographic heritage can determine not only the actual foods she consumes but also the manner in which and occasions on which she eats them. A thorough nutrition assessment can help to identify a client's unique cultural food practices. A local registered dietition may be able to provide helpful information for the nurse who is unfamiliar with the cultural food behaviors of a community.

Many cultures have certain food taboos that restrict consumption of particular foods, such as pork products by Jews who follow kosher dietary laws. Cultural health beliefs can also strongly influence food practices. During childbearing, in particular, pregnant and lactating women may have strict rules on acceptable food intake.

Many cultural food patterns do not follow what is commonly known as the "basic four food groups": meats, dairy products, fruits and vegetables, and breads and cereals. Certain cultures lack certain food groups as a result of the agricultural capabilities of the particular country. Nurses should not assume that an individual's diet is unbalanced because it does not meet the "basic four." Many Asians have lactose intolerance and avoid dairy products but are able to obtain adequate dietary calcium from tofu, fish paste made from small whole fish, and soups made from fish bones. Table 14–6 presents food plans for selected cultural groups.

Nurses should become familiar with the cultural food practices of the community in which they work. Knowledge of ethnic and other food habits promotes communication between the caregiver and the client. Cross-cultural and subcultural nutrition counseling can be challenging because it requires that counselors accept values, customs, and behaviors of a culture or subculture that may be very different from their own. When recommending dietary changes, consider advising only those that are essential to good health. Cultural and other food practices that are neutral or beneficial to the client's health should be praised and supported. For example, maintaining good nutrition through use of culturally specific or more nutritious fast food items should be accepted. If the client's beliefs and values conflict with the information provided by the caregiver, she may not follow the caregiver's recommendations.

Anthropometric Measurements

Anthropometry is the measurement of physical characteristics of the body. These physical findings can be used to assess a client's growth and development by comparison with a standard, or to evaluate individual fluctuations in body composition. Height and body weight measurements are most commonly obtained during pregnancy. To assess the pattern of weight gain, the preconception weight and current body weight are recorded at all prenatal visits (Fig. 14–5).

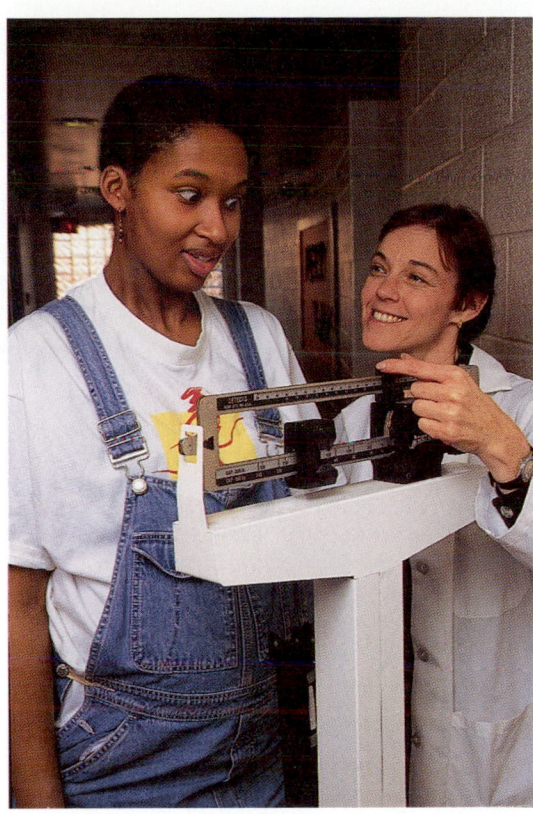

FIGURE 14–5. Obtaining a weight measurement of a pregnant client as part of nutrition screening and assessment.

The pattern of weight gain during pregnancy should be followed closely to monitor rapid fluctuations in body weight. A sudden increase in weight gain could indicate excessive calorie intake or edema. Figures 14–1 and Figure 14–2 provide tools for calculating BMI and evaluating prenatal weight gain.

Biochemical Indexes

Biochemical data can be used to detect a nutrient deficiency before clinical signs become apparent. Many tests can be influenced by gender, age, nutritional status, or disease state. These factors should therefore be considered in the interpretation of the results. Routine nutrition-related laboratory tests conducted during prenatal visits include urinary analysis for the presence of glucose, ketones, and protein and a complete blood count, which includes measures of iron status such as hemoglobin and hematocrit. The hemoglobin level and hematocrit are obtained on the first prenatal visit and, if within normal limits, again in the third trimester. Pregnant women may develop a physiologic anemia in the second trimester and need supplementary iron and folic acid. If the client is found to be anemic, hemoglobin levels and hematocrits are obtained more frequently. In some instances where

nutritional deficiency is suspected, serum iron studies or other more sophisticated blood tests are also done.

Physical Examination

Nursing assessment can identify clinical signs of a nutrient deficiency. Special attention is given to the skin, gums, tongue, eyes, and hair because these parts of the body have the most rapid cell turnover (mucosal and epithelial tissues) and, therefore, are most susceptible to changes in nutritional status. For example, skin pallor during pregnancy may be related to iron deficiency.

▶ Nursing Diagnoses

Once a complete assessment of dietary, anthropometric, biochemical, and clinical data is conducted, nursing diagnoses are developed, and a plan for intervention can then be initiated. Examples of possible nursing diagnoses that are based on nutrition screening and assessment include:

Problem-oriented diagnoses:

- Altered nutrition: less than body requirements related to nausea and vomiting
- Altered nutrition: risk for more than body requirements related to observed higher baseline weight at the beginning of the pregnancy

Wellness-oriented diagnoses:

- Asset in nutrition, related to knowledgeable consumption of food
- Asset in nutrition, related to knowledgeable habits about foods and eating behaviors

▶ Nursing and Collaborative Management

Planning nutritional interventions involves the pregnant woman, her family, and the nurse. Another member of the interdisciplinary team who is particularly important in nutritional planning is the nutritionist. Collaboration helps to ensure that a realistic plan for the pregnant client and her family is developed.

Dietary Counseling

Dietary counseling should be directed toward the needs identified during screening and assessment. On the basis of this information, short-term objectives and long-term goals that represent input from the client and health care team can be developed. Specific goals and objectives should reflect a realistic assessment

▶ **TABLE 14-6**

Selected Cultural Food Patterns

Foods	Preparation
Chinese Dietary Habits	
Meats: Pork (favorite), lamb, goat, and poultry. Entire animal is eaten, including organs, brain, spinal cord, skin, and coagulated blood.	Quantity is small and is usually cut into small thin slices about 2 inches long and cooked in sesame or peanut oil with soy sauce, spices, and a little water and served mixed with vegetables. Many methods for preserving and drying. Sweet and pungent pork or duck is a favorite (meat cubes rolled in batter and fried in oil, then simmered in sauce made of pineapple, green peppers, molasses, brown sugar, vinegar, and seasonings).
Fish: Fish and shellfish liked.	Fish is frequently baked with native spices or prepared in sweet-and-sour dishes. Many dried.
Other proteins: Hen, duck, and pigeon eggs in abundance when affordable; soybean products; legumes	Eggs are preserved and dried; also combined with chicken, mushrooms, and bean sprouts and served with soy sauce (looks like vegetable omelet), termed *egg foo yong*. Egg roll served at beginning of meal is made of shrimp or meat and chopped vegetables rolled in thin dough and fried in deep fat. Soybeans used as sauce, as milk for infants in China, and in many products. Legumes as substitute for meat.
Vegetables: Many plants such as carrots, onions, leeks, peas, cabbage, white turnips, corn, cucumbers, green and yellow beans, squash, shepherd's purse, radish leaves, sprouts (bean, bamboo, etc.), some white but more sweet potatoes	Cut into uniform pieces and simmered or steamed with eggs or meat or added to meat and widely used in soups.
Fruits: Kumquat is favorite	Preserved dessert.
Cereals and breads: Rice used freely. Some wheat, barley, corn, and millet seed. Noodles are popular. Rice is main dish; others are side dishes.	Rice is used as main dish, plain or fried. Millet seed is made into cakes or used in a gruel. Noodles are small and fried. Steamed bread is eaten at breakfast.
Milk: Very little and generally not used. Given to children and invalids	
Cheese: Little used	
Fats: Chief oil is peanut oil. Some soy oil, rice oil, sesame oil, or lard. Practically no butter or cream	Used in cooking.
Seasonings: Sesame seed, salt, ginger, garlic, fresh herbs, red pepper	
Beverage: Tea is the national beverage.	Beverage at all meals, when affordable.
Japanese Dietary Habits	
Meats: The Buddhist tradition of not eating meat conforms with the physical necessities of agriculture. The Japanese consume very little meat, except beef. Since World War II, however, protein intake has steadily increased.	Quantity is small. Usually cut into small pieces and served mixed with vegetables and cereal products.
Fish: Liked and one of the staple foods.	Prefer fish, shellfish, and other marine life to meats of all types. Certain kinds of raw fish are considered great delicacies. Others cooked or dried.
Other proteins: Soybean preparations used freely. Eggs used when available.	Variety of soybean preparations.
Vegetables: Prefer plants such as seaweed, bamboo shoots, onions, large radishes, dried mushrooms (shiitake), and beans. Potatoes and others when available	Pickled is the favorite form. Others cooked with meat or fish.
Fruits: Principal fruit is nasi (tastes somewhat like pear, shaped like an apple; yellow, rough skin). Some persimmons and mulberries. Tangerines in mountain regions. Postwar increase in variety	Dessert.
Cereals and breads: Rice is main food. Some barley, oats, and rye	Rice is mixed with barley by farmers and the poorer classes. Wheat bread, especially in urban communities.
Milk: Enjoy when available; mainly import evaporated or dry milk power	Mostly for children.
Cheese: Very little	
Fats: Soy oil. Rice oil. Suet when available. Practically no butter or cream	Used in cooking.
Seasonings: Salt, sake (liquor distilled from rice)	
Beverages: Tea, sake	Tea freely used when affordable.

▶ **TABLE 14-6** *(continued)*

Selected Cultural Food Patterns

Foods	Preparation
Cuban Dietary Habits	
Meats: Beef, pork, lamb, veal, poultry, sausages	Pork is either roasted or fried. Beef and chicken are used in soups, stewed, roasted, broiled, or barbecued. The sausages are used with beans.
Fish: All varieties of fish (fresh, salted, smoked, and canned)	Fried, boiled, marinated, roasted, or grilled.
Other proteins: Beans (black, red, kidney, navy, yellow, lima, green); split peas; eggs	Black beans with rice and roast pork is a favorite dish and is eaten on Christmas day. Eggs are eaten daily: fried, scrambled, or in dessert.
Vegetables: Native tubers such as *yuca, ñame, malanga* (white and yellow), *boniato* (white yams), *chayote, berenjena*, plantain, potatoes, lettuce, tomatoes, carrots	The tubers are boiled and served with *mojo* (made with sour orange, crushed garlic, sliced onions and hot oil), or mashed with butter and milk. Fried ripe or green plantains are a favorite side dish.
Fruits: Anona, mamey, guanábana, chirimoya, papaya, banana, *zapote, marañón*, mangoes, grapefruit, oranges (sweet and sour), coconuts, *caimito*.	Eaten fresh, in juice, or in desserts such as pastes, jellies, puddings.
Cereals: Rice, cornmeal, cornstarch, imported breakfast cereals, such as oatmeal, corn flakes	The favorite is white (long grain) steamed rice; sometimes *bijol* is added to make it yellow as in *arroz con pollo* (yellow rice with chicken). White rice is eaten daily for dinner and supper.
Milk: Fresh cow's milk (whole, skimmed), condensed, evaporated, dry; sour cream; goat's milk for the sick, usually	Adults use it in coffee; children use as beverage. Also used in cream sauces, gravies, desserts, etc.
Cheese: Gouda, cream, *queso de mano*	The native cheese is *queso de mano* (hard cheese) made from milk, lactate of calcium, and salt, which looks like compressed cottage cheese; usually eaten with guava paste.
Fats: Pork lard, olive oil, peanut oil, soy oil, butter, margarine, and shortening	Pork lard is most popular. Oil is used in salads and beans.
Desserts: Fruits, ice cream, cakes, pies, custards, puddings; guava, prune and mango pastes; *morón* cookies, *terrejas, boniatillo, buñuelos, cafiroleta*	Eaten after each meal and also as snacks. *Raspadura* is very sweet and the most typical native dessert.
Seasonings: Oil, vinegar, cumin, oregano, *bijol*, salt, pepper, garlic, onion, green peppers	
Beverages: Coffee, beer, wines, tea, carbonated beverages	Dark strong coffee served demitasse, with or without sugar.
Spanish–American–Mexican Dietary Habits	
Meats: Chicken, pork chops, wieners, cold cuts, and hamburger	Used only once or twice a week.
Other proteins: Eggs, beans	Eggs used frequently and usually fried. In rural areas, chickens are kept for their eggs. Beans usually eaten mashed and refried with lard.
Vegetables: Potatoes, red and green chilies, fresh and canned tomatoes, pumpkin, corn, field greens, onions, carrots	Potatoes are basic item, usually fried; may be used three times a day. Chilies are popular at each meal. Fresh tomatoes are very popular. Other vegetables used frequently.
Fruits: Bananas, melons, peaches, canned fruit cocktail, oranges, apples	Oranges, apples used occasionally as snacks. Others are the more popular fruits.
Cereals and breads: Oatmeal, enriched white flour, packaged breakfast cereals, macaroni, white bread, tortillas, sweet rolls	Sugar-coated packaged cereals are popular; oatmeal used occasionally. Macaroni is fried and served with beans and potatoes. Tortillas are homemade daily. Both purchased and homemade breads are used frequently. Purchased sandwich bread is a status symbol.
Milk: Limited availability, expensive	
Cheese: Limited amounts used	
Fats: Lard, salt pork, bacon fat	Used liberally. Most foods are fried.
Beverages: Soft drinks; other sweets very popular	
Greek Dietary Habits	
Meats: Lamb is main meat. Some beef, goat, mutton, pork products; poultry is popular	Meat is either cut into small pieces or ground. Poultry is cooked into broth. Lamb is cooked on skewers or cut up and browned in oil or fat with rice or flour and vegetables.
Fish: Saltwater fish (fresh, smoked or salted), shellfish, smoked roe, squid, and octopus	Fish is fried or steamed with vegetables. Used frequently.

(continued)

► **TABLE 14–6** *(continued)*
Selected Cultural Food Patterns

Foods	Preparation
Greek Dietary Habits *(continued)*	
Other proteins: Eggs, white beans, and legumes	Legumes are boiled, mashed or stewed and eaten either hot or cold. Soup made of dried beans, onions, celery, and carrots is a national dish. Eggs are popular.
Vegetables: Cabbage, cauliflower, cucumbers, eggplant, greens, okra, onions, peppers, some potatoes, vine leaves, zucchini, tomatoes, salad greens	Vegetables are boiled or fried in a small amount of olive oil and served hot or cold. Many vegetables are stuffed. Potatoes or vegetables are cooked with meat or fish. Lemon juice is used to dress salads and cold foods.
Fruits: Apricots, cherries, dates, oranges, lemons, figs, grapes, melons, nuts, plums, peaches, pears, quinces, and raisins	Fruits in season are eaten raw, grapes are pressed into wine or dried as raisins. Fruit for dessert.
Cereals and breads: Maize, rice, and wheat	Maize is used in polenta; rice is an ingredient for *pilawi* and stuffing for vegetables; wheat is made into bread. Bread used abundantly, and white is preferred.
Milk: Cow's, goat's, and sheep's milk	Milk is boiled for children. Fermented milk or *yaourti* is eaten as dessert or with pastry.
Cheese: Soft and mild, hard and dry cheese	Cheese is popular.
Fats: Olive oil, seed oils, salted black olives, and little butter	Olive oil is used to dress salads and hot or cold vegetables and in cooking.
Seasonings: Caraway and pumpkin seeds, herbs, honey, nuts (hazel, pignolia, and pistachio), and sesame	Seeds are eaten between meals, and nuts are served as dessert.
Beverages: Coffee and wine	Coffee (American) is the beverage served in the mornings. At other meals it is made and served Turkish style. Wine is served at meals.

Reproduced, with permission, from Mahan, L.K., & Escott-Stump, S.E. (1996). Food, nutrition, and diet therapy (9th ed.). Philadelphia: W.B. Saunders.

of the client's needs and abilities based on a thorough review of the health, social, and dietary data. These goals and objectives should be stated clearly in the health record to provide a means of evaluating the client's progress, and as a channel of communication among health care professionals to ensure continuity of care.

The nurse should emphasize the positive aspects of the client's diet and help her to correct nutritional deficiencies. Nutritional recommendations should incorporate any assessed nutritional deficiencies, income of the family, and cultural food preferences. Clients should be given information about the dietary requirements of pregnancy. If supplementation is required (e.g., iron and folic acid), the reason for the supplementation and any discomforts that might occur, such as constipation, should be given. The nurse monitors nutritional intake throughout pregnancy, facilitates appropriate dietary planning, assists the client in planning her own diet, and encourages positive self-care practices. Moreover, referral to such programs as the Special Supplemental Food Program for Women, Infants, and Children (WIC) assists the low-income family to obtain the food needed for good nutrition for pregnant and lactating women, infants,

 *Client Teaching*

Nutrition Education: Poor Weight Gain

For the pregnant client who is at risk for poor weight gain, the nurse can suggest the following interventions:

- Make an appointment with a registered dietitian to evaluate your diet
- Eat 5–6 meals/snacks per day
- Avoid low kilocalorie foods such as diet drinks and fat-free foods
- Add condiments such as olive oil, canola oil, mayonnaise, and salad dressings to foods
- Choose healthy snacks such as nuts, dried fruits, and low-fat milkshakes
- Evaluate your physical activities to determine if you are burning excessive kilocalories
- Eat your largest meal during the day when you are the most hungry

 *Commonly Asked Questions*

Now that I am pregnant should I be "eating for two"?

Although your nutrient needs have increased, you do not need to be eating for two adults. Considering the small size of the developing baby you only need to increase your normal food intake by 300 kcal per day. This is approximately the amount of kilocalories in the combination of the following three foods: one glass of skim milk, one ounce of chicken, and one small orange.

I am already overweight. Why do I have to gain weight during pregnancy?

The recommended weight gain during pregnancy is based on the normal bodily changes that occur during pregnancy such as an increase in blood and fluid volume, and the new products of conception such as the placenta and the developing fetus. The recommended weight gain for an overweight (15–25 lbs) or obese (15 lbs) pregnant woman does not promote storage of additional body fat but is sufficient for the development of a normal healthy baby.

If I take a prenatal vitamin and mineral supplement do I still have to eat a healthy diet?

A vitamin and mineral supplement should be a "supplement" to the diet and not serve as a replacement to a variety of healthy foods. The prenatal supplements lack the kilocalories that are contained in foods like protein, lipids, and carbohydrates. Supplements cannot replace healthy foods like whole grain breads, cereals and grain products, fruits and vegetables, lean meats, fish and poultry, and low-fat diary products.

The nurse has told me that I have iron deficiency anemia. What changes should I make in my diet?

In addition to taking a daily iron supplement you should increase your intake of foods high in iron. These foods include organ meats (liver, kidney, brains), red meats, egg yolks, poultry, whole grain cereals, dark green vegetables, dried fruits, and dried beans. Consider taking your iron supplement with a fruit juice high in vitamin C such as orange juice or grapefruit juice as this helps to improve your body's use of iron.

---

and young children (see Public Health Nutrition Programs).

Nutrition Education

Nutrition education involves teaching clients to make knowledgeable decisions about their nutritional health. It may occur on an individual basis or among groups. Many perinatal clinics provide nutrition education classes targeted toward the needs of the prenatal client. The following are possible nutrition education topics:

- Recommendations for weight gain during pregnancy
- Vitamin and mineral supplementation
- Control of common gastrointestinal problems, such as nausea, vomiting, constipation
- Preparation of easy, nutritious snack foods
- Increasing calcium, iron, and folic acid in the diet
- Food assistance programs

Group classes are often popular because they provide expectant mothers with an opportunity to share information and ask questions in a supportive atmosphere. Nutrition education programs are also an effective use of the nurse's and nutritionist's time, as many clients have similar needs that can be discussed in a group rather than focused on individually.

▶ Evaluation

Nutritional assessment and management are ongoing processes that require continuous reassessment of the client's nutritional status, redefinition of goals and objectives, and evaluation of the changes implemented. Good nutritional practices during pregnancy help to ensure a healthy newborn and an uncomplicated postpartum recovery. There is little question that nutrition profoundly affects pregnancy and the fetus. The objective of nursing management is to promote the best possible level of health for the childbearing individual and family through positive nutritional practices. These practices motivate the family to maintain a healthy diet throughout the family life span.

► HEALTHY EATING GUIDE FOR PREGNANCY

Food guides or plans which are based on the United States Department of Agriculture (USDA) Food Guide Pyramid are appropriate for pregnant women (see Fig. 14–3). As demonstrated in Table 14–2, these plans recommend a wide variety of food from all the food groups such as grain products, vegetables, fruits, dairy products, and meat and protein containing foods. The food guide should be tailored to the specific nutritional needs, likes, and dislikes of the client. A thorough dietary assessment can provide essential information about the client's present eating habits. For instance, if the nurse, doing a nutrition assessment, learns that the client avoids dairy products because of a lactose intolerance, the nurse should recommend alternative sources of calcium such as leafy greens, sardines, and calcium-fortified orange juice. Calcium supplementation may also be advised. Food guides which reflect different cultural food practices may be available from the local public health department or the WIC program.

► PUBLIC HEALTH NUTRITION PROGRAMS

Women of low socioeconomic status are at high risk for delivering premature and low-birth-weight infants as a result of several factors, including inadequate health care, poor sanitation and housing, and inadequate diet. The WIC program was established in 1972 to improve the nutritional status of low-income women and therefore help to reduce infant mortality and morbidity, and to promote good health from conception through early childhood. The program, funded by the USDA, serves to provide food and nutrition education to low-income pregnant women classified as being at medical or nutritional risk. Also eligible are lactating women, infants, and children up to 5 years of age who meet the medical and financial criteria. The monthly food package for pregnant women includes vouchers to purchase such foods as milk, cheese, eggs, vitamin- and mineral-fortified cereals, fruit juice, dried peas and beans, and peanut butter. To be eligible to receive the food package, the applicant must first meet financial eligibility guidelines as determined by the annual federal poverty income guidelines. Screening also requires a physical examination by a private or clinic physician and a nutrition assessment by a WIC nurse or nutritionist. Factors indicating nutritional risk include nutritional anemia, age (less than 18 or greater than 35), short interconceptional period, and previous history of delivering a premature or low-birth-weight infant. Once the applicant is certified, she must receive regular medical checkups and attend nutrition education classes given by the WIC nurse or nutritionist. The food package is designed to serve as a supplement to foods already in the diet, with an emphasis on increasing the intake of both energy and the essential nutrients during pregnancy.

The WIC program helps to promote better pregnancy outcomes and healthier children while being cost effective. Owen and Owen (1997), in a review of research examining the impact of the WIC program, concluded that WIC participation decreases the prevalence of low-birth-weight and very-low-birth-weight infants born to low-income WIC mothers. The U.S. General Accounting Office reports that WIC is a cost-effective program because for every dollar spent on WIC, between $2.89 and $3.50 was saved during the first eighteen years of life (U.S. General Accounting Office, 1992). The promotion of healthy nutrition and early and frequent prenatal visits increases the likelihood of high-risk mothers achieving a more healthy maternal and fetal outcome.

► Food Stamp Program

The Food Stamp Program is available to low-income individuals who meet financial guidelines determined by the federal poverty level. Each month, eligible participants receive food stamps (coupons) with which they purchase food. The value of the stamps depends on the size of the family and the available income. Food stamps can be used to purchase any food except pet food and any beverages except alcoholic beverages.

The Food Stamp Program and WIC, in addition to other such programs, allow the health care professional to refer clients to other agencies for food assistance. Many public health clinics employ social workers who refer clients to the appropriate programs. The initial nutrition assessment should include questions related to the economic resources available for food purchases so as to identify those individuals eligible for food assistance. Many prenatal clinics routinely screen for eligibility for the WIC program. By establishing a system of referral to local agencies that provide food and nutrition services, the health care center can provide more comprehensive services.

► MANAGEMENT OF NUTRITIONAL RISK FACTORS DURING PREGNANCY

Management of individuals who are at risk for nutritional problems during pregnancy is the joint responsibility of the interdisciplinary perinatal team. Important members of this team are nurses and nutritionists, who collaborate to provide comprehensive nutritional care to the high-risk mother and her family.

Later chapters of this text discuss nutritional management of clients with specific health care problems such as diabetes mellitus (Chapter 19), hypertension (Chapter 19), and anemia during pregnancy (Chapter 16). This section briefly describes care of the woman who is at risk because of her weight and nutritional considerations in the care of a a woman with multiple pregnancies and a pregnant adolescent.

► Obesity, Underweight, and Weight Gain

Obesity

Nutritional management of obese women during pregnancy has historically been an area of controversy, particularly with respect to recommended weight gain. Obesity is defined as a prepregnancy BMI greater than 29.0. Overweight is defined as a prepregnancy BMI of more than 26.0 to 29.0. Obesity during pregnancy is associated with both increased maternal mortality and morbidity and increased fetal morbidity (Suitor, 1997). The following risks associated with obesity during pregnancy are of critical importance in determining prenatal care:

- Gestational diabetes
- Urinary tract infections
- Inadequate weight gain
- Wound infection
- Thromboembolism
- Pregnancy-induced hypertension
- Fetal monitoring difficulties
- Prolonged labor
- Fetal macrosomia
- Birth trauma

Some researchers believe that the recommended 7-pound increase in maternal fat stores in preparation for the last trimester may be unnecessary in obese women. No research, however, has clearly demonstrated that fat deposition among obese women during pregnancy is unnecessary. Although the ideal weight gain for obese pregnant women appears to be less than that recommended for normal-weight women, pregnancy is not the time to diet or lose weight. When kilocalorie intake is less than the body's requirements, ketones become the chief energy source. The long-term effect of maternal ketosis on fetal development is unknown, but there is some evidence it may lead to neurologic damage to the fetus. Ketones do cross the placental barrier and will be used for energy by the fetus who is not receiving adequate supplies of glucose and amino acids. In addition, insufficient caloric intake can also lead to inadequate intake of essential vitamins and minerals.

The recommended weight gain for an overweight woman is 15 to 25 pounds (7 to 11.5 kg), and that for obese women is 15 pounds (6.8 kg). Nutritional management of obese pregnant women requires special considerations. Many women, particularly those who were dieting, are reluctant to accept the recommendation for a 15- to 20-pound weight gain. In addition, the mother may experience lack of support by family members who fail to understand the need for weight gain in an obese person. Before providing nutrition education it is valuable to assess the client's attitudes and beliefs about weight gain. During the initial assessment, the nurse or nutritionist should also inquire about the client's weight and diet history. Such information as recent weight loss or weight gain prior to conception, or fad diets currently or previously followed, aids in the development of an appropriate nutritional care plan. The client is also advised that liquid diets, diet pills, herbal weight loss supplements, or any fad diet are unsafe during pregnancy.

To aid the client and family in understanding nutrient and kilocalorie needs during pregnancy, a diagram illustrating the components of weight gain is helpful. The overweight client is then able to visualize that the recommended 20-pound weight gain does not accumulate into 20 pounds of body fat, but is used in normal maternal and fetal growth and development. The pattern of weight gain recommended is as follows: no weight gain during the first trimester (as opposed to a 3-pound weight gain in a normal-weight woman) and an approximately half-pound increase in weight each week during the second and third trimesters. To promote adequate weight gain, total kilocalorie intake should be 300 kcal per day above the level that would otherwise maintain the client's present body weight. In general, pregnancy is not the time to diet, but obese women may need strong support and close supervision to achieve the recommended weight gain.

Underweight Before Pregnancy

Underweight for height is defined as a prepregnancy BMI less than 19.8. Several complications are associated with the pregnancies of underweight women, such as low birth weight, prematurity, low Apgar scores, and iron deficiency anemia in the mother. The recommended weight gain for underweight women is 28 to 40 pounds (13 to 18 kg). This recommendation is made to reduce the risk of delivering an infant with intrauterine growth retardation. Like the obese mother, the underweight woman may be reluctant to increase her body weight, preferring a slim body profile. Attitudes toward weight gain should be explored during the initial nutrition assessment to identify women who are at risk for poor weight gain or who are at risk for eating disorders. Under ideal conditions, underweight women should achieve an ideal body weight prior to conception to ensure the availability of optimal nutrient stores.

▶ Multiple Gestation

In multiple fetuses there is a significant increase in requirements for nutrients and energy. The rate and total amount of weight gain in multiple pregnancies should exceed that of singleton pregnancies due to greater increases in maternal, placental, and fetal tissues. The rate of weight gain should be based on

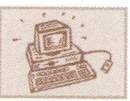

Research Abstract

Factors Influencing Poor Weight Gain During Pregnancy

Inadequate weight gain during pregnancy is associated with preterm births and intrauterine growth retardation. There are many factors that influence gestational weight gain. In general, preconception weight, height, age, race, education, and cigarette smoking have been shown to be predictors of total weight gain. Researchers are keenly interested in identifying factors associated with poor weight gain because they may promote understanding of determinants of gestational weight gain.

This study examined baseline factors that are the best predictors of poor weight gain among pregnant Hispanic women. The sample was comprised of 8,736 women receiving care in California public health clinics participating in the Prematurity Prevention Project. Instrumentation for the study included a psychosocial questionnaire, administered by a trained project staff member, and client medical records. Prepregnancy weight was self-reported at the first client visit and maternal weight was collected at each prenatal visit. Poor total weight gain (at a mean gestational age of 35 weeks) was defined as less than 21 lb for women with a BMI of less than 26 and less than 10 lb for women with a BMI of 26 or greater. Data analyses included descriptive statistics and multiple regressional analysis.

Poor weight gain occurred in 29% of the women. Maternal height, primiparity at any age, education, being divorced, experiencing a family member's death during the pregnancy, and maternal place of birth in the United States were positively associated with weight gain during pregnancy. Factors negatively associated with weight gain included: prepregnancy BMI of less than 26, being multiparous and younger than 20 years or older than 29.1 years, being single, experiencing depression during the pregnancy, and being physically abused by the father.

The researchers noted that the study results may not be generalizable to all Hispanic women. This sample included predominately low-income Mexican immigrants attending public health clinics in Los Angeles.

Application to Practice

Psychosocial assessment of pregnant women can provide valuable information related to factors that influence maternal weight gain. In particular, information regarding financial support, physical and emotional problems, and physical abuse should be carefully evaluated.

Source: Siega-Riz, A.M., & Hobel, C. (1997). Predictors of poor maternal weight gain from baseline anthropometric, psychosocial, and demographic information in a Hispanic population. Journal of the American Dietetic Association, 97(11), 1264–1274.

maternal prepregnancy BMI. Normal weight women with a twin gestation should be encouraged to gain 1.5 pounds/week during the second half of pregnancy. Underweight women with a twin gestation should experience a 1.75 pound/week weight gain after 20 weeks' gestation (Lantz, Chez, Rodriguez, & Porter, 1996). Guidelines for appropriate weight gain in triplet gestation have not been established. In general, weight gain should be encouraged by promoting a healthy diet plan.

▶ Eating Disorders

Anorexia nervosa, bulimia nervosa, and binge disorders are examples of eating disorders that can lead to poor nutrition, fetal growth retardation, and life-threatening maternal and fetal conditions such as electrolyte imbalance and organ damage. (See Chapter 7 for discussion of these eating disorders.) The client should be asked about present and past practices used to control weight, although many clients may be reluctant to admit to these problems. Being underweight prior to pregnancy or a history of large weight fluctuations may indicate an eating disorder. Clients with eating disorders, however, may or may not be underweight. Clients routinely should be advised against such practices as self-induced vomiting and use of enemas or any unprescribed medications during pregnancy. Eating disorders are complex problems that should not be ignored. Clients with eating disorders should be referred to health care professionals specializing in their treatment.

▶ Adolescent Pregnancy

Adolescence is a period of the human life cycle in which rapid physical growth occurs and nutrient requirements increase. A teenager who conceives within 4 years of menarche (average onset: 12.7 years of age) and thus has a young gynecologic age is considered to be at high nutritional risk, as she must meet not only her own nutrient needs but also those of the developing fetus. These young pregnant adolescents have high neonatal mortality rates, and give birth to more preterm and low-birth-weight infants than older women (National Academy of Sciences Institute of Medicine, 1990a, 1990b). Pregnant adolescents are also at higher risk for pregnancy-induced hypertension and anemia (Scholl, Hediger, & Belsky, 1994).

Many other factors may place a pregnant teenager at nutritional risk. One is related to weight gain during pregnancy. Teenagers frequently have a low prepregnancy weight and gain less than 16

pounds during pregnancy. Poor weight gain during pregnancy is positively associated with low-birth-weight infants. Adequate weight gain also lowers fetal mortality rates.

Research studies have indicated that the energy needs of the pregnant teenager vary between 38 and 50 kcal/kg per day. Different patterns of physical activity can influence the variation in energy requirements. Because of the extensive tissue growth and development that occur during pregnancy, high protein intake is advised. For 15- to 18-year-olds, the RDA for protein is 1.5 g of protein per kilogram of body weight, and for younger females, 1.7 g of protein per kilogram of body weight.

In addition to the physiologic and nutritional demands of pregnancy, the erratic eating habits of pregnant teenagers also contribute to their nutritional risk. Food patterns commonly observed include frequent meal skipping (particularly breakfast) and consumption of foods high in salt and sugar and low in vitamins and minerals. Limited financial resources to purchase healthy foods may also have harmful effects on the diet. Lack of knowledge concerning the diet may make it difficult for the individual to make healthy food choices. Pregnant teenagers who are financially eligible will benefit by being referred to WIC, which provides nutritional counseling and food vouchers that allow the individual to buy nutritious foods.

To reduce perinatal risks, pregnant teenagers should receive early and ongoing nutrition assessment and intervention. Attention should be focused on promoting healthy eating habits and preventing consumption of harmful substances. For example, if snacking is a major feature of the diet, the nurse should emphasize nutritious snack foods such as fresh fruits, cheese, fresh vegetables with yogurt dip, granola bars, and peanut butter.

▶ Bedrest

A healthy diet while on bedrest can be challenging to pregnant women because food shopping and cooking are restricted. Several simple suggestions can be valuable to clients, as follows:

- Have the client either prepare the grocery list for the person who will be responsible for doing the shopping or phone a grocery store that delivers. Some stores offer free delivery as a community service to the homebound; other stores charge for home delivery.
- Include foods on the list that are easy to prepare and can be eaten cold or at room temperature.
- Select foods that can be microwaved.

- Consume a high-fiber diet rich in fruits, vegetables, and whole grain breads and cereals to prevent constipation due to lack of physical activity.
- Ask a friend or family member to collect menus from local restaurants that offer home delivery. However, remember that prepared "take-out" foods can be expensive; this option may cost too much for many families. The nurse needs to know about local religious or community groups that provide meals for people who are ill at home. Referral to such groups can provide a temporary and needed service for pregnant women who are on bedrest and who do not have other sources of support.
- Keep an ice chest or cooler in the room with cold drinks, fruit, and sandwiches to have food readily available.
- Eat small frequent meals and snacks to stimulate the appetite and promote better digestion.

Critical Thinking in Care Planning

Care of the Adolescent Client at Risk for Inadequate Weight Gain During Pregnancy

Jennifer Boyd is a 16-year-old primipara who is 14 weeks' pregnant. During the assessment, Jennifer tells the nurse that she is fearful of gaining too much weight because she does not want to "become fat." She states, "I am afraid I will not lose the weight after my baby is born." She describes her typical diet as consisting of a glass of orange juice and a piece of toast for breakfast, a hot dog on a roll with a Coke for lunch and pasta with tomato sauce and bread and skim milk for dinner. This morning, she skipped breakfast.

Jennifer lives at home with her mother and her ten-year-old brother. Her mother works full time and is responsible for the food shopping and cooking. Jennifer is income and medically eligible for the WIC program, which is available at the prenatal clinic.

The physical examination reveals that Jennifer has lost two pounds since conception. Her prepregnancy weight was 120 lbs and her height is 5'6". Hemoglobin and hematocrit are normal, but her urine is positive for acetone and protein. Jennifer reports that she was feeling nauseous for the first several weeks of her pregnancy but within the last week she started to feel better with an increase in appetite.

▶ Assessment

- 16-year-old primipara at 14 weeks' gestation experiencing poor weight gain
- Lost 2 pounds since conception
- Client states, "I do not want to become fat."

- Vital signs: weight, 120 lbs; height, 5'6"
- Lab values: Hgb = 13g/dl, Hct = 39%, urine = + for acetone
- Medically and income eligible for WIC

Nursing Diagnosis

Altered nutrition: less than body requirements related to nausea and vomiting during the first trimester and personal attitudes toward weight gain

Expected Client/Family Outcomes	Nursing Action/Intervention	Evaluation
By the end of the visit, the client will:		
• Identify nausea and vomiting as a common occurrence during the first trimester of pregnancy.	Explain the influence of maternal hormone production on appetite and gastrointestinal changes in the first trimester. *Rationale* The nausea and vomiting (due to changes in maternal hormone production) experienced during the first trimester may have contributed to the weight loss. These symptoms usually cease after 12 weeks.	When asked, the client is able to identify nausea and vomiting as a common problem during pregnancy.
• Describe the reasons why weight gain during pregnancy is essential to the health of the baby and identify the constituents of weight gain.	Discuss body image during pregnancy and explain the components of gestational weight gain. *Rationale:* Client's negative attitudes towards weight gain may have influenced her total food intake.	Client gains 1 to 2 lbs by the next one-week visit and urinalysis is normal.
• Identify healthy food choices for meal and snack time.	Assist client in developing sample menu plan. *Rationale:* Consumption of nutritious foods will ensure adequate dietary intake.	Client follows a nutritious menu plan.

(continued)

Critical Thinking in Care Planning *continued*

Expected Client/Family Outcomes	Nursing Action/Intervention	Evaluation
• Discuss the benefits of changing eating habits to increase kilocalorie intake.	Recommend 5–6 feedings/day. *Rationale:* Consumption of 5–6 small meals/day encourages intake of a variety of nutritious foods.	Client eats 5–6 small nutritious meals/day and reports increased levels of energy.
• Identify effects of physical exercise on kcal intake.	Evaluate kcal expenditure in physical activity and assess kcal and nutrient intake in a 24-hour recall. *Rationale:* Effect of physical activity on kcal and nutrient intake can be assessed through a 24-hour recall and modifications in the diet and/or activity can be made as necessary.	Client brings 24-hour recall to next one-week visit and states the effects of physical activity on nutrient intake.
• Discuss the benefits of participation in WIC for herself and her baby.	Refer to nutritionist with WIC program. *Rationale:* The WIC program can provide dietary counseling and vouchers to purchase nutritious foods.	The WIC program sends notification of client's enrollment in the program.

Chapter Highlights

▶ Weight gain during pregnancy is a result of growth of the fetus, placenta, amniotic fluid, uterus, and breasts.

▶ The recommended weight gain for pregnant women of normal preconceptual weight is 25–35 pounds over the course of pregnancy.

▶ Kilocalories provide the mother and fetus with the necessary energy requirements and it is recommended that an additional 300 kcal per day above normal prepregnant levels be consumed by pregnant women.

▶ Proteins, carbohydrates, and lipids are essential in meeting the body's requirements for kilocalories.

▶ Vitamins and minerals play an essential role in promoting the use of energy from proteins, carbohydrates, and lipids; in building new tissue; and in acting as regulating agents in metabolic processes in the body.

▶ The nurse needs to assess the client's use of substances such as caffeine, alcohol, and non-food items related to the practice of pica due to their potential and established teratogenic effects on the fetus and counsel the pregnant woman and her family in choosing healthy nutritional patterns.

▶ Nutrition screening and assessment involves the entire perinatal interdisciplinary team and serves several purposes: it allows for early detection and treatment of nutrition-related abnormalities; it establishes baseline data for evaluation of the client's health status; and it promotes development of intervention strategies.

▶ Nutrition assessment consists of collection of dietary data, anthropometric measurements, physical examination, and laboratory studies.

▶ Nutritional interventions involve the pregnant woman, her family, the nurse, and the interdisci-

Chapter Highlights continued

plinary team and include dietary counseling and nutrition education.

▶ Referral of the pregnant client to the WIC and Food Stamp Program can improve both maternal and fetal outcome.

▶ Management of nutritional risk factors during pregnancy include problems of obesity, overweight, and underweight; incidence of multiple gestation; presence of eating disorders such as anorexia nervosa, bulimia nervosa, and binge eating; adolescent pregnancy; and effects of bedrest on adequate nutrition.

After reading the vignette at the beginning of this chapter, use what you have learned to answer these questions:

1. What nutritional practices might affect Erika Watson's gaining enough weight during pregnancy?

2. What strategies can Susan Rosengarten, MSN, NP, use to help Erika Watson understand the dietary requirements of pregnancy and comply with a healthy nutritional plan?

3. In what ways does collaboration among interdisciplinary health care team members enhance dietary counseling of pregnant clients like Erika Watson?

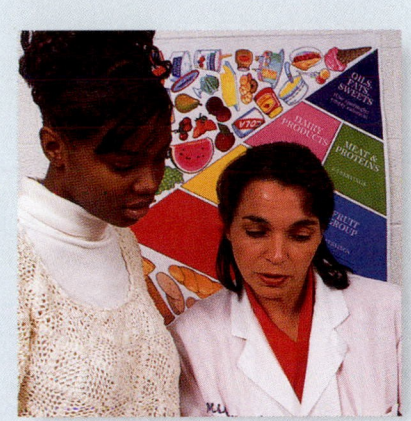

Critical Thinking Questions

▶ References

Centers for Disease Control (1992). Recommendations for the use of folic acid to reduce the number of cases of spina bifida and other neural tube defects. *Morbidity/Mortality Report, 41* (no RR-14).

Fenster, L., Eskenazi, B., Windham, G.C., & Swan, S.H. (1991). Caffeine consumption during pregnancy and fetal growth. *American Journal of Public Health, 81*(4), 458–461.

Godel, J.C. (1992). Smoking and caffeine and alcohol intake in a northern population: Effect on fetal growth. *Canadian Medical Association Journal, 147*(2), 181–188.

Horner, J. (1991). Pica practices of pregnant women. *Journal of the American Dietetic Association, 91*, 34–38.

Lantz, M.E., Chez, R.A., Rodriguez, A., & Porter, K.B. (1996). Maternal weight gain patterns and birth weight outcome in twin gestation. *Obstetrics and Gynecology, 87*, 551–556.

MRC Vitamin Study Research Group. (1991). Prevention of neural tube defects: Results of the Medical Research Council Vitamin Study. *Lancet, 388*(8760), 131–137.

National Academy of Sciences. (1989). *Recommended dietary allowances* (10th ed.). Washington, DC: National Academy Press.

National Academy of Sciences Institute of Medicine, Subcommittee on Nutritional Status and Weight Gain During Pregnancy. (1990a). *Nutrition during pregnancy. Part I. Weight gain.* Washington, DC: National Academy Press.

National Academy of Sciences Institute of Medicine, Subcommittee on Nutritional Status and Weight Gain During Pregnancy. (1990b). *Nutrition during pregnancy. Part II. Nutrient supplements.* Washington, DC: National Academy Press.

National Academy of Sciences Institute of Medicine, Subcommittee on Nutritional Status and Weight Gain During Pregnancy. (1992). *Nutrition during pregnancy and lactation. An implementation guide.* Washington, DC: National Academy Press.

Owen, A.L., & Owen, G.M. (1997). Twenty years of WIC: A review of some effects of the program. *Journal of the American Dietetic Association, 97*(7), 777–782.

Rothman, K.J., Moore, L.L., Singer, M.R., Nguyen, U.S., Mannion, S., & Milunsky, A. (1995). Teratogenicity of high vitamin A intake. *New England Journal of Medicine, 333*, 1369–1373.

Scholl, T.O., & Hediger, M.L. (1994). Anemia and iron deficient anemia: Compilation of data on pregnancy outcome. *American Journal of Clinical Nutrition, 59*(2S), 492S–500S.

Scholl, T.O., Hediger, M.L., & Belskey, D.H. (1994). Prenatal care and maternal health during adolescent pregnancy: A review and meta-analysis. *Journal of Adolescent Health, 15*(6), 444–456.

Siega-Riz, A.M., & Hobel, C. (1997). Predictors of poor maternal weight gain from baseline anthropometric, psychosocial, and demographic information in a Hispanic population. *Journal of the American Dietetic Association, 97*(11), 1264–1274.

Smithells, R.W., Sheppard, S., Schorah, C.J., Sellar, M.J., Nevin, N.C., Harris, R., Read, A.P., & Fielding, D.W. (1965). Folic acid metabolism and human embryopathy. *Lancet, 1,* 1254.

Suitor, C.W. (1997). *Maternal weight gain: A report of an expert work group.* Arlington, VA: National Center for Education in Maternal and Child Health.

U.S. Food and Drug Administration. (1996). Food labeling: health claims and label statements—folate and neural tube defects. *Federal Register 61,* 8752–8780.

U.S. General Accounting Office (1992). *Early Intervention: Federal investments like WIC can produce savings* (GAO/HRD) Publication No. 92-18). Washington DC: U.S. Government Printing Office.

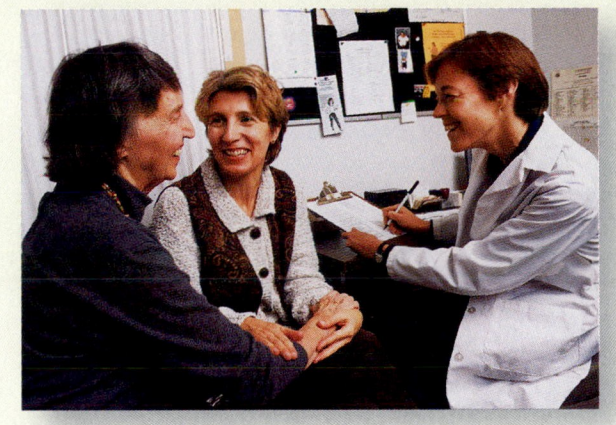

Jeanne Goodwin, age 36, is accompanied by her mother, Rachel Ackerman, to her prenatal visit. Jeanne is 8 weeks' pregnant with her third child. While talking with Ann Salzman, CNM, MSN, Jeanne states, "Sometimes I feel a little overwhelmed with the thought of caring for another child. When I think of my mother raising five children," she continues, touching her mother's hand, "I don't know how she did it."

Rachel looks at her daughter sympathetically and grasps her hand. The nurse asks, "Are you afraid that you may not live up to your expectations of being as good a mother as your own?" Jeanne nods alowly and replies, "Yes. I find myself, especially with this pregnancy, wanting to be like my mother, but I don't always know how to do that." Rachel smiles, "Jeanne, you're doing better than you think." She then looks at the nurse and asks, "What can I do to help my daughter deal with these concerns?" ■

15

The Expectant Family: First Trimester

Although much current medical thought stresses an understanding of the state of the fetus in weeks of gestation, trimesters are still a simple and fairly accurate way for practitioners to view the pregnant woman and family. Unique, broad changes in physiologic, psychologic, and sociocultural factors of the woman, embryo/fetus, and family occur in each of the three trimesters that encompass the prenatal period. Each trimester is quite distinct in its specific characteristics and manifestations and the impact it has on the family. In addition, each trimester has its unique "flavor" and is different from the other trimesters in both quantitative and qualitative aspects. To focus on the prenatal period in total is to ignore specific nuances, in terms of both biophysical and psychosocial function, of the mother, father, and family.

The first 12 weeks of pregnancy are generally referred to as the first trimester. From the moment of conception, changes begin to take place in almost every system in the woman's body. Physiologic adaptation to pregnancy is necessary to sustain the growing products of conception for a total period of about 40 weeks.

In addition, psychologic changes begin to affect not only the woman, but also the father and the entire nuclear and extended family. Psychologic, sociologic, and cultural factors have a major impact on family well-being, transition to parenthood, and ability to relate to and parent the newborn.

Prenatal care is defined as a series of interventions received by a woman during her pregnancy with the goal of promoting a favorable outcome for mother, family, and baby. It is an essential determinant of birth outcome, second only to socioeconomic status. Initiation of prenatal care during the first trimester is essential, as many vital changes in the mother and embryo/fetus occur during this time.

Assessment is integral to the clinical reasoning process. Diagnoses, goals, and interventions evolve from assessment and require the nurse to make clinical decisions. Interventions stem from well-constructed goals, and evaluation provides feedback to determine efficacy of the interventions in meeting goals. The nurse has a major role in delivery of health care to women and families during the first trimester.

▶ PHYSIOLOGIC CHANGES DURING THE FIRST TRIMESTER

The first trimester is a critical period both for development of the embryo/fetus, and for initiation of physiologic changes in the mother's body systems. A healthy beginning at this stage sets the tone for subsequent trimesters.

▶ Growth and Development of the Embryo/Fetus

Prenatal care always includes the changes occurring in the embryo/fetus, as well as the changes taking place in the mother. Growth and development of the embryo/fetus have already been discussed in Chapter 13. During the first trimester, rapid cell division occurs in the embryo. By the end of the first lunar month, the foundation for all major organ systems has been laid, the heart begins to beat, and many other changes are taking place. Environmental insults, such as the use of drugs by the mother, can affect the formation of the organ systems in the developing embryo/fetus. By the end of the first trimester, developmental "milestones" include maturation of the fetal gallbladder, spleen, and pancreas. Fingernails and toenails are present, and the external genitalia may often be identified as male or female (Knuppel, 1994). To support the developing pregnancy, the placenta is also forming during the first trimester.

▶ Maternal Physiologic Adaptation

From the time of conception, physiologic changes take place in the woman's body. These changes support and nourish the products of conception; prepare the expectant mother's body for labor, delivery, and lactation; and help to maintain a state of maternal and fetal wellness. The nurse can help the family prepare for and cope with these changes to promote a healthy outcome for mother and fetus. Maternal physiologic responses to the first trimester are summarized in Table 15–1.

▶ The Placenta

The placenta is a complex organ that is fetal in origin but depends almost completely on maternal blood.

Placental Hormones
The placenta acts as an endocrine gland during pregnancy, and produces estrogens, progesterone, human chorionic gonadotropin, and human placental lactogen. Major effects of these hormones are summarized in Table 15–2. Placental hormones promote maternal and fetal development during pregnancy. Some hormonally induced changes also account for maternal discomforts during pregnancy. Placental hormones

▶ **TABLE 15-1**

Summary of Physiologic Changes in the First Trimester

Organ	Change
Reproductive System	
Uterus	Uterus increases in size through hypertrophy and hyperplasia of cells (size doubles by 10 weeks)
	Uterus softens and enlarges asymmetrically until 10 weeks; the growth of the uterus is greater in the fundus
	Uterus changes position; rises out of pelvis and can be felt above the symphysis pubis (Fig. 15–1)
	Number of muscle fibers increases
	Muscle fibers elongate and widen
	Braxton Hicks contractions (irregular, painless contractions of the uterus without cervical dilation) begin, but are usually not felt
	Endometrium changes to decidua (see Fig. 13–4)
Cervix	Cervix softens
	Vascularity increases
	Vasocongestion causes bluish color (**Chadwick's sign**)
	Cervical glands hypertrophy
	Cervical glands increase activity; **leukorrhea** (a whitish or yellowish vaginal discharge) occurs
	Mucous plug forms (acts as a barrier to protect the fetus from infection) (Fig. 15–2)
	Lengthens
Vagina	Vascularity increases
	Chadwick's sign
	Vagina softens
	Glycogen content of epithelium increases
	pH becomes acidic (3.5–6.0) which helps to control the growth of harmful bacteria
	Changes cause predisposition to yeast *(Candida albicans)* infections
Fallopian tubes	Few structural changes occur
	Epithelium flattens
	Site of fertilization (distal one third) produces ductal fluid to nourish fertilized ovum and help cleavage
Ovary	Ovulation stops after conception
	Corpus luteum enlarges to about one-third the size of the ovary
	Corpus luteum most active during the first 6 to 7 weeks of pregnancy
	Corpus luteum secretes hormones to support pregnancy until the placenta develops (including estrogens, progesterone, and relaxin)
Breasts	Mammary ducts and alveoli hypertrophy
	Breasts swell, become tender
	Blood flow increases
	Montgomery tubercles (hypertrophic sebaceous glands scattered in the areola) become pronounced
	Pigment of nipple and areola begins to darken
	Little or no breast secretion occurs
Cardiovascular System	Cardiac output begins to increase due largely to an increase in stroke volume
	Blood volume begins to increase
	Resting pulse increases (about 8 beats per minute over nonpregnant rate)
	Blood pressure remains unchanged
	Physiologic systolic flow murmur may develop because of increased plasma volume
	Leukocyte count increases
	Neutrophil count rises
	Lymphocytes and monocytes remain unchanged
	Red blood cells show little or no change
	Blood clotting factors increase starting at about the third month of pregnancy: Factor I (plasma fibrinogen), factors VII, VIII, IX, and X
Respiratory System	
Lungs	Tidal volume increases
	Total oxygen-carrying capacity of red blood cells increases
	Inspiratory capacity begins to increase
	Woman breathes more deeply to compensate for the increased oxygen demands of fetus and maternal organs
Respiratory passages	Lungs perform more efficiently
	Respiratory rate shows little or no change
	Hormonally induced vasocongestion and edema of mucous membranes cause nasal stuffiness, nosebleeds, discharge, and general feelings of congestion

(continued)

▶ **TABLE 15-1** *(continued)*

Summary of Physiologic Changes in the First Trimester

Organ	Change
Urinary System	Kidneys increase in size and weight
	Glomerular filtration rate increases by 50%
	Renal plasma flow increases by 25 to 50%
	Ureters, renal pelves, and renal calyces dilate, contributing to stasis of urine
	Woman is prone to urinary tract infections
	Excretion of such substances as glucose and water-soluble vitamins increases
	Blood urea nitrogen and serum creatinine levels decrease
Musculoskeletal System	Clinical changes are minimal
Integument	
Skin	Pigmentation begins to increase
	Linea nigra, a dark line from the symphysis pubis to the top of the fundus, appears
	Areola and nipples darken
	Increased blood flow to skin gives feelings of warmth
	Telangiectases (vascular spiders), small dilated end-arterioles related to increased estrogen production, may develop
	Some skin conditions improve; some worsen
	Allergic sensitivity increases
	Activity of sebaceous and sweat glands increases
Hair	New hair continues to grow at usual pace
	Hair does not fall out as fast, and thus seems thicker
	Growth of fine and downy hair begins to increase
Nails	Nails begin to grow faster
	Nails soften
Gastrointestinal System	Hyperemia of tissues in mouth begins in response to elevated hormones
	Gums become extra sensitive to irritants
	Changes are mostly hormonally induced; uterus as yet too small to cause changes related to expanding size
	Motility and tone of gastrointestinal tract decrease
	Stomach takes longer to empty
	Pepsin and hydrochloric acid levels decrease
	Time for absorption of nutrients increases
	Iron absorption from small intestine increases
	Water absorption from large intestine increases
	Nausea and vomiting are experienced by 50 to 88% of pregnant women
	Appetite changes
	Ptyalism (excessive salivation) is experienced
	Taste and smell are altered
	Nutritional requirements change
Endocrine System	See Table 15–2
Pituitary	Anterior pituitary enlarges slightly
	Hypothalamus inhibits luteinizing and follicle-stimulating hormones
	Hormones are secreted to foster development of pregnancy and development of breasts
Thyroid	Thyroid enlarges
	BMR[a] increases
	Free T_3 and T_4 do not rise significantly; total T_3 and T_4 begin to rise[a]
Parathyroids	Parathyroids enlarge
	Parathyroid hormone level may decrease
Adrenals	Adrenal cortex begins to hypertrophy
	Adrenocorticotropic hormone and cortisol decrease
	Aldosterone increases
Pancreas	Insulin production decreases in response to fetal demands for glucose
Placenta	Placenta develops and becomes fully functional

[a]T_3, triiodothyronine; T_4, 3, 5, 3′, 5′ = tetraiodothyronine (thyroxine); BMR, basal metabolic rate.

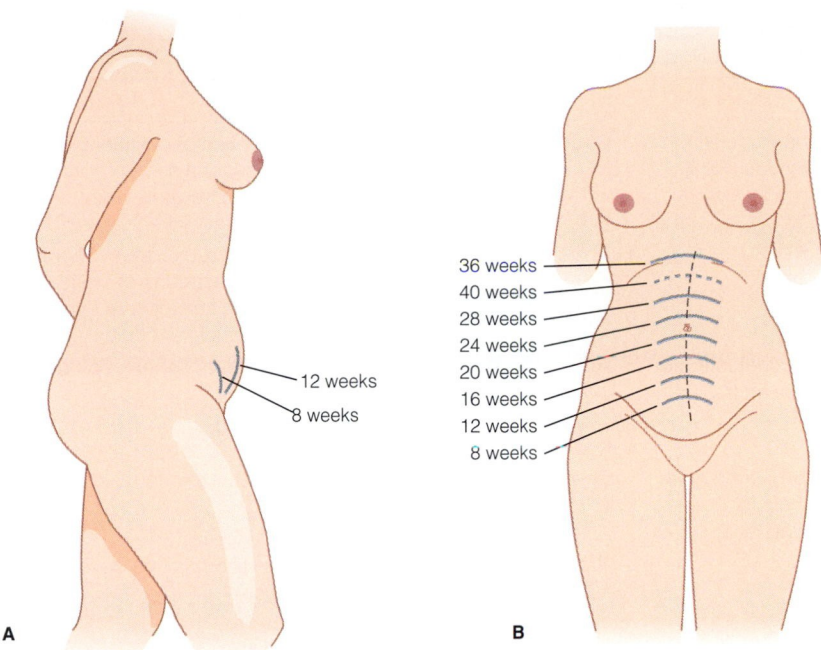

FIGURE 15–1. Position of the uterus. **A.** Height of the fundus at 8 and 12 weeks. **B.** After the first trimester the uterus grows beyond the pelvis into the abdominal cavity.

and their interactions are extremely complex and not completely understood.

Estrogens. Estrogens are steroid hormones secreted largely by the ovary in early pregnancy. The estrogen secretion by the corpus luteum is dependent on the maternal precursors, cholesterol and acetates.

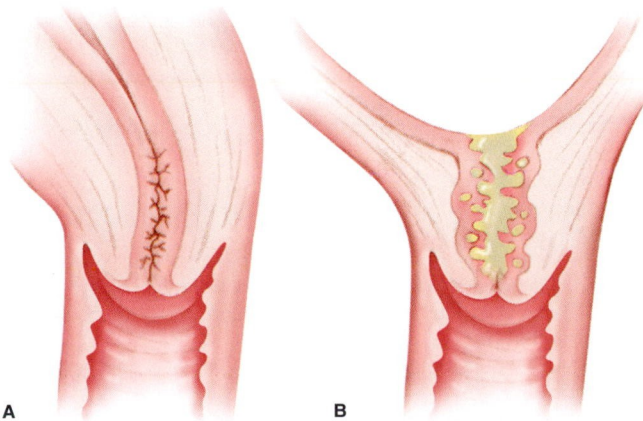

FIGURE 15–2. A. Cervix of a nonpregnant woman. **B.** Cervix of a pregnant woman. Note the elaboration of the mucosa into a honeycomb-like structure, filled with a tenacious mucus—the so-called mucous plug.

By the seventh week of gestation, more than half of the estrogens are secreted by the placenta; as pregnancy advances, the placenta secretes most of the body's estrogens. Placental production is dependent on fetal androgens secreted by the fetal liver and adrenals, as well as by androgens in the maternal circulation. The fetal–placental unit is thus important in controlling both the secretion of estrogen and the environment of pregnancy. During pregnancy, estrogen secretion increases about 1000 times above the nonpregnant level of the premenopausal woman (Cunningham et al., 1997).

More than 25 types of estrogen have been found in maternal urine. The most common in pregnancy are estrone, estradiol, and estriol. Estriol, the predominant estrogen produced by the placenta, has many functions (see Table 15–2). Large amounts of estriol are secreted during normal pregnancy. Estriol produced by the placenta is found in maternal blood and urine and in amniotic fluid. For this reason, estriol levels, especially those in maternal urine and serum, are indicators of placental and fetal well-being. For example, decreasing serial urinary estriol levels suggest fetal jeopardy. Today, more direct and accurate measures, such as the nonstress test, are available for fetal assessment in high-risk situations (see Chapter 18).

Progesterone. Progesterone is a steroid hormone secreted by the corpus luteum for about the first 7

▶ **TABLE 15-2**

Examples of Hormonal Effects During Pregnancy

Gland	Hormone	Target Organ	Major Effects
Anterior pituitary (adenohypophysis)	Follicle-stimulating hormone (FSH)	Ovary	Acts in maturation of ovarian follicle Stimulates estrogen secretion from follicular fluid Suppressed during pregnancy
	Luteinizing hormone (LH)	Ovary, uterus, breasts	Stimulates ovulation Maintains the corpus luteum of pregnancy for about 7 weeks Stimulates progesterone secretion Prepares uterus for fertilized ovum Prepares breasts for lactation
	Adrenocorticotropic hormone (ACTH)	Adrenal cortex, placenta (role of placental ACTH unclear)	Stimulates adrenal cortex to produce cortisol
	Thyrotropin (thyroid-stimulating hormone, TSH)	Thyroid	Stimulates the thyroid to release thyroxine
Anterior pituitary of mother and fetus (myometrium and endometrium)	Prolactin	Breasts	Maternal prolactin fosters development of breast in preparation for lactation
Posterior pituitary (neurohypophysis)	Oxytocin	Smooth muscle of uterus and breasts	Stimulates contractions of the uterus during labor, delivery, and involution Stimulates contractions of the breast during lactation
Thyroid	T_3, T_4[a]	Body cells	Serum protein-bound iodine increases Increases basal metabolic rate Increases use of nutrients
Adrenal cortex	Cortisol	Body cells	Assists in regulation of glucose in maternal blood by stimulating the liver to synthesize carbohydrates from noncarbohydrates such as amino acids Increases concentration of amino acids in the blood by stimulating degradation of proteins within maternal cells (amino acids and glucose are needed by the mother and fetus for growth and development)
	Aldosterone	Kidneys, blood	Regulates sodium content of blood Causes retention of sodium and water when blood sodium levels are low May counteract some effects of progesterone, because progesterone stimulates sodium and water loss by the kidney Helps to increase blood volume
Ovaries, placenta (after 7 weeks of gestation)	Estrogen (estriol is predominant, but many forms of estrogen exist)	Multiorgan effects (especially uterus, skin, stomach, breasts)	Stimulates development of uterine lining Stimulates hypertrophy of uterine muscles and development of additional blood supply; increases uteroplacental blood flow Suppresses secretion of FSH and LH by anterior pituitary Promotes metabolism of nutrients Decreases secretion of hydrochloric acid and pepsin by the stomach Promotes sodium and water retention by kidney Produces increased pliability of connective tissue with relaxation of joints and ligaments Stimulates growth of breasts and development of duct system Stimulates production of melanocyte-stimulating hormone Contributes to integumentary changes, such as darkening of skin pigment Implicated in development of vascular spiders and palmar erythema
	Progesterone (placental synthesis depends on maternal precursor, lipoprotein cholesterol)	Multiorgan effects (especially uterus, breasts, smooth muscle)	Suppresses FSH and LH by the anterior pituitary gland Maintains corpus luteum of pregnancy until placenta is functional Develops decidual cells of uterus; maintains uterine lining for implantation and early pregnancy Stimulates uterine enlargement in early pregnancy

▶ **TABLE 15-2** *(continued)*

Examples of Hormonal Effects During Pregnancy

Gland	Hormone	Target Organ	Major Effects
			Aids in formation of placenta
			Increases vascularity of cervix
			Increases absorption of nutrients
			Stimulates storage of fat
			Relaxes smooth muscle; decreases uterine contractility; promotes vasodilation; decreases tone of bladder and ureters; reduces motility and tone of gastrointestinal tract, including gallbladder
			Stimulates sodium excretion (naturesis)
			Promotes lobular-alveolar system of breasts and mammary growth
			Resets three maternal hypothalamic centers, resulting in increase in basal body temperature until midpregnancy; an increase in fat storage; stimulation of respiratory center to facilitate pulmonary transfer of carbon dioxide
			May also prevent rejection of fetus by mother's body
	Relaxin	Pelvic joints, blood	Relaxation of pelvic joints; regulation of uteroplacental blood flow
Placenta	Human chorionic gonadotropin (hCG)	Ovary	Synthesized in syncytiotrophoblasts
			Found in maternal urine and blood; basis for many pregnancy tests
			Highest levels occur by about 10 weeks of pregnancy and decrease to lowest level by 20 weeks
			Maintains corpus luteum during early pregnancy
			Promotes testosterone synthesis and secretion and sexual differentiation in males
			Used in diagnosis of pregnancy or high-risk conditions such as hydatidiform mole
			May directly stimulate thyroid activity
	Human placental lactogen (hPL)	Body cells	Secreted by chorionic villi
			Influences growth and development of fetus and placenta
			Stimulates growth of breasts
			Influences metabolic processes
			Promotes lipolysis and increases free fatty acids, thus offering an energy source for maternal metabolism and fetal nutrition
			Spares glucose and protein by inhibiting uptake of glucose and also gluconeogenesis
			Effects raise levels of maternal insulin, which promotes protein synthesis, thus creating a source of amino acids for transport to fetus
			Possibly serves as a "backup" mechanism; may not be needed for successful pregnancy outcome

[a]T_3, triiodothyronine; T_4, 3, 5, 3′, 5′ = -tetraiodothyronine (thyroxine).

weeks of pregnancy to help develop the maternal decidual cells and maintain the corpus luteum itself. After the seventh week of gestation, the placenta is the major source of progesterone. Unlike estrogen, progesterone requires no fetal precursors. Instead, maternal cholesterol, which enters the trophoblast as a low-density lipoprotein, is needed for progesterone synthesis. Ten times more progesterone is secreted by the placenta than by the ovary when a woman is not pregnant. Progesterone is also produced in greater quantities than estrogens in the course of pregnancy; levels rise during pregnancy and peak at term.

Reduction of myometrial contractility during pregnancy is one effect of progesterone. Because of this, progesterone withdrawal was thought to be necessary for the onset of labor. Currently no evidence supports this theory. Progesterone withdrawal may be only one step in the complex events leading to labor.

Human Chorionic Gonadotropin. Human chorionic gonadotropin (hCG) is a protein hormone secreted by the syncytiotrophoblast early in pregnancy. It helps sustain the corpus luteum, which in turn secretes the progesterone and estrogen necessary for early pregnancy. This hormone is in maternal blood and urine as early as 8 days after conception and reaches its highest level toward the end of the first trimester, at about 8 to 10 weeks. Thereafter, hCG levels sharply decline.

Human Placental Lactogen. Human placental lactogen (hPL), a protein hormone, may be detected in the syncytiotrophoblast as early as 2 to 3 weeks after conception (Cunningham et al., 1997). This hormone is referred to as human chorionic somatomammotropin and chorionic growth hormone because it promotes the growth of the fetus, breasts, and uterus during pregnancy (see Table 15–2).

Human placental lactogen is thought to affect growth of the fetus and the placenta, because the level of hPL in the maternal circulation is directly related to fetal and placental weight. The level of hPL increases as pregnancy progresses and peaks at about 35 weeks of gestation. The placenta is the chief source of hPL in the healthy, pregnant woman.

Human placental lactogen is believed to have no role in human lactation, because lactation occurs when production of hPL has stopped.

▶ Other Hormones: Prostaglandins

Prostaglandins are derived from arachidonic acid, an unsaturated fatty acid. Their exact function is unknown. They are in most body tissues and, during pregnancy, in high concentrations in the amnion, chorion, and decidua. Prostaglandin synthesis is greatest in the amnion. Prostaglandin E (PGE) and prostaglandin F (PGF) are believed to have an important role during labor; however, an antagonistic relationship seems to exist between prostaglandins E and F. When concentrations of PGE are elevated, blood vessels dilate. When PGF is elevated, blood vessels constrict. Both prostaglandins contract smooth muscle and are metabolized in the lungs. Tissue levels of prostaglandins remain constant throughout pregnancy.

▶ Signs and Symptoms of Pregnancy

During the first trimester, indicators of pregnancy become apparent and the woman may experience certain related discomforts. Indicators of pregnancy are classified as signs and symptoms. Symptoms are subjective feelings or sensations experienced by the woman; signs are observed by others. For conceptual ease, symptoms and signs of pregnancy are divided into three groups: presumptive, probable, and posi-

tive. The student should learn to identify and describe them because the terms are widely used. Table 15–3 summarizes the symptoms and signs of pregnancy.

Presumptive Indications
Presumptive indicators of pregnancy are so called because they can be caused by factors other than pregnancy. Most presumptive indicators become apparent during the first trimester.

Presumptive Symptoms. Amenorrhea is often the earliest presumptive symptom. Menses cease after conception in response to the increasing progesterone level produced by the corpus luteum. In a woman who has regular menstrual cycles, this is a dependable symptom but is not a positive symptom of pregnancy; other factors, such as endocrine problems, emotional stress, chronic disease, certain drugs, and tumors, can be responsible. In exceedingly rare instances, women may have unexplained cyclic bleeding during pregnancy and therefore cannot depend on the absence of vaginal bleeding as a sign of pregnancy.

Nausea and vomiting, also presumptive symptoms, are experienced by about 50% of women. They are most severe during the first trimester, between 2 and 12 weeks; however, nausea and vomiting can be symptoms of such conditions as gastrointestinal viruses and emotional stress.

Breast changes, primarily tenderness (mastodynia), are early presumptive symptoms of pregnancy. Factors that contribute to tenderness include hormonal influences on the mammary ducts and alveolar system of the breasts and increases in blood circulation to the area. These changes, however, may also occur with other conditions, such as chronic cystic mastitis, or prior to menstruation.

Urinary frequency, caused by pressure of the enlarging uterus on the bladder, is also a symptom of urinary tract infections.

Fatigue is a presumptive symptom reported by many women throughout the first trimester. Stress, illness, and lifestyle changes affecting sleep habits are examples of conditions that can also produce fatigue.

Quickening, the first sensation of fetal movement, is a presumptive symptom that usually is experienced during the second trimester. Primigravid women tend to experience quickening around 18 to 20 weeks; multigravid women feel quickening earlier, about 14 to 16 weeks. As peristalsis and "gas" may produce similar sensations, quickening is not a dependable sign of pregnancy; nevertheless, it is helpful in identifying how far a pregnancy has progressed.

▶ **TABLE 15-3**

Symptoms and Signs of Pregnancy

Symptom/Sign	Physiologic Base	Cause Other Than Pregnancy
Presumptive Symptoms		
Amenorrhea	Increased progesterone; inhibition of FSH and LH	Endocrine disorders, malnutrition, emotional factors, systemic disease, early menopause
Nausea/vomiting	Unknown cause; may be related to altered carbohydrate metabolism, increased levels of hCG, decreased gastrointestinal motility, and other factors	Gastrointestinal disorders, acute infections, emotional factors
Breast tenderness	Development of duct system influenced by increased hormone levels	Premenstrual symptoms, chronic cystic mastitis
Urinary frequency	Pressure of enlarging uterus on bladder	Urinary tract infections, stress, tumors
Fatigue	Unknown cause	Stress, anemia, infections, other illnesses
Quickening	Fetal movements felt by mother	Gastrointestinal activity
Presumptive Signs		
Increased basal body temperature	Increased metabolic activity	Infections
Linea nigra	Increase in melanocyte-stimulating hormone	
Melasma (chloasma)	Cause unclear, possibly increased estrogen, progesterone, melanocyte-stimulating hormone	Certain contraceptives
Striae	Separation of collagen tissues beneath skin; may be hormonally related; cause unknown	Obesity
Colostrum secretion	Hormonal stimulation (increased prolactin levels)	Pituitary tumors
Enlargement of secondary breast tissue	Hormonal stimulation	Breast cysts, tumors
Probable Signs		
Chadwick's sign	Increased vascularity of vagina, cervix, and vulva	Hyperemia of pelvic organs as a result of non-pregnancy-related hormonal influences
Goodell's sign	Pelvic vasocongestion	Oral contraceptives
Ladin's sign	Anterior uterine softening at midline	
McDonald's sign	Flexibility of uterus where uterus and cervix join	Myomas, tumors
Hegar's sign	Hyperemia of pelvic organs	Anatomically soft walls of nonpregnant uterus
Braun von Fernwald's sign	Hormonal influences, implantation	Myomas, tumors
Piskacek's sign	Softening over implantation site in cornua of uterus	Myomas, tumors
Uterine enlargement	Growing products of conception	Tumors
Braxton Hicks contractions	Irregular contractions of uterus	Hematomas, soft myomas
Uterine souffle	Whooshing sound caused by maternal blood moving into placental vessels and sinuses	
Ballottement of uterus	Movement of fetus during examination	Ascites, ovarian cysts, tumors
Positive pregnancy tests	Human chorionic gonadotropin in urine and blood	Disease states, such as choriocarcinoma, hydatidiform mole
Positive Indications		
Fetal heartbeat heard	Fetus	
Fetal movements felt by examiner	Fetus	
Fetal outline seen	Fetus	

Presumptive Signs. Increased basal body temperature that continues longer than 3 weeks may be considered a presumptive sign if the temperature is conscientiously charted. A low-grade, elevated temperature could also be a sign of infection.

Several changes are also noted in the skin. Linea nigra may be observed.

Melasma, also called **chloasma,** is darkening of the skin on the face (forehead, nose, cheekbones). It usually appears during the second trimester, after 16 weeks. Certain illnesses or medications, however, can also cause changes in skin pigmentation.

Striae gravidarum, often called "stretch marks," are reddish or purplish streaks that develop in the skin over the maternal abdomen, breasts, thighs, and hips, possibly as a result of hormonal influences and the loosening and stretching of connective tissue. Striae are a presumptive sign that usually appears during the second or third trimester; however, stretch marks may also result from such conditions as marked obesity and swelling.

The breasts are the site of several changes. In response to hormonal stimulation during early pregnancy, the Montgomery tubercles (sebaceous glands) in the areola enlarge at about 6 to 8 weeks of gestation.

Colostrum is secreted (see Chapter 17) from the breasts usually beginning during the second trimester, about 16 weeks. Secretion of fluid from both breasts, however, occurs in other conditions, for example, prolactin-secreting pituitary tumors.

Enlargement of secondary breast tissue and its increased pigmentation can be seen along the nipple line. Hypertrophied axillary breast tissue may be identified as a lump in the armpit. Although normal presumptive signs of pregnancy, these can be confused with true breast pathology. Any breast or axillary lump, therefore, needs careful, expert evaluation.

Probable Indications

Probable symptoms and signs of pregnancy are the result of physiologic changes in the pelvic organs and hormonal influences. Although they aid in the diagnosis of pregnancy, these indicators, like presumptive ones, do not definitively identify pregnancy.

Probable Symptoms. Probable symptoms are the same as presumptive symptoms.

Probable Signs. Several probable signs of pregnancy can be observed during the first trimester. Many are identified during a pelvic examination (see Assessment of Physiologic Change in the Mother, later in this chapter). The probable signs include changes in the pelvic organs and positive pregnancy tests.

Among the changes that occur in the pelvic organs are changes in color, consistency, and size. For example, the mucous membranes of the vulva, vagina, and cervix become bluish (**Chadwick's sign**) as a result of hyperemia and proliferation of cells. In addition, there is softening of the cervix (**Goodell's sign**) related to vasocongestion and hypertrophy of the cervical glands. The anterior part of the uterus also softens at the midline where the uterus and cervix join (**Ladin's sign**). The softening occurs at about 6 weeks and is probably related to hormonal changes (Fig. 15–3).

The uterus also becomes easily flexed at the site where it is joined by the cervix (**McDonald's sign**). Moreover, the isthmus of the uterus widens to the

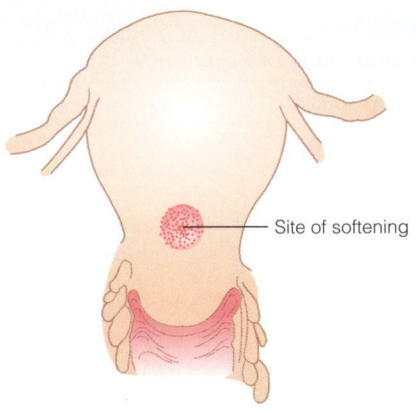

FIGURE 15–3. Anterior of uterus depicting area where softening (Ladin's sign) occurs at about 6 weeks. *(Reproduced with permission, from DeCherney, A.H., & Pernoll, M.L. (Eds.) (1994). Current obstetric & gynecologic diagnosis & treatment (8th ed.). Norwalk, CT: Appleton & Lange, p. 186.)*

point that it can be compressed on bimanual examination (**Hegar's sign**). Unilateral softening of the uterus may be detected at 4 to 5 weeks, with development of a palpable groove lengthwise between the soft and firm parts (**Braun von Fernwald's sign**). This sign is related to softening of the uterus at the site of implantation. Uterine asymmetry may occur in the cornual area, an implantion site, and become apparent at 6 weeks of gestation (**Piskacek's sign**). By 10 weeks, the uterus enlarges symmetrically.

Abdominal enlargement is a probable sign that becomes noticeable after 7 weeks. Painless uterine contractions (Braxton Hicks contractions) may be felt during the second and third trimesters. Another probable sign is uterine souffle, the "shooshing" sound made as maternal blood fills the blood vessels and sinuses in the placenta. It can be heard through the abdomen after 16 weeks. The rate of uterine souffle is the same as that of the mother's pulse.

Ballottement is a maneuver to detect pregnancy in which the examiner places two fingers in the vagina and pushes the fetal body upward. The fetus is felt to rise and then fall like a heavy body in water. Later in pregnancy, ballottement may be done abdominally.

A positive pregnancy test is another probable sign. Currently used laboratory tests show positive results when hCG is present in the maternal blood and urine during the first trimester. The tests are probable indicators because false-negative and false-positive results can occur (see box entitled Conditions Contributing to False-Negative or False-Positive Pregnancy Test Results). Because the tests are not 100% accurate, they are used as adjuncts to a health history and physical examination in diagnosing pregnancy. In the past, biologic animal assays were used to detect

► **CONDITIONS CONTRIBUTING TO FALSE-NEGATIVE OR FALSE-POSITIVE PREGNANCY TEST RESULTS**[a]

FALSE-NEGATIVE RESULTS (TEST FAILS TO DETECT PREGNANCY)

- Test misread by examiner
- Test done too early or too late in pregnancy
- Urine too dilute (possibly because a random sample rather than a first-morning urine used)
- Urine stored too long or improperly
- Missed or impending spontaneous abortion
- Ectopic pregnancy
- Drug interference

FALSE-POSITIVE RESULTS (TEST INACCURATELY READ AS PREGNANT)

- Test misread by examiner
- LH cross-reaction
- Protein in urine
- Blood in urine

- Lipemia or turbidity (in serum specimen)
- Continuing cyst of the corpus luteum
- Recent pregnancy (less than 10 days after pregnancy terminated)
- Residue on glassware used for test (especially detergent)
- Premature menopause
- Certain drugs, for example, aldomet, marijuana, phenothiazines, antidepressants
- hCG treatment, e.g., fertility treatment injections
- Thyrotoxicosis
- Malignant tumors that secrete hCG (e.g., ovarian and breast tumors, melanoma)

[a]Directions for performing each pregnancy test must be read and followed carefully, as false results can often be attributed to improper testing procedures. Certain tests may also require use of a stopwatch for precision in timing. Tests indicating surprising results should be repeated.
Adapted from Hatcher, R.A. et al. (1992). *Contraceptive technology: 1990–1992.* (15th ed.). New York: Irvington.

hCG. In most cases, however, they have been replaced by simpler, less expensive chemical tests.

Detection of Human Chorionic Gonadotropin in Blood or Urine. Pregnancy tests for urinary hCG may be performed as a single service for minimal or no charge at women's health centers; as part of comprehensive assessment for a first prenatal visit; as part of assessment of the woman with amenorrhea; and at home using over-the-counter test kits.

Blood (serum) tests for hCG are performed in a laboratory, clinic, or office as part of comprehensive client evaluation.

In the healthy woman, the hormone hCG is produced only during pregnancy. Low levels are present after fertilization, but increase rapidly after implantation when trophoblastic cells proliferate and produce greater amounts. Under healthy conditions, hCG levels follow a predictable pattern. As shown in Figure 15–4, hCG levels rise rapidly during early pregnancy,

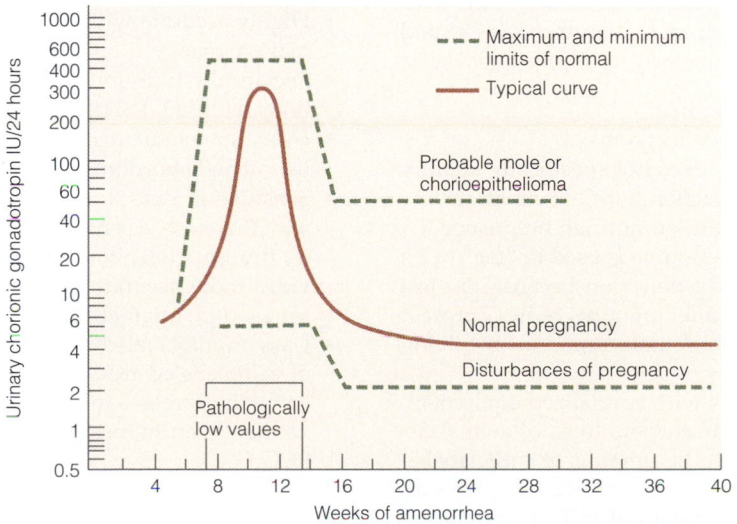

FIGURE 15–4. Human chorionic gonadotropin levels during pregnancy. *(Reproduced, with permission, from Hatcher, R.A. et al. (1988). Contraceptive technology: 1988–1989 (14th ed.). New York: Irvington, p. 381.)*

peak about 60 to 70 days after conception, and then drop to a lower level for the rest of pregnancy.

Tests for hCG in blood or serum are based on the principle that hCG, or a subunit of hCG, is recognized by an antibody to the hCG molecule. The hCG molecule has an alpha subunit and a beta subunit. The alpha subunit of hCG is similar in molecular structure to such hormones as luteinizing hormone (LH). For this reason, pregnancy tests that detect the whole hCG molecule, which includes the alpha subunit, may pro-duce false-positive results. Tests that detect the beta subunit have less incidence of false-positive results, because the beta subunit is specific for pregnancy and does not crossreact with other hormones in the body. (See box entitled Major Types of Pregnancy Tests Based on Detection of Human Chorionic Gonadotropin in Blood or Urine.)

Home pregnancy test kits are currently available without prescription to consumers and can be purchased in pharmacies and supermarkets. They are

---

▶ MAJOR TYPES OF PREGNANCY TESTS BASED ON DETECTION OF HUMAN CHORIONIC GONADOTROPIN IN BLOOD OR URINE

TESTS FOR HUMAN CHORIONIC GONADOTROPIN

Immunoassay (IA) (test "tube" or slide; serum or urine)
- Accurate within 7 to 28 days of conception
- Tests for the hCG molecule; does not specifically identify the beta subunit, so cross-reaction with LH can occur
- Readily accessible; widely used as a pregnancy test in routine situations
- Does not require radioisotopes and sophisticated laboratory analysis
- Based on antigen–antibody reaction (Most tests are positive if the solution stays homogeneous and no agglutination occurs; most are negative if agglutination is noted; directions *must* be read carefully, as not all tests are conducted or read in the same way.)

Examples
- Latex agglutination inhibition test (LAI), which uses a specimen from the client, a reagent containing hCG, antibody, and latex particles bound to hCG as the antigen (slide test)
- Hemagglutination inhibition test (HAI), which uses a specimen from the client, a reagent containing hCG antibody, and reagent-containing animal erythrocytes coated with hCG as the antigen (tube test)

Radioreceptor Assay (RRA) (serum)
- Accurate within 14 days of conception
- Tests for the hCG molecule; does not specifically identify the beta subunit, so cross-reaction with LH can occur
- Used for early confirmation of normal pregnancy (A small amount of radioactive isotope is used to "tag" hCG; this method allows for early detection because the test can be positive with the smaller amounts of hCG present in early pregnancy or with high-risk conditions involving low levels of hCG.)
- Requires laboratory analysis with specialized equipment
- Uses hCG receptors from the corpora lutea of animal tissue and radiolabeled hCG (The amount of radiolabeled hCG that remains unbound to the specific receptor sites increases in relation to the amount of hCG in the client's serum.)

TESTS FOR BETA SUBUNIT OF HUMAN CHORIONIC GONADOTROPIN

Enzyme-Linked Immunoassay (EI)/Enzyme-Linked Immunosorbent Assay (ELISA) (urine or serum)
- Accurate within 12 days of conception
- Specific for the beta subunit of hCG; no cross-reactions with LH, FSH, or other hormones
- Particularly helpful for testing perimenopausal women who normally have higher levels of LH and might otherwise have a positive result based on cross-reaction with this hormone
- Urine tests usually positive when maternal serum levels are at least 25 mIU/mL, but do not quantitate level of beta subunit
- Results have less interference from urinary blood or protein if present
- Uses a monoclonal antibody specific for the beta subunit of hCG and an antigen–enzyme conjugate (A simple color change takes place when the beta subunit is present.)
- Method used in newer home pregnancy kits

Radioimmunoassay (RIA)
- Highly accurate within 7 days of conception during normal pregnancy
- Specifically tests for beta subunit of hCG; no cross-reactions with LH, FSH, or other hormones
- Used for evaluating abnormal pregnancy, for example, threatened abortion, hydatidiform mole
- Sensitive in detection and quantification of beta subunit and, therefore, a sensitive indicator of trophoblastic activity (Information about the exact level of beta subunit provides more accurate interpretation of any findings from ultrasound, often also done for high-risk evaluation.)
- Uses a radiolabeled hCG In a fixed amount (The amount of radiolabeled hCG that can bind to the anti-hCG in a solution decreases in relation to the amount of hCG in the woman's serum, permitting quantitative measurement of hCG.)

urine tests for hCG that can be performed by the client in the privacy of her home. Some home tests involve simple color changes as the result of monoclonal antibody reactions. Others are hemagglutination inhibition tests that use sheep erythrocytes, antibodies to hCG, and a sample of the woman's urine. Pharmaceutical research has focused on the development of consumer tests that are increasingly easy to use.

Although consumer tests have advantages such as privacy and early detection, many occasionally produce inaccurate results, especially if they are not done correctly. False-negative results tend to occur more frequently than false-positive results, because the test is often not sensitive enough to identify hCG early in pregnancy when urinary levels are low.

Positive Indications

Positive indications of pregnancy clearly demonstrate the presence of a fetus and cannot be due to other conditions. Positive confirmation of pregnancy is made solely on objective signs. New methods of assessment make early first-trimester diagnosis possible. Although many symptoms suggest pregnancy, only a few definite positive signs exist: detection of fetal heart tones, palpation of fetal movements, and visualization of the fetus.

With the use of a fetoscope, fetal heart tones can be auscultated at about 16 to 20 weeks, or later if the woman is obese or if implantation was anterior. Blood flow through the fetal heart can be identified with a Doppler instrument as early as 8 weeks.

Fetal movements can be palpated by the examiner after 18 weeks. The gestational sac may be visualized on ultrasound as early as 4 weeks and 3 days from the last menstrual period (Jurkovic, Gruboeck, & Campbell, 1995).

Clear demonstration of the presence of a fetus, for example, on ultrasound, ends any controversy about whether a pregnancy exists. Sources, however, differ with regard to whether other signs are presumptive, probable, or positive. For example, sometimes, all subjective signs are called "presumptive," and objective signs, "probable." At other times, signs may be classified as "presumptive" or "probable" according to their reliability in diagnosing pregnancy. An important consideration is that the woman who demonstrates only presumptive signs of pregnancy should begin prenatal care. This will help to ensure early, consistent health care for the mother and fetus.

▶ PSYCHOLOGIC AND SOCIOCULTURAL DIMENSIONS OF THE FIRST TRIMESTER

Concurrent with the changes in maternal and fetal body systems are changes in the psychologic processes of mother, father, siblings, and extended family members. Those changes enable both the mother and father to parent their newborn. The family, as a whole, alters in structure and function to enable it to incorporate a new member. In addition, the family's social network changes in anticipation of the new family member. The family's cultural background has a major effect on how changes occur.

▶ Psychologic Changes in the Mother

Considerations Before Pregnancy Is Diagnosed

Although pregnancy begins with conception, some time passes before pregnancy testing indicates that pregnancy is probable. Some women claim to have had no idea they were pregnant in the early stages; others "know" within days of conceiving. They detect subtle changes, such as breast enlargement, during the beginning of their pregnancy.

During their reproductive years, sexually active women may experience a "false alarm" when their menstrual period is delayed and they suspect that they are pregnant. On the other hand, a woman who frequently has irregular menses may doubt that she is pregnant when menses is delayed. Women experience various reactions during this time of uncertainty. Whether they respond with hopeful excitement, a sense of fatigue, or a feeling of dread depends on many factors:

1. Whether the pregnancy was planned
2. Whether the pregnancy is wanted (It is important to realize that "unplanned" does not necessarily mean "unwanted.")

Women's Health

In using home pregnancy tests, women should observe these guidelines (Cunningham et al., 1997):

- Follow product directions carefully
- Repeat negative tests within a week if amenorrhea persists
- Schedule an appointment for clinical examination as appropriate

3. Economic status of the family
4. Number and ages of other children in the family
5. Support that the mother perceives from her significant others, especially her husband or partner and her mother
6. Woman's cultural and religious background
7. Whether the couple has had difficulty conceiving or a history of infertility

Research is lacking concerning the psychologic aspects of the postconception and early first-trimester periods, possibly because women are not readily accessible to researchers within the health care system.

Most women seek confirmation of pregnancy at some point during the first trimester. Some may first use home pregnancy tests; others go to a clinic or private office setting for diagnosis of pregnancy. Occasionally, women deny the symptoms of pregnancy until the second or even third trimester. Indeed, nearly every experienced labor and delivery nurse has worked with a client who arrived at term in the delivery suite saying she never knew she was pregnant. Denial that extends into the mid-second or third trimester is not normal. These clients need to be carefully evaluated to identify high-risk psychologic or social conditions. It is important to distinguish between clients who knew they were pregnant but did not come for prenatal assessment and clients who maintain they never knew they were pregnant.

Reactions After Pregnancy Is Diagnosed

Specific maternal concerns differ in each of the three trimesters. During the first trimester, a woman's concerns are focused mainly on herself, on early physical changes she experiences, and on her feelings about the pregnancy. The infant-to-be is of less concern at this stage, unless the woman perceives herself to be at some degree of risk.

Occupational environment and personal habits can place a developing embryo/fetus at risk (see Chapter 13). Indeed, pregnant women are advised to avoid exposure to chemicals and other agents that may damage a fetus or harm pregnancy. Some women inaccurately believe they will make appropriate changes once they become pregnant. By the time the pregnancy is diagnosed, however, the foundation for the fetal organ systems has often been laid. The sense of unreality about the first trimester, therefore, can contribute to teratogenic problems.

Ideally, women contemplating childbearing should avoid substances and circumstances that could jeopardize pregnancy. In reality, this often does not happen. The nurse must address client concerns related to lifestyle, occupation, and environment during the first trimester. Nurses working with nonpregnant, sexually active clients of childbearing age also must counsel clients on promoting a healthy pregnancy.

Currently, most adult women in the United States have some type of employment. During the first trimester, women who are employed experience little change in their general feelings of well-being. If the nature of the job and work environment present no problems related to pregnancy, then employment during the first trimester is no problem.

As early as the first trimester, women who plan to continue employment after childbirth may be concerned about their jobs and careers. Employment status should be part of the prenatal history taken at the first visit. Employment options can be discussed if problems are identified. With delivery many months away, the newly expectant mother has time to think and plan employment changes.

Acceptance of Pregnancy

During the first trimester, women normally experience ambivalence about being pregnant. Some reasons for initial ambivalence during the first trimester include shock at the major changes in life that will take place, potential economic hardships related to the cost of childbearing and childrearing, potential impact on career goals, potential housing problems, feelings of not being ready, degree of discomfort experienced, and feelings of being "fat" (Beck, 1993).

By the end of the first trimester, most women accept pregnancy (Rubin, 1984), although ambivalence is normal at times throughout pregnancy. For example, women who experience physical discomfort such as hemorrhoids or women who face potential difficulties in finding child care may ask themselves why they wanted to be pregnant. Normal ambivalence during the first trimester may, however, signal unresolved conflicts and family problems during the later trimesters.

According to Lederman (1996) ambivalence may be assessed according to the following criteria: (1) how honestly ambivalence is expressed, (2) the reason for it, (3) the intensity of ambivalence, and (4) how long ambivalence is sustained throughout pregnancy.

Women may be at psychologic risk if they are not able to share their doubts about being pregnant, have a lifestyle that may be negatively affected by childbirth, and have vigorous, continuing personal conflict over having a child. Lack of acceptance of pregnancy, expressed in various ways during prenatal visits, may alert the nurse to high-risk psychologic and social conditions (see box entitled Maternal Indicators of Acceptance of Pregnancy). The nurse may state the concern directly or discuss it in an indirect or general

▶ MATERNAL INDICATORS OF ACCEPTANCE OF PREGNANCY

ACCEPTANCE

- Overall feelings of happiness and enjoyment of pregnancy
- Good tolerance of physical discomforts or few discomforts
- Minor degree of ambivalence during the first trimester
- Minor to moderate mood swings
- Feelings that she and her family can handle pregnancy and childbearing; feelings of self-confidence and hope

LACK OF ACCEPTANCE

- Overall feelings of despair or hopelessness
- Feelings of being overwhelmed by changes related to pregnancy (physical, lifestyle)
- Feelings that her world will change for the worse because of the pregnancy (marriage dissolve, career end)
- Persistent regret at becoming pregnant
- Persistent feelings of being ill; excessive subjective physical discomforts

manner. At times, a discussion of feelings during prenatal visits and identification of community resources such as prenatal support groups (usually advertised as early-pregnancy classes) or infant care services can help allay client concerns. Persistent ambivalence indicates the client's need for counseling, social service interventions, or both, and referral for follow-up assessment and intervention is appropriate.

There is a difference between ambivalence toward a pregnancy and rejection of the fetus. Ambivalence about pregnancy usually evolves into acceptance and preparation for the coming baby; however, rejection of the fetus presents a potential threat to the mother–infant relationship.

Maternal Role Attainment

During the first trimester, a woman begins to move into the role of mother. According to Rubin (1984), most of her activities at this stage involve replication. At the very beginning of pregnancy, this may include direct copying of practices and behaviors of other pregnant women or of women who have successfully borne children. Opinions and recommendations of professionals, such as the nurse, also may be modeled. The newly pregnant woman searches for models and "tries on" the behaviors. This process is also called **mimicry.** The woman may be eager to wear maternity clothes, although her regular clothing still fits. Mimicking models gives the woman stable guidelines during a time of uncertainty.

Role models also give the newly pregnant woman guidelines for the experiences of pregnancy. Although they may not yet coincide with her real experiences, the models give the mother-to-be some feeling of control over the unexpected. In general, the most important model is the pregnant woman's own mother.

Role playing, another replicative behavior, occurs in both first and successive pregnancies. It begins during the first trimester and continues into the second.

Instead of a model, the pregnant woman finds a partner with whom to practice role behavior. For example, the pregnant woman may offer to babysit to interact with a baby or child, or she may "mother" a pet. The responses of the partner signal acceptance or rejection of the mothering behaviors, and then new behaviors can be tried. Multiparous women tend to explore role behaviors related to having two or more children of different sexes.

Fantasies

During the first trimester, the woman has vague fantasies, both daydreams and nightdreams, about babies and childbearing (Sherwen, 1991). During the second and third trimesters, fantasies become increasingly vivid and provide important clues to the progress of pregnancy and the woman's feelings about it.

Relationship with Mother

For the expectant mother, the process of rethinking her relationships with her parents begins during the first trimester. Research has demonstrated that the woman's own mother is her primary role model (Lederman, 1996). If conflicts exist in the relationship between the newly pregnant woman and her mother, reconciliation may be attempted in the first trimester. Other research confirmed the intergenerational attachment relationship between the pregnant woman and her mother (Zachariah, 1994).

Relationship with Fetus

The use of ultrasound has tended to change the vague relationship that women once had with their fetus during the first trimester. Generally, the sensation of fetal movement during the second trimester made the fetus "real" for the mother and ushered in the phase of maternal–fetal interactions. Ultrasound used in first-trimester fetal diagnosis, for specific indications, makes visualization of the fetus possible before fetal movements are felt. Studies have shown however, that maternal–fetal attachment increases over time (Lee, 1994; Muller, 1996). As yet, the effects of ultrasound visualization on maternal–fetal interaction and attachment have not been extensively documented; the practice of using ultrasound solely to foster attachment is controversial.

Body Image

An increase in size of a woman's body during pregnancy represents growth of the child within her. In the pregnant woman's perceptions of the body, these changes in size and weight pertain to the baby, while she herself remains "unchanged."

During the first trimester when growth is not obvious, real physical evidence of a baby is lacking. Although women experience breast fullness, it is similar to that experienced during the premenstrual period. Even a positive pregnancy test does not mean "baby." To the woman, the test results may represent her physiologic situation, not the baby's. Often she has a slight loss of weight or appetite during the first trimester. Because weight gain, not loss, is most often associated with pregnancy, loss of weight may increase the woman's uncertainty about the reality of a baby (Lederman, 1996).

Changes in body boundary occur with growth of the woman's body. No change in size, however, occurs during the first trimester, and body boundaries also tend to remain unchanged.

▶ Psychologic Changes in the Father

Expectant fathers undergo unique psychologic processes during pregnancy, although much remains unknown. During the first trimester, the expectant father is thought to progress through three stages (Herzog, 1982).

1. During the getting ready period, the father and his partner know that they will try to make a child. Emotionally, fathers have the feeling of starting something new and have a sense of urgency to "get on with it."
2. When pregnancy is medically confirmed, the man who desired pregnancy may experience feelings of joy, manliness, and increased sexual interest in his partner. The man who did not want pregnancy may react negatively and respond with anger, the feeling of being "trapped," and resentment.
3. At the end of the first trimester, fathers perceive a great change in their lives. Feelings of "having to give" and nurturing the mother and fetus emerge.

Attachment

During pregnancy, paternal–fetal attachment is a major predictor of attachment after birth (Ferketich & Mercer, 1995). The father's relationship with the infant at birth is dependent on the relationship he had with his own father and the support of his partner (Anderson, 1996).

Fantasies

Expectant fathers have fantasies about pregnancy and the infant-to-be, much as the expectant mother does. Early literature found that toward the end of the first trimester, expectant fathers begin to have new and different fantasies and night dreams. Sexual fantasies are prevalent. Other fantasies include nurturing, birds nesting, eggs hatching, and images of water. Night dreams reflect a fear of being excluded by the pregnancy (Gurwitt, 1982).

Couvade Syndrome

The man's experience of the couvade syndrome (see Chapter 4) includes mild to severe symptoms that increase as pregnancy progresses. They may include weight gain and gas pain, although almost any symptom is possible. The couvade syndrome may become evident in some fathers during the first trimester, especially when the pregnancy is probable or confirmed.

Concerns

Specific paternal concerns during the first trimester need to be researched. The woman's career or employment status is one important concern. The father, who may feel that his provider role is vital, will be affected by his partner's concerns about her career and employment. If the couple decides that the woman will stay home during pregnancy or after the baby is born, or during both times, the father will usually become the primary breadwinner for the family. In the United States today, no mandatory employment policy guarantees a long-term paid parental leave from employment for either mother or father. Therefore, worry about absorbing the high costs of a new family member and maintaining the family's lifestyle may affect the father-to-be. In addition, the expectant father may be concerned over the nature of his partner's work or work environment.

▶ Psychologic Changes in the Family

During the first trimester, the family is usually eager to confirm the woman's pregnancy. Aside from curiosity, the possibility of a child raises such issues as inheritance and continuation of the family name. In families where children are greatly wanted and valued, news of pregnancy may make the expectant couple the focus of enthusiastic family attention. Feeling attachment to the embryo/fetus during the first trimester, however, may be difficult for family members. The developing baby is not a reality to the expectant father or other family members until fetal movements are evident and the mother's abdomen begins to grow during the second trimester (Erickson, 1996; Lee, 1994).

Physiologic changes in the mother during the first trimester have an impact on the family. For example, the couple's sexual relationship may be affected if the expectant mother does not feel well. In addition, if the mother is nauseous or fatigued, her daily activities may be interrupted, and consequently, family members may have additional responsibilities. Therefore, role changes for significant others, especially for members of the extended family, begin during the first trimester, although the reality of the baby is tentative.

In contrast, some couples may not tell extended family members about the pregnancy in its early stages. Young children may not be made aware of it or may not understand what pregnancy means.

Despite the sense of unreality, psychologic conflict can emerge during the first trimester. Although both mother and father may desire the pregnancy and an infant, a couple may be ambivalent during the first trimester. Fear and uncertainty about changes they must undergo to become parents and conflicts about leaving their current lives behind become apparent.

Ideally, the pregnant couple begins a new relationship with the broader community during the first trimester. For example, they may come to health care providers for pregnancy diagnosis and early prenatal care.

▶ The Siblings' Experience

Relationships between parents and children begin to change as early as the first trimester. Physical discomforts, such as nausea and fatigue, affect the amount of energy the expectant mother has to devote to care of other children. Although young children may not understand the normal physical changes of pregnancy, they are aware of changes in their mothers, especially those changes that affect activities of daily living. The child may instigate attention-getting behaviors, such as tantrums, that also release frustration at changes he or she cannot understand or control.

Programs to prepare a child for the birth of a sibling are reported in the literature. Most do not begin during the first trimester. To be effective, sibling edu-cation must be based on the child's age and stage of cognitive development (see Chapter 17).

Children older than 5, during the first trimester, can usually comprehend the event of pregnancy, although the concept of "months ahead" is vague for many 5- to 7-year-olds. Parents also need to tailor explanations of the event based on the child's level of cognitive development.

Many parents do not tell their toddler or preschool child about pregnancy during the first trimester, because the child may not understand the concept of a nonvisible baby growing inside the mother. Ultrasound photos also have little meaning. More extensive preparation for the very young child may best occur after the pregnancy is visible.

Secrets about early pregnancy are not necessary. After discussion of sibling growth and development, parents should be encouraged to present information about the baby at a time they feel is best for themselves and their children.

Parents need to understand how changes in their own behavior may be perceived, especially by young children. For example, quiet activities can be suggested for times when a mother's first-trimester fatigue alters a usually vigorous schedule.

▶ The Grandparents' Experience

Pregnancy confers the status of grandparent on the parents of the expectant couple. Research has begun to focus on the special needs of grandparents during pregnancy. As discussed earlier, both the expectant mother and father look to their own parents, especially the parent of the same sex, for support and role modeling. Often grandparents are informed about the pregnancy during the first trimester. Their reaction to the news depends on several factors:

- How ready the grandparent perceives the expectant couple to be for parenthood
- The expectant grandparent's ability to deal with personal transitions, such as the change from parent to grandparent
- Whether the expectant grandparents have other grandchildren
- The relationship between the expectant couple and the grandparents (Strom & Strom, 1992)

The nature of the role that grandparents will finally assume with their grandchildren is highly dependent on the family's cultural and socioeconomic background (Carlson, 1993). The nurse needs to thoroughly assess the extended family system, as well as the nuclear family, to determine interventions to facilitate the grandparents' transition.

► Sociocultural Dimensions

Within the scope of any textbook, it is impossible to discuss all cultural groups. Indeed, religious and ethnic beliefs are part of cultural considerations. An individual may belong to several groups at one time. For example, a client may be a Catholic, Protestant, or Jewish Lebanese-American. Actual practices may evolve from a combination of Middle Eastern, American, and religious influences.

A family's culture greatly affects perceptions and behaviors related to childbearing. Cultural ideas and practices may or may not be consistent with those valued by nurses. Indeed, North American nurses themselves may be considered a cultural group. For example, early prenatal care delivered by a physician or nurse-midwife is a cultural value that nurses support. Nurses base this belief on scientific research and clinical experience in working with healthy and high-risk clients. On the other hand, other cultural groups may or may not value early prenatal care (especially that given by a male physician or nurse) for reasons as valid in their cultural belief system as scientific research is in nursing's belief system (Kavanaugh & Kennedy, 1992). In addition, many religious and ethnic groups are represented within the nursing culture. Therefore, although early prenatal care may be valued by nurses in general, Chinese and Irish nurses, for example, may view first-trimester prenatal options differently.

The nurse must strive to understand the cultural backgrounds of clients and identify specific beliefs and practices related to childbearing. The nurse must determine how cultural groups that are different from the "typical" (e.g., dominant) North American culture perceive pregnancy and prenatal care.

Culturally sensitive care evolves from basic respect for clients and curiosity about their cultural background, as well as their personal history. Among the cultural factors that challenge nursing skills are differences in language, dress, religion, support systems, and attitudes toward personal hygiene and health care.

Although some clients may come for preconception care, the initial contact between the client and the prenatal health care system is more often in the first trimester. The type and nature of the care may determine whether the client continues to seek prenatal care. In providing culturally sensitive care at any time, the nurse must understand certain factors:

- All cultures have specific attitudes and practices related to childbearing. They affect daily activities, diet, and relationships with others.
- Each culture has its own relationship system: who is related to whom and the nature of that relationship vary with the culture.

- What constitutes "marriage" varies among cultures. For example, the Koran, the Islamic holy book, allows a man to have more than one wife, provided he can treat each the same.
- Cultures tend to prescribe particular male and female roles for childbearing, as well as daily living. These roles, such as the father's lack of participation in birth, may be expected and accepted by members of that culture.
- Cultures tend to have their own ceremonies and rituals related to childbearing.
- Cultural views tend to affect whether or not women seek early or any prenatal care from physicians and nurses. Prenatal care may be sought from "traditional" caregivers, such as a lay midwife or lay healer.
- The role of nurses varies widely around the world. In some countries, nursing is not considered a profession but a menial type of work done by the least advantaged of that society. Nurses need to understand cultural views of nursing to plan effective care.
- Differences in language between health care providers and clients can be a barrier to culturally sensitive care. Use of interpreters, a kind tone of voice, and real interest in the client can be helpful. Teaching sheets can be written in the client's language.

This chapter focuses on an African-American family's experience of pregnancy as an example of how pregnancy is perceived from a cultural perspective. On one hand, there are countless ways in which members of a given African-American family, or any ethnocultural family, may experience pregnancy. On the other hand, there tend to be experiences that are unique and culture-bound to a given ethnocultural group. Although the latter may have the potential for creating stereotyping, relating those experiences is a way to illustrate unique differences. Later chapters of the text will explore how families from other cultural groups perceive pregnancy and the postpartum/newborn period. Stereotyping should, however, be avoided; prenatal care needs to be based on each client's unique perceptions and needs.

Socioeconomic Influence

Socioeconomic level has a distinct impact in addition to culture. Childbearing is a very expensive process. Families who perceive themselves financially stressed may respond to the prospect of pregnancy, childbirth, and childrearing with despair or panic, especially if the mother's income is needed and jeopardized by the pregnancy. Public assistance, the Food Stamp Program, the Special Supplemental Food Program for

Women, Infants, and Children (WIC), and other programs do not cover the increasingly high costs associated with having children. Lack of insurance and ability to pay for private care greatly limits where and when pregnant women seek prenatal health care. Even in areas where some sort of prenatal care may be available to women regardless of their ability to pay, transportation and other obstacles may make access difficult. Other financially related concerns may include obtaining maternity clothing, loss of employment due to pregnancy or childbirth, living in an environment with inadequate material resources, or increasing financial responsibilities related to a new baby.

Cultural Focus: The African-American Family

Variations in African-American families are influenced by geographic location in the United States (e.g., urban North, rural South), level of acculturation, religious background, and socioeconomic status (Patterson, 1993). Socioeconomic status is especially important to consider. Persons of different cultural backgrounds who live in poverty share similar social problems. Nurses should base care on the unique needs and patterns of each client and her family (Jezewski, 1993; Wenger, 1993).

Although every African-American family must be assessed during pregnancy to discover its unique characteristics, certain cultural traditions and patterns may help the nurse understand the family's responses to pregnancy and childbirth. African-American families possess many adaptive strengths that help bring about a positive pregnancy outcome. These strengths include strong kinship bonds, flexibility in family roles, and a high value on religion, education, and work.

Kinship Bonds. Strong kinship bonds have helped African Americans survive extremely difficult conditions since the days of slavery (Boyd-Franklin, 1989). Reliance on the kinship network has been an important source of support (Morgan, 1996). This kinship is not always drawn along "blood lines," that is, with those to whom they are related. Families may evolve complex patterns of coresidence and kinship-based exchange networks that link various domestic units. In addition, the family units often have broad household boundaries and strong bonds to three generations of households. People in this network are involved in many cooperative domestic exchanges. A large number of people inside and outside the "nuclear family" may operate within the boundaries of the complex family network. Thus, not only do the pregnant woman's partner, parents, and children affect the course of the childbearing cycle, uncles, aunts, preachers, male and female friends, brothers, sisters, and cousins may also have influence. Far from being disorganized, as nursing students who make home visits into such flexible families fear, these networks are often organized. They can provide lifelong relationships that offer stability for family members (Boyd-Franklin, 1989).

Family Roles. The role of the African-American man may be difficult. He may demand and receive recognition as head of the household; yet, this recognition is often tied to his ability to provide for his family, which may be difficult in the prevailing social structure. In response to this situation, some men are said to become peripheral to (i.e., exist outside) their family. Current investigators believe this peripheral relationship has been overstated, because the great investment African-American men have in the family is often overlooked. For example, the role behaviors of adolescent fathers include provision of child care and participation in pregnancy (Dallas & Chen, 1996).

African-American men and women may have great role flexibility in childrearing and household responsibility. They may comfortably reverse roles, especially concerning care of children. Such a pattern has important implications for the nurse providing prenatal care to the couple.

Members of the extensive kinship network may assume roles usually reserved for nuclear family members (Morgan, 1996). For example, during childbearing and childrearing, a maternal or paternal aunt or grandmother may share or assume responsibility for child care. A child or infant may be adopted informally and reared by extended family members who have resources not available to the child's parents or who live in a different environment. Thus, the term *significant others* sometimes takes on a different meaning for an African-American family, and genograms often do not conform to blood lines.

The nurse who explores role responsibilities with the expectant family must recognize that the family system may function well, despite its flexible boundaries and role patterns. For example, that a teenage

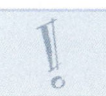

Nursing Alert

The rates of low-birth-weight and preterm delivery are twice as high for African Americans as they are for whites in the United States.

African-American mother does not learn to care for her newborn infant may not be a major problem if, in her family system, this will not be her responsibility. Her own mother, aunt, or sister may actually "mother" the newborn, and the biologic mother's role may be to resume her life as a student. The nurse should determine who will fulfill what roles in care of the newborn and work within the structure of the unique family system of her pregnant client.

Religion. Religion and the church tend to be strong influences and to serve numerous functions for the African-American community. The religious system provides support in ministers, deacons, deaconesses, and other church members. Spirituality influences the health and well-being of African Americans (Morgan, 1996). Spiritual comfort and support are gained from religious beliefs. In addition, numerous church activities may provide a social life for members of the entire family.

A strong church influence is important during pregnancy, as it is throughout life. The church and its members may promote physical health by encouraging young pregnant women to enter early prenatal care and maintain a lifestyle that can foster a healthy pregnancy outcome. For example, church members may provide transportation to prenatal facilities; collaborating with health care providers, church members have provided space within church properties for mobile prenatal clinics and educational programs related to childbearing.

The African-American Family's Experience of Pregnancy.
Numerous factors may influence how African-American women and their families accept pregnancy and prenatal care, for example, social and economic circumstances. It has been demonstrated that African-American women who received inadequate care during their first pregnancy are more likely to receive inadequate care in their second pregnancy (McDermott, Drews, Adams, Berg, Hill, & McCarthy, 1996). Satisfaction with her own education and career, along with satisfaction with her partner's education and job, generally fosters a woman's acceptance of pregnancy. A woman married to a man with less education and no stable employment may accept or resent pregnancy, depending on such factors as the number of previous pregnancies, timing of the pregnancy, and the family's economic status. These attitudes are similar among most women.

Although menstruation is a time when some African-American women view themselves as "sick," pregnancy is seen as a state of wellness. This may be one reason why many African-American women do not seek early prenatal care; they do not see early care as important because they are healthy. Prenatal care is preventive care, and preventive care is an unfamiliar concept to some who enter the health care system only in a health crisis. Other factors that may prevent some African-American women from obtaining early prenatal care are an indifferent, inaccessible health care system and the stereotyping of pregnant African-American women (Murrell, Smith, Gill, & Oxley, 1996). Because low-income African-American women have a high incidence of maternal, fetal, and infant morbidity and mortality, reaching this population is a major responsibility of nurses. Early prenatal care must become meaningful for the low-income African-American woman, and health care services made accessible so that she seeks early prenatal care.

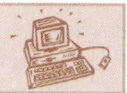

Research Abstract

Factors Influencing Prenatal Care of African-American Women

The purpose of this research was to describe and analyze the beliefs, practices, and values of African-American women about prenatal care. Four major themes were identified from the African-American women in the study: (1) cultural care meant protection and sharing; (2) factors that influenced their health and well-being were spirituality, kinship, and economics; (3) prenatal care was viewed by the women as essential but there was distrust of noncaring professionals and barriers to such care; and (4) folk health beliefs and practices were widely used by women in the African-American community.

Application to Practice

It is important for nurses to understand the cultural values and beliefs of African-American women related to prenatal care. Culturally congruent prenatal care may help to motivate African-American women to obtain early prenatal care and in the end improve pregnancy outcomes.

Source: Morgan, M. (1996). Prenatal care of African American women in selected USA urban and rural contexts. Journal of Transcultural Nursing, 7(2), 3–9.

▶ NURSING AND COLLABORATIVE ASSESSMENT

Assessment during the first trimester not only confirms the fact of pregnancy, it also lays foundations for interventions that will hopefully steer the pregnancy to a healthy outcome for all involved.

During the first prenatal visit, the nurse assesses the health of the expectant mother and her family by compiling a comprehensive data base, which includes a health history, physical examination, and laboratory studies. The assessment process is guided by several principles:

- Childbearing is a normal, although not always comfortable, developmental stage for the family.
- Assessment should focus on the whole client and her significant others and include psychologic and cultural as well as physiologic aspects.
- Childbearing couples need comprehensive information, so that they can make informed decisions regarding their care. In providing information, nurses should avoid technical jargon and use terms that families can readily understand.
- Risks and benefits of interventions should be explained and informed consent should be obtained before any procedure.
- The childbearing family's self-care practices should be fostered. Participation in self-care necessitates family participation in planning of care.
- Many of the assessment techniques available to assess the expectant client or embryo/fetus may carry some type of risk to physical or emotional well-being; the costs of some tests outweigh benefits. Tests should be performed only when indicated; healthy, normal women should not be treated as if they were high risk.
- Childbearing families need advocates who will support them in a nonjudgmental way. Nurses can serve as advocates for the family with other care providers.

Initial assessment of the healthy pregnant client is similar to assessment of the well woman, as described in Chapter 7, but special attention is given to factors related to childbearing and early parenting. This type of detailed assessment is done during the first visit, regardless of the trimester in which the client comes for her initial visit. In some cases women move or change care providers during their pregnancies. Certain laboratory tests may not need to be repeated if clinical documentation can be provided; however, a comprehensive history and a physical examination are performed for any "new" client. Results are recorded in the client's chart and may also be communicated during discussion with other health care professionals working with the client.

In an uncomplicated pregnancy, first-trimester prenatal visits are usually scheduled about 4 weeks apart. Ideally, the client and her family are assessed about three times during the first trimester.

During return prenatal visits, the health history is updated to reflect the client's and family's current status, and a physical examination is done. Various laboratory tests, such as hemoglobin and glucose assessment, may be part of routine assessment as pregnancy progresses. From thorough assessment at the first and subsequent visits, diagnoses can be determined and strategies for the client's nursing, medical, and self-care management developed or modified (see box entitled Assessment Focus at First Prenatal Visit and Return Visits).

Collaborating with other health care providers, the nurse has an important role in initial and ongoing assessment of the pregnant client. During the first visit, the nurse establishes a trusting relationship with the client and family and anticipates their needs at various stages of the pregnancy, such as information necessary for improving self-care or making informed decisions.

▶ Prenatal Health History

During the first prenatal visit, health care providers obtain and record information about the current and past health status of the expectant mother and her family. By collaborating on a health history outline, nurses, physicians, and other prenatal health care providers can avoid asking the client the same questions.

Information from the health history helps the physician or nurse to individualize the prenatal physical examination, to document the normal progress of pregnancy, to identify any risk factors, and to develop a plan of care. Assessment should be done in a private setting and begin with identification of the client's reason for her visit (Fig. 15–5).

A thorough health history for a first prenatal visit is similar to the health history taken during a well-woman visit. Table 7–1 is a sample outline for a comprehensive health history. A variety of health history formats may be used to meet the goal of comprehensive assessment. At the first prenatal visit, however, particular attention is paid to the reproductive history (Table 15–4); physical or psychosocial changes characteristic of pregnancy; and the existence of physical,

▶ ASSESSMENT FOCUS AT FIRST PRENATAL VISIT AND RETURN VISITS

FOCUS DURING FIRST PRENATAL VISIT

- Existence of pregnancy
- Past and present maternal health status through health history, physical examination, and laboratory data
- Risk factors for childbearing and early parenting, including physical, psychologic, and sociologic factors
- Signs and symptoms of pregnancy
- Well-being of embryo/fetus
- Psychosocial adaptation to pregnancy
- Cultural, socioeconomic, or other factors that influence health care practices
- Client/family strengths and resources
- Client/family educational needs

FOCUS DURING RETURN VISITS

- Maternal health status through updated health history, physical examination, and laboratory testing as indicated
- Risk factors (new or ongoing)
- Progress of pregnancy
- Fetal well-being
- Progression of psychosocial adaptation to pregnancy
- Cultural, socioeconomic, or other factors that influence health care practices as pregnancy progresses
- Client/family strengths and resources
- Client/family educational needs

psychologic, socioeconomic, medical, lifestyle, environmental, or occupational factors that could affect pregnancy, positively or negatively. Adequate nutrition is critical to the well-being of the expectant mother and embryo/fetus and is one of the most important aspects of prenatal assessment. (Prenatal nutrition is discussed in detail in Chapter 14.) Terms related to gravidity and parity are employed to interpret the reproductive history. In addition, numeric scoring systems are frequently used in clinical practice to summarize current and past pregnancies.

Gravidity and Parity

Gravidity is the state of being pregnant. A gravid woman is a pregnant woman. The word *gravida* refers to a pregnancy regardless of its duration. A woman's gravidity relates to the total number of her pregnancies, regardless of their duration.

- A **primigravid** woman is a woman pregnant for the first time.
- A **multigravid** woman is a woman who has been pregnant more than one time.

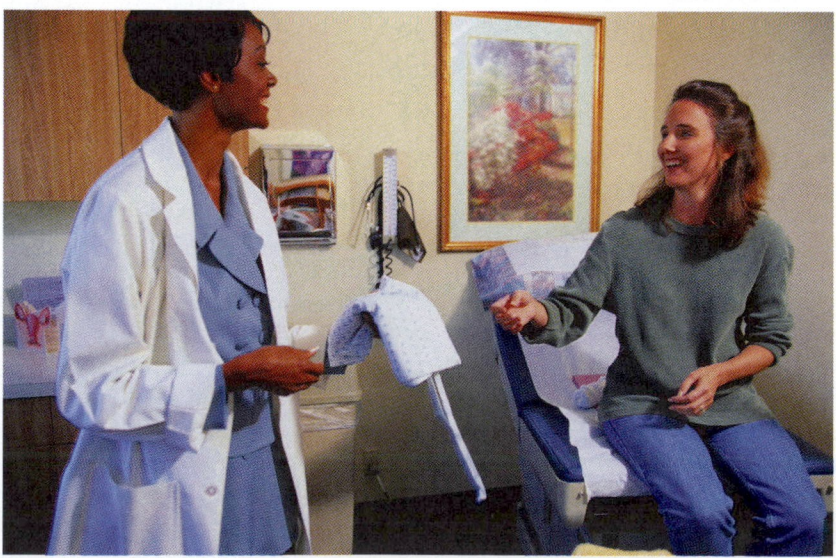

FIGURE 15–5. The nurse conducts the prenatal health history in collaboration with the client as one of the components of the assessment process during the first trimester.

▶ **TABLE 15–4**

Sample Outline for a Reproductive History During the First Prenatal Visit

Area	Inquiries
Suspicion of pregnancy	Sexual activity, missed menses, home pregnancy test
Planned/unplanned pregnancy	Reaction of self and significant others to possibility of pregnancy
Menstrual history	Date when last menstrual period began; history of regular/irregular menses; atypical bleeding or other vaginal discharge; treatments
Family planning history	Birth control practices (attitude toward birth control, type of methods used, length of time used, complications related to the methods); any infertility treatments used to facilitate conception; length of time trying to achieve pregnancy
Obstetric history	Previous pregnancies (planned, unplanned); outcome of previous pregnancies (live, stillborn, aborted, premature); dates and types of deliveries, including length and course of labor; infant's birth weight, sex, and status; obstetric or neonatal complications and treatments; reaction of self and significant others to obstetric events
Gynecologic history	
Breasts	Changes related to early pregnancy, such as increase in size, tenderness; history of breast disease of any kind, including types and dates of treatment; continued practice of breast self-examination; recent screening for breast disease; family history of breast cancer (maternal relatives or sister)
Genitalia	Vaginal discharge (nature, amount, duration, foul odor); itching, burning, lesions; gynecologic problems of infectious (sexually transmitted diseases) or noninfectious (e.g., endometriosis, fibroids) origin, including dates and treatments; date of last Pap test; understanding and practice of genital self-examination
Sexual history	Recent change in sexual patterns (especially in relation to suspicion of pregnancy); pain or vaginal bleeding after intercourse; sexual orientation (heterosexual, bisexual); history of multiple sexual partners or sexual partners with other high-risk behaviors, such as intravenous drug use; concerns related to sexuality and pregnancy
Sources and dates of current or previous reproductive care	Private physician, certified nurse-midwife, clinic staff, others

Parity refers to the number of past pregnancies that have reached viability and have been delivered, regardless of the number of children involved. For example, the birth of triplets increases the parity by only one. The term *para* refers to past pregnancies that have reached viability.

- A **nulliparous** woman is a woman who has never delivered a child that reached viability.
- A **primiparous** woman is a woman who has had one pregnancy that terminated at the stage when the child was viable.
- A **multiparous** woman is a woman who has had two or more pregnancies that terminated at the stage when the children were viable.

Gravida and *Para* terminology are combined.

- A woman pregnant for the first time is primigravid and is described as gravida 1, para 0.
- If a woman aborts before viability, she remains gravida 1, para 0.
- If she delivers a fetus that has reached viability, she becomes primiparous, regardless of

whether the child is alive or dead. She is now gravida 1, para 1.
- During a second pregnancy the woman is gravida 2, para 1.
- After she delivers the second child past the point of viability she is gravida 2, para 2.
- A woman with two abortions and no viable children is gravida 2, para 0. When she becomes pregnant again she is gravida 3, para 0. When she delivers a viable child she is gravida 3, para 1.
- Multiple births do not affect the parity by more than one. A woman who has viable triplets in her first pregnancy is gravida 1, para 1.

GTPAL is the acronym for a five-digit numeric scoring system used to summarize a client's obstetric situation. It differs from the two-digit scoring system (above) because it provides more detailed information about parity.

G Gravidity (total number of pregnancies)
T Term births
P Premature births
A Abortions
L Living children

► Assessment of Physiologic Change in the Mother

During the initial prenatal visit, a complete physical examination of the mother is done. The physical examination, which includes pelvic assessment, provides objective data. The nurse prepares the mother for the procedure and supports her throughout.

The pelvis is assessed for abnormalities. Changes related to pregnancy are assessed through inspection and bimanual examination. The staff nurse prepares the couple and assists the examiner, who may be a physician, a certified nurse-midwife, or an advanced practice nurse with specialized education in prenatal physical assessment.

Uterus

To maintain pregnancy and accommodate the developing fetus, the uterus undergoes many changes, for example, in size and shape. The changes are important to assess, as they help to detect pregnancy and determine the length of gestation.

Hegar's sign (Fig. 15–6) is apparent at 4 to 6 weeks of gestation. Braun von Fernwald's sign (Fig. 15–7), is detectable at 4 to 5 weeks. Additional uterine changes that should be assessed are Piskacek's sign and McDonald's sign. (See earlier section Signs and Symptoms of Pregnancy.) Nurses should be prepared to explain these signs to clients who ask about them.

During the first trimester, uterine enlargement is noted during bimanual pelvic examination. By 8 weeks of gestation, the uterus can be palpated abdom-

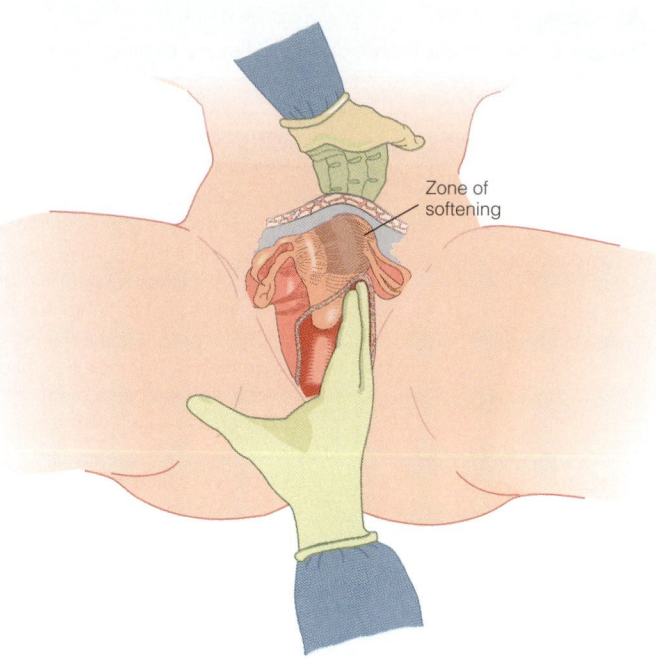

FIGURE 15–7. Assessment to determine Braun von Fernwald's sign. *(Adapted, with permission, from DeCherney, A.H., & Pernoll, M.L. (Eds.) (1994). Current obstetric & gynecologic diagnosis & treatment (8th ed.). Norwalk, CT: Appleton & Lange, p. 187.)*

inally 1 to 2 cm above the symphysis (see Fig 15–1). The uterus in early pregnancy is pyriform, or pear-shaped, but by the end of the first trimester becomes ovoid or globular.

Cervix

By about 2 to 4 weeks of gestation, under the influence of estrogen and progesterone, the cervix increases in anteroposterior diameter. Cervical appearance is altered in pregnancy by an outward extension of columnar epithelial tissue where normally squamous epithelium is present (Cunningham et al., 1997).

Additional cervical changes that should be noted include Chadwick's sign and Goodell's sign (Fig. 15–8) (see Signs and Symptoms of Pregnancy earlier in chapter). In addition Ladin's sign is detectable by about 6 weeks (see Fig. 15–3).

Vagina

The vaginal tissue undergoes increased vascular congestion in pregnancy and becomes bluish violet (Chadwick's sign) at 6 to 8 weeks of gestation. The rugae, or folds, of the vagina become more prominent in nulliparous women. In comparison, the vaginal rugae of multiparous women are smoother or flatter, and the entire vaginal canal may be widened. Estrogenic influences cause vaginal smooth muscle hypertrophy, loos-

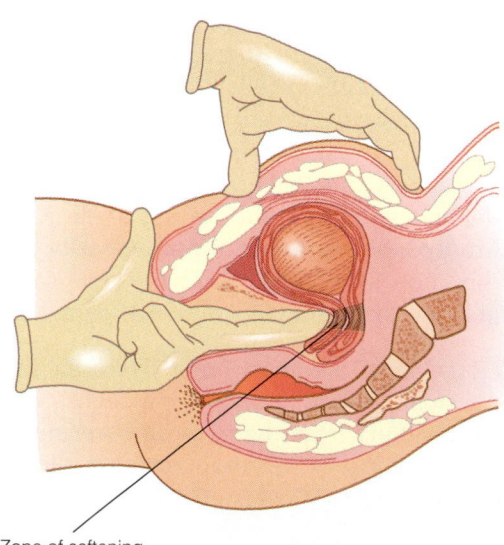

FIGURE 15–6. Assessment to determine Hegar's sign. *(Adapted, with permission, from DeCherney, A.H., & Pernoll, M.L. (Eds.) (1994). Current obstetric & gynecologic diagnosis & treatment (8th ed.). Norwalk, CT: Appleton & Lange, p. 187.)*

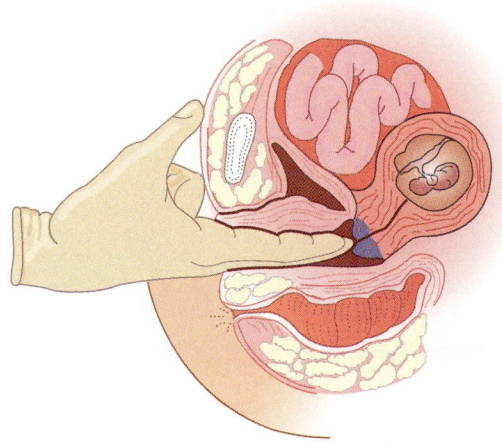

FIGURE 15–8. Assessment to determine cervical softening (Goodell's sign). *(Adapted, with permission, from DeCherney, A.H., & Pernoll, M.L. (Eds.) (1994).* Current obstetric & gynecologic diagnosis & treatment *(8th ed.). Norwalk, CT: Appleton & Lange, p. 186.)*

ening of connective tissue, and increased thickening, acidity, and production of vaginal mucous discharge.

Pelvic Measurements

Measurement of diameters (distances) between bony structures of the pelvis is called **pelvimetry** (Cunningham et al., 1997). It is done to assess whether the expectant mother's pelvic canal is adequate for passage of the fetus. A maternal pelvis that is too small or abnormally shaped can alert health care providers to potential difficulties in labor. Pelvimetry during the first trimester is a clinical examination.

Clinical pelvimetry provides estimates of the size of the true pelvis (see Pelvic Outlet later in chapter). Prior to clinical pelvimetry, the examiner measures the tip of the middle or longest finger and the fist across the knuckles, as they will be used as the measurement instruments. Experienced examiners will come to know their own measurements and will not need to determine them prior to each clinical pelvimetry evaluation. Measurements of the distance between bones of the pelvis in anteroposterior (front to back), transverse (sideways), and oblique (diagonal) directions indicate the interior width of the bony passage through which the fetus will pass.

Bimanual pelvic examination is part of routine assessment during the first trimester, whereas external abdominal assessment is done during the second and third trimesters. Therefore, clinical pelvimetry is performed by the physician or advanced practice nurse (often a nurse-midwife) as part of the pelvic examination during the first trimester and usually on the first prenatal visit. Staff nurses need to be able to explain

the procedure and provide support to the client during examination.

Pelvic Anatomy

Prenatal pelvic assessment is based on an understanding of normal female pelvic anatomy, especially in relation to childbearing. For successful vaginal delivery, the fetus must descend through a bony ring in the mother's pelvis (Fig. 15–9). The sacrum, coccyx, and two innominate bones (hip bones) form the normal adult pelvis. The innominate bone is composed of the ilium, ischium, and pubis, or pubic bone. (Note that each side of the pelvis is made up of similar bones.) At the back, the two large innominate bones connect to the sacrum at the iliums. In the front, the innominate bones join at the symphysis pubis.

Men and women have the same number of pelvic bones; however, a female pelvis is shaped somewhat differently, which has special importance for childbearing.

The pelvis is divided into two sections, commonly called the false pelvis and the true pelvis. The **linea terminalis** is the bony line that divides the two; the **false pelvis** lies above the linea terminalis, the **true pelvis** below. The false pelvis has little obstetric importance. The fetus passes through the bony canal of the true pelvis; the shape and size of bones of the true pelvis are therefore of great significance for labor and delivery.

The True Pelvis. The upper portion of the true pelvis is bounded by the sacral promontory, linea terminalis, and upper margins of the pubic bones. The lower part of the true pelvis is bounded by the lower

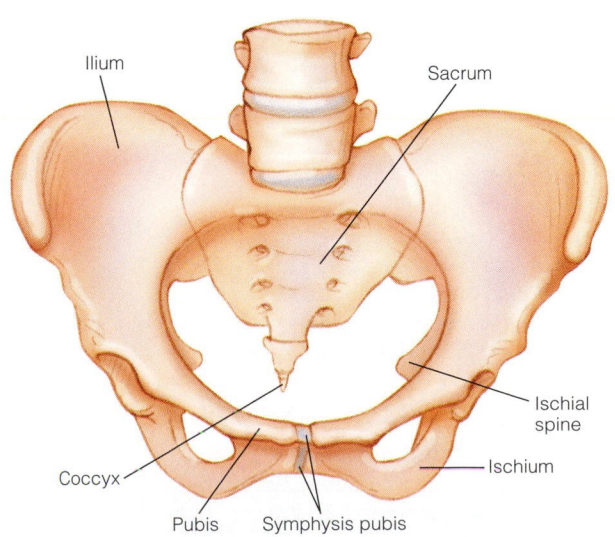

FIGURE 15–9. Normal pelvis.

margins of the ischial tuberosities and the end of the coccyx. The anterior parts of the sacrum and coccyx form its borders in the back. In front, the true pelvis is bordered by the pubic bones, the ascending upper rami of the ischial bones, and the obturator foramina, between the pubic and ischial bones. On the sides, the true pelvis is bordered by the sacroiliac notches and ligaments, as well as by the inner surface of the ischial bones. (See Chapter 6 for discussion of the shapes of the true pelvis.)

For conceptual ease, the true pelvis is divided into three imaginary planes: the pelvic inlet; the midpelvis, or pelvic cavity; and the pelvic outlet. Certain distances between bony "landmarks" within these planes are considered necessary if the fetus is to fit through the maternal passageway during labor and delivery. Pelvimetry focuses on measurements of distances within the true pelvis. The box entitled Summary of Important Diameters of the True Pelvis in Assessing Adequacy for Childbearing summarizes the planes and diameters of the true pelvis.

Pelvic Inlet. The **pelvic inlet,** or **superior strait,** is the upper entrance to the true pelvis. It is bordered in the back by the sacral promontory, on the sides by the linea terminalis, and in the front by the upper part of the symphysis pubis and horizontal rami of the pubic bones.

The inlet has three anteroposterior diameters (Fig. 15–10). The **true conjugate** (conjugate vera), which in the typical woman is at least 11.5 cm, is measured from the upper margin of the symphysis pubis to the sacral promontory.

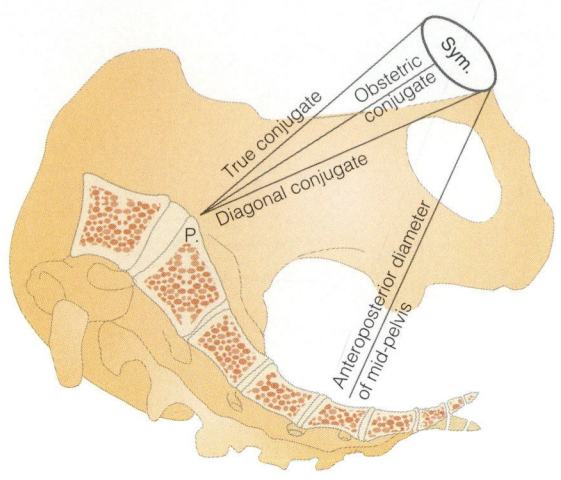

FIGURE 15–10. Three anteroposterior diameters of the pelvis: the true conjugate, the more important obstetric conjugate, and the clinically measurable diagonal conjugate. The anteroposterior diameter of the midpelvis is also shown. P = sacral promontory, Sym = symphysis pubis. *(Adapted, with permission, from Cunningham, F.G. et al. (1997). Williams obstetrics (20th ed.). Stamford, CT: Appleton & Lange, p. 61.)*

The **diagonal conjugate** is measured from the lower margin of the symphysis to the sacral promontory and is at least 12.5 cm. The diagonal conjugate is the only pelvic inlet distance that can be measured with clinical pelvimetry. To estimate the diagonal conjugate, the examiner extends the middle finger of the hand toward the sacral promontory, pushing the tissue between the index finger and thumb against the pubic symphysis (Fig. 15–11A). The distance between the tip of the examining finger and the point of pres-

---

► SUMMARY OF IMPORTANT DIAMETERS OF THE TRUE PELVIS IN ASSESSING ADEQUACY FOR CHILDBEARING

PELVIC INLET

- Anteroposterior diameters:
    True conjugate: 11.5 cm
    Obstetric conjugate: 11 cm
    Diagonal conjugate: 12.5 cm
- Transverse diameter: about 13.5 cm
- Oblique diameters (left and right): about 12.5 cm
- Posterior sagittal diameter: about 4.5 cm

PELVIC CAVITY (MIDPLANE/MIDPELVIS)

- Plane of greatest dimensions:
    Anteroposterior diameter: 12.75 cm
    Transverse diameter: 12.5 cm

- Plane of least dimensions:
    Anteroposterior diameter: 12.0 cm
    Transverse diameter: 10.5 cm
    Posterior sagittal diameter: 4.5–5.0 cm

PELVIC OUTLET

- Bi-ischial or intertuberous diameter: 10 cm
- Obstetric anteroposterior diameter: 11.5 cm
- Transverse diameter: 11.0 cm
- Posterior sagittal diameter: 9.0 cm
- Anterior sagittal diameter: 6.0 cm

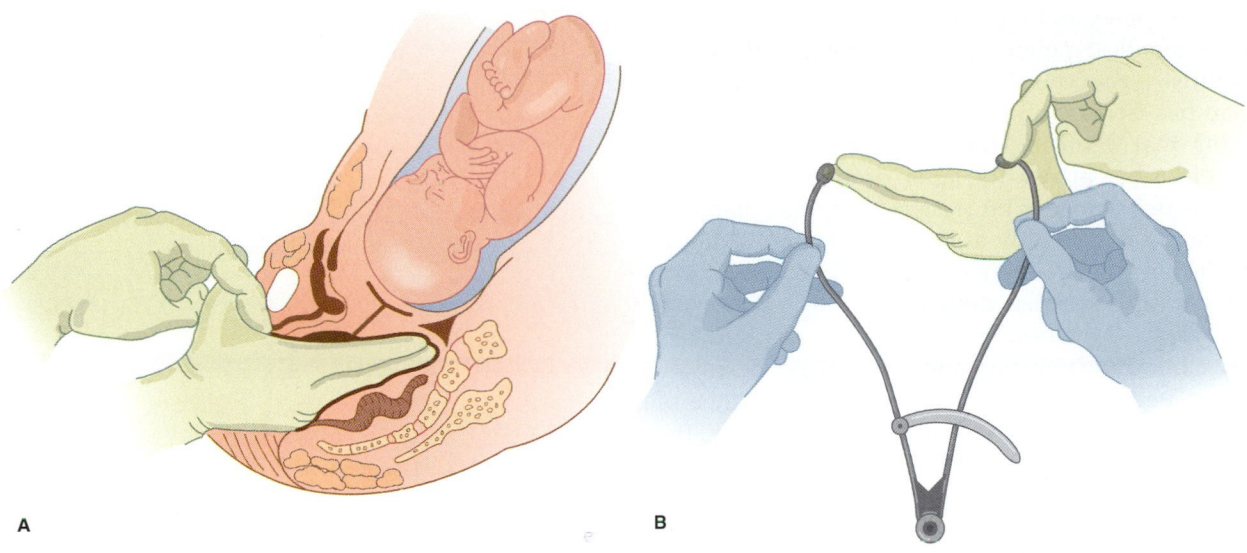

FIGURE 15–11. Measurement of the diagonal conjugate. **A.** Determining length of conjugate on examiner's hand. **B.** Measuring this length on the examiner's hand.

sure against the symphysis pubis is then measured (see Fig. 15–11B). The symphysis pubis is thicker in the middle than at the top or bottom. Subtracting 1.5 to 2 cm from the diagonal conjugate (to account for a shorter front-to-back diameter and the angle of the bone) gives an indirect estimation of the actual anteroposterior diameter of the pelvic inlet; this diameter is called the **obstetric conjugate** and is about 11 cm. The obstetric conjugate is important because it is the smallest front-to-back distance through which the fetal head must pass in moving through the pelvic inlet.

Other measurements of the pelvic inlet are the transverse diameter, the diagonal diameters, and the posterior sagittal diameter. The transverse diameter (about 13.5 cm) is the largest diameter of the pelvic inlet and is located at right angles to the true conjugate. The transverse diameter is the distance measured between the linea terminalis on each side of the pelvis. The diagonal (oblique) diameters of the pelvic inlet are about 12.5 cm and cannot be measured clinically. The posterior sagittal diameter of the pelvic inlet extends from the point where the anteroposterior and transverse diameters cross each other to the middle of the sacral promontory (about 4.5 cm).

Pelvic Cavity. Between the pelvic inlet and outlet is the **pelvic cavity,** pelvic canal, **midpelvis,** or midplane of the pelvis. The diameters of greatest dimensions (largest distance) and diameters of least dimensions (shortest distance) are in this portion of the pelvis.

As expected, the plane of greatest dimensions is the roomiest part of the pelvic canal. It is bounded in the front by the midpoint of the posterior surface of the pubis, on the sides by the upper and middle thirds of the obturator foramina, and in the back by the junction of the second and third sacral vertebrae. The plane has little obstetric management importance; because it is large, it can readily accommodate an average-sized, normal fetus. From front to back (from the midpoint of the posterior surface of the pubis to the junction of the second and third sacral vertebrae), the plane of greatest dimension measures about 12.75 cm. The widest distance between the lateral parts of the plane, the transverse diameter, is about 12.5 cm.

The plane of least dimensions is important in obstetrics because it has the least amount of room. As the narrowest part of the bony maternal passageway, the plane of least dimensions can be a place where labor fails to progress. The plane extends from the top of the subpubic arch, through the ischial spines, to the sacrum, at or near the point where the fourth and fifth sacral vertebrae join. From front to back, this plane is bordered by the lower boundary of the symphysis pubis, the white line on the fascia over the obturator foramina, the ischial spines, the sacrospinous ligaments, and the sacrum.

The anteroposterior, transverse, and posterior sagittal diameters of the plane are important. The anteroposterior diameter, about 12.0 cm, extends from the lower boundary of the symphysis pubis to the junction of the fourth and fifth sacral vertebrae. The transverse (interspinous) diameter stretches between the ischial spines and measures about 10.0 or 10.5 cm. It is the smallest pelvic distance through which the fetus must pass. The distance can be decreased if a woman has ischial spines that are especially sharp or large or that protrude into the pelvic cavity; they could place her at risk for labor problems related to adequate pelvic size. The posterior sagittal diameter of the cavity is generally at least 4.5 cm, and extends from the bispinous diameter to the junction of the fourth and fifth sacral vertebrae.

Pelvic cavity measurements are not easily determined clinically; however, adequacy of pelvic cavity size may be estimated by noting the prominence of the ischial spines. During vaginal examination, the ischial spines are palpated for prominence and distance. Spines that are flat or blunt are optimal for birth, whereas prominent or encroaching spines can decrease the size of the pelvic cavity. The distance between the two ischial spines is estimated by placing one examining finger on one spine and extending the other finger to the opposite spine. The length of the

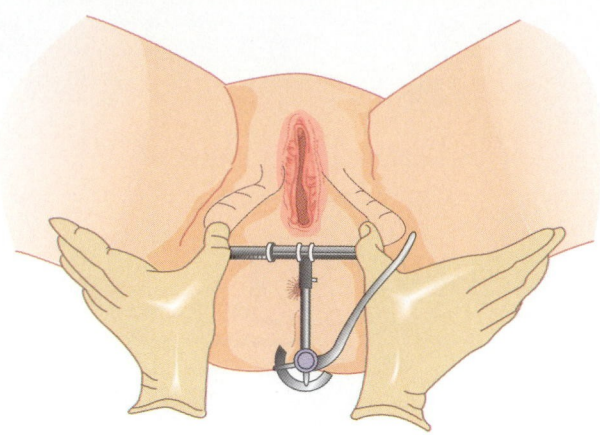

FIGURE 15–13. Measuring distance between the ischial tuberosities (bi-ischial diameter), using a pelvimeter. *(Adapted, with permission, from Benson, R.C. (1983).* Handbook of obstetrics & gynecology *(8th ed.). Los Altos, CA: Lange Medical Books.*

sacrospinous ligament is also determined by following the ligament to the point of insertion on the sacrum. This measurement is the same as the width of the sacrosciatic notch. A length of two to three fingerbreadths indicates a good anteroposterior diameter of the midpelvis. If the sacrosciatic notches are narrow, the midpelvis may be inadequate for a vaginal delivery. The shape of the sacrum is determined by moving the examining fingers down the sacrum to the coccyx. The sacrum should feel hollow, not flat or curved, and the coccyx should feel movable, not fixed.

Pelvic Outlet. The **pelvic outlet,** the lower border of the true pelvis, is described as two triangles (Fig. 15–12). The transverse diameter of the outlet forms the common base of the triangles. The transverse diameter of the outlet is the distance between the inner parts of the lowest aspect of the ischial tuberosities. This distance is also called the bi-ischial or intertuberous diameter and is about 10 cm (Fig. 15–13). The anterior triangle has the transverse diameter as the base, the subpubic angle as the apex, and the pubic rami and ischial tuberosities as the sides. The posterior triangle has the transverse diameter as the base, the sacrococcygeal joint as the apex, and the sacrotuberous ligaments as the sides.

To estimate the transverse diameter of the pelvic outlet, the examiner places the closed fist between the ischial tuberosities and measures the distance between the knuckles of the first and last fingers (Fig. 15–14). The anteroposterior diameter of the outlet can also be estimated (11.5 cm). The shape of the outlet is determined by palpating the pubic rami and noting the angle of the rami. Pubic rami are short and concave; a subpubic angle of more than 90° suggests

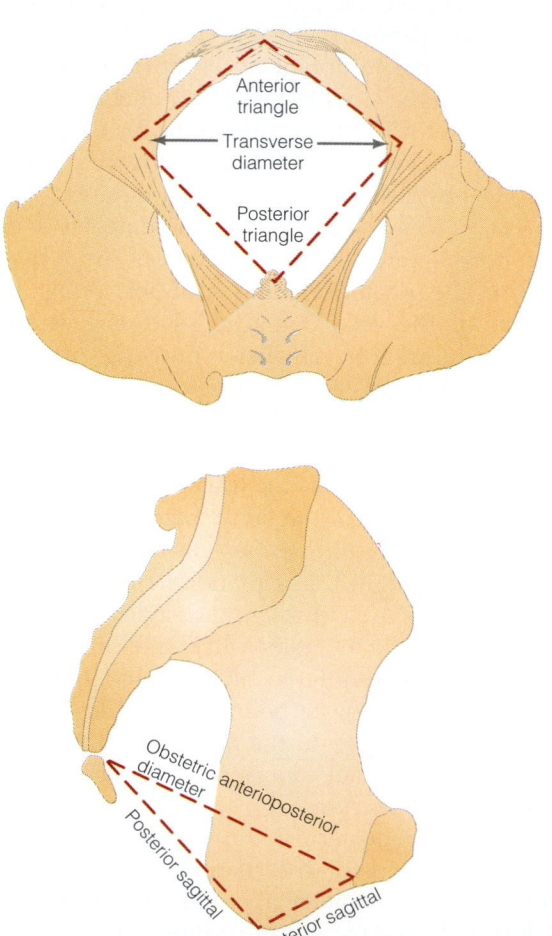

FIGURE 15–12. Pelvic outlet.

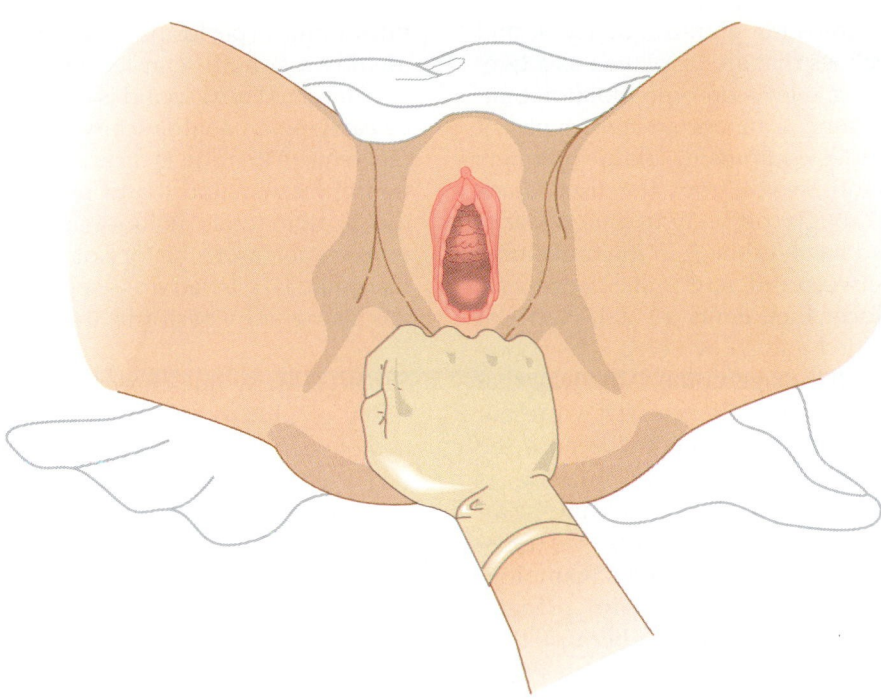

FIGURE 15–14. Assessment of the pelvic outlet using the examiner's hand as a measurement tool.

inadequacy of the outlet. The examiner also determines if the coccyx is movable by placing firm but gentle pressure on the coccyx with the examining fingers. A coccyx that is not movable can reduce the diameter of the outlet.

Advantages and Limitations of Pelvimetry

Theoretically, the goal of first-trimester pelvic measurement is to determine whether the passage provided by the bony pelvis will accommodate the descending fetus at term. Internal examination of bony pelvic structures provides a way to identify a woman whose pelvis is normally shaped or abnormally narrowed or contracted. If a woman's pelvis does not have certain measurements, then she is thought to be at risk of not being able to deliver vaginally. Prenatal health forms often have space for inclusion of clinical pelvimetry measurements; however, assessment of pelvic measurements early in the first trimester is not firm confirmation of pelvic disproportion. Whether a healthy woman delivers vaginally depends on factors at term, such as size and position of the fetus in relation to the maternal pelvis.

Discomforts Related to Clinical Pelvimetry

Clinical pelvimetry generally takes only a few moments during a bimanual pelvic examination. The woman may sense pressure as the examiner presses against bones and soft tissues. The healthy woman will not experience any acute physical pain. Explaining the procedure and sharing the results help to allay client anxiety.

▶ Assessment of Pregnancy

Ultrasound

Ultrasound (sonography) is a technique that involves the use of high-frequency sound waves. **Ultrasound** is defined as any sound with a frequency of greater than 20,000 Hz (undetectable by the human ear). The sound waves bounce off tissues of differing acoustic density. A frequency range of 3.5 to 5 MHz is usually used in obstetrics, although it may be higher. Today, ultrasound is a valuable, widely used means of fetal and maternal assessment. However, there is controversy about the routine use of ultrasound during pregnancy (Cunningham et al., 1997).

Ultrasound may be used to assess the pregnant client, developing fetus, or both. It is also used to visualize internal maternal and fetal structures to guide other diagnostic procedures, such as chorionic villus sampling (see later discussion) and amniocentesis (Harrington & Campbell, 1993) (see Chapter 17).

Pulse echo imaging and Doppler systems are two classifications of ultrasound used often in obstetrics.

Pulse echo systems transmit high-frequency sound pulses and receive echoes that are displayed as a two-dimensional image on a television-type monitor. Static scanners and real-time scanners are two types of pulse echo ultrasound equipment. Static scanners emit a pulse of sound waves from the transducer. These waves move through soft body tissues. Some of the energy is reflected back (echoed) to the transducer when an interface between different tissue densities is reached. The transducer then emits a small electrical voltage that is magnified and shown on a screen. Static scanners give a "still" image in the same way that a photograph freezes a moment in time. They present still views from several different points, because the transducer, which is responsible for the imaging, is moved across the woman's abdomen. Real-time scanners show movement as it happens, because the transducers send out many pulse echo systems (Cunningham et al., 1997). In clinical practice with prenatal clients, real-time scanners are often used because they allow fetal movements, as well as heart and breathing activity, to be observed.

Pulse echo scanning may be done by an ultrasound technician, nurse, or physician. The American College of Obstetricians and Gynecologists recommends that this test be done by "a trained professional" (American College of Obstetricians and Gynecologists, 1993). Final interpretation of ultrasound tests is done by a physician. Pulse echo ultrasound scanners may be located in hospital outpatient clinics or in physicians' offices. Ultrasonography is also considered a subspecialty of radiology, and diagnostic ultrasound may be performed in radiology departments.

Basic and Targeted Ultrasound. Basic and targeted ultrasound provide different types of information. The basic ultrasound is used most frequently in the first trimester to assess the presence of an intrauterine pregnancy, gestational sac location, the number of fetuses, fetal heart activity, and fetal crown–rump length. The gestational sac, embryonic poles, yolk sac, fetal heart, and crown–rump length can accurately predict gestational age within 4 days. With recent advances in ultrasound imaging, the gestational sac can be detected within the uterine cavity as early as 4 weeks and 3 days after the last menstrual period (Jurkovic, Gruboeck, & Campbell, 1995). A yolk sac without an embryo indicates a missed abortion. Fetal death at any time throughout pregnancy may also be confirmed. Basic ultrasound is also used to determine location of the placenta, maturity, and abnormalities of the placenta. Placental circulation may also be evaluated early in pregnancy (Merce, Barco, & Bau, 1996). The amount of amniotic fluid, abnormalities in gross fetal anatomy, and maternal pelvic pathology can also be assessed. Repeat (serial) ultrasounds, performed when indicated, can help identify a growth-retarded fetus.

Targeted ultrasound is done if a client is thought to be carrying an anatomically or physiologically abnormal fetus. Attention is directed toward specific evaluation of fetal anatomy and physiology. Indications for the examination include abnormalities on clinical examination and a history of offspring with anomalies that could be viewed on sonogram. A specialist in high-risk sonography performs this examination.

Safety. Many questions have been raised about the safety of ultrasound. Pregnancy is a physically vulnerable period for the developing fetus. Salvesen and Eiknes (1995) reviewed the epidemiological studies of human exposure to diagnostic ultrasound during pregnancy. They found no associations between ultrasound exposure in utero and childhood malignancies, neurological problems, dyslexia, and delayed speech. They did find that there were some issues, such as low birth weight after frequent Doppler ultrasound exposure, that needed further testing.

Ultrasound, specifically indicated, is thought to benefit the mother and fetus because the information provided can be important to diagnosis and treatment. For example, screening for chromosomal trisomies of the fetus can be done as early as the tenth week of pregnancy using ultrasound. Trisomy 21 (Down syndrome) and other chromosomal defects may be first identified by an increased **nuchal translucency** thickness (opaque thickness in the neck of the fetus > 3 mm). Some clinicians advocate screening for nuchal translucency thickness based on advanced maternal age in order to predict fetal chromosomal trisomies (Nobel, Abraha, Snijders, Sherwood, & Nicolaides, 1995; Pandya, Snijders, Johnson, De Lourdes Brizot, & Nicolaides, 1995). Others believe that while the efficacy of the test in a research setting is

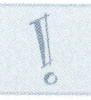

Nursing Alert

A study entitled the Routine Antenatal Diagnostic Imaging with Ultrasound (RADIUS) concluded that routine ultrasound screening for low-risk women did not improve pregnancy outcome. Furthermore, the study suggested that savings for perinatal care could be about $1 billion if there was a decrease in ultrasound screens during routine pregnancy (Berkowitz, 1993).

good, the effectiveness in everyday usage is much less impressive (Kornman, Morssink, Beekhuis, De Wolf, Heringa, & Mantingh, 1996).

Controversy does exist over whether ultrasound should be routinely used for all pregnant women. Questions also arise about the cost effectiveness of a screening process that does not improve outcome.

Transabdominal Approach. This approach is used during the first, second, and third trimesters. The transabdominal approach is difficult during the first trimester because the uterus has not yet grown out of the pelvis, making the embryo, as well as maternal pelvic structures, difficult to visualize. To obtain clearer images during the first trimester, women are required to drink one to two quarts of clear fluid to fill the urinary bladder and thereby push the uterus higher into the abdomen where it can be more accurately scanned. The test is performed with the woman lying on her back. Side-lying positions may be requested to provide better visualization of certain structures. A transducer is passed over the women's abdomen and images of internal structures are produced on a monitor. Unfortunately, a highly distended bladder can be very uncomfortable or embarrassing for the woman. Although the transabdominal approach may be used during the first trimester, it is more frequently used during the second and third trimesters, when the uterus is an abdominal organ.

Transvaginal Approach. This approach is used for first-trimester ultrasound. Transvaginal ultrasonography allows small, deep pelvic organs, such as the ovaries, to be visualized more clearly, because these structures are close to the transducer probe. Factors such as greater distance or the presence of other body tissues can affect the quality of sonographic pictures; accurate diagnosis depends on clear pictures (Harrington & Campbell, 1993).

A transvaginal approach is especially useful with obese clients, whose thick abdominal layers cannot be adequately penetrated by the ultrasound when a transabdominal approach is used. Transvaginal ultrasonography facilitates earlier detection of ectopic pregnancies. Serious complications, such as tubal rupture resulting from ectopic tubal pregnancy, may then be prevented. In addition, transvaginal ultrasonography can be used to monitor the developing embryo, help identify abnormalities, and help establish gestational age.

Transvaginal ultrasound is performed with the client in lithotomy position. A small reversed Trendelenburg tilt to the examining table allows the slight amount of peritoneal fluid to pool in the pelvis and create tissue/fluid interfaces. These interfaces enhance visualization and help the examiner to identify normal or pathologic structures in the pelvis and fetus (Fig. 15–15).

After being coated with a special coupling gel, the transvaginal probe is covered with a protective

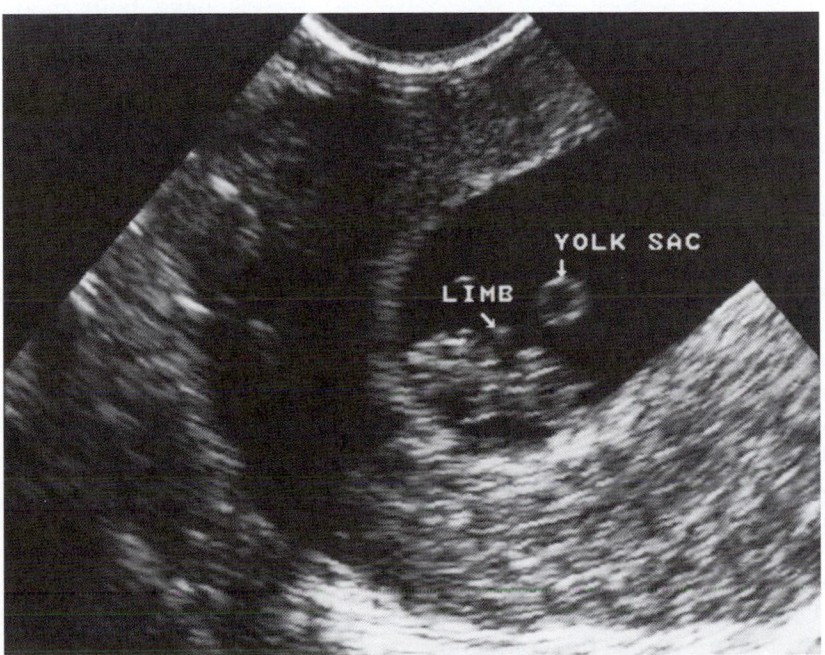

FIGURE 15–15. Transvaginal ultrasound image at 7 to 8 weeks of gestation, demonstrating yolk sac and limb of embryo. *(Reproduced, with permission, from Fleischer, A.C. et al. (1991). The principles and practice of ultrasonography in obstetrics and gynecology (4th ed.). Norwalk, CT: Appleton & Lange, p. 48.)*

sheath. A condom, the finger of a clean rubber surgical glove, or a probe cover provided by the manufacturer may be used. Gel is also used to lubricate the covered probe to promote conductivity and client comfort. The probe is placed in the vagina by the person performing the sonogram; however, the client may insert the probe if she chooses. During the examination the angle or position of the probe may be changed and the electrical control panel adjusted to provide nearly complete access to the whole pelvis.

Transvaginal ultrasound takes about 10 minutes, although it can vary, depending on whether pathology is identified. The procedure should not be physically painful; the client may experience a sense of pressure as the probe is moved. Discomfort relates mostly to being in the lithotomy position or to a pathologic condition.

Doppler Ultrasound. Unlike ultrasound techniques that provide actual images of body structures, Doppler ultrasound provides information about blood moving within living blood vessels and body organs. Sound waves of known frequency are directed at blood vessels containing moving red blood cells. The waves "bounce off" the blood cells and return at a different frequency. The change in frequency depends on how fast the red blood cell is moving. The difference between the ultrasound wave frequency "sent out" and the frequency "received back" is called the Doppler shift (Boemi et al., 1996).

Blood cells at a vessel's center travel faster than those near the sides. At any time within a blood vessel, red blood cells are moving at different speeds. Therefore, at any one time during the cardiac cycle, a range of shifted frequencies exists within each blood vessel. Special Doppler imaging equipment can sample blood flow in the entire vessel or in specific areas within the vessel. In obstetrics, circulation is assessed using transducers with frequencies from 2 to 8 MHz. Several types of Doppler instruments may be used, as described below:

- *Continuous wave.* Continuous-wave (CW) Doppler instruments send a continuous beam of ultrasonic waves. The velocity of red blood cells in the path of the beam is then recorded. This type of Doppler evaluation is commonly used in prenatal clinics or private offices to electronically monitor fetal heart rate and detect blood flow through the fetal heart. Continuous-wave Doppler instruments are used during the first trimester because flow of blood through the fetal heart may be detected around 8 weeks, whereas auscultation of fetal heart sounds is not possible until 17 to 20 weeks. It

has also been shown that transvaginal Doppler auscultation of the fetal heart is more sensitive than transabdominal auscultation (Mitra, Laurent et al., 1996). Doppler readings may be affected by such factors as the mother's breathing or fetal position or movements.

To take a CW Doppler reading, the transducer head is coated with gel and then positioned against the woman's abdomen. With simple, hand-held Doppler instruments, fetal heart rate activity may be heard and counted. More sophisticated fetal heart rate monitors provide recorded tracings of fetal heart rate and amplify the sound of fetal heart tones. Fetal heart tones may be monitored externally with a belt holding the transducer against the mother's abdomen or internally with the probe fastened to the presenting part of the fetus.

- *Pulsed wave.* Pulsed-wave Doppler instruments differ from CW instruments by sending out pulses of waves each second rather than a continuous beam of ultrasound waves. These pulses of sound waves bounce off different areas within the blood vessel, depending on how far they have traveled. If the returning waves are sampled at different time intervals as they return to the transducer head, velocity of flow in specific areas of the blood vessel can be measured.
- *Duplex scanning.* The combination of the pulsed Doppler with real-time ultrasound is known as duplex scanning. Modern transducer heads have both modalities within a single unit. By use of real-time ultrasound, specific blood vessels can be located. The velocity of blood flow within the vessels can then be determined using the pulsed Doppler instrument. Structures such as the uterine placental vessels, umbilical vein, fetal aorta, carotid arteries, and the fetal heart can be precisely imaged, and blood velocity can be quantified. For example, increasing resistance to blood flow in these vessels has been measured with duplex scanners and is associated with such problems as fetal intrauterine growth retardation.
- *Color flow.* Color flow imaging is an extension of duplex scanning. For example, a specific area of a blood vessel is first imaged with real-time ultrasound. With the pulsed Doppler instrument, multiple samples of velocity of blood flow are taken within the visualized area of the blood vessel. A mean velocity of each sample is calculated and assigned a color by the machine. The result is the blood vessel's image, portrayed in color on a monitor screen. Direction and mean velocity of blood flow are repre-

sented by color changes during the cardiac cycle. Color coding facilitates identification of the blood vessels and the actual direction of flow (Hung, Ng, Pan, Yang, & Shu, 1997).

Although Doppler ultrasound signals are easy to record from the expectant woman and fetus during pregnancy, interpreting and understanding the significance of the findings are more difficult. Results can be affected by such factors as the problems in obtaining measurements of the same place in the same blood vessel or in having measurements taken by different operators (Weiner, Reichler, Zlozover, Mendelson, & Thaler, 1993).

Client Reactions. A wide variety of client and family reactions, ranging from excitement to fear, may be expected in relation to ultrasound. Client reactions may relate to the reason for the ultrasound study. For example, the first-trimester client who will have Doppler ultrasound done during her prenatal visit may excitedly bring the expectant father to hear the heartbeat. Clients referred for ultrasound to assess for a blighted ovum or a missed abortion may respond with fear. When maternal or fetal abnormalities are detected or when fetal death is confirmed, clients react with grief.

Role of the Nurse. Providing information and support to the client and her family before, during, and after ultrasound studies is an important role of the nurse. Several questions need to be addressed.

- Why is the procedure being done?
- Is the procedure safe?
- Who will perform the ultrasound?
- Where will the ultrasound be done?
- What will the ultrasound be able to show?
- Is any preparation necessary?
- What does the procedure entail?
- What will the client feel during the ultrasound?
- How may the client deal with any discomfort (e.g., breathing, imagery)?
- How long will the ultrasound study take?
- How much time can the client expect to commit to the ultrasound (includes waiting and follow-up testing)?
- Who will interpret the ultrasound findings?
- When will the client be informed of the results?
- Should a relative or friend accompany the client? (Especially in high-risk conditions, presence of a significant other is helpful in ensuring that the client returns home safely.)
- What specifically does the client question and fear in relation to the ultrasound?

- Will photos of the fetus be given to the client? (Photos are often desired by clients having ultrasound for gestational dating or other nonthreatening conditions, but may also be desired by clients with abnormal fetuses.)

Advance staff planning can clarify ways in which collaboration can provide information and deal with client concerns and feelings. Ways to support clients who receive bad news need to be planned. Interdisciplinary staff conferences may also help health care providers to deal with their own feelings about diagnosis of fetal abnormalities.

Staff nurses in prenatal and labor and delivery settings may frequently use Doppler ultrasound in assessing and monitoring fetal heart rate patterns. Familiarity with the equipment and procedure, as well as with principles of basic Doppler ultrasound, is necessary.

Estimating Delivery Date

The average pregnancy has a gestation of 266 days or 38 weeks postconception. The estimated delivery date (EDD), previously referred to as expected date of confinement (EDC), can be arrived at using a variety of methods.

Nägele's Rule. **Nägele's rule** is the most frequently used method of estimating delivery: subtract 3 months from the first day of the last normal menstrual period (LMP) and then add 1 year and 7 days to that date. For example, if the woman's LMP began December 20, subtracting 3 months provides a date of September 20, to which 7 days are added to derive the EDD of September 27 of the following year:

Estimated delivery date (EDD) =
First day of LMP − 3 months (+) 1 year + 7 days
(12/20/99)   (9/20/99)   (9/27/00)

Fundal Height Measurement. The fundal height is considered a gestational estimation but may be inaccurate if there is a multiple gestation, intrauterine growth retardation, or maternal obesity. Estimation of the delivery date may be guided by fundal height if the LMP is unknown; however, other clinical data should be obtained for confirmation. McDonald's method of fundal height determination corresponds to the gestational week within a 2- to 4-week range after 22 to 24 weeks. With McDonald's method, the fundal height is measured in centimeters with a tape measure, from the superior border of the symphysis pubis to the fundus. At 12 weeks of gestation, the fundus is level with the symphysis. Before the fundus reaches the umbilicus (at 22 to 24 weeks), 4 cm is added to the measurement to determine gestation. To

▶ **TABLE 15-5**

Selected Sonographic Findings in First Trimester

Findings	Gestational Age (weeks)	
	Transabdominal	Transvaginal
Gestational sac and yolk sac	6	5
Fetus	7	6
Fetal heart activity	7	6

Source: Chin, 1997.

ensure accuracy, measurement should be consistent (e.g., a tape measure instead of fingerbreadths) and the same practitioner should perform the initial and subsequent assessments if possible.

Sonogram. Sonographic determination of gestation can be done through transabdominal or transvaginal ultrasound in the first trimester. The dimensions of the gestational sac and yolk sac, the presence of the fetus, assessment of fetal heart activity, and the crown–rump measurement can be obtained. Table 15–5 describes selected sonographic findings in the first trimester.

▶ Determination of Risk Status

Pregnancy may carry some risk of perinatal morbidity or mortality. Thus, the expectant mother and her family should be screened for potential risk factors during the initial prenatal visit and at each subsequent visit, because risk factors may emerge during the course of pregnancy. Research has indicated that perinatal morbidity and mortality are affected by such factors as maternal socioeconomic status, quality of prenatal care, age, nutrition, past obstetric history, current pregnancy problems, and associated illness (Cunningham et al., 1997). Risk assessment during pregnancy is therefore based on the evaluation of physiologic, psychosocial, socioeconomic, lifestyle, and environmental factors that may affect perinatal outcome. As indicated in Table 15–6, risk factors are also related to specific pregnancy problems.

Management Guidelines

Once high-risk status has been determined, appropriate nursing and collaborative management can be initiated to promote maternal, fetal, and family well-being. A plan of care, based on the unique needs and condition of each family, is developed. The primary objective of management is to provide appropriate

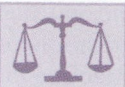

Ethical Decision Making

In evaluating the risk status of pregnant women, the nurse needs to be aware of numerous factors that may affect perinatal outcomes and must consider the following questions:

1. Should all women of childbearing age be considered potentially pregnant, especially in light of the ethical implications of this classification on vendors who sell women cigarettes or alcohol, pharmacists who sell women over-the-counter medications, and pediatricians who immunize adolescents of childbearing age for rubella?

2. Should women be required to document their nonpregnant status before buying certain potentially toxic products or engaging in activities potentially detrimental to an embryo or fetus?

and timely preventive or restorative care with a minimum of technologic intervention and financial or emotional cost. Management strategies may include health education, continued observation, further assessment procedures, specific interventions, or referrals to regional antenatal centers that specialize in management of pregnant clients with specific high-risk conditions. Management guidelines for the client identified as high risk are discussed in later chapters of this text.

Screening Tools

Various screening tools, such as risk rating scales or questionnaires, are available to determine risk status during pregnancy. The usefulness of any risk screening tool in a particular situation depends on the ability of the tool to predict outcome criteria (maternal complications, fetal problems, or neonatal status).

Unfortunately, no screening tool identifies all possible problems with complete certainty. Scoring systems predict approximately half the problems experienced during pregnancy. Screening tools do, however, have several advantages. For example, many high-risk conditions are actually identified through use of the tools. In addition, uniform data can be obtained for populations of pregnant clients. Uniform data can then assist in diagnosis and management of high-risk conditions and in better definition

► **TABLE 15–6**

Specific Pregnancy Problems and Related Risk Factors

Problem	Risk Factor
Preterm labor	Age below 16 or over 35 Low socioeconomic status Maternal weight below 50 kg (110 lb) Poor nutrition Previous preterm birth Incompetent cervix Uterine anomalies Smoking Drug addiction and alcohol abuse Pyelonephritis, pneumonia Multiple gestation Anemia Abnormal fetal presentation Preterm rupture of membranes Placental abnormalities Infection
Polyhydramnios	Diabetes mellitus Multiple gestation Fetal congenital anomalies Isoimmunization (Rh or ABO) Nonimmune hydrops Abnormal fetal presentation
Intrauterine growth retardation (IUGR)	Multiple gestation Poor nutrition Maternal cyanotic heart disease Chronic hypertension Pregnancy-induced hypertension Recurrent antepartum hemorrhage Smoking Maternal diabetes with vascular problems Fetal infections Fetal cardiovascular anomalies Drug addition and alcohol abuse Fetal congenital anomalies Hemoglobinopathies
Oligohydramnios	Renal agenesis (Potter's syndrome) Prolonged rupture of membranes Intrauterine growth retardation Intrauterine fetal demise
Postterm Pregnancy	Anencephaly Placental sulfatase deficiency Perinatal hypoxia, acidosis Placental insufficiency
Chromosomal abnormalities	Maternal age 35 years or more at delivery Balanced translocation (maternal and paternal)

Reproduced, with permission, from DeCherney, A.H., & Pernoll, M.L. (Eds.) (1994). Current obstetric & gynocologic diagnosis & treatment (8th ed.). Norwalk, CT: Appleton & Lange, p. 276.

of high-risk indicators among differing socioeconomic groups (Cunningham et al., 1997).

Biochemical Techniques. The initial biochemical screening during the first trimester of pregnancy provides baseline data and allows for early intervention to ensure optimal maternal and fetal well-being. After the initial confirmation of pregnancy, the fol-

lowing tests may be routinely ordered: urinalysis, complete blood count (CBC), blood typing and Rh determination, rubella titer, serology for syphilis, gonorrhea culture, and Papanicolaou (Pap) smear. The prenatal assessment is an ongoing process and some screening tests warrant repetition at specific times as the pregnancy progresses. Subsequent prenatal visits include urinalysis for albumin and glucose and periodic determinations of hemoglobin and hematocrit. More extensive screening may also be warranted on the basis of maternal history and clinical indications; for example, if glucose is found in the urine, serum glucose testing may be ordered.

- *Urinalysis.* A freshly voided urine sample is tested for glucose, protein, and ketones at each prenatal visit to identify complications of pregnancy. A clean-catch technique may be used if microscopic examination and culture are to be done to screen for asymptomatic bacteriuria. A single specimen with a colony count of 100,000 (10 mL) or more per milliliter is considered asymptomatic bacteriuria.
- *Blood studies.* A variety of blood studies are performed at the initial prenatal visit. Additional studies may be ordered if there are specific indications. (See box entitled Selected Blood Studies Performed at the First Prenatal Visit.)
- *Cytology.* At the first prenatal visit, a Pap smear is taken to detect cytologic abnormalities (see Chapter 7).
- *Cultures.* In some settings, cervical cultures for *Neisseria gonorrhoeae* (gonorrhea) and chlamydia may be routinely performed. In other settings, the tests are done only for clients at risk or with a history of the diseases. On the basis of the client's history or observations made by the examiner during the vaginal examination, cultures for other organisms, such as *Gardnerella, Trichomonas,* or herpes virus, may be done.

Identifying Psychosocial Risk Factors in a Family

The nurse can help the family cope with various psychosocial tasks of pregnancy through counseling and support of family members. Thorough prenatal assessment during the first trimester allows the nurse to identify normal and abnormal patterns of adaptation. Focusing on the following specific areas will identify psychosocial risk factors:

- *Patterns of Self-Perception/Concept.* Pregnancy can bring changes in both the mother's and father's self-image. The nurse should assess whether the expectant couple views the preg-

► SELECTED BLOOD STUDIES PERFORMED AT THE FIRST PRENATAL VISIT

CBC AND DIFFERENTIAL ANALYSIS

- Screening tool for blood disorders and infections (see Appendix B for normal laboratory values during pregnancy)
- White blood cell count: elevation indicative of infection
- Hemoglobin below 11 to 12 g/100 mL and hematocrit of 33 to 36% indicate anemia

BLOOD TYPING AND Rh DETERMINATION

- Used to identify specific type (A, B, O, or AB) and presence of the Rh factor or antibodies to prevent isoimmunization during future pregnancies (occurs when the mother is Rh negative and the fetus is Rh positive)
- Paternal blood may be tested for Rh factor if the mother is Rh negative

RUBELLA (GERMAN MEASLES) SCREENING

- Routinely performed to determine past maternal rubella infection or adequate immunization
- Serum antibody titer to determine level of immunity is evaluated (titer less than 1:8 is considered indicative of maternal susceptibility to rubella or lack of immunity; titer of 1:8 to 1:32 indicates past rubella exposure; and titer greater than 1:32 indicates immunity)

SYPHILIS SCREENING

- Venereal Disease Research Laboratories (VDRL) test: nontreponemal antibody screening test (note: certain chronic diseases can produce false-positive results for the VDRL and this test may be negative in the early infectious phase of syphilis)
- Reactive plasma reagin (RPR) test: nontreponemal antibody screening test
- Fluorescent treponemal antibody absorption (FTA-ABS) test: treponemal antibody test (more sensitive to spirochete infections)
- *T. pallidum* immobilization (TPI) test: treponemal antibody test (more sensitive to spirochete infections)

HUMAN IMMUNODEFICIENCY VIRUS (HIV) SCREENING

- HIV screening should be offered to all prenatal clients

---

nancy as reinforcing or as threatening to their self-image. The nurse may then intervene to validate the positive aspects or offer guidance to alter threats to self-image.

- *Cognitive/perceptual aspects.* The mother's cognitive ability and sensory perceptions are variable and need to be assessed individually to establish a realistic plan of prenatal care.
- *Behavioral aspects.* The first trimester is typified by uncertainty, ambivalence, and the need for attention and reassurance.
- *Coping/stress tolerance.* Pregnancy can be a stressful event, because of the many changes that take place within the woman and within the family. Pregnancy may tax the financial and physical resources of the family. The nurse must evaluate the stress perceived by family members during pregnancy, as well as the effectiveness of coping patterns.
- *Roles/relationships.* The transition to motherhood and fatherhood is accompanied by changes in roles and relationships within the family, within employment situations, and within the societal structure. The nurse assesses the ways in which the expectant family is adapting to pregnancy and identifies potential conflicts in roles and relationships.

Cultural Assessment of the Family

The cultural and spiritual needs of the expectant family should be assessed, because various beliefs and practices influence the couple's interpretation of and receptiveness to health care. These influences can then be incorporated into a care plan tailored to the unique needs of the client and family.

► Prenatal Diagnostic Assessment

Fetal assessment during the first trimester may be done through a variety of means, including measuring fundal height and using Doppler ultrasound and ultrasound imaging, which have been discussed. Chorionic villus sampling (CVS), however, is a first-trimester procedure for fetal assessment done specifically for diagnosis when chromosomal abnormalities are a risk factor for the fetus.

Chorionic Villus Sampling

Chorionic villus sampling is a first-trimester procedure performed to obtain fetal cells for diagnosis of chromosomal and congenital abnormalities. It is indicated for women of advanced maternal age; women with a previous history of a fetus or child with a genetic disorder; couples who express or carry a genetic abnormality; and any other women for whom there is reason to suspect a genetically abnormal fetus.

In the United States, desire to know the sex of the fetus does not justify this invasive procedure; however, sex of the fetus is determined by CVS. Members of some cultures, such as Asian or Indian, may nevertheless request the procedure for the purpose of determining the sex of the fetus. As health care providers, it is the nurse's responsibility to make certain that clients are provided with the necessary information to make informed choices about this procedure.

Chorionic villi, which are of fetal origin, reflect the chromosomes, enzymology, and DNA content of the fetus. Identification of chromosomal disorders such as trisomy 21, trisomy 18, translocations, X-linked disorders such as Tay-Sachs disease, and hematologic diseases such as sickle cell anemia and thalassemia is possible through the use of CVS. Unlike amniocentesis CVS cannot detect neural tube defects because the level of alpha-fetoprotein, which may determine neural tube defects, can only be tested using serum or amniotic fluid.

Advantages. Chorionic villus sampling may be done between 9 and 12 weeks' gestation, as compared to amniocentesis, which is usually performed between 15 and 18 weeks' gestation. Test results from CVS are available within a few days, as compared with the 3 to 4 weeks usually needed for results from amniocentesis. Normal findings help allay clients' anxieties about certain genetic disorders. Abnormal results permit clients who choose to continue the pregnancy to receive special support and have time to prepare for the baby. Some clients, on the other hand, elect to terminate the pregnancy. First-trimester terminations are medically safer, quicker, and easier than second trimester terminations. Because first-trimester pregnancy is less visible, the client may have greater privacy in decision making than during the second trimester.

Disadvantages/Risks. There have been reports of unusual clusters of limb defects in newborns of mothers who underwent CVS, especially prior to 10 weeks' gestation (Hsieh, Shyu, Sheu, Lin, Chen, & Huang, 1995). Although the relationship between CVS and limb defects in the newborn is unclear, the following statements have been made by the American College of Obstetricians and Gynecologists (1995):

1. Chorionic villus sampling is a relatively safe procedure when performed at 10 to 12 weeks and is an acceptable alternative to amniocentesis.
2. Chorionic villus sampling is not recommended prior to 10 weeks.

3. Genetic counseling should be provided prior to performing the procedure.
4. Women should be counseled that the estimated risk of limb defects may be about 1 in 3000 births.

Other possible risks of the CVS procedure include spontaneous abortion, ruptured amniotic sac, intrauterine growth retardation, and Rh isoimmunization. Results of the testing may also be inaccurate. A 1.7% discrepancy rate between the apparent villus karyotype and the fetus has been reported.

Chorionic villus sampling does not ensure that the fetus will be completely healthy, as other conditions can develop during gestation or delivery, and certain abnormalities, such as neural tube defects, are not detected.

Procedure. The client who elects CVS receives genetic counseling. The procedure, its risks, and its benefits are explained, and the client signs a consent form. At the time the test is scheduled, the client should be made aware of the time commitment necessary to permit her to make appropriate adjustments in her usual schedule and responsibilities. Preparation, procedure, and recovery may require 2 hours, although the procedure takes only 20 minutes. Delays in the testing center may prolong this time. The client should be informed of the need for rest at home after the procedure.

Transcervical and transabdominal approaches have been used for CVS. The transcervical approach is easier when the placenta is located posteriorly, while the transabdominal approach appears easier when the placenta is anterior (Cunningham et al., 1997). For twin gestations, a transcervical approach for both fetuses is not recommended (De Catte, Liebaers, Foulon, Bonduelle, & Van Assche, 1996).

In the transcervical approach (Fig. 15–16), the client is placed in lithotomy position, a pelvic examination is done, and a speculum is inserted into the vagina so that the cervix can be seen. A slender catheter is passed through the cervix. Under direct visualization with real-time ultrasound, a small sample of chorionic villi is aspirated through the catheter into a syringe. In the transabdominal approach, the skin on the maternal abdomen is cleansed with a standard surgical preparation solution. An 18 to 20 gauge needle is inserted into the chorionic bed under ultrasonic guidance. The specimen for either procedure is inspected carefully for villi and the aspirated villi are put into a sterile medium for cytogenic analysis (Cunningham et al., 1997).

Because first trimester cells divide rapidly, time is not needed for them to grow in a laboratory.

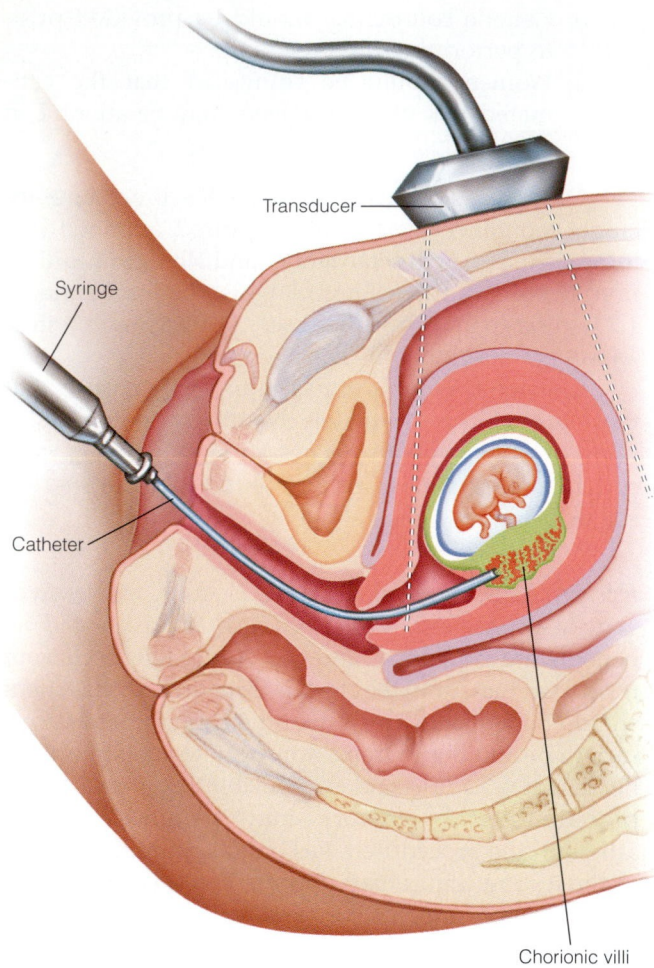

Transducer

Syringe

Catheter

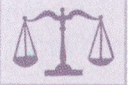
Chorionic villi

FIGURE 15–16. Chorionic villus sampling using transcervical approach.

appear, heavy bleeding or the passage of amniotic fluid, clots, or tissue is not normal and should be reported to the physician at once. A clear or pink-tinged specimen may be discarded, whereas tissue passed may be sent for laboratory analysis.

Chorionic villus sampling is an outpatient procedure, and the client leaves for home if her vital signs are stable, she is not experiencing cramping, and she is having no vaginal discharge other than spotting. The nurse remains accessible to the client and provides an opportunity for the client to express her feelings. A client with associated complications is kept in the antenatal testing unit until she is stable or, if necessary, admitted.

After the procedure the client is advised to avoid sexual activity for 48 hours and to contact her physician if bleeding, cramping, or flulike symptoms are experienced. She returns for examination and ultrasound 1 week later, returns for an ultrasound examination at 16 weeks (to evaluate fetal and placental development), and avoids heavy or vigorous physical activity. Clients should plan to rest for the remainder of the day.

▶ Supportive Measures During Diagnostic Assessment

The purpose of diagnostic assessment during the first trimester is secondary prevention, that is, early identification of abnormalities. Many clients do not have uncomfortable symptoms during the early stages of

Preliminary laboratory reports can be obtained within 24 to 48 hours and confirmed reports within 5 to 10 days of CVS.

Role of the Nurse. Working collaboratively with the physician in an antenatal testing unit, the nurse has several important roles, including client education, assessment, and support. The nurse's role involves teaching the client and her partner about CVS, its risks and benefits; acting as a client advocate for the couple when they make an informed decision regarding the procedure; and caring for the client before, during, and after CVS. In addition, the nurse's role may involve teaching about choices the woman may face if an abnormality is detected.

After the procedure, the client's blood pressure and pulse are taken. If vital signs are normal, the client may void in a collection container in the bathroom. Although a small amount of spotting may

Ethical Decision Making

Ultrasound and chorionic villus sampling are two diagnostic tools that may be used in the first trimester of pregnancy. Concerns continue to be raised about potential long-term effects of these tests and the nurse needs to consider the following questions:

1. How much technology should be used routinely?
2. Should all pregnant clients be assessed as potentially high risk?
3. If the client states that she would at no time consider terminating the pregnancy, should she still be offered tests for chromosomal abnormalities?

disease processes; therefore, diagnosis may be delayed. Prompt treatment may help cure or control pathologic conditions.

All diagnostic tests can be a source of misinterpretation and worry for the client and her family. Unfortunately, no one test can answer all questions about the well-being of the developing fetus or a complicated maternal condition. In addition to providing teaching about the test and support during procedures, health care providers need to make sure that clients receive test results as soon as possible to reduce anxiety.

▶ Nursing Diagnoses

The first trimester assessment process provides extensive information about the client and her family. Diagnoses are then developed from the subjective and objective data collected and reflect conclusions about the client and her family. Despite changes and discomforts related to early pregnancy, the first trimester is part of a healthy life process. Nursing diagnoses, therefore, focus on wellness and on the need to identify potential risk factors. Examples of nursing diagnoses include:

Physiologic
Problem-oriented diagnoses:

- Fatigue, related to demands of pregnancy during first trimester
- Altered nutrition: less than body requirements, related to first-trimester nausea and vomiting

Wellness-oriented diagnoses:

- Asset in health of mother, related to normal physical changes in the first trimester
- Progressive normal embryo/fetal growth and development, related to maternal health and nutritional status during the first trimester

Psychosocial
Problem-oriented diagnoses:

- Anxiety, related to—
  - Initial encounter with the health care system
  - Financial pressures related to economic impact of childbearing
- Knowledge deficit, related to—
  - Lack of understanding about first-trimester changes
  - Lack of information about first-trimester discomforts
  - Lack of understanding about early prenatal assessment techniques

- Lack of information about the nature and extent of services available in the prenatal health care system

Wellness-oriented diagnoses:

- Potential asset in self-care practices, related to early initiation of prenatal care

Cultural
Problem-oriented diagnoses:

- Social isolation, related to cultural differences in perception of roles during early pregnancy
- Impaired social interaction, related to differences in language between client and care providers

Wellness-oriented diagnoses:

- Positive self-concept, related to congruence between cultural beliefs and—
  - Achievement of pregnancy
  - Expectations of prenatal care

▶ NURSING AND COLLABORATIVE MANAGEMENT

After assessment, including examination, during the first visit, the nurse and examiner collaborate to develop a plan of care. On the basis of assessment, specific diagnoses are identified, behavioral outcomes projected, health care interventions planned, and evaluation criteria noted. Client participation in development of the care plan is important. In this way a plan of care that is realistic, feasible, and acceptable for each client is devised.

The care plan is recorded in the client's chart, reviewed before each prenatal visit, and updated as necessary. At times generic care plans that provide general approaches to client care may be available. Childbearing families are never identical, however, and generic care plans must always be individualized to meet each family's needs.

Goals for nursing care during the first trimester are established after a thorough analysis of assessment data. First-trimester goals set the tone for the health care that is delivered throughout the prenatal period.

▶ Keeping Professionally Current

Publications related to principles, practice, ethical issues, and research in antenatal care are increasingly available. Optimal prenatal care requires that nurses, as well as other health care providers, keep up with current advances that affect practice. Attending professional meetings, in-service programs that focus on different childbearing topics, and "journal club" meetings where staff present relevant articles help nurses provide state-of-the-art care.

▶ Establishing a Philosophy of Care with Well-Defined Goals

Prenatal health care providers should collaborate to develop a philosophy of care with well-defined goals and objectives. The process of establishing goals and carrying out care for the client and family during the first trimester has many aspects:

- Preparing the client and family for prenatal health care
- Evolving a data base for diagnosis development
- Supporting the client
- Recognizing cultural influences
- Facilitating informed decision making
- Promoting psychologic adaptation to early pregnancy
- Facilitating family attachment
- Meeting early-pregnancy educational needs
- Promoting nutritional well-being
- Assisting the client to cope with first-trimester discomforts
- Promoting client safety
- Evaluating antenatal care
- Ensuring appropriate client referral/removing barriers to care
- Contributing to general prenatal public health

Ways in which the philosophy is incorporated into routine client care should be outlined. For example, staff can show their commitment to childbearing as a normal, family-centered process by encouraging family members to attend all prenatal visits, participate in prepared childbirth activities, and be present for labor and delivery.

Preparing the Client and Family for Prenatal Health Care

Preparation of the client and her family for prenatal health care involves orienting them to health care providers and the prenatal health care system. Indeed, the initial contact may influence a client's willingness to continue early prenatal care; the first visit begins a pattern for the client–health provider relationship (see the box entitled Outline of a Prenatal Visit). It is important to realize the variations among prenatal care facilities.

During the initial visit, the first-trimester client should be oriented to the prenatal facilities, the per-

sonnel who will provide care, what to expect during each visit, and the scheduling of prenatal visits.

Prenatal Facilities. Giving careful directions to the client about how to get to the clinic or office, including transportation or parking arrangements, minimizes stress. Many obstetric centers routinely offer tours of the facilities at the first visit.

Personnel. Primary prenatal care is delivered by certified nurse-midwives, physicians, or house–staff physicians (under supervision of attending physicians in clinic settings). Nurse practitioners, clinical nurse specialists, prenatal staff nurses, dietitians, nutritionists, social workers, and chaplains are also part of the prenatal care team. Student participation, under instructor and staff supervision, is often welcomed.

Prenatal settings, whether a private obstetric practice or clinic, vary widely with respect to the type and number of health care personnel interacting with the client. In addition, personnel and the primary care provider may vary from visit to visit. The client needs to be informed of the identity of all personnel directly involved in her care. A nurse has a particularly important role in group practice and clinic settings, as she or he may be the only health care provider the client sees consistently at each prenatal visit throughout pregnancy. Therefore, the nurse can do much to ensure continuity of care.

Expectations of Visit. To prepare a client for prenatal care, it is helpful to provide her with information about many topics:

- Name and location of the prenatal care facility
- Directions to facility from major travel routes
- Description of center, range of services offered
- Specific focus of facility, for example, a birth center specializing in low-risk healthy clients or a tertiary care center focusing on high-risk care
- Philosophy of the staff
- Personnel who work with childbearing clients
- Usual pattern of visits, frequency of visits based on client's individual needs
- Length of visits
- What client may expect at visits
- Who is encouraged to attend visits with client; policy related to children accompanying clients
- Cost of care, method of payment accepted, provisions for clients unable to pay
- Who other than client is to be contacted for information about care (name, telephone number, address)

▶ OUTLINE OF A PRENATAL VISIT

APPOINTMENT

- Directions to facilities
- Information about length of visit
- Expectations for reimbursement

WAITING AREA

- Assessment begun (self-report forms, e.g., demographic information, health history)
- Health promotion: teaching materials available, e.g., posters, audiovisual programs, pamphlets, other literature

BEFORE CLIENT UNDRESSES FOR EXAMINATION

- Nurse and physician or certified nurse-midwife meets with client (separately or together)
- Assessment continued: review of client's self-report form, history taken; blood pressure, pulse, respiration, temperature, weight; in some settings, fingerstick for hemoglobin/hematocrit analysis; assessment data recorded
- Diagnoses made: information shared between nurse and physician or nurse-midwife prior to further examination

PREPARATION OF CLIENT FOR EXAMINATION

- Gown given
- Location for clothing shown (locker, closet, or hooks in examining room)
- Anticipatory guidance given
- Client instructed in collection of urine specimen
- Urine sample tested in unit or sent to laboratory

MEETING BETWEEN CLIENT AND PHYSICIAN OR NURSE-MIDWIFE

- Assessment continued: physical examination performed with female staff member in room
- Diagnoses made
- Teaching performed (In some settings, client may dress before meeting for postexamination interview.)

Note. Client may meet again with nurse for continued teaching on topics such as nutrition

SCHEDULING OF NEXT ANTENATAL APPOINTMENT

- Client referred to laboratory for further testing, e.g., blood sampling (Blood samples may be drawn by staff in some prenatal settings.)

The client coming for her initial visit may be advised of what to expect over the telephone and/or sent written information. Nurses should be aware of client responsibilities, such as employment or her need to be home when children return from school. Every effort is made to fulfill all health care needs in one visit, especially for clients who must take time from work or who live at a distance from the care facility.

Scheduling of Prenatal Visits. The client must be informed of the need for prenatal visits at least every 4 weeks during the first trimester. More frequent visits can be scheduled to meet client needs. Clients should also be given telephone numbers to call for advice and for answers to any questions they may have between visits.

Evolving a Data Base for Diagnosis Development

A comprehensive data base is established during the first visit, using the assessment process, which first identifies the reason for the client's visit (e.g., confirmation of pregnancy or continuing prenatal care) and includes a complete history and physical examination

with appropriate laboratory tests. The history is updated at subsequent visits throughout pregnancy. In history taking, a collaborative approach is used by health care providers.

Staff nurses participate in prenatal physical assessment and testing. Prior to the examination, the nurse ensures that equipment is prepared for the client. The box entitled Facilities and Equipment for Prenatal Examination lists suggested facilities and equipment for prenatal examination. The client is asked to void and instructed in the collection of urine samples. An empty bladder facilitates accurate pelvic assessment and minimizes discomfort. The nurse may perform urine tests to confirm pregnancy and to detect protein, glucose, and ketones in the urine. The nurse may also label and send specimens for laboratory urinalysis, culture, and sensitivity. The nurse provides the client with support and anticipatory guidance for pelvic examination.

Prior to the client's examination by the advanced practice nurse (nurse-midwife or women's health practitioner) or physician, the nurse takes and records the client's weight, blood pressure, pulse, respirations, and temperature. The nurse makes certain to bring any abnormalities in history or physical assessment to

► FACILITIES AND EQUIPMENT FOR PRENATAL EXAMINATION

FACILITIES

- Private examining area (ideally, private room)
- Adequate ventilation, temperature control
- Handwashing facilities in room
- Toilet facilities
- Writing surface for charting
- Examination table with stirrups for pelvic examination
- Movable light in working order

EQUIPMENT

- Clean barrier (paper or cloth) for examining table
- Examination gloves

- Specula in a variety of sizes
- Water-soluble lubricant for vaginal/rectal examinations
- Culture tubes, slides, and fixative for cultures and smears
- Stethoscope (considered a personal item and not shared among personnel)
- Sphygmomanometer
- Fetoscope (however, does not detect fetal heart rate during first trimester)
- Doppler device (may detect fetal blood flow through fetal heart during first trimester)
- Hand mirror for educational examination
- Emergency equipment (including oxygen and suction)

---

the attention of the advanced practice nurse or physician before assessment begins. In some settings, nurses may draw blood samples from fingersticks (for hemoglobin or hematocrit) or from the cephalic or brachial veins near the antecubital fossa. Nurses may perform hemoglobin or hematocrit testing in the prenatal setting or prepare and send blood tubes to specified laboratories for further analysis. Staff nurses may also perform tuberculosis screening, for example, with mantoux testing, for clients who are not known to be positive.

The nurse assists the client in getting onto the examining table, positioning properly for examination, and getting up from the table. A female staff member remains in the examining room throughout physical assessment as witness to proper conduct of the examination.

During the pelvic examination, the nurse helps the examiner as needed. For example, the nurse makes sure that equipment, such as the speculum, is accessible to the examiner.

Supporting the Client

Nursing strategies to provide support to the client during prenatal visits include remaining accessible and using therapeutic communication skills. The nurse stays with the client during her examination and is available to answer any questions. Attention should be directed to the client and her partner or toward collaboration with other staff in working with the client. Communication skills such as attentive listening and interest in client well-being promote the nurse–client relationship and are essential to the assessment process.

Some clients are frightened and uncomfortable during pelvic examinations. Identifying reasons for the fear, providing anticipatory guidance, using an educational approach to the examination, and, when needed, providing the comfort of a hand to hold during the exam can help to reduce anxiety.

Recognizing Cultural Influences

Success of any prenatal care strategy depends on the nurse's ability to recognize the client's cultural background and incorporate appropriate measures into care. Stereotyping, however, must be avoided. The nurse needs to identify individual prenatal cultural influences on each family. An open-minded, flexible approach and willingness to learn about different childbearing practices are essential for culturally sensitive care. In general, support may be given to any practices that do not jeopardize the health and safety of the client, the fetus, or the family.

Nurses need to be aware of how prenatal care and scheduling may conflict with the client's cultural background. For example, some expectant fathers, such as men from Orthodox Jewish or Moslem groups, may not wish to be present while their wives are immodestly garbed and positioned during pelvic examination. In addition, clients should not be pressured to attend prenatal visits at times that conflict with religious or cultural practices.

Several strategies may be used to communicate with clients who do not speak English. Clients should be encouraged to bring adult family members or friends who can serve as interpreters at their prenatal visits. In certain ethnic areas, staff who speak the language of the surrounding community are hired. Staff who act as interpreters must be individuals who are able to discuss with the client intimate topics related to pregnancy in a culturally appropriate context. Prenatal literature may be translated into a variety of languages; however, translations should be done only by individuals who have a strong command of the language and an understanding of prenatal care.

Facilitating Informed Decision Making

The client and her family have the right and responsibility to make informed decisions about pregnancy and prenatal care. The pregnant client's rights and responsibilities can be discussed. Risks and benefits of all pregnancy and birth options should be explained.

During the initial visit, the family's plans for birth are discussed. Specific aspects of the birth plan are finalized during the third trimester. In the first trimester, the client usually selects caregivers and a setting that will make desired aspects of childbirth possible. The nurse orients the client and her family to the childbearing setting and provides referrals for the client whose birth plan would be better implemented elsewhere.

The client must understand that no birth plan can be guaranteed. The need for alternative plans in case of complications must also be considered, as must the setting in which those alternative plans will take place.

Clients may have to make decisions about altering their lifestyle. For example, if the woman's daily activities at home or at work involve potential teratogens, she must make an informed choice about the activity. Nurses therefore need to be able to identify risks and reassure clients whose activities do not place them at risk during pregnancy.

Promoting Psychologic Adaptation to Early Pregnancy

Mixed feelings occur during early pregnancy among expectant mothers and fathers, even those who desire pregnancy. They may feel overwhelmed. Clients' concerns may include uncertainty about ways to inform others about the pregnancy, their own physical well-being, and early-pregnancy changes and discomforts such as nausea and fatigue. Among the nursing strategies that promote psychologic adaptation and parental role attainment are the following:

- Provide opportunities for the couple to discuss concerns during prenatal visits.
- Encourage clients to telephone if they have questions or concerns between visits.
- Reassure the couple about normal feelings and uncertainties.
- Reassure the couple that they have a lot of time to prepare emotionally for the baby.
- Encourage the client to talk with her own mother, sister, or other female relatives and friends, as evolving her own concept of the

maternal role is an important part of maternal role attainment and prenatal adaptation.
- Encourage similar behaviors for the expectant father. Unlike men in previous generations, expectant fathers in the United States today are encouraged to be nurturing and expressive. Therefore, some expectant fathers may find their own fathers or men of older generations surprised or reluctant to discuss paternal feelings.
- Inform the couple about early-pregnancy classes, which can provide an environment of group support and information.
- Assist the couple to identify whom they are concerned about informing of the pregnancy.
- Discuss ways that news of the pregnancy can be shared.
- Provide referrals for couples who need counseling.

Facilitating Family Attachment

As early as the first trimester, the nurse encourages behaviors that permit family members to support each other throughout pregnancy and develop feelings of closeness. This encouragement may be needed at a time when the expectant parents are ambivalent about the pregnancy and siblings may have not yet been told. Prenatal visits should be scheduled at convenient times for the entire family. The nurse may also assist the couple in planning how and when to inform siblings about the pregnancy.

Meeting Early-Pregnancy Educational Needs

Providing the client and family with information is one of the most important nursing responsibilities during prenatal care. Education focuses on health promotion, for example, teaching the client how to maximize feelings of wellness during the first trimester; on primary prevention, for example, teaching the client to avoid hazardous substances and situations; and on secondary prevention, for example, teaching the client to identify warning signs during pregnancy. All clients, including pregnant nurses, physicians, and others with backgrounds in obstetrics, should be given basic information.

Client education takes place throughout the prenatal visit. It focuses on explanations of current and future changes related to pregnancy. Waiting areas can be used for visual and audiovisual displays. Pamphlets and other printed literature should also be there for clients to take home. During physical assessment and an educational session afterward, teaching strategies, based on behavioral objectives, can be implemented on a one-to-one basis. The box entitled Client Teaching Guidelines During the First Trimester

► CLIENT TEACHING GUIDELINES DURING THE FIRST TRIMESTER

- Normal physiologic changes in first trimester
- Normal fetal growth and development
- Client safety
    Hazards during pregnancy
    Use of drugs and alcohol, smoking
    Threats to safety and security (seat belts, environmental hazards related to lifestyle, and high-risk behaviors)
- Pets
- Warning/danger signs of pregnancy
- Nutrition and weight management
- Dental health
- Discomforts of pregnancy during first trimester
- Sexuality

- Normal psychologic reactions to first trimester—client, expectant father and family; informing others of pregnancy; worries and concerns; adaptation
- Self-care practices to promote wellness
    Breast care
    Relaxation and stress reduction
    Posture and movement
    Exercise
    Clothing
    Food preparation
    Gardening activities
    Bathing and swimming
    Personal hygiene
    Travel

summarizes the topics that should be discussed during education sessions.

All pregnant clients and family members have questions. Although some clients bring specific questions to prenatal visits, others are too shy to ask or they "forget" when they are in the presence of a nurse, nurse-midwife, or physician. Encouragement and sufficient time are needed for clients to ask their questions. Clients can be encouraged to write down questions when they occur at home and bring them to prenatal visits.

Many pregnant women share concerns about certain topics. The nurse may anticipate these concerns and initiate discussion. Moreover, clients should leave any prenatal visit with a clear idea of whom to call about questions and concerns they may have between visits.

Promoting Nutritional Well-Being

As discussed in Chapter 14, nutritional counseling is one of the most important aspects of prenatal management. The types of foods selected and the time of day when foods and beverages are ingested may vary in response to pregnancy-related discomforts. For example, a first-trimester client experiencing nausea may tolerate only simply prepared foods without heavy spices, sauces, or odors. Small portions, spaced between periods of nausea, may ensure adequate intake.

Nutritional assessment begins at the initial visit and continues at each visit throughout pregnancy for every client. In establishing nursing diagnoses related to positive nutritional practices and well-being, the nurse assesses such parameters as the client's weight in relation to her height; current and past weight management practices; pattern of prenatal weight gain; hemoglobin and hematocrit levels; skin eruptions possibly related to poor diet; usual dietary intake; pattern of intake; and consumption of nonfood items. It is important to remember that clients whose weight is within normal limits, as well as wealthy or financially disadvantaged clients, may not eat a nutritionally adequate diet for pregnancy.

Nutritional management counseling should be tailored to the diets of the individual client and her family. In counseling the client, the nurse should keep in mind the price of foods, as well as their availability, and be prepared to counsel clients from a variety of cultural and financial backgrounds.

Management encompasses identifying the client at nutritional risk for physical, educational, psychologic, or financial reasons. Some women maintain their prepregnancy weight by constant dieting and may be extremely anxious about "losing" their figures and "getting fat." Nutritional counseling related to healthy prenatal patterns and weight management is necessary. Clients who gain more than the recommended weight between visits should be advised against vigorous dieting or exercising to "make up" for the gain. Referral to social services may make nutritional supplements available to financially disadvantaged women through such programs as the Special Supplemental Food Program for Women, Infants, and Children.

Assisting the Client to Cope with First-Trimester Discomforts

Discomforts during pregnancy evolve from such factors as hormonal changes and the growing uterus. A client's fear and anxiety may magnify perceptions.

 *Commonly Asked Questions*

Why am I so tired all the time, especially when I'm not doing anything differently?

Fatigue is normal during the first trimester and occurs regardless of the woman's activity level. The cause of fatigue has never been clearly identified. Fatigue is thought to occur in response to hormonal levels, physical changes, psychologic changes, and other factors.

Does "morning sickness" occur only in the morning?

No. Nausea and vomiting, "morning sickness," can occur at any time. Although most women experience episodes of nausea and vomiting during the first trimester, some women report that periods of nausea continue into the second and third trimesters.

Will cutting back on fluids help having to urinate frequently?

Frequency of urination occurs as the uterus enlarges and presses on the bladder. Urinary frequency will occur regardless of fluid restriction. Greater amounts of fluid do produce more urine and more frequent urination. Because of the risks of dehydration and the importance of fluids for normal pregnancy development, however, a daily fluid intake of 6 to 8 glasses of noncaffeinated beverages is recommended.

Are bleeding gums anything to be concerned about?

Gum changes during pregnancy are thought to occur because of increased hormone levels. During pregnancy, gums may be more sensitive to irritants in the mouth; however, bleeding need not occur and may be a sign of poor dental hygiene or periodontal (gum) disease. Any pregnant woman with bleeding gums needs to be evaluated by a dentist. It is also important to remember to inform the dentist of pregnancy, as pregnancy usually does not "show" during the first trimester. Dentists need to be aware that the client may be pregnant, because some dental medications and procedures may be contraindicated during pregnancy.

If I want to be in good physical condition should I start exercising vigorously now?

No. Pregnancy is no time to begin vigorous exercise programs, especially for the woman unaccustomed to heavy exercise; however, mild exercise such as walking is encouraged.

Will my working harm my pregnancy?

Employment alone is no reason to quit work during the first trimester. Daily activities at home and at work should, however, be evaluated. Any activity that poses a risk to safety and health, such as exposure to potentially teratogenic chemicals, should be avoided. This may involve a change in employment status or a transfer to another type of employment.

Before I was pregnant, my husband and I thought we wanted a baby so very much. Now that I am pregnant, we are both uncertain. Are these feelings normal?

Yes. Most women and men have mixed feelings about having a baby, especially during the first trimester of pregnancy. These feelings are normal and expected.

Is it too early to start thinking about plans for childbirth?

No. It is a good idea to begin thinking about the type of delivery you would like and to make certain that the health care providers and childbirth setting you select will support your decisions, such as for a birthing room delivery. Your actual birth plan, that is, your written plan for the birth experience, can be finalized during the third trimester.

Is it all right to have wine with dinner during the first trimester?

Wine, beer, or other alcoholic beverages are never recommended at any time during pregnancy, because of the potential for harm to the developing embryo and fetus. No safe level of alcohol has been established during pregnancy.

Careful assessment helps the nurse differentiate between normal discomforts related to healthy first-trimester changes and high-risk conditions. Through anticipatory guidance and counseling, the nurse can help the client cope with discomforts as temporary, although unpleasant, manifestations of pregnancy. Discomforts related to the first trimester are described below. Although discomforts such as varicose veins, hemorrhoids, and heartburn can occur during the first trimester, they are more frequent later in pregnancy. Therefore, such discomforts are discussed in Chapters 17 and 18.

Nausea and Vomiting—"Morning Sickness."
Nausea and vomiting, also referred to as **morning sickness,** occur in about 50 to 80% of pregnant women. As discussed earlier, these symptoms usually appear shortly after the first missed menses and end by the 12th week of gestation. Nausea with or without vomiting can occur at any time of the day.

No known treatment relieves nausea and vomiting for all women during the first trimester. The nurse must therefore thoughtfully assess the client to identify her unique reaction to this discomfort and suggest interventions that will be specifically helpful to her.

Many women benefit from knowing that nausea and vomiting are normal during pregnancy. It is necessary, however, for the nurse to realize that nausea and vomiting are real discomforts that occur when many other changes are taking place.

Ptyalism.
Ptyalism, an uncommon discomfort during pregnancy, usually occurs in women who also experience nausea, possibly because of the difficulty in swallowing anything while nauseous. Avoidance of swallowing increases the amount of saliva, which, in turn, may increase nausea. Although higher estrogen levels are suspected as the cause, this symptom is not well understood. Treatment varies, but includes encouraging women to swallow consciously, practice good oral hygiene, use mouthwash, suck hard candy, and chew gum. Ingestion of starch may stimulate salivary glands and should be discouraged.

Altered Taste.
During the first trimester, a woman may experience a bitter or sour taste in her mouth. The nurse can advise her to brush her teeth well, use mouthwash, chew gum, or suck hard candies (particularly mint or "tart" candies) in an effort to relieve the symptoms.

Bleeding Gums.
Beginning in the first trimester, hyperemia of the gums, perhaps related to increased estrogen secretion, may cause those tissues to be more friable. Periodontal disease may be accelerated during pregnancy and contribute to tooth loss. Bleeding gums during pregnancy are common; however, with a well-balanced diet, regular dental examinations, prophylactic professional cleanings, and conscientious home care (regular brushing, flossing, and gum stimulation), the incidence of sore, inflamed, bleeding gums (gingivitis) can be reduced or eliminated. Nurses should never ignore this condition, but instead refer clients who report bleeding gums for dental evaluation.

Breast Tenderness.
Breast tenderness, caused by elevated estrogen and progesterone levels, is particularly noticeable in the first trimester of pregnancy. Although tenderness usually resolves within the first trimester, the breasts often continue to enlarge throughout pregnancy. The mother should be encouraged by the nurse to wear a well-fitting support

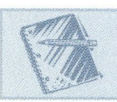 *Client Teaching*

Interventions to Relieve Nausea and Vomiting

The nurse can suggest the following strategies to the expectant mother to help relieve nausea and vomiting:

- Increase your intake of dry carbohydrate foods, such as plain crackers or dry cereal, which are easily digested. If the nausea occurs in the morning, keep soda crackers at your bedside and eat one or two before arising.
- Eat 5 to 6 small, frequent meals each day.
- Avoid greasy, fatty foods.
- Avoid fluids during meals.
- Drink fruit juices and milk between meals to meet fluid needs.
- Avoid odors that cause nausea and vomiting. Select menus that you can tolerate preparing. To decrease odors, improve ventilation by opening windows or turning on stove fans. Avoid using artificial room deodorants as their smell can increase, rather than relieve, nausea. Enlist the help of other family members in meal preparation.
- Change positions slowly, especially when getting out of bed in the morning.

brassiere. Warm showers may also provide the mother with some relief.

Urinary Frequency. Urinary frequency is a common discomfort during the first trimester of pregnancy. It begins around the 6th week and usually subsides as the uterus rises out of the pelvic cavity, around the 12th week. Urinary frequency may again be normally experienced during the third trimester, when the baby "drops" or "lightens". Urinary frequency is sometimes accompanied by leakage of urine, especially when the mother coughs or sneezes late in the pregnancy. The expectant mother can be reassured that these symptoms will subside when the pregnancy is completed. She can also be taught to perform Kegel exercises, contracting the muscles of the pelvic floor for 5 seconds frequently during the day (may be as many as 100 times per day). Kegel exercises tighten the pubococcygeal muscle, maintain good perineal muscle tone, and strengthen the urinary sphincter. Fluid intake should not be decreased to relieve frequency.

Urinary frequency can be a sign of urinary tract infection. Any reports of frequency therefore need to be evaluated carefully. Women must be taught about signs of urinary tract infection and advised to call their health care provider should the signs appear.

Nasal Stuffiness and Epistaxis. Increased estrogen levels during pregnancy can cause edema of the mucous membranes of the nasal cavity. Nasal stuffiness and discharge and epistaxis (nosebleeds) may occur. The expectant mother should be advised by the nurse to avoid the use of nasal decongestants and sprays, as well as other medications. Humidifiers, cool mist vaporizers (without medications added), or normal saline drops may relieve some of these symptoms.

Increased Vaginal Secretions (Leukorrhea). Leukorrhea begins during the first trimester. Some clients become distressed about this condition; others may worry they have an infection. Before advising the client, the nurse needs to identify why the client feels she may be infected and assess for signs of infection, for example, burning, itching, change in color of vaginal discharge, foul odor of the discharge, and temperature elevation. The client is advised to call her health care provider should any of these signs occur.

Pregnant women should be advised not to wear tampons to absorb secretions, because of the risk of infection. Good personal hygiene, including daily washing of the perineal area with water and a mild soap, is usually sufficient to control leukorrhea. Cotton underpants or absorbent external minipads may promote comfort.

Women's Health

Douching is not recommended for the pregnant woman who is experiencing leukorrhea. She may experience sensitive allergic reactions to the douching solution. In addition, during pregnancy, women are more susceptible to air and fluid embolisms resulting from vaginal instillation of air or fluid under pressure.

Fatigue. Early in the first trimester, the woman may begin to experience fatigue, which is possibly related to the physiologic and psychologic changes taking place. Fatigue can be an upsetting symptom, especially when a woman becomes tired out of proportion to her activities.

Before a woman's fatigue can be identified as a normal manifestation of pregnancy, anemia must be ruled out. Women may need to be treated for anemia.

The goals of nursing management for first-trimester fatigue help the woman to deal with related concerns and relieve or minimize fatigue. The best treatment for fatigue in a healthy woman is more frequent rest periods during the day; however, nurses need to be realistic and creative in their counseling. Evaluating daily activities at work and at home can aid in planning rest periods or relaxation exercises that are acceptable to the client. Indeed, even during a work day, brief relaxation exercises, such as closing the eyes and visualizing oneself in a restful environment, can promote feelings of well-being. Although rest means inactivity, relaxation involves knowledge of the muscular system and the ability to learn ways to release tension. Encouraging family members to assist the woman with specific tasks, such as laundry or shopping, not only promotes her rest, but fosters family communication.

Promoting Client Safety

Management includes a focus on client safety throughout pregnancy. To meet the goal of promoting safety during the first trimester, strategies are devised to prevent client injuries during prenatal visits and to teach the client about safety outside the office or clinic. For example, the nurse assists the client during the physical examination to prevent falls from the examining table. In addition, the nurse counsels the client about the importance of using seat belts in automobiles or about the importance of maintaining a clear pathway between her bed and the bathroom and, at bedtime, leaving a night light on, thereby helping to prevent falls while the client walks sleepily during the night.

Throughout the assessment process, the nurse helps the client identify threats to safety posed by her lifestyle or environment and to design ways to avoid or minimize them. Counseling relates to the client's daily activities, such as food preparation, caring for pets (especially cats), and gardening. Care strategies may include referring the client to a smoking cessation group. Occasionally, a client may need to change her work responsibilities to avoid teratogenic exposure or other high-risk situations. The nurse verifies for the client the need for a work transfer or a leave of absence for pregnancy-related reasons.

Promoting a client's safety includes educating her about warning and danger signs related to pregnancy (Table 15–7). Clients who experience any of these signs are advised to contact their health care provider without delay.

▶ **TABLE 15–7**

Warning/Danger Signs in Pregnancy

Sign	Characteristics
Headache	Persistent
	Severe
	Otherwise unusual
Altered vision	Blurring
	Double vision
	Seeing spots
Nausea	Persistent
	Intense
	Interfering with food or fluid intake
Vomiting	Intense
	Frequent
	Interfering with food or fluid intake
Epigastric pain	
Abdominal pain	Intense
	Persistent
	Unusual
Muscular irritability/ seizures	
Signs of infection	Fever of 101°F or above
	Burning with urination
	Flank pain
	Diarrhea
	Other
Vaginal bleeding	
Other vaginal discharge (not leukorrhea)	Gush of fluid
	Leakage of fluid
Decrease or cessation of fetal movement	

Evaluating Prenatal Care

Evaluation is part of the nursing process and enables the nurse to identify effective care strategies as well as strategies that need to be changed. Strategies that result in a healthy outcome for the mother, infant, and family are regarded as effective; however, despite the best strategies, the outcome at times may be poor. During the first trimester, the effectiveness of interventions may be reflected in a client's regular attendance at prenatal visits, behaviors that indicate prescribed strategies have been carried out, and the client's meeting with sources of referral.

Evaluating the effectiveness of teaching is at times difficult. Learning objectives need to focus on behaviors that can be observed. For example, a weight gain of a pound and a half between monthly visits during the first trimester or a client's report of a diet that is well balanced indicates her ability to meet nutritional needs of pregnancy.

Ensuring Appropriate Client Referral and Removing Barriers to Care

Through the assessment process the nurse frequently identifies client needs that require specialized referrals, such as social services or nutritional counseling. Working with the physician or nurse-midwife, the nurse can ensure that appropriate referrals are made for such services as ultrasound and CVS.

Nurses need to be knowledgeable about possible referral, including the nature and scope of services offered, the quality of the services, how clients can receive the services, and the costs involved.

Numerous barriers prevent clients from receiving early prenatal care during the first trimester. Some evolve from the client or family and some from the health care system.

As discussed earlier, socioeconomic factors, such as lack of insurance, inability to pay for health care, or lack of free prenatal services, limit access to prenatal care for economically disadvantaged women. Limited, expensive, or unsafe transportation and long waits in prenatal clinics make regular trips for prenatal care unfeasible. For example, the woman who has to travel for 2 hours to receive care and who has other responsibilities, such as preschool or school-aged children, may simply not be able to attend a prenatal visit that will keep her away from home after the school bus comes. Certain cultural groups may not value or accept the need for prenatal care during the first trimester.

Nurses can do much to help surmount barriers to early prenatal care, as shown in these examples:

1. Prenatal sessions can be scheduled to include evening or weekend hours. In this way, work-

ing women do not have to choose between their jobs and their health care.

2. Through professional nursing organizations, direct contact with legislators, and networking with private corporations, nurses can seek support to provide funds to make prenatal care accessible to all women.

3. Through roles as authors, speakers, producers, and consultants to the media, nurses can raise public awareness about the importance of early prenatal care.

4. By providing a welcoming and supportive attitude at all prenatal contacts, nurses can encourage clients to keep their first and subsequent prenatal visits.

5. By assessing barriers to prenatal care that individual clients may face, nurses can provide appropriate referrals to resources, for example, to social services or to prenatal clinics closer to the client's home. Nurses may also initiate change to reduce barriers in their own settings.

Contributing to General Prenatal Public Health

The growing importance of primary health care is particularly evident during childbearing. Public education campaigns are effective in teaching people of childbearing age about preconceptional and early prenatal health. Nurses will play an increasingly vital role in public education by serving as expert consultants to the media, schools, and community groups, as speakers on topics related to preconceptional and prenatal health, and as authors and producers of articles and programs. Through professional organizations, lobbyists, and direct contact with legislators, nurses can have further meaningful impact on prenatal health care.

Critical Thinking in Care Planning

Care of the Family During the First Trimester

Rosa and Anthony Martucci, ages 30 and 31, respectively, have come to the obstetrician's office because they suspect that Rosa is pregnant. They have been married for 2 years and this is their first pregnancy. Rosa was born in the Dominican Republic and came to the United States with her mother and older sister when she was 8 years old. She has a master's degree in business administration and is employed as a computer analyst. She expects to return to work after the baby is born. Anthony, an engineer, was born in the United States and is of Italian descent. The couple's religious affiliation is Roman Catholic.

Present Health Status

Rosa states that she has been in excellent health. She has regular health examinations, the last being 6 months ago when she was found to be in good health. She states that she is 2 weeks late with her period. A home pregnancy test performed 4 days ago was positive. Rosa admits that she is "compulsive" about not gaining weight. She tries to eat a well-balanced diet, avoiding red meat and caffeine. She also walks about 3 miles a day. Rosa states that she has recently been bothered by a "sour taste in her mouth from some foods" and tingling and fullness of her breasts. She also does not feel as energetic as she did prior to missing her period.

Anthony states that he has no health problems. He also tries to eat a balanced diet and exercise regularly.

Past Health Status

Childhood Illnesses

Rosa reports that her mother told her she had the childhood diseases measles, mumps, chickenpox, and rubella before the age of 12. She has no history of scarlet fever or strep infections.

Immunizations

She was immunized for diphtheria, pertussis, and tetanus (DPT), polio, and smallpox. Her last tetanus booster was 6 months ago.

Allergies

She has no known allergies to foods or medications. She occasionally complains of sinus congestion after cutting the lawn.

Hospitalizations and Other Illnesses
None.

Accidents and Injuries
None.

Medications

Acetaminophen approximately once a month for premenstrual headache. Occasionally takes decongestant for sinus congestion.

Habits

Client is in bed by 10 PM and arises at 6 AM during the work week. On weekends, she goes to bed "later and gets up later." She eats three meals a day, with no snacking. She does not smoke cigarettes, has never experimented with drugs, and has not consumed caffeinated or alcoholic beverages since hoping to become pregnant. She admits that her mother believes in certain cultural folklore with respect to pregnancy. "Certain foods should be avoided so that the baby will not be born with marks." Rosa, herself, does not ascribe to these beliefs, but tries to keep her mother happy when she is in her company.

Review of Systems

General

Height 5 ft 6 in. Usual minimum–maximum weight 118 to 120 pounds. Rosa states that she watches her weight carefully. Since missing her menses, she feels somewhat fatigued.

Integument

Denies rashes, bruising, color changes. States that sometimes her skin feels dry, especially in the winter. Skin lotions help the dryness.

Nails

No peeling, cracking, splitting, or biting of nails.

Critical Thinking in Care Planning continued

Hair

Does not use dyes, hairsprays, or gels. No loss of hair. Washes hair daily with baby shampoo.

Head

Complains of headache about once a month, over the eyes. Headache occurs 1 week prior to menstruation and is relieved by Tylenol Extra-Strength, 1 tablet.

Eyes

Reports visual acuity in both eyes. Denies blurred vision, infection, double vision, cataracts, or problems with night vision.

Ears

No discharge, pain, tinnitus, or history of hearing loss.

Nose and Sinuses

States that she occasionally has sinus congestion after cutting grass, which is relieved by a decongestant. Denies sinus pain, nasal discharge, problems with olfaction.

Mouth

Sees dentist every 6 months; has not had a cavity in 6 years. No history of gingivitis or bleeding gums. No swelling of mouth, lips, or tongue. Flosses teeth every day; brushes teeth three times a day.

Throat

No history of hoarseness or frequent sore throats.

Neck

Denies stiffness, pain, limitation of motion.

Lymph Nodes

Denies node enlargement or tenderness.

Respiratory

No history of bronchitis, pneumonia, tuberculosis, asthma, or emphysema. No history of difficult breathing, cough, hemoptysis, orthopnea, or night sweats. Mantoux test done last summer—negative.

Cardiovascular

No palpitations, cyanosis, precordial pain, edema, or varicose veins. No history of heart disease, rheumatic fever, or high blood pressure.

Gastrointestinal

No diarrhea, constipation, hemorrhoids, jaundice, or food intolerances. Lately she has experienced a sour taste in her mouth with some nausea in the morning.

Urinary

No history of kidney or bladder infection, hematuria, urgency, frequency, nocturia, incontinence, polyuria, or venereal disease.

Musculoskeletal

Reports occasional lower back pain when sitting at her desk, relieved by getting up and walking for a few minutes. No problems with range of motion.

Extremities

No history of arthritis, deformities, varicosities, phlebitis, discoloration, limited range of motion, or coldness. No joint pain, swelling, or redness.

Neurologic

No episodes of fainting, weakness, difficulty with balance, disorientation, hallucinations, depression, tremors, numbness, speech disorders, or tingling. No history of seizures, aphasia, loss of memory, paralysis, pain, or paresthesias. States she rarely has mood swings.

Hematopoietic

Denies history of blood disease, bleeding tendency, or transfusions. Blood type O+.

Endocrine

No polyuria, polydypsia, or polyphasia. No problems with thyroid, heat or cold intolerances, or hirsutism.

Reproductive Data

Menstrual History

Menarche 13 years. Since onset, menstrual cycle is 26 to 28 days, duration 5 to 7 days. No cramping; complains of headache 1 week before menses and breast tenderness. No dysmenorrhea, menorrhagia, infection, or pruritis. Has had Pap smear within last year. Denies use of tampons. Last menstrual period October 9 (6 weeks ago).

(continued)

Critical Thinking in Care Planning *continued*

Obstetric History
Has never been pregnant.

Presumptive Signs
Tingling and fullness of breasts, nausea, fatigue, amenorrhea.

Breasts
No masses or discharge. Self-examines breasts every month 1 week after menses. Experiences fullness in breasts prior to menses. Now feels fullness and tingling of breasts.

Nutritional History
Tries to eat a nutritionally sound diet, but admits to being very weight conscious. For breakfast, she eats a bowl of oatmeal with one cup of milk and a glass of water, fruit; for lunch, cottage cheese, decaffeinated tea with skimmed milk; and for dinner, two portions of vegetables, one small slice of fish or chicken, salad with dressing, and one glass of skimmed milk. Drinks water between meals; tries not to snack.

Family History
Significant family health histories include hypertension (both Rosa's mother and Anthony's father are being treated for chronic hypertension).

Social Data

Support Systems
Rosa feels that her husband is her greatest support. She would like them to experience the pregnancy, labor, and delivery together. She is close to her sister and her mother, and states she never knew her father. Her husband's family is close knit and he counts on them for emotional support during periods of crisis. Rosa and Anthony have a few close friends at their places of employment and some others maintained since school.

Home Environment
The couple recently purchased a one-family home, which has eight rooms, including three bedrooms and a spacious kitchen. Rosa states that she worries about the mortgage payments and feels she needs to return to work shortly after the baby is born. Her mother has agreed to come to live with them so that she can care for the baby, allowing Rosa to return to work.

Economic Status
The couple is in the middle-income socioeconomic group with potential for advancement in their careers. They both believe that the two incomes are necessary to maintain their household.

Occupational History
Rosa is a computer analyst and Anthony is an engineer. She experiences backache when sitting for prolonged periods. Both admit to stress in their employment, but also like their jobs.

Cultural Affiliations
The couple denies any customs that might affect their response to pregnancy. Rosa does admit that her mother has certain health beliefs regarding pregnancy. These include that pregnancy is a "hot" condition so that vitamins or iron tablets, which are considered "hot" medications, should be avoided. Rosa's mother also believes that antacids should be taken in the first 6 months of pregnancy so that the baby will not be "marked," and that the postpartum woman should not leave the house for 40 days after the birth of the baby. Rosa states that she herself does not hold to these beliefs, but that there may be some conflicts with her mother because she will come to live with them.

Sexual History
Rosa states that they both feel good about themselves and their sexual relationship. They feel they have a loving relationship. Both deny any problems with sexuality. Rosa used a diaphragm for 1 year. She stopped using the diaphragm 2 months ago. Both admit that the pregnancy was planned. Rosa states that she has some ambivalent feelings because of her career and wonders how she is going to handle motherhood and employment. She also has fears and anxieties regarding the pregnancy.

Exercise and Activity
The couple enjoys movies, music, and going out to dinner for relaxation. Both exercise daily; Rosa walks 3 miles a day.

Critical Thinking in Care Planning continued

Stress
Rosa states that when she experiences stress, she walks or reads a book. At work, she will close her eyes for a minute in an attempt to relax. Anthony states that if he feels stressed at work, he "takes a walk" during lunch break.

▶ Assessment

- Presumptive signs of pregnancy; tingling and fullness of breasts, nausea, fatigue, amenorrhea
- Early prenatal care:
  - regular health examination
  - regular exercise: walks 3 miles
  - no use of drugs, e.g., cigarettes, caffeine, alcohol
- Normal growth and development of embryo/fetus and placenta
- Physical examination revealing uterine enlargement and changes consistent with early pregnancy
- Normal maternal assessment data:
  - low risk history
  - vital signs: T 98°F, P 72, R 18, BP 110/70

- height, 5 ft 6 in.
- weight, 118 pounds
- urinalysis (protein, blood, glucose, acetone) negative
- blood studies: hematocrit 39, hemoglobin 13%, serology negative, glucose 80
- Physical examination: all systems within normal limits
- Discomforts related to pregnancy:
  - nausea in morning
  - fatigue
  - breast tenderness, tingling
  - sour taste in mouth

Nursing Diagnosis

Health seeking behaviors, related to pregnancy

Expected Client/Family Outcomes	Nursing Action/Intervention	Evaluation
Client and her support person will: • Be prepared for physical assessment prior to first examination.	Teach couple about physical examination including the pelvic examination. *Rationale:* Preparing couple will alleviate anxiety associated with a new process.	If asked, client is able to report that she has received teaching in preparation for the examination. Client behaviors may include familiarity with the procedure.
• Describe health care setting and program by end of first visit.	Introduce couple to personnel and setting; provide literature about the prenatal program. *Rationale:* Orientation of couple to health care personnel and setting helps establish a trusting relationship and alleviates fear of unknown.	Client completes tour and orientation program provided by staff. Client discusses program with the nurse or other health care provider.
• Identify physical changes that occur during first trimester by end of first visit.	Teach couple basic physiologic changes during first trimester and reasons for these changes. *Rationale:* Education regarding physiologic changes helps couple cope with changes and alleviates fear of the unknown.	When asked, client is able to discuss physiologic changes that occur during the first trimester by end of first visit.
• Identify warning signs of pregnancy complications by end of first visit.	Teach couple warning signs of pregnancy complications. Provide couple with outline of warning signs, including instructions of what to do and whom to call if they occur. *Rationale:* Knowledge of warning signs allows couple to seek prompt treatment.	When asked, client is able to describe warning signs of pregnancy complications by end of first visit. Client leaves

(continued)

Critical Thinking in Care Planning continued

Expected Client/Family Outcomes	Nursing Action/Intervention	Evaluation
		first visit with a written outline of warning signs of pregnancy complications and instructions about what to do and whom to call if they occur.
• Identify physical changes of second trimester by end of first trimester.	Teach couple regarding basic physiologic changes that occur in second trimester, including growth and development of fetus. *Rationale:* Anticipatory guidance helps couple cope with changes in second trimester.	By end of first trimester, client is able to discuss changes that occur during second trimester.
• Identify resources for information about pregnancy by end of first visit.	Explore with couple community resources related to pregnancy; provide list of resources. *Rationale:* Couple often requires information and support beyond the scope of prenatal services.	By end of first visit, client is able to identify appropriate resources. Client leaves first visit with a written list of resource agencies and programs.
• State purpose, procedures, and time required for first-trimester screening and assessment by end of first visit.	Inform couple of screening procedure; give relevant information concerning purpose, procedure, and time required. *Rationale:* Anticipatory guidance relieves anxiety.	Couple is able to make informed decisions. Couple describes and schedules screening procedures for first trimester; they realistically plan to fit procedure into their schedule.
Couple determines husband's participation in procedures during first trimester.	Give husband the option of remaining with his wife throughout prenatal examination. *Rationale:* Clients have right to make informed decisions about degree of participation of support persons.	Couple makes decision about husband's level of involvement.

Nursing Diagnosis

Potential asset in health care during pregnancy, related to positive health practices

By end of first trimester, client will continue prenatal self-care practices, such as pregnancy exercise.	Encourage client to continue to exercise, but allow for fatigue. Encourage couple to continue prenatal care; teach that their continued positive health care practices are an asset to pregnancy. *Rationale:* Effective coping with changes occurring during pregnancy is helped by positive health care practices prior to pregnancy. Couple should be given positive feedback as motivation to continue health care practices.	For a typical 24-hour period, client is able to describe healthy self-care practices, such as exercise, rest, and nutrition.

Critical Thinking in Care Planning continued

Expected Client/Family Outcomes	Nursing Action/Intervention	Evaluation
	Teach couple self-care practices specific to pregnancy. *Rationale:* Self-care allows people to participate in their health care. Participation helps people feel in control of their lives.	

Nursing Diagnosis

Potential asset for healthy newborn, related to normal development of fetoplacental unit

Throughout first trimester, client will: • Avoid potentially hazardous behaviors and substances related to intake or environment. • Identify deviations from healthy prenatal development. • Identify health-promoting behaviors.	Encourage client to continue activities that foster fetal development: to obtain adequate rest and nutrition and avoid harmful substances and exposure to infections and teratogens. Teach couple about fetal growth and development during the first trimester. *Rationale:* Teratogens have the greatest impact during the first trimester; safe practices are the responsibility of the client, but health care providers need to offer client the necessary information.	Client is able to identify any hazards in home or workplace. Client is able to identify positive health care practices: nutrition, rest, exercise. Couple describes their fetus during first trimester.

Nursing Diagnosis

Potential asset for healthy mother, related to normal pregnancy development

Throughout first trimester, client will: • Be screened for normal prenatal development. • Identify warning signs of pregnancy. • Identify health-promoting behaviors.	Discuss with client the pregnant patient's rights and responsibilities. Participate in screening hemoglobin, hematocrit, glucose, vital signs, urinalysis, height, weight, pelvic exam for size of uterus, clinical pelvic measurements. Teach couple about normal pregnancy changes during first trimester. Teach couple warning signs of pregnancy. *Rationale:* Preparing couple will minimize anxiety related to uncertainty; an understanding of warning signs of pregnancy will help clients promote their own health by early identification and follow-up of problems. Ongoing screening ensures early identification of risks.	Couple discusses pregnant patient's rights and responsibilities with understanding. Client regularly attends prenatal visits. Couple reports normal changes to nurse as they occur. Couple will verbally identify warning signs of pregnancy.

(continued)

Nursing Diagnosis

Knowledge deficit, related to comfort measures to manage normal physiologic pregnancy changes

Expected Client/Family Outcomes	Nursing Action/Intervention	Evaluation
Client will describe comfort measures for nausea, fatigue, breast tenderness, and sour taste by end of visit.	Teach client to eat dried soda crackers before arising in the morning; to decrease fluids during mealtimes. Reassure her that symptoms usually abate by end of first trimester. *Rationale:* :Eating dried carbohydrates and decreasing fluids during meals may help alleviate nausea. Nausea and vomiting abate by second trimester.	When asked, client is able to identify normal discomforts of pregnancy.
	Counsel client to elevate feet and close her eyes for a few minutes every hour during work, and to get 8 hours of sleep every night. *Rationale:* Method of closing eyes alleviates stress. Increasing rest periods may help with fatigue.	Client relates discomfort she is experiencing and comfort measures that were successful.
	Counsel client to wear support bra and take warm showers in effort to provide comfort for breast tenderness. *Rationale:* Warm showers and support bra provide comfort for breast tenderness.	Client leaves visit with written outline of normal discomforts related to pregnancy.
	Teach client to brush teeth as desired, use mouthwash, chew gum, or suck on hard candy. *Rationale:* Use of oral hygiene interventions will improve sour taste in mouth.	Client is able to identify specific relief measures she may use for discomforts related to first trimester. Client leaves visit with written outline of home relief measures to use for discomforts related to first trimester.

Chapter Highlights

► The first trimester of pregnancy is a critical period for development of the embryo/fetus and for initiation of physiologic changes in the mother's body systems.

► Maternal physiologic changes occur in the reproductive (uterus, cervix, vagina, fallopian tubes, ovary, and breasts), cardiovascular, respiratory, urinary, integumentary, gastrointestinal, and endocrine systems.

► The placenta acts as an endocrine gland during pregnancy, and produces estrogens, prog-

esterone, human chorionic gonadotropin, and human placental lactogen.

► Presumptive, probable, and positive symptoms and signs are used to identify pregnancy.

► Pregnancy brings change to the entire family system, and involves not only the mother-to-be, but the expectant father, siblings, and other family members.

► The woman's concerns tend to focus on herself and the early physical changes of pregnancy as

Chapter Highlights *continued*

well as her initial attempts to move into the role of the mother.

▶ The expectant father also progresses through a variety of stages during the first trimester and may experience couvade symptoms, such as weight gain and gas pains.

▶ Relationships between expectant parents and siblings begin to change during the first trimester due to the physiologic and psychologic alterations that occur within the childbearing family.

▶ Expectant parents look to their own parents as role models and as sources of support.

▶ Since a family's culture affects childbearing behaviors, nurses must strive to understand the cultural backgrounds of their clients and identify specific practices related to childbearing.

▶ Comprehensive assessment in the first trimester includes physical, psychosocial, socioeconomic,

and cultural dimensions and focuses on the client, her family, significant others, and home and work environments.

▶ Assessment of pregnancy is obtained through the use of ultrasound (both pulse echo imaging and Doppler) and estimation of delivery date through Nägele's rule, fundal height measurement, and sonograms.

▶ If certain risk factors are identified during prenatal assessment, several laboratory and diagnostic tests, such as urinalysis, blood studies, cytology, cultures, and chorionic villus sampling, may be performed.

▶ Nursing care during the first trimester is tailored to the unique needs of each client and should include physiologic, psychologic, and sociocultural aspects of the childbearing family.

After reading the vignette at the beginning of this chapter, use what you have learned to answer these questions:

1. What are the benefits and potential drawbacks of Jeanne Goodwin using her mother as a role model in responding to the experiences of pregnancy?

2. What strategies can Ann Salzman, CNM, MSN, suggest to help Jeanne Goodwin and her mother build on their relationship as a way for Jeanne to strengthen her sense of herself as a mother?

3. How might a client's desire to achieve an acceptable maternal role affect her physiologic and psychologic adaptation to the first trimester of pregnancy?

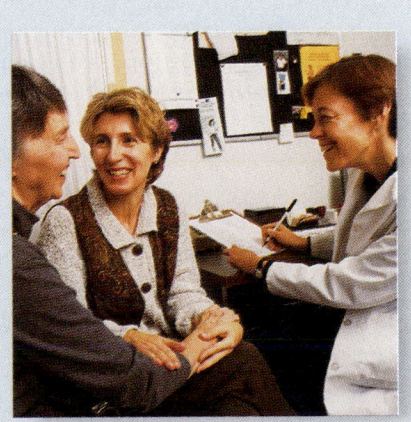

Critical Thinking Questions

► References

American College of Obstetricians and Gynecologists. (1993). *Ultrasonography in pregnancy* (Technical Bulletin No. 187). Washington, DC: Author.

American College of Obstetricians and Gynecologists. Committee on Genetics. (1995). *Chorionic villus sampling* (Committee Opinion No. 169). Washington, DC: Author.

Anderson, A.M. (1996). The father-infant relationship: becoming connected. *Journal of Pediatric Nurses, 1*(2), 83–92.

Beck, B. (1993). Body image and pregnancy: Building the mind–body connection: A guide for health care professionals. *Journal of Perinatology, 13,* 300–304.

Berkowitz, R.L. (1993). Should every pregnant woman undergo ultrasonography? *New England Journal of Medicine, 329,* 874–880.

Boemi, G., Bruno, M.T., La Ferrera, G., Butera, L., Pulvirenti, G., Lanzone, A., & Mancuso, S. (1996). Maternal renal and interlobar arteries waveforms evaluation with Doppler ultrasound in pregnancy-induced hypertension. *Fetal Diagnosis and Therapy, 11*(2), 132–136.

Boyd-Franklin, N. (1989). *Black families in therapy.* New York: Guildford.

Carlson, G. (1993). When grandmothers take care of grandchildren. *MCN, American Journal of Maternal Child Nursing, 18,* 206–207.

Chin, H. G. (1997). *On call obstetrics and gynecology.* Philadelphia: W.B. Saunders.

Cunningham, F.G., MacDonald, P.C., Gant, N.F., Leveno, K.J., Gilstrap, L.C., Hankins, G.D.V., & Clark, S.L. (1997). *Williams obstetrics* (20th ed.). Stamford, CT: Appleton & Lange.

Dallas, C., & Chen, S.C. (1996). Adolescent fatherhood in the black culture: An integrative review. *ABNF Journal, 7*(5), 118–123.

De Catte, L., Liebaers, I., Foulon, W., Bonduelle, M., & Van Assche, E. (1996). First trimester chorionic villus sampling in twin gestations. *American Journal of Perinatology, 13*(7), 413–417.

Erickson, M. (1996). Predictors of maternal-fetal attachment: An integrative review. *Online Journal of Knowledge Synthesis for Nursing, 3*(32), 1–26. Available: http://www.stti.iupui.edu/publications/journal/

Ferketich, S.L., & Mercer, R.T. (1995). Paternal-infant attachment of experienced and inexperienced fathers during infancy. *Nursing Research, 44*(1), 31–37.

Gurwitt, A.R. (1982). Aspects of prospective fatherhood. In S. Cath, A.R. Gurwitt, & J.M. Ross (Eds.), *Father and child: Developmental and clinical perspectives* (pp. 160–172). Boston: Little, Brown.

Harrington, K., & Campbell, S. (1993). Fetal size and growth. *Current Opinion in Obstetrics and Gynecology, 5*(2), 186–194.

Herzog, J.M. (1982). Patterns of expectant fatherhood: A study of the fathers of a group of premature infants. In S. Cath, A.R. Gurwitt, & J.M. Ross (Eds.), *Father and child: Developmental and clinical perspectives* (pp. 50–68). Boston: Little, Brown.

Hsieh, F.J., Shyu, M.K., Sheu, B.C., Lin, S.P., Chen, C.P., & Huang, F.Y. (1995). Limb defects after chorionic villus sampling. *Obstetrics and Gynecology, 85*(1), 84–88.

Hung, J.H.H., Ng, H.T., Pan, Y.P., Yang, M.J., & Shu, L.P. (1997). Color Doppler ultrasound, pregnancy-induced hypertension and small-for-gestational-age fetuses. *International Journal of Gynecology and Obstetrics, 56*(1), 3–11.

Jezewski, M. (1993). Culture brokering as a model for advocacy. *Nursing Health Care, 14,* 78–85.

Jurkovic, D., Gruboeck, K., & Campbell, S. (1995). Ultrasound features of normal early pregnancy development. *Current Opinion in Obstetrics and Gynecology, 7*(6), 493–504.

Kavanaugh, K., & Kennedy, P. (1992). *Promoting cultural diversity.* Newbury Park, CA: Sage.

Knuppel, R.A. (1994). Maternal-placental-fetal unit: Fetal and early neonatal physiology. In A.H. DeCherney & M.L. Pernoll (Eds.), *Current obstetric and gynecologic diagnosis and treatment* (8th ed.) (pp. 155–182). Norwalk, CT: Appleton & Lange.

Kornman, L.H., Morssink, L.P., Beekhuis, J.R., De Wolf, B.T., Heringa, M.P., & Mantingh, A. (1996). Nuchal translucency cannot be used as a screening test for chromosomal abnormalities in the first trimester of pregnancy in a routine ultrasound practice. *Prenatal Diagnosis, 16,* 797–805.

Lederman, R.P. (1996). *Psychosocial adaptation in pregnancy: Assessment of seven dimensions* (2nd ed.). New York: Springer.

Lee, T.Y. (1994). Maternal-fetal attachment in normal and previously-infertile Chinese women. *Nursing Research (China), 2*(1), 67–77.

McDermott, J.M., Drews, C., Adams, M., Berg, C., Hill, H.A., & McCarthy, B.J. (1996). Factors associated with inadequate prenatal care during the second pregnancies among African-American women. *Journal of Nurse Midwifery, 41*(5), 368–376.

Merce, L.T., Barco, M.J., & Bau, S. (1996). Color Doppler sonographic assessment of placental circulation in first trimester of normal pregnancy. *Journal of Ultrasound in Medicine, 15*(2), 135–142.

Mitra, A.G., Laurent, S.L., Moore, J.E., Blanchard, G.F., Jr., & Chescheir, N.C. (1996). Transvaginal versus transabdominal Doppler auscultation of fetal heart activity: a comparative study. *American Journal of Obstetrics and Gynecology, 175*(1), 41–44.

Morgan, M. (1996). Prenatal care of African American women in selected USA urban and rural cultural contexts. *Journal of Transcultural Nursing, 7*(2), 3–9.

Muller, M.E. (1996). Prenatal and postnatal attachment: A modest correlation. *Journal of Obstetric, Gynecologic, and Neonatal Nursing, 25*(2), 161–166.

Murrell, N.L., Smith, R., Gill, G., & Oxley, G. (1996). Racism and health care access: A dialogue with childbearing women. *Health Care for Women International, 17*(2), 149–159.

Nobel, P.L., Abraha, H.D., Snijders, R.J., Sherwood, R., & Nicolaides, K.H. (1995). Screening for fetal trisomy 21 in the first trimester of pregnancy: Maternal serum free beta-hCG and fetal nuchal translucency thickness. *Ultrasound in Obstetrics and Gynecology, 6*(6), 390–395.

Pandya, P.P., Snijders, R.J., Johnson, S.P., De Lourdes Brizot, M., & Nicolaides, K.H. (1995). Screening for fetal trisomies by maternal age and fetal nuchal translucency thickness at 10 to 14 weeks of gestation. *British Journal of Obstetrics and Gynecology, 102*(12), 957–962.

Patterson, K. (1993). Experience of risk for pregnant black women. *Journal of Perinatology, 13,* 279–284.

Rubin, R. (1984). *Maternal identity and maternal experience.* New York: Springer.

Salvesen, K.A., & Eiknes, S.H. (1995). Is ultrasound unsound—A review of epidemiological studies of human exposure to ultrasound. *Ultrasound in Obstetrics and Gynecology, 6*(4), 293–298.

Sherwen, L. (1991). Fantasy state during pregnancy: A psychoanalytic account. *Journal of Perinatal Psychology, 6,* 55–71.

Strom, R., & Strom, S. (1992). *Achieving grandparent potential: Viewpoints on building intergenerational relationships.* Newbury Park, CA: Sage.

Weiner, Z., Reichler, A., Zlozover, M., Mendelson, A., & Thaler, I. (1993). The value of Doppler ultrasonography in prolonged pregnancies. *European Journal of Obstetrics and Gynecology and Reproductive Biology, 48*(2), 93–97.

Wenger, A. (1993). Cultural meaning of symptoms. *Holistic Nursing Practice, 7,* 22–35.

Zachariah, R. (1994). Maternal-fetal attachment: Influence of mother-daughter and husband-wife relationships. *Research in Nursing and Health, 17,* 37–44.

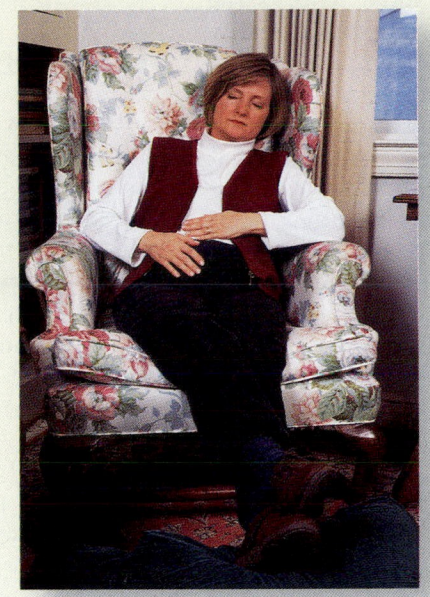

Laura O'Connor is 12 weeks' pregnant with her third child. During her last prenatal visit, Laura reported to the nurse practitioner that she had been feeling more tired than usual. A complete blood count revealed Laura's hemoglobin level at 10 g/dL and a hematocrit of 30%. Additional laboratory testing confirmed that Laura is experiencing iron-deficiency anemia. She is counseled to take ferrous sulfate tablets, 60 mg, once a day.

After a few days of taking the oral iron supplement before breakfast, Laura experiences nausea and constipation, especially in the late morning and early afternoon. She worries that her discomfort is interfering with her desire to eat and gain the necessary weight for her baby's growth. She is also concerned that coping with the effects of the treatment is affecting the care of her older children. She remembers that the nurse practitioner had suggested that she eat certain foods that are high in iron and thinks to herself, "Maybe if I eat these foods instead of taking these iron pills, I will feel better and the anemia will be treated." ∎

16

The Expectant Family at Risk: First Trimester

During the first trimester of pregnancy, a woman's body undergoes many physiologic changes as the embryo grows and develops into a fetus. At the same time psychologic changes are occurring as the reality of approaching motherhood is validated.

Complications in the first trimester are often approached differently from complications in subsequent trimesters. Many women may not realize that they are pregnant when help is sought for a health care need. As a result they often do not present themselves in a maternity or obstetric setting and may be quite amazed to learn that they are pregnant.

If problems are so severe that viability of the embryo or first-trimester fetus is questioned, very little can usually be done. Perinatal medicine has not advanced to the point where treatment in such situations is definitive. A waiting and watching approach may develop. Sometimes, symptoms are so severe that the mother's life is endangered and pregnancy termination is elected. When medical conditions exist prior to the pregnancy, the mother's symptoms often become increasingly critical as the pregnancy progresses. For these clients, however, the first trimester often is relatively free of problems compared with later trimesters.

It is somewhat difficult to characterize specific conditions as complications that occur during the first trimester of pregnancy because many continue into the second and third trimesters. Two categories of conditions that occur during the first trimester are discussed in this chapter: hemorrhagic conditions, specifically spontaneous abortion and ectopic pregnancy; and metabolic conditions, including hyperemesis gravidarum, anemia, and thyroid disorders.

The nurse plays an important role in assisting the client and her family to deal with such complications in a positive manner. The nurse's ability to make clinical judgments is crucial, as care derived from such judgments may be lifesaving. Assessment skills are important in providing data on the nature and extent of the problem so that appropriate care can be planned, implemented, and evaluated for effectiveness. Both physical and emotional supportive measures are needed to assist the pregnant woman and her family in understanding and coping with the high-risk condition occurring during the first trimester.

▶ HEMORRHAGIC CONDITIONS

Vaginal bleeding during pregnancy, except for very light spotting, is a serious complication that demands immediate attention. The two major causes of bleeding in early pregnancy are spontaneous abortion and ectopic pregnancy.

▶ Spontaneous Abortion

Abortion is the termination of a pregnancy before the fetus is viable. A fetus of less than 20 weeks' gestation or weighing less than 500 g is considered an abortus, even though the exact age when a fetus is sufficiently developed to survive is difficult to determine.

The term *abortion* may be used by health care personnel to describe either a spontaneous or an induced event. A **spontaneous abortion** is the expulsion of the products of conception occurring naturally and without external cause. An **induced abortion** is one that is artificially initiated by the use of medications or mechanical means for therapeutic or personal reasons. Laypeople, however, commonly use the word *miscarriage* to describe a spontaneous abortion and may become upset at the use of the word *abortion* to describe an event over which they had no control.

As many as one in five pregnancies ends in a spontaneous abortion. Many pregnancies may not be identified before the abortion occurs, however, so the rate may actually be higher. Most occur during the first 12 weeks of gestation. The incidence decreases rapidly thereafter. The incidence increases from 12% in women less than age 20, to 26% in those over age 40 (Cunningham et al., 1997).

Types
The types of spontaneous abortion include threatened, incomplete, complete, inevitable, missed, and habitual.

Threatened Abortion. A **threatened abortion** is suggested when a woman experiences vaginal spotting or bleeding early in pregnancy (Fig. 16–1A). Often, but not always, uterine cramping and backache are reported. The bleeding is usually slight, but may continue for several days or weeks. No cervical dilation is present. Threatened abortion is estimated to occur in about 20% of all diagnosed pregnancies. Of this percentage, approximately half abort (Cunningham et al., 1997).

Incomplete Abortion. An **incomplete abortion** occurs when cervical dilation results in partial expulsion of the products of conception, with some of these products retained in the uterus (Fig. 16–1B). The placenta is more likely to be retained after the 10th week of pregnancy. When tissue remains in utero, the uterus is unable to contract completely, and blood vessels leading to the placenta are not adequately

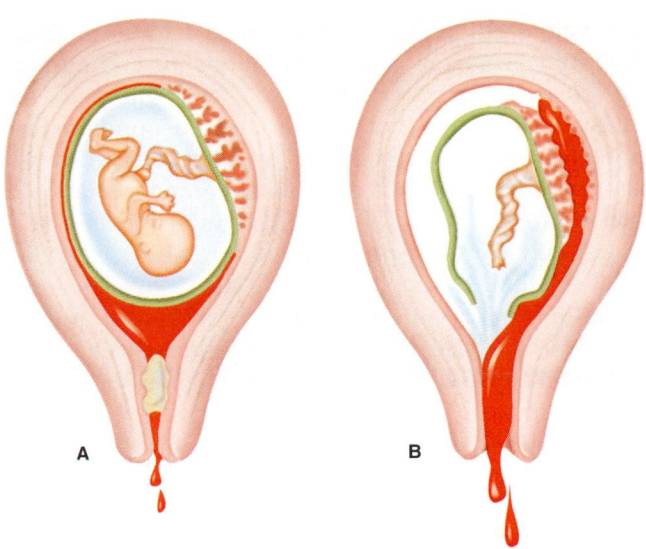

FIGURE 16–1. Two types of spontaneous abortion. **A.** Threatened abortion. **B.** Incomplete abortion.

compressed by uterine muscle fibers. Excessive vaginal bleeding results. Retained tissue also increases the risk of infection.

Complete Abortion. All products of conception are entirely expelled in a **complete abortion.** Very few physical complications occur with a complete abortion, but emotional support is necessary.

Inevitable Abortion. An **inevitable abortion** occurs when the cervix has begun to dilate, uterine contractions are uncomfortable, and vaginal bleeding increases. Tissue may not have been passed. The membranes rupture as the process proceeds. Ultrasound may reveal the gestational sac in the dilated lower uterine segment. This type of spontaneous abortion cannot be prevented.

Missed Abortion. The fetus dies in a **missed abortion,** but continues to be retained in the uterus 8 weeks or longer. Clinical assessment indicates that the uterus has stopped enlarging; it may become smaller as amniotic fluid is absorbed and the fetus degenerates. The woman loses a small amount of weight and has a brownish vaginal discharge. Pregnancy symptoms, such as nausea and breast tenderness, disappear. A pregnancy test may become negative as the placenta stops producing gonadotropin. Fetal heart tones are absent. Infrequently, a coagulation defect—disseminating intravascular coagulation (DIC)—develops (Chapter 19). Rarely, a fetus is retained long enough that it calcifies.

Habitual Abortion. When a woman has three or more consecutive spontaneous abortions, it is termed **habitual abortion.** It is an extremely distressing experience. Possible causes include chronic pelvic infection, reproductive hormonal imbalances, inherited chromosomal anomalies, autoimmune disease, and structural defects in the reproductive tract.

Etiology

About 50% of spontaneous abortions result from chromosomal abnormalities in the embryo or fetus. The most common chromosomal defects are autosomal trisomies (Ransom & McNeeley, 1997). There is not much known about paternal factors that contribute to spontaneous abortion (Cunningham et al., 1997). The maternal factors associated with spontaneous abortion include the following:

- *Infections.* Maternal infections that have been associated with spontaneous abortion include herpes simplex, syphilis, and vaginal colonization with group B streptococci (Cunningham et al., 1997).
- *Progesterone deficiency.* An insufficient quantity of progesterone secreted by the corpus luteum may cause inadequate endometrium to maintain the pregnancy (Ransom & McNeeley, 1997).
- *Autoimmune factors.* Immunological factors have been implicated in recurrent spontaneous abortion. The presence of anticardiolipin antibodies, which belong to a family of autoantibodies known as antiphospholipid antibodies, are believed to cause spontaneous abortion through increased blood coagulation at the site of the placenta (Ament, 1994).
- *Drugs and environmental chemicals.* Drugs that have been associated with spontaneous abortion include chemotherapy for cancer treatment and some antibiotics. Cigarette smoking and alcohol consumption have also been linked to spontaneous abortion. Examples of environmental chemicals are organic solvents, mercury, and toulene.

The associations that have been made between cigarette and alcohol consumption and spontaneous abortion show that the risk is greater with increasing consumption (Armstrong, McDonald, & Sloan, 1992). Mills and co-workers (1993) did not find any evidence that moderate caffeine intake increased the risk of abortion, although this relationship has been reported elsewhere (Armstrong, McDonald, & Sloan, 1992).

Evaluation of workplace exposure to reproductive hazards is difficult because multiple agents and exposure to nonoccupational hazards may be involved. There is evidence that there may be an association between occupational exposure to certain glycol ethers and adverse reproductive outcomes (Snow, 1994). An increased risk for spontaneous abortion has also been reported among dental assistants exposed to 3 or more hours of nitrous oxide in offices without scavenging equipment (Rowland, Baird, Shore, Weinberg, Savitz, & Wilcox, 1995).

Exposure to any environmental agent that is potentially harmful to a pregnancy should be considered threatening until the relationship of the substance to fetal loss and fetal development can be determined.

Often the cause of a spontaneous abortion is not known. Cunningham and coworkers (1997) described maternal conditions that are suspected causes, but for which evidence is not totally convincing: congenital anomalies of the uterus; debilitating systemic disease, such as metabolic disorders or severe nutritional deficiencies; psychologic stress; and physical trauma.

Nursing and Collaborative Assessment

Observing signs and symptoms is an essential element in the assessment of spontaneous abortion. The classic symptom for all spontaneous abortion is vaginal bleeding, which may be dark spotting and progress to frank, bright red bleeding.

Careful assessment is required to determine whether the cause of the bleeding is a threatened abortion. It must be differentiated from other possible causes of bleeding, including cervical polyps, hydatidiform mole, ectopic pregnancy, carcinoma of the cervix, and normal implantation of the blastocyst (Gilbert & Harmon, 1993). (See Table 16–1 for assessment techniques for spontaneous abortion.)

Assessment to differentiate spontaneous abortion from other possible causes of bleeding is done. For example, a speculum is used to examine the cervix and vagina for polyps; a Pap smear is done to help determine cervical carcinoma; ultrasound examination rules out an ectopic pregnancy and will reveal an intrauterine gestational sac; serial ultrasounds determine lack of fetal growth; and serial radioimmunoassay tests determine the level of human chorionic gonadotropin (hCG) (Gilbert & Harmon, 1993).

A pelvic examination will determine signs of cervical dilation. Assessment is also done for signs and symptoms of intrauterine infection, including a fever higher than 100.4°F (38°C), a white blood cell count greater than 16,000, foul-smelling vaginal discharge, general malaise, and urinary urgency or frequency. Other blood values, including hemoglobin and hematocrit, may indicate anemia resulting from blood loss (Gilbert & Harmon, 1993). In general, anemia in women is reflected in a hemoglobin of less than 12.0 g/dL, and during pregnancy, a hemoglobin of less than 11.0 g/dL.

When a woman is bleeding vaginally, the nurse should ask her how many weeks pregnant she is; if tissue or amniotic fluid was discharged; and what other symptoms, such as cramps or abdominal pain, are present. Determining the parents' responses to the vaginal bleeding is also important. Are they sad or frightened? Do they blame themselves or each other?

Nursing Diagnoses

Once the assessment data have been collected and analyzed to determine the cause of vaginal bleeding, the nurse formulates appropriate nursing diagnoses that will become the basis of the plan of care. Examples of nursing diagnoses are:

Problem-oriented diagnoses:

- Anxiety, related to threat of pregnancy loss
- Dysfunctional grieving, related to inability to express feelings for lost pregnancy

▶ **TABLE 16-1**

Assessment Techniques for Spontaneous Abortion

Technique	Purpose
Pelvic examination	Determination of cervical dilation; presence of vaginal polyp
Ultrasound	Visualization of an intrauterine gestational sac with central echoes from the embryo
Serial ultrasound	Determination of fetal growth or lack of fetal growth for gestational age
Serial radioimmunoassay	Determination of human chorionic gonadotropin (hCG) level
Serum progesterone values	Determination of presence of a live intrauterine pregnancy
Hemoglobin and hematocrit	Determination of anemia resulting from bleeding
Leukocyte count	Determination of elevated white blood cell count (greater than 16,000) resulting from infection
Vital signs	Determination of fever (greater than 100.4°F or 38°C) resulting from infection
Other	Analysis of client reports about experience of foul-smelling vaginal discharge, urinary urgency or frequency, and general malaise

Wellness-oriented diagnoses:

- Asset in grieving, related to ability to express feelings concerning pregnancy loss to significant others

Nursing planning and implementation is based on the prognosis of the pregnancy and the nursing diagnoses. The nurse plans holistically, taking into account the psychosocial needs of the family as well as the physical needs of the mother. Anticipatory guidance should be given to every pregnant woman about the occurrence of bleeding during pregnancy.

Nursing and Collaborative Management

When bleeding occurs, the woman should contact her health care provider. The severity of a client's symptoms determines the aggressiveness of treatment for vaginal bleeding. If vaginal examination determines that the cervix remains closed, watching and waiting is a general guide to care. The woman is usually advised to stay in bed, as bedrest may help maintain the pregnancy. If pain accompanies bleeding, the prognosis is less hopeful; however, the condition may resolve without additional threat of abortion. Intercourse or orgasm should be avoided for 2 weeks after any bleeding.

Ultrasound assessment is done regularly to help determine the pregnancy's continuing viability. The nurse explains to the woman that ultrasound reliably establishes the presence of a gestational sac.

If symptoms persist, the woman may be advised to resume normal activities in an attempt to hasten the process of abortion. Because most abortions result from fetal abnormalities, many clinicians question whether any attempt should be made to retain a pregnancy when symptoms of abortion are present.

If abortion proceeds, it is important that all of the products of conception be expelled because retention of the products of conception can lead to hemorrhage. Intravenous oxytocin (Pitocin) in solution may be given to promote expulsion. If the cervix is not partially dilated, prostaglandin E_2 vaginal suppository or gel, or laminaria dilators, may be used (Gilbert & Harmon, 1993). If these measures are ineffective, the products of conception must be removed surgically. A uterine curettage is most often done.

Inspection for complete expulsion is important. The client, whether at home or hospitalized, should be instructed to save all clots and tissues that are passed so that they can be inspected.

Inevitable and incomplete abortions, on the other hand, require prompt nursing action. Hemorrhage is a priority. Vital signs are monitored frequently, and the amount and character of vaginal bleeding are continually assessed. Is blood dark brown or bright red? Is bleeding heavy, moderate, or light? All clots and tissues are saved for examination.

The woman must be carefully observed for signs of shock, such as dizziness, light-headedness, decreased blood pressure, and increased pulse. Rho(D) immune globulin must be given within 72 hours after delivery of the fetus if the mother's blood type is Rh negative. Nursing responsibilities also include continued observation for signs of infection and reporting any that are detected.

Uterine cramping is uncomfortable for a woman experiencing an abortion. The nurse's calm, supportive approach may help promote relaxation. Slow, rhythmic back rubs and abdominal breathing also promote relaxation. The nurse can be supportive by reassuring the woman that she is managing well. Comfort measures—ice chips if allowed, cool, smooth linens, and comfortable positioning—may all prove helpful. Analgesics may be prescribed to lessen the discomfort.

Nursing management must also address the psychologic needs of a family experiencing a spontaneous abortion. Vaginal bleeding after pregnancy is

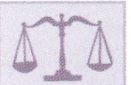 *Ethical Decision Making*

Mary Clark is 10 weeks' pregnant. She was placed on bedrest one week ago because of vaginal bleeding. The obstetrician diagnosed a threatened abortion and suggested that she stay home from work and on bedrest. Mary has no health or sick leave benefits. She insists that although she wants this pregnancy desperately, she also needs to continue working. She also wonders whether there might be "something wrong" with the fetus.

As the nurse caring for this client, consider the following questions:

1. If, after a reasonable period of bedrest, Mary is still experiencing vaginal bleeding, cramping, or both, should she be encouraged to become more active in an attempt to speed up the spontaneous abortion?
2. What are the factors in Mary's situation that contributed to your decision?
3. If Mary's situation had been different, would you have made another decision? If so, what would the decision have been?

confirmed is frightening for the woman and her family. Waiting and watching is often difficult, although it may be the only treatment suggested by the clinician. Because many, if not most, women and persons close to them are somewhat ambivalent at the diagnosis of a pregnancy, loss of the pregnancy may cause significant guilt. Before they have accepted being pregnant, the pregnancy is lost. The guilt is often expressed in terms of wishing and wondering if the mother should have done things differently. Should I have eaten better? Did playing tennis or jogging cause the abortion?

Anger and disappointment are often common emotions expressed after a spontaneous abortion. This is particularly true when the pregnancy is planned. Often a woman prepares for pregnancy long before it occurs. She may begin paying close attention to her diet, drinking more milk, and eating fresh vegetables. She stops taking all prescription or over-the-counter drugs and stops smoking. To this woman, the fetus is much more than a mass of cells. The fetus is already an infant to whom definite attachment has begun.

Nursing research (Bansen & Stevens, 1992; Beil, 1992) has explored responses of women and their families to spontaneous abortion. These studies show that all mothers mourn the involuntary loss of a pregnancy, but with varying degrees of intensity. The fetus has not yet taken on specific physical characteristics or gender for the family. They must, therefore, grieve for their fantasies of the unseen, unborn child. The significance of the loss may be unrecognized by the woman as well as her family. Grief may last from 6 months to a year, or even longer. Men's experiences with their partners' miscarriage include seeking help and accepting as they move through the grieving process (Miron & Chapman, 1994).

Feelings of anger, disappointment, and sadness are commonly experienced by the couple. The couple may want and need to express the intense feelings that are evoked by the loss of their child, but may believe that family, friends, and often health care personnel are uncomfortable or unable to provide emotional support after a spontaneous abortion. No societal customs, such as a funeral or period of mourning, exist to acknowledge the loss. Anniversaries of the abortion may precipitate feelings of loss (Jones, 1997).

The nurse can help the woman deal with her feelings and grief. Open-ended questions and active listening help initiate emotional healing. The nurse should recognize that a range of feelings are commonly experienced by women after a spontaneous abortion and permit the client to acknowledge and deal with her feelings. Empathetic listening is an essential therapeutic intervention.

Often restlessness, malaise, insomnia, and a general feeling of dissatisfaction follow spontaneous abortion. Women need to know that these feelings are normal. Support groups are available to help women cope (Steele & Knight, 1995; Walters & Nelson, 1997). If grieving is unresolved over a long period or dealing with the abortion is particularly traumatic, counseling services may be suggested.

The woman's partner and other family members may also experience grief. For them to acknowledge and express their feelings is important, especially if they are a source of support for the primary client.

The importance of advising the client about what to expect regarding medical intervention, pelvic examination, and laboratory testing cannot be overstated. Spontaneous abortion is a frightening experience; however, the client can be helped to regain a sense of control by understanding the expected sequence of events and the prognosis for future pregnancies.

Research Abstract

Men's Experiences with Their Partner's Miscarriage

The purpose of this qualitative study was to investigate men's experiences with their partner's miscarriage. Eight men whose partners had experienced 10 miscarriages were interviewed. The men described four sequential phases that they had experienced: recognizing signs, confirming the news, working through it, and getting on with life. The four concepts that emerged from the data were: (1) living the feelings, (2) waiting, (3) seeking help, and (4) accepting. Supporting was the basic social process that emerged.

Application to Practice

It is important that fathers' as well as mothers' experiences with miscarriage are considered by the nurse. Fathers need nursing support to work through their feelings during this crisis.

Source: Miron, J., & Chapman, J.S. (1994). Supporting men's experiences with the event of their partner's miscarriage. Canadian Journal of Nursing Research, *26(2), 61–72.*

The grief caused by the death of a baby can affect families for years and influence attitudes toward subsequent pregnancies (Walters & Nelson, 1997). The woman may delay verifying the pregnancy or seeking prenatal care until the first trimester has passed. She may not tell her family or friends about the pregnancy to avoid "jinxing" the outcome, or remain detached from the fetus to prevent hurt if the pregnancy is lost.

▶ Ectopic Pregnancy

An **ectopic pregnancy** is any pregnancy that occurs when the fertilized ovum implants in tissue other than the lining of the uterus. Ectopic pregnancy is classified as tubal, ovarian, cervical, or abdominal, depending on the implantation site. The majority of ectopic pregnancies, close to 98%, implant in the fallopian tube. Rare sites of implantation include the abdomen (0.75 to 1%), ovary (1%), and cervix (less than 1%) (Fig. 16–2). This section focuses on tubal ectopic pregnancies, as they are by far the predominant form.

Ectopic pregnancy is a serious problem that accounts for 10% of maternal mortality (Cunningham et al., 1997). It is the leading cause of pregnancy-related death during the first trimester (Powell &

Spellman, 1996). The incidence is about 16 per 1000 pregnancies, with the rate of ectopic pregnancies increasing four times over the past 20 years (Ransom & McNeeley, 1997). In addition, rates are higher for nonwhite women and increase with age in both white and nonwhite women (Cunningham et al., 1997).

The increase in ectopic pregnancies among women of childbearing age is attributed to the following factors:

- Pelvic inflammatory disease (PID) and endometriosis (Cunningham et al., 1997)
- Use of intrauterine devices (IUDs) (Cunningham et al., 1997)
- Tubal surgery (Cunningham et al., 1997)
- Congenital tubal anomalies such as diverticula, accessory tubes, and excessively long tubes
- Tubal tumors
- History of previous ectopic pregnancy
- Abdominal or pelvic surgery
- Appendicitis
- Therapeutic abortion
- Infertility

Infertility is also a contributing factor in ectopic pregnancy. Fortunately, the rise in incidence has been offset by decreases in morbidity and mortality because of improved diagnostic techniques and better

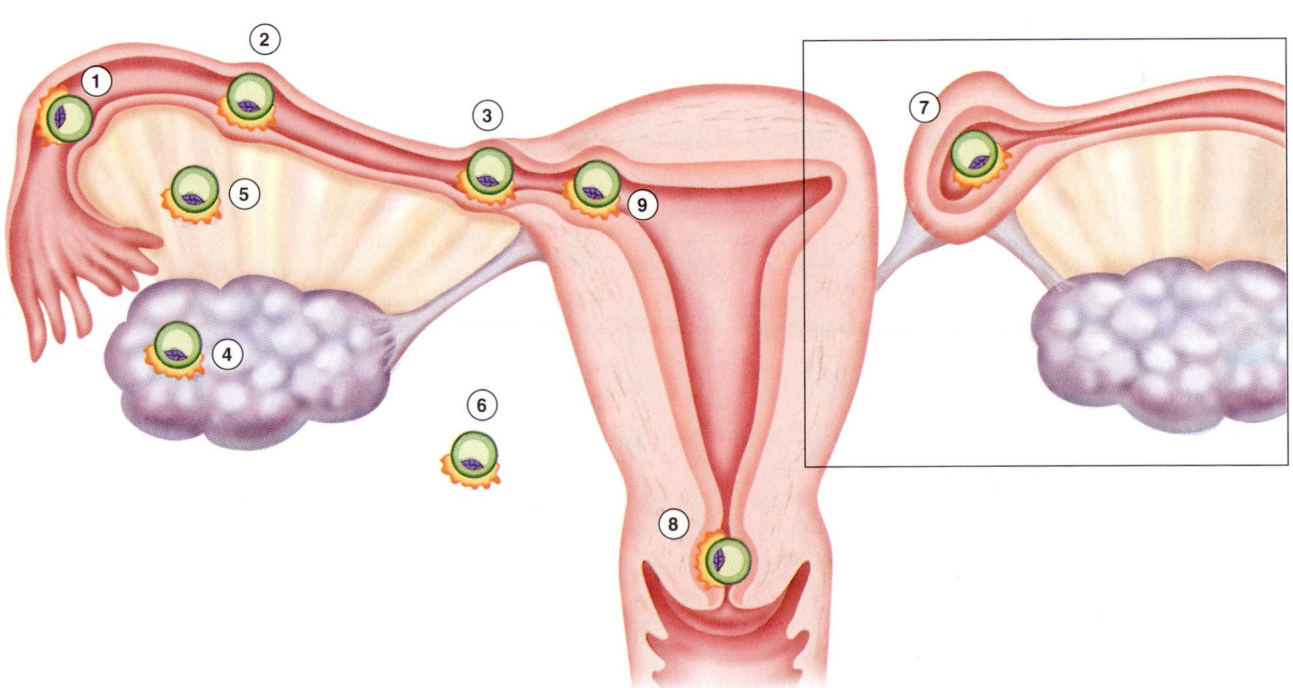

FIGURE 16–2. Implantation sites of ectopic pregnancy in order of frequency. **(1)** Ampulla of tube. **(2)** Remainder of tube. **(3)** Interstitial portion of tube. **(4)** Ovary. **(5)** Broad ligament (intraligamentary). **(6)** Surface of peritoneum (abdominal). **(7)** Rudimentary horn. **(8)** Cervix. **(9)** Tubouterine junction (angular).

access to health care. However, although the mortality has been reduced for white women, the death rate for nonwhites is still twice that of white women. Furthermore, nonwhite adolescents are almost five times as likely to die of ectopic pregnancy (Bernstein, 1995).

Only the uterus is theoretically capable of sustaining an implanted fertilized ovum. Rarely are pregnancies carried to term in the abdomen. Other sites of implantation eventually rupture. The timing of the rupture depends on the implantation site. In the fallopian tube, the specific site's stretchability determines the rupture's timing. The ampulla of the fallopian tube is the most common site and usually ruptures between 6 and 12 weeks of gestation. The second most common site, the isthmic portion of the tube, generally ruptures during the first 6 weeks of the pregnancy. The rupture occurs as the fertilized ovum erodes and degenerates the tube at the site of the placental insertion. The erosion of blood vessels results in bleeding, from scanty discharge to frank hemorrhage. Nourishment for the embryo's development is also severely limited. Any stress such as intercourse, straining due to constipation, or a vaginal examination further weakens the structure. Eventually, however, as a result of overdistension, the tube ruptures spontaneously. Hemorrhage is internal.

Nursing and Collaborative Assessment

Unfortunately, ectopic pregnancy is not frequently diagnosed prior to rupture because the indications are not that different from those of an intrauterine pregnancy. The classic clinical symptoms—abdominal pain, amenorrhea, and abnormal vaginal bleeding—may or may not be present. The woman often does present with a history of infertility, PID, current IUD use, or tubal surgery.

Initially after fertilization, the usual signs of pregnancy such as amenorrhea, breast tenderness, and a positive pregnancy test can occur; however, women with irregular menstrual periods may not recognize any abnormality or delay in their menstrual periods. The more common signs of pregnancy, such as breast enlargement and nausea, may not be present because of the early stage of gestation and low production of hormones associated with pregnancy. Thus, many women do not realize they are pregnant.

Pain is the most common complaint and a valuable diagnostic clue. The pain usually occurs early, probably as a result of fallopian tube distension. Pain may be experienced for a week or longer, but some clients report acute pain of less than 1 day's duration. The pain is often described as vague, colicky, or cramping. Frequently it is localized to the right or left pelvic area or may be bilateral. Intermittent vaginal spotting also may occur as the uterine decidua is

Nursing Alert

Women in their reproductive years with pelvic pain and menstrual irregularity should be evaluated for ectopic pregnancy. Ectopic pregnancy accounts for 10% of maternal deaths. If the fallopian tube is affected, early diagnosis allows for a more conservative surgical approach and the preservation of the affected tube.

sloughed off. The discharge is generally dark in color. Profuse or bright red vaginal bleeding is uncommon with an ectopic pregnancy.

More notable symptoms develop if the ectopic pregnancy ruptures. Characteristically these symptoms include abdominal pain, unilateral palpable pelvic mass, dizziness, and ensuing hypovolemic shock. Referred shoulder pain may occur if blood pools under the diaphragm. Vaginal examination may be very painful if extensive blood has collected in the vaginal cavity. Hemoglobin and hematocrit levels may be low. If rupture and subsequent bleeding are more gradual, the client may have vague abdominal discomfort or fullness, nausea, vomiting, and diarrhea. Diagnosis, therefore, is somewhat difficult.

Other disorders with similar presenting symptoms include salpingitis (inflammation of the fallopian tube), abortion, ruptured corpus luteum cyst, appendicitis, twisted ovarian cyst, gastrointestinal disturbance, endometriosis, and discomfort from an IUD (Saint-Louis, Mendez, & Penalver, 1996). It is important that the diagnosis be accurately differentiated from other disorders. Diagnosis is further complicated if a client goes to a variety of health care locations, unaware of the real cause of her symptoms. Table 16–2 summarizes problems that may be confused with ectopic pregnancy.

The combined use of ultrasound technology, serum progesterone evaluation, and radioimmunoassay of the beta subunit of hCG (beta-hCG) is increasingly helpful in early diagnosis of an ectopic pregnancy (Tanabe, 1994). A positive pregnancy test (beta-hCG) rules out other conditions and narrows the focus of investigation. The accuracy of diagnosis using only ultrasound varies from 70 to 94%; however, transvaginal ultrasound has improved diagnosis. With a normal pregnancy, a gestational sac in the uterus is visible 5 to 6 weeks after the last menstrual period. A positive pregnancy test and the inability to

▶ **TABLE 16–2**

Differential Diagnosis of Ectopic Pregnancy

Problem	Symptoms
Salpingitis	Spotting, bilateral pain and tenderness, temperature exceeding 100.4°F (38°C), negative urinary pregnancy test, negative serum hCG.
Abortion	Uterine bleeding more profuse, pain generally less severe, cramps likely to be rhythmic and located in middle of abdomen.
Ruptured corpus luteum and follicular cyst	Negative serum hCG, diagnosis frequently made during laparoscopy.
Appendicitis	Signs and symptoms of pregnancy lacking, pain localized higher in abdomen, pain during vaginal manipulation of cervix less severe.
Twisted ovarian cyst	No signs of pregnancy, mass more discrete.
Gastrointestinal disturbances	Nausea, vomiting, diarrhea, abdominal pain without pregnancy symptoms present. (If pregnancy symptoms are present, investigate further.)
Endometriosis	Pelvic pain that begins 1–2 days prior to menses, infertility.
Intrauterine device discomfort	Very difficult to differentiate as cramping, bleeding, pelvic pain (often unilateral) are common in both ectopic pregnancy and discomfort from an intrauterine device. (Use of an intrauterine device does *not* prevent tubal pregnancy.)

visualize an intrauterine gestation by ultrasound lead to a presumptive diagnosis that is close to 100% accurate.

Hemoglobin, hematocrit, and leukocyte values may also be useful in diagnosing suspected ectopic pregnancies. Hemoglobin and hematocrit values may show a slight reduction after the hemorrhage that accompanies the rupture of the ectopic pregnancy. After the first few hours, the hemoglobin and hematocrit may drop significantly because of acute hemorrhage. In about half the women with ruptured ectopic pregnancies, the leukocyte count is normal. In the other half, leukocytosis of up to 30,000 μL may occur.

Prior to instituting specific diagnostic procedures, a routine pelvic examination is performed. Because the procedure may be painful, the examination must be done with care.

Culdocentesis may be used to confirm ectopic pregnancy, especially when ultrasound is not available. In culdocentesis, the physician inserts a needle through the posterior vaginal wall into the cul-de-sac of Douglas (a section of the peritoneal cavity behind the uterus) and aspirates fluid. Aspiration of nonclotting blood may indicate a ruptured ectopic pregnancy. Clear fluid rules out a ruptured ectopic pregnancy. Lack of fluid does not provide diagnostic data (Ransom & McNeeley, 1997).

A laparoscopy may be performed if a definite diagnosis cannot be made using other methods (see Chapter 10).

Figure 16–3 describes a protocol for diagnosis of suspected ectopic pregnancy. Table 16–3 summarizes assessment techniques for ectopic pregnancy.

Nursing Diagnoses

After assessment of the woman with an ectopic pregnancy, nursing diagnoses are formed that will become the basis of the plan of care. Examples of nursing diagnoses include:

Problem-oriented diagnoses:

- Risk for infection, related to surgical incision from salpingostomy, salpingotomy, and salpingectomy
- Anticipatory grieving, related to perceived loss of pregnancy
- Fluid volume deficit, related to loss of blood from ruptured ectopic pregnancy

Wellness-oriented diagnoses:

- Functional grieving, related to positive social support
- Spiritual strength, related to maintenance of belief system during treatment for ectopic pregnancy

Medical Treatment

Once the medical diagnosis is determined, the products of conception are removed surgically. Sometimes the affected tube must be removed, although an attempt may be made to save it by resection in order to maintain fertility. Table 16–4 presents the medical and surgical therapies used to resolve an ectopic pregnancy.

Nursing and Collaborative Management

Assessment and nursing diagnoses are the basis for planning and intervention for families experiencing

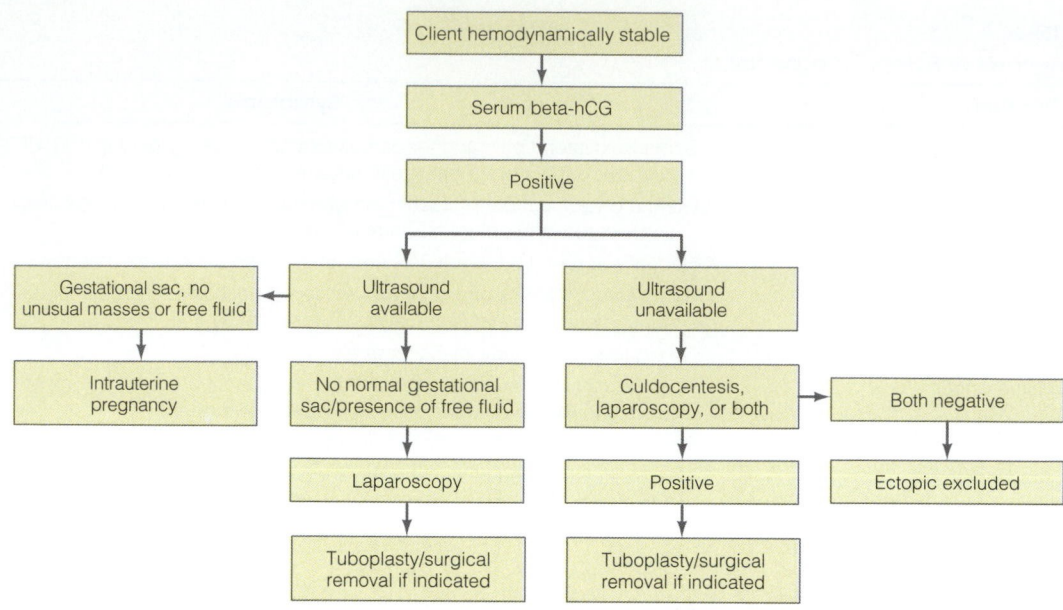

FIGURE 16–3. Protocol for diagnosing suspected ectopic pregnancy in hemodynamically stable woman. If client is unstable, surgery is performed without delay. *(Reproduced, with permission, from Patrick, J. (1985). Ectopic pregnancy.* Topics in Emergency Medicine, 7, *30. © 1985 Aspen Publishers, Inc.)*

an ectopic pregnancy. Approximately 85% of the deaths resulting from ectopic pregnancy are caused by blood loss. The remaining deaths occur from a variety of other causes including pulmonary edema and air embolism.

▶ **TABLE 16–3**

Assessment Techniques for Ectopic Pregnancy

Technique	Purpose
Pelvic examination	Palpation of pelvic mass and state of cervix; determination of presence of pain and location
Abdominal palpation	Palpation of pelvic mass and enlargement of uterus; determination of presence of pain and location
Radioimmunoassay (hCG)	Determination of positive pregnancy test
Ultrasound	Visualization of gestational sac to rule out intrauterine pregnancy
Serum progesterone levels	Determination of presence of live intrauterine pregnancy
Laparoscopy	Visualization of peritoneal cavity and organs
Culdocentesis	Aspiration of fluid from peritoneal cavity to rule out ruptured ectopic pregnancy
Hemoglobin, hematocrit	Determination of anemia resulting from blood loss
Leukocyte count	Determination of elevated white blood cell count (leukocytosis)

The large number of deaths resulting from ectopic pregnancy reinforces the necessity of "thinking ectopic." The diagnosis must be expeditiously sought every time it is suspected. Women at increased risk must be educated to seek care promptly when symptoms are present. Education and prompt action by health care professionals should aid in reducing the mortality from this dangerous complication of pregnancy.

The main concern with ruptured ectopic pregnancy is hemorrhage. A central venous line may be used to monitor the extent of blood loss. In addition, vital signs are frequently assessed and skin color and urinary output are monitored. Blood transfusion and intravenous therapy are necessary to replace fluids.

Some moderate vaginal bleeding is expected, and pads must be counted to determine the extent of bleeding. Maintaining bedrest is essential.

Postoperative nursing care after surgery for a ruptured ectopic pregnancy is similar to nursing care for any client experiencing abdominal surgery. The incision must be assessed for redness, edema, discharge, and intactness. The physician will usually prescribe broadspectrum antibiotics prophylactically. Pain medication is needed to control discomfort.

Early ambulation and adequate rest should be encouraged. To prevent paralytic ileus, oral intake is avoided until bowel function returns to normal. If the client is Rh negative and has not been sensitized, she should receive Rho(D) immune globulin, because isoimmunization may follow ectopic pregnancy.

▶ **TABLE 16–4**

Medical and Surgical Therapies: Ectopic Pregnancy

Therapy	Uses	Procedure
Salpingostomy	Unruptured ectopic pregnancy; no previous salpingitis; future pregnancies desired	Linear incision over site of pregnancy through which products of conception are removed; hCG levels followed until negative
Methotrexate	Unruptured ectopic pregnancy; hemodynamically stable; no history of hepatic or renal disease; future pregnancies desired	Administered parentally, orally or by injection into the amniotic sac; post-medication ultrasound examinations to document amniotic sac resolution; hCG levels followed until undetectable
Salpingotomy	Unruptured ectopic pregnancy larger than 2 cm in length; no previous salpingitis; future pregnancies desired	A longitudinal incision is made in fallopian tube and the products of conception are removed with forceps and gentle suction; the incision is sutured
Salpingectomy	Ruptured or unruptured ectopic pregnancy; severe damage of tube or if hemostasis is unattainable	Removal of tube through operative laparoscope; cornual resection

Sources: Cunningham et al., 1997; Powell & Spellman, 1996; Weinman, 1996.

Reconstructive tubal surgery is an option when the woman's condition becomes stable.

Rupture of an ectopic pregnancy can be an overwhelming event to the childbearing family. Not only does the woman undergo surgery, but she loses a baby and her fertility status may be permanently altered, especially if the other fallopian tube is not intact. The couple needs time to sort out what has happened and work through their grief.

Many couples develop attachment to their babies very early and experience much sadness when an embryo is lost. The nurse can encourage the client and her family to verbalize their feelings by asking open-ended questions. The couple should be assured that their grief is normal and also be allowed to grieve privately. The nurse can help to decrease feelings of guilt or blame by empathetically explaining the causes of ectopic pregnancy. Pregnancy may tax the family's ability to cope under the most favorable conditions. If there are problems with the pregnancy, the family's coping abilities are further stressed (Bachman & Lind, 1997). Support groups offer ongoing help to the family. Many men are likely to experience the same reactions to ectopic pregnancy as their female partner, but feel that their role is to "be strong." Particular attention should be paid to their concerns.

Couples also need information about their chances for a subsequent successful pregnancy. The success of future pregnancies depends on the specifics of the woman's reproductive history and whether at least one fallopian tube remains to transport a fertilized ovum to the uterus.

In addition, the couple needs specific information during the recovery period. The couple can be advised that intercourse may be resumed once the incision has healed. It will probably be 6 to 8 weeks before a normal menstrual period occurs. The couple is advised to use contraceptives for at least three menstrual periods before attempting another pregnancy, and should realize the risk of another ectopic pregnancy. They should also be counseled to obtain early prenatal care with a subsequent pregnancy (Ransom & McNeeley, 1997).

▶ METABOLIC CONDITIONS

Few metabolic conditions completely prevent pregnancy, but many can complicate its course. An understanding of the interaction of pregnancy and the specific disease state is essential to nursing care of the high-risk pregnant woman. Interdisciplinary collaboration also is required to provide optimal care of the woman experiencing a complication of pregnancy.

This section discusses several metabolic complications of pregnancy that require observation or intervention during the first trimester, specifically hyperemesis gravidarum, anemia and hemoglobinopathies, and thyroid disorders. Although management of these conditions is included as a part of first-trimester concerns, treatment of these conditions continues throughout the period of gestation.

▶ Hyperemesis Gravidarum

Hyperemesis gravidarum, also called pernicious vomiting of pregnancy, is severe (excessive) vomiting that results in maternal dehydration, weight loss, and nutritional deficiencies. It begins most frequently during the first trimester of pregnancy (Hod, Ovietor, Kaplan, Friedman, & Ovadia, 1994).

Nausea and vomiting are fairly common during early pregnancy. Although troublesome and distressing, these symptoms usually respond to such measures as eating small, frequent meals and avoiding strong odors. Hyperemesis, however, persists beyond the first trimester. Fortunately, it affects only about 1 of every 1000 women, and its incidence is decreasing (Cowan, 1996). The condition appears to recur in subsequent pregnancies and is more common among women who have a multifetal pregnancy.

Etiology

The etiology of hyperemesis gravidarum is not well understood. It is likely that it is caused by a combination of factors. It appears to be related to high or rapidly increasing levels of hCG or estrogens (Cunningham et al., 1997). Much attention has been given to the increased level of hCG in women with this condition. The increase is especially apparent in gestational trophoblastic disease, an abnormality in the chorionic villi (see Chapter 19), when hyperemesis gravidarum also exists; however, dehydration from the excessive vomiting may influence the elevated hCG levels.

Evidence of transient hyperthyroidism has been encountered among women with hyperemesis gravidarum. It is possible that hCG may overstimulate the thyroid. Symptoms of hyperemesis have been shown to resolve following administration of propylthiouracil.

Psychologic and social factors, such as family conflict, may also play a role. These factors are given increasing credence, especially as more is learned concerning the relationship of other eating disorders to emotional and social causes.

Nursing and Collaborative Assessment

The clinical picture of a pregnant woman suffering from hyperemesis gravidarum varies based on the severity of the complication. Nausea progressively worsens and may persist all day so that eventually nothing can be retained by mouth. Weight loss results, along with stomach pain and heartburn. Dehydration and starvation eventually occur. Symptoms include fluid and electrolyte imbalance, hypotension, elevated hematocrit, hypokalemia, and decreased urine output. Eventually protein and vitamin deficiencies become apparent. These symptoms should be differentiated from other causes of nausea and vomiting such as hepatitis, gastroenteritis, cholecystitis, and pancreatitis. Left untreated, hyperemesis gravidarum can be fatal, although symptoms may cease at any point and health be restored. Interestingly, the disease is not associated with increased incidence of spontaneous abortion or prematurity. A lower incidence of fetal

loss has been documented in women experiencing nausea and vomiting during pregnancy (Hod et al., 1994).

Nursing Diagnoses

Several nursing diagnoses may apply to the woman with hyperemesis gravidarum. They include:

Problem-oriented diagnoses:

- Fluid volume deficit, related to persistent vomiting
- Altered nutrition for mother and fetus: less than body requirements, related to persistent vomiting
- Altered oral mucous membrane, related to dehydration

Wellness-oriented diagnoses:

- Potential asset in resolution of vomiting, related to home management of hyperemesis gravidarum

Nursing and Collaborative Management

Care of the client experiencing hyperemesis begins after other causes of nausea and vomiting are diagnostically ruled out. Once this is done, the following principles of care are stressed:

1. Hospitalization is often required to change the woman's environment and institute a course of treatment. A change in environment is sometimes necessary if psychosocial factors are contributing to the condition. Hospitalization may also be required if the woman is severely dehydrated and needs fluid replacement; however, many women with hyperemesis gravidarum are successfully managed at home (see Chapter 20).

2. Intravenous therapy is initiated to treat dehydration. Generally, the woman will receive approximately 3000 mL intravenously in the first 24 hours. Glucose, vitamins, and electrolytes added to the intravenous solution help to restore electrolytes and nutrients. Intake and output need to be carefully monitored as the body's depleted fluid reserves are restored. Adequacy of hydration is assessed by measuring urinary output; 1000 mL in each 24 hours is desired (Cowan, 1996).

3. Small frequent feedings as tolerated by the woman are usually possible within 48 hours of admission. Special attention is paid to how the food is served, being sure it is arranged attractively and that cold food is cold and hot food is hot. Options other than oral food intake con-

sist of high-calorie tube feedings (Newman, Fullerton, Anderson, 1993; Wolkomir, 1996) or, in severe cases, hyperalimentation. Mouth care is also important, as the mouth may be very dry.

4. Sedatives may be given to relax the hyperactive gastrointestinal tract.

5. Acupressure has also been used successfully for nausea and vomiting of pregnancy (Belluomini, Litt, Lee, & Katz, 1994).

Supportive, therapeutic measures to deal with the emotional component of the disease are helpful. A therapist or counselor will often be involved in this process. The nurse, however, can offer an unhurried willingness to listen and do much to maintain a relaxed, nonstressful environment. The pregnant woman's acceptance of her situation and the pregnancy itself is essential to a favorable outcome of the condition. Assisting the woman in problem-solving and coping with a future child may be an effective strategy.

▶ Anemia

Anemia is a decrease in both the circulating red blood cell mass and the cells' capacity to carry oxygen to vital organs of the mother and the fetus. Although a minor increase in the oxygen-carrying ability of each cell is possible in response to a decrease in red blood cell mass, this compensatory mechanism is soon overwhelmed. Cardiac output must then increase to maintain adequate oxygen delivery to the tissues.

Both red blood cell and plasma volumes increase during pregnancy. The plasma volume begins to increase about the 6th week of pregnancy and continues until term. Around the 6th month of gestation, the red blood cell volume begins to increase; however, this increase is not as great proportionately as the expansion of plasma volume. The result is a fall in the hematocrit and hemoglobin of a pregnant woman. Because the magnitude of this plasma volume change varies among pregnant women, a range of hemoglobin levels is seen during pregnancy. In addition, altitude may cause a variation in hemoglobin level. For example, a woman residing at sea level would be considered anemic if her hemoglobin were below 12 g/dL in the nonpregnant state or less than 11 g/dL during pregnancy or the puerperium (Cunningham et al., 1997; Hoffman, 1993).

Etiology

Anemia may be caused by pregnancy, as with iron deficiency anemia or folic acid deficiency anemia, or it may be one type of hemoglobinopathy. Anemia, how-

ever, may be an indicator of nutritional, social, and/or environmental problems that also affect pregnancy. It is questionable if treatment of the anemia alone will always increase the favorable outcome of the pregnancy.

The hemoglobin level of most iron-sufficient pregnant women is usually 11 g/dL or higher. The incidence of all types of anemia during pregnancy is variable, depending on whether supplemental iron or other supplements are taken during pregnancy.

Iron-Deficiency Anemia

Iron-deficiency anemia accounts for more than 75% of all anemia that develops during pregnancy. A woman needs a total of about 1300 mg of iron during her pregnancy. This includes the amounts necessary for increasing maternal blood volume (approximately 800 mg) and for fetal and placental development (approximately 500 mg) (Cunningham et al., 1997).

Fortunately, the body is more capable of absorbing iron during pregnancy because of its improved iron-binding capacity (approximately three times that in the nonpregnant state). Despite the intake of 15 mg or more iron daily and the increased iron-binding capacity of the body, the balance between iron need and availability is tenuous. This is especially true during the second half of pregnancy, when the need for iron is the greatest. Many women, however, begin pregnancy in an anemic state and their situation is even more risky. Those particularly at risk include adolescents, poorly nourished clients and followers of fad diets, women with multiple gestations, and women whose pregnancies are closely spaced. The dietary habits of such women rarely include amounts of iron adequate for pregnancy.

Nursing and Collaborative Assessment. Assessment of iron-deficiency anemia begins with a systematic health history that includes a record of hematologic diseases and a dietary history. The family's socioeconomic status is also assessed, as well as eating habits, pica practices, and any history of dieting.

A nutritional history is helpful in identifying the woman at risk for developing anemia during pregnancy. In clients with mild to moderate anemia, symptoms are generally not detectable except by hemoglobin and hematocrit tests. Severe anemia may be more apparent.

In a method commonly used to provide an overview of the woman's dietary patterns, the woman recalls foods consumed during the previous 24 hours. She should be encouraged to list everything ingested at mealtime and between meals. The 24-hour recall is further evaluated to determine usual variations in food intake throughout the week (see Chapter 14).

Other important information to gather includes general food habits, preparation methods, size of portions, seasonings used, and general likes and dislikes. The woman's usual ingestion of foods rich in iron, including liver, red meat, legumes, green vegetables, whole grains, and shellfish, should be assessed (Table 16–5).

Approximately 25% of pregnant women with iron deficiency and anemia are found to practice pica (see Chapter 14). Screening for this practice is necessary during the assessment process.

As iron-deficiency anemia may result from decreased intake of necessary nutrients, the food consumed should be compared with intakes recommended during pregnancy to determine any area of deficiency in amount or quality of nutrients. The total intake of calories and protein can also be determined using standard nutritional guides.

The woman with iron-deficiency anemia usually comes to the health care provider with skin pallor and complaints of fatigue, listlessness, weight loss, and weakness. The classic symptom of pallor may, however, be absent because of the hyperemia of the skin that is normally seen during pregnancy. Other physical signs of iron-deficiency anemia include infections due to a decrease in immunocompetence, which occurs in severe anemia, and changes in the structure and function of epithelial tissues.

Routine laboratory tests begin with a complete blood count, which identifies anyone with low hemoglobin and hematocrit levels so that further testing is initiated. The physiologic changes of normal pregnancy result in lower hemoglobin and hematocrit levels making lab values difficult to interpret (Long, 1995). If the hemoglobin level is below 11 g/dL or if the hematocrit is below 32%, the woman is determined to be anemic. Additional laboratory work to diagnose anemia in the pregnant client includes red blood cell indices, reticulocyte count, serum iron and total iron-binding capacity, transferrin saturation, and serum ferritin level.

▶ **TABLE 16–5**

Iron Content of Selected Foods

Food	Serving Size	Iron (mg/serving)
Oysters	¾ cup	10.0
Beef liver	3 oz	8.0
Pinto beans	1 cup cooked	6.1
Navy beans	1 cup cooked	5.1
Lentils	1 cup cooked	4.2
Spinach	1 cup	4.0
Chipped beef	3 oz	4.0
Clams	3 oz	3.5
Lean beef, pork, lamb	3 oz	3.0

With severe deficiencies, the red blood cells become microcytic and hypochromic, and the serum iron level decreases. A decrease in transferrin saturation is also noted. Serum ferritin values offer a fairly precise measurement of the available iron stored (Cunningham et al., 1997). These values should be obtained at 6- to 8-week intervals.

Nursing Diagnoses. Several nursing diagnoses can be made after comprehensive assessment of the client with iron-deficiency anemia. Examples of these diagnoses are:

Problem-oriented diagnoses:

- Altered nutrition: less than body requirements, related to inability to purchase food
- Risk for infection, related to decrease in immunocompetence

Wellness-oriented diagnoses:

- Health seeking behavior, related to consumption of ethnic foods high in iron
- Asset in self-care, related to adequate public resources to obtain food

Nursing and Collaborative Management. Oral iron supplements, such as ferrous sulfate 60 mg one to three times per day, are successful in treating most iron-deficiency anemias during pregnancy. Iron supplements may be given parenterally (e.g., Inferon) for severe anemia or when the oral iron supplements cause vomiting, diarrhea, or other side effects the pregnant client cannot tolerate.

Because of the increased iron requirements during pregnancy and the fact that most women enter pregnancy with low iron reserves, most pregnant women receive prophylactic iron supplementation throughout their pregnancy. This treatment is somewhat controversial, however, especially because deleterious effects of mild anemia have not been documented.

The nurse can assist the client in devising a dietary plan as rich in iron as possible. The diet should include foods known to be high in iron, taking into consideration the preferred foods of the client. Iron-fortified foods, especially cereals, may be an economic way of further fortifying the diet with iron.

Diet therapy alone is generally not sufficient to meet the iron needs of women experiencing iron-deficiency anemia. Ingestion and absorption of amounts of iron adequate to overcome the deficit are difficult; however, most anemic clients respond readily to iron therapy. Oral administration is preferred because of its simplicity and safety. One study found that the treatment effect of weekly iron supplementation was similar to that of daily supplementation (Ridwan, Schultink, Dillon, & Gross, 1996). The nurse can be instrumental in encouraging the client to take the iron supplements as prescribed. Ingesting the iron with beverages high in vitamin C, such as orange juice, improves absorption.

Gastrointestinal side effects, such as nausea, vomiting, constipation, and diarrhea, are common with iron supplementation. Consequently, many women tolerate oral supplements poorly, especially in early pregnancy with the tendency for nausea that already exists.

A woman should be advised that her stools may turn dark green or black from supplementary iron that is not absorbed from the gastrointestinal tract. If constipation occurs, the client should increase fluid and fiber in her diet to increase stool bulk and facilitate its passage. Exercise helps prevent constipation.

A body usually responds rapidly to iron supplementation. A rise in hemoglobin and hematocrit levels should be obvious after 2 weeks of therapy, and they should continue to increase to normal levels if an underlying condition does not exist.

Folic Acid Deficiency Anemia (Megaloblastic Anemia)

During pregnancy, increased maternal red blood cell production and fetal demands can result in folic acid or folacin deficiency. (See Chapter 14 for discussion of the physiologic function of folic acid.) Folic acid deficiency is the most common cause of megaloblastic anemia during pregnancy. Megaloblastic anemia is a disorder of red blood cell production that demonstrates as an alteration in cell morphology. Besides anemia, other symptoms include a sore tongue, stomatitis, anorexia, nausea, and vomiting (Cunningham et al., 1997).

Folic acid plays an additional role in pregnancy that at present is not entirely understood. Many complications including abruptio placentae, spontaneous abortion, and pregnancy-induced hypertension have been related to folic acid deficiency, although evidence is not conclusive. Fetal growth and development do not appear to be affected by maternal folate deficiency, with the exception of neural tube defects (Cunningham et al., 1997).

Nursing and Collaborative Assessment. Folic acid deficiency may be determined by assessing maternal nutrition, signs and symptoms related to folate deficiency, and laboratory values.

A 24-hour dietary recall is requested from the client. In addition, how the woman prepares her food is investigated. Overcooking with large volumes of water or canning destroys as much as 80% of the available folic acid in food substances. Moreover, microwave cooking destroys more folic acid in foods than conventional cooking.

The nurse also explores signs and symptoms related to folate deficiency. They include nausea, vomiting, pallor, anorexia, soreness of the tongue, and stomatitis.

Laboratory values that are assessed include hemoglobin, hematocrit, red blood cell indices such as mean corpuscular volume, peripheral blood smears, and serum folate levels. (Appendix B lists normal laboratory values during childbearing.) The mean corpuscular volume may be elevated. Smears of the peripheral blood will demonstrate macrocytes (an immature form of the red blood cell). A folate level less than 5 mg/mL is indicative of folic acid deficiency (Cunningham et al., 1997).

Nursing Diagnoses. Once the assessment data are collected and analyzed, nursing diagnoses can be formulated for the client experiencing folic acid deficiency anemia. Examples of diagnoses are similar to those outlined for iron-deficiency anemia.

Nursing and Collaborative Management. During pregnancy, the recommended daily dietary allowance for folic acid increases from 180 to 400 µg because of the increased production of red blood cells. Treatment for a deficiency consists of oral folic acid supplementation of 0.5 to 1.0 mg per day beginning in the second trimester. Clients respond readily to therapeutic dosages.

Dietary instruction on the inclusion of foods containing high levels of folic acid in the diet is also

Women's Health

To minimize the gastrointestinal side effects of iron supplementation, the nurse can suggest the following interventions to the pregnant client with iron-deficiency anemia:

- Take a reduced dosage of the iron preparation since a lower dosage is less likely to cause side effects
- Take the preparation with or shortly after meals or before bedtime
- Use coated tablets, time-released capsules, or liquid preparations to decrease gastrointestinal distress (note: coated tablets are not absorbed as well as uncoated tablets)

important. Good sources of folic acid include green leafy vegetables, fish, meat, poultry, eggs, milk, and legumes. Cooking habits should be explored as part of the nutritional history. Excessive cooking of vegetables is common in some groups. The nurse should encourage the client to steam vegetables in small amounts of water to ensure retention of both folic acid and essential vitamins. Augmentation of iron intake is usually recommended to coincide with folic acid augmentation, as iron-deficiency anemia is often found with folic acid deficiency.

Sickle-Cell Anemia

Hemoglobinopathies are hereditary disorders characterized by an abnormal form of hemoglobin. There are several specific types of hemoglobinopathies, including sickle-cell anemia (hemoglobin S disease), hemoglobin C disease, and thalassemia.

Hemoglobin is an iron-containing protein molecule that is produced by red blood cells. The primary physiologic function of hemoglobin is to transport oxygen in arterial blood. In its predominant form, a molecule of hemoglobin (hemoglobin A) consists of four globulin chains: two alpha and two beta chains. Variations in the structure of hemoglobin also exist. For example, fetal hemoglobin, which is normally present in the fetus and in early infancy, consists of two alpha chains and two gamma chains (rather than beta chains); in addition, there are delta chains which may combine with alpha chains. Variations in the sequencing and varieties of amino acids in the protein strand result in great differences in the physiologic functioning of the hemoglobin. For example, alterations of the amino acids on the beta chains may cause hemoglobin S and C diseases. Thalassemias, in contrast, are characterized by normal globin chains, but a decreased rate of chain synthesis. Any of the abnormalities can alter oxygen-carrying capacity and the impact on pregnancy can be fatal.

Sickle-cell anemia, the most common hemoglobinopathy in the United States, is a disorder in which valine is substituted for glutamine at position 6 on the beta chain. The disease is genetically transmitted as a recessive trait almost exclusively among the African-American population.

In the heterozygous form, known as sickle-cell trait, the person is a carrier of the disease. Even though approximately 25 to 50% of the hemoglobin is abnormal, enough normal hemoglobin is produced to compensate for the defect and signs and symptoms do not present. Approximately 8% of African-Americans are heterozygous carriers of the disease. The homozygous form of the disorder, sickle-cell anemia, occurs in 1 in 500 African-Americans.

Sickle-cell anemia results in defective hemoglobin molecules. The red blood cells become elongated, crescent-shaped, and interlock with one another in the presence of decreased oxygenation. Their shape is distorted into a sickled or holly leaf–shaped cell. Small blood vessels become clogged by these sickle cells, and blood supply to various parts of the body is compromised. Infections and dehydration greatly increase the chances of sickling. When sickled red blood cells obstruct blood flow to tissues, further hypoxia and the resultant sickling occur. In addition, these sickled red blood cells have a life span of 15 to 20 days, in contrast to the normal life span of 120 days. Decreased serum red blood cell values result. The disease is inherited at birth, but does not become apparent until about 4 months of age when fetal hemoglobin has been replaced by the abnormal adult hemoglobin.

The course of the disease is one of episodes of acute crisis. These episodes may follow infections causing dehydration, respiratory infections resulting in hypoxia, or strenuous exercise causing hypoxia. Air pollution and anesthesia are other causes of inadequate oxygenation that may result in crisis. In some situations, no specific cause can be found. Symptoms of a crisis include pain in extremities, acute abdominal pain, hepatomegaly, and splenomegaly. The symptoms result from pooling of sickled cells in blood vessels and subsequent tissue hypoxia.

As treatment has improved, more adults are surviving the disease and reaching reproductive age. During pregnancy, both mother and fetus are at risk. Maternal complications include pneumonia, postpartum infections, anemia, congestive heart failure, and pregnancy-induced hypertension (Cunningham et al., 1997). A maternal mortality rate of 1.1% suggests the serious consequences of pregnancy to the client with sickle-cell anemia. There is an increased risk of fetal wastage, preterm delivery, and intrauterine growth retardation (DeCherney & Pernoll, 1994). This fetal wastage is due to increases in the numbers of spontaneous abortions, fetal deaths, and low-birth-weight infants. Uterine hypoxia resulting from slow circulation of sickled red blood cells in the uterine blood vessels is cited as a cause. Despite these mortality rates, improvement in health care and expert assessment and intervention have significantly improved maternal and fetal outcomes.

Genetic Considerations. Genetic counseling is invaluable to couples at risk for passing the sickle-cell trait to their offspring. If one parent is known to carry the trait, the other should also be screened for its presence. The parents' chances of producing a normal offspring need to be accurately determined and

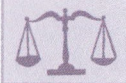

Ethical Decision Making

In consideration of the significant risks of sickle-cell anemia to both the expectant mother and fetus, the nurse needs to examine the following issues:

1. Should a woman with sickle-cell anemia become pregnant?
2. If she does, when does concern about her health take precedence over fetal well-being?

explained. If both parents carry the sickle-cell trait, the child has a 25% chance of having sickle-cell disease (SS) and a 50% chance of being a carrier of the disease (SA). If one parent has sickle-cell disease, the child will be a carrier or have the disease, depending on the other parent (Fig. 16–4).

Heterozygous

Parent HbA₁/S

Gametes	A₁	S
A₁	A₁A₁ Normal	A₁S Carrier
S	A₁S Carrier	SS Affected

(HbA₁/S)

Homozygous/Heterozygous

Parent Hb S/S

Gametes	S	S
A₁	A₁S Carrier	A₁S Carrier
S	SS Affected	SS Affected

(HbA₁/S)

Homozygous

Parent Hb S/S

Gametes	S	S
A₁	A₁S Carrier	A₁S Carrier
A₁	A₁S Carrier	A₁S Carrier

(HbA₁/A₁)

FIGURE 16–4. Genetic transmission of sickle-cell trait.

The fetus' genotype can be determined through chorionic villi sampling or amniocentesis. The results determine whether the fetus is unaffected, a carrier, or affected. If it is determined the fetus is homozygous and has sickle-cell anemia, the partners should be counseled concerning the child's condition and resultant handicaps. The parent's beliefs and values must be the priority as decisions concerning carrying the pregnancy to term are made.

The nurse can serve as a support person to couples trying to sift through the information given to them by the genetic counselors. Often, the parents need additional emotional resources as the reality of the situation becomes apparent.

Because of the severe complications pregnancy superimposes on a woman already debilitated from sickle-cell anemia, additional pregnancies are often not recommended. Sterilization may be considered or a very reliable method of birth control recommended. The methods recommended are a progestin-only oral contraceptive or a barrier contraceptive, such as the diaphragm or condom. An IUD is not recommended, as it would increase the risk of infection or heavy uterine bleeding. Oral contraceptives containing estrogen are contraindicated because sickle-cell anemia predisposes the client to heart disease and vascular occlusion may be intensified by the estrogen (DeCherney & Pernoll, 1994).

A better prognosis resulting from increasingly individualized, comprehensive prenatal care will give clients with sickle-cell anemia more alternatives with respect to childbearing decisions. In the past, recommendations for terminating the pregnancy might have been made to protect the mother's life and health. Now these high-risk mothers are identified early and managed comprehensively. The possibilities of positive outcomes for mother and infant increase with comprehensive management.

Nursing and Collaborative Assessment. The health history is an important assessment tool in caring for pregnant women with sickle-cell anemia. Complications that the client has experienced should be documented in the history. During prenatal visits, the nurse should carefully investigate all problems that have arisen. Review of old information or new teaching concerning the disease is important to establish the client's knowledge base. The client also should be assessed for nausea and vomiting, which may result in dehydration.

The nurse assists in many diagnostic tests and often may interpret the results of the test to the client. In most instances, the diagnosis of sickle-cell anemia will have been made prior to pregnancy. A sickling test or Sickledex is commonly used for screening purposes. If the test is positive, hemoglobin electrophoresis is necessary to differentiate between the homozygous and heterozygous forms of the disease and to determine the percentage of abnormal hemoglobin.

Throughout the pregnancy, maternal and fetal assessments are made frequently. Urine cultures should be obtained monthly even if the mother is asymptomatic because of her predisposition to urinary tract infections. Fetal well-being must be assessed frequently to identify any difficulties. The fetal hemoglobin from uncontaminated cord blood can be checked for the presence of sickle-cell trait or sickle-cell anemia. The nonstress test evaluates the fetus' response to movement. The fetal heart rate normally increases with fetal movement (a reactive stress test). It is a convenient and accurate technique to assess fetal well-being in this situation. A nonreactive stress test indicates the need for further evaluation. Placental function tests may be indicated. Placental dysfunction resulting from placental infarction is common in clients with sickle-cell anemia. Placental infarction can result in fetal death and preterm labor.

The problems associated with sickle-cell anemia may be worsened by the stress of labor. The increased need for oxygen by the cells may increase the risk of a painful sickle-cell crisis. Determination of hemoglobin and hematocrit levels is important to the accurate assessment of this situation. The hemoglobin level usually does not fall below 7 g/dL if the woman has adequate nutrition and is free of infection (Cunningham et al., 1997). These women are also at risk for congestive heart failure because of numerous occlusions of pulmonary arteries by sickled cells. Cardiac enlargement often results. Vital signs should be assessed, along with signs of dyspnea, cyanosis, and edema.

The risk of infection for the client with sickle-cell anemia is increased in both the intrapartum and postpartum periods. Anemia results in improper oxygenation of tissues, allowing bacteria to become established. The client should be assessed for urinary tract infections, pyelonephritis, and, pneumonia, which are frequently complications of sickle-cell anemia. During the postpartum period, the nurse should also carefully assess for thrombophlebitis, which may result from the increased viscosity of sickle cells.

Nursing Diagnoses. After careful assessment, nursing diagnoses can be formulated for the pregnant woman with sickle-cell anemia. Nursing diagnoses include:

Problem-oriented diagnoses:

- Impaired gas exchange, related to altered oxygen-carrying capacity of the blood
- Impaired physical mobility, related to pain or discomfort

Wellness-oriented diagnoses:

- Family coping: potential for growth related to family members using available support systems.
- Health-seeking behaviors, related to asking for information about sickle-cell disease and pregnancy

Nursing and Collaborative Management. One of the first concerns of management is counseling of the pregnant family. Counseling includes emphasizing the importance of attending all prenatal visits. It also focuses on optimal nutrition and the need for rest. The nurse should teach the mother the importance of avoiding symptom-relief measures that are generally acceptable to sickle-cell clients except during pregnancy. In particular, pain medications must be prescribed by a physician; home or over-the-counter remedies should not be used.

Folic acid supplementation is needed because of the greatly increased production of red blood cells during pregnancy. Iron therapy may be prescribed as iron deficiency may occur. Careful monitoring for infection is of utmost importance because infection is a stress or leading to vascular stasis. Fluid intake should be encouraged to prevent dehydration. If a crisis occurs, immediate hospitalization is generally required to reduce the risk of morbidity.

Prophylactic exchange transfusion of red blood cells to prevent maternal and fetal complications remains controversial. This technique results in withdrawal of 75 to 85% of the recipient's blood and injection of an equal amount of donor blood. The end result is a decrease in the concentration of hemoglobin that sickles. The pregnant client exists on normal transfused cells rather than her own abnormal hemoglobin. Severe complications can occur, however, including maternal and neonatal hepatitis, hemolytic disease of the newborn, and sensitization of the mother. At present, it appears that this treatment is best reserved for clients with worsening anemia, infection, or cardiovascular insufficiency rather than for prophylactic use (Cunningham et al., 1997).

The anemia associated with sickle-cell disease often results in a painful labor. Support provided by the nurse or significant other in constant attendance by the bedside is important. Use of psychoprophylactic techniques to cope with contractions is helpful. Use of analgesics also may be indicated to decrease discomfort. Acetaminophen is preferred over salicylates for relief of moderate pain. Large dosages of salicylates may result in acid overload. An epidural can be offered in most situations. Oxygen is given at 3 to 6 L/min to decrease risk of hypoxia to the fetus. The client should also be adequately hydrated with intravenous solutions. Blood should be typed and cross-matched in advance so that transfusions are available as needed. Strict aseptic technique must be used during delivery to prevent infection. Broad-spectrum antibiotics often are given prophylactically. The client should remain in left lateral position. The fetus should be continuously monitored electronically. The pediatrician or neonatologist and high-risk nursery should be notified when labor begins so that they are available if problems develop.

The mother is monitored during the postpartum period because an acute sickling crisis can develop and recovery is often prolonged. Congestive heart failure, severe anemia, infection, or pulmonary edema may develop. The risks of further pregnancies also must be explained to the woman and her partner.

Hemoglobin C Disease

Other hemoglobinopathies may result in complications during pregnancy. This is particularly a problem if the hemoglobinopathy is combined with sickle-cell trait. In **hemoglobin C disease,** lysine replaces glutamine at position 6 on the beta chain. As a result, the amount of normal hemoglobin is reduced. Rarely does a woman inherit two genes for hemoglobin C production. In about 1 in 2000 pregnancies, however, an African-American woman inherits sickle-cell hemoglobin C disease (Cunningham et al., 1997).

Nursing care of women with this disorder is similar to the client with sickle-cell anemia. As with sickle-cell anemia, this condition increases the rate of perinatal mortality resulting from spontaneous abortion and pneumonitis caused by embolization of necrotic bone marrow. Successful pregnancy outcome in women with sickle cell-hemoglobin C (Hemoglobin SC) disease increases significantly with individualized prenatal care.

Thalassemia

Thalassemia is a form of anemia that results from an alteration in the gene that normally controls the rate of the polypeptide chain synthesis. Either alpha or beta chains may be involved, leading to alpha or beta thalassemia. Symptoms vary significantly depending on whether the homozygous or heterozygous form is present. Individuals who are heterozygous for alpha or beta thalassemia are said to have thalassemia minor. Individuals who are homozygous for alpha or beta thalassemia are said to have thalassemia major. Persons of Mediterranean, Central African, or Asian descent are most frequently affected.

The most commonly encountered thalassemia condition is sickle-beta thalassemia, in which sickle-cell trait is combined with an underproduction of normal beta chains of hemoglobin. Clinical manifestations of this disorder vary depending on the differing proportions of sickle-cell trait and the beta chains. The course of this condition in pregnancy is similar to that of Hemoglobin SC disease.

Homozygous alpha thalassemia is generally not compatible with life and results in intrauterine death. Homozygous beta thalassemia (Cooley's anemia) is a severe form of anemia, and persons with this condition rarely survive to the reproductive years. Pregnancy has not been reported as those who do survive to the reproductive years are usually sterile.

Heterozygous thalassemia of either the alpha or the beta type is not a serious condition. Affected clients have no unusual fertility problems and their pregnancies follow a normal course. Heterozygous beta thalassemia is the form of thalassemia most commonly found in pregnant women. For this reason, assessment and management for heterozygous beta thalassemia are discussed here.

Nursing and Collaborative Assessment. The client is assessed for an increase in hemoglobin A_2 and in hemoglobin F. Hemoglobin A_2 increases 3.5% above normal and hemoglobin F increases 2 to 5% with heterozygous beta-thalassemia. A mean corpuscular volume less than 80 indicates that the client should be further assessed through electrophoresis. Prenatal nutritional assessment also is important for these clients, as they are at risk for iron deficiency.

Nursing and Collaborative Management. Mothers with heterozygous beta thalassemia are generally considered low-risk depending on the degree of anemia present. They are managed similarly to all normal pregnant women. When placed on iron supplementation, clients with anemia caused by beta thalassemia do not respond to the supplementation. This is one way in which heterozygous beta thalassemia is differentiated from other anemias. Hemoglobin A_2 levels should be rechecked again in 2 to 4 weeks.

▶ Thyroid Disorders

Thyroid disease is quite common in women. The estimated prevalence rate of both hyperthyroidism and hypothyroidism is approximately 1 to 2%. When caring for pregnant clients with thyroid disease, the following principles should be kept in mind:

1. Signs and symptoms of a diseased thyroid can be mimicked by the pregnancy itself.
2. Pregnancy alters standard thyroid function tests.
3. Placental transfer of most thyroid hormones is minimal.
4. Antithyroid drugs are easily passed to the fetus.
5. Clients with thyroid abnormalities should be closely monitored.

Hyperthyroidism

Hyperthyroidism is the second most common endocrine disorder in pregnancy next to diabetes. It occurs in approximately 1 in every 500 pregnancies. Assessment of thyroid function is somewhat difficult during pregnancy as the pregnancy itself results in physiologic changes indicative of hyperthyroidism. The gland enlarges by about 50% during the prenatal period, and by term, the pregnant woman's basal metabolic rate has increased by approximately 25%.

In severe cases, hyperthyroidism causes anovulation and infertility. As the woman's metabolism increases with hyperthyroidism, so does metabolism of secreted sex hormones. In addition, excessive synthesis of a globulin that binds the sex hormones eventually decreases blood concentrations of these hormones and, therefore, their availability. In milder cases, hyperthyroidism increases the incidence of premature delivery, small-for-gestational-age neonates, fetal death, and preeclampsia (Popovich & Moore, 1993).

Nursing and Collaborative Assessment. Symptoms of hyperthyroidism indicate the need for further diagnostic assessment. These symptoms include tachycardia, weakness, increased appetite, heat intolerance, sweating, enlarged thyroid, exophthalmos, nervousness, weight loss, and fine tremors. The woman may also demonstrate pronounced palmar erythema and resting pulse rate greater than 100 beats per minute, a wide pulse pressure, and atrial arrhythmias. Laboratory tests will indicate an increased basal metabolic rate and increased serum thyroxine level. Laboratory analysis for hyperthyroidism includes measurement of circulating levels of T_4 (thyroxine) and resin T_3 (triiodothyronine) uptake to obtain a rough estimate of the metabolically active T_4. The normal value for free thyroxine index ranges from 2.5 to 3.5 µg/dL (Popovich & Moore, 1993). Radioactive iodine cannot be used in testing or as a therapeutic agent because it may affect the functioning of the fetal thyroid gland.

Nursing Diagnoses. After careful assessment, nursing diagnoses can be formulated. They include:

Problem-oriented diagnoses:

- Activity intolerance, related to imbalance between oxygen supply and demand
- Sleep pattern disturbance, related to psychologic stress of pregnancy and biorhythm imbalance

Wellness-oriented diagnoses:

- Potential for activity tolerance related to treatment
- Asset in family coping, related to knowledge of physiologic changes

Nursing and Collaborative Management. Hyperthyroidism in pregnancy can be treated with antithyroid drugs or surgery. With either method of treatment, the client's condition must first be controlled with medical therapy to avoid any risk of thyroid storm. Thyroid storm is a rare occurrence in which the client presents with an extremely high fever, severe dehydration, sweating, tachycardia, and possible heart failure. Further, the woman may appear confused and disoriented. The drug of choice during pregnancy is propylthiouracil (see box entitled Drug Guide: Propylthiouracil (PTU)). rather than methimazole, another drug commonly used to treat hyperthyroidism.

Fetal hypothyroidism is a major concern in managing the pregnant hyperthyroid client, as it is possible that the antithyroid drugs will cross the placenta and block the development and function of the fetal thyroid gland. At present, the best method to prevent this occurrence seems to be maintenance of the client on as low a dosage of antithyroid medication as possible, so that thyroid function values are in the upper range of what is considered normal for a nonpregnant woman.

Another concern for the fetus is hyperthyroidism, which occurs in about 1% of fetuses whose mothers have hyperthryoidism. Hyperthyroidism occurs as a result of the transfer of high titers of thyroid-stimulating immunoglobulins from mother to fetus. Again, thyroid function tests should be performed on the newborn immediately after birth and if clinically indicated by the observation of irritability or tachycardia in the neonate over the next several weeks.

A subtotal thyroidectomy to remove part of the woman's malfunctioning thyroid may also be initi-

▶ DRUG GUIDE: PROPYLTHIOURACIL (PTU)

ACTIONS/INDICATIONS

Inhibits synthesis of thyroid hormones by interfering with incorporation of iodine into hormone precursors; PTU has no effect on hormones already formed in the thyroid gland. Inhibits the synthesis of thyroid hormones. Palliative treatment of hyperthyroidism.

DOSAGE AND ROUTE

Administered orally only, 300 to 450 mg every 8 hours. Clients with severe disease may require 600 to 1200 mg/day initially. Thyrotoxic crisis: 200 mg every 4 to 6 hours until control is achieved.

CONTRAINDICATIONS AND PRECAUTIONS

Use with caution in clients taking other drugs known to cause agranulocytosis and anticoagulants. May induce goiter and hypothyroidism in fetus; thus value of drug therapy should be evaluated in pregnancy. Use cautiously with breastfeeding.

ADVERSE REACTIONS

Skin: Rash, urticaria, pruritus, hair loss, skin pigmentation. *GI:* Nausea, vomiting, loss of taste. *MS:* Arthralgia, myalgia. *CNS:* Drowsiness, vertigo. *Hematologic:* Agranulocytosis, myelosuppression, thrombocytopenia, hypoprothrombinemia. *Other:* Drug fever, lupuslike syndrome.

DRUG INTERACTIONS

Produces additive bone marrow depression with antineoplastic medications; additive antithyroid effects with lithium; increased risk of agranulocytosis with phenothiazides. Warfarin: Propylthiouracil may potentiate its effect.

NURSING IMPLICATIONS

1. Teach client to administer drug at the same time each day relative to meals.
2. Drug may be withdrawn 2 to 3 weeks before delivery to prevent excess drug passage across placenta.
3. Monitor neonatal thyroid function closely if mother breastfeeds.

ated for treatment of hyperthyroidism. The surgery removes the need for PTU drug therapy but does present some problems of its own. First, surgery is always a risk to an individual, but the risk is compounded by the presence of a fetus (Burrow & Ferris, 1995). Second, risks associated with subtotal thyroidectomy, such as laryngeal nerve paralysis and hypoparathyroidism, are rare but disabling. Burrow and Ferris (1995) suggested that surgery be reserved for those instances of hypersensitivity to antithyroid drugs or cases in which drug therapy is ineffective. After surgery, the client must be carefully assessed for hypothyroidism. If laboratory values indicate the presence of decreased thyroid functioning, thyroxine replacement therapy should begin.

Nursing care for a pregnant client experiencing hyperthyroidism includes client education and support.

Hypothyroidism

Hypothyroidism in pregnancy is quite rare, as this condition generally results in infertility until treated. The general metabolic depression characteristic of hypothyroidism affects the reproductive system, resulting in anovulation. In mild forms of the condition, however, conception can occur.

Consequences of maternal hypothyroidism include a higher-than-expected incidence of spontaneous abortion, fetal death, and gestational hypertension (Lenung, Millar, Koonings, Montoro, & Mestman, 1993). An increased frequency of congenital anomalies also has been suggested, but this is not universally accepted. The reason for any increased perinatal mortality or fetal anomalies is unclear, because the fetal thyroid functions independently of the maternal system and transfer of thyroid hormone through the placenta is minimal. Fetal effects include spontaneous abortion, fetal goiter, cretinism, and fetal anomalies. Newborns are now routinely screened to detect low thyroxine levels.

Nursing and Collaborative Assessment. The usual symptoms of hypothyroidism may be difficult to distinguish from physiologic changes in pregnancy. Typical symptoms include fatigue, weight gain, dry skin, constipation, and cold intolerance. If these clinical signs are present or the maternal history is suggestive of hypothyroidism, thyroid function studies should be done. These include T_4, T_3, and thyroid-stimulating hormone levels. The laboratory diagnosis of hypothyroidism is made if the T_4 level is between 4 and 8 µg/dL, like that found in the normal nonpregnant woman. The hypothyroid pregnant woman also demonstrates a reduction in T_3 resin uptake (less than 20%) to a level lower than that found in the normal pregnant woman. The thyroid-stimulating hormone level is higher than normal (Popovich & Moore, 1993). Testing to determine uptake of radioactive iodine is contraindicated, as radioactive iodine is also taken up by the fetal thyroid and may cause fetal anomalies.

Nursing and Collaborative Management. Treatment of hypothyroidism consists of supplemental hormone replacement. Serum levels of thyroid hormones should be restored or maintained at normal. Controversy exists over the necessity of increasing supplemental thyroid hormone in pregnancy. Burrow and Ferris (1995) recommended increasing dosages, but Girling and deSwiet (1992) found that 80% of their clients needed no change in thyroid supplementation. Individual monitoring of client levels of thyroid hormones is important. There is no evidence to suggest that replacement therapy with thyroid medication suppresses fetal thyroid function.

Critical Thinking in Care Planning

Care of the Client Experiencing a Spontaneous Abortion

Susie Ottosen is 25 years old and pregnant for the first time. At 9 weeks of gestation, she notices dark brown vaginal spotting about the size of a dime. By 11 AM the next day, the vaginal bleeding is bright red and the size of a half dollar. Susie immediately telephones her obstetrician. About 3 hours later, mild cramping begins. The cramping becomes increasingly uncomfortable. Until now, this planned pregnancy had been without complication.

Susie and Matthew have been married for 4 years and Susie conceived 6 months after she stopped taking birth control pills. She had experienced some minor discomforts of pregnancy including sore breasts, fatigue, and urinary frequency. There is no family history of spontaneous abortion. She has taken no medication since stopping her birth control pills. Susie is employed as a retail clerk in a woman's clothing store.

While speaking with her obstetrician, Susie describes the classic symptom of threatened spontaneous abortion—vaginal spotting. She is told to stay in bed and avoid intercourse or orgasm. The spotting, however, rapidly increases as the day goes on, and cramping becomes more intense. She again calls her obstetrician, who suggests that she be hospitalized.

On admission to the hospital, Susie's bleeding and cramping increase, and she experiences a spontaneous abortion. Blood tests indicate that she is Rh negative; she reports that her husband is Rh positive.

Matthew and Susie are extremely upset about the loss of their baby and find it hard to discuss the event with their parents. Susie expresses her concern to the nurse that she may have done something to cause her to lose the baby.

▶ Assessment

- Vaginal bleeding at 9 weeks of gestation; uterine cramping
- Client's blood reveals that she is Rh negative; she reports her husband is Rh positive
- Uterine cramping, which becomes increasingly uncomfortable
- Client has suffered spontaneous abortion; pregnancy was planned
- Client and husband experience difficulty in discussing loss with other family members
- Client expresses guilt about the relationship of her actions to the loss of the pregnancy

Nursing Diagnosis

Altered peripheral tissue perfusion, related to uterine cramping and bleeding

Expected Client/Family Outcomes	Nursing Action/Intervention	Evaluation
During hospitalization: - Client's vital signs will remain within normal range.	Assess history of present pregnancy; health status, infections, activities; and vital signs. *Rationale:* History may provide clues to possible cause of abortion.	Vital signs remain within normal limits.
- Client will maintain bedrest, report any increase in amount of vaginal bleeding.	Encourage bedrest. *Rationale:* Decreased physical activity may help to maintain pregnancy.	Client maintains bedrest.

(continued)

Critical Thinking in Care Planning continued

Expected Client/Family Outcomes	Nursing Action/Intervention	Evaluation
	Monitor blood loss. Note amount and character of blood loss. Observe for signs of shock: decreased blood pressure, rapid pulse, low urine output, cool and clammy skin, dizziness. *Rationale:* Amount of blood lost is used to assess for hypovolemic shock and monitor extent of bleeding.	Blood loss is accurately assessed. Client reports any signs of increased bleeding. No additional signs of shock are apparent.
	Obtain hematocrit, hemoglobin, and blood type. Encourage client to ingest iron supplements as prescribed. *Rationale:* If anemia occurs after abortion, iron stores need to be rebuilt.	Blood values remain within normal limits.
	Administer Rho(D) immune globulin. *Rationale:* If sensitization is possible in the Rh-negative client, Rho(D) immune should be given. Leakage of fetal blood into the maternal circulation is possible.	Rho(D) immune globulin is given if client is Rh negative and if father's blood type is Rh positive or unknown.
	Save all tissue and clots for inspection. Prepare client for possible dilation and curettage. *Rationale:* Determination must be made as to whether all of the products of conception have been expelled. If products of conception are not completely expelled, medical intervention to remove them is necessary.	Embryo/fetus and membranes have been passed or client has been prepared for dilation and curettage.

Nursing Diagnosis

Pain, related to uterine cramping.

Expected Client/Family Outcomes	Nursing Action/Intervention	Evaluation
During hospitalization: • Client will use controlled breathing and relaxation techniques. • Client copes effectively with discomfort until relief is achieved.	Maintain calm, supportive approach. Remain with client or ensure that significant other is present. *Rationale:* Stress, anxiety, and fear produce muscle tension, adding to pain's discomfort, and should therefore be reduced.	Client is not left alone.
	Explain what to expect with a threatened abortion. *Rationale:* Explanations reduce anxiety related to uncertainty.	Appropriate explanations are given.
	Teach relaxation techniques and controlled abdominal breathing. *Rationale:* Relaxation techniques help relieve discomfort.	Client demonstrates relaxation and breathing techniques.
	Include client and family in decision making. *Rationale:* Informed decision making keeps client and family in control.	Relevant participation by client and family is achieved.
	Administer analgesics as prescribed. *Rationale:* Analgesics reduce discomfort.	Pharmacologic agent is administered as needed.
	Encourage position changes. Administer back rubs as needed. *Rationale:* Comfort measures provide nonpharmacologic relief of discomfort.	Client indicates a reasonable degree of comfort.

Critical Thinking in Care Planning continued

Nursing Diagnosis

Dysfunctional grieving, related to loss of desired pregnancy.

Expected Client/Family Outcomes	Nursing Action/Intervention	Evaluation
Prior to discharge: • Client and family will initiate grieving process. • Client identifies support system (both personal and professional). • Client maintains positive self-image.	Determining personal meaning of this pregnancy to client and her family. *Rationale:* Such information provides insight into the extent of the loss.	Client and her family are able to talk about her feelings.
	Accept feelings as client and family experiences them. Facilitate client and family grieving. Offer information concerning the miscarriage *Rationale:* Attachment begins early in pregnancy. Grieving is a natural phenomenon after such a loss.	Grief is resolved as evidenced by continuation of normal activities and family's statements.
	Contact clergy, social worker, or other support people as appropriate. *Rationale:* Professional support people are trained to help women and families work through losses.	Professional support people or family are available for client and her significant others.
	Arrange for products of conception to be baptized and buried if client wishes. *Rationale:* Spiritual needs of family and client must be met.	Spiritual needs of client and her family are met concerning the abortion.
	Ensure that future childbearing potential is discussed. *Rationale:* Client and her family must be realistic in planning future pregnancies. Knowledge helps with grief resolution and reduces anxiety, guilt, and blaming.	Future childbearing possibilities are clearly discussed by client and her family.

Nursing Diagnosis

Knowledge deficit, related to care after abortion.

| During hospitalization and after discharge:

• Client will experience normal recovery. | Assess for symptoms of infection and treat appropriately:

• Temperature elevated over 100°F.
• Foul-smelling vaginal discharge.
• Urinary urgency and frequency.
Rationale: Infection can readily occur after abortion. Careful assessment of symptoms can allow for early detection of infection. | No signs of infection are apparent. Temperature is within normal range. Vaginal discharge is without foul odor. No urinary frequency or urgency is experienced. |
| | Assess for increased vaginal bleeding. *Rationale:* Increased vaginal bleeding indicates retention of fragments of conception. | Bleeding within normal amount. |

(continued)

Critical Thinking in Care Planning continued

Expected Client/Family Outcomes	Nursing Action/Intervention	Evaluation
	Teach importance of using effective contraception for 4 to 6 months before attempting another pregnancy. *Rationale:* Allows regeneration of endometrial lining.	No pregnancy within 4 to 6 months.
	Stress need for gynecologic follow-up in 2 to 3 weeks. *Rationale:* Important to assure normal recovery.	Visits women's health nurse practitioner or physician 2 to 3 weeks after abortion.

Chapter Highlights

▶ The types of spontaneous abortions include threatened, incomplete, complete, inevitable, missed, or habitual.

▶ Nursing care of women experiencing spontaneous abortions consists of observing vital signs and indicators of shock and infection in the women as well as addressing the psychologic needs of the family in their attempt to cope with this event.

▶ Ectopic pregnancies occur when the fertilized ovum implants in tissue other than the lining of the uterus.

▶ The majority of ectopic pregnancies implant in the fallopian tube, which may rupture from overdistenstion, thus causing severe hemorrhage.

▶ Women at increased risk for ectopic pregnancy need to be educated about the importance of seeking care promptly when symptoms are present so as to reduce the mortality associated with this complication.

▶ The care of a pregnant woman experiencing hyperemesis gravidarum includes intravenous therapy to treat dehydration, small frequent feedings, sedatives to relax the gastrointestinal tract, and maintenance of a relaxed environment.

▶ Two types of anemias that may occur during pregnancy are deficiency anemias, such as iron-deficiency anemia and folic acid deficiency anemia, and hemoglobinopathies, such as sickle-cell anemia, hemoglobin C disease, and thalassemia.

▶ Management of iron-deficiency and folic acid deficiency anemia is primarily centered on iron and folic acid supplementation through both pharmacologic agents and development of dietary plans that contain adequate amounts of these minerals.

▶ Nursing care of the pregnant client with sickle-cell anemia includes proactive counseling during prenatal visits, promotion of optimal nutrition, and development of strategies to prevent infection and ensure adequate rest.

Chapter Highlights continued

▶ The goals of treatment for women experiencing hyperthyroidism in pregnancy are alleviation of the symptoms produced by the disorder and client education about the relationship of the condition to pregnancy.

▶ The monitoring of levels of thyroid hormones is an important component of nursing care for pregnant clients experiencing hypothyroidism due to supplemental hormone replacement therapy.

After reading the vignette at the beginning of this chapter, use what you have learned to answer these questions:

1. Why is it important that Laura O'Connor's iron-deficiency anemia be treated aggressively before her pregnancy advances into the second and third trimesters?

2. What strategies can the nurse practitioner suggest to help Laura O'Connor manage the side effects of oral iron supplementation?

3. What nursing interventions can be developed to help Laura O'Connor and her family plan meals to meet Laura's nutritional requirements?

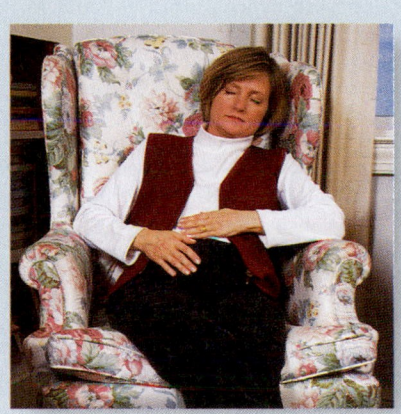

Critical Thinking Questions

▶ References

Ament, L.A. (1994). Anticardiolipin antibodies. A review of the literature. *Journal of Nurse Midwifery, 39*(1), 19–24.

Armstrong, B.G., McDonald, A.D., & Sloan, M. (1992). Cigarette, alcohol, and coffee consumption and spontaneous abortion. *American Journal of Public Health, 82,* 85–87.

Bachman, D.H., & Lind, R.F. (1997). Perinatal social work and the high risk obstetrics patient. *Social Work in Health Care, 24*(3/4), 3–19.

Bansen, S.S., & Stevens, H.A. (1992). Women's experiences of miscarriage in early pregnancy. *Journal of Nurse Midwifery, 37*(2), 84–90.

Beil, E.R. (1992). *Miscarriage: An examination of the influences of selected variables on grief.* Unpublished doctoral dissertation, University of Maryland, Baltimore, MD.

Belluomini, J., Litt, R.C., Lee, K.A., & Katz, M. (1994). Acupressure for nausea and vomiting of pregnancy: A randomized blinded study. *Obstetrics and Gynecology, 84,* 245–248.

Bernstein, J. (1995). Ectopic pregnancy: A nursing approach to excess risk among minority women. *Journal of Obstetric, Gynecologic, and Neonatal Nursing, 24*(9), 803–810.

Burrow, G.N., & Ferris, T.F. (1995). *Medical complications during pregnancy* (4th ed.). Philadelphia: W. B. Saunders.

Cowan, M.J. (1996). Hyperemesis gravidarum: Implications for home care and infusion therapies. *Journal of Intravenous Nursing, 19*(1), 46–58.

Cunningham, F.G., MacDonald, P.C., Gant, N.F., Leveno, K.J., Gilstrap, L.C., Hankins, G.D.V., & Clark, S.L. (1997). *Williams obstetrics* (20th ed.). Stamford, CT: Appleton & Lange.

DeCherney, A.H., & Pernoll, M.L. (Eds.). *Current obstetric and gynecologic diagnosis and treatment* (8th ed.). Norwalk, CT: Appleton & Lange.

Gilbert, E.S., & Harmon, J.S. (1993). *Manual of high-risk pregnancy.* St. Louis: C.V. Mosby.

Girling, J.C., & deSwiet, M. (1992). Thyroxine dosage during pregnancy in women with primary hypothyroidism. *British Journal of Obstetrics and Gynecology, 99,* 368–370.

Hod, M., Ovietor, R., Kaplan, B., Friedman, S., & Ovadia, J. (1994). Hyperemesis gravidarum. A review. *Journal of Reproductive Medicine, 39,* 605–612.

Hoffman, J.A. (1993). Iron deficiency anemia: An update. *Journal of Perinatal and Neonatal Nursing, 6,* 13–20.

Jones, M. (1997). Women with special needs, mothers who need to grieve: The reality of mourning the loss of a baby. *British Journal of Midwifery, 5*(8), 478–481.

Leung, A.S., Millar, L.K., Koonings, P.P., Montoro, M., & Mestman, J.H. (1993). Perinatal outcome in hypothyroid pregnancies. *Obstetrics and Gynecology, 81,* 349–353.

Long, P.J. (1995). Issues and opinions. Rethinking iron supplementation during pregnancy. *Journal of Nurse Midwifery, 40*(1), 36–40.

Mills, J.L., Holmes, L.B., Aarons, J.H., Simpson, J.L., Brown, Z.A., Jovanovic-Peterson, L.G., Conley, M.R., Graubard, B.I., Knopp, R.H., & Metzger, B.E. (1993). Moderate caffeine use and the risk of spontaneous abortion and intrauterine growth retardation. *Journal of the American Medical Association, 269,* 593–597.

Miron, J., & Chapman, J.S. (1994). Supporting men's experiences with the event of their partner's miscarriage. *Canadian Journal of Nursing Research, 26*(2), 61–72.

Newman, V., Fullerton, J.T., & Anderson, P.O. (1993). Clinical advances in the management of severe nausea and vomiting during pregnancy. *Journal of Obstetric, Gynecologic, and Neonatal Nursing, 22*(6), 483–490.

Popovic, D., & Moore, L. (1993). Pregnancy in women with thyroid disease: A delicate balance. *Journal of Perinatal and Neonatal Nursing, 7*(3), 29–38.

Powell, M.P., & Spellman, J.R. (1996). Medical management of the patient with an ectopic pregnancy. *Journal of Perinatal and Neonatal Nursing, 9*(4), 31–43.

Ransom, S.B., & McNeeley, S.G. (1997). *Gynecology for the primary care provider.* Philadelphia: W.B. Saunders.

Ridwan, E., Schultink, W., Dillon, D., & Gross, R. (1996). Effects of weekly iron supplementation on pregnant Indonesian women are similar to those of daily supplementation. *American Journal of Clinical Nutrition, 63*(6), 884–890.

Rowland, A.S., Baird, D.D., Shore, D.L., Weinberg, C.R., Savitz, D.A., & Wilcox, A.J. (1995). Nitrous oxide and spontaneous abortion in female dental assistants. *American Journal of Epidemiology, 141*(6), 531–538.

Saint-Louis, H., Mendez, L.E., & Penalver, M. (1996). Managing the gynecologic causes of severe abdominal pain. *Journal of Critical Care, 11*(12), 793–800.

Snow, J.E. (1994). Occupational exposure to glycol ethers: Implications for occupational health nurses. *AAOHN Journal, 42*(9), 413–419.

Steele, R., & Knight, B. (1995). Burying a baby after miscarriage. *Modern Midwife, 5*(2), 30–31.

Tanabe, P. (1994). Commentary on ectopic pregnancy. *ENA's Nursing Scan in Emergency Care, 4*(2), 1.

Walters, C., & Nelson, P. (1997). Never too late . . . support groups . . . the death of a very young baby. *Nursing Times, 93*(8), 26–27.

Weinman, S.A. (1996). Drug update: Nonsurgical treatment of an ectopic pregnancy with methotrexate. *Journal of Emergency Nursing, 22*(6), 597–599.

Wolkomir, M.S. (1996). Primary care update. Managing nausea in pregnancy: Your first- and second-line options. *Consultant, 36*(2), 298, 303, 307.

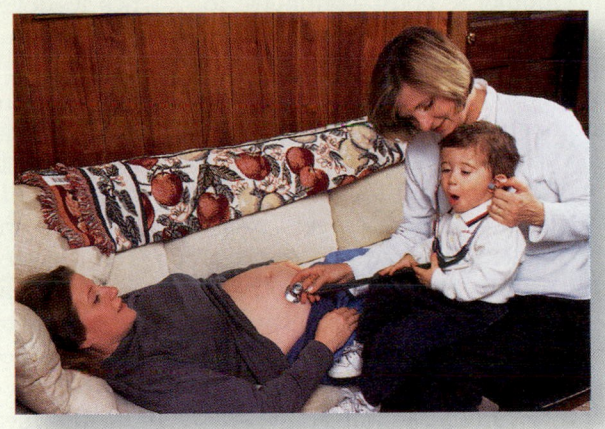

Melissa Hamilton is 20 weeks' pregnant with her second child. Her 4-year-old son Kevin, having been told about the baby by his parents, seems excited and happy about his new sister. However, Melissa lately notices that Kevin seems alternately curious and confused about her changing shape. Melissa tries to explain to him that the baby is growing inside her stomach, but he either giggles or talks about something unrelated to the baby.

Melissa discusses Kevin's response with Linda Doherty, RN, and states that she is concerned that he may become frustrated with trying to understand the changes occurring in their family. Through an innovative sibling education program, the nurse visits Melissa and Kevin at home and helps Kevin listen to the baby's heartbeat through a stethoscope pressed against the midline of Melissa's abdomen. When he hears the heartbeat, Kevin's eyes widen and his mouth opens. "Mommy, I hear my baby sister inside your tummy!" Melissa, smiling, asks, "What else can I do to prepare Kevin for the rest of the pregnancy and the baby's birth?" ∎

17

The Expectant Family: Second Trimester

The second trimester begins with the 13th week of gestation and extends through the end of the 24th week. The expectant mother's body continues to change. Changes provide for the growth and increasing needs of the still immature fetus, the continuation of pregnancy for an additional trimester, and the maintenance of the mother's own state of wellness.

During the second trimester, major changes also occur in the family, its members and social network. For the expectant parents and family members, pregnancy and the baby no longer seem unreal. Moreover, as pregnancy becomes readily identifiable to others, societal and cultural expectations of family behaviors during pregnancy are activated, and family members attain a different status. Accomplishment of certain psychologic, social, and cultural tasks during the second trimester will allow the family to move into their new lifestyle and prepare for their newest member, the infant.

By the beginning of the second trimester, the woman with an uncomplicated pregnancy optimally will have seen her health care provider two or three times. During the second trimester the healthy woman is assessed every 4 weeks. The nurse monitors fetal and maternal adaptations to pregnancy and identifies clients at risk. Assessment goals are pursued.

The clinical nursing process continues to provide an ideal means for organizing information and implementing nursing strategies. Health promotion, primary prevention, and secondary prevention remain essential to nursing care during the second trimester. Goals of nursing care that were established during the first trimester continue; however, changes in management related to nursing care goals reflect unique adaptations of the second trimester.

▶ PHYSIOLOGIC CHANGES DURING THE SECOND TRIMESTER

During the second trimester, maternal physiologic changes continue to take place as the fetus continues to grow and develop. As first-trimester discomforts fade, the healthy expectant mother develops a sense of physical well-being that is unequaled in either early or late pregnancy.

▶ Growth and Development of the Fetus

During the second trimester, major body systems of the fetus become functional (see Chapter 13). By the end of the 16th week of gestation, the fetus looks like a very thin baby; the head accounts for one third of the total length. The musculoskeletal system continues to develop, with advancing ossification of bone and movement of the arms and legs. The fetus begins holding the head in a more erect position, as the back and neck muscles develop. Fetal movements (quickening) may be first felt by the mother during the fourth month. Lanugo begins to develop over the fetal body. Blood vessels can be seen through the transparent skin, and pads develop on the fingers and toes. The digestive system begins functioning during the fourth month. The fetus swallows amniotic fluid, which contains skin cells, hair, and vernix caseosa, and produces **meconium,** the first stool of the newborn, in the intestinal tract.

By the 20th week of gestation, subcutaneous deposits of brown fat develop in the neck, chest, and inguinal areas. Glands in the skin begin to produce vernix caseosa to help protect the skin from the amniotic fluid. Lanugo increases. The mother feels many fetal movements, as the activity level and strength of the fetus continue to increase. Maximum brain growth begins with the fifth month. By the sixth month of gestation, the alveoli of the lungs begin to develop, and mature hemoglobin can be identified in fetal blood. Grasp, startle, and blink reflexes are present, and the fetus makes muscular breathing movements. By the second trimester, organ systems are formed. The fetus remains vulnerable, especially to environmental insults that could impair function of the brain or other organ systems. The pregnant woman must therefore continue to pay attention to potential effects of environmental and lifestyle factors such as drug use and alcohol consumption.

▶ Maternal Physiologic Adaptation

In the second trimester, physiologic changes in the mother occur along with and in response to the increasing needs of the fetus. Table 17–1 summarizes physiologic changes that take place during the second trimester.

▶ PSYCHOLOGIC AND SOCIOCULTURAL DIMENSIONS OF THE SECOND TRIMESTER

The expectant mother, father, and family undergo distinct psychologic changes during the second trimester. Many of the changes begun during the first trimester are facilitated as the pregnancy and fetus become "real" to family members and society at large.

▶ **TABLE 17-1**

Summary of Physiologic Changes in the Second Trimester

Organ	Changes
Reproductive System	
Uterus	Continues to enlarge, mainly by hypertrophy of cells
	Uterine wall thins, softens
	Fetus is palpable abdominally
	Uterus becomes ovoid
	By the end of trimester, fundus is felt above the umbilicus (Fig. 17–1)
	Braxton Hicks contractions are felt
Cervix	Continues to lengthen, reaching greatest length between 20 and 25 weeks
	Mucous plug is in place (see Fig. 15–2)
	Muscle cells hypertrophy
Vagina	Mucosa thickens
	Smooth muscle cells hypertrophy
	Walls elongate and loosen
	Leukorrhea continues
	pH is acidic, 3.6–6.0
Ovary	Corpus luteum degenerates
Breasts	Mammary ducts and alveoli continue to hypertrophy
	Areolae and nipples enlarge and pigment deepens
	Colostrum (precursor of milk composed mainly of serum and white blood cells) secretion begins
Cardiovascular System	Blood volume expands rapidly (red blood cells and plasma) (Fig. 17–2)
	Hemoglobin may decrease as a result of a greater expansion of plasma than red blood cells; physiologic anemia of pregnancy
	Cardiac output reaches a peak of 30 to 40% above non-pregnant output (Fig. 17–3)
	Stroke volume increases 30% over non-pregnant level
	Heart rate increases about 10 to 15 beats per minute
	Blood pressure remains the same or decreases slightly (highest reading in sitting position; lowest reading in left side-lying position)
	Supine hypotension may occur, especially in late second trimester
	Pulmonary and peripheral vascular resistance decreases 40 to 50%
Respiratory System	Oxygenation of blood increases
	Woman breathes more deeply
	Tidal volume and minute volume increase
	Oxygen consumption by organ systems, fetus, and placenta increases by about 15%
	Expanding uterus displaces diaphragm and causes rib cage to expand and to flare
	Thoracic, rather than abdominal, breathing takes place by 24 weeks
	Nasal congestion continues
	Shortness of breath develops
Urinary System	Size and vessel tortuosity of bladder increase
	Physiologic edema occurs in bladder tissue
	Urinary frequency decreases
	Kidneys increase in size
	Kidneys and ureters, especially on right side, dilate
	Mother is susceptible to urinary tract infections
	Glomerular filtration rate rises about 50% to process wastes from mother and fetus
	Renal plasma flow remains elevated at first trimester's level
	Excretion of glucose, amino acids, polypeptides, electrolytes, and water-soluble vitamins increases
Musculoskeletal System	Sacroiliac, sacrococcygeal, and pubic joints relax
	Woman's center of gravity shifts as a result of expanding uterus
	Gait widens
	Physiologic lordosis develops
	Pressure and strain on round ligament cause abdominal and inguinal pain
Integument	
Skin	Pigment deepens, especially on areolae, nipples, vulva, and perineal area
	Chloasma (melasma) is observed
	Linea nigra is apparent
	Vascular spiders may develop
	Palmar erythema (redness of the palms of the hands that may occur due to high estrogen levels) may appear
Hair	Hair continues to thicken
Nails	Softer and rate of growth increases

(continued)

► **TABLE 17-1 (continued)**

Summary of Physiologic Changes in the Second Trimester

Organ	Changes
Gastrointestinal System	
Mouth and gums	Hyperemia continues
	Sensitivity to irritants continues
	Epulis, small vascular swellings on the gum, may form
Esophagus and stomach	Esophagus shifts to side and stomach is pushed upward
	Angle at which esophagus enters stomach changes
	Stomach capacity decreases
	Cardiac valve works less efficiently with resulting gastric reflux; some women experience heartburn
	Secretion of hydrochloric acid and pepsin in stomach decreases
Liver	Changes occur in function, e.g., increased serum alkaline phosphatase, decreased plasma albumin and plasma globulins
Gallbladder	Capacity increases
	Empties more slowly
	Woman becomes predisposed to gallstones
Pancreas	Hypertrophy, hyperplasia, and hypersecretion occur in beta cells of the islets of Langerhans
	Physiologic demands of pregnancy can cause gestational diabetes or aggravate existing diabetes mellitus
Intestines	Food remains longer in the intestines
	Absorption of nutrients and water increases
Endocrine System	
Pituitary	Suppression of luteinizing and follicle-stimulating hormones continues
	Prolactin production increases
Thyroid	Vascularity increases
	Increased T_3 and T_4 levels reflect increase in thyroxine-binding globulin
	Basal metabolic rate increases; dietary iodine continues to be important
Parathyroids	Parathyroid hormone increases
Adrenals	Adrenocorticotropic hormone levels increase
	Cortisol level rises because metabolic clearance is lower
	Aldosterone level increases
Placenta	Fully formed and functioning by 14th to 16th week

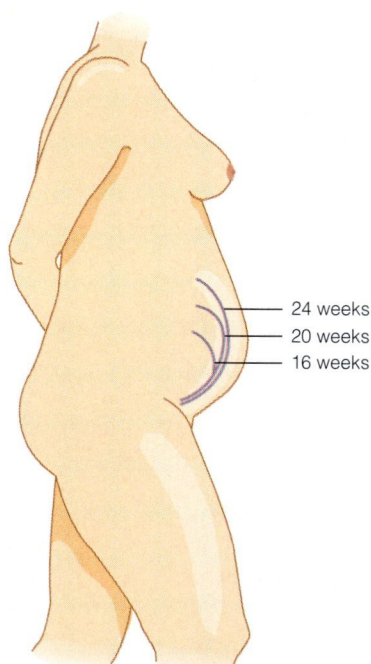

FIGURE 17–1. Height of the fundus during second trimester at 16, 20, and 24 weeks.

24 weeks
20 weeks
16 weeks

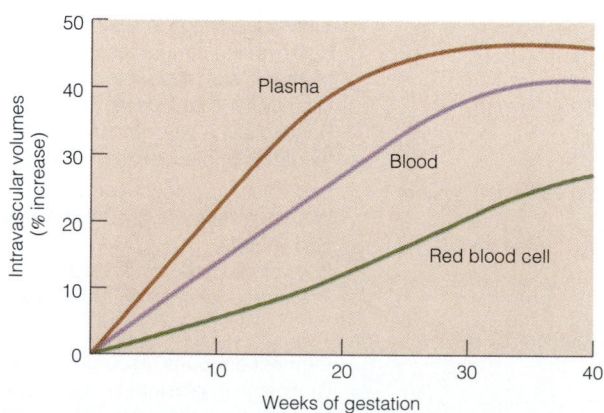

FIGURE 17–2. Increases in plasma, blood, and red blood cell volumes during pregnancy. *(Reproduced, with permission, from Burrow, G.N., & Ferris, T.F. (1989). Medical complications during pregnancy (3rd ed.). Philadelphia: W.B. Saunders, p. 181.)*

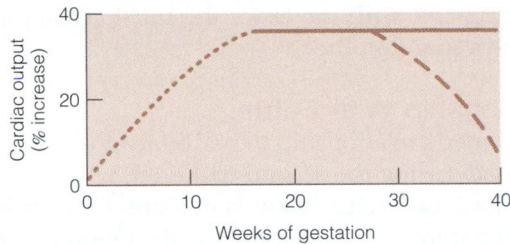

FIGURE 17–3. Cardiac output during pregnancy. *(Reproduced, with permission, from Burrow, G.N., & Ferris, T.F. (1989). Medical complications during pregnancy (3rd ed.). Philadelphia: W.B. Saunders, p. 181.)*

▶ Psychologic Changes in the Mother

For most low-risk expectant mothers, the second trimester is a happy, content period, marked by confirmation of the pregnancy, presence of a live fetus, and developing affection for the fetus. The uncertainty and ambivalence of the first trimester are generally resolved, and the expectant mother moves toward achieving the changed lifestyle of "woman and child." Discomforts of the first trimester, such as nausea and fatigue, subside, and the mother usually feels physically well.

Many women continue to work during the second trimester. Indeed, for a healthy woman, work in itself is no problem at any time during pregnancy (Piotrkowski & Hughes, 1993). During the second trimester, however, employed women are concerned with whether and when maternity leave should be taken, how to find child care, how significant others feel about her working before and after the baby is born, and what effects working will have on the baby and family. Although they will not deliver for several months, women who intend to return to work may want to discuss and plan future employment.

Acceptance of Pregnancy

In a classic study, Caplan (1969) noted that by the middle of the second trimester, the pregnant woman's feelings of ambivalence usually give way to joy over being pregnant. He felt that "quickening," the first sensation of fetal movements, was the event that ushered in this change. For the pregnant woman, quickening meant that a real baby, not just a "pregnancy," existed.

Lederman (1996) did not find complete joy and acceptance during the second trimester in her sample of healthy pregnant women. She found that the expectant woman's ambivalence could be repeated occasionally throughout the pregnancy as a wish not to be pregnant. This wish may reflect the woman's uncertainties about motherhood. All of the women in Lederman's sample were primiparous; however, adding another child to a family is also a great step in the family life cycle. According to Lederman (1996), ambivalence about pregnancy can range from low to high. Although occasional, low levels of ambivalence are common, persistent, high levels of ambivalence may signal emotional difficulties. Each expectant client and her family needs to be assessed with care.

Maternal Role Attainment

During the second trimester, replication, which begins in the first trimester, continues. Rubin (1984) believes that each stage of the pregnancy cycle involves new models for replication. Once a stage is completed, former models are no longer relevant and, psychologically, the woman moves on. For example, the woman who has completed the prenatal role must progress into the role of woman in labor.

During the second trimester, activities begin to be unconsciously integrated into the woman's personality system; they become part of her. Like Caplan, Rubin (1984) sees the presence of a "real" fetus/baby and fetal movement as the catalyst for **internalization.** This leads to fantasy, which is another method of role attainment during the second trimester.

Fantasies

Fantasies, both daydreams and night dreams, become an important part of the expectant mother's prenatal experience during the second trimester. A woman's life history and attitudes toward the pregnancy can influence both her dreams and the course of labor. The "real" fetus/baby who provides stimuli through fetal movement initiates maternal fantasies. The fantasies and dreams may help a woman attain the maternal role and work through unresolved problems in her life (Sherwen, 1991). A pregnant woman's concerns may be revealed openly in her daydreams and night dreams. This information can provide the nurse with many insights into the pregnant woman's current concerns.

Descriptions of second-trimester fantasies tend to confirm this trimester as a relatively happy, content phase of childbearing. In Rubin's (1984) study, the infant-to-be is first imagined to be like a 6-month-old baby floating peacefully in space. The expectant woman may fantasize about a baby of a specific sex, as indicated by dreams of dressing the baby, and later the child, in gender-specific clothing. By the middle of the second trimester the age of the baby in the mother's fantasies begins to vary. The expectant woman may fantasize about her child (either sex) as an adolescent, as a school-aged child, or as an infant usually not younger than 6 months.

Fantasies during the second trimester are therefore important in (1) helping the pregnant woman attain the maternal role, (2) helping the pregnant woman "bind in" to her future child, and (3) providing clues to the woman's concerns about her pregnancy, significant others, and life events.

Relationship with Mother

In the second trimester, the expectant woman's adaptation is influenced by her relationship with her own mother—the grandmother. Five components of the relationship develop as pregnancy progresses (Lederman, 1996): availability of the grandmother, grandmother's reaction to the pregnancy, grandmother's respect for her daughter's autonomy, willingness of the grandmother to reminisce, and empathy with the grandmother.

Availability of the Grandmother. In ideal situations, pregnancy and childbirth provide the expectant mother and grandmother with an opportunity to move their relationship to a higher level. In healthy relationships the expectant woman's own mother is interested in her daughter and able to provide emotional support. The original mother–child relationship has evolved into a relationship between two adults, which will remain close despite their living at a distance.

Grandmother's Reaction to the Pregnancy. Ideally, the grandmother reacts to the pregnancy by accepting her daughter as a mother as well as being enthusiastic about the grandchild.

Grandmother's Respect for Her Daughter's Autonomy. In a healthy, autonomous relationship, the expectant mother and grandmother relate to each other as two independent adults. The grandmother's belief in her daughter's independence and maturity strengthens decision making by the pregnant woman and promotes her confidence in herself as a mother (Lederman, 1996).

Willingness of the Grandmother to Reminisce. The expectant mother's early childhood experiences and the grandmother's childbearing experiences are topics shared between expectant mothers and their own mothers. When done in a positive manner, this form of close communication tends to increase the ego strength and self-confidence of the mother-to-be.

Empathy with the Grandmother. In a relationship that includes mutual sharing, the expectant woman may also be supportive of her own mother. She can empathize with her mother's experiences in parenting and with the tasks she must accomplish to become a grandmother.

Relationship With Fetus

The mother's relationship to her infant-to-be is greatly enhanced during the second trimester, when the presence of a "real" fetus/baby is evident. Quickening or ultrasound images encourage the development of this relationship.

Prenatal attachment can be seen in maternal behaviors such as:

- Identifying the fetus as a separate individual
- Imagining the attributes of the fetus (e.g., hair, eye color, personality)
- Imagining the role of the mother
- Selecting names for the baby
- Talking to the fetus
- Touching and stroking fetal parts as they are outlined against the abdomen
- Considering feeding methods and calling the fetus by a pet name

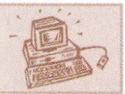

Research Abstract

Changes in Maternal–Fetal Attachment During Pregnancy

The purpose of this research was to determine if differences exist in maternal–fetal attachment over the first and second trimesters of pregnancy. The sample consisted of 40 Chinese women who had a normal pregnancy and 37 who had a history of infertility. The results of the study indicated that maternal–fetal attachment scores, as measured by the Cranley Maternal–Fetal Attachment Scale, increased from the first to the second trimesters for both groups.

Application to Practice

Since it has been shown that maternal–fetal attachment increases over time, nurses can plan nursing interventions to educate clients about attachment. Evaluation of attachment behaviors for both normal and previously infertile couples should continue throughout pregnancy.

Source: Lee, T.Y. (1994). Maternal–fetal attachment in normal and previously-infertile Chinese women. Nursing Research (China), 2*(1),* 67–77.

Speculation is growing that the fetus, in some manner, also establishes a relationship with the mother before birth.

Body Image

The woman's body image changes during the second trimester as the signs of pregnancy become increasingly obvious. After quickening the woman may begin to view the fetus as separate from her body (Berk, 1993). Moreover, she wears maternity clothes from necessity, not to validate pregnancy, as in the first trimester.

Body image during the second trimester is more gratifying and stable than in the first trimester. The growth of the uterus is obvious to others; however, the woman's abdomen does not enlarge enough to cause discomfort, as in the third trimester. Abdominal prominence and weight gain represent "baby" to the woman and she searches her body for additional physical signs of pregnancy.

The concept of body boundary can be studied in at least two ways: (1) the degree to which the body is perceived by the woman as an effective barrier, and (2) the amount of space the body is perceived to occupy. The expectant woman's perception of her body boundary as a protective barrier or container for the fetus increases during the second trimester (Berk, 1993). She also begins to see her body as potentially vulnerable to the environment.

Perception of body space, or how far the pregnant woman's body boundary seems to extend into her environment, is another way to assess body boundary and body image. Toward the end of the second trimester, the woman's body size is actually quite large. Her movement, therefore, may be affected and she may feel increasingly vulnerable. Some women may try to restrict their social activities because of this, although there is no physiologic reason for doing so.

▶ Psychologic Changes in the Father

During the second trimester, a father-to-be who is "tuned in" to his feelings about pregnancy may report a variety of couvade symptoms (Clinton, 1986). He also enters the stage of turning toward his own father and the fathering role. He looks to his own father for a role model. The psychologic experiences of expectant mothers and fathers are similar in that they reestablish relationships with the parent of the same sex (Zachariah, 1994) and they are oriented toward getting to know the fetus (Sandelowski & Black, 1994).

Couvade Syndrome

During the second trimester, men in one study reported a large number of couvade symptoms—an average of 12.4 per month. This was more than what was reported during the first or third trimester or postpartum. Symptoms included stomachache and weight gain (Clinton, 1986).

Although the couvade syndrome occurs widely in the United States, some men may worry that they are silly or abnormal. Nurses should assess for the couvade syndrome and provide reassurance that mild symptoms are real and normal.

Body Boundaries

The father's perceptions of his own body boundaries may begin to blur as his partner's pregnancy becomes increasingly evident (Fawcett, 1978). The significance of this change is unclear.

▶ Psychologic Changes in the Family

The second trimester is often a happy time for the healthy pregnant client and her family. The visible pregnancy does, however, produce concerns, such as anxiety about medical care, childbirth, and future pregnancies. Stress can result from biologic, psychologic, interpersonal, and sociocultural factors. For example, the biologic stress of the growing pregnancy, the psychologic stress of accomplishing maternal tasks, the interpersonal stress of moving into new roles, or conflict arising from cultural expectations or financial concerns may become apparent during the second trimester. Although stress may be present in some form throughout pregnancy, the nature of stress changes in each trimester.

▶ The Siblings' Experience

The physical and psychologic changes occurring in the mother during the second trimester make pregnancy obvious to even a young child. Although the mother feels physically well, the child may feel deprived of the mother's attention as she psychologically focuses on her pregnancy and fetus.

How the child experiences the mother's pregnancy depends largely on his or her stage of development. Three major developmental patterns may affect a sibling's experience of pregnancy:

- *Stage of psychosocial development.* According to Erikson (1963), the growing child evolves behaviors that allow him or her to interact in social situations with others. This process begins in infancy with parents and family and expands to others outside the family as the child grows to adolescence and adulthood. For conceptual ease, psychosocial development is subdivided into six stages.

- *Stage of cognitive development.* According to Piaget (1970), cognitive development relates to ways in which a child develops thinking processes and the ability to solve problems. Cognitive ability begins in infancy and continues to develop through adulthood.
- *Separation–individuation.* As described by Mahler, Pine, and Bergman (1975), separation–individuation is the process by which a child becomes an independent and interdependent individual. Not only is the person able successfully to function alone, but she or he can live and work with others.

All three developmental patterns begin in infancy and develop through childhood, adolescence, and adulthood. All involve mental and interactional processes; however, each pattern focuses on different, yet essential aspects of development. Along with physiologic maturation, they describe how children grow and develop.

Table 17–2 summarizes developmental patterns during childhood. Nurses need to understand developmental patterns to provide appropriate guidance to parents who are preparing a sibling for the new baby. An outline of developmental patterns is included in this chapter, because the second trimester is the time when children become aware of the mother's changing shape.

Guidelines for Preparation of Siblings

There is no "best" time for telling siblings about a pregnancy and birth. Sibling preparation is a topic of great concern to the healthy pregnant couple. Although negative sibling reactions to the prospect of a new baby have been discussed in the popular press and professional literature, many siblings respond to the news of the coming baby with interest and curiosity (Gullicks & Crase, 1993). Through anticipatory guidance and counseling the nurse can provide guidelines:

- Recognize the normal psychologic changes related to childbearing. By understanding the inward focus of women during the second trimester, couples can take steps, such as providing extra attention, to ensure that the child does not feel rejected or left out.
- Identify ways in which psychologic changes related to pregnancy can conflict or coincide with the child's developmental patterns.
- Consider the child's age. As noted in Table 17–2, a child less than 3 years old may not understand the meaning of pregnancy or the abstract concept of future. Chronologic age, however, does not always coincide with developmental patterns. Discussion therefore needs to be based on assessment of each sibling.
- Realize the need of the sibling to continue to feel loved, wanted, and valued. This is important regardless of the age of the child, although the manner of expression varies with the child's developmental pattern.
- Realize that children should not be expected to shoulder adult responsibilities. Expectant parents need to understand that what may appear to be a small contribution to them, such as bringing a tired mother a glass of juice, may actually be seen as a large contribution by the child.
- Understand that news of a new baby may not be greeted with joy by the sibling. School-aged children may wonder what their own role will be, especially if they have no other siblings. Adolescents may be uncomfortable at the confirmation of their parents' sexuality or may worry about changes in their family. Strategies that include attention, loving support, and developmentally appropriate discussion can help a child to receive a sibling positively.
- Appreciate the value of sibling preparation aids, such as books and sibling preparation classes.

Prenatal classes for siblings, delivered at a level the child can comprehend, might cover how a baby develops, what happens when the baby is born, where the child's mother (and father) will go when it is time for the baby to be born, who will remain with the child at home or at the birth center, what the new baby will be like, what it will be like for the child to be a "big" brother or "big" sister, and what it will be like to have the new brother or sister.

Classes may be informal or formal, depending, for example, on parental support of sibling education (provided by the parents with or without assistance from health care providers), characteristics of the siblings, the setting for prenatal care and childbirth, the philosophy of the health care providers, and whether the sibling will be present at the birth. Sibling teaching may be done on an individual basis during prenatal visits and through scheduled sibling tours and classes.

▶ The Grandparents' Experience

During the second trimester, the couple's parents must also accept the reality of the pregnancy and their coming grandchild. When feasible, the nurse can encourage the pregnant couple to bring the expectant

▶ **TABLE 17-2**

Summary of Developmental Patterns Affecting a Sibling's Experience of Pregnancy

Psychosocial Development (Erikson)

Basic Trust Versus Mistrust (birth to 1 year)	Infant gains basic sense of security in self and in surroundings. Infant needs to "receive and accept" attention, love, food, and so on. Infant has difficulty coping with decreased attention from primary caregiver (usually mother). Development of trust is the successful completion of this stage and is highly dependent on the caregiver. Mother's attention to another pregnancy creates a need for additional attention from others (such as father or grandparent).
Autonomy Versus Shame and Doubt (1 year to 3 years)	Child learns to control own body. Child develops a sense of "self." Child starts to balance autonomy with parents' wishes. Child needs much attention from caretakers to develop autonomy and avoid feelings of shame and doubt.
Initiative Versus Guilt (3 years to 6 years)	Child is becoming the type of person he or she will be later in life. Child wants to be like parents. Sexual curiosity develops; notes differences between parents. Child needs to maintain a sense of worth and initiative, while recognizing she or he is not a grownup. Child starts to develop a conscience. Child without adequate support can develop feelings of guilt. Child notices mother's pregnancy as a manifestation of being a woman. Child may ask sexually oriented questions, although she or he will not understand detailed answers. Child may make contact with others outside family if in a preschool program.
Industry Versus Inferiority (6 years to 12 years)	Child wants to learn all he or she can about the world. Child makes contact with people outside the family, especially through school, and develops friendships. Child is interested in making and collecting things; participation in team efforts becomes important. Child may worry about whether her or his efforts are valued; may have worries about being not good enough. Child is likely to be interested and pleased about mother's pregnancy and birth of baby, and may understand changes in mother. Child, especially between ages 8 and 12, usually relates well to friends. Peer groups lessen the need for mother's attention. Child with a sense of "industry" may want to help prepare for the baby; can do simple chores, help select baby's name, and so on.
Identity Versus Identity Diffusion (12 years to 18 years)	Adolescent solidifies continuing personal sense of self. Adolescent may be threatened by "identity diffusion"; that is, he or she feels unable to keep an independent sense of self, but gains identity only through cliques, organizations, or identification with "heroes." Adolescent with healthy sense of self may be excited about mother's pregnancy. Adolescent with fragile sense of self may be angry, ashamed, or jealous of mother's pregnancy. Adolescents will have stated or unstated questions about pregnancy and relationships. Parents may initiate discussion of sexuality, love, and marital bond with adolescents. Mother's pregnancy presents opportunity to help adolescent incorporate a model of mature sexual love, childbearing, and birth into his or her own identity.

Cognitive Development (Piaget)

Sensorimotor Period (birth to 2 years)	Child progresses through action sequences in which the result of a behavior stimulates repetition of that behavior (especially when behavior is pleasing). Child learns to gain desired results by various willed activities. Action sequences are carried out in actual behavior alone; child does not think about them in complex manner. Child cannot really grasp cognitively the meaning of pregnancy. Child's experience of pregnancy is at a feeling level.
Preoperational Stage (2 years to 7 years)	More complex thinking can take place, especially for the preschool and school-aged child. Thinking is very concrete. Child tends to believe that everyone sees the world the same as he or she does (egocentrism). Child tends to think that real events have intentional causes, for example, the child causes rain by putting on a raincoat (called animism). Child views pregnancy in a simplistic, concrete way.

(continued)

▶ **TABLE 17–2 (continued)**

Summary of Developmental Patterns Affecting a Sibling's Experience of Pregnancy

Preoperational Stage (continued)	Child is usually unable to understand abstract explanations of pregnancy.
	The 2- to 3-year old can perceive the growth of the mother's abdomen; however, understanding that there is a growing baby inside may be difficult. This becomes easier for children of 6 or 7.
	Time (past and future) is still a difficult concept, especially for children 2 to 5 years of age.
	Patience and repetition ("talks" with parents, age-appropriate sibling preparation books, and so on) needed to help child understand about future baby.
	Child may repeatedly ask the same questions.
	Questions need to be answered simply and concretely; explanations should be based on what a child can see.
Concrete Operations (7 years to 11 years)	Child develops reasoning ability.
	Child can conceive of events that would be impossible in the real world.
	Child has a better perception of time; he or she can go back in time or reverse the directions of a thought sequence.
	Child is less egocentric.
	Thought still depends on concrete experiences.
	Parents can discuss pregnancy and birth with child; explanations should be concrete and direct.
	Child will have specific questions about childbirth.
	Child may participate in preparation for baby.
Formal Operations (11 years onward)	Child can reason abstractly about things and events that cannot be represented in reality.
	Child is able to understand relationships beyond events and things represented in reality.
	Child can appreciate alternatives in any situation.
	Child can understand adult-type explanations about pregnancy and birth.
	Child can understand abstract notions, such as parental motivations for having another child.
	Child can participate in preparation for the baby; can assume greater responsibilities.
Separation–Individuation (Mahler)	
Symbiosis (pregnancy to after birth)	Closeness, "bondedness."
	Not applicable to sibling, as child must be at least 10 or 11 months old before sibling is born.
	Mother who remains in close symbiosis with baby as he or she develops may have difficulty attaching to the fetus in a future pregnancy.
Rapprochement (18 months to 2 years)	Child is aware of her or his growing separation and autonomy from parents.
	Child desires autonomy but may fear loss of mother; may cry when well-liked babysitter arrives and mother leaves.
	Child has little tolerance for frustration.
	Child wants mother to participate in all activities even though he or she no longer requires this participation.
	Child may have "arguments" or tantrums if mother does not provide enough attention.
	Child may become more demanding as mother becomes more emotionally unavailable in relation to pregnancy; developmental phases of child and mother may thus be in conflict.
	Parents need to ensure that child receives adequate attention; parents need support to deal with demanding child behaviors.
Separation–Individuation (2 years to 3 years)	Continues; the child perceives self as a separate individual.
	The more separate and individuated the child is from the mother, the better is the child's ability to cope with pregnancy and a new sibling.

Source: Erikson, 1963; Piaget, 1970; Mahler, Pine, & Bergman, 1975.

grandparents to prenatal visits (Fig. 17–4). A class for expectant grandparents may be offered, focusing on such topics as changes in obstetric care, the importance of the grandparenting role, and the bridging of generation gaps (Biasella, 1993). Literature can be made available at the classes or in waiting rooms. Grandparent support groups may provide an enjoyable setting for the sharing of thoughts and feelings about this developmental step.

Roye and Balk (1997) described a special program geared toward pregnant teenagers and their mothers in a large inner-city municipal hospital in New York. Through a series of classes, scheduled on the same day as the prenatal care appointments and taught by pediatric nurse practitioners or certified nurse-midwives, and meetings with a social worker, teens and their mothers not only received prenatal education and support but continued with the program until the child turned 3 years old or the mother turned 19. Benefits of this supportive program were reported to include better coping on the part of the grandmothers and improved relationships and communica-

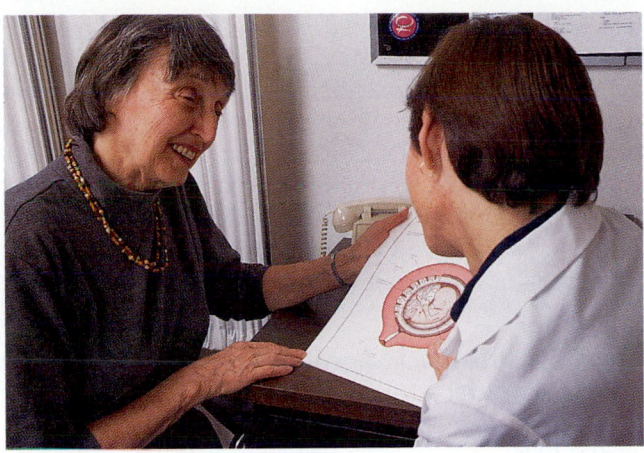

FIGURE 17–4. The nurse can be very helpful in providing information about the physiologic changes that occur during pregnancy with the expectant grandmother.

tion between grandmothers and their daughters; grandmothers also felt that the entire family had been helped by such a program.

Expectant grandparents may need information about the psychologic changes of pregnancy and their own importance to their expectant daughter or son. In working with grandparents-to-be, the nurse must remain sensitive to cultural patterns of communication between the expectant parents and grandparents, especially with respect to presence during physical examination (Strom & Strom, 1992).

► Sociocultural Dimensions

Cultural patterns exist in nearly every family and affect internal family dynamics and interactions with others in the environment. Health care providers working with a family during a woman's second trimester must understand cultural proscriptions surrounding family members during childbearing. In addition, nurses should be aware of the influence of socioeconomic factors on the childbearing family.

In Chapter 15, the African-American family was used to illustrate how membership in a specific cultural group may affect perceptions and practices during pregnancy and childbirth. In this chapter, the Japanese-American family is considered as one example of East Asian cultural groups.

Socioeconomic Influence

Stress concerning finances may increase during the second trimester. Some issues of concern are potential loss of the mother's job or position as the pregnancy becomes more evident, increasing need for such resources as maternity clothing, lack of adequate

insurance, and loss of the mother's job-related benefits. There is also a recognized correlation between poverty and culture (Klainberg, Holzemer, Leonard, & Arnold, 1998). Economically disadvantaged people face major stresses during pregnancy related to poverty.

Cultural Focus: East Asian Cultural Groups

Japanese, Chinese, Korean, and Vietnamese are a few of the many cultural groups that originated in East and Southeast Asia; these groups comprise numerous subgroups. In addition to readily apparent differences in physical characteristics and language, East Asians differ greatly from other cultural groups in the United States, especially in philosophic approaches to life. These approaches are generally influenced by traditional belief systems, for example, Confucianism and Buddhism (D'Avanzo, 1992; Spector, 1996).

East Asian philosophic systems do not tend to stress the individual's independence and autonomy, but rather emphasize that the wishes of the individual are replaced by those of the family. The East Asian family may adhere to the tradition of specific hierarchic roles with formal rules of behavior for all members. Each person's response and loyalty to this code may be more a reflection of the family than of the individual. The extended family, then, is responsible for maintaining the status of the family. All relationships, such as those among husband and wife and parents and children, have particular definitions. Males may be valued more than females, and there may be different expectations for men and women (McGoldrick, Giordano, & Pearce, 1996).

In addition to the broad distinction between East Asian and Western cultures, each of the many East Asian groups is unique. East Asian groups differ in vital developmental aspects of life, such as language, history, and social and economic backgrounds (McGoldrick et al., 1996; Spector, 1996). People need to be assessed individually; however, an understanding of common features of family structure gives the nurse a starting point for a plan of care. Planning is then tailored to the specific needs of each family and client. Further assessment is based on key factors, including the family's social class, geographic origin, birthplace, and generation of family members living in the United States. Broad cultural concepts are most applicable when considering recent immigrants and others with strong traditional ties. Although East Asians born in the United States may be more assimilated into the "American" culture, they may retain deep cultural ties to their East Asian heritage.

Time. In the United States, the primary family unit is the nuclear family, which has a time-limited life span. In other words, the nuclear family dissolves when children grow to adulthood and have their own families and when their parents die. For the East Asian, the family may not be time limited; it may extend both backward and forward in time. The individual is seen as the product of all the generations of his or her family. Because of the extended sense of family existence, an individual's behaviors reflect not only on him- or herself, but on all past and future generations of the extended family. Thus, East Asians may perceive responsibility that goes far beyond personal concerns (McGoldrick et al., 1996).

Marriage. Marriage and choice of a partner may also be different for an East Asian person. The family of both partners may greatly influence the choice of partners. This may also be true among East Asians living in the United States. Marriage is often viewed as a continuation of the man's family line. The woman is considered to have left her family of origin on her marriage and to have been absorbed into her husband's family. In this arrangement her status as a young wife may be low.

Family Roles. Within the traditional East Asian family, roles are clearly defined. The father is the leader. He makes decisions, is responsible for the "success or failure" of the family's well-being and status, and enforces family rules. His authority was traditionally unquestioned by other family members. To his children, he may be a stern disciplinarian.

The mother, on the other hand, nurtures husband and children. East Asian women have not been free to engage in the same kinds of work and activities as men. Children establish the strongest emotional tie to their mother. This emotional tie has importance later in the mother's life, in case the father dies and the oldest son becomes the family leader. The oldest son's great emotional attachment to his mother influences his behavior to fulfill her wishes. Thus, East Asian women often have much power over their daughters-in-law.

Children in East Asian families may also have defined roles. The most important role may be that of eldest son, who is groomed to become the family leader and often has authority over other children. He also has much responsibility and is expected to be a role model. In traditional Asian families, daughters are not valued as highly as sons, possibly because they join their husbands' families at the time of marriage. The daughter's role is primarily caretaker of the home. Some change and loosening of tradition have occurred as attitudes toward women change. Daugh-

ters now have some freedom in choice of a partner and career.

One consideration for maternity nursing may be the East Asian husband's lack of involvement during pregnancy and birth. This separation of men's and women's roles is mutually agreeable in traditional families. Although traditional patterns of interaction are being influenced by increased contact with the West, they nevertheless remain.

Family Dimensions. Among other important dimensions of East Asian family life are the concepts of obligation, shame, and communication (McGoldrick et al., 1996). These concepts may affect the nurse's interactions with East Asian families during pregnancy.

To maintain harmony in relationships with others, the concept of obligation is vital. Obligation arises through ascribed roles or status and through helpful or kind actions toward another person. This person then incurs obligation. The greatest obligation of the East Asian is often to parents.

Shame and shaming reinforce societal expectations and proper behavior in traditional East Asian society. The desire to avoid "loss of face" is a powerful motivating force.

For East Asian cultures, what may be communicated between people is determined by specific characteristics of those individuals. Some characteristics that determine individuals' relationships to each other and their manner of verbal and nonverbal communication are age, sex, education, occupation, social status, family background, marital status, and parenthood. Ambiguous situations in which the East Asian may not know the attributes of the person to whom he or she is speaking may cause anxiety. Often, this anxiety is due to the fear of making a social error in speech and thus losing face. In such situations, the East Asian may withdraw, be silent, and watch for cues from the unknown individual. In particular, the East Asian may feel that to ask questions is to present a challenge to a person in authority. Thus, questioning is avoided. In addition, the nurse working with East Asian clients must appreciate the importance of harmony in their relationships. Directness may lead to disagreement, disharmony, and loss of face for both client and health care provider. Direct confrontation is therefore avoided whenever possible (McGoldrick et al., 1996).

Family Transition. Transition to the culture of the United States can be difficult. East Asian family members may experience conflict and grief-type reactions.

The reactions may comprise six stages (McGoldrick et al., 1996):

1. Cultural shock, resulting from differences between what was expected in the United States and what really exists, especially if expectations were for a better economic life
2. Disappointment about what exists
3. Grief at separation and loss of what was left behind
4. Depression because of the current family situation
5. Acceptance of the current situation
6. Mobilization of family resources and energy to cope with the new environment

The last stage may be difficult, as the family may try to use familiar traditional problem-solving methods that worked in their former culture, but may not be effective in the United States. The nurse must keep this in mind when attempting to use crisis intervention techniques.

Not all families or all family members pass through the six stages. Ideally, the acculturated family comes to value both the old and the new culture.

Role of the Nurse. The nurse must assess the unique nature of any pregnant East Asian family to avoid stereotyping. The extent of the East Asian family's acculturation in the United States affects nursing actions.

Nurses in prenatal clinics may attempt to counsel a traditionally oriented pregnant East Asian woman on prenatal diet and medications. If this woman follows traditional family practices, she may not be the correct person for the nurse to address concerning family or individual dietary changes. The husband's role as leader of the family may require him to "approve" dietary changes. The husband may decide whether it is necessary to consult his mother, as she has a major influence on the manner in which the husband may make family decisions.

The nurse who works with an ethnic or cultural population must learn about specific cultural family patterns. If not, the nurse's culturally ignorant behaviors might have undesired results.

Cultural Focus: The Japanese-American Family

Among Japanese-American families, adherence to traditional cultural beliefs and practices varies depending on how many generations of the family have lived in the United States. The majority of third-, fourth-, and fifth-generation Japanese-Americans are well assimilated into the dominant North American culture; however, the extent of assimilation may vary with socioeconomic status, geographic location, and in what country the person has been educated.

In an early study, Okamoto (1978) interviewed women from various generations about their attitudes and beliefs about pregnancy, birth, and childbearing. She concluded that Japanese-Americans have managed pregnancy and birth in a variety of ways. Certain aspects of traditional Japanese beliefs, affiliations, and practices are retained; others are replaced by those of their sociocultural environment. Each woman interviewed, regardless of her generation, kept some ethnic affiliation and identity. Ethnicity was demonstrated in food preparation, use of the Japanese language in the home, and participation in traditional rituals or practices related to pregnancy and birth. Although this sample represented three generations with diverse levels of acculturation, all women retained a strong affiliation to the Japanese identity.

In general, Japanese-American women sought and received prenatal care similar to that obtained by members of the dominant culture. All generations saw pregnancy and birth as natural events. Moreover, Japanese-American women in this sample seemed to take a more active, pragmatic interest in health education concerning the pregnancy cycle than many members of the dominant culture.

In many ways, Japanese-American families see pregnancy as North American families of the dominant culture do; however, as pregnancy involves the extended family, being of Japanese background may produce some changes in the psychologic processes involved in becoming parents. For example, because of the importance of the father and grandparents during pregnancy, the nurse should assess the cultural orientation and level of assimilation not only of the expectant mother, but also of her partner and both maternal and paternal families of origin.

Specific cultural practices place emphasis on rest and warmth during pregnancy. For example, pregnant Japanese women may wear knee socks for warmth. Beginning around the fifth month, traditional women may use a white abdominal binder (*obi*) as an undergarment to promote warmth.

During the second trimester, when the pregnancy becomes apparent, culturally related conflicts may arise between generations. Other potential problems in the Japanese-American family during pregnancy may be geographic separation of the nuclear family from families of origin. If unable to be united with their families, Japanese-Americans may experience a sense of isolation.

► NURSING AND COLLABORATIVE ASSESSMENT

Several goals are developed to guide assessment during the second trimester, with the intent of monitoring fetal and maternal adaptations to pregnancy and identifying risk at an early stage. Assessment may focus on several aspects of the childbearing family.

- Maternal adaptation to pregnancy
- Development of new risk factors
- Effects of existing risk factors on the pregnant family
- Fetal well-being
- Psychosocial status and adaptation to pregnancy
- Educational needs
- Resources available to the pregnant client and her family

For women who begin prenatal care during the second trimester, the approach to assessment during the initial visit is the same as that described during first-trimester assessment. A woman may not begin care until the second trimester for a variety of reasons: lack of awareness of her pregnancy, travel or residence during early pregnancy in an area where prenatal care was inaccessible, financial concerns, fear of the health care system, or fear of confirmation of pregnancy.

Reasons for delay in seeking care are assessed by the nurse. Nursing diagnoses and interventions are based on the unique needs of the client during the second trimester.

► Assessment of Maternal Adaptations to Pregnancy

Updating the Health History

Ideally, the collaborative approach taken by health care providers during the first trimester will continue during the second, with the documentation and recording of current physiologic and psychosocial changes and the related interventions.

The care plan was based in part on information received from the client's initial history, taken by the nurse-midwife, physician, or staff nurse. During subsequent visits in the second trimester, a woman's history and care plan (e.g., with respect to nutrition and exercise/activity) are revised in response to changes.

Physiologic Assessment

Prenatal visits are recommended every 4 weeks during the second trimester for the healthy low-risk client (Cunningham et al., 1997). During each prenatal visit, a standard set of parameters are assessed to obtain information about maternal physiologic adaptations to pregnancy and fetal well-being (Table 17–3).

Knowledge about normal and abnormal findings and their relation to physiologic adaptations is necessary so that effective interventions can be planned and implemented. Table 17–4 presents an overview of

---

► TABLE 17-3

Physiologic Parameters Assessed During the Second Trimester

Assessment Parameter	Frequency of Assessment	Purpose
Vital signs, including blood pressure, pulse, respiration	Monthly	Detect any changes from normal/baseline that may indicate development of complications (e.g., preeclampsia)
Uterine growth, measured by fundal height; fetal well-being, measured by fetal heart tones and, after quickening, fetal movement	Monthly	Assess for disproportionate enlargement, which may indicate multiple gestation, inadequate fetal nutrition, and so on; assess location and quality of fetal heart tones (fetal heart tones and activity indicate fetal well-being)
Maternal weight and nutritional status	Monthly	Assess pattern of weight gain and nutritional adequacy and detect fluid retention
Urinalysis for protein and glucose	Monthly	Detect development of complications (e.g., preeclampsia and need for diabetic screening) However, glucosuria can be an unreliable diagnostic finding
Suggested blood studies		
Alpha-fetoprotein	16–18 weeks	Screen for neural tube defects
Glucose	24–28 weeks	Screen for diabetes

▶ **TABLE 17–4**

Selected Clinical Findings During the Second Trimester

Body System	Clinical Findings
Integumentary	Darkened breasts and areolae, chloasma; linea nigra; increased perspiration; stretch marks; hot flashes (cutaneous flushing of skin); hair seems to thicken and nails grow faster
Cardiovascular	Increase in heart rate of on average 10–15 beats per minute over nonpregnant rate
	Decrease in blood pressure from baseline during first 24 weeks of on average 5 mm Hg systolic and 10 mm Hg diastolic
	Supine hypotension may occur and be accompanied by nausea, lightheadedness, tachycardia, sweating
	Increased splitting of heart sound with loudness of S_1, S_2; systolic murmur may be heard
	Dependent edema of the legs; edema that disappears after elevating legs; hemorrhoids; varicose veins in legs, vulva
Respiratory	Dyspnea on exertion; respiratory rate 16–24 per minute
Hematologic	Hgb 12 g/dL or greater; Hct 35%; below 11 g/dL usually due to iron deficiency
Gastrointestinal	Constipation
	Pyrosis (heartburn)
	Hypercholesterolemia; lipid intolerance
Musculoskeletal	Backache, especially in lower sacral area
	Pregnancy "waddle"; loosening of pelvic joints
Urinary	Nocturnal voiding
	Trace glycosuria
	Trace proteinuria
	BUN 8.17 ± 1.5 mg/100 mL
	Serum creatinine 0.46 ± 0.13 mg/100 mL
Reproductive	Progressive enlargement of uterus
	Round ligament pain
	Braxton Hicks contractions
	Vaginal leukorrhea
	Breasts—fullness, tingling, and heaviness; colostrum may appear; everted nipples
Neurologic	Alert, appropriate
	Normal (+1 to +2) deep tendon reflexes in all four extremities

nursing assessment of maternal physiology during the second trimester.

Risk Assessment

Assessment of risk factors continues at each prenatal visit because high-risk conditions can appear at any time during pregnancy. Early identification of the woman with a complication is necessary to minimize poor maternal or neonatal outcome. The nurse assesses risk factors from information obtained through interviews, physical examinations, laboratory studies and prenatal diagnostic studies. Second-trimester risk assessment focuses on current pregnancy risk factors and any changes in physiologic, psychosocial, demographic, lifestyle, or socioeconomic factors (see box entitled Second Trimester Risk Factors).

Biochemical Screening Techniques

Urinalysis. At each prenatal visit during the second trimester, a freshly voided urine specimen is assessed for the presence of protein, glucose, and ketones by use of a dipstick. If a UTI is suspected through the report of symptoms, such as painful and frequent urination, fever, or flank back pain, a clean-catch urine specimen should be obtained for microscopic study and culture.

During pregnancy, normal protein loss through the kidneys is up to 200 mg per 24 hours. Proteinuria of more than 500 mg per 24 hours may indicate a disease process (Moore, 1994). Trace to 1+ proteinuria on a urine sample may be considered negligible. Readings of 2+ and above require further assessment. Preexisting signs, such as elevated blood pressure, excessive weight gain, and generalized edema, are likely to be present if PIH exists, because proteinuria occurs late in the course of the disorder (see Chapter 19). A 24-hour urine collection test to measure the total amount of protein being lost may be performed for the client who has 2+ proteinuria.

Slight glycosuria may be present because of physiologic decrease in the renal threshold for glucose during pregnancy. About 50% of women excrete glucose in the urine at some point during pregnancy (Moore, 1994).

Blood Studies. Blood glucose screening is performed between 24 and 28 weeks of gestation to detect the development of gestational diabetes. Women who have had gestational diabetes with previous pregnancies may be screened earlier. If early screening results are normal, subsequent screening is done at 24 to 28 weeks (American College of Obstetricians and Gynecologists, 1994). A random blood glucose sample and a 1-hour abbreviated glucose tolerance test are two approaches used in screening for gestational diabetes. A random blood glucose level greater than 120 mg/dl indicates the need for a full glucose tolerance test. The 1-hour abbreviated glucose tolerance test assesses blood glucose 1 hour after a 50-g standard oral glucose solution is ingested. A value of 140 mg/dl or greater (or as specified by unit protocol) is considered a positive result and indicates the need for a 3-hour glucose tolerance test (Cunningham et al., 1997).

▶ SECOND TRIMESTER RISK FACTORS

SOCIOECONOMIC FACTORS

Lack of money and/or health insurance or other essential resources
Poor living conditions
Threats to safety and security
Inadequate nutrition

MATERNAL/FETAL HEALTH FACTORS

Physiologic or mental conditions, such as cardiovascular or pulmonary disease, chronic hypertension, depression, or retardation
Seizure disorder
Sexually transmitted diseases or other infections, for example, urinary tract infection (UTI) or febrile illnesses
Abnormal weight loss or gain
Malignancy
Surgery during pregnancy
Major congenital anomalies of the reproductive tract
Pregnancy-induced hypertension (PIH)/albuminemia
Personal or family history of genetic or congenital abnormalities

PREGNANCY STATUS

Late or no prenatal care
Abnormal uterine or fetal growth
Exposure to environmental hazards and teratogens
Multiple fetuses
Vaginal bleeding
Rh isoimmunization
Preterm labor
Premature rupture of membranes
Cervical dilation/effacement

PSYCHOSOCIAL FACTORS

Problems accepting pregnancy or adapting to the changes
Lack of understanding or acceptance of need for prenatal care; inability or refusal to participate in healthy practices
Lack of partner, friends, or family support
Severe stress at home or work
Conflict with predominant culture

LIFESTYLE

Smoking
Alcohol/drug use
Multiple sexual partners
Sexual partners with high-risk lifestyle, e.g., substance abuse

Psychosocial Assessment

Thorough psychosocial assessment with follow-up at each prenatal visit is an essential aspect of prenatal care during the second trimester (see box entitled Components of Second-Trimester Psychosocial Assessment). Attentive listening to the woman's concerns assists the nurse in individualizing nursing interventions during the second trimester and throughout pregnancy.

Cultural Assessment

Assessment of the client's cultural beliefs and her responses to pregnancy and prenatal care continues throughout pregnancy. The healthy, low-risk client usually feels well during the second trimester. The perception of the client and family about health care during periods of wellness may be influenced by their religious and cultural practices. By interviewing the client and observing her responses to health care, the nurse can identify cultural influences on family behavior during the second trimester.

▶ Assessment of Fetal Well-Being

Assessment of fetal well-being during the second trimester includes low-risk and high-risk assessment. Low-risk assessment involves physical examination techniques such as measurement of fundal height and fetal heart rate (Table 17–5). Maternal reports of lifestyle behaviors and reports of fetal activity after quickening are also useful indicators of fetal health. High-risk assessment involves screening for abnormalities (e.g., genetic disorders). Techniques such as diagnostic ultrasound, maternal serum screening for alpha-fetoprotein levels, amniocentesis, and percutaneous umbilical blood sampling (PUBS) are used to screen for abnormalities and assess fetal well-being.

Fundal Height

During a routine prenatal visit, assessment of uterine size and palpation of the fetus can provide important information about fetal well-being. One method of evaluating fetal growth is measurement of uterine

► COMPONENTS OF SECOND-TRIMESTER PSYCHOSOCIAL ASSESSMENT

PSYCHOLOGIC FACTORS

General emotional status
Previous history of emotional problems
Level of stress

SOCIOECONOMIC, CULTURAL, AND ENVIRONMENTAL FACTORS

Family integrity, structure, and level of functioning
Cultural, community, and family support systems
Economic status of family
Availability of adequate housing and food
Access to appropriate prenatal care
Knowledge about and accessibility of community resources
Employment outside of the home, nature of job
Cultural beliefs and practices affecting reproduction
Lifestyle
Health beliefs and practices
Work and home environment

ADAPTATION TO PREGNANCY

Feelings at this time about pregnancy
Anxiety in relation to concern about fetus, maternal well-being, and physical testing
Sexual functioning: changes in, feelings about, and problems with
Perception of pregnancy affecting present activities and responsibilities
Perception of physiologic changes and body image
Accomplishing "tasks of pregnancy"

COPING PATTERNS

Ability of client and her partner to cope with stressful situations
Effectiveness of coping methods (Do they result in positive outcomes? If not, what follows?)

NETWORK OF SUPPORT

Father's present attitude toward pregnancy
Amount of emotional support from parents, siblings, other family members, and friends
Accessibility of family, distance client lives from family
Amount and types of support client expects from family and friends during pregnancy, childbirth, and early parenting

---

► TABLE 17–5

Pregnancy Milestones in the Second Trimester

Milestone	Time Frame
Quickening	
Placenta in anterior part of uterus	19 weeks—primigravidas 17.5 weeks—multiparas
Placenta in posterior part of uterus	18 weeks—primigravidas 16.1 weeks—multiparas
Fetal heart tones	16–20 weeks—unamplified auscultation 8–10 weeks—Doppler ultrasound
Fundal heights and estimated gestation	12 weeks—at level of symphysis pubis 16 weeks—halfway between symphysis pubis and umbilicus 20 weeks—one to two fingerbreadths below umbilicus 24 weeks—one to two fingerbreadths above umbilicus

size. By the second trimester, the fundus is palpable above the maternal symphysis pubis (see Fig. 17–1). Pelvic examination is not usually performed as part of the ongoing assessment in the second trimester.

Fundal height is usually measured in centimeters by use of a tape measure. The nurse first explains the procedure to the client. While preparing the client, the nurse can obtain information about the tone, irritability, and consistency of the uterus. The examiner measures the distance between the upper border of the maternal symphysis pubis, over the midline of the abdomen, to the top of the uterine fundus. This measurement is then inserted into McDonald's formula:

$$\frac{\text{distance in centimeters} \times 8}{7} = \text{total weeks of gestation}$$

This finding should correlate with gestation after 22 to 24 weeks. If a difference exists between actual findings (in centimeters) and gestational age, further assessment is necessary to rule out conditions that could alter fundal height. Fundal height may be altered by increased uterine size as a result of polyhydramnios, hydatidiform mole, and multiple gestation or by decreased size as a result of oligohydramnios or intrauterine growth retardation.

Uterine Activity

Uterine activity is also assessed during each second-trimester visit. Normally, it consists of mild, low-intensity Braxton Hicks contractions, which are characterized by irregular, painless tightening of the uterus. As pregnancy progresses, Braxton Hicks contractions increase in frequency and intensity.

Women should be taught the distinction between false and true contractions so that the onset of labor can be recognized. This is particularly important during the second trimester because of problems related to preterm birth.

Fetal Heart Tones

Fetal heart tones can be detected as early as 8 weeks with Doppler ultrasound amplification (Cunningham et al., 1997). Without amplification, fetal heart tones can be auscultated at 16 to 20 weeks' gestation. Fetal heart sounds during the second trimester are usually detected at the midline of the maternal abdomen or slightly to the left or right of the midline, depending on fetal position. The average fetal heart range is 120 to 160 beats per minute; a fetal heart range of 150 to 160 may be common during the second trimester. The baseline fetal heart rate generally decreases as pregnancy advances and the fetus matures.

Quickening

Quickening may be used to determine gestational age in conjunction with other assessments. Quickening may be perceived by the mother between the 17th and 20th weeks of pregnancy as a gentle fluttering feeling in the abdomen. Quickening alone, however, cannot be used as positive identification of gestational age.

▶ Prenatal Diagnostic Assessment

Diagnostic Ultrasound

Ultrasound's major uses during the second trimester are in fetal assessment, visualization of internal structures during invasive diagnostic procedures and treatments, and identification of maternal abnormalities (Fig. 17–5). For example, gestational age may be calculated based on biparietal diameters of the fetal head. Fetal growth can be followed by serially estimating fetal weight and plotting the values against gestational age. This is done in cases of suspected intrauterine fetal growth retardation (Sokol, Jones, & Pernoll, 1994).

Fetal evaluation for structural malformations, estimation of fetal head size, and identification of the symmetry and proportional growth of the fetal brain

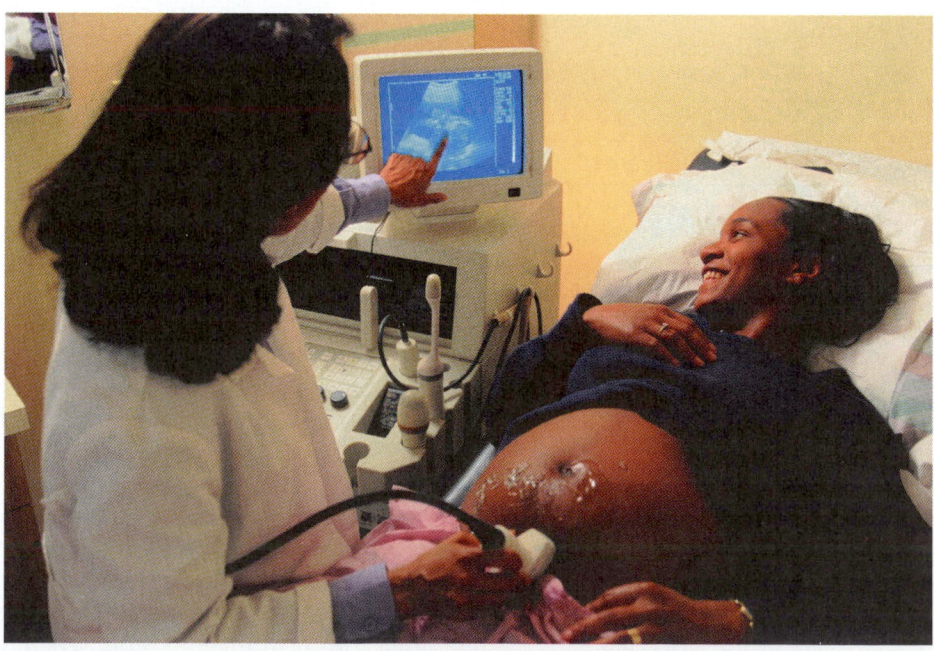

FIGURE 17–5. Diagnostic ultrasound is used as a prenatal assessment tool during the second trimester for purposes of evaluation of fetal well-being and identification of maternal abnormalities.

and liver are among the factors that provide information about fetal well-being. The box entitled Indications for Ultrasound Diagnosis in the Second Trimester summarizes the conditions or risk factors for which ultrasound can be used as a screening and evaluation tool.

Assessment for Neural Tube Defects

Neural tube defects are potentially major central nervous system malformations that occur when the embryonic neural tube does not develop normally. The neural tube may not close properly, or it may close normally but then overdistend and rupture. The brain, spinal cord, and overlying tissues may be affected.

Neural tube defects may be closed, that is, covered by skin or a thick membrane, or "open" as in cases when neural tissue is totally exposed or covered only by a thin, transparent membrane. The three most common neural tube defects are anencephaly, spina bifida, and encephalocele.

"Open" neural tube defects leak **alpha-fetoprotein (AFP),** a glycoprotein normally found in pregnancy. It is synthesized in the embryonic yolk sac, developing gastrointestinal tract, and fetal liver. It is found in fetal serum, amniotic fluid, and maternal serum. Concentrations of AFP in the fetal serum and amniotic fluid decrease rapidly after 15 weeks' gestation while those in the maternal serum continue to rise until late in pregnancy.

Maternal Serum Alpha-fetoprotein Screening (MSAFP).

Alpha-fetoprotein in the maternal serum is the basis for screening for neural tube defects (elevated levels) and Trisomy 21 (low levels) in the second trimester of pregnancy. Because levels of AFP change during pregnancy, calculation of correct gestational age is important for interpretation of findings. Maternal serum screening is most sensitive at 16 to 18

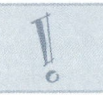

Nursing Alert

The American College of Obstetricians and Gynecologists (1996) recommends that all pregnant women should be offered maternal serum alpha-fetoprotein screening. However, this screening should be coordinated to include quality control, counseling, and follow-up.

weeks' gestation, although it can be performed from 15 to 22 weeks' gestation (Cunningham et al., 1997). Several factors may produce an abnormal AFP level in maternal serum (see box entitled Conditions Associated with Abnormal Maternal Serum Alpha-Fetoprotein Concentrations).

Serum screening is followed with ultrasound if abnormal AFP results are reported. Neural tube defects may be seen on ultrasound. In addition, conditions that may affect AFP levels, such as gestational age, other congenital anomalies, and multiple gestation, may be identified.

Low AFP levels have been connected with an increased risk of Trisomy 21, and further diagnostic tests, such as amniocentesis, may be indicated. To increase the sensitivity and specificity of MSAFP as a screening tool for Trisomy 21, new tests, the double marker test and the triple test, were developed. The double marker test adds human chorionic gonadotropin hCG testing to AFP testing. The median gonadotropin level doubles in mothers with a fetus with Trisomy 21 (Haddow, 1995), and hCG is the most sensitive maternal marker for the detection of the syndrome (American College of Obstetricians and

---

▶ **INDICATIONS FOR ULTRASOUND DIAGNOSIS IN THE SECOND TRIMESTER**

- Estimation of gestational age for women with uncertain clinical dates
- Evaluation of fetal growth
- Estimation of fetal weight
- Measurement of fetal femur length and nuchal skin fold thickness
- Vaginal bleeding of undetermined etiology
- Suspected multiple gestation
- Adjunct to amniocentesis or PUBS
- Adjunct to cervical cerclage placement

- Significant uterine size/clinical dates discrepancy
- Suspected hydatidiform mole
- Suspected uterine abnormality
- Suspected polyhydramnios or oligohydramnios
- Presentation with premature ruptured membranes
- Premature labor
- Abnormal serum alpha-fetoprotein value
- Serial evaluation of fetal growth in multiple gestation

Source: Sokol, Jones, & Pernoll, 1994; Vintzileos, 1998.

► CONDITIONS ASSOCIATED WITH ABNORMAL MATERNAL SERUM
ALPHA-FETOPROTEIN CONCENTRATIONS

ELEVATED LEVEL

Neural tube defects
Pilonidal cysts
Esophageal or intestinal obstruction
Liver necrosis
Cystic hygroma
Sacrococcygeal teratoma
Abdominal wall defects (omphalocoele, gastroschisis)
Urinary obstruction
Renal anomalies (polycystic or absent kidneys)

Congenital nephrosis
Osteogenesis imperfecta
Congenital skin defects
Cloacal exstrophy
Low birthweight
Oligohydramnios
Multiple gestation
Decreased maternal weight
Underestimated gestational age

LOW LEVEL

Chromosomal trisomies
Gestational trophoblastic disease
Fetal death

Increased maternal weight
Overestimated gestational age

Reproduced, with permission, from Cunningham, F.G. et al. (Eds.) (1997). *Williams obstetrics* (20th ed.). Stamford, CT: Appleton & Lange, p. 922.

Gynecologists, 1996). The triple test adds unconjugated estriol measurements to AFP screening and hCG screening. Lower levels of maternal serum unconjugated estriol have been found in fetuses with Trisomy 21 (Cunningham et al., 1997).

Role of the Nurse. Alpha-fetoprotein testing programs are collaborative endeavors. Nurses work closely with clients, obstetricians, genetic counselors, ultrasonographers, and perinatologists. The nurse's role differs among settings, depending on the nurse's specialized educational background and whether the client will be cared for in a high-risk testing unit or a low-risk environment. Advanced practice nurses may provide genetic counseling or assist in the coordination of prenatal testing.

Staff nurses must be knowledgeable about the screening programs, about the advantages and limitations of AFP screening, about procedures that will be recommended for clients with positive results, about options available to clients, about the staff who will work with the client, and about support resources. They may also be responsible for obtaining blood samples. In particular, nurses who work in a prenatal testing setting must be sensitive to clients' unique concerns related to AFP screening and receiving care in an unfamiliar setting. Nurses also need to provide support to clients during the difficult period of waiting for test results.

All staff need to be prepared to deliver emotional support for the client with prenatal diagnosis of a fetus with a neural tube defect. Procedures and protocols must be ready for implementation in advance of any client care. Options available to the client are discussed, and the client makes her own decision. Support groups for clients who decide to terminate pregnancy and also for clients who decide to continue the pregnancy can be important sources of assistance.

Amniocentesis

Amniocentesis involves the transabdominal withdrawal of fluid from the amniotic sac (Fig. 17–6). The development of the amniocentesis procedure and the successful cultivation of amniotic cells for genetic determination have made it possible to identify some abnormal fetal conditions, for example, a genetic abnormality or a neural tube defect. News of a genetically normal fetus may allay anxiety. Information about an abnormal fetus may be used by the client to make an informed choice to terminate the pregnancy or to prepare for the birth of an infant with special needs. Amniocentesis is an invasive procedure that is performed only for specific reasons. The following are indications for amniocentesis (Cunningham et al., 1997):

- Maternal age 35 years or greater
- Previous chromosomally abnormal offspring
- Chromosomal abnormality in either parent, including balanced translocation carrier state, aneuploidy, and mosaicism
- Trisomy 21 or other chromosomal abnormality in a close family member

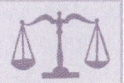

Ethical Decision Making

Maria Santiago is a 16-week primigravid who experienced a spontaneous abortion in her first pregnancy. As a component of her prenatal care, Maria has been advised to undergo diagnostic testing, specifically ultrasound and alpha-fetoprotein screening, to assess the well-being of her fetus. Maria refuses to participate in these tests on the basis of her religious beliefs. She also states that she does not consider abortion as an option in the event of abnormalities being detected in the fetus. If you were the nurse caring for Maria, consider the following issues:

1. Should routine ultrasound and alpha-fetoprotein screening be done for all pregnant women?

2. Do potential but unknown risks justify benefits of information gained from routine ultrasound?

3. Does prenatal diagnosis allow the client or couple to receive help and support throughout pregnancy even if they decide not to terminate a pregnancy with an abnormal fetus?

4. How would you reconcile the mother's autonomy in this decision with that of your desire to provide the best care for her and her baby?

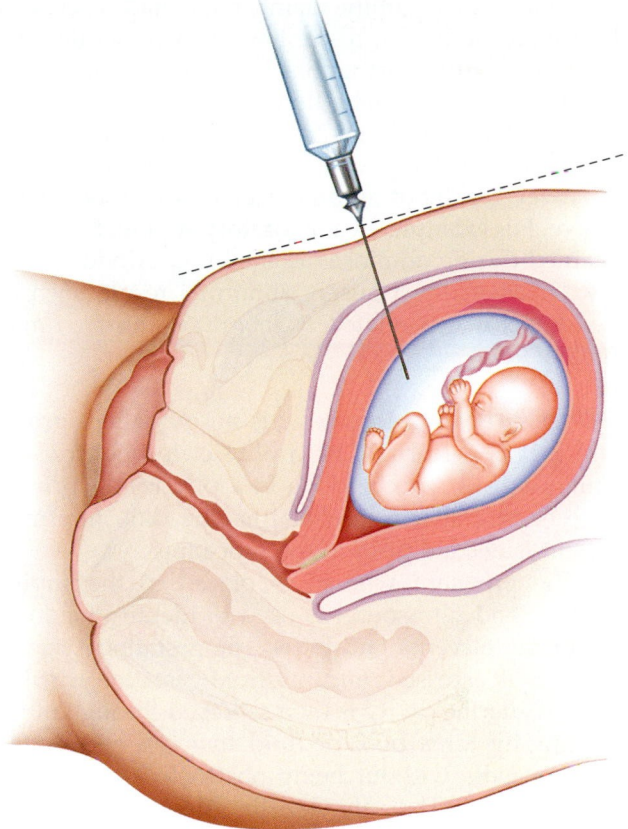

FIGURE 17–6. Amniocentesis: cross-sectional view.

- Pregnancy after three or more spontaneous abortions
- Previous fetus/infant with multiple major malformations
- Risk of a serious X-linked hereditary disorder
- Risk of a serious autosomal or X-linked recessive disorder
- Risk of a neural tube defect (e.g., personal or family history, exposure to drugs such as valproic acid and aminopterin, maternal conditions such as diabetes mellitus)
- Elevated maternal serum AFP level, obtained by routine screen

Amniocentesis for prenatal diagnosis of genetic abnormalities or neural tube defects is usually performed between 15 and 18 weeks of gestation, when enough amniotic fluid is present for aspiration. Using continuous ultrasound, some centers are able to per-

form this before 15 weeks (Sokol et al., 1994). Results of cell cultures usually take about 2 to 4 weeks. Scheduling the procedure is therefore important so that adequate time is left for the couple to consider reproductive options.

Analysis of amniotic fluid and cultured fetal cells drawn during one amniocentesis can provide information to diagnose chromosomal abnormalities and biochemical disorders. Amniotic fluid analysis can also give information about general fetal well-being, as in the case of a fetus compromised by Rh isoimmunization, in which a known Rh-negative mother has a high antibody titer (1:8 to 1:16). Approximately 50 to 100 mL of amniotic fluid is withdrawn and placed in collection tubes. The tubes must be covered with opaque material to prevent the breakdown of bilirubin by light rays. The fluid is analyzed for optical density, which measures the quantity of bilirubin in the fluid. Elevated levels indicate hemolysis. The levels are plotted on optical density graphs according to gestational age. The placement on the graph gives an indication of the extent of hemolysis and fetal compromise. Intrauterine exchange transfusions may then be done to correct fetal anemia, if needed.

Women are also referred for amniocentesis to detect neural tube defects. The procedure is indicated if a woman or a family member has had a fetus or child with the defect, if she has elevated serum AFP levels, or if either partner has a neural tube defect.

Analysis of amniotic fluid does not screen for all possible abnormalities; a "clean" report is *not* a guarantee that the baby will be normal in every way. Moreover, results of an amniocentesis may be inconclusive. For example, in a laboratory setting, fetal cells obtained during amniocentesis may not divide properly. Occasionally, a falsely abnormal result, such as pseudomosaicism related to laboratory artifact, may emerge.

Procedure. Amniocentesis is an outpatient procedure that is performed by a physician (obstetrician). Amniocentesis may be done in a physician's private office or in a special prenatal testing unit. Informed consent is needed prior to the procedure.

The pregnant woman is placed in the supine position, and ultrasound is used to identify the location of the placenta and fetus. The gestational age of the fetus is assessed, and multiple gestation is ruled out. The uterine cavity is then searched through ultrasonography for a pool of fluid that can be reached with a needle without being obstructed by the placenta or fetus. The safety of the procedure and the success of obtaining a specimen of blood are enhanced by the use of sonography (Sokol et al., 1994). A specimen contaminated with blood may alter results, especially if maternal and fetal blood mix.

Once a pool of amniotic fluid is located, the insertion site is marked on the abdomen. The abdomen is then washed with an iodine solution and draped, to create a sterile field. This reduces the risk of introducing infection into the uterine cavity. The physician may inject a local anesthetic subcutaneously around the intended puncture site. A 20- or 22-gauge needle, 3 to 6 in. long (depending on the thickness of the abdominal wall and location of the pool), is then inserted into the uterine cavity; up to 30 mL of amniotic fluid may then be withdrawn (Cunningham et al., 1997). The woman may feel pressure and slight cramping at the puncture site. The character of the amniotic fluid is assessed for the presence of blood, discoloration, or foul odor. The fluid is transferred from the syringe to specimen tubes and sent to the clinical laboratory for culture and analysis.

The client is discharged approximately 30 minutes after the procedure if no complications occur. She is instructed to keep the puncture site clean and to report any complications such as vaginal discharge, severe, persistent cramping, and onset of fever. Normally, the client may experience some mild cramping for several hours. After the procedure she is instructed

to rest, but may resume normal light activity after the cramping subsides (Sokol et al., 1994).

Risks. Three major risks are associated with amniocentesis (Cunningham et al., 1997):

- Trauma to the fetus, placenta, umbilical cord, or maternal structures
- Infection
- Premature labor and spontaneous abortion

Hemorrhage can result from perforation of the placenta. A hematoma may develop at the perforation site, and the transfer of nutrients between the placenta and uterus may be decreased. Uteroplacental insufficiency and intrauterine growth retardation may result. In addition, placental hemorrhage and transfer of fetal blood to the mother may cause maternal isoimmunization in the Rh-negative mother carrying an Rh-positive fetus, possibly resulting in hemolytic disease of the fetus. In such instances, anti-Rho globulin is administered to nonsensitized Rh-negative women to prevent isoimmunization from taking place (Steyn, Pattison, & Odendaal, 1992).

The risk of injury to the fetus and umbilical cord is minimal with an experienced physician, using a well-guided needle insertion. At times, even the most skillful clinician cannot obtain enough fluid, and another puncture is necessary. Repeated punctures may increase the risk of fetal injury. Most reported cases of injury occur late in pregnancy (Cunningham et al., 1997).

Infection can result when pathogens are inadvertently introduced into the uterine cavity, as may occur when surgical aseptic technique is broken. Amnionitis, with complications such as preterm labor and delivery, may occur. Signs and symptoms of infection include fever, chills, uterine cramping, and possibly prurulent discharge at the puncture site.

Role of the Nurse. The nurse is an essential member of the interdisciplinary health care team during amniocentesis. A primary nursing role during this procedure is that of support person and advocate for the pregnant client. The nurse ensures that the client understands the procedure, its significance, and the risks and benefits to her and her fetus. The client undergoing amniocentesis is frequently anxious and fearful about the procedure itself and the results it might yield, and the nurse must be able to anticipate these feelings and respond through both verbal and nonverbal methods.

The nurse may also be responsible for preparing the client and the equipment for the procedure and assisting the physician during the actual technique. The client's vital signs must be monitored before, during, and after the procedure and the nurse implements actions to relieve the client's physical discomfort, particularly after the withdrawal of the amniotic fluid. The procedure is then documented in the client's record.

Percutaneous Umbilical Blood Sampling

Percutaneous umbilical blood sampling (PUBS), or cordocentesis, provides direct access to the fetal circulation. With this technique, fetal blood samples may be taken or treatments, such as direct blood transfu-

sions, may be given to the fetus (Sokol et al., 1994) (Fig. 17–7). Percutaneous umbilical blood sampling is currently the primary method of fetal blood sampling. The following are some indications for use of PUBS in assessment and diagnosis (Bell & Weiner, 1993):

- Coagulation abnormalities
- Hemophilias, such as hemophilia A and hemophilia B
- Hemoglobinopathies
- Congenital infections, such as toxoplasmosis and rubella

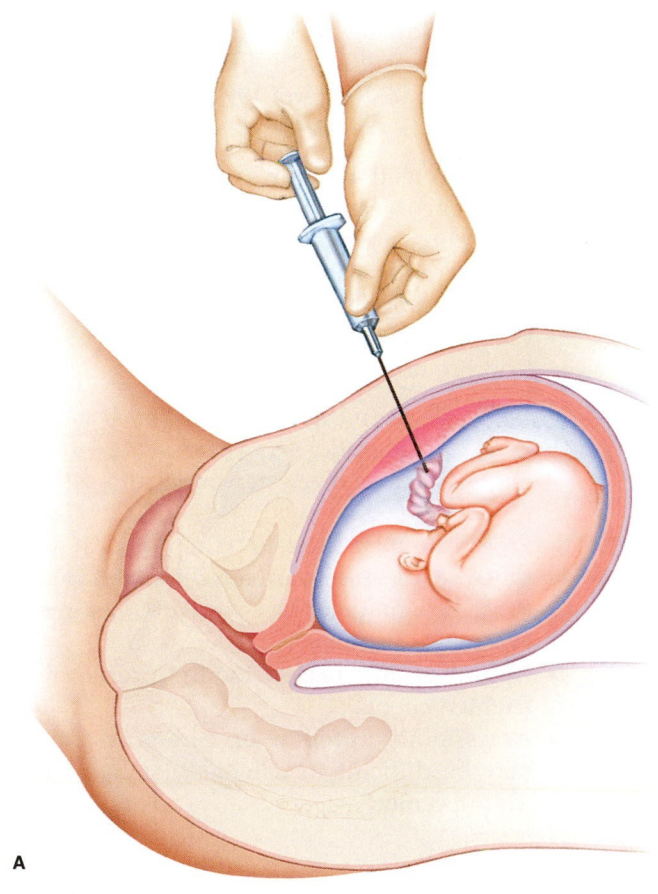

A

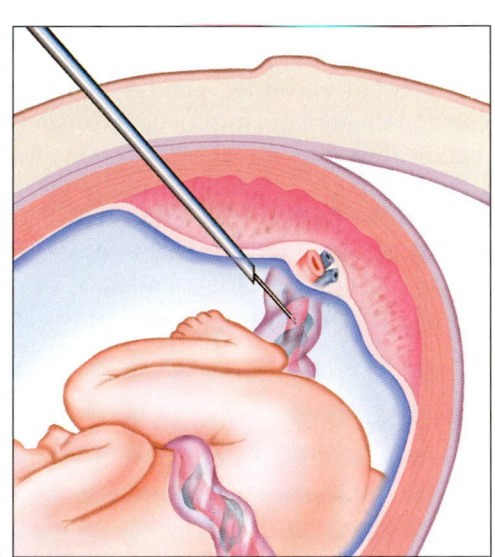

B

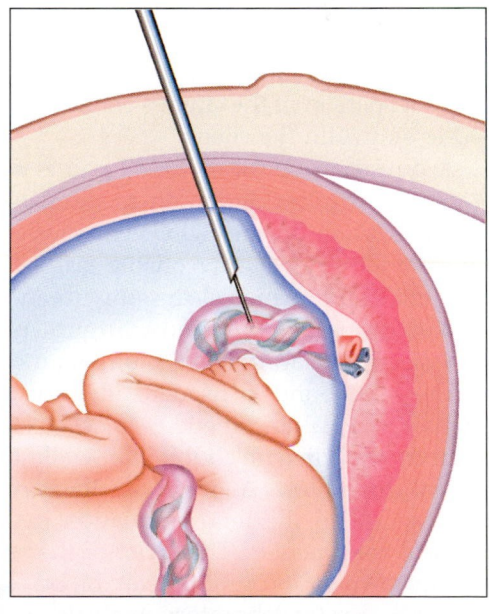

C

FIGURE 17–7. Percutaneous umbilical blood sampling. Access to the umbilical artery or vein varies, depending on both the placental location and the position of cord insertion into the placenta. **A.** With an anterior placenta, the needle may pass through the placenta. **B.** With a posterior implantation, the needle usually passes through the amniotic fluid before penetrating an umbilical vessel. **C.** With a lateral or fundal placenta, the needle may pass through the placenta and amniotic cavity to enter the umbilical vessel.

- Metabolic or cytogenetic abnormalities that cannot be identified by amniocentesis or other types of screening
- Karyotyping, for example, when results of amniocentesis are inconclusive, when fetal anomalies or severe growth retardation exists, or when rapid results are necessary
- Rh disease
- Blood gas concentration
- Immune deficiency
- Administration of blood products for treatment of fetal anemias and Rh disease
- Administration of medications to fetus

This list is not all-inclusive, as the indications for PUBS are continually developing.

PUBS has expanded possibilities for fetal assessment and treatment. Improved ultrasound guidance of needle insertion in the cord has enhanced the safety of this technique. Contraindications to PUBS include fetal distress; infection; cases in which delivery and neonatal care would be more effective or would be associated with lower risk; and lack of client acceptance of the procedure or willingness to come for follow-up care.

Procedure. Informed consent is needed prior to the procedure. The client must understand the reason for PUBS and the risks, benefits, and nature of follow-up care. Preprocedure counseling usually involves the client's meeting with a genetic counselor.

Percutaneous umbilical blood sampling is an outpatient procedure that is performed with sterile technique. To prevent supine hypotension, the client with a greatly enlarged uterus is positioned on her left side. A support person of the client's choice may be encouraged to stay with the client.

A physician performs PUBS and is assisted by a nurse and an ultrasonographer. Ultrasound is used for visualization during PUBS. The mother may need a full bladder, depending on the size of the uterus. The client's abdomen is cleansed with an iodine solution and draped, as with any surgical procedure. A sterile sleeve is placed over the ultrasound transducer, and the ultrasound is used to identify the area for puncture. A local anesthetic is injected by the physician into the client's abdominal wall, to minimize physical discomfort. A spinal needle may be used to obtain access to the fetal circulation by way of the umbilical cord vessels. The stylet of the spinal needle is withdrawn, appropriate fetal blood samples are taken and sent for laboratory analysis, and any treatments are administered. Obtaining fetal blood samples takes about 10 minutes. Physical discomfort is minimal and is similar to the sense of pressure with

possible cramping experienced with amniocentesis. After the procedure, the client is monitored until the fetus is noted to be normally reactive.

Care after PUBS is similar to care after amniocentesis; however, the risk of infection is greater for PUBS than for amniocentesis. The physician may prescribe antibiotics prophylactically for the client. In addition, the client is advised to check her temperature twice daily and to contact her health care provider promptly if her temperature exceeds 100°F. She is advised to return at specified intervals for evaluation, which may include ultrasound. Further assessment and treatment are prescribed according to individual needs and conditions.

Risks. The following are some risks and special considerations associated with PUBS (Ghidini, Sepulveda, Lockwood, & Romero, 1993):

Risks
- Injury to fetal structures
- Placental or fetal hemorrhage, placenta abruptio
- Thrombus of umbilical vessel
- Fetal arrhythmias
- Chorioamnionitis
- Preterm labor
- Rupture of amniotic membranes
- Fetal death

Special Considerations
- High-risk specialized personnel and setting are required.
- Procedure may need to be repeated at another time if cord vessels are too difficult to reach.
- Procedure may not be covered by insurance.
- Procedure is expensive.
- Nature of and reason for the procedure may frighten clients.
- Accessibility to follow-up care is essential, but may be difficult for clients who live far from testing center.

Role of the Nurse. As with each of the techniques for second-trimester assessment, the nurse caring for a client undergoing PUBS has important roles in educating and supporting the client before, during, and after the procedure. Working with the physician and the genetic counselor, the nurse makes certain that the client understands the reason for the procedure, the procedure itself, its risks and benefits, and any interventions that will be offered based on the results of PUBS. The nurse also makes sure that the client understands postprocedure instructions and is able to perform self-care practices, such as recognizing and reporting complications and returning for follow-up care.

Prior to and after the procedure, nurses monitor the client's vital signs. During the procedure the nurse assists the physician performing PUBS and provides support to the client and her support person. The nurse assesses fetal monitor tracings done after the procedure, promptly reports signs of fetal distress, and undertakes emergency measures, such as position changes and administration of oxygen, according to the unit's protocols. The nurse is responsible for ensuring that emergency equipment is accessible and in working order. The nurse's role may also involve telephone outreach to clients after their discharge home.

Nurses have important roles in coordinating care for the client undergoing PUBS. Nurses who work in high-risk prenatal settings may network with nurses in the referral site. Staff education, including invitations to visit the test center, can ensure continuity of care and understanding of the testing process.

▶ Psychologic Concerns Related to Assessment

Second-trimester assessment can be an exciting and pleasant process for the low-risk, healthy client and her family. The expectant parents may look forward to hearing the fetal heartbeat, to confirming that pregnancy is progressing normally, and to discussing concerns and plans with their health care providers. Some clients, however, may fear physical examination or worry about their own health or the health of their fetus. Nurses should evaluate each client's unique responses to the assessment process and make certain that clear explanations are given to allay anxiety. Test findings should be promptly communicated and healthy clients assured that they are progressing normally.

Some clients may be terrified of the high-risk screening procedures done during the second trimester to evaluate the fetus. In addition, waiting days or weeks for test results may be especially stressful for clients. Nurses need to be sensitive to the concerns of clients and their families, to ensure that families receive test results without delay, and to refer the client to a support group if appropriate (French, Kurczynski, Weaver, & Pituch, 1992).

Research supports the importance of prompt communication of test results. In their research with second-trimester women, Heidrich and Cranley (1989) found that women who underwent genetic amniocentesis had lower attachment scores before the procedure than other second-trimester women stud-

ied; however, a month after normal results, these women had attachment scores that did not differ significantly from the scores of the other women in the study. Such findings support clinical reports that suggest women withhold personal investment in the fetus and in the pregnancy until a normal result has been received.

Nurses, physicians, and other health care providers who participate in high-risk assessment need to be prepared to intervene with clients who do have abnormal results. Several strategies can be employed with these clients:

- Remain accessible to the client.
- Support the client through further evaluation procedures when indicated.
- Encourage verbalization.
- Be able to answer questions.
- Discuss options regarding the pregnancy and future treatment.
- Coordinate care to minimize delays in testing, especially when advancing pregnancy makes time a concern.
- Help clients meet their spiritual needs during this time.
- Obtain support for clients from other sources.

Many communities have support groups for people who have experienced prenatal or neonatal loss or for those who have children with special needs. Representatives of these groups can provide a strong and supportive community network for clients. Representatives from pastoral care may also be helpful, and clients may welcome the special support they can provide.

▶ Nursing Diagnoses

Nursing diagnoses for the healthy client during the second trimester are based on careful assessment data. They include:

Physiologic
Problem-oriented diagnoses:

- Constipation, related to second-trimester changes in gastrointestinal system
- Fatigue, related to dietary intake of needed iron

Wellness-oriented diagnoses:

- Asset in health of mother and fetus, related to physiologic adaptation in the second trimester
- Progressive normal fetal growth and development, related to maternal health-promoting behaviors during the second trimester

Psychosocial

Problem-oriented diagnoses:

- Altered maternal role performance, related to lack of maternal role model (grandmother)
- Decisional conflict, related to
    Career conflicts
    Need for income from work

Wellness-oriented diagnoses:

- Positive family coping during the second trimester, related to adequate support from significant others and few role conflicts
- Beginning maternal–fetal attachment, related to statements about perception of fetal movement (quickening)

Cultural

Problem-oriented diagnoses:

- Altered family process, related to cultural differences in perception of roles during pregnancy and parenting

Wellness-oriented diagnoses:

- Positive partner self-concept, related to congruence between perceptions of appropriate maternal and paternal role behavior

---

► NURSING AND COLLABORATIVE MANAGEMENT

Throughout pregnancy, the plan of care, based on the nursing process, provides an important tool for implementing management strategies. Through the collaboration of health care providers, relevant diagnoses are identified and a comprehensive care plan developed. Implementation strategies may vary as pregnancy progresses, individualizing care to each family.

By the second trimester, progress has been made in establishing a trusting relationship among the childbearing family, the nurse, and other health care providers. This relationship is critical to effective nursing care.

► Continuing a Philosophy of Care with Well-Defined Goals

The philosophy, goals, and objectives for continuing prenatal care should be discussed with clients. The plan of nursing care for the second trimester includes:

- Preparing the client and family for continued care

- Continuing assessment and updating the data base for diagnosis development
- Continuing to support the client
- Continuing to recognize cultural influences
- Continuing to encourage informed decision making
- Promoting psychologic adaptation to midpregnancy
- Fostering family attachment during midpregnancy
- Meeting educational needs
- Promoting nutritional well-being
- Helping the client cope with second-trimester discomforts
- Promoting client safety
- Evaluating prenatal care
- Ensuring appropriate client referral

During interviews at subsequent visits, the nurse assesses the client's understanding of these important components and makes certain that care provided is individualized, as well as congruent with philosophy, goals, and objectives.

Preparing the Client and Family for Continued Care

Before the end of each prenatal health care visit, the next visit should be scheduled and the client informed about what to expect at that meeting. The client should be introduced to new staff members involved in her care and should be informed about any changes in policies or protocols that affect her.

Updating the Data Base for Diagnosis Development

At each visit during the second trimester, the client's history is updated. Complete physical examination is performed on the first visit. During the low-risk woman's subsequent visits, physical assessment focuses on assessment parameters outlined in Table 17–3. Other health aspects are evaluated further if indicated.

Components of each second-trimester visit include continued interdisciplinary assessment, anticipatory guidance and education based on the unique needs of each family during the second trimester, supervision in self-care procedures, and referrals to appropriate resources. All relevant information gathered during the assessment process, interventions, responses to interventions, and evaluation of client responses continue to be recorded clearly in the client's chart. Health care providers review the chart prior to seeing the client at each visit and update the records during the visit or shortly after seeing the client.

Continuing to Support the Client

The nurse's supportive role remains unchanged throughout the second trimester. Continued contact at numerous prenatal visits provides the opportunity for development of a strong and trusting nurse–client relationship. By getting to know the client, the nurse is able to anticipate times when the client will need special support. Nursing strategies to support the client include remaining accessible, encouraging verbalization, providing anticipatory guidance, and acting as the client's advocate in the health care system.

As discussed earlier, clients may undergo diagnostic testing during the second trimester. Nursing interventions help clients cope with stress related to the tests.

Continuing to Recognize Cultural Influences

Throughout the second trimester the nurse continues to recognize the client's cultural background and adapt prenatal care appropriately. For example, the nurse may continue to provide nutritional teaching based on culturally prescribed dietary patterns identified at the first prenatal visit. With an understanding of the cultural backgrounds of clients, the nurse can identify potential areas of conflict.

Continuing to Encourage Informed Decision Making

By the second trimester, the client ideally has decided on the birthing facility and selected caregivers. The childbearing family is encouraged to think about the birth plan, although this is not finalized until the third trimester. The need for the client to make informed decisions related to aspects of prenatal care continues, especially in regard to prenatal tests such as ultrasound, genetic amniocentesis, and AFP screening. The nurse ensures that the client is fully informed about the risks and benefits of any second-trimester screening procedure. The client can then make an informed decision about the test.

Promoting Psychologic Adaptation to Midpregnancy

Psychologic adaptation normally takes place throughout pregnancy. During the second trimester, nurses can do much to assist families in meeting psychologic tasks of pregnancy. Experiencing pregnancy together and preparing for a new family member require new family patterns of interpersonal interaction and adaptation. A basic, yet essential, care strategy is to encourage couples to share their feelings and concerns with each other. Through anticipatory guidance and teaching about physiologic and psychologic changes, nurses can also do the following:

- Identify and discuss clients' concerns about such topics as sexuality.
- Identify clients' concerns about body image, which is affected by the rapidly changing shape during the second trimester.
- Explain normal psychologic processes of the second trimester.
- Prepare or help the couple cope with tensions in other family members related to "moving up" a generation. These tensions may manifest during the second trimester when the pregnancy is visible.
- Discuss changing interpersonal family relationships and clients' reactions to them.
- Discuss the importance of thinking about characteristics they would like to have as parents and changes parenthood may bring.
- Reassure clients about normal fantasy processes.
- Explore paternal reactions to pregnancy during the second trimester and explain the couvade symptoms that may normally occur.
- Encourage sharing of feelings between the expectant father and his own father.

Ambivalence about pregnancy usually resolves by the end of the first trimester, although some ambivalence may continue in the second trimester. Through assessment of second-trimester psychologic adaptation, the nurse can identify high-risk situations that require further counseling and referral (see box entitled Behaviors Indicating High-Risk Psychologic Adaptation During the Second Trimester).

Fostering Family Attachment During Midpregnancy

During the second trimester, pregnancy becomes visible and more "real" to family members. Support of positive family dynamics during pregnancy by health care professionals may potentially increase the quality of family–fetal attachment (Fuller, Moore, & Lester, 1993). Attachment can be fostered by encouraging the client to bring significant others to prenatal visits, by including them in teaching about pregnancy, and by helping them to hear the fetal heartbeat and to feel fetal body parts or movements. Understanding the importance of a woman's relationship with her own mother during pregnancy, the nurse may encourage the client to share her thoughts about pregnancy with her own mother if possible.

Expectant parents are frequently concerned about encouraging siblings to accept the pregnancy and new

▶ BEHAVIORS INDICATING HIGH-RISK PSYCHOLOGIC ADAPTATION DURING THE SECOND TRIMESTER

MATERNAL AMBIVALENCE TOWARD THE PREGNANCY, THE FETUS, OR BOTH

No questions asked about pregnancy, labor and delivery, and infant care; plans about these topics remain fuzzy and vague

No interest in the fetus; not interested in listening to the fetal heartbeat, feeling fetal parts, or discussing fetal growth

Unrealistic expectations of labor, delivery, and postpartum

Past negative experiences with pregnancy or labor and delivery

Denial of pregnancy and of fetal movement actually felt by caregiver

Pregnancy and parenthood seen as interfering greatly and negatively with lifestyle and self-image

Continuation of activities that could damage self or fetus, for example, heavy drinking and drug use

Reporting persistent and many physical complaints

HIGH STRESS EXPERIENCED BY THE PREGNANT FAMILY OR MEMBERS

Reports of high-stress life events

Ineffective means of coping with stress

LACK OF NUCLEAR AND EXTENDED FAMILY SUPPORT SYSTEMS

Lack of support from expectant father

Lack of support from own parents, siblings, and family members

Feelings of isolation

---

baby. The nurse can encourage the couple to express their thoughts; provide anticipatory guidance about normal sibling reactions, based on the age and developmental level of the child; suggest ways in which siblings can be made to feel included in decisions about the baby (e.g., helping to select items for the baby); encourage the couple to bring siblings to prenatal visits; and include siblings in teaching about the developing baby. Finally, the second trimester is an appropriate time to establish support groups for expectant parents, who are then able to share thoughts and concerns and to network with others who are also experiencing the same phase of pregnancy.

Meeting Educational Needs

Throughout pregnancy, education continues to be a major focus of nursing care. Education is based on each family's individual needs, rather than on a set schedule of content; family participation in determining educational needs is encouraged.

As the second trimester progresses, the client may enroll in prepared childbearing classes. The nurse should be informed about available programs and refer clients based on an understanding of each client's unique needs.

Promoting Nutritional Well-Being

Nutrition is a major focus of nursing care throughout pregnancy because of its importance to fetal growth and development and to maternal health status.

Weight management may be a problem during the second trimester, because women tend to feel well. Excess intake causes many women at this time to gain weight rapidly. Dietary changes may also be necessary to minimize second-trimester discomforts such as heartburn, described later in this chapter.

Assisting the Client to Cope with Second-Trimester Discomforts

A sense of well-being usually characterizes the second trimester of pregnancy. By this time some distressing first-trimester symptoms, for example, nausea, fatigue, and urinary frequency, have subsided. Although the uterus rises out of the pelvis and the woman begins to look pregnant, uterine enlargement has not yet produced the uncomfortable changes of the third trimester.

The discomforts experienced by the expectant mother during the second trimester are not necessarily restricted to this stage of pregnancy. Some women may develop these discomforts earlier or later in their pregnancies. Nursing assessments must therefore be individualized.

Many remedies for physical discomforts can be purchased over the counter. The pregnant client should be advised that many of these medications should not be used during pregnancy. The pregnant client should be advised to check with her health care provider before using any relief remedy in topical, tablet, liquid, inhalant, or any other form.

Heartburn. Gastric reflux affects up to 80% of women during pregnancy. During the second and

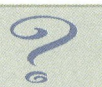

Commonly Asked Questions

When will I first feel the baby move?

Women having their first baby usually feel first fetal movements around 17 to 20 weeks of gestation. Women who have already borne a child may experience these movements around 16 weeks or, in some cases, earlier. These movements often feel like a "fluttering" sensation. Experiencing fetal movements for the first time is called *quickening*.

How often should I feel the baby move?

After quickening occurs, fetal movements are felt about once or twice daily. By 22 to 24 weeks, fetal movements are frequently felt. During the second trimester, fetal movements most often feel like "kicks" and "punches." A pregnant woman who has already experienced quickening should call her health provider without delay if fetal movement decreases or stops or if marked increases in fetal movement are noted.

If fetal organ systems are formed during the first trimester, are there any restrictions on medications during the second trimester?

Yes. Fetal organ systems, for example, the lungs and central nervous system, continue to develop throughout pregnancy. Many medications cross the placenta and affect the maturing fetus; therefore, no medication should ever be taken during pregnancy unless it is prescribed by the obstetric health care provider or unless the health care provider in another specialty (e.g., dentist, ophthalmologist) is informed that the client is pregnant.

If I eat a lot over the weekend, is it harmful to "fast" to make up for excess weight gain?

Possibly. Bingeing and fasting are never healthy dietary patterns and should be avoided throughout pregnancy. Such conditions as electrolyte imbalance and ketosis can result from fasting and adversely affect the fetus. Any day of heavy eating should be followed by a return to a normally prescribed dietary pattern. Pregnant women should seek nutritional counseling if they are unable to maintain healthy eating patterns during pregnancy.

Is it safe to have vaginal intercourse during the second trimester?

Yes. In general, there is no reason for the healthy pregnant woman not to continue sexual activity during the second trimester. Indeed, many women experience increased libido in this stage of pregnancy.

Is it safe to take a bath during the second trimester?

Yes. Tub bathing can be relaxing during pregnancy and may be recommended as long as membranes are intact and bath water does not fill the vagina. Bath water should not, however, exceed 102°F to avoid raising the core body temperature.

Can I use a sauna during the second trimester?

Use of saunas is not recommended. Intense heat can produce increased body temperature and generalized vasodilation. The shunting of blood to the skin can lower blood pressure. Increased sweating can contribute to dehydration and electrolyte imbalance.

Is swimming hazardous during the second trimester?

Swimming, like tub bathing, may be encouraged as long as membranes are intact; however, concern about the water quality itself should be raised and areas at high risk for pollution avoided. Diving is not recommended, because of the possibility of trauma.

May I travel during the second trimester?

There is no reason why the healthy, low-risk woman cannot travel by plane, car, or train during this stage of pregnancy and enjoy vacation or business trips. Changing position while in transit, stopping or getting up to walk every hour and a half, maintaining adequate fluid intake, and wearing clothing that does not constrict or inhibit circulation from the lower extremities promote well-being. Before undertaking any long trip, it is wise to investigate the nature and availability of prenatal health care. Trips to areas of the world where there are poor facilities, high incidence of disease, and lack of available health care are not encouraged during pregnancy. Vacations that involve unusually strenuous or stressful activities, as well as activities that require balance for safety, should be avoided.

Should I quit my job?

A healthy pregnant woman who does not work in an emotionally or physically hazardous environment may continue to work throughout the second trimester. Women who do work in high-risk areas may need to use special precautions, transfer from the area, or stop working in that environment.

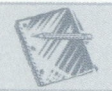

Client Teaching

Interventions to Relieve Heartburn

The nurse can suggest the following strategies to the expectant mother to help relieve heartburn:

- Eat smaller, more frequent meals
- Avoid fried, fatty, or spicy foods or any foods that increase heartburn
- Eliminate beverages with meals
- Eat the last meal of the day at least 3 hours before bedtime
- Drink milk
- Avoid lying down immediately after a meal
- Keep your head elevated when lying down, especially if heartburn episodes are frequent or severe (this may help counteract the effects of gravity on gastric reflux)
- Maintain good posture to provide more room for the stomach to function
- Try sips of water during heartburn episodes to "clear" the esophagus
- Take antacids such as magnesium trisilicate (Gelusil), magnesium hydroxide (Maalox), and calcium carbonate (Tums) if prescribed by your health care provider
- Avoid taking sodium bicarbonate since excessive intake can affect acid-base balance and contribute to the development of such conditions as metabolic alkalosis

third trimesters, the altered position of the stomach, the relaxation of the cardiac valve, and the progesterone-induced decrease in muscle tone and motility of the gastrointestinal tract combine to make pyrosis (heartburn) a common discomfort. If reflux becomes so severe that the client is at risk of aspiration or mucosal damage or is unable to perform daily activities, further evaluation is necessary; however, the healthy client who experiences occasional reflux can be assured that this condition is normal during pregnancy and will subside after delivery.

Constipation. Constipation is a change in the client's normal bowel patterns and includes decreased frequency of bowel movements, increased stool consistency, and increased difficulty with defecation. Normal bowel patterns vary considerably among people.

In general, constipation clinically becomes problematic during the second and third trimesters of pregnancy. As discussed earlier, pressure and displacement of the intestines by the enlarging uterus, decreased gastrointestinal tone and motility, and increased absorption of water from the stool contribute to this condition. Constipation is also a side effect of iron supplementation, which may be recommended during the second trimester. Prior to counseling the expectant mother, the nurse should discuss previous bowel patterns with the client to identify whether constipation exists.

Hemorrhoids. A combination of factors, such as increased pressure of the expanding uterus on the hemorrhoidal veins, the influence of progesterone on the walls of blood vessels and on the large intestine, conditions predisposing to constipation, and straining during bowel movements, contribute to the development of hemorrhoids during the second and third trimesters. Although hemorrhoids subside and may disappear after pregnancy, they can be a source of considerable discomfort as pregnancy progresses. The expectant mother may experience itching and throbbing rectal pain that increases after a bowel movement or after long periods of sitting or standing. Irritation of swollen hemorrhoids may produce bleeding.

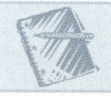

Client Teaching

Interventions to Relieve Constipation

The nurse can suggest the following strategies to the expectant mother to help relieve constipation:

- Drink 6 to 8 glasses of water or other noncaffeinated fluids per day
- If heartburn is a problem, drink fluids between meals
- Eat foods that contain roughage, bulk, and natural fiber, such as prunes, figs, and bran
- Exercise, such as walking at a moderate pace for a mile a day
- Do not use laxatives, suppositories, or stool softeners without checking with health care provider
- Establish regular bowel patterns; do not postpone bowel movements

Pregnancy-related hemorrhoids are rarely "cured" during pregnancy, although relief may be obtained with the following measures:

- Follow strategies to decrease constipation (see Client Teaching feature)
- Avoid straining during bowel movements
- Take warm baths (not to exceed 102°F) to increase circulation and provide topical relief (e.g., full baths or partial sitz baths)
- Apply ice packs or astringent solutions (witch hazel) to reduce the hemorrhoids
- Assume certain positions to relieve pressure and facilitate circulation, including resting in bed with hips and legs elevated and lying on the left side with a pillow between the legs
- Gently replace the hemorrhoids into the rectum
- Take stool softeners as prescribed
- Use nonsteroidal ointments (e.g., Preparation H) or sprays to reduce swelling and provide analgesis as prescribed

Faintness or Dizziness. Faintness or dizziness is caused by sudden changes in position, being in warm, crowded areas, or standing for prolonged periods. Faintness or dizziness is attributed to postural hypotension, which causes pooling of blood in the dependent veins in the legs when the pregnant woman stands too long or stands suddenly. The gravid uterus also may place pressure on the vena cava when the expectant mother lies in a supine position. The result is supine hypotensive syndrome.

The nurse should encourage the expectant mother to move slowly, avoid sudden changes in position, avoid warm crowded areas if possible, lie on her side rather than supine, and lower her head or lie down on her side if she feels faint.

Round Ligament Pain. Early in the second trimester, the expectant mother may experience round ligament pain. As the uterus enlarges, the round ligaments stretch and lengthen. This results in a throbbing or sharp pain from the fundus to the pubic bone. The pain may extend or localize in the inguinal area. Pathologic conditions, such as appendicitis, may present with similar types of pain. Therefore, the client needs to be examined before the normal diagnosis of pregnancy-related round ligament pain can be confirmed.

Unfortunately, round ligament pain cannot be prevented or "cured." Reassurance that this is a normal discomfort related to healthy pregnancy may, however, help many women. In addition, to obtain some relief the woman should be advised to take warm baths (not to exceed 102°F), apply a heating pad, support the uterus with pillows while lying on the left side, wear a nonconstricting yet supportive maternity girdle, and avoid further stretching of the ligaments when getting out of bed by first rolling on the side and then pushing upward with the hands.

Promoting Client Safety

Nursing goals to promote safety continue to focus on prevention of client injuries during the prenatal visit and teaching related to safety. During the second trimester, safety and safe passage for self and fetus become emotionally important to the pregnant woman. The mother may be very receptive to alteration of potentially harmful activities, such as smoking or ingestion of alcohol.

During the second trimester, the woman's center of gravity and balance change as the uterus enlarges in size and weight. This physiologic alteration can place the woman at risk of injury during activities that require balance or quick movements, such as skating and skiing. The nurse helps the client to identify which of her activities can be safely continued and which hold risk of injury.

Some second-trimester clients avoid using seatbelts for fear of harming the fetus. However, clients may be more severely injured if they are in an accident while not wearing seat restraints, even if the car has an air bag. Indeed, research has shown that automobile broadside collisions are associated with fetal and maternal death (Aitokallio-Tallberg & Halmesmaki, 1997). The nurse advises the client about the importance of motor vehicle safety throughout pregnancy.

At each visit, the nurse helps the client recognize potential safety hazards related to lifestyle or environment and develop ways to minimize or avoid these. Warning or danger signs of pregnancy are reviewed at each visit (see Table 15–7). Signs and symptoms of preterm labor are also presented.

Evaluating Prenatal Care

During the planning phase of care, desired maternal and fetal outcomes are stated in measurable, behavioral terms. Throughout pregnancy, evaluation continues to reflect the degree to which these behavioral objectives are met. Evaluation, related to outcome behaviors identified in the care plan, is recorded in the client's chart.

Ensuring Appropriate Client Referral

In addition to the types of referrals described in Chapter 15, nurses frequently refer second-trimester clients to childbirth education classes. In addition, through assessment, the nurse may identify clients at social or emotional risk and refer them to a social service or counseling resource.

Critical Thinking in Care Planning

Care of the Family During the Second Trimester

Yuri Yamaguchi is a 28-year-old Japanese-American woman who teaches home economics in the local high school. Her husband, Hideo, is a 29-year-old math teacher in the same school. They are in the second trimester of pregnancy with their second child. Their first child, Kenji, is a healthy 4-year-old boy.

The Yamaguchis live with Hideo's mother and father in a two-family house in the town where they teach. Hideo's mother emigrated to the United States as a young child, prior to the second World War. She has tried to follow Japanese culture in her lifestyle and takes great pride in teaching her grandson about Japanese ways. Hideo's father was born in the United States.

Yuri has had prenatal care since early in the first trimester. The pregnancy was planned, and although Hideo's parents would like another grandson, Yuri and Hideo express no sex preference for their second child.

The pregnancy is progressing normally. During her prenatal visit, Yuri tells the nurse, "I'm starting to look so fat; my clothes look terrible on me."

▶ Assessment

- Vital signs: temperature 98.6°F, pulse 72, respirations 15, blood pressure 106/68
- Uterine size appropriate for gestation
- Fundus felt slightly above umbilicus
- Urinalysis negative for glucose, protein, acetone
- Continued growth and development of fetus
- Fetal heart tone: 160 regular
- Quickening felt by mother at 20 weeks
- Gained 2 pounds in 1 month
- 24-hour recall of diet reveals adequate nutrient intake when iron and folacin supplements are used

- Additional laboratory values reveal deficiency in iron and folic acid
- Client expresses reluctance to gain weight
- Client expresses delight at fetal movement
- Client refers to fetus alternately as "she" or "he" and gives fetus a pet name
- Client describes a dream about having a baby
- Client describes inability to discuss pregnancy thoroughly with 4-year-old son
- Traditional mother-in-law lives with family
- Couple states that paternal grandmother wants them to adhere to traditional Japanese birth and childbearing practices

Nursing Diagnosis

Potential asset for healthy mother, related to normal physiologic indices

Expected Client/Family Outcomes	Nursing Action/Intervention	Evaluation
The client will: • Continue positive health care practices throughout second trimester.	Provide positive reinforcement regarding health care practices. *Rationale:* Positive feedback is a teaching technique that supports people's efforts and encourages learning.	If asked, client reports that she is engaging in positive health-related behaviors, such as moderate exercise.
• Identify physiologic changes occurring during this stage of pregnancy by end of initial second-trimester visit.	Teach family members expected physiologic changes throughout second trimester; focus on pregnant woman and fetus. *Rationale:* Enlargement of uterus and onset of quickening make fetus a reality to family members so that teaching can be focused on fetus as well as the mother.	Indices such as blood pressure and uterine growth remain within normal limits throughout second trimester. Client describes how fetus will

Critical Thinking in Care Planning continued

Expected Client/Family Outcomes	Nursing Action/Intervention	Evaluation
	Give anticipatory guidance on physiologic changes expected during third trimester. *Rationale:* Anticipatory guidance alleviates uncertainty and helps family members cope with ongoing changes of pregnancy.	look during second trimester. Client relates subjective experiences of second-trimester pregnancy to physiologic changes.
• Identify behaviors that do not promote optimum childbearing health by end of initial second-trimester visit. • Identify health-promoting behaviors for third trimester by end of second trimester.	Prepare couple and family members for second-trimester visits and testing. *Rationale:* Client preparation for assessment procedures ensures understanding of specific techniques and implications of testing and enables client to understand importance of positive health care practices.	Client identifies physiologic changes that occur in third trimester and states ways in which she will cope with the associated discomforts. Client can discuss her own behaviors and differentiate between health-promoting behaviors and behaviors that negatively affect her and her fetus. Client discusses intentions to continue self-care practices during third trimester and acknowledges need to alter practices that negatively alter own or fetus' health.
• Continue to use childbearing resources throughout second trimester of pregnancy.	Advise client to review sources of support and seek out additional resources. *Rationale:* Use of childbearing resources enables client to cope with changes that occur during second trimester.	Client makes resource list after discussion with the nurse, evaluates those resources that have been helpful, and indicates which resources she and her family will continue to use during this phase of pregnancy. Client questions nurse about new or additional resources as needed.

(continued)

Critical Thinking in Care Planning *continued*

Nursing Diagnosis

Potential asset for healthy newborn, related to normal fetal growth parameters

Expected Client/Family Outcomes	Nursing Action/Intervention	Evaluation
Throughout the second trimester, the client will:	Support health-promoting behaviors: nutrition, exercise, stress reduction, rest, and avoidance of drugs, alcohol, and cigarettes. Evaluate quickening felt by the mother. *Rationale:* Holistic nursing views pregnancy as a normal state; low-risk clients should not receive high-risk care.	When asked, client describes quickening and health care practices such as nutrition, exercise, rest, and avoidance of alcohol and drugs.
• Identify behaviors that will continue to foster healthy fetal development.		
• Identify deviations from healthy fetal prenatal development (e.g., cessation of fetal movement).	Advise client to contact health care providers without delay if fetal movement decreases or ceases. *Rationale:* All clients must be able to identify warning signs, as prompt treatment often improves outcome.	When asked, client can identify the warning signs of pregnancy.
	Measure fundal height with tape measure and explain procedure to client and other family members. Assess fetal heart rate. *Rationale:* Assessment of fundal height and fetal heart activity confirms presence of live fetus.	Client discusses physiologic significance of evaluation of fundal height and fetal heart rate and expresses joy with the ability to see and feel the fetus.
• Continue to avoid situations and substances that are potentially hazardous to the health of the fetus.	Teach health-promoting behaviors and effects on fetal development during second trimester. *Rationale:* Anticipatory guidance reduces anxiety, and social support given by the nurse relates to positive health care practices.	When asked, client can identify hazardous situations and substances in her own environment. Client identifies methods and strategies for avoiding hazardous situations and substances.
	Teach about assessment techniques during second trimester. *Rationale:* Explanations of risks and benefits of various procedures allow couple to make informed decisions and cope with uncertainty about the unknown.	Couple describes assessment procedures performed during second trimester and understands the risks and benefits related to each.

Nursing Diagnosis

Potential asset in maternal and fetal health, related to adequate nutrient intake

The client will:	Explore with client and family dietary intake practices. *Rationale:* Nutrition during pregnancy is an important component in optimal maternal–fetal health status.	Client lists nutrients needed during pregnancy.
• State need for additional nutrients during pregnancy by end of visit.		
	Reassess nutritional intake through 24-hour recall and dietary diary. *Rationale:* 24-hour recall and dietary diary provide comprehensive assessment. Planning with clients instead of for clients helps ensure motivation toward positive health care practices.	Client identifies from 24-hour dietary recall assets and deficiencies in her diet. Client plans nutritious diet.

Critical Thinking in Care Planning continued

Expected Client/Family Outcomes	Nursing Action/Intervention	Evaluation
	Knowledge and anticipatory guidance help to motivate client toward continued positive health practices.	Client's 24-hour recall and diary reflect adequate folic acid and iron intake through food and supplementation. Client relates necessary nutrients to the four food groups, taking into account her cultural preferences.
• Continue to eat nutritionally sound diet and continue iron and folacin supplementation as prescribed.	Explain and support client's prescribed supplementation of folacin and iron. *Rationale:* Iron and folacin supplement dietary intake to meet prenatal nutrition requirements.	When asked, client identifies foods containing iron and folacin. Client also reflects knowledge in cooking practices, such as those designed to maximize folic acid retention in food. Client can identify reasons for laboratory studies such as those for hemoglobin and hematocrit values.

Nursing Diagnosis

Altered health maintenance, related to possible negative perceptions of pregnant body

The client will:	Explore with client her feelings with regard to nutrient intake and perceptions of body image. Explore with client factors that influenced her body image prior to and during pregnancy. *Rationale:* Body image and body boundary are important parameters for assessment when providing nursing care for pregnant family. Perception of body image is developmental and occurs prior to pregnancy. During the second trimester, the woman's body image changes as a result of changes in the gravid uterus and normal weight gain. Strengthening of expectant family's support networks facilitates psychologic adjustment during pregnancy.	Client discusses feelings about body image prior to pregnancy as well as during pregnancy.
• Discuss feelings about weight gain and body image by end of visit.		
• Describe normal weight gain parameters.	Encourage client to continue to eat a well-balanced diet. *Rationale:* Good nutrition promotes maternal–fetal well-being.	Client continues to gain weight normally and maintains adequate intake.

(continued)

Critical Thinking in Care Planning continued

Expected Client/Family Outcomes	Nursing Action/Intervention	Evaluation
• Participate in discussion of weight-related issues in prenatal classes.	Encourage discussion of weight-related issues during prenatal classes. *Rationale:* Group discussion helps client to deal with feelings also shared by others.	Client and husband attend prenatal classes. Client participates in group discussion about weight-related issues.

Nursing Diagnosis

Potential asset in mother–child attachment, related to positive binding in of mother to fetus

The client and her family will continue attachment behaviors to fetus throughout second trimester.	Discuss with client and husband the psychosocial processes that occur during this and later stages of pregnancy. *Rationale:* Binding in of the mother to fetus helps the mother to identify a maternal role and attain a maternal identity.	Family members jointly assess fetal movements. Family members palpate fetal movements, talk about coming baby. Family members begin to seek resources connected to child care (e.g., books, groups, and other resources).
	Explore with husband paternal attachment behaviors and his feelings regarding the pregnancy and his role as father. *Rationale:* Fathers also begin attachment and role assumption during pregnancy.	Husband discusses his feelings about pregnancy and baby and evolving role as father.
	Explore with couple maternal and paternal fantasies. *Rationale:* Fantasies foster parental attachment and role assumption.	Couple discusses their fantasies about the fetus and acknowledges the function of fantasies in attaining the maternal and paternal roles.

Nursing Diagnosis

Altered family processes, related to knowledge deficit of 4-year-old son

The client and family will: • Identify ways to teach a 4-year-old about pregnancy and newborn by next prenatal visit.	Explore with parents problems that they have in explaining the pregnancy to their child. *Rationale:* Children differ in their ability to understand and cope with pregnancy based on their developmental level.	When asked, client and family identify strategies to teach child that are appropriate to developmental level.
	Explain the psychosocial and cognitive development of a 4-year-old. *Rationale:* Teaching of children should be age appropriate.	Client and family describe the psychosocial and cognitive abilities of their child.

Expected Client/Family Outcomes	Nursing Action/Intervention	Evaluation
	Encourage client and husband to bring their child with them to prenatal vists and suggest enrolling child in preparation class. *Rationale:* Involvement in the pregnancy through accompanying parents during prenatal visits and attending preparation class helps the child to understand and look forward to birth of newborn.	Parents bring their child with them to the next prenatal visit and enroll him in a sibling preparation class.
• Identify informational resources available to help parents teach children about pregnancy by end of visit.	Give parents list of books and videos that can be used to assist them in teaching their child about pregnancy.	Parents buy books appropriate to the child's developmental level.

Nursing Diagnosis

Decisional conflict in parenting, related to cultural beliefs of paternal grandmother

The client and her family will:	Reassess family function and family dynamics. *Rationale:* Acculturation affects how family members cope with pregnancy.	Parents and grandmother discuss cultural rituals and beliefs regarding family and pregnancy.
• Discuss their feelings about cultural beliefs by end of second trimester.		
• Discuss potential conflicts that may arise related to beliefs by next prenatal visit.	Reassess potential family conflict based on cultural differences. *Rationale:* Cultural prescriptions influence family members' roles and attitudes.	When asked, family members identify differences in beliefs between culture of origin and Western cultural norms.
• Identify strategies for resolving culturally based conflicts by end of second trimester.	Help family members identify potential conflicts and strategies to deal with conflicts, such as compromise. *Rationale:* The family controls relationships of its members so that conflict resolution is dependent on strategies they can use to foster positive relationships.	Family members acknowledge conflicts between cultures. Family members plan strategies for conflict resolution.
	Encourage communication among family members. *Rationale:* Effective communication helps to promote understanding and resolve conflicts about cultural differences.	Family members communicate with each other.

Chapter Highlights

▶ In the second trimester, physiologic changes in the mother occur rapidly in most organ systems, including the reproductive, cardiovascular, and gastrointestinal systems.

▶ During the second trimester, the woman continues to move through the process of role attainment, as her relationship with her own mother becomes increasingly important.

▶ The woman's relationship with her fetus is enhanced by quickening, continued fetal activity, and the enlarging uterus.

▶ The expectant father also passes through the psychologic stages of midpregnancy and becomes increasingly concerned with his relationship to his own father and may experience a large number of couvade symptoms.

▶ A sibling's reactions to pregnancy depend on the age of the child, the stages of psychosocial and cognitive development, and the degree of separation–individuation.

▶ Whenever appropriate and possible, the participation of expectant grandparents in the pregnancy can be fostered through methods such as encouraging the grandparents to attend prenatal visits, providing literature, and organizing expectant grandparents programs.

▶ Socioeconomic factors, especially financial stress, have a profound effect on an expectant family's adaptation to the second trimester.

▶ Assessment of the client and her family continues into the second trimester with prenatal visits every 4 weeks and includes physiologic, psychosocial, and cultural dimensions

▶ Low-risk assessment of the second trimester client involves physical examination techniques such as measurement of fundal height and fetal heart rate and maternal reports of quickening.

▶ Diagnostic tests and procedures such as ultrasound, alpha-fetoprotein screening, amniocentesis, and percutaneous umbilical blood sampling may be used in diagnosis and treatment of many high-risk conditions.

▶ Nurses caring for clients undergoing diagnostic procedures have important roles in educating and supporting clients before, during, and after the procedures.

▶ Second trimester management focuses on monitoring pregnancy progress, guidance, and teaching.

After reading the vignette at the beginning of this chapter, use what you have learned to answer these questions:

1. Given Kevin Hamilton's age, what developmental patterns should be considered in evaluating his experience of pregnancy?

2. What guidelines can Linda Doherty, RN, suggest to help the Hamiltons strengthen their attachment to each other and prepare for the addition of a new family member?

3. How do sibling responses to the changes occurring during the second trimester affect the physiologic and psychologic adjustment of the family to the pregnancy experience?

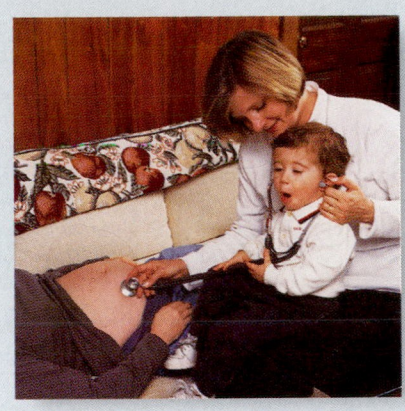

Critical Thinking Questions

▶ # References

Aitokallio-Tallberg, A., & Halmesmaki, E. (1997). Motor vehicle accident during the second or third trimester of pregnancy. *Acta Obstetricia et Gynecologica Scandinavica, 76*(4), 313–317.

American College of Obstetricians and Gynecologists. (1994). *Antepartum fetal surveillance* (Technical Bulletin No. 188). Washington, DC: Author.

American College of Obstetricians and Gynecologists. (1996). *Management of isoimmunization in pregnancy* (Education Bulletin No. 227). Washington, DC: Author.

Bell, J.G., & Weiner, S. (1993). Has percutaneous umbilical blood sampling improved the outcome of high-risk pregnancies? *Clinics in Perinatology, 20,* 61–80.

Berk, B. (1993). Body image and pregnancy: Building the mind–body connection: A guide for health care professionals. *Journal of Perinatology, 13,* 300–304.

Biasella, S. (1993). A comprehensive perinatal education class. *AWHONN Clinical Issues in Perinatal and Women's Health Nursing, 4*(1), 5.

Caplan, G. (1969). *Concepts of mental health and consultation.* Washington, DC: U.S. Department of Health, Education, and Welfare.

Clinton, J. (1986). Expectant fathers at risk for couvade. *Nursing Research, 35,* 290–295.

Cunningham, F.G., MacDonald, P.C., Gant, N.F., Leveno, K.J., Gilstrap, L.C., Hankins, G.D.V., & Clark, S.L. (1997). *Williams obstetrics* (20th ed.). Stamford, CT: Appleton & Lange.

D'Avanzo, C.E. (1992). Bridging the cultural gap with Southeast Asians. *MCN, American Journal of Maternal Child Nursing, 17,* 204–208.

Erikson, E. (1963). *Childhood and society.* New York: Norton.

Fawcett, J. (1978). Body image and the pregnant couple. *MCN, American Journal of Maternal Child Nursing, 3,* 227–233.

French, B.N., Kurczynski, T.W., Weaver, M.T., & Pituch, M.J. (1992). Evaluation of the Health Belief Model and decision-making regarding amniocentesis in women of advanced maternal age. *Health Education Quarterly, 19,* 177–186.

Fuller, S.G., Moore, L.R., & Lester, J.W. (1993). Influence of family functioning on maternal-fetal attachment. *Journal of Perinatology, 13,* 453–460.

Ghidini, A., Sepulveda, W., Lockwood, C.J., & Romero, R. (1993). Complications of fetal blood sampling. *American Journal of Obstetrics and Gynecology, 168,* 1339–1344.

Gullicks, J.N., & Crase, S.J. (1993). Sibling behavior with a newborn: Parents' expectations and observations. *Journal of Obstetric, Gynecologic, and Neonatal Nursing, 22,* 438–444.

Haddow, J.E. (1995). Prenatal screening for Down syndrome. *Contemporary Obstetrics and Gynecology, 40,* 43.

Heidrich, S.D., & Cranley, M.S. (1989). Effect of fetal movement, ultrasound scans and amniocentesis on maternal-fetal attachment. *Nursing Research, 38,* 81–84.

Klainberg, M., Holzemer, S., Leonard, M. & Arnold, J. (1998). *Community health nursing: An alliance for health.* New York: McGraw-Hill.

Lederman, R.P. (1996). *Psychosocial adaptation in pregnancy: Assessment of seven dimensions* (2nd ed.). New York: Springer.

Lee, T.Y. (1994). Maternal-fetal attachment in normal and previously-infertile Chinese women. *Nursing Research (China), 2*(1), 67–77.

Mahler, M., Pine, F., & Bergman, A. (1975). *The psychological birth of the human infant.* New York: Basic Books.

McGoldrick, M., Giordano, J., & Pearce, J.K. (1996). *Ethnicity and family therapy.* New York: Guilford Press.

Moore, P.J. (1994). Maternal physiology during pregnancy. In A.H. DeCherney & M. Pernoll (Eds.), *Current obstetric and gynecologic diagnosis and treatment* (8th ed.) (pp. 146–154). Norwalk, CT: Appleton & Lange.

Okamoto, N. (1978). The Japanese American. In A. Clark (Ed.), *Culture, childbearing, health professionals* (pp. 200–258). Philadelphia: F.A. Davis.

Piaget, J. (1970). *Genetic epistemology.* New York: Columbia University Press.

Piotrkowski, C.S., & Hughes, O. (1993). Dual-earner families in context: Managing family and work systems. In F. Walsh (Ed.), *Normal family processes* (pp. 185–207). New York: Guilford Press.

Roye, C.F., & Balk, S.J. (1997). Caring for pregnant teens and their mothers, too. *MCN, American Journal of Maternal Child Nursing 22*(3), 153–157.

Rubin, R. (1984). *Maternal identity and maternal experience.* New York: Springer.

Sandelowski, M., & Black, B.P. (1994). The epistemology of expectant parenthood [including commentary by R.T. Mercer, V. Bergum, M.C. Stanton, with author response]. *Western Journal of Nursing Research, 16*(6), 601–622.

Sherwen, L. (1991). Fantasy state during pregnancy: A psychoanalytic account. *Journal of Perinatal Psychology, 6,* 55–71.

Sokol, R., Jones, T.B., & Pernoll, M.L. (1994). Methods of assessment for pregnancy at risk. In A.H. DeCherney & M. Pernoll (Eds.), *Current obstetric and gynecologic diagnosis and treatment* (8th ed.) (pp. 275–305). Norwalk, CT: Appleton & Lange.

Spector, R.E. (1996). *Cultural diversity in health and illness* (4th ed.). Stamford, CT: Appleton & Lange.

Steyn, D.W., Pattinson, R.C., & Odendaal, H.J. (1992). Amniocentesis—still important in the management of severe rhesus incompatibility. *South African Medical Journal, 82,* 321–324.

Strom, R., & Strom, S. (1992). *Achieving grandparent potential: Viewpoints on building intergenerational relationships.* Newbury Park, CA: Sage.

Vintzileos, A.M. (1998). Evidence-based fetal surveillance. In *Proceedings of the 6th annual perinatal ultrasound symposium* (pp. 60–67). New Brunswick, NJ: UMD New Jersey.

Zachariah, R. (1994). Maternal-fetal attachment: Influence of mother-daughter and husband-wife relationships. *Research in Nursing and Health, 17,* 37–44.

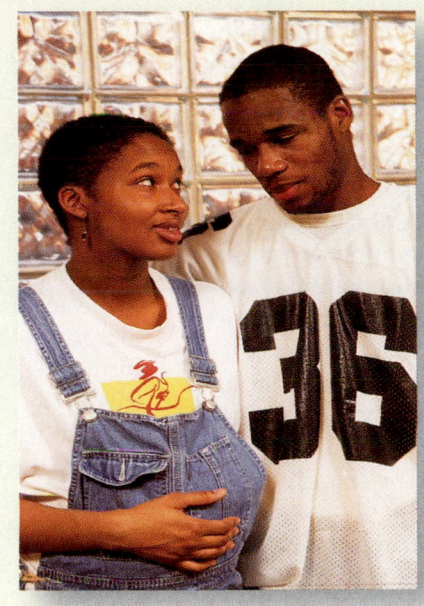

Tamika and Rashid Dengler are attending their weekly prenatal visit at their obstetrician's office. Tamika is 37 weeks' pregnant with their first child. After Tamika's health history is updated, the nurse asks the couple to review the birth plan they had prepared a few weeks' earlier. As they read the birth plan, the nurse notices that Rashid appears uneasy and seems unable to look directly at Tamika. Tamika states, "Everything here looks fine, except that I would like to have my sister, as well as my mother, with us during labor and delivery." Rashid glances nervously at Tamika, whose eyes widen in surprise. She asks, "Rashid, what is it? You do understand that I need my mother and my sister there, don't you?" The nurse asks, "Rashid, are you uncomfortable with having other family members with you during labor? Do you want to talk about the concerns you have about this experience?" ∎

18

The Expectant Family: Third Trimester

The third trimester of pregnancy encompasses the period from the beginning of the 25th week to full-term delivery, which usually occurs anytime from the beginning of the 38th week of gestation through the end of the 42nd week. Although the third trimester includes specific physiologic changes necessary to allow the fetus to fully mature and the mother to enter into labor and the puerperium, pregnancy is a continuous process. Many changes discussed in the third trimester actually begin during the first trimester and continue throughout the second. The nurse must realize that body changes are complex and that body systems, as well as psychosocial and environmental factors, are interrelated.

The third trimester differs in many ways from the preceding two trimesters. The pregnancy is obvious to everyone because of the woman's size. Labor and delivery are no longer far off. The family must actively prepare for the new baby.

By the beginning of the third trimester of pregnancy, the low-risk, healthy expectant mother and her partner will have seen the health care provider five to six times. Around 36 weeks, clients and health care provider meet on a weekly basis. By collaborating with other health care providers, the nurse ensures that comprehensive third-trimester assessment is performed. The nurse's role includes client interviews for the purpose of updating the health history and assessment of the family's readiness for labor, delivery, and the postpartum period. The nurse also participates in aspects of physical assessment of the expectant mother and the fetus, such as measuring the client's blood pressure and taking the fetal heart rate. In addition, the client continues to be assessed for emergence of high-risk conditions.

Nursing care during the third trimester continues to focus on monitoring the progress of the pregnancy and developing fetus; anticipatory guidance and teaching become especially important so that clients can participate actively in labor and delivery and prepare for the newborn. The increase in frequency of prenatal visits provides an excellent opportunity to strengthen the ongoing relationship between the third-trimester family and their health care providers. Nursing care focuses on specific care goals relevant for the third trimester.

▶ PHYSIOLOGIC CHANGES DURING THE THIRD TRIMESTER

Maternal physiologic adaptation during the third trimester of pregnancy supports the final phases of intrauterine fetal development. During that time, physiologic adaptation also prepares the expectant mother for labor, delivery, and lactation.

▶ Growth and Development of the Fetus

The third trimester of pregnancy is highlighted by rapid growth and maturity of fetal organ systems (see Chapter 13). During the seventh lunar month, the fetal lungs are capable of gas exchange and the alveoli continue to manufacture surfactant. As the third trimester progresses, increasing amounts of surfactant are produced, preparing the fetus for respiration after birth. The central nervous system also matures during this time, with the maturation process continuing after birth. The cerebral cortex proliferates, and myelin, the fatty sheath that transmits nerve impulses, is laid down around the neurons. By the 28th week of gestation, there is a growth spurt with respect to brain size, surface area, and cells. At this time the senses of the fetus begin maturing. The fetus can taste, hear, smell, and perceive light.

Beginning in the seventh lunar month, subcutaneous fat (white fat) forms under the skin of the fetus. By 30 weeks of gestation, the quantity of white fat constitutes about 8% of the fetal weight, so that the skin becomes smooth and the legs and the arms fill out. The lanugo begins to disappear in the eighth lunar month. By the 28th week of gestation, the bone marrow is producing red blood cells.

The ninth and tenth lunar months are times of slower fetal growth. Although the rate of growth slows, weight increases are greater. In the last few weeks of gestation, about 14 g of white fat is laid down each day. The body of the fetus, as well as the extremities, appears plump. The fingernails are well developed. The tenth lunar month is considered the "finishing" period, as the fetus prepares for adaptation to the extrauterine environment.

During the tenth lunar month, the fetus is usually positioned head down in the pelvis in preparation for labor and delivery. The fetus has developed biorhythms, such as sleep–wake cycles, so that a distinct pattern of behavior has been established by birth. At term the average newborn weighs 3400 g (7½ pounds).

▶ Maternal Physiologic Adaptation

A great deal of physiologic adaptation is required as the end of pregnancy approaches because the expectant mother's body must simultaneously nourish a rapidly enlarging, active fetus and prepare for childbirth and lactation in the near future. Table 18–1 summarizes physiologic changes of the third trimester.

▶ **TABLE 18-1**

Summary of Physiologic Changes in the Third Trimester

Organ	Changes
Reproductive System	
Uterus	Enlarges to its greatest size
	Average weight increases 20-fold from a prepregnant weight of 50 to 1100 g
	Volume increases from 10 mL prior to pregnancy to 4 to 8 L at term
	Myometrium distends
	Uterine walls thin and soften
	The position of the uterus changes:
	• By 8 months, height of fundus is three quarters of way between umbilicus and ensiform cartilage
	• Toward end of ninth month, fundus reaches ensiform cartilage
	• **Lightening,** the presenting part of the fetus descending into pelvis, occurs 1 to 2 weeks before term (especially in primigravidas)
	Braxton Hicks contractions increase in strength and frequency
Cervix	**Effacement,** cervical thinning and shortening, occurs prior to or during labor
	Cervical ripening, the process by which the cervix softens and thins, occurs late in the third trimester
	Mucous plug may be expelled causing small capillaries to rupture and stain the mucus with blood; referred to as the **bloody show**
Vagina	Continues to relax and distend as a result of physiologic changes
	Epithelial cells continue to change
	Growth of *Lactobacillus,* which maintains acidic environment, increases
	Leukorrhea increases
	Hyperemia of connective tissue continues
Breasts	Enlarge
	Colostrum is present
Cardiovascular System	Cardiac output remains elevated up to 40% over prepregnant level and is distributed to organs (Fig. 18–1)
	Maternal blood volume increases 30 to 50% over nonpregnant level or about an additional 1500 mL
	Circulation to decidua, myometrium, placenta, kidneys, and skin increases
	Heart is pushed upward and to left
	Heart rate continues to be increased about 15 beats over nonpregnant level
	Stroke volume continues to be elevated over nonpregnant level until term, when decrease begins
	Cardiovascular workload peaks at beginning of third trimester, presenting a risk to women with preexisting cardiac disease
	Supine hypotensive syndrome, a decrease in venous return from the lower portion of the body, may occur when mother lies on her back from pressure of gravid uterus on aorta (Fig. 18–2)
Respiratory System	Changes are due to displacement by uterus and to hormonal factors
	Diaphragm rises about 4 cm
	Anteroposterior and transverse chest diameters increase
	Ribs flare; rib cage expands
	Oxygen consumption increases substantially (Fig. 18–3)
Urinary System	Some dilation of renal calyces, pelves, and ureters occurs, especially on right side
	Urinary frequency results from pressure of presenting part of fetus settling into pelvis
	Physiologic hypervolemia occurs
	Fluid and electrolyte balance continues to be affected by complex hormonal interactions, increased glomerular filtration rate, decreased renal vascular resistance, decreased plasma albumin concentration, and other factors
	Glycosuria may occur
Musculoskeletal System	Joints continue to relax and become mobile, especially the sacroiliac, sacrococcygeal, and pubic joints
	Center of gravity continues to shift forward
	Lordosis progresses
	Balance is altered
	Walking and changing positions become more difficult
	Women waddle, develop wide gait
	Numbness and tingling in upper extremities, carpal tunnel syndrome, and diastasis recti (separation of the rectus muscles along the midline of the abdomen) may develop
Integument	
Skin	Striae gravidarum may increase and become more pronounced
	Sweat and sebaceous gland activity increases
	Vascular spiders and palmar erythema may be present or develop
	Skin pigmentation darkens

(continued)

▶ **TABLE 18-1** *(continued)*

Summary of Physiologic Changes in the Third Trimester

Organ	Changes
Hair	Continues to seem thicker Some women may have hair loss
Nails	Continue to grow faster than in nonpregnant state Continue to be softer and break more easily than in nonpregnant state
Gastrointestinal System	
Mouth and gums	Hyperemia continues Gums continue to be sensitive to irritants
Esophagus and stomach	Gastric reflux continues or increases Stomach capacity decreases because of enlarging uterus Hydrochloric acid and pepsin remain lower than in prepregnant state
Liver	Is pushed upward and to right by uterus No change occurs in liver size or morphology Alterations in liver function continue
Gallbladder	Capacity continues to be greater Continues to empty more slowly than in nonpregnant state Predisposition to gallstones continues
Pancreas	Responds to greater demands for glucose metabolism Production of insulin increases Gestational diabetes may develop
Intestines	Pushed upward and to side Decreased motility and tone continue and foster increased absorption of nutrients and water Changes predispose to constipation
Endocrine System	
Pituitary	Continues to be enlarged Prolactin level increases until about 36 weeks, then decreases Follicle-stimulating and luteinizing hormone levels remain suppressed Growth hormone level decreases Oxytocin production increases Melanotropic hormone level increases
Thyroid	May be palpable Vascularity and hyperplasia increase Basal metabolic rate increases Free T_3 and T_4 levels remain within normal nonpregnant limits; thyroid-binding globulin level remains elevated
Parathyroids	Calcium and phosphorus metabolism increases
Adrenals	Adrenocorticotropin level continues to be elevated Concentration of cortisol rises, although rate of cortisol secretion does not Aldosterone level continues to be elevated
Placenta	Remains fully functional to term Grows in size and weight

▶ **PSYCHOLOGIC AND SOCIOCULTURAL DIMENSIONS OF THE THIRD TRIMESTER**

During the third trimester of pregnancy, the contentment of the second trimester gives way to a period of ambivalence and activity. The family, as a whole and as individuals, must now prepare for the imminent addition of a new member.

▶ **Psychologic Changes in the Mother**

The second trimester is generally a calm period for the pregnant woman. The third trimester, unlike the second, is emotionally turbulent. The woman is faced with the impending birth and a new baby; her lifestyle will soon change. She is not as physically comfortable as she was during the second trimester.

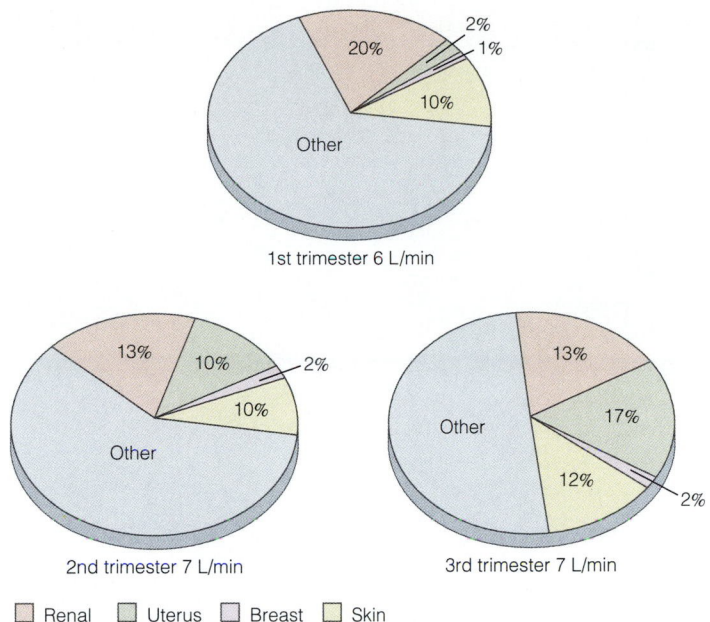

1st trimester 6 L/min

2nd trimester 7 L/min

3rd trimester 7 L/min

☐ Renal   ☐ Uterus   ☐ Breast   ☐ Skin

FIGURE 18–1. Distribution of increased cardiac output during pregnancy. "Other" (denoted in circles) refers, for example, to coronary, splanchnic, skeletal, and cerebral systems. Little change in blood distribution occurs in the first trimester; however, cardiac output in a woman who is not pregnant is 5 L/minute, compared with 6 L/minute during first trimester. *(Adapted, with permission, from Burrow, G.N., & Ferris, T.F. (1989). Medical complications during pregnancy (3rd ed.). Philadelphia: W.B. Saunders, p. 183.)*

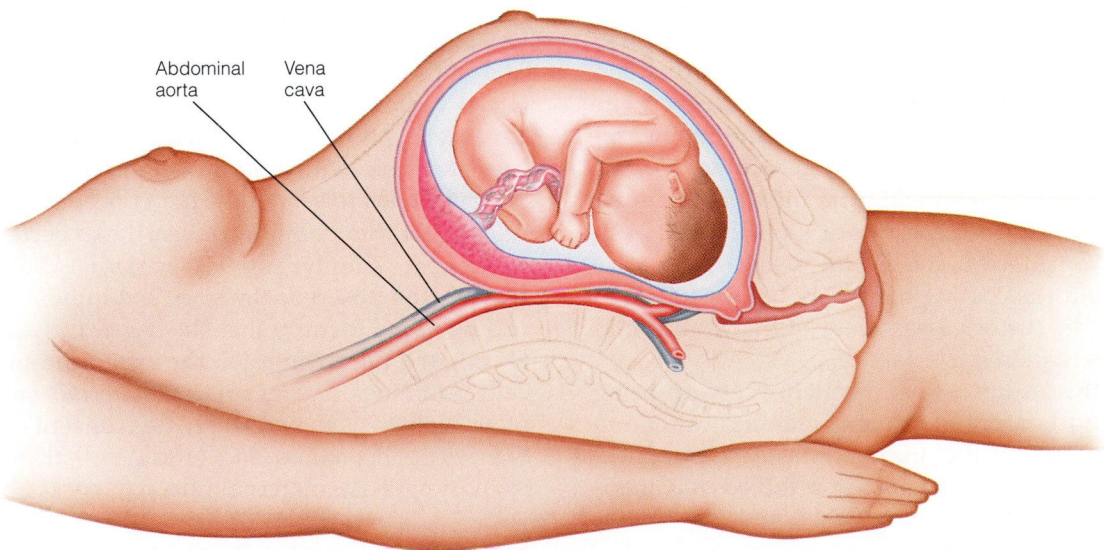

Abdominal aorta

Vena cava

FIGURE 18–2. Supine hypotensive syndrome. When the woman lies on her back, the large, heavy uterus compresses the vena cava and abdominal aorta against the spinal column, thereby interfering with circulation.

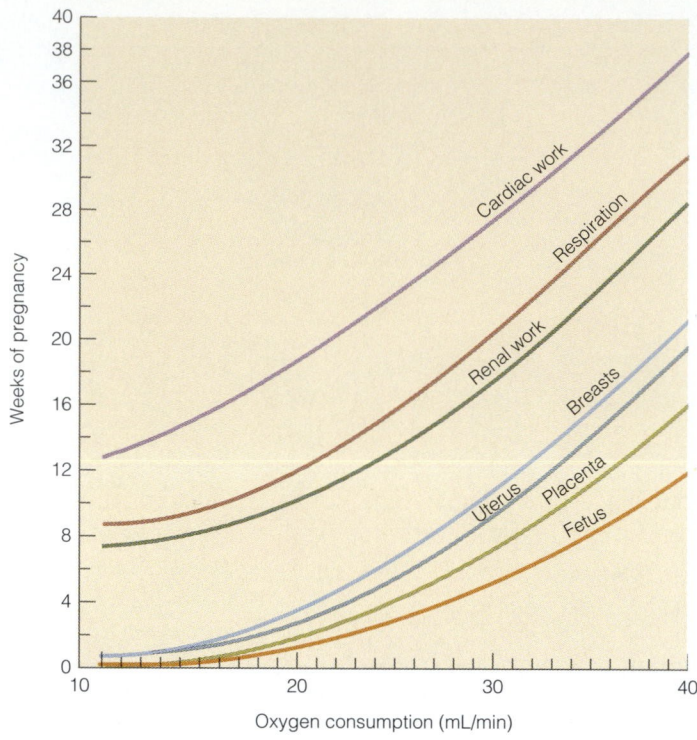

FIGURE 18–3. Increase in oxygen consumption among body organs during pregnancy.

Time needs to be scheduled for prenatal visits at 2-week and then 1-week intervals. As she approaches her due date, the woman must complete many psychologic preparations to move into the changed lifestyle of mother and child.

Acceptance of Pregnancy

By the third trimester, the pregnant woman normally may again have negative feelings about "being pregnant." She is anxious for the pregnancy to end and often becomes tired of her pregnant body and the restrictions it places on her; however, the mother-to-be should demonstrate general acceptance of the fetus. Rejection of the fetus during the third trimester is an ominous sign for the future mother–child relationship. Women who consistently express negative feelings about the coming baby may be considered at emotional risk; further assessment of the woman and her family situation is warranted.

A mother's intense ambivalence about being pregnant and becoming a parent may indicate unresolved conflicts in the third trimester (Lederman, 1996). Severe conflicts that are not resolved may interfere with her acceptance of the newborn.

Maternal Role Attainment

By the third trimester, the expectant mother has taken on enough of the maternal role that she may give birth and be able to nurture her newborn; however, maternal role assumption and maternal role competence are developmental processes that continue after the birth of the infant (Mercer & Ferketich, 1994, 1995). Dedifferentiation and fantasy are among the activities of maternal role assumption in the third trimester.

Dedifferentiation

The stage of maternal role assumption that Rubin (1984) calls dedifferentiation occurs during the third trimester. The woman still tries to "match" or "replicate" her role with role models in the environment. She continues to search for her concept of the "ideal" mother. At this point, however, the expectant mother no longer simply mimics maternal behaviors of women she observes. Instead, she builds on the core of a maternal identity that she has already developed. During the third trimester, the expectant mother critically examines and evaluates maternal behaviors of other women as they relate to her concept of the ideal. She rejects behaviors and attitudes that do not "fit" her vision of the maternal role.

Fantasies

During the third trimester, fantasies (daydreams and night dreams) are felt more as real experiences than as unreal imaginary events. Fantasies may have greater meaning for the woman during the third trimester. Third-trimester fantasies may be accompanied by worry, anxiety, and fear, despite the woman's attempts to orient herself to the "real world" and to keep her mind off unpleasant thoughts. The pregnant woman may fear for herself and for her infant during the coming labor and delivery; she may also hope and wish for her child to be born and the tiresome burden of pregnancy to end (Sherwen, 1991).

Sherwen (1991) reported on a survey of fantasies experienced by pregnant women in their third trimester. Women recorded their night dreams and daydreams during a 6-week interval. Fantasies fell into certain thematic categories or groupings and seemed to be associated with positive emotions, such as pleasure, joy, and peace, or with negative emotions, such as fear, guilt, and panic. Sherwen classifies these third-trimester maternal fantasies into eight categories:

1. *Fantasies about having an abnormal infant.* The woman delivers a deformed infant, an infant of abnormal size or with extraordinary ability such as flying, or multiple infants, or she experiences delivery complications that will affect the infant.
2. *Fantasies about being attacked.* The mother, or a symbol, is attacked in some manner.
3. *Fantasies about being enclosed or drowning.* In these fantasies, mostly night dreams, the woman is inside a tunnel, a car, a small room, or another type of enclosure. Sometimes she tries or is unable to get out.
4. *Fantasies about losing things.* During the third trimester, women frequently report unpleasant fantasies about losing objects or people who are important to them, especially the infant-to-be.
5. *Fantasies about being unprepared.* In this recurring fantasy, the woman is unprepared for labor.
6. *Fantasies about sexual encounters.* Sexual fantasies can evoke positive or negative emotions, depending on such factors as who the fantasized partner is.
7. *Fantasies about restoration.* These fantasies are unusual because they deal primarily with death; however, they are accompanied by positive feelings. During pregnancy women may have an opportunity to rework and resolve old crises through fantasy. The pregnant woman who reports having this type of fantasy seems to be resolving the loss of someone close to her. In addition, these dreams seem to provide a link among generations and a means to con-

nect the infant-to-be with ancestors. Women restore the family chain that has been broken by death, and add another link to the chain with a new baby.
8. *Everyday fantasies.* These fantasies deal with the concerns, plans, and problems faced by any family having a new baby. Some common themes are life changes and restructuring of living space for the new baby; characteristics of the new baby-to-be, for example, sex, health, hair and eye color, beauty, and family resemblances; strategies for coping with labor; checklists of chores for preparation; living with and caring for the baby-to-be, for example, loving, playing with, or feeding the baby; reactions of the father or significant others to the baby; the expectant mother's own childhood experiences; and the baby in different stages of growth and development.

Sherwen (1987) regards the presence of such everyday fantasies as "bonding clues." As these fantasies seem to be instrumental to "binding in" to the child, their absence or suppression may indicate a block in maternal attachment to the fetus.

Through exploration of maternal fantasies during the third trimester, the nurse may gain much insight into the pregnant woman's current concerns. Fantasies may be unsettling to the expectant mother. The nurse should be aware of their often disturbing nature and be prepared to discuss them with the client when asked.

Relationship with Mother

As labor approaches, the expectant mother strives for a positive balance in her relationship with her own mother, and in many cases, the mother–daughter relationship improves (Lederman, 1996). The expectant woman's perception of her mother as reassuring, tolerant, and supportive of her contributes to her self-esteem and modifies her anxiety in the days before delivery. Indeed, as Lederman (1996) observed, a poor relationship with mother and unresolved conflicts by the end of the third trimester can be manifested by such childbirth problems as prolonged labor.

The expectant mother often depends on her own mother to provide support to her and to her family, although the nature and extent of desired support depends on the mother–daughter relationship. She may also experience conflict between her partner's and her parents' involvement surrounding birth and early parenting, particularly if she is having her first baby and her mother is becoming a grandparent for the first time. Research has noted that there are positive intergenerational attachment relationships between the pregnant woman and her mother (Zachariah, 1994). Open discussion with significant others, clarification of roles and responsibilities, and avoidance of using mother or husband as scapegoat in dealings with the other person can foster harmony in the third trimester.

Relationship with Fetus

During the third trimester, the woman's desire for pregnancy to end and her perception of pregnancy as a burden conflict with her attachment to her fetus. However, as pregnancy goes to term, the expectant mother becomes increasingly aware of the fetus and fetal activity patterns.

Toward the end of the third trimester, the mother becomes eager and ready to have and hold the infant (Lederman, 1996). Both high-risk and low-risk pregnant women demonstrate attachment to their fetuses (Mercer & Ferketich, 1994).

Body Image

During the third trimester, the woman perceives many differences in the size of her body, her body boundaries, and the space her body occupies. The size of the body in the third trimester begins to be cumbersome to the pregnant woman. The pregnant woman becomes progressively less tolerant of abdominal growth, is increasingly anxious about how much more childbearing will demand of her body, and generally feels irritable. Many women view third-trimester body changes, such as stretch marks, as unpleasant. They may wish to be rid of the pregnancy, but not the child. Examples of negative third-trimester body images, such as lack of pride in the body or concerns over body predictability, have been presented in the literature (Berk, 1993; Lederman, 1996). Some women, however, may delight in the body changes and maintain a positive body image during the third trimester, viewing all of pregnancy as a time of beauty. Women's perceptions of their bodies may reflect complex factors such as their overall self-image, whether they feel their partners consider them beautiful, and what the cultural standards of beauty are. Furthermore, body satisfaction during the third trimester of pregnancy has been associated with the woman's intent to breastfeed her infant (Foster, Slade, & Wilson, 1996).

Body Boundaries. During the third trimester, the woman's thinning abdominal walls and increased size make her feel that her fetus is more vulnerable to external influences. She feels that her body, as a barrier, is more fragile and may express this feeling in fantasies.

Body Size and Position. The woman's experience of her body in space changes radically after the second trimester (Berk, 1993). As the woman approaches the end of pregnancy, she becomes more preoccupied with her body's position in space. Contributing factors include the change in balance resulting from the increased size and the shift of body weight, decreased mobility, and perceptions of the body as vulnerable. In a classic study, Fawcett (1977) found that both women and their husbands may have an increase in their perceived body space, compared with perceptions of body space in the first and second postpartum month.

Preparation for Labor

The pregnant woman must take specific steps, including concrete actions and imaginary rehearsals, in preparation for labor and parenting. Maternal preparation includes nesting behaviors (practical activities such as taking childbirth classes and preparing infant clothes) as well as gearing up psychologically for labor. From her research, Lederman (1996) identified three ways that women may plan for labor:

1. Practical activity, for example, gathering information about labor and delivery, taking prenatal classes, talking to other women, reading books and viewing films, preparing a layette for the baby, arranging for additional help in the home after the birth, and arranging transportation to the place for birthing
2. Imaginary rehearsals
3. Dreaming about labor

Third-trimester activities have the overall goal of helping the expectant mother prepare psychologically for the end of pregnancy and the birth of the infant. By 38 weeks of gestation, the low-risk healthy pregnant woman is psychologically as well as physiologically ready for her baby.

▶ Psychologic Changes in the Father

The nature of paternal feelings and psychologic experiences during the third trimester has not been documented well in research. The expectant father may have his most negative feelings during the third trimester of his partner's pregnancy. The last half of the third trimester can be a stressful time for expectant fathers. Many expectant fathers experience a loss both of personal freedom and of the partner's time and attention. Some fathers report feeling they are in the background, outside the maternal–fetal dyad. Expectant fathers also may report a need for increased attention, which they generally do not feel they receive.

Fantasies

Like the expectant mother, the expectant father has specific fantasies during the third trimester. Dreams begin to include the baby's coming and the birth process.

Sherwen (1986) found that, in comparison to non-expectant men, expectant third-trimester fathers had more fantasies oriented in the present. The extent of the father's involvement in his partner's pregnancy also affected the nature of his fantasies. The more involved the father was in the pregnancy, the more positive were his fantasies.

Like maternal fantasies, paternal fantasies during the third trimester can be grouped into major themes, which Sherwen (1987) identified:

1. Anxiety about upcoming events (e.g., being a good father, the condition of his wife, cesarean delivery, lack of money)
2. Happiness about coming events
3. Fear of injury or trauma to the self, spouse, or significant other (e.g., wife being mugged or attacked)
4. Fantasies about the father's winning or coming into large sums of money
5. Concerns about being prepared
6. Concerns about loss and/or death
7. Fantasies about "creative" acts or dependents he must care for (as acquiring and caring for a dog)
8. Concerns about the reactions of others, especially the father's father, to the child

Fantasy themes can give the nurse clues to a father's current concerns and provide a basis for anticipatory guidance.

Couvade Syndrome

Many expectant fathers experience couvade symptoms during the third trimester (Clinton, 1986; Fawcett & York, 1986). Examples of couvade symptoms during this trimester include unintentional weight gain, gastrointestinal discomforts, and difficulty in concentrating.

Attachment to Fetus

The process of paternal attachment to the coming baby is likely to be somewhat different from maternal attachment, as the expectant father does not carry the fetus in his body and experience prenatal physical changes. There is, however, little doubt that fathers do attach to their fetuses prenatally.

The concept of paternal–infant bonding is not new; however, there is a lack of research describing the factors that influence the father–infant relation-

ship from the father's perspective (Anderson, 1996). Expectant fathers may approach delivery with preconceived ideas about the "scientific" importance of attending delivery to foster their attachment to their infant. They may worry about not being good fathers if they do not attend every prenatal class or labor and delivery. Through individual client teaching and prepared childbirth classes, nurses can discuss attachment with expectant fathers.

Preparation for Parenthood

In general, expectant fathers come to terms with the reality of a baby in a process similar to the way in which the expectant mother identifies with the maternal role. Expectant men prepare for fatherhood by reading and planning, fantasizing and thinking about the baby and the changes in their lifestyle, attending classes, talking to other fathers, and being exposed to television, radio, magazines, and other types of media (Fig. 18–4) (Lederman, 1996). Men who relate poorly to their wives may have difficulty accepting the responsibilities of fatherhood.

Although the modern American father is currently expected to be involved in childbearing and childrearing, specific roles are as yet unclear. Men are also greatly affected by their families' cultural background and expectations for the role of the father. Research has shown that mothers have a significant influence in assisting the father–infant relationship after birth (Anderson, 1996). Through thoughtful discussion of paternal concerns, the nurse can assist the couple in evolving their new roles as parents.

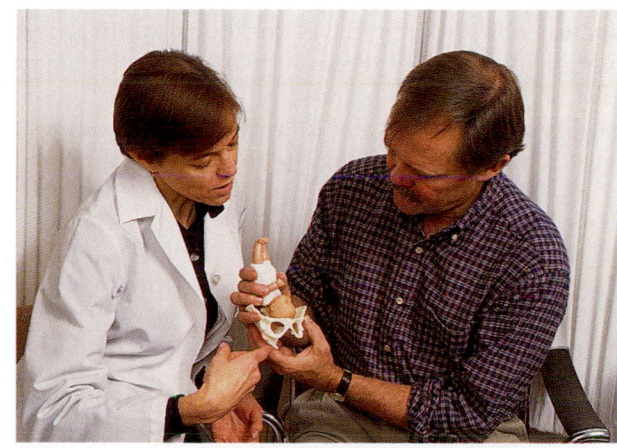

FIGURE 18–4. An expectant father can prepare for parenthood by discussing his questions about the labor and birth experience with the nurse.

▶ Psychologic Changes in the Family

During the third trimester, concerns of the family and, in particular, the expectant mother may place stress on the pregnancy and affect pregnancy outcome. This may happen during a first or subsequent pregnancy.

Stress or negative emotional states can be higher during the end of pregnancy than at other times during the childbearing cycle. Most pregnancy-related concerns seem to be voiced during the third trimester.

Many studies on stress and pregnancy outcome have been done during the third trimester. Among the stress-producing factors identified by these studies are fear of damage to the self, childbirth, effects of birth on the baby, finances, family, future pregnancies, negative self-concept, previous loss of a fetus, terminating work, major life changes, and concern about pain in labor and delivery.

Denial of stressful concerns may also be damaging to the pregnancy. The stressful problems do not simply disappear and may result in increased obstetric complications. Family-centered nursing care focuses on encouraging the family and the pregnant woman to deal with stressful pregnancy-related concerns.

▶ The Siblings' Experience

Third-trimester pregnancy can have a major impact on siblings (Gullicks & Crase, 1993). The mother has become large and noticeably pregnant. Third-trimester discomforts, as well as the mother's size, may restrict her usual schedule. The mother may wish to engage in quiet rather than physically demanding activities. Her attention may be directed more toward preparation for the baby and less toward entertaining the older sibling(s).

Most children are aware of their mothers' pregnancies. All children have questions, although the level of questions and the child's ability to comprehend and to verbalize vary with the child's age and developmental level. The following may be topics of concern to children during the third trimester:

- What does the baby look like?
- What does the baby do?
- What will become of me when Mommy goes to have the baby?
- What will happen when Mommy is having the baby?
- Will Mommy be all right? Will she come back to me?
- Will I still be loved as much?
- Will the baby use my things (blanket, toys, and so on)?

- Can I choose the baby's name?
- Will I get to help?
- Will I know who is going to take care of me?
- Can I stay home and "help" Mommy?

Negative sibling responses to late pregnancy and birth include sleep disturbances, frequent crying, and regressive behaviors, especially in relation to toilet training (Gullicks & Crase, 1993). In addition to being a potential source of disturbance, however, advancing pregnancy and the prospect of a new baby can be a source of great interest, particularly to firstborn children (Fig. 18–5) (Gottlieb & Mendelson, 1990).

As the pregnancy becomes increasingly visible, the older child or children need reassurance of their parents' love. Indeed, a strong and loving parent–child relationship can help the sibling, as well as the parent, get ready for the baby. Expectant parents also need to feel that they are adequately preparing siblings for the arrival of the baby (Gullicks & Crase, 1993).

Siblings' lives will be greatly affected by a new baby and family member. The activities for most families change because of infant care concerns. Many families cannot afford separate bedrooms for each child. The sibling(s) may therefore be expected to share a bedroom, time, and often toys with the new family member.

Parents may also want to reuse infant furniture, clothing, and accessories, especially if the new baby is the same sex as a sibling. During the third trimester, the sibling may make the transition from crib to bed, and the bedroom furniture may be rearranged. Although most young children want to feel "grown up," they may still miss the crib or feel upset that their possessions are being passed along. Gentle parental

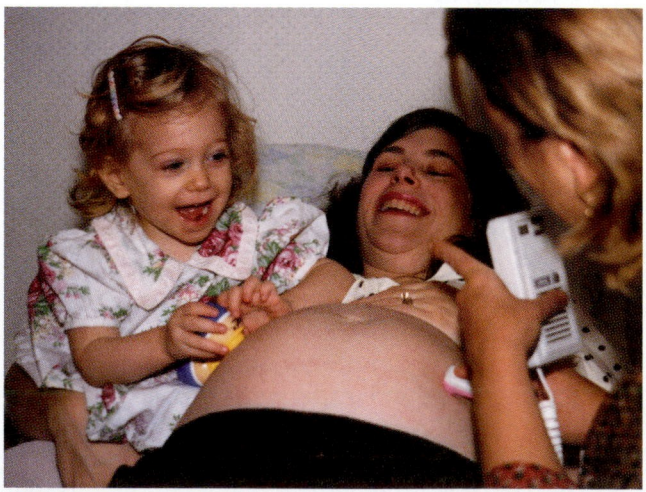

FIGURE 18–5. Firstborn children may be greatly interested in advancing pregnancy.

strategies that allow the sibling to feel she or he is "giving" items to the baby or no longer "wants" them are necessary to make a smooth transition and to maintain the sibling's feelings of love and belonging.

In families with two or more siblings, parents may require help in daily activities from the older siblings. School-aged and adolescent expectant siblings may need to help care for younger children in the family or help in meal preparation or other household chores; however, their contributions should be age appropriate. Children often want to help and view their contributions as important in preparation for the baby. The nurse can help parents to base their expectations on what a child, and not an adult, can emotionally and physically contribute.

With the addition of a new baby to the family, the status and roles of siblings change. As plans are made for the baby during the third trimester, siblings in families where there are already two or more children may compete with each other over who will do what for the baby. By providing anticipatory guidance, nurses can help parents prepare each child in the family for the new baby.

▶ The Grandparents' Experience

During the third trimester, as the time for birth of the infant draws closer, expectant grandparents may participate actively in making plans for the new baby. They may assist the expectant parents with care of older siblings, may make arrangements to stay with the children while the mother delivers and recovers, and may contribute to overall preparations. During the third trimester, expectant grandmothers, especially the woman's mother, may share experiences and demonstrate support by participating in prenatal rituals, for example, a baby shower for the parents-to-be.

During the third trimester, expectant grandparents may have concerns, such as the health of the expectant mother and baby and the safety of labor and delivery. Moreover, the third trimester, especially the last month of pregnancy, may seem long for them.

Becoming a grandparent and moving up a generation can be important to older adults. Types of experiences that grandparents go through during the third trimester are (Strom & Strom, 1992):

- Enhancement of overall quality of life, physical and mental health, and adjustment to old age
- Strengthening the sense of identity and feelings of personal meaning
- Recognition as a valued elder who is a resource person for children and who identifies with grandchildren

- Assurance of immortality through continuation of the family line and through contact with the grandchild
- Reinvolvement with a personal past as grandchildren evoke memories of early life and experiences with the grandparent's own grandparents
- Opportunity to indulge grandchildren and, especially for the grandfather, to be lenient without worrying about "spoiling" the grandchildren

Unlike their own parents who may have been able to help when the now-expectant parents were born, contemporary grandparents may not be accessible or they may not have regular child care responsibilities among their life goals. Such grandparents may thus have to deal with adult children who wish they would be around to help them, not only with child care, but also in their preparations for delivery during the third trimester.

Moving up a generation evokes fears of getting older and dying for some expectant grandparents. For others, there may be role conflicts. For example, in the past they were responsible for teaching their child; now their child assumes that responsibility. As a result of changes in social structure and the increase in technology in the United States, health care workers, rather than grandparents, may be seen as the experts on pregnancy and parenthood. Indeed, the information shared by grandparents about pregnancy and childbirth may be regarded by their children as outdated, rather than valuable. Increasing emphasis on paternal involvement in pregnancy and birth may strengthen the marital bond during advancing pregnancy, yet make the expectant grandparents feel distanced. Although expectant parents may welcome contact with their own parents, grandparents' suggestions may be regarded as interference. Expectant and new parents may be caught in conflicts between suggestions of their parents, those of health providers, and their own wishes. Such conflicts may be minimized if expectant grandparents are prepared through clarification of changes in childbearing and childrearing.

In contrast, growing numbers of grandparents actually assume total care of an infant or child at some time during the child's life. Such societal issues as the increase in substance abuse, human immunodeficiency virus (HIV) infection, poverty, and homelessness may make a child's parent unable to care for the child. Child welfare agencies are mandated to place children with relatives whenever possible; most often the relative is a grandparent. Researchers are just beginning to describe problems and concerns of caretaking grandparents which include social isolation and role restriction (Kelley, 1993). Nurses who work with expectant grandparents may need to consider this greatly changed role expectation.

Childbirth education programs for expectant grandparents can ease the transition to grandparenthood. Most expectant grandparent programs are offered during the third trimester. Considering the important role of the parent's parents in maternal and paternal role development, grandparent preparation might be encouraged earlier in the pregnancy.

At times an expectant grandmother, rather than an expectant father, will plan to be the woman's support person during labor. Among certain ethnic groups, an expectant grandmother or another female relative may be the primary support person. Women who do not have support from the expectant father and wives of men who cannot be present for births, such as military servicemen or men who must travel, may look to their own mother for support. In accepting this responsibility, the expectant grandparent may also need support, education, and guidance. The grandparent may be encouraged to attend prenatal visits and also to accompany the expectant mother to prepared childbirth classes.

► Sociocultural Dimensions

The cultural orientation of the expectant family is reflected in their preparation for birth. How birth is viewed and the rituals and customs that surround it differ among cultural groups. The nurse might expect a third-generation white middle-class American family and a first-generation Filipino-American family to have different expectations of childbearing. Cultural sensitivity and appreciation of differing beliefs and traditions are essential components of holistic care. In addition, nurses must be aware of the influence of socioeconomic factors on the childbearing family during the third trimester.

Socioeconomic Influence

Socioeconomic concerns can have great importance during the third trimester. For clients, the realization in the third trimester that birth is near is accompanied by the realization of the need to acquire infant clothing and accessories. Most families have financial concerns caused by the coming infant; these can become sources of conflict. Clients who live in poverty have difficulty meeting basic needs; other clients, even those with adequate incomes, may perceive themselves to be in financial jeopardy.

Health care and delivery are also expensive. It is not unusual to find that an expectant family has no or inadequate insurance coverage for maternity care. Women may depend on public assistance to help them gain financial access to prenatal care, which

takes place on a weekly basis during the third trimester. These women may have to travel long distances to reach health care providers who will provide services without charge. Some clients who are unable to buy insurance or qualify for public assistance are forced to forego prenatal care, even in late pregnancy.

To help meet family expenses, women may choose to work until delivery; however, the woman's cumbersome size and other physiologic changes during the third trimester may make certain jobs difficult, especially if long periods of standing, lifting, or heavy physical activity are required. The prospect of decreased family income can be stressful, especially if maintaining the family's lifestyle depends on income contributed by the expectant mother.

Hispanic Cultural Groups

Hispanic subgroups comprise the second largest emerging minority group in the United States. Hispanic-Americans, also referred to as Latino-Americans, originated in such Spanish-speaking areas as Mexico, Puerto Rico, Cuba, and countries in Central and South America (Spector, 1996). It is estimated that by the year 2000, Hispanics will be the largest minority group in the United States (Burk, Wieser, & Keegan, 1995). They represent a complex cultural tradition. Care must be taken to identify the unique characteristics of each Hispanic cultural group. Indeed, even the Spanish language varies according to such factors as geographic area. This chapter focuses on the Chicano family as one example of a Hispanic group.

Cultural Focus: The Chicano Family

Chicano refers to all Americans of Mexican descent. Mexican-American is another term used to identify this group (Burk, et al., 1995). Chicano families constitute one of the largest ethnic groups of childbearing families in the United States.

Many Chicanos were born either in Mexico or to parents born in Mexico: however, many Chicanos are also descendants of early settlers in California and the southwestern region of the United States (Burk, et al.,

Women's Health

Data have shown that women in both rural and urban settings receive inadequate prenatal care (Alexy, Nichols, Heverly, & Garzon, 1997). Lack of prenatal care increases the risk of giving birth to low-birth-weight infants by threefold.

1995). Many Hispanic cultural traditions may be practiced by this group, because they have met barriers to full assimilation into the dominant culture in the United States. Although Chicanos hold all types of employment, many have found themselves relegated to low-paying jobs. Unemployment remains high. Depending on the amount of time lived in the United States and the opportunity to learn English, Chicanos may be bilingual, speak English to some degree, or speak no English.

Many Chicanos are *mestizos*—of Mexican and American Indian descent. Both these heritages are fused in their cultural practices. Although the predominant religion is Roman Catholic, the American Indian belief system is often evident (McGoldrick, Giardano, & Pearce, 1996).

Family Patterns. Broad cultural generalizations cannot explain all the unique behaviors in any Chicano family. Each family within a culture has its own private reality. The nurse must remember to assess and treat each family as unique, regardless of the cultural heritage. Cultural norms and patterns merely provide a framework to use to organize thoughts.

Many Chicano immigrants to the United States in the past 30 to 40 years were poor or working class families from rural or semirural areas of northern and central Mexico (McGoldrick et al., 1996). The following descriptions relate to these families. Like many other groups, Chicano nuclear families are closely surrounded by an extended family, which may include grandparents, uncles, aunts, cousins, and even *compadres* (children's godparents). Cousins, perhaps even third or fourth cousins, are very close to each other. Boundaries among these individuals are flexible, and many family functions, such as the care and discipline of children and financial or emotional support, are shared. The extension of kinship ties is called *familism* (McGoldrick et al., 1996). To help the kinship network function, affiliation and cooperation among individuals are stressed; confrontation and competition are discouraged. Chicanos generally perceive membership in some kind of family, so that all life cycle events and rituals, such as birth, are *family* events that affirm family unity.

The family protects the individual but expects loyalty. Autonomy and individuality are not emphasized, but honesty and dignity are very important. Although the extended family is cohesive, nuclear families live in separate dwellings, thereby preserving their boundaries and identity. The Chicano nuclear family is typically large and may include four or five children (McGoldrick et al., 1996).

Marital Relationships. The roles of husband and wife in Chicano culture are often set by tradition, the husband being the provider and protector and the wife homemaker and caretaker. Male dominance (*machismo*) is the ideal male role. Within individual families, couples often arrange their own balance of power and control. Indeed, the wife is often very powerful, as she exerts much psychologic control as the "self-sacrificing" mother. Research demonstrates that, in fact, gender roles in today's Chicano families appear to be more democratic. Women make decisions within the family and seek employment outside of the home (Burk et al., 1995).

Many newly married couples live with the husband's family, and the mother-in-law–daughter-in-law relationship is important. The success of the marriage may be affected by how well these two women work out their respective role relationships.

Parent–Child Relationship. Traditionally, the romantic ties of marriage are not viewed as important as the parent–child relationship in the Chicano family. Preservation of the marriage is important, and children validate the marriage. Motherly love is seen as stronger than marital love; the father is also involved with his children. As the parent–child relationship is primary, the couple has little freedom from parental functions throughout the childbearing and childrearing phases of the family life cycle.

Chicano children tend to leave their family at an older age than children of other cultural groups. Thus, the Chicano couple has a long period of parenthood. A primary focus throughout life is parenting and then grandparenting.

Traditional parental roles are complementary: the father disciplines and controls, the mother nurtures and supports. Both parents are respected by the children. Parent–child interaction is hierarchical, with children having lower status. Chicano parents are very nurturing and generally relaxed in their childrearing. Chicano children also receive nurturance and support from extended family members.

Sibling Roles. Ties among brothers and sisters in Chicano families may be very strong. Siblings and cousins are often constant companions during childhood. Competition and fighting among siblings are discouraged; cooperation, sharing, and sacrifice are stressed. As they grow to adulthood, Chicano siblings maintain close ties and become part of the extended family network. Life cycle events of one sibling, such as birth, will affect the other siblings and their nuclear families.

Spiritual Dimensions. Health care providers must appreciate the importance that spiritual dimensions and religion often hold for Chicano families. Families frequently have shrines in their homes and participate in religious rituals, for example, in relation to health and illness (Spector, 1996).

The Chicano Family's Experience of Pregnancy.

The traditional Chicano family may have a variety of cultural beliefs related to pregnancy. For example, while pregnant, Chicano women may follow a series of "pregnancy rules" (Poma, 1987). The rules are a series of prescriptions and taboos for the pregnant woman to follow, especially during her first pregnancy. These rules, which are believed to protect the fetus and provide for easy delivery, evolved from practices of traditional midwives *(parteras)* and folk healers. Some of the activities used to prepare a woman for labor, delivery, and birth are described here (Burk et al., 1995; Poma, 1987).

1. *Control of the environment.* The pregnant woman should avoid cool, moving air, especially night air. Moonlight is thought particularly hazardous, and the sun's rays, coming through glass, are also seen as dangerous. Pregnant women should not sit in drafts or by closed windows. Bathing in water, however, is encouraged during pregnancy.

2. *Food taboos and prescriptions.* Consuming or avoiding certain foods calls attention to the status of pregnancy for Chicano women. Cravings must be satisfied, or the infant may be marked by the food that was craved. Pica is not a common practice, but takes the form of eating ashes or dirt when it does occur. Women may avoid drinking to prevent the baby from growing too large and being hard to deliver.

3. *Control of the gastrointestinal tract.* Chicano women treat nausea and vomiting by drinking flour and water, flour and lemon juice, or chamomile tea. Heartburn is believed by some to predict a long-haired baby and is treated with baking soda and commercial antacids. (This practice is at odds with the current recommendation to avoid baking soda, which may cause acid–base imbalances.) Constipation is treated with over-the-counter medications and herbal teas (said to cause "violent purges" and used with care). During pregnancy, Chicano women may readily take vitamin and iron preparations, which they believe will enrich their blood.

4. *Sleep and exercise.* Chicano women believe that sleeping on their back will protect the fetus. It is believed that activity helps the mother to keep the fetus from becoming too big and aids delivery. Chicano women remain very active and mobile and avoid only the heaviest chores during pregnancy. Massage is thought to help put the fetus in a good position for delivery. Reaching high, crossing legs, and sitting in tailor position are believed to cause knots in the umbilical cord and are therefore avoided.

5. *Affective states.* The pregnant woman tries to avoid feelings of rage or anger, as they may harm the pregnancy. The pelvic examination is frightening and may cause the woman shame. It is also not acceptable to her partner and should be performed in complete privacy and only when necessary. Sexual relationships are maintained throughout pregnancy to keep the birth canal well lubricated.

6. *Rituals.* Baby showers are not held until delivery is near. To have one earlier is perceived as bad luck. Chicano women also undertake the prediction of their baby's sex.

Maintaining a balance between "hot" and "cold" or "wet" and "dry" elements is believed to foster good health in general (Spector, 1996). Treatments may be based on restoring the body's balance. For example, delivery, considered a "hot" experience, would be balanced by eating "cold" foods. Hot and cold refer to specific substances, not their temperature or the amount of spice used. Rules related to hot and cold differ from person to person; however, an understanding of the nature of the concept is important to health care providers working with Chicano clients.

▶ NURSING AND COLLABORATIVE ASSESSMENT

During the third trimester, client visits are more frequent. Health care providers monitor changes related to pregnancy and assess the expectant family's readiness for labor, delivery, and early parenting. Targets of assessment during the third trimester include the following:

- Maternal adaptations to the third trimester
- Development of new risk factors, including those associated with preterm birth, gestational diabetes, and pregnancy-induced hypertension
- Effects of existing risk factors on the pregnant family during the third trimester
- Fetal well-being
- Psychosocial status and adaptations to the third trimester
- Educational preparation and readiness for labor, delivery, and early parenting

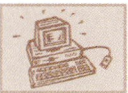

Research Abstract

Providing Culturally Relevant Prenatal Care to Hispanic Women

The purpose of this comparative study was to examine the number of prenatal visits and the pregnancy outcomes of Mexico-born Hispanics and U.S.-born Hispanics. Medical records of 783 women living in California were reviewed. The results demonstrated that more prenatal visits did not improve the outcome during pregnancy, labor, or the postpartum period. The researchers concluded that culturally relevant care is needed to improve pregnancy outcomes with this population.

Application to Practice

This study demonstrates that early and consistent prenatal care does not always prevent poor pregnancy outcomes, such as low-birthweight infants. Nurses need to focus on providing models of care that center on cultural relevance so that positive pregnancy outcomes can be achieved.

Source: Goss, G.L., Lee, K., Koshar, J., Heilemann, M.S., & Stinson, J. (1997). More does not mean better: Prenatal visits and pregnancy outcome in the Hispanic population. Public Health Nursing, 14(3), 183–188.

- Development of a birth plan
- Resources available to the pregnant client and her family during the last trimester

▶ The Woman Who Begins Prenatal Care During the Third Trimester

Women may delay prenatal care until the third trimester because they lack the finances, have no access to prenatal care (e.g., lack transportation or live a significant distance from facilities), fear the health care system, or do not value wellness-oriented prenatal services. Other reasons may also be given.

The comprehensive assessment approach used during the initial visit in the first trimester is employed for the client who seeks care for the first time during the third trimester. Reasons for the delay in seeking care are identified. Nursing diagnoses, interventions, and assessment methods are based on the special needs of the client during the third trimester.

▶ Assessment of Maternal Adaptations to Pregnancy

Updating the Health History

Using a collaborative approach, health care providers update the health history at each prenatal visit throughout the third trimester. Assessment identifies client and family strengths as well as potential or actual risk factors during the third trimester.

Physiologic Assessment

For the low-risk client, assessment during the third trimester usually takes place according to the following schedule: every 4 weeks for the first 28 weeks, every 2 to 3 weeks until 36 weeks of gestation, and every week from 36 weeks to labor. Women who are considered at risk are seen more often.

The nurse bases her assessment of the mother's physiologic state on knowledge of changes that normally occur during the third trimester and high-risk conditions that may be present at this time. Table 18–2 outlines physiologic parameters assessed during the third trimester, and Table 18–3 summarizes selected clinical findings.

During the third trimester the fetus assumes position for delivery; by term, full growth and development are attained. Around 32 weeks of gestation, fetal presentation and position and engagement of the fetus are assessed at each visit through the use of Leopold's maneuvers, described later in this chapter. The uterus continues to enlarge steadily, and fundal growth and fetal size are assessed at each visit. Ultrasound evaluation of the fetus and amniotic fluid may be recommended if marked differences exist between uterine or fetal size and dates of the pregnancy. In this way conditions such as fetal intrauterine growth retardation may be identified.

Near term some clinicians perform pelvic examinations at each prenatal visit to assess the readiness of the cervix for delivery and engagement of the presenting part in the pelvis. Others see little need for third-trimester pelvic examination unless there is specific indication, for example, contractions that might be related to preterm labor.

Risk Assessment

Risk assessment is continued at each prenatal visit, because high-risk conditions such as preeclampsia

▶ **TABLE 18-2**

Physiologic Parameters Assessed During the Third Trimester

Assessment Parameter	Frequency of Assessment	Purpose
Vital signs, including blood pressure, pulse, respirations	Each visit	Detect any changes from normal/baseline that may indicate development of complications (e.g., preeclampsia); determine maternal adaptation to third trimester
Uterine growth, measured by fundal height	Each visit	Assess for disproportionate uterine enlargement, which may indicate multiple gestation, polyhydramnios, inadequate fetal nutrition, and other conditions
Uterine characteristics such as present contractility, soreness, irritability	Each visit	Assess for signs of infection, preterm labor, and so on
Abdominal muscle tone	Each visit	Assess for poor muscle tone, contributing to discomforts such as low back pain
Fetal presentation, engagement, lie, and position, measured by Leopold's maneuvers	Each visit	Identify potential labor and delivery problems related to fetal presentation, position, or lie (especially when engagement has occurred)
Fetal heart rate auscultated with fetoscope or assessed with Doppler; fetal movements felt by examiner, reported by mother	Each visit	Fetal heart tones, fetal movement, and activity indicate fetal well-being
Maternal weight and nutritional status	Each visit	Assess nutritional patterns and detect fluid retention
Urinalysis for protein, glucose, ketones	Each visit	Detect development of complications, such as preeclampsia and diabetes
Suggested blood study for		
Hemoglobin or hematocrit	Early in third trimester (some facilities routinely screen more often)	Detect anemia of pregnancy
Serum glucose	28 weeks, if not done during second trimester	Screen for diabetes
Rh antibody titer (in unsensitized Rh-negative clients)	28 weeks	Identify clients at risk for Rh hemolytic disease
Suggested cultures		
Chlamydia trachomatis	Once in third trimester if mother was infected or at risk	Detect Chlamydia trachomatis infection
Group B streptococcus	35 to 37 weeks	Detect Group B streptococcus infection

may develop during the third trimester. Prompt identification and intervention can often minimize complications and foster delivery of a healthy infant.

As prematurity remains the most significant perinatal problem, risk assessment for preterm delivery is essential. The nurse assesses socioeconomic status, past history, daily habits, and current prenatal events; however, signs and symptoms of preterm labor are reviewed with all third-trimester women, because many women who deliver prematurely have no identifiable risk factors.

The third-trimester expectant woman and her partner are also assessed for risk factors that may indicate a potential problem with accepting or caring for the newborn. Socioeconomic status and related living conditions can present great risks to family health during pregnancy and after childbirth. Financially impoverished clients may not be able to provide adequate nutrition, shelter, or clothing for themselves or an infant. Through prenatal assessment, nurses identify clients in such high-risk situations and make appropriate referrals.

Biochemical Screening Techniques

Urinalysis. During third-trimester visits, urine is assessed for protein, glucose, and ketones, as during the second trimester; these signs may indicate the onset or progression of high-risk conditions.

▶ **TABLE 18-3**

Selected Clinical Findings During the Third Trimester

Body System	Clinical Findings
Integument	Striae gravidarum over abdomen, breasts, and thighs Pruritis of the skin and vulva Chloasma, vascular spiders, or hemangiomas may develop or increase
Cardiovascular	Continued increase in heart rate of, on average, 10–15 beats per minute above baseline Return of blood pressure to baseline from decrease during first 24 weeks of gestation Supine hypotensive syndrome—drop in systolic and diastolic blood pressure from baseline if client is in supine position Leg cramps Varicosities of the legs and vulva
Respiratory	Shortness of breath, difficulty breathing (dyspnea)
Hematologic	White blood cell count 5000–12,000 μL (Counts as high as 16,000 μL have been seen in the third trimester.) Hgb 11 g/dl or greater; Hct 32% or greater Rh-negative mother, Rh-positive father, antibody screening negative
Gastrointestinal	Pyrosis (heartburn) Increased flatulence
Musculoskeletal	Low backache Diastasis recti
Urinary	Frequency of urination similar to that of first trimester Edema of legs and ankles
Reproductive	Braxton Hicks contractions Round ligament pain Effacement of cervix Vaginal leukorrhea Fullness and heaviness of breasts; presence of colostrum
Neurologic	Alert, appropriate Continued normal reflexes in all four extremities Possible numbness and tingling of fingers and toes (paresthesias); carpal tunnel syndrome

Blood Studies. Blood studies include determination of hemoglobin and hematocrit, antibody screening, and glucose screening. Around 32 weeks, a hemoglobin or hematocrit level is drawn to assess for anemia. This may be the point in pregnancy when the hemoglobin and hematocrit levels are at the lowest levels. A hemoglobin value below 11 g/dL or a hematocrit below 32% is considered anemic.

Screening for antibodies is done to identify hemolytic disease in the fetus and newborn (see Chapter 32). The Rh (rhesus) system is no longer limited to Rh-positive and Rh-negative blood group factors, as many other red blood cell antigens have been recognized. Exposure to any antigen, for example as a result of a blood transfusion, may trigger an antibody reaction if that antigen does not already exist on the client's red blood cells. Most red blood cell antigens occur rarely or do not severely affect the fetus, that is, cause hemolytic disease; however, others, for example, the D (Rh$_o$) antigen, can be a major cause of hemolytic disease in the fetus and newborn. (See Chapter 32 for further discussion of blood incompatibilities.) Pregnant women should therefore be screened at their initial visit for ABO and Rh types and the presence or absence of antibodies in their serum. Ideally, this visit would take place in the first trimester.

Antibody screening is done again around 28 weeks of gestation if the expectant father is Rh positive and the unsensitized expectant mother is Rh negative or if the expectant father is unavailable for testing. Antibody screening may be done earlier and more frequently if additional risk is suspected.

Serum glucose screening is usually performed between the 24th and 28th weeks.

Other studies that may be done in the third trimester include testing for *Chlamydia trachomatis*. Screening for chlamydia should be done at the initial visit and again in the third trimester if there is a history of previous infection (American College of Obstetricians and Gynecologists, 1994b). Some practitioners also recommend screening cultures for group B streptococcus at 35 to 37 weeks gestation (American College of Obstetricians and Gynecologists, 1996).

Psychosocial Assessment

During the third trimester the client and her family actively prepare for the birth of the baby and their changing roles within the family structure. Fears and worries regarding the labor and delivery process surface during this trimester. Family members also accomplish certain psychosocial developmental tasks discussed earlier in this chapter. The nurse assesses accomplishment of family tasks, feelings toward the pregnancy and fetus, maternal and paternal fears and fantasies, and adaptation to parental roles.

Preparation of siblings for the baby's arrival is important during the third trimester. The nurse assesses such factors as the age, developmental level, and number of siblings, as well as the family's cultural background and the parents' involvement in sibling preparation.

Assessment of Plans for Birth and Early Parenting

The goal of assessment of the client's plans for birth and early parenting is to identify client preparation for childbirth, the puerperium, and care of a neonate. Through assessment the nurse can ensure the following:

- The client's birth plan remains feasible within the selected birthing environment.
- The client has a basic understanding of the labor and delivery process and what to expect in the selected birthing environment.
- The client receives educational preparation regarding labor and delivery techniques (e.g., prepared childbirth classes).
- The client is prepared for alternatives in the event of emergency.
- The client is prepared for postpartum changes and care.
- The client is able to care safely for a newborn with existing resources.
- The client who requires supplementary services is able to receive them.
- The client has identified options in infant feeding methods.
- The client can identify health care and community resources related to childbearing.

Cultural Assessment

During the third trimester, the nurse assesses cultural values and beliefs related to late pregnancy, to the labor and delivery experience, and to early childrearing practices. For example, some Orthodox Jewish sects follow a traditional and strict interpretation of Jewish law (Lutwak, Ney, & White, 1988). Tsniut is one category and refers to laws of modesty. A Jewish man who observes Tsniut will not directly view his wife while she is immodestly exposed, for example, during pelvic examinations. For this reason, the couple may not want the expectant father to be present

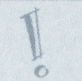

Nursing Alert

When assessing the expectant mother's adaptation to the parental role, the nurse must be aware of the following psychosocial problems that may be exhibited by the client during the third trimester:

- Unsuitable responses to pregnancy and prenatal care
- Growing apprehension about the changes occurring during this period and the prospect of labor and birth
- Failure to make plans for the baby after birth (e.g., clothes, living space)
- Rejection of pregnancy

If these problems are noted, the nurse needs to provide the client with knowledgeable support and guidance to help her understand the basis of these feelings and to resolve them successfully so as to ensure a successful pregnancy outcome.

throughout prenatal physical assessment. Nevertheless, they may share a loving relationship. This type of religious belief contrasts with current prenatal philosophy and practice that encourage and expect both partners will want to share all aspects of prenatal care, labor, and delivery. As illustrated by this example, what may appear as new and family centered to American nurses may actually be regarded as odd and unacceptable to clients from different backgrounds.

▶ Assessment of Fetal Well-Being

Fundal Height

Measurement of fundal height with a tape measure is one method used to assess fetal growth during the third trimester (Fig. 18–6). Between 22 and 34 weeks, the measurement of the fundal height in centimeters should correlate with the gestational age in weeks. After 36 weeks, the presenting part may descend into the pelvis, and fundal height may decrease.

Leopold's Maneuvers

Fetal lie, presentation, position, and engagement of the presenting part of the fetus into the pelvis can be

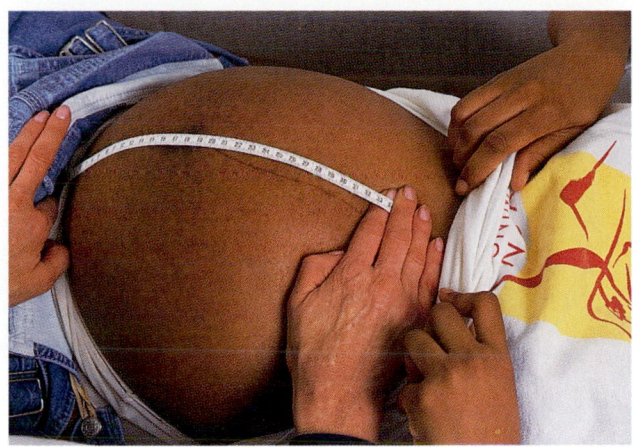

FIGURE 18–6. The height of the fundus is measured at prenatal visits during the third trimester.

determined by abdominal palpation of the mother through use of **Leopold's maneuvers.** Abdominal palpation also provides other information, such as uterine irritability, tone, tenderness, and current contractility, fetal movement, and estimation of fetal size. To prevent discomfort related to a full bladder during abdominal examination, the client is asked to void. The expectant mother then lies on her back on the examining table with the shoulders raised by a pillow and the knees drawn up slightly (Fig. 18–7).

After explaining the procedure, the examiner performs Leopold's maneuvers (Fig. 18–8), by assessing the part of the fetus located in the fundus, the location of the back of the fetus, the presenting part, and whether the part is engaged in the pelvis. During abdominal palpation, the examiner also makes the observations noted earlier.

First Maneuver. The examiner stands at the mother's side and palpates the fundus with the fingertips of both hands to assess which fetal part is in the fundus. The fetal head feels firm and round and is

gently movable. When pressing down on the head, the examiner will feel the head move against the fingertips. This is referred to as **ballottement.** If the fetal breech (sacrum) is found in the fundus, the fetal part will feel large and nodular with less movement; there will be no ballottement.

Second Maneuver. After identifying which part of the fetus lies in the fundus, the examiner places the palms of the hands on either side of the maternal abdomen and exerts gentle pressure. Through this maneuver, the examiner determines where the back and small parts (feet and hands) of the fetus are located. The back feels like a hard, consistent structure, whereas the small parts feel like nodules. If the expectant mother is obese or there is a large amount of amniotic fluid, the back may be felt by putting pressure on the side of the abdomen with one hand, while palpating with the other.

Third Maneuver. The third maneuver is done to determine the presenting part of the fetus. The lower uterine segment, just above the symphysis pubis, is held between the thumb and fingers of one hand. This maneuver is similar to the first maneuver in that the fetal head feels hard and globular, whereas the breech feels large and nodular. An attempt is also made to move the presenting part (usually the head) from side to side to determine whether it is free (floating) or in the pelvis and fixed (engaged). After completion of the third maneuver, the examiner has located the fetal head, breech, back, and extremities. The fourth maneuver than provides information regarding the attitude of the head.

Fourth Maneuver. During the fourth maneuver, the examiner stands at the mother's shoulder and faces toward her feet. The fingertips of each hand gently move down the uterus toward the symphysis pubis. When the head is the presenting part, one hand is stopped sooner than the other hand by a rounded

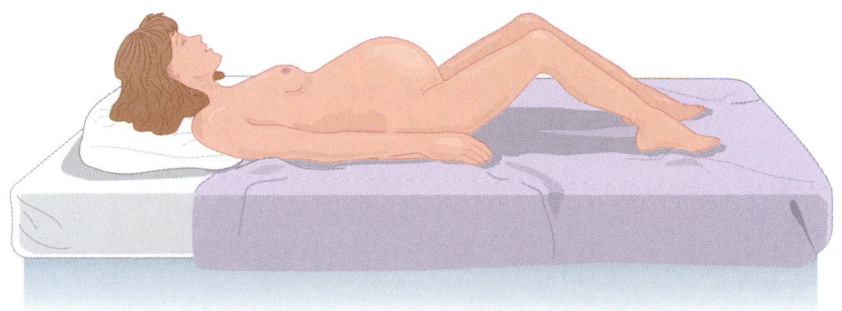

FIGURE 18–7. Position of mother for abdominal palpation.

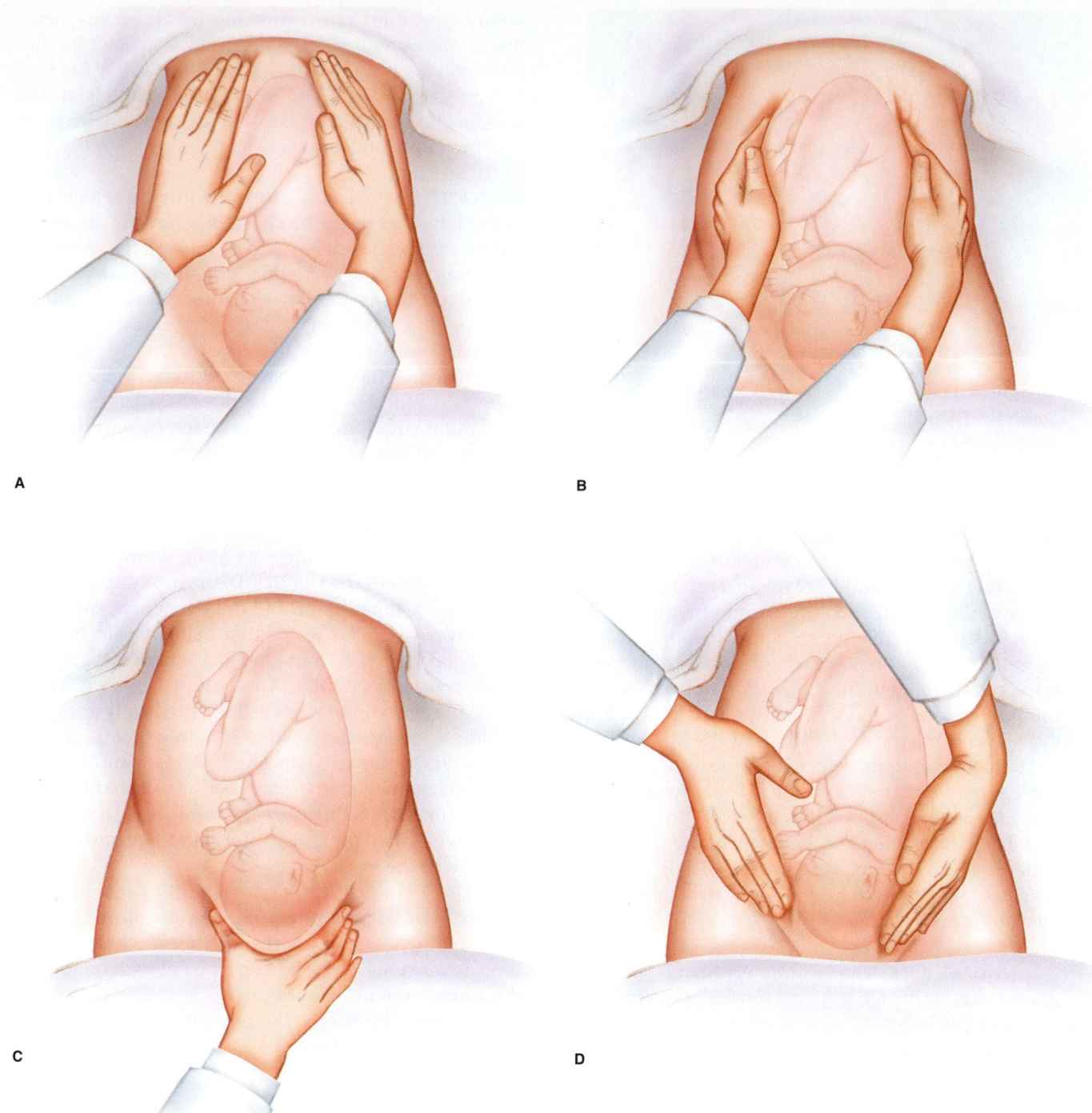

A

B

C

D

FIGURE 18–8. Leopold's maneuvers to determine fetal lie, presentation, position, and engagement. **A.** First maneuver. **B.** Second maneuver. **C.** Third maneuver. **D.** Fourth maneuver. *(Reproduced, with permission, from Cunningham, F.G. et al. (1997). Williams obstetrics (20th ed.). Stamford, CT: Appleton & Lange, p. 258.)*

body, the cephalic prominence. When the fetal head is flexed, the forehead is the cephalic prominence and is found on the same side as the fetal small parts. If the fetal head is extended, the occiput is the cephalic prominence and can be felt on the same side as the fetal back. A fetal attitude of flexion is the most desirable for the labor and delivery process.

While palpating the maternal abdomen, the nurse has an opportunity to teach the client and her support person about fetal growth, lie, position, and presentation. The expectant father and siblings can also participate in this assessment as part of the plan of care.

Assessment of Fetal Movement

Fetal movement is an indication of fetal well-being in the third trimester. Movements are considered to be an indirect measure of central nervous system function, as coordination of fetal movements involves complex neurologic control. Fetal movement can be monitored subjectively by the mother and recorded. This is frequently referred to as keeping a fetal "kick count." One approach has the mother note the time required for ten movements to occur daily (Fig. 18–9). The expectant mother begins to count movements at 8 AM and indicates in her record the time when the tenth movement is felt. If ten movements are not felt by 8 PM, or if it takes twice as long to feel ten movements as it did on previous days, the mother reports these findings to the health care provider. If the mother were not to begin timing until 9 AM, she would continue until 9 PM, 12 hours later. Another way of measuring fetal activity is to have the expectant mother set aside time each day or evening to count fetal movements. Fetal activity, with this method, is defined as three or more movements in 1 hour. If fewer than three movements occur, the expectant mother should report these findings (Pernoll & Taylor, 1994).

Monitoring of fetal movements provides information about fetal well-being. Although evidence of an active fetus is reassuring, an inactive fetus is not necessarily an ominous sign. Reduction in activity may instead reflect a normal fetal state such as sleep (Cunningham et al., 1997). Some clinicians feel that the absolute number of fetal movements per day is less important than the degree of change in fetal movements (Marnoch, 1992). Using this criterion, the mother would report findings if the number of fetal movements decreases. Monitoring of fetal movements is a highly subjective measure of assessment that depends on client perceptions, understanding, and actual use of the procedure. Errors in interpretation can result from lack of client perception of all types of movement and lack of attention to recordkeeping as a result, for example, of distractions from everyday activity.

The opportunity for the expectant mother and her partner to participate in the assessment of the fetus is one positive aspect of monitoring of fetal movements. They are also able to become more aware of the fetus; this may foster attachment behaviors. Persistent focusing on the presence or absence of fetal movement may also cause anxiety about fetal well-being. Although counting fetal movements may be used as one means of fetal surveillance, other tests are used to identify the compromised fetus. These tests should not be done routinely with all pregnancies, but are helpful in estimating fetal well-being in pregnancies considered at risk. Additional tests, described later, include the nonstress test, the contraction stress test, and the fetal biophysical profile.

Fetal movement record

	M	Tu	W	Th	F	Sat.	Sun.	
8 AM								
10 AM								
12 PM								
2 PM								
4 PM								Name:
6 PM								Date:
8 PM								EGA:

FIGURE 18–9. Fetal movement record. EGA: estimated gestational age. *(Reproduced, with permission, from DeCherney, A.H., & Pernoll, M.L. (Eds.). (1994). Current obstetric & gynecologic diagnosis & treatment (8th ed.). Norwalk, CT: Appleton & Lange, p. 288.)*

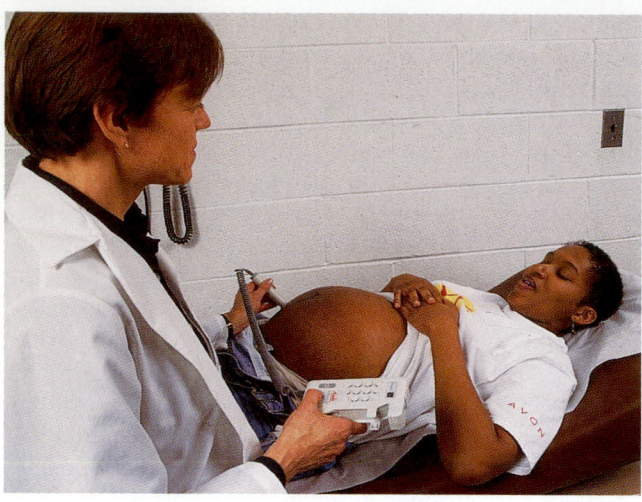

FIGURE 18–10. Assessing fetal heart activity through the use of a Doppler device.

Electronic Fetal Monitoring

Electronic fetal monitoring records fetal heart activity through use of Doppler ultrasound (Fig. 18–10). At the same time, uterine activity is assessed with a tocotransducer. This apparatus is held painlessly in place by a belt or adhesive pad placed on the expectant mother's abdomen. The tocotransducer records the duration and frequency of uterine contractions at the same time that the ultrasound transducer records the fetal heart rate. In this way the response of the fetus to any contractions, including the rhythmic, usually painless contractions experienced during pregnancy, can be assessed; in addition, information about fetal activity during contraction-free periods can be provided. Electronic fetal monitoring can be used for fetal surveillance during pregnancy, as well as during labor (Sokol, Jones, & Pernoll, 1994).

In the nonstress test, the contraction stress test, and the fetal biophysical profile, a fetal heart tracing must be obtained with an electronic fetal monitor. The nurse needs to know certain parameters of the fetal heart rate tracing when interpreting test results:

1. The **baseline fetal heart rate** is usually in the range of 120 to 160 beats per minute (BPM). By evaluating the fetal heart rate (FHR) for a 10-minute period, the nurse can determine the FHR baseline of the individual fetus.
2. The FHR has variability, or fluctuations, if the fetus has normal neurologic functioning. The beat-to-beat variability of the FHR can be 6 to 25 BPM. Lack of variability or decreased variability may indicate fetal sleep state or fetal distress. When an external fetal heart monitor is used, FHR variability may be artificially increased (Cunningham et al., 1997). This parameter is therefore less reliable as an indicator of fetal distress in the prenatal period when noninvasive external electronic fetal monitoring must be used.
3. The FHR will accelerate above the baseline in response to fetal movement. This is referred to as a *reactive pattern* of the FHR and is an indication of fetal well-being.
4. The FHR may fall below the baseline in response to uterine contractions. This is referred to as *fetal heart rate deceleration* and may be classified as follows:

   - *Early decelerations* occur early in the contraction, usually in the latter stages of labor, in response to pressure on the fetal skull. Transient decelerations occur at the beginning of the contraction and do not indicate fetal distress.
   - *Variable decelerations* occur any time during the contraction and are associated with cord compression. These can sometimes be relieved by turning the mother from back to side (especially onto her left side) or from side to side (Cunningham et al., 1997). If they are not relieved, they may indicate fetal distress.
   - *Late decelerations* occur late in the contraction (after the acme) and indicate uteroplacental insufficiency. These can be an ominous sign.

The Nonstress Test. The **nonstress test** (NST) has become a widely used method for assessment of fetal health. The NST uses electronic fetal monitoring to assess FHR acceleration in response to fetal movement. The basis of this test is the knowledge that the FHR accelerating above the baseline with fetal movement is an indication of an intact fetal autonomic nervous system. Loss of fetal acceleration with movement may indicate fetal central nervous system depression from hypoxia. Normal fetal sleep cycles as well as gestational age may influence the results of the NST (Cunningham et al., 1997).

The expectant mother is placed in the left lateral or semi-Fowler position to prevent maternal supine hypotension. A reclining chair may also be used as a comfortable alternative. External fetal monitoring equipment is applied to the maternal abdomen and a FHR tracing is obtained. The externally placed detector most often used is an ultrasound transducer, because both phonocardiography and fetal electrocardiography can be unsatisfactory in tracing the FHR through maternal tissue (Cunningham et al., 1997). Fetal movements are noted with an external tocotransducer, which is secured to the maternal abdomen.

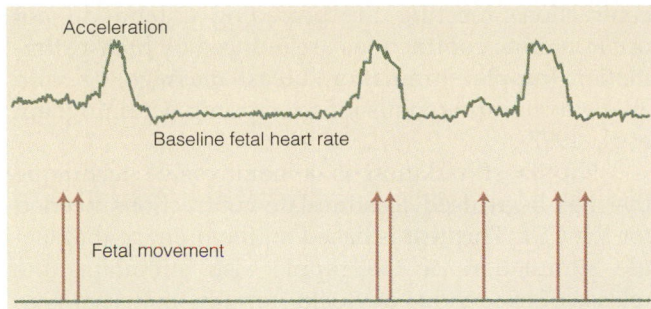

FIGURE 18–11. Reactive nonstress test: normal finding. *(Reproduced, with permission, from Oxorn, H. (Ed.). (1986). Oxorn-Foote human labor and birth (5th ed.). Norwalk, CT: Appleton & Lange, p. 599.)*

Fetal movements can be recorded by the mother using a remote event marker that she presses each time she senses movement (Sokol et al., 1994). The event marker records the movement on the same moving paper strip on which the FHR is recorded. The nurse also monitors fetal activity and writes "FM" (fetal movement) on the strip when movement is noted.

Results of the nonstress test are interpreted with respect to the pattern, reactive or nonreactive. Several different protocols have been used to define a reactive test; each prescribes a certain number of FHR accelerations in a defined period; each identifies particular values of the amplitude and duration of FHR accelerations (Cunningham et al., 1997). According to the American College of Obstetricians and Gynecologists (1994a), the NST is considered reactive (normal) when there are two or more FHR accelerations of 15 beats/minute or more, each lasting 15 seconds or more, during a 20 minute observation period. Furthermore the baseline fetal heart rate should be in the normal range with no periodic decelerations (Fig. 18–11). The recommendation further states that accelerations should be accepted with or without fetal movements and that a 40 minute tracing should be performed before assessing the pattern as nonreactive.

The NST is considered nonreactive (abnormal) when fewer than two accelerations occur during a 20 to 40 minute period. If accelerations do occur, the test is considered nonreactive when their amplitude is less than 15 beats/minute and their duration is less than 15 seconds (Sokol et al., 1994) (Fig. 18–12).

Because the normal fetus has sleep-wake cycles, the fetus may be asleep when the NST is performed. The following fetal stimulation techniques may be used to produce fetal movements:

- Instructing the mother to drink juice to raise her blood sugar level.

- Manipulating the fetus (done by either the mother or the nurse).
- Performing fetal auditory stimulation (acoustic stimulation) that consists of ringing a bell next to the mother's abdomen or using loud speakers to deliver varying levels of sound (Kisilevsky, Muir, & Low, 1989).
- Conducting vibroacoustic stimulation, a technique that consists of holding an artificial larynx against the maternal abdomen over the area of the fetal head (after the baseline FHR has been documented) (Sleutel, 1989, 1990; Zimmer & Dixon, 1993). The vibrating sound (100 to 110 dB at 1000 Hz in open air) provides both an auditory and vibratory stimulus that causes the healthy fetus to react. Fetal reactions can be so pronounced that FHRs may remain elevated for up to an hour or longer, possibly reflecting a change in the fetal state of arousal (Sleutel, 1990). No long-term effects of vibroacoustic stimulation have been documented.

Problems can occur in interpretation of the NST. With a true false-normal test, a reactive pattern is identified but the fetus dies before the next testing date or delivery. This occurs rarely and may be due to problems not identified by the NST. For example unrelated events (such as trauma, drug use, placental abruption, complications during labor) may cause fetal death after the test date. Certain high-risk conditions such as diabetes, postmaturity, and intrauterine growth retardation require at least twice weekly testing to assess fetal status.

In as many as 50 to 80% of cases, the NST can be falsely abnormal; that is, a fetus with a nonreactive NST has a normal outcome. Lack of agreement about what actually represents normal fetal reactivity is one reason for the high false-abnormal rate. Studies have demonstrated that nonreactivity of the test may be a

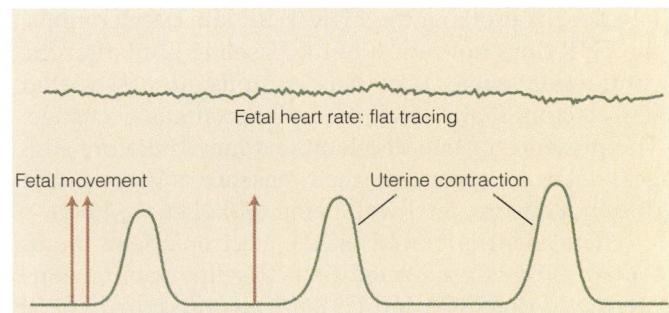

FIGURE 18–12. Nonreactive nonstress test: abnormal finding. *(Reproduced, with permission, from Oxorn, H. (Ed.). (1986). Oxorn-Foote human labor and birth (5th ed.). Norwalk, CT: Appleton & Lange, p. 605.)*

function of gestational age rather than of fetal jeopardy. They conclude that such tests should not be performed prior to 30 weeks of gestation. Further, they suggest that extending test duration when accelerations are absent initially, accepting lower thresholds for reactivity, or both may reduce errors in the interpretation of test results (Cunningham et al., 1997; Pillai & James, 1990). Using fetal stimulation techniques, such as vibroacoustic stimulation, may also elicit fetal reactivity. In addition, variation among individuals who interpret tests can account for some differences.

The NST is considered a noninvasive test. Attention to maternal position should avoid or promptly correct supine hypotensive syndrome, which could be a risk related to the procedure. Like any fetal surveillance test, the NST carries a potential emotional risk, as clients may be anxious about fetal well-being, especially if the test is read as nonreactive. Anticipatory guidance, emotional support, and strategies to foster fetal reactivity and minimize false-abnormal results can address these possible problems.

The Contraction Stress Test. A **contraction stress test** (CST) is a third-trimester assessment method that is performed when the NST is nonreactive and when the expectant mother is at risk because of such conditions as hypertension, insulin-dependent diabetes, and renal disease. Scheduling of the CST is based on clinical evaluation of the client late in the third trimester. The test may be performed weekly or more frequently if the client has a change in status or a high-risk condition such as diabetes. While the NST is a test of fetal condition, the CST is a test of uteroplacental function (Cunningham et al., 1997). The CST subjects the fetus to uterine contractions that compress the arteries supplying the placenta, thus reducing placental blood flow and the flow of oxygen to the fetus. The fetus with adequate oxygen reserve will tolerate transient reductions in the flow of oxygen; the heart rate will remain relatively unchanged. When the fetus has minimal metabolic reserve, contractions will cause late decelerations of the FHR. With late decelerations, the FHR does not return to the baseline until after the contraction ends. Late decelerations are associated with factors that reduce uteroplacental gas exchange. The presence of late decelerations may therefore suggest fetal compromise; their absence suggests, but does not ensure, fetal well-being (Sokol et al., 1994).

The client is placed on the electronic fetal monitor. An NST is performed first. Baseline spontaneous uterine contractions and FHR are recorded for 15 to 30 minutes. If spontaneous uterine contractions lasting 40 to 60 seconds and recurring approximately three times in 10 minutes are detected, the responses of the FHR to the contractions are evaluated. If spontaneous

contractions meeting the preceding criteria do not occur, uterine contractions are induced by breast stimulation (nipple stimulation/breast massage) or with an oxytocin intravenous infusion pump (Cunningham et al., 1997).

Nipple stimulation is a noninvasive technique that has been used to stimulate contractions needed for the CST. This test is based on the premise that tactile stimulation of the nipple also stimulates the release of exogenous oxytocin from the maternal posterior pituitary gland. Studies have indicated that the nipple stimulation test is comparable to the oxytocin challenge test in obtaining contractions needed for the CST (Cunningham et al., 1997).

Protocols for the nipple stimulation test may vary. According to a recommendation by the American College of Obstetricians and Gynecologists (1994a), the following procedure should be followed:

- Woman should rub one nipple through her clothing for 2 minutes or until a contraction begins.
- The technique should be restarted after 5 minutes if the first nipple stimulation does not produce three contractions in 10 minutes.
- Bilateral stimulation may also be tried to stimulate uterine contractions.
- Once the contractions begin, the nipples, breasts, or both are massaged intermittently so that the desired contractions are stimulated.

If no contractions result, oxytocin infusion may be used (Sokol et al., 1994). The CST takes about 1 to 2 hours.

Nipple stimulation and breast massage make use of the body's own natural resources; however, hyperstimulation of the uterus (contractions lasting 90 seconds or more) has been reported in some studies in which nipple stimulation was used (Cunningham et al., 1997).

In the absence of spontaneous uterine contractions for the CST, oxytocin may be administered intravenously. A dose of 0.5 mU per minute may be used to begin the test. A controlled-rate infusion pump is used to regulate the infusion of oxytocin in normal saline or Ringer's lactate solution. The oxytocin infusion should be "piggybacked" to a main intravenous line. In case of complications related to oxytocin infusion, the medication can be easily discontinued while the vein is kept open and accessible. There is greater risk of inadvertently giving the client a bolus of oxytocin when the infusion is piggybacked higher in the tubing. The following guidelines are observed in administering the oxytocin challenge test:

- The dose, administered in milliunits, is increased every 15 to 30 minutes until at least three contractions, lasting 60 seconds, occur per 10 minutes. Typical rate of oxytocin infusion used to elicit contractions is 4 to 5 mU per minute (rarely, the client will require more than 8 mU per minute to stimulate contractions).

- Oxytocin infusion is stopped once satisfactory contractions occur.

The procedure is discontinued if no contractions occur by the end of 30 minutes and the infusion has been working properly, if contractions occur more often than every 2 minutes or last longer than 60 seconds, if uterine tetany takes place, or if continued FHR decelerations are noted (Sokol et al., 1994). After the test,

the client is not discharged until contractions are at least 10 minutes apart.

Interpretations of the CST are summarized in Table 18–4. Categories such as positive (abnormal), negative (normal), suspicious, hyperstimulated, and unsatisfactory have been used and are based on frequency of contractions and FHR decelerations; however, concern related to accuracy of results, especially false-positive readings, has prompted additional categorization of the CST into reactive negative, nonreactive negative, reactive positive, and nonreactive positive. These categories, also included in Table 18–4, are based on the presence or absence of FHR accelerations as well as decelerations (Sokol et al., 1994).

▶   **TABLE 18–4**

Interpretations of the Contraction Stress Test

CST results may be interpreted according to frequency of contractions and FHR decelerations:

Positive: abnormal	Consistent and persistent late decelerations of the FHR occur with 50% or more of the contractions. A true positive CST indicates fetal compromise related to uteroplacental insufficiency.
Negative: normal	No late decelerations of the FHR take place, and at least three contractions, each lasting at least 40 seconds, occur within 10 minutes. Usually FHR reactivity (accelerations of the FHR with fetal movement) are also seen on the tracing. About 80 to 85% of CSTs are negative. A negative CST usually indicates that fetal well-being related to uteroplacental function will continue for at least another week. The negative CST may therefore be repeated weekly unless complications emerge and either require testing at a shorter interval or necessitate other types of interventions.
Suspicious	Inconsistent late decelerations of the FHR take place but do not continue with subsequent contractions. About one fifth of suspicious tests become positive on repeated testing. The test is usually repeated within 24 hours of obtaining suspicious test results. Timing of the repeated test is based on clinical assessment; the test may be repeated the same day. For example, when variable decelerations occur, ultrasound may be indicated to assess whether cord compromise, related to oligohydramnios or fetal presentation, is present.
Hyperstimulated	Contractions occur more often than every 2 minutes or last longer than 90 seconds. Late decelerations of the FHR with this excessive uterine activity do not necessarily indicate uteroplacental insufficiency. Caution should be used when administering oxytocin by intravenous infusion or when exogenous oxytocin is supplied through nipple stimulation. Excessive uterine activity may cause fetal compromise because of decreased oxygen. In this situation, the test itself may cause the compromise. The hyperstimulation test may be repeated within 24 hours and with careful observation.
Unsatisfactory	This term refers to a test that cannot be read adequately. For example, inability to stimulate at least three contractions within 10 minutes or unsatisfactory tracings, related to such factors as positioning or fetal movement, may account for unsatisfactory test results. Attentive, one-to-one nursing care with appropriate positioning and adjustment of the transducer may avoid an unsatisfactory test result. The unsatisfactory test may be repeated within 24 hours.

CST results may be interpreted according to presence or absence of FHR accelerations as well as decelerations:

Reactive negative	Normal accelerations of the FHR (more than 15 BPM, lasting 15 seconds) occur with fetal movement and no FHR decelerations. Results indicate a normal, healthy fetus with good oxygen reserve (Fig. 18–13).
Nonreactive negative	There is an absence of accelerations of the FHR following fetal movement and no late decelerations occur with contractions. This pattern is observed in only 0.4% of CSTs and could be related to subtle late decelerations that are being missed, a congenital anomaly of the fetus, or maternal therapy with a central nervous system depressant (Fig. 18–14).
Reactive positive	Normal accelerations of the FHR following fetal movement occur with the presence of late decelerations with some uterine contractions (Fig. 18–15). These reactive positive tests are often false-positive tests and thus require careful assessment. The test may be repeated or an alternative method of fetal assessment, such as the fetal biophysical profile, may be considered.
Nonreactive positive	Fetal heart rate accelerations following fetal movement are absent and persistent late decelerations occur with uterine contractions (Fig. 18–16). The nonreactive positive CST is more accurately indicative of fetal compromise. The false-positive rate is less than 5%. If this interpretation is made on the CST, delivery is usually needed for the near-term fetus. If the fetus is very immature, a biophysical profile may be done to document fetal status.

Sources: Sokol et al., 1994; Cunningham et al., 1997.

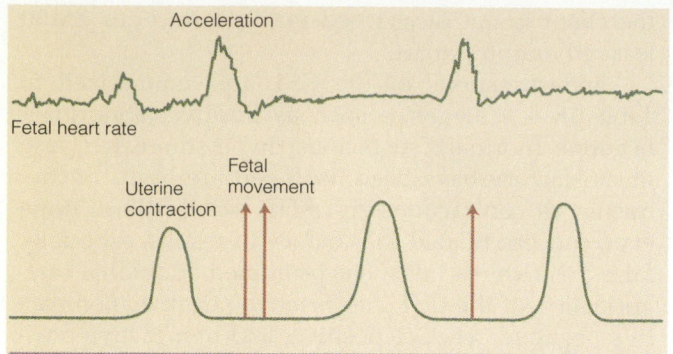

FIGURE 18–13. Reactive negative contraction stress test that shows normal acceleration of the fetal heart with movement; no decelerations are present. *(Reproduced, with permission, from from Oxorn, H. (Ed.). (1986). Oxorn-Foote human labor and birth (5th ed.). Norwalk, CT: Appleton & Lange, p. 605.)*

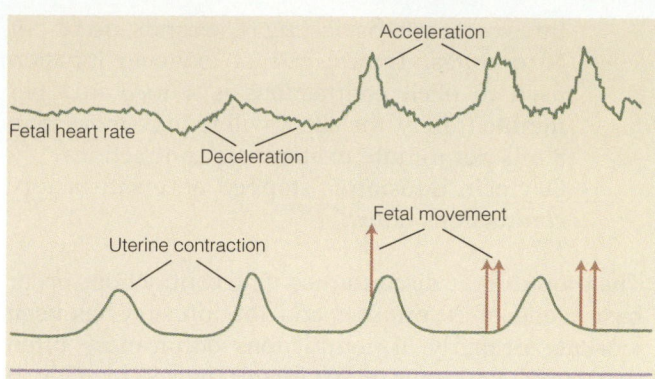

FIGURES 18–15. Reactive positive contraction stress test. *(Reproduced, with permission, from Oxorn, H. (Ed.). (1986). Oxorn-Foote human labor and birth (5th ed.). Norwalk, CT: Appleton & Lange, p. 607).*

The CST is a valuable technique for assessing fetal well-being; however, results that do not accurately reflect fetal status, that is, false results, can occur.

A negative test generally indicates that the uteroplacental unit will continue to support fetal life for at least a week longer. There is, however, no absolute assurance that the fetus will be well. A test is said to have a false-negative or false-normal result when fetal death occurs within 7 days of the test. Fetal death within that time could occur as the result of many factors. New complications or unrelated conditions, such as trauma, abruptio placentae, and drug abuse, could arise after the test. Problems in test administration or interpretation or lack of sensitivity of the test to actual fetal status could also contribute to a false-negative result.

Unfortunately, the CST can have a high rate of false-positive or false-abnormal results, as high as 50 to 75% (Cunningham et al., 1997). A false-positive test occurs when an abnormal test result is then followed by normal FHR patterns in labor and normal fetal outcome. False-positive results can reflect several conditions, such as problems in interpretation of test results or technical difficulties in obtaining tracings. Categorization of CSTs based on the presence or absence of FHR accelerations, as well as decelerations, has promoted better specificity and reliability of the test, but problems remain. Positive test results pose difficult management questions: Should delivery take place without delay? What happens if a normal fetus is delivered too early? Other tests, for example, a fetal biophysical profile or ultrasound, may be used for assessment of fetal well-being.

Certain risks and contraindications are associated with the CST, because oxytocin can cause powerful uterine contractions. Contraindications to the CST include (Sokol et al., 1994):

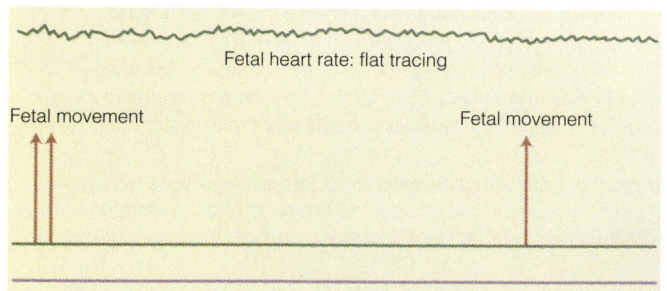

FIGURE 18–14. Nonreactive negative contraction stress test.

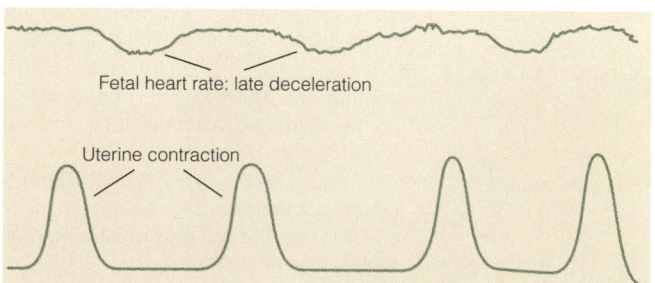

FIGURE 18–16. Nonreactive positive contraction stress test. *(Reproduced, with permission, from Oxorn, H. (Ed.). (1986). Oxorn-Foote human labor and birth (5th ed.). Norwalk, CT: Appleton & Lange, p. 607.)*

- Predisposition to uterine rupture
- Predisposition to premature labor (especially in women who have a history of preterm birth or who are carrying more than one fetus)
- Bleeding (e.g., in placenta previa)

Fetal Biophysical Profile. The **fetal biophysical profile,** first developed by Manning and associates (1987) to assess fetal well-being, consists of five parameters: FHR reactivity, fetal breathing movements, gross fetal body movements, fetal tone, and volume of amniotic fluid. Fetal heart rate reactivity is measured with the NST, and the other four parameters are measured with real-time ultrasound scanning.

The basic premise behind the biophysical profile is that multiple variable assessment of fetal biophysical activities is a more reliable test of fetal well-being than the examination of a single fetal parameter, such as FHR (Sokol et al., 1994). One purpose of the biophysical profile is the identification of fetuses with chronic asphyxia or congenital anomalies. See box entitled Advantages and Limitations of the Fetal Biophysical Profile. Indications for biophysical profile testing include postdate pregnancy, maternal hypertension (chronic or pregnancy induced), diabetes mellitus, premature rupture of membranes, vaginal bleeding, maternal reports of decreased fetal movement, maternal Rh sensitization, and maternal history of previous fetal death. Life's complexities make absolute prediction of good health impossible. There-

fore, the biophysical profile may be most useful in identifying a fetus that is in jeopardy, rather than in predicting future fetal well-being. Indeed, research has shown that there is a relationship between scores on the biophysical profile and fetal blood pH values (Manning, Snijders, Harmon, Nicolaides, Menticoglou, & Morrison, 1993). Others, however, found that fetal morbidity such as growth retardation was more determined by gestational age than prenatal tests, including the biophysical profile (Weiner et al., 1996).

Assessment of the five parameters of the fetal biophysical profile are summarized below:

1. *Fetal heart rate reactivity.* The FHR is considered reactive when there are movement-associated FHR accelerations of at least 15 beats per minute above baseline and 15 seconds in duration over a 20-minute period (American College of Obstetricians and Gynecologists, 1994a). A score of 2 is given if FHR reactivity is noted; a score of 0 means that the FHR is nonreactive.
2. *Fetal breathing movements.* Assessment is based on the assumption that the presence of fetal breathing movements (chest wall and diaphragmatic movements that mimic respiratory movements) (Cunningham et al., 1997) indicates fetal well-being and their absence may indicate hypoxemia. Fetal breathing tends

---

▶ **ADVANTAGES AND LIMITATIONS OF THE FETAL BIOPHYSICAL PROFILE**

ADVANTAGES

- Noninvasive.
- Results are available as soon as test is completed and interpreted.
- Testing can be done on outpatient basis, thereby reducing hospital admissions and associated financial and emotional costs.
- Provides other types of useful information, e.g., fetal number, placental location, risk of intrauterine growth retardation, and congenital anomalies.
- May help in monitoring clients with premature rupture of membranes for impending infection, thereby preventing neonatal or maternal sepsis.
- May decrease false-positive or false-negative results associated with the NST.
- Indicates current fetal well-being, especially in high-risk groups, thereby allowing for conservative treatment and avoidance of certain interventions, e.g., early delivery, iatrogenic prematurity, and cesarean delivery.

LIMITATIONS

- Duration and frequency of hypoxemia and effects on the fetus are unknown.
- Exogenous factors can affect the central nervous system and change fetal activities and test results.
- Each variable is given equal weight; it is possible that certain variables are indeed more important than others.
- Testing intervals are arbitrary.
- Long-term development outcomes of fetuses with low scores are unknown.
- Research related to use of this technique and meaning of scores is lacking.
- May not accurately predict continued fetal well-being.

Compiled courtesy of N. Hoffman, MSN, RN.

► FACTORS INFLUENCING FETAL BREATHING MOVEMENTS

- Fetal breathing movements have been shown to increase during the second and third hours after maternal meals and at night (1 AM to 7 AM) during maternal sleep due to increased blood glucose levels after eating and stable blood glucose levels during sleep (Gebauer & Lowe, 1993).
- Fetal breathing movements may not be regarded as a sign of well-being in diabetic mothers because hyperglycemia can increase them (Devoe, Youssef, Gardner, Dear, & Murray, 1992).
- Fetal breathing movements may be decreased as a result of such conditions as hypoxemia, hypoglycemia, nicotine use, or ingestion of alcohol.

to occur periodically after 28 weeks and becomes increasingly regular in frequency and uniformity between the 33rd and 36th week of gestation (Badalian, Chao, Fox, & Timor-Tritsch, 1993). To earn a score of 2, the fetus must have at least one episode of fetal breathing at least 60 seconds long within a 30-minute observation period. The failure to meet this criteria is scored 0 on the fetal biophysical profile. Several factors can alter fetal breathing movements (see box entitled Factors Influencing Fetal Breathing Movements). The episodic nature of fetal breathing movements, the multiple factors that can affect them, and the long period that may be necessary for documentation of a normal pattern detract from the usefulness of this parameter in identifying the fetus in jeopardy.

3. *Fetal body movements.* The presence of at least three discrete episodes of fetal movements within a 30-minute observation period is given a score of 2. Simultaneous limb and trunk movements are counted as a single movement. For decreased fetal movements, which is recorded as two or fewer discrete fetal movements in 30 minutes, a score of 0 is given (Gebauer & Lowe, 1993). Factors to be considered when assessing this parameter include: differences in fetal movements in certain abnormal conditions such as intrauterine growth retardation and diabetes; need to distinguish fetal rest periods from those related to a compromised uterine environment; and relationship between fetal movements and time elapsed since maternal consumption of a meal (fetal activity is greatest 1 to 3 hours after eating).

4. *Fetal tone.* In utero, although the fetus is normally in flexion, the arms, legs, trunk, and head may be flexed and extended at certain times. The fetus earns a score of 2 when there is at least one episode of active extension with return to flexion of fetal limb(s) or trunk. A score of 0 is given for slow extension with return to partial flexion, fetal movement not followed by return to flexion, limbs or spine in extension, and an open fetal hand (Strong, Jordan, & Marden, 1992).

5. *Amniotic fluid volume.* Amniotic fluid should be evident throughout the uterine cavity (by 36 weeks, the volume is about 1000 mL). Assessment of this parameter has been demonstrated to be an effective method of predicting fetal distress (Tongsong & Srisomboon, 1993) since oligohydramnios has been associated with fetal anomalies (Manning et al., 1987). A score of 2 indicates that at least one pocket of amniotic fluid that measures 1 cm in two perpendicular planes has been identified. A score of 0 indicates that either fluid is absent in most areas of the uternine cavity or that the largest pocket of fluid measures 1 cm or less in the vertical axis (Sokol et al., 1994).

Table 18–5 describes the interpretations of scores for the five parameters of the fetal biophysical profile. Each of the five parameters of the fetal biophysical profile contributes either 2 or 0 points to the total score. A score of 10 is a perfect score; a score of 0 is the worst score. A score of 8 or 10, with a normal amount of amniotic fluid, indicates a healthy fetus. No interventions would be indicated other than repeat testing at weekly intervals. Testing at twice weekly intervals would be appropriate for high-risk conditions. A score of 8 with oligohydramnios or a score of 4 or 6 is equivocal. An equivocal test score is interpreted as possibly abnormal. The false-positive rate in the equivocal group has been estimated to be 44% (Sokol et al., 1994). Some clinicians recommend repeating the test within 24 hours; however, others advocate extending testing after any equivocal or abnormal test result (Sokol et al., 1994). In this way a sleeping fetus may be distinguished from an asphyxiated fetus;

▶ **TABLE 18–5**

Fetal Biophysical Profile[a]

Fetal heart rate activity	Reactive pattern: at least 2 FHR accelerations of ≥ 15 BPM and ≥ 15 seconds' duration, associated with fetal movement in 20-minute period	Nonreactive pattern: fewer than 2 FHR accelerations of ≥ 15 BPM and 15 seconds' duration associated with fetal movement in 40-minute period
Fetal breathing movements	Present: presence of at least one episode of fetal breathing of ≥ 60 seconds' duration within a 30-minute period	Absent: absence of fetal breathing movements or the absence of an episode of fetal breathing movements of ≥ 60 seconds' duration during a 30-minute period
Gross fetal body movement	Present: presence of at least three discrete episodes of fetal movement within a 30-minute period; simultaneous limb and trunk movements are counted as a single movement	Decreased: two or fewer discrete fetal movements in a 30-minute period
Fetal tone	Upper and lower extremities in full flexion; trunk in position of flexion and head flexed on chest; at least one episode of extension of limbs with return to position of flexion, extension of spine with return to flexion, or both	Decreased: limbs in position of extension or partial flexion; spine in extension; fetal movement not followed by return to flexion; fetal hand open
Volume of amniotic fluid	Fluid evident throughout uterine cavity; largest pocket of fluid greater than 1 cm in vertical diameter	Decreased: fluid absent in most areas of uterine cavity; largest pocket of fluid 1 cm or less in vertical axis; crowding of fetal small parts

[a]Normal: score = 2, abnormal: score = 0. The intermediate score of 1 is not used with this scoring system.
Reproduced, with permission, from Oxorn, H. (Ed.). (1986). Oxorn-Foote human labor and birth (5th ed.). Norwalk, CT: Appleton & Lange, p. 609.

impending fetal death between the time of the nonreassuring result and the repeat test done on the following day can be avoided. A score of 0 or 2 is abnormal and indicates the need for assessment for immediate delivery. The abnormal rating (0 or 2) has a low false-positive rate and is considered a reliable measure of severe fetal compromise.

Despite the useful information provided by the biophysical profile, management decisions for client care cannot be based solely on the composite scores of this test. There is a wide variation in normal fetal biophysical performance (Cunningham et al., 1997).

Several variations of the biophysical profile have been developed; their use varies among prenatal testing units (Sokol et al., 1994). In one variation, NST testing is combined with ultrasonic assessment of amniotic fluid. An index of 5 cm or less for amniotic fluid is considered abnormal (Nageotte, Towers, Asrat, & Freeman, 1994). This modified biophysical profile is considered an acceptable alternative to the full biophysical profile (American College of Obstetricians and Gynecologists, 1994a).

Nursing Role in Electronic Fetal Monitoring.
In many prenatal testing settings, nurses may perform NSTs and CSTs, do initial assessment of the tracings, and initiate appropriate strategies for nonreassuring findings. By remaining with the client during the tests, the nurse is in a unique position to document maternal and fetal events during each procedure and to make certain that the tests are administered correctly. The tests are also evaluated by a physician, ide-

ally on the same day. A collaborative approach that incorporates test interpretation by the nurse and physician can offer the client a better assessment than one individual reading. Interpretation of prenatal tests requires education and skill on the part of nurses and physicians. False-positive or false-negative readings, related to inaccurate interpretation, may result in failure to diagnose fetal compromise or in unnecessary interventions. As in any area of practice, nurses are accountable for their interpretation of tests. In addition, nurses involved in prenatal testing need to make certain that procedures for test administration and interpretation are developed and followed, that all personnel performing the tests are qualified to do so, and that the prenatal settings allow for adequate staffing for the tests.

The nursing role in antepartal fetal assessment involves client teaching and psychosocial support for the client and her family.

The nurse assesses the client's understanding of the test, provides teaching about the test, and notes the client's response to teaching. Topics for teaching related to prenatal testing include the following:

- Type of test (NST, CST, fetal biophysical profile)
- Reason for test; implications of the test for fetal well-being
- Nature of the test
- Length of the test; total time commitment needed for the test
- Site of the test
- Personnel who will conduct the test

- Significant other who may accompany client during test
- Discomforts related to the test
- Possible complications related to the test; reassurance related to lack of risks of NST
- Interpretation of test results; need for any further testing (what the test can and cannot indicate)
- Cost of test
- Posttest teaching:
  - Signs and symptoms of labor (especially for CST)
  - Advice *not* to try nipple stimulation at home to induce contractions or labor

The client's response to potential or actual high-risk status is assessed. Clients referred for prenatal testing may be terrified about the health of the fetus; they may also worry about the possibility of fetal death during pregnancy, fetal compromise during labor, or premature birth. Some clients may have experienced fetal loss during previous pregnancies. The need for bedrest may interfere with the usual schedule or perception of self as healthy and may add to the stress of prenatal testing.

Tests should be conducted with respect for the client's reaction to the nature of the test and her need for privacy. For example, many clients may feel shy about nipple stimulation for CST. Calm explanation of the physiologic rationale for the test and provision of privacy can do much to promote emotional comfort. A private room or room dividers such as curtains or screens, as well as restriction of personnel coming to see the client during the test, may be used. A sheet may be used to cover the client during the NST or CST.

Clients undergoing prenatal tests may have blocks of free time, especially during NSTs. This provides a special opportunity for the nurse to undertake assessment of client and family responses to pregnancy and testing and to provide appropriate teaching.

▶ Assessment of Fetal Maturity

Delivery may be recommended when prenatal testing indicates the fetus is seriously compromised. The fetus therefore needs to be assessed for maturity and ability to survive outside the uterus. Amniocentesis, ultrasound, and magnetic resonance imaging are examples of tests for fetal maturity that can be used during the third trimester.

Amniocentesis

Amniocentesis may be used in the third trimester to estimate the maturity of the fetal lungs. Type II pneu-monocyte cells of the fetal lung alveoli produce surfactant (a phospholipid that maintains alveolar patency and lowers surface tension in the lungs). Surfactant appears in the amniotic fluid by 24 to 26 weeks of gestation. As the fetus approaches maturity, the amounts of surfactant in the amniotic fluid increases. Lecithin (phosphatidylcholine) is a major component of the pulmonary surfactant and constitutes about 80% of the phospholipids. Other phospholipids include phosphatidylglycerol, the phospholipid that has the second largest concentration in surfactant; phosphatidylinositol; and sphingomyelin. Measurements of the ratio of amniotic fluid lecithin to sphingomyelin and of phosphatidylglycerol concentration have been used to assess the maturity of the fetal lungs (Pernoll & Taylor, 1994).

Lecithin:Sphingomyelin Ratio. Mean proportions of lecithin and sphingomyelin do not differ markedly until about the 30th week of gestation. The level of sphingomyelin stops rising at week 32, whereas the level of lecithin rises gradually above that of sphingomyelin. In assessing fetal maturity, a **lecithin:sphingomyelin (L:S) ratio** equal to or greater than 2:1 indicates a positive result, that is, fetal lung maturity with little likelihood of immaturity-related respiratory distress syndrome in the newborn. A ratio of 1.5:1 to 1.9:1 indicates the possibility of mild to moderate respiratory distress in the newborn. A ratio of 1.0:1 to 1.49:1 usually reflects immaturity of the fetal lungs and a possibility of moderate to severe respiratory distress in the newborn. A ratio less than 1.0:1 indicates immaturity of the lungs and predicts severe respiratory distress in the newborn (Pernoll & Taylor, 1994).

About 5 mL of amniotic fluid is needed for measurement of the L:S ratio. Phospholipid is extracted from the amniotic fluid and evaluated by thin-layer chromatography. This method assesses the size and density of the lecithin and sphingomyelin "spots," which then indicate the stage of fetal lung maturity (Pernoll & Taylor, 1994).

The reliability of the L:S ratio may at times be questioned. Contamination of amniotic fluid by blood or meconium may alter the L:S ratio and produce inaccurate results.

Certain high-risk conditions alter fetal lung maturation; therefore the L:S ratio must be interpreted with caution. For example, misleading results may be obtained from expectant mothers with diabetes. In this situation, fetal lungs may be immature despite an L:S ratio of 2:1. Other factors may influence neonatal respiratory distress, such as sepsis, despite a mature L:S ratio (Low, Pangiotopoulous, & Derrick, 1994).

Phosphatidylglycerol Test. Phosphatidylglycerol (PG) has become another indicator of fetal lung maturity. PG is found in amniotic fluid late in gestation, after 35 weeks; its concentration in amniotic fluid then gradually increases to term. Phosphatidylglycerol is found solely in amniotic fluid, in lungs, and in semen. Therefore, contamination of the amniotic fluid by blood or meconium does not influence the test results because these substances contain no PG. Further, the presence of PG in the amniotic fluid in the vagina when membranes are ruptured usually indicates low risk for respiratory distress syndrome of the newborn (Cunningham et al., 1997).

The test for PG indicates a more mature surfactant complex than that found in the L:S ratio, because PG appears late in gestation. It has been noted that PG was absent in cases where the L:S ratio indicated pulmonary maturity and respiratory distress occurred (false-positive result). Conversely, when PG was present, respiratory distress syndrome did not develop (Cunningham et al., 1997). The absence of PG is not necessarily an indication that respiratory distress *will* develop; its absence indicates that respiratory distress syndrome *may* develop (Cunningham et al., 1997). Unless there is at least 0.5% PG in amniotic fluid, elective delivery is discouraged (Pernoll & Taylor, 1994).

Problems with Amniotic Fluid Analysis for Fetal Maturity. Use of analyses such as the L:S ratio has declined in certain high-risk situations. For example, intervention may be necessary regardless of the risk of respiratory distress syndrome in cases where severe hemorrhage or fulminating preeclampsia threatens the mother's life. The development of ultrasound has also made more precise dating of gestation and fetal maturity possible, so that amniotic fluid analysis need not be the sole method of assessment of fetal maturity.

Risks. Risks associated with amniocentesis include bleeding, infection, and premature labor. Maternal supine hypotension may be avoided through proper positioning, as for any examination. The large size of the fetus and fetal movements during the third trimester contribute to a greater risk of trauma to the fetus; however, the use of ultrasound to guide amniocentesis promotes safety of the procedure. Nevertheless, when amniocentesis is performed during the third trimester, the newborn is assessed carefully for any evidence of trauma.

Diagnostic Ultrasound

During the third trimester, ultrasound is used to provide information about maternal and fetal structures and fetal activity and to guide invasive procedures such as amniocentesis. The following are indications for third-trimester ultrasound:

- Estimation of gestational age for uncertain clinical dates
- Verification of dates for women who are to have scheduled elective cesarean delivery or induction of labor
- Assessment of fetal growth
- Vaginal bleeding of undetermined etiology
- Determination of fetal presentation
- Adjunct to amniocentesis
- Significant difference between uterine size and clinical dates of gestation
- Suspected fetal death
- Biophysical assessment for fetal well-being (FHR reactivity, fetal breathing movements, gross body movements, fetal tone, amniotic fluid volume)
- Suspected polyhydramnios or oligohydramnios
- Suspected abruptio placentae
- Follow-up evaluation of placental location for identified placenta previa
- Serial evaluation of fetal growth in multiple gestation

Fetal Measurements Obtained During Ultrasound. Certain fetal parameters are used to assess fetal growth and gestational age through ultrasonic evaluation. Among these are fetal biparietal diameter, cephalic index, circumference of the head, abdominal circumference, head circumference: abdominal circumference ratio, and femoral length and are described below:

1. *Biparietal diameter.* The **biparietal diameter** (BPD) is the widest diameter of the fetal skull; it is the most widely used determinant of fetal growth and gestational age. Between 14 and 28 weeks of gestation, the BPD is accurate to within plus or minus 7 to 10 days. After 28 weeks of gestation, the accuracy is only within 3 weeks. The BPD may be difficult to measure late in pregnancy because of fetal position or engagement of the fetal head in the maternal pelvis. It has been estimated that if serial BPD alone were used to determine fetal growth, some 20 to 50% of growth-retarded fetuses would not be detected (Jacobsen, G, 1992). This is especially true when fetuses have unusual head shapes (flattened or elongated).

2. *Cephalic index.* The **cephalic index** (CI) is the ratio of the BPD to the occipitofrontal diameter

(OFD) (diameter that extends from a point just above the top of the nose to the most prominent portion of the occiput) of the fetal skull. This parameter provides a means of quantifying fetal head shape. The CI remains constant throughout fetal development, and the normal shape index is 79 ± 8%. A CI less than 71% indicates a flattened BPD; a CI greater than 87% indicates an elongated shape. In the first case, the BPD would underestimate, rather than properly reflect, gestational age. In the second case, the BPD would overestimate gestational age. In cases where the CI is out of the normal range, the BPD should not be used for gestational age or estimates of fetal weight (Chang, Robson, Boys, & Spencer, 1992; Harrington & Campbell, 1993; Jacobsen, 1992). Tables relating BPD with period of gestation may vary in the actual values presented; however, these tables are used frequently with different populations of expectant mothers.

3. *Circumference of head.* The OFD also may be used to estimate the head circumference (HC) in an effort to calculate gestational age:

$$(BPD + OFD) \times 3.14/2 = HC \text{ (cm)}$$

4. *Abdominal circumference.* To estimate abdominal circumference (AC), the anteroposterior abdominal diameter (APAD) and the transverse abdominal diameter (TAD) are measured at the level of the umbilical vein or fetal liver. The formula used to calculate abdominal circumference is

$$(APAD + TAD) \times 3.14/2 = AC \text{ (cm)}$$

Abdominal circumference is used mainly as an estimate of intrauterine growth retardation rather than as an estimate of gestational age (Harrington & Campbell, 1993). The optimal time for measuring AC is at 34 weeks ± 1 week (Hearn-Stebbins, 1995).

5. *Head circumference:Abdominal circumference ratio.* The head circumference:abdominal circumference (HC:AC) ratio is used as an indicator of fetal growth and nutrition, rather than of gestational age. The adequacy of liver stores of glycogen primarily determines liver size and, therefore, abdominal circumference. The HC:AC measurement directly compares brain size with liver size. Before 36 weeks of gestation, the HC:AC ratio is greater than 1.0; that is, the HC is greater than the AC. After 36 weeks of gestation, the ratio is less than 1.0; the HC is less than the AC. Disproportionate HC:AC ratios may indicate problems with

fetal growth. A low HC:AC may indicate a large baby, for example, a fetus of a diabetic mother. A high ratio may indicate intrauterine growth retardation. The HC:AC may be calculated by the following formula (Harrington & Campbell, 1993; Sokol et al., 1994):

$$HC:AC = \\ [(BPD + OFD) \times 3.14/2]:[(APAD + TAD) \times 3.14/2]$$

6. *Femoral length.* Femoral length (FL) is used as an estimate of gestational age. It is less affected by changes in growth than the head or abdomen; thus, FL is considered a useful aid in determining gestational age and in identifying the fetus with abnormal growth. Femoral length is the length of the shaft of the femur (excluding the femoral head). Femoral length increases in a linear fashion with gestational age; FL should be measured after 13 weeks of gestation, because before that time FL measurements are unreliable (Tahilramaney, Platt, & Golde, 1991).

Assessment of Amniotic Fluid. Measurement of amniotic fluid volume through ultrasound is considered one of the important fetal assessment tools (Cunningham et al., 1997). Assessment of amniotic fluid may be done alone or with other parameters of the biophysical profile. Oligohydramnios or polyhydramnios may indicate problems with the fetus (see Chapter 19). The **amniotic fluid index (AFI)** is a method of approximating the volume of amniotic fluid in the uterus (Fresquez, 1997).

The uterus is divided into four quadrants with the umbilicus at the center. The ultrasound transducer is moved over the four quadrants. The deepest vertical pocket of amniotic fluid in each quadrant is identified. A pocket of amniotic fluid that has multiple loops of cord is not measured. The AFI is determined by adding the measurements from the four quadrants. The generally accepted norms range from an AFI of greater than 5 and less than 20 cm. Oligohydramnios is an AFI of 5 cms or less and polyhydramnios is an AFI of 20 cm or more (Fresquez, 1997).

The AFI value may be influenced by several factors. For example, maternal hydration or dehydration may affect the volume of amniotic fluid. High altitudes may also increase the index without related fetal compromise. It is recommended that borderline values be repeated before interventions are undertaken (Cunningham et al., 1997).

Role of the Nurse. Clients having third-trimester ultrasound are generally at risk for some real or potential problem. The nurse needs to recognize that anxiety and emotional pain may be experienced by the client and her partner. The nurse provides anticipatory guidance and teaching about the procedure; encourages the client and her partner to remain together during the test; promotes the client's physical comfort during the procedure through such techniques as proper positioning; identifies maternal and fetal structures seen on the monitor (may be done by the person performing the ultrasound); remains accessible to and supportive of the client regardless of the outcome of the test; and makes certain that clients are appropriately referred for additional counseling when needed.

Current Imaging Techniques: Magnetic Resonance Imaging

Magnetic resonance imaging (MRI) is an assessment technique that provides computer-derived images based on the detection of energy in the nuclei of atoms within the body. MRI depends on the physical property of magnetism, which is possessed by some of the nuclei of the body's atoms, and is based on the principle that protons within the nucleus of the atom have magnetic spins with different energy levels. In the normal state all energy seeks the lowest level. MRI creates an intense magnetic field that raises the energy of the protons within the nucleus of the atoms. The magnetic field is then turned off. As the protons revert to their original state, energy is released; the magnetic moments are detected and translated into images by the computer. Not all nuclei within the body have magnetic moments; therefore, such structures as bone are not seen on MRI, although soft tissues in the reproductive system are well visualized. In this way, MRI differs from x-ray studies that provide information about bony structures and their relationships. MRI studies are interpreted by a physician specially educated in MRI. Uses for MRI during pregnancy include the following (Cunningham et al., 1997).

- Replacement for x-ray diagnostic imaging
- Adjunct to ultrasound (MRI offers additional information on fetal development, growth, or structures, such as the central nervous system and subcutaneous tissues, which are not seen well on ultrasound.)
- Identification of soft tissue relationships between the fetus and the birth canal (MRI is thus helpful in identifying whether a client carrying a fetus in a breech position would be at risk during a vaginal delivery.)
- Confirmation of fetal anomalies, such as anomalies associated with oligohydramnios (Unlike ultrasound, MRI does not need amniotic fluid to visualize the fetus.)

- Diagnosis of ectopic pregnancy in complicated situations
- Definition of the size of the pregnant uterus and the position of the placenta; assessment of areas of poor placental perfusion or infarction

Risks/Limitations. At present there are no documented adverse reactions or harm to a human mother or fetus as a result of the use of MRI; however, ample study of the safety of MRI has not yet been done, and caution in using this technique should be taken, MRI is used only when other more traditional methods cannot provide the same information and maternal or fetal condition provides a strong indication for the test. Limitations of the test include higher cost than other diagnostic tests such as ultrasound and problems with obtaining images because of fetal movement. Because MRI is a fairly new technique, there is a lack of well-documented imaging parameters. This situation at times complicates diagnosis.

Role of the Nurse. High-risk clients undergoing MRI during pregnancy require support and teaching. Although MRI is not physically painful, the client's positioning in the unit, along with the reason for the test, may be stressful and upsetting to her. Nurses can do much to ensure that staff members conducting the test provide reassurance to the client during this potentially frightening procedure, that results of the test are communicated promptly, and that the client receives adequate and appropriate support if pathology is diagnosed.

► Nursing Diagnoses

Third-trimester assessment continues to enrich the data base for diagnosis development. Nursing diagnoses for the low-risk client during the third trimester evolve from the client's adaptation to the changes of advanced pregnancy, responses to screening procedures, and preparations for childbirth and early parenting. Nursing diagnoses include:

Physiologic

Problem-oriented diagnoses:

- Sleep pattern disturbance, related to fetal activity, shortness of breath, pressure on bladder
- Impaired physical mobility, related to relaxation of joints and muscles and altered balance

Wellness-oriented diagnoses:
- Asset in health of mother and fetus, related to normal physical changes in the third trimester

Physiologic

Problem-oriented diagnoses:

- Anxiety, related to:
    Third-trimester discomforts
    Financial pressures associated with costs of childbearing and potential loss of income
    Impending labor and delivery
    Caring for a first or additional child
    Third-trimester diagnostic techniques
    Diagnostic tests for fetal well-being
    Having a normal fetus and infant
- Knowledge deficit, related to:
    Lack of understanding about third-trimester changes
    Lack of preparation for labor and delivery
    Lack of understanding about fetal assessment techniques
- Altered sexuality patterns, related to:
    Physical changes in third trimester
    Fear of hurting fetus
    Lack of comfort during third trimester

Wellness-oriented diagnoses:

- Positive parental self-image, related to support from extended family and friends
- Potential for positive sibling interaction, related to sibling preparation during the third trimester

Cultural

Problem-oriented diagnoses:

- Altered family processes, related to cultural differences in perception of roles during third trimester of pregnancy, labor, delivery, and early parenting

Wellness-oriented diagnoses:

- Positive self-care practices, related to incorporation of cultural beliefs and practices into plan of care

▶ NURSING AND COLLABORATIVE MANAGEMENT

Throughout pregnancy, the plan of care serves as a vehicle to express management strategies. The client's chart and care plan are always reviewed by the nurse and the examiner prior to meeting with the client at each prenatal visit.

Some management strategies, such as preparation of the client for childbirth and early parenting, assume special importance during the third trimester as delivery approaches. Many strategies change as

pregnancy progresses, although particular goals continue. For example, knowledge deficits related to pregnancy may continue as a diagnosis throughout pregnancy. Nursing care related to knowledge deficits in the third trimester focuses on assessment of client responses to teaching during the first and second trimesters, client mastery of topics covered at prior visits, and client initiatives in addressing knowledge deficits; identification of specific subjects for third-trimester teaching and educational preparation for labor, delivery, and parenthood; development or continuation of intervention strategies that best meet the unique educational needs of the client; and identification of ways in which the client's mastery of the subjects taught may be evaluated (return demonstrations of proper body mechanics when bending, breathing exercises for labor and delivery, and so on).

For the low-risk healthy family, the third trimester is a time of expectation and increasing readiness for childbirth. Nursing care during the third trimester focuses on goals that foster healthy fetal, maternal, and family development and that prepare the family for labor, delivery, and early parenting.

▶ Continuing a Philosophy of Care with Well-Defined Goals

As discussed in Chapters 15 and 17, every prenatal care facility should have a philosophy of care with clearly defined goals and objectives related to care of the childbearing family. All staff members need to be well informed about the philosophy, goals, and objectives and to be able to translate them into practice:

- Preparing the client and family for continued care
- Preparing the client for intrapartum care and early postpartum care
- Updating the data base for diagnosis development
- Continuing to support the client
- Continuing to recognize cultural influences
- Assisting the client to finalize birth plans
- Discussing alternatives in the event of high-risk intrapartum, postpartum, or neonatal conditions
- Promoting psychologic adaptation to late pregnancy
- Fostering family attachment during late pregnancy
- Meeting educational needs and promoting preparation for labor, delivery, and early parenting
- Promoting nutritional well-being

- Assisting the client to cope with third-trimester discomforts
- Promoting client safety
- Evaluating prenatal care
- Ensuring appropriate client referral

Preparing the Client and Family for Continued Care

Around 28 weeks of gestation, the client's prenatal visits increase to every other week; at about 36 weeks of gestation, the client begins weekly visits. The client may be seen more often, if needed. Before the end of each visit, the client continues to make future appointments. Third-trimester clients often schedule several advance appointments to be better able to make their own plans, such as transportation and child care, and to ensure they will not have difficulty finding an available appointment at a convenient time. (First- or second-trimester clients who need to make plans 2 months ahead may also do this.) Frequent prenatal visits can be difficult to manage, especially for clients who are employed, live at a distance, or have other regularly scheduled responsibilities. Attention therefore needs to be paid to making certain that appointments progress on time. Flexible scheduling of prenatal sessions, including evening hours, does not force the working client to choose between prenatal care and a paycheck.

Preparing the Client for Intrapartum Care and Early Postpartum Care

During the third trimester, the nurse ensures that the client and her family are prepared for intrapartum care and for early postpartum care. Clients who attend childbirth preparation classes at the same facility where they will deliver may receive information about intrapartum and postpartum care through their prepared childbirth classes. In some settings members of the nursing staff may also be certified childbirth educators and teach the childbirth preparation classes. Many clients, however, attend childbirth education programs elsewhere in the community; therefore, as part of third-trimester care, the nurse makes certain that the client is informed about what to expect in the particular setting during labor and delivery and what she, her family, and her newborn will experience after birth there.

As part of a birth center experience, clients become well educated about all aspects of the center before delivery. Birthing areas are usually adjacent to prenatal assessment areas, and clients have ample prenatal opportunity to become familiar with them and to select the room they wish to use for labor and delivery, if available. Clients who come for prenatal care in private office or clinic settings usually have little contact with the intrapartum facilities, although many have toured the facilities in selecting their birthing environment. During the third trimester, clients should therefore be encouraged to tour the facility again, as new questions may arise with advanced pregnancy. Prenatal nurses should make certain that clients do not see the intrapartum facility for the first time when they arrive in labor.

During the third trimester, the client should be prepared for changes that will take place in her body after delivery and in the early postpartum period, although postpartum teaching will also be given in the postpartum setting or in the home after early discharge. For example, such topics as postpartum lochial discharge (which can be a source of surprise and anxiety to the unprepared woman), the components of postpartum assessment, care of the newborn, and contact between mother, family members, and the newborn should be discussed.

Updating the Data Base for Diagnosis Development

Assessment strategies for the third-trimester client were discussed in an earlier section. Screening for high-risk conditions continues to be a major focus of third-trimester assessment, because high-risk conditions such as pregnancy-induced hypertension can emerge suddenly and jeopardize maternal and fetal well-being. Assessment continues to identify client and family strengths and assets, so that successful self-care practices can be reinforced, independence fostered, and the family included in care decisions. Through assessment the nurse collaborates with other health care providers in updating or formulating new nursing diagnoses and evaluating client responses to previous strategies. As the third trimester progresses, new diagnoses also include readiness of the client for labor, delivery, and early parenthood.

The format for repeat prenatal visits remains similar throughout pregnancy, although certain screening tests, such as hemoglobin/hematocrit, repeat testing for syphilis or other infections (in women at risk), irregular antibody screen, and Rh antibody testing for Rh-negative women, may be done during the third trimester. In some settings, pelvic examinations are again begun around 36 weeks of gestation to assess cervical ripening and dilation and fetal station. In other settings, pelvic examinations are not routinely done for the low-risk client until labor begins.

Continuing to Support the Client

Support of the pregnant family remains essential throughout pregnancy. The nurse should continue to remain accessible and to anticipate client concerns, such as late-pregnancy discomforts, altered physical appearance, weight gain, increased feelings of vulnerability, and lack of confidence in ability to cope with labor, delivery, or a new family member. During the third trimester, many couples need to be reassured that their fetus is developing normally and that their concerns are also normal. By 40 weeks of gestation, the low-risk client will ideally have made about 15 visits. Thus, during pregnancy, and especially the third trimester, the nurse frequently has more contact with the client than do some members of the client's own family.

Third-trimester diagnostic testing focuses on assessment and fetal well-being and maintenance of the pregnancy to term. Such assessment measures as the NST, the CST, and the fetal biophysical profile may be particular sources of anxiety to couples who are fearful about the health of their developing fetus. Lack of conclusive results or the need for repeat tests contributes to stress. Nurses have an important role in providing emotional support to expectant families throughout the diagnostic process.

Continuing to Recognize Cultural Influences

The client's cultural background must be integrated into any management strategy. This is especially important during the third trimester, as the nurse provides anticipatory guidance and counseling for intrapartum, postpartum, and neonatal care.

The health care system and lifestyle of women in the United States at times are in conflict with beliefs and practices of other cultures. Clients should be encouraged to discuss ways in which their own cultural expectations differ from health care practices in the United States. Interpreters for non-English-speaking clients should be present for each visit and should accompany clients on tours of the birthing facility.

Special arrangements may need to be made prenatally to accommodate cultural variations within the intrapartum and postpartum settings. For example, some facilities do not have arrangements for kosher diets. Jewish clients who follow kosher dietary practices need to be prepared to bring their own foods and beverages. During the third trimester, the nurse, working with an interpreter whenever necessary, can assist the couple to develop a birth plan that reflects their cultural beliefs. In this way staff can work with the client toward realizing a satisfying birthing experience within the health care delivery system.

Cultural conflict during the third trimester is not restricted to religious or ethnic groups, but may affect women whose lifestyles or responsibilities conflict with past beliefs regarding late-trimester behavior. Identification of conflict is part of the assessment. For example, in the United States women traditionally were expected to leave their jobs well in advance of delivery. A woman who works because of necessity, work responsibilities, or need to maximize maternity leave after birth of the infant may experience personal or interpersonal conflict related to her continued working. In this type of situation, nursing strategies include supporting the client's decision to continue working.

Assisting the Client to Finalize Birth Plans

During the third trimester, the nurse serves as a consultant to the client in finalizing a **birth plan,** a list of options preferred for the client's labor and delivery experience. The expectant couple is encouraged to discuss a draft of their birth plan with health care providers around 34 weeks of gestation, although some couples may choose to do this sooner. After discussion, the birth plan is modified as necessary.

The nurse advises the couple in developing a plan that is consistent with available facilities. For example, siblings may be welcomed to attend birth in a birth center; however, "special" permission may be needed in advance in hospital settings. A birth plan including a sibling that is "approved" in advance may prevent client disappointment or conflict with staff at the time of labor.

Questions that may be written for the woman and her family to consider include:

- Would you like to do something special with the lighting? the music? What roles do you wish your partner/support person[s] to take during labor and at the actual delivery?
- Do you have children who will be present at this birth? How will they be supported?
- Do you have special fears or desires you would like to discuss?
- What room do you prefer for the birth?
- Do you wish to have pictures taken of the birth?

A woman should feel free to list anything that will assist staff at the birth facility to make the birth experience what the mother would like it to be (see box entitled Sample Birth Plan).

A copy of the client's written birth plan is placed in the client's chart, and one copy is kept by the parents. When feasible, clients may request that staff who may substitute for their prenatal caregivers review the birth plan and discuss any areas of disagreement. The birth plan ideally then becomes standing orders for the midwife or physician who will attend the birth. The couple is therefore "spared" the necessity of re-explaining their birth plans or negotiating with intrapartum staff during labor, especially if attended by staff who did not work with them prenatally.

▶ SAMPLE BIRTH PLAN

During labor and delivery I would like my husband and sister to be present with me. My sister will bring her camera and take photos. I want to stay out of bed as long as I am able and would prefer to be able to walk, to use the jetted tub for relaxation, or to be up in the chair in the birthing suite. I would like to be able to listen to the tapes that we will bring and do not want the television to be on at any time. My husband and I have attended the prepared childbirth classes, but I know we will need "on the job" teaching which I would like from the staff. If all goes well, my husband would like to cut the cord. Please delay the baby's eye antibiotic long enough for me to be able to look into the baby's eyes. After delivery I would like to introduce the baby to his or her grandparents and three-year-old brother and to spend time with my family in the birthing suite.

In the event that I require transfer I would like my husband and the nurse-midwife to remain with me through delivery. If I need a cesarean delivery, I would like to remain awake, if feasible, to have a low transverse skin incision if circumstances allow, and, if the baby's condition permits, to see and touch the baby as soon as possible.

Currently, childbirth education supports shared decision making between clients and health care providers, as evidenced by the implementation of birth plans. A goal of birth plans is to meet the unique needs of each family for a personally satisfying childbirth, while fostering mutual participation and sharing of information between expectant families and their health care providers.

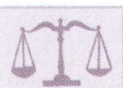 *Ethical Decision Making*

Consider a situation in which you are caring for an expectant client who has a history of high-risk labor and delivery and she is in the process of finalizing her birth plan. In discussing alternatives with the client that may need to be implemented in the event of a high-risk condition emerging during the intrapartum period, the following issues should be examined:

1. Should this well, pregnant woman with her history be encouraged to choose a high-risk health care facility for the birth of her baby or can she be managed in a low-risk environment if her problem is unlikely to recur?
2. What type of strategies would you implement to promote both the family's decision-making processes related to their choice in birthing facilities and a successful maternal-fetal outcome?

Discussing Alternatives in the Event of High-Risk Intrapartum, Postpartum, or Neonatal Conditions

During the third trimester, health care providers and the client should discuss alternatives in the event high-risk intrapartum, postpartum, or neonatal conditions emerge. The client should also be encouraged to develop an alternative birth plan to be included in the chart with the original birth plan. If feasible at the time, the alternative birth plan would be used in the event of unexpected outcomes. For instance, if an unplanned cesarean delivery becomes necessary, the client may request that her partner remain with her.

Promoting Psychologic Adaptation to Late Pregnancy

During the third trimester, nurses continue to have an important role in helping families to meet emotional tasks of late pregnancy and to complete their preparations for childbirth and early parenting. Continuing to encourage couples to share their feelings with each other remains a basic management strategy. Other components of psychosocial care are important during the third trimester:

- Meeting with the client (and family members, if present) prior to physical examination by the midwife or physician at each visit. The nurse assesses the progression of the client's and family's preparation for childbirth and parenting, provides anticipatory guidance and counseling, formulates or revises nursing diagnoses, and communicates any client care problems to the physician or certified nurse-midwife for collaborative follow-up.
- Reassessing family functioning in late pregnancy. Psychosocial factors, such as acceptance of the coming infant, are crucial during the

third trimester, when birth of the baby is imminent. Through observation, interview, or the use of screening tools the nurse may identify whether the third-trimester family is continuing to adapt normally or whether high-risk psychosocial conditions have emerged.

- Explaining normal psychologic processes of the third trimester. For instance, as the woman continues to focus inward, family members may feel increasingly isolated from her.
- Providing anticipatory guidance and teaching. Topics include rearrangement of time and space for a new infant or additional child, the mother's employment plans, the family's plans for care of the new mother and infant at home, paternal feelings of being "left out" of the mother–infant dyad, feelings of paternal attachment to the fetus and infant, and sexuality during the third trimester.
- Discussing changing interpersonal family relationships and the client's own reactions as delivery approaches.
- Fostering the expectant grandmother's involvement in the pregnancy by continuing to encourage the client to bring her to prenatal visits and by encouraging the client to share her feelings with her own mother.
- Reassuring the client about normal fantasy processes. As discussed earlier, dreams and concerns about an abnormal infant are normal for women during the third trimester. They can, however, be extremely upsetting to clients who worry that these fantasies are prophetic. Clients and families may greatly benefit from the nurse's anticipating these concerns, identifying the nature of maternal and paternal fantasies, and providing appropriate reassurance.
- Exploring paternal reactions to pregnancy during the third trimester. Expectant fathers should be encouraged to discuss concerns related to pregnancy, feelings about the pregnant partner, sexuality during late pregnancy, the paternal role during labor and delivery and early parenting, and couvade symptoms that normally may occur during the third trimester.
- Assisting the expectant couple to cope with stress in themselves and other family members, related to the birth of the baby in the near future.
- Encouraging sharing of feelings between the expectant father and his own father, as this relationship assumes special importance as childbirth approaches.
- Encouraging the expectant couple to discuss plans for integrating the newborn into the family and providing anticipatory guidance as appropriate.

Through assessment of third-trimester psychologic adaptation, the nurse can identify high-risk situations that require additional counseling and referral.

Fostering Family Attachment During Late Pregnancy

During the third trimester, attachment to the fetus normally progresses, not only for the expectant mother, but for the expectant father, grandparents, and siblings. Nurses can assess attachment behaviors by encouraging clients to talk about their fetuses. They can also encourage clients to focus on the fetus as a separate being. Facial expression, tone of voice, and nature of description provide clues to maternal and paternal attachment as well as to psychologic adaptation in the third trimester.

Including significant others in prenatal visits, identifying fetal parts, encouraging family members to listen to the fetal heartbeat, and providing learning materials, such as charts, to illustrate fetal growth and development are activities that reinforce the reality of the developing baby and promote attachment on the part of family members. Failure to attach to the fetus by the third trimester indicates an emotionally high-risk situation in need of further assessment.

Meeting Educational Needs and Promoting Preparation for Labor, Delivery, and Early Parenting

Throughout the third trimester, educational preparation remains an essential component of nursing care. Education during the third trimester assumes special importance, as the expectant couple must learn not only about third-trimester adaptations, but also about labor, delivery, the early postpartum period, and the newborn. Before the end of pregnancy, the family should have resources mobilized for independent self-care practices in late pregnancy and after returning home with the newborn.

Third-trimester education includes advice and teaching about items that will be needed for care of the newborn. To avoid confusion and additional stress in the busy days after childbirth, expectant families may be encouraged to prepare items that will be used for the new baby. Some families may be reluctant to bring major baby items into the home before the baby is born because of fears that "all will not be well." Such beliefs may be culturally supported. The families may, however, plan, select, and order items such as a crib that can be delivered after the baby is born. (See box entitled Items for Care of the Newborn.)

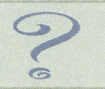

Commonly Asked Questions

How often should I feel the baby move?

About ten fetal movements are usually felt in a 6-hour period; however, a fetus normally has different activity periods during a 24-hour period. The health care provider should be consulted promptly if a change in the usual patterns of fetal movements, for example, a marked decrease or increase in fetal movements or their absence, is noted.

What can I do to get to sleep at night? I can't seem to get comfortable and I'm tired all day. Is a glass of wine or a beer advisable?

Sleeplessness is a common problem during the third trimester. Helpful strategies include preparing a restful environment before sleep (comfortable room temperature, smoothed bed, soft lights or no light, restful music, tapes of waves, rain, or other relaxing sounds); engaging in relaxation techniques (back rub from partner, relaxation exercises such as imagery); reading nonstressful material; trying to put stressful topics aside at least half an hour before sleep; avoiding stressful confrontations with others before bedtime if possible; drinking a glass of warm milk; avoiding caffeinated foods and beverages, such as chocolate and caffeinated coffee or tea; trying not to focus on insomnia. *Alcoholic beverages of any kind are never recommended during pregnancy because of potential hazards to the fetus.*

Should I abstain from intercourse during the third trimester? Does sexual intercourse hurt the baby?

There is no reason why the healthy woman with intact membranes should not have intercourse during pregnancy. Sexual intercourse does not hurt the baby.

Is swelling in my feet normal during the third trimester?

Many women normally experience swelling in their feet during the third trimester, especially if they sit or stand for long periods. The large uterus tends to slow circulation from the legs and contributes to the swelling. Sudden swelling in the legs should be reported promptly to the health care provider, particularly if accompanied by swelling of the hands, face, or lower back, headache, altered vision, abdominal pain, or nerve or muscular irritability.

Can I take a bath or go swimming during the third trimester?

Yes, as long as membranes have not ruptured. During late pregnancy, women need to be especially careful not to fall, as increased size and altered center of gravity and balance make trauma a real risk. Skid protectors should be used in bathtubs and showers; women who have difficulty getting in or out of the bathtub may find showering safer.

Is there any problem with traveling for business or vacation until my due date?

Possibly. A due date is calculated for the 40th week of gestation; however, many women deliver at term up to 2 weeks earlier. Planning vacation trips at the end of pregnancy is therefore not advised. Women who must travel should bring a copy of their prenatal health records with them. Strenuous, stressful trips are not recommended during the third trimester, nor is travel to areas of the world where obstetric health care is inaccessible, where there is poor sanitation, and where there is a high incidence of infectious disease.

My dreams are so vivid. Sometimes the baby I dream about doesn't look normal. Is this a cause for worry?

These types of dreams are upsetting, but common occurrences in the third trimester. They have no relationship to a couple having a handicapped infant. Talking about the dreams with the health care provider or a supportive significant other may help to decrease anxiety.

At times I feel like my husband is withdrawing from me. He seems so interested in his new hobby. Is this normal?

Yes. During the third trimester, expectant fathers may focus on their own concerns, and may worry about providing for the enlarged family and coping with additional responsibilities. In addition, expectant fathers may fulfill their own desires to create by undertaking a hobby or acquiring a pet at this time. Sharing your feelings about this with your husband may be helpful.

Why is a birth plan important?

A birth plan gives the expectant family a chance to think in advance about what would make their

(continued)

Commonly Asked Questions continued

childbirth experience especially meaningful and what they would like to avoid. Finalizing plans in consultation with health care providers during the third trimester and having those plans incorporated into your chart minimize confusion or negotiations at the time of labor and delivery.

What can I do to prevent stretch marks?

Unfortunately, there is currently no known treatment that prevents stretch marks. Moisturizers may prevent dry skin and associated itching.

My hips seem to feel "loose"; sometimes I also have a feeling of pelvic pressure. What can I do for relief?

These are normal symptoms during the third trimester and are related to relaxation of joints and increasing weight of the uterus. Many women expe-

rience these symptoms at night in relation to sleeplessness when they cannot seem to get comfortable in bed. Strategies that provide some relief include wearing a support garment, such as a maternity girdle, using good body mechanics, and assuming a side-lying position, with pillows between the legs and supporting the abdomen, when in bed.

During this trimester I have been having a heavy, clear to whitish vaginal discharge like I did during my first trimester. Is this normal?

Leukorrhea, which can manifest as a heavy, clear to whitish vaginal discharge, is a normal but common discomfort, especially during the first and third trimesters of pregnancy. Examination is important, however, to confirm that the discharge is indeed normal leukorrhea.

Items used for infants vary among cultures and among different socioeconomic groups within the same culture. Creativity, resourcefulness, and access to community groups or programs that assist the disadvantaged are important for nurses working with clients who are experiencing economic hardship. Nurses need to be aware of the cost and alternative sources of infant items, for example, borrowing or buying used items and attending yard sales.

Specialized prepared childbirth programs enhance teaching that takes place during prenatal visits in the third trimester. Although prenatal education classes may be available throughout pregnancy, many couples attend series that begin late in the second trimester or early in the third trimester. Nurses are often consulted by clients and other health care providers for referrals to prepared childbirth programs. Childbirth education programs vary greatly; nursing referrals are therefore based on the individual needs and preferences of each family. Nurses working with third-trimester clients may also be asked to discuss or explain topics presented in these classes.

During third-trimester prenatal visits, the nurse explains current physiologic and psychosocial adaptations related to the third trimester. The nurse continues to provide anticipatory guidance to relieve potential client anxiety about her normal, low-risk status and to inform her of what she may expect at future visits or in the intrapartum unit. The healthy client

needs to understand that the need for increasing the frequency of prenatal visits during the third trimester reflects standard protocols of care rather than problems with her pregnancy.

In the United States, obstetric care for the healthy childbearing family is completed with the final postpartum checkup, usually scheduled around 6 to 8 weeks after delivery. The prenatal nurse advises the client about the importance of this visit, and encourages the family to call with any questions that may arise.

Promoting Nutritional Well-Being

Throughout pregnancy, nutrition remains an essential component of management because of its impact on fetal development and maternal adaptation.

During the third trimester, nutritional status continues to be reflected by such factors as general appearance, the client's pattern of weight gain, fetal growth, previous weight management history and patterns, hemoglobin/hematocrit, usual dietary intake, and consumption of nonfood items.

Weight gain may be perceived by the client as problematic during the third trimester. Careful assessment is needed to diagnose that weight gain is not due to fluid retention related to pathologic conditions, for example, pregnancy-induced hypertension. Dietary counseling can also help the client cope with third-trimester discomforts, such as constipation.

▶ ITEMS FOR CARE OF THE NEWBORN

CRIB OR CRADLE WITH WELL-FITTING STURDY MATTRESS

To promote infant safety, the source and composition of the mattress need to be considered, especially if the mattress is not new. If a crib or cradle cannot be obtained, a large dresser drawer or heavy-duty plasticized laundry basket may be padded and placed on the floor for the infant. A heavy, folded blanket placed inside a pillow case can serve as a mattress. Pillows should not be used as "crib" mattresses, because their softness does not provide adequate support for the infant.

CARRIAGE OR STROLLER THAT WILL SUPPORT THE INFANT WHEN LYING FLAT

An "umbrella"-type stroller is easy and lightweight. The infant and young child will use this for a longer period than a heavy carriage; however, not all umbrella-type strollers provide adequate support for the newborn.

STRAP-ON INFANT CARRIER

CAR SEAT

If the infant will travel in an automobile, a car seat is necessary. A car seat can be used as an infant feeding seat and can foster an infant's interest in the environment by providing a wide viewing area. Any infant seat support should have shoulder restraints to prevent injury related to falls.

CLOTHING

- 6 undershirts, 2 with cuffs (The 6- to 12-month size allows room for growth and saves the additional cost of infant wear.)
- 6 receiving blankets
- 6 "stretchies" or other types of seasonal infant outfits
- 1 or 2 infant sweaters or sweatshirts
- 2 infant hats (in hot weather, for sun protection; in cool weather for protection and warmth)
- 1 infant snowsuit or heavy outerwear (in cold climates)

BEDDING ITEMS

- 1 heavy blanket
- 2 or 3 infant crib sheets
- 2 crib pads (cotton on one side, plastic or rubber on the other side)

DIAPER BAG

This does not have to be a special "diaper" bag, but could be any spacious bag made of canvas or other sturdy material.

DIAPERS

- 1 large (48 count) box or package of disposable diapers, if these are to be used

- 36 diapers, if cloth are to be used and laundered at home (More may be obtained, depending on how often laundry will be washed.)
- 12 thin "birdseye" diapers (These are versatile for folding and dry more quickly than heavier diapers.)
- 36 diaper liners
- 1 deep diaper bucket for soiled diapers and neutralizing solution such as baking soda (one-half cup dissolved in warm water)
- Diaper service (If this service will be used, initial delivery will be scheduled before infant is born or comes home.)
- 4 diaper pins (2 for use, one extra set) (Avoid plastic heads, as they tend to break with frequent use. Pins may be stored open in a bar of soap. The soap allows pins to slide easily into diaper fabric. *Pins must be kept out of reach of other children and of the infant.*)
- 6 or 12 (one package) cloth diapers for clients who use disposable diapers (These make excellent shoulder or crib sheet protectors.)
- 3 to 6 pairs of plastic pants
- 1 container of diaper wipes to be used to clean infant when away from home. (For a less expensive alternative, cut a disposable cloth in two, soap one piece, wet the other piece, and place in separate plastic bags or containers to use when traveling.)

ITEMS RELATED TO INFANT FEEDING

- 6 baby bibs (plastic lined, remove after feeding)
- 6 baby bottles with nipples, 8-oz size (Bottles may also be obtained by breastfeeding mothers who will be expressing milk for infant feeding.)
- 1 manual breast pump for breastfeeding mothers (cylinder type, e.g., Kanason); for bottle-feeding mothers, 1 week's supply of infant formula, as prescribed by the pediatrician (When finances are a major concern, formula may be purchased in advance at intervals and in accordance with the family's budget. Many retailers will accept returned formula if in unused condition with seals intact, should this become necessary. Powdered formula is the most economical, because the client needs to mix only what will be consumed.)
- 1 small nipple brush for cleaning bottle nipples
- 1 bottle brush
- 3 pacifiers

MILD SOAP FOR LAUNDERING INFANT CLOTHING

White vinegar (one-half cup in rinse water) may be used to soften baby clothes.

INFANT BATH ITEMS

- Special infant bathing tubs are an unnecessary expense for the family with financial concerns. Once the umbilical cord stump has dried and healed, a large plastic dishpan,

(continued)

▶ ITEMS FOR CARE OF THE NEWBORN *(continued)*

used exclusively for the infant, or a clean bathroom tub may be used.

- Mild soap for use on infant's skin
- 2 bath towels, 3 thin washcloths (easier to use with an infant), 1 hand towel (to be placed under the infant in the bath to prevent sliding)

INFANT SKIN CARE ITEMS

- Emollient (Avoid baby oils, make certain to remove before reapplying.)
- 1 box of cornstarch
- White petroleum jelly without additives (especially for use with circumcised male infants)

- Paper nail file for fingernails (Avoid scissors or metal files to prevent injury.)

STORAGE ITEMS, E.G., DRESSER AND CABINET

- If lack of furniture is a problem, heavy-duty cartons, available free from supermarkets or other stores, can be obtained, covered with contact paper for a bright look and stacked sideways to form open shelves.

Courtesy of Kathleen Y. Donnelly, RN.

Assisting the Client to Cope with Third-Trimester Discomforts

The third trimester is an uncomfortable time for most women. Many discomforts are related to the large size of the uterus and to continuing hormonal changes. Discomforts experienced during the second trimester may continue through the third trimester. In addition, the woman may experience edema of the lower extremities, varicose veins, lower backache, shortness of breath, and tingling or numbness in the fingers.

The discomforts that the expectant mother experiences during this stage of pregnancy may cause anxiety. Simple explanations of the basis of the discomforts and measures of relief can help relieve her worries.

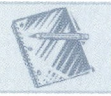 *Client Teaching*

Edema of the Feet, Ankles and Lower Legs

The nurse can suggest the following strategies to the expectant mother to help relieve or prevent edema:

- Avoid prolonged sitting or standing
- Avoid restrictive clothing around the legs
- Avoid knee-high stockings
- Drink 6 to 8 glasses of noncaffeinated beverages/day
- Rest with legs elevated or on left side

Edema of the Feet, Ankles, and Lower Legs. Edema of the feet, ankles, and lower legs is a common discomfort during the third trimester. Women may experience a sense of tightness or pulling in the swollen areas. Shoes worn prenatally may become tight and no longer fit. Some women report an increase in shoe size at this time. Edema of the feet, ankles, and lower legs results from sodium and water retention, which is influenced by such factors as estrogen, cortisol, prolactin, and human placental lactogen. In addition, the pregnant uterus presses on the veins in the legs and impairs return of blood flow from the legs. Posture also influences ankle edema. Sitting or standing for prolonged periods results in increased edema.

Urinary Frequency. As discussed previously, the presenting part of the fetus may settle into the pelvis during the last month of pregnancy, placing pressure on the bladder. The woman again experiences urinary frequency. Nursing interventions focus on evaluation of the woman to make certain that the urinary frequency is a normal manifestation of third-trimester pregnancy and not a sign of urinary tract infection or other pathology. Fluids should not be restricted. Other than reassuring the woman of the normalcy of this condition and its indication that pregnancy will soon be completed, there are no measures that can provide adequate relief.

Nocturia. In addition to the nuisance of urinary frequency during the third trimester, the woman may experience increased production of urine at night or during prolonged rest periods, especially when in a side-lying position. This condition complicates insomnia for some women and may lead to sleep deprivation. Explanations of this normal condition may help relieve anxiety. Although reducing fluid intake after dinner may provide a small amount of relief, women should be careful to space a fluid intake of six to eight full glasses of noncaffeinated beverages throughout the day. In addition, care should be taken to avoid falls when getting up during the night. There should be a clear path to the bathroom; a nightlight is also helpful.

Insomnia. Insomnia during the third trimester may be attributed to several factors, such as difficulty in finding a comfortable position as a result of the enlarged uterus, fetal activity, heartburn, nocturia, and emotional concerns. For a woman accustomed to falling asleep on her abdomen, the third trimester requires changes in a life-long practice.

Varicose Veins. Varicose veins in the legs, vulva, and rectum may be especially problematic during the third trimester, although they also cause discomfort earlier in pregnancy. Discomfort from varicosities may be experienced as a dull, throbbing-type pain. Varicose veins are aggravated by venous congestion, which worsens because of pressure from the expanding uterus. Progesterone, which relaxes smooth muscles and the walls and valves of veins, may also contribute to the development of varicosities. Unfortunately varicose vein formation may also be familial. The expectant mother should be advised to avoid restrictive clothing around the legs; to avoid prolonged sitting and standing; to wear supportive pantyhose, which should be put on before getting up in the morning; to keep the legs uncrossed when sitting; to rest with legs elevated or in a left side-lying position (placing a pillow between the legs may also provide relief for varicosities of the vulva and rectum); to provide support for vulvar varicosities (this may be done by using a sanitary belt to hold a foam rubber pad in place); and to call her health care provider if signs of phlebitis (areas of hardness, redness, swelling, increased pain) should occur.

Lower Backache. Lower backache is very common as pregnancy progresses because of the compensatory changes in posture resulting from the enlarging uterus. As discussed previously, musculoskeletal changes in the third trimester result in a progressive lordosis.

The mother should be taught to use correct body mechanics, including positions for sitting, standing, and lifting; to avoid back strain from improper or excessive lifting; to wear low-heeled shoes to reduce back strain; to practice pelvic tilt exercises (see Chapter 9) to help strengthen the muscles supporting the uterus; and to use a well-fitting, nonconstricting maternity girdle to provide support.

Leg Cramps. Sudden, painful leg cramps may occur during the third trimester. The physiologic reason is unclear. Explanations attributing leg cramps to calcium–phosphorus metabolism or pressure from the enlarging uterus on pelvic blood vessels have never been supported. Several measures may provide relief. Dorsiflexing the foot ("toes pointed toward the nose") may relieve cramping. Pressing the bottom of the foot against a firm flat surface, such as the footboard of the bed or the floor, is also helpful. Good body mechanics should be employed to facilitate circulation. An adequate diet that includes calcium is always advised.

Shortness of Breath. During the third trimester the expectant mother may experience shortness of breath as the uterus pushes the diaphragm upward. The nurse may advise the woman to avoid hyperventilation and consciously try to regulate her breathing when she realizes she is hyperventilating; to practice correct body mechanics to allow for maximum

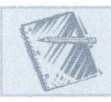 ## Client Teaching

Insomnia

The nurse can suggest the following strategies to the pregnant client to help relieve insomnia:

- Have a warm drink before bedtime. Alcoholic beverages, including wine and beer, should not be recommended, because of potential effects on the fetus.
- Avoid stimulation found in caffeinated foods such as chocolate and coffee.
- Seek quiet activities before bedtime. (For some women, reading a textbook has an excellent sedative effect!)
- Never take sleeping pills or other medications without first consulting your health care provider.
- Attempt relaxation techniques such as deep breathing or visualizing yourself in a quiet and peaceful environment.
- Have your partner provide a backrub to promote relaxation.

expansion of the lungs; to use two or more pillows at night to identify a comfortable position; and periodically to stand and take a deep breath while stretching the arms overhead.

Carpal Tunnel Syndrome.

Carpal tunnel syndrome is a condition in which feelings of tingling, numbness, and burning are felt in the fingers and hands. It is thought to result from edema, which compresses the median nerve within the carpal tunnel at the wrist. The woman's posture, such as holding the shoulders too far back and flexing the head forward to counterbalance the heavy uterus and curved back of late pregnancy, contributes to this condition. Discomfort may be present on awakening. Relief measures include raising the affected hand above the head and flexing and slowly extending the fingers upward to relieve symptoms, paying attention to good posture and, if necessary, using a splint, applied to the slightly flexed wrist and worn during sleep.

Promoting Client Safety

Safety continues to be an important aspect of nursing care during the third trimester. As delivery approaches, the woman continues to be concerned about safety for herself and her fetus.

The woman's large size and altered center of gravity and balance make trauma related to falls a concern during the third trimester. Often, normal physiologic changes will provide women with clues regarding activities they can no longer undertake; however, women should be advised to avoid activities that require balance, such as climbing ladders or using a chair as a ladder at work or at home. Recreational sports that require balance and speed, such as skiing, are not recommended during late pregnancy. Health care providers may need to provide the expectant mother's employer with written verification of the need for her to refrain from certain work-related activities that jeopardize the safety of the woman or her fetus during late pregnancy.

Showering and bathing are permitted as long as membranes remain intact; however, the third-trimester pregnant woman's large size makes getting out of a tub difficult. Special care must be taken to avoid falls. Early in pregnancy, skid protectors, available inexpensively in hardware stores, bath shops, and other retail settings, can be applied to the bottom of tubs and showers to make these surfaces less slippery when wet.

Seat belts should continue to be used during travel, although during the third-trimester women may need to shift position frequently to remain comfortable.

At each visit, the nurse continues to assist the client in identification of safety concerns and potential safety hazards related to lifestyle or environment. The nurse also assists the client in developing ways to minimize or avoid these. Warning or danger signs of pregnancy continue to be reviewed.

As discussed in Chapter 19 high-risk conditions such as pregnancy-induced hypertension and premature labor can appear during the third trimester and present severe complications. Signs and symptoms of preterm and term labor are discussed with the client. As term approaches, signs and symptoms of normal labor are presented, along with appropriate strategies.

The nurse continues to provide positive reinforcement and support for self-care practices that promote wellness, such as breast self-examination and good nutritional patterns.

Discussion of safety issues includes plans for care of the newborn. During the third trimester, the nurse discusses the importance of always using an infant car seat when traveling in an automobile, as the family may wish to obtain a seat prior to the baby's birth. In many states, use of an infant car seat is state law. Many hospitals or charitable groups provide infant seats at minimal or no charge. The nurse can identify and appropriately refer clients in need of these services.

Expectant parents may "babyproof" their home during late pregnancy. Many people enjoy all preparations for the newborn, and the postpartum period is often too hectic for some parents to make this aspect of safety a priority. (Ideally, parents who have young children will have done this already.) The infant develops so rapidly within the first year that potential hazards can become actual hazards suddenly (see box entitled Ways to "Babyproof" a Home).

Concerns for safe passage for self and fetus are especially important during the third trimester as delivery approaches. By encouraging the client to express her concerns and by listening intently, the nurse encourages the client to express her fears related to safety, provides relevant teaching, and offers appropriate reassurance.

Evaluating Prenatal Care

Third-trimester evaluation continues to address the extent to which behavioral objectives are achieved. For example, meeting self-care objectives related to third-trimester edema of the legs and feet would be noted by a decrease in swelling after implementation of such strategies as resting on the left side, elevating the legs, and no longer wearing knee-high stockings with constricting bands. The value the client places on prenatal care is evidenced by verbal reports, regular attendance at prenatal visits, and willingness to

► WAYS TO "BABYPROOF" A HOME

- Walk through each room in your home. Look carefully from the floor to the ceiling in each room. Are there any potential or real hazards to the safety of an infant? Assume that babies are curious; will pull, chew, or swallow anything; and have no "judgment."
- Place protectors on each electric outlet.
- Examine the area around the baby's crib or cradle. Remove wires, extension cords, and other items that could be pulled or could fall into the baby's crib.
- Examine all baby toys carefully. Do not use any toys with sharp or removable pieces that could cut the baby or be swallowed by the baby. Do not use any large toys or objects that could possibly smother an infant. For example, large stuffed animals or crib bumpers are not appropriate for use with the newborn.
- Reduce the temperature of the hot water so that it is not able to scald directly from the tap.

- Use cribs with slats that are less than 2⅜ in. apart to avoid head injuries. Check cribs that are more than 2 years old for dangers that might result in injuries.
- Remove all medications, matches, household cleaners, and other chemicals from areas accessible to young children (this becomes important as the child develops).
- Place guard rails on any windows that can be opened.
- Discuss plans for supervision of pets around the newborn.
- Make certain that the infant can rest in a crib or cradle inaccessible to pets.
- Repair peeling paint or plaster on ceiling or walls near the infant's personal areas.
- Use only products that are nontoxic to infants and young children. Follow the manufacturers' directions carefully; contact manufacturers for additional product information related to use around children.

---

implement prescribed care strategies. Evaluation, related to outcome behaviors identified in the care plan, continues to be carefully documented in the client's chart.

Prenatal written records, kept in the client's chart, allow for continuity of care by intrapartum and postpartum staff who may not have known the client personally before her delivery, as frequently happens in hospital settings.

Ensuring Appropriate Client Referral

Except for routine well-woman examinations or in situations where family practitioners provide care across the life span, the healthy family will have the most contact with pediatric health care providers after the postpartum period. In many situations, this relationship extends until the child reaches young adulthood. Prenatal nurses and physicians should encourage clients to select and to meet with their pediatric health care provider prior to the birth of the infant. Health care providers should also be prepared to provide referrals for pediatric care.

As discussed earlier, nurses frequently provide referrals to educational programs for childbirth preparation and early parenting and to other care providers such as social service workers.

Critical Thinking in Care Planning

Care of the Family During the Third Trimester

Belinda and Luis Mendez are a Chicano couple who are expecting their second child in 10 weeks. They have an 8-year-old daughter, Yolanda, who was born after a difficult labor at 38 weeks' gestation. She is currently at the appropriate developmental level and attends public school.

Belinda (34 years old) is a loan officer at a local bank and plans to return to work 6 weeks after delivery. Luis (40 years old) is a partner in a law firm. Luis' father, who has a small apartment in the Barrio, keeps in constant touch with the family.

Since early in her first trimester, Belinda has received care from a certified nurse-midwife at a birth center. Luis, who did not attend the first delivery, would like to be present at the birth. Yolanda is attending the sibling preparation program at the birth center and would also like to be with her parents when the baby is born.

Although Belinda has had a normal pregnancy, she has been experiencing backache and inability to "fit into her shoes." At the current visit she is upset because she has had dreams of her baby being malformed.

▶ Assessment

- Client reports lower backache especially when sitting and standing too long; ankle edema, "can't even get my shoes on anymore."
- Weight gain appropriate for gestation: Hgb 12.5 g/dl, HCT 36%.
- Client reports that diet includes nutrients from all food groups in the food pyramid.
- Client states that she and her husband have chosen to breastfeed their baby.
- Client reports being upset by having several dreams of her baby being born malformed: "I dream about having a little boy with no ears and a strange nose."
- Father states "I hate to hear that she has dreams like that. I've been very worried about this baby being normal throughout the pregnancy."

- Couple expresses fear regarding labor and delivery.
- Couple attends prepared childbirth classes.
- Client practices relaxation exercises several times each day.
- Client reads literature concerning labor and delivery.
- Client describes own previous negative labor experiences and negative experiences of family members and friends.
- Couple states that they would like their daughter to attend the birth and daughter expresses excitement about seeing the baby born.
- Daughter has begun to attend sibling classes, but has several questions.
- Client's husband states that his father, who was born in Mexico, keeps telling him that "it is not manly to be around women in labor."

Nursing Diagnosis

Pain, related to physiologic response during the third trimester

Expected Client/Family Outcomes	Nursing Action/Intervention	Evaluation
By end of visit, the client will: • Identify changes in body mechanics that will decrease discomfort.	Reinforce pelvic tilt exercises and use of proper body mechanics when standing, bending, and lifting. *Rationale:* Physiologic changes that occur as pregnancy progresses produce predictable discomforts. Knowledge of physiologic changes allows client to remedy the discomforts.	Client describes changes in body mechanics that will decrease discomfort (e.g., postural changes, demonstration of pelvic tilt exercises, and proper body mechanics).

Critical Thinking in Care Planning continued

Expected Client/Family Outcomes	Nursing Action/Intervention	Evaluation
• Describe the physiologic basis for discomforts in late pregnancy.	Teach couple possible factors that could cause back pain during late pregnancy: gravid uterus, stretching of abdominal muscles, increased curvature of spine. *Rationale:* Discussion of discomforts and their physiologic bases can reduce stress. Reinforcement facilitates learning.	Client discusses with the nurse the basis for backache and ankle edema.
• Implement self-care practices to increase comfort.	Encourage client to wear comfortable clothing and shoes; take frequent rest periods with legs elevated; avoid prolonged standing and sitting; use techniques of leg extension and foot dorsiflexion for leg cramps; check for physiologic alterations that might produce same symptoms (e.g., pregnancy-induced hypertension, phlebitis). *Rationale:* Comprehensive assessment includes ruling out pathophysiology.	Client relates changing self-care practices to increased comfort (e.g., resting with legs elevated, stooping instead of bending).

Nursing Diagnosis

Potential asset for lactation, related to nutritional status of the mother

By end of seventh month, the family will: • Describe the physiology of lactation.	Assess family's knowledge of lactation. Assess family's knowledge about nutrition for breastfeeding. *Rationale:* Good maternal nutritional status promotes lactation and infant nutrition.	Family members point to diagram of the breast, identify the anatomy, and discuss basic physiology of lactation. Family members can identify techniques to promote lactation.
• Describe culturally acceptable, nutritious diet that will facilitate lactation.	Teach maternal nutrient needs during lactation: increase protein by 20 g per day; increase vitamins and minerals; increase calories by 500 g per day. Plan with family a sample daily diet that will facilitate lactation, taking into consideration cultural food preferences. *Rationale:* Prenatal nutritional counseling will influence the adequacy of the diet during lactation.	Client and family members describe types and amounts of nutrients necessary to maintain lactation. Family members plan diet that fits their cultural background and meets requirements of lactation.
• Identify community resources that foster nutrition and lactation.	Provide list of community resources such as LaLeche League or lactation consultants that assist in the breastfeeding experience. *Rationale:* Support systems in community and family are often instrumental in success of breastfeeding.	Client and family leave visit with list of appropriate community resources, such as LaLeche League. Family members identify resources that are accessible in the neighborhood.

(continued)

Critical Thinking in Care Planning continued

Nursing Diagnosis

Altered family processes, related to maternal fantasies of the third trimester

Expected Client/Family Outcomes	Nursing Action/Intervention	Evaluation
By eighth month of pregnancy, the family will: • Identify maternal fantasies as normal aspect of pregnancy.	Inform couple that it is normal to have such fantasies, especially during the third trimester. *Rationale:* Women's night dreams and other fantasies increase during the third trimester and are often about frightening situations.	When asked, family members discuss fantasies.
• Discuss feelings about fantasies together and with nurse and other members of health care team and family.	Encourage couple to relate any daydreams or night dreams about pregnancy, childbirth, or infant. *Rationale:* It is common for both men and women to fantasize during pregnancy.	Family members discuss positive and negative reactions to fantasies.
• Identify underlying concerns that might be connected with maternal fantasies.	Explore with couple their feelings concerning their fantasies. *Rationale:* Fantasies may be connected to some underlying concern.	Family members link fantasies with concerns such as child care.
• Identify coping strategies to manage concerns that might be connected with maternal fantasies.	Assist couple in identifying strategies to cope with any concerns that might be connected with specific fantasies (e.g., "talking it out"). *Rationale:* Discussion of fantasies and coping strategies can reduce anxiety.	Family members devise plan for managing identified concerns such as child care preparation classes and parenting support groups.

Nursing Diagnosis

Self-esteem disturbance, related to fear of labor and delivery

By eighth month of pregnancy, the family will: • Express their fears concerning labor and delivery. • Discuss specific fears concerning labor and delivery.	Encourage couple to express their fears regarding labor and delivery. Encourage couple to identify specific fears such as pain and loss of control. *Rationale:* Fear of the unknown or previous negative experiences cause anxiety. Allowing family to communicate their fears in a nonthreatening atmosphere fosters identification of fears and problem-solving processes.	Family members identify and discuss labor and delivery fears with nurse.
• Discuss previous labor and delivery experience.	Explore with couple previous labor and delivery experiences and methods they used to cope with them (e.g., breathing, support systems). Review with couple knowledge gained in childbirth education classes. *Rationale:* In the teaching-learning process, it is important to identify what learner knows and any apprehension he or she may have about labor and delivery.	Family members discuss positive and negative aspects of previous birth experience.

Critical Thinking in Care Planning *continued*

Expected Client/Family Outcomes	Nursing Action/Intervention	Evaluation
• Identify several strategies to cope with fear of labor and delivery experience.	Review family's birth plan. *Rationale:* Decision-making process involved in developing birth plan helps family to identify strategies that will help them cope with the labor and delivery experience.	Couple identifies coping strategies from content learned in childbirth education. Couple describes birth plans.

Nursing Diagnosis

Self-esteem disturbance, related to cultural conflict

By end of eighth month, husband will identify cultural conflicts concerning paternal participation in childbirth experience.	Explore with husband his cultural beliefs and practices. Encourage open communication between husband and his own father. *Rationale:* Acculturation is an important factor to be considered when caring for the childbearing family. Men from the expectant grandfather's culture did not traditionally attend births. Families may be influenced by attitudes of significant others.	Client's husband describes his relationship with his own father, his cultural background, and family expectation of roles.

Nursing Diagnosis

Potential asset in sibling bonding, related to total family participation in the childbearing experience

By end of eighth month, the family will: • Identify their respective roles in childbearing experience.	Explore with family their perceptions of their roles during the childbearing experience. *Rationale:* The third trimester is seen as the most appropriate time to begin preparation of siblings for childbirth.	Family decides that daughter will witness birth.
• Discuss their daughter's role in birthing process. • Evaluate their daughter's preparedness concerning birthing experience.	Explore with daughter what was learned in sibling preparation class. Use a model and a doll to reinforce learning at daughter's developmental level. Explore with daughter her feelings and wishes with regard to participation in birth experience. *Rationale:* Strategies used for teaching children about birth should be age appropriate (e.g., books, dolls, movies).	Through play, daughter will demonstrate knowledge of the birth and readiness to participate.
• Identify resources that will facilitate a positive experience for sibling.	Refer family to other community resources that prepare siblings for birth experience. Explore possibility of having a separate support person for daughter present at the birth. *Rationale:* Referring family to appropriate community resources assists in sibling and family coping. Children need support persons during new and different procedures or experiences. Parents involved in delivery cannot also attend to child.	Family members identify specific support person for child during the birth process.

 *Chapter Highlights*

► Physiologic changes in the third trimester of pregnancy support the final phases of intrauterine fetal development and prepare the mother and fetus for labor, delivery, and lactation.

► Changes in the mother's body during the third trimester are initiated by hormones and the greatly expanded uterus, which mechanically displaces or strains body structures.

► The third trimester is an emotionally turbulent time for the pregnant woman and she is faced with several psychologic preparatory activities, such as demonstrating active acceptance of the fetus, building on the core of maternal identity, exploring maternal fantasies, strengthening her relationship with her mother, establishing a close relationship with her fetus, and preparing for labor.

► The expectant father may experience the greatest amount of stress during the third trimester since he feels a loss both of personal freedom and of the partner's time and attention and is engaged in the attachment process with his infant as well as preparing for his role as parent.

► As the third trimester progresses, siblings need reassurance of their parents' love so as to facilitate the family's preparation for the baby and parents need to feel that they are adequately preparing siblings for the infant's arrival.

► During the third trimester, expectant grandparents may participate actively in making plans for the new baby and assisting the parent with care of older siblings, activities that can enhance the childbearing experience for these family members.

► The goals of the third-trimester assessment are to identify normal third-trimester adaptation, recognize high-risk conditions, evaluate fetal well-being, and determine readiness for labor and delivery.

► Assessment of maternal adaptations to the third trimester includes an updated health history, physiologic evaluation, risk assessment, biochemical screening tests, and psychosocial and cultural assessment.

► Assessment of fetal well-being during the third trimester is based on fundal height, Leopold's maneuvers, assessment of fetal movement, and electronic fetal monitoring.

► Assessment of clients at risk include procedures such as the nonstress test, the contraction stress test, the fetal biophysical profile, amniotic fluid analysis, ultrasonic assessment of fetal growth, and magnetic resonance imaging.

► Nursing responsibilities in third-trimester assessment include technical aspects, psychosocial support, teaching, and advocacy.

► Third-trimester management for the healthy, low-risk client includes assessment every other week and then weekly until delivery, anticipatory guidance, and teaching.

► Educational preparation focuses on adaptations during late pregnancy and on topics related to labor and delivery, the postpartum, and newborn care.

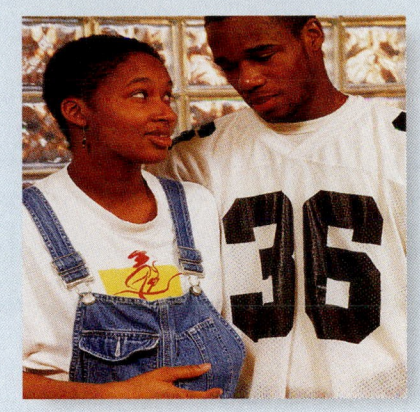

After reading the vignette at the beginning of this chapter, use what you have learned to answer these questions:

1. What factors may be involved in Rashid Dengler's reluctance about having other family members present during Tamika's labor and delivery?

2. What actions can the nurse take to ease the differences in Tamika and Rashid Dengler's expectations of the labor and delivery experience?

3. What strategies can the nurse use to prepare this couple both physically and emotionally for labor, delivery, and the postpartum period?

Critical Thinking Questions

▶ References

Alexy, B., Nichols, B., Heverly, M.A., & Garzon, L. (1997). Prenatal factors and birth outcomes in the public health service: A rural/urban comparison. *Research in Nursing and Health, 20*(1), 61–70.

American College of Obstetricians and Gynecologists. (1994a). *Antepartum fetal surveillance* (Technical Bulletin No. 188). Washington, DC: Author.

American College of Obstetricians and Gynecologists. (1994b). *Gonorrhea and chlamydial infections* (Technical Bulletin No. 190). Washington, DC: Author.

American College of Obstetricians and Gynecologists, Committee on Obstetric Practice. (1996). *Prevention of early onset group B streptococcal disease in newborns* (Committee Opinion No. 173). Washington, DC: Author.

Anderson, A.M. (1996). The father-infant relationship: becoming connected. *Journal of Pediatric Nurses, 1*(2), 83–92.

Badalian, S.S., Chao, C.R., Fox, H.E., & Timor-Tritsch, I.E. (1993). Fetal breathing-related nasal fluid flow velocity in uncomplicated pregnancies. *American Journal of Obstetrics and Gynecology, 169*, 563–567.

Berk, B. (1993). Body image and pregnancy: Building the mind–body connection: A guide for health care professionals. *Journal of Perinatology, 13*, 300–304.

Burk, M.C., Wieser, P.C., & Keegan, L. (1995). Cultural beliefs and health behaviors of pregnant Mexican-American women: Implications for primary care. *Advanced Nursing Science, 17*(4), 37–51.

Chang, T.C., Robson, S.C., Boys, R.J., & Spencer, J.A. (1992). Prediction of the small for gestational age infant: Which ultrasonic measurement is best? *Obstetrics and Gynecology, 80*, 1030–1038.

Clinton, J. (1986). Expectant fathers at risk for couvade. *Nursing Research, 35*, 290–295.

Cunningham, F.G., MacDonald, P.C., Gant, N.F., Leveno, K.J., Gilstrap, L.C., Hankins, G.D.V., & Clark, S.L. (1997). *Williams obstetrics* (20th ed.). Stamford, CT: Appleton & Lange.

Devoe, I., Youssef, A.A., Gardner, P., Dear, C., & Murray, C. (1992). Refining the biophysical profile with a risk-related evaluation test performance. *American Journal of Obstetrics and Gynecology, 167*, 346–351.

Fawcett, J. (1977). The relationship between identification and patterns of change in spouse's body images during and after pregnancy. *International Journal of Nursing Studies, 14*, 199–213.

Fawcett, J., & York, R. (1986). Spouses' physical and psychological symptoms during pregnancy and the postpartum. *Nursing Research, 35*, 144–148.

Ferketich, S.L., & Mercer, R.T. (1995). Paternal-infant attachment of experienced and inexperienced fathers during infancy. *Nursing Research, 44*(1), 31–37.

Fresquez, M. (1997). *Ob/gyn limited ultrasound* (videotape series). Baltimore: Williams & Wilkins.

Foster, S.F., Slade, P., & Wilson, K. (1996). Body image, maternal-fetal attachment, and breastfeeding. *Journal of Psychosomatic Research, 41*(2), 181–184.

Gebauer, C.L., & Lowe, N.K. (1993). The biophysical profile: Antepartum assessment of fetal well-being. *Journal of Obstetric, Gynecologic, and Neonatal Nursing, 22*, 115–124.

Goss, G.L., Lee, K., Koshar, J., Heilemann, M.S., & Stinson, J. (1997). More does not mean better: Prenatal visits and pregnancy outcome in the Hispanic population. *Public Health Nursing, 14*(3), 183–188.

Gottlieb, L., & Mendelson, M. (1990). Parental support and first-born girls adaptation to the birth of a sibling. *Journal of Applied Developmental Psychology, 11*, 29–48.

Gullicks, J.N., & Crase, S.J. (1993). Sibling behavior with a newborn: Parents' expectations and observations. *Journal of Obstetric, Gynecologic, and Neonatal Nursing, 22,* 438–444.

Harrington, K., & Campbell, S. (1993). Fetal size and growth. *Current Opinion in Obstetrics and Gynecology, 5*(2), 186–194.

Hearn-Stebbins, B. (1995). Fetal growth assessment: A literature review. *Journal of Diagnostic Medical Sonography, 11*(4), 176–187.

Jacobsen, G. (1992). Detection of intrauterine growth deviation. A comparison between symphysis-fundus height and ultrasonic measurements. *International Journal of Technology Assessment in Health Care, 8*(Suppl. 1), 170–175.

Kelley, S. (1993). Caregiver stress in grandparents raising grandchildren. *Image, 25,* 331–337.

Kisilevsky, B.S., Muir, D.W., & Low, J.A. (1989). Human fetal responses to sound as a function of stimulus intensity. *Obstetrics and Gynecology, 73,* 971–976.

Lederman, R.P. (1996). *Psychosocial adaptation in pregnancy: Assessment of seven dimensions* (2nd ed.). New York: Springer.

Low, J.A., Pangiotopoulos, C., & Derrick, E.J. (1994). Newborn complications after intrapartum asphyxia with metabolic acidosis in the term fetus. *American Journal of Obstetrics and Gynecology, 170,* 1081.

Lutwak, R.A., Ney, A.M., & White, J.E. (1988). Maternity nursing and Jewish law. *MCN, American Journal of Maternal Child Nursing, 13,* 44–46.

Manning, F.A., Morrison, I., Harman, C.R., Lange, I.R., & Menticoglou, S. (1987). Fetal assessment based on fetal biophysical profile scoring. Experience in 19,221 referred high-risk pregnancies. II. An analysis of false-negative fetal deaths. *American Journal of Obstetrics and Gynecology, 157,* 880–884.

Manning, F.A., Snijders, R., Harman, C.R., Nicolaides, K., Menticoglou, S., & Morrison, I. (1993). Fetal biophysical profile score 6: Correlation with antepartum umbilical venous pH. *American Journal of Obstetrics and Gynecology, 169,* 755–763.

Marnoch, A. (1992). An evaluation of the importance of femoral maternal-fetal movement counting as a measure of fetal well-being. *Midwifery, 8,* 54–63.

McGoldrick, M., Giordano, J., & Pearce, J.K. (1996). *Ethnicity and family therapy.* New York: Guilford Press.

Mercer, R.T., & Ferketich, S.L. (1994). Predictors of maternal role competence by risk status. *Nursing Research, 43*(1), 38–43.

Mercer, R.T., & Ferketich, S.L. (1995). Experienced and inexperienced mothers' maternal competence during infancy. *Research in Nursing and Health, 18*(4), 333–343.

Nageotte, M.P., Towers, C.V., Asrat, T., & Freeman, R.K. (1994). Perinatal outcome with the modified biophysical profile. *American Journal of Obstetrics and Gynecology, 170,* 1672–1676.

Pernoll, M.I., & Taylor, C. (1994). Normal pregnancy and prenatal care. In A. H. DeCherney & M. L. Pernoll (Eds.), *Current obstetric and gynecologic diagnosis and treatment* (8th ed.) (pp. 183–201). Norwalk, CT: Appleton & Lange.

Pillai, M., & James, D. (1990). The development of fetal heart rate patterns during normal pregnancy. *Obstetrics and Gynecology, 76,* 812–815.

Poma, P.A. (1987). Pregnancy in Hispanic women. *Journal of National Medical Association, 79,* 929–935.

Rubin, R. (1984). *Maternal identity and maternal experience.* New York: Springer.

Sherwen, L.N. (1986). Third trimester fantasies of first-time expectant fathers. *Maternal-Child Nursing Journal, 15,* 153–170.

Sherwen, L.N. (Ed.). (1987). *Psychosocial dimensions of the pregnant family.* New York: Springer.

Sherwen, L. (1991). Fantasy state during pregnancy: A psychoanalytic account. *Journal of Perinatal Psychology, 6,* 55–71.

Sleutel, M.R. (1989). Vibroacoustic stimulation and fetal heart rate in nonstress tests. *Journal of Obstetric, Gynecologic, and Neonatal Nursing, 19,* 199–204.

Sleutel, M.R. (1990). An overview of vibroacoustic stimulation. *Journal of Obstetric, Gynecologic, and Neonatal Nursing, 18,* 447–452.

Sokol, R., Jones, T.B., & Pernoll, M.L. (1994). Methods of assessment for pregnancy at risk. In A.H. DeCherney & M. Pernoll (Eds.), *Current obstetric and gynecologic diagnosis and treatment* (8th ed.) (pp. 275–305). Norwalk, CT: Appleton & Lange.

Spector, R.E. (1996). *Cultural diversity in health and illness* (4th ed.). Stamford, CT: Appleton & Lange.

Strom, R., & Strom, S. (1992). *Achieving grandparent potential: Viewpoints on building intergenerational relationships.* Newbury Park, CA: Sage.

Strong, T.H., Jr., Jordan, D.L., & Marden, D.W. (1992). The fetal recoil test. *American Journal of Obstetrics and Gynecology, 167,* 1382–1383.

Tahilramaney, M.P., Platt, L.D., & Golde, S.H. (1991). Use of femur length measured by ultrasonography to predict fetal maturity. *Journal of Perinatology, 11,* 157–160.

Tongsong, T., & Srisomboon, J. (1993). Amniotic fluid volume as a predictor of fetal distress in post-term pregnancy. *International Journal of Gynaecology and Obstetrics, 40,* 213–217.

Weiner, Z., Divon, M.Y., Katz, N., Minor, V.K., Nasseri, A., & Girz, B. (1996). Multivariant analysis of antepartum fetal test in predicting neonatal outcome of growth retarded fetuses. *American Journal of Obstetrics and Gynecology. 174,* 338.

Zachariah, R. (1994). Maternal-fetal attachment: Influence of mother-daughter and husband-wife relationships. *Research in Nursing and Health, 17,* 37–44.

Zimmer, E., & Dixon, M. (1993). Fetal vibroacoustic stimulation. *Obstetrics and Gynecology, 81,* 451–457.

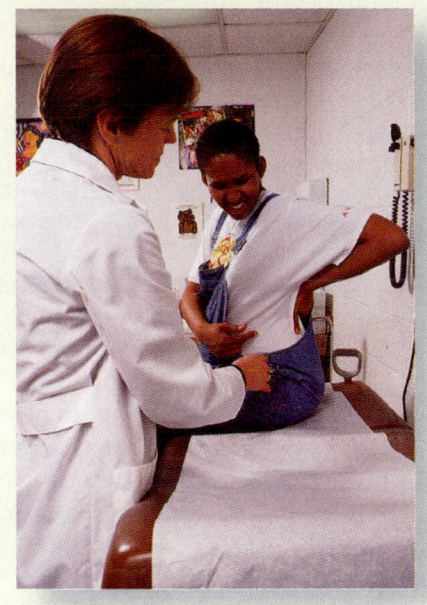

Tamika Dengler, 32 weeks' pregnant with her first child, is attending her scheduled prenatal visit at her obstetrician's office. As Ann Salzman, CNM, MSN, is preparing to begin Tamika's physical examination, she asks her how she is feeling. Tamika replies, "Generally, I feel fine. But," she continues, "in the last few days, it seems that I'm urinating more than usual and my back is a little sore." As Tamika is speaking, she places the palm of her hand against her lower back and frowns.

The nurse observes the location of the pain and asks, "Are you experiencing any other symptoms such as urgency or pain when you urinate?" Tamika states that she does feel a burning sensation on urination. The nurse smiles and states, "Let's take your vital signs and then I'd like you to give me a urine specimen. You may have a urinary tract infection." Tamika replies, "Is an infection like that dangerous? What can I do to prevent it from hurting my baby?" ■

19

The Expectant Family at Risk: Second and Third Trimesters

Most women experience normal pregnancy, deliver healthy infants, and suffer no ill effects. Pregnancy is, nonetheless, a period of heightened vulnerability. All body systems are affected by pregnancy. Nurses working with prenatal clients should know the signs and symptoms associated with low-risk pregnancy and recognize those outside the range of normal. Table 15–7 lists the common danger signs of pregnancy that nurses and their clients need to know. Once conditions are recognized, nurses are involved actively in their management.

Numerous high-risk maternal conditions are associated with adverse fetal and maternal outcomes. Some are associated with pregnancy—for example, pregnancy-induced hypertension, bleeding disorders in pregnancy, premature labor, intrauterine growth retardation, multiple gestation, and postmaturity. Others result from concurrent medical problems—for example, all types of infection, chronic hypertension, cardiac disease, and diabetes mellitus, although diabetes may only emerge during pregnancy. In general, the nurse must remember that pregnant women can experience the same medical or surgical problems as nonpregnant women. In such cases fetal well-being is potentially in jeopardy.

Under optimal conditions pregnancy is a period of psychologic upheaval, taxing the woman's and her family's ability to adapt. Every high-risk condition has psychosocial implications for the client and her family. The client's high-risk status can affect her lifestyle, her stress level, and the status of the newborn. In addition, the frequent assessments necessary in high-risk pregnancy are constant reminders that problems exist. The nurse can assist the family to adapt to the high-risk situation and to participate in therapies that will promote a positive outcome for mother and neonate.

Nursing strategies always include an emphasis on psychosocial and cultural as well as physiologic aspects of client care. For conceptual ease, specific high-risk conditions occurring during the second and third trimesters of pregnancy are discussed in this chapter. Psychosocial implications of high-risk pregnancy are discussed in Chapter 12.

▶ HYPERTENSIVE DISORDERS

Hypertensive disorders of pregnancy are a leading medical cause of maternal deaths in the Western world. Pregnancy-induced hypertension is also the most frequently reported risk factor in the United States. It occurs most often among women with a predisposition for chronic hypertension. Hypertension prevalence is known to be greater among women of

color. Thus, these women are at higher risk for becoming hypertensive with pregnancy.

▶ Definition and Classification

Hypertension in pregnancy is operationally defined as a blood pressure of at least 140/90 mm Hg (Cunningham et al., 1997).

The hypertensive diseases of pregnancy have been classified in the United States by the Working Group on High Blood Pressure in Pregnancy, convened by the National High Blood Pressure Education Program of the National Heart, Lung, and Blood Institute. Their definition identifies four categories of hypertension associated with pregnancy: (1) pregnancy-induced hypertension, with subcategories of preeclampsia and eclampsia; (2) chronic hypertension; (3) chronic hypertension with superimposed preeclampsia; and (4) transient or gestational hypertension (National High Blood Pressure Education Program, 1990).

Pregnancy-Induced Hypertension

Pregnancy-induced hypertension (PIH) refers to conditions characterized by an abnormal rise in blood pressure during pregnancy. **Preeclampsia** is a progressive form of PIH characterized by proteinuria and/or generalized edema that occurs initially after 20 weeks of gestation. It is a disease that primarily affects primigravid women at the extremes of reproductive age. Multigravid women with multiple gestation, diabetes, vascular disease, or chronic renal disease are also at risk (Cunningham et al., 1997). Preeclampsia may be mild or severe, although the distinction between the two is inexact. What appears to be mild preeclampsia can swiftly become a critical condition.

Eclampsia is a critical condition in which preeclamptic signs are accompanied by grand mal seizures, coma, and/or shock precipitated by the PIH. A correlation between severity of hypertension and seizure activity has not been documented. Seizures may occur in the antepartum, intrapartum, or early postpartum period (Lubarsky, Barton, Friedman, Nasreddin, Ramadan, & Sibai, 1994). Eclampsia is rare among women in whom preeclampsia is promptly diagnosed and treated, and the greatest morbidity and mortality associated with PIH are attributed to eclampsia.

Chronic Hypertensive Disease in Pregnancy

Chronic hypertension is diagnosed prior to the 20th week of gestation or persists beyond 6 weeks postpartum (James, Steer, Weiner, & Gonik, 1994). Blood pressure elevations are noted on at least three separate occasions and may occur in the presence of diabetes mellitus or other chronic medical conditions.

Chronic Hypertension with Superimposed Preeclampsia

This disorder occurs when chronic hypertension is complicated by further increases in blood pressure during pregnancy.

Transient or Gestational Hypertension

When a previously normotensive woman experiences an elevation in blood pressure after 20 weeks of gestation, or in the intrapartum or early postpartum period without proteinuria or other signs and symptoms of PIH, transient or gestational hypertension is said to occur. Blood pressure usually does not exceed 140/90 mm Hg and returns to normal within 10 days after delivery.

▶ Pregnancy-Induced Hypertension

Pregnancy-induced hypertension is a major cause of perinatal and maternal mortality. It is often associated with intrauterine growth retardation and an increased tendency toward mental retardation in surviving offspring. If detected and managed early, its negative impact may be minimized or avoided.

Theories of Causation

Over the years, numerous theories for the etiology of PIH have been proposed. Theories have attributed PIH to abnormal immunologic responses of the woman, hereditary factors, overall physiologic and psychologic stress, placental parasites, nutritional excesses or deficiencies (especially protein deficiency) and endocrine disturbances. To date, the actual cause of PIH remains unknown (Cunningham et al., 1997).

Risk Factors

Several risk factors for PIH have been identified.

1. *Parity.* Primigravid women or women pregnant for the first time after an abortion are more susceptible to PIH than multiparous women.
2. *Family history.* Increased risk if blood relatives had PIH.
3. *Multiple pregnancy.* The incidence of PIH is six times greater with twin gestation. Risk increases with more fetuses.
4. *Diabetes.* Women with diabetes have increased incidence of PIH.

5. *Trophoblastic disease.* Increased risk is related to excessive trophoblastic tissue. Onset of PIH prior to 20 weeks gestation is suggestive of a hydatidiform mole.
6. *Fetal hydrops* (profound fetal edema reflecting fetal–maternal blood incompatibility). This is associated with a tenfold increase in incidence of PIH.
7. *Chronic hypertension or renal disease.* There is an increased risk of PIH, fetal death, and abruptio placentae with both disorders. PIH may occur earlier than usual when these conditions are present.
8. *Age extremes.* Women younger than 16, or older than 35, are at increased risk.
9. *Previous PIH.* Severe preeclampsia or eclampsia predisposes to reccurrence of PIH.
10. *Poor pregnancy outcome.* Poor outcome may be indicative of underlying risk.
11. *Malnutrition.*

Pathophysiologic Processes of Pregnancy-Induced Hypertension

Decreased levels of prostaglandins, unusual sensitivity to angiotensin II, impaired glomerular perfusion, and decreased uteroplacental perfusion are evident in preeclampsia. It is by no means clear in what sequence these processes take place.

Vasospasm is basic to the disease process of preeclampsia and accounts for the development of arterial hypertension. Vasospasm takes place throughout the arterial system, including the arteries of major organs, such as the uterus and placenta. Over time the vascular walls are damaged. In clients experiencing PIH, angiotensin II, which normally is increased during pregnancy, but to which these individuals are more sensitive, makes intravascular endothelial cells contract, creating leaks through which platelets and fibrin pass to be deposited subendothelially. Injury to the blood vessels thus may decrease platelet and fibrinogen levels. Red blood cells may be damaged or destroyed as they move through narrowed parts of blood vessels. Vascular changes and local tissue hypoxia account for the lesions, hemorrhage, infarction, and necrosis that have been observed in many organs throughout the body including the ocular retinas, placenta, liver, lungs, and brain. The progression of preeclampsia to eclampsia may be caused by the formation of cerebrovascular occlusion by these lesions. This can lead to cerebrovascular accident (stroke). Vascular damage accounts for the presence of abnormally high levels of protein in the urine of patients with preeclampsia.

The characteristic renal lesion in preeclampsia is glomerular endothelial cell swelling with fibrin deposits. Glomerular capillary lumens become narrowed and glomerular filtration is reduced. Renal tubules demonstrate ischemia and deposition of protein materials. Serum blood urea nitrogen (BUN) and creatinine levels rise, sodium is retained, and urine output decreases. The sodium retention may contribute to the increased sensitivity to angiotensin II and the increased extracellular fluid volume. In severe cases arterial thrombosis can lead to renal cortical necrosis. The glomerular lesions usually heal once the pregnancy ends, but some clients demonstrate glomerular damage even years later.

As in any hypertensive state, the workload of the heart is increased. Clients with preeclampsia do not demonstrate the typical pregnancy-related 2000-mL increase in blood volume, probably because of the contracted vascular bed and the increased vascular permeability and extravasation of fluid into the extravascular compartment. They experience hypovolemia and hemoconcentration. Feedback from pressoreceptors in the vital organs demands increasing cardiac output to ensure maintenance of homeostasis.

The presence of generalized edema reflects vascular damage, decreased glomerular filtration, and hypertension. Implications include the development of increased central nervous system irritability reflecting cerebral edema, the onset of retinal edema, the development of dyspnea related to pulmonary edema, and the onset of congestive heart failure.

Probably because of the leakage of blood components into the extravascular space, a consumptive coagulopathy similar to disseminated intravascular coagulation may be observed. This contributes to a heightened vulnerability to hemorrhage.

In severe PIH liver function may be altered. Hepatic edema, subcapsular edema, or hemorrhage may account for the right upper quadrant or epigastric pain in severe preeclampsia. This pain may indicate that seizures are about to occur. Placental vasospasm and the development of infarcts can result in intrauterine growth retardation and fetal hypoxia. Vasospasm of cerebral vasculature probably accounts for the persistent headaches or visual disturbances associated with severe preeclampsia.

Sequelae of PIH represent serious threats to maternal and fetal well-being. They include abruptio placentae; retinal detachment; acute renal failure; cardiac failure; cerebral hemorrhage; maternal death; and fetal growth retardation, hypoxia, and death. About 70% of fetal deaths are due to large placental infarcts, markedly small placental size, and abruptio placentae.

Symptoms subside as soon as the placenta is delivered. The vascular bed will dilate in early postpartum and the hematocrit will fall. These women are unusually sensitive to blood loss at delivery. It is important to note that preeclampsia as well as eclampsia can emerge intrapartally or postpartally, even if there is no evidence of symptoms prenatally. The first 48 hours after delivery is a period of great risk.

Signs and Symptoms

Assessment is based on an understanding of signs and symptoms of PIH. Signs and symptoms of PIH include elevated blood pressure, edema, proteinuria, impending eclampsia, and eclampsia.

Blood Pressure. Identification of blood pressure elevation was described earlier in the chapter.

Edema. Many women develop some generalized edema during pregnancy; however, edema that occurs in association with hypertension or proteinuria indicates that pathophysiologic processes are occurring. Preeclampsia may be indicated by the presence of dependent edema on arising, a woman's inability to remove rings from her fingers, and a weight gain exceeding 1.5 kg per week during the third trimester (Fig. 19–1). Edema is described on a scale of 1+ to 4+, as explained in Table 19–1.

Proteinuria. **Proteinuria** is defined as the presence of 300 mg or more of protein in a 24-hour urine collection, or a concentration of 1 g/L or more in at least two random samples collected at least 6 hours apart (Cunningham et al., 1997). This is reflected in a 1+ to 2+ result with the standard turbidimetric (dipstick) method of testing. In contrast, trace protein in urine in the absence of hypertension, edema, or both represents a normal physiologic adaptation to pregnancy and is not a cause for concern.

Impending Eclampsia. Preeclampsia may progress to eclampsia, the convulsive phase of PIH. In severe cases, clients may experience frontal or sometimes occipital headache that is not relieved by analgesics, visual disturbances (e.g., blurring, visual spots or "floaters"), right upper quadrant or epigastric pain, nausea, or vomiting, and may exhibit hyperreflexia, altered sensorium, irritability, onset of fever, cyanosis, pulmonary edema, or oliguria (Cunningham et al., 1997). These symptoms herald the progression of preeclampsia to eclampsia.

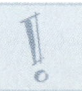

Nursing Alert

Proteinuria is a late sign in the course of preeclampsia and represents an increased risk of fetal mortality.

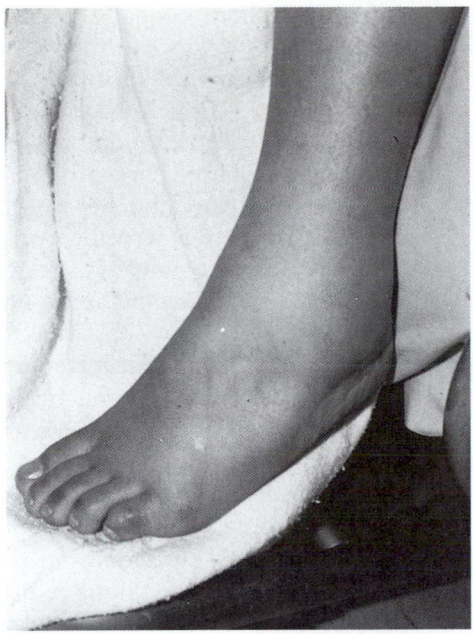 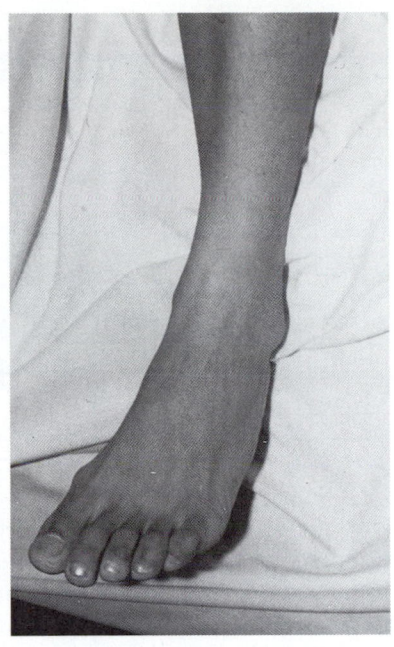

A   B

FIGURE 19–1. A. Severe edema in a young primigravida with antepartum eclampsia and a markedly reduced blood volume compared with normal pregnancy. **B.** The same woman 3 days after delivery. The remarkable clearance of pedal edema, accompanied by diuresis and a 28-pound weight loss, was spontaneous and unprovoked by any diuretic drug therapy. *(Reproduced, with permission, from Cunningham, F.G., & Pritchard, J.A. (1984). How should hypertension during pregnancy be managed? Experience at Parkland Memorial Hospital. Medical Clinics of North America, 68, 505–526.)*

Eclampsia. Eclampsia is marked by the occurrence of tonic–clonic seizures or vascular collapse. In the event of seizures, the following signs are observed: a prodromal facial twitching lasting only a few seconds, a tonic contraction of the entire body lasting about 20 seconds, and a convulsion lasting about a minute. During this time, the woman may not breathe. After the convulsion, the client may fall into a coma lasting minutes or hours. Eclampsia is an obstetric emergency.

Nursing and Collaborative Assessment

Preeclampsia. All clients are screened for signs and symptoms of preeclampsia at each prenatal visit, especially during the second and third trimesters.

▶ **TABLE 19-1**

Assessment of Pitting Edema

1+	Edema is minimal at pedal and pretibial sites.
2+	Edema of lower extremities is marked.
3+	Edema is evident in face, hands, lower abdominal wall, and sacrum.
4+	Generalized massive edema (anasarca) is evident with ascites (abdominal distension resulting from the accumulation of fluid in the peritoneal cavity).

Chapters 15, 17, and 18 outline routine assessment parameters during prenatal visits.

In assessing the client with preeclampsia, attention is focused on the following areas:

- Blood pressure monitoring
- Presence of protein in urine
- Presence and degree of edema
- Pattern of weight gain
- Deep tendon reflexes
- Fetal growth, activity, and heart rate
- Presence of warning signs such as headache, visual disturbances, and right upper quadrant or epigastric pain

Serum glucose may be assessed, as diabetic clients have a higher incidence of preeclampsia than nondiabetic women.

For severe preeclampsia, complete blood chemistry, serum liver and renal function tests, 24-hour urine collection for protein and creatinine clearance, and serial hematocrit levels are obtained. Screening for the presence of disseminated intravascular coagulopathy is also done. Blood specimens are sent for determination of prothrombin time, partial thromboplastin time, platelet count, fibrinogen levels, and the presence of fibrin split products. Laboratory findings in PIH are summarized in Table 19–2.

▶ **TABLE 19–2**

Laboratory Findings in Pregnancy-Induced Hypertension

↑	Serum uric acid
↑	Blood urea nitrogen
↑	Serum creatinine
↓	Serum albumin
↓	Globulin
↑	Hematocrit
↓	Platelets
↑	SGOT (serum glutamic-oxaloacetic transaminase)
↑	SGPT (serum glutamic-pyruvic transaminase)
↑	Serum bilirubin
↑	Burr cells (fragmented red blood cells)

If the preeclamptic client is hospitalized, her sensorium, affect, and vital signs, including blood pressure, pulse, respirations, and deep tendon reflexes, are assessed and recorded every 4 hours, or more frequently if she is unstable. Fetal heart rate is recorded at the time maternal vital signs are assessed. Continuous fetal monitoring may be used to assess fetal status. The maternal lungs are assessed for rales, indicating pulmonary edema. Nail beds are assessed for cyanosis. The woman is asked if she experiences any of the symptoms of impending eclampsia described previously. If the client is stable, a late-night assessment may be eliminated in order not to interrupt her sleep.

Prior to term, fetal assessment for the preeclamptic client may include evaluation of fetal activity records, nonstress tests, contraction stress tests, ultrasound with Doppler studies of the placenta and fetal blood vessels, and biophysical profile. Tests for fetal maturity, such as amniocentesis for the lecithin: sphingomeylin ratio and phosphatidylglycerol, may be performed in order to plan delivery (see Chapter 18).

Eclampsia. If eclampsia occurs, the nurse notes the onset, course, and duration of the convulsions. Vital signs are monitored every 5 minutes until stable and every 15 minutes afterward. The client's lung fields are assessed for pulmonary edema. Blood is obtained for typing and cross-matching. Studies are the same as for severe preeclampsia. Fetal heart rate is determined and continuous fetal monitoring is initiated.

Nursing and Collaborative Management

Preeclampsia. Early detection and management of preeclampsia are associated with the greatest success in reducing risks and progression of this condition. Delivery is the most effective treatment for PIH. Management goals focus on maintaining pregnancy until the fetus is mature. In cases of severe preeclampsia or eclampsia, however, an immature neonate who

receives excellent neonatal intensive care may have a better chance of survival than if not delivered.

Disease severity is the critical indicator for hospital admission. In circumstances of mild preeclampsia without fetal deterioration, some providers may elect to allow a reliable woman to remain at home on bedrest. The client and her family must understand the need for bedrest as indicated, must be able to recognize and report symptoms related to progression of the disease process, and must make certain that the client is assessed by her health care providers as appropriate. Two to three examinations are provided weekly, often in the home by home health nurses. Hospitalization and more aggressive therapy is indicated for worsening disease.

Modified bedrest in the left lateral position may be advised for the client with mild preeclampsia. This position decreases pressure on the vena cava and is believed to improve venous return and placental and renal perfusion. With increased renal perfusion, excess fluid is mobilized, urine output increases, and blood pressure may stabilize or decrease. Dietary restrictions are no longer advised, and the client may follow a reg-

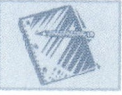 *Client Teaching*

Home Treatment for Mild Preeclampsia

The nurse can suggest the following strategies for the client experiencing preeclampsia:

- Try to stay in bed as much as possible and lie on your left side. You may notice an increase in voiding after you have been on bedrest for one or two days. This is normal and a positive sign.

- Eat a well-balanced diet with moderate salt intake and increase your fluid intake to 6 to 8 8-oz glasses per day.

- Try to keep a quiet environment with minimal stimulation. Excess stimuli can aggravate PIH.

- See your health care provider at least one or two times a week for a blood pressure check and to check on your baby's well-being. It is important that you keep these appointments.

- If you experience any of the following symptoms, inform your health care provider: headache, visual disturbances, abdominal or epigastric pain, or increased swelling.

ular, well-balanced diet as tolerated. Home management should also include frequent observation of mother and fetus, daily urine protein analysis (notify provider if 2+ or more), home blood pressure monitoring by the woman (Fig. 19–2), and teaching that includes the danger signs of a worsening condition. Emotional support is an important component of home management. The home health nurse collaborating with the primary provider should facilitate appropriate referrals for support services as needed.

Clients who have more than mild signs and symptoms of preeclampsia are hospitalized. Those with severe preeclampsia are very ill and require careful observation. The hospitalized client is kept on bedrest, although whether or not bedrest is complete will depend on her actual situation. The client is protected from central nervous system stimuli such as loud noise and bright light, which may aggravate central nervous system irritability. In some facilities the client is sedated; however, sedatives do not prevent seizures, and oversedation can further compromise the fetus.

Magnesium sulfate is the treatment of choice to prevent convulsions (see box entitled Drug Guide: Magnesium Sulfate) (Karch, 1998). Reflexes and respiratory status are assessed and blood levels of magnesium sulfate monitored to ensure that the therapeutic level is not exceeded. Therapeutic blood levels of MgSO$_4$ are 4–8 mg/dl (Cunningham et al., 1997). Loss

of deep tendon reflexes can occur over 10 mg/dl and respiratory arrest may develop if levels exceed 12 mg/dl. The drug is usually withheld if the client's respiratory rate is less than 12 per minute. Intake and output are recorded. A Foley catheter provides accurate output measurements. An hourly output of less than 25 to 30 cc should be reported. Magnesium sulfate is excreted renally, and diminished output can predispose the woman to magnesium toxicity.

When magnesium sulfate is prescribed, calcium gluconate must be available at the bedside to counter potential toxic effects. The emergency cart and defibrillator are close at hand and checked daily. Wall suction and oxygen should be available in the maternity unit for immediate use.

If diastolic pressure exceeds 110 mm Hg, an antihypertensive drug, such as hydralazine, may be administered intravenously to lower diastolic pressure to between 90 and 100 mm Hg. This is a short-term intervention. In preeclampsia, placental perfusion is already compromised. Decreasing maternal blood pressure can further reduce placental perfusion and stress the fetus (Cunningham et al., 1997). Fetal heart rate and maternal vital signs are assessed continuously during therapy.

Intravenous routes are maintained, and fluid therapy is calculated to avoid cardiac overload. Ringer's lactate is often used. Daily weights may be recorded to assess fluid retention. Hemodynamic monitoring with a central venous pressure line or, more commonly, pulmonary artery (Swan–Ganz) catheter may be performed.

If preeclampsia is severe, the decision may be to deliver the child as soon as the woman is stabilized. If clinically indicated, vaginal delivery may be attempted through induction with intravenous oxytocin. Cesarean delivery is performed if induction is unsuccessful.

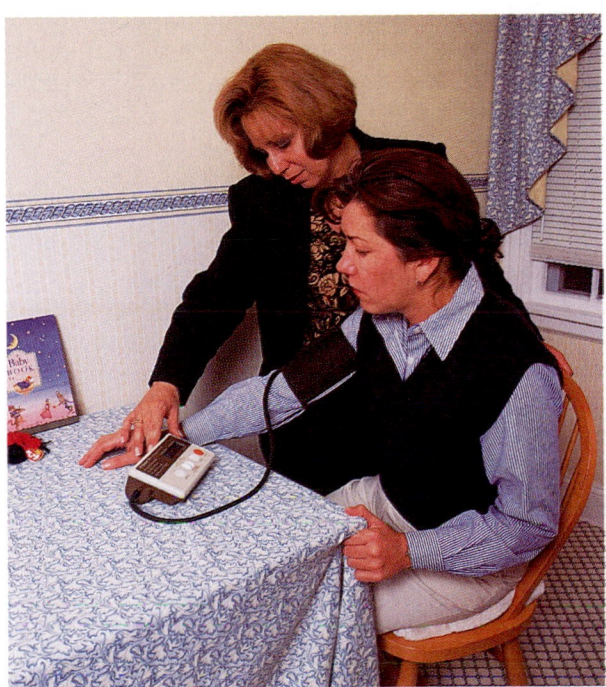

FIGURE 19–2. Home blood pressure monitoring by woman experiencing mild preeclampsia.

Nursing Alert

Signs of magnesium sulfate toxicity:

- Respirations < 12/minute
- Absence of deep tendon reflexes
- Serum MgSO$_4$ levels > 8 mg/dl
- Diminished sensorium, drowsiness
- Urine output < 30ml/hr

► DRUG GUIDE: MAGNESIUM SULFATE (EPSOM SALT, MgSO₄)

ACTIONS/INDICATIONS

Competes with calcium to block release of acetylcholine causing smooth muscle relaxation. Results in decrease in activity of the CNS, motor neurons, and heart. Used for prevention and control of seizures by causing vasodilatation and prevention of uterine contractions in preterm labor by relaxing uterine muscle.

DOSAGE

Administered parenterally. IV loading bolus (4 g over 20 minutes) is given, followed by continuous infusion (2–3 g/hr) via infusion pump. Therapeutic blood levels are 4–8 mg/dl (Cunningham et al., 1997).

CONTRAINDICATIONS AND PRECAUTIONS

Use with caution in clients with impaired renal function. Contraindicated in clients with heart block or myocardial damage.

ADVERSE REACTIONS

Result from magnesium intoxication (overdose). Flushing, sweating, hypotension, depressed reflexes, flaccid paralysis, hypothermia, circulatory collapse, depression of cardiac function, CNS depression, fetal respiratory paralysis.

DRUG INTERACTIONS

- Barbiturates, opiates, general anesthetics, and other CNS depressants: Additive central depressant effects.
- Neuromuscular blocking agents: Additive neuromuscular blocking effect; use concomitantly with extreme caution.

NURSING IMPLICATIONS

- Assess for magnesium toxicity: absent or weak patellar reflex, respirations below 12 per minute, urinary output of less than 25 to 30 ml./per hour.
- Assess vital signs every 30 minutes.
- Assess patellar reflexes at least every 4 hours.
- Draw serum magnesium levels as ordered, usually every 4 to 6 hours.
- Assess fetal heart rate every 15 minutes.
- Place resuscitation equipment in room.
- Place calcium gluconate in room to be readily available if client displays magnesium toxicity.

Eclampsia. Client safety is the primary management concern during eclamptic seizures. The nurse should remain with the client and summon help. Siderails need to be up and padded to prevent injury. The nurse needs to note the timing and sequence of events and record the episode as soon as possible. After seizure activity has ceased, the nurse assesses the client's airway and suctions secretions as needed. Oxygen is administered by mask.

Labor is induced or a cesarean delivery is performed as soon as the client is conscious and oriented. The client and fetus are monitored throughout labor and delivery and the nurse prepares for delivery of the neonate as determined by the interdisciplinary perinatal team. In general, vaginal delivery presents a lower risk than cesarean delivery.

Special Management Considerations

Several approaches to preventing preeclampsia in high-risk women have been proposed. A few studies have examined the use of low-dose aspirin therapy (LDAT) during the second and third trimesters as a means to decrease the incidence of PIH and reduce the risk of low birth weight. The findings, however, have been inconclusive.

Another prevention modality under study is calcium supplementation after the 20th week of gesta-tion. Sanchez-Ramos, Briones, Kaunitz, Delvalle, Gaudier, and Walker (1994) and additional research studies have concluded that calcium supplementation in high-risk pregnant women reduces the risk of PIH. Additional studies are currently underway.

Care Plan

Nursing care for a client with PIH is outlined in the care plan at the end of this chapter.

HELLP Syndrome

A severe consequence of preeclampsia may be the development of the HELLP syndrome, a potentially fatal condition characterized by *h*emolysis, *e*levated *l*iver enzymes, and *l*ow *p*latelet count. Its pathophysiology is depicted in Figure 19–3. Arteriolar vasospasm is the underlying factor in the sequence of events. The precise cause of hepatic failure is unknown, but it may be the formation of microemboli in the hepatic vasculature, causing ischemia and tissue damage. Delivery is the only definitive treatment for HELLP syndrome; however, the symptoms may persist for several days after delivery. Management of the altered hemodynamic status and clotting represents the major challenge in medical management of the HELLP syndrome.

► Chronic Hypertension

Hypertensive cardiovascular disease is marked by the formation of fatty deposits within the arterial walls. This increases vascular resistance to the flow of blood and increases the work of the heart. Tissue perfusion throughout the body is diminished as a result, and over a period of years all organs will be adversely affected. Hypertensive cardiovascular disease is a continued elevation of blood pressure of 140/90 or higher before pregnancy or before the 20th week of gestation in the absence of trophoblastic disease.

Many factors are associated with the development of hypertensive cardiovascular disease. Major factors include family history of hypertension, race (increased prevalence among African-Americans), a sedentary lifestyle, use of tobacco, excessive use of alcohol, obesity, a diet high in cholesterol and triglycerides, a stressful lifestyle and inappropriate means of coping, and a history of PIH. The client with chronic hypertension may have an underlying predisposing condition such as renal disease.

It is difficult to distinguish chronic hypertension from PIH, particularly in a woman who has not received early prenatal care. Because blood pressure may normally decrease in the first and second trimesters, blood pressure measurements for the woman with chronic hypertension may appear normal. Typically, as pregnancy progresses the blood pressure returns to its hypertensive state.

Nursing and Collaborative Assessment

Chronic hypertensive disease, in contrast to preeclampsia, is suggested by the observation of hemorrhages and exudates in the optic fundi; plasma creatinine concentrations greater than 1 mg/dL; plasma urea nitrogen concentrations greater than 20 mg/dL; and the presence of other predisposing chronic diseases such as diabetes, connective tissue disease, or renal disease.

Complications of chronic hypertension in pregnant women include abruptio placentae, intrauterine growth retardation, and superimposed preeclampsia.

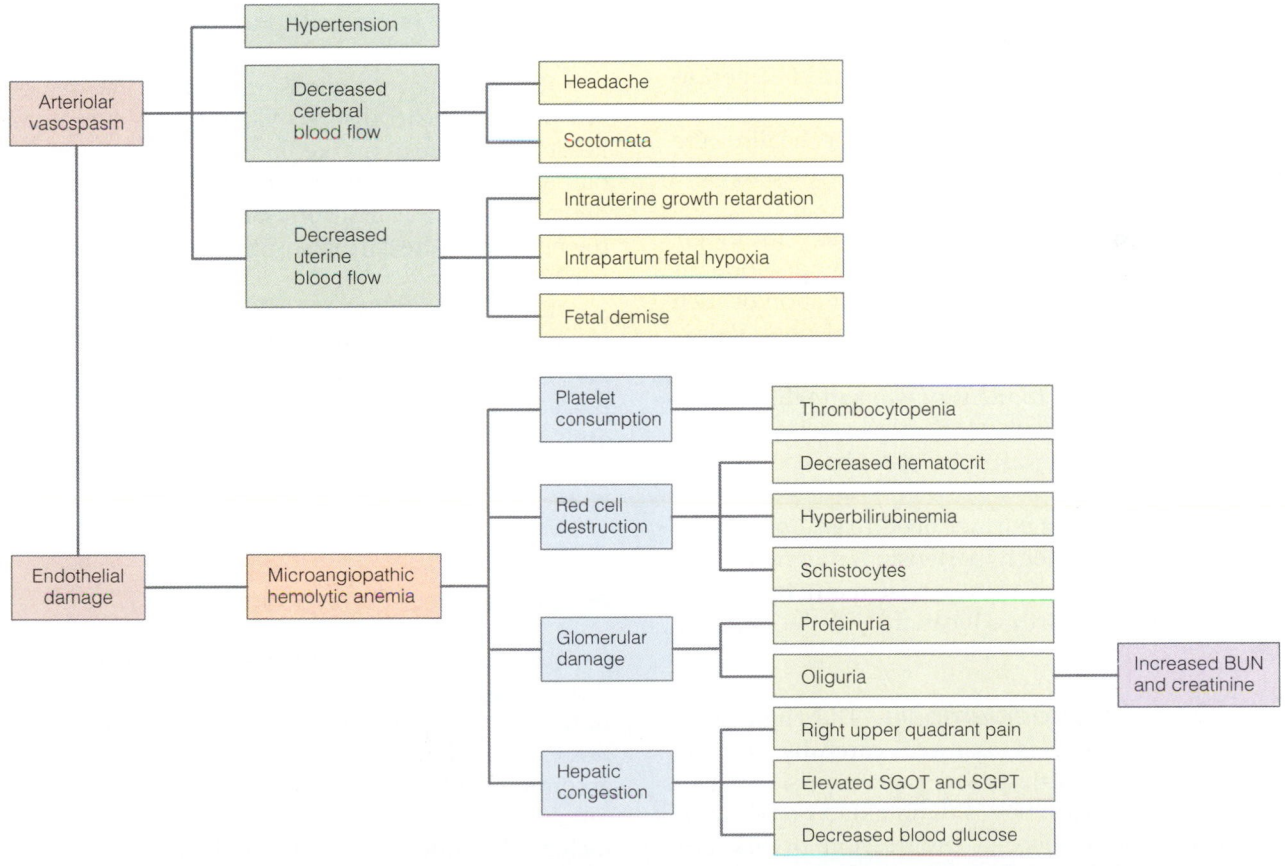

FIGURE 19–3. Physiologic alterations occurring in the HELLP syndrome. BUN: blood urea nitrogen; SGOT: serum glutamic-oxaloacetic transaminase; SGPT: serum glutamic-pyruvic transaminase. *(Reproduced, with permission, from Whittaker, A.A. et al. (1986). Hemolysis, elevated liver enzymes, and low platelet count syndrome. Nursing care of the critically ill obstetric patient. Heart and Lung 15:402–408.)*

Nursing and Collaborative Management

Some experts believe that chronic hypertension is best left untreated during pregnancy unless diastolic pressure exceeds 110 mm Hg. Otherwise, treatment could mask the onset of preeclampsia until that disease process is well advanced. Furthermore, control of chronic hypertension does not seem to reduce the client's risk of developing PIH (Cunningham et al., 1997).

According to a different perspective, the client with chronic hypertension should be treated during pregnancy just as she would be routinely. Blood pressure is evaluated weekly. Tests to assess fetal well-being are performed (see Chapters 17 and 18).

The most frequently used anti-hypertensive medications today are methyldopa and hydrazaline. Labetalol and nifedipine are becoming more common as well (James et al., 1994). The woman remains at home as long as her blood pressure is controlled; hospitalization is indicated when better control needs to be established.

The nurse needs to review the client's regimen for maintenance of her condition with her, including explicit teaching about the medication regimen and observation of untoward effects. Reinforcement and clarification are provided as needed. Blood pressure is carefully assessed at each contact. The nurse carefully observes the client for the development of superimposed preeclampsia and for evidence of fetal distress. The client is instructed to contact her health care provider without delay if any of the warning signs of pregnancy occur.

Pregnancy is not the appropriate time to undertake a weight control program, but moderation in sodium intake is appropriate, as is elimination of such hazardous substances as smoking and alcohol. Relaxation techniques can be taught. The client's life situation may be reviewed to identify ways in which overall stress can be reduced. Moderate exercise such as walking can be undertaken in the absence of preeclampsia.

The client and her partner need reassurance that, with good control of her hypertension, pregnancy can progress normally. They can exercise many options in planning their childbirth education and the delivery itself.

Superimposed Preeclampsia. The client with chronic hypertension is assessed carefully for the development of superimposed preeclampsia, which occurs in 25% of cases. She is maintained on her anti-hypertensive medication. If progression of the disease is observed, hospitalization may be warranted. If the preeclampsia worsens during a course of bedrest, the fetus may need to be delivered without delay.

▶ HEART DISEASE

▶ Types of Heart Disease

Heart disease is the leading medical cause of maternal mortality. Cardiac disease affects approximately 1% of all pregnant women, with rheumatic heart disease and congenital heart disease accounting for most of the cases (Cunningham et al., 1997). Mitral stenosis is the most common lesion present in women with rheumatic heart disease (Kennedy, 1995).

▶ Pregnancy Risks for Mother and Infant

The likelihood of a favorable outcome for the mother with heart disease and her fetus depends in part on the functional capacity of her heart. The New York Heart Association (NYHA) has classified individuals with heart disease on the basis of past and present disability. See Table 19–3 for a description of the classes. Mortality risk associated with pregnancy for NYHA classes I and II is considered to be less than 1%. Classes III and IV carry a 4 to 7% mortality risk and pregnancy is generally not recommended (Cunningham et al., 1997).

Risk for the mother is related to the degree of symptomatic heart disease. Clients with symptomatic heart disease are at markedly increased risk for maternal morbidity and mortality due to the increased demands of the heart from larger blood volume and the need for more cardiac output during normal pregnancy.

Risks to the fetus include spontaneous abortion, intrauterine growth retardation, premature delivery, and intrauterine death. An additional risk is inheritance of congenital heart disease. Genetic counseling and fetal echocardiography are recommended to determine the risk and/or presence of congenital heart disease in the fetus.

▶ Signs and Symptoms

One of the following confirms the presence of heart disease in pregnancy: a diastolic, presystolic, or continuous heart murmur; unequivocal cardiac enlargement; a loud, harsh systolic murmur especially if accompanied by a thrill; and severe arrhythmia (Cunningham et al., 1997). Additional observations may include distended neck veins and pulmonary rales.

Cardiac decompensation, or congestive heart failure, occurs when the heart cannot keep up with the load placed on it. Normal homeostatic mechanisms, such as increasing heart rate, are mobilized without

▶ **TABLE 19-3**

Classification of Functional Capacity in Individuals with Heart Disease

Class I	*Uncompromised:* These individuals have no symptoms of cardiac insufficiency or anginal pain. Physical activity is not restricted.
Class II	*Slightly compromised:* These individuals with cardiac disease experience discomfort in the form of fatigue, palpitation, dyspnea, or angina if they undertake ordinary physical activity. Physical activity is slightly limited.
Class III	*Markedly compromised:* These individuals experience fatigue, palpitation, dyspnea, or angina when they undertake less than ordinary activity. Physical activity is markedly restricted.
Class IV	These individuals are unable to perform any physical activity without discomfort. Symptoms of cardiac insufficiency or angina may occur even at rest.

Source: American Heart Association, New York City Affiliate, 1994.

success. Venous blood backs up into the general circulatory system and into the pulmonary circulation. This accounts for the observation of progressive symptoms including generalized edema, distension of neck veins, dyspnea, pulmonary rales, and frequent moist cough (Table 19–4). Heart rate increases to the extent that the electrical conduction system develops irregularities. The woman experiences palpitations, and ectopic beats can be observed on cardiac monitoring.

▶ **Collaborative Assessment and Management**

Mortality risk in pregnancy for the woman with heart disease is based on her potential inability to adapt to the physiologic demands of pregnancy. The importance of preconceptional counseling for these women cannot be overstated. Preconceptional counseling provides an opportunity to discuss the risks for both client and fetus with the woman and her family; appropriate measures should be performed to establish a functional class; a full history and physical examination with laboratory workup, EKG, and echocardiogram provide baseline data for further evaluation; and referrals for evaluation by a cardiologist, a maternal-fetal medicine subspecialist, genetic counselor, anesthesiologist, cardiothoracic surgeon, and others as appropriate should be arranged. A team approach is essential. Medical problems that are correctable should be treated before pregnancy is attempted and anticoagulation therapy should be adjusted from coumarin to heparin to avoid the risk for fetal warfarin syndrome (Corbett, 1995) (see box entitled Drug Guide: Heparin). Prior medical and sur-

gical records should be obtained and become part of a prenatal record that is available to all members of the health care team.

Once pregnancy is established, the focus of management is on minimizing any extra cardiac demands on the pregnant woman. Cardiac status is assessed carefully at each prenatal visit to identify signs of cardiac compromise. Nutritional counseling focuses on a low sodium diet to prevent excessive blood volume (McAnulty, Metcalfe, & Ueland, 1995). Recommended weight gain depends on the woman's current health status. Prenatal vitamins, iron, and folate are given as necessary to avoid anemia. Anemia triggers a homeostatic response to increase cardiac output, a physiologic response that the heart cannot accommodate. Isometric exercise is advised against and aerobic exercise is limited. The client should avoid heat and humidity. Rest is advised and afternoon naps encouraged. At least 10 hours of sleep per night is recommended. Heavy housework and lifting children should be avoided. Prevention of infection is encouraged and prompt treatment is necessary if infection does occur. Urine is screened monthly for asymptomatic bacteriuria. Pharmacologic management may include diuretics, glycosides, and antiarrhythmic therapy (Table 19–5). Close attention is paid to leg care because of the risk of thromboembolus. The client is counseled to avoid passive sitting and standing. Support hose are recommended. Because of inferior vena cava compression by the gravid uterus, the supine position should be avoided. The client should be provided with honest informed answers to questions to help alleviate unnecessary fears and emotional stress.

Vaginal delivery is the preferred method of delivery for the pregnant cardiac client, with cesarean section reserved for obstetric indications. Strategies to avoid cardiac strain include effective analgesia, the lateral position, and a shortened second stage of labor. Breathing and relaxation techniques, soothing music, massage, and an atmosphere of professional calm and competence reduces anxiety and contributes to the physical and emotional well-being of the client. Prophylactic antibiotic therapy is recommended to pre-

▶ **TABLE 19-4**

Signs and Symptoms of Cardiac Decompensation

Symptoms	Signs
Shortness of breath	Cyanosis
Angina	Cardiac arrhythmias
Palpitations	Abnormal heart sounds
Syncope	Cardiomegaly
Cough	Hepatomegaly
Fatigue	Neck vein distension
	Peripheral edema
	Pulmonary rales

▶ DRUG GUIDE: HEPARIN

ACTIONS/INDICATIONS

Inhibits thrombus and clot formation through the inactivation of thrombin and the potentiation of antithrombin III. Indicated for prophylaxis and treatment of various thromboembolic disorders, venous thrombosis, pulmonary embolism. Also treatment of atrial fibrillation with embolization, diagnosis and treatment of disseminated intravascular coagulation, and treatment of peripheral arterial embolism.

DOSAGE

Administered by IV infusion, intermittent IV injection, or deep SC injection for full-dose therapy and deep SC injection for low-dose therapy. *Full-dose therapy: IV infusion:* Initial bolus dose of 5000 U by direct IV, then 20,000 to 40,000 U in 1000 mL isotonic sodium chloride solution over 24 hours. *Intermittent IV injection:* Initial dose of 10,000 U followed by 5000 to 10,000 U every 4 to 6 hours. *Deep SC:* Initial dose of 10,000 to 20,000 U IV, usually preceded by bolus dose of 5000 U IV, then 8000 to 10,000 U every 8 hours or 15,000 to 20,000 U every 12 hours. Follow PTT (partial thromboplastin time) for adjustment of doses in all regimens. *Low-dose therapy:* 5000 U SC every 8 to 12 hours. *Disseminated intravascular coagulation:* 50 to 100 U/kg by IV infusion or IV injection every 4 hours. If no improvement after 4 to 8 hours, heparin therapy should be discontinued.

CONTRAINDICATIONS AND PRECAUTIONS

Hypersensitivity to pig or beef proteins. Use with caution in cases in which the risk of hemorrhage is increased, such as dissecting aneurysm; ulcerative GI lesions; diverticulitis; hemorrhagic blood dyscrasias; menstruation; ovulation; threatened abortion; subacute bacterial endocarditis; increased capillary permeability; arterial sclerosis; severe hypertension; renal, hepatic, or biliary disease; eye, brain, or spinal cord surgery; continuous tube drainage from any orifice; and spinal tap or spinal anesthesia.

ADVERSE REACTIONS

Most common: minor bleeding. *Less common:* CV—major hemorrhage; hematologic—thrombocytopenia, localized or disseminated thromboses (white clot syndrome); GI—elevated liver enzymes; local reactions—with deep SC injection, local irritation, erythema, mild pain, hematoma, ulceration, or cutaneous and subcutaneous necrosis; other—hypersensitivity reactions, osteoporosis, and spontaneous fractures in clients receiving $\geqq$10,000 U/day for 3 or more months.

DRUG INTERACTIONS

- Aspirin, nonsteroidal anti-inflammatory agents, dipyridamole: Inhibit platelet function and may increase risk of hemorrhage.
- Streptokinase, urokinase: May increase risk of bleeding.
- Dihydroergotamine: May potentiate antithrombogenic effects of heparin.
- IV nitroglycerin: May antagonize anticoagulant effect of heparin.
- Probenecid: Enhances the duration and intensity of effects produced by heparin.

NURSING IMPLICATIONS

- Assess blood coagulation studies. If not within therapeutic range, contact physician.
- Assess for signs of bleeding (e.g., epistaxis, blood in urine, ecchymosis).
- Observe needle sites for hematoma, swelling, heat, redness, and pain.
- Teach client and her partner the signs of hemorrhage and the rationale for the treatment.

---

vent subacute bacterial endocarditis at time of delivery in women with prosthetic heart valves or grafts. When the cervix is fully dilated and the fetus is engaged, prompt forceps delivery is indicated unless an easy, spontaneous vaginal delivery is imminent (Cunningham et al., 1997). Epidural anesthesia is preferred because it generally offers greater hemodynamic stability. However, hypotension is potentially lethal in the pregnant cardiac client, and great care must be taken to avoid it. Blood loss should be minimized. Fundal massage and intravenous oxytocin are suggested. Oxytocin should be administered slowly to avoid hypotension. Early ambulation reduces the increased risk for deep-vein thrombosis and thromboembolism in the postpartum period.

Although pregnancy in class III and IV heart disease is contraindicated, women markedly compromised may become pregnant and wish to continue the pregnancy. Management of these clients includes bedrest throughout the pregnancy. Hospitalization is usually required. The focus of care for women in cardiac failure (class IV) is medical rather than obstetric. Delivery for any woman in frank failure carries with it a high mortality rate.

▶ Nursing Diagnoses

Examples of nursing diagnoses for the client with heart disease are:

► **TABLE 19-5**

Medications Commonly Used in Care of the Pregnant Woman with Heart Disease

Medication	Purpose	Nursing Implications
Cardiac glycoside: digoxin (Lanoxin, Lanoxicaps)	Increases cardiac output	Assess apical pulse rate for 1 full minute and withhold medication if heart rate is less than 60. Monitor for presence of arrhythmias. Provide foods rich in potassium. Withhold medication if gastrointestinal disturbances develop.
Thiazide diuretic: hydrochlorothiazide (HydroDiuril, Hydrochlor)	Treatment of edema associated with congestive heart failure	Encourage client to eat potassium-rich foods. Record weight daily. The client may experience photosensitivity. Last daily dosage should be no later than 3 PM to avoid nocturia. Medication should be taken after meals to reduce gastric irritation.
Anticoagulant: heparin	Anticoagulant	Medication is incompatible with most antibiotics. Assess for evidence of hemorrhage. Rotate subcutaneous injection sites.
Antibiotic prophylaxis: benzathine penicillin, ampicillin, or gentamycin	Prevention of valvular infection for women with rheumatic heart disease	Antibiotics can cause local or generalized hypersensitivity response. Gentamycin is incompatible with other drugs in solution. Client should be questioned regarding medication allergies.
Iron supplement: FeSO$_4$	Prevention of anemia	Dietary fluids and roughage will prevent constipation.

Problem-oriented diagnoses:

- Decreased cardiac output, related to heart disease during pregnancy
- Activity intolerance, related to compromised cardiac status during pregnancy
- Altered family processes, related to pregnant cardiac client's inability to care for family
- Fear in client and family, related to maternal and fetal outcome complicated by cardiac disease during pregnancy

Wellness-oriented diagnoses:

- Potential asset in maintenance of cardiopulmonary functioning during pregnancy, related to functional ability of heart

► DIABETES MELLITUS

Diabetes mellitus is regarded as a major health care complication of pregnancy. Diabetic mothers, especially those whose disease is uncontrolled, are subject to increased morbidity and mortality. Since the discovery of insulin in 1922, maternal mortality rates have declined from almost 50% to less than 5% as compared to a rate of 1 to 2% in the nondiabetic pop-

ulation. According to Cunningham and associates (1997) 2 to 4% of pregnancies are complicated by overt diabetes mellitus. In 90% of these cases the diabetes is a consequence of the metabolic changes of pregnancy; this is termed gestational diabetes. In only 10% of cases is the diabetic condition pregestational.

► Effect of Pregnancy on Carbohydrate Metabolism

Pregnancy causes alterations in carbohydrate metabolism that serve to ensure satisfactory growth of the fetus and establish a maternal energy store (see Chapter 14 for discussion of carbohydrate metabolism during pregnancy).

In the second and third trimesters, there is an increase in placental hormones (human placental lactogen, progesterone, estrogen). These hormones are antagonistic to the effects of insulin, resulting in an increase in insulin requirements and maternal fasting glucose levels. Diminished glucose tolerance may be manifested by glucosuria and slight ketonuria. The exaggerated rate and amount of insulin release and the decreased sensitivity to insulin is referred to as the "diabetogenic effect" of pregnancy.

Client Teaching

Cardiac Disease During Pregnancy

The nurse can suggest the following self-care practices to the pregnant client experiencing cardiac disease:

- Avoid fatigue. It is important to rest frequently during the day and get adequate sleep at night to avoid overstressing the heart.
- Eat a well-balanced diet that is low in sodium and take prenatal vitamins every day to avoid anemia.
- Observe for symptoms that might indicate your heart is being compromised such as fatigue, shortness of breath, chest pain, or cough.
- Prevent infection by avoiding crowds, maintaining good personal hygiene, and washing your hands frequently.
- Keep all of your prenatal appointments that are scheduled by your health care provider.

▶ Pregestational Diabetic Conditions

Pathophysiology

Diabetes mellitus is a complex syndrome, a major feature of which is impaired carbohydrate metabolism. This manifests as hyperglycemia. In the face of excess serum glucose the body is actually starving, as the problem lies in the transport and utilization of carbohydrate molecules. The pancreatic hormone insulin effects this activity. In diabetes, insulin production is impaired, and many diabetic people are dependent on exogenous insulin. Use of fat and protein stores for energy in the absence of carbohydrates leads to a state of ketoacidosis. Because of increased serum osmolality with increased glucose levels, fluids are drawn from cells and the interstices into the vascular bed. Because of the osmotic pressure exerted by glucose in the urine, polyuria is a prominent feature. With intercellular dehydration the individual experiences profound thirst.

Diabetic individuals have accelerated atherosclerotic microvascular disease in which capillary basement membranes thicken. Neuropathy is a serious complication as the disease progesses. With a higher level of glucose in the extracellular fluid, which is conducive to the growth of microorganisms, diabetic individuals are prone to infection. Decreased capillary exchange makes healing difficult. Neuropathy decreases the sensation of peripheral trauma. As a result, undetected skin wounds can quickly lead to gangrenous conditions that may require amputation.

There are two types of diabetes: type I (or insulin-dependent) and type II (non–insulin-dependent). In type I diabetes, the pancreatic beta cells in the islets of Langerhans are smaller and fewer than normal and they produce virtually no insulin. The etiology is unknown, but onset is often sudden. Genetic, environmental, and autoimmune factors may play a role in its development. In type II diabetes, the pancreas is unable to meet increased demands for insulin over time, as is the case in obesity-related type II diabetes, or pancreatic function diminishes over time. There is a familial tendency for type II diabetes.

With insulin deficiency, glucose is not transported from the extracellular into the intracellular compartment, and the cells must oxidize fats and proteins for energy. This results in tissue wasting. As serum glucose level rises, cellular water is pulled into the blood. The hyperosmotic pressure of glucose in the urine accounts for decreased renal tubular resorption of water. Extracellular dehydration develops. The four cardinal symptoms of diabetes, in response to these processes, are polyphagia, polyuria, polydipsia, and weight loss.

Impact of Pregnancy on Preexisting Diabetes

A classification system (White's classification) for diabetes that complicates pregnancy was first developed in 1949, and revised in 1978. The system was adapted by the American College of Obstetricians and Gynecologists for clarification of the relationship between diabetes and pregnancy (Table 19–6).

The normal changes in carbohydrate metabolism that occur during pregnancy make control of preexisting diabetes more difficult. Insulin resistance increases. Nausea and vomiting increase the risk of hypoglycemia and insulin shock. Ketoacidosis develops more easily. Any infection can lead to the rapid onset of ketoacidosis. Some preexisting complications of diabetes are affected by pregnancy while others are not. Purdy and associates (1996) has suggested a significant worsening of renal disease.

▶ Pathogenesis of Gestational Diabetes

Gestational diabetes occurs when the pancreas cannot meet the added demands of pregnancy. Factors indicating risk for gestational diabetes include prior gestational diabetes; prior delivery of or current evidence of a macrosomic infant (greater than 90th percentile weight for gestational age); family history of diabetes; unexplained fetal death; prior delivery or current evidence of an infant with a congenital anomaly; maternal obesity, hypertension, or glycosuria; polyhydramnios; recurrent urinary tract infection or vaginitis; and large or poor weight gain during pregnancy. Half of women who develop gestational diabetes exhibit none of these risk factors (Coustan, 1996). For that reason the American Diabetes Association advocates universal screening by means of an oral carbohydrate load followed by assessment of serum glucose level.

Nursing Alert

Fetal risk is most closely related to the degree of glycemic control achieved during pregnancy. Pregestational diabetics are at highest risk for fetal morbidity and mortality (Buchanan & Coustan, 1995).

▶ Diabetic Emergencies

Ketoacidosis

The development of ketoacidosis is associated with a fetal mortality rate of 50 to 90%. It develops over hours or days when insulin levels are inadequate. As fats are metabolized for energy, ketones are produced faster than the body can catabolize them. Metabolic acidosis occurs and, in severe cases, results in diabetic coma. The need for insulin is increased by such factors as pregnancy, trauma, infection, development of insulin resistance, and psychologic stress. Women treated for premature labor with beta-sympathomimetic drugs may develop ketoacidosis (Cunningham et al., 1997). Signs and symptoms of early and late ketoacidosis are presented in Table 19–7.

Hypoglycemia

Hypoglycemia is the most common cause of coma in diabetic clients; nearly all insulin-dependent diabetic clients experience hypoglycemia at some time. It is especially likely when a woman is trying to maintain strict euglycemic control during pregnancy. Onset is rapid, occurring in minutes. Hypoglycemia may result from decreased food intake, vomiting, increased exertion, or modification of insulin dose. Change to a more purified form of insulin or to human-derived insulin can result in hypoglycemia. Signs and symptoms are listed in Table 19–7.

▶ Effects of Diabetes on Maternal–Infant Outcomes

There are numerous adverse effects of diabetes on pregnancy. Burrow and Ferris (1995) report a 15 to 31% incidence of hypertensive disorders in pregnant diabetics. It is found in at least one-third of women with preexisting vascular disease. Infection is more frequent and more severe, and diabetic women are at higher risk for urinary tract infection than nondiabetic pregnant women. There is an increased risk of cesarean delivery because of dystocia. Polyhydramnios plus a larger-than-usual fetus can lead to cardiopulmonary

---

▶ TABLE 19–6

Classification of Diabetes Complicating Pregnancy

		Pregestational Diabetes		
Class	Age at Onset	Duration (years)	Vascular Disease	Therapy
A[a]	Any	Any	None	A-1, diet only
B	>20	<10	None	Insulin
C	10–19 or	10–19	None	Insulin
D	<10 or	>20	Benign retinopathy	Insulin
F	Any	Any	Nephropathy	Insulin
R	Any	Any	Proliferative retinopathy	Insulin
H	Any	Any	Heart disease	Insulin

	Gestational Diabetes		
Class	Fasting Plasma Glucose		Postprandial Plasma Glucose
A-1	<105 mg/dL	and	<120 mg/dL
A-2	>105 mg/dL	and/or	>120 mg/dL

[a]Chemical diabetes.

Reprinted, with permission, from the American College of Obstetricians and Gynecologists. (1986). Classification of diabetes in pregnancy (ACOG Technical Bulletin No. 92). Washington, DC: Author.

► **TABLE 19-7**

Signs and Symptoms of Ketoacidosis and Hypoglycemia

	Onset	Signs and Symptoms	
		Early	Late
Ketoacidosis	Slow, over hours or days	Polyuria Polydipsia Malaise	Rapid, deep breathing Hypothermia Acetone breath Nausea and vomiting Abdominal pain Coma Death
Hypoglycemia	Rapid, within minutes	Tachycardia Diaphoresis Tremor Hunger Pallor Dizziness Irritability Nausea Headache Paresthesia	Confusion Strange behavior Stupor Convulsions Stroke syndrome Coma

symptoms in the mother. Diabetic women demonstrate less of the normal increase in cardiac output that normally accompanies pregnancy. This may contribute to the diminished uteroplacental perfusion observed in diabetic women, and to decreased fetal oxygenation. Diabetic women also demonstrate a greater incidence of postpartum hemorrhage. According to Boden (1996), women with gestational diabetes are more likely than the general population to develop type II (or non–insulin-dependent) diabetes.

In addition, diabetes has adverse effects on the fetus. If the disease is not well controlled the fetal death rate is significantly higher than among the general population. Reece and Eriksson (1996) reported that the incidence of congenital anomalies is 6 to 10% when the woman is diabetic. Congenital malformations have also emerged as a significant contributor to perinatal loss. Malformations account for 40% of perinatal mortality. Infants of diabetic mothers are subject to a higher morbidity rate. This may result from birth trauma because of their tendency toward macrosomia, or it may result from respiratory distress or metabolic imbalance disorders such as hypoglycemia and hypocalcemia.

Women with vascular complications that compromise uteroplacental blood flow may have small-for-gestational-age infants. Infants of diabetic mothers are born prematurely more often than the general population. There is an increased incidence of fetal distress during labor among infants of diabetic mothers. Tachypnea, polycythemia, and hyperbilirubinemia occur more frequently than in the general population.

These infants have an increased incidence of respiratory distress syndrome even at term. Common congenital malformations that are seen in the infant of the diabetic mother are neural tube defects, caudal regression syndrome (hypoplasia of the sacrum and lower extremities), and cardiac and other vascular defects. Neurologic symptoms such as seizure activity are observed in children of diabetic women more often than among the general population. Finally, the children of diabetic mothers are at increased risk of developing obesity and diabetes. See Chapter 32 for further discussion of the effects of diabetes on the newborn. Problems related to maternal diabetes can be minimized in the newborn if maternal glucose levels are well controlled prior to and throughout pregnancy.

► ## Collaborative Assessment

Several sources recommend screening all pregnant women between the 24th and 28th weeks of pregnancy using a 50-g oral glucose load followed by a serum glucose determination 1 hour later. The woman need not be fasting for the screening test. However, sensitivity is improved in the fasting state. If the test is given without regard for fasting, 140 mg/dL is the upper limit of normal. If the test is given when the woman is fasting, the upper acceptable limit is 135 mg/dL. Clients who exceed these limits should be further evaluated with a 3-hour glucose tolerance test (GTT). If the screening value exceeds 190 mg/dL, a fasting blood glucose test should be done prior to the GTT.

For the 3-hour GTT, the woman consumes 200 g of carbohydrates per day for 2 days. She then fasts from the midnight prior to the test. A fasting serum specimen is drawn. She ingests a 100-g carbohydrate load and specimens are drawn at 1, 2, and 3 hours. If any two readings exceed the upper limit of normal, a diagnosis of gestational diabetes is made. The normal plasma glucose levels (mg/dL) are 105 (fasting), 190 (1 hour), 165 (2 hours), and 145 (3 hours) (Cunningham et al., 1997).

A useful way to assess the degree of glycemic control for the preceding 4 to 8 weeks is to measure hemoglobin A_{1c}, or glycosylated hemoglobin. During the lifetime of a red blood cell, glycolysation occurs in proportion to the average plasma glucose concentration to which the cell is exposed. The lower the value, the stricter the glycemic control that was maintained over the previous 1 to 2 months, and the better the indication. Assessment of hemoglobin A_{1c} is particularly useful when the woman is planning to conceive.

On a daily basis, home monitoring of serum glucose levels has replaced urine testing for glucose, as home urine testing for glucose is unreliable in diabetes. Home serum glucose monitoring involves obtaining a capillary sample on a test strip by fingerstick and use of a reflectance meter (Fig. 19–4). Some brands of test strip can be read by comparison with a color chart. Accuracy of the reading depends on cleanliness of the fingerstick site and timing of the procedure. The best site is the midlateral aspect of a large finger pad. This procedure may be done as many as eight to ten times per day. Both pregestational and gestational diabetic clients monitor serum glucose levels. In addition, urine is tested at home daily for the presence of ketones by use of reagent strips.

Fetal well-being is assessed using maternal monitoring of fetal activity, serial ultrasonography for assessment of fetal growth, nonstress tests weekly or twice weekly during the third trimester, contraction stress tests, and fetal biophysical profile. Near term, tests for fetal maturity, such as amniocentesis for phosphatidylglycerol and lecithin:sphingomyelin ratio, may be performed. (See Chapter 18 for discussion of these tests.) Ominous developments in the diabetic pregnant woman include urinary tract infection with fever exceeding 39°C, diabetic acidosis, development of PIH, and neglect of the diabetic condition or inability to manage the disease.

► Collaborative Management

The objectives of management are to avoid the increased risk of intrauterine death in late pregnancy, to minimize the risk of complications in the mother, and to educate the mother in self-care practices regarding nutrition, glucose testing, and treatment. Abnormal carbohydrate metabolism must be detected precisely, serum glucose levels must be carefully regulated, the woman must be educated in self-care practices, and the woman and her neonate must be cared for by a skilled, experienced team.

Diet

Usually gestational diabetes can be controlled by diet alone; however, insulin treatment also may be needed to gain control of serum glucose levels. Excess weight gain must be avoided. Optimally, ideal weight is attained prior to conception. Although an adequate weight gain for the diabetic client is as important as for the nondiabetic client (see Chapter 14), the diet of the pregnant diabetic is more carefully controlled. Optimal outcomes are observed with a total gain of 25 to 30 pounds. In obese women, a gain of 15 to 16 pounds is associated with the best outcomes; in underweight women, a gain of 30 pounds is associated with the best outcomes.

Total caloric intake is the same in the first trimester as in the nonpregnant state. During the second and third trimesters, the woman needs 15 kcal per pound of ideal body weight plus 300 kcal. The Recommended Dietary Allowances (RDAs) for the pregnant diabetic woman are similar to those for women who are not diabetic.

The primary goal of diet therapy is to promote normal blood glucose levels while meeting the elevated nutrient requirements of pregnancy. Specific dietary recommendations are based on the classification of the disease, the preexisting body weight, and calculated calorie needs.

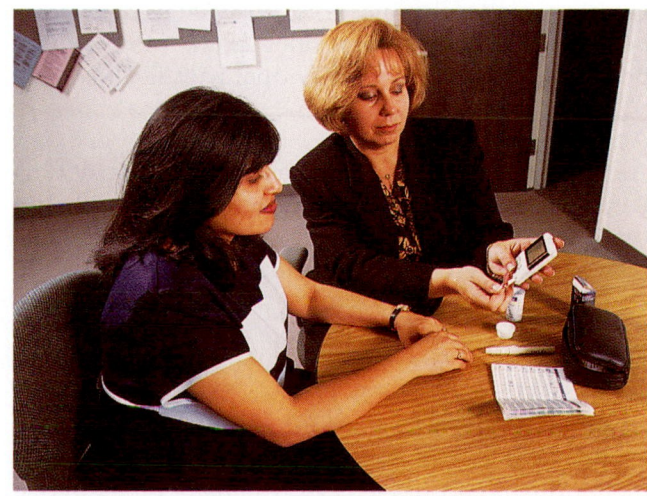

FIGURE 19–4. Pregnant woman performing home serum glucose monitoring.

Insulin-Dependent Diabetes Mellitus. For the pregnant woman with insulin-dependent diabetes mellitus (IDDM), adequate nutritional care should begin before conception. Because of the need for rigid control of blood glucose levels, the diabetic diet during pregnancy may be more restrictive than the diet to which the client was previously accustomed. In particular, special attention must be paid to the blood glucose fluctuations that occur during pregnancy.

Daily energy requirements to achieve the recommended weight gain are 300 kcal/day above the RDA. To obtain an accurate estimation of the client's kilocalorie requirements, the nurse or registered dietician conducts a thorough nutrition assessment. Once the diet has been prescribed, weight gain and blood glucose levels are carefully monitored to determine whether the diet meets the individual's energy needs.

"Carbohydrate counting" has replaced the exchange list previously used for dietary planning. A consult with a dietician or nutritionist is recommended for accurate assessment of the needs of the individual client.

Non-Insulin-Dependent Diabetes Mellitus.
Pregnant women with non–insulin-dependent diabetes mellitus (NIDDM) ideally have been adhering to a diabetic diet prior to conception. Like clients with IDDM, clients with NIDDM should be reeducated about the need for more rigid control of blood glucose levels during pregnancy. The dietary principles are the same as those outlined for the individual with IDDM.

Gestational Diabetes. In gestational diabetes, adequate blood glucose control is essential to avoid the need for insulin. The nurse must carefully provide dietary instruction to the woman with gestational diabetes, who often has no prior knowledge of the diabetic diet. The diet composition is the same as that described earlier for the individual with IDDM.

Activity
Along with dietary management, physical activity is increased as tolerated to promote improved carbohydrate transport and metabolism. The most desirable activities are aerobic: three times per week, about 20 minutes per session. Walking at a rate of 2 miles per hour for 30 minutes is an appropriate form of exercise. Activity is not promoted if serum glucose levels exceed 250 mg/dL, and ketones are present in the urine. Exercising with elevated glucose levels actually causes further secretion of glucose. Blood glucose monitoring is encouraged before and after the exercise period, with the addition of carbohydrate snacks as required.

Insulin
If dietary management and increased activity are not adequate to bring about a normal serum glucose level, insulin is prescribed (Table 19–8). The most commonly used delivery method is the subcutaneous injection. Another method is the insulin pump, which delivers a continuous subcutaneous insulin infusion at a basal rate with a bolus before meals and snacks. There is no significant difference in metabolic control using either method. However, clients using pumps must be extremely attentive to self-blood glucose monitoring.

Women are taught how to adjust insulin dosage on a day-to-day basis in accordance with their serum glucose levels. Since the advent of human insulin, almost all diabetics have had their insulin type changed to human. It is less allergenic, but more potent, than beef or pork insulin.

Many congenital anomalies in fetuses of diabetic women are believed to be preventable if diabetes that is overt prior to pregnancy is well controlled before conception. Ideally, the pregnant woman will maintain a glucose level of 60 to 100 mg/dL in the fasting state, not to exceed 120 mg/dL after a meal. Women whose disease is being managed with oral antidiabetic medications should be switched to insulin as soon as pregnancy becomes a possibility, because oral medications have been found to be teratogenic in research animals.

Hospitalization
Hospitalization is required whenever strict glycemic control is not maintained. Other indications include hyperemesis gravidarum, development of hypertension, any evidence of infection, ketoacidosis, onset of labor, or evidence of fetal distress.

Preparation for Delivery
In the past, induced or cesarean delivery at 37 weeks of gestation was routine because there is an increased incidence of late fetal demise among infants of diabetic mothers. This practice contributed to the higher-than-usual incidence of prematurity among infants of diabetic mothers. Now, with greater capabilities to monitor fetal well-being, a pregnancy without complications and with normal fasting and postprandial glucose values is allowed to continue from 38 to 40 weeks. The route of delivery is controversial. In the well-controlled client with a soft cervix that is partially effaced and dilated, labor may be induced with oxytocin and artificial rupture of membranes. Cesarean delivery is favored when antepartum testing is suggestive of fetal distress, when the cervix cannot be ripened with prostaglandin gel, or when fetal macrosomia is suspected. Failed induction or fetal distress in labor is also an indication for cesarean deliv-

▶ **TABLE 19–8**

Nursing Considerations When Using Various Types of Insulin

Type	Peak Effect (Duration)	Pregnancy Considerations	Nursing Implications
Regular insulin Bovine Porcine Concentrated	1–2 hours (5–6 hours)	Insulin requirements decrease in first trimester, then increase to two to three times prepregnancy dose. Postpartum requirements drop drastically for 48 hours. Use of insulin in gestational diabetes reduces macrosomia. Insulin does not cross placenta.	Client may experience allergic reaction. Resistance to insulin with foreign protein contaminants is possible. Breastfeeding is safe. Neonate must be assessed for hypoglycemia. Drug must be refrigerated. Check expiration date. Establish site rotation chart. Regular, intermediate, or long-acting insulin can be mixed if in the same concentration. Regular insulin may be given intravenously.
Prompt insulin zinc suspension (Semilente)	2–8 hours (12–16 hours)		
NPH (isophane insulin suspension)	6–12 hours (24–28 hours)		
Insulin zinc suspension (Lente), globin zinc, protamine zinc insulin suspension	6–12 hours (24–28 hours)		
Extended insulin zinc suspension			
Human insulin Regular NPH	2½–5 hours (8 hours) 4–12 hours (24 hours)	Human insulins may lead to hypoglycemic response in same dosages as porcine or bovine products because of absence of allergic resistance.	Instruct women on need to increase serum glucose surveillance when changing from porcine or bovine to human-origin or purified insulins.

ery. A neonatologist should be present at the delivery. It may be necessary to refer a woman to a regional perinatal center for delivery if neonatal intensive care is not available in her community birthing facility.

The metabolic changes that occur during labor and delivery are dramatic; therefore, glucose levels should be monitored every 1 to 3 hours during labor. An intravenous infusion should be continuous, with the type of solution dependent upon maternal glucose levels.

Nursing Alert

Women with diabetes mellitus should be aware that oral hypoglycemics are usually discontinued during pregnancy and insulin used instead. Insulin administration and blood sugar monitoring may be unfamiliar to the woman in this situation.

During postpartum recovery, the parameters of glycemic control can be relaxed and glucose values of 150 to 200 mg/dL are acceptable. Some women may require little or no insulin for the first 24 to 48 hours. Frequent blood glucose monitoring is used to adjust the dose. The woman is usually stabilized within a few days after delivery.

Breastfeeding is safe for the diabetic woman and her infant and should be encouraged. Because of the increased energy needs of lactation, careful attention should be given to caloric intake. The prenatal diet should be continued with snacks redistributed to compensate for the infant's feeding schedule. Insulin requirements in the breastfeeding mother may drop because of the loss of carbohydrate to produce breast milk. Frequent monitoring for hypoglycemia is necessary, especially during night feedings.

▶ ### Nursing Assessment and Management

The nurse who has contact with pregnant clients must be knowledgeable about gestational diabetes, including risk factors and laboratory values. In a woman with preexisting diabetes, assessment includes:

- Onset, duration, and course of diabetes
- Presence of diabetic complications affecting vital organs, peripheral nerves, or vasculature
- Prepregnancy treatment regimen for diabetes, including a review of how insulin is administered and how glucose and ketone levels are monitored
- Prepregnancy weight
- Obstetric history of past and current pregnancies and history of infertility
- Nausea and vomiting
- Socioeconomic constraints on the therapeutic regimen
- Recent hypoglycemia or ketoacidosis
- History of infections
- Contraceptive history

Physical assessment includes, in particular, pulse, respirations, and blood pressure; fetal heart rate; evidence of PIH; weight; pedal pulses; skin integrity at injection sites; vaginal bleeding or abdominal tenderness; and vaginal discharge suggestive of monilia. Persily and associates (1996) found that home visiting by a perinatal clinical nurse specialist facilitates continued control of diabetes.

The pregnant woman with diabetes has several specific needs:

- *Need to perform continued self-assessment.* The nurse instructs the client on the danger signs of pregnancy that require immediate attention. Nausea and vomiting can result in hypoglycemia. Evidence of infection such as burning on urination, fever, vaginal discharge or pruritis, and a cough can herald ketoacidosis. If the woman has decreased peripheral sensation, she must inspect her feet each day for lesions that can become infected. Vaginal bleeding or abdominal pain can signal abruptio placentae. Signs and symptoms of PIH are assessed. The client is instructed on early signs and symptoms of hypoglycemia and ketoacidosis. Using the woman's equipment, the nurse should review assessment of serum glucose level and of urinary ketone level by demonstration and assessment of return demonstration. After quickening occurs, the nurse will instruct the woman on surveillance of fetal activity.
- *Need to meet nutritional requirements of the disease and of pregnancy.* The nurse reviews dietary habits with the client and assesses food preferences, for example, ethnic food customs. The nurse also initiates a referral for dietary counseling. As a team, the client, nurse, and nutritionist can plan a diet that meets caloric needs and is also sensitive to the client's preferences. On each contact between the nurse and client there may be a need for dietary review and for clarification about carbohydrate counting. Particularly for the woman with gestational diabetes, a large amount of material must be learned fairly quickly so that strict euglycemia can be maintained. Literature that is accurate, clear, and in the client's first language, preferably, will reinforce the nurse's teaching.
- *Need for initial instructions in the administration of insulin.* Insulin requires refrigeration. It is injected subcutaneously, and the sites are rotated to prevent skin toughening, which impairs absorption. Sites include the hips, thighs, abdomen, upper arms, and subscapular areas. Most insulin preparations are available in a concentration of 100 units/mL, and insulin syringes are calibrated in units. The nurse instructs the woman in drawing up the proper dosage and self-administration.
- *Need of both the client and her family to know how to prevent and recognize hypoglycemia and ketoacidosis early, and what to do should these conditions arise.* Hypoglycemia is best prevented by compensating for activity with increased food intake and by eating one or two evening snacks. Ketoacidosis develops more slowly. The client is taught to prevent ketoacidosis by diligently monitoring her serum glucose level and adjusting the insulin dosage accordingly. If ketoacidosis develops, emergency care is required to find and treat the cause.
- *Need to understand the tests she will undergo throughout her pregnancy.* The client will be expected to undergo testing for fetal well-being once or twice per week, or even daily in some instances. The nurse can explain the procedures and their rationale. If the client understands the need for careful fetal monitoring for an optimal outcome, she is more likely to value the benefits of frequent testing than be frightened by it.
- *Need of both the woman and her partner for support throughout the pregnancy.* Diabetic individuals are susceptible to "burnout" because of the unrelenting need to carry out a tedious health maintenance regimen. The pregnancy complicated by diabetes is characterized by vulnerability and uncertainty. Scare tactics are counterproductive in motivating diabetic clients. More effective strategies include helping the woman to identify support people in her network of social contacts and support services whose assistance she may need, for example, a 24-hour telephone contact with a nurse

who can provide guidance when urgent questions arise about her diabetes management regimen. Praise from the nurse for her self-care is highly motivating.

- *Need for a sense of mastery.* Rather than being controlled by her disease, the pregnant diabetic woman needs to have her autonomy enhanced. The nurse can facilitate this by fully incorporating the woman into the planning of her care. A diabetic self-care regimen is a way of life; as such, it must be comfortable to the individual. This is particularly critical with diet planning, as food has other psychosocial meanings.
- *Need of both woman and her partner to deal with anxiety.* Past coping patterns may be useful now. Support groups for couples experiencing high-risk pregnancies or close friends as well as the nurse may support expression of feelings by the couple. Familiarity with the facility in which she will give birth and childbirth preparation appropriate to high-risk parents can allay fear of the unknown. The nurse can encourage relaxation strategies, such as diversional activities or meditation.

▶ BLEEDING DURING THE SECOND AND THIRD TRIMESTERS

Second- or third-trimester vaginal bleeding complicates an estimated 3.8 to 4% of pregnancies. Bleeding may vary from a small amount to hemorrhage. Hemorrhage continues to be a major reason for maternal deaths because of the need for prompt blood replacement. Hemorrhage during the second and third trimesters jeopardizes maternal and fetal well-being and more than quadruples the rate of premature delivery and perinatal mortality. In addition, maternal isoimmunization can occur as a result of bleeding (see later discussion in this chapter).

Five conditions most often account for second- or third-trimester bleeding: abruptio placentae, placenta previa, uterine rupture, disseminated intravascular coagulation, and gestational trophoblastic disease. Each is considered in the following discussion. Major signs and symptoms of the conditions are compared in Table 19–9. Placental bleeding, for example abruptio placentae or placenta previa, is the most common source of heavy bleeding.

▶ Abruptio Placentae

Abruptio placentae is the partial or complete separation of a normally implanted placenta from the uterine wall prior to delivery, usually occurring after 20 weeks of gestation. It accounts for about 30% of cases of third-trimester bleeding. The incidence of abruptio placentae has been reported to be 1 in 150 to 200 deliveries (Cunningham et al., 1997). The risks to the woman and her fetus are determined by the severity of hemorrhage, extent of separation of the placenta, overall maternal and fetal health status prior to the abruption, and effectiveness of interventions. Fetal death is not uncommon in extensive abruptions. In deliveries where the infant survives, there is an increased incidence of neurologic damage to the infant secondary to fetal anoxia or factors that caused the abruption.

Abruptio placentae can be complete or partial. The initial event is a tearing and bleeding in the inner layer of the endometrium (the decidua basalis). A hematoma forms and compresses the adjacent placenta. Placental function is destroyed locally, causing further separation of the placenta. As bleeding contin-

Client Teaching

Diabetes During Pregnancy

The nurse can suggest the following self-care practices to the pregnant client experiencing pregestational or gestational diabetes:

- Monitor your blood glucose daily since the dosage and frequency of insulin will change significantly as you progress through your pregnancy.
- As part of a moderate exercise program, walk 20 to 30 minutes each day. Be sure to check your blood sugar before and after your walk.
- Monitor the amount of insulin and syringes you keep at home to avoid running out.
- Carry glucose monitoring strips and your insulin supplies as well as a supply of carbohydrate with you when away from home for the day. Six jelly beans are a quick sugar source if you feel "shaky."
- Let your health care provider know if your face, fingers, or feet swell early in the day, as you may need your blood pressure checked.
- Drink 6 to 8 8-oz glasses of water and avoid coffee, tea, or colas to help prevent a urinary tract infection. Report any burning or frequency of urination.

▶ **TABLE 19–9**

Signs and Symptoms in Five Hemorrhagic Conditions of Pregnancy

Abruptio Placentae	Placenta Previa	Uterine Rupture	Disseminated Intravascular Coagulation	Gestational Trophoblastic Disease
Onset sudden	Bleeding frank, bright red	Rapid onset of symptoms of shock	Petechiae	Brown vaginal spotting over several weeks
Dark vaginal bleeding possible	Spontaneous cessation of bleeding possible	Frank or concealed vaginal bleeding possible	Prolonged oozing from puncture sites	Vaginal expulsion of vesicles
Extreme abdominal tenderness possible	Abdominal pain infrequent	Bright red bleeding	Bruising	Onset of anemia
Rigid, boardlike abdomen possible	Anemia possible	Fetal distress	Bleeding from mucous membrane	Fundal heights exceeding norm for gestational age
Abdominal distension possible	Fetal distress possible	Parts of fundus not palpable in complete rupture	Alteration in laboratory indices of clotting ability	Absent fetal movement, heart sounds
Fetal distress possible	Shock possible			Nausea
Hypovolemic shock possible				Onset of PIH
Occurrence in presence of PIH possible				Possible discomfort from uterine overdistension; rarely, rupture

ues, placental function is compromised, resulting in fetal hypoxemia. The gravid uterus is unable to contract to stop the bleeding. Most often bleeding continues until the fetus is delivered or the mother dies.

The site of separation is clinically significant. Marginal placental separations that involve the veins at the edge of the placenta or the intervillous space are less serious than central separations. When the placenta abrupts centrally, arteries are disrupted and a high-pressure arterial bleed occurs. The result is a substantially larger retroplacental hemorrhage.

Abruptio placentae is associated with two types of bleeding, external and internal. Frank vaginal bleeding will not be seen if the margin of the placenta remains completely attached to the uterine wall or if the fetal head is tightly engaged. This is referred to as concealed hemorrhage. Vaginal bleeding will be detected if some of the bleeding occurs external to the amniotic membranes (external hemorrhage).

Often, the cause of abruption is not known. Predisposing or related factors include trauma, a short umbilical cord, the presence of a uterine tumor or anomaly, uterine pressure on the vena cava, smoking, ethanol consumption, or use of cocaine. Abruptio placentae may also follow sudden decompression of the uterus, as when membranes rupture in the case of polyhydramnios, precipitous delivery, or the birth of the first of twins. As many as half of all cases occur in women with hypertension, either chronic or pregnancy induced.

Disseminated intravascular coagulation (DIC) is a consumptive coagulopathy that is a serious conse-

quence of abruptio placentae (see discussion later in this chapter). The blood clotting process is triggered intravascularly and retroplacentally.

Renal failure can occur in severe cases of abruptio placentae when hypovolemia is not aggressively treated. Renal cortical or cortical necrosis results from hypoperfusion of the kidneys.

Uteroplacental apoplexy, or **Couvelaire uterus,** occurs in severe abruptio placentae when blood extravasates into the uterine musculature, beneath the uterine serosa, into the connective tissue of the broad ligaments, and even into the peritoneal cavity. Formerly it was believed that Couvelaire uterus required hysterectomy to prevent postpartum hemorrhage because such a uterus would be unable to contract. Now, with suturing followed by administration of intravenous oxytocin postpartally, hemorrhage and the need for hysterectomy are rare.

Collaborative Assessment

Signs and symptoms can vary markedly in abruptio placentae and do not reliably indicate the degree of danger to the fetus. Commonly observed signs and symptoms include:

- Vaginal bleeding
- Uterine tenderness
- Back pain
- Stress
- Increased frequency of contractions
- Uterine hypertonicity and rigidity
- Premature labor

- Abnormal blood coagulation studies
- Fetal distress
- Fetal death

Hemorrhagic shock depends on the degree of blood volume loss. Signs and symptoms of early and late shock are contrasted in Table 19–10. The heart rate increases and the pulse becomes thready. Blood pressure remains normal until hypovolemia is severe, at which time a dropping blood pressure is observed. A drop of 20 mm Hg in systolic pressure or an increase of 20 beats per minute in heart rate generally signifies a 20% blood loss. Other signs include pallor, diaphoresis, and orthostatic hypotension. Individuals in hypovolemic shock experience a sense of foreboding or anxiety. With significant blood loss oliguria develops because of a decrease in renal perfusion. Postpartum pituitary necrosis (Sheehan's syndrome) may follow hypovolemic shock as a result of pituitary ischemia. This may be evidenced by lack of postpartum milk production.

Any bleeding in the latter half of pregnancy must be evaluated by inspection, assessment for possible hemorrhage, and by such studies as ultrasound. Contrary to a popular belief, pain is not totally reliable as a means of differentiating between abruptio placentae and placenta previa. Pain is more commonly associated with abruption and less commonly associated with placenta previa, but exceptions occur. Pain is more likely with concealed abruption as there is no relief of the pressure exerted by the entrapped blood.

Collaborative Management

Treatment depends on the status of the mother and fetus. If the bleeding is heavy, blood and intravenous fluid replacement is started immediately. Oxygen is administered. An indwelling catheter is inserted to assess urinary output. Central venous pressure may be measured. Fetal monitoring is initiated and the fetus is delivered as soon as possible. The woman is screened for DIC.

If blood loss is minimized and the fetus is immature but stable, close observation while the mother is hospitalized on bedrest may be prescribed. Mother and fetus are carefully monitored. "Expectant management" plans for the possibility of an emergency cesarean delivery are developed.

Nursing Assessment and Management

The nurse assesses the client with respect to the following: risk factors such as cocaine use; amount and nature of bleeding (dark red vaginal bleeding); blood pressure, pulse, respirations; fundal height, which is marked with a pen (increasing size indicates bleeding); reports of uterine pain; uterine contractions or

▶ **TABLE 19–10**

Signs and Symptoms of Early and Late Hypovolemic Shock

Assessment Parameter	Early Shock	Late Shock
Blood loss	15%	30–40% or more
Pulse rate	Slight increase	>120 or higher
Respiratory rate	Normal	30–40
Blood pressure	Normal	Decreased
Postural hypotension	Absent	Present
Capillary refill	Normal	Prolonged
Pulse pressure	Normal or widened	Narrowed
Level of consciousness/ behavior	Slightly anxious	Agitated/confused
Urine output	30–35 mL/h	5–15 mL/h or less

tonus; fetal heart rate patterns and fetal activity; evidence of coagulopathy; intake and output; reaction to blood products; and reaction of the client and her partner to this emergency.

The woman with abruptio placentae has specific needs that require nursing action:

- *Need for restoration of blood volume.* An intravenous route with a large-gauge (18-g) needle is established. Blood and fluid replacement is started. Intake and output are monitored. Urine output must exceed 30 mL per hour to avoid renal necrosis from hypoperfusion.
- *Need for oxygen.* The nurse positions the woman on her left side. Oxygen is administered by mask as needed.
- *Need for safety in preparation for delivery.* The physician is notified immediately of the woman's condition. The delivery room is set up for an assisted vaginal delivery and for cesarean delivery with possible hysterectomy. No vaginal or rectal examination is performed until the location of the placenta is known. Fetal monitoring is initiated with an external monitor until placenta previa is ruled out. Position of the fetus is assessed. If surgery is likely the woman is placed on NPO (nothing by mouth) status and the neonatal interdisciplinary team is contacted. Blood samples are obtained for typing and cross-matching and for evaluation of clotting status.
- *Need for support.* The family will be very anxious during this emergency. There may not be time to provide lengthy explanations of procedures or to encourage expression of feelings; however, the staff can allow the woman's

husband or other support person to remain with her as much as possible. Procedures can be simply explained. A calm manner communicates competence. Continuity of nursing care throughout the experience promotes security. Touch communicates caring. False reassurance that everything will be fine is to be avoided, because an emergency delivery attended by a neonatal interdisciplinary team clearly demonstrates that a serious, potentially life-threatening condition exists.

► Placenta Previa

Normally the placenta implants in the upper body of the uterus. In **placenta previa,** the placenta implants over or very near the cervical os. Placenta previa is described by degree:

1. Total placenta previa exists when the placenta totally covers the os.
2. Partial placenta previa exists when the placenta partially covers the os.
3. Marginal placenta previa exists when the edge of the placenta is at the margin of the internal os.
4. Low-lying placenta is the designation when the placenta is implanted in the lower uterine segment close to the internal os. Up to half of pregnant clients may have a low-lying placenta before 30 weeks; however, in many cases this does not become a clinical problem, because the placenta migrates away from the internal os as the cervix enlarges.

The degree of placenta previa changes as cervical dilation progresses, influencing assessment of the problem. Cervical softening and dilation causes the cervix to pull away from the placenta. This results in bleeding and potential jeopardy to the fetus. The lower segment of the uterus is unable to contract effectively to compress the torn vessels. Because of this, low-lying placentae in general are also associated with increased risk of postpartum hemorrhage.

Placenta previa is reported to occur in 1 in 200 pregnancies. The etiology of placenta previa is unknown. Factors associated with this condition include multiparity, advanced maternal age, cigarette smoking or cocaine use, uterine anomaly, history of placenta previa, history of cesarean delivery or other uterine surgery, intrauterine growth retardation, placenta accreta (a condition in which the placenta invades the myometrium and cannot easily be separated), breech and transverse lie, and large placenta (occurring in such conditions as multiple gestation and fetal erythroblastosis).

Collaborative Assessment

Collaborative assessment focuses on identification of signs and symptoms that indicate placenta previa. The most characteristic observation is the sudden onset of bright red bleeding, generally in the third trimester. The woman may discover heavy bleeding by awakening in a pool of blood. Usually this bleeding is painless and may or may not be accompanied by contractions. The initial bleeding may stop spontaneously but suddenly resume later. Sometimes, hemorrhage does not occur until labor begins. Women are assessed for signs and symptoms of hemorrhage (see Table 19–9), the nature of apparent bleeding, and the time of onset. Women with total placenta previa tend to bleed earlier and more severely during pregnancy.

Ultrasound is used to confirm placenta previa. If this is not possible, then careful vaginal examination is done in the delivery room. A double setup, that is, a setup for the vaginal examination and for cesarean delivery, is used in case hemorrhaging occurs and immediate cesarean birth is required.

Placenta previa is rarely complicated by consumptive coagulopathy. Cesarean delivery and blood replacement have reduced the incidence of shock and its sequelae in the event of placenta previa. The major cause of perinatal death is prematurity.

Collaborative Management

The goals of collaborative management are to minimize effects of blood loss, to deliver a healthy newborn, and to treat emotional crisis in the client and her family.

Cunningham and colleagues (1997) identify four groups of women with placenta previa, each of whom is managed differently:

1. Women whose fetus is premature but the condition of mother and fetus is stable
2. Women who are within 3 weeks of term
3. Women who are actually in labor
4. Women who are hemorrhaging so extensively that they must be delivered despite fetal immaturity

For the first group, close observation and a regimen of restricted activity and bedrest are often enough. The woman may be hospitalized for observation until bleeding has stopped for 24 hours even after ambulation. The woman is instructed to avoid sexual intercourse. She is taught symptoms that need immediate intervention, and her proximity to emergency care and transportation is evaluated. Droste and Keil (1994) found that women with complete placenta previa managed at home had the same outcomes as those hospitalized until delivery.

When bleeding is heavy, blood is replaced to maintain an adequate hemoglobin level. Women in

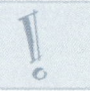

Nursing Alert

Vaginal examinations are avoided in women with vaginal bleeding since, if placenta previa exists, examination could cause further separation of the placenta from the cervix, lacerate the placenta, and result in more bleeding.

the first group who have less than 30% previa may deliver vaginally, with constant monitoring. If bleeding is controlled and there is no fetal distress, women who are preterm and not in labor may be managed with bedrest until the fetus is mature. Preterm labor in the woman who is otherwise stable may be managed with tocolysis to suppress contractions and betamethasone to promote fetal lung maturity.

For the other three groups, cesarean delivery is indicated, even when the fetus is dead, because of the potential danger to the mother of hemorrhage. With blood replacement and cesarean delivery the maternal mortality rate in placenta previa is low.

Nursing Assessment

For the client experiencing placenta previa, the nurse assesses the following parameters:

- Onset, duration, and amount of bleeding
- Vital signs and other evidence of hypovolemic shock
- Presence of pain
- Uterine contractions or tonus
- Fetal heart rate
- Fetal lie
- Length of gestation
- Laboratory values, including hemoglobin and hematocrit and clotting factors
- Maternal understanding of the problem and coping behaviors

Postpartally the nurse pays particular attention to assessment of postpartum hemorrhage. Contraction by the uterus is less effective than usual in compressing uterine vessels exposed at the placental site. In addition, the woman with placenta previa is more prone to intrauterine infection.

Nursing Diagnoses

Nursing diagnoses for the woman with partial placenta previa include, but are not limited to, those listed here:

Problem-oriented diagnoses:

- Altered tissue perfusion, related to placenta previa
- Anxiety, related to vaginal bleeding
- Fear of death, related to vaginal bleeding

Wellness-oriented diagnoses:

- Asset in physiologic integrity, related to minimal blood loss from partial placenta previa

Nursing Management

Nursing management addresses the following client needs:

- *Need for safety.* The woman is placed on NPO status until it is determined that immediate delivery is not necessary. Enemas, rectal or vaginal examinations, and the insertion of any object into the vagina are prohibited unless a double setup is prepared. The nurse prepares the client for ultrasonography. The interdisciplinary neonatal team is contacted when delivery is imminent. If delivery is not indicated and the woman is discharged, the nurse reinforces teaching about the signs and symptoms that require immediate attention as well as the client's access to transportation and emergency care.
- *Need for rest.* The nurse explains the role of bedrest in the treatment of placenta previa. Resting in a semi-Fowler's position allows the fetus to act as a tamponade, thereby slowing bleeding. For the client who is discharged prior to delivery, health care providers must consider whether the woman's life circumstances permit adequate rest at home. If there are other children, another caretaker needs to be identified.
- *Need for alleviation of stress.* The woman realistically may be worried about such problems as her own health, the health of her fetus, and the implications of being on bedrest. The nurse can help the client identify sources of support and strategies that have helped her cope with stressors in the past. Accurate information about the situation, how it is usually handled, and access to health care experts can help the woman further deal with her concerns. It is true that the fetus is in greater-than-usual jeopardy, and false reassurance must be avoided.

▶ Uterine Rupture

Rupture of the uterus is an uncommon emergency that is associated with high rates of maternal and perinatal mortality. Without immediate surgical intervention, as many as three fourths of all infants may die from hypoxia. Maternal deaths are most often due to hemorrhage. In rare cases, severe hemorrhage does not occur if major arteries are not involved and the uterus contracts well after fetal expulsion into the peritoneal cavity. Uterine rupture is usually associated with prior uterine surgery or cesarean delivery and abdominal trauma, but it can also be caused by inappropriate use of the drug oxytocin to stimulate or increase uterine contractions. Other associated factors include prolonged labor, multiparity, polyhydramnios, macrosomia, fetal anomalies, a transverse fetal position, obstetric trauma, development of a pathologic uterine retraction ring, and overdistension of the lower uterine segment.

Nursing and Collaborative Assessment

Rupture occurs most often during labor but it has been known to rarely occur spontaneously during pregnancy. The client is assessed for signs and symptoms of complete rupture, which include the following:

- Profuse bright red bleeding into the vagina (not universal, as covert bleeding into the peritoneum may occur)
- Sharp abdominal pain (related to covert bleeding into the peritoneum)
- Palpation of the fundus, which is firm and rounded, alongside the fetus
- Rapid onset of hypovolemic shock
- Rapid onset of fetal distress or cessation of fetal heart tones
- Uterine hypertonicity

If the rupture is incomplete, the following signs and symptoms are observed.

- Abdominal tenderness and pain that progresses (however, a great deal of pain may not always be present)
- Small amount of vaginal bleeding, although this is not universal
- Development of a palpable retraction ring across the lower uterine segment
- Distension of the lower uterine segment
- Failure of labor to progress even though contractions continue
- Early evidence of the onset of hypovolemic shock, such as maternal anxiety

These signs and symptoms may indicate impending uterine rupture:

- Severe lower abdominal pain
- Failure of labor to progress
- Formation of a retraction ring

- Palpable or visible distension of the lower uterine segment
- Uterine tetany

Collaborative Management

Uterine rupture necessitates emergency cesarean delivery and, frequently, hysterectomy. Antibiotics are administered. Packed red blood cells are infused as quickly as possible, with Ringer's lactate solution for fluid replacement via a second infusion system. Intravenous oxytocin may be administered to contract the uterus until it is removed.

Nursing Management

It may well be the nurse who observes the preceding signs and symptoms of impending or actual uterine rupture. Immediate action to stabilize the woman is mandatory. The nurse notifies obstetric and neonatal medical staff and calls for assistance to obtain a large supply of blood. Blood and fluid replacement is started immediately. Surgical setups for cesarean delivery and hysterectomy are readied. Vital signs and evidence of shock are monitored every 2 to 3 minutes. Fetal monitoring is initiated, if not established prior to the emergency.

Because time is crucial to survival in this emergency, explanations are given succinctly and without delay. Continuity of nursing care can promote security in a crisis situation. Afterward, the woman and her close family members will need support and counseling to help them cope with the emergency events they have experienced, particularly if fetal impairment or loss or hysterectomy occurred.

▶ Disseminated Intravascular Coagulation (DIC)

Disseminated intravascular coagulation (DIC) is a complex condition in which the formation of blood clots and the lysis of clots are triggered throughout the vascular bed. When the coagulation mechanism is upset in this manner, the risk of obstetric hemorrhage is increased.

Pregnancy normally induces a state of hypercoagulability in which coagulation factors are increased. The alteration prepares a woman for hemostasis during labor and delivery. (All pregnant women are at some increased risk for DIC.) Conditions such as abruptio placentae, fetal demise, hydatidiform mole (gestational trophoblastic disease), PIH, sepsis, hemorrhage, and saline abortion increase the potential for DIC to occur.

The coagulation mechanism is activated by the release of thromboplastin at sites of tissue destruction.

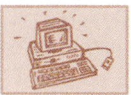

Research Abstract

Implications of Bedrest for the High-Risk Pregnant Woman

A focused qualitative study was designed to investigate the experiences of 24 high-risk pregnant women on prolonged bedrest. The 24 women involved were confined to bedrest at home or in the hospital, from 7 to 50 days. The majority of participants were white, married, well-educated women who had planned this pregnancy. The age range was from 18 to 36 years. Ten were primiparas, and 14 were multigravida. Diagnoses were varied as follows: placenta previa (n = 7), premature rupture of membranes (n = 4), pregnancy-induced hypertension (n = 5), and preterm labor (n = 8). Twelve were in a hospital on bedrest, 3 were at home, and 9 had been in bedrest in both places.

The methodology involved diary keeping by the subject, field notes, and an interview. The focus was on the emotional and psychologic aspects of bedrest.

The researchers used a stress process model to classify data. Themes of stressors fall into three categories: situational, environmental, and family. Some situational themes were assumption of the sick role, uncertainty as to the fetus' "well-being," and lack of control. Environmental stressors included feeling like a prisoner, "missing out," and "feeling bored." Family stressors were concerns about children and role reversal. Stress manifested itself in women's emotional reactions, such as guilt, anger, depression, and loneliness. Socially, stress manifested as altered relationships with others. The physical side effects of stress and prolonged bedrest included altered wake and sleep cycles, digestive changes, muscle wasting, weakness, and fatigue.

Mediators for stress included tangible physical or emotional support by family, friends, and health care providers. Answering questions was seen as the most significant contribution of the nurse. Expression of a sense of caring by the nurse was also highly important. Many women found that educating themselves about their high-risk condition was helpful.

Application to Practice

This focused study provides qualitative data about the stressors experienced by the high-risk antepartum client confined to bedrest, and what nursing can do to help the client cope with this situation.

Source: Gupton, A., Heaman, M., & Ashcroft, T. (1997). Bedrest from the perspective of the high-risk pregnant woman. Journal of Obstetric, Gynecologic, and Neonatal Nursing, 26(4) 423–430.

Fibrinogen is converted to fibrin, causing a state of hypofibrinogenemia (depletion of fibrinogen). Platelets and fibrin are consumed by the formation of large numbers of microemboli, which are tiny clots, throughout the vascular bed. Clots are lysed (or dissolved), resulting in increased levels of fibrin split products. Fibrin split products have anticoagulant properties. The increase in fibrin split products, decrease in number of platelets, and reduction of fibrinogen combine to result in generalized hemorrhage. The woman may bleed extensively, for example, from venipuncture sites, and she may demonstrate petechiae and oozing from mucous membranes and gums. Hematomas may develop. The disseminated microemboli can cause ischemia of vital organs, resulting in any number of organic dysfunctions.

Collaborative Assessment

Women at risk for DIC are assessed for signs and symptoms of generalized bleeding and screened periodically for its development. Table 19–11 summarizes blood tests which are commonly used to assess for DIC. In areas where laboratory analysis is readily available, clotting time and bleeding time tests have been widely replaced by the determination of the prothrombin time, partial thromboplastin time, platelet count, and measurement of products of fibrin degradation (fibrin split products).

Collaborative Management

The objectives of treatment include prompt identification of DIC, elimination of the causative factor, stabilization of hypovolemic shock, and treatment of the DIC.

Duffy (1995) identifies steroids, platelets, fresh frozen plasma and cryoprecipitate as interventions to correct the coagulopathy. Cardiovascular support is necessary in a woman with severe shock. Delivery of the infant is essential to management.

If the causative factor has been eliminated and no liver damage has occurred, plasma factors are likely to return to normal levels within 48 hours and the coagulation defects will resolve spontaneously. Platelet counts should return to normal by 7 days. However, platelets may be administered separately. Cryoprecipitate may be used in the presence of very low fibrinogen levels. Salicylates are contraindicated because they promote bleeding.

Complications of DIC, such as acute renal failure and infarction of other vital organs, must be diagnosed and treated promptly. The neonate may be compromised if hypoxia is experienced in utero.

Nursing Assessment

In assessing the client at risk for DIC, the nurse:

- Screens the client for factors indicating risk and presence of DIC
- Monitors laboratory data (see Table 19–11)
- Observes for petechiae, gingival bleeding, oozing of blood caused by the pressure exerted on the arm when the blood pressure is taken, excessive bleeding after injections or venipuncture, and bruising
- Records intake and output and assesses for edema
- Auscultates the lungs and notes respirations
- Assesses the client's level of consciousness

- Checks urine and stool for the presence of blood
- Takes the vital signs every 2 hours when the client is stable
- Looks for signs of early shock, such as tachycardia, central venous pressure, diaphoresis, and anxiety

Nursing Management

Nursing care focuses on the following parameters:

- DIC is a grave obstetric emergency necessitating intensive care by the interdisciplinary team. If DIC is demonstrated and bleeding occurs, fetal oxygenation is maintained by positioning the woman on her left side and administering oxygen by mask. The nurse administers blood products as prescribed by the physician. A large (16- or 18-gauge) needle or catheter is used. If hemorrhage has occurred, lactated Ringer's solution is usually given intravenously in addition to blood products. The client is observed for signs of cardiac overload as well as transfusion reactions.
- Activities that might cause bleeding are modified. The nurse instructs the client to use a soft-bristle toothbrush or even gauze sponges, rather than a regular toothbrush, to clean her teeth. The blood pressure cuff is inflated no more than 20 mm Hg above expected systolic pressure. Women with DIC are prone to skin breakdown, and must be turned gently. If evidence of shock is observed, the physician is contacted immediately.
- The seriousness of DIC will probably be evident to the client, who may be gravely ill, and her family. Fear for the sake of the woman and

► **TABLE 19–11**

Laboratory Findings in Disseminated Intravascular Coagulation (Consumptive Coagulopathy)

Test	Normal Nonpregnancy Value	Normal Pregnancy Value	Value in DIC
Platelets	130,000–400,000	75,000–320,000	Reduced
Burr cells	Absent	Absent	Present
Prothrombin time	9.5–11.3	Normal	Prolonged
Partial thromboplastin time	60–70 sec	Shortened	Prolonged
Activated partial prothrombin time	25–45 sec	Shortened	Prolonged
Bleeding time	7–8 min	Normal	Prolonged
Thrombin time	15–20 sec	Shortened	Prolonged
Total bilirubin	0.2–0.9 mg/dL	Slightly increased	Increased
Fibrin split products	Absent	Absent	Present
Fibrinogen	150–400 mg/dL	Slightly increased; 300–600 mg/dL	Decreased

fetus, and anxiety related to the whole situation, can be anticipated. Women may experience emotional crises related to the high-risk condition and to their pregnancy. The client needs adequate opportunities to express these feelings. She and her partner need to understand her condition, the tests, her inability to prevent DIC, and its tendency to resolve over time. Family members can be involved in the woman's care. This client is never left unattended by health care providers when she is in labor or when actively bleeding. After the birth, the nurse can promote family integrity to the extent that the woman and her newborn can tolerate it. If the newborn should not survive, family members will need to express their grief (see Chapter 12 on family response to neonatal death).

▶ Gestational Trophoblastic Disease (GTD)

Gestational trophoblastic disease (GTD) begins with a fertilized ovum that has implanted in the endometrium. In normal pregnancy, the trophoblast (outer cellular lining of the morula) will eventually form the placenta. In GTD cellular differentiation is halted and trophoblastic tissue proliferates.

Human chorionic gonadotropin (hCG) is produced by the trophoblast and is the hormone that provides the basis for pregnancy testing. There is a direct relationship between serum hCG levels and the amount of trophoblastic tissue. Therefore, hCG is considered a highly specific tumor marker for GTD.

There are two categories of GTD:

1. *Hydatidiform mole (molar pregnancy).* The presence or absence of an embryo or fetus is used to differentiate between the two types of hydatidiform mole.
   a. Complete mole: The chorionic villi change into masses of clear vesicles that resemble grapes. In this type of molar pregnancy, it is hypothesized that an "empty egg," one devoid of chromosomes, is fertilized (Cunningham et al., 1997). The normal sperm then reproduces itself, producing a 46XX or 46XY abnormal zygote. The zygote eventually degenerates as the chorionic villi begin to proliferate rapidly.
   b. Partial mole: In this type of molar pregnancy, part of a fetus or at least an amniotic sac is present and the hydatidiform changes are less aggressive. The usual chromosomal content of a partial mole is 69XXX, 69XXY,

or 69XYY, with the duplicate set of chromosomes paternal in origin. Very rarely, a normal twin can coexist with a partial mole and be born alive.
2. *Gestational trophoblastic tumors.* In 20% of women with complete mole, gestational trophoblastic tumors will develop (Cunningham et al., 1997). These tumors have the potential to become choriocarcinoma, an invasive malignancy which can metastisize.

Hydatidiform mole occurs once in 1000 pregnancies in the United States and Europe. The incidence among women over 45 is 10 times greater than that among women aged 20 to 40. There is a slightly increased incidence of hydatidiform mole among women who have had a previous molar pregnancy. Maternal mortality in hydatidiform mole is virtually zero when prompt diagnosis and appropriate therapy are carried out.

Choriocarcinoma is rare, occurring in an estimated 2 to 5% of cases of gestational trophoblastic disease, and the etiology of the malignant transformation of the trophoblast is unknown. Choriocarcinoma is characterized by a rapidly growing mass invading uterine muscle and blood vessels, causing hemorrhage and necrosis. Sepsis may develop. The most common sign is irregular bleeding associated with uterine subinvolution. Complaints associated with pathologic changes at metastatic sites may precede identification of the choriocarcinoma. The growth may perforate the uterus, leading to peritoneal hemorrhage.

Nursing and Collaborative Assessment

Typically, molar pregnancy becomes evident later in the first trimester or in the second trimester. Assessment for molar pregnancy includes the following observations:

- Uterine bleeding is the most outstanding sign of molar pregnancy. Marked hemorrhage can occur, but more typically dark brown spotting occurs for weeks or months. Iron deficiency anemia commonly accompanies this bleeding.
- Uterine size is an important index. In a molar pregnancy, the fundal height often exceeds that expected for the date.
- Fetal activity and fetal heart tones are usually absent.
- Molar pregnancy may be accompanied by hyperemesis gravidarum.
- Pregnancy-induced hypertension often accompanies a molar pregnancy, and in this one exception it develops earlier than the usual 20 weeks of gestation.

- Very high serum hCG levels may be noted 100 days or more after the last menstrual period.
- Pulmonary embolism may occur if trophoblastic material escapes the uterus in the venous outflow. Death and even local infarct are rare, but the tissue can establish itself and proliferate in this distal site as invasive mole or choriocarcinoma.
- Plasma thyroxine levels may be elevated.
- The grapelike vesicles may be passed vaginally, especially around the fourth month of pregnancy.
- Ultrasound confirms the diagnosis of molar pregnancy.

Assessment for metastatic disease may include a preevacuation chest x-ray. Computed tomography or magnetic resonance imaging may be performed, if indicated. Many women have not heard of molar pregnancies. Clients may react with horror, fear, or grief. The nature and extent of psychologic reactions to this condition will need to be assessed.

Nursing and Collaborative Management

Management addresses the objectives of immediate evacuation of the mole and follow-up for the prevention and early detection of malignant transformation.

Most often, vacuum aspiration performed by the physician is the method used to evacuate the mole. An intravenous line is inserted using an 18-gauge needle. General anesthesia is administered and the cervix is dilated. Two to four units of packed red blood cells are available. Intravenous oxytocin is administered to contract the uterus during the procedure. Curettage follows the evacuation, and the tissue obtained is submitted for histologic evaluation. Occasionally, hysterotomy is the method selected for evacuation. As with vacuum aspiration, oxytocin is infused and curettage follows the evacuation.

Hysterectomy may be elected, especially if the woman is over 40 or desires no more children. Choriocarcinoma is a more likely sequela among older and high-parity women.

The follow-up protocol is of critical importance for women experiencing molar pregnancy. Serum hCG levels are assayed every 1 to 2 weeks until normal nonpregnancy levels are achieved. The assay is repeated monthly for 6 months and then every 2 months for 1 year. A rise or a plateau in the hCG level necessitates further diagnostic assessment and usually treatment.

Pregnancy should be avoided during the 1-year follow-up period since use of hCG levels cannot be used as a diagnostic tool to confirm pregnancy. Pregnancy would obscure the evidence of choriocarcinoma. Any of the birth control methods in current use may be prescribed. However, oral contraceptives are recommended. Not only do they provide the most effective method of protection from pregnancy, they also inhibit luteinizing hormone (LH), which can react with hCG to cause a falsely elevated reading.

In addition, a baseline x-ray of the lungs is obtained postpartally and compared to the preevacuation x-ray. If hCG levels plateau or rise, the x-ray is repeated. Some protocols call for repeat chest x-rays every 2 months for 1 year.

If hCG levels do not regress normally, curettage or hysterectomy is performed. If that does not effect a cure or if there is evidence of metastasis to the lungs, chemotherapy is initiated.

The nurse addresses client needs that are similar to those observed in other hemorrhagic conditions. The client is prepared for the diagnostic and therapeutic procedures she is about to undergo. She needs education and support to participate in the year-long follow-up protocol.

Unique to GTD is the concept that pregnancy was associated with something other than a fetus and that cancer may result. Depending on the explanation of molar pregnancy provided by health care professionals, the woman's self-esteem can suffer from the awareness that the products of conception were so abnormal. The nurse can reassure the woman and her partner that this condition cannot be prevented, given current knowledge.

If the woman initially became aware of the disease because she passed a vesicle, the nurse needs to be sensitive to what a frightening or startling event this can be. A couple may have objections to abortion; therefore they need to understand that the life of a fetus is not at stake. If contraception during the 1-year follow-up protocol is objectionable, the nurse can emphasize that future reproductive integrity as well as preservation of the woman's life is the goal of follow-up care. In addition, ethicists from a religious background similar to that of the client may be consulted.

▶ INFECTIONS

Infection can affect the progress and outcome of pregnancy. Specific effects depend on type of organism, body systems involved, and severity of infection. Infection places the fetus at risk for sepsis, low birth weight, prematurity, congenital anomalies, or death. Implications of various infections for pregnancy are summarized in Table 19–12.

▶ **TABLE 19–12**

Implications of Maternal Infections for Pregnancy and the Neonate

Infection	Agent	Implications for Pregnancy
Asymptomatic bacteriuria, cystitis, acute pyelonephritis	Commonly *Escherichia coli, Proteus, Klebsiella*	Maternal hormones relax urinary tract, making ascent of bacteria easier. Risk of premature delivery. Sulfonamides in late pregnancy may cause hyperbilirubinemia and kernicterus in the neonate. Breastfeeding safety depends on drug therapy used.
Human immunodeficiency virus	Human immunodeficiency virus (HIV)	Transplacental infection may occur. Infected infant develops failure to thrive, hepatosplenomegaly, interstitial pneumonia, recurrent infections, and neurologic abnormalities. Infants are often SGA and may evidence Epstein–Barr virus. Neonatal/infant mortality rate 81%. Breastfeeding is contraindicated except in third world countries. Mother must learn appropriate, sometimes complex, infant care.
Bacterial vaginitis	*Gardnerella vaginalis*	Ampicillin or sulfa-containing vaginal creams may be used. Breastfeeding safety depends on particular drug therapy.
Chlamydia	*Chlamydia trachomatis*	Infants may develop conjunctivitis or pneumonia. Prematurity and fetal demise may occur. Breastfeeding safety depends on particular drug therapy.
Chorioamnionitis	Diverse organisms	Fetus can be severely compromised. Preterm labor may occur. Breastfeeding is safe when woman is febrile, depending on the drug therapy used.
Cytomegalovirus	Cytomegalovirus	Neonate may develop learning disabilities, mental retardation, cerebral palsy, and deafness as well as anemia and hyperbilirubinemia. Breast milk should be pumped and discarded during infectious period.
Gonorrhea	*Neisseria gonorrhoeae*	Infection at birth may cause ophthalmia neonatorum and subsequent blindness in the neonate. Breastfeeding safety depends on particular drug therapy.
Group B Streptococcus	β-hemolytic streptococcus (*Streptococcus agalactiae*)	Asymptomatic, colonized women are at risk for premature labor, maternal fever, endometritis, chorioamnionitis, and bacteremia. Neonatal infection occurs up to 3 months after birth involving pneumonia, respiratory distress syndrome, meningitis, and sepsis.
Hepatitis B	Hepatitis B virus	Infection of the fetus can result in prematurity and chronic liver disease. Breast milk should be pumped and discarded during infectious period.
Herpes	Herpesvirus type 2	Infection is contracted by the neonate during vaginal delivery. May cause death or neurologic damage. Primary infection, especially in the third trimester, may cause intrauterine growth retardation or prematurity. Breastfeeding is safe with good maternal handwashing.
Human Papilloma Virus (HPV)	Papilloma virus	Podophyllin, which is used in nonpregnant women, may be teratogenic. Local treatment such as laser or cryosurgery may be used. Neonatal infection is possible. There are no restrictions on breastfeeding. Increased risk of future cervical dysplasia.
Moniliasis	*Candida albicans*	An infant who comes into contact with the microorganism in the birth canal may develop oral thrush.
Rubella	Rubella virus	Early in pregnancy neonatal infection may result in such anomalies as congenital heart disease and cataracts, intrauterine growth retardation, mental retardation and cerebral palsy, diabetes, deafness, glaucoma, and a progressive encephalitis. Breast milk should be pumped and discarded during the infectious period.
Syphilis	*Treponema pallidum*	Disease may be transplacentally passed to the fetus. Result may cause second-trimester abortion, fetal death at term, or a congenitally infected infant. Breastfeeding is safe after treatment.
Toxoplasmosis	*Toxoplasma gondii*	Infection is associated with increased incidence of abortion, prematurity, fetal death, neonatal death, and severe congenital anomalies involving convulsions, coma, microcephaly, hydrocephalus, blindness, deafness, and severe retardation. Breastfeeding safety depends on particular drug therapy.
Trichomoniasis	*Trichomonas vaginalis*	The most commonly used drug, metronidazole, is potentially teratogenic. Breastfeeding safety depends on particular drug therapy.
Tuberculosis	*Mycobacterium tuberculosis, M. africanum, M. bovis*	Congenital infection can occur. The focus of fetal infection is the liver or lymph nodes. Mother and infant must be separated until treatment begins. Mother and baby must be strictly isolated. The pregnant woman taking INH must take pyridoxine. Breast milk should be pumped and discarded during infectious period. Breastfeeding during INH therapy is controversial.
Varicella	Human alpha herpes virus 3 (herpes zoster virus)	Infection can cause teratogenicity, fetal death, abortion. Herpes zoster immunoglobulin is recommended for the high-risk infant after exposure. Breast milk should be pumped and discarded during infectious period.

▶ Infection of the Urinary Tract

During pregnancy, anatomic and physiologic changes in the urinary tract predispose the woman to urinary tract infection (UTI) (see Chapters 15, 17, and 18). Under the influence of elevated serum progesterone levels the renal pelves and ureters dilate. Peristalsis decreases, allowing urinary stasis. Increased uterine and vaginal secretion promotes leukorrhea, harboring gram-negative coliform microorganisms near the urethral meatus. As the uterus expands, the ureters may be compressed. Torsion on the bladder makes it more susceptible to injury. These changes mean that pregnant women are at greater risk for bacteriuria. Ascending infection of the urinary tract develops more easily in pregnant than nonpregnant women.

Ascending UTI results in acute pyelonephritis, which is one of the most common medical complications of pregnancy and affects about 2% of pregnant women (Cunningham et al., 1997). This condition is occasionally associated with septic shock, spontaneous abortion, fetal death, and premature delivery.

Asymptomatic bacteriuria occurs in as many as 7% of all pregnant women. It is most common among economically disadvantaged, multiparous, minority women, especially those with sickle cell trait, but it can be observed in any woman (Cunningham et al., 1997).

Nursing and Collaborative Assessment

Infection is confirmed if there are more than 100,000 organisms of the same type per milliliter of a clean-catch midstream urine specimen or 20,000 to 50,000/ml without symptoms (Rouse, Andrews, Goldenberg, & Owen, 1995). Because of the prevalence of bacteriuria among pregnant women and the grave implications of pyelonephritis for the fetus, a urine culture for screening purposes may be performed at the first prenatal visit. Urine cultures at least once per trimester may be recommended for high-risk clients. Even in the absence of symptoms, bacteriuria is potentially harmful: in many women it persists past delivery and is often associated with the development of chronic lesions in the urinary tract (Cunningham et al., 1997).

Signs and symptoms of cystitis, or bladder infection, include urinary frequency, urgency, dysuria, hematuria, and pyuria. In ascending UTI, and even occasionally in cystitis, flank pain or costovertebral angle tenderness is a prominent feature. When the kidneys are palpated, the individual experiences sharp, intense pain. Signs and symptoms of cystitis are discussed further in Chapter 29, along with preventive measures.

The woman with acute pyelonephritis experiences fever and chills or hypothermia, lumbar pain, anorexia, nausea, and vomiting. Tachycardia and hypotension may occur if bacteremia or bacterial toxemia has developed.

In addition to urine cultures and monitoring for signs and symptoms, assessment parameters include temperature, pulse, respirations, blood pressure, and intake and output. Fetal monitoring is performed. Pyelonephritis can be confused with conditions such as chorioamnionitis and preterm labor; therefore, careful assessment is necessary.

Nursing Diagnoses

After careful assessment, nursing diagnoses related to UTI may be developed:

Problem-oriented diagnoses:

- Altered urinary elimination, related to infection
- Pain, related to infection
- Risk for injury to urinary tract structure, related to infection

Wellness-oriented diagnoses:

- Potential for continued positive role performance, related to relief of discomfort from UTI

Nursing and Collaborative Management

Pregnant women should be instructed routinely about strategies that can lower their risk of UTI. Such strategies include:

- Use of cotton-crotch undergarments
- Avoidance of chemical irritants such as feminine hygiene sprays and bubble bath
- Adequate fluid intake
- Frequent urination
- Urination after sexual intercourse

Women who are pregnant are instructed to seek health care immediately if burning occurs on urination.

Many women with asymptomatic bacteriuria or overt lower-tract infection develop pyelonephritis (Cunningham et al., 1997). This can be prevented by the treatment of bacteriuria with antibiotics, even prior to the occurrence of symptoms.

Women with cystitis and pyelonephritis are advised to increase their intake of clear, noncaffeinated fluids to 16 cups per day. Cranberry juice is often used to acidify the urine, making it less habitable to microorganisms.

Women who develop pyelonephritis are often hospitalized during the acute phase of the illness.

Dehydration is treated with intravenous fluids. Acetaminophen may be prescribed to lower fever and a cooling blanket may be applied to reduce high fevers. Analgesics are used to relieve pain. If the client is not febrile, a heating pad may provide some topical pain relief.

Intravenous therapy with medications such as ampicillin or cephalosporins may be initiated. Changes in antibiotics are made if culture and sensitivity results indicate a need to do so. Intravenous antibiotic therapy for 72 hours should result in abatement of the woman's symptoms. At that time, oral antibiotics can be used and the client continues her treatment for 14 days. The urine should be recultured at the end of her course of medication. Cultures must be negative to consider the problem resolved. The client is instructed on the importance of continuing treatment for the prescribed period, although she may begin to feel well. Failure to complete antibiotic treatment can lead to recurrent infection and growth of antibiotic-resistant organisms.

► Chorioamnionitis

Chorioamnionitis is infection of the chorion, amnion, amniotic fluid and, by association, the fetus. Normally a mucous plug in the cervix protects the uterine contents from infection, and amniotic fluid has some bacteriostatic properties. But most cases of chorioamnionitis occur with prolonged rupture of membranes and are caused by the normal flora of the genital tract. Risk factors include frequent vaginal exams with rupture of membranes, internal monitoring, long labors and cervical cerclage (Burrow & Ferris, 1995).

Nursing and Collaborative Assessment

Early signs and symptoms may be nonspecific, including fever and tachycardia. Preterm labor is a possible manifestation of chorioamnionitis. Later, uterine tenderness develops, and may be accompanied by malodorous discharge. When the membranes rupture, the amniotic fluid is cloudy and foul smelling.

Nursing and Collaborative Management

Delivery of the infant and intravenous antibiotic therapy for the mother and, if needed for the infant are the major medical interventions. Cesarean delivery is performed when the fetus is stressed, or if an effective labor pattern cannot be achieved. But surgery in the presence of infection is always more dangerous than usual in terms of wound healing, abscess formation, secondary infections, and septicemia.

Antibiotic therapy is instituted typically during the intrapartum period since these drugs cross the placenta and achieve peak levels an hour after parenteral administration to the mother, providing more effective protection against neonatal sepsis.

Nursing responsibilities include monitoring for signs of infection, administration of antibiotic therapy as ordered with assessment of the woman's response, promotion of generous fluid intake and continual assessment of maternal and fetal status. Specific observations include vital signs, intake and output, and symptoms of drug toxicity. Oxytocin may be used to induce labor; otherwise, the nurse prepares for cesarean delivery as indicated.

► TORCH Infections

TORCH is an acronym for a variety of organisms, most of which can cross the placenta and damage the fetus. It stands for *t*oxoplasmosis; "*o*ther" infections (including those caused by type B hepatitis virus, varicella, and syphilis); *r*ubella; *c*ytomegalovirus; and *h*erpes.

Toxoplasmosis

Toxoplasmosis is caused by a protozoan and can be transferred hand to mouth after handling cat feces or contaminated soil and by consuming undercooked meat. The infection can also be transmitted transplacentally. The embryo or fetus is affected if the woman contracts the disease during her pregnancy.

Infection in a healthy woman usually is without symptoms. If pregnant, there is a direct relationship between the time in pregnancy at which the mother becomes infected and the incidence of fetal infection. If the woman is infected in the first trimester, the chance of fetal infection occurring is 15%. This rises to 60% in the third trimester. The most severe infection occurs before the sixth month; however, the severity of infection for the fetus diminishes throughout pregnancy (Burrow & Ferris, 1995). The perinatal mortality rate in maternal toxoplasmosis is 10 to 15%, but 85% of infants who survive show psychomotor retardation by age 4. Half have visual problems within the first year.

Nursing and Collaborative Assessment.

Assessment for risk of toxoplasmosis may be done with a blood test to identify the presence of antibodies. Ideally, serologic assessment would be performed prior to pregnancy to distinguish women who are already immunized against the disease from women who remain at risk. Serial surveillance with blood tests around 8 weeks, 6 months, and at delivery may be done for women who live in areas where there is a high incidence of toxoplasmosis (Burrow & Ferris, 1995).

Nursing and Collaborative Management. Women with toxoplasmosis who are not pregnant are advised to avoid pregnancy for 1 year. If the woman is already pregnant, the health care provider discusses the options for treatment and, if infection occurred in the first trimester, for termination of the pregnancy. If the woman chooses to continue the pregnancy, treatment is oral sulfadiazine for 28 days. Pyrimethamine, a folic acid antagonist, is contraindicated during the first trimester because it is teratogenic. In the second and third trimesters, sulfadiazine is administered in conjunction with pyrimethamine. Folic acid is given concurrently to prevent bone marrow suppression. The nurse instructs the woman about her medication regimen, including timing and dosage, storage of the drugs, side effects to observe, and duration of treatment. See Chapter 9 for discussion of the actions through which the risk of toxoplasmosis can be lessened.

Other Infections

Hepatitis. The "other" category includes hepatitis B (HBV). It is transmitted to the fetus usually through contact with maternal body fluids at the time of delivery. Individuals at risk for HBV include parenteral drug users or their sexual partners, women with multiple sexual partners, and health care professionals who handle blood or body fluids. Outbreaks have also occurred in relation to tattoos and acupuncture.

Signs and symptoms of HBV include jaundice, lethargy, anorexia, vomiting, and fever. Intervention is usually supportive. No antiviral treatment exists at this time.

Infants who subsequently test positive for HBV surface antigen are rarely symptomatic. If acute hepatitis does develop, its course is usually benign. Such infants may be chronic antigen carriers.

Women in high-risk groups should be screened early in pregnancy. An effective vaccine exists for HBV and it is recommended that individuals at risk be immunized; however, vaccination during pregnancy is avoided. On exposure, clients should be offered hepatitis B immunoglobulin prophylaxis. Infants of women who test positive for HBV antigen should be given a dose of hepatitis B immunoglobulin within 24 hours after birth. The hepatitis B vaccine series should be started at the same time and continued at 1 month and 6 months after initial dose.

Varicella. Varicella, caused by the varicella-zoster virus, is also one of the "other" TORCH infections.

The occurrence of varicella–zoster viral infections such as shingles and varicella (chickenpox) during pregnancy can result in congenital malformations of the infant's skin, peripheral nervous system, autonomic nervous system, and musculoskeletal system. The infant can develop encephalitis.

Maternal signs and symptoms include eruption of vesicles along nerves arising from posterior ganglia. There is regional itching and pain. Malaise and gastrointestinal distress may occur before outbreak of vesicles. Newborns of women who develop chickenpox within the 5 days preceding or the 2 days following delivery should receive prophylaxis. There is no evidence that prophylaxis is effective in protecting the fetus if administered to the mother earlier in pregnancy. Drugs used against herpes zoster include vidarabine and acyclovir. Safety of these drugs for use by pregnant women has not been established. Chickenpox vaccination is now available and should be recommended to non-immune women prior to conception.

Syphilis. Syphilis, another infection in the "other" TORCH category, is a sexually transmitted disease caused by the spirochete *Treponema pallidum* (see Chapter 5). In the United States, syphilis is most prevalent among individuals of reproductive age. If a pregnant woman with syphilis is untreated, there is a significant risk of second-trimester miscarriage, fetal death, and/or the development of congenital syphilis. Lesions associated with congenital syphilis include interstitial changes in the lungs, liver, spleen, pancreas, and long bones. Because of the severe effects of untreated syphilis on the developing fetus, as well as on the woman, a blood test to screen for this disease is performed at the first prenatal visit.

Rubella

Rubella is decreasing in incidence in the United States. Since the early 1960s, infants have been immunized routinely around 15 months of age. Women in the health care professions are screened and immunized. Despite these efforts, about 6 to 25% of women are still susceptible to rubella (U.S. Centers for Disease Control and Prevention, 1994). Rubella titers ideally should be part of the initial well-woman assessment. Immunizations should be offered to nonpregnant women who are not immune, along with counseling to avoid pregnancy for 3 months.

Pregnant women who are not immune should be advised to avoid, when possible, travel to areas where people are not routinely immunized and to avoid contact with infected individuals. For example, a pregnant nurse who is not immune should not care for a newborn with congenital rubella. In the early postpartum period, prior to discharge, immunization should be offered to women who are not immune.

The effect of maternal rubella on the fetus can be serious, depending on gestational age at the time of the infection. Rubella during the first trimester of pregnancy can cause severe defects to the fetus and spontaneous abortion. By the fifth month of pregnancy, exposure to rubella carries significantly less risk to the fetus.

The most common anomalies include defects of the eyes, heart, ears, and central nervous system; intrauterine growth retardation; hematologic deficits; hepatosplenomegaly; chronic diffuse interstitial pneumonitis; osseous changes; and chromosomal abnormalities (Table 19–13).

Nursing and Collaborative Assessment.
Rubella serum antibody levels are routinely assessed at the first prenatal visit (see Chapter 15) so that immunization status can be determined.

Nursing and Collaborative Management.
There is no treatment for rubella. The dilemma faced by women who know that they have been exposed during the first trimester is whether or not to terminate the pregnancy. There is currently no method for early assessment of the extent of damage to the fetus, and although half of fetuses infected in the first month are seriously damaged, half are not. First-trimester rubella has been considered an indication for therapeutic abortion, but the decision depends on other factors in the woman's situation. She and her partner need complete information about the implications of rubella for her pregnancy. If she decides to continue the pregnancy her decision may be negatively regarded by some health care professionals. Whatever the woman and her partner decide, they need support and acceptance by professional nurses throughout their experience.

Cytomegalovirus

Cytomegalovirus (CMV) is a common cause of perinatal infection, affecting 0.5 to 2% of all neonates (Cunningham et al., 1997) (see Chapter 5).

Neonatal effects of CMV may be transient, as in patent ductus arteriosus. They may be reparable, as in hypospadias; however, they may constitute major handicaps. All infected infants need to be followed, as sensorineurologic problems can arise as much as 7 years later. The degree of damage is not related to gestational age at the time of infection.

Prenatal screening is not cost effective as there is no treatment or vaccine. Abortion is not an appropriate measure after CMV infection because the risk of fetal infection and the severity of fetal illness or its sequelae are not predictable. Strategies for the prevention of this disease have not been devised, although it is common practice in neonatal intensive care units to avoid assigning pregnant nurses to care for CMV-infected infants. Because of the prevalence of CMV and the rarity of symptoms there is no way to identify and break the chain of transmission. Treatment and vaccination are in the research stage.

Herpes Simplex

All herpetic infections are potentially life threatening to neonates. Herpes simplex, particularly genital herpes, has reached epidemic proportions in the United States (see Chapter 5). Herpes transmission occurs as the infant travels through the birth canal of an infected mother, either during active primary or recurrent infection; less commonly, the virus ascends the vaginal canal and cervix after rupture of membranes. Transplacental transmission can occur but rarely does. In some cases asymptomatic women shed herpes virus, placing their infants at risk. For mothers who have had active herpes in the last month of pregnancy, cesarean delivery is common practice. Even with positive cultures or visible lesions, however, a woman with premature rupture of membranes is allowed to deliver vaginally if a length of time identified by the

▶ **TABLE 19–13**

Common Findings in Neonates with Congenital Rubella[a]

Eye lesions
  Cataracts
  Glaucoma
  Microphthalmia
  Other abnormalities
Heart lesions
  Patent ductus arteriosus
  Septal defects
  Pulmonary artery stenosis
Sensorineural deafness
Central nervous system defects
  Meningoencephalitis
Small-for-gestational age
Hematologic deficits
  Thrombocytopenia
  Anemia
Liver alterations
  Hepatosplenomegaly
  Jaundice
Chronic diffuse interstitial pneumonia
Osseous changes
Chromosomal abnormalities

[a]Infants born with congenital rubella can be contagious to susceptible adults, infants, and children. They may shed the virus for several months after birth.
Adapted, with permission, from Cunningham et al. (1997). Williams obstetrics (20th ed.). Stamford, CT: Appleton & Lange, p. 1303.

institution has passed. The rationale is that after 8 or 12 hours the fetus cannot be protected from the virus by cesarean delivery, so there is no point in subjecting the woman to abdominal surgery. Women who do not test positive for herpes or demonstrate lesions during the last month of pregnancy can deliver vaginally.

Women who know they have herpes should see their health care provider for culturing as soon as symptoms recur. Cultures from the lesion are performed weekly from the 32nd week of pregnancy, but the emergence of clinical symptoms supersedes a recent negative culture in determining activity of the disease. If a woman's sexual partner has recurrent genital herpes, precautions should be taken, particularly during the last 6 weeks of pregnancy, so that the woman does not acquire a primary infection close to delivery. Primary infections are more easily contracted by neonates. This means that the couple should use condoms during sexual activity and abstain when his disease is active.

Primary herpes infection has been associated with spontaneous abortion and premature birth. The incidence of neonatal herpes is about 1 in 7500 live births. Neonatal herpes is usually disseminated, affecting the liver, adrenals, and central nervous system. As many as 60% of neonates with disseminated herpes die (Martens, 1994).

► *Chlamydia trachomatis*

Approximately 50 to 60% of the neonates delivered vaginally to women with chlamydia are infected with the disease (James et al., 1994). When the *Chlamydia trachomatis* organism is transmitted to the eyes by venereal transmission or by fetal descent through the birth canal of an infected woman, a keratoconjunctivitis called trachoma may develop. Trachoma is the leading cause of preventable blindness in the world. Inclusion conjunctivitis develops within the first two weeks of life. Infants at risk should be followed for 3 weeks. Eye prophylaxis such as erythromycin ointment is effective in preventing trachoma. Neonates may also develop chlamydial pneumonia after exposure to *C. trachomatis*. Any woman with a sexually transmitted disease and her sexual partner should be screened for chlamydia, and treated if necessary. (See Chapter 5 for further discussion.) The recommended drug for chlamydial pneumonia is erythromycin (U.S. Centers for Disease Control and Prevention, 1998).

► *Candida albicans*

Candida albicans infection, or yeast infection, is commonly transmitted to the fetus during descent through the birth canal. The infant may develop oral thrush or yeast infection of the diaper area. Treatment with nystatin suspension or ointment is indicated, but this problem is generally minor. Vaginal yeast infection is fostered by physiologic changes of pregnancy, and is discussed in Chapter 5.

► Tuberculosis

Tuberculosis results from infection by *Mycobacterium tuberculosis*. Transmission is by droplets. Tuberculosis generally, but not always, involves the pulmonary system.

Pregnant women with tuberculosis may be asymptomatic. Symptomatic individuals may demonstrate malaise, fatigue, loss of appetite, weight loss, and 103 to 104°F fever. Body temperature tends to increase in the afternoon, and night sweats are characteristic. Production of blood-streaked sputum is a later-stage development.

Tuberculosis screening of antenatal women is routine. If the screening test is positive, chest x-ray may be done to confirm the presence of active tuberculosis. The pregnant woman's abdomen and pelvis must be well shielded by lead aprons when the chest x-ray is performed. If active tuberculosis is established or strongly suspected, isoniazid (INH) and rifampin are administered daily with ethambutol added initially when drug resistance is suspected. Isoniazid is associated with an increase in fetal malformations, particularly neurotoxicity. Pyridoxine should be administered simultaneously to prevent their development. Prophylactic chemotherapy is not administered until after delivery.

► Group B Streptococcus

Group B streptococcus (GBS) is a bacteria found in 10 to 30% of all healthy adults (Mitchell, Steffenson, Hogan, & Brooks, 1997a). It normally colonizes in the rectum and vagina and does not produce symptoms unless it spreads to other areas such as the uterus. Group B streptococcus can result in spontaneous abortion, fetal death, preterm birth, and infections such as chorioamnionitis and endometritis. The risk to the neonate includes significant infection causing death in 5 to 15% of infected infants. Onset of infection occurs within the first few days of life for 80% of these infants (Mitchell, Steffenson, Hogan, & Brooks, 1997b). Initial signs of distress are typically respiratory compromise, meningitis, and sepsis.

Currently the U.S. Centers for Disease Control and Prevention (1996) have recommended two approaches to reduce the risk and occurrence of GBS infection. One approach is to culture all pregnant women between 35 and 37 weeks of gestation. Women who test positive should be given penicillin intrapartally. Another approach is to give penicillin during the intrapartum period to all women with risk factors for GBS regardless of whether cultures were obtained. Those risk factors include:

- Previous infant with GBS disease
- GBS bacteriuria during pregnancy
- Delivery before 37 weeks' gestation
- Intrapartum fever of 100.4°F or above
- Rupture of membranes over 18 hours

These approaches have been found to significantly reduce early-onset GBS disease in the neonate (Mitchell, Steffenson, Hogan, & Brooks, 1997a, 1997b).

▶ Human Immunodeficiency Virus

Human immunodeficiency virus infection is a condition of immune system suppression caused by the human immunodeficiency virus (HIV) (see Chapter 5). The disease remains dormant in cells of the immune and other systems for a period of months to years after infection. Currently there is no proven cure for HIV infection. HIV infection is both an acute and chronic disease, which eventually progresses to death in virtually every case.

Vertical (perinatal) transmission of HIV infection is a major and growing problem, especially in populations where high-risk behaviors such as intravenous drug use or sexual relationships with multiple partners occur. The percentage of acquired immunodeficiency syndrome (AIDS) cases in women increased from 8% in 1987 to 18% in 1995 and continues to rise (Ungvarski, 1997). An infected woman has a 15 to 25% chance of passing the infection to her child (U.S. Centers for Disease Control and Prevention, 1998). The majority of pediatric AIDS cases in the United States are perinatal in origin (Ungvarski, 1997).

Most mothers who are seropositive passively transfer maternal HIV antibodies to their fetus or neonate. In addition, they can be infected by the mother with the HIV virus during the perinatal period through the transplacental route, during the birth process, or through breastfeeding. Although all fetuses receive HIV antibodies from their infected mother, it is not known why or how some of these fetuses actually become infected with HIV and some do not. Experts believe that the passively transferred maternal HIV antibody could persist in the infant for up to 15 months of life. At this point, infants who are not truly infected will convert to a seronegative status. Infants who are HIV infected will remain seropositive, and may begin to manifest symptoms of HIV disease, progressing eventually to AIDS. Thus, infants who are

seropositive perinatally should be tested at regular intervals for persistence of antibodies or any other abnormalities associated with HIV infection. An infant who does not have symptoms and who has converted to a seronegative status can be considered unlikely to be infected with HIV. See Chapter 32 for additional discussion about nursing care of infants infected with HIV.

Recent clinical studies have shown a significant reduction in perinatal transmission to 8% with the maternal use of zidovudine during pregnancy, and is currently recommended for HIV-positive women after the first trimester of pregnancy (Ungvarski, 1997).

▶ Additional Nursing Management Considerations in Perinatal Infection

Women with perinatal infections need emotional support and physical assistance. The woman needs to understand her illness and its implications. In some cases, she must be isolated from her neonate. In some instances the course of pregnancy is markedly altered by development of an infection, as when herpes necessitates a cesarean delivery.

The U.S. Centers for Disease Control and Prevention (CDC) advocate universal precautions in all client care settings. Such measures as using gloves when coming into contact with blood or body fluids are essential. Rooms must be thoroughly cleaned after use. Ideally, a woman with a perinatal infection would labor, deliver, and recover in the same room, for the protection of other clients.

Specific isolation practices may be necessary. For example, enteric precautions are implemented when a client has hepatitis, and respiratory isolation is necessitated by tuberculosis. Isolation can be perceived by the client as alienation, particularly during such a social life event as birth. If possible, the infant of a woman with an infection should be isolated with her. If the infection or severity of maternal or neonatal illness requires separation of mother and infant, other family members can be encouraged to visit and handle the infant as appropriate.

Anxiety often develops when expectant mothers learn that they are carriers of disease, or if after delivery, the infant is discovered to have acquired one. Before birth there may be constant worry that the infant will be ill. If the infant is ultimately found to have been infected, with negative consequences, the family can experience feelings of guilt, recrimination, and hopelessness.

Nurses can provide instruction on points identified earlier, with the goal of prevention. They can teach women the signs and symptoms they should report to their health care providers throughout pregnancy. For a number of the TORCH infections, however, there is little beyond general hygiene measures that an individual can do to control transmission. The family, particularly the woman, needs continual reassurance that they have responded appropriately to the threat of infection. Women with chronic viral infections do need to understand potential risks and what can be done to minimize them before they undertake pregnancy.

▶ ABNORMALITIES OF AMNIOTIC FLUID PRODUCTION

▶ Polyhydramnios

Polyhydramnios, or hydramnios, is an excessive quantity of amniotic fluid. This has arbitrarily been defined as more than 2000 mL. Normally the amount of amniotic fluid is believed to increase steadily until 33 weeks of gestation, and then to decrease progressively to term. During the last half of pregnancy amniotic fluid is produced by amniotic and fetal skin transfer of water and other molecules. During the second trimester, the fetus swallows, urinates, and inspires amniotic fluid. These processes probably regulate the amniotic fluid volume.

Polyhydramnios occurs in 0.4 to 1.5% of pregnancies, and is associated with various maternal and fetal complications of pregnancy, such as diabetes, multiple gestation, anencephaly, and esophageal atresia. It has been observed that when fetal swallowing is impaired, as in esophageal atresia, polyhydramnios develops. In anencephaly and spina bifida there is increased transfer of fluid across exposed meninges. Anencephalic fetuses lack antidiuretic hormone, so that they urinate excessively; this also contributes to polyhydramnios. In twin pregnancy, one fetus is thought to have benefit of more of the fetal circulation than the other, and to have increased urine output. The relationship of polyhydramnios to maternal diabetes is not understood.

The incidence of polyhydramnios is greater than can be explained by pregnancy complications alone. Recent data analysis suggests a relationship between polyhydramnios and maternal smoking during pregnancy. Several biologic mechanisms are hypothesized: human placental lactogen that regulates fluid flux across placental membranes is decreased in smokers; increased angiotensin-converting enzyme in the lungs of smokers enhances activation of the angiotensin system; and nicotine results in atrophic and hypovascular changes in the placenta.

Nursing and Collaborative Assessment

Signs and symptoms of polyhydramnios include a sensation of pressure, maternal dyspnea, and vulvar edema. Assessment includes:

- Vital signs, especially presence of respiratory difficulty
- Weight gain
- Measurement of uterine size
- Fetal heart rate, lie, and activity
- Evidence of uterine compression on venous return
- Possible ultrasound assessment of amount of amniotic fluid

Acute polyhydramnios is associated with a twofold increase in the incidence of premature labor. The client is also assessed for signs and symptoms of maternal hazards, including preterm labor, abruptio placentae, uterine dysfunction, uterine rupture, and postpartum hemorrhage.

Nursing and Collaborative Management

Mild or moderate polyhydramnios is not treated. In severe cases, marked by maternal dyspnea, amniocentesis can relieve maternal distress. An 18-gauge intravenous catheter is placed abdominally under local anesthesia. Sonographic visualization guides the procedure so that the placenta or the fetus is not punctured. Removal of up to 1500 to 2000 mL of fluid usually relieves symptoms temporarily. Amniocentesis can be repeated as maternal discomfort dictates. The risks associated with this procedure include chorioamnionitis, abruptio placentae, initiation of preterm labor, and puncture of a fetal vessel.

The nurse needs to understand and clarify for the client that restriction of salt or fluid intake, or the use of diuretic drugs, plays no known role in the prevention or relief of polyhydramnios. The nurse answers the woman's questions about the condition and teaches her the changes to observe, including uterine hyperirritability, dyspnea, vaginal bleeding, and abdominal pain. Rest in the left lateral position may be advised to promote the client's comfort; however, bedrest does not usually decrease polyhydramnios.

▶ Oligohydramnios

A lower-than-normal volume of amniotic fluid is termed oligohydramnios. Operationally, this is defined in accordance with gestational age of the fetus. The average amount of amniotic fluid at 40 weeks is 800 mL. At 42 weeks, the average is 350 mL. Complications arise most commonly when there is less than 200 mL of amniotic fluid. Severe oligohydramnios is characterized by sonographic evidence of no echo-free space between fetal limbs and the uterine wall, or by the inability to identify more than two pockets of amniotic fluid at least 1 cm in diameter. Nuclear magnetic resonance imaging has also been used to assess amniotic fluid volume (see Chapter 18).

Oligohydramnios is associated with postmaturity and may occur in conjunction with congenital obstruction of the urinary tract or renal agenesis. Failure to excrete urine contributes to a decrease in total amniotic fluid volume.

Fetuses born with renal agenesis have an array of characteristics referred to as Potter's syndrome, including flat nose, recessed chin, flattened ears, pulmonary hypoplasia, and limb positional defects such as talipes equinovarus (club foot). These symptoms all reflect fetal compression by the uterus and possibly the lack of a growth hormone in amniotic fluid. Adhesions also can form between the fetus and the membranes.

Oligohydramnios may also be associated with a slow leak in the chorionic membranes. Loss of fluid in this manner is usually followed by premature labor.

Other complications of oligohydramnios include pulmonary hypoplasia and umbilical cord compression. Inspiration of amniotic fluid promotes alveolar maturity and chest wall expansion. In the absence of adequate fluid, the lungs may not develop normally.

The umbilical cord may be compressed because amniotic fluid is not present to cushion the cord from the pressure of the fetus's body. Cord compression is associated with fetal distress. Variable decelerations and other stress patterns that may be associated with oligohydramnios are managed in part by amnioinfusion, a procedure that infuses sterile saline into the uterus. There is no other general treatment approach to oligohydramnios.

► SPONTANEOUS ABORTION/ INCOMPETENT CERVIX

Unplanned labor and parturition before the age of viability or before 20 weeks of gestation is termed spontaneous abortion. Miscarriage is the term often used by clients to avoid confusion with elective abortion, the process in which pregnancy is voluntarily terminated (see Chapters 8 and 16). During the second trimester spontaneous abortion may occur as a result of incompetent cervix.

Incompetent cervix is the most common structural defect predisposing to spontaneous abortion, although it does not occur often. **Incompetent cervix** is defined as an anatomic defect of the cervix result-

ing in painless dilation without uterine contractions. The membranes may prolapse through the opened cervix and into the vagina. The membranes may also rupture, and delivery may ensue so prematurely that the infant does not survive. Cervical dilation usually occurs between the 16th and 20th weeks of gestation, although the condition may take place earlier or later. The condition tends to recur in future pregnancies.

Incompetent cervix may be caused by cervical trauma. The woman frequently has a past history of a traumatic delivery, dilation and curettage, or cervical biopsy conization. Abnormal cervical development may also play a role. For example, exposure to diethylstilbestrol (DES) is related to abnormal cervical development. Increasing weight and pressure of the fetus during advancing pregnancy result in dilation of the incompetent cervix. By 16 weeks' gestation, the products of conception are large enough to efface and dilate the cervix.

Spontaneous abortion occurring as a result of incompetent cervix differs from first-trimester spontaneous abortion. Incompetent cervix is a structural defect that results in the loss of the products of conception, while the majority of first-trimester spontaneous abortions are related to chromosomal abnormalities in the embryo or fetus. Pregnancy loss from incompetent cervix occurs much less frequently, and is managed differently than first-trimester abortion. (See Chapter 16 for a complete discussion of first-trimester spontaneous abortion.)

Treatment for incompetent cervix is accomplished between 14 and 20 weeks gestation. The cervix is sutured to prevent opening. This surgical approach, called **cerclage,** is performed by a physician if the cervix is less than 4 cm dilated and no signs of other high-risk conditions, such as bleeding, ruptured membranes, and uterine contractions, are present. Cunningham and associates (1997) report that bulging membranes are related to a high failure rate in cerclage. Ideally, the sutured cervix remains closed until near term, when the sutures are removed in preparation for vaginal delivery or when cesarean delivery takes place. In some cases, cerclage may be considered a risk factor for preterm labor or premature rupture of membranes, especially in more advanced pregnancy. Bedrest, rather than cerclage, may then be used, particularly beyond 20 weeks of gestation. However, successful cerclage has been reported in women who were between 21 and 24 weeks of gestation and who presented with advanced cervical changes.

Prior to cerclage, vaginal examination and ultrasound are done to assess the degree of cervical effacement and dilation and to confirm the presence of a living fetus with no major anomalies. In addition, cervical smears are done to make certain that cervical cells are normal and that no infection, such as chlamydia or gonorrhea, is present. The client is advised not to have vaginal intercourse for at least 1 week before and after cerclage; however, restrictions on sexual activity are based on the client's individual condition.

The McDonald technique and the Shirodkar technique are two surgical procedures currently performed by physicians to treat incompetent cervix. Both reinforce the cervix with an encircling purse-string suture. After the McDonald procedure, the suture must be removed at term to allow for vaginal delivery. Sutures from the Shirodkar technique remain intact, so that future pregnancies will be possible without further surgical manipulation of the cervix. Cesarean delivery is performed at term. However, sutures can also be removed by the physician for vaginal delivery.

Postoperatively, the most common complications are rupture of the membranes and uterine contractions. Bedrest for 24 hours and close monitoring to detect uterine contractions are recommended. If the membranes rupture, the physician must be notified. The sutures must be removed by the physician and the woman delivered because of the risk of sepsis. If uterine contractions begin and the membranes remain intact, the woman is placed on bedrest and medication may be prescribed to arrest preterm labor.

During labor, a woman who has had cerclage may at first progress slowly as a result of the fibrotic changes that take place in the cervix after the procedure. This may be followed by a sudden delivery. Postdelivery, the client is assessed for cervical lacerations, as this is a common complication.

Incompetent cervix, by its very name, suggests that the client is less than adequate in her ability to carry a pregnancy to term. This negative connotation reinforces the tendency of the woman to feel she is a failure, especially if the fetus was otherwise normal. The situation is particularly difficult if a previous pregnancy ended because of incompetent cervix.

Although success rates of 85 to 90% have been achieved with cerclage, clients may be anxious about the outcome of their pregnancy and the sudden transition to high-risk status. Restrictions of daily activities may be a burden, especially for the employed woman. Family concerns are similar to those experienced by women after spontaneous abortion. Grief over loss of the pregnancy, worry over future pregnancies, and desire to identify reasons why the condition existed are all common feelings.

The nurse's role includes anticipatory guidance and support of the client undergoing this high-risk procedure. In addition, careful physical assessment and prompt reporting of complications are necessary.

▶ PRETERM LABOR AND BIRTH

Any true labor experienced before the end of the 37th week of gestation and after 20 weeks is called **preterm labor. Preterm birth** is delivery after the age of viability or potential for survival but before completion of 37 weeks of gestation. The age of viability is difficult to define, because technology and expert care have made survival of younger and sicker infants possible.

Prematurity accounts for 66% of all neonatal deaths (Cunningham et al., 1997) and despite technologic advances, the incidence of preterm births in the United States has not decreased.

▶ Preterm Labor

Clients in whom preterm labor will subsequently occur must be identified with a reasonable degree of discrimination if preventive interventions are to be used appropriately. The symptoms of preterm labor are summarized below.

- Uterine contractions, 5 to 8 minutes apart or less; pain may or may not be present; contractions are unrelieved by rest
- Low backache or pain, unrelieved by rest
- Pelvic pressure; discomfort may radiate to inner thighs
- Menstrual-type cramps
- Intestinal cramping, with or without indigestion or diarrhea
- Alteration in usual nature of vaginal discharge, particularly the onset of mucoid, watery, or blood-tinged discharge
- Gush or trickle of fluid from vagina (ruptured membranes)

Particular attention should be focused on early diagnosis, because the majority of women in preterm labor do not recognize their symptoms. Delayed recognition of symptomatology causes women to present for care after their labor is too far progressed for effective management. Several modalities for early diagnosis have been identified, yet the predictive ability of most modalities is low (Cunningham et al., 1997). However, several factors do correlate strongly with subsequent preterm labor, as listed in the box entitled Risk Factors for Preterm Labor.

Reducing risk factors for preterm labor is a valuable approach in its management. Maternal infection has been strongly associated with the incidence of

► RISK FACTORS FOR PRETERM LABOR

- Placenta previa
- Abruptio placentae
- Chorioamnionitis
- Antiphospholipid antibody syndrome
- Poor nutrition
- Poor weight gain
- Substance abuse (including tobacco)
- < 18 years of age
- > 40 years of age
- Poverty

- Short stature
- Psychologic stress
- Urinary tract infection
- Group B streptococcus
- DES exposure
- Multiple gestation
- Uterine fibroids
- > 2 second-trimester abortions
- > 3 first-trimester abortions
- PIH

preterm labor and recent research has studied elevated levels of Interleukin-10 and Interleukin-3 as indicators of eventual preterm labor (Gibbs & Eschenbach, 1997; Romero et al., 1993). Client teaching to prevent maternal infection can reduce this risk factor.

Antiphospholipid antibody syndrome (APS) is currently being researched as to its relationship to preterm labor as well as other complications of pregnancy. Early identification of APS and treatment with prednisone, low dose aspirin and/or heparin therapy will hopefully decrease the incidence of preterm labor in women with APS (Hewell & Hammer, 1997).

Intensive client education is provided for those women identified at risk for preterm labor. Symptomatology associated with preterm labor is taught and women are instructed to contact their health care provider if problems are encountered. Home uterine activity monitoring is often used, with daily telephone contact with a perinatal nurse.

The problem of preterm labor is complex. To date, the most effective means of treatment is identification of women at risk as well as diagnosing preterm labor very early in its inception. A wide array of efforts is needed, including teenage pregnancy prevention; health education focused on decreasing the incidence of infectious diseases; universal access to early and comprehensive prenatal services; and preconceptional counseling, screening, and early intervention for medical conditions that complicate pregnancy. Pregnant women also need nutrition education early in pregnancy. Eligibility for nutritional supplementation programs such as the Special Supplemental Food Program for Women, Infants, and Children (WIC; see Chapter 14) should be determined. Midwifery practices have demonstrated decreased incidence of prematurity and low birth weight among traditionally underserved populations, reflecting the benefit of client teaching and supervision for prevention of problems associated with preterm labor.

Nursing and Collaborative Assessment

Preterm labor may be difficult to distinguish from false labor prior to significant changes in cervical effacement and dilation. Uterine contractions alone may be confused with Braxton Hicks contractions and result in an incorrect diagnosis of false labor. The onset of labor is usually confirmed if uterine contractions are occurring with a frequency of at least once every 10 minutes and a duration of 30 seconds or more or if there is progressive cervical dilation. In the presence of uterine irritability, monitoring with external electronic tocography is advised to assess uterine activity.

Following stabilization of an acute episode of preterm labor in the hospital, assessment of uterine activity may be done while the client is maintained on therapy at home. For clients able to participate responsibly in their own care, home therapy is much less financially and emotionally burdensome than hospitalization. Clients may be taught to assess their own uterine contraction patterns and are advised to contact their health care provider if contractions increase in frequency or intensity or if other signs of preterm labor emerge.

When indicated, perinatal nursing services may be employed to assess uterine activity while the client remains in her home. Nurses with special background in antenatal testing or labor and delivery remain in telephone contact with clients on a daily or more frequent basis. In addition to assessing a client's reports of her condition and responses to therapy, the nurse evaluates tracings of uterine activity.

The client who is managed at home is provided with a tocodynamometer. She is instructed how and when to record uterine activity. The client fits the speaker part of her telephone into a device on the recorder. She pushes a button, which causes the data to be swiftly transmitted to the antenatal testing center, and printed for the nurse to read at once. The nurse then can provide counseling to the client, confer

Nursing Alert

The initial signs of preterm labor are often subtle and frequently do not resemble full-term labor symptoms. Clients at risk should be counseled regarding these indications and urged to contact their health care provider if they occur.

with the physician at the testing center on interpretation of strips, and refer the client to her obstetrician if nonreassuring patterns are identified.

At times, antenatal testing for clients being treated for preterm labor may be done by the nurse through home visits. Although home monitoring services are much less expensive than hospitalization, clients may have problems in securing approval for reimbursement from certain insurance sources.

Nursing and Collaborative Management

Care of the client at risk for preterm labor requires collaboration and a close working relationship among health care providers, client, and family. The client at risk for preterm labor is instructed on surveillance for and prevention of labor. Teaching also focuses on reducing risk factors.

The nurse instructs the woman to limit activity and increase daytime rest. Active sports, heavy housework, and lifting children should be avoided. Daytime rest is increased to 2 to 3 hours or more if uterine activity does not abate. She is also instructed to drink 8 to 10 cups of nonalcoholic, noncaffeinated beverages per day and to urinate every 2 hours. Additional amounts of fluids may be prescribed if contractions occur. Intercourse, sexual arousal, and breast or nipple manipulation are contraindicated, because these activities affect the release of oxytocin. Clients who are not on prescribed bedrest may attend prepared childbirth classes, but are advised to participate only in breathing exercises. The nurse working with the client on bedrest is encouraged to provide individualized educational materials for the home. Hospital-based childbirth education programs available for high-risk women may be able to establish an outreach program for homebound clients.

If home care measures are ineffective in preventing increased uterine activity, the woman is hospitalized. Various strategies for management of preterm labor exist. However, all will include some combination of bedrest, hydration, and pharmacologic intervention with tocolytic agents.

Tocolytics are potent drugs used to inhibit uterine contractions. Several medications are currently in use, including beta-adrenergic agents such as ritodrine hydrochloride (Yutopar) and terbutaline sulfate (Brethine); magnesium sulfate; prostaglandin synthetase inhibitors such as indomethacin (Indocin); and calcium channel blockers such as nisedepine (Procardia). Mixed results in the efficacy of these agents have led to controversy. No one drug has been shown to be totally safe and effective when used in the management of preterm labor. Beta-adrenergic agents have cardiovascular and metabolic side effects that include pulmonary edema and chest pain, cardiac arrhythmias, a widening of pulse pressure, and significant glucose intolerance in both mother and fetus (see box entitled Drug Guide: Terbutaline Sulfate).

Magnesium sulfate has been used extensively for the management of PIH. More recently it has been recognized as an effective tocolytic agent. Although serious maternal and neonatal side effects are uncommon, magnesium toxicity is a concern. Absence of patellar reflex and respiratory depression may signal impending respiratory arrest or cardiovascular collapse (see box entitled Drug Guide: Magnesium Sulfate earlier in chapter). The tachyarrhythmias seen with beta-sympathomimetic drugs are not seen with magnesium sulfate.

Calcium antagonists for the control of premature uterine contractility are still experimental and have not been approved by the FDA for use as a tocolytic. To date no fetal effects have been reported in humans. Mothers may experience mild discomfort from facial flushing, transient tachyarrhythmias and palpitations, light-headedness, headache, peripheral edema, nausea, and cramps.

Fear of fetal and neonatal effects has limited the use of prostaglandin synthetase inhibitors (PGSIs). Premature closure of the ductus arteriosus and persistent fetal circulation are associated with the use of PGSIs in pregnancy. Elevated bilirubin levels, altered platelet function, and urinary effects have also been reported in infants. Long-term effects remain unknown. Maternal side effects are primarily gastrointestinal and may be decreased by administering the medication with an antacid or after meals. Increased bleeding may occur during labor and the postpartum period because PGSIs alter platelet function. Antipyretic effects may mask signs of infection, particularly in the woman with ruptured membranes.

Following stabilization on one of the parenteral tocolytic agents, the client may be weaned to oral ritodrine or terbutaline and discharged for home care. Although acute episodes of preterm labor may be effectively managed with any of the tocolytic drugs, long-term maintenance with oral beta-mimetic agents

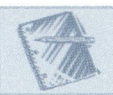

Client Teaching

Preterm Labor

The nurse can suggest the following self-care practices to the pregnant client experiencing preterm labor:

- Signs of labor may not be obvious. If you experience any of the following symptoms, notify your health care provider: constant low backache, menstrual-like cramps, pelvic pressure, intestinal cramping, change in vaginal discharge, vaginal bleeding, fluid from the vagina, or fever.
- If you are experiencing preterm labor, restrict your activities as instructed. Bedrest and home monitoring are vital to prevention of and/or determining early onset preterm labor.
- Never hesitate to contact your health care provider if you "sense" something is wrong with your baby.

is associated with a breakthrough of uterine activity in as many as 50% of women treated. After prolonged and continuous high-dose therapy, the beta receptors in the body become desensitized. Continuous, subcutaneous, low-dose bimodal delivery of terbutaline using a portable infusion pump may be used to prevent loss of sensitivity to the drug.

The effectiveness of tocolysis is most profound if treatment begins within 24 to 72 hours from the onset of labor. Long-term tocolysis is most effective if initiated before advanced cervical dilation and effacement have occurred. Advanced dilation is defined as greater than 3 cm dilated and 50% effaced.

Although the incidence of preterm delivery and sequelae have not markedly changed with the use of tocolytics, it is suggested that treatment does allow a 48-hour window of opportunity for more aggressive use of glucocorticoids to stimulate lung maturity and reduce the severity of respiratory distress syndrome. Transfer of the laboring woman to a tertiary care center is also facilitated.

Bedrest is the most widely used first-level intervention for the management of preterm labor. As much as 10 to 20 weeks of inactivity may be necessary to achieve a term delivery. Although decreased

---

▶ DRUG GUIDE: TERBUTALINE SULFATE

ACTIONS/INDICATIONS

Stimulates beta-2 receptors of sympathetic nervous system causing relaxation of uterine muscle. Also causes bronchodilation and, at high doses, cardiac effects. Used for prevention and treatment of preterm labor.

DOSAGE

May be given IV, SC infusion, or oral route. SC infusion and oral are preferred routes.
SC infusion: 0.25 mg every 1–3 hrs.
Oral: 2.5–5 mg every 2–4 hrs.
Lowest dose possible used to minimize adverse reactions and still maintain therapeutic effect. When changing from SC to oral route, give oral dose 30 minutes prior to discontinuing SC therapy.

CONTRAINDICATIONS AND PRECAUTIONS

Contraindicated before 20 weeks' gestation and if continuation of pregnancy is hazardous to maternal-fetal health. Should not be used with maternal conditions such as uncontrolled diabetes, hyperthyroidism, uncontrolled hypertension, cardiac dysrhythmias, and asthmatics using beta-mimetic or steroid agents. Currently not FDA approved for use as tocolytic agent but widely used.

ADVERSE REACTIONS

Dose related: Most common are maternal-fetal tachycardia, palpitations, cardiac arrhythmias, chest pain, widening of pulse pressure, dyspnea, restlessness, headache, flushing, hypokalemia, and maternal-fetal hyperglycemia.

DRUG INTERACTIONS

- Corticosteroids: Concurrent administration may cause pulmonary edema.
- Other beta agonists: May increase adverse reactions, particularly cardiac effects.
- Beta blockers: Antagonizes therapeutic effects of terbutaline.

NURSING IMPLICATIONS

- Assess therapeutic effect on uterine contractions.
- Monitor maternal vital signs and fetal heart rate q15–30 minutes.
- Assess for significant adverse reactions: Maternal heart rate >110, respirations >24, systolic BP <90, FHR >160, chest pain, dyspnea, elevated glucose levels.

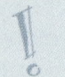

Nursing Alert

Tocolytic therapy is contraindicated in the presence of certain complications, including fetal anomalies and fetal distress, hemorrhage, severe maternal illness that is progressing during pregnancy, or severe PIH. Premature rupture of membranes is also considered a contraindication for tocolytic therapy, but there may be exceptions if the woman is hospitalized and under strict supervision.

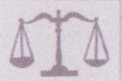

Ethical Decision Making

Ms. Reyes, a 34-year-old gravida 7, para 4 presents to Labor and Delivery complaining of ruptured membranes. An ultrasound confirms membrane rupture and a pregnancy of 21 weeks' gestation, with a living fetus. Ms. Reyes is admitted for observation, monitoring, and hydration. She is on bedrest with bathroom privileges and continues to leak clear fluid with ambulation, but she has no contractions. Extended hospitalization is probable.

After four days of hospitalization, Ms. Reyes is found weeping and packing her suitcase. She states that she cannot find child care any longer for her four preschool children, and she must return home. When questioned, she states she has no close family that could help at home and she is the only source of financial support. The physician explains to her that she is putting herself and the baby at risk for infection, preterm labor, prolapsed cord, and delivery of a nonviable infant. She insists on signing out AMA, stating, "I have four small children at home who need me more."

1. Whose rights are paramount here: the mother or the fetus? Does the mother have the right to endanger the life of the fetus knowingly?
2. Should the hospital intervene on behalf of the fetus? Does a fetus of 21 weeks have the right to be protected legally?
3. Is Ms. Reyes morally justified in putting the needs of her other children first?
4. What could you, as her nurse, do that could make a difference in the outcome?

activity improves uterine blood flow and reduces pressure on the cervix, women on prolonged bedrest undergo physiologic changes related to recumbency that may be made worse by the normal vascular system changes of pregnancy. In addition to the concern related to potential physiologic complications, health care providers are troubled by the fact that loss in physical strength and endurance may affect a woman's return to activities of daily living and infant care. Although exercise is a component of most bedrest protocols in the hospital, limited research has been done on the relationship between exercise and uterine activity. Researchers have found that a regular exercise program for women with preterm labor on long-term bedrest resulted in minimal changes in the frequency of uterine contractions. Preliminary findings suggest that closely monitored preterm labor clients may be able to safely participate in a conditioning exercise program of isometric and isotonic muscle contractions.

The client being treated for preterm labor needs much support. She may require guidance in planning for outside assistance in maintaining her home and tending to the needs of her family. Furthermore, she needs assistance in dealing with boredom and social isolation that occur during weeks or months of inactivity.

Women in preterm labor may feel emotionally unprepared, as they have not completed psychologic processes of the third trimester. The anticipation associated with delivery of a premature infant can also be frightening for a couple. A tour of the neonatal intensive care unit at the hospital in which the mother will deliver may prove reassuring. If restricted activity prevents a tour, photographs of the unit and the equipment may provide anticipatory guidance. Photographs are often available from the Parent Support Coordinator or Social Worker at the intensive care unit.

▶ Preterm Delivery

In the case of preterm labor and delivery, the more immature the fetus, the greater the risks of labor and delivery. The blood vessels within the preterm infant's head are fragile, and intracranial hemorrhage is a risk when the infant is exposed to pressure changes or hypoxia during labor and birth. Some perinatal centers perform cesarean deliveries of all fetuses below an established gestational age to avoid head trauma.

If delivery will be vaginal, labor must not be forceful. Oxytocics are generally contraindicated. Continuous electronic monitoring is performed. Trauma, such as tugging on the infant in either vaginal or cesarean delivery, is avoided. If the infant is born vaginally, a liberal episiotomy further reduces head trauma. An interdisciplinary neonatal team should be on hand to resuscitate the infant if necessary. The infant will probably be placed in a special care nursery for observation and treatment as needed. (See Chapter 33 for a complete discussion of the complications of prematurity.)

In a situational crisis like preterm birth, individuals may need assistance to develop, maintain, or utilize a support system. Nursing care includes determining what premature delivery of the infant means to the woman and her partner, how they perceive the events that led up to the delivery, what role in this sequence the woman ascribes to herself, what blaming behaviors are going on in the family system, how the family has coped with crises in the past, and what resources, particularly in the form of support persons, they can identify (see Chapter 12).

Where parents' perceptions of events surrounding the birth are inaccurate, correct information is required. The woman may feel guilty that she could not protect her infant or carry out her reproductive role, or that she does not have her fantasized infant. Nursing care that provides education and support can promote positive maternal perceptions despite prematurity. Clients may also be referred to support groups.

► Rh ISOIMMUNIZATION

Rh isoimmunization is a hemolytic disease arising from incompatibility of Rh factors of maternal and fetal blood which causes an antigen–antibody reaction and destruction of fetal red blood cells. The most lethal form of hemolytic disease of the newborn (HDN), erythroblastosis fetalis, causes the fetus to experience severe anemia, hypoxia, cardiac failure, and fetal death. The incidence of HDN is at an almost irreducible minimum in the United States. Women at risk, however, may go undetected. Further reduction in the incidence of HDN can only be accomplished through early identification, appropriate management and follow-up, and client education. Nurses play a key role in this effort.

HDN is theoretically possible with the following sequence of events: (1) an antigen in the fetus that is absent in the mother; (2) transfer of fetal blood into mother's circulation; (3) sensitization of mother's blood as the result of an antigen–antibody response against the fetal blood antigen; (4) transport of the maternal antibody across the placenta to the fetus; and (5) reaction between maternal antibody and fetal antigen on the fetal cell surface that results in the destruction of fetal red blood cells.

Sensitization usually occurs when an Rh-negative woman is pregnant with an Rh-positive fetus. When the fetus is delivered, fetal erythrocytes enter the maternal circulation. The mother forms antibodies to the Rh complex of antigens. In subsequent pregnancies where the fetus is Rh-positive, Rh antibodies from the sensitized woman's circulation cross the placenta and enter the fetal circulation, where they cause the destruction of fetal red blood cells. Hemolytic diseases of the newborn are discussed in detail in Chapter 32.

Although sensitization occurs most frequently in the early postpartum period following either vaginal or cesarean delivery, other circumstances can result in isoimmunization. Examples are ectopic pregnancy, spontaneous and therapeutic abortion, any occurrence that breeches the integrity of the placenta and causes bleeding, or transfusion of an Rh-negative woman with Rh-positive blood.

An individual's Rh type is genetically determined. Among the several Rh factors (C, Cw, c, D, d, E, and e), the D antigen, also designated Rho(D), Rh(D), DD, or Dd, is the antigen implied when discussing Rh status. Rh type is either homozygous (DD) or heterozygous (Dd). The D allele is autosomal dominant. Therefore, only the person who is homozygous dd will be Rho(D)-negative. The mother who is Rho(D)-negative (dd) can only be sensitized by a Rho(D)-positive (Dd or DD) fetus.

In the United States, 85% of the population is Rh positive. Hemolytic disease of the fetus or newborn occurs in 1.5% of pregnancies, and this particular blood incompatibility accounts for 75% of all maternal–fetal incompatibilities. The incidence of Rh isoimmunization has been reduced drastically in the United States since the availability of Rho(D) immune globulin (RhoGAM).

► Collaborative Assessment

Screening criteria for Rh isoimmunization are well standardized and constitute the foundation for assessment. At the initial prenatal visit, each pregnant woman should be evaluated for ABO blood group, Rh status, presence or absence of antibodies, and an IgG antibody titer. Various tests are used to determine the presence of antibodies in the mother, including saline agglutination, albumin agglutination, and antiglobulin testing (indirect Coombs' test). The indirect Coombs' test is the most commonly used in clinical practice. This test can measure the number of antibodies in the maternal blood. A sample of maternal blood is diluted with a specific quantity of known washed Rh-positive red blood cells (RBCs). Anti-human globulin from animal sources is added. If the woman's serum contains antibodies, the Rh-positive RBCs will clump. The dilution at which the Rh-positive RBCs clump gives the titer of maternal antibody. Negative titers are accurate indicators that a fetus is not at risk. Rh-negative status or positive titers require further evaluation.

If the mother is Rh-negative, her charts should be clearly labeled and Rh-status added to the care plan. Rh status of her male partner should also be determined. When question of paternity is at issue, it is in the best interest of the fetus to assume that the father of the baby is Rh-positive.

Further screening of the mother is warranted when the father is Rh-positive. Titers are determined monthly through the second trimester and every two to four weeks through the third trimester. If titers exceed a laboratory's own critical titer, then spectrophotometric analysis of amniotic fluid for the presence of bilirubin (ΔOD450) is the most sensitive index of severity of fetal hemolysis. Amniotic fluid analysis is based on the following pathology: Rh isoimmunization results in hemolysis of fetal RBCs. The destruction of RBCs releases bilirubin into the amniotic fluid. Bilirubin causes a peak in the otherwise smooth slope of the optical density curve at the 450-nm wavelength. The size of the peak, when correlated with the gestational age, provides an indication of the degree of hemolysis.

▶ Collaborative Management

The nonsensitized Rh-negative mother may receive a prophylactic dose of Rho(D) immune globulin (RhIG) in the 28th week of pregnancy. This practice is not without its critics. Some practitioners feel that prophylaxis provides benefit to only a small percentage of treated individuals and does not warrant the cost of mass inoculation. It is also noted that the most common cause of Rh-sensitization is the failure to appropriately administer RhIG in the postpartum period. Other risks associated with administration of a blood product (RhIG is produced from plasma) also raise questions of efficacy.

If Rh sensitization has occurred, the need for fetal exchange transfusion is determined using ΔOD450 values, ultrasound, and percutaneous umbilical blood sampling (PUBS). PUBS is a technique that provides direct access to the fetal circulation. Not only does PUBS permit sampling of fetal blood, but it also allows for intrauterine fetal transfusions. PUBS has effectively replaced intrauterine intraperitoneal exchange transfusion and may eliminate the need for spetrophotometric analysis of amniotic fluid. See Chapter 17 for discussion of the risks from PUBS.

Ideally, fetal maturity of 36 to 37 weeks is achieved before delivery. Management during delivery depends on the status of the fetus.

▶ Nursing Assessment and Management

Rho(D) immune globulin (RhIG) is administered to the Rh-negative client within 72 hours of maternal exposure to antigens, specifically after abortion, transfusion, premature separation of the placenta, amniocentesis, ectopic pregnancy, or birth of an Rh positive infant. Even though the postpartum administration of RhIG has significantly reduced the incidence of Rh-isoimmunization, 10 to 15% of postpartum mothers at risk do not receive adequate protection. This is likely due to antepartal sensitization, undetected or forgotten Rh-positive fetuses in previous pregnancies, transfusions, or insufficient dose of postpartum RhIG. The standard dose of RhIG contains at least 300 µg of RhIG and inactivates a fetal–maternal transfusion of at most 15 mL of RBCs (30 mL of whole blood). The nurse present at delivery should verbally inform the postpartum staff of excessive bleeding that may result in the need for an adjusted dose. A woman's candidacy for postpartum administration of RhIG is based on the following parameters: an Rh-negative mother, an Rh-positive fetus, and a negative direct Coombs' test on cord blood (indicates that an antigen–antibody response has not already occurred). The nurse initiates the blood studies necessary to establish candidacy, evaluates the results, and administers the appropriate dose of RhIG within 72 hours of delivery. An in-house registry of all Rh-negative women with date and time of RhIG administration may help avoid oversights.

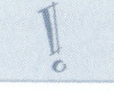

Nursing Alert

All Rh-negative women should be counseled to receive RhIG after any pregnancy, even a first-trimester abortion.

Women's Health

Nurses working with women of childbearing age need to assume responsibility for the education of the Rh-negative woman. She needs instruction about when and why RhIG is administered. Her awareness that she will be responsible for informing health care providers of her need for RhIG after exposure to the Rh-positive antigen for the rest of her childbearing years may be the single best prevention modality.

The sensitized woman provides an additional challenge to the nurse in terms of assessment and management. To participate successfully in her own care, she needs to understand the regimen of testing she will undergo. The woman and her partner will need psychosocial support throughout the regimen of monitoring and treatment for erythroblastosis fetalis. Serial amniocentesis and intrauterine transfusion are stressful. This couple requires childbirth education appropriate for high-risk pregnancy and may appreciate the opportunity to become familiar with the neonatal intensive care unit and personnel.

▶ ABO Incompatibility

ABO incompatibility most typically results when a type O woman is pregnant with a type A or B fetus. Development of the disease during a current pregnancy is not related to its occurrence in subsequent pregnancies. The antigens of the ABO group are not limited to the surface of the fetal RBC, but are found in many tissues and may be secreted in saliva and gastric juices. Therefore, a person may become sensitized to A and B antigens without being exposed to A or B RBCs. This "naturally" occurring sensitization accounts for the fact that ABO incompatibility can occur in a primigravidous woman and affect the first fetus. The hemolytic disease that results is mild compared with Rh incompatibility, and antenatal treatment is not warranted. The neonate is monitored for the development of hyperbilirubinemia (see Chapter 32).

The presence of ABO incompatibility can be beneficial when it co-exists with Rh incompatibility. Maternal ABO antibodies destroy the transfused fetal RBCs before sensitization to the Rh surface antigen can occur.

▶ THROMBOPHLEBITIS AND DEEP VEIN THROMBOSIS

Superficial thrombophlebitis is an inflammatory process involving clot formation within a superficial vein. **Deep venous thrombosis** (DVT), a clot in the deep veins, does not involve an inflammatory process. A potentially fatal complication of DVT is pulmonary embolus (PE). Factors associated with increased risk during pregnancy include:

- Maternal age greater than 35
- Obesity
- Immobilization
- Cardiopulmonary disease
- Diabetes mellitus
- Prior history of thromboembolism
- Method of delivery, with cesarean delivery being associated with a three times greater risk than vaginal delivery

DVT is less common than superficial vein involvement.

Pregnancy is a hypercoagulate state because of an increased production of procoagulant factors and a decrease in anticoagulant factors. In addition, venous stasis tends to occur in the lower extremities and groin as a result of compression by the gravid uterus. Activity, hydration, and avoiding restrictive clothing or positions that compromise venous return are usually adequate to protect all but high-risk women from thromboembolic events.

Signs of superficial thrombophlebitis include tenderness, redness, and induration directly over the superficial vein. Signs of DVT include calf tenderness, particularly on ambulation; swelling, confirmed by calf measurements or swelling of one leg in relation to the other; redness and warmth; and pain in the back of the calf. In many clients with confirmed DVT, however, all of the preceding signs and symptoms may be absent.

▶ Collaborative Assessment

The diagnosis of both these conditions may be confirmed by noninvasive tests or invasive tests. Doppler flow studies and impedance plethysmography (IPG) are the most common noninvasive tests.

Doppler studies involve a combination of ultrasound imaging and Doppler analysis of blood flow. Ultrasound is used to visualize veins and to detect their compressibility. If a vein cannot be compressed when the transducer of the duplex scanner is pressed against the skin, thrombosis is likely.

During IPG, the rate of emptying of the deep veins in the calf is measured after occlusion of the deep veins in the thigh by inflation of a thigh cuff. A clot in deep veins above the knee will cause obstruction of outflow of venous blood from the affected calf. Venous emptying time of the calf veins thus increases.

An invasive test sometimes used in diagnosis of superficial thrombophlebitis and DVT is venography. During this procedure, radiopaque dye is injected into a vein in the foot. The dye is then followed by x-ray as it travels through the deep veins of the leg into the pelvis. Clots in deep or superficial veins may be directly seen. This method is less popular during pregnancy because of exposure of the fetus to radiation.

Clot fragments from deep veins may break off, travel up the inferior vena cava to the right side of the heart, and then proceed into the lungs. The clot may block or reduce the flow of blood from the right side of the heart into that part of the lung. This condition is called a pulmonary embolism. The client may not be able to maintain adequate oxygen levels in the blood because of poor perfusion of the affected part of the lung. If the clot is large enough, the client may go into sudden right-sided heart failure.

Signs of pulmonary embolism include dyspnea, tachypnea, sudden chest pain, tachycardia, cardiac arrhythmias, apprehension, and hemoptysis. Death may result from hypoxia, cardiac failure, or cardiac arrhythmias. Pulmonary embolism ranks as the second most common cause of maternal death (Burrow & Ferris, 1995). DVT is known to precede pulmonary embolism in many of these cases. As with DVT, clinical signs and symptoms of pulmonary embolism may be absent.

▶ Collaborative Management

Collaborative management of superficial thrombophlebitis and DVT is the same except for anticoagulation therapy. Anticoagulation is rarely necessary for superficial venous thrombosis. Therapeutic measures include the following:

- Bedrest with elevation of the affected leg, as indicated.
- Moist heat to relieve pain and inflammation.
- Bed cradle to keep covers away from the leg.
- Custom-measured compression stockings; prophylactic use of compression stockings in high-risk clients.
- Anticoagulation with heparin, given intravenously at first. Heparin therapy is monitored by the partial thromboplastin time (PTT). The dose should be titrated to keep the PTT approximately twice the control value. Platelet counts should be monitored routinely. In rare cases, heparin may induce platelet aggregation and result in low platelet counts. These platelet aggregates may block both arteries and veins in other areas of the body. This condition is referred to as heparin-induced thrombocytopenia. Once PTT levels have stabilized and the client's clinical condition permits, the client is switched from intravenous to subcutaneous heparin therapy for the duration of the pregnancy. As the client's estimated date of delivery (EDD) approaches, plans may be made for a controlled delivery. Induction allows the practitioner to stop subcutaneous heparin and start low-dose (5000 units every 12 hours or an adjusted dose to keep the PTT at 1.3 times control) intravenous heparin until delivery. When labor is spontaneous, subcutaneous heparin is stopped and the PTT gradually decreases. Heparin therapy is prescribed with caution during pregnancy. Recognized complications of long-term therapy include osteoporosis. Oral anticoagulants, such as warfarin, are contraindicated during pregnancy because of fetotoxicity (Clarke-Pearson, 1994). Women with DVT above the knee who cannot receive anticoagulants may have a filter placed in the inferior vena cava to trap clots.
- Blood studies including PTT, complete blood count, and platelets.

▶ Nursing Assessment

Nursing assessment includes evaluating the potential for DVT based on the family and medical history. The woman is monitored for evidence of thrombophlebitis and DVT at each antenatal visit and daily during the postpartum period. Women on anticoagulant therapy should be observed for bleeding gums, bruising, and prolonged oozing from puncture sites. Frequent assessment for postpartum hemorrhage is essential. Silent bleeding may be evidenced by hematomas.

▶ Nursing Diagnoses

Nursing diagnoses are developed on the basis of comprehensive assessment. Examples of nursing diagnoses for a woman with venous disease are:

Problem-oriented diagnoses:

- Risk for peripheral neurovascular dysfunction, related to DVT

- Pain and discomfort, related to superficial thrombophlebitis

Wellness-oriented diagnoses:

- Progressive home maintenance management, related to assistance from others

▶ Nursing Management

Nursing management includes the following measures:

- Anticipatory guidance, support, and education about anticoagulation therapy, associated signs of complications, and risks.
- Monitoring laboratory values during heparin therapy.
- Emergency measures if pulmonary embolism is suspected (assessment of mental status, nature, onset and severity of pain, skin color, respiratory status, pulse, blood pressure; notification of physician without delay; oxygen therapy as ordered; possible admission of client to intensive care unit). Other diagnostic measures may be performed by the physician and include arterial blood gas determination, chest x-ray, ventilation perfusion scan, and possibly pulmonary angiography.
- Teaching for prevention of venous disease or its recurrence, including advising the client to rest on her left side at night and at intervals during the day; to elevate her legs when possible; and to avoid salicylates, which promote bleeding if the woman is on anticoagulation therapy.
- Educating clients about risks, signs, and symptoms of venous disease and the need to seek care promptly if signs and symptoms occur.

▶ MULTIPLE GESTATION

Twin births account for 1 in 80 to 95 live births in the United States. Triplet and greater multiple births are far less common. However, in 1993, the rate for multiple births exceeded 100,000. There were 96,000 twin live births, 3834 triplets, 277 quadruplets, and 57 quintuplets (Cunningham et al., 1997). Multiple gestations arise either from fertilization and division of one ovum (monozygotic twinning) or fertilization of more than one ovum (dizygotic twinning) during a single ovulatory cycle. (See Chapter 13 for additional discussion of multiple gestation.)

Factors associated with dizygotic twinning include increased maternal age, increased parity, a positive family history of twins, optimal nutrition, increased levels of follicle-stimulating hormone and luteinizing hormone, increased coital frequency early in marriage, pregnancy within 1 month of stopping oral contraception, use of infertility drugs (such as clomiphene citrate and Pergonal), and in vitro fertilization. In contrast, monozygotic twinning seems to occur independent of race, heredity, age, and parity, although there may be some relation to therapy for infertility. The significant rise in higher-order births can be attributed to the use of fertility treatments, particularly by older, white, well-educated women.

▶ Collaborative Assessment and Management

Routine ultrasound is able to defect multiple gestation 87% of the time prior to delivery (Cunningham et al., 1997). Other factors that may be present in the woman's reproductive history to assist with diagnosis include a maternal family history for dizygotic twinning, recent use of fertility drugs, and self-report of increased sensation of fetal movement or feeling larger than normal for the length of gestation. Clinical signs that increase the health care provider's index of suspicion are listed below.

- Uterus larger than normal for dates
- Fetal parts palpable in all four quadrants
- Fetal movement reported in all four quadrants
- Excessive nausea and vomiting
- Anemia
- Two or more distinct fetal heart sounds
- Dyspnea
- Shortness of breath
- Pedal edema
- Backache
- Onset of PIH
- Polyhydramnios
- Abnormal alpha-fetoprotein (AFP) levels
- Visualization of more than one fetus on ultrasound

Biochemical testing, while not conclusive, further alerts the practitioner to the possibility of a twin gestation. Serum chorionic gonadotropin, placental lactogen, and AFP levels are all higher in twin pregnancies than in singleton gestations. Definitive diagnosis can be made by careful ultrasonography using at least two views. However, the incidence of twin gestation on early ultrasound may be greater than at term because of the "vanishing twin" syndrome. Spontaneous abortion of one member of a multiple gestation may be attributed to blighted ovum or reabsorption of a gestational sac. Ultrasonic refraction errors or physiologic conditions, such as bicornuate uterus, that mimic multiple gestation may yield a false diagnosis.

Morbidity and mortality are also much higher among multiple fetuses. Twins account for 10% of all preterm deliveries and 25% of all preterm deaths. Two thirds experience intrauterine growth retardation. This contributes to the increased incidence of fetal death, fetal distress in labor, and perinatal asphyxia. Twins experience a higher incidence of developmental problems including learning disabilities, motor skill deficiencies, hand-eye coordination difficulties, and speech problems. The incidence of major and minor congenital anomalies in twins is double that found among singletons and is more common among monozygotic twins. The long-term effects of multifetal gestation other than twins has not been extensively researched, as the increased incidence is a relatively new phenomenon. However, early statistics suggest a direct relationship between the number of fetuses per pregnancy and morbidity and mortality for both the mother and her fetuses.

Other complications unique to monozygous twins include "twin-to-twin transfusion syndrome," in which vascular communication develops between the twins. The donor fetus is hypotensive, anemic, severely growth retarded, and oligohydramniotic. The recipient is hypervolemic, polycythemic, heavier, and polyhydramniotic. Although there is no treatment for this problem, diagnosis via ultrasound allows the neonatal team to be prepared for two very sick infants. In 80% of cases in which this complication arises, at least one twin does not survive.

Twins who share an amniotic sac are at risk for becoming entangled in each other's umbilical cord. The rate of fetal death among monoamniotic twins exceeds 50%.

Maternal complications of multifetal pregnancies include an increased incidence of hyperemesis gravidarum, iron and folate deficiency anemias, PIH, placenta previa, and abruptio placentae.

Early diagnosis by ultrasonography allows for more intensive prenatal care of the mother of multiple fetuses. She can be educated as to possible complications in multifetal pregnancies, her role in prevention of complications, and early recognition and reporting of complications. Bedrest is widely observed to be useful in promoting fetal weight gain and prolonging pregnancy, although the amount of bedrest is controversial.

Strategies generally employed in preventing preterm labor may not be successful in multiple gestation. Fetal well-being is assessed regularly. Nonstress tests (NSTs) are begun at 30 to 34 weeks and may be repeated as often as twice a week; however,

they must be interpreted with caution, as nonreactive NST is common among fetuses of less than 32 weeks of gestation. A nonreactive NST in either fetus is followed by a contraction stress test. Serial ultrasound measurements are performed to measure growth. Severe distress and compromised growth are indications for preterm delivery. The method of choice is likely to be cesarean.

In the presence of a reactive NST, vaginal delivery is attempted as long as the multiples are mature and the presentation of each twin is favorable. There is an increased frequency of abnormal presentations with multiples (Fig. 19–5). The tendency towards fetal distress in labor makes it necessary to monitor each fetus electronically. The mother is attended by a nurse throughout labor. An intravenous route is established and packed red cells are kept on hand. The primary nurse is responsible for notifying the appropriate attendants when delivery is imminent. An anesthesiologist should be present at delivery in the event that intrauterine manipulation or cesarean delivery is necessary. Two or more neonatal resuscitation teams and two or more obstetricians are desirable, although not always possible. The second twin may require a cesarean delivery after the vaginal birth of the first. Early detection of multiple gestation prenatally allows the provider and family to prepare for this possibility. Houlihan and Knuppel (1996) state that triplet or more gestations should be delivered by cesarean birth.

▶ Nursing Assessment
and Management

The nurse evaluates the woman's reproductive history and clinical presentation as previously discussed. Over the course of the pregnancy, special attention is paid to fetal growth, maternal weight gain, maternal nutritional status, hematocrit and hemoglobin levels, the presence of associated risk factors, and the occurrence of signs and symptoms of preterm labor.

Nursing interventions include instruction regarding complications of pregnancy and the importance of early reporting. The need for adequate rest is reinforced. The woman expecting multiples can be counseled toward good nutrition, increasing her protein, calcium, iron, and folate intake beyond the RDAs for normal pregnancy. Women with multiple fetuses are at higher risk for malnutrition than those with a single fetus (Casele, Dooley, & Metzger, 1996). The recommended weight gain for women expecting twins is about 50% greater than that for a singleton birth. A total weight gain of about 40 pounds is appropriate.

The woman expecting multiples is at increased risk for preterm labor, hyperemesis gravidarum, and

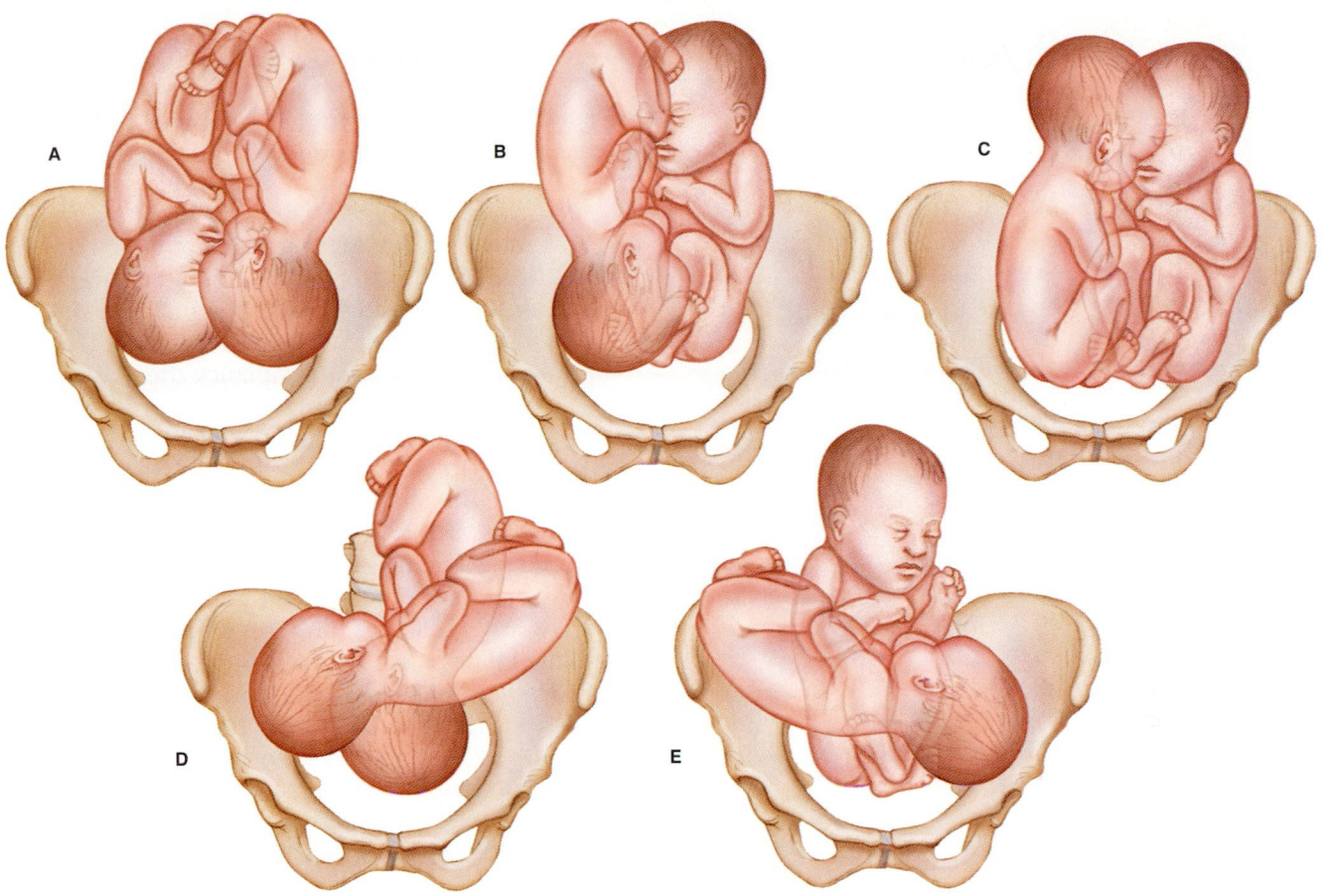

FIGURE 19–5. Examples of twin presentations. **A.** Two vertexes. **B.** One vertex, one breech. **C.** Two breeches. **D.** One vertex, one transverse. **E.** One transverse, one breech.

PIH. She requires instruction in early detection and health maintenance related to these complications. Increased surveillance requires antenatal visits every 2 weeks during the second trimester and weekly during the third.

With the significant increase in pregnancies that produce multiple fetuses, both the family and health care providers are faced with issues that have not been addressed before. The health risk to mother and fetuses is dramatically increased, as is the financial, psychologic, and emotional needs of the family unit. Ethical issues such as selective termination of a certain number of the fetuses in a multiple pregnancy is one that parents and health care professionals may face.

The family expecting multiples may be stressed by the greater financial responsibilities, by anticipation of the greater workload of child care, and by the awareness that this pregnancy is high risk. If they are

taught about potential risks to the mother and infants, particularly the risk of prematurity, expectant families will be concerned about their infants' survival. These families need anticipatory guidance about the birth itself and all of the people who may be involved. For example, one mother expecting twins asked if she faced two separate labors.

Parents of multiples face numerous practical considerations, such as obtaining double nursery furnishings and equipment, breastfeeding, and the risks and benefits of fostering twins' togetherness or separateness. The nurse can help by referring parents to the local chapter of a national group known variously as Parents of Twins or Mothers of Multiples. La Leche League supports mothers of multiples who wish to breastfeed. Publications such as "Twins" are written for families. Mothers of multiples who have attended the same antenatal clinic or delivered in the same facility may also be introduced to one another.

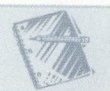

Client Teaching

Multiple Gestation

The nurse can suggest the following self-care practices to the woman expecting multiples:

- Nutrition is very important for you and the babies' health. Eat high-quality foods that will give you the most benefit. Increase your intake of protein, fiber, water, fruits and vegetables, and calcium-containing foods.
- Eat three balanced meals and three snacks each day. Take your prenatal vitamin daily.
- Walk 20–30 minutes every day (unless you start to feel short of breath).
- Whenever possible, rest on your left side. This increases blood flow to the babies. Allow yourself frequent rest periods during the day, but try to maintain as much activity as you are comfortable with without getting overfatigued.
- Wear low-heeled, soft-soled shoes to help your balance.
- Do not lift anything heavy.
- Avoid long periods of sitting in one position.
- See your health care provider at least every two weeks after the first trimester. Be sure to report unusual symptoms immediately: bleeding, clear vaginal discharge, frequent urination, fever, nausea and vomiting, swelling of the face, feet, or hands, persistent headaches, and abdominal pain or cramps.

▶ POSTTERM PREGNANCY

A **postterm pregnancy** is one that continues past the estimated date of delivery (EDD). Given the error in calculating EDD, the end of 42 weeks of gestation is commonly considered the point at which a pregnancy is postterm.

The incidence of prolonged pregnancy is reported to be 3.5 to 14.9% of all pregnancies; however, accurate diagnosis of postterm pregnancy depends on accurate dating of the pregnancy. Strategies for determining the EDD are described in Chapter 15 and are based on a detailed menstrual history, assessment of

uterine growth, dates of quickening and first fetal heart tones, and ultrasonography.

Factors associated with postterm pregnancy include anencephaly and fetal adrenal hypoplasia. Women who have experienced one postterm pregnancy are at increased risk in subsequent pregnancies. However, the etiology of postterm pregnancy is not really known because the mechanism for the initiation of labor is not completely understood.

Findings associated with postmaturity include oligohydramnios and meconium staining. Possible sequelae of the postterm pregnancy are classified as the postmaturity syndrome. The infant is wrinkled with peeling skin, alert facies, creases covering the surface of the soles, and the absence of vernix and lanugo. The infant may demonstrate respiratory distress, hypoglycemia, polycythemia, and temperature instability. Postmature infants have increased morbidity and mortality. They have been observed to have lower Brazelton scores, and to experience increased childhood illness and hospitalization, decreased social maturity, more sleep disorders, and more reading difficulties at age 6. In addition, the infants are rated "difficult" by their mothers more often than controls.

The underlying pathology in postmaturity syndrome is impaired uteroplacental perfusion, or placental insufficiency, often attributed to placental aging. This theory, however, has not been well documented in research (Cunningham et al., 1997). Oligohydramnios is another factor that contributes to postmaturity syndrome. Cord compression can occur due to decreased amniotic fluid and cause fetal jeopardy.

▶ Nursing and Collaborative Assessment

The challenge in postterm pregnancy lies in identifying infants at risk for postmaturity syndrome. Perhaps as few as 30% of pregnancies identified as postterm truly exceed 40 weeks of gestation, and only 10 to 20% of babies born are postmature. Therefore routine induction between 40 and 42 weeks of gestation, though practiced widely, does not always reflect the needs of the client.

When pregnancy extends beyond 41 weeks the woman is asked to count fetal movements several times each day: greater than 3 fetal movements per hour, or more than 10 in 3 hours, is a common standard of fetal well-being. The woman keeps a chart and contacts her midwife or obstetrician immediately should activity levels drop.

The NST is a standard measure of fetal well-being; however, there are findings indicating that the contraction stress test (CST) is more sensitive in predicting risk of postmaturity syndrome. The nipple stimulation CST is an inexpensive, efficient variation on the oxytocin challenge test (see Chapter 18).

The fetal biophysical profile is ascertained by ultrasound and NST. It includes assessment of amniotic fluid volume, fetal activity, tonus, respiratory effort, and fetal heart rate reactivity (Chapter 18). This method has potential as an indicator of postmaturity.

▶ Nursing and Collaborative Management

Management of postmaturity begins with accuracy in dating the pregnancy. Once dates are well established and postmaturity is suspected, monitoring fetal well-being becomes critical. This monitoring is time consuming and often an intrusive ordeal for postterm clients. One fourth to one third of women whose pregnancies are postterm are considered by health care professionals to be "noncompliant" because they do not fully participate in the surveillance protocol.

When pregnancy extends beyond the due date, particularly when women feel they know precisely when they conceived, stress increases. In a study of 30 expectant mothers who were at least 3 days overdue, reactions included the feeling that they would be pregnant forever. Sleep difficulties, the desire to be induced, a tendency to hang on physicians' and nurses' every word for reassurance, seeking reassurance about delivery from other mothers, fussing with the baby's clothes and equipment, overexertion with housework, and increased discomfort were common activities and complaints. Interventions by health care professionals that were most helpful included discussion of the women's feelings, discussion of the expected time range of the birth, allowing the mother to listen to the fetal heart tone, and discussion of comfort measures. The investigator concluded that women at risk for postmaturity have an intense need for someone to acknowledge that a postterm pregnancy is stressful.

The nursing presence is never more appreciated than during labor. In cases of postmaturity, labor is generally induced. Electronic fetal monitoring and close supervision are indicated. The woman's ability to focus on and work with contractions may be overwhelmed during induction, so her need for support and, in turn, her coach's need for support are greater than normal. Postmature infants are at risk for being stressed during labor. If the fetus is stressed, cesarean delivery will be performed. The team on hand to tend to the newborn should anticipate the possible need for resuscitation.

▶ OTHER MEDICAL AND SURGICAL CONDITIONS

Pregnant women can experience any medical or surgical illness that afflicts women of childbearing age. In addition, it is not uncommon to encounter women with such conditions as asthma, epilepsy, or renal disease in maternity settings. Women can experience emergencies such as appendicitis, for which surgery is required. Several important considerations are necessary for assessment and management.

1. During pregnancy many conditions are more difficult to diagnose because of normally occurring physiologic alterations of pregnancy, for example, edema and trace protein in the urine. For a nonpregnant woman with renal disease, these observations may be early evidence of the disease's progression.

2. Some complications of pregnancy mimic medical or surgical conditions in nonpregnant women. For example, abruptio placentae must be differentiated from appendicitis.

3. It may be more difficult to treat a medical or surgical complication because of the fetotoxic effects of usual strategies such as certain drug therapies. In extreme instances, the woman may be forced to choose between treating her own life-threatening illness and avoiding harm to her fetus. Treating cancer during pregnancy is an example. With the proliferation of fetal monitoring capabilities and neonatal intensive care units, this type of choice need not be made as often as it was two decades ago. But, in general, medications are used with extreme caution during pregnancy.

4. Some surgeries can be accomplished during pregnancy with a minimal increase in risk to the mother or fetus. General anesthesia need not threaten fetal well-being.

5. Pathophysiologic processes that do threaten fetal survival include hypoxia, acidosis, and hypotension. Hypertension is equally threatening to the fetus but the effects occur more slowly. As a consequence, uteroplacental perfusion is decreased and the risk of abruptio placentae is increased.

▶ TRAUMA

Trauma refers to client injury that is inflicted by the client herself or by other living or nonliving sources. Trauma can be caused accidentally or deliberately, and is the largest cause of death in women of child-bearing age. Physiologic changes and psychosocial stress related to pregnancy may put the client at risk for injury. Trauma during pregnancy involves both the expectant woman and the fetus; however, actual injury to the woman or fetus depends on the type of trauma and the maternal and fetal organs that are affected. Although the pregnant woman may sustain many types of trauma, the following injuries are seen frequently in clinical practice.

1. *Abdominal trauma.* The pregnant woman is at high risk during the second and third trimesters due to the enlarged uterus. The third trimester poses the greatest risk to the fetus, because there is less amniotic fluid than in the second trimester and the fetus is larger. During the first trimester, the embryo or fetus is protected by the bony pelvis. Blunt abdominal trauma occurs as the result of such conditions as auto accidents (in which the woman is thrown from the vehicle or against its steering wheel or dashboard) and interpersonal conflict in which the woman is punched or kicked. Injuries include fracture of the fetal skull, feto-maternal transfusion, and placental abruption. Severity of injuries does not necessarily predict whether abruptio placentae will occur. Careful observation of mother and fetus after trauma is critical. The most common causes of penetrating abdominal trauma are bullet wounds and stab wounds.

2. *Thermal trauma.* Thermal injury results from burns. Although pregnancy may not be affected if less than one third of the mother's body is burned, actual injury and threat to pregnancy depend upon the extent of the burns and circumstances in which they occurred. In addition to requiring care according to protocols for burn victims, pregnant women need attention to oxygenation, electrolyte balance, and fluid replacement. Respi-ratory or cardiac arrest and fluid and electrolyte imbalance present life-threatening conditions to both mother and fetus. The fetus is particularly susceptible to maternal hypotension because of uterine hypoperfusion. Fetal monitor tracings may show signs of fetal hypoxia even when maternal vital signs are normal.

3. *Pelvic fractures.* Pelvic fractures can occur as the result of such conditions as automobile accidents or falls. Pelvic fractures can present major problems at any time during pregnancy. In late pregnancy, when the fetal head is engaged in the pelvis, fetal skull fractures may also result.

4. *Physical abuse.* Approximately one third of all injuries to pregnant women are intentionally inflicted, and this statistic may be higher during the postpartum period (Cunningham et al., 1997). Women who are physically abused during pregnancy are at high risk for preterm labor, low-birth-weight infants, and chorioamnionitis, in addition to the damage inflicted by the abuse.

Comprehensive assessment of pregnant clients who sustain trauma requires understanding of principles of trauma, normal changes associated with pregnancy, and fetal physiology. The specialty of trauma is a branch of critical care and requires special nursing and medical expertise. Whenever feasible, the client should be taken to a trauma center capable of caring for a high-risk obstetric client and a neonate requiring sophisticated intensive care, or transferred to this type of trauma center when she is stable enough to survive transport. The goals of care focus on thorough assessment to identify the impact of injury on the expectant mother and her fetus and to implement strategies designed to stabilize the client, prevent impairment or death, and restore health. Assessment and management are based on protocols that have been published by groups such as the American College of Surgeons.

Critical Thinking in Care Planning

Care of a Client Experiencing Pregnancy-Induced Hypertension

Janet Orson, age 33, gravida 2 para 1, is 28 weeks' pregnant. She and her husband, Steven, have a healthy 2-year-old son, Jason. Her current obstetric history was normal, but it took 2 years to conceive this pregnancy. At 5 ft. 2 in., Janet weighed 132 pounds prior to pregnancy. She has gained weight appropriately. On her most recent prenatal visit her blood pressure was 122/78, her urine was negative for protein, and her 1+ pedal edema was relieved by elevation. One day in the 28th week, after walking 2 blocks, Janet suddenly experienced extreme edema of the lower extremities, dyspnea, "heartburn," and headache. The next morning in her obstetrician's office, her blood pressure was 240/170 and her urine was 4+ for protein. She has gained 10 pounds within 2 weeks. On immediate admission to the perinatal center, vital signs were blood pressure 252/178, temperature 36.5°C, pulse 94, and respirations 18. Fetal heart rate was 136. The fetus was active. Admission weight was 161 pounds. Pretibial edema was marked. Her face was swollen. Janet was apprehensive, complained of headache, and said "everything looks so dark." She had not voided since arising other than 15 mL in her obstetrician's office on the day of admission.

▶ Assessment

- Sudden onset of hypertension accompanied by edema, proteinuria, headache, epigastric pain, visual changes, low urine output.

- Vital signs: BP = 252/178
  Urine = 4+ protein
  T = 36.5°C
  P = 94
  R = 18

Nursing Diagnosis

Risk for maternal and fetal injury, related to abnormal cardiovascular adaptation, as evidenced by elevated blood pressure, proteinuria, edema, and related symptoms

Expected Client/Family Outcomes	Nursing Action/Intervention	Evaluation
Client will demonstrate stabilized cardiovascular status prior to delivery.	Maintain client on bedrest in left lateral position. *Rationale:* Left lateral position enhances circulation.	Client remains stable until delivery.
Client will experience decreased blood pressure, decreased edema, and increased urine output within 48 hours of delivery.	Assess vital signs, level of consciousness, skin temperature and moisture, and deep tendon reflexes every 30 minutes until stable. *Rationale:* Status can change quickly. Fever and altered sensorium can precede convulsions.	Client experiences reduction in blood pressure and return to normal within 12 hours.
Client's preeclampsia will not progress to eclampsia.	Review laboratory data: • CBC with platelets • PT	

(continued)

Critical Thinking in Care Planning continued

Expected Client/Family Outcomes	Nursing Action/Intervention	Evaluation
Client will demonstrate normal blood pressure by sixth postpartum week.	• PTT • Ca • SGOT, BUN *Rationale:* Preeclampsia is associated with consumptive coagulopathy. Initiate intravenous route. Administer magnesium sulfate as ordered. *Rationale:* Intravenous magnesium sulfate is treatment of choice for prevention of convulsions. Maintain intake and output record. *Rationale:* All clients with IVs and all clients who are critically ill require assessment of intake and output. Administer antihypertensives as ordered. *Rationale:* Elevation in blood pressure is responsible for many of the complications accompanying PIH. Assess patellar reflexes at least every 4 hours, respiratory status every 30 minutes. *Rationale:* Magnesium toxicity is evidenced by respiratory and neurologic depression. Keep calcium gluconate at bedside. *Rationale:* Calcium gluconate is the antidote for excess magnesium sulfate. Keep emergency cart and airway at bedside. *Rationale:* Respiratory depression may require emergency resuscitation. Assess lungs, mucous membranes, neck veins, and presence of edema for evidence of cardiac failure. *Rationale:* Hepatomegaly can lead to congestive heart failure. Briefly explain nature of the disease process, purpose of treatment, and the symptoms that should be reported immediately. *Rationale:* Understanding promotes client cooperation and reduces stress. If the client reports evidence of a change in status, prompt intervention is possible.	Client experiences no adverse reaction to medication. Client demonstrates return to normal blood pressure on her 6-week postpartum visit.

Critical Thinking in Care Planning continued

Nursing Diagnosis

Risk for maternal and fetal injury, related to hypoxia, maternal convulsions, and decreased uteroplacental perfusion

Expected Client/Family Outcomes	Nursing Action/Intervention	Evaluation
During hospitalization: • Fetus will not demonstrate ominous fetal heart rate.	Assess fetal heart rate every 15 minutes until client's vital signs are stabilized. *Rationale:* Fetal hypoxia may accompany seizures. Prepare client for fetal electronic monitoring; assess baseline variability and fetal heart rate pattern with uterine contractions. *Rationale:* Monitoring establishes fetal heart rate patterns and effects of decreased uteroplacental perfusion. Prepare client for immediate delivery if fetal status deteriorates. *Rationale:* If fetal status deteriorates, immediate delivery is often needed.	Fetus does not demonstrate ominous fetal heart patterns.
• Client will deliver a viable neonate.	Administer nonstress tests twice weekly until delivery. Take kick counts every shift. Determine presence of meconium with rupture of membranes. *Rationale:* Tests provide information on fetal well-being.	Client delivers a viable neonate.
• Client will not experience seizure or cerebrovascular accident.	Assess client's level of consciousness, deep tendon reflexes, affect, headache, and reports of visual changes every 4 hours. *Rationale:* Neurologic signs may herald eclamptic convulsions. Place client in a dark, quiet room. Plan nursing activities with minimal disturbance. Sedate client as ordered; remove prostheses. Restrict visitors. Remove telephone from room. *Rationale:* Convulsions can be triggered by neurologic stimuli. Keep bed at lowest level. Siderails should be up and padded. *Rationale:* In a safe environment, the client will not incur trauma should convulsions occur. Keep emergency oxygen kit and suction set at bedside; test equipment each shift. *Rationale:* Progression of preeclampsia requires treatment as an emergency. Treat fetal bradycardia with oxygen and left lateral position. *Rationale:* Oxygen and maternal position will prevent fetal deterioration. Give client brief, clear rationale for actions. *Rationale:* Understanding can reduce stress and promote rest.	Client does not experience convulsions. Client does not sustain trauma.

(continued)

Critical Thinking in Care Planning *continued*

Expected Client/Family Outcomes	Nursing Action/Intervention	Evaluation
	Assess client for and teach her signs of labor. Assess client for hemorrhage and evidence of abruptio placentae during labor. *Rationale:* Abruptio placentae is a complication of PIH.	

Nursing Diagnosis

Activity intolerance, related to an increase in edema on exertion

Client will avoid activity until postpartum recovery is evident. Client will demonstrate stabilized or improved pattern of urine output prior to delivery.	Monitor respiratory status and maintain client on strict bedrest in left lateral position as described above. Explain need for restrictions and position call bell and table with oral fluids within client's reach. Advise client to call for bedpan to maintain bedrest. *Rationale:* This regimen minimizes cardiovascular and neurologic stress and promotes uteroplacental perfusion.	Client carries out regimen of rest until evidence of postpartum recovery allows increased activity.

Nursing Diagnosis

Altered tissue perfusion, related to pathophysiology of PIH, as evidenced by weight gain, proteinuria, pitting edema

Client will demonstrate output commensurate with intake and reduced pretibial edema 48 hours after delivery.	Implement strict intake and output (indwelling catheter may be used). Record weight daily. Monitor BUN, creatinine, uric acid. Monitor urine protein every 4 hours. Adjust fluids based on output. Use Ringer's lactate for intravenous infusions. *Rationale:* With evidence of proteinuria and oliguria indicative of renal damage, and liver involvement that restricts circulation, fluid overload is a possible sequela.	Fluid load does not increase prior to delivery. Fluid balance restoration starts by 48 hours postpartum. Renal function is within normal limits by 6th postpartum week.

Critical Thinking in Care Planning *continued*

Nursing Diagnosis

Anxiety, related to sudden development of threat to fetal well-being

Expected Client/Family Outcomes	Nursing Action/Intervention	Evaluation
During hospitalization: • Client will experience reduction in anxiety with orientation to unit and information about her condition and that of her fetus. • Client will form a positive relationship with her primary nurse.	Assess sensorium, hyperirritability, hyperreflexia, and clonus. *Rationale:* Agitation may accompany PIH. Determine client's level of comprehension of explanations. Address specific concerns of client. *Rationale:* Understanding the situation will foster relief of anxiety, which will promote physical relaxation. Explain procedures prior to implementation. Provide anticipatory guidance with respect to NICU. *Rationale:* Anticipation and understanding of events decrease client's fears. Assess sources of support. Advise family to contact clergyman. *Rationale:* Mobilization of support can reduce anxiety.	Child at home is cared for. Family member stays with client. Client develops rapport with primary nurse. Client becomes familiar with procedures. Client uses hospital resources (e.g., social services) and chaplain, as needed. Client understands that health care team is prepared to support preterm infant.

Nursing Diagnosis

Self-esteem disturbance, related to obstetric emergency

During hospitalization and at the 6-week postpartum checkup: • Client will verbalize belief that she acted appropriately regarding this complication. • Client will grieve loss of expected pregnancy, labor, and delivery experience appropriately.	Assess client's beliefs about her condition; clarify reality. Observe family interactions. Provide positive reinforcement for client's prenatal course and actions. *Rationale:* High-risk clients may blame themselves or each other for the threat to their fetus. Help couple reconstruct experience during postpartum. *Rationale:* Couple needs to incorporate the experience into their life. Help client talk to older child on telephone daily. *Rationale:* Satisfying interaction with other child(ren) promotes self-esteem as mother.	Client expresses satisfaction that she acted appropriately. Family members, especially husband, are supportive. Client grieves her high-risk experience appropriately.

Chapter Highlights

▶ Four categories of hypertension associated with pregnancy are pregnancy-induced hypertension, chronic hypertension, chronic hypertension with superimposed preeclampsia, and transient or gestational hypertension.

▶ Preeclampsia is a progressive form of pregnancy-induced hypertension characterized by proteinuria and/or generalized edema that occurs after 20 weeks of gestation.

▶ Eclampsia is a critical condition in which preeclamptic signs are accompanied by grand mal seizures, coma, and/or shock caused by pregnancy-induced hypertension.

▶ Preconceptual counseling of the pregnant woman with cardiac disease is essential in helping the client adapt to the physiologic demands of pregnancy.

▶ Pregestational and gestational diabetes mellitus are major health care complications of pregnancy and can lead to diabetic emergencies such as ketoacidosis and hypoglycemia.

▶ Collaborative management of the pregnant client with diabetes focuses on diet, activity patterns, use of insulin to control serum glucose levels when dietary management and activity are not successful, hospitalization in the event of emergencies, and preparation of the client for delivery.

▶ The five conditions that most often result in second- or third-trimester bleeding are abruptio placentae, placenta previa, uterine rupture, disseminated intravascular coagulation, and gestational trophoblastic disease.

▶ The goals of management for clients experiencing hemorrhage during the second and third trimesters are to minimize the effects of blood loss in the mother, to deliver a healthy newborn, and to interact with the client and family so as to relieve the emotional crisis they experience in this situation.

▶ Infections such as urinary tract infections, chorioamnionitis, TORCH infections, *chlamydia trachomatis, candida albicans,* tuberculosis, group B streptococcus, and human immunodeficiency virus have a significant impact on the progress and outcome of pregnancy and require intervention on the part of the nurse in educating women and their families about the signs and symptoms of the various conditions.

▶ Two forms of abnormal amniotic fluid production are polyhydramnios, an excessive quantity of amniotic fluid, and oligohydramnios, a lower-than-normal volume of amniotic fluid.

▶ The nurse's role in managing a client experiencing incompetent cervix, an anatomic defect of the cervix resulting in painless dilation without uterine contractions, consists of anticipatory guidance and support of the client undergoing cerclage.

▶ The most effective means of treatment of women experiencing preterm labor is identification of women at risk as well as diagnosis of the condition early in its inception.

▶ Careful screening of Rh-negative women and prompt intervention with administration of Rho(D) immune globulin within 72 hours of maternal exposure to antigens can significantly reduce the incidence of Rh-isoimmunization.

▶ Nursing care of clients experiencing either superficial thrombophlebitis or deep vein thrombosis consists of education about anticoagulation therapy, monitoring of laboratory values during heparin therapy, initiation of emergency measures if pulmonary embolism is suspected, and teaching for prevention of venous disease.

▶ For families expecting multiples, nurses can provide important information concerning complications of pregnancy, importance of reporting signs of preterm labor, need for adequate rest, and promotion of good nutrition.

Chapter Highlights continued

▶ In cases of postmaturity, the nurse is instrumental in educating the client and family about the methods of monitoring fetal well-being and supporting them in handling the stress associated with this condition.

▶ The goals of care for a pregnant client experiencing trauma are to identify the impact of injury on the mother and fetus and implement strategies to stabilize the client, prevent death, and restore health.

▶ Client education is a major nursing management strategy that results in client compliance and risk reduction and includes health maintenance strategies, therapeutic drug administration, warning signs of potential complications, and the importance of close supervision throughout a high-risk pregnancy.

After reading the vignette at the beginning of this chapter, use what you have learned to answer these questions:

1. How can Ann Salzman, CNM, MSN, inform Tamika Dengler about the risks related to urinary tract infections without alarming her about her own health or the health of her baby?

2. What educational strategies can Ann Salzman, CNM, MSN, share with Tamika Dengler that will help her avoid the risk of developing a urinary tract infection?

3. What effect may a condition such as a urinary tract infection have on a client's physiologic and psychologic adaptation to the third trimester of pregnancy?

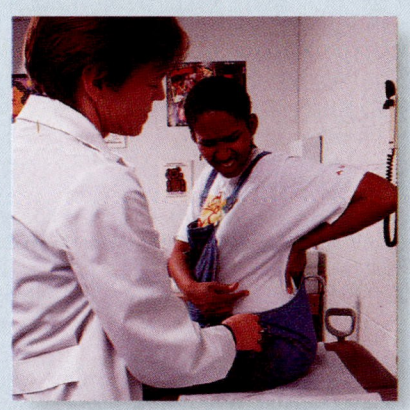

Critical Thinking Questions

► References

Boden, G. (1996). Fuel metabolism in pregnancy and in gestational diabetes mellitus. *Obstetric and Gynecologic Clinics of North America, 23*(1), 1–10.

Buchanan, T., & Coustan, D.V. (1995). Diabetes mellitus. In G.N. Burrow & T.F. Ferris (Eds.), *Medical complications during pregnancy* (4th ed.) (pp. 29–61). Philadelphia: W.B. Saunders.

Burrow, G.N., & Ferris, T.F. (1995). *Medical complications during pregnancy* (4th ed.). Philadelphia: W.B. Saunders.

Casele, H.L., Dooley, S.L., & Metzger, B.E. (1996). Metabolic response to meal eating and extended overnight fasting in twin gestation. *American Journal of Obstetrics and Gynecology, 175*(4 Pt 1), 917–921.

Clarke-Pearson, D.L. (1994). Venous thromboembolic disease in pregnancy. In F.P. Zuspan & E.J. Quilligan (Eds.), *Current therapy in obstetrics and gynecology* (4th ed.) (pp. 300–323). Philadelphia: W.B. Saunders.

Corbett, J.V. (1995). Anticoagulants during pregnancy. *MCN, American Journal of Maternal-Child Nursing, 20*(1), 56.

Coustan, D.R. (1996). Screening and testing for gestational diabetes mellitus. *Obstetric and Gynecologic Clinics of North America, 23*(1), 25–136.

Cunningham, F.G., MacDonald, P.C., Gant, N.F., Leveno, K.J., Gilstrap, L.C., Hankins, G.D.V., & Clark, S.L. (1997). *Williams obstetrics* (20th ed.). Stamford, CT: Appleton & Lange.

Droste, S.K., & Keil K. (1994). Expectant management of placenta previa: Cost-benefit analysis of outpatient treatment. *American Journal of Obstetrics and Gynecology, 170*, 1254–1257.

Duffy, T.P. (1995). Hematologic aspects of pregnancy. In G.N. Burrow & T.F. Ferris (Eds.), *Medical complications during pregnancy* (4th ed.) (pp. 62–82). Philadelphia: W.B. Saunders.

Gibbs, R.S., & Eschenbach, D.A. (1997). Use of antibiotics to prevent preterm birth. *American Journal of Obstetrics and Gynecology, 177*(2), 375–380.

Gupton, A., Heaman, M., & Ashcroft, T. (1997). Bedrest from the perspective of the high-risk pregnant woman. *Journal of Obstetric, Gynecologic, and Neonatal Nursing, 26*(4), 423–430.

Hewell, S.W., & Hammer, R.H. (1997). Antiphospholipid antibodies: A threat throughout pregnancy. *Journal of Obstetric, Gynecologic, and Neonatal Nursing, 26*(2), 162–168.

Houlihan, C., & Knuppel, P.A. (1996). Intrapartum management of multiple gestations. *Clinical Perinatology, 23*(1), 91–96.

James, D.K., Steer, P.J., Weiner, C.P., & Gonik, B. (Eds.). (1994). *High risk pregnancy: Management options.* Philadelphia: W.B. Saunders.

Karch, A.M. (1998). *Lippincott's nursing drug guide.* New York: J.B. Lippincott.

Kennedy, B.B. (1995). Mitral stenosis: Implications for critical care obstetric nursing. *Journal of Obstetric, Gynecologic, and Neonatal Nursing, 24*(5), 406–412.

Lubarsky, S.L., Barton, J.R., Freidman, S.A., Nasreddin, S., Ramadan, M.K., & Sibai, B.M. (1994). Late postpartum eclampsia revisited. *Obstetrics and Gynecology, 83*, 502.

Martens, K.A. (1994). Sexually transmitted and genital tract infections during pregnancy. *Emergency Medicine Clinics of North America, 12*(1), 91–113.

McAnulty, J.H., Metcalfe, J., & Ueland, K. (1995). Cardiovascular disease. In G.N. Burrow & T.F. Ferris (Eds.), *Medical complications during pregnancy* (4th ed.) (pp. 123–154). Philadelphia: W.B. Saunders.

Mitchell, A., Steffenson, N., Hogan, H., & Brooks, S. (1997a). Group B streptococcus and pregnancy: Update and recommendations. *MCN, American Journal of Maternal-Child Nursing, 22*, 242–248.

Mitchell, A., Steffenson, N., Hogan, H., & Brooks, S. (1997b). Neonatal group B streptococcal disease. *MCN, American Journal of Maternal-Child Nursing, 22*, 249–253.

National High Blood Pressure Education Program Working Group Report on High Blood Pressure in Pregnancy. (1990). *Am J Obstet Gynecol, 163*, 1691–1712.

Persily, C.A. (1996). Relationship between the perceived impact of gestational diabetes mellitus and treatment adherence. *Journal of Obstetric, Gynecologic, and Neonatal Nursing, 27*(7A), 601–607.

Persily, C., Brown, L., & York, R. (1996). A model of home care for high risk childbearing families: Women with diabetes in pregnancy. *Nursing Clinics of North America, 31*(2), 327–332.

Purdy, L.P., Hantsch, C.E., Molitch, M.E., Metzger, B.E., Phelps, R.L., Dooley, S.L., & Hou, S.H. (1996). Effect of pregnancy on renal function in patients with moderate to severe diabetic renal insufficiency. *Diabetes Care, 19*(10), 1067–1074.

Reece, E.A., & Eriksson, U.J. (1996). The pathogenesis of diabetes-associated congenital malformations. *Obstetric and Gynecologic Clinics of North America, 23*(1), 29–45.

Romero, R., Yoon, B.H., Mazor, M., Gomez, R., Diamond, M.P., Kenney, J.S., Ramirez, M., Fidel, P.L., Sorokin, Y., & Cotton, D. (1993). The diagnostic and prognostic value of amniotic fluid, white blood cell count, glucose, interleukin-6 and gram stain in patients with preterm labor and intact membranes. *American Journal of Obstetrics and Gynecology, 169*(4), 805–816.

Rouse, D.J., Andrews, W.W., Goldenberg, R.L., & Owen, J. (1995). Screening and treating of asymptomatic bacteriuria of pregnancy to prevent pyelonephritis. A cost-effectiveness and cost-benefit analysis. *Obstetrics and Gynecology, 86*, 119.

Sanchez-Ramos, L., Briones, D.K., Kaunitz, A.M., Delvalle, G.O., Gaudier, F.L., & Walker, C.D. (1994). Prevention of pregnancy induced hypertension by calcium supplementation in angiotensin-II sensitive patients. *Obstetrics and Gynecology, 84*(3), 349–353.

Ungvarski, P.J. (1997). Update on HIV infection. *American Journal of Nursing, 97*(1), 44–51.

U.S. Centers for Disease Control and Prevention. (1994). Rubella and congenital rubella syndrome. United States: January 1, 1991–May 7, 1994. *Morbidity and Mortality Weekly Report, 43*, 391.

U.S. Centers for Disease Control and Prevention. (1996). Prevention of perinatal group B streptococcal disease: A public health perspective. *Morbidity and Mortality Weekly Report, 45*(RR-7), 1–24.

U.S. Centers for Disease Control and Prevention. (1998). 1998 guidelines for treatment of sexually transmitted diseases. *Morbidity and Mortality Weekly Report, 47*(RR-1), 1–111.

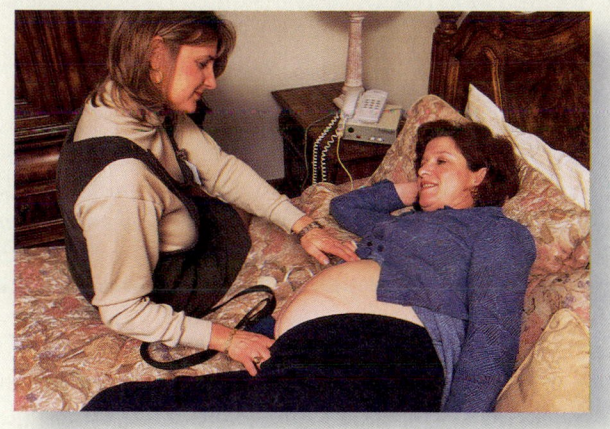

Maureen Brandon is 30 weeks' pregnant with her second child. When she was pregnant with her older daughter Amanda, now 3 years old, Maureen went into preterm labor at the end of the 34th week of gestation. Based on her medical history and some physical findings, Maureen is placed on bedrest at home and qualifies for weekly home care visits through her husband's health plan.

Joyce Keegan, NP, MSN, the perinatal home care nurse, is conducting her weekly assessment of Maureen's status. As she is measuring the fundal height, she asks Maureen if she has any questions about her care. Maureen replies, "When Amanda was born, I had no idea I was in labor until my contractions were occurring every 6 minutes. I'm really worried that I may not recognize the signs of preterm labor with this baby either. How can I prevent this from happening again?" ∎

20

Community-Based Nursing During Pregnancy

Community-based care for low-risk and high-risk clients is a growing trend in the United States. Economics, technology, and public policy all have an impact on delivery of nursing care to clients in the community.

As health care institutions implement measures to control costs, childbearing clients and their infants are being discharged earlier to the home setting. The nurse serves as a link between institutional and community-based care and provides services to low- and high-risk prenatal families.

This chapter provides the reader with a broad perspective of community-based care for the childbearing family during pregnancy. It concludes with a discussion of the role of the community nurse who cares for these families in a complex and changing health care delivery system.

▶ OVERVIEW

Nurses have provided home care for centuries. For years nursing care in the home focused on the poor and sick. As early as the first century, nurses in the Roman Empire organized to care for the sick. Nurses in Paris visited patients at their homes in the 1600s. Nurses visited families stricken with cholera and smallpox in Ireland and England in the 1800s. Florence Nightingale was the first to organize systematic home care for families, and this evolved into district visiting nursing programs.

In 1893 Lillian Wald expanded the home nursing services of the Henry Street Settlement House to include preventive care. In the 1930s, home nursing became known as public health nursing and focused on prevention as well as treatment for illness. The objectives of public health nursing were to educate families, individuals, and community members about their own health, living conditions, and health and social programs.

Consistently throughout the history of public health nursing, also called community health nursing, maternal and infant home visits have been an integral part of the nurse's scope of practice. The 1970s, however, marked a sharp decline in the support of maternal–infant home visits. This was a result of cost-cutting decisions, a decline in infant mortality, and little empirical data supporting the benefits of home visits. The 1980s, however, brought a dramatic change. Infant mortality began to climb. The incidence of preventable diseases, such as acquired immunodeficiency syndrome (AIDS), began to rise. Public awareness of health risks, such as smoking and drugs, increased. Government agencies and nursing leaders looked again to community-based care settings as a strategy to meet maternal–child public health needs. Nursing research, validating the cost effectiveness and clinical benefits of community-based nursing, stimulated support of such maternal–infant programs (Goodwin, 1992).

In 1989 Title V of the Social Security Act was amended by Congress to authorize funding for home nursing visits for pregnant women and infants. State Medicaid programs began compensating for maternal and infant home visits. Community-based nursing care of high-risk maternity clients also developed in the 1980s, with the development of uterine monitoring devices and the expansion of infusion therapy services at home.

▶ MODELS FOR COMMUNITY-BASED NURSING PROGRAMS

▶ Hospital-Based Programs

Hospital-based programs for perinatal home care are increasing. This may be due to the fact that, with the decrease in hospital stays, revenue has also decreased. Hospitals have realized that community-based care has great revenue potential and promotes continuity of care for clients who are discharged from the hospital. Hospitals also have a large physician base for client referrals and experienced perinatal nurses may wish to make the transition from inpatient to community care (Goodwin, 1994). Physicians are more likely to refer clients to a program that is staffed with nurses they know and trust from the hospital setting (Dahlberg & Koloroutis, 1994).

▶ Home Care Agencies

Many existing home care agencies now offer perinatal nursing care in addition to already existing services, such as hospice care and infusion therapy. In this model, nurses are usually paid on a per-case basis. Some agencies have negotiated contracts with insurance companies; clients are referred through these companies or health maintenance organizations (HMOs) (Goodwin, 1994).

▶ Privately Owned Programs

Privately owned community-based programs are considered small businesses, some of which are owned by nurses. These nurses possess business skills, as well as a proficient nursing knowledge base from which protocols for the agency can be developed. States regulate reimbursement policies, and they vary according to the nurse practice acts of each state. These agencies may contract directly with hospitals, insurance companies, or physicians to provide services (Goodwin, 1994).

▶ FACTORS AFFECTING COMMUNITY-BASED CARE

In today's economic and political environment, the survival of many health care institutions, hospitals, community-based agencies, HMOs, and long-term care facilities depends on providing the most appropriate level of care in the most efficient and timely manner. More specifically, there has been great concern nationally about evolving a means of health care delivery that will decrease costs without sacrificing health care quality or access. Health care delivery through community-based care is seen as one means to accomplish this goal; however, delivery of comprehensive community-based health care is profoundly complex and involves the development of public policy.

▶ Health Policy and Community-Based Care

Health policy development has been of great concern to the federal government since the implementation of Medicaid and Medicare. Public monies are being allocated to care for the poor and the elderly. One only need read the daily newspaper to realize that there is a growing national concern for cost containment of medical services and health care. Hospital expenses, in particular, have risen faster than other health care costs. Reasons given for the rise include technologic sophistication, professional salaries, institutional maintenance functions, and insurance costs. Policy makers have believed that institutional care, especially the acute care hospital, was in need of cost containment policies. Community-based nursing services that could prevent or shorten hospitalization have been seen as a primary means of containing costs. Nurses must be in the forefront of developing national health policy and standards of care for nursing services delivered in the community.

▶ Economics of Community-Based Care

One way in which the major payers of health care— the federal and state governments and large employ- ers—have attempted to control spiraling costs is by shifting from a retrospective to a prospective form of payment for health and illness services. That is, instead of reimbursing physicians, hospitals, and so on for services already given to a client, a fixed amount of money is paid, in advance, for specific necessary services required for a specifically diagnosed condition. An example of this approach is seen in one type of insurance reimbursement called the **health maintenance organization (HMO).** The HMO pays the health care provider a set amount of money per client in advance, regardless of the health care services that are actually used by the client. Another prospective payment approach is **diagnostic-related groups (DRGs).**

Diagnostic-related groups were legislated as a part of the Social Security Act amendments of 1983 and were intended to change reimbursement for services to Medicare clients. Under this law, hospitals would receive payment prospectively for services to Medicare clients on the basis of 467 diagnostic related groups. This meant that each diagnosis included in the list of 467 had a price tag connected to it. The hospital received a set amount of money, in advance, for treating a client with a particular diagnosis. It is easy to see that the less time a client stayed in the acute care setting, the greater the financial reward to the hospital (less time equals less daily service and more money left from the advance payment for that

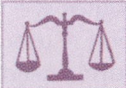

Ethical Decision Making

Despite the benefits of community-based perinatal nursing care for childbearing families, agencies that provide these services may be forced to limit care to clients because of economic considerations. If you were a nurse employed by an agency that is facing this situation, how would you respond to the following questions:

1. If there is insufficient money for community-based care, why are clients being discharged early from the hospital?
2. How can a nurse ethically balance the needs of clients for home care with the agency's need for financial solvency?
3. If the agency goes bankrupt because of nonpayment, who will deliver care to the clients?

specified DRG). Thus, this legislation provided a major incentive for hospitals to reduce their lengths of stay and discharge the clients as soon as possible.

Although originally connected with Medicare and the federal government, DRGs were often adopted by other insurers. This prospective system of payment under DRGs had three major effects on delivery of health care:

1. It increased admissions to community-based care services.
2. It intensified the trend toward discharge of sicker, more acutely ill clients.
3. It resulted in earlier discharge of low- and high-risk mothers and neonates from birthing institutions.

This fact, coupled with the development of new technology, has created the "high-tech" service category in community-based care delivery and expanded maternal–infant home nursing services.

▶ COMMUNITY-BASED CARE FOR THE PREGNANT FAMILY

▶ Low-Risk Pregnant Family

Research demonstrates that women receiving prenatal home nursing visits are more likely to attend childbirth classes, improve their diets, and communicate with family, friends, and health care providers about their pregnancies and personal lives than women who do not receive home nursing visits (Dineen, Rossi, Lia-Hoagberg, & Keller, 1992). Community-based nursing care is not the standard for low-risk prenatal clients. It would, however, provide optimal levels of preventive care to families in their familiar environment. In particular, families who do not feel comfortable with traditional office or clinic-based prenatal care would benefit from home visits.

Some insurance companies and HMOs have implemented prenatal home care services for maternity clients who have traditionally poor postpartum outcomes, such as low-birth-weight infants and preterm births, while other insurance companies offer prenatal nursing visits to all their pregnant clients. These visits include general prenatal teaching and comprehensive risk assessment. Maternity clients with identified risks, such as substance abuse or inadequate nutrition, are connected with the appropriate community resources. Community-based nurses assist clients in making the appropriate appointments with their health care providers.

Nurses can realistically assess the pregnant client and her family in the home and provide nursing care based on that assessment. For example, assessment of the nutritional status of the woman in the home allows the nurse to assist with planning a realistic diet based on the true picture of what is available in the home. In addition, teaching can also be more effective in the home environment away from the many distractions in the health care facility.

One innovative means of delivering prenatal care in the community is to have mobile units or vans go to specific neighborhoods. Residents are enlisted to identify and reach out to pregnant women in need of prenatal care.

▶ High-Risk Pregnant Family

An increase in technology and a decrease in the hospitalization of high-risk obstetrical patients has led to a need for high-risk perinatal nurses in the community setting (Fig. 20–1). Skilled nursing care has been shown to have a positive effect on pregnancy outcomes in high-risk situations such as hyperemesis gravidarum, preterm labor, pregnancy-induced hypertension, and gestational diabetes (Arnold & Bakewell-Sachs, 1991; Olds, Henderson, Tatelbaum, & Chamberlin, 1986). Standards have been developed by the Association of Women's Health, Obstetric and Neonatal Nurses (AWHONN) and include competencies for nurses who care for high-risk antepartum women (AWHONN, 1998).

Preterm Labor
Prematurity (delivery that occurs between 20 and 37 weeks of gestation) is the major cause of neonatal morbidity and mortality. Preterm birth prevention programs have reduced early delivery by identifying those at risk, providing client education, promoting frequent prenatal visits, and conducting cervical examination and assessment of uterine contractions.

During the prenatal period, the health care provider identifies the woman at risk for preterm labor (see Chapter 19). Once a woman is identified as being at risk, antepartum home care may be initiated. During the initial encounter with the client, the perinatal nurse should obtain a thorough history, which should include demographic data, past obstetrical and medical histories, life style patterns, emotional status, environmental assessment, social support systems, and the woman's understanding of the plan of care. Prenatal education, including self-palpation of uterine contractions and signs and symptoms of labor, is also begun during the initial visit. Home uterine activity monitoring (HUAM) is usually initiated when the woman at risk is at approximately 20 weeks of gestation. The monitor consists of an electronic

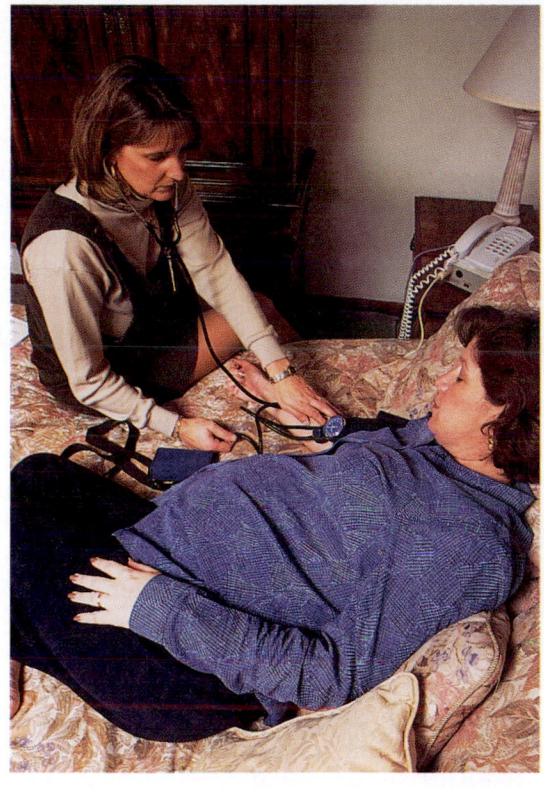
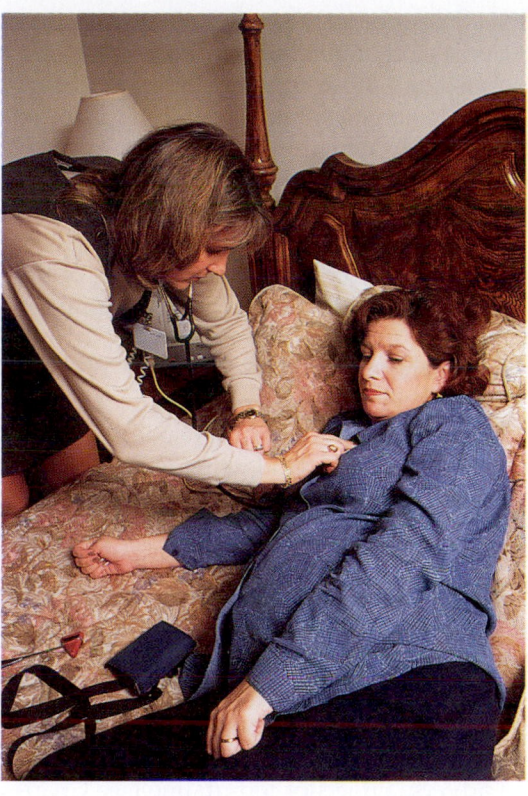

A   B

FIGURE 20–1. The perinatal community-based nurse provides care for the high-risk pregnant client. **A.** Blood pressure assessment. **B.** Auscultation of heart rate.

recorder and a contraction sensor that the woman wears around her abdomen. Typically, the woman will monitor uterine activity for 60 minutes twice a day. The data is transmitted from the recorder via the telephone to a receiving center. At the receiving center, a perinatal nurse reviews the data for evidence of preterm labor (such as contractions or uterine irritability) (Fig. 20–2). The perinatal nurse can then question the woman regarding fetal activity and any other signs or symptoms of labor. Each woman has a contraction threshold (determined by the physician). If the client exceeds her threshold, the perinatal nurse advises her to drink fluids, empty her bladder, and remonitor for an hour. If she continues to go over threshold, the nurse notifies the physician for further orders. Typically, the woman will be sent to the hospital for further evaluation, including cervical status. When preterm labor is detected early enough, tocolysis can be started to prevent its progressing. It is not yet known whether it is the uterine activity monitoring, the daily contact with an experienced perinatal nurse, or a combination of both that contributes to the effectiveness of preterm prevention programs. Many women report that they felt better just knowing their nurse was only a phone call away.

In many cases, there are no known factors that would place a woman at risk for preterm labor. The first indication may be when the woman calls her health care provider with suspicions that labor is starting. In this situation, tocolysis is started in the

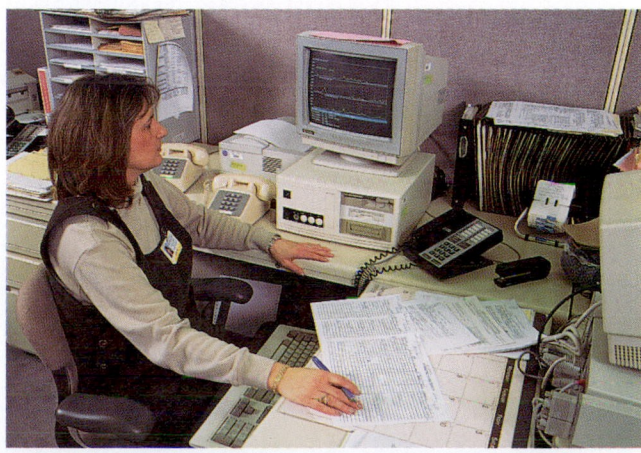

FIGURE 20–2. The perinatal coordinator can receive and assess data generated by home uterine activity monitoring from clients in remote sites.

hospital and, after stabilization, plans for home care are made. Prior to discharge, the perinatal home care nurse visits the client and discusses the plan of care. This plan may include tocolytic agents that may be administered orally. It has been reported that approximately 40–50% of women will have a recurrence of preterm labor within a 3-week period when on oral tocolytics. Some of the potential causes of oral tocolytic failure are noncompliance, side effects of the medication, and drug tolerance. The continuous terbutaline infusion pump is an alternative to oral terbutaline when there is a recurrence of preterm labor or when the woman cannot tolerate the side effects (Fig. 20–3). The perinatal nurse usually initiates pump therapy in the hospital following an episode of increased uterine activity. The nurse programs the pump to deliver a continuous low dose of terbutaline (basal rate) subcutaneously. A bolus dose (a larger amount of medication) may also be programmed to be delivered either on demand, or on a schedule. The amount of medication that is administered by the pump is much lower than the typical oral dosage. The nurse instructs the woman regarding pump functions, changing the syringe, changing the site, signs and symptoms of adverse effects of terbutaline (see Chapter 19), how to administer a bolus dose, and how to take her pulse, since tachycardia is a side effect of terbutaline. The woman will also be placed on HUAM, if she was not prior to her hospitalization.

Once uterine activity stops, the woman is discharged home, with weekly visits by the perinatal home care nurse. At each visit, an assessment is performed to determine the effectiveness of the terbutaline pump therapy, and to determine maternal and fetal well-being (Fig. 20–4). Adjustments may be made to the basal or bolus rates based on HUAM and signs and symptoms of preterm labor reported by the woman.

Many women who are at risk for preterm delivery are given corticosteroids to mature the fetal lungs. Corticosteroid administration before preterm delivery is associated with a large reduction in the incidence of early neonatal death and neonatal respiratory distress syndrome. Betamethasone is the corticosteroid used for antenatal therapy (NIH Consensus Conference, 1995). Two doses of 12 mg each are given intramuscularly 24 hours apart. To obtain maximum results, delivery should be delayed for at least 24 hours after administration of the drug. The effects of the betamethasone last 7 days; therefore, the treatment should be repeated every week until 34 weeks of gestation. The perinatal home care nurse may be responsible for administering the betamethasone to the woman who is home on complete bedrest.

Gestational Diabetes

Since gestational diabetes is a much more common condition during pregnancy than pregestational diabetes, screening for gestational diabetes has become a standard component of prenatal care (see Chapter 19). Once a diagnosis of gestational diabetes has been established, the perinatal nurse can play a key role in helping the pregnant woman manage this complication. Home serum glucose monitoring, along with nutritional counseling by a dietician, should be started immediately. During the initial encounter, a thorough history and assessment should be obtained. Factors such as lifestyle and stress management are important when caring for the diabetic client, since these factors could significantly affect glucose metab-

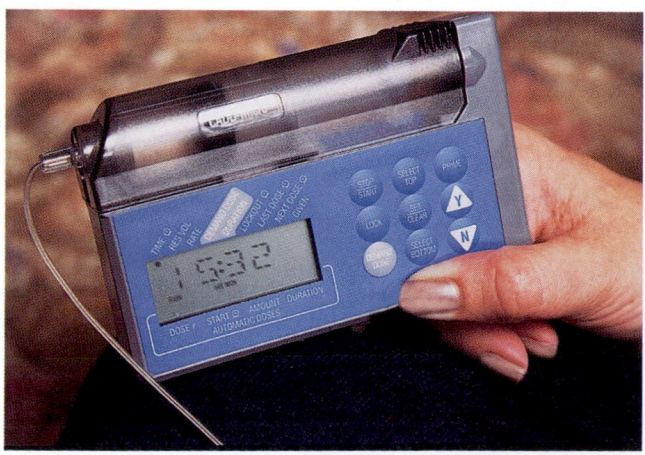

FIGURE 20–3. Terbutaline pump used in community-based settings.

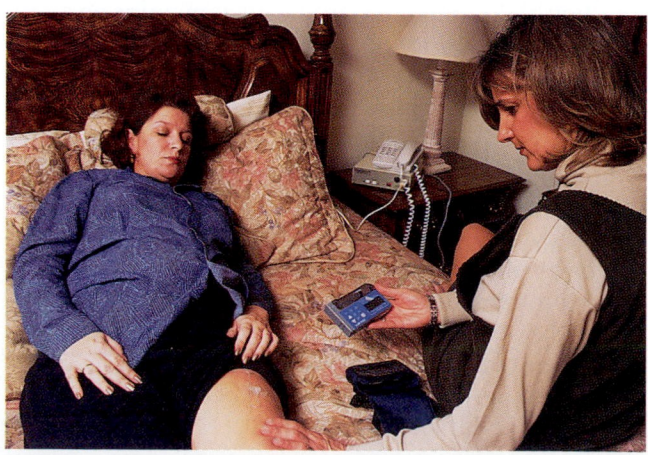

FIGURE 20–4. A perinatal nurse monitoring a high-risk pregnant client on home terbutaline therapy.

olism. Client education should include an overview of diabetes, the different types of diabetes and their effects on the growing fetus, the use of equipment such as the glucometer and urine dipsticks, signs and symptoms of hypoglycemia and hyperglycemia, fetal kick counts, and the possible need for insulin (Grohar, 1994). Routinely, home serum glucose monitoring should be done four times a day: a fasting blood glucose prior to breakfast, 2 hours after breakfast, 2 hours after lunch, and 2 hours after dinner. Optimal blood glucose values during pregnancy are: fasting levels: < 100 mg/dL; 2 hours after meals: < 120 mg/dL. Many newly diagnosed gestational diabetics have daily contact with a perinatal nurse to report their blood glucose levels and fetal activity. During these daily telephone calls, the nurse can answer any questions the woman may have regarding her glucose levels as well as her diet. The perinatal nurse usually makes weekly or biweekly reports to the physician. Diet alone may be adequate to control the blood glucose level. However, if this modality is unsuccessful in managing the condition, the physician may prescribe insulin. Since corticosteroids alter blood glucose levels, diabetic women who are receiving betamethasone as a part of preterm labor management may also need insulin. Human insulin, rather than bovine or porcine insulin, is recommended for use during pregnancy since it is less likely to cause an allergic reaction. Instruction on insulin therapy, including mixing insulin and self-administration, are often the responsibility of the perinatal nurse. Many women need a mixture of an intermediate insulin, such as NPH, and rapid acting regular insulin (Mandeville & Troiano, 1992). Oral hypoglycemics are usually discontinued during pregnancy in favor of insulin. A family member should be instructed on how to use a glucagon (a glucose bolus) emergency kit in the event that the client loses consciousness due to low blood sugar.

Fetal kick counts should be started at 28 weeks' gestation and reported to the perinatal nurse or the physician. Weekly or biweekly nonstress tests or biophysical profiles are usually begun at 30 to 32 weeks of gestation to assess fetal well-being. Fetal growth is also assessed to rule out intrauterine growth retardation or macrosomia (Mandeville & Troiano, 1992).

Pregnancy-Induced Hypertension

Pregnancy-induced hypertension (PIH) is defined as hypertension accompanied by proteinuria and edema after the 20th week of pregnancy. Hypertension in pregnancy is defined as a blood pressure of at least 140/90 mm Hg. Home care of the client with PIH should be made on an individual basis, but she must be considered to be in stable condition to be cared for at home (Grohar, 1994). The following criteria should

Women's Health

The use of home serum glucose monitoring during pregnancy has been instrumental in both enhancing the diabetic client's sense of independence and autonomy and lessening the need for hospitalization for diabetic emergencies.

guide home care: gestational age of more than 20 weeks; blood pressure less than 150/100 mm Hg; proteinuria less than 100 mg/L on urine dipstick or less than 1 g/24 hours; absence of marked edema and clonus; absence of PIH-related headache with visual disturbance and epigastric pain; laboratory values within normal limits; and the ability to use electronic blood pressure equipment (Helewa, Heaman, Robinson, & Thompson, 1993).

Once a physician determines the client can be cared for at home, the perinatal nurse plans physical and educational interventions based on the physician's orders. Parameters for blood pressure, pulse, weight gain, fetal kick counts, and laboratory values are usually set by the physician. An initial assessment should include a thorough history and physical examination. The physical assessment should include: blood pressure in both sitting and left lateral positions; fetal heart rate; fundal height; client's weight; and urine dipstick. Educational interventions include: an overview of PIH and its effects on the client and the fetus; a review of signs and symptoms of a worsening condition that may need immediate attention, such as an increase in blood pressure, headache, visual disturbances, epigastric pain, decreased fetal movement, abdominal pain, vaginal bleeding or signs of labor; a review and reinforcement of the prescribed activity level (many clients are placed on strict bedrest); use of the equipment necessary for care, such as an automated blood pressure machine and urine dipsticks for protein; and the necessity of daily weights and fetal kick counts. The frequency of nursing visits is based on the client's assessment and understanding of the plan of care. At each visit, a complete assessment is performed. Daily telephone contact is encouraged to review signs and symptoms of PIH and evaluate the blood pressure, pulse, urine dipstick, fetal movement, and activity level (Grohar, 1994).

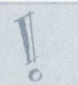

Nursing Alert

In caring for the pregnant client with PIH at home, the perinatal nurse must be certain to explain and reinforce the reasons for the prescribed bedrest since a woman with mild preeclampsia may not experience any debilitating symptoms and thus may not comply with this restriction on her activity.

▶ ROLE OF THE NURSE DELIVERING CARE IN THE COMMUNITY

Community-based care for childbearing families requires that the nurse be skilled in maternal–child health nursing practices as well as community practice (Bailey, 1994). The professional nurse who delivers care in the community has a vital role in assuring quality care in both low- and high-risk situations. These nurses support clients in adapting care practices begun in the hospital to the home environment

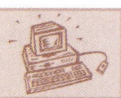

Research Abstract

Client Satisfaction with Community-Based Antepartum Programs

The Antepartum Home Care Program in Winnipeg, Canada, was developed to provide a safe, acceptable alternative to hospitalization for women with various antepartal complications. Goals of the project included reducing hospital antepartum care costs and offering a service that was less disruptive to the family and that encouraged greater participation in self-care. Pregnant women who met certain physical, psychosocial, and geographic criteria were referred to the program by their physicians or the hospital's antepartum unit. As part of the program, the women received daily home visits from a specially trained public health nurse who also had perinatal nursing experience. Home visits included physical assessment; review of the woman's record and of her progress toward health; and teaching such topics as pregnancy complications, self-monitoring regimens, and general childbirth education. In addition, homemaker services were arranged for women who were unable to comply with prolonged rest and/or who had no other sources of support.

Clients' satisfaction with the Antepartum Home Care Program was investigated in this descriptive study. A convenience sample of 66 pregnant women completed a home care program evaluation questionnaire, devised for this study. Ninety-eight percent (n = 65) of the women reported that the care they received in this program met their expectations. Most of the women were very satisfied with the teaching and the physical and emotional care they received through the home care program. Results of the study indicated that antepartum home care was acceptable to the clients surveyed.

Application to Practice

Hospitalization was a traditional way of caring for high-risk pregnant clients. Such issues as cost and the client's separation from her family, however, fostered the development of prenatal home care for appropriate high-risk clients. Maintaining high quality while containing costs is always a challenge, and evaluation is necessary for any program. Assessment of client satisfaction is a core component of program evaluation; this study illustrates one approach to identifying client responses to an innovative home care program. Surveys such as this help identify factors that contribute to a program's success, areas that need further refinement, and directions for further research about client's responses to prenatal home care. More studies of this type are needed as increasing numbers of high-risk pregnant women are cared for at home.

Source: Heaman, M., Robinson, M.A., Thompson, L., & Helewa, M. (1994). Patient satisfaction with an antepartum home-care program. Journal of Obstetric, Gynecologic, and Neonatal Nursing, 23*(8), 707–713.*

using creative techniques. The nursing role incorporates health promotion, direct care, epidemiology, counseling, and political involvement. The nurse should be conversant with systems theory. This will support the nurse's assessment of both the community and the family. Continuing education is always necessary to provide up-to-date information and skills that affect practice (Bailey, 1994).

The nurse should understand the ethnic, political, and demographic makeup of the community that his or her agency serves. Community resources (financial, support, therapeutic, and informational) should be identified for the family by the nurse.

The nurse acts as a client advocate in using the political system to influence health care policy. For example, nurses who care for childbearing families may contact legislators to influence health policy for preventive childbearing services as well as high-risk services.

The community nurse must become experienced with establishing a role on the interdisciplinary health care team. The nurse may coordinate care with occupational therapists, physical therapists, nutritionists, and home health care aides.

The home health care aide is one team member who has had an increasing role with both low- and high-risk pregnant women and their families. Programs have been developed to prepare already skilled homemaker-home health aides to work specifically with these clients.

Home health aides perform homemaker tasks such as meal preparation for pregnant clients with activity restrictions or medical complications (Fig. 20–5). These home aides perform homemaker tasks as well as assisting with the personal care needs of the expectant mother.

▶ Working for Change

Community-based care for childbearing families has become a priority for the health care system. Nurses are the primary care providers who assume responsibility for home care of mothers, infants, and families. Many low- and high-risk care activities, especially health promotion for healthy childbearing families, should be available in the home. Without, however, a payment system directed toward preventive services and direct reimbursement to nurses for delivery of care in the community, the needs of many childbearing families will go unmet. The nurse must take an active role in changing health policy.

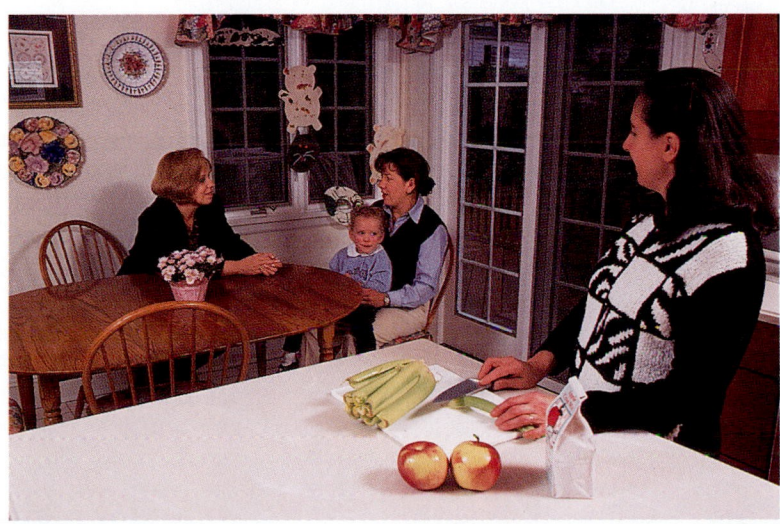

FIGURE 20–5. The community-based nurse and home health care aide collaborate in the care of a high-risk pregnant client and her family.

Critical Thinking in Care Planning

Care of the Client Experiencing Preterm Labor

William and Missy Trevor are expecting their first baby. At 25 weeks of gestation, Missy begins having uterine contractions. In the emergency room, she is found to have 2 cm cervical dilation and 50% effacement. Ultrasound confirms that Missy is 25 weeks' pregnant. The physician determines that Missy is at risk for preterm labor, but that she can be managed at home on modified bedrest and tocolytic therapy (terbutaline) with weekly antepartum visits.

▶ Assessment

- Cervical dilation 2 cm

- Effacement 50% in 25-week pregnancy

Nursing Diagnosis

Knowledge deficit, related to prevention of recurrent preterm labor and home management of pump

Expected Client/Family Outcomes	Nursing Action/Intervention	Evaluation
Client will experience no episodes of recurrent preterm labor. Client will recognize signs and symptoms of preterm labor. Client will state appropriate times to call physician for complications of preterm labor.	Teach client signs and symptoms of preterm labor (cramps, pelvic pressure, backache, vaginal discharge, rupture of membranes, diarrhea) and importance of early detection. *Rationale:* Many women do not know the signs and symptoms of labor. If early treatment is sought, it may be possible to stop labor.	The client states signs and symptoms for which she will observe. The client seeks prompt attention for preterm labor.
Client's uterine activity will remain within prescribed baseline. Decreased uterine activity will be maintained by adjustments of basal rate and bolus doses of terbutaline.	Instruct client on proper procedures for home monitoring to identify changes in contractility patterns not perceived by client. *Rationale:* Changes in contractility patterns are more easily observed if client is aware of and is able to monitor the activity.	Client is able to correctly monitor uterine contraction patterns.
	Adjust pump dosages based on uterine activity data, client symptoms, and physician orders. *Rationale:* Infusion pump helps prevent exceeding therapeutic levels.	Client maintains appropriate dosage schedule.
	Teach client safe operation of terbutaline pump, syringe, and site changes. Instruct client to observe site daily for signs of infection. *Rationale:* Safe operation of pump and site care ensures effective delivery of medication and minimizes risk of infection.	Client is able to describe operation procedures for use of the pump and care of the injection site.

Critical Thinking in Care Planning continued

Expected Client/Family Outcomes	Nursing Action/Intervention	Evaluation
	Instruct client of importance of bedrest and sexual abstinence to reduce risk of recurrence of preterm labor. *Rationale:* Exertion and sexual activity may stimulate uterine contractions.	Client does not engage in strenuous exertion and avoids sexual activity.

Nursing Diagnosis

Decreased cardiac output, related to terbutaline therapy

Client will not experience cardiovascular complications. Client's pulse will remain under 120 beats/min. Client will not demonstrate altered lung perfusion values.	Instruct client on cardiovascular side effects of terbutaline: shortness of breath, chest pain, headache, hypotension, dizziness. *Rationale:* Awareness of side effects of terbutaline therapy prevents occurrence of adverse reactions. Instruct client not to administer boluses if pulse >120 beats/min. Auscultate heart and lung sounds at each visit. Instruct client in orthostatic hypotension prevention. *Rationale:* Interventions to minimize side effects of terbutaline promotes compliance with treatment.	Client states the side effects of terbutaline therapy. Client describes precautions to be observed and interventions to perform to minimize the side effects of terbutaline.

Nursing Diagnosis

Ineffective management of therapeutic regimen, related to error in medication delivery due to operation errors

Client will demonstrate correct operation of terbutaline pump. Client will have access to nursing advice about operation of pump 24 hours/day.	Instruct client on basic operations necessary for delivery of prescribed basal rate/bolus dose of terbutaline. *Rationale:* Client education about operation of terbutaline pump minimizes medication error. Ensure 24-hour availability of nursing personnel to provide telephone assistance with pump operation. *Rationale:* Referral to 24-hour assistance promotes reassurance in client about correct operation of pump. Replace pump immediately if malfunction occurs. *Rationale:* Prompt intervention in the event of pump malfunction can prevent significant interruption of terbutaline treatment.	Client is able to describe the correct operation of terbutaline pump. Client keeps telephone number of nursing service within easy reach. Client understands importance of notifying the nurse immediately if pump malfunction occurs.

(continued)

Critical Thinking in Care Planning continued

Expected Client/Family Outcomes	Nursing Action/Intervention	Evaluation

Nursing Diagnosis

Risk for infection, related to impaired skin integrity at subcutaneous injection site

Client will demonstrate principles of asepsis. Client will rotate site every 72 hours. Client will remain free of infection.	Instruct client in principles of aseptic technique. *Rationale:* Effective practice of aseptic technique minimizes risk of infection at site of injection. Teach client to change SC site every 72 hours and to alternate between right and left anterior thighs. *Rationale:* Site rotation minimizes tissue breakdown and risk of infection. Instruct client to inspect site twice daily for signs of infection: pain, redness, edema, or drainage at the site. *Rationale:* Awareness of the signs of infection alerts client to contact health care provider and prevent complications.	Client states the principles of asepsis. Client demonstrates ability to change injection sites every 72 hours. Client is able to describe signs of infection at injection site.

Nursing Diagnosis

Constipation, related to bedrest and side effects of terbutaline

Client will report regular bowel elimination.	Provide information regarding dietary measures to promote gastrointestinal motility. Instruct client to drink 8–12 glasses of noncaffeinated fluid per day. Instruct client to report constipation to physician. *Rationale:* Client education about methods through which constipation can be relieved can contribute to client's ability to cope with bedrest regimen.	Client discusses methods to use if she experiences constipation.

Nursing Diagnosis

Anxiety, related to stress of preterm labor and effects of terbutaline on fetus

Client will express feelings and needs openly. Client will actively identify stress factors that are changeable.	Encourage verbalization of feelings regarding potential pregnancy outcomes, role and relationship changes, financial burden. *Rationale:* Listening is often an effective comfort measure. Assist client to identify factors or coping patterns that may be used to reduce overall stress. *Rationale:* Client may have a pattern of successful coping during crisis; if not, nurse can make appropriate recommendations.	Client verbalizes fears and anticipates events appropriately. Client and her partner demonstrate positive coping.

Critical Thinking in Care Planning continued

Expected Client/Family Outcomes	Nursing Action/Intervention	Evaluation
Client will state awareness of increased uterine activity associated with times of emotion.		
Family will show interest in plan of care.	Instruct client to be aware that signs of preterm labor may increase during periods of heightened emotion. *Rationale:* Knowledge of connection between stress and increased uterine activity helps client to manage emotional health positively.	

Nursing Diagnosis

Altered family processes, related to bedrest and immobility of client with preterm labor

Client is able to access family and community support for home management.	Assess client support and facilitate problem-solving abilities to meet home management challenges. *Rationale:* Use of family and community resources minimizes disruption in family roles and responsibilities.	Social support system is mobilized; household and other responsibilities are addressed.
Family members express confidence in ability to assist client with care.		
Client expresses satisfaction with adaptations in family roles.	Encourage family input into plan of care. *Rationale:* Involvement of all family members in care promotes integration and self-reliance.	Client and family report individual and joint participation in care.

Chapter Highlights

▶ Three models of community-based nursing programs that provide perinatal services are hospital-based programs, home care agencies, and privately owned programs.

▶ Development of health policy for perinatal nursing services delivered in the community and economic structures such as health maintenance organizations and diagnostic-related groups are two factors that are influencing the growth of community-based care.

▶ Community-based care for the low-risk pregnant family consists of prenatal teaching and comprehensive risk assessment.

▶ Skilled nursing care delivered within the community setting has a positive effect on pregnancy outcomes in high-risk situations such as preterm labor, gestational diabetes, and pregnancy-induced hypertension.

▶ The nursing role in community-based care for low- and high-risk pregnant clients and families incorporates health promotion, skilled nursing interventions, counseling, and advocacy.

After reading the vignette at the beginning of this chapter, use what you have learned to answer these questions:

1. What benefits does a high-risk pregnant client like Maureen Brandon gain in receiving community-based care within her home?

2. What educational strategies can Joyce Keegan, NP, MSN, use to help Maureen Brandon recognize the signs of preterm labor?

3. To what community resources can Maureen Brandon and her family be referred to help them cope with her high-risk status?

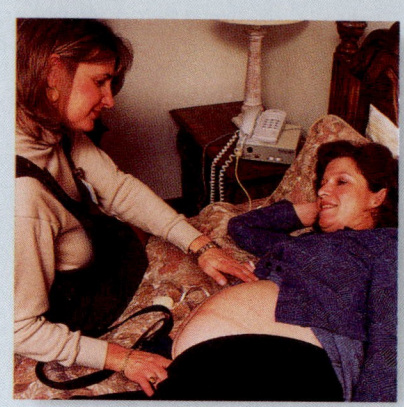

Critical Thinking Questions

▶ References

Arnold, L.S., & Backewell-Sachs, S. (1991). Models of perinatal home follow-up. *Journal of Perinatal and Neonatal Nursing, 5,* 18–26.

Association of Women's Health, Obstetric, and Neonatal Nurses. (1998). *Standards and guidelines for professional nursing practice in the care of women and newborns* (5th ed.). Washington, DC: Author.

Bailey, C. (1994). Education for home-care providers. *Journal of Obstetric, Gynecologic, and Neonatal Nursing, 23*(8), 714–719.

Dahlberg, N.L., & Koloroutis, M. (1994). Hospital-based perinatal home-care program. *Journal of Obstetric, Gynecologic, and Neonatal Nursing, 23*(8), 682–686.

Dineen, K., Rossi, M., Lia-Hoagberg, B., & Keller, L.O. (1992). Antepartum home-care services for high-risk women. *Journal of Obstetric, Gynecologic, and Neonatal Nursing, 21,* 121–125.

Goodwin, L. (1992). Home fetal assessment. *Journal of Perinatal and Neonatal Nursing, 5,* 33–45.

Goodwin, L. (1994). Essential program components for perinatal home care. *Journal of Obstetric, Gynecologic, and Neonatal Nursing, 23*(8), 667–673.

Grohar, J. (1994). Nursing protocols for antepartum home care. *Journal of Obstetric, Gynecologic, and Neonatal Nursing, 23*(8), 687–694.

Heaman, M., Robinson, M.A., Thompson, L., & Helewa, M. (1994). Patient satisfaction with an antepartum home-care program. *Journal of Obstetric, Gynecologic, and Neonatal Nursing, 23*(8), 707–713.

Helewa, M., Heaman, M., Robinson, M.A., & Thompson, L. (1993). Community-based home-care program for the management of pre-eclampsia: An alternative. *Canadian Medical Association Journal, 149,* 829–834.

Mandeville, L., & Troiano, N. (1992). *High risk intrapartum nursing.* Philadelphia: J.B. Lippincott.

NIH Consensus Conference. (1995). Effects of corticosteroids for fetal maturation on perinatal outcomes. *Journal of the American Medical Association, 273*(5), 413–417.

Olds, D.L., Henderson, C.R., Tatelbaum, R., & Chamberlain, R. (1986). Improving the delivery of prenatal care and outcome of pregnancy: A randomized trial of nurse home visitation. *Pediatrics, 77,* 16–28.

IV

Birth

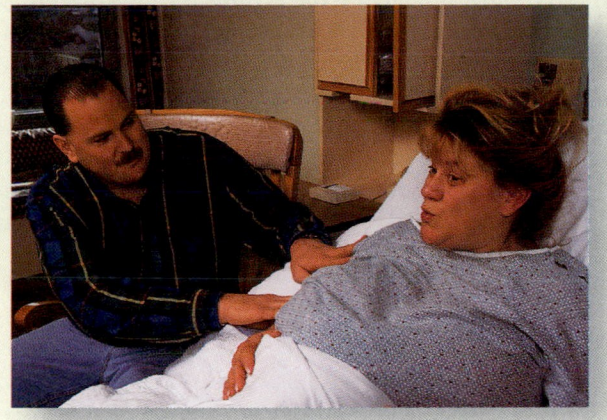

Cathleen Harris, a 30-year-old multigravida, is in labor with her second child. The latent phase of her labor lasted approximately 6 hours and she is now, 2 hours later, in the active phase. Her contractions are occurring every 2 minutes and each lasts for 1 minute. Her cervix is 9 cm dilated and 90% effaced.

Cathleen's husband Bill is at her side and gently rubs her shoulder. After experiencing a particularly strong contraction, Cathleen lays her head against the pillow and moans. Bill asks, "Are you all right?" Cathleen closes her eyes and does not respond. Bill then states, "Cathy, let's try some more breathing. It might ease the pain a little." Cathleen opens her eyes and, looking at Bill, begins to breathe first slowly and then more quickly as she experiences another contraction. Cathleen tells Bill that the breathing takes her mind off the pain briefly, but she is afraid that she will not be able to tolerate it for much longer. Bill asks Margaret Kiely, RN, "What else can I do to help her get through this?" ∎

21

Physiology of Labor and Birth

The processes of labor and birth require complex physiologic responses by the mother and fetus, among them the initiation of uterine contractions, effacement and dilation of the cervix, and fetal accommodation and passage through the maternal pelvis and birth canal. This chapter examines physiologic responses during the labor and delivery processes, beginning with theories of labor onset and ending with the initial postpartum recovery of the mother.

► ONSET OF LABOR

► Hypotheses

Several mechanisms have been hypothesized to influence the initiation of labor, among them the uterine stretch mechanism and both maternal and fetal hormonal stimulation. To date, biomedical research has been unable to document a single cause-and-effect relationship between any of these mechanisms and the onset of labor. It seems most likely that a combination of factors is responsible for labor onset. Research in this area concentrates almost exclusively on possible physiologic mechanisms, with a notable absence of investigation into any psychologic components. As hormonal response to emotion and emotional response to hormonal shifts have been documented in other contexts, it appears that there may be causes of onset that are as yet unexplained.

Uterine Stretch Mechanism
One of the earliest hypotheses about labor onset proposed that distension of the uterus eventually results in increased irritability and contractility. The increased irritability of the uterus may be heightened by an increase in oxytocin levels or may cause an increase in production of the hormone. Support for this hypothesis came from the observation that some mothers with multiple gestations or polyhydramnios experience preterm labor and delivery. The physiologic secretion of oxytocin during labor may, however, vary; in fact, oxytocin may be secreted more in the expulsive phases of labor than in the early phases. This would seem to contradict the uterine stretch–oxytocin relationship.

Hormonal Stimulation
Hormonal stimulation hypotheses focus on the interplay among the mother, fetus, and placenta. Maternal, fetal, and placental hormones, possibly controlled by fetal adrenal cortisol activity, are believed to contribute to the onset of labor. Specific hypotheses involve (1) oxytocin, (2) prostaglandins, (3) fetal cortisol, and (4) estrogen and progesterone.

Oxytocin. Oxytocin has been postulated to be a primary factor in the initiation of labor because it is known to be a potent uterotonin (uterine muscle contractant), it is found naturally in humans, and it is effective in inducing labor at term. Other arguments for the role of oxytocin in the initiation of labor include the significant increase in the number of oxytocin receptors in the uterine tissue near term. These receptors must be present for oxytocin to act to contract the uterus. Other evidence, however, suggests that the uterine receptors do not sensitize the uterus to oxytocin until after the onset of labor (Cunningham et al., 1997). Yet other findings suggest that the uterine tissue may in fact synthesize oxytocin at the end of gestation, contributing to the initiation of labor (Lefebvre, Giaid, Bennett, Lariviere, & Zingg, 1992).

In general, physiologic evidence for the role of oxytocin in the initiation of labor is inconclusive. Animal and human research has demonstrated increased levels of oxytocin during labor; however, research has been unable to document a rise in oxytocin immediately prior to the onset of labor. Some argue that oxytocin has little importance in the initiation of labor and that its major role occurs during labor and delivery.

Prostaglandins. Estrogen appears to stimulate prostaglandin production. Prostaglandins stimulate the uterus and can induce effective uterine contractions at any stage during the pregnancy. Infusion of one of the prostaglandin compounds, prostaglandin $F_{2\alpha}(PGF_{2\alpha})$ can result in cervical effacement throughout pregnancy; however, the amounts of prostaglandins necessary to induce labor are significantly higher than those found naturally in maternal tissue and fetal membranes (Cunningham et al., 1997). Research has documented that the amounts of prostaglandins found in maternal tissue at term are ineffective in inducing contractions (Challis, 1994).

Cortisol. Animal studies have demonstrated that a sharp increase in the rate of production of cortisol by the fetal adrenal acts on the placenta, reducing progesterone formation and increasing production of prostaglandins. The same findings, however, are not conclusive in humans. Specifically, no significant increase in cortisol concentrations in fetal blood has been found before the onset of labor. Further, there is no evidence of a decline in human maternal plasma progesterone levels before or during labor (Cunningham et al., 1997). Thus, the role of cortisol as an initiator of labor is inconclusive.

Estrogen and Progesterone. In animals, estrogen increases the number of uterine receptor sites for oxytocin. Progesterone (also in animal studies) acts to quiet the uterine response (Blackburn & Loper, 1992). In humans, the balance between estrogen and progesterone serves to stabilize and maintain the pregnancy. In the past it was believed that a decrease in progesterone levels at term allowed estrogen to excite the contractile response of the uterus. Newer studies, however, have failed to consistently document decreased progesterone in maternal blood, leaving this hypothesis of labor onset in question (Cunningham et al., 1997).

▶ Interplay Among Factors Affecting Labor Onset

As the preceding discussion indicates, research has been unable to document any single hypothesis regarding the onset of labor. Each of the hormones discussed can influence uterine contractions; however, each taken separately fails to explain the initiation of labor. A variety of factors, both maternal and fetal, act in concert to initiate labor in the low-risk pregnant woman. Further research will likely focus on the interactions among various factors that may combine to trigger the onset of labor.

▶ FACTORS INFLUENCING THE OUTCOME OF LABOR

Traditionally, the "three P's"—passage (pelvis), passenger (fetus), and powers (contractions)—were considered to be the major factors determining the outcome of labor and delivery. The fourth "P", the maternal psyche, is an important factor affecting labor and delivery; therefore psychologic influences on labor and delivery are also discussed briefly in this section. For additional discussion, the reader is referred to Chapter 24.

▶ Passage

Bony Pelvis
The bony pelvis of the pregnant woman is assessed in relation to the size, lie, and presentation of the fetus. As the pelvic structure is relatively unyielding (except for the coccyx, which may be somewhat movable) and is the passage through which the fetus must descend for a successful vaginal delivery, internal and external pelvic diameters are measured.

Ideally, skeletal assessments are made at least twice during pregnancy, after a detailed history is taken to identify factors that may have impact on the development of the pelvis. Conditions such as rickets,

polio, and trauma resulting in pelvic fracture or a history of previous cephalopelvic disproportion may affect delivery outcome. An initial assessment is performed in the first trimester to identify any gross abnormalities or obvious barriers to vaginal delivery (see Chapter 15). Assessment of the pelvis is essential for estimating successful passage of the fetus during labor and delivery (see section on Passenger). Usually, the smallest diameter of the fetal skull will descend in the largest diameters of the true pelvis.

The anatomy, diameters, and planes of the pelvis are described in Chapter 15. This section highlights several key anatomic landmarks.

The portion of the pelvis below the linea terminalis is termed the true pelvis. It is composed of the pelvic inlet, cavity, and outlet.

Pelvic Inlet. The pelvic inlet is bounded anteriorly by the pubic bones, laterally by the linea terminalis, and posteriorly by the sacral promontory. The important measurements of this structure are the obstetric conjugate, the anatomic or true conjugate, the diagonal conjugate, the internal obstetric conjugate, the transverse diameter, and the right and left oblique diameters (see Chapter 15).

Pelvic Cavity. The pelvic cavity consists of a curved cavity between the inlet and outlet with a straight anterior wall bounded by the pubis; a curved posterior wall bounded by the sacrum, which is roughly twice the length of the anterior wall; and side walls bounded laterally by the ischium and part of the ilium. Pelvic planes are imaginary surfaces used to describe points of critical dimension. The two planes are the plane of greatest dimension (the anteroposterior diameter and the transverse diameter) and the plane of least dimension (the anteroposterior diameter, the transverse diameter, and the posterior sagittal diameter) (see Chapter 15).

Pelvic Outlet. The pelvic outlet is made up of an anterior and a posterior triangular plane, sharing a common base. The diameters of the pelvic outlet are the obstetric anteroposterior diameter, the transverse diameter, the posterior sagittal diameter, and the anterior sagittal diameter (Fig. 21–1) (see Chapter 15).

The following pelvic measurements determine whether the pelvis is adequate to allow passage of the fetus:

- Obstetric conjugate of the inlet
- Distance between the ischial spines
- Subpubic angle and transverse diameter
- Posterior and sagittal diameters of the three planes
- Curve and length of the sacrum

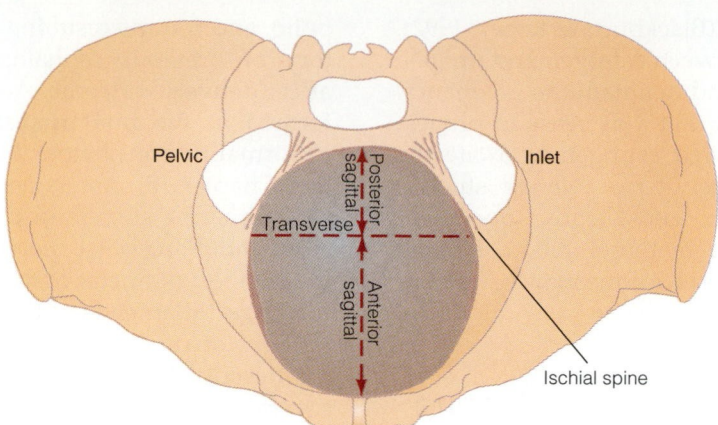

FIGURE 21–1. Pelvic cavity: plane of least dimensions. The anterior-posterior view showing anterior-posterior and transverse diameters. *(Reproduced, with permission, from Oxorn, H. (Ed.). (1986). Oxorn-Foote human labor and birth (5th ed.). Norwalk, CT: Appleton & Lange, p. 31.)*

Vagina

Bounded by the vulva, the uterus, the bladder, and the rectum, the vagina is composed of muscular tissue with a mucosal overlay. This tube, 6 to 8 cm long, with the cervix at one end and the introitus or vaginal opening in the perineum at the other, is extremely elastic and readily distends to accommodate passage of the fetus.

▶ Passenger

Fetus

The fetal head is the most important parameter of the fetal body because it is the largest and least yielding fetal part. It is also most frequently the part that presents first in the maternal pelvis.

Fetal Skull. The fetal skull is made up of three parts: the face, the vault, and the base. The bones of the face are heavier than those of the vault and are fused. The vault is composed of two frontal bones anteriorly, two parietal bones on the sides, and one occipital bone posteriorly. The bones of the vault are not fused. Instead, they are separated from each other by membranes that allow the head to change shape as it descends through the maternal pelvis. The base consists of two temporal bones.

The skull **sutures** are membrane-occupied spaces between the bones of the vault. The sutures in the cranial vault allow for molding of the fetal skull during labor and delivery. The **sagittal suture** is located between parietal bones and follows the anteroposterior direction of the skull. The **frontal suture** is an anterior continuation of the sagittal suture, and is

found between the two frontal bones. The **coronal sutures** are found between the parietal and frontal bones, extending transversely on both sides of the anterior fontanelle. The **lambdoidal sutures** are located between the occipital bone and the two parietals, extending transversely on either side of the posterior fontanelle (Fig. 21–2).

The **fontanelles** are membrane-covered spaces found where the sutures intersect. The **anterior**

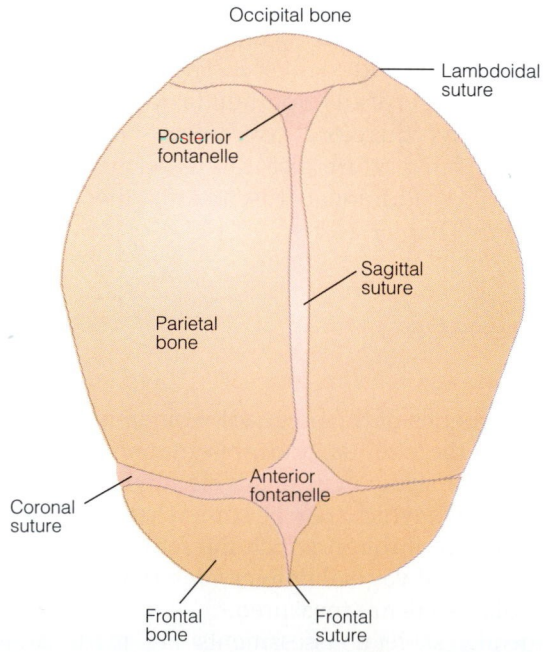

FIGURE 21–2. Superior view of the fetal skull. *(Adapted, with permission, from Oxorn, H. (Ed.). (1986). Oxorn-Foote human labor and birth (5th ed.). Norwalk, CT: Appleton & Lange, p. 43.)*

fontanelle, or **bregma,** is located at the anterior junction of the sagittal and coronal sutures. It is diamond-shaped and measures on average 3 × 2 cm. The anterior fontanelle remains open for 12 to 18 months after birth to allow for growth of the brain. The **posterior fontanelle,** or **lambda,** is located at the posterior junction of the lambdoidal and sagittal sutures. It is triangular, measures on average between 0.5 and 1 cm at its widest diameter, and closes 6 to 10 weeks after birth (see Fig. 21–2).

Landmarks of the Fetal Skull. Certain landmarks of the fetal skull are important in describing the relationship of the fetal presenting part to the maternal pelvis during delivery. These landmarks are referred to as **denominators:**

- *Occiput.* Region in the back of the head, behind and inferior to the posterior fontanelle.
- *Brow.* Region bounded by the anterior fontanelle and the coronal sutures superiorly and by the orbital ridges inferiorly.
- *Vertex.* Located between the anterior and posterior fontanelles and bounded laterally by the parietal bones.
- *Mentum or chin.* Guiding point for face presentations (see later), which occur when the head is in complete extension.

Additional denominators that are not landmarks of the fetal skull are discussed later in this chapter.

Diameters of the Fetal Skull. The diameters of the fetal skull are important in judging the ability of the fetus to fit through the maternal pelvis. The most important dimensions are the anteroposterior and transverse diameters.

The anteroposterior diameter of the fetal skull that presents to the maternal pelvis depends on the extension or flexion of the fetal head and consists of three sub-diameters:

- Suboccipitobregmatic diameter (9.5 cm): extends from the undersurface of the occipital bone to the center for the anterior fontanelle; shortest anteroposterior diameter of the head; and presents to the maternal pelvis when the fetal head is well flexed (Fig. 21–3A)
- Occipitofrontal diameter (11.5 cm): extends from a point just above the top of the nose to the most prominent portion of the occiptial bone (Fig. 21–3B)
- Occipitomental diameter (12.5 cm): extends from the chin to the most prominent portion of the occiput and is found when the head is extended (Fig. 21–3C)

Of the two transverse diameters, the biparietal is longer, measuring 9.5 cm. It extends from one parietal prominence to the other (Fig. 21–4).

The bitemporal diameter of the fetal skull extends between the lateral sides of the temporal bones and measures 8 cm (see Fig. 21–4).

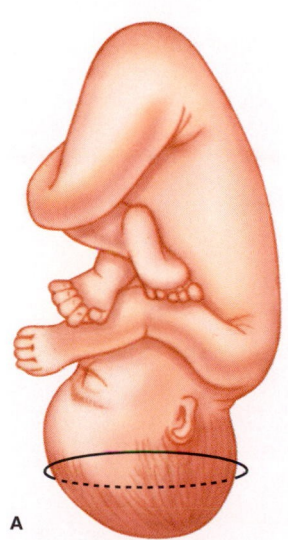 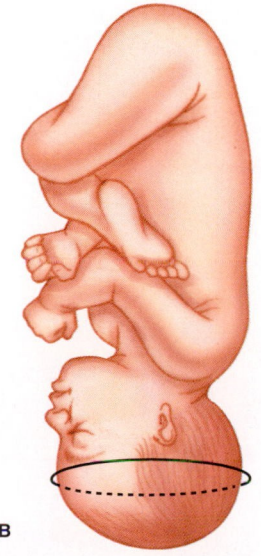 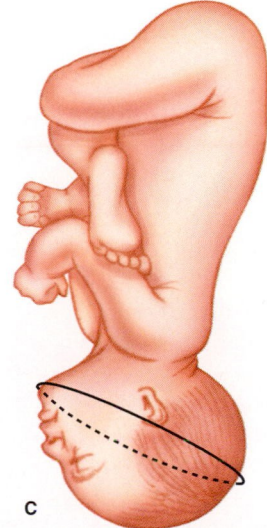

FIGURE 21–3. Anteroposterior diameters of the fetal skull. **A.** Suboccipitobregmatic diameter. **B.** Occipitofrontal diameter. **C.** Occipitomental diameter.

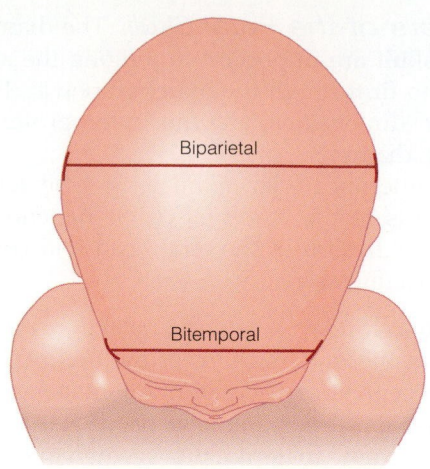

FIGURE 21–4. Transverse diameters of the fetal skull.

Fetopelvic Relationships

Attitude. **Attitude** is the relationship of the fetal parts to each other. The typical fetal attitude is one of **flexion,** whereby the arms and legs are folded in front of the body, the back is curved forward, and the head is bent on the chest. This attitude occurs as a result of growth of the fetus and the process of fetal accommodation to the uterine cavity. The extent of flexion of fetal parts, especially the head, determines which diameter will enter the maternal pelvis.

Lie. **Lie** is the relationship of the long axis of the fetus to the long axis of the mother, and can be longitudinal, transverse, or oblique. Longitudinal lies are present in more than 99% of term pregnancies. In a longitudinal lie, the head or buttocks may enter the

maternal pelvis first. A transverse lie finds the long axis of the fetus at right angles to the long axis of the mother. In this lie, the shoulder of the fetus enters the maternal pelvis first. A transverse lie is rare, and the fetus cannot be delivered vaginally in this position. Occasionally, the long axes of the mother and fetus cross at a 45° angle, forming an oblique lie. This lie becomes either longitudinal or transverse during the course of labor.

Presentation. **Presentation** describes the manner in which the fetus enters the pelvic inlet of the mother. This part of the fetus is termed the presenting part. In longitudinal lies, the presenting part is either the head or the fetal pelvic parts; these are termed cephalic and breech presentations, respectively. In a transverse lie, the presenting part is the shoulder, arm, or trunk; this is termed a shoulder presentation.

Cephalic presentations are classified according to the attitude of the fetal head. If the head is flexed, the occiput is the presenting part. This is referred to as a vertex or occiput presentation (Fig. 21–5A). The **vertex presentation** is the most efficient presentation for delivery and also the most common, occurring in 95% of all term pregnancies. A face presentation occurs when the fetal head is completely extended, with the widest part of the face presenting for delivery (Fig. 21–5B). When the fetal head is partially extended, the presenting part is the brow; this is referred to as a brow presentation (Fig. 21–5C).

Breech presentations are classified according to the attitude of the fetal hips and knees. In a complete breech presentation, the fetus presents buttocks first with flexion at both the hips and the knees (Fig. 21–6A). In a frank breech presentation, the thighs are

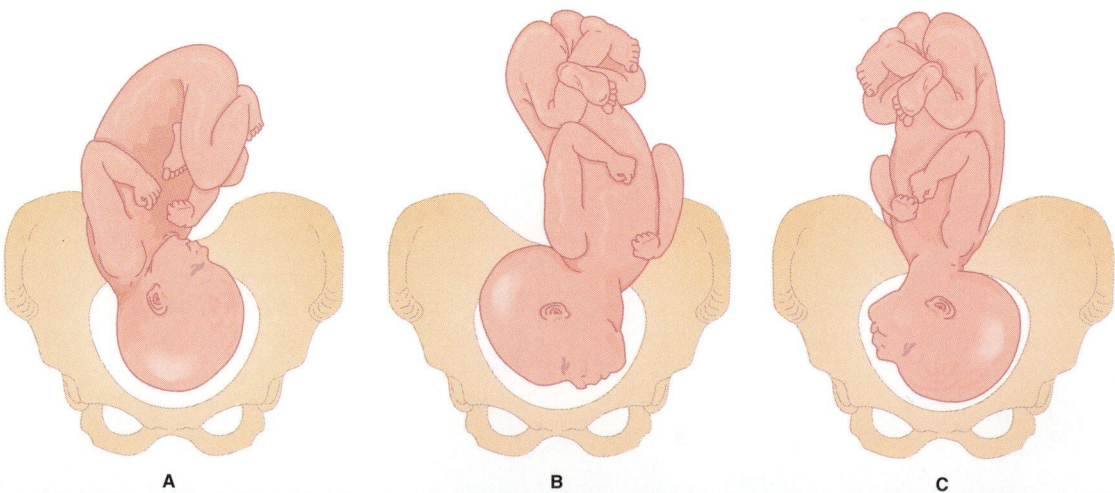

FIGURE 21–5. Cephalic presentations. **A.** Vertex/occiput presentation. **B.** Face presentation. **C.** Brow presentation.

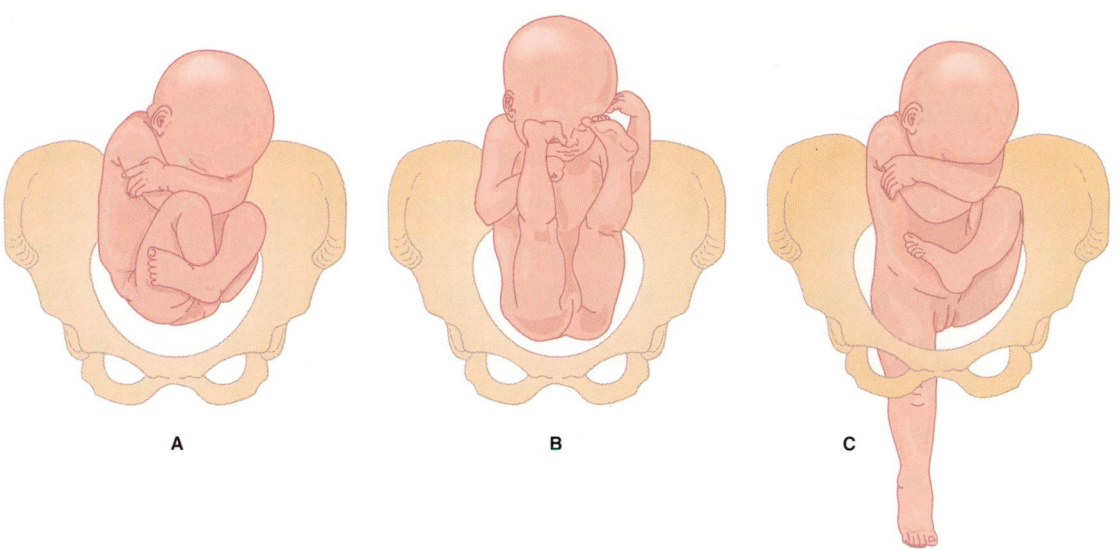

FIGURE 21–6. Breech presentations. **A.** Complete breech. **B.** Frank breech. **C.** Footling breech.

flexed and the legs extend over the anterior surfaces of the fetal body (Fig. 21–6B); the presenting part is still the buttocks. An incomplete or footling breech presentation occurs when the presenting part is one or both feet, with extension at both the hips and knees (Fig. 21–6C).

A shoulder presentation (also called a transverse lie) occurs when the long axis of the fetus is perpendicular to the long axis of the mother (Fig. 21–7). The most frequent presenting part is the shoulder; however, the fetus may also present the trunk or arm. Shoulder presentations, which occur in less than 1% of deliveries, are serious malpresentations. Unless the fetus changes to a longitudinal lie, vaginal delivery cannot occur. (See Chapter 25 for a discussion of complications of childbirth.)

Position. **Position** refers to the relationship of landmarks (denominators) of the fetal presenting part to the sides, front, or back of the maternal pelvis. Each

presentation has its own denominator. Table 21–1 lists the fetal denominators for each presenting part.

When describing the fetal position in the mother's pelvis, three sets of terms are used: (1) denominator; (2) right or left, depending on which side of the mother's pelvis the denominator is in; and (3) anterior, posterior, or transverse, according to whether the denominator is located in the front, back, or side of the mother's pelvis. Eight positions (Fig. 21–8) are possible for each fetal presentation:

Vertex Presentations

- Left occiput anterior (LOA)
- Left occiput posterior (LOP)
- Right occiput anterior (ROA)
- Right occiput posterior (ROP)
- Right occiput transverse (ROT)
- Left occiput transverse (LOT)
- Occiput anterior (OA)
- Occiput posterior (OP)

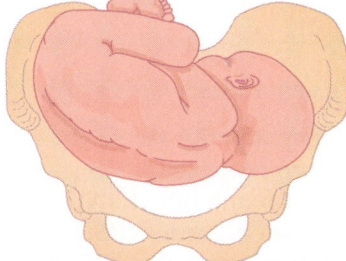

FIGURE 21–7. Shoulder presentation (transverse lie). *(Adapted, with permission, from Oxorn, H. (Ed.). (1986). Oxorn-Foote human labor and birth (5th ed.). Norwalk, CT: Appleton & Lange, p. 57.)*

▶ **TABLE 21–1**

Denominators for Fetal Presenting Parts

Presenting Part	Denominator
Vertex (occiput)	Occiput (O)
Face	Mentum (chin) (M)
Brow	Frontum (forehead) (Fr)
Buttocks	Sacrum (S)
Feet	Sacrum (S)
Shoulder, arm	Scapula (Sc)

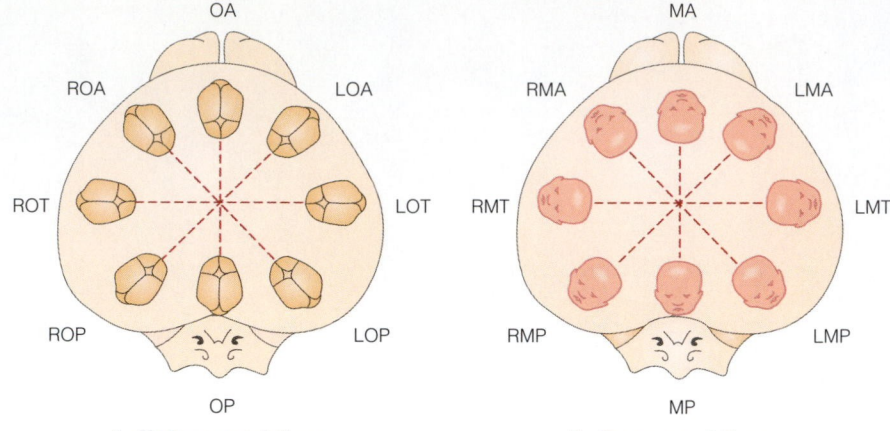

A. Vertex presentations

B. Face presentations

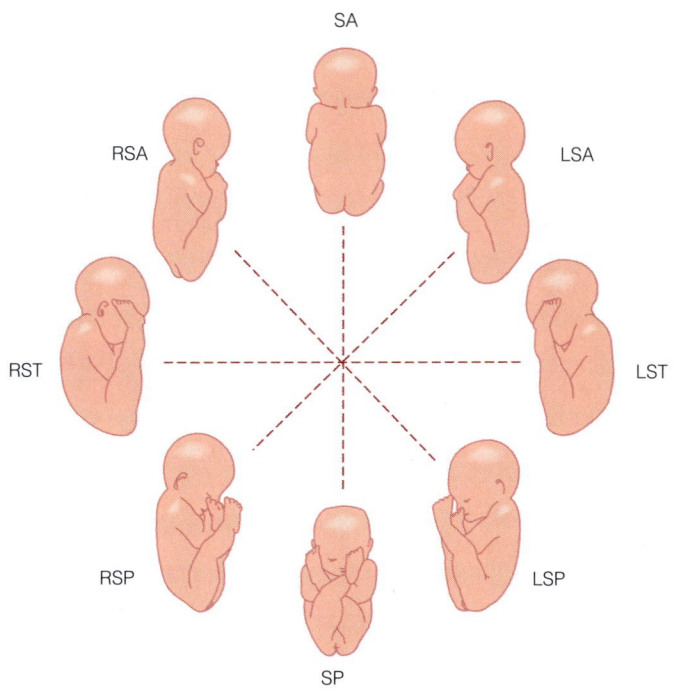

C. Breech presentations

FIGURE 21–8. Fetal positions. *(Reproduced, with permission, from Oxorn, H. (Ed.). (1986).* Oxorn-Foote human labor and birth *(5th ed.) Norwalk, CT: Appleton & Lange, p. 59.)*

Face Presentations

- Left mentum anterior (LMA)
- Left mentum posterior (LMP)
- Right mentum anterior (RMA)
- Right mentum posterior (RMP)
- Right mentum tranverse (RMT)
- Left mentum transverse (LMT)
- Mentum anterior (MA)
- Mentum posterior (MP)

Breech Presentations

- Left sacrum anterior (LSA)
- Left sacrum posterior (LSP)
- Right sacrum anterior (RSA)
- Right sacrum posterior (RSP)
- Right sacrum transverse (RST)
- Left sacrum transverse (LST)
- Sacrum anterior (SA)
- Sacrum posterior (SP)

Brow presentations are rarely described in this manner, because they usually convert to a vertex or face presentation during labor.

▶ Powers

Three variables—uterine contractions, intraabdominal pressure, and passive counterpressure of the pelvic floor—constitute the powers, or energy component, of birth. These powers may be further described as primary (involuntary) or secondary (voluntary).

The uterus is a muscular organ composed of three layers: the outer (maternal side) layer, or perimetrium; the middle, thickest layer, or myometrium; and the internal (fetal side) layer, or endometrium. The myometrium is itself structured in three interlacing layers that encircle the uterus. Each muscle cell in the myometrium has a double curve so that the interlacing of the cells forms a figure-eight configuration. The muscle fibers of the myometrium are permeated in all directions by blood vessels.

The musculature of the myometrium has a unique characteristic termed **brachystasis,** the ability to contract in response to a stimulus and to shorten and thicken progressively with each stimulus. The meshlike structure of the musculature of the myometrium acts to exert pressure on uterine blood vessels, and is believed to aid in lessening the blood loss that would otherwise result from disruption of multiple small vessels.

Uterine contractions are primary or involuntary. Several mechanisms seem to enhance involuntary labor contractions. The first of these mechanisms is oxytocin, which is thought to enhance rhythmic labor contractions. At term, when the cervix is ripe (softened and in the earliest stage of dilation and effacement), the uterus is sensitive to oxytocin, although the degree of sensitivity varies with the individual.

The second mechanism involves pacemakers in the uterus, which are thought to help initiate rhythmic uterine contractions.

The third mechanism is the mechanical stretching of the cervix. This appears to cause an increase in prostaglandin levels in women at term, and prostaglandins are capable of causing contractions of the uterus. It is not known whether the natural softening of the cervix elicits a similar response.

All three mechanisms—hormonal stimulation, pacemaker cell activity, and cervical change and consequent prostaglandin response—may act together to establish rhythmic contractions. The uterine contractions provide the power that shortens, thickens, and straightens the body of the uterus and further dilates and effaces the cervix.

Dilation is the widening of the cervical os from an opening that will not admit a finger to an opening that is 10 cm when fully dilated. Effacement is the thinning and shortening of the cervical os from a 2.5-cm structure to a part of the lower uterine segment. Ideally, the cervix is ripe when labor begins. A ripe cervix is soft, is less than 1.3 cm long, and admits a finger easily.

Completion of the first stage of labor (from 0 to 10 cm dilation with full effacement) is followed by the second stage of expulsion, which is characterized by the overwhelming urge of the laboring client to exert abdominal muscle pressure with each contraction, or to "push." This is considered the secondary power of labor. The pelvic floor exerts a passive counterpressure as the fetal presenting part encounters resistance and is guided to the vaginal opening.

▶ Psyche

The physical process of labor and delivery is affected by the level of excitement, tension, and fear experienced by the client and her family and by the degree to which the client's self-esteem is threatened or supported. Somatic manifestations of fear—elevated blood pressure, increased heart and respiratory rates—should not be confused with normal excitement. The nurse should be aware that baseline vital signs, taken when the client first enters the birthing area, may be affected by anxiety and therefore less reliable than those read when the client has calmed. Fear and panic are extreme responses to real or perceived threats to bodily or psychic integrity. Labor can be experienced as a loss of control, particularly by the primiparous client or the client without childbirth preparation. Psychologic aspects of labor and delivery are further discussed in Chapter 24.

▶ MECHANISMS OF LABOR

The terms mechanisms of labor and **cardinal movements of labor** are used to describe the simultaneous accommodation of the fetal anatomy to the maternal pelvis and birth canal and passage of the fetus from the abdominal site to the outside world. Although the mechanisms are traditionally described in a "list" fashion, such a presentation may be misleading as several of the mechanisms occur either at the same time or in an overlapping time frame (Fig. 21–9).

The relatively unyielding planes of the maternal pelvis require that the fetus accommodate to the pelvic contours. In 95% of deliveries, presentation involves the fetal head; therefore, in the description of

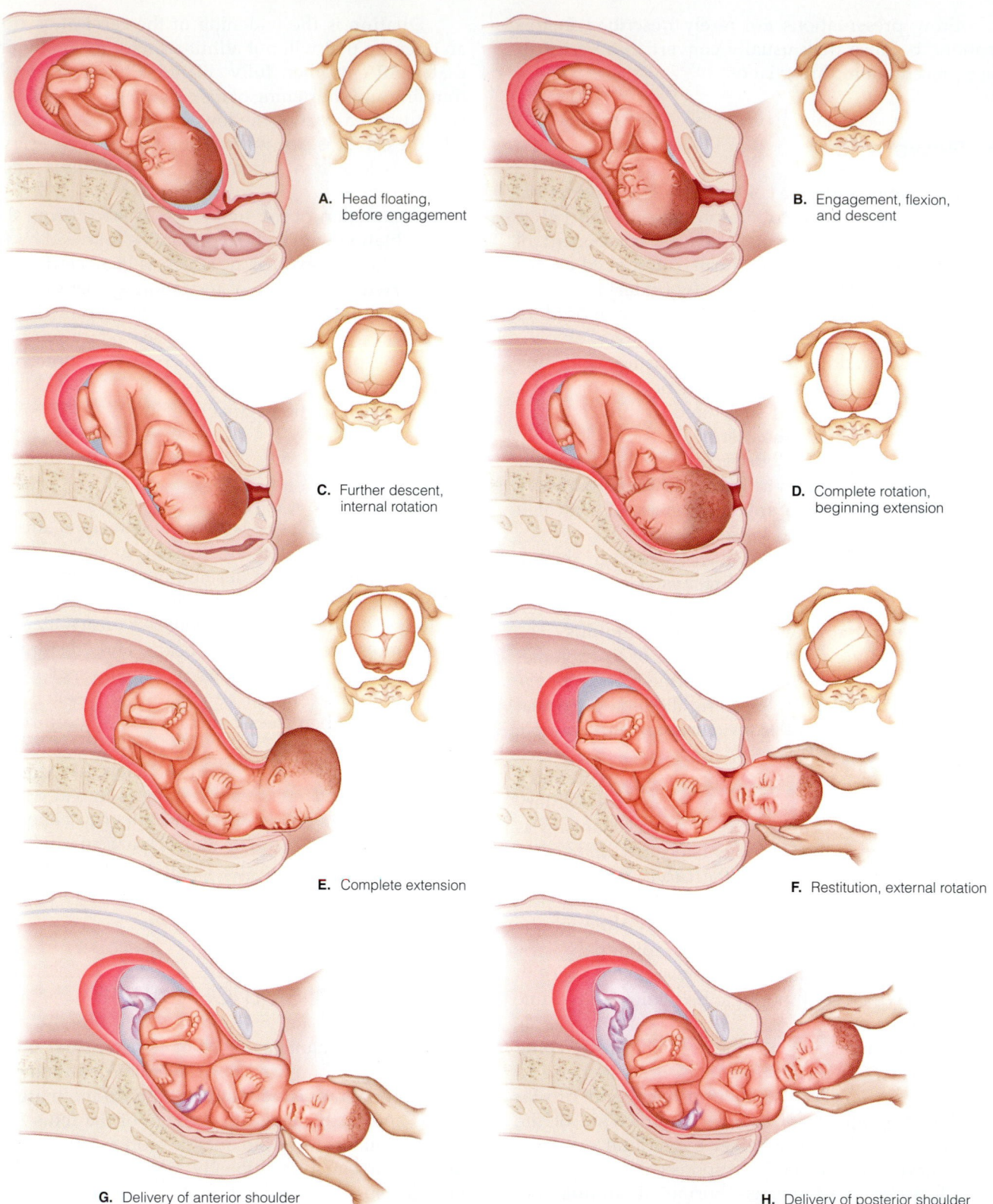

A. Head floating, before engagement

B. Engagement, flexion, and descent

C. Further descent, internal rotation

D. Complete rotation, beginning extension

E. Complete extension

F. Restitution, external rotation

G. Delivery of anterior shoulder

H. Delivery of posterior shoulder

FIGURE 21–9. Mechanisms of labor: left anterior occiput position. *(Adapted, with permission, from Cunningham, F.G. et al. (Eds.). (1997). Williams obstetrics (20th ed.). Stamford, CT: Appleton & Lange, p. 320.)*

the mechanisms that follows, fetal skull designations, particularly the occiput, are used to indicate the fetal presenting part during descent.

▶ Descent

The fetus descends throughout labor. Descent is a variable of normal labor that is continuous and measurable; progress can be measured against a known standard.

The ease with which the fetus is born is a result of the interaction between fetal accommodation and maternal internal structures. The progress of fetal movement through the maternal pelvis is monitored by the stations of descent.

Measurement of the **stations of descent,** in centimeters, reflects the progress of the descending fetal presenting part to the maternal ischial spines. On this scale, the point where the presenting part reaches the ischial spines is identified as zero. Measurements above the ischial spines are denoted in negative numbers and those below, in positive numbers, depending on how many centimeters above or below the ischial spines the presenting part is located.

Some practitioners divide the stations above and below the ischial spines into fifths (Fig. 21–10). Thus, when the presenting part is at a −5 station, it is at the level of the pelvic inlet. When the presenting part is at zero station, it is at the level of the ischial spines. Below the spines, the presenting part is considered at +1, +2, +3, and so on. At +5, crowning occurs and birth is imminent.

Protocols for recording station may vary according to established custom; for example, some institutions use a −3 to +3 notation, arbitrarily dividing the area above and below the ischial spines into thirds. Therefore, if the presenting part is at the level of the pelvic inlet, it is recorded as −3 station; if it has descended one-third the distance between the pelvic inlet and the ischial spines, it is noted as −2 station; two-thirds the distance is noted as −1 station. If the presenting part has descended one-third or two-thirds the distance between the ischial spines and the pelvic outlet, it is noted to be at +1 or +2 station, respectively. When the presenting part is on the perineum, its station is +3.

The station of the presenting part is an estimation in centimeters. Some authorities believe that to avoid confusion between the "thirds" and the "fifths" systems, the designation of station should be a fraction, with the station the numerator and the system the denominator (eg, −5/5 or −3/3) (Cunningham et al., 1997).

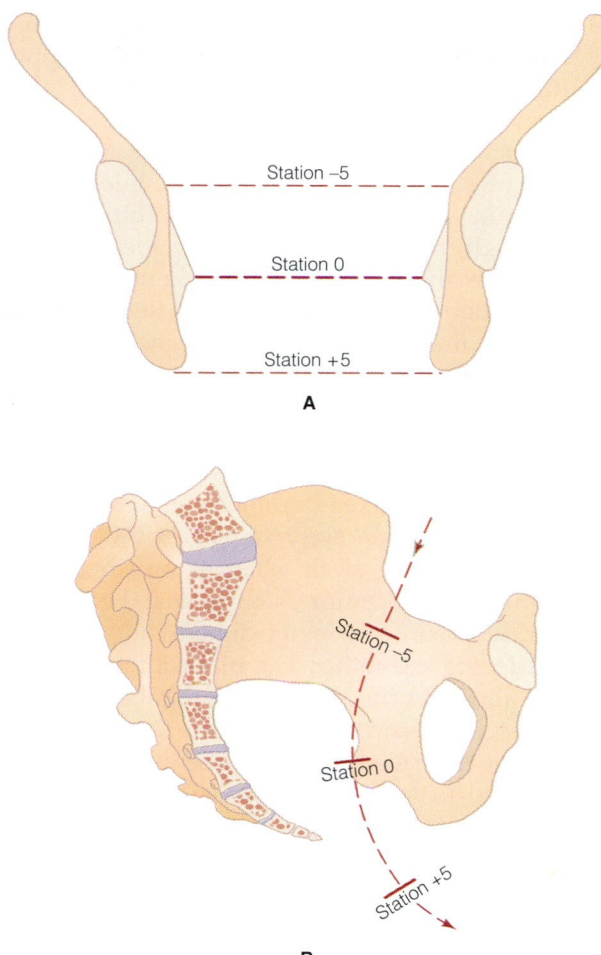

FIGURE 21–10. Stations of descent. **A.** Anteroposterior view. **B.** Lateral view. *(Adapted, with permission, from Oxorn, H. (Ed.). (1986). Oxorn-Foote human labor and birth (5th ed.). Norwalk, CT: Appleton & Lange, p. 69.)*

The station is assessed by vaginal examination and the use of Leopold's maneuvers. It is assessed at the same point in the contraction cycle each time an examination is done because the fetus may advance and recede with each contraction.

▶ Flexion

Flexion of the fetal head is necessary to bring the smaller suboccipital diameter into and out of the midpelvis of the mother. Flexion occurs when the fetal head meets resistance from the bony pelvis and soft tissue. Two additional factors make extreme flexion of the fetal head possible: (1) The fetus has the typical receding chin that characterizes the neonate. The mandible recedes even further in response to pressure and permits hyperflexion of the head. (2) The hormone relaxin may contribute to the process described, permitting a degree of hyperflexion that will never again be possible after birth.

Flexion of the fetal head should occur as the fetus in vertex presentation enters the pelvic inlet. Flexion allows the largest transverse diameter (biparietal) to pass through the pelvic inlet after the fetus has entered, with the sagittal suture in a transverse or oblique relationship to the pelvic inlet. Refer to Figure 21–9, which illustrates the mechanisms or cardinal movements of labor.

The dimensions of the fetal presenting part and of the pelvis of the mother must always be studied in relation to each other, not separately. The pelvis of the mother is relatively fixed in dimension, with the only pelvic accommodation occurring when the coccyx is movable. The fetal skull changes in dimensions throughout labor as compression against the maternal pelvis causes narrowing in one dimension with consequent widening in another. The joints of the fetal skull (sutures) allow for this accommodation both through compression and through override. This process of skull change is termed **molding.** The degree of molding is related to such factors as length of labor and size of the fetal head in relation to maternal structures.

When the fetal head is in flexion (truly, hyperflexion) the chin of the fetus is tucked down so that in a

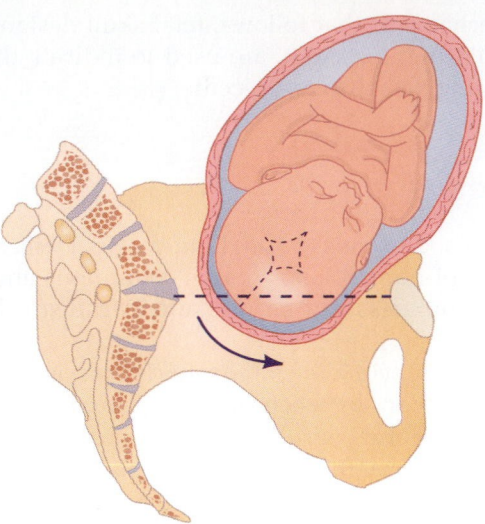

FIGURE 21–12. A less optimal position for descent occurs when the fetal head is not parallel to the planes of the maternal pelvis during engagement.

vertex presentation when descent and degree of dilation permit, the posterior fontanelle can be palpated on vaginal examination.

▶ Engagement

When the presenting part of the fetus has entered the true pelvis, **engagement** has occurred. Specifically, in a vertex presentation, engagement occurs when the largest transverse diameter (biparietal) of the fetal head has passed through the maternal pelvic inlet.

The fetal head engages most often with its anteroposterior diameters in the transverse diameter of the pelvis (Fig. 21–11). Thus, the most common position of the fetal head during engagement is the left occiput transverse position, with the biparietal diameter parallel to the planes of the pelvis. In this position, the smallest diameter of the head (suboccipitobregmatic) enters the widest diameter of the pelvic inlet (transverse). It is thus the best position for an effective descent. A less optimal position for descent occurs when the fetal head is not parallel to the planes of the pelvis on engagement (Fig. 21–12).

The head may enter the pelvic inlet in positions other than vertex, for example, brow or face presentations. Brow presentations often convert spontaneously to vertex and can initially be considered on the normal continuum. If conversion does not occur, a cephalopelvic disproportion may result in dystocia or an abnormality in the labor process (see Chapter 25). Face presentations rarely convert and lie outside the normal continuum.

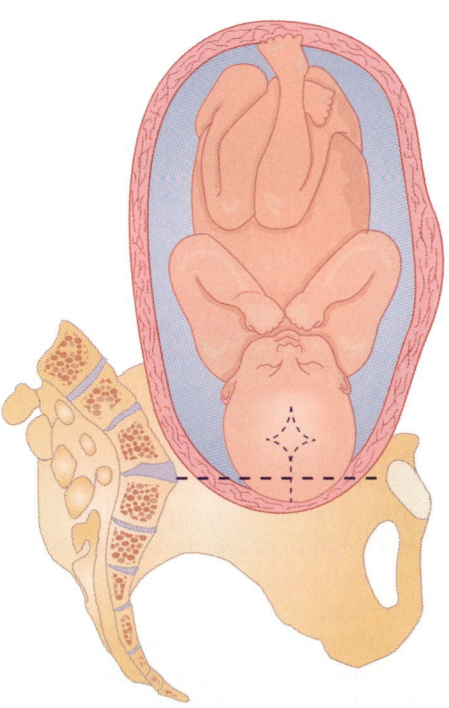

FIGURE 21–11. Engagement of the fetal head in the transverse diameter of the maternal pelvis.

► Internal Rotation

Internal rotation of the fetal head results in alignment of the anteroposterior diameter of the fetal head with the anteroposterior diameter of the maternal pelvis. Usually this rotation brings the fetal head from a LOA or ROA position into a direct anterior position, resulting in an OA position; that is, the fetus is looking down to the floor if the mother is on her back. In about 4% of cases, the fetus enters the pelvis in a LOP or ROP position and rotates into a direct OP position; that is, the fetus is looking up to the ceiling if the mother is lying on her back.

Internal rotation is caused by a combination of (1) the powerful pressure exerted by uterine contractions on the fetus, (2) the curved shape of the pelvic floor, and (3) the relationship of the vertex to the projection of the ischial spines in the midpelvic cavity.

The ischial spines act as guides or tracks, aiding the fetal skull to assume the position that will facilitate birth. Because the fetal skull and fetal shoulders are at right angles to each other, the ischial spines aid the body of the fetus in passage through the pelvis. As internal rotation takes place (a 45° turn) the pelvis of the mother compels the limbs and body of the fetus to assume the most compact shape possible. Once complete internal rotation occurs the fetus has usually descended to the pelvic floor (see Fig. 21–9).

► Extension

The birth of the head occurs by extension in OA position and by flexion, then extension in the OP position. In the OA position the resistance of the pelvic floor from its anatomic curve directs the head upward toward the vaginal outlet, causing extension of the fetal head. The back of the fetal head in the suboccipital region moves under the symphysis pubis and acts as a pivotal point for the extension. Additional pressure from the contracting uterus and from maternal pushing helps to extend the head further until it emerges through the vulvovaginal opening. In the OP position the sinciput moves beneath the symphysis pubis and becomes the pivotal point for delivery of the head. The head remains flexed as it (occiput) distends the vulvovaginal opening. In effect the back of the head is born first and then extension takes over and the front (face) of the head is born (see Fig. 21–9).

► Restitution

After the birth of the infant's head (with the sagittal suture parallel to the mother's long axis) the head rotates 45°, returning to the position it assumed when it first entered the pelvis. This maneuver, known as **restitution,** restores the normal anatomic alignment of the infant's neck and shoulders (see Fig. 21–9).

► External Rotation

External rotation occurs as the shoulders (which are still in the pelvis) rotate 45° to bring them in line with the anteroposterior diameter of the pelvis. When the shoulders rotate, the head rotates another 45° into the LOT or ROT position (see Fig. 21–9).

► Expulsion

The birth of the shoulders is by lateral flexion. The anterior shoulder is usually born first and is seen at the anterior portion of the vulvovaginal opening. Like the head in the OA position, the anterior shoulder moves under the symphysis pubis. With the continued forces of maternal pushing and contractions, the posterior shoulder distends the perineum and is born by lateral flexion following the pelvic curve. The remainder of the body follows the same curve and is readily born, as it is much smaller and more flexible than either the head or shoulders.

► PREMONITORY PHASE

Occasionally, it is difficult for the woman to determine if labor has truly begun. It is important for the nurse to distinguish between false and true labor. True labor includes a premonitory phase and results in dilation and effacement of the cervix. False labor, on the other hand, does not dilate or efface the cervix.

Signs that the onset of labor is imminent may be noted subjectively by the mother or may go unnoticed. Primigravid women may experience lightening, or descent of the presenting part of the fetus into the pelvis, more frequently than multigravid women. Lightening is more common when the fetus presents in a vertex position, the mother has good abdominal muscle tone, and there is no cephalopelvic inlet disproportion. The expectant mother reports relief from pressure on the upper abdomen and diaphragm and, quite possibly, an easing of the problem of heartburn. Pelvic pressure, frequent urination as a result of bladder compression, increase in leg cramps, and the characteristic waddling gait are other symptoms that accompany lightening. This initial uterine/fetal descent may occur several weeks before the onset of labor; the indeterminate time frame makes lightening a weak predictor of labor.

The Braxton Hicks contractions that have "exercised" the uterine musculature throughout pregnancy become more perceptible to the mother near term. As anxiety heightens awareness and impatience magnifies each somatic change, the pregnant woman may experience the Braxton Hicks contractions as painful. Multiparous women report that these preparatory contractions become more uncomfortable with each succeeding pregnancy, probably as a result of loss of uterine tone. Braxton Hicks contractions are irregular and experienced primarily in the abdomen.

Many women experience a rush of energy several days before the onset of true labor. In the 72-hour period before onset the woman at term often can be found cleaning, washing windows, waxing floors, or rearranging the nursery. Such "nesting behavior" is also exhibited in species other than humans and appears to be a deep-seated, biologically patterned response to impending birth. Because sleep is often difficult as the woman nears term (as a result of the need to void frequently, difficulty in breathing, fetal activity, and the general discomfort of a cumbersome body), this short period of intense physical activity further depletes energy stores. Prenatal teaching must include caution against overdoing. Walking or short periods of light activity might be suggested as a substitute. The mother who is made aware of the significance of the energy burst can use this time to review preparations for the trip to the hospital and to practice prepared childbirth techniques.

A slight weight loss of 1 to 4 pounds may directly precede labor as the hormonal balance between progesterone and estrogen causes a shift in electrolytes.

An increase in vaginal mucous secretions may be confused with amniotic leakage. The increase is caused by congestion of tissues. A "bloody show" of pink-stained mucus may be present for several days preceding labor onset.

Nursing Alert

Due to the pelvic pressure of lightening and the more relaxed pelvic joints that occur during the premonitory phase, a woman may report that she feels slightly unstable when walking. The nurse should reinforce safety precautions with the client, with a special emphasis on the need to exercise caution so as to minimize the risk of falls.

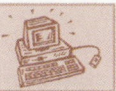

Research Abstract

Relationship Between Maternal Sleep and the Onset of Labor

The purpose of this study was to examine the relationship between the quality of maternal sleep prior to the onset of labor and length of labor. Ninety-nine women completed the Visual Analog Sleep Scale each morning for two weeks prior to their due date. Following delivery, the women completed the Perception of Labor and Delivery Scale. Researchers examined data about the women's labor. The results showed that, although the women reported high sleep disturbances, there were no significant relationships between sleep quality and length of labor or maternal perceptions of labor.

Application to Practice

Nurses may use these findings to provide anticipatory guidance to mothers about the possibility of disturbed maternal sleep prior to labor. Mothers can be taught relaxation techniques to enhance sleep. They may also reassure mothers that it has been shown that sleep disturbances prior to labor do not interfere with the progress of labor.

Source: Evans, M.L., Dick, M.J., & Clark, A.S. (1995). Sleep during the week before labor: Relationships to outcomes. Clinical Nursing Research, 4(3), 238–252.

In summary, there are several signs of the premonitory stage of labor. The nurse should make the pregnant couple aware of these signs, but should explain that the signs may not be experienced by all women.

▶ STAGES AND PHASES OF LABOR

For purposes of assessment, labor is divided into stages and phases using the variables of time, effacement/dilation of the cervix, and changes in maternal behavioral responses. Each stage and phase have characteristic landmarks and parameters that are useful in determining progress or lack of progress. Patterns of labor are highly individual. The nurse should listen carefully to the woman who reports that her labors in the past have "gone from 3 to 10 cm in 90 minutes." What appears to be a history of abnormally long or startlingly short labors may reflect inherited pelvic anatomy and, for that individual woman, a normal pattern.

▶ First Stage

The **first stage of labor** begins with the onset of true labor and ends when cervical dilation is accomplished. It is made up of two phases: the latent phase and the active phase.

The **Friedman curve** (Friedman, 1982) is a graphic representation of these phases in the normal progress of labor. On this graph, cervical dilation, in centimeters, is the vertical axis, and time, in hours, is the horizontal axis (Fig. 21–13). The Friedman curve has been useful for more than 20 years. The nurse who is caring for more than one woman during labor may find the graphic method an aid to early identification of a trend toward deviation from normal.

Latent Phase

The **latent phase** begins with the onset of true labor and ends when the cervix dilates approximately 3 cm. The latent phase has traditionally been considered to be longer for primigravid women (8.6 hours) than for multigravid women (5.3 hours, with outer limits of normal of 20 hours for primigravid women and 14 hours for multigravid women).

Contractions during the latent phase are widely spaced (15 to 30 minutes) and of mild to moderate intensity. The Friedman curve is nearly flat during the

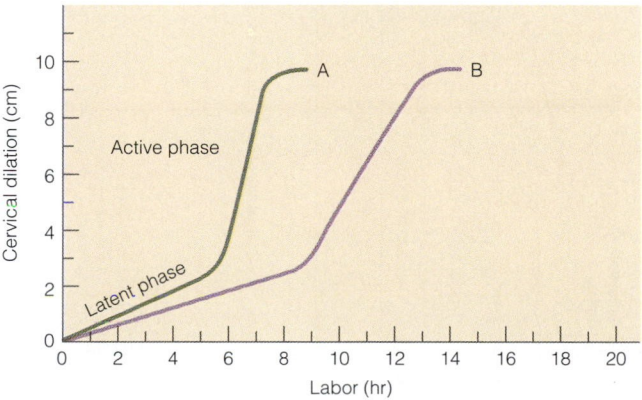

FIGURE 21–13. Friedman's curve, showing first stage of labor for **(A)** a multiparous woman and **(B)** a primigravid woman. *(Reproduced, with permission, from Oxorn, H. (Ed.). (1986). Oxorn-Foote human labor and birth (5th ed.). Norwalk, CT: Appleton & Lange, p. 120.)*

latent phase. Nulliparous women frequently assume that because of the relative comfort of the latent phase, the remaining labor will not be difficult. The nurse caring for the nulliparous client supports the client in building confidence in her ability to accomplish the tasks of labor: "You have certainly managed the contractions very well so far. I'm sure that as labor becomes more intense you will do equally well." Such comments imply that the client retains the control essential to her self-image and self-confidence (the word *manage* is chosen deliberately).

Active Phase

Once the cervix is dilated to 3 cm, the woman enters the **active phase** of labor. The active phase lasts from the end of the latent phase until full dilation of the cervix. Contractions grow stronger and longer (30 to 60 seconds). They are more frequent, occurring every 2 to 3 minutes. The Friedman curve during the active phase becomes a nearly vertical incline until the second stage of labor is almost reached, when the curve flattens again. The active phase is further subdivided into the acceleration phase, phase of maximum slope, and deceleration phase.

Acceleration Phase. A prelude to the intense activity that follows, the **acceleration phase** is characterized by an intense increase in the rate of dilation from approximately 3 cm to 4 to 5 cm.

Phase of Maximum Slope. The greatest increase in the rate of cervical dilation is referred to as the **phase of maximum slope**. Rapid cervical dilation during this phase averages 3 cm per hour. An increase of less than 1.2 cm in a primigravid woman or 1.7 cm in a multiparous woman is considered abnormal. The use of such fractional measurements may give the impression that complete precision in measuring cervical dilation is possible; however, normal variations occur among laboring women.

Deceleration Phase. Also termed the transition phase, the **deceleration phase** is characterized by cervical dilation of 8 to 10 cm. Effacement of the cervix is either complete or almost complete, with only a rim remaining (similar to the mouth of a balloon) on vaginal examination. The rim may completely encircle the os, or may be partial if a portion of the cervix is trapped between the presenting part (particularly in a vertex presentation) and the pubic arch. Contractions are moderate to strong and occur at 1- to 2-minute intervals.

Behavior of the laboring woman often changes markedly in transition. Although earlier in labor she may have welcomed the soothing touch of her support person or the nurse as backrubs and a cool washcloth on the forehead provided comfort, the woman now tends to be irritable and dislikes being touched. Nausea and vomiting may add to her discomfort. She concentrates totally on the labor process and may experience a loss of control with subsequent panic as contractions increase in intensity. The so-called "bloody show" becomes more profuse during this phase.

If relaxation techniques have been learned, the laboring woman may sleep in the brief intervals between contractions to conserve strength. The first stage of labor ends with complete effacement and dilation of the cervix. The longest period of labor is over, and preparation of the birth passage has been completed. The nurse should be aware that sedation may prolong the latent phase. Figure 21–14 illustrates the progress of rotation of an occipitoanterior position in the successive phases and stages of labor.

Rupture of Membranes

The membranes that constitute the sac containing the fetus and amniotic fluid are subject to extreme pressure in the lower uterine segment as the presenting part of the fetus descends into the pelvis. A pocket of fluid is trapped and applies pressure against the cervix. Membranes may rupture any time during labor or in the prelabor period before admission. Characteristically, however, rupture occurs at the height of a moderate to strong contraction, with the

fetal presenting part well engaged and descended. The membranes can also be ruptured artificially through the procedure of amniotomy.

▶ Second Stage

The **second stage of labor** begins at full dilation, that is, 10 cm, and ends with delivery of the neonate.

Delivery of the Newborn

At full dilation and effacement with the fetal presenting part (vertex) at +5 station, caput (fetal scalp) will be visible with each contraction. The mother feels an uncontrollable involuntary urge to push out the contents of the uterus. The perineum distends further with each contraction, bulging as the presenting part applies pressure. Labia minora and labia majora disappear with distension and rectal mucosa often protrudes with the effort of expulsion. The fetal head advances with each contraction, then slips back in the resting plateau. Each advance moves the fetus farther until the widest diameter of the fetal skull (biparietal) is rimmed by the introitus, and with the next contraction or two, the head emerges.

Duration of Second Stage

The Friedman graphic analysis of normal labor indicates that on average the second stage of labor lasts about 1 hour in primigravid women and about 20

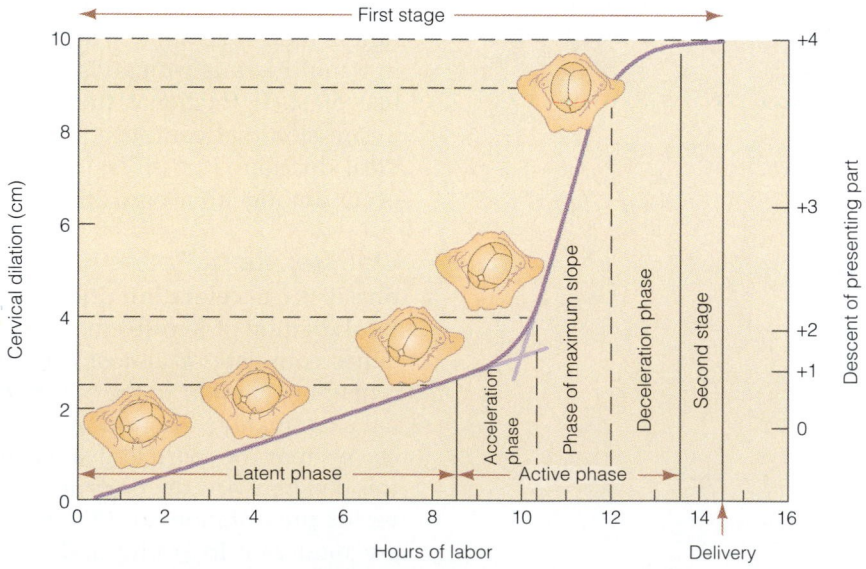

FIGURE 21–14. Progress of rotation of occipitoanterior presentation in the successive stages of labor. *(Reproduced, with permission, from DeCherney, A.H., & Pernoll, M.L. (Eds.). (1994). Currrent obstetric & gynecologic diagnosis & treatment (8th ed.). Norwalk, CT: Appleton & Lange, p. 211.)*

minutes in multigravid women. Both time designations represent means, not absolutes. In primigravid women, second-stage labor can last up to 2 hours and still be considered "normal" if there is a measurable rate of descent and no indication of fetal distress.

▶ Third Stage

The **third stage of labor** encompasses the time between delivery of the neonate and expulsion of the placenta. With the birth of the neonate the formerly distended uterus contracts, beginning the process of placental disengagement. The sight of the newborn and the first sounds may also form a powerful primary stimulus to the production of maternal oxytocin, which in turn promotes further contraction of the uterus.

Separation of the Placenta

The placenta may safely remain attached to the uterine wall for as long as 30 minutes before being termed *retained.* In most births, placental separation occurs 5 to 10 minutes after delivery of the neonate.

Failure of the placenta to fully separate, or retention of placental fragments, may require manual removal under anesthesia. The totally retained placenta is a rare complication. Retention of placental fragments, although not common, occurs more frequently than total retention and may cause immediate or delayed hemorrhage (see Chapter 29).

The separated placenta presents in one of two ways. In the Schultze mechanism, dubbed "shiny Schultze," the placenta first separates from the uterine wall at its center with the edges releasing last so that the shiny membranous fetal side is seen first, trailing the membranes (Fig. 21–15). In the Duncan mechanism, dubbed "dirty Duncan," the maternal side presents first, indicating that separation has occurred first at an edge and progressed. The maternal surface that has adhered to the uterine wall is rough and bumpy in appearance (Fig. 21–16).

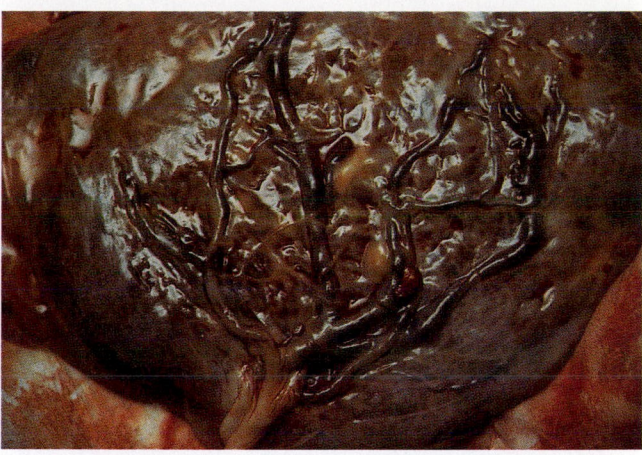

FIGURE 21–15. Fetal surface of the placenta. *(Photo courtesy of Harriette Hartigan/Artemis.)*

▶ Fourth Stage

The **fourth stage of labor** has traditionally been identified as the period after or within 4 hours of delivery of the placenta. In practice it is viewed as the period required for stabilization of the mother's physical and emotional state after the stresses of labor and delivery. In the hospital setting, this postdelivery period may therefore be very short and encompass only the time required for hygienic care and assessment of the mother's status before transport to a postpartum unit, or it may include a stay of several hours in a delivery recovery area.

With the fourth stage of labor the mother's body systems begin a phase of physiologic restoration. The final outcome of the adjustments will be return of the woman's body to a physiologic state similar to the prepregnancy state.

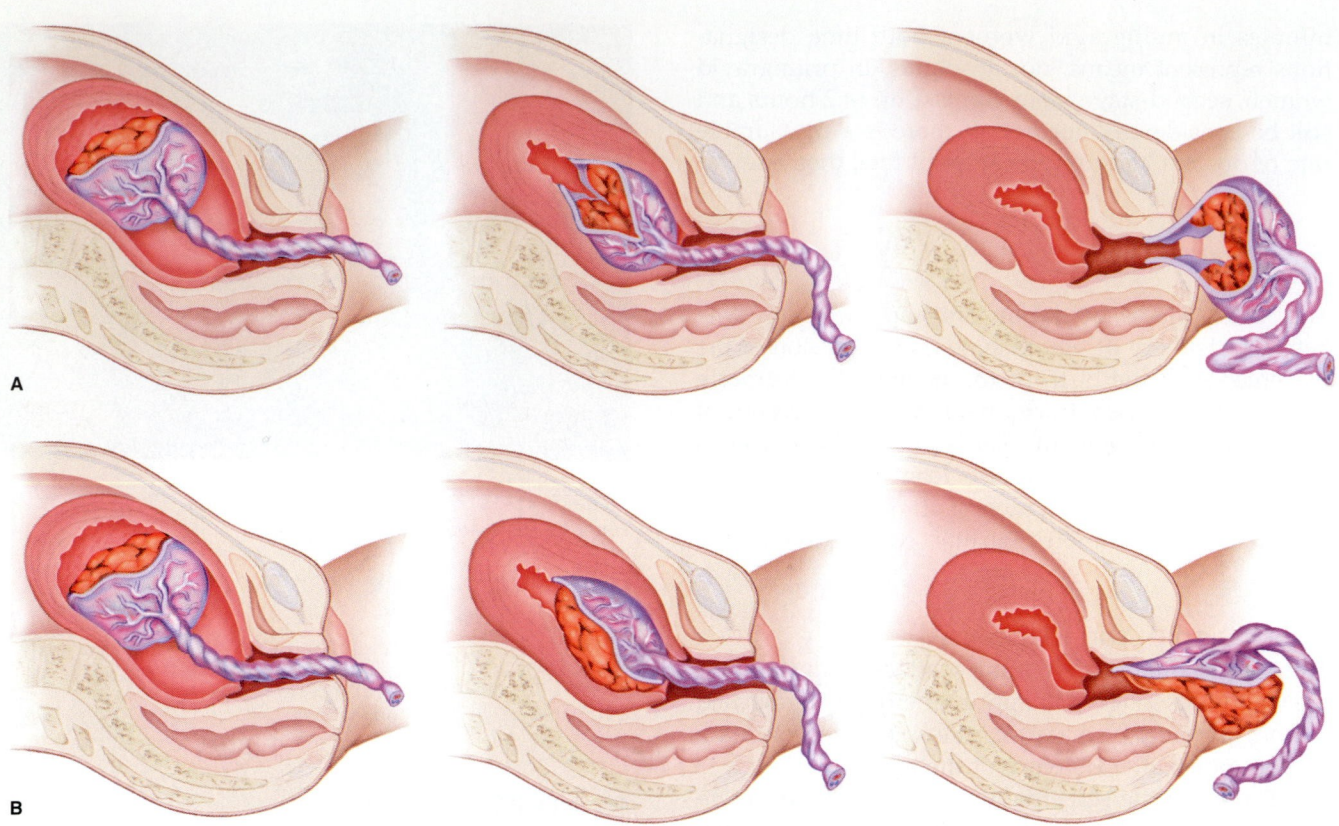

FIGURE 21–16. Placental separation. **A.** Schultze mechanism. **B.** Duncan mechanism.

Chapter Highlights

▶ Contributing factors to the onset of labor include the uterine stretch mechanism and maternal and fetal hormones.

▶ Progress of labor is influenced by the four P's: passage, or true pelvis, consisting of the pelvic inlet, pelvic cavity, and pelvic outlet; passenger, or fetus (fetal skull and fetopelvic relationships); powers, the uterine contractions, intraabdominal pressure, and counterpressure of the pelvic floor; and psyche, the maternal psychologic responses.

▶ Fetal attitude, lie, presentation, and position describe fetopelvic relationships in terms of the fetus in relation to himself, herself, or the maternal pelvis.

▶ The most frequent fetal presentation is the vertex (or occiput) presentation, with the head flexed and the occiput presenting.

▶ The mechanisms or cardinal movements of labor are descent, flexion, engagement, internal rotation, extension, restitution, external rotation, and expulsion.

▶ Progress of the descending fetal presenting part to the maternal ischial spines is measured using a scale termed stations of descent.

▶ Common signs of labor onset include lightening (descent of the fetus into the pelvis), more pronounced Braxton Hicks contractions, and experience of a heightened level of energy ("nesting behavior") in the 2 to 3 days before onset of true labor.

▶ The first stage of labor begins with the first true labor contraction and ends with complete dilation of the cervix.

▶ The Friedman curve divides the first stage of labor into the latent and active phases.

▶ The second stage of labor begins with complete dilation and effacement of the cervix and ends with the birth of the baby.

▶ The third stage of labor begins with the birth of the baby and ends with delivery of the placenta.

▶ The fourth stage of labor is the period after or within 4 hours of delivery of the placenta and is viewed as the time required for stabilization of the mother's physical and emotional state after the stresses of labor and birth.

▶ Nursing care of the woman and her family during labor and birth is based on a thorough knowledge of maternal physiology and the stages and phases of labor.

After reading the vignette at the beginning of this chapter, use what you have learned to answer these questions:

1. In what ways can Margaret Kiely, RN, intervene to help Cathleen and Bill Harris manage the fear and discomfort they are experiencing during labor?

2. What information can the nurse provide this couple to promote their understanding of the mechanisms of labor and the factors that may affect its outcome?

3. How does successful management of the first stage of labor prepare Cathleen and Bill Harris for the later stages of labor and birth of their baby?

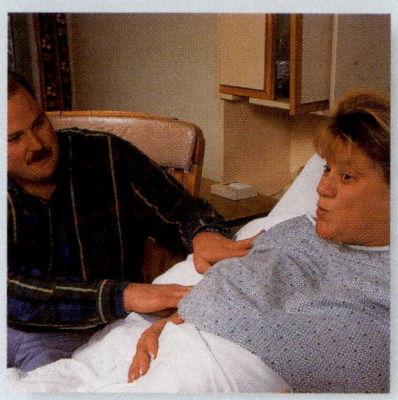

Critical Thinking Questions

▶ # References

Blackburn, S.T., & Loper, D.L. (1992). *Maternal, fetal, and neonatal physiology.* Philadelphia: W.B. Saunders.

Challis, J.R.G. (1994). Characteristics of parturition. In R.K. Creasy & R.R. Resnick (Eds.), *Maternal fetal medicine* (3rd ed.) (pp. 52–68). Philadelphia: W.B. Saunders.

Cunningham, F.G., MacDonald, P.C., Gant, N.F., Leveno, K.J., Gilstrap, L.C., Hankins, G.D.V., & Clark, S.L. (1997). *Williams obstetrics* (20th ed.). Stamford, CT: Appleton & Lange.

Evans, M.L., Dick, M.J., & Clark, A.S. (1995). Sleep during the week before labor: Relationship to outcomes. *Clinical Nursing Research, 4*(3), 238–252.

Friedman, E. (Ed.) (1982). *Obstetric decision making.* St. Louis: C.V. Mosby.

Lefebvre, D.L., Giaid, A., Bennett, H., Lariviere, R., & Zingg, H.H. (1992). Oxytocin gene expression in rat uterus. *Science, 256,* 1553–1555.

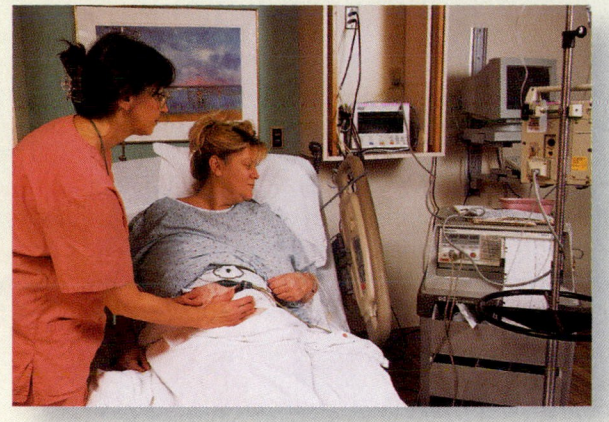

Cathleen Harris is admitted to the labor and delivery unit in the latent phase of the first stage of labor. This is Cathleen's second pregnancy. Margaret Kiely, RN, introduces herself to Cathleen and her husband, Bill. After the nurse obtains Cathleen's health history, she monitors the fetal heart rate and fetal presentation and assesses Cathleen's vital signs. Cathleen is also placed on a tocodynamometer to monitor the uterine contractions.

The nurse places her hand on the tocodynamometer on Cathleen's abdomen and observes the tracing of the fetal heart rate as well as the duration and intensity of a contraction on the monitor. Cathleen also looks at the monitor and then glances at the nurse. She states, "When I was in labor with my son Andrew, I wanted to understand the information that was being recorded, but I was so focused on the contractions and what was about to happen that I didn't ask any questions. Can you tell me what these readings mean to me and my baby?" ∎

22

Assessment of the Family During Labor and Birth

Women come to a birthing facility at different phases in the laboring process and with different levels of wellness. Accurate initial and ongoing maternal and fetal assessment during labor by the professional nurse is critical to the well-being of the mother and her fetus. "The touch of a caring hand is needed as well as the ultrasonic . . . probe" (Creasy, 1986). Assessment is the basis for diagnostic decision making and guides appropriate nursing interventions. In addition to using the assessment skills of observation, palpation, and auscultation, the nurse watches for subtle clues that may indicate a problem. The continual presence of the nurse with the laboring woman permits ongoing assessment and the opportunity to individualize care for the woman and her family.

▶ THE DELIVERY TEAM

The delivery team consists of many different professionals and may vary considerably among various birth sites, institutions, and communities (Table 22–1). The nurse, as part of the team, works with each of the other members to effect the best outcome for mother, baby, and family.

▶ **TABLE 22–1**

Members of the Delivery Team

Team Member	Role
Perinatologist/ maternal–fetal medicine obstetrician	Most medical technically prepared team member; a physician trained in the obstetric care of the high-risk woman and fetus. Usually works in a subspecialty facility and takes referrals from all other personnel (usually other obstetricians, family practitioners, or nurse-midwives) when the mother or fetus has had or is having considerable problems. Also may care for the low-risk woman.
Neonatologist	Pediatric physician trained in the care of sick neonates who works in a subspecialty center, and usually receives referrals from obstetricians, perinatologists, and sometimes nurse-midwives.
General obstetrician	Physician who in the United States cares for most women during their childbearing years. May work in a variety of settings, but most often at a basic or specialty facility. Can handle all normal pregnancies and most complications of pregnancy and birth. In cases of high-risk mothers or neonates, will either consult with or directly refer the client to the perinatologist.
Family practitioner	Modern and more educated version of the general practitioner or family doctor. Trained to handle normal births, minor complications, normal newborns, and general family health care. May act in the same capacity as the obstetricians and pediatricians in communities in which these practitioners are not available.
Pediatrician	Physician trained in the care of children; the member of the delivery team who examines the neonate after birth and cares for the normal neonate in the birthing institution and community.
Pediatric nurse practitioner (PNP)	Nurse with additional education in the care of children. Many PNPs have master's degrees and also function as advanced practice nurses. Affiliated with a pediatrician. May perform all the normal newborn examinations and provide care in the birthing institution or community. Cares for the normal newborn and also handles minor illnesses of childhood.
Family nurse practitioner (FNP)	Nurse with additional education who provides care for all family members. Also provides care of the infant after birth and during the life span.
Certified nurse-midwife (CNM)	Individual educated in the two disciplines of nursing and midwifery who possesses evidence of certification according to the requirements of the American College of Nurse-Midwives. Education can be at the certificate, master's, or doctoral level. In collaboration with a physician, cares for the woman during her pregnancy, birth, and postpartum and also does family planning and well-woman gynecology. May work in a variety of settings ranging from own midwifery private practice to a physician's private practice, as either a partner or an employee of the physician, and in a variety of health care agencies.
Maternity clinical nurse specialist (CNS) Woman's Health Nurse Practitioner	Registered nurse with master's level advanced practice preparation in the care of women during the childbearing cycle. Advanced practice nurse (APN) designates a nurse who has expertise in a defined area of knowledge and practice. It is mastery of the domain of maternity nursing that allows the APN to coordinate care for childbearing clients in a variety of settings.
Maternity (OB) nurse	Registered nurse with additional formal or informal education in the care of the mother and fetus during the prenatal, intrapartum, and postpartum periods. May work in a variety of settings, although most work in hospitals. Role is to provide nursing care needed to give the woman and her family a safe and positive birth experience.

► ASSESSMENT OF THE WOMAN AND FETUS IN LABOR

Throughout the prenatal course, the nurse has acted as a facilitator to client care. In doing so, the focus has been on health promotion and prevention of complications to help clients enter into labor and delivery with a high level of wellness.

► Admission to the Birthing Facility

Most couples who arrive at the birthing facility for delivery are excited that the birth of their baby is imminent and anxious that everything will go well. The nurse can relieve much of this anxiety by ensuring that the couple understands the events of labor and delivery and care that will be provided. From the outset, the childbearing couple needs to feel that the birthing facility and staff are there for them, not that they are strangers with others in control. This tone is set by the nurse who welcomes the couple into the system. Nursing assessment, which includes obtaining the health history and performing a physical examination, is done in this same empathic manner throughout labor and delivery. An assessment of the couple's preparation and expectations for their experience is particularly important.

Informed Consent

Informed consent should be obtained prior to any procedures. This requires that the client be given information about the reasons for the care she will be given, including the potential benefits and risks and possible alternatives. Informed consent should be obtained before any medications are given that may affect the client's ability to make decisions.

Health History

When the couple contacts the delivery team, an assessment must be made about whether the expectant mother is in labor, her risk status, and her birthing plans. The information obtained in the history helps determine her progress in labor and who on the health care team needs to be notified (Fig. 22–1). The client's medical history is important because some medical conditions, such as diabetes and cardiac disease, may necessitate specific interventions during labor. Ideally, much information is obtained during the prenatal period and recorded on the prenatal record. If this is not the case, the labor and delivery nurse obtains the history.

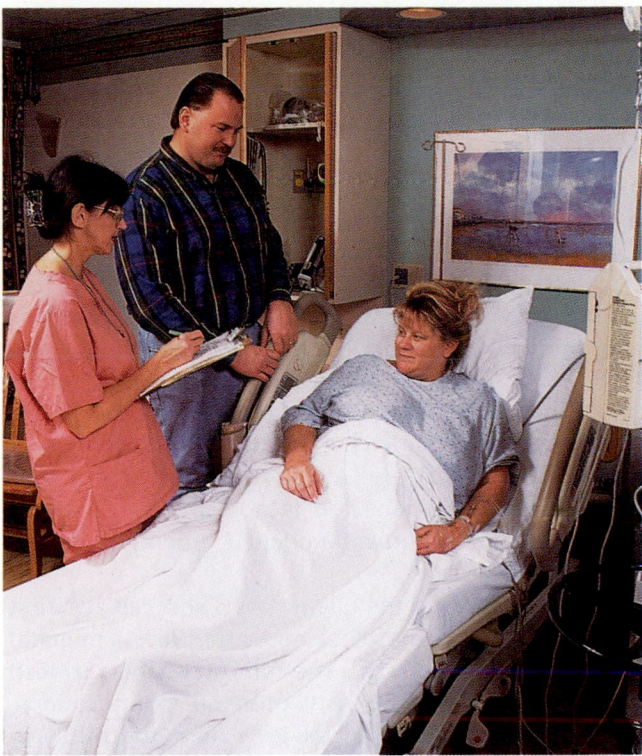

FIGURE 22–1. The labor and delivery nurse obtains the health history from the childbearing couple at their arrival at the birthing facility.

Demographic and Descriptive Data. The labor and delivery nurse introduces herself and asks the mother and her support person their names and how they would like to be addressed while in labor. Other important descriptive data are the age of the client (may determine risk status), ethnic and religious group, and estimated date of delivery (EDD). The EDD can be obtained from the prenatal record. If the prenatal record is not available and the mother knows the date of her last menstrual period, the nurse can calculate the EDD by using Nägele's rule (see Chapter 15). The prenatal record should also be checked for blood type, Rh factor, serology, and hepatitis screen.

The reason for admission is stated in the client's own words and should include at least the following:

- *Contraction pattern.* Time and date of onset, frequency, duration, intensity, change of pattern, and degree of discomfort felt by client.
- *Amniotic membranes (bag of waters).* Intact or ruptured; if ruptured, color and odor of fluid, date and time the membranes ruptured, and anything unusual surrounding the event.
- *Bleeding/bloody show.* Date, time, color, and amount; bright red bleeding, date, time,

amount, circumstances, associated pain, and other associated symptoms or problems, for example, nausea, vomiting, diarrhea, and pain (location).

The client should be asked when she last ate or drank anything prior to labor onset. The woman should also be asked if she has any allergies to medications or foods.

Obstetric History. The client's obstetric history is important because it gives the nurse an idea of the client's risk status and the other personnel (e.g., obstetrician, perinatologist, pediatrician, neonatologist, certified nurse-midwife) who should be notified, and it affects the plan of care. A good prenatal record provides this information; if it is not already available, this information should be elicited quickly but completely, if possible.

The nurse asks the client when she had her first prenatal visit and the place and provider of prenatal care. The course of the present pregnancy is also important information. Any prenatal complications, hospitalizations, and special tests alert the nurse to potential problems during the labor and delivery period.

Information about the client's present and past pregnancies adds information about her risk status and helps the nurse determine which members of the delivery team need to be notified.

Maternal–Fetal Examination

A physical examination of the woman and fetus is performed when the mother is first seen in labor by the nurse or other professional; elements of the examination are repeated during the course of labor. In addition, other factors that affect the progress of the labor, such as the woman's psyche and cultural background, are assessed.

During labor, the changes that the mother and fetus experience are so interconnected that they cannot be considered two distinct entities. Thus, assessment and care are of the maternal–fetal dyad rather than the mother and fetus separately.

► Fetal Assessment

Fetal Heart Rate

Fetal heart rate (FHR) should be evaluated early in the admission process. FHR is the number of times the fetal heart beats per minute. Auscultation with a fetoscope, a hand-held Doppler ultrasound instrument, or electronic fetal monitor (EFM) are the basic techniques used to assess FHR. Each method has its advantages and limitations, necessitating individualized decision

making. The method and frequency of FHR monitoring are determined following consideration of maternal–fetal risk factors and stage of labor.

Auscultation. Auscultation of the FHR is an auditory assessment procedure that allows evaluation of the FHR both during and immediately following the stress of a uterine contraction. Auscultation between contractions provides the baseline FHR. Intermittent auscultation of the FHR at 15-minute intervals during the active phase of the first stage of labor and at 5-minute intervals during the second stage, with a 1:1 nurse:fetus ratio, has been shown to be equivalent to EFM (American Academy of Pediatrics and American College of Obstetricians & Gynecologists, 1992).

Because the FHR can be heard most clearly at the fetal back, the nurse should perform Leopold's maneuvers to identify the fetal presentation and position before listening (see Chapter 18). The nurse should listen and count the rate for one full minute. Checking the rate before, during, and for at least 15 seconds after the contraction is important to determine that there are no decelerations or irregularities. Listening to the FHR during a contraction and immediately after enables the nurse to evaluate how the fetus reacts to the contraction. If tachycardia, bradycardia, irregular beats, or decelerations are heard, EFM should be used for continual monitoring of the FHR.

A handheld Doppler ultrasonic device may be used in place of the fetoscope to assess the FHR. With a Doppler device, nurses can easily listen to the fetal heart throughout a contraction.

Electronic Fetal Monitoring. Fetal heart rate can also be measured with the electronic fetal monitor. Electronic fetal monitoring is an auditory and visual assessment procedure that provides data for the evaluation of uterine activity and fetal heart responses, including baseline FHR, fetal heart variability, and FHR changes over time. The FHR can be assessed during labor indirectly (externally) and directly (internally). The indirect method is accomplished using an ultrasonic transducer. A spiral scalp electrode is used for direct monitoring. Uterine contractions may be monitored externally with a tocodynamometer or internally with an intrauterine pressure catheter.

External EFM is accomplished with the use of an ultrasonic transducer that emits continuous high-frequency sound waves. When the transducer is placed correctly on the maternal abdomen, the ultrasound strikes the moving fetal heart and directs a signal back to the transducer. A continuous recording of the FHR and any changes that may occur in response to the contraction is printed out on the upper part of the strip chart. The ultrasound signal can be affected by minor changes in the position of the transducer or the fetus. Changes in the direction of the sound beam during uterine contractions may distort the tracing and mask periodic changes in the FHR. Ultrasound cannot assess short-term variability or beat-to-beat changes in the FHR because it reflects only mechanical movement of the fetal heart. An approximation of short-term variability can be made with monitors that have autocorrelation capability.

The ultrasonic transducer is applied to the maternal abdomen after determining the placement of the fetal back through use of Leopold's maneuvers. A water-soluble gel is applied to the underside of the transducer for conduction of the fetal heart sounds, and the transducer is kept in place with an elastic belt or a stretchable cloth binder.

Uterine contractions can be monitored externally by using a tocodynamometer, which is a pressure device. It is placed on the client's abdomen directly over the fundus, the area of greatest contractility, and kept in place with an elastic belt or a binder, similar to the ultrasound transducer. During a uterine contraction, pressure is exerted against the pressure–sensing button on the underside of the tocotransducer. The pressure from the tightening uterus creates an electrical signal that is transmitted to the monitor and recorded on the lower part of the graph paper. Both frequency and duration of the contraction, but not intensity, are displayed. Absolute intensity can be assessed only with the intrauterine pressure catheter.

Internal monitoring of the FHR is accomplished through use of an internal spiral electrode which is attached to the skin of the fetal scalp or buttocks. The spiral electrode gives an exact reading of FHR variability. To attach the spiral electrode, the cervix must be dilated at least 2 to 3 cm and the presenting fetal part must be accessible by vaginal examination.

Frequency, duration, and intensity of uterine contractions and resting tone of the uterus may be assessed through use of an intrauterine catheter inserted vaginally directly into the uterine cavity. The fluid-filled plastic catheter is compressed during uterine contractions and this pressure is reflected on the monitor strip chart in the form of millimeters of mercury (mm Hg). Table 22–2 is a comparison of various methods of FHR assessment.

Parameters of Fetal Heart Rate Tracing.
Several parameters of the FHR tracing are assessed, such as baseline FHR, baseline beat-to-beat variation, FHR accelerations, and FHR decelerations.

The baseline FHR is the average rate assessed between contractions. The baseline FHR is usually between 120 and 160 beats per minute. The baseline

▶ **TABLE 22–2**

Comparison of Various Methods of Fetal Heart Rate Assessment

Method	Benefits	Risks
Fetoscope	Easily portable, noninvasive	Intermittent auscultation may miss subtle changes; need to listen to FHR during contraction and immediately after contraction
Doppler stethoscope	Magnifies beat	Same as above
Ultrasonic transducer	Continuous record, noninvasive	Equipment may inhibit maternal movement and encourage supine position
Internal fetal scalp electrode	True fetal electrocardiogram, less inhibition of maternal movement	Dilation must be 2–3 cm, membranes ruptured, station –1 or lower; possibility of maternal or fetal infection

FHR is the least sensitive indicator of fetal distress. A compromised fetus could have a normal baseline rate. Conversely, changes in the baseline may be considered a possible sign of fetal distress. The baseline fetal heart rate is assessed using the following criteria:

- Normal range: 120–160 beats per minute
- Tachycardia
  - Mild: 161–180 beats per minute
  - Severe: >180 beats per minute
- Bradycardia
  - Mild: 100–119 beats per minute
  - Moderate: 70–99 beats per minute
  - Severe: <70 beats per minute

The normal FHR has a beat-to-beat variability of 6 to 25 beats per minute. This beat-to-beat variability in labor indicates that the fetus has an intact central nervous system that is capable of controlling the FHR during contractions.

Variability of the baseline FHR is a more significant parameter of fetal well-being than is assessment of the baseline alone. Baseline variability of the FHR may be divided into two types: short-term variability and long-term variability.

Short-term variability (STV) is the normal variance between successive cardiac cycles. It is the change in FHR from one beat to the next. For example, when the fetal heart beats 130 times over the course of a minute, there are times in that minute when the heart rate is 124 or 136. Only the spiral electrode can accurately assess STV.

Long-term variability (LTV) is the rhythmic fluctuation in the heart rate and appears as waves on the FHR tracing. The usual frequency is 3 to 5 cycles per minute. All monitors can present evidence of LTV whether the woman is monitored internally or externally.

When the amplitude of the cycle exceeds 25 beats per minute, the LTV is said to be increased. Possible explanations include mild fetal hypoxia, fetal hemorrhage, and compression of the umbilical cord.

A decrease in the LTV may be related to fetal hypoxia, physiologic sleep cycle, central nervous system–depressing drugs, or parasympatholytic or sympatholytic drugs.

Another pattern to evaluate is a baseline FHR that is persistently flat, although within the normal range. A persistently flat baseline FHR is usually defined as **absent variability** and is considered nonreassuring and a sign of potential fetal distress. This pattern may be caused by congenital anomalies of the cardiac or central nervous systems, prematurity, or hypoxia and acidosis, or it may be idiopathic (Tucker, 1992). Figure 22–2 illustrates FHR variability.

When a fetus is healthy, the FHR accelerates above the baseline in response to fetal movement. Fetal heart rate accelerations occurring in the prenatal period or in early labor represent intact neurologic functioning of the fetus. They can occur during labor before or after variable decelerations and may be the earliest indicator of possible partial cord compression.

A decrease in the FHR below the baseline in response to uterine contractions is termed an FHR deceleration. Fetal heart rate decelerations are classified according to their shape and their timing relative to uterine contractions (Fig. 22–3). The following classification is used (Tucker, 1992):

- *Uniform.* The FHR pattern related to the uterine contraction. Subcategories would be early decelerations and late decelerations.
- *Variable.* There is no relationship between the uterine contraction and the FHR.

Early decelerations of the FHR have the following characteristics (Benson & Pernoll, 1994):

1. The curve has a uniform shape that remains the same from contraction to contraction.
2. The patterns of the FHR and the contraction are similar.
3. The onset of the deceleration occurs early in the contraction.
4. The nadir of the deceleration occurs at the peak of the contraction.
5. FHR returns to baseline at the same time the contraction ends.
6. The lowest amplitude is proportional to the strength of the contraction.
7. Baseline FHR usually does not fall below 100 beats per minute.
8. Baseline STV is maintained.

Early decelerations usually occur in the later stages of labor and do not indicate fetal distress. They

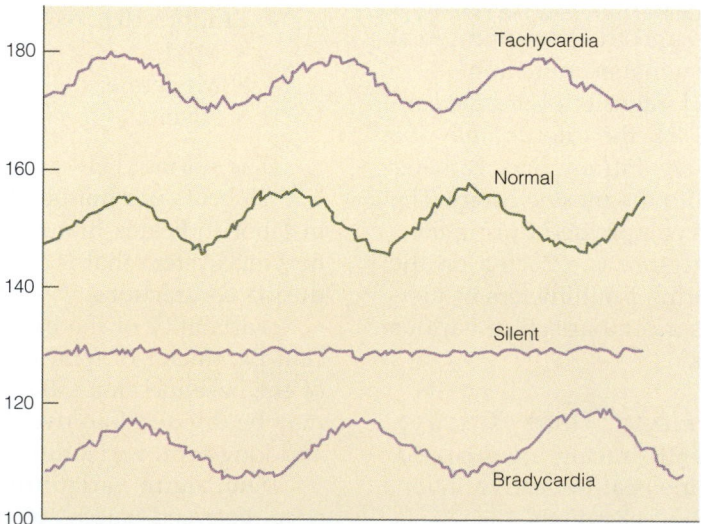

FIGURE 22–2. Fetal heart rate variability. *(Reproduced, with permission, from Oxorn, H. (Ed.). (1986). Oxorn-Foote human labor and birth (5th ed.). Norwalk, CT: Appleton & Lange, p. 623.)*

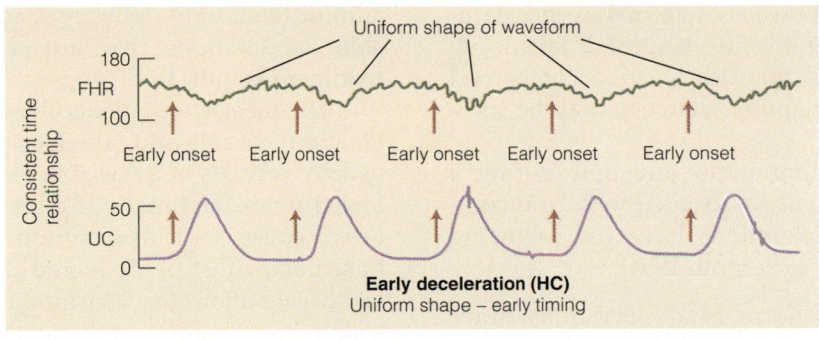

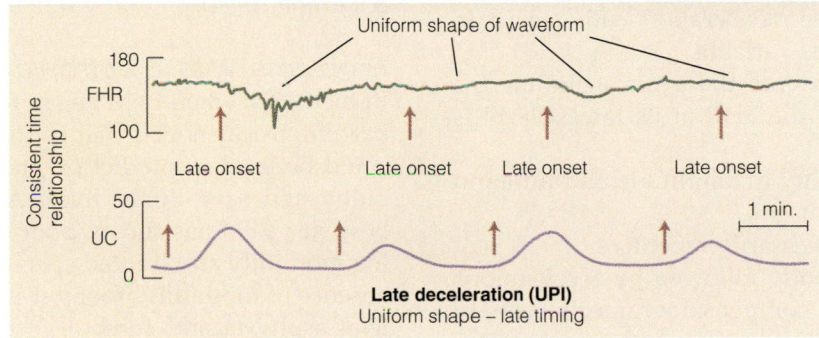

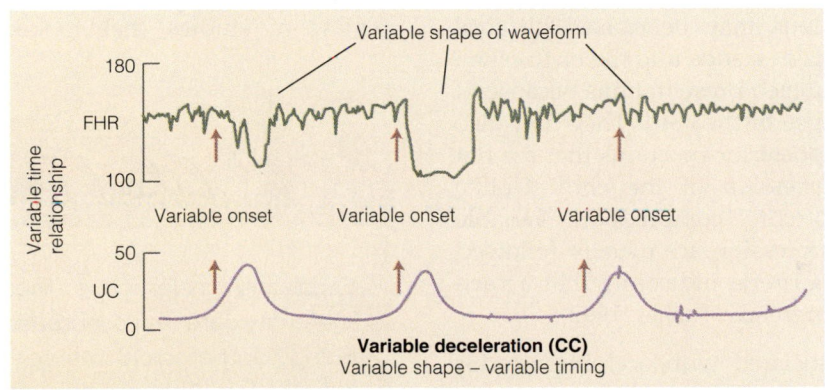

FIGURE 22–3. Fetal heart rate decelerations. *(Adapted, with permission, from Hon, E.H. (1968). An atlas of fetal heart rate patterns. New Haven, CT: Harty.)*

usually occur as a result of pressure on the fetal skull, and no treatment is indicated.

Late decelerations of the FHR are usually an ominous sign. They have the following characteristics (Tucker, 1992):

1. The curve has a uniform shape that mirrors the shape of the contraction.
2. The onset of the deceleration occurs late in the uterine contraction (at or after the peak).
3. FHR does not return to baseline until after the uterine contraction ends (usually more than 20 seconds after uterine pressure returns to its resting tone).
4. The amplitude of deceleration is usually proportional to amplitude of contraction.
5. The pattern may be subtle, and the FHR may be within the normal range.

Late decelerations of the FHR may indicate uteroplacental insufficiency, which causes a reduction in fetal PO_2. Uteroplacental insufficiency may be caused by maternal supine hypotension, maternal dehydration, hyperstimulation of the uterus with oxytocic agents, postmaturity, and abruptio placentae.

If late decelerations are noted, the nurse turns the mother on her left side and discontinues the use of oxytocic agents for stimulation of labor. Administration of oxygen to the mother increases maternal oxygen saturation of hemoglobin and is also helpful. If late decelerations persist over 30 minutes or are accompanied by decreased FHR variability, delivery may be indicated.

Variable decelerations occur any time during a contraction and are usually associated with cord compression. Variable decelerations have the following characteristics (Benson & Pernoll, 1994):

1. The shape and form of decelerations differ from one deceleration to the next.
2. The onset of the deceleration with regard to the contraction is variable.
3. The interval between the peak of the uterine contraction and the FHR at its lowest level is variable.
4. There is variability in amplitude and duration of deceleration.
5. They are not necessarily repetitive.
6. They are frequently followed by accelerations of the FHR, a compensatory mechanism to increase the flow of oxygen to the fetus.

Variable decelerations may be caused by cord compression as the fetus descends into the birth canal. They may occur with breech presentations because of the possibility of prolapse of the cord. They may also be noted with occipitoposterior positions that are not accompanied by compression of the cord. Unlike decelerations with no cord compression, variable decelerations with compression are usually followed by FHR accelerations. Criteria indicating that a variable deceleration is benign are (Tucker, 1992):

- Deceleration associated with occipitoposterior positions
- FHR deceleration lasting no longer than 45 seconds on a repetitive basis
- Abrupt return of the FHR to the baseline
- Baseline rate that does not increase
- Baseline variability that does not decrease

One of the most important criteria used to evaluate potential problems with variable decelerations is the baseline variability. A decrease in the baseline variability when variable decelerations are present indicates potential fetal compromise.

Management varies according to the interpretation of the cause of variable decelerations and the stage of labor. If the mother is in early labor and the cause is thought to be cord compression, then delivery by cesarean section may be indicated. If, however, the mother is in the second stage of labor, vaginal delivery may proceed. If the nurse suspects a prolapsed cord, the mother may be placed in a knee–chest position, to take pressure off the cord; oxygen is administered until delivery is accomplished. For variable decelerations that are considered benign, no treatment is indicated.

The most ominous deceleration pattern is a combination variable and late deceleration pattern, which usually consists of a variable onset of the pattern, followed by development of a late deceleration pattern. Most fetuses with this pattern are severely compromised and must be delivered if the interventions for late decelerations (e.g., turning mother on side) do not lead to improvement in the fetal heart pattern (Benson & Pernoll, 1994).

Problems with Electronic Fetal Monitoring.
In the 1960s, when EFM began to be used in the intrapartum, it was hoped that continual FHR monitoring could be used to predict or prevent neurologic morbidity and save infant lives. After 25 years of use, however, EFM has shown poor sensitivity in identifying morbidity and limited specificity in predicting the absence of morbidity. Today it is recognized that both fetal asphyxia and cerebral ischemia may exist well before the intrapartum and neonatal periods. A review of studies that looked for an association

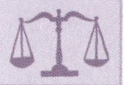 *Ethical Decision Making*

Escalating malpractice litigations, related to maternity care, have increased the use of technology and medical interventions that may not be needed. The medical community believes that if a negative outcome occurs, the physician can state that all available interventions were employed; the physician, therefore, is not at fault. If you were the nurse caring for a woman who refuses an electronic fetal monitor after being told that there is a possibility of risk to her fetus, how would you respond to the following issues:

1. Should the ethical principle of respect for autonomy of the mother override the ethical value of altruism and the principle of beneficence in concentrating on the welfare of the fetus?
2. Should the ethical principle of autonomy outweigh the malpractice issues perceived by the physician and other members of the delivery team?

between FHR, as measured by EFM, and neonatal neurologic abnormalities, showed no specific FHR pattern or group of patterns that can predict brain damage. There is no evidence that EFM is more effective than FHR auscultation in reducing poor fetal outcomes (Albers, 1994). Furthermore, use of EFM focuses the nurse's attention more on technology than on caring (Albers, 1994; Rosen & Dickinson, 1993).

Fetal Presentation

Fetal presentation, position, lie, attitude, and descent are usually determined by means of Leopold's maneuvers, uterine measurements, and vaginal examination, in that order. The nurse or other health care professional should not rely solely on vaginal examination, as a great deal of information can be overlooked, such as estimated length of gestation, multiple-fetus gestation, estimated fetal weight, polyhydramnios, and uterine abnormalities. Leopold's manuevers are used in the intrapartum period to determine fetal presentation, position, and lie. Vaginal examination includes assessment of presenting part, station, and position.

It is important to note when assessing fetal station that if extensive formation of caput or molding of the head has occurred, the fetal head may not be engaged even though the vertex is at 0 station. An unengaged head in a nulliparous woman in early labor may indicate cephalopelvic disproportion or malpresentation. Generally, the higher the station at the beginning of labor, the longer the labor is likely to be. High station when the amniotic membranes rupture can be associated with prolapse of the umbilical cord.

Fetal Oxygenation

Although the assessment of fetal cardiac function has become more sophisticated and more accurate with the advent of electronic internal and external monitors, the instrumentation provides data that may be far from definitive. Variations of rate, baseline, and reactivity may be a fetal response or a characteristic of the equipment. When such a question arises, it is often necessary to obtain a blood sample from the fetal presenting part for pH analysis. There is always a correlation between FHR changes and pH shifts. Fetal blood is collected when membranes are ruptured, the cervix is dilated at least 3 to 4 cm, and station is −1, 0, or lower. Using sterile technique and an endoscope for direct visualization, the clinician collects a blood sample in long, heparinized capillary tubes. Normal fetal scalp blood has a pH of 7.25 or higher. Fetal hypoxia and acidosis are suspected when fetal blood pH falls below 7.20. pH values of 7.20 to 7.24 are considered preacidotic. Blood loss resulting from fetal sampling may be significant and difficult to control. The sampling site is at risk of neonatal infection. For these reasons, sampling is undertaken only to clarify a confusing or nonreassuring FHR pattern.

Signs and Symptoms of Fetal Distress

Throughout a woman's labor, the nurse assesses the fetus for signs of distress (see box entitled Signs and Symptoms of Fetal Distress).

▶ Maternal Assessment

Important maternal assessment data are obtained by monitoring maternal vital signs (Table 22–3); measuring contractions; performing a vaginal examination including the cervix (dilation and effacement) and amniotic membranes; and evaluating the bladder and psyche.

Maternal Contractions

The primary power of labor comes from the uterine contractions, which efface and dilate the cervix and move the fetus through the birth canal. Measuring contractions helps determine the progress of labor. They are measured either by palpating the uterus during contractions or by using an electronic fetal monitor. The frequency, duration, intensity, and pattern of contractions are documented (Fig. 22–4).

Frequency. Frequency of contractions is recorded in minutes. While palpating with fingertips over the

---

▶ SIGNS AND SYMPTOMS OF FETAL DISTRESS

- Ominous FHR changes or patterns (e.g., late or severe variable decelerations accompanied by a decrease in or lack of variability and progressive acceleration in the baseline FHR that are indicative of hypoxia).

- Fetal scalp blood pH below 7.20.
- Meconium-stained amniotic fluid with a vertex presentation (staining with a breech presentation is usually not considered ominous).

▶ **TABLE 22-3**

Assessment of Maternal Vital Signs During Labor

Vital Sign	Frequency of Assessment	Findings	Implications
Blood pressure	On admission and 1 to 2 hours if normal	Systolic 100–120 Diastolic 60–80	If blood pressure is abnormal (30 mm Hg systolic and/or 15 mm Hg diastolic over baseline or below 90/60), repeat reading with woman on left side
Temperature	On admission and 4 hours	98 to 99.6°F (36.2 to 37.6°C); slightly elevated throughout labor	Elevated temperature may indicate dehydration or infection
Pulse	On admission and 1–2 hours	60–100 beats/minute	Pulse may indicate stress, pain, infection, hemorrhagic shock, or dehydration
Respirations	On admission and 1–2 hours	14–20 breaths per minute; more rapid respirations during contractions may be found	Respirations above or below baseline may be associated with abnormal breathing patterns or hyperventilation

client's fundus, frequency is measured from the beginning of one contraction to the beginning of the next. When the fetal monitor is used, the contractions are usually measured from the peak of one contraction to the peak of the next. This peak method, however, cannot be used when recording manually.

Duration. Duration is recorded in seconds and is measured from the beginning of the contraction until the end of that same contraction.

Intensity or Quality. Intensity, too, is recorded either manually or electronically. Using the manual

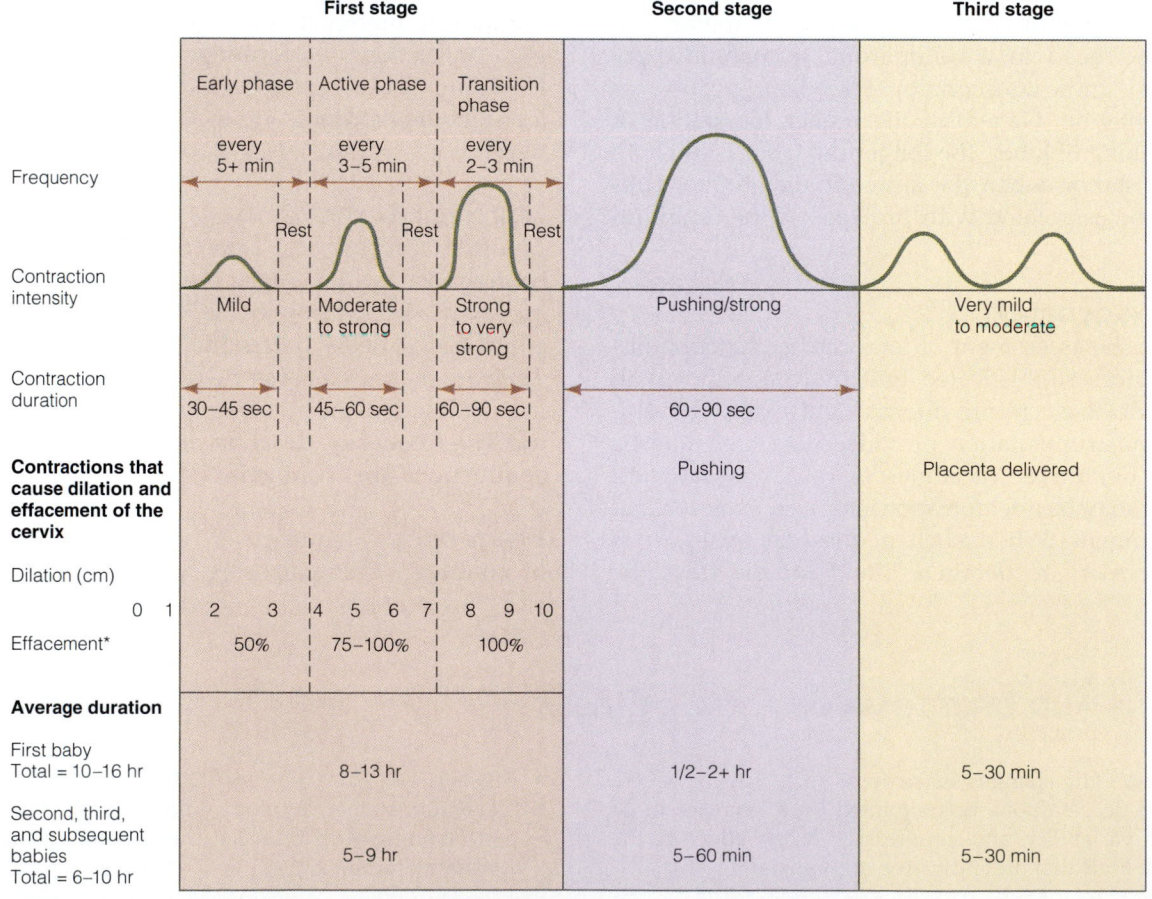

FIGURE 22–4. Contraction patterns in first, second, and third stages of labor. *Primigravidas may be 100% effaced before labor begins.

method, the nurse places the pads of his or her fingers on the uterine fundus to determine if the contraction feels mild, moderate, or strong. Experience is required for the nurse to accurately assess intensity. The following correlation offers a good rule of thumb in evaluating the contracted uterus:

- *Mild.* Feels like the tip of the nose.
- *Moderate.* Feels like the chin.
- *Strong.* Feels like the forehead.

An exact determination of contraction intensity is achieved only by using the electronic fetal monitor and the intrauterine pressure catheter. This method produces an exact pressure recording on the monitor strip. The normal resting tone (between contractions) is usually less than 15 mm Hg of pressure. The intensity ranges from 30 to 100 mm Hg during the peak of contractions, depending on the stage and phase of labor.

Some practitioners use the external monitor to estimate the intensity of contractions. The nurse can estimate that one contraction appears more intense than another, provided the woman does not change position or push during this period. It is also important to listen to the client. She is often most accurate in assessing the strength of the contractions.

Pattern.

The pattern of contractions is important because it may indicate the stage of labor, whether the woman or fetus is having difficulty, and possible dysfunctional labor.

On average, labor starts with contractions of mild intensity, 10 to 20 minutes in frequency and 30 seconds in duration. As labor proceeds, the contractions become progressively more frequent, of longer duration, and stronger. The pattern may show a smooth, progressive change or the labor may start off immediately with contractions 3 to 4 minutes in frequency.

Other Factors Affecting Contraction Patterns.

Contraction frequency, duration, and intensity may be affected by a number of other variables. These include rupture of the membranes, medications, change in position, and the mother's fear or anxiety. Amniotomy, or artificial rupture of the amniotic membranes, sometimes arrests labor and sometimes accelerates labor (Rosen & Peisner, 1987; Rouse, McCullough, Wren, Owen, & Hauth, 1994). Medications may decrease the frequency and intensity of contractions in labor. The position the woman assumes during labor does affect the frequency and quality of the contractions. The most effective position is upright (either sitting, standing, or walking); the next is side lying (preferably on her left side). In

Women's Health

The level of a woman's anxiety and fear experienced during labor and birth can have a direct effect on the intensity of contractions. To help a client cope with these feelings, the nurse should share information about the progress of labor with the woman and her partner, advise her about the physical and psychosocial feelings she may experience, and invite the couple to ask questions about the assessments that need to be conducted.

the upright or side-lying position, the contractions may occur less frequently but the strength or intensity of the contraction may be greater and, therefore, more effective for the progress of labor. Women are usually more comfortable and require less medication in upright positions. There is evidence that women who ambulate for a significant amount of time during labor have decreased rates of cesarean deliveries as compared to those who do not ambulate (Albers et al., 1997).

Vaginal Examination

The nurse-midwife, physician, or staff nurse may perform vaginal examinations throughout the course of labor. No examination is done if frank bleeding is present.

The vaginal exam may be stressful for a laboring woman and her support person and should be done only often enough to ensure safe conduct of labor. By being with the woman continually and following the progress of her labor (evaluating uterine contractions, bloody show, and the woman's responses to labor), fewer vaginal examinations are necessary.

The vaginal exam is done during labor to determine cervical effacement and dilation, fetal presentation, position, and station. If an examination is to be done, the nurse should explain the evaluation, why it is being done, and how it might feel. To prepare for the exam, the woman empties her bladder. The nurse then cleans the perineal area. Other steps that the nurse should take throughout the exam include helping the woman to relax and breathe, speaking and acting very gently, and explaining what is being done. The results of the exam and what they mean in terms of labor progress and management are communicated to the woman.

Cervix. The cervix is assessed using the following parameters:

- *Location of the cervical os with respect to the fetal head.* Posterior, midposition, anterior.
- *Effacement.* Thickness or thinness of the endocervical canal denoted in percentages (see inside back cover). Uneffaced = approximately 2 cm long and thick; 25% effaced = 1.5 cm long and thinning; 50% effaced = 1 cm long; 75% effaced = 0.5 cm long; 100% or completely effaced = no endocervix remains, cervix feels paper thin.
- *Dilation.* The diameter of the cervical opening from the margin of the cervix on one side to the opposite side, expressed in centimeters (0–10 cm) (see inside back cover). When the cervix has opened enough to permit passage of the fetal head (average 10 cm), it is said to be fully dilated.

The nulliparous woman usually effaces first and then starts to dilate as effacement nears completion. The multiparous woman usually dilates and effaces simultaneously. Women often enter labor already dilated about 2 cm or more, particularly if they are multiparous. Figure 22–5 illustrates dilation of the cervix in the primigravid woman.

Membranes. With the fingers in the cervix, the examiner assesses the membranes to determine whether they are ruptured or intact.

Spontaneous rupture of membranes (SROM) leads to a gush, trickle, or seepage of fluid from the vagina. **Premature rupture of membranes** (PROM) occurs spontaneously before the onset of labor. Of women who have PROM at term, 80% go into labor within 24 hours. The incidence of SROM before the onset of contractions is 8% (Cunningham et al., 1997).

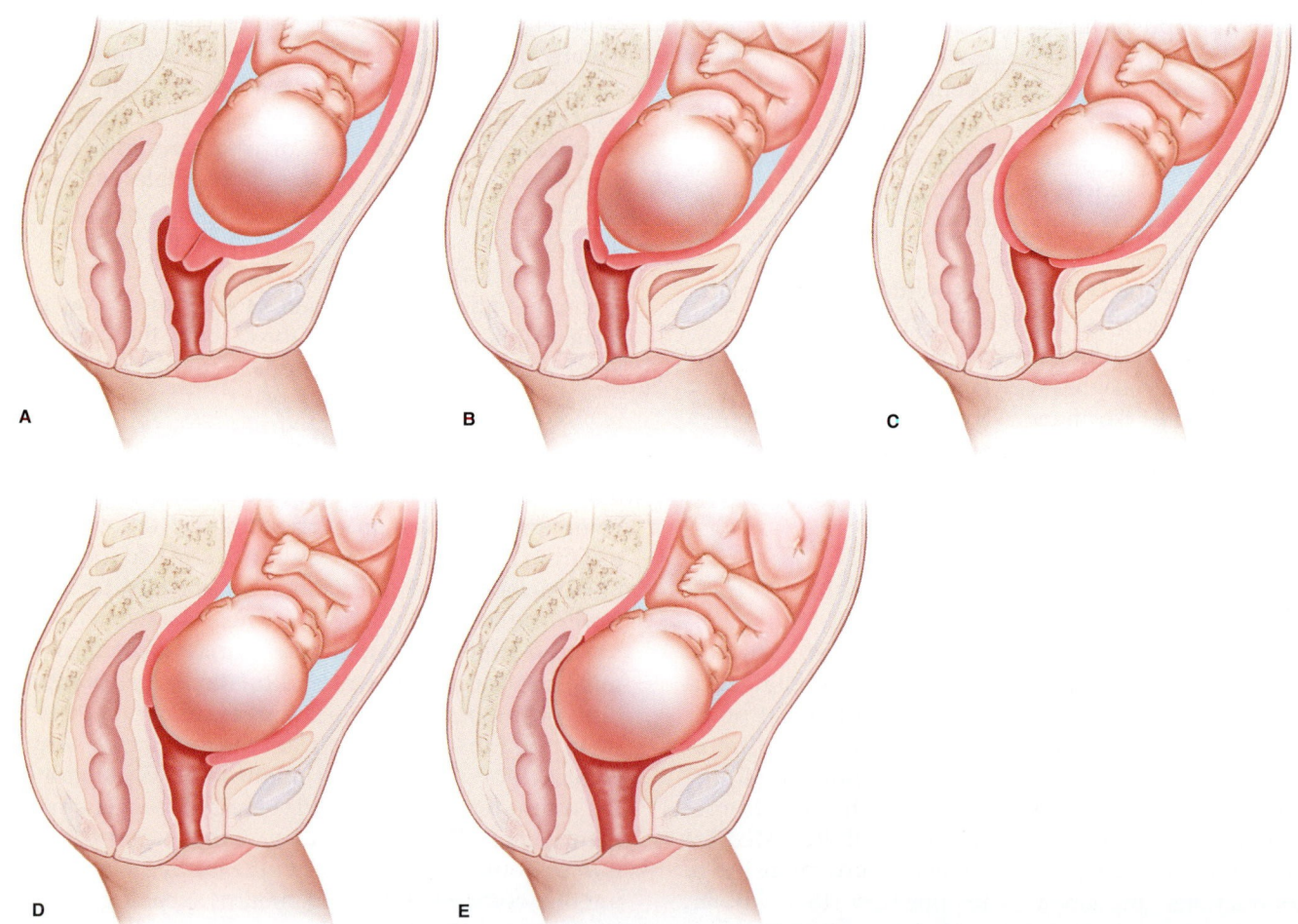

FIGURE 22–5. Cervical effacement and dilation of the cervix in a primigravid woman. **A.** Cervix thick and closed. **B.** Cervix effaced. **C.** Cervix effaced and dilated 2 to 3 cm. **D.** Cervix half open. **E.** Cervix fully dilated and retracted.

Assessment of the membranes is important because once the uterine and fetal seal to the outside world is broken, the environment of the fetus and mother is open to infection. PROM is associated with infection, incompetent cervix, increased maternal age and parity, trauma, manipulation of the amniotic membranes, malpresentation of the fetus, prematurity, floating presenting part, prolapse of the cord or limb, and increased perinatal mortality and morbidity (DeCherney & Pernoll, 1994).

To assess whether the membranes have ruptured, the examiner may complete the following:

1. *History.* Information is obtained as to time, amount, color, and odor of fluid loss and last sexual intercourse (loss of semen from the vagina can sometimes be mistaken for rupture of membranes).
2. *Tests.* The fluid may be tested with nitrazine paper. A color code is used to determine any pH changes. Presence of amniotic fluid indicates a pH of 7.0 to 7.5 and turns the paper dark blue. The examiner must take care to avoid touching the nitrazine paper onto the cervix or any other fluids, as this will give a false reading. In a separate step, a few drops of fluid are allowed to dry undisturbed on a clean glass slide and then are examined under a microscope on low power. The presence of ferning indicates amniotic fluid.
3. *Sterile speculum examination.* Sterile gloves, nitrazine pH paper, clean glass slide, and microscope are required equipment. Wearing the sterile gloves and using a sterile speculum (using no lubricating jelly), the examiner inserts the speculum into the vagina and locates the cervix. The woman is asked to cough or bear down (while abdominally moving the fetal head up) and the examiner observes the fluid that escapes onto the lower blade of the speculum. The speculum is not routinely used in the exam.

Bladder

On admission and periodically throughout labor, the mother's urine should be evaluated for ketones, glucose, and protein. Ketonuria may be an indication of dehydration or exhaustion. Glycosuria is common because of the increased glomerular filtration rate in the proximal tubules and the inability of these tubules to increase absorption of glucose. Slight proteinuria (trace, 1+) is common in labor. Proteinuria of 2+ and above is abnormal and indicative of preeclampsia.

Retention of urine can occur during labor because of hypotonus of the bladder, pressure of the present-ing part on the bladder neck or urethra, or analgesia or regional anesthesia. For these reasons, women should be encouraged to void frequently during labor, at least every 2 hours. Periodically throughout labor, the nurse should palpate the suprapubic region to detect any distension and, if distension is present, encourage the woman to void.

Psyche

The psyche is an important dimension to assess when planning care for the laboring woman and her support person(s). Research with women in labor or anticipating labor indicates that body image, value of self as indicated by assertiveness, and tolerance of self are indicators that yield important data (Lederman, 1996) that may have an effect on labor progress. The ability to trust—both the efficiency of her own body and the abilities of the caregivers—is another indication of the client's psyche. The mind–body continuum is nowhere more evident than during labor and delivery.

Psychosocial dimensions of labor and birth are discussed in depth in Chapter 24.

Cultural Influences

Culture also influences the process of labor and delivery, and may be considered a component of the mother's "psyche." The folklore of childbirth helps the nurse understand the client and family members' reactions to labor and birth. The nurse must realize that the very familiarity that allows him or her to function smoothly may be frightening to the client and family, who are not familiar with the "culture" of the health care institution.

Previous chapters have reviewed the family life of different cultural groups found in the United States. The Puerto Rican family is discussed here.

Cultural Focus: The Puerto Rican Family

The Puerto Rican family represents a complex cultural tradition that covers the spectrum of racial differences. Although racial and cultural ancestry may be a mixture of African, Taino Indian, Corsican, and Spanish, ethnic identification is Puerto Rican (Garcia-Preto, 1996; Spector, 1996). Thus, families who identify their background as Puerto Rican may differ as much from each other as do members of different cultural subgroups.

Puerto Rican families also differ on the basis of the economic life in which the family participated when in Puerto Rico. Families have different characteristics, structural organizations, and even different communication patterns depending on whether they came from agrarian groups (sugar cane workers or coffee growers), middle-class groups, or upper-class groups (Garcia-Preto, 1996). Although Puerto Ricans cannot be viewed as one distinct cultural group, some values present in all classes and groups can be characterized as Puerto Rican. These include the belief in spirituality, dignity of the individual, and respect for authority.

1. *Belief in spirituality.* The Puerto Rican family places an emphasis on spiritual values and often is willing to sacrifice material goods for spiritual goods. Family members live in the present; the future and past are seen as less important in the scheme of things. Though not resigned, families accept "fate." Many Puerto Ricans are Roman Catholic. Many individuals believe in spirits and spiritualism. They believe, for example, that mental illness is caused primarily by evil forces. There are also "good" spirits who influence human behavior (Spector, 1996).

2. *Dignity of the individual.* Puerto Rican family members define self-worth in terms of inner qualities that give them self-respect and earn them the respect of others (Garcia-Preto, 1996). This form of individualism is called *personalism* or *personalismo.* This focus on inner qualities allows a person to experience self-worth regardless of whether she or he is rich or poor. *Personalismo* also enhances self-disclosure of the individual (Burk, Wieser & Keegan, 1995).

3. *Respect for authority.* Respect is vital in the interpersonal relationships of the Puerto Rican family and plays a major role in maintaining social networks. Failure to show proper respect to a Puerto Rican man insults his manliness, his self-esteem, and even his family integrity. Respect is learned in the family, and extends to the outside society. Respect also incorporates tactfulness and discourages confrontation (Burk et al., 1995).

Family Structure. The focus in Puerto Rican families is on the extended rather than the nuclear family. Relationships are often intense, and members experience a deep sense of family commitment, obligation, and responsibility. Individuals may seek advice from family members about health care before going to see a traditional health care provider (Spector, 1996).

Traditionally, Puerto Rican families have been patriarchal. The father's responsibility is to protect and provide for his family. *Machismo* (maleness, virility) is a desirable trait for the man to possess.

The role of the woman is to care for the home and keep the family together. She is expected to perform household tasks and childrearing (without her husband's help) and is further expected to respect him.

Yet, the Puerto Rican woman can often become the "power behind the scenes" in the family system.

Traditionally, Puerto Rican couples marry early and have large families. Children are valued, and parents (especially the mother) often feel obligated to sacrifice for their children. During infancy, children receive much love and attention from all adults in the family. After age 2, children are trained by their mother and grandmother. Children are trained to show gratitude and respect and are not seen as autonomous individuals by their parents. Discipline may include spanking, and parents may hesitate to reward their children's good behavior for fear that they will lose respect (Garcia-Preto, 1996).

The extended family includes not only those individuals related by blood or marriage, but also *compadres* (godparents) and *hijos de crianza* (informally adopted children). The extended family is a source of strength for the nuclear family, and can provide much needed emotional and physical support. For example, female extended family members often help the Puerto Rican woman during childbearing and childrearing, as the Puerto Rican man is not expected to perform domestic tasks. Birth is a major life event for the extended family and is joyfully celebrated by the family and community.

Emigration and the Puerto Rican Family. Many families from the island of Puerto Rico emigrate to the United States seeking economic opportunity. Emigration may have several negative effects on the family. If the family lived in poverty in Puerto Rico, it is likely that they will be poor in America. Moreover, they are often the targets of racism.

Cultural values and attitudes are not reinforced by the dominant culture of the United States, and families may experience culture shock. For example, sex roles may be reversed, with the woman supporting the family economically. Children may learn English before their parents, thus gaining power over parents and losing respect for them. Finally, emigration to the mainland may separate the nuclear family from the extended family, increasing feelings of loss and isolation. Some Puerto Rican families thus opt to return to Puerto Rico, and movement between the island and the mainland is common.

Birth Experience. Puerto Rican women may have fears about the labor process, their ability to parent a newborn, and their change in body image. Pain during labor is seen as a means of achieving the goal of giving birth as soon as possible. Many Puerto Rican women do not see the necessity of the father's presence at delivery. This may reflect traditional masculine and feminine roles in the Puerto Rican family.

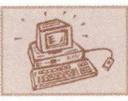

Research Abstract

Cultural Expectations of Women in Labor

This qualitative study was conducted to determine the expectations of Latina women regarding support from their partners during the labor experiences. The partners in this study were not limited to the fathers of the babies or husbands.

The sample consisted of 10 pregnant Latina women, aged 18 to 40, from a large California university medical center. All the women participated in childbirth education classes held in Spanish.

In-depth structured interviews were done to provide an opportunity for the women to describe their needs relative to support during the labor process. The interviews were conducted once during the woman's third trimester of pregnancy and once postpartum, before her discharge from the hospital.

Data analysis revealed that three themes emerged from the prenatal interviews. The first theme centered on the women's desire for their partner to be with them throughout the labor and delivery. The second theme revealed the women's wishes for communication with their partners in the form of understanding words and encouragement. In the third theme, the women expressed the wish that their partners would demonstrate love to them while they labored. The three themes—presence at the bedside, communication, and showing love—were repeated in the postpartum interviews.

Application to Practice

This study is an important step in providing information relative to cultural expectations of laboring women. Nurses need to provide culturally sensitive care to women and their partners during the labor and delivery experience. More studies need to be done to determine if there are differences in the expectations of women and their partners based on cultural variations.

Source: Khazoyan, C.M., & Anderson, N.L.R. (1994). Latinas' expectations for their partners during childbirth. MCN, American Journal of Maternal-Child Nursing, 19, 226–229.

Chapter Highlights

► The professional nurse is an integral part of the delivery team and provides care to the woman and her partner in the birthing facility.

► The nurse is responsible for establishing an environment for labor and birth in which the woman and her partner are treated with respect and kindness and in which they can actively participate.

► The initial intrapartum assessment includes taking a medical and obstetric health history; conducting a physical examination of the mother and fetus; and assessing the psyche of the laboring woman and her support person.

► Fetal assessment during labor and birth consists of monitoring the fetal heart rate through either auscultation or electronic fetal monitoring; determining the fetal presenting part, station, and position; and evaluating fetal cardiac function.

► Maternal assessment data during labor and birth are obtained by monitoring vital signs; measuring the frequency, duration, and intensity of maternal contractions; performing a vaginal examination including dilation and effacement of the cervix; determining the status of the amniotic membranes; and evaluating the bladder.

► Cultural beliefs about labor and birth influence a woman's and family's experience of this process and are an important component of nursing assessment.

► The nurse's continual assessment of the woman's responses to labor adds necessary information for evaluating the labor and birth process.

After reading the vignette at the beginning of this chapter, use what you have learned to answer these questions:

1. How does the explanation of the assessment data that are being obtained help Cathleen Harris in her experience of labor?

2. How can Margaret Kiely, RN, develop and maintain a trusting relationship with Cathleen Harris so as to promote her sense of competency during labor?

3. By what methods can the nurse achieve a balance between the humanistic and technical aspects of care during labor and delivery?

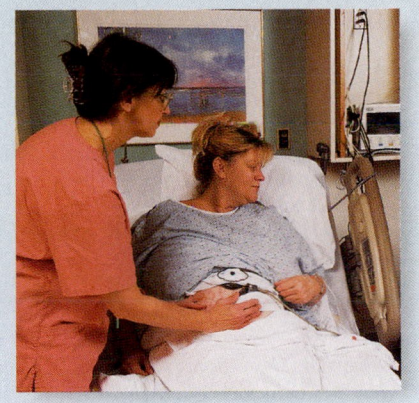

Critical Thinking Questions

► References

Albers, L.L. (1994). Clinical issues in electronic fetal monitoring. *Birth, 21*(2), 108.

Albers, L.L., Anderson, D., Cragin, L., Daniels, S.M., Hunter, C., Sedler, K.D., & Teaf, D. (1997). The relationship of ambulation in labor to operative delivery. *Journal of Nurse Midwifery, 42*(1), 4–8.

American Academy of Pediatrics and American College of Obstetricians and Gynecologists. (1992). *Guidelines for pediatric care* (3rd ed.). Washington, DC: Authors.

Benson, R.C., & Pernoll, M.L. (1994). *Handbook of obstetrics and gynecology* (9th ed.). New York: McGraw-Hill.

Burk, M.E., Wieser, P.C., & Keegan, L. (1995). Cultural beliefs and health behaviors of pregnant Mexican-American women: Implications for primary care. *Advances in Nursing Science, 17*(4), 37–52.

Creasy, R. (1986). *Prenatal risk assessment and perinatal outcome.* Paper presented at March of Dimes Conference, New York City.

Cunningham, F.G., MacDonald, P.C., Gant, N.F., Leveno, K.J., Gilstrap, L.C., Hankins, G.D.V., & Clark, S.L. (1997). *Williams obstetrics* (20th ed.). Stamford, CT: Appleton & Lange.

DeCherney, A.H., & Pernoll, M.L. (Eds.). (1994). *Current obstetric and gynecologic diagnosis and treatment* (8th ed.). Norwalk, CT: Appleton & Lange.

Garcia-Preto, N. (1996). Puerto Rican families. In M. McGoldrick, J. Giordano, & J.K. Pearce (Eds.), *Ethnicity and family therapy,* (2nd ed.) (pp. 106–115). New York: Guilford Press.

Khazoyan, C.M., & Anderson, N.L.R. (1994). Latinas' expectations for their partners during childbirth. *MCN, American Journal of Maternal-Child Nursing, 19,* 226–229.

Lederman, R.P. (1996). *Psychosocial adaptation in pregnancy: Assessment of seven dimensions* (2nd ed.). New York: Springer.

Rosen, M.G., & Dickinson, J.C. (1993). The paradox of electronic fetal monitoring: More data may not enable us to predict or prevent infant neurologic morbidity. *American Journal of Obstetrics and Gynecology, 168,* 745–751.

Rosen, M.G., & Peisner, D.B. (1987). Effects of amniotic membrane rupture on length of labor. *Obstetrics and Gynecology, 70,* 604.

Rouse, D.J., McCullough, C., Wren, A.L., Owen, J., & Hauth, J.C. (1994). Active-phase labor arrest: A randomized trial of chorion-amnion management. *Obstetrics and Gynecology, 83,* 937–940.

Spector, R.E. (1996). *Cultural diversity in health and illness* (4th ed.). Stamford, CT: Appleton & Lange.

Tucker, S.M. (1992). *Pocket guide to fetal monitoring.* St. Louis: Mosby-YearBook.

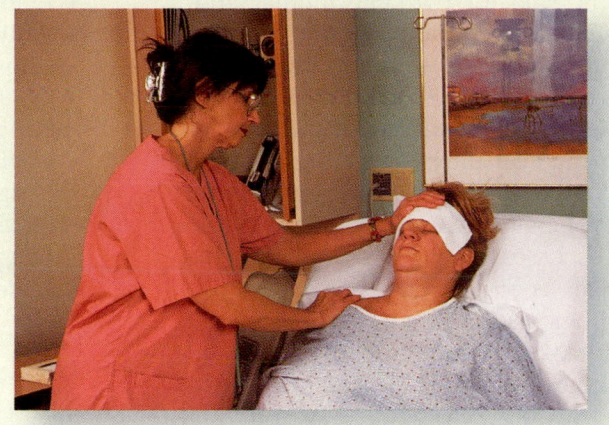

Cathleen Harris, a 30-year-old multigravida, was admitted to the labor and delivery unit 7 hours ago. Contractions are occurring every 8 minutes and her cervix is 5 cm dilated. Cathleen is restless and, with help from her husband Bill, changes her position in bed often.

After Cathleen experiences a strong contraction, Margaret Kiely, RN, notices that Cathleen is perspiring and has pushed the bed linens away from her body. She fans her face with her hand. Cathleen groans softly and states, "If only I could rest for a few minutes." The nurse moistens a washcloth with cool water and gently holds it against Cathleen's forehead. Cathleen closes her eyes and states, "That feels good. I thought I would be able to handle the pain better this time. I really didn't want to have an epidural again, like I had when my son Andrew was born, but I don't know if I can tolerate the pain." ∎

23

Pain Management

Medication administered during labor must relieve a woman's pain, but not interfere with labor or her participation. It must be safe for both the mother and fetus, prevent fetal depression, and be readily accessible for administration and effective for an indeterminate time (Cunningham et al., 1997). All medications predispose the maternal–fetal dyad to side effects or to the potential for medical intervention. Anesthesia and analgesia also increase the maternal mortality rate (Atrash, Koonin, Lawson, Franks, & Smith, 1990).

This chapter discusses the factors affecting the woman in labor, theories of pain, and nonpharmacologic and pharmacologic methods of pain relief. It also explores the considerations that must be weighed when deciding which anesthesia should be used during labor.

A woman's need for pain relief depends on the timing and length of labor; both are unpredictable. Nurses should be advocates for the laboring woman and ensure that she is aware of all methods that will assist her during labor and birth. An informed client is better able to make choices.

▶ HISTORICAL PERSPECTIVES

Pain dominates illness and childbirth. For centuries women were assisted by herbs, potions, home remedies, and alcohol. Public support for pain-free birth grew with Queen Victoria's use of chloroform during the birth of her children in 1853 and 1857. The use of morphine and scopolamine began in the early 20th century; however, women tended to become sleepy and forgetful. Experimentation with regional anesthesia has continued until the present. It is the preferred choice for a pain-free labor and birth. Alternative methods for achieving pain relief include hypnosis and psychoprophylaxis.

▶ FACTORS AFFECTING THE WOMAN IN LABOR

For most women, labor is a normal physiologic process that requires comprehensive care from support persons and the health care team. Women anticipating labor often wonder what the extent of their pain will be. Each woman's labor is different and interpreted differently. Her pain is influenced by variables that are specifically related to the childbearing process and by others that are not. The extent of pain a woman experiences is influenced by the following:

- Parity and age
- Racial, cultural, and ethnic factors
- Coping mechanisms
- Relaxation methods
- Emotional factors
- Attitude
- Knowledge level
- Confidence
- Support systems
- Environment
- Fatigue
- Nausea, vomiting, and diarrhea
- Length of labor
- Maternal and fetal positions

Nursing interventions may help a woman and her family cope with labor and the extraneous circumstances surrounding labor and birth. Each of the influences listed is discussed below.

▶ Parity and Age

A multiparous woman's cervix softens before labor onset; therefore, it is not as sensitive as the cervix of a primiparous woman. The intensity of uterine contractions is greater in the primiparous woman, especially during early labor, although not in the later stages.

Among primiparous women, younger women experience a shorter, less painful labor than older women.

Although research demonstrates these variations, no assumption can be made that parity and age automatically increase or reduce pain. The nurse must be aware of each client's needs and comfort levels. Realizing that labor may progress more slowly because of parity and age, the nurse should intervene earlier for a primiparous woman. Comfort measures include positioning, breathing exercises, and application of heat or cold.

▶ Racial, Cultural, and Ethnic Factors

The data from many studies suggest that racial, cultural, and ethnic differences influence the expression of pain. Expression is based on surrounding attitudes of pain rather than the actual experience (Bonica & McDonald, 1995). No client, however, should be typecast; the nurse accepts a woman's reports of pain and provides relief measures. Accurate assessment of the progress of a woman's labor and her pain tolerance helps the nurse to determine dysfunctional labor and avoid labels that imply cultural causes.

▶ Coping Mechanisms

Each person has ways of dealing with stress to help make pain manageable; however, when threatened, an individual has difficulty coping and pain surfaces. The nurse should observe how a woman relieves her pain and assess the effectiveness of the method. In this way, the nurse gives the woman an opportunity to first use pain relief methods familiar to her.

▶ Relaxation Methods

Women who demonstrate an ability to relax during contractions improve their comfort during labor. They develop an increased pain threshold, reduce their anxiety, lower catecholamine response, stimulate uterine blood flow, and reduce muscle tension. Relaxation is evident with the woman's using a specific breathing technique during contractions (Lowe, 1996).

▶ Emotional Factors

Fear of the unknown is a powerful negative influence on the client and her family. Ignorance of the birth event and misinformation can increase pain. Women, however, can prepare for labor and reduce uncertainty; they can learn to distance themselves from pain, by means of distraction, and refocus their attention (Bonica, 1994).

Grantly Dick-Read first discussed women's fear of labor and the fear-tension-pain syndrome. One aspect of the syndrome is having one's feelings or wishes ignored or dismissed as unimportant. In addition, being misunderstood or not understood because of a language difference is frustrating and can lead to fear-tension-pain syndrome. An interpreter should assist if needed.

Open communication with the woman and her support persons can address the problem of fear. The nurse should introduce herself or himself to the client and explain any procedure that is planned and why it is needed. The nurse must try to understand why a woman is afraid and explain why cooperation is necessary. During the second stage of labor, for example, a woman may fear pushing because she is afraid of passing a stool or tearing the birth area. Childbirth education can be extremely effective in relieving fears.

▶ Attitude

Women who look forward to becoming mothers approach labor in a better frame of mind. Because they do not view the experience negatively, pain can be lessened. Laboring women who believe that pain is tolerable will manage their actions more positively.

The nurse provides reinforcement and compliments women on their positive approach. Some pro-fessionals believe the term *pain* should be avoided. Generally, "work" or "labor" is appropriate terminology. Assessment continues and the nurse assists the woman with whatever measures she requests, such as changes in position, breathing exercises, and hot or cold compresses.

▶ Knowledge Level

Research has indicated that women who are better educated about childbirth tend to be more secure and sure of themselves. Those who participate in childbirth education better understand what is happening, are less anxious, and require less pain medication.

The nurse consistently informs the client and her partner about the progress of labor and any plans that are made, and reinforces the couple's knowledge. Lack of knowledge is a major obstacle to safe, effective care and control. Information must be actively provided to all women.

▶ Confidence Level

Having confidence in one's own abilities permits an individual to perform at an optimum level. A woman's confidence in her ability to handle pain is a critical variable in her description of labor pain (Lowe, 1991). Reinforcement increases a woman's ability to cope and reaffirms her ability to handle the stress and pain of labor. The nurse must support the plans of a woman and her partner and offer suggestions if necessary.

▶ Support Systems

The people with a laboring woman can make a difference in how she feels and copes with labor. A support person has been shown to reduce the need for medical and surgical interventions among laboring women (Kennell, Klaus, McGrath, Robertson, & Hinkley, 1991). In addition to providing support and comfort, support persons may coach breathing patterns and interpret actions or requests as needed. The nurse provides support persons with information and is a role model for them.

Nurses must remember the wide variety of family structures; for example, the father of the infant is not always a support person. Occasionally, it is necessary for a support person to leave for a brief period and another to attend the woman. Recognizing and respecting the family unit are unifying forces within a family. The birth experience also usually strengthens and enriches a family. Chapter 24 discusses in greater detail the psychologic dimensions of labor and delivery.

► Environment

Many hospitals provide birthing suites so that women may labor and deliver in a homelike environment, which is more relaxing. At the same time, medical intervention is available if it is required.

The nurse must ensure that the surroundings are clean, safe, private, quiet, free from unpleasant odors, and aesthetically pleasing. Television and music may provide diversion. A restful, soothing atmosphere should prevail.

► Fatigue

How fatigue is handled depends on the stage of labor, maternal and fetal health, the wishes of the woman, and the need for her cooperation. The extent of a woman's fatigue is influenced by the amount of sleep lost; the fluid and calories she is permitted; the number of calories consumed during labor; her ability to work with the forces of labor; rest during labor; her general condition; and the extent to which information from childbirth classes is implemented.

If the latent phase of labor is longer than average or if it is difficult to distinguish true from false labor and the woman has not slept for awhile, the obstetrician may prescribe medication. Meperidine (Demerol) or a tranquilizer may be given to help her sleep for several hours. Medication will arrest false labor or permit the woman to sleep if she is in the early latent phase of labor. Sometimes medication is used with hypertonic or dysfunctional contractions. In such cases, the goal of medication is to decrease or temporarily stop labor with the hope that when it resumes, the pattern of contractions will be more normal.

If a woman sleeps between contractions, the nurse gently reorients her to her surroundings when she awakens so that she is not startled and does not lose control.

Hypnosis may also be used to promote sleep. The client, however, must have previously been prepared for hypnosis and the practitioner must know the procedure well. In addition, techniques such as acupressure may be used to eliminate or relieve pain and to help the woman sleep. To avoid the extreme effects of fatigue, the woman should have adequate fluids and caloric intake and change her positioning often.

► Nausea, Vomiting, and Diarrhea

Many women have nausea, vomiting, or diarrhea, or all of these symptoms, during the transition phase of labor. These symptoms are also side effects of meperidine, which the woman may be taking for analgesia. Fluids, calories, and electrolytes, which are needed for labor, may be depleted. If the woman can take oral fluids, the nurse may suggest high-calorie ones, for example, clear juices. If she is receiving intravenous fluid, the nurse monitors the fluid intake, urine output, and additional fluid requirements.

In some cases, an antiemetic medication, hydroxyzine (Vistaril) or promethazine (Phenergan), may be given alone or with an analgesic.

Diarrhea usually subsides with the birth of the baby.

► Length of Labor

When women have a long labor, not surprisingly they experience more fatigue and stress. Consequently, their pain threshold is affected. A large baby or a pelvis that is small or abnormally shaped can interfere with the progress of labor; additional discomfort and fatigue may result. Again, the mother will need assistance coping with pain.

The duration of labor varies greatly. The first stage for primiparous women averages 8.6 hours (range 6–18 hours), and for multiparous women, 5.3 hours (range 3–10 hours). The second stage for primiparous women averages 1 hour (range 30 minutes to 3 hours), and for multiparous women, 20 minutes (range 5–30 minutes). Third stage is usually completed in 30 minutes for both groups. Labors that are longer than these averages may be normal and uncomplicated. Before a dysfunctional labor is identified, the contractile pattern, maternal and fetal conditions, and the woman's response to labor interventions, as well as the length of labor, must be evaluated.

► Maternal and Fetal Positions

The position a woman assumes during labor and the fetal position in utero greatly affect her comfort.

Maternal Position
The best maternal positions to assist the first stage of labor are standing and walking; these are followed (in descending order) by sitting, lying on the left side, and lying on the right side. Standing and sitting reduce low-back pain and, compared with supine or

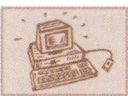

Research Abstract

Benefits of an Upright Position During Labor

The object of this study was to describe the benefits of an upright position in the laboring woman during second stage labor and to reduce fetal stress and maternal pain.

The project was sponsored by the Association of Women's Health, Obstetric, and Neonatal Nursing National Research Utilization Project on Second Stage Labor Management. Data were submitted by 33 labor and delivery unit coordinators from 40 hospitals in the United States and 2 from Canada in the year-long project.

The study concluded that the upright position facilitates fetal descent and increases pelvic inlet and outlet capacities. Uterine contractions are stronger and fetal oxygenation is higher. Women who were upright reported less pain with sitting or standing positions. Analgesia need and use was less.

Some site coordinators reported an increased number of women sitting upright as long as they were stable from their epidural. Other hospital units were not able to incorporate this position with their clients due to risk of hypotension and lack of leg strength and mobility. However, there was mention of a more individualized approach with epidural medication that permitted laboring women to move about more freely. Women receiving intrathecal narcotic analgesia were found to be active participants and moved about without risk of postural hypotension.

Application to Practice

This study demonstrates that women are comfortable in the upright position and require less analgesia while in labor. However, hospital practices and protocols hindered effective implementation of the program's guidelines. Nurses can help clients through individualized approaches to care, rather than strict adherence to long-standing policies. Research on these issues is recommended.

Source: Shermer, R.H., & Raines, D.A. (1997). _Positioning during the second stage of labor: Moving back to basics._ Journal of Obstetric, Gynecologic, and Neonatal Nursing, _26_(6), 727–734.

side-lying positions, reduce front and back contractions.

Women should avoid the supine position because it is uncomfortable, causes less efficient uterine contractions, and may induce supine hypotensive syndromes (see Fig. 18–2). This syndrome, caused by pressure exerted by the uterus and fetus on the inferior vena cava and abdominal aorta, results in decreased maternal blood pressure and fetal oxygen supply.

Ambulation during labor can be a positive influence on a woman's perception of pain. In addition, the possibility of cord prolapse is decreased if a low-risk client with the fetal presenting part well engaged is permitted to walk with assistance. If a mother chooses to remain in bed and indications require bedrest, changes in her position will help relieve pain.

Squatting, assuming a knee–elbow position, or sitting with a support person or pillow behind her may also help the laboring woman.

Fetal Position

Pressure caused by the fetus if it is in the left occiput posterior (LOP), right occiput posterior (ROP), or occiput posterior (OP) position may result in maternal back pain. In such cases, the back of the fetal head (occiput) presses against the mother's sacrum, which has a large nerve supply. The back pain may be controlled when the mother stands, lies on the side opposite the fetal back, or positions herself on her hands and knees while being massaged from her back to front and the side where the fetal back is positioned. The latter two positions encourage the fetus to rotate to the anterior position, thereby relieving maternal pain.

▶ PAIN

Pain has two parts: (1) the output with sensory receptors and (2) the processing or reaction to the pain

(Lowe, 1996). The first component is a physiologic reaction that results from a stimulus and response of one's sensory receptors and the second aspect identifies and responds to the pain (Lowe, 1996).

Pain is highly subjective. It is described as an unpleasant sensation, emotion, affect, or feeling that may or may not produce suffering (Lowe, 1991). Pain is whatever an individual says it is. The nurse should never deny, admonish, or belittle a woman with pain, but rather acknowledge the pain and help overcome it.

Pain is often the first sign that labor is progressing. Labor pain is frequently described as sharp, intense, tiring, aching, torturing, or nagging. Early reports of labor pain ranked it among the most intense pain.

Analgesia occurs naturally during labor in the form of beta-endorphins. These polypeptides are produced by the placenta as a result of the stress of labor; they increase with labor and correspond with the woman's pain perception (Mokriski, 1993). Beta-endorphins are more potent than morphine. They increase tolerance to pain while contractions are occurring; their concentration decreases between contractions. Although they help a laboring woman, the level of beta-endorphins in the amniotic fluid increases to more than 20 times the normal level during labor, which may provoke fetal distress.

In the first stage of labor, pain is due primarily to dilation and effacement of the cervix and lower uterine segment (LUS) and to subsequent distension and stretching or tearing of these structures during contractions. Second-stage labor pain may cause the woman to forcefully bear down; lacerations may result. Pain in this stage is related to stretching of the lower vagina, vulva, and perineum. Pain may occur with tearing of fascia and subcutaneous tissues, from pressure of the perineum on skeletal muscles, and with pressure and distension caused by the presenting part (Figs. 23–1, 23–2, and 23–3).

In addition, distension of the bladder or lower uterine segment, uterine muscle hypoxia, vaginal tissue lacerations, and emotional tension caused by fear and anxiety may produce pain. Pain increases cardiac output, decreases uterine blood flow, and causes tachycardia, cardiac arrhythmias, tachypnea, hyperventilation, and sweating.

▶ Theories of Pain

Specificity Theory

Pain is a specific sensation that travels via a pathway from the skin and spinal cord to the thalamic pain center (Melzack & Wall, 1965).

Pattern Theory

All nerve fiber endings are similar; pain results when total cell output exceeds a certain level because of excessive receptor stimulation or pathology. Excessive

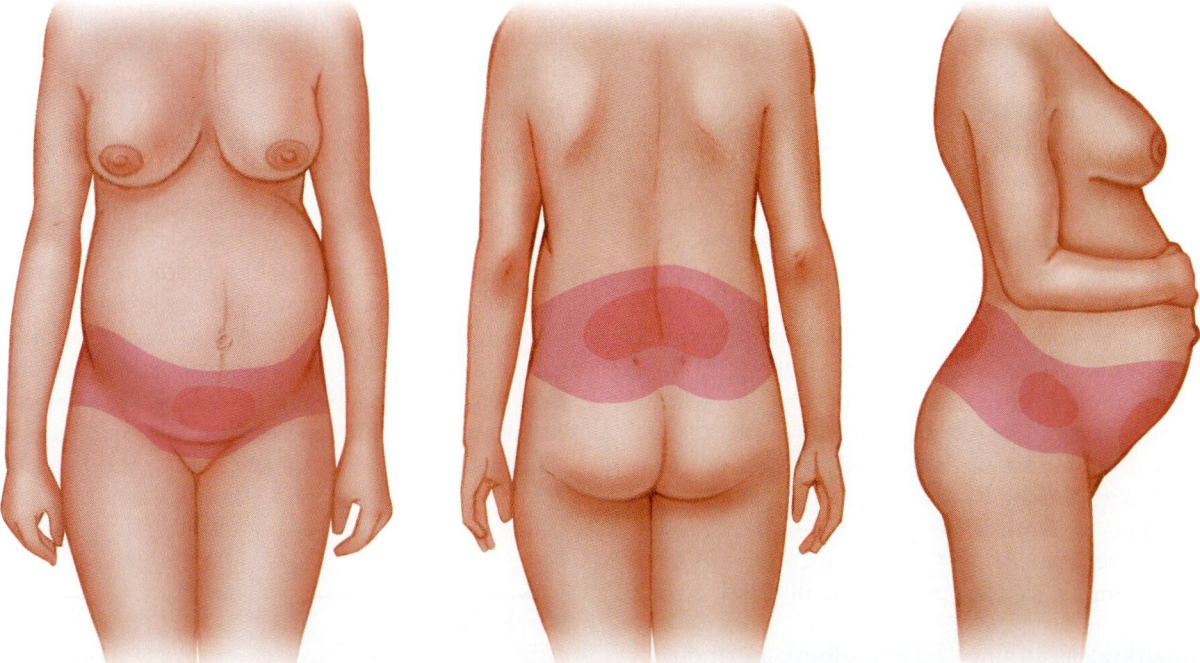

FIGURE 23–1. Distribution of pain during the early phase of the first stage of labor. Graduated shades of color indicate intensity of pain. *(Adapted, with permission, from Bonica, J.J., & McDonald, J.S. (Eds.). (1995). Principles and practice of obstetric analgesia & anesthesia (2nd ed.). Baltimore: Lea & Febiger.)*

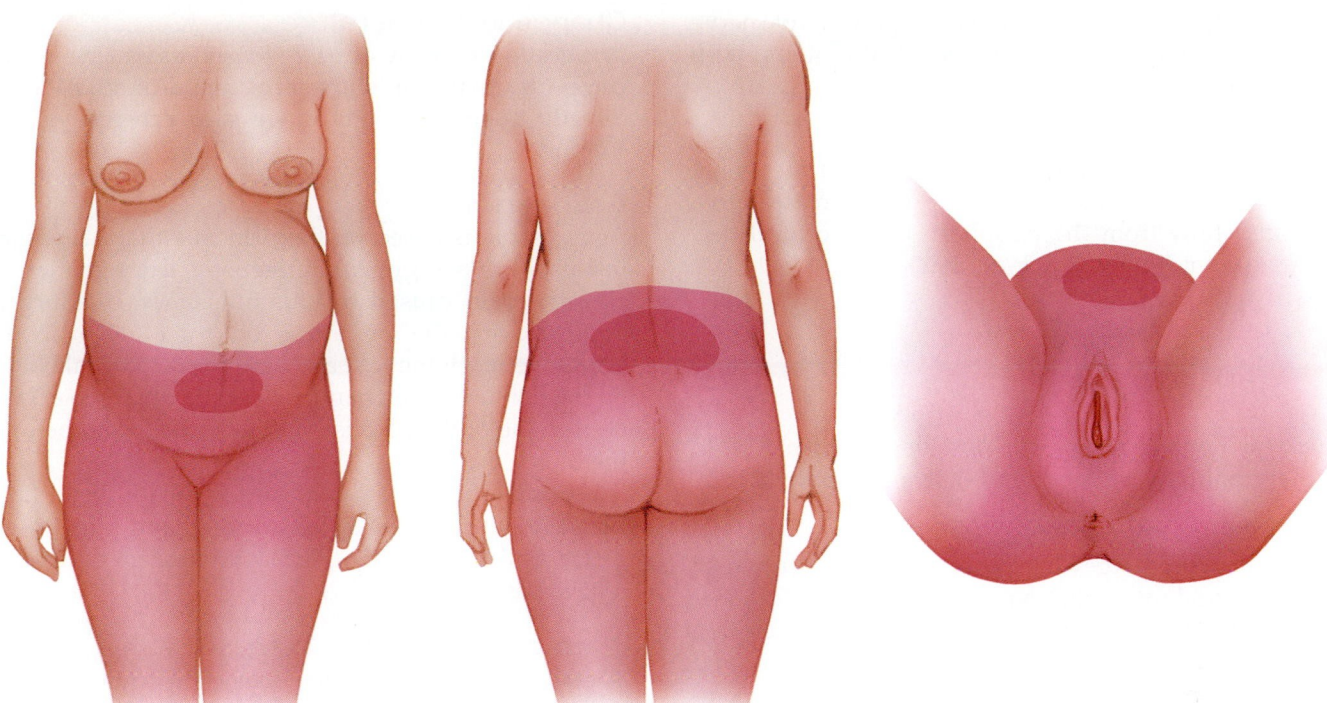

FIGURE 23–2. Distribution of labor pain during the latter phase of the first stage and early phase of the second stage. *(Adapted, with permission, from Bonica, J.J., & McDonald, J.S. (Eds.). (1995). Principles and practice of obstetric analgesia & anesthesia (2nd ed.). Baltimore: Lea & Febiger.)*

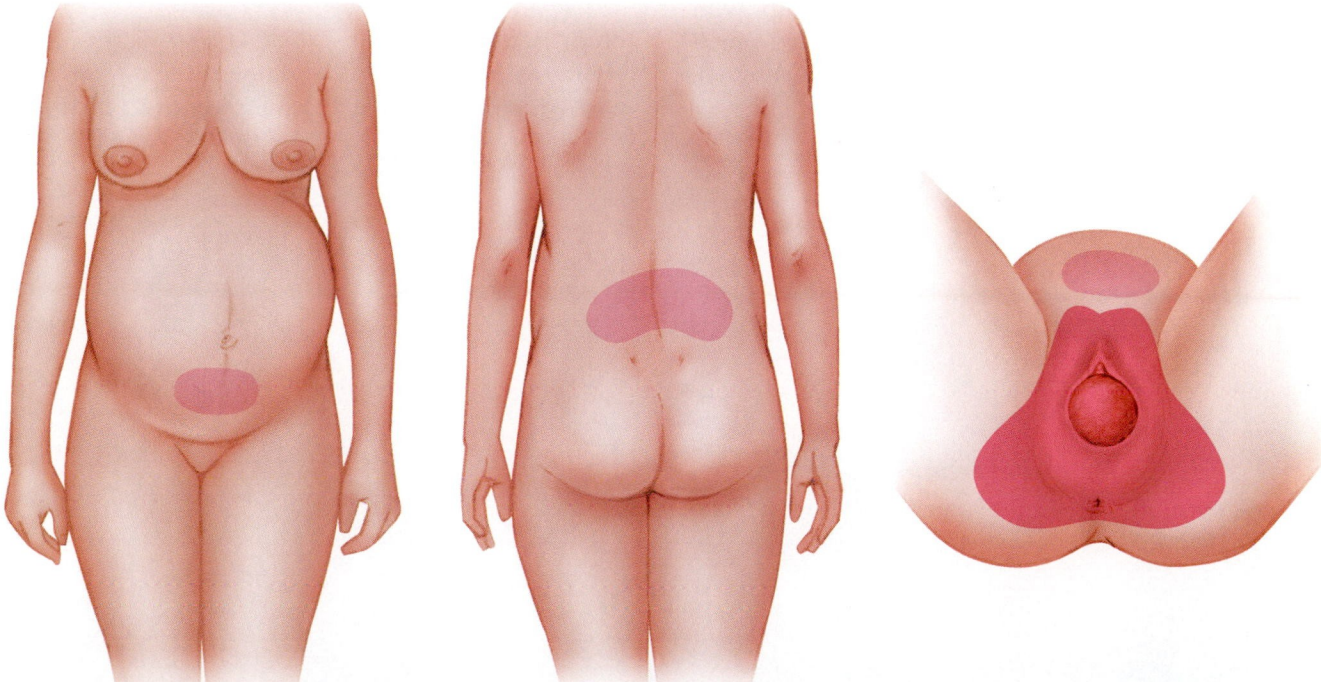

FIGURE 23–3. Distribution of labor pain during the latter phase of the second stage and actual delivery. *(Adapted, with permission, from Bonica, J.J., & McDonald, J.S. (Eds.). (1995). Principles and practice of obstetric analgesia & anesthesia (2nd ed.). Baltimore: Lea & Febiger.)*

peripheral stimulation initiates a pattern of nerve impulses, which is interpreted centrally as pain (Melzack & Wall, 1983).

Gate Control Theory

A neural mechanism in the dorsal horn of the spinal cord acts like a gate to increase or decrease nerve impulse flow from the periphery to the central nervous system (Melzack & Wall, 1965, 1983).

► Nonpharmacologic Methods of Pain Relief

Several nonpharmacologic options are available to relieve pain during labor and delivery (Simkin, 1995).

Hydrotherapy (Water Therapy)

A woman submerges herself in a warm bath, which causes local vasodilation and muscle relaxation. Although blood pressure is lowered, perineal trauma is reduced, emotional experiences are better, and intervention is avoided, further research is recommended to evaluate hydrotherapy. Jet hydrotherapy (whirlpool bath) also promotes relaxation, relieves pain, and stimulates cervical dilation.

A randomized study of laboring women (n = 393 in the treatment group and n = 392 in the control group) demonstrated less narcotic and epidural usage in the treatment group who used a whirlpool bath during labor. The whirlpool group had less instrumentation at delivery and had more intact perinea. There was no difference between the group with maternal or newborn infections with ruptured membranes (Rush, Burlock, Lambert, Loosley-Millman, Hutchison, & Enkin, 1996).

Change in Temperature

Application of heat directly to an area using a hot compress, bath, or shower or application of cold directly to an area with an ice pack can relieve discomfort.

Acupressure

Acupressure is based on the principle that pain is an imbalance of energy within the body. During labor, to ease the pain caused by this imbalance, pressure is applied with the fingertips on three major body points: between the first and second metacarpal bones on the dorsum of the hand; below the tibial tuberosity on the side of the tibialis anterior muscle; and behind the tibia.

Counterpressure using acupressure or direct firm massage with the fist or heel of the hand (Fig. 23–4), tennis balls, or a can filled with frozen fluid also relieves discomfort.

Therapeutic Touch

Therapeutic touch operates on the principle that the human body is an energy field. Pain relief may be mediated through a person, such as the nurse, who transmits energy (recuperative powers) to the pregnant woman's body. Pain may be alleviated.

Imagery/Visualization

In imagery/visualization, a laboring mother pictures the birth in a positive light. She visualizes her vagina gently and easily opening to allow fetal passage. Music often accompanies imagery.

Hypnosis

Hypnosis reduces the sensation of pain for some women in labor and undergoing cesarean birth. It is

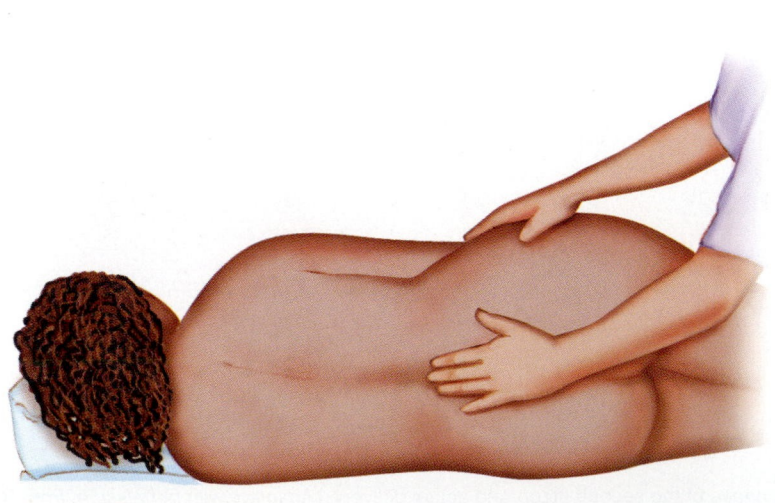
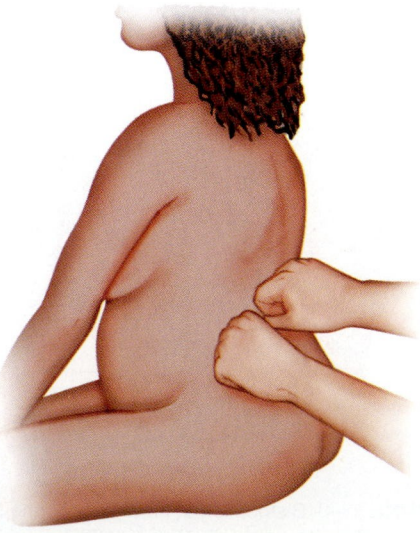

FIGURE 23–4. Massage techniques for back labor.

not effective for everyone and only carefully selected women benefit. Hypnosis is reversible. There are no known adverse effects, such as hypotension, uteroplacental perfusion, itching, nausea, and neonatal respiratory depression. Complications include acute anxiety and frank psychosis. The woman must be prepared prenatally for hypnosis during a series of sessions. The depth of her trance increases with each session. Oster (1994) described hypnosis as a model of psychologic preparation that permitted the mother's active participation in the birth process. This method was even applied postpartally as well as during other painful procedures.

The nurse or a support person can perform some or all of these techniques. Having the support person assist the woman strengthens the bond between them.

The gate control theory may be implemented to interrupt pain impulse transmission.

Acupuncture

In acupuncture, needles may be inserted at selected points to interrupt transmission of pain; its use has been documented to help control pain in China and the Far East. It is least effective in controlling pain in the lower part of the body. Success rates seem to depend on careful client selection, high client motivation, and cultural conditioning.

Effleurage

Rhythmic stroking and massage of the abdomen **(effleurage)** during a contraction have some minor effect on pain transmission. Effleurage is better tolerated in early labor (Fig. 23–5).

Abdominal Pressure

During the latter part of the first stage of labor, effleurage no longer helps. Instead, stimulation of abdominal pressure points is effective; firm downward pressure or deep massage is applied to the area of greatest pain intensity. The woman or her partner positions the hands over the area of acute pain, either above the pubic bone or over the anterior-superior borders of the ilia (Fig. 23–6).

Transcutaneous Electrical Nerve Stimulation

In transcutaneous electrical nerve stimulation (TENS), large nerve fibers in the skin are stimulated using cutaneous electrodes, which blocks pain transmission in the dorsal horn (spinal gate). Surface TENS electrodes are placed over dermatomes at the T10–L1 level along the back and sacrum (Fig. 23–7). With stimulation of the upper electrodes and increased stimuli from the woman during contractions, a tingling sensation occurs with pain relief. Some relief is provided for the first stage of labor; it is less effective

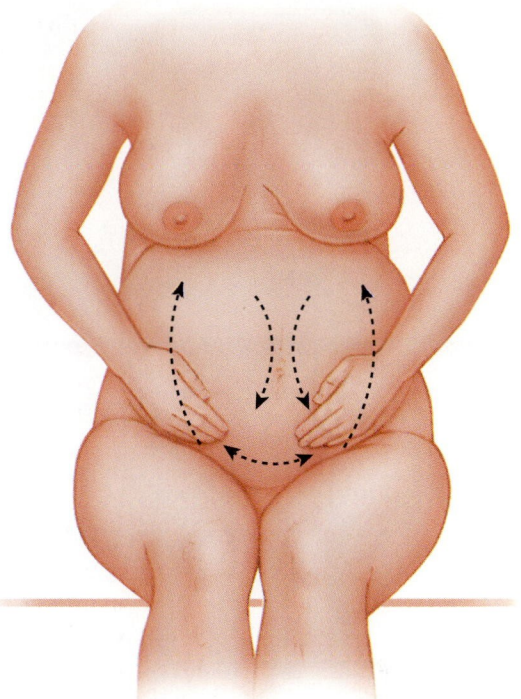

FIGURE 23–5. Direction of abdominal effleurage for the latent and active phases of the first stage of labor.

in the second stage. TENS decreases the need for narcotic analgesia; it is noninvasive and safe for both the woman and her fetus. Some women, however, cannot tolerate the stimulation. Other drawbacks of TENS are interference with fetal heart rate (FHR) monitoring and expense of the equipment.

Biofeedback

Biofeedback techniques, in which a person responds to a painful stimulus by using specific relaxation responses, have been used to relieve the discomfort of labor and delivery. A variety of techniques have been used.

Comfort Measures

Reducing stress often reduces pain. Bed linens must be clean and dry and not restrict the woman's movement. Massage of the lower back, thighs, or legs is often welcome until transition. Placing a cool washcloth on the forehead or sponging the face and neck is refreshing. The woman may rinse her mouth with water or mouthwash. Healthy laboring women may drink water or juice or take ice chips to relieve mouth dryness. Perineal care maintains medical asepsis and is comforting. Caregivers should demonstrate respect for the client's modesty with appropriate draping and curtaining at all times. These basic comfort measures carry a message of caring.

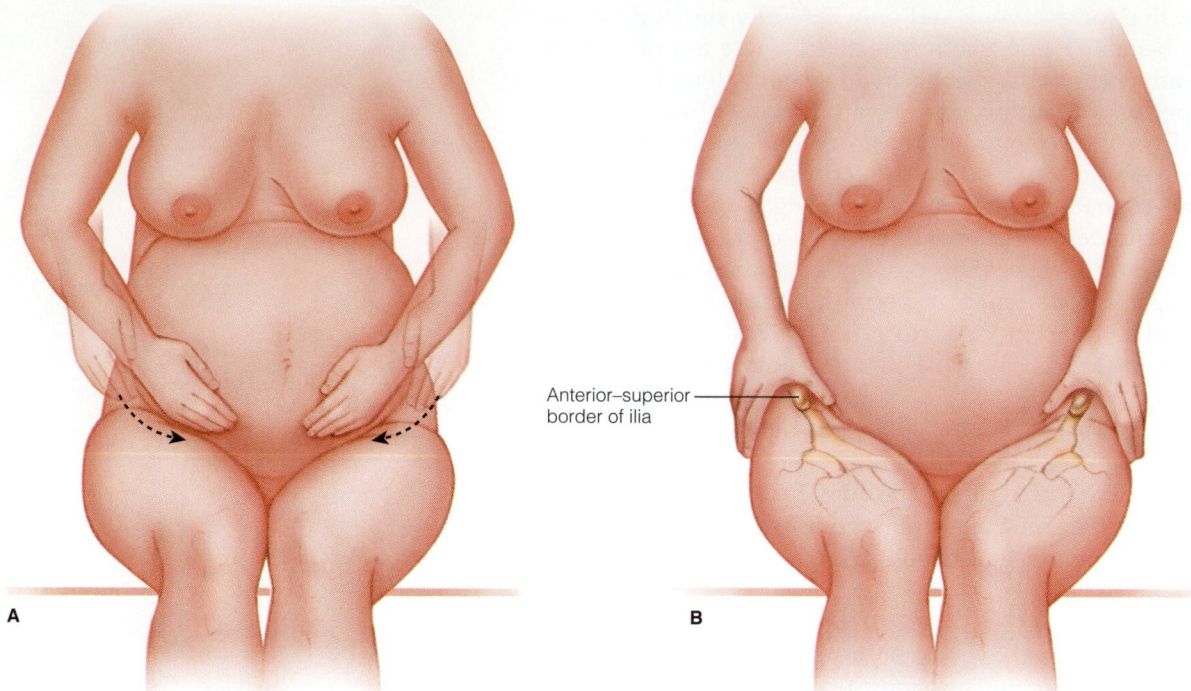

A

B

Anterior–superior border of ilia

FIGURE 23–6. Use of abdominal pressure points during transition. **A.** Pressure applied above the pubic bone. **B.** Pressure applied over the anterior-superior border of the ilia.

Distraction

The creativity of a labor and delivery nurse may be challenged by the distraction method of pain control. Many clients enjoy watching television during the latent phase; others prefer listening to music. Earphones may be used to listen to a radio. The nurse should interview and observe each client to determine individual preferences for distraction. Would the woman prefer silence? Music? Conversation? Viewing the monitoring screen? Many women find the sound of the fetal heartbeat, amplified by the monitor, reassuring and hypnotic. Others, however, become anxious with the variability of the FHR.

Application of Childbirth Education

The nurse should identify how the couple was prepared for childbirth (see Chapter 9). What method did they learn? In addition, different breathing techniques can be taught in the intrapartum period. During the first stage, the practiced technique should be encouraged.

For example, the Dick-Read method employs deep breathing, both abdominal and chest, and shallow breathing. In the Lamaze method, the woman breathes at a slow pace and changes to a modified pace as the first stage progresses. The Bradley method, on the other hand, involves breath control and abdominal breathing during the first stage.

If the couple has not attended childbirth education classes, controlled relaxation techniques can be taught by an experienced nurse. They may reduce pharmacologic interventions.

Each of the aforementioned methods uses basically the same pushing technique during the second stage of labor. The woman takes one or two cleansing breaths, pushes at the peak of the contraction, and uses the cleansing breath again at the end.

Recommendations have changed over the years about the force used in pushing and the length of time the breath is held. Today instruction is flexible: the woman may push for the length of time and with the force that feels right for her. Some women naturally push about 10 seconds, take a deep breath, and push again, continuing the pattern until the contraction ends.

▶ Pharmacologic Methods of Pain Relief

Pharmacologic as well as nonpharmacologic interventions may be required during labor, although judi-

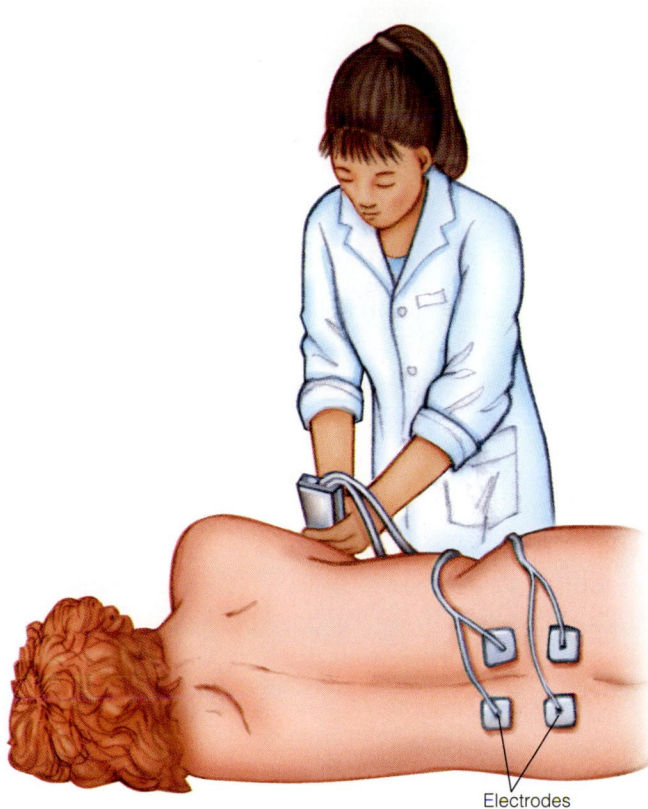

FIGURE 23–7. Use of transcutaneous nerve stimulation for pain relief in labor. *(Adapted, with permission, from Ottoson, D., & Lundeberg, T. (1988).* Pain treatment by transcutaneous electrical nerve stimulation: A practical manual. *Heidelberg: Springer Verlag, p. 108.)*

cious use of medications is necessary. Analgesics, tranquilizers, sedatives, or anesthetics may be used. **Analgesia** is the reduction of pain without loss of consciousness; **anesthesia** is the loss of sensation, either complete or partial, with or without loss of consciousness. Overlap exists in the use of these terms.

Nonpharmacologic and pharmacologic methods of pain management lessen the perceived pain of labor or block the pain pathways during labor and delivery. The perceived pain and discomfort differ according to the stage of labor. Figures 23–1, 23–2, and 23–3 illustrate pain pathways in the first and second stages of labor.

Nursing Alert

The nurse should caution the woman against long hard pushing during labor as it may lead to fetal bradycardia and trauma to maternal body tissues.

Analgesia

Analgesics, Tranquilizers, and Sedatives.

Before administering systemic medication to a laboring woman, the nurse must assess maternal and fetal status. Any medication will affect the woman, fetus, and labor. Consequently, the nurse checks maternal respiration, pulse and blood pressure, and FHR prior to administering medications. Any change in the mother may produce fetal hypoxia.

Pain medication can affect the progress of labor; contractions may occur farther apart and become less intense. In general, medications should be timed so that they are not given too early, thereby slowing labor and delivery, or too late, not giving the mother and fetus ample time to metabolize and excrete the medication. Medications such as meperidine can cause respiratory depression in the newborn.

Meperidine is an analgesic used frequently during labor. The tranquilizers often given are antianxiety agents, such as hydroxyzine (Vistaril); benzodiazepines, such as diazepam (Valium); and phenothiazines, such as promethazine (Phenergan). Generally, they are given intramuscularly and can be repeated if the woman is restless or uncomfortable. Tranquilizers alone do not provide analgesia but, together with narcotics, may provide sedation. They may produce additional maternal and fetal depression. Barbiturate sedatives such as secobarbital (Seconal) and pentobarbital (Nembutal) are rarely used during labor, as they actually antagonize analgesic effects. Table 23–1 is an overview of common analgesics given during labor.

Women's Health

In light of the various viewpoints expressed by health care professionals and the general public about the use of analgesia and anesthesia during labor, women may experience feelings of incompetency and guilt if they either choose or require these pharmacologic methods of pain relief during the intrapartum period. The nurse needs to be aware of these feelings and encourage the client and her partner to view the use of analgesia or anesthesia not as a failure on the part of the couple to cope with labor but as a means of ensuring a positive outcome for the woman and her baby.

► **TABLE 23-1**

Common Analgesics Used During Labor

Drug Name	Indications	Administration	Onset and Duration of Action	Intended Effects
Analgesics				
Meperidine (Demerol)	Maternal desire for pain relief; early labor, to help sleep	IM or IV: 25–100 mg in active labor Epidurally: up to 100 mg has been used intrathecally: 10–20 mg	IV: immediate effect lasting 1–4 h IM: 15–30 min to take effect, lasting 2–3 h intrathecally: lasts ½ to 2½ h	Sedation of mother and good (but not complete) pain relief without loss of consciousness; analgesics rarely relieve all the painful feelings of contractions; usually relieve the pain associated with the beginning and end but not the peak of contractions
Butorphanol (Stadol)	Pain relief during labor; avoid in opioid-addicted clients	30–40 times more potent than meperidine IM: 1–2 mg IV: 0.5–1 mg	IM: maximum analgesia in 30 min; duration 0.5–2 h	Same as for meperidine
Nalbuphine (Nubain)	Pain relief during labor; avoid in opioid-addicted clients	IV: 1 mg at 6- to 10-min intervals PCA: 2–4 mg IV loading dose and 1 mg IV on demand at 6–10 min IM: 5–10 mg	Onset 2–15 min; duration 1–4 h	Decreased pain
Fentanyl (Sublimaze)	Pain relief during labor	100 times as potent as meperidine IV: 25–50 µg IM: 50–100 µg epidurally: 100–200 µg intrathecally: 25 µg	Rapid, within 10 min IM and 1–2 min IV; duration up to 2 h	Decreased pain
Sufentanil (Sufenta)	Pain relief during labor	10 times as potent as fentanyl; potency inhibits use systemically epidurally: 10–30 µg intrathecally: 3–15 µg	Immediate action lasting less than 1 h	Decreased pain
Bupivacaine (Marcaine)	Pain relief during labor	Intermittent injections impractical with short duration of action intrathecally: 2.5 mg	Onset 15–20 min; duration 60–100 min	Decreased pain
Alfentanil (Alfenta)	Pain relief during labor	80 times as potent as morphine; one third as potent as fentanyl and lasts 30% as long; not appropriate systemi-cally as neurobe-havioral score was affected in monkeys; 10–30 mg/kg epidurally: some use when delivery remote	Immediate effect, peaks within 1–2 min; duration 10–15 min	Decreased pain
Morphine	Rarely used in normal labor; used to inhibit premature labor; used postcesarean for pain relief	IM: 5–10 mg IV: 2–5 mg Epidurally: up to 5 mg Intrathecally: 0.2–1 mg	Immediate to within 15–20 min (IM); lasts up to 3–4 h to 24 h (epidurally); titration difficult with slow onset	Attempt to inhibit premature labor

Effects on Labor	Maternal Effects	Placental Transfer	Fetal Newborn Effects
In early labor, there may be a decrease in intensity and frequency of contractions; excessive doses prolong labor; repeated injections may be necessary	Respiratory and circulatory depression, dizziness, confusion, nausea, vomiting, cough suppression, gastrointestinal stasis, lowered blood oxygen; with potential respiratory depression in the mother or fetus have available resuscitative equipment and personnel and naloxone (Narcan) 0.4 mg IM/IV to counteract drug effects	Within 30 seconds of IV dose	Effects dependent on dose or administration relative to time of birth, size, health, and fetal age; respiratory depression; fetus/newborn cannot easily metabolize the medication; naloxone (Narcan) 0.1 mg/kg given to infant to counteract immediate respiratory depression; some deficiency exists for a day or so but does not affect neonatal feeding, weight gain, or development; controversy surrounds reports of neurobehavioral changes from systemic drugs
Does not interfere with labor	No excessive sedation or somnolence; adequate pain relief with few side effects	Rapid	Neonatal respiratory depression less than with meperidine; care must be taken that drug is not given with meperidine as it antagonizes effects of meperidine; sinusoidal FHR pattern after administration
Decreased pain	Increased sedation and limited ceiling effect; with PCA, less nausea and vomiting and less sedation; prophylactic nalbuphine seems unable to prevent pruritus	Rapid	With this dosage, there is ceiling effect for neonatal respiratory depression
Sometimes pain persists	Studies show no nausea, vomiting, or sedation; repeated injections or constant infusion may be necessary; may cause drowsiness, hypotension, bradycardia	Rapid within 1 min	Minimal respiratory depression
Decreased pain	May cause drowsiness, hypotension, bradycardia	Rapid	Fetal depression; caution if fetus premature; may cause developmental delays
Decreased pain	Decreased pain; cardiotoxicity	Rapid	Unclear
Decreased pain	Drowsiness, hypotension, bradycardia	Rapid	Some fetal depression; developmental delays
Inhibits premature labor	Drowsiness, hypotension, respiratory depression, pruritus, nausea, vomiting; large doses required for analgesia; hypotensive action compromises IV use	Rapid	Same as for meperidine but a greater effect on respiratory depression

(continued)

► **TABLE 23–1** *(continued)*

Common Analgesics Used During Labor

Drug Name	Indications	Administration	Onset and Duration of Action	Intended Effects
Tranquilizers				
Hydroxyzine (Vistaril)	Tense, anxious mother; administered with meperidine to potentiate analgesia and to counteract nausea and vomiting	IM only: 25–100 mg	Onset 15–30 min; duration 2–4 h	Sedation of mother; lessens anxiety; raises pain threshold; muscle relaxant; potentiates narcotics and barbiturates; antinauseant
Promethazine (Phenergan)	Same as for hydroxyzine	IM or IV: 25–50 mg	Rapid onset; duration 6–8 h	Same as for hydroxyzine
Diazepam (Valium)	Same as for hydroxyzine; used to treat preeclampsia in some countries	IM: 15–20 mg IV: 5–15 mg	Rapid onset; duration 1–1½ h	Same as for hydroxyzine
Sedatives				
Secobarbital (Seconal)	Helps woman who may be in false or prolonged labor to sleep; helps calm anxious woman; rarely used today	PO, IM, or IV: up to 100 mg	PO: 30–60 min IM: about 15 min IV: 30–60 seconds	Sedation of woman in early latent phase when delivery remote
Pentobarbital (Nembutal)	Same as for secobarbital	Same as for secobarbital	Same as for secobarbital	Same as for secobarbital

Narcotic Analgesics. Fentanyl (Sublimaze), sufentanil (Sufenta), alfentanil (Alfenta), nalbuphine (Nubain), and butorphanol (Stadol) are among the narcotic analgesics. All narcotics as well as tranquilizers cross the placenta and may cause neonatal respiratory depression.

Anesthesia

Common anesthetic methods used in labor and delivery include local, regional (paracervical, pudendal, epidural, and spinal), and general (gas, volatile, intravenous). The same drug, administered by alternate routes and doses, may produce the anesthetic effect. The anesthetic should be simple to use and safe, preserve maternal and fetal health, and be administered by a competent practitioner (e.g., anesthesiologist or nurse anesthetist) with expertise in obstetric anesthesia. It should not interfere with the progress of labor. Although the staff nurse does not administer anesthesia, she or he is responsible for closely monitoring the mother and fetus, especially during labor when the nurse is the primary care provider.

Local Anesthesia. Local infiltration of anesthetic into the subcutaneous and intramuscular tissue of the perineum is the simplest method for delivery. It has minimal side effects on the mother and fetus. The site of the episiotomy is numbed for incision and repair (Fig. 23–8). In addition, it may be useful surrounding the episiotomy if anesthesia is inadequate. Local infiltration of the perineum with 0.5 to 1% lidocaine or 1 to 2% 2-chloroprocaine is insufficient for labor but effective for delivery.

Local anesthetic agents may also be used by peripheral nerve block and intraspinally during labor and following cesarean section. The three most commonly used are lidocaine, 2-chloroprocaine, and bupivacaine (Table 23–2).

Regional Anesthesia. **Regional anesthesia** causes loss of sensation along nerve pathways of a particular organ and surrounding tissues. Paracervical, pudendal, epidural, and spinal blocks are examples of regional anesthesia that may be administered.

Effects on Labor	Maternal Effects	Placental Transfer	Fetal Newborn Effects
Unknown	Drowsiness, confusion, drop in blood pressure, urinary retention, dry mouth, fat embolism, amnesia, pain at injection site	Rapid	Unclear but possible CNS depression and hyperbilirubinemia
Possible depression of uterine contractions	Same as for hydroxyzine, except no fat embolism	Rapid	Loss of FHR beat-to-beat variability
Unknown	Same as for promethazine with muscle relaxation	Rapid	Hyperbilirubinemia, hypothermia, hypotonia, hypoactivity, loss of FHR beat-to-beat variability
May stop false labor; may slow early labor	Decreases pulse, blood pressure, and general responsiveness; reduces anxiety and allows rest, but client may have difficulty dealing with contractions as this is not a pain reliever	Seconds to minutes	Drug accumulates in tissue; may cause CNS depression (especially when given with narcotic); no effective antidote; have resuscitative equipment and personnel available
Same as for secobarbital	Same as for secobarbital		Same as for secobarbital

The **paracervical block** can be used to relieve the discomfort of labor when the cervix is dilated about 5 to 6 cm, but not more than 8 cm, as the risk of intrafetal injection rises (Flynn, 1993) (Fig. 23–9). Lidocaine or another local anesthetic agent is injected directly into the cervix at 3 and 9 or 4 and 8 o'clock positions (Fig. 23–10). Paracervical block does not relieve perineal pain; therefore, additional anesthesia, such as a pudendal block, may be needed for delivery.

Although pain relief is achieved during the first stage of labor with only rare maternal complications, paracervical blocks may cause fetal bradycardia associated with fetal asphyxia (Costello, 1993). Recommendations are to avoid this block if the fetus is stressed, uteroplacental insufficiency is suspected, or if delivery is complicated, as in breech and multiple gestations (Costello, 1993). Nursing care involves careful monitoring of the fetal heart rate.

A **pudendal block** involves injection of a local anesthetic agent, such as lidocaine, in the vicinity of each of the two pudendal nerves as they pass between the ischial spines (Fig. 23–11). The pudendal nerves are approached either through the vagina (transvaginal), which is more common (Fig. 23–12), or through the perineum (transcutaneous).

Bilateral pudendal blocks take effect within 3 to 4 minutes and relieve most of the discomfort from perineal distension during second-stage labor and at delivery. They permit the use of low-forceps or vacuum extraction. Before administration of a pudendal block, the infiltration of the fourchette, perineum, and vagina with the anesthetic (e.g., 1% lidocaine solution) at the site of a possible episiotomy is often done. This allows an episiotomy to be made without pain if delivery takes place before the pudendal block has time to become effective (Cunningham et al., 1997). If administered too late, anesthesia is inadequate. It may interfere with maternal pushing; in rare cases, convulsions may occur with intravascular injection of the anesthetic agent, and a hematoma or abscess may form. Pudendal block is not recommended for midforceps deliveries, uterine manipulation, or repair of deep vaginal or cervical lacerations (Costello, 1993).

Common Anesthetics Used During Labor

Type of Anesthetic	Indications	Administration	Onset and Duration of Action
Local	Numbs tissue at site of episiotomy incision and for repair of laceration	Interstitially, directly into tissue to be repaired; carbocaine (Mepivacaine) and lidocaine (Xylocaine) are amide-type local anesthetics; 1% solution up to 200 mg or 20 mL; ester-type local anesthetic 2-chloroprocaine (Nesacaine)	Onset 1–10 min; duration 1 h
Regional Paracervical block	For pain relief in first-stage labor; not commonly used	5 mL of local anesthetic used per site, given into 3 and 9 or 4 and 8 o'clock positions of lateral vaginal fornices when cervix is dilated about 5–6 cm, but not more than 8 cm	Onset within 2–5 min; duration depends on drug used, varies from 45 min to 3 h; injection may be repeated in 30 min
Pudendal block	Given into pudendal nerve via transvaginal or transcutaneous approach; may be used for outlet forceps or difficult delivery, large or extensive incision, laceration, and repair	Same as for local agent; other agents include 2-chloroprocaine, bupivacaine, and mepivacaine	Same as for local agent
Epidural block	In active labor for pain relief from contractions and pelvic pressure/pain, at woman's request after 4 cm and contractile pattern well established; in second stage, for delivery, especially if manipulation or forceps anticipated; also for cesarean birth	Given by anesthesiologist into epidural space at L-2, L-3, L-4, or L-5 while woman lies on her side with legs drawn up in fetal position or in sitting position; combination of opioids with local anesthetics for improved relief; bupivacaine (0.06–0.5%) never more than 20 mg at any one time; lidocaine 1–2%; 2-chloroprocaine 2–3%; and combinations of fentanyl, sufentanil, or alfentanil with bupivacaine	Epidural may take 30 min to administer; onset varies from rapid to slow depending on medication; can be within minutes to 20 min lasting up to 100 min; medication may be given in one bolus injection through catheter or by continuous infusion via catheter attached to infusion pump, where constant and specific amount of medication is given
Spinal block	For delivery or if excessive manipulation or forceps anticipated; also for cesarean birth	Given by anesthesiologist into spinal column at L-2, L-3, L-4, or L-5 while woman lies on her left side in fetal position; generally fentanyl, sufentanil, morphine, tetracaine (Pontocaine) 1% 6–8 mg, or lidocaine 5% 50–70 mg	Onset within 3–5 min; duration 1–3 h or longer depending on medication
General Nitrous halothane (Fluothane), oxide enflurane (Ethrane), isoflurane (Florane)	Complete loss of sensation and consciousness for cesarean birth, difficult birth, uterine relaxation, or postpartum uterine manipulation	Volatile anesthetics used to supplement nitrous oxide during maintenance of general anesthesia	Rapid onset; duration varies with length and dose of anesthetic
Intravenous thiopental (Pentothal), ketamine (Ketalar)	Rapid induction of general anesthesia, usually followed by inhalation agents	Pentothal: usually given in a dose less than 4 mg/kg maternal weight so side effects to woman and fetus are minimized Ketamine: given in dose less than 1 mg/kg maternal weight with same anesthetic effect; can also be used as alternative to inhalation anesthesia in a dose 0.25 mg/kg body weight	Immediate

Intended Effects	Effects on Labor	Maternal Effects	Placental Transfer	Fetal/Newborn Effects
Numbs site	None known, especially as it is given at delivery	When used locally, rare maternal side effects, including cardiac depression, CNS depression, restlessness, dizziness, and, in large doses, convulsions; amide-type anesthetics penetrate tissue better and act more rapidly and longer than ester-type drugs	2–3 min	None if given after birth and rare even before birth; may cause bradycardia, tachycardia, fetal acidosis, and, in high blood levels, convulsions; metabolism of amide drugs requires liver enzymes that are not mature in the fetus
Pain relief from uterine contractions and dilating cervix	Rare, but might slow labor	Pain relief for first-stage labor only; rare systemic effects	Rapid, as close to uterus and placenta	Bradycardia in 2–70% of cases; convulsions, death if injected into fetus and vaginal area; fetal risk if given during bradycardia
Numbs lower vagina and perineum	Given in second-stage labor; woman may have decreased bearing down reflex; fails to provide adequate analgesia if given too late	See Effects on Labor	Same as for local agent	Same as for local agent
Pain relief in lower part of body	If given too early, improperly, or in too large a dose, labor may slow or stop; labor stimulant (oxytocin [Pitocin]) may be necessary; decreases the urge to push, may necessitate forceps; with combination of opioids and anesthetics, lack of motor block, and woman has increased chance of pain-free and unparalyzed delivery	Frequent vital signs needed because of hypotensive effect (prehydration with 500–1000 mL lactated Ringer's); fetal monitor to detect labor or fetal adverse effects; IV fluids needed for hypotension, oxytocin, forceps	7–15 min depending on agent used	FHR decelerations resulting from maternal hypotension
Numbs body from waist to feet	High doses may stop labor; pain relief obtained	Loss of sensation, motor function, and pushing reflex; forceps may be needed; hypotension (prehydration needed as with epidural), headache; some nausea, vomiting, pruritus, urinary retention; possible infection at puncture site and meningitis	Rapid	Epidural and spinal opioids pose no risk to fetus or neonate because the doses of opioids are small
Complete anesthesia; loss of consciousness with complete muscle relaxation	Labor stops if given during first stage; reserved for delivery only	Complete loss of consciousness, no pain felt, extreme uterine relaxation, cardiovascular depression, hypotensive effect, increased bleeding, aspiration of vomitus, rarely death	Rapid	Depending on drug, dose, and length of anesthesia, respiratory depression, decreased alertness, decreased orientation, decreased responsiveness to visual and auditory stimuli, poor consolability, and irritability
Rapid induction of general anesthesia	Minimal when recommended doses used	Pentothal: Possible hypotension and laryngospasm
Ketamine: Little effect on maternal CNS with recommended doses; stimulates maternal cardiovascular system and may be used with maternal hypotension and hemorrhage; avoid with maternal hypertension	Rapid	Pentothal: Severe fetal depression when rapid delivery occurs after injection
Ketamine: Avoid using with fetal distress; if dose recommendation exceeded, maternal respiratory depression and increased neonatal muscle tone threatening infant ventilation

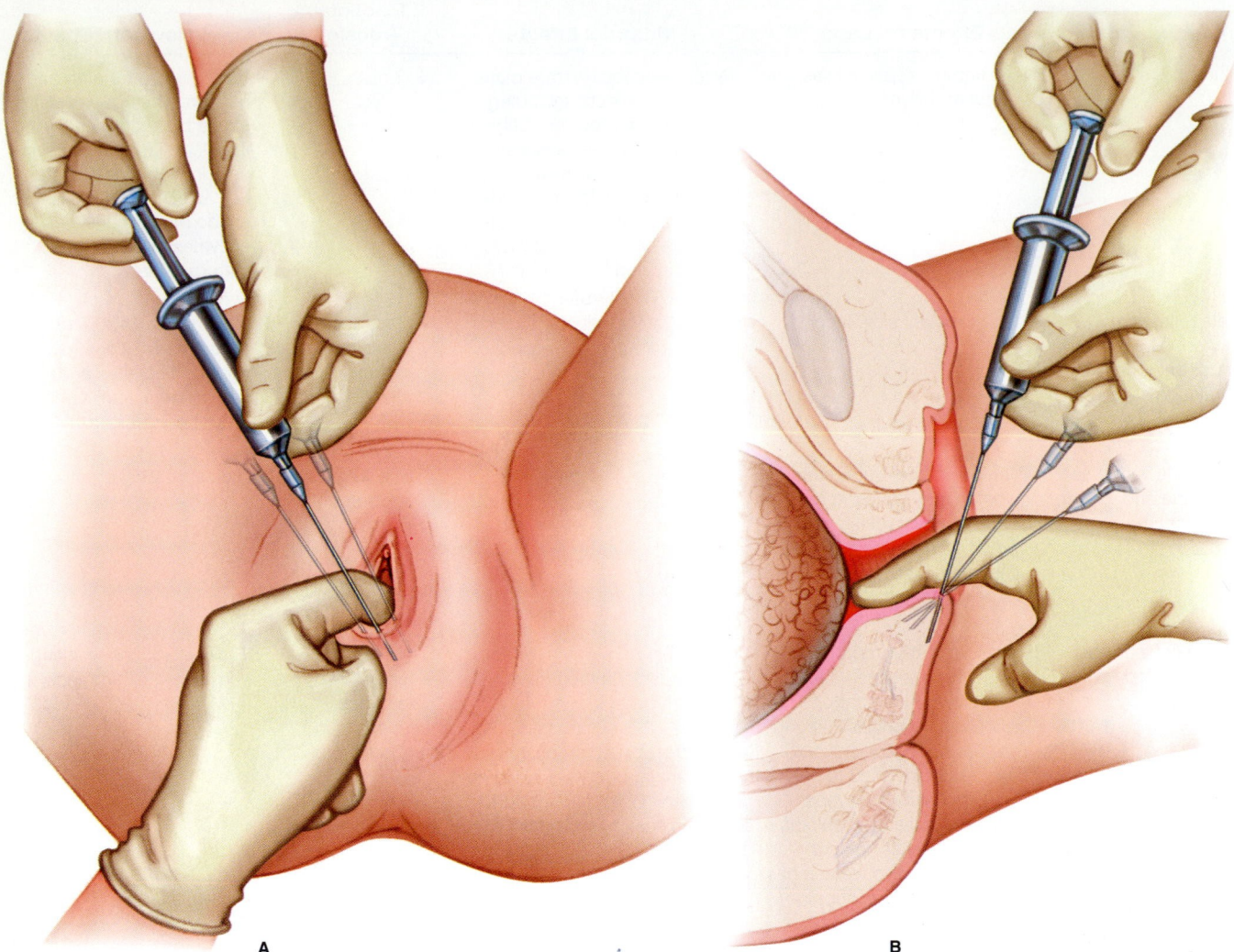

FIGURE 23–8. Technique of local infiltration for episiotomy and repair. **A.** Anterior view. **B.** Sagittal view showing fanwise pattern of injections.

An **epidural block** is a regional anesthesia used for vaginal and cesarean births. The terms *epidural, peridural,* and *extradural* are used interchangeably. The anesthetic drug is usually injected through a catheter that is inserted into the epidural space (Fig. 23–13). It is common in obstetric analgesia today, but may not be available in every institution.

The epidural space is a potential, not actual, space located between the dura (the fibrous membrane covering the spinal cord and cerebrospinal fluid) and the vertebrae. The epidural space holds blood vessels, lymphatics, areola tissue, and an internal venous plexus.

The anesthetic is placed outside the dura, not in the subarachnoid space where spinal anesthetics are inserted (see Fig. 23–13). The anesthetic blocks nerve fibers that transmit pain.

An epidural is used once labor is firmly established and progressing and the client requests pain relief. Epidural analgesia is now more site specific, extending from T10 to L1 in the first stage of labor. It extends to the sacral sections in the second and third stages (Bonica, 1994; Cunningham et al., 1997). For abdominal delivery, the block extends from the 8th thoracic level to the first sacral dermatome (Fig. 23–14). Continuous epidural infusions are often used during labor. When compared with intermittent injections, continuous infusions improve maternal analgesia and fetal safety.

Prior to epidural insertion, the nurse administers intravenous fluids to expand the woman's circulating volume. For epidural insertion, the woman may sit on the side of the bed or lie on her side. If she is sitting, the nurse or the woman's partner supports her

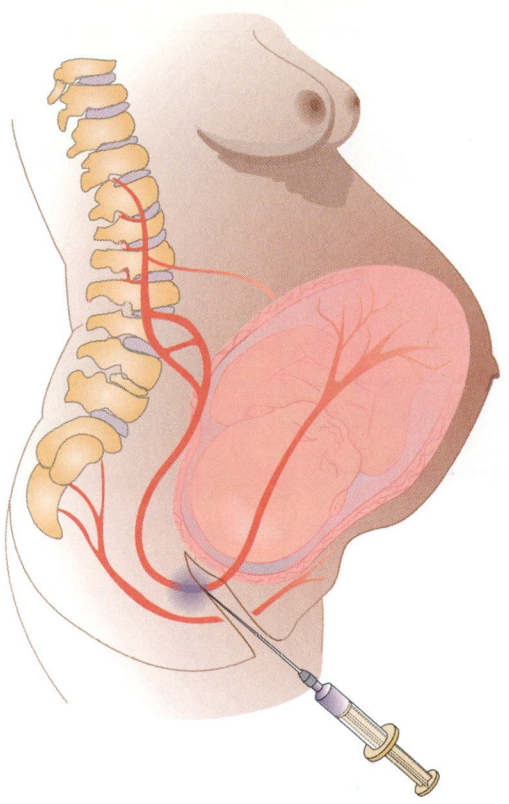

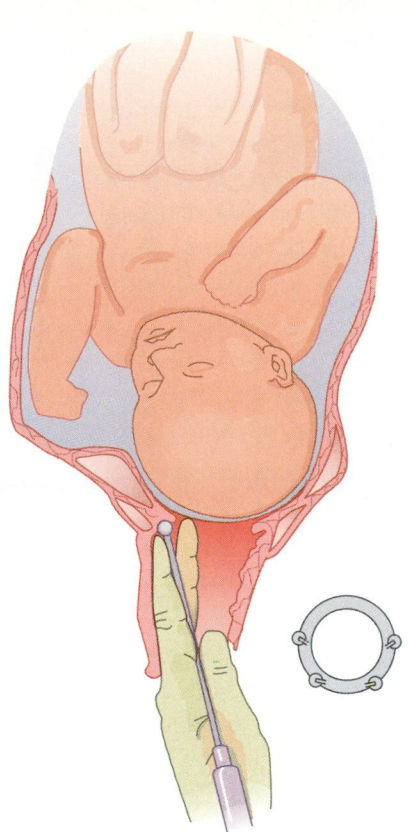

FIGURE 23–9. Paracervical block. Sensory pathways and site of interruption, in relation to fetus.

FIGURE 23–10. Technique of paracervical block. *(Reproduced, with permission, from Zuspan, F.P., & Quilligan, E.J. (1988).* Douglas-Stromme operative obstetrics *(5th ed.). Norwalk, CT: Appleton & Lange, p. 134.)*

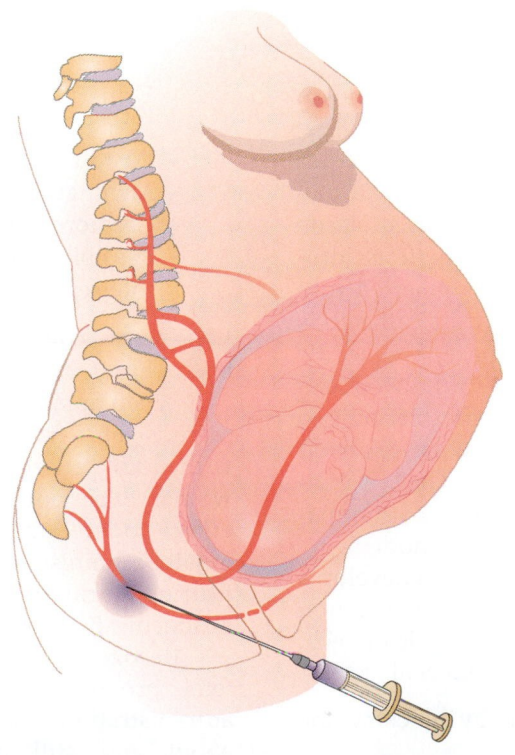

FIGURE 23–11. Diagram of site for pudendal nerve block.

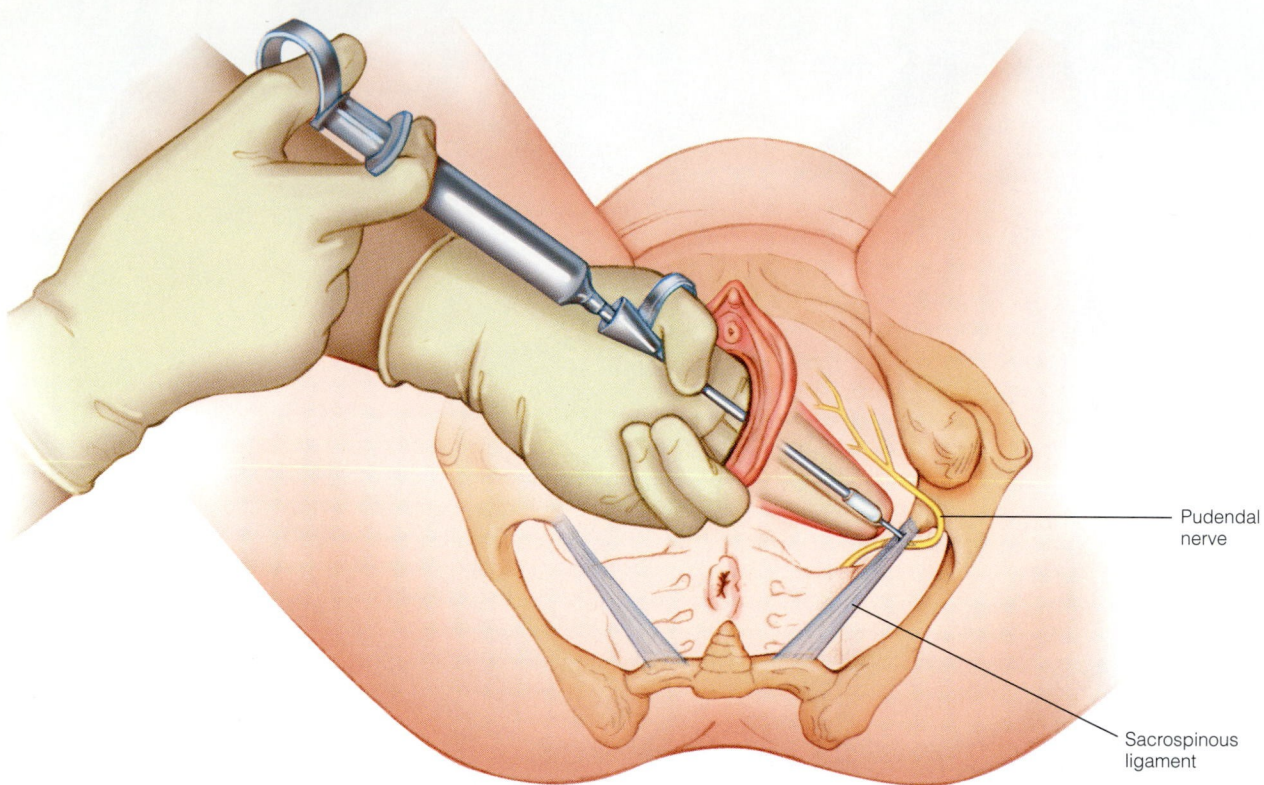

FIGURE 23–12. Technique of transvaginal pudendal block showing the needle extended beyond the needle guard and passing through the sacrospinous ligament to reach the pudendal nerve. *(Reproduced, with permission, from Cunningham, F.G. et al. (1997). Williams obstetrics (20th ed.). Stamford, CT: Appleton & Lange, p. 389.)*

shoulders while she bends at the waist. If the woman lies on her side, she flexes her spine and puts a pillow under her head, but not under her shoulders. After cleaning the area with a solution such as povidone-iodine (Betadine), the administrator places a sterile towel under the woman. A local anesthetic is infiltrated and then the epidural needle is inserted into the epidural space L2–3 or L3–4. A thin catheter is passed through the needle into the space. The needle is withdrawn and the catheter taped to the woman's back. She resumes a comfortable position. Periodic to continuous local anesthetic medication is delivered into the catheter via a volumetric pump. The box entitled Administration of Epidural Anesthesia summarizes the procedure involved with this method.

If the dura is punctured, the woman can develop a headache (nursing care is described in the next section with side effects of spinal anesthesia). Complications of epidural anesthesia include (Cunningham et al., 1997):

- Maternal hypotension caused by blocking the sympathetic tracts
- High or total spinal anesthesia

- Urinary retention
- Headache
- Postdural puncture seizures
- Meningitis
- Cardiorespiratory arrest
- Possible slowing of labor and delivery
- Interference with maternal pushing

Long-term complications include headaches and backaches (Cunningham et al., 1997).

When opiates are injected into the epidural space, there is relief from pain. Opiates are generally given with local anesthetics, such as bupivacaine. The woman experiences quick pain relief, decreased shivering, and reduced motor blockage. Side effects of opiate administration with epidural block include pruritus, urinary retention, nausea, vomiting, and headaches (Cunningham et al., 1997).

Recognizing that the upright position facilitates fetal progress through the birth canal, epidural administration can now enable the woman to walk about and still be comfortable. Monitoring for hypotension, motor function, FHR, and uterine con-

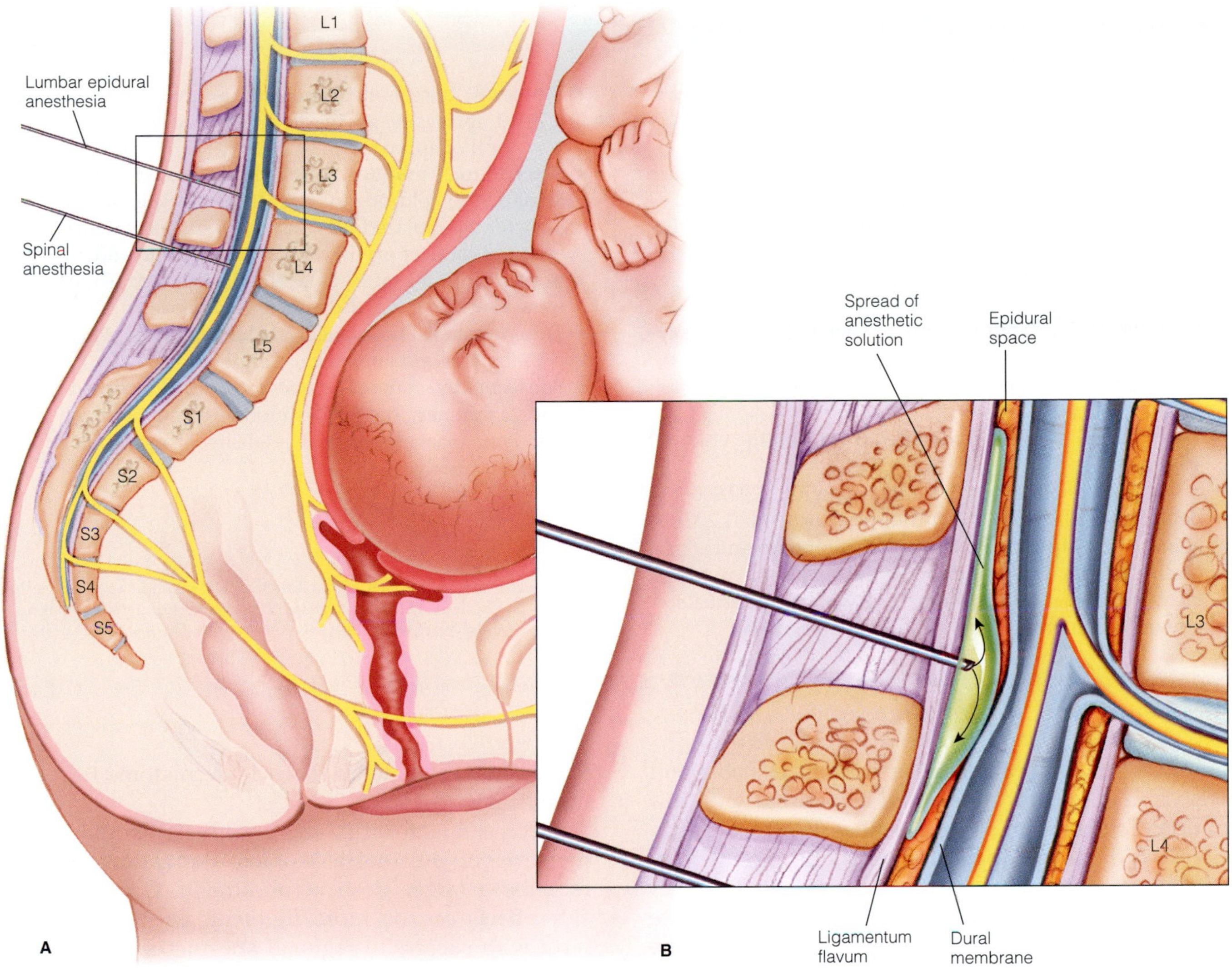

Lumbar epidural
anesthesia

Spinal
anesthesia

Spread of
anesthetic
solution

Epidural
space

Ligamentum
flavum

Dural
membrane

A

B

FIGURE 23–13. A. Placement of epidural and spinal anesthetics. **B** illustrates needle in epidural space, located between the dura and vertebrae. The slight bulge illustrates the dura being pushed away from the tip of the needle by the force of the injection.

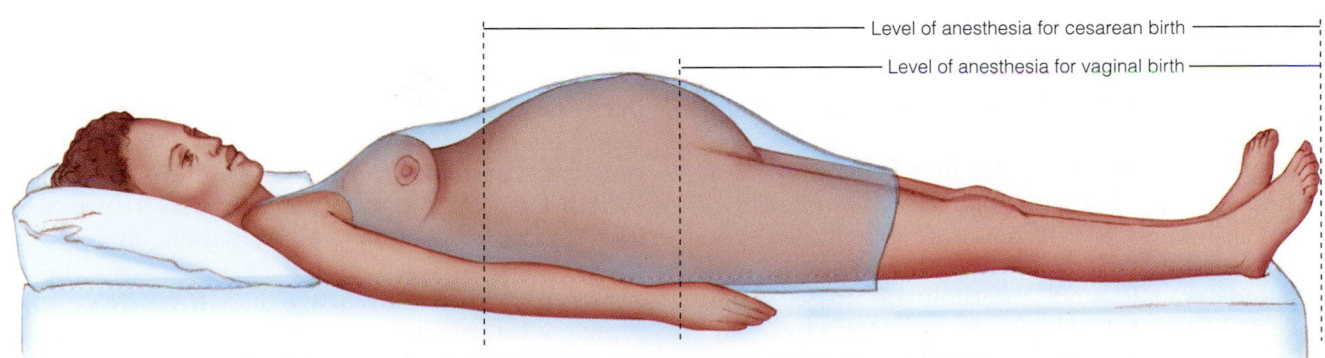

Level of anesthesia for cesarean birth

Level of anesthesia for vaginal birth

FIGURE 23–14. Anesthesia levels for vaginal and cesarean births. *(Adapted, with permission, from Ross Products Division, Abbott Laboratories, Columbus, OH 43216 from CEA #17, Regional.)*

▶ ADMINISTRATION OF EPIDURAL ANESTHESIA

- Informed consent is obtained, and the obstetrician consulted.
- Monitoring includes the following:
  - Blood pressure every 1 to 2 minutes for 15 minutes after giving a bolus of local anesthetic.
  - Continuous maternal heart rate monitoring during induction of anesthesia.
  - Continuous FHR monitoring.
  - Continual verbal communication.
- Hydration with 500 to 1000 mL of Lactated Ringer's solution.
- The woman assumes a lateral decubitus or sitting position.
- The epidural catheter is threaded 3 cm into the epidural space.
- A test dose of 3 mL of 1.5% lidocaine with 1:200,000 epinephrine or 3 mL of 0.25% bupivacaine with 1:200,000 epinephrine is injected after careful aspiration and after a uterine contraction (to minimize the chance of confusing tachycardia that results from pain with tachycardia secondary to intravenous injection of the test dose).

- If the test dose is negative, one or two 5-mL doses of 0.25% bupivacaine are injected to achieve a cephalad sensory level of approximately T10.
- After 15 to 20 minutes, the block is assessed using loss of sensation to cold or pinprick. If no block is evident, the catheter is replaced. If the block is asymmetric, the epidural catheter is withdrawn 0.5 to 1.0 cm and an additional 3 to 5 mL of bupivacaine is injected. If the block remains inadequate, the catheter is replaced.
- The woman is positioned in the lateral or semilateral position to avoid aortocaval compression.
- Subsequently, maternal blood pressure is recorded every 5 to 15 minutes. The FHR is monitored continuously.
- The level of analgesia and intensity of motor block are assessed hourly.

Reproduced, with permission, from Glosten, B. (1994). Local anesthetic techniques. In Chestnut, D.H. (Ed.). *Obstetric analgesia: Principles and practice.* St. Louis: Mosby-YearBook, p. 354.

---

tractions are performed. If the woman is stable and wishes to ambulate, she should be assisted with this option (Youngstrom, Baker, & Miller, 1996).

To provide prolonged analgesia, the anesthesiologist may administer a narcotic through the catheter before it is removed. The narcotic interrupts opiate pain receptors at the level of the cord. This is done often following a cesarean birth.

For a **spinal block,** also called a subarachnoid block, anesthetic is injected through the second, third, or fourth interspace. It is used for vaginal or cesarean delivery (see Fig. 23–13). The needle is inserted below the spinal cord, not into it, as some women fear. Although the needle is inserted at the lumbar level, the sensory blockage is felt higher, to the level of the fourth thoracic dermatome (T4). The drug acts on the spinal nerve roots and prevents both nerve transmission and sensation of pain. The effect begins with the toes and spreads to the perineum and, then, the legs and abdomen.

Single injections of opioids may be administered any time during labor, although they are more effective in early labor. Sometimes, a double-needle technique is used to allow simultaneous injection of subarachnoid opioids and insertion of an epidural catheter. If the spinal opioids are ineffective, the epidural catheter is in place for additional analgesics.

A low spinal block, also referred to as a modified saddle block, is used for vaginal deliveries. Anesthesia extends to the tenth thoracic dermatome (level of umbilicus).

For cesarean birth, the anesthetic should reach the level of the fourth thoracic dermatome, which requires a larger dose of anesthetic. Consequently, side effects can be more frequent. During cesarean birth with successful regional anesthesia, the mother is awake and aware, yet feels no pain. Additional oxygen may be given by mask, but she is not intubated. An intravenous infusion is kept running for fluid and electrolyte therapy; it is also an available route for intravenous medications.

Occasionally, a woman feels pressure as the baby is delivered or pressure and nausea as the uterus is manipulated. Some women feel cold. After the cesarean delivery, shivering may occur, possibly related to loss of body heat from extensive sympathetic nerve blockade. After the procedure, warmed blankets will promote client comfort. In the recovery room, the woman will first feel touch. Then, motor function, position sense, temperature sensation, superficial pain, and autonomic activity return. (See Chapter 26 for additional information on cesarean delivery.)

Some women who have had a cesarean birth receive intravenous narcotic medications for 24 to 48 hours. They control the medication with a patient-controlled analgesia (PCA) pump. The pump, which operates on a time mechanism, administers a preset

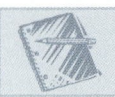

Client Teaching

Strategies for Pain Management

To help clients choose the pain relief measures that would be appropriate for them during labor, the nurse can suggest the following strategies:

- Call the childbirth education department at your hospital to learn about the program of prepared childbirth classes offered.
- Talk with your obstetrician or nurse-midwife about your options for pain relief measures while in labor.
- Explore with your obstetrician or nurse-midwife his or her views on natural childbirth.
- Ask to speak with nurses in labor and delivery at your selected birthing facility about the pain relief measures available to you.
- Make your own decision about what you want for pain relief or what measures you wish to use during labor, based on your education in childbirth preparation.

dosage in a predetermined period. The woman uses the machine switch to administer medication as needed. A safety mechanism prevents delivery of the medication outside the designated period.

The side effects of spinal anesthetics include:

- Hypotension
- **Spinal headache**
- Bladder dysfunction postdelivery
- Total spinal blockade with respiratory paralysis

A spinal, or postpuncture, headache is severe and often associated with neck stiffness when the woman is upright. Treatment and prevention are controversial. Keeping the client flat in bed has generally been ineffective. Vigorous hydration with intravenous or oral fluids may be of value, but the procedure still lacks conclusive empiric documentation. Providing abdominal support with a tight binder or girdle when the client is upright has resulted in some relief.

Fortunately, most spinal headaches resolve by themselves, usually within 3 to 5 days, using conservative therapy. Those that do not can be treated with an epidural blood patch. In the procedure, 10 mL of maternal blood is injected into the epidural space to seal the leak.

General Anesthesia. **General anesthesia** is rarely used for routine vaginal delivery, as it depresses the maternal and fetal central nervous systems, may cause maternal aspiration, and prevents the woman from participating in the birth and immediate bonding process. It is usually reserved for emergency cesarean and some operative vaginal deliveries. Nitrous oxide, volatile anesthetics, or intravenous drugs may be used. The time between induction of anesthesia and delivery is kept as short as possible.

Following general anesthesia, the nurse must closely monitor the woman for vomiting, aspiration, and respiratory depression. The newborn is also watched for respiratory depression.

Nitrous oxide is the only anesthetic gas currently used for maternity clients in the United States. By itself, it is not a potent or complete anesthetic and must be supplemented with a volatile anesthetic to ensure relief from pain.

Volatile anesthetics include halothane (Fluothane), enflurane (Ethrane), and isoflurane (Florane). These agents readily cross the placenta and can produce severe fetal depression.

Intravenous anesthetics are usually used in combination with inhalation agents, for example, thiopental (Pentothal) and ketamine (Ketalar).

General anesthesia usually involves a combination of several agents. After preoxygenation, the woman is rendered unconscious by a rapidly acting drug such as thiopental or ketamine. She then receives a rapid-acting muscle relaxant such as succinylcholine (Anectine) to permit placement of a cuffed endotracheal tube in the trachea. The tube ensures an open, clear airway and protects against pulmonary aspiration. Anesthesia is maintained with various inhalation agents. When the woman awakens following the birthing procedure, she is extubated, her upper airway reflexes are responsive, and she has no residual muscle weakness.

Table 23–2 describes anesthetics used in labor and delivery. The nurse should know about each medication or anesthetic agent used in labor and birth: the indications, dosages, and routes of administration, onset and duration of action, intended effects, effects on labor, maternal side effects, placental transfer times, and potential fetal and newborn effects. Debate continues concerning the safety of anesthetics for a pregnant woman and her fetus. Analgesia or anesthesia should be given judiciously. The nurse works with the woman, her family, and the interdisciplinary team to help a client select the pain relief measure most appropriate for her. These issues are outlined in the

▶ ADVANTAGES, LIMITATIONS, AND POTENTIAL COMPLICATIONS OF GENERAL AND REGIONAL ANESTHESIA FOR CESAREAN BIRTH

GENERAL ANESTHESIA

Advantages

- Pain-free induction of anesthesia and delivery
- Can be induced rapidly; useful in emergencies requiring immediate delivery (e.g., massive bleeding, severe fetal distress)
- Level of anesthesia readily controlled
- Associated with less hypotension and cardiovascular instability than regional analgesia
- Better control of airway and ventilation
- Preferable in clients with such conditions as gross neurologic problems, infections, or blood clotting problems
- Can be administered by a nurse anesthetist as well as by physicians
- May be preferred by some clients who do not want to be awake for abdominal delivery
- Used if regional analgesia is inadequate for birth

Limitations

- Client not awake for birth; loss of experience of being aware of baby's birth
- Client may be "groggy" in recovery room; possible delay in bonding
- In some settings, fathers not allowed in delivery room if mother asleep, thus, limitation of father's birth experience
- A less vigorous, sleepy baby at birth

Potential Complications

- Pneumonitis from aspiration of gastric contents (see text for medications to prevent this)
- Potential respiratory depression
- Problems with accessing and maintaining patent airway
- Tension pneumothorax related to positive-pressure ventilation
- Possible injury to teeth and mouth during intubation
- Neonatal depression

REGIONAL ANALGESIA: SPINAL

Advantages

- Client awake and able to experience birth; able to share birth with support person
- Pain-free birth; mild discomfort when administered
- Client able to breathe on own
- Oxygen administered by face mask; avoids risk of failed intubation, a complication related to general anesthesia
- Decreased risk of aspiration of gastric contents, as client remains awake
- Safer for emergency birth if client has recently eaten
- Does not irritate respiratory system
- Less neonatal drug depression than with general anesthesia

Limitations

- Requires skilled operator for administration
- Almost always given in single dose, which produces 1½–4 hours of analgesia; complications prolonging surgery may then necessitate general anesthesia
- Less likely to be given via spinal catheter than epidural because of greater risk of spinal headache
- Requires slightly more time to establish than general anesthesia
- Absolute contraindications—refusal; uncorrected hypovolemia; apparent clinical coagulopathy; infection at insertion site
- Relative contraindications—potential hypovolemia; laboratory coagulopathy; systemic infection; neurologic disease; back pain; fetal distress; severe preeclampsia
- Nausea and shivering related to the surgery may be experienced during the cesarean birth

Potential Complications

- Hypotension
- Hypovolemic shock
- Possibility of spinal headache, which may last up to 4 days postpartum (see text for treatment measures)
- Postspinal backache or soreness at site of injection
- Total spinal anesthesia with respiratory paralysis (occurs rarely)
- Vasopressor-induced hypertension from interaction of vasoactive drugs and ergot derivatives

REGIONAL ANALGESIA: EPIDURAL

Advantages

- Similar to advantages for spinal anesthesia
- Early breastfeeding
- Decreased stress response
- Lower risk of deep leg venous thrombosis
- Can be administered in single, repeated, or continuous dosages via catheter placed into epidural space
- With indwelling epidural catheter, length of procedure is not a problem
- Less incidence of headache
- Hypotension occurs less rapidly than with spinal anesthesia
- Easier to control than spinal
- Provides a route for administration of postpartum analgesics, such as the opioids
- Less blood loss than with general anesthesia

Limitations

- Similar to limitations for spinal anesthesia
- Time needed to initiate epidural block for effective analgesia
- Absolute contraindications—same as for spinal anesthesia

> ► ADVANTAGES, LIMITATIONS, AND POTENTIAL COMPLICATIONS OF GENERAL AND REGIONAL ANESTHESIA FOR CESAREAN BIRTH (continued)

- Relative contraindications—aspirin therapy; neuromuscular diseases, e.g., multiple sclerosis; spinal deformity or previous spinal surgery; systemic infection

Potential Complications
- Hypotension
- Nausea and vomiting
- Accidental misplacement of anesthetic and overdose into intravenous line can cause major problems such as cardiac arrest or convulsions

- Injection into subarachnoid space may cause total spinal anesthesia
- Intraoperative discomfort may occur and adjunctive medications may be necessary
- Specific complications relate to the drug used
- Epidural hematoma at site of injection
- Infection
- Nerve injury (rare, because any pressure on spinal cord or nerve roots is so painful that it is an unlikely occurrence)

box entitled Advantages, Limitations, and Potential Complications of General and Regional Anesthesia for Cesarean Birth.

Traditionally, women are permitted nothing by mouth (NPO) prior to general anesthesia. It remains important, however, to decrease the chances of gastric acid aspiration. Several methods are helpful. For example, sodium citrate (Bicitra), an antacid, is taken orally; 10 to 30 mL quickly increase gastric pH. A second dose is recommended if more than one hour has passed since the first dose and when anesthesia is to be given (Cunningham et al., 1997).

In addition, a histamine-blocking agent, such as ranitidine (Zantac), may be given intravenously with sodium citrate about 2 hours before elective use of general anesthesia. Ranitidine can also be given the night before surgery. This combination maintains gastric pH above 2.5 for a longer time and does not increase gastric volume.

Effervescent cimetidine (Tagamet) 400 mg/ sodium citrate 0.9 M in 15 mL of water also alkalinizes gastric contents. It maintains the gastric pH higher than if an antacid were used. It is effective for more than 1 hour after ingestion.

For women fasting before an elective cesarean birth, omeprazole taken in 40-mg capsules at bedtime and in the morning reduces gastric volume and acidity (Malinow, 1993). It inhibits the activity of the acid pump, which is found at the secretory surface of the gastric parietal cell. Gastric acid formation is blocked (Skidmore-Roth & McKenry, 1997).

The antiemetic metoclopramide (Clopar) may be given prior to anesthesia for urgent cesarean birth. It increases the tone of the lower esophageal sphincter within 2 to 5 minutes of intravenous administration and promotes gastric emptying, thereby lowering the chance of reflux and regurgitation.

► DECIDING WHICH ANESTHESIA

The type of anesthesia used for a cesarean birth depends on whether the delivery is an emergency or elective procedure. Obstetric emergencies, such as massive bleeding and severe fetal distress, necessitate immediate cesarean delivery with the fastest mode of anesthesia, usually general anesthesia. In some situations, such as failure to progress in labor or failure of labor induction, immediate delivery is not crucial. The woman may have a working epidural already in place; therefore, this method is used (Table 23–3).

Client preference also influences the type of anesthesia selected. (Some women do not wish to be awake during the surgery.) General anesthesia, however, is not encouraged because of maternal and fetal complications. Another influence is that not every hospital has staff round-the-clock who are able to provide regional as well as general obstetric anesthesia. The obstetrician, anesthesiologist, or nurse anesthetist works closely with the woman and her support person(s) to help her select the best method.

Ideally, anesthesia should be discussed prenatally with each client, as should the possibility of cesarean birth. A client will then have an opportunity to express her concerns related to anesthesia. Families, too, can help select the anesthesia if maternal and fetal safety allows. In collaboration with the obstetrician, anesthesiologist, or nurse anesthetist, the nurse can provide information about anesthetic options. Nurses must be knowledgeable about the topics related to anesthesia, because variation among hospitals can be great. Some hospitals, for example, permit a support person to be present if a woman receives general anesthesia; others do not.

▶ **TABLE 23-3**

Epidural Analgesia Following Cesarean Birth

Purpose	Relief of postpartum pain after cesarean or difficult vaginal delivery.
Placement of epidural catheter	During labor; before cesarean birth.
Administration of analgesic	Administered by clinician skilled in epidural management. One dose of epidural narcotic (e.g., morphine 4 to 5 mg) is usually given to cesarean clients at the time the abdomen is being closed or before the epidural catheter is removed. Pain is minimized, because the effects of epidural analgesia take hold as the effects from the epidural anesthesia wear off.
Action	Thought to act directly on spinal cord opiate receptors; block pain sensation without impairing motor, sensory, or sympathetic function. Systemic absorption plays little role in analgesia.
Example of analgesics used	Preservative-free morphine (Duramorph). Drug choice is based on client assessment and is made by the anesthesiologist. The usual dose of epidural morphine is 4 to 5 mg; no more than 10 mg per 24 hours is recommended. No restriction in breastfeeding is necessary, because of the low dose of epidural morphine used.
Contraindications	Allergy to the analgesics used (absolute contraindication). *Epidural morphine should not be used when staffing is inadequate to provide careful monitoring of respiratory adequacy for 24 hours after administration.* All clients receiving epidural morphine analgesia are at risk for respiratory depression and *must* be evaluated closely and carefully for 24 hours after the last injection.
Effectiveness	Varies according to the analgesic used. Effects of epidural morphine begin within 30 to 60 minutes and may last through the first 18 to 24 hours. Postpartum pain is usually minimal. "Breakthrough" pain may occur in some clients. Reasons for breakthrough pain include administration of too little of the narcotic analgesic or local anesthetic dissipation before the onset of morphine analgesia. Administration of additional parenteral narcotics to relieve breakthrough pain can raise the chance of respiratory depression and other adverse effects.
Side effects	• **Respiratory depression** (rate less than 12 per minute) or obstruction occurring as early as 30 minutes to 2 hours or as late as 16 hours after administration. Generally seen as a general decrease in rate, respiratory depression is more common 6–12 hours after administration. It is recommended that a physician evaluate the client in the first 24 hours before additional narcotics are given. Depression is treated with naloxone (Narcan) 0.4 mg IV if respirations are less than 10 per minute. • **Pruritus (itching)** is the most common side effect and is usually experienced on the face or upper body. Pruritus may begin within 3 hours and last up to 10 hours after administration. Generally, it is not severe and can be treated with either naloxone (Narcan) 0.04–0.2 mg IV, nalbuphine (Nubain) 5–20 mg IV, hydroxyzine (Vistaril) 50 mg IM, or diphenhydramine (Benadryl) 25–50 mg IM. • **Nausea and vomiting** may occur, but are less frequent than pruritus and occur in 10–30% of cases. It is uncertain if this results from the medication or from the labor itself, hypotension, other medications, or psychologic factors. It is treated with either nalbuphine (Nubain) 5–10 mg IV, naloxone (Narcan) 0.1–0.2 mg IV, or droperidol (Inapsine) 2 mg IM, or 0.625 mg IV. • **Urinary retention** may occur with epidural morphine. It is usually not a problem, because the cesarean client has a Foley catheter after the surgery. • **Herpes simplex labialis.** Some reports exist. It probably arises as a result of scratching to relieve pruritus and leads to reactivation of the virus.
Nursing interventions	For clients receiving postcesarean epidural analgesics, such as epidural morphine. • Make certain that risks and benefits are discussed prior to surgery. This is usually a physician's responsibility; however, nurses also need to be able to answer clients' questions and help clarify and dispel misconceptions. After the cesarean, nurses may need to present information about epidural analgesia again and to advise clients to report side effects. • Make sure resuscitation equipment is accessible and working; oxygen and suction materials should be at the client's bedside; keep naloxone (Narcan) available for management of narcotic complications; make certain a physician skilled in epidural analgesia and management of complications is readily available. • Assess client's level of pain. • Check respiratory rate, depth, and pattern for a full minute every 15 minutes for the first hour, every hour for the next 24 hours, and then every 2 to 8 hours (close assessment for first 24 hours). • Assess other parameters indicating respiratory status, such as level of alertness and agitation. • If respirations are suppressed, inform physician without delay; give naloxone (Narcan) as ordered. • Assist client to assume semi-Fowler position to minimize chance of respiratory depression. If appropriate, apply apnea monitor/pulse oximeter to aid nursing observations (however, apnea monitors curtail client movements, interfere with normal activities, tend to give many false alarms, and can be a source of stress). • Maintain intravenous infusions for 24 hours in case of need for resuscitation measures. • Assess presence and degree of itching. Reassurance alone may be adequate for mild itching. Cool compresses may provide some relief. If severe itching occurs, naloxone (Narcan) and or diphenhydramine (Benadryl) may be used for control.

▶ **TABLE 23-3** *(continued)*

Epidural Analgesia Following Cesarean Birth

	• Observe for nausea and vomiting, between 4 and 7 hours after administration. Droperidol (Inapsine) or other antiemetics given intravenously may decrease nausea, yet maintain analgesia. • Maintain indwelling Foley catheter for 12 to 24 hours after cesarean to minimize complications related to urinary retention. • Continue usual postcesarean care (turning, blood pressure assessments, fundal checks, and so on).
Benefits	Prolonged pain relief Early ambulation, better ability to turn, cough and deep breathe because of less discomfort; therefore, decreased risk of postoperative complications related to pain-induced restricted mobility (e.g., atelectasis, pneumonia, thrombophlebitis). Lower doses of narcotic are needed to control postcesarean pain when the epidural rather than systemic route is used. Decreased need for sedation or other analgesics. Potential benefits to attachment, related to greater feelings of maternal well-being and ability to care for her newborn.
Drawbacks related to epidural morphine analgesia	Potential complications (see Side Effects). Need for careful, frequent monitoring, especially during first 24 hours. Need for adequate staffing and staff expertise to provide monitoring and to intervene appropriately should complications arise. Need for presence in the hospital of a physician skilled in the management of epidural analgesia and its complications.

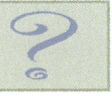

Commonly Asked Questions

I want to try to go natural, but if the pain gets too bad during labor, can I have something to help me?

Of course. There are many different pain medications and ways of giving them, and we will discuss these options with you so as to determine what is best for you and your baby. We will work with you to help make you as comfortable as possible during your labor. You can let us know when you feel that the contractions are becoming too much to handle.

What if I change my mind again and don't want medications after I receive the first dose?

If you do not wish to have medications, you will not receive them. You will only get what you are comfortable with. We will give you as much or as little of the medications as is safe and effective for you and your baby.

Will the medications hurt my baby?

The medication dosage is specific to help you with your contractions but not harm your baby. We will check your baby through fetal heart rate monitoring as well as check your vital signs and your contraction patterns during your labor to make sure that the medication is not producing harmful side effects.

What if I want to breastfeed my baby right after delivery? Will the baby be too sleepy from the pain medications?

We will continue to monitor you and the baby during your labor as well as check that you receive only the amount of medications you need. Some babies are sleepy and slow to nurse, but the nurses here and on the postpartum unit will help you with breastfeeding.

Care of the Client in Labor

It is 6 AM and Brenda Kiernan, a 26-year-old gravida 1, para 0, has just been admitted to the labor and delivery unit of the local community hospital. She has been having contractions since 11 PM the previous evening. Contractions are now 5 minutes apart. She is examined and her cervix is 3 cm dilated and 100% effaced, and the fetus is at 0 station. Her membranes are intact. She desires an epidural for her pain.

▶ Assessment

- Client states she is uncomfortable, tired, feels warm and sweaty, and is experiencing significant pain.
- Client reports that the mucus plug was passed at 5 a.m., but states that her water has not broken yet.
- Vital signs:
  - Blood pressure: 126/78
  - Temperature: 98.8°F
  - Pulse: 78

- Respirations: 26
- Height: 5 feet 6 inches
- Weight: 165 pounds
- Contractions: every 5 minutes for 45 seconds; 50 mm Hg
- Cervix: 3 cm dilated, 100% effaced
- Fetus: ROA position
  138 FHR

Nursing Diagnosis

Pain, related to uterine contractions

Expected Client/Family Outcomes	Nursing Action/Intervention	Evaluation
Client will demonstrate effective breathing pattern during contractions within 30 minutes.	Review client's practiced breathing pattern. *Rationale:* The nurse needs to be familiar with what the client was taught and has practiced. This helps the client incorporate the learning into actual experience.	Client demonstrates her breathing technique. Client seeks help in getting comfortable during labor.
Client will be more in control of contraction discomfort and have a decreased respiratory rate within 30 minutes.	Coach client on effective breathing regimen to use during contractions. *Rationale:* When a client has not mastered a specific method of childbirth preparation, the nurse can provide the teaching. Effective teaching helps the client become more independent and comfortable.	Client's respiratory rate decreases to 18 per minute. Client and coach work on breathing technique during each contraction. Client becomes more comfortable with each contraction.

Nursing Diagnosis

Knowledge deficit, related to unfamiliarity with the labor experience

Client will ask questions about her care and what to expect during labor.	Explain procedures and review the labor process. *Rationale:* An informed client experiences less pain, is more comfortable during labor, and is more receptive to teaching.	Client is able to explain what is happening with her labor.

Expected Client/Family Outcomes	Nursing Action/Intervention	Evaluation
Client will tell staff when she needs immediate assistance with pain relief.	Keep the client and her coach informed about her condition and progress. *Rationale:* Explanations keep the client involved and informed.	Client informs the nurse when she feels her contractions change and become more uncomfortable.

Nursing Diagnosis

Fear, related to the unknown experience of labor and birth

Client will be able to respond to directions and questions within 1 hour.	Encourage the support person to use massage techniques to help relax the client. *Rationale:* Relaxation exercises decrease pain and relax the client, which lessens anxiety and fear.	Client breathes more slowly and becomes more relaxed with each contraction.
Client will tell the support person and nurse what will help her the most within 1 hour.	Encourage the support person to reinforce the teaching given to the client. *Rationale:* Education improves knowledge base and decreases fear.	Client asks questions and explains answers to the support person.

Chapter Highlights

► All women experience labor differently and the pain associated with labor is influenced by variables such as parity and age; racial, cultural, and ethnic factors; coping mechanisms; relaxation methods; emotions; attitude; knowledge level; confidence; support systems; environment; fatigue; nausea, vomiting, and diarrhea; length of labor; and maternal and fetal positions.

► Pain is highly subjective and the nurse should never deny or minimize the pain a woman in labor is experiencing but, rather, help the woman overcome it.

► Nonpharmacologic methods of pain relief include hydrotherapy; change in temperature; acupressure; therapeutic touch; imagery; hypnosis; acupuncture; effleurage; abdominal pressure; transcutaneous electrical nerve stimulation; biofeedback; comfort measures; distraction; and application of childbirth education principles.

► Pharmacologic methods for pain relief, such as analgesia and anesthesia, vary depending on the client's needs as well as the physiologic state of the mother and fetus.

► Common anesthetic methods used in labor and delivery include local, regional (paracervical, pudendal, epidural, and spinal), and general (gas, volatile anesthetics, and intravenous anesthetics).

► The nurse must ensure that a woman has information concerning the available pain relief methods available during labor so that she can make an informed decision in selecting the appropriate method.

► After the client has made a decision about the use of pain relief methods, the nurse incorporates the assessment of maternal and fetal needs into a plan for effective pain management.

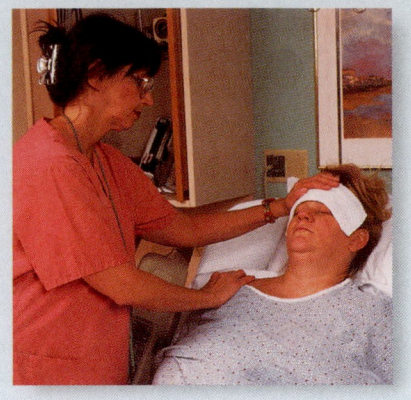

After reading the vignette at the beginning of this chapter, use what you have learned to answer these questions.

1. What factors may influence Cathleen Harris' response to the pain she is experiencing during labor?

2. What other measures can Margaret Kiely, RN, provide to ease Cathleen Harris' discomfort?

3. How can the nurse help Cathleen and Bill Harris make informed decisions about the methods of pain relief available to them during the labor process?

Critical Thinking Questions

▶ References

Atrash, H.K., Koonin, L.M., Lawson, H.W., Franks, A.L., & Smith, J.C. (1990). Maternal mortality in the United States, 1979–1986. *Obstetrics and Gynecology, 76*(6), 1055–1060.

Bonica, J.J. (1994). Labour pain. In P.D. Wall & R. Melzack (Eds.), *Textbook of pain* (pp. 615–641). New York: Churchill-Livingstone.

Bonica, J.J., & McDonald, J.S. (1995). *Principles and practice of obstetric analgesia and anesthesia* (2nd ed.). Baltimore: Williams & Wilkins.

Costello, D. (1993). Peripheral nerve blocks for labor and delivery. In M.C. Norris (Ed.), *Obstetric analgesia* (pp. 297–306). Philadelphia: J.B. Lippincott.

Cunningham, F.G., MacDonald, P.C., Gant, N.F., Leveno, K.J., Gilstrap, L.C., Hankins, G.D.V., & Clark, S.L. (1997). *Williams obstetrics* (20th ed.). Stamford, CT: Appleton & Lange.

Flynn, R. (1993). Epidural anesthesia for cesarean section. In M.C. Norris (Ed.), *Obstetric analgesia* (pp. 391–417). Philadelphia: J.B. Lippincott.

Kennell, J., Klaus, M., McGrath, S., Robertson, S., & Hinkley, C. (1991). Continuous emotional support during labor in a US hospital: A randomized controlled trial. *Journal of the American Medical Association, 265*(17), 2197–2201.

Lowe, N.K. (1991). Maternal confidence in coping with labor: A self-efficacy concept. *Journal of Obstetric, Gynecologic, and Neonatal Nursing, 20*(6), 457–463.

Lowe, N.K. (1996). The pain and discomfort of labor and birth. *Journal of Obstetric, Gynecologic, and Neonatal Nursing, 25*(1), 82–92.

Malinow, A.M. (1993). General anesthesia for cesarean delivery. In M.C. Norris (Ed.), *Obstetric analgesia* (pp. 365–390). Philadelphia: J.B. Lippincott.

Melzack, R., & Wall, P.D. (1965). Pain mechanisms: A new theory. *Science, 150*(3699), 971–979.

Melzack, R., & Wall, P.D. (1983). *The challenge of pain.* New York: Basic Books.

Mokriski, B.L.K. (1993). Physiologic adaptation to pregnancy: The healthy parturient. In M.C. Norris (Ed.), *Obstetric analgesia* (pp. 3–33). Philadelphia: J.B. Lippincott.

Oster, M.J. (1994). Psychological preparation for labor and delivery using hypnosis. *American Journal of Clinical Hypnosis, 37*(1), 12–21.

Rush, J., Burlock, S., Lambert, K., Loosley-Millman, M., Hutchison, B., & Enkin, M. (1996). The effects of whirlpool baths in labor: A randomized, controlled trial. *Birth, 23*(3), 136–143.

Shermer, R.H., & Raines, D.A. (1997). Positioning during the second stage of labor: Moving back to basics. *Journal of Obstetric, Gynecologic, and Neonatal Nursing, 26*(6), 727–734.

Simkin, P. (1995). Reducing pain and enhancing progress in labor: A guide to nonpharmacologic methods for maternity caregivers. *Birth, 22*(3), 161–171.

Skidmore-Roth, L., & McKenry, L. (1997). *Mosby's drug guide for nurses* (2nd ed.). St. Louis: Mosby-YearBook.

Youngstrom, P.C., Baker, S.W., & Miller, J.L. (1996). Epidurals redefined in analgesia and anesthesia: A distinction with a difference. *Journal of Obstetric, Gynecologic, and Neonatal Nursing, 25*(4), 350–354.

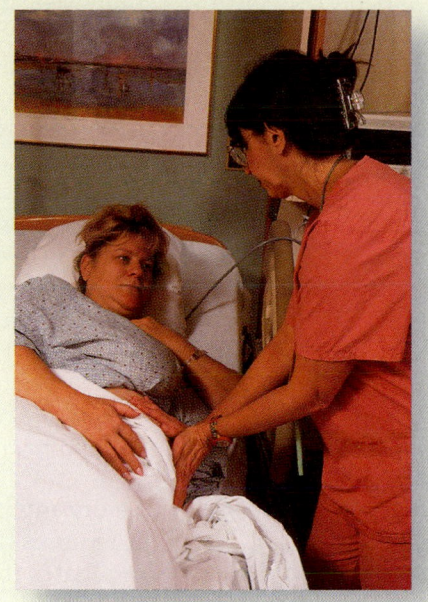

Cathleen Harris, who was admitted to the labor and delivery unit 7 hours earlier, sighs deeply as she experiences a contraction. This is her and her husband Bill's second pregnancy. Contractions are occurring every 3 minutes and last for 35 seconds. Her cervix is 7 cm dilated and 75% effaced.

Margaret Kiely, RN, approaches the bed in which Cathleen is lying on her left side. She states, "I'd like to palpate your abdomen to check your contractions." Cathleen nods her head and moves her gown aside to allow the nurse to place her fingers on Cathleen's abdomen. Cathleen asks, "Would it be all right if I kept my hand on my stomach while you do the procedure this time?" ■

24

Care of the Family During Birth

Childbearing is a significant life event, and families seek the assistance of the health care team to help them achieve a safe, satisfying birth experience. Nurses, in the multifaceted role of manager, coordinator, advocate, and facilitator of labor and delivery are also responsible for the health of the family structure. Maternity nurses base their care on principles that support the coping strengths of the family and promote healthy role definition and self-concept.

The nurse is an advocate for the family and coordinator of the delivery team. Nursing care during labor and delivery means one-to-one care for the woman giving birth and her support persons. The nature of the care will vary, depending on the risks and strengths the woman brings to her labor, the wishes of the mother and family, the events of labor, and where the labor and birth takes place.

The focus of this chapter is on care that is given during the stages of labor, including the psychosocial and cultural dimensions of the family. The procedures discussed may not occur in all instances and situations. It should be emphasized that labor and delivery is a normal physiologic process; however, nurses must be aware of the interventions that may be implemented during this time.

▶ NURSING CARE DURING THE FIRST STAGE OF LABOR

During the first stage of labor, the nurse determines whether the mother is in true or false labor, obtains informed consent, and evaluates maternal and fetal progress in labor. Several procedures may be performed during the first stage of labor; however, they are not used in all cases or in all settings. As with delivery of care throughout pregnancy, during the intrapartal period the nurse maintains conscientious adherence to universal precautions against the human immunodeficiency virus (HIV). Because the nurse may be exposed to maternal body fluids and blood (and potentially to HIV), a special reminder to use universal precautions is warranted. It is also important for the nurse to assess the psychosocial responses of the mother and father to the first stage of labor so that appropriate support and care are provided to the couple.

▶ False or True Labor

Women frequently have difficulty knowing if true labor has begun. Most pregnant women, particularly nulliparous women, fear they will mistake false labor as real. Because onset of labor symptoms may be mild

and perceptible only to the woman experiencing them, partners, family, and friends tend to regard the mother as the "expert" in determining whether labor has indeed finally begun. Clients, therefore, should be taught the difference between true and false labor and given information such as that in Table 24–1. The family should be advised to contact their health care provider if questions arise relative to labor's onset.

Early labor does not always follow the textbook picture. For example, contractile patterns are occasionally irregular and do not progress in a regular series, but still may indicate true labor. Therefore, clients should be advised to contact their health care provider when any signs of labor occur.

▶ Informed Consent

Before any intervention, informed consent is obtained. It requires that first a verbal explanation be provided of what is to be done including the risks, benefits, and alternatives of the procedure or medication. Occasionally, audio- or videotapes may be used to ensure consistent, accurate information for the consent, with time provided after the presentation for the client to ask questions. The client signs the consent form after her questions are answered. The conversation is documented in the client's chart. Ideally, obstetric explana-

---

▶ **TABLE 24–1**

Differences Between False and True Labor

False Labor	True Labor
Contractions are mainly abdominal.	Contractions are felt in abdomen and spread to lower back.
Contractions are irregular and may disappear during sleep or with activity.	Contractions may be widely spaced and somewhat irregular at onset. They usually progress with increasing intensity and progressively shortened resting interval. They do not decrease with activity.
Vaginal mucus is clear or slight threads of pink. Mucous plug may be expelled.	Mucous plug may be expelled. Mucus has definite pink tinge.
Fetus is more active or unchanged.	Fetal activity may lessen, but should never disappear.
Membranes are intact.	Membranes may rupture with "gush" of amniotic fluid or slow continuous seepage.
Cervix may be ripe and slightly dilated on sterile vaginal examination.	Cervical dilation and effacement are palpable on sterile vaginal examination and continue to progress.

tions should be given prenatally when the woman is not as anxious or preoccupied with labor and has time to think and read about issues of particular concern (in some states, the law requires that these consents be given prenatally when possible).

Whatever format is used, certain elements of informed consent must be explained:

- Procedure and its purpose (in a way that the client can understand)
- How it will feel
- Benefits and risks to mother and fetus
- Alternatives to the place, procedure, or medication and their benefits and risks
- How complications can be treated
- Information that the client is free to withdraw consent at any time.

The consent form is written in the client's primary language with the purpose, benefits, and risks carefully explained. It must have the client's signature, date of consent, and the signature of a witness certifying that the client was given a fair explanation and appeared to understand it.

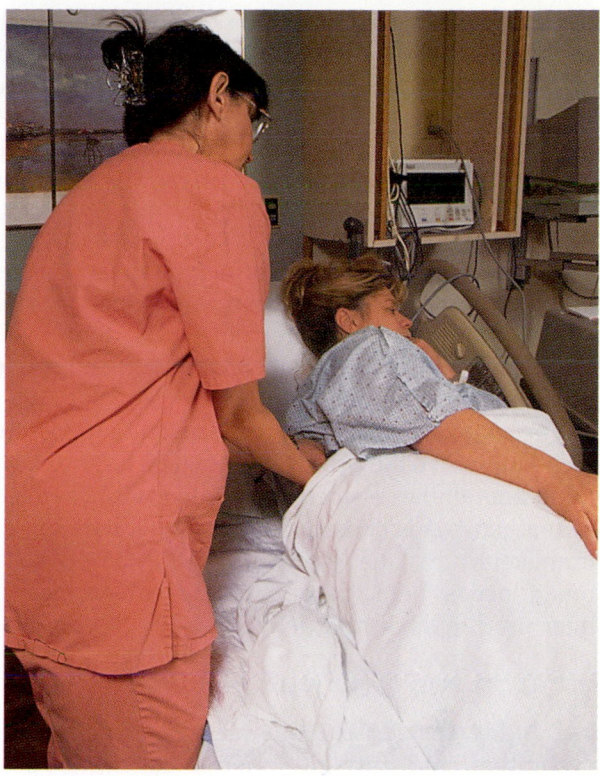

FIGURE 24–1. Administering a sacral backrub to the client can help relieve some of the discomfort experienced during the first stage of labor.

▶ Maternal and Fetal Progress in Labor

Throughout the first stage of labor, the nurse assesses maternal progress in labor by observing maternal vital signs and perineal signs. In addition, maternal behaviors, for example, facial expressions, positioning, remarks or noises, restlessness, and response to comfort measures and coaching, are observed. As labor progresses, a vaginal examination is done, contraction pattern monitored, and maternal hydration and elimination assessed.

The nurse may need to change the client's environment to facilitate labor. For example, additional coaching may help her to breathe more effectively, her position may need to be changed, the temperature of the room adjusted, or medications given for nausea or pain. Additional measures that may increase her comfort are providing ice chips, mouth care, cool washcloth, back rub (Fig. 24–1); cleaning body area soiled from blood, feces, or vomitus; changing bedclothes or underpads; and having someone remain with the woman.

Research has demonstrated that expectant fathers feel most helpful to their wives during labor (Nichols, 1993). Therefore, the support person's needs, including rest, nourishment, and encouragement, must be considered.

In monitoring fetal progress, the nurse must assess the heart rate (FHR), presentation, and position (see Chapter 22). In addition, the amniotic fluid is assessed for color and odor.

▶ Procedures

Certain procedures and treatments may be done during the first stage of labor; however, they are not done for all clients.

Shaving Pubic Hair

The major indication for shaving pubic hair is cesarean delivery; hair is removed from the abdomen to just below the pubic hair line. Some practitioners believe that removing hair reduces the possibility of infection, as hair carries bacteria and may interfere with the incision, repair, or healing. For vaginal births, shaving hair has been shown to increase the possibility of infection, not decrease it.

In the past, complete preparation for birth involved shaving the entire mons, perineal, and rectal areas. Then, shaving hair from the clitoral area to the rectum ("miniprep") generally replaced complete preparation. Often, shaving is not done at all.

When shaving is needed, equipment includes a shaving kit, sharp razor blade, special soap or Betadine, sponges, towels, and gloves. Wearing gloves, the nurse cleanses the skin and leaves it soapy for shaving. Where skin is not taut, it is held tightly in one direction while shaving the hair in the opposite direction. Since this procedure is often embarrassing to the client, the nurse needs to ensure privacy and support.

Evacuation of the Lower Bowel/Enema

Enemas are no longer used routinely in most facilities, although an enema or rectal suppository may be used to evacuate stool in the rectum. It is done if the woman requests it because of constipation and if there are no contraindications.

The woman may insert a rectal suppository, which eliminates the problem of watery fecal contamination and embarrassment associated with enemas.

If an enema is chosen, a Fleet enema may be self-administered by the woman, or the nurse if the woman needs help. Large volume enemas are no longer used in labor and delivery.

Hydration and Calories

Oral Nourishment. Fluids and nutrients prevent dehydration and provide calories to the laboring woman. The policy of prohibiting oral intake for women in labor has been questioned (Sharp, 1997). Oral nourishment may be taken by the woman as she feels the need.

Oral fluids may be taken throughout labor but they are usually limited to water, ice chips, and high-calorie clear fluids, as tolerated.

Intravenous Fluids. Although it is typical in many health care facilities to start an intravenous infusion routinely for all women in labor, there is seldom any real need for this intervention during normal labor (Cunningham et al., 1997). Intravenous infusion provides fluids and calories to the laboring woman via a vein, usually in the hand or arm. Infusion is beneficial when a woman does not want or is unable to drink or is vomiting. It is also necessary when epidural anesthesia is used.

When intravenous fluids are indicated, a nurse or other professional inserts a small catheter into the vein of the hand or forearm and connects it to tubing attached to a bag filled with sterile fluid (usually normal saline or lactated Ringer's solution—an electrolyte solution). The use of 5% dextrose in water (D_5W) is not recommended because it results in an increased incidence of hypoglycemia in the newborn. The nurse should have the proper solution ready along with Betadine or bacteriocidal cleansing wipes, tubing, tape, blood tubes for the laboratory tests, and protective pads to place under the intravenous site to prevent any blood from spilling on the floor or bedding. Having someone assist when inserting the IV line is helpful.

Inserting the line is painful and may cause bruising. The woman is at risk for infection at the site or in the vein. An intravenous infusion is also uncomfortable because it restricts movement of the affected limb and of the woman in general.

Bathing

Bathing during labor, either in a shower or tub, is a noninvasive means of providing comfort (Schorn, McAllister, & Blanco, 1993).

A woman may immerse herself in warm water, comfortable to her touch, or let warm water from the shower cover her body while she stands or sits in the shower. How long she remains is often up to the woman and the comfort afforded by the hydrotherapeutic effects of the water.

Induction or Augmentation of Labor

Induction of labor is the process of starting labor artificially with medications, primarily oxytocin (see box entitled Drug Guide: Oxytocin). **Augmentation** is the stimulation of labor once it has begun naturally; oxytocin or breast stimulation may be used. Prostaglandins, specifically PGE_2, are widely used in Europe for labor induction and have recently become available in the United States (Reilly, 1994).

Induction. To determine whether the client's condition is favorable for induction, a scoring system, for example, the Burnett scale or Bishop score, is often used. Cervical dilation, effacement, position, and consistency are noted, as well as the station of the fetal head. On the Burnett scale each item is rated from 0 to 2, with a total score of 0 to 5 indicating risk to mother and fetus, and 5 to 10 increasing the chance of delivery within 6 hours if adequate oxytocin is given. In the Bishop scoring system, a score of ≥ 9 indicates that labor may be induced with only a small chance of failure (Reilly, 1994).

If an induction is indicated, an external fetal monitor is applied and an intravenous line is started. Two intravenous bags are required, one containing oxytocin and the other, with no drug, is set up in case the oxytocin must be stopped or other medications need to be administered to the woman. The intravenous line to the oxytocin should be attached to an infusion pump to ensure that the correct amount of drug is administered. The bag containing the oxytocin must be labeled with the name of the drug and the number of units.

Augmentation. Augmentation may be achieved artificially using the same procedure described for

▶ DRUG GUIDE: OXYTOCIN

ACTION/INDICATIONS

Synthetically produced hormone similar to endogenous hormone produced by the posterior pituitary gland. Stimulates contraction of the uterine smooth muscle. Also facilitates milk ejection in lactating women. Induction of labor in clinical situations where prolongation of labor may be harmful to fetus, mother, or both. Augmentation of contractions in first and second stages of labor if labor is prolonged or dysfunctional uterine inertia occurs. Management of postpartum bleeding. Promotion of milk ejection in lactating women.

DOSAGE

Administered intravenously, intramuscularly, or as a nasal mist. Dosage determined by uterine response. *Induction of labor:* 1 mU/min, increased at 15-minute intervals by 1 mU/min until desired response. *Augmentation of labor:* 2 mU/min. *Postpartum bleeding:* 10 to 40 U added to 1000 mL nonhydrating diluent to control uterine atony. *Induction of milk ejection:* nasal preparation (40 USP units/mL) administered as spray or 1 drop in one or two nostrils 2 to 3 minutes before breastfeeding.

CONTRAINDICATIONS/PRECAUTIONS

Contraindicated for induction of labor in cases of cephalopelvic disproportion, unfavorable fetal position, or uterine scarring from previous surgery or when vaginal delivery is contraindicated. Use caution in fetal distress, partial placenta previa, prematurity, overdistension of uterus, grand multiparity, or history of uterine sepsis of traumatic delivery.

ADVERSE REACTIONS

Maternal

With large doses or in sensitive clients, hyperstimulation of uterus with strong and prolonged contractions, which could result in uterine rupture, postpartum hemorrhage, abruptio placentae, or impaired fetal blood flow. Also, hypotension, tachycardia, cardiac arrhythmias, and water intoxication.

Fetal

With excessive maternal doses, sinus bradycardia, cardiac arrhythmias, brain damage, intraventricular hemorrhage, and death from asphyxia.

DRUG INTERACTIONS

Severe hypotension can occur if oxytocin administration follows treatment with vasoconstrictive drugs. Concurrent use with cyclopropane may produce hypotension and bradycardia.

NURSING IMPLICATIONS

Labor and Delivery

- Assess and record maternal blood pressure and vital signs, intake–output ratio, nature of uterine contractions, and fetal heart rate and tone.
- Careful control and monitoring of infusion are essential.
- Use Y-connection so that infusion with oxytocin can be discontinued while keeping vein open.
- If contractions occur at less than 2-minute intervals or last 90 seconds or longer, or if monitor records contractions at about 50 mm Hg, stop infusion to prevent fetal anoxia, turn client on left side, give oxygen if necessary, and report.

Postpartum

- During delivery, IV oxytocin may be continued or IM oxytocin is easily injected deep into deltoid muscle; massage injection site for quick absorption.
- Fundus should be checked frequently during first few hours postpartum and several times daily thereafter.

General

Oxytocin administration should be supervised by persons having thorough knowledge of the drug and the skill to identify complications.

---

induction, without the scoring system. Augmentation can also be done "naturally" by nipple stimulation. The procedure is similar to the antepartal contraction stress test (see Chapter 18); however in this case stimulation is continued until a reliable labor pattern is established.

Benefits. Induction may help women whose deliveries are postdates or for women with pregnancy-induced hypertension, Rh incompatibility, or diabetes. Fetuses who are intrauterine-growth-retarded are also benefited because the risk of induction is less than that of letting the pregnancy continue.

The benefits of induction and augmentation are similar, but with augmentation, because labor has already started, complications are less probable. Augmentation accomplished by nipple stimulation also has a decreased risk, as no drugs are involved.

Risks. Induction and augmentation are sometimes contraindicated when a mother has a contracted pelvis, scarred uterus, overdistended uterus (multiple fetuses or polyhydramnios), grand multiparity, prematurity, or acute fetal distress. Complications from these procedures include hypertonic uterus and hypertonic contractions, fetal distress, uterine rupture, iatrogenic prematurity of the fetus, and neonatal jaundice. In addition, breast stimulation for augmentation has only recently been used on a large scale so that the best procedures, the precautions, and risks are not well documented.

Amniotomy

Artificial rupture of the fetal membranes (amniotomy) is done during labor to prevent the fetus from aspirating amniotic fluid with meconium at delivery (the exact mechanism or timing of this complication is not clear), to permit internal fetal monitoring, or to induce or augment labor. It is contraindicated when the presenting part is not engaged, when the woman is not in active labor (unless it is done for induction), funic (cord) presentation occurs, or placenta previa occurs.

The nurse explains the procedure to the woman, listens to the FHR and, as with any contact with blood or bodily fluids, uses universal precautions. The physician or nurse-midwife performs a vaginal examination and then ruptures the forewaters with the amniohook or Allis clamp, keeping the hand in the vagina and slowly letting the fluid out (Fig. 24–2). The color, consistency, and volume of fluid are noted. The nurse evaluates the FHR, places a clean pad under the woman, and charts the date, time, and results of the procedure and the FHR before and after the procedure. If an electronic monitor was used, the date, time, and results of the procedure are also noted on the graph paper.

Benefits. Amniotomy permits internal electronic monitoring and scalp pH sampling. In addition, the practitioner can view the amniotic fluid directly to ascertain that there is no meconium, which, if present, might indicate fetal distress. Amniotomy may also enhance the contracting ability of the uterus.

Risks. Risks include possible prolapse of the umbilical cord and infection. Some studies have shown that early rupture of membranes can lengthen the labor, lower the fetal scalp pH, increase the number of FHR decelerations, increase caput succedaneum, and increase cranial bone disalignment (Cunningham et al., 1997).

Spontaneous Rupture of the Membranes. Membranes rupture as a natural event during labor. After rupture, the nurse should immediately assess the FHR and amniotic fluid, noting the fluid's color and odor, if present, and estimating the quantity. A vaginal examination may also be done to rule out a prolapsed cord.

Fetal heart rate is of primary concern. A forceful gush of amniotic fluid could permit a loop of umbilical cord to slide between the fetal presenting part and the maternal pelvis. Subsequent cord compression would compromise oxygenation of the fetus, resulting in fetal bradycardia.

In addition, the mother's wet bed linens and bed clothes should be changed to ensure the mother's

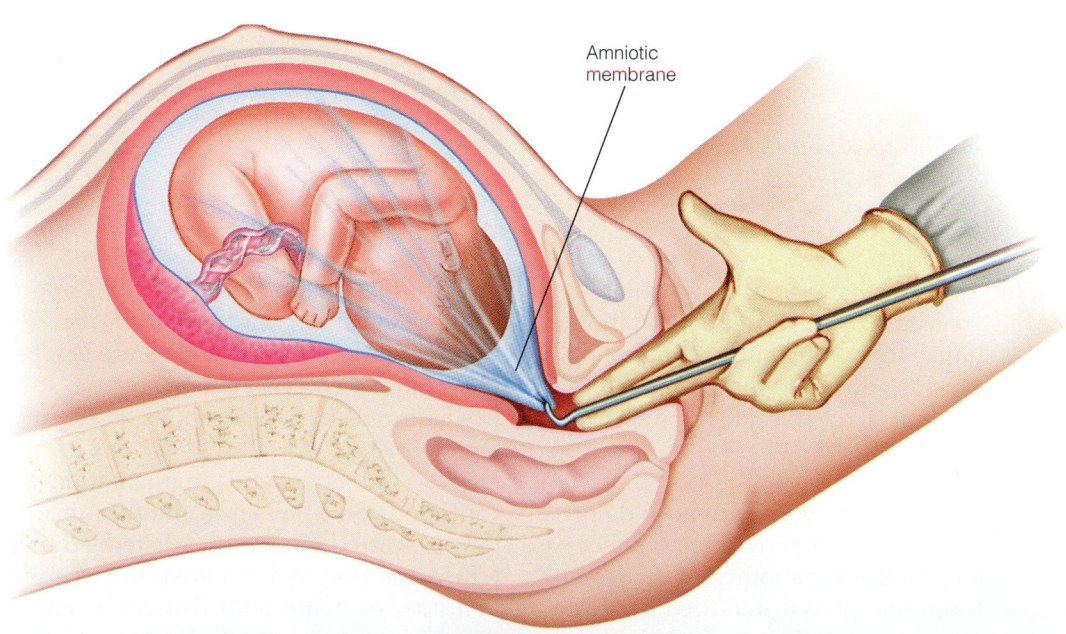

Amniotic membrane

FIGURE 24–2. Amniotomy.

comfort. Charting involves the date and time of membrane rupture, the color and consistency of the fluid, and the FHR. This information is placed on the client's chart and graph paper if an electronic monitor is used.

Positioning for Labor

Nursing care during the intrapartum period includes helping a mother assume positions for labor and birth (Fig. 24–3). The choice of position is determined by custom, comfort, fetal status, force of uterine contractions, and location of the discomfort.

During labor, a woman should not lie on her back for prolonged periods because of the negative effects of supine hypotension syndrome on both mother and fetus. In terms of efficiency of uterine contractions and overall reported maternal comfort, the best positions for labor are (in descending order) upright, sitting, lying on left side, and lying on right side. Ambulation has also been noted to be effective in progress of labor (Albers et al., 1997).

A woman is encouraged to take the position of greatest comfort and not to feel confined to one position. The electronic fetal monitor is adjusted to meet the client's comfort; the woman *is not* positioned to facilitate use of the machine. If monitoring is continuous the woman should be able to move about in or around the bed or to a nearby chair. When internal electronic monitoring is used, telemetry should not prevent her from walking. If a client is walking during active labor, she should be accompanied by someone who can assist her during contractions.

Benefits. When a woman assumes comfortable positions, particularly those in which she is walking, uterine contractions are more efficient, leading to shorter labor. Less pain medication is needed. An upright position during labor produces fewer side effects in the fetus; complications such as hypoxia, bradycardia, and acidosis are noted if a woman is supine or in a dorsal position and less frequently noted when she is upright.

Risks. The physiologic and physical safeness of a position during a particular phase in labor determines maternal risk. More research is needed regarding how positions influence the progress of labor; however, it is known that lying flat in bed throughout labor is the least helpful physiologically, in terms of fetal and maternal outcomes.

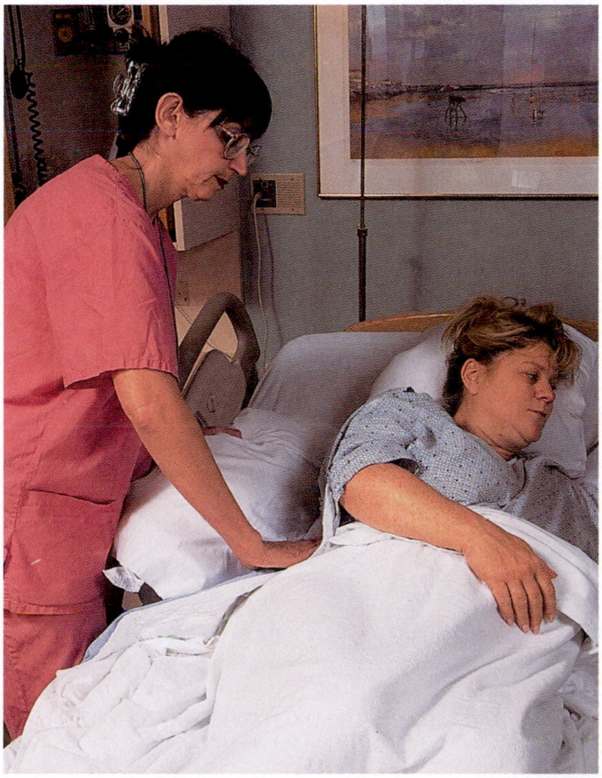

▶ Maternal Psychosocial Reactions

Maternal reactions to labor are unique and varied. Past experiences, cultural background, relationship with significant others, fatigue, personality, and parity all contribute to the expectant mother's responses. Variations also occur in relation to frequency, intensity, and timing of the mother's psychologic reactions. Common reactions to labor include excitement and uncertainty; anxiety and fear; recruitment and use of support; use of role models; alterations in body image; expression of pain; maintenance of control; and hostility and aggression. The nurse needs to understand these reactions to interpret a woman's progress in labor and to provide supportive care during the intrapartum period. Table 24–2 outlines maternal behavioral characteristics during the first stage of labor. These guidelines are generalizations that help assess progress in labor and strengthen therapeutic decision making.

Maintenance of Control

A well-substantiated, recurring theme in the literature is the need for control or mastery in the psychologic task of childbirth. Control in childbirth is defined as a woman's perception of active participation and involvement in the birth process (Evans & Jeffrey,

FIGURE 24–3. The nurse helps the client in labor to assume a side-lying position to promote efficiency of contractions and maternal comfort.

► **TABLE 24-2**

Behavioral Characteristics Demonstrated by Women During the First Stage of Labor

Behavior	Latent	Active	
		Early	Transition
Nonverbal			
General	Makes decisions readily	Makes decisions slowly, may ask support person to help determine choices	Does not make or has difficulty making decisions
	Anxiety mild to severe		Anxiety may be severe
	Excited labor has begun	Anxiety level either diminishes or escalates	Increased dependency
	Hypervigilant		Does not want to be left alone
	Functions independently	Demonstrates dependency	Irritable, especially when touched
	Tolerates being alone for intervals of time	Desires presence of others; does not tolerate being alone very well	Withdrawn
	Can be distracted—reads, plays cards, watches TV	Distraction becomes increasingly less possible	Responds slowly to auditory stimuli directed toward her
	Sociable	Less sociable	Hiccups
	Demonstrates awareness of activities beyond immediate environment	Withdraws awareness to immediate environment	
	Responsive to auditory stimuli	Responds to auditory stimuli directed toward her; may not respond to other auditory stimuli in room	
	Use of role models as a standard for behavior and progress		
Response to uterine contractions	Continues previous activity	Anticipates onset	Disoriented as to onset and completion
	May pause, cease conversation, and feel contraction	Ceases all other activity	Self-control tenuous
		Increasing body tension	Body very tense
	Easily distracted from focus on contraction	Squeezes support person's hand, siderail, pillow, and so on	Vicelike grasp
	Tolerates external stimuli; usual breathing pattern	Implements control of breathing	May refuse to grasp another's hand, preferring an inanimate object
	Pain: generally not identified or designated as cramping located more in lower back	Evidences increasing discomfort located in the pelvic area; may rub lower back, which aches	May hyperventilate
	Cultural norms affect the expectation and expression of pain		Evidences extreme discomfort located in pelvic area; if back ached previously, now very intense; indicates sensations of internal pressure
Facial cues			
Eyes	Open	Begins to close eyes between contractions	Closes eyes
	Follows activities in environment	Opens eyes with onset of contraction, then closes; looks toward activity in environment, then closes	May open eyes at onset of contraction, then close
	Maintains eye contact when interacting with others		Does not visually indicate awareness of activity in environment
		May make initial contact while interacting with others, then closes eyes	Closed, no contact when interacting with others
Expression	Generally smiles spontaneously	Forced smile, if any	Grimaces
	Facial muscles relaxed	Facial muscles may be tense	Facial muscles fixed and tense
	May demonstrate anticipation, excitement, or fear	Takes on a serious demeanor	May clench teeth
		May reflect pain	Serious
			May reflect pain
			Worried or startled expression
Posture	Alert	Body tension noticeable	Body tension very noticeable, difficulty relaxing
	Generally relaxed body	Flexes or extends extremities depending on position	Increasing flexion of extremities depending on position
			May brace body

▶ **TABLE 24-2 (continued)**

Behavioral Characteristics Demonstrated by Women During the First Stage of Labor

Behavior	Latent	Active	
		Early	*Transition*
Movement	Purposeful Normal pace Moves during and between contractions Able to control body movement Alters position without assistance	Purposeful or aimless More slowly paced Moves between contractions Less sense of control of body movement May use help to move Reflects a feeling of body heaviness Restlessness may begin	Purposeful motion may occur Very slowly paced Moves between contractions with encouragement Minimal sense of control of body movement When necessary to move, usually needs help and considerable urging Reflects a feeling of extreme body heaviness Movement appears to take much effort Marked restlessness may be noted
Verbal			
Quantity	Very verbal Complete sentences Elaborate	May talk between, not during, contractions Fewer, more fragmented, partial sentences Less elaboration	Speaks only to impart messages Short fragments of sentences Separate words No elaboration
Quality	Normal tone Distance appropriate Normal pace or very rapid	Quiet, subdued tone Not distance appropriate Normal pace	Some normal tones Whispers, shouts Not distance appropriate
Content	Seeks information about self, baby, others, environment, procedures Discusses previous labors Shares information about self Social talk	Seeks information about self, baby, procedures Asks for help Tells what she wants done Answers questions briefly Cries out in pain, may moan or groan	Cries for help at once Commands Protests pain is too much May scream, moan, or groan May ask to go home or tell others to go away
Subject	Self Self in relation to others Others	Self Self in relation to others	Self Self in relation to others
Orientation to time			
Past	30%	20%	1%
Present	58%	72%	98% right now!
Future	12%	8%	1%

1995; Knapp, 1996). During labor, women try to regulate their behavior, emotions, body functions, interpersonal relations, and ability to manipulate the environment. Many stressors simultaneously affect a woman's ability to maintain control in labor. Examples of such stressors are pain, sensory overload, sleep loss, a strange environment, new role requirements, and the physiologic changes resulting from the labor process.

During early labor, an observer may not realize when a contraction occurs, unless the woman mentions the contraction or the uterus is monitored for activity. When anxiety level is not too high, women watch television, read, play cards, and interact socially during early labor. They converse in normal tones and in a normal manner.

Women search for information as a means to help maintain control. They seek information by asking about themselves, the baby, other people, procedures, and the environment. Information is taken in visually, as women follow all of the activity around them (Evans & Jeffrey, 1995).

In early labor women make decisions readily, and most women want this responsibility. As labor progresses to the active phase, women expend increasing energy to maintain control. Control may become tenuous, and some women experience dependent behavior or loss of control as labor intensifies. Awareness and focusing attention become increasingly restricted as efforts to maintain control become more difficult. Once the active phase of labor begins, women respond to questions directed toward them, but they generally do not respond to other activity within their immediate vicinity. They continue to withdraw, turn inward, and shut out extraneous stimuli, and they respond more slowly to activities directed toward them.

The woman's search for information as a means of maintaining control continues into active labor. Requests for information now tend to focus more narrowly on self, baby, and procedures. Women begin to close their eyes between contractions, opening them at the onset of a contraction to inform others that a contraction has begun, then closing them again.

Nursing Interventions

There are several nursing strategies to help the woman cope with her labor. Strategies for the woman experiencing anxiety include assessing her level of anxiety; identifying factors such as past experiences, fear, and pain that contribute to anxiety; educating the woman about institutional routines and procedures; providing options and informed consent; intervening in a nonjudgmental manner; providing supportive nursing interventions to the woman and family members; and intervening in a timely fashion before the cycle of fear, pain, and tension becomes established.

The nurse also identifies cultural factors that influence selection of support persons during labor. The nurse should be instrumental in establishing institutional policies that allow for flexibility in attendance of significant others during labor and at birth. The nurse assists the support person by providing rest and nourishment, as well as encouragement.

Gathering data about the laboring woman's expectations is part of a nurse's assessment. This information helps the nurse to identify actual and potential stressors that affect the mother's psychosocial and physical reactions during the intrapartum experience. Other nursing strategies include assessing the possible influences of expectations and of role models on the course of the mother's labor; assessing coping methods that the mother used in previous labors; maintaining a nonjudgmental attitude toward the mother's chosen coping strategies (such as screaming); and assisting the mother to feel comfortable adopting coping mechanisms that work for her.

Women commonly experience alterations in their body image during pregnancy. Each woman has a personal space or body boundary that she may perceive as being threatened by caregiving procedures (e.g., vaginal examinations). A nurse who understands how alterations in body image affect women during labor and why a woman reacts as she does is better able to assist the woman in regulating nonproductive behavior. Strategies to assist the mother in coping with alterations in body image include assessing the mother's response to stimuli, such as pain; teaching the mother about the procedures that may be used during labor and delivery prior to their use; getting permission and alerting the mother before touching her for a procedure; and performing nursing interventions in such a way that the mother maintains a sense of being intact and in control.

The nurse should also understand the varied reactions a woman can have to childbirth pain (Fig. 24–4). The nurse assesses the pain experience to identify when intervention is needed. Knowledge of childbirth pain and the relationship of pain to the physical changes that occur during labor provides a basis for determining progress or failure to progress in labor. Understanding pain variations and their causes also helps the nurse to accept each woman's expression of pain in a positive, nonjudgmental manner and to give the support each family needs throughout the childbirth experience (see Chapter 23).

Strategies for helping the mother maintain control during the labor process include assessing the mother's expectations, level of awareness, and focus of attention during labor; reducing surrounding stimuli in the environment that may cause sensory overload; and keeping the mother and her support person informed of the progress of labor and procedures that may be done. The nurse also promotes maternal decision making during labor by providing choices and flexible standards. It is also important for maternal control to help the mother focus attention on a contraction and support the mother and support person in the use of childbirth preparation techniques.

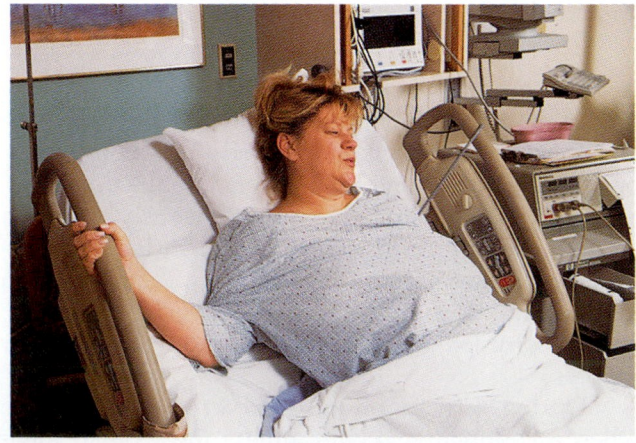

FIGURE 24–4. During the first stage of labor, the woman may express the pain she is experiencing by body movements such as grasping the bed rail during a contraction.

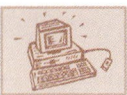

Research Abstract

Women's Evaluation of Labor and Delivery Nurses

With the advanced technology available in obstetrics today, such as central monitoring stations and automated vital sign machines, it is easy for nurses to rely on machines when caring for women in labor. This qualitative study documented women's evaluations of their labor and delivery nurses. Sixty-one women were interviewed, using tape recorded, open-ended questions. Ninety percent evaluated their nurses favorably, 10% unfavorably. Nurses were evaluated favorably because of their positive participation (80%), acceptance (78%), information giving (75%), encouragement (65%), presence (53%), and competence (7%). The authors concluded that, although technical competence is important, manner, provision of supportive care, and acceptance of each woman as a unique human being may be the nurse's most important characteristics.

Application to Practice

Nursing care that is sensitive, personal, and supportive is a major factor that contributes to the quality of the childbearing couple's experience of labor and delivery. The various physiologic and psychosocial responses and changes that occur in women during labor require that nurses be both technically competent and emotionally interactive with their clients so that an effective integration of the two aspects is achieved and the goal of a positive labor and delivery outcome is attained.

Mackey, M.C., & Stepans, M.E.F. (1994). Women's evaluation of their labor and delivery nurses. Journal of Obstetric, Gynecologic, and Neonatal Nursing, 23(5), 413–420.

▶ Paternal Psychosocial Reactions

Many types of families exist, and paternal involvement may be nonexistent; however, most women in labor are accompanied by the child's father. Common responses to labor as experienced by the father include level of involvement during childbirth; provision of supportive actions to the woman; control; providing protective actions; anxiety; guilt; anger and hostility; neglect of personal needs; and pride and self-esteem and are discussed below. Table 24–3 presents selected nursing interventions designed to help fathers manage these responses positively.

Level of Paternal Involvement

Paternal participation during childbirth has become accepted and, to some extent, expected practice. An expectant father attends labor and delivery to provide support to his partner and to see his baby born. Unfortunately, some men feel pressured to attend and are therefore doing so to avoid guilt feelings. The father should be regarded as a unique human being who is sharing a challenging experience with his partner. Unlike mothers, fathers may choose how involved they will be during this important event. As a result, their levels of participation during birth differ. Indeed, some fathers will not wish to be present during labor and delivery for cultural or other reasons.

Fathers usually want to know as much as possible about what the mother experiences. They may have attended childbirth classes and demonstrate an understanding of the birth process. They usually seem to enjoy coaching, caregiving, and supporting the mother. They want to share as much as possible and participate as equal partners in the experience. A few fathers identify completely with the mother, internalize the experience, and may actually experience labor with the mother. Fathers should be included in the labor experience and need support in their role as coach (Chandler & Field, 1997).

Some fathers tend to be observers. Although they are delighted with the thought of becoming a father, they may be unable to imagine themselves actually involved in the birth process. Others may accompany the mother during childbirth but do not become obviously involved in the event. They talk and interact with the mother while she is comfortable and needs distraction. When the mother withdraws and focuses inward, these fathers also seem to withdraw.

Supportive Actions

Fathers provide various forms of support for the laboring woman, for example, by their presence, touch, praise, verbal coaching, helping, and caring (Chou, Chao, & Yee, 1994) (Fig. 24–5). However, fathers do not always use the most effective coaching techniques, and their interactions may not be helpful to the laboring woman.

Involved fathers generally coach the woman during labor. Most often these fathers coach relaxation and breathing techniques, because that is what most have learned in prenatal classes. If an electronic

▶ **TABLE 24-3**

Nursing Interventions for Care of the Father During the First Stage of Labor

Responses	Nursing Interventions
Level of paternal involvement	Assess the father's desired level of involvement and respect his choices in participation
	Support his chosen level of involvement in a nonjudgmental manner
	Care for the father's needs during labor and delivery
Supportive actions	Avoid competition with the father in supporting the mother
	Do not expect the father to perform the nursing role (e.g., do not leave fathers alone with the mothers for extended periods)
	Offer the father respite from his role as the support person for the mother (e.g., encourage him to take a break, let him know that you will stay with the mother in his absence, assure him that someone will call him if there is a change in the mother's or baby's status)
	Offer nourishment
	Praise his role as support person
	Inform the father of the progress of labor and the procedures to be performed
	Make him feel valuable
Control	Prepare the father for changes in the mother's behavior
	Anticipate factors such as fear that might cause him to feel out of control
	Modify surrounding stimuli
	Inform the father of the progress of labor and the procedures to be performed for the mother
	Give positive reinforcement for his participation, regardless of the level
Protective actions	Nurture the father
	Communicate potential maternal behavioral changes that may occur during the progress of labor
	Explain procedures carefully
	Respect the father's coping style
	Respect the couple's birth plan
	Provide care that attempts to meet the couple's expectations
Anxiety	Assess the father's level of anxiety
	Orient him to the labor and delivery areas
	Explain procedures and the progress of labor
	Answer questions
	Support the father in his role as support person
	Maintain a nonjudgmental attitude concerning the father's display of anxiety
Guilt	Assess the cultural background of the father
	Assess the father's satisfaction or dissatisfaction with previous birth experiences
	Allow him to verbalize his feelings
	Support the father's chosen level of involvement in the birthing experience
Anger and hostility	Assess the father's reasons for anger, including feelings of helplessness
	Provide him with comfort and support
	Maintain a nonjudgmental attitude toward paternal behaviors
	Allow the father to verbalize his feelings
Attention to own needs	Encourage breaks and reassure the father that you will remain with the mother and call if anything happens
	Provide a comfortable chair
	Offer nourishment
	Show the father how to use proper body mechanics
	Minimize surrounding stimuli in the environment such as sights, sounds, or odors as much as possible
	Reassure the father that his responses are normal
Pride and self-esteem	Provide the father with positive reinforcement for his role in supporting the mother
	Value the father as a person
	Focus on successful supportive interventions

monitor is being used, fathers quickly learn to use the monitor to help their coaching. If a monitor is not in use, fathers may write down the time each contraction begins. As labor progresses fathers frequently identify the contraction pattern. They recognize when a contraction is beginning and start coaching in anticipation of the next contraction.

Control

Fathers also want to be in control during the childbirth situation. Regardless of how well prepared a father is, the childbirth situation is unfamiliar and strange, especially for first-time fathers. As a result fathers do not always know what is expected of them.

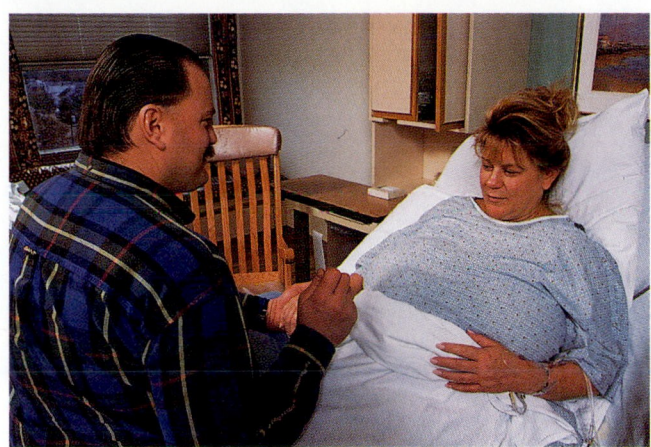

FIGURE 24–5. The father is providing support to the mother during labor by helping her to focus on a family photo that is meaningful to both of them.

In Western countries, fathers may act as protectors and providers for their partners. In the birth setting, the woman's responses to labor may be overwhelming, and the father may perceive that he has little control over rules and events deemed routine by caregivers. To retain control, fathers seek information.

Fathers' ability to maintain control varies widely. Some fathers remain calm throughout labor. They may be effective in coaching their partners. Other fathers may consciously give control of their partners' care to others.

There are times when the father loses control, often in response to his partner's loss of control. In such instances the father may persist in use of measures that are not helpful. He may be unable to change his coaching techniques, either because he does not recognize a need to or because he does not know any other technique. This type of behavior often continues until the couple receives help.

Protective Actions

Fathers try to protect their partners during childbirth. The father may request physical care for the woman, pain relief, and assistance with labor. As the demands of labor become all consuming, the father may communicate the woman's wishes to the caregiver or even demand that something be done. These demands often occur in relation to requests for pain relief, perceived failure to make progress toward delivery, or perceived risk.

The father protectively seeks information and asks questions about procedures, equipment, and caregivers. He asks questions to assure himself that the best available care is being given. He monitors equipment to be sure it functions as explained (Chou, Chao, & Yee, 1995).

Protective reactions also include defending goals set for the labor experience prior to its onset. For example, expectant parents sometimes plan not to use analgesics or anesthetics during labor. The mother may be afraid that she may change her mind once labor begins. As a precaution she may ask the father to promise that he will not let her use medications even if she asks for it. Should labor fail to progress as expected, or if she has unbearable pain or fatigue, the woman may change her mind and ask for medication. The father, based on his promise, may then refuse to allow the medication to be given. It is important to remember in such cases that the father is not acting harshly. Caregivers need to consider his promise as well as the woman's distress and preexpectations. In other cases the father evaluates the situation and encourages the use of medication. This type of situation also may occur in relation to other interventions such as use of fetal monitors.

Anxiety

During labor, fathers experience a range of emotions related to the partner's birth experience and to the experience of becoming a father.

Fathers concerned for the well-being of their partners and babies frequently are anxious during labor. Anxiety occurs at all levels of intensity. Mildly anxious fathers may seek information as a way to manage their anxiety. They may be unsure about what to do and what they are allowed to do in the unfamiliar birthing environment. These fathers respond positively to reassurance and encouragement from caregivers. They welcome instruction about what they can do to be of assistance.

As his partner's labor intensifies, an anxious father may become disorganized, particularly when his efforts to help seem to be ineffective. Such fathers respond well to caregivers' redirecting their activities and helping them to understand that changes in interventions are needed as labor progresses.

Guilt

Fathers may feel guilty when they observe their partners in distress, particularly if the father was the one who suggested having the baby. Guilt may be verbalized openly or expressed nonverbally, for example, by crying.

Fathers also may feel guilty because of messages received from caregivers. Caregivers may inappropriately convey a value judgment about how involved the "ideal" father should be in childbirth. This judgment fails to consider the capability of each father as an individual, as well as his cultural background. As a result, a father who is not totally involved in active coaching may feel guilty and stressed.

Anger and Hostility

Fathers may react with anger and hostility during labor. These strong emotions tend to erupt when the father has done all he can to help his partner and sees few results for his efforts. The father does not know how to help and begins to feel inadequate and powerless. If this continues, he may become frustrated and angry, striking out at others. His anger may be directed at his partner, or he may accuse the nurse and other caregivers of not helping enough.

Attention to Own Needs

Fathers often pay little attention to their own physical and emotional needs during the childbirth experience. They feel that they should support their partners. Many fathers choose not to take a break for rest or nourishment because they are concerned something will happen while they are away or that their partner will be upset if they go.

All fathers become fatigued without sleep or food over an extended period. Standing near the bedside or sitting in an uncomfortable chair for hours is fatiguing. Fathers may also remain in awkward positions as they give sacral pressure or hold their partners without admitting their own discomfort. Fathers also may be unaware of the effects unaccustomed sights, sounds, or odors have on them until they become nauseated or emotionally upset.

Pride and Self-Esteem

Fathers experience a sense of pride and self-esteem when they feel they are needed and helpful during labor. A father who coaches his partner while providing her physical comfort and psychologic support has a sense of achievement during labor (Fig. 24–6). He realizes he is able to help when his partner needs him and thus shares a mutually satisfying experience. Other fathers who accompany their partners but do not actively participate also experience a sense of pride. A sense of achievement and self-esteem results from each father giving what he is able to do successfully.

▶ NURSING CARE DURING THE SECOND STAGE OF LABOR

Nursing management for the childbearing family during the second stage of labor involves support and care through the so-called expulsive stage and culminates with the long-awaited birth of the baby (Fig. 24–7). As with the first stage of labor, certain procedures may or may not be performed, depending on the birth setting, the wishes and needs of the mother, the needs of the fetus and family, and the treatment modalities of the practitioner. As with the first stage of labor, nurses also need to be aware of the psychosocial responses of the mother and father to the second stage and develop strategies to support families during this process.

▶ Maternal and Fetal Physiologic Responses

Contractions in the second stage are intense, strong, and frequent and may reach a maximum duration of 90 seconds. To assess intensity and duration of a contraction palpation is used. If a monitor is used, the monitor tape alone is not sufficient, as the involuntary urge to bear down or push may distort the tracing through artifacts (false marking on the tape) or positioning.

Bloody show increases as capillaries are torn during fetal descent. It must be emphasized that a flow of blood, spurting blood, or clotted blood is not normal and requires that the nurse further assess the client and report the findings.

As the fetal head compresses the rectum, the laboring woman perceives the pressure as an urge to defecate. If feces are present in the rectum and descending colon, defecation frequently occurs, which

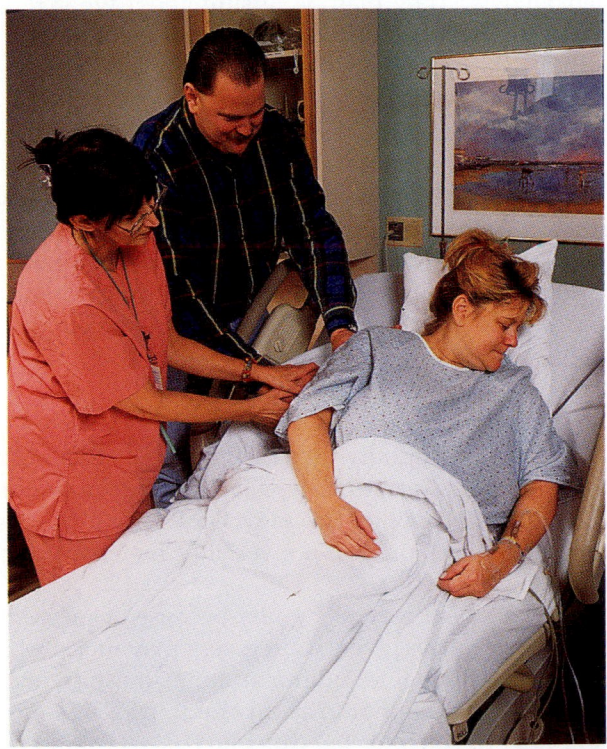

FIGURE 24–6. The nurse guides the father in performing comfort measures for the mother during labor such as supporting her back during contractions so as to alleviate discomfort.

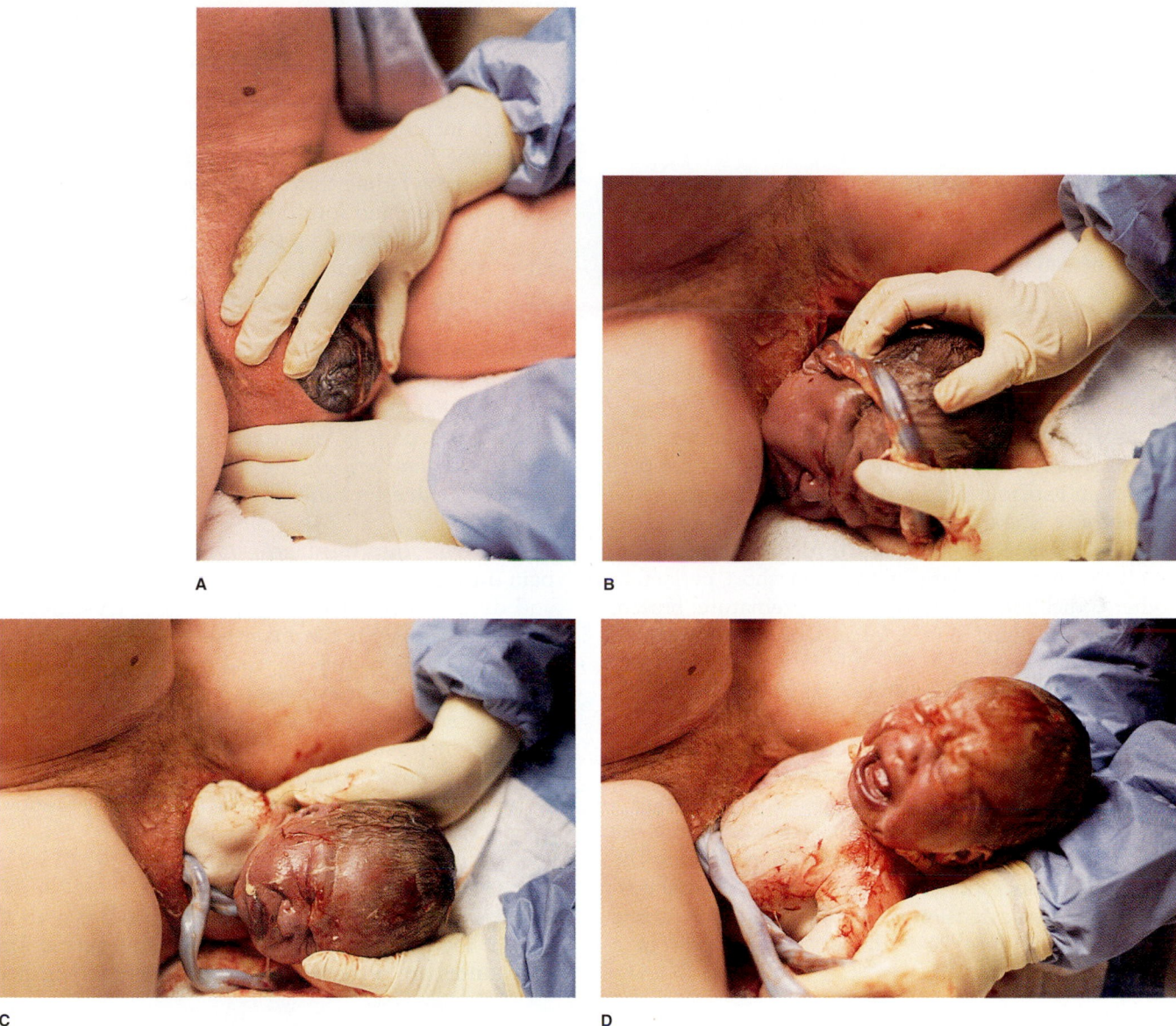

FIGURE 24–7. Sequence of delivery. **A.** Fetal head distends perineum and appears at introitus. **B.** Delivery of fetal head begins. **C.** Completion of delivery of fetal head. **D.** Shoulders are delivered. *(Photos courtesy of Harriette Hartigan/Artemis.)*

may embarrass the mother. She is given hygienic care and padding is quickly replaced between contractions.

Although formerly detailed bearing down instructions were given to a mother, the developing trend is to allow a mother to set her own bearing down pattern. The support person quietly encourages the woman throughout her natural bearing down efforts. Research has shown that women, when allowed to follow their own body sensations to push during labor, have an increased sense of accomplishment (Bergstrom, Seidel, Skillman-Hull, & Roberts, 1997). They may also have shorter labors than those

who are recumbent and given instructions. The support person may alert the women (who may sleep between contractions) to the onset of a contraction. The mother may require physical support of her back as she attempts to bear down. The involvement of support persons, including the nurse, in this final predelivery stage will continue during delivery (Gagnon, Waghorn, & Covell, 1997).

Assessment of fetal well-being during the second stage of labor is continuous. Although the body of the fetus is generally well adapted to withstand the stress of labor, a primary goal of those caring for mother and baby is to minimize intrapartum risk and maximize health. This goal is achieved when caregivers have employed every means available to ensure that no sign of distress, regardless of how fleeting, is ignored and that the client remains alert and informed.

► Procedures

Two procedures that may be done during the second stage of labor are an episiotomy and a forceps/vacuum extraction. The nurse provides continuity of care throughout the birthing process and during operative obstetric procedures.

Episiotomy

An **episiotomy** is an incision into the perineum to facilitate delivery of the fetus and to protect the perineum and surrounding muscle and fascia from tears. Episiotomy should not be routinely performed. It may be indicated when a fourth degree laceration is likely because of a large fetus or a short perineum. Other indications are to deliver a premature, breech, or distressed fetus, and a forceps or vacuum extractor delivery.

Two types of episiotomies that are often used are median (midline) and mediolateral (Fig. 24–8). The incision for the midline episiotomy is made from the fourchette straight down toward the rectum but not including it. The mediolateral episiotomy is either a right-angle or left-angle incision extending from the fourchette at a 45-degree angle into the perineum. The mediolateral incision is designed to decrease the possibility that an extension of the incision will tear into the rectum. Figure 24–9 demonstrates repair of a median episiotomy.

Benefits. Evidence is growing that routine episiotomy is not beneficial to the mother or baby (Labrecque, Baillargeon, Dallaire, Tremblay, Pinault, & Giugras, 1997). Benefits often listed of routine episiotomy include preventing trauma to the fetal head, shortening the second stage, preventing ragged lacerations, and avoiding third-degree lacerations (into the anal sphincter) and fourth-degree (into the rectum).

The two types of episiotomies also have advantages and disadvantages. Practitioners in different parts of the world have preferences. Most European practitioners prefer the mediolateral episiotomy; most American practitioners, the median. The median is more anatomically sound in that the muscles are separated rather than cut across. It is easier to repair, heals better, pain is less, dyspareunia less common, and blood loss is less. The mediolateral episiotomy has fewer extensions into the rectum.

Risks. The disadvantages of episiotomy include pain during the procedure, its repair, and postpartum and dyspareunia for months afterward. Dyspareunia may interfere with the maternal–infant relationship and disrupt the couple's sexual relationship. In addition, episiotomies may extend, by laceration, into the anal sphincter (third degree) or rectum (fourth degree), increasing the risk of infection or loss of sphincter control, or development of a fistula from the rectum into the vagina. These latter complications may occur from lacerations as well.

Forceps and Vacuum Extraction

Forceps and vacuum extraction methods are used to extract the fetal head from the maternal pelvis. The procedures are done when the fetal head is engaged

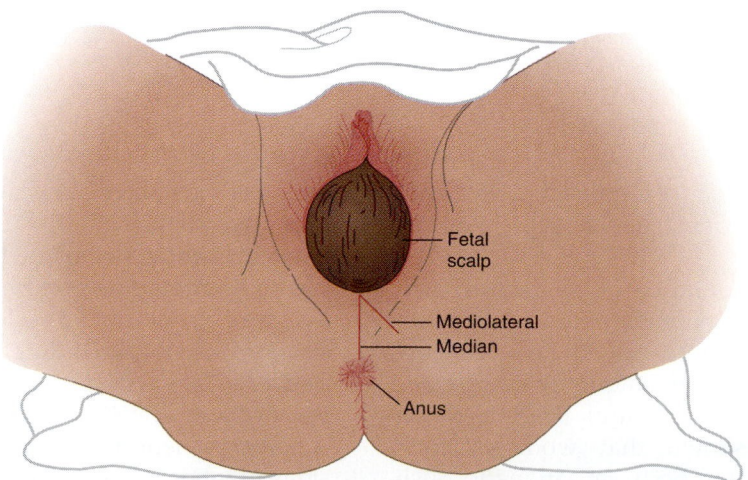

FIGURE 24–8. Episiotomy incisions: mediolateral and median (midline). *(Adapted, with permission, from Benson, R.C. (Ed.). (1983). Handbook of obstetrics and gynecology (8th ed.). Los Altos, CA: Lange Medical Books, p. 166.)*

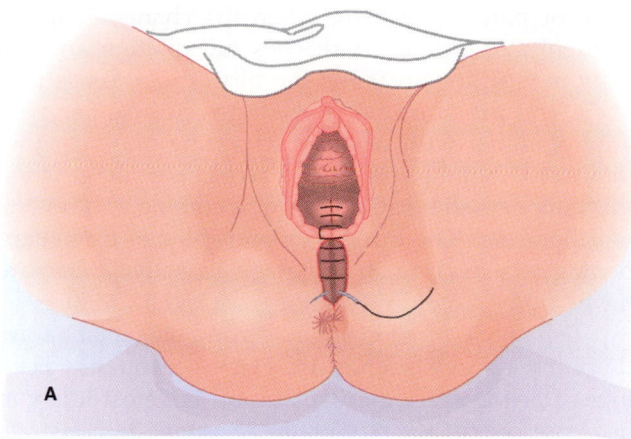

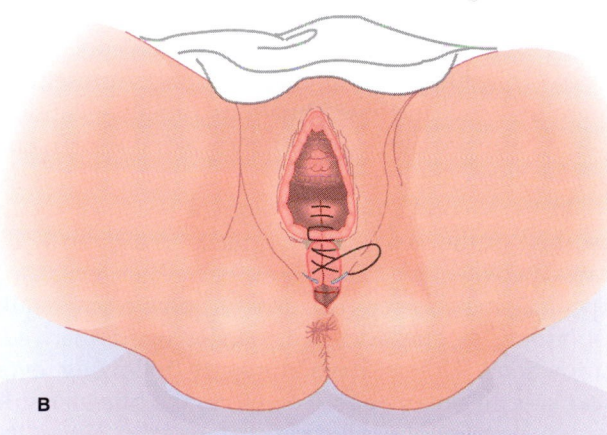

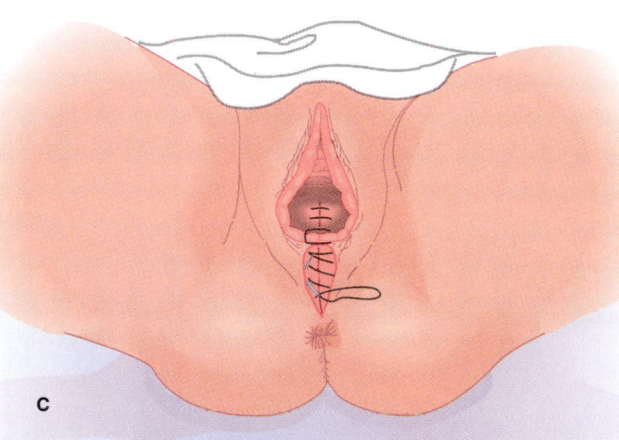

FIGURE 24–9. Median episiotomy repair. **A.** After closure of the vaginal incision and reapproximation of the cut margins of the hymenal ring, the suture is tied and cut. Next, three or four sutures are placed in the fascia and muscle of the incised perineum. **B.** A continuous suture is now carried downward to unite the superficial fascia. **C.** Completion of the repair.

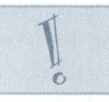

Nursing Alert

Median episiotomies have been associated with third and fourth degree lacerations in women having their first baby. The incidence of severe perineal tears could be decreased if the use of episiotomies was reduced.

and is arrested in the pelvis (Cunningham et al., 1997). They are not done to shorten the second stage of labor. When either procedure is required, it must first be explained to the client.

Forceps are made of stainless steel and can be used for extraction and rotation of the fetal head. Vacuum extractors include a suction cup attached to a suction pump for the extraction of the head.

The woman is moved to the delivery room and placed in lithotomy position. The nurse drapes the client and cleans her perineum. The physician may order a catheterization done to reduce bladder trauma. In addition, the nurse monitors the FHR and uterine contractions throughout the procedure.

The nurse passes the requested vacuum extractor or forceps and provides water-soluble lubricant to the physician for the forceps blades. With the forceps method, the physician places one and then the other blade of the forceps over the fetus's parietal bones and locks the blades together. Traction is applied during contractions until the head is low enough to permit an episiotomy. The episiotomy is done, and the forceps are removed when the biparietal bones pass through the vulvar ring. With the vacuum method, the suction cup is placed on the fetal head over the bony area and suction is gradually applied. Suction is released when the fetal head is on the pelvic floor.

Benefits. Forceps or vacuum extraction is useful primarily with a vaginal delivery (to avoid cesarean delivery) in cases of maternal exhaustion, fetal distress, or if it is undesirable for the mother to push (e.g., the client with cardiac disease, hypertension, or tuberculosis), or if the second stage of labor fails to progress.

Risks. The woman should have an adequate pelvis, the bladder and rectum should be empty to avoid injury, an accurate diagnosis of fetal presentation and position should be made, anesthesia should be available and adequate, lacerations should be minimal and repaired properly, and asepsis should be maintained. The mother may develop bruising or hematoma from the manipulation. In addition, the fetus may have soft tissue damage to the face, fracture of the skull, tentorial tears, shoulder dystocia, and brain hemorrhage.

▶ Delivery of the Neonate

Once the fetal head has emerged, the clinician quickly explores the fetal neck to ascertain that the cord has not become looped around the neck during labor. If it has, the cord is slipped over the head if length permits, clamped, and cut to prevent tearing the cord or rupturing the placenta, or manipulated over the fetal shoulders to permit delivery through the looped cord. The body of the neonate is delivered with the next one or two contractions. A gush of amniotic fluid follows expulsion of the fetal body and limbs.

The neonate's nares and mouth may be suctioned as soon as the head emerges, particularly if the physician or midwife has time to wait for external rotation before delivery of the shoulders and body. Suctioning helps prevent neonatal aspiration of mucus, amniotic fluid (particularly if meconium stained), and debris from the first inspirations. The umbilical cord is double clamped and cut between clamps. With the first cries of the neonate, the second stage of labor ends.

With delivery, the parents have their first opportunity for neonatal–parental attachment. The neonate may be placed on the mother's abdomen while the cord is cut. Skin-to-skin contact facilitates attachment.

Birth of the baby culminates the long waiting period of pregnancy. The fantasized infant now becomes a reality. The nurse, as a parent advocate, can ensure that parents have an opportunity for privacy to become acquainted with their baby. Once neonatal respirations have been established, the many technical aspects of newborn care (e.g., infant identification, eye prophylaxis, weighing) can be delayed until after this initial acquaintance period. (See Chapter 30 for further discussion of care of the infant immediately after birth.)

▶ Maternal Psychosocial Reactions

Relief often accompanies the onset of the second stage of labor. The woman knows that the baby will be born soon and the discomforts of labor will end. At this time pushing to deliver the baby is encouraged. This active form of participation also contributes to the woman's feelings of relief.

Sometimes women react to the inner sensations that occur at the onset of second-stage labor with surprise or panic, especially when the changes happen suddenly. As the cervix reaches full dilation and the baby moves downward in the birth canal, sensations of extreme pressure and stretching occur. Women who are unfamiliar with what is happening may fear that they are "coming apart." If a woman is alone when this happens, she fears the baby is coming and no one will help her. The nurse can prevent this from happening by ensuring that women in active labor are never alone (Gagnon, Waghorn, & Covell, 1997).

Behaviors of women in second-stage labor are uninhibited, and feelings are expressed openly. Feelings of helplessness and frustration are most likely to be expressed as anger. Women also may demonstrate lack of modesty at this time. Most women become very warm when labor is intense and they may remove any covering in an attempt to cool themselves. This happens no matter who is present or where they are. In these situations caregivers should maintain the woman's privacy by making certain curtains or doors are closed.

In the second stage, the woman becomes totally absorbed in the task of giving birth. She often withdraws between contractions, closing her eyes and appearing to be asleep (Fig. 24–10). Some women talk, responding to questions with single words between contractions. Others have difficulty following even short specific commands. Therefore, the nurse should present instructions as simple steps and allow the woman to focus on and complete each part successfully.

Even women who adapted well early in labor may find second-stage sensations difficult. Self-control is often tenuous and the caregiver's help is needed to prevent loss of perceived control. At this

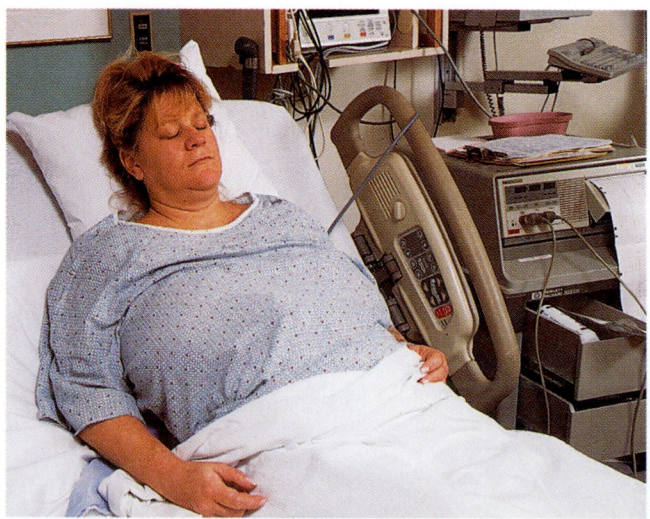

FIGURE 24–10. Resting between contractions.

point, women usually respond when "talked through" a contraction. With each contraction constant repetition of what to do helps them to remain in control. Difficulty also is experienced in control of body movement. Assistance is needed for turning or moving; these activities require energy and concentration that overwhelm the woman.

Throughout the second stage most women focus on what is happening to themselves rather than on the baby. Completely absorbed with the expulsive effort, they may close their eyes. Many women who desire to watch the baby's birth need to be reminded to open their eyes.

Nursing Interventions

Strategies supportive of the mother in the second stage of labor include talking the mother through a contraction; giving the mother simple instructions; removing distractions to the mother's concentration during pushing; assuring the mother that she will not be left alone during the second stage; calming the mother's fears concerning body intactness; performing desired comfort measures; and informing the mother that labor is nearly over.

▶ Paternal Psychosocial Reactions

Fathers tend to interact with their partners during the second stage of labor much as they did earlier. Those who coached, actively continue. They praise their partner's pushing efforts, doing all they can to encourage her. Less assertive fathers sometimes feel they are in the way once pushing begins and will watch from a distance.

Birth is a very emotional time for fathers as well as mothers. For some men, fatherhood becomes a reality only as the birth of the baby takes place. Suddenly they realize the extent of the responsibility that fathering entails. Some fathers express their feelings openly, sharing their joy and delight with their partners. They are proud of their partners' efforts and proud to be fathers. Other fathers do not express their feelings openly. Their inner feelings may be expressed in a quick look shared with their partners. Occasionally a father may feel faint at the time of delivery, and the nurse should be alert to this possibility. As a rule, fathers who are overwhelmed tend to look away. They relax visibly once assured that both mother and baby are well.

Nursing Interventions

Strategies to support the father during the second stage of labor include encouraging him to change into delivery room attire in ample time (if birth occurs in a hospital setting and the hospital requires this); allowing him to choose his level of involvement; encouraging him and praising his efforts; keeping him informed on the progress of the birth; and allowing him to freely express emotion.

▶ NURSING CARE DURING THE THIRD STAGE OF LABOR

Nursing care during the third stage of labor entails care and support of the client during delivery of the placenta.

After birth, the placenta begins to separate from the uterine wall. Signs of separation include a change in the shape of the uterus from ovoid to globular; a trickle or gush of blood; lengthening of the umbilical cord; rise of the fundus, which occurs as the placenta descends; and failure of the cord to retract when the uterus is pushed upward.

The nurse assesses the fundus for contractility, the vaginal discharge for evidence of excessive bleeding (bright red blood gushing from the vagina), and the maternal vital signs.

The placenta, after delivery, is carefully examined to ascertain whether any fragments remain attached to the uterus. The umbilical cord is inspected to determine placement, length, the presence of one vein and two arteries, and evidence of a knot or bleeding within the cord. A cord abnormality directs the nurse to examine the neonate for defects or damage associated with the cord problem.

To facilitate uterine contraction after the third stage of labor, pharmacologic agents, such as oxytocin (Pitocin) (see box entitled Drug Guide: Oxytocin), ergonovine (Ergotrate), and methylergonovine (Methergine), are often used to promote the firm contractions that help to minimize maternal blood loss. After delivery of the placenta, oxytocin may be added to an intravenous solution (10–40 U/1000 mL). The IV is regulated to the lowest possible rate that will maintain contractility of the uterus. Before

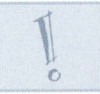

Nursing Alert

Oxytoxics such as oxytocin, ergonovine, and methylergonovine may be contraindicated for use after the delivery of the placenta if the woman exhibits an elevated blood pressure.

administration of oxytoxics, the nurse assesses maternal blood pressure. Oxytocin alone must never be relied on to maintain contraction of the uterus; in the third and fourth stages, it is always coupled with gentle, guarded fundal massage. Ergonovine and methylergonovine may also be ordered after delivery of the placenta to stimulate contraction of the uterus.

▶ NURSING CARE DURING THE FOURTH STAGE OF LABOR

The fourth stage of labor is when a mother's body systems stabilize, usually within 1 to 4 hours of the delivery. The nurse monitors the beginning indicators of stabilization.

The cardiovascular system quickly adjusts to the loss of pressure from the gravid uterus, but the mother should be reminded not to rise too quickly from a supine to sitting position, as hypotension and dizziness or syncope may result. A chill causing a brief episode of shivering is common in the fourth stage and appears to result from physical and emotional factors. It is hypothesized that loss of the fetal body heat, relaxation of large pelvic blood vessels, and the sudden emotional calm after the "storm" cause this reaction. A warm blanket and a warm drink usually bring relief.

Postdelivery, the fundus is palpated gently but firmly to assess firmness and promote contraction (Fig. 24–11). The nurse should refrain from forcefully expressing uterine contents unless uterine relaxation is a persistent problem. Such manipulation may disturb clotting, which is the beginning of healing at the site where the placenta had been attached. Lochial color, odor, consistency, and amount are also assessed. Maternal vital signs are taken every 15 minutes during the first hour postpartum until stable. Parental acquaintance with the newborn may continue. In addition, the individual who has supported the mother throughout labor and delivery may be encouraged to obtain food and rest at this time.

▶ Maternal Psychosocial Reactions During the Third and Fourth Stages of Labor

Immediately after delivery mothers want to know if the baby is healthy and normal. The first cry, awaited in silence, is greeted with smiles, excitement, and joyful tears. Mothers may reach down to touch the baby even before the cord is cut. Some mothers, fatigued after a long labor with little sleep, fall asleep after

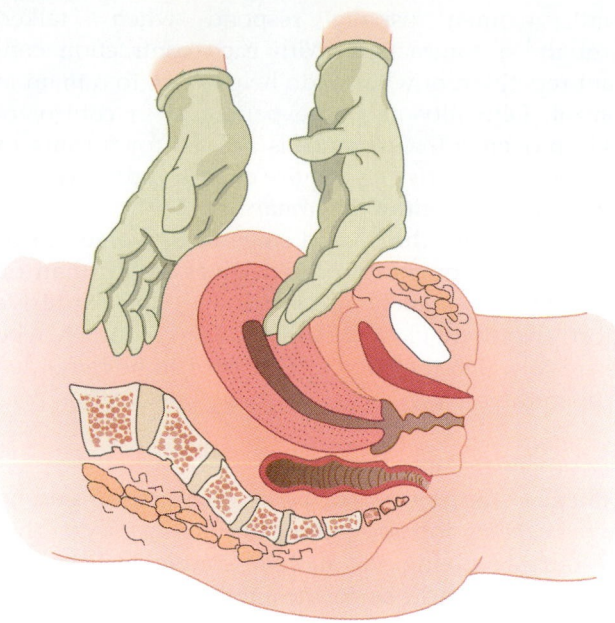

FIGURE 24–11. Palpating the uterus to assess its firmness and to promote contraction.

learning the baby is healthy. Others experience an emotional high; in a state of elation they are very excited and talkative. They may hug and kiss the father telling him they could not have made it through the labor without his help. They also express pride in the baby, ask questions, and exclaim over the baby's sex, size, and appearance.

In the immediate postdelivery period, most mothers want to hold the baby. Those planning to breastfeed begin at this time while the baby is awake and alert. Mothers try to make eye contact as they hold their baby. The baby can be placed skin to skin on the mother's body and a warm blanket placed over both to prevent chilling. The mother explores the face and hands with her fingers. She may offer the father an opportunity to hold the baby also. She then will share her observations of the baby with the father as they both observe the baby or as she watches the father and baby interact.

Nursing Interventions

Strategies related to maternal reactions in the immediate postdelivery period focus on bonding with the infant and include encouraging the mother to hold and inspect the baby; delaying routine newborn care such as eye prophylaxis so the mother and her support person have time with the baby; putting the baby to breast for those mothers who choose breastfeeding; and encouraging the new family to remain together.

▶ Paternal Psychosocial Reactions During the Third and Fourth Stages of Labor

When the delivery is over the father watches the newborn and may hold the baby. Some fathers participate in delivery by cutting the cord. Fathers will try to make eye contact with the baby while holding and talking to the baby. Fathers also share their observations about the baby with the mother. Once they are sure that mother and baby are settled, fathers will attend to their own physical needs.

Nursing Interventions

Strategies related to paternal reactions also focus on beginning bonding behaviors. Specifically, these include allowing the father to hold the baby as soon as possible after delivery (after breastfeeding has been initiated and mother is ready); encouraging the father to support and nurture the mother as she makes the acquaintance of the baby; supporting the father as he makes the acquaintance of the baby; and encouraging the father to meet his own needs after the initial interaction period with infant and mother.

▶ OTHER FAMILY MEMBERS' REACTIONS TO LABOR AND DELIVERY

When significant others accompany the childbearing parents, the nurse needs to consider the entire group when care is provided.

Institutional visitation policies vary as to when and who is permitted to be present during childbirth. Siblings attend births most often in the home or in an alternative birthing center. The number of hospitals allowing children to be present during birth is increasing. Hospital policies regarding the presence of grandparents during childbirth tend to be more flexible, as the term *adult significant other* is not restricted to the expectant father.

▶ Grandparents

A grandparent, particularly the woman's own mother, may attend childbirth; in some cases, a grandparent (usually the mother's mother) may be the only support person present. Grandparents may come to the birth experience with little knowledge of what to expect about current birthing practices. Much of what they know about childbirth is based on their own

experiences a generation ago. Their experiences may have occurred in a different setting and at a time when mothers were heavily sedated and delivered with a general anesthetic so that they were not awake for the birth of their babies. It is likely that the grandmother experienced her labor apart from significant others, although if she and her partner had attended childbirth education classes they may have been allowed to remain together. The father and family usually waited in a separate room and wondered what was happening. It is also possible that the grandparents' birth experiences occurred in another culture or country where birth practices differ.

Grandparents can be very supportive and nurturing toward the childbearing parents. They may provide temporary relief for the father, allowing him to meet his own personal needs. They also encourage and express pride in the childbearing parents. Their presence has a calming and stabilizing effect.

Nursing Interventions

Strategies related to grandparents' experiences during childbirth depend on the level of participation that the family has chosen. If grandparents are present during the labor and delivery, specific nursing strategies include educating the grandparents about current birthing care and equipment; encouraging their support of the childbearing couple; allowing grandparents to talk about their own birthing experiences; and allowing the grandparents to be alone with the childbearing couple with and without the baby present.

▶ Siblings

Parents sometimes wish to include their children in the birth experience and children may request to be present. Siblings who attend the birth should be given the freedom to regulate how much or how little they participate in the birth. They should have another adult support person (other than their mother or father) to interpret labor and birth events, respond to their needs, and accompany them as they come and go from the birthing room. Young children with a short attention span often come and go frequently. They play in an adjacent room or nearby in the birthing room, even on the mother's bed when allowed. In early labor the mothers sometimes play with the children. As labor intensifies, some mothers continue to make an effort to interact with their children between contractions. Other mothers are too involved in coping with the labor and need to be free of distraction from their children.

Siblings often act in a nurturing manner toward their mothers during labor. They may wipe their mother's face with a cool cloth, give her ice chips or water, pat her arms or legs, or copy other adult actions.

Young children may become bored or tired during labor. They may continue their usual routine of eating, sleeping, or playing. When delivery is imminent, they are awakened or brought back to observe the birth of the baby.

Siblings, like their parents, have varied emotional reactions. Children's reactions depend on such factors as age, stage of development, and preparation for the event.

Nursing Interventions

Strategies with regard to siblings' experiences during childbirth depend on the level of participation that the family has chosen and the age of the siblings. Specific strategies include supporting the sibling according to his or her developmental level; allowing the sibling(s) to come and go from the birthing site as he or she desires; advising parents prenatally to arrange for a support person to be available for the sibling(s) throughout labor and delivery; answering the sibling's questions and explaining the sights and sounds that accompany the birth; and allowing the sibling(s) to see and interact with the baby when she or he is ready.

▶ CULTURAL ASPECTS OF CHILDBIRTH

Chapters 15, 17, 18, and 22 presented the family structure of several different cultural groups. These cultural groups were chosen as examples of the varied people that a nurse will meet in the course of delivering health care to individuals and families. The following paragraphs examine birth experiences in the United States and Canada.

▶ Birthing Experience in the United States

The birth experience in the United States has been studied in comparison to that of other countries. Several features of the birth event are common to all birth situations, regardless of the country or cultural group, and may serve as a basis for describing childbirth in the United States. These features are the group's definition of the event, modes of preparation for the birth, the nature of the birth territory, the use of medication in childbirth, and the technology of birth.

Definition of the Event

How a society or cultural group conceptualizes birth is the best indicator of what its birthing system is like. The definition of the birth event provides participants with a shared view regarding the course and management of events and guides them in conducting the process of birthing.

In the United States today at least two opposing views or definitions of the birth event are demonstrated. On one hand, birth is seen as a high-tech medical event; on the other, it is a highly natural event. In either case, the family, as a whole, should have a positive birth experience.

Preparation for Childbirth

Society prepares a woman and her family for the experience of childbirth in two ways. The first is the manner in which girls and boys are socialized into the roles of parents and prepared for the event of pregnancy. The second concerns the knowledge that couples, once pregnant, are expected to acquire for the birth itself.

In the United States, much information is transmitted to the family through formal channels connected with the health care delivery system (i.e., clinics, physician's offices, birth centers, prepared childbirth classes). Information also comes informally to the family. Often, this information has a cultural "flavor" and contributes to the variability in perceptions of different cultural groups, even when these groups have been acculturated into the dominant culture.

Information coming from these formal or informal channels may or may not help prepare the family members for the realities of the birth situation. For example, prepared childbirth philosophy may present an idealized picture of the birth experience. Couples who do not experience their concept of an ideal birth may feel guilty and disappointed, believing that they have failed. On the other hand, sometimes information received through informal channels may be so negative about the birth experience that the couple is terrified and is unable to cope with labor and delivery. Information that is either too positive or too negative can be equally detrimental to the expectant couple's experience of childbirth.

Childbirth Territory

Societies also prescribe an appropriate place for giving birth. Two types of birth environments may be identified: (1) specifically designated and specialized, or (2) unspecific, within the family's own environment. Thus, the woman and her support persons may go to a special facility to give birth (i.e., a hospital or birth center) or the family may experience the birth in their routine environment (i.e., their own home or other familiar setting).

Use of Medication in Childbirth

The use of medication in labor provides an indication of how much a society sees fit to intervene in the process of childbirth. In general, medications affect the course of labor (speed it up, slow it down) or provide pain relief for the laboring woman.

Medication use in the United States is fairly common, but may depend on the location of the birth, preparation of the woman and her support persons for the labor, and other techniques used to moderate the surrounding stimuli of labor. Medication use during the process of birth is still quite controversial in the United States. Many individuals feel that pharmacologic intervention is overused, whereas others believe that the benefits of medication use outweigh the risks. Couples need to understand the advantages and risks of medications during labor and take decision-making responsibility for medication use.

Technology of Childbirth

Birth, like other events in a society, is seen as having a variety of equipment and instruments necessary for managing the process in a culturally appropriate manner. Birth technology in the United States is highly advanced, with new, more sophisticated equipment being constantly developed. Birthing instruments (forceps, electronic monitoring, and so on) represent the American belief in the necessity of medical intervention during the birth process; however, not all individuals in the United States today believe in the appropriateness of use of extensive birth technology. Many believe that the benefits of this technology and equipment in the United States are likely to remain a controversial issue for many years to come.

▶ Birthing Experience in Canada

Health care delivery in Canada is currently under close scrutiny as health care professionals and policy makers contemplate models for reform in the United States health care delivery system. A consideration of birthing practices in Canada will assist with this process.

Major shifts have been occurring in the way Canadians view childbirth. The disease/medical model is being replaced by a belief that pregnancy and childbirth are normal, safe events. Movements to reduce the rates of cesarean delivery and the use of unnecessary medical technology are ongoing.

In-hospital birth centers in Ontario have successfully provided a safe, satisfying, and cost-effective alternative to traditional hospital care for women experiencing an uncomplicated pregnancy and birth. Shifts in medical and nursing practices have been observed in the labor and delivery departments of the hospitals that have an in-hospital birth center.

In January 1994 the Ontario government announced that it would fund the operation of three free-standing (out of hospital) birth centers across the province. These birth centers are staffed by midwives and governed by a board of directors (Sutton et al., 1993).

Canada is the last industrialized country in the World Health Organization to have provisions for regulated midwifery. Until recently, midwifery was practiced outside the health care system, without legislation to govern and protect. After much work Ontario became the first province in Canada to pass modern midwifery legislation, the Midwifery Act, in November 1991. Governments in Alberta and British Columbia are also committed to recognition of the profession and the integration of midwives into the health care system. In Quebec, legislation has been passed to allow midwifery practice in a series of ministry-funded pilot projects. Manitoba is also actively investigating the issues. Interest and activity in other provinces continue to grow (Allemang et al., 1993).

The Ontario model of midwifery is quite unusual. Aspects of other countries' models of practice were considered and rejected or used in the development of the Ontario model. Midwifery care is based on respect for pregnancy as a state of health and childbirth as a normal process. The fundamental underpinnings of midwifery in Ontario are continuity of caregiver, informed consent, and choice of birth place. Midwives have privileges to care for their clients in the hospital, community, or home. In the hospital they have both admitting and discharging privileges and report to the department of OB/GYN service or family practice until a department of midwifery can be established. The Ministry of Health funds a nonprofit organization which identifies agencies to fund individual midwives (Sutton et al., 1993). Midwives are salaried for their practice. Research has clearly shown the effectiveness of nurse midwifery programs for positive client outcomes as well as being an appropriate use of health care dollars (Harvey, Jarell, Brant, Stainton, & Rach, 1996).

▶ DIAGNOSTIC DECISION MAKING

The nurse is an integral member of the health team that manages the family during labor and delivery. The nurse carefully assesses the physiologic and psychosocial needs of the woman, her fetus and newborn. Possible nursing diagnoses for labor and delivery include:

Physiologic
Problem-oriented diagnoses:

- Risk for injury, related to augmentation of labor
- Pain, related to physiologic response to labor

Wellness-oriented diagnoses:

- Normal progress during labor and delivery, related to positive health care practices during pregnancy
- Asset in maternal and fetal health during intrapartum period, related to normal progression of labor as evaluated by Friedman's curve

Psychosocial
Problem-oriented diagnoses:

- Anxiety, related to situational crisis
- Powerlessness, related to lack of control during labor

Wellness-oriented diagnoses:

- Enhanced self-esteem, related to perceived control in labor and delivery and effective use of childbirth preparation techniques

- Enhanced paternal self-esteem, related to active participation during labor and delivery

Cultural
Problem-oriented diagnoses:

- Self-esteem disturbance, related to incongruence between cultural beliefs and childbirth practices in health care settings

Wellness-oriented diagnoses:

- Asset in maternal coping, related to presence of culturally appropriate labor social support

Once the nursing diagnoses have been developed, an individualized plan of care for the woman and her partner experiencing the birthing process can be formulated. The goals and outcome criteria that form the basis of nursing care serve as the framework for the specific nursing interventions for the childbearing couple. Continuous evaluation of the plan of care and effectiveness of the nursing strategies during the intrapartum period ensures a positive outcome for the family. Figures 24–12 and 24–13 present examples of clinical pathways for vaginal delivery for the mother and infant, respectively.

Target Postdelivery LOS = 24–48 hours

Date of Birth: _____   Time of Birth: _____

Category	Prenatal record to L&D by 36 weeks	Labor, delivery, recovery	0–12 hours	13–24 hours	Within 2 hrs. of discharge	Home
Laboratory/ Diagnostic Tests	H + H; Type + Screen; Rubella; RPR; HBSAG	CBC per order; MS BOS per order; RPR	H + H or CBC if ordered; Determine RhoGAM and rubella status	RhoGAM if Rh negative and baby Rh positive; RPR results; Rubella if not immune		
Treatments/ Assessments		Receive medical records from MD's office by 36 weeks; Assessment, vital signs and EFM per patient care standard	Post partum assessment per patient care standard; Peri care; Hygiene + comfort measures; Anesthesia follow-up if indicated	Assess parenting skills; Postpartum assessment per patient care standard; Peri care; Hygiene + comfort measures; Anesthesia follow-up if indicated		Follow-up phone call at 3–5 days postdischarge by maternity nurse to assess; Assessment by HHC nurse
Medications/ IVs	Prenatal vitamins	Analgesia/anesthesia per order; Pitocin per order	IV discontinued; Analgesics as needed for pain	Stool softener as ordered; Analgesics as needed for pain		
Consultations	Social work per guidelines		Lactation consult if breastfeeding problem (per BF Care Plan and Supplementation Policy/Procedure); Social work PRN; Pediatrician visit with mother			Lactation consult if breastfeeding problem; Social work consult if needed
Activity		OOB unless contraindicated	OOB with assistance; Shower; Voiding without difficulty; Rest	OOB with assistance; Voiding without difficulty; Rest	Escort mother and baby to car	
Nutrition		Clear liquids per order; Ice	Regular diet	Regular diet	Regular diet	
Education/ Discharge Planning	Childbirth preparation classes; Parentcraft classes; Breastfeeding class if BF; Orient to discharge program tour; Contraceptive planning; Select pediatrician; Preparing for Your Baby's Birth at Jefferson; "Baby Talk" video	Comfort measures and relaxation techniques; Orient to EFM; 2nd stage pushing; Initial breastfeeding instruction if breastfeeding; Breastfeeding	Handwashing; Orient to baby's crib; Infant positioning, feeding, changing	Sitz bath; Infant care class; Discharge planning; Infant safety; S&S of dehydration and infection; Circumcision care if baby circumcised; Breast pump if needed	Discharge instructions; Gift pack; Infant car seat requirement; Smoke detector; Follow-up appointments; Educational needs summary	Reinforce teaching of infant and self-care by HHC nurse
Home Care	Referral to home care			Notify home care of delivery	Home care contact in hospital	Scheduled home care visits 24–48 hours postdischarge; Earlier home care if needed; 2nd home care visit if needed
Variances	Order / Reason / Order / Reason / Order / Reason					

RN Signature: _____

Target discharge status = Minimal vaginal bleeding; Demonstrates parenting skills; Minimal physical discomfort

Confirmed postdelivery by obstetrician: _____

Signature _____   Date _____

FIGURE 24–12. Clinical pathway: vaginal delivery: mother. (*Courtesy of Thomas Jefferson University Hospital, Jefferson Health System, Philadelphia, PA.*)

Target LOS = 24–48 hours

Date of Birth: _____ Time of Birth: _____

	0–6 hours	7–12 hours	13–18 hours	19–24 hours	Within 2 hrs. of discharge	Home 24–48 hrs. postdischarge
Laboratory/ Diagnostic Tests	Coombs; Maternal Hep B status			Coombs results; Maternal RPR status at delivery ← – – – PKU and bilirubin at age 24 hours – – –		PKU, if initial PKU done before 24 hrs; Bilirubin if > 5 at age 24 hours or if baby jaundiced by home health nurse; report results to pediatrician
Treatments/ Procedures	Stabilization; Baby ID; Vital signs as per patient standard; Weight = ___ gm; Bath	Circumcision permit		Circumcision care if circumcision done		
Medications/IVs	Triple dye to cord; Vitamin K; Erythromycin ointment to eyes	HBIG if mother Hep B positive or status unknown; Hep B vaccine				
Consultations						
Activity	Radiant warmer until stable temp	Open crib	Open crib	Open crib	Open crib	
Nutrition	Breastfeeding/or glucose H₂0	Breastfeeding per policy/care plan or formula at least q 4 hrs	Breastfeeding/or formula at least q 4 hrs	Breastfeeding/or formula at least q 4 hrs	Breastfeeding/or formula	
Assessments	Apgar at 1 and 5 minutes; Gestational age; Nursing assessment for VS, feeding, voiding, bonding	I + O; Nursing assessment for VS, feeding, voiding, bonding	I + O; Assess circumcision site	Physician assessment of body systems; Nursing assessment for VS, feeding, voiding, stooling, bonding		HHC nurse assessment of physical environment and baby including VS, feeding, voiding, stooling, bonding, jaundice
Education/ Discharge Planning	See clinical pathway/mother			Instructions to parents		
Home Care						
Variances Order Reason Order Reason						

RN Signature: _____

Target discharge status = Feeding well; Maintaining temperature; Voiding and stooling adequately; Bonding

Confirmed by pediatrician:

Signature _____ Date _____

FIGURE 24–13. Clinical pathway: vaginal delivery: infant. (*Courtesy of Thomas Jefferson University Hospital, Jefferson Health System, Philadelphia, PA.*)

Chapter Highlights

▶ During the first stage of labor, the nurse determines whether the mother is in true or false labor; obtains informed consent; monitors maternal and fetal progress in labor; performs procedures such as providing adequate hydration and calories and helping the woman assume a comfortable position for labor; and assesses the psychosocial responses of the mother and father in order to provide supportive care to the couple.

▶ Nursing care during the second stage of labor consists of evaluating maternal and fetal physiologic responses to labor; assisting in procedures such as an episiotomy or forceps/vacuum extraction; ensuring the safe delivery of the neonate and promoting early parent–child attachment; and acknowledging maternal and paternal psychosocial reactions to this stage of labor.

▶ The focus of nursing care during the third stage of labor is on support of the client during delivery of the placenta and assessment and intervention to facilitate contraction of the uterus.

▶ During the fourth stage of labor, nursing interventions include palpation of the fundus to promote uterine contraction; evaluation of the lochia; assessment of maternal vital signs; and promotion of parental acquaintance with the newborn.

▶ As participants in the birthing experience, family members such as grandparents and siblings need preparation and support for the actions they will observe and the emotions they will feel during this event.

After reading the vignette at the beginning of this chapter, use what you have learned to answer these questions.

1. How do the actions of Margaret Kiely, RN, and Cathleen Harris promote Cathleen's sense of control during the labor process?

2. What behavioral characteristics would be important for Margaret Kiely, RN, to assess to evaluate Cathleen's adaptation to the progress of labor?

3. What nursing interventions can the nurse use to encourage both Cathleen and Bill Harris' involvement in the subsequent stages of labor?

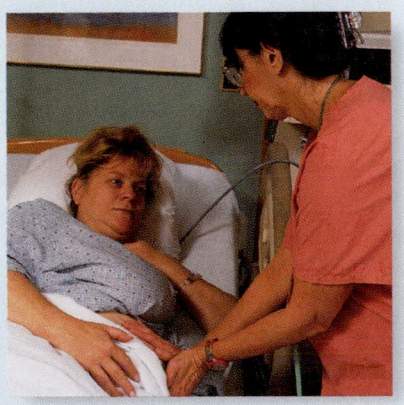

Critical Thinking Questions

► References

Albers, L.L., Anderson, D., Cragin, L., Daniels, S.M., Hunter, C., Sedler, K.D., & Teaf, D (1997). The relationship of ambulation in labor to operative delivery. *Journal of Nurse-Midwifery. 42*(1), 4–8.

Allemang, E. et al. How midwifery care will fit into Ontario's health care system. *Ob/Gyn Women's Health Care, 5,* 478–481.

Bergstrom, L., Seidel, J., Skillman-Hull, L., & Roberts, J. (1997). "I gotta push. Please let me push!" Social interactions during the change from first to second stage labor. *Birth, 24*(3), 173–180.

Chandler, S., & Field, P.A. (1997). Becoming a father: First time fathers experience of labor and delivery. *Journal of Nurse-Midwifery, 42*(1), 17–24.

Chou, F.H., Chao, Y.M., & Yee, D.H. (1994). The lived experience of expectant fathers throughout labor and birth. *Nursing Research, 2*(4), 359–370.

Chou, F.H., Chao, Y.M., & Yee, D.H. (1995). The nursing needs of expectant fathers accompanying wives throughout labor and birth. *Nursing Research, 3*(4), 376–386.

Cunningham, F.G., MacDonald, P.C., Gant, N.F., Leveno, K.J., Gilstrap, L.C., Hankins, G.D.V., & Clark, S.L. (1997). *Williams obstetrics* (20th ed.). Stamford CT: Appleton & Lange.

Evans, S., & Jeffrey, J. (1995). Maternal learning needs during labor and delivery. *Journal of Obstetric, Gynecologic, and Neonatal Nursing, 24*(3), 235–240.

Gagnon, A.J., Waghorn, K., & Covell, C. (1997). A randomized trial of one to one nurse support of women in labor. *Birth, 24*(2), 71–80.

Halldorsdottir, S., & Karlsdottir, S. (1996). Journeying through labour and delivery: Perceptions of women who have given birth. *Midwifery, 12*(2), 48–61.

Harvey, S., Jarell, J., Brant, R., Stainton, C., & Rach, D. (1996). A randomized, controlled trial of nurse-midwifery care. *Birth, 23*(3), 128–135.

Knapp, L. (1996). Childbirth satisfaction: The effects of internality and perceived control. *Journal of Perinatal Education, 5*(4), 7–16.

Labrecque, M., Baillargeon, L., Dallaire, M., Tremblay, A., Pinault, J.J., & Gingras, S. (1997). Association between median episiotomy and severe perineal lacerations in primaparous women. *Canadian Medical Association Journal, 156*(6), 797–802.

Mackey, M.C., & Stepans, M.E.F. (1994). Women's evaluation of their labor and delivery nurses. *Journal of Obstetric, Gynecologic, and Neonatal Nursing, 23*(5), 413–420.

Nichols, M.R. (1993). Paternal perspectives of the childbirth experience. *Maternal-Child Nursing Journal, 21*(3), 99–108.

Reilly, K.E. (1994). Induction of labor. *American Family Physician, 49*(6), 1427–1432.

Schorn, M.N., McAllister, J.L., & Blanco, J.D. (1993). Water immersion and the effect on labor. *Journal of Nurse-Midwifery, 38,* 336–342.

Sharp, D.A. (1997). Restriction of oral intake for women in labor. *British Journal of Midwifery, 5*(7), 408–412.

Sutton, W. et al. (1993). Free-standing birth centres: The Toronto Birth Centre Model. *Ob/Gyn Women's Health Care, 5,* 478–481.

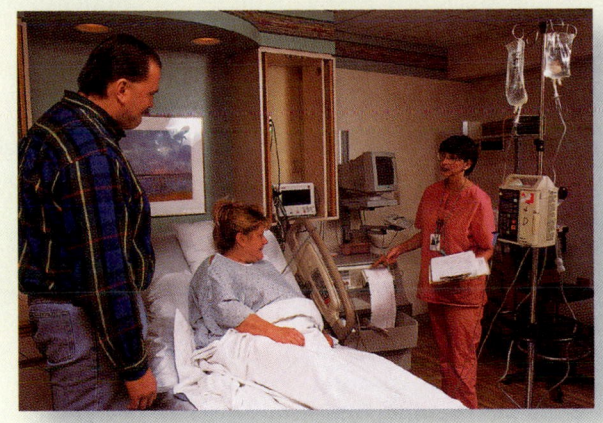

Cathleen Harris, a 30-year-old multigravida, was admitted to a labor and delivery unit 9 hours ago. For the first 2 hours of active labor, her contractions occurred every 3 minutes and lasted for 35 seconds. Her cervix is now 7 cm dilated and 75% effaced. At the beginning of the third hour of labor, however, Cathleen experiences only one contraction during a 10-minute period. Cathleen's contractions and the fetal heart rate are being monitored by a tocodynamometer.

As Margaret Kiely, RN, observes the monitor, Cathleen, noticeably worried, asks, "Why have my contractions slowed down?" The nurse informs Cathleen and her husband Bill that, although the intensity of the contractions has decreased to 20 mm Hg, the fetal heart rate is strong and is recorded at 140 beats per minute. Cathleen and Bill look at each other, and Bill smiles reassuringly at his wife. Cathleen asks, "What will happen if my contractions continue to decrease? Can this condition hurt our baby?" ∎

25

Care of the Family at Risk During Birth

Labor is a complex process that requires the harmonious interaction of four factors: the powers, the passenger, the passage, and the psyche. The powers refer to the forces of the uterine contractions. Uterine contractions need to be strong and coordinated so they can produce effacement and dilation of the cervix and facilitate the descent of the fetus through the maternal pelvis. The passenger is the fetus. The fetus must be of an appropriate size for the pelvis, and positioned to allow for movement into and down through the pelvis. The passage includes the bony pelvis and soft tissues. For labor to occur, the pelvis must be of adequate size and free from obstacles that would retard the descent of the fetus. The psyche refers to the psychologic aspects of labor. How the laboring woman adapts psychologically to labor and childbirth can have an effect on the labor process itself. If any of the factors, singularly or in combination, are abnormal or fail to function properly, complications can occur.

In addition other problems, which may or may not interfere with the process of labor itself, may emerge or become critical during labor and delivery. For example, problems with the cord, amniotic fluid, or placenta may become acute during labor or delivery. The delivery of multiple fetuses may also become a problem at this time.

Complications that arise during labor or delivery can put the mother at risk. Both her health and safety can be adversely affected. The prognosis for a favorable outcome for the fetus as well may be questionable. To ensure the best possible outcome for both mother and fetus, the nurse who cares for the woman in labor must have a thorough knowledge of normal labor. Frequent assessments of the laboring woman's progress must be made, with particular emphasis on any deviations from the normal course of labor. Continuous communication between the nurse and nurse-midwife or physician is essential so that if complications do occur and obstetric intervention is necessary, the proper steps can be taken.

▶ DYSTOCIA

Normal labor, or **eutocia,** follows a fairly predictable course. (The normal processes of labor and delivery were discussed earlier in Chapter 21.) Any deviation from this normal pattern results in **dystocia,** the term used to describe a difficult labor. The term is not precise. For example, Notzon and others (1994) described 15 different ICD-9 codes describing cesarean delivery for dystocia, including arrest of descent and failure to progress. Indeed, dystocia is the most frequent indication of cesarean delivery in the United States (Cunningham et al., 1997). When complications occur during the labor process that either prevent a vaginal delivery or make the vaginal route hazardous for the mother or fetus, cesarean delivery is chosen.

▶ Classification

Dystocia can be classified according to which of the three physiologic factors—powers, passenger, or passage—is involved. Dystocia related to the powers is uterine dystocia. Dystocia related to the passenger is fetal dystocia, and dystocia related to the passage is pelvic dystocia.

▶ DYSTOCIA RELATED TO THE POWERS

Uterine contractions need to be strong, coordinated, and intermittent to be effective. When the uterine contractions fail to meet these criteria, they cannot effect cervical dilation and fetal descent, and uterine dystocia occurs.

▶ Dysfunctional Labor Patterns

A dysfunctional labor pattern is one in which the pattern of the uterine contractions is not normal. This abnormal pattern prevents labor from progressing as expected. Several dysfunctional labor patterns have been identified. They include hypertonic uterine dysfunction, hypotonic uterine dysfunction, and precipitous labor.

Hypertonic Uterine Dysfunction

The labor pattern identified as hypertonic uterine dysfunction is characterized by an increase in the frequency of contractions, but a decrease in the intensity. The resting tone of the uterus is also increased (Fig. 25–1).

During labor, the contractions occur at more frequent intervals, but little intrauterine pressure is built up during the contraction. Without the increase in pressure, not enough force is exerted on the cervix by the presenting part of the fetus for dilation to occur. The increased resting tone indicates the uterine muscle remains in a state of tension. This inhibits resumption of the blood flow to the fetus, which has been interrupted by the contraction.

The increased frequency of contractions in hypertonic uterine dysfunction may be linked to the action of the uterine pacemakers. Normally, the uterus has two pacemakers situated near the end of each fallopian tube. The pacemakers are responsible for initiating a contraction that spreads in a coordinated fashion

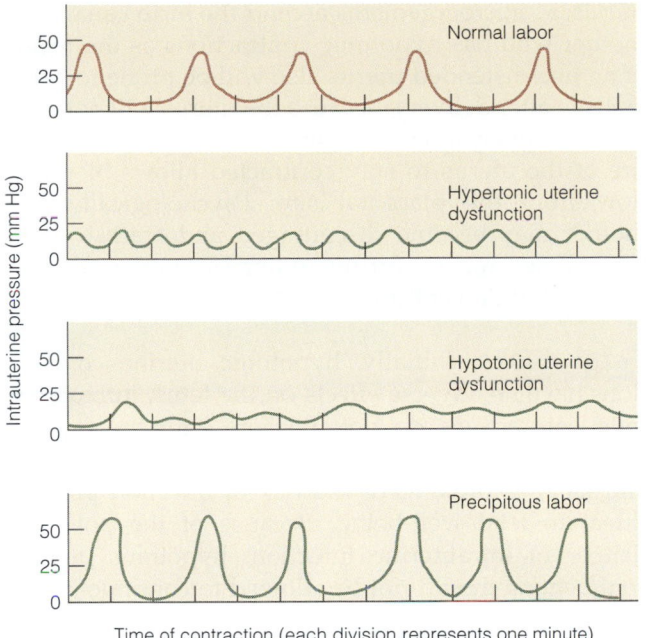

FIGURE 25–1. Patterns of normal and abnormal contractions: normal labor, hypertonic uterine dysfunction, hypotonic uterine dysfunction, and precipitous labor.

from fundus to cervix. For reasons not completely understood, other pacemakers may appear in the uterus, initiating contractions that are uncoordinated in their actions. The uterine musculature responds by contracting as if in a spasm and without purpose.

Although the mechanism is unknown, a relationship has been noted between this contractile pattern and the mother's feelings of fear and tension. Very anxious primiparous women commonly experience hypertonic labor. Hypertonic uterine dysfunction usually occurs in the latent phase of labor when contractions are just beginning. In conditions where there is hypertonus of the uterus, abruption of the placenta should be investigated as a possible cause (Cunningham et al., 1997).

Maternal Risks. Pain and fatigue are two problems facing the mother who is experiencing hypertonic uterine contractions. The pain is out of proportion to the intensity of the contractions, caused by hypoxia of the muscles, and is brought on by the frequency of the contractions. Hypoxia is compounded by the diminished resting tone between the contractions. The frequency with which the contractions occur provides the woman with little time to rest. She hardly has time to recover from one contraction before another contraction begins. If the labor is allowed to continue in this manner, the mother soon becomes exhausted. Discouraged by the lack of prog-

ress and the painful contractions, the mother and her labor partner experience increasing anxiety and may have difficulty coping with the situation.

Fetal Risks. Fetal distress resulting from hypoxia is the major concern with hypertonic uterine dysfunction. Frequent contractions, coupled with a decreased resting tone, keep the uterine musculature in a state of tension. This tension results in a decrease in the amount of oxygenated blood available to the uterine muscle and, in turn, a decrease in the amount of blood circulating in the placenta. With decreased blood flow, oxygen transport to the fetus diminishes, and hypoxia occurs. If these abnormal contractions are allowed to continue for an extended period, prolonged pressure will be exerted on the fetal skull. This pressure may cause excessive molding of the fetal head, a swelling of the head called **caput succedaneum,** or even cephalhematoma. A **cephalhematoma** is a localized collection of blood from damaged vessels that appears between the skullbone and its periosteum.

Nursing and Collaborative Assessment. Because hypertonic contractions place the mother and fetus at risk, the nurse must continually monitor both the mother and the fetus. Frequent assessment of the uterine contractions and fetal heart tones is made. This provides for early detection of signs of possible complications. Monitoring uterine contractions for frequency, duration, and intensity may be done by the nurse or nurse-midwife. The intensity of the uterine contractions can be assessed manually by palpating the uterus with the fingertips throughout a contraction. If the membranes are ruptured, a catheter can be used to measure the intrauterine pressure directly. A fetoscope or an electronic fetal monitor may be used to assess fetal heart tones. If labor is prolonged, dehydration may become a problem. Maintaining accurate records of intake and output then becomes necessary.

Nursing Diagnoses. Nursing diagnoses related to hypertonic uterine dysfunction are developed after careful assessment. Examples of diagnoses include:

Problem-oriented diagnoses:

- Pain, related to hypertonic uterine contractions
- Fatigue, related to the increase in the frequency of contractions
- Impaired fetal gas exchange, related to fetal hypoxia

Wellness-oriented diagnoses:

- Effective coping and management of anxiety during hypertonic uterine contractions, related to effective relaxation techniques

Nursing and Collaborative Management.
The nurse may help to reduce the anxiety experienced by the client and the labor partner by offering clear explanations about the nature of the contractions and the interventions that the nurses and midwife or physician are using to manage the condition. Both the labor partner and nurse should support the mother in her efforts and provide encouragement. Comfort measures such as back rubs and effleurage may help the client to relax.

The aim of medical treatment is to stop the abnormal contractions so that both the uterus and the mother can rest. Sedation in the form of a short-acting barbiturate may promote rest, relieve pain, and stop the abnormal uterine activity. Tocolytic agents such as ritodrine have been used, presumably with some success, especially in other countries.

The physiologic demands of labor require adequate hydration, so intravenous fluids are given. During the rest period, intake and output should be monitored. Assessment of urine for signs of ketones, which would indicate a fluid or electrolyte imbalance, is also performed. After the rest period, the majority of clients go into efficient labor and proceed to delivery. For those who continue with hypertonic contractions and show signs of fetal distress, cesarean delivery is performed.

Hypotonic Uterine Dysfunction

Hypotonic uterine dysfunction (see Fig. 25–1) is characterized by a decrease in the number of contractions to less than two per 10-minute interval. The intensity of the contraction is less than 25 mm Hg, and the resting tone falls below 8 mm Hg. These contractions are not effective because the intrauterine pressure is not sufficient to provide enough force for cervical dilation and fetal descent.

One cause of hypotonic uterine dysfunction is overdistension of the uterus. Muscle fibers that are overstretched do not contract efficiently. Polyhydramnios (excessive amniotic fluid), multiple gestation, or a parous uterus, which is one that has been through previous pregnancies, may cause overdistension. Another cause is fetopelvic disproportion, in which the fetus is too large for the pelvis. Another major cause of hypotonic uterine dysfunction is the excessive use of narcotic analgesics, anesthetics, or sedatives in early labor. These drugs slow the progress of labor, especially if they are administered before the cervix has dilated to 3 to 4 cm.

Maternal Risks. Hypotonic contractions are not usually painful. If, however, they cause prolonged labor, premature rupture of the membranes can occur, increasing the risk of infection developing within the uterus, as microorganisms ascend the birth canal. The mother who has hypotonic contractions as the result of an overdistended uterus also will be prone to hemorrhage after delivery, because the uterus will not contract effectively after the delivery of the placenta. Failure of the uterus to stay contracted allows blood to flow from the placental site. Psychologically, the mother may become discouraged and fearful when labor slows and no further progress in cervical dilation or fetal descent occurs.

Fetal Risks. Initially, hypotonic uterine contractions have no adverse effects on the fetus. Infrequent, mild contractions do not interfere with the oxygen supply to the fetus. If membranes rupture, however, and labor is prolonged, the risk of infection poses a threat to fetal well-being. Because of the potential danger of intrauterine infection, hypotonic uterine contractions should not be allowed to continue indefinitely.

Nursing and Collaborative Assessment.
Hypotonic uterine dysfunction appears most often during the active phase of labor. Contractions that have been normal become less frequent and are of decreased intensity and shorter duration. Progress in labor is halted.

Nursing assessment includes the frequent monitoring of contractions, fetal heart tones, and maternal vital signs. As labor continues, the nurse must be alert to signs of infection, such as elevated temperature and chills.

Nursing Diagnoses. Examples of nursing diagnoses related to hypotonic uterine dysfunction include:

Problem-oriented diagnoses:

- Ineffective individual coping, related to lengthy labor
- Risk for infection, related to premature rupture of the membranes

Wellness-oriented diagnoses:

- Asset in physiologic integrity, related to prevention of maternal and fetal infection

Nursing and Collaborative Management.
The client should be offered an explanation of the abnormal contraction pattern and of the planned interventions. An understanding of the treatment plan enhances the client's participation in the labor process.

Stimulation or augmentation of labor may be needed if the hypotonic contractions do not improve in quality; however, fetopelvic disproportion must be ruled out first. Induction of intense uterine contractions when the fetus is too large for the pelvis is dangerous for both the mother and the fetus. Both amniotomy and the intravenous infusion of oxytocin may be used to augment labor. Prostaglandins are also used for this purpose in countries other than the United States. (See Chapter 24 for an in-depth discussion of induction or augmentation of labor.)

Precipitous Labor

Labor lasting less than 3 hours is considered a precipitous labor. This pattern is characterized by the occurrence of more than five contractions in a 10-minute period (see Fig. 25–1). Intrauterine pressures may reach 50 to 70 mm Hg. Along with the frequent intense contractions, women who experience precipitous labor may demonstrate abnormally low resistance of their soft tissues. This permits the fetus to pass easily through the pelvis.

Maternal Risks. With little resistance of the soft tissues and an effaced and dilated cervix, maternal complications are rare. Studies have indicated that the maternal and fetal risks are no greater than the average labor. If the tissues do offer resistance and the cervix is long and thick, lacerations of the cervix, vagina, and vulva may occur. Forceful, intense contractions might also be responsible for a hypotonic uterus after delivery resulting in hemorrhage.

Fetal Risks. The fetus may experience hypoxia as a result of the frequent, intense contractions. Trauma to the fetal head may occur if there is resistance during passage through the pelvis. Precipitous labor may lead to a birth that is unattended and the newborn may suffer from a lack of immediate care at delivery.

Nursing Diagnoses. Examples of nursing diagnoses related to precipitous labor include:

Problem-oriented diagnoses:

- Risk for fetal trauma, related to resistance during passage through the pelvis
- Anxiety, related to concern for fetal well-being during rapid progression of labor

Wellness-oriented diagnoses:

- Potential for successful coping with precipitous labor, related to receiving clear explanations about the situation

Nursing and Collaborative Assessment and Management. Rapid labor usually results in a rapid, spontaneous delivery. The nurse-midwife or physician and nurse should be prepared for the delivery. An unassisted delivery will leave the newborn without care during the critical first few minutes of life. Pregnant women at risk for a rapid labor may be identified during the nursing assessment. A history of a previous precipitous labor should alert the nurse to the possibility that a rapid labor may be repeated. During labor, the nurse should observe the client for rapid cervical dilation and fetal descent as well as frequent, intense contractions. These may signal a precipitous labor. If delivery is imminent and the nurse does not have time to contact the nurse-midwife or physician for the delivery, she or he should be prepared to deliver the fetus.

Psychologically, this type of labor may be very stressful for the client. She may have difficulty coping with the discomfort caused by the intense contractions. The rapid progress of labor may make her feel that she has lost control. Both the nurse and the labor partner need to convey a sense of calm to the client. The nurse must assure the client that she will not be left alone. Clear, concise explanations can help relieve anxiety as well as gain the client's trust. Including the labor partner in explanations that are given will help to allay any fears related to the health and safety of both the mother and the fetus.

▶ Abnormal Labor According to Friedman's Curve

Traditionally, labor is divided into four stages (as discussed in Chapter 21). Three of the four stages are useful in assessing progress in labor: the first, second, and third. The fourth stage, which relates to the immediate postpartum period, is not relevant in this discussion.

The first stage begins with the onset of labor and ends with full cervical dilation. The first stage is further divided into two phases: the latent phase and the active phase. The latent phase includes the time from the onset of contractions until the rate of cervical dilation accelerates, usually around 3 to 4 cm. The active phase begins with the accelerated rate of dilation and continues until the cervix is fully dilated. The second stage of labor extends from full dilation of the cervix to the birth of the infant. The third stage refers to the period from birth of the infant to delivery of the placenta. Each of these three stages is monitored to assist in making a diagnosis of dystocia related to the powers.

The Friedman graph may be used to assess progress in labor (see Chapter 21). Using the relationships of cervical dilation and fetal descent against elapsed time in labor, the practitioner can determine if

▶ TYPES OF DYSFUNCTIONAL LABOR

1. Preparatory division
   Prolonged latent phase
2. Dilational division
   Protracted active dilation
   Protracted descent
3. Pelvic division
   Prolonged deceleration phase
   Secondary arrest of dilation
   Arrest of descent
   Failure of descent
4. Precipitous disorders
   Precipitous labor
   Precipitous delivery

cervical dilation and fetal descent are occurring at a normal rate, too fast, too slow, or not at all.

Plotting a graph of the client's progress in labor and then comparing it with Friedman's curve are useful in assessing the normalcy of labor. Based on his analysis of labor, Friedman described nine types of dysfunctional labor. They are classified as (1) disorders of the preparatory division of labor, (2) disorders of the dilational division of labor, (3) disorders of the pelvic division of labor, and (4) precipitous disorders (see box entitled Types of Dysfunctional Labor).

The following discussion focuses on disorders of the preparatory, dilational, and pelvic divisions of labor. Precipitous labor has been described in the preceding section.

Preparatory Division of Labor

The preparatory division of labor includes the latent and active phases described earlier. The abnormal labor pattern that may occur during this time is the prolonged latent phase.

Prolonged Latent Phase. A latent phase is necessary to the labor process, helping to establish the pattern of labor contractions. Prolongation of this phase can, however, indicate underlying problems. A latent phase lasting longer than 20 hours in a nulliparous woman and 14 hours in a multiparous woman is generally considered to be prolonged.

One cause for a prolonged latent phase might be false labor. As described in Chapter 24, true labor is differentiated from false labor by the presence of cervical effacement and dilation. Absence of these processes indicates that true labor has not started. An "unripe" cervix (one that is long, thick, and closed) may be another cause. Before it can dilate, the cervix must ripen or become soft, shorten, and thin out.

This process takes time and will prolong the latent period.

Fetopelvic disproportion occurs when the fetus is too large for the pelvis; malposition occurs when the presenting part of the fetus is entering the pelvis in an awkward manner. When either of these occur, the presenting part of the fetus cannot descend and create the pressure on the cervix necessary for dilation. Medication may be another cause of a prolonged latent phase. Administration of narcotic analgesics too early in the labor process may slow labor. Meperidine (Demerol), for example, when administered at the appropriate time, helps with cervical relaxation; however, given too early in labor, it disrupts the labor pattern, prolonging labor.

Although a long latent phase is worrisome, it usually does not endanger the mother or fetus. Rest is prescribed for false labor or an unripe cervix and for those clients who have received too much medication. Maternal posturing, or having the client periodically assume various positions (e.g., lateral, Sims', and knee-chest) may help to move the fetus from a malposition to a more favorable position. Barring absolute fetopelvic disproportion, in which there is no possibility for a vaginal delivery, contractions may be augmented with oxytocin.

Dilational Division of Labor

The dilational division of labor includes the phase of maximum slope of dilation. The disorders of this division are protracted active phase dilation and protracted descent. A protracted disorder is one in which progress is slower than normally expected.

Protracted Active Dilation. During the active phase of labor, once the cervix has started to dilate, dilation should continue at a rate of at least 1.2 cm per hour in a nulliparous woman and 1.5 cm per hour in a multiparous woman. Failure to progress in this manner results in protracted active phase dilation. A client with this condition has mild to moderately intense contractions and some cervical dilation takes place, but the rate of dilation is slower than normal and indicates that some problem is present. Assessment of the relationship of the fetus to the pelvis is necessary. A major disproportion would necessitate a cesarean delivery. If no disproportion is found, labor is allowed to continue as long as some progress is being made and the fetus is in no distress.

Protracted Descent. Protraction disorders also are evident in fetal descent. Normally, the rate of descent in a primiparous woman is 1.0 cm per hour, and in a multiparous woman, 2.0 cm per hour. Progress that is slower than this rate is termed protracted descent. Fetopelvic disproportion and inefficient uterine contractions are the principal causes of protracted descent. Both possibilities must be assessed and appropriate action taken to correct the problem.

Pelvic Division of Labor

The deceleration phase, the second stage of labor, and the phase of maximum slope of descent are included in Friedman's pelvic division of labor. The abnormal labor patterns that may occur include prolonged deceleration phase, secondary arrest of dilation, arrest of descent, and failure of descent.

Conditions in which either cervical dilation or fetal descent stops after having initially progressed are referred to as arrest disorders. Once dilation or descent has started, it should continue until completion unless complications arise and interfere with the progress. The diagnosis of arrest of dilation is made only after there has been no progress for 2 hours. Vaginal examinations to determine cervical dilation should be performed by the same person during this time so documentation of no progress can be made. Arrest of descent can be diagnosed when the presenting part of the fetus shows no progress in moving down the pelvis for at least an hour. The examination to determine progress should also be made by the same individual.

Prolonged Deceleration Phase. Cervical dilation that shows no progress for 3 hours or more in a nulliparous woman and 1 hour or more in a multiparous woman is indicative of prolonged deceleration phase. Fetopelvic or cephalopelvic disproportion may be suspected; if found to be the cause, cesarean deliv-

ery is recommended. In the absence of fetopelvic or cephalopelvic disproportion, additional labor may be warranted unless fetal distress is evident.

Secondary Arrest of Dilation. Cessation of the active phase progression for more than 2 hours in a nulliparous woman or 1 hour in a multiparous woman indicates secondary arrest of dilation. Again, cephalopelvic disproportion is suspected. If no cephalopelvic disproportion or fetal distress is found, oxytocin augmentation and rest constitute the treatment of choice.

Arrest of Descent. Fetal descent that stops and shows no progression in fetal station for an hour or more is termed arrest of descent. In the absence of cephalopelvic disproportion, stimulation of uterine contractions may effect a vaginal delivery.

Failure of Descent. Cephalopelvic disproportion is the usual cause of the presenting part's failure to descend during the deceleration phase and the second stage of labor. Cesarean delivery is most often indicated to manage failure of descent.

► Development of Pathologic Uterine Rings

During the course of normal labor, the uterus differentiates into two distinct segments, the upper or active segment and the lower or passive segment (Fig. 25–2). With each contraction, the muscle fibers in the upper segment shorten to maintain the downward

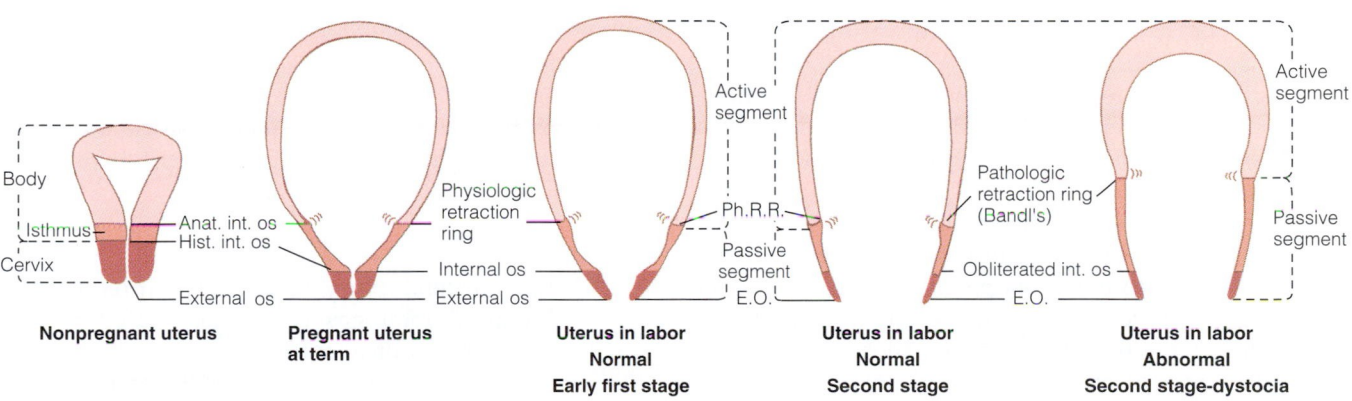

FIGURE 25–2. Sequence of development of segments and rings in the uterus in pregnant women at term and in labor. Note comparison between the uterus of a nonpregnant woman, the uterus at term, and the uterus during labor. The passive lower segment of the uterine body is derived from the isthmus; the physiologic retraction ring develops at the junction of the upper and lower uterine segments. The pathologic retraction ring develops from the physiologic ring. (Anat. int. os = anatomic internal os; Hist. int. os = histologic internal os; Ph.R.R. = physiologic retraction ring; E.O. = external os. *(Reproduced, with permission, from Cunningham, F.G. et al. (1997). Williams obstetrics (20th ed.). Stamford, CT: Appleton & Lange, p. 264.)*

pressure that is needed. Continued shortening causes thickening. The lower segment becomes thinner and more distended as the muscle fibers there stretch. The boundary between the two is termed a **physiologic retraction ring.**

Pathologic retraction rings may develop, however. They are an exaggeration of the normal physiologic ring and cause uterine dystocia. Bandl's ring is the most common type of pathologic retraction ring. A **constriction ring,** a rare development, is more easily managed.

Bandl's Ring

Bandl's ring forms when the labor is obstructed, meaning that fetal descent stops because of fetopelvic or cephalopelvic disproportion or some other complication preventing the fetus from moving down the pelvis. Contractions continue in the presence of obstructed labor. The upper segment of the uterus overretracts while the lower segment overdistends. Labor is further impeded as part of the fetus becomes trapped above the ring and part below. Without intervention, uterine rupture may occur. Development of Bandl's ring necessitates a cesarean delivery.

Constriction Ring

Constriction rings are rare and localized. Usually they conform to a depression in the baby, such as the neck. Descent of the fetus is prevented. Unlike Bandl's ring, where the obstruction to the passage of the fetus comes first and is the cause of the ring, the constriction ring is the cause of the obstruction. Relaxation of the ring by analgesia, anesthesia, or both is the treatment of choice, permitting a vaginal delivery.

▶ DYSTOCIA RELATED TO THE PASSENGER

During labor, the fetus, aided by the force of the uterine contractions, enters the pelvis and undergoes a series of maneuvers called the mechanisms of labor. (See discussion in Chapter 21.) These movements allow the fetus to move down the pelvis to delivery.

The easiest way to accomplish these maneuvers is for the fetus to enter the pelvis head first in what is called a vertex or cephalic presentation. With the head flexed on the chest, the smallest diameter of the fetal head is able to enter the pelvic inlet. This anterior–posterior diameter, called the suboccipito-bregmatic diameter, extends from the lower edge of the occipital bone to the anterior fontanelle and averages 9.5 cm at term.

At the midpelvis, the fetal head must rotate to an anterior position facing the mother's spine. This posi-tion is necessary because the narrowest transverse diameter in the pelvis is at the midpelvis and the fetal head must rotate to pass through this area. The rotation at midpelvis is most easily accomplished if the head enters the pelvic inlet in a transverse or side-to-side position. The biparietal diameter, the largest transverse diameter of the fetal head, is the distance between the parietal eminences (the points at which the parietal bones are farthest apart) and averages 9.5 cm at term. Any deviation with regard to presentation or position results in dystocia.

Malpresentation and malposition of the fetus make movement through the pelvis difficult and, in some instances, impossible. The second most common cause of dysfunctional labor is malpresenta-tions. Labor complicated by malpresentation or malposition is termed **fetal dystocia.** Fetal dystocia can also be caused by fetal conditions contributing to felopelvic and cephalopelvic disproportion and shoulder dystocia.

▶ Malpresentation

When the presenting part entering the pelvic inlet is other than the completely flexed head of the fetus, **malpresentation** is said to occur. Abnormal presenta-tions may involve other parts of the fetal skull, such as the brow or face. These presentations are a result of the fetal head being extended rather than flexed. Dystocia occurs because the fit in the pelvis is less than ideal, making the passage through the pelvis more difficult. If the adaptation of the presenting part to the cervix is less than symmetric, the efficiency of labor is reduced. Malpresentation also may occur when a part other than the fetal head presents, as in shoulder and breech presentations. Table 25–1 summarizes the techniques used to assess malpresentation.

Nursing Diagnoses

Nursing diagnoses related to fetal dystocia are developed after careful assessment of the mechanisms of labor. Examples of diagnoses include:

Problem-oriented diagnoses:

- Risk for fetal injury, related to malpresentation
- Impaired fetal gas exchange, related to prolapse of umbilical cord
- Fatigue, related to prolonged labor caused by malposition
- Fetal trauma, related to fetal hydrocephalus

Wellness-oriented diagnoses:

- Effective maternal coping, related to adequate support of partner

► **TABLE 25-1**

Techniques Used to Assess Fetal Malpresentation

Assessment Technique	Possible Finding
Leopold's maneuvers	Ballottement at the fundus indicating breech presentation
Auscultation of fetal heart	Heart heard in upper quadrants for breech presentation, in lower quadrants for brow or face presentations
Inspection of abdomen	Maternal abdomen is unusually wide from side to side, fundus scarcely above umbilicus in a transverse lie
Vaginal examination	Palpation of portion of fetal head between orbital ridge and anterior fontanelle in brow presentation; mouth, nose, malar bones, and orbital ridges in face presentation (mouth and malar prominences form a triangle); fetal lower extremities and buttocks and anus in breech (anus on line with ischial tuberosities)
Sonography, x-ray pelvimetry, or computed tomographic pelvimetry	Determination of fetal position
Fetal heart rate monitoring	Variable deceleration rate indicating possible prolapsed cord associated with breech presentation

Brow Presentation

A moderate extension of the fetal head as it enters the pelvis results in a **brow presentation** (Fig. 25–3). The verticomental diameter, which is the distance between the vertex at the top of the head and the chin, enters the pelvis first. This measurement is the largest anteroposterior diameter of the head and averages 13.5 cm. Brow presentations are rare, occurring in 1 in 1000 to 3000 deliveries (DeCherney & Pernoll, 1994). Frequently as the descent in the pelvis progresses, the brow presentation spontaneously converts to an occiput or face presentation for delivery. Pressure of the head against the bony maternal pelvis causes the head either to flex or to hyperextend before delivery occurs.

Etiology. A persistent brow presentation is associated with factors that delay or prevent engagement. In the mother, factors associated with brow presentation include too small a pelvis for the size of the fetus, tumors in the lower segment of the uterus, or a placenta that has implanted low in the uterus rather than in the fundus where implantation normally occurs.

Fetal factors include those conditions that prevent flexion of the head, for example, having the umbilical cord wrapped around the neck. Fetal anomalies involving the fetal head need to be considered.

Nursing and Collaborative Management. Nursing interventions are aimed at supporting the client and helping her to cope with a difficult and prolonged labor. Both the client and her labor partner need to be kept informed of the progress of labor. Frequent assessment of both mother and fetus must be carried out throughout the labor. Comfort measures such as back rubs, frequent mouth care, and change of position may help the mother relax. Intervention is not necessary if cervical dilation and fetal descent

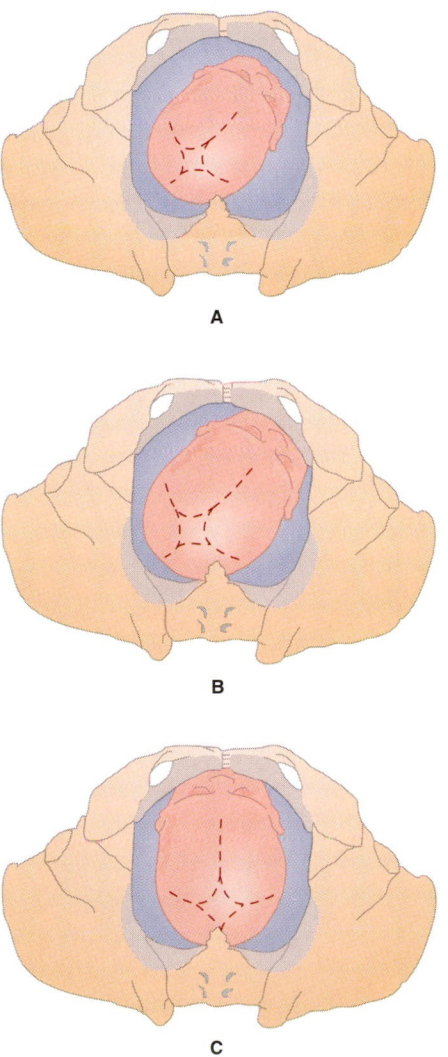

FIGURE 25–3. Brow presentation (left frontum anterior), vaginal view. **A.** Onset of labor. **B.** Descent. **C.** Internal rotation—left frontum anterior to frontum anterior. *(Adapted, with permission, from Oxorn, H. (Ed.). (1986). Oxorn-Foote human labor and birth (5th ed.). Norwalk, CT: Appleton & Lange, p. 211.)*

progress satisfactorily and there is no fetal or maternal distress. If, however, fetal distress or arrest of descent occurs, prompt cesarean delivery is recommended.

Face Presentation

A **face presentation** is a vertex presentation with the fetal head hyperextended so that the face enters the pelvic inlet first (Fig. 25–4). The part of the face that presents is the area between the glabella (directly above the root of the nose) and the chin. It is the submentobregmatic diameter and measures about 9.6 cm. Face presentations occur in about 0.2% of deliveries (DeCherney & Pernoll, 1994).

Etiology. As with the brow presentation, anything that interferes with the engagement of the fetal head in flexion can be a causative factor. A frequent cause is fetopelvic disproportion. Face presentation is common among anencephalic fetuses.

Nursing and Collaborative Management. The nurse closely monitors the progress of the labor and the status of the fetus during labor. The client and her labor partner both need to be supported as they

cope with the long and difficult labor that may occur with a face presentation.

Vaginal delivery for a face presentation is possible if certain conditions exist. First, the chin (mentum) of the fetus must be in the anterior position (Fig. 25–4D). In an anterior position, the fetal face is looking toward the mother's umbilicus, with the back of the head resting on either the left or right side of the pelvis. Second, the contractions must be forceful enough to propel the fetus through the pelvis. And, finally, there must be no pelvic contracture. The fetus must be able to enter and move through the pelvis. If the chin presents and stays in a posterior position, spontaneous vaginal delivery is impossible. When the face reaches the midpelvis, internal rotation occurs and the chin rotates posteriorly 45° into the hollow of the sacrum. Flexion cannot take place, nor can the fetus advance any further in the pelvis. With the arrest of descent, cesarean delivery is required.

Shoulder Presentation

Shoulder presentation, also known as transverse lie, occurs when the long axis of the fetus is at a right angle to the long axis of the mother. In essence, the

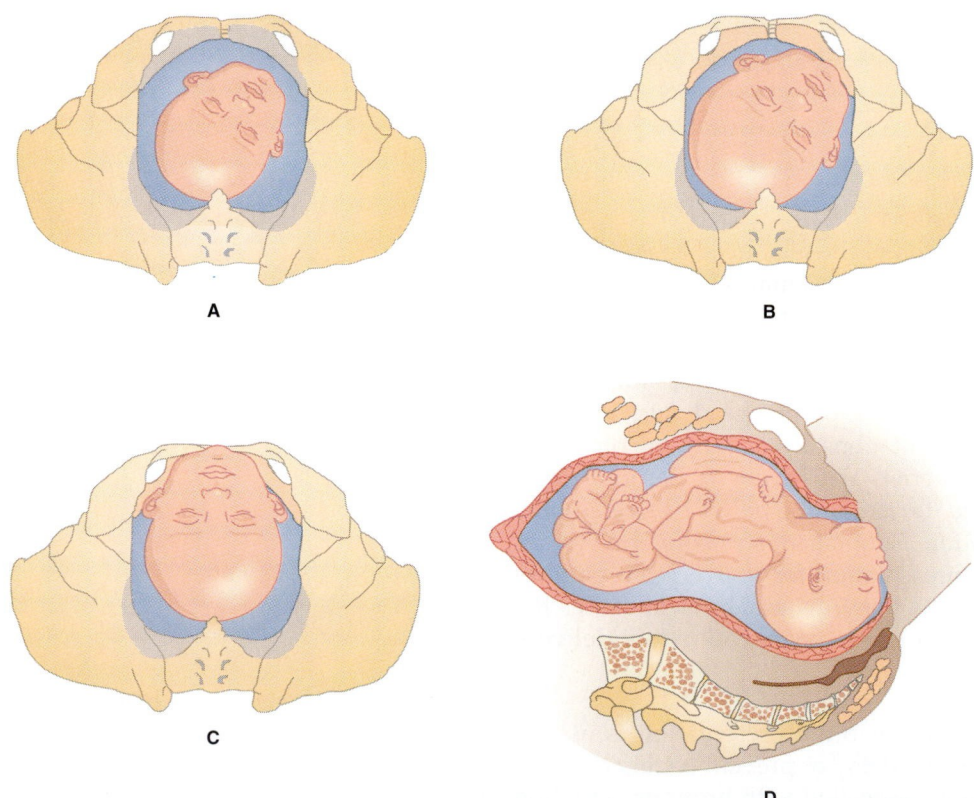

FIGURE 25–4. Face presentation (left mentum anterior), vaginal and lateral views. **A.** Onset of labor. **B.** Extension and descent. **C.** and **D.** Internal rotation—left mentum anterior to mentum anterior (**C.** vaginal view; **D.** lateral view). *(Adapted, with permission, from Oxorn, H. (Ed.). (1986). Oxorn-Foote human labor and birth (5th ed.). Norwalk, CT: Appleton & Lange, p. 187.)*

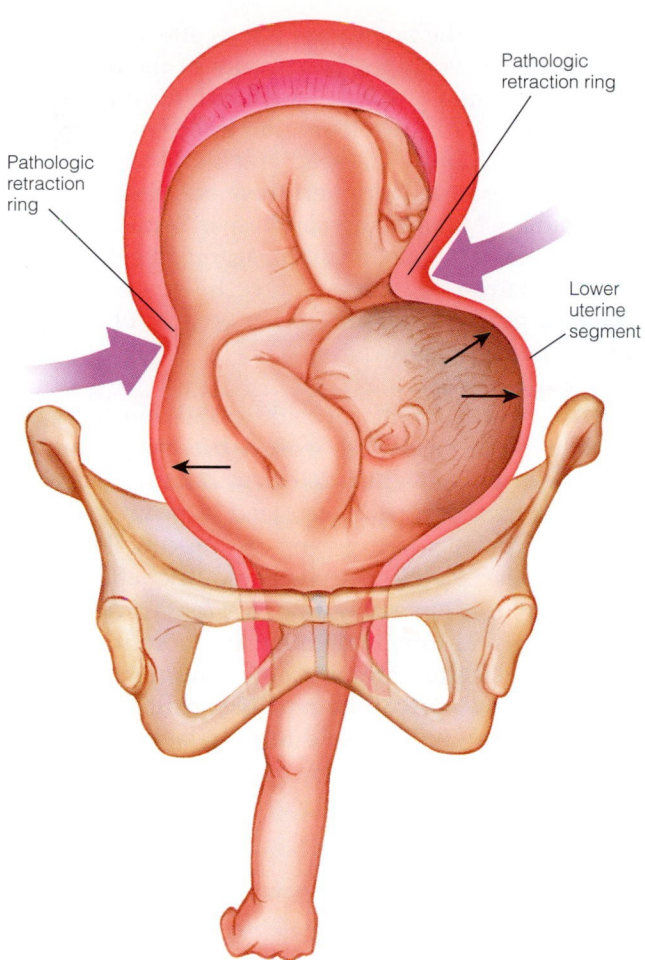

FIGURE 25–5. Neglected shoulder presentation. A thick muscular band forming a pathologic retraction ring has developed just above the very thin lower uterine segment. The force generated during a uterine contraction is directed at and above the level of the retraction ring, serving to stretch further and possibly to rupture the very thin lower segment below the retraction ring.

fetus is lying across the mother's abdomen and the shoulder is the presenting part that dips into the pelvis. The fetus may lie directly across the maternal abdomen or obliquely. The incidence of shoulder presentation is about 1 in 300 deliveries (DeCherney & Pernoll, 1994).

Etiology. Shoulder presentation is more common in multiparous than primiparous women because the abdominal and uterine muscles tend to be weakened after several pregnancies and deliveries. Other causes include placenta previa, preterm fetus, contracted pelvis, and an abnormal uterus.

Nursing and Collaborative Management. Delivery of a full-term fetus in a shoulder presentation is not considered possible, as the fetus cannot

move through the pelvis in this position. Moreover, labor with shoulder presentation can result in risk to the mother from spontaneous rupture of the uterus, and significant risk to the fetus (Fig. 25–5). When conditions make a safe vaginal delivery questionable, cesarean delivery is necessary.

The couple may be anxious and fearful about the complication and possible cesarean delivery. The nurse supports the couple and provides factual information concerning the problem and its management. In addition, the nurse helps prepare the client and her support person for cesarean delivery, should it be necessary.

Compound Presentation

In **compound presentation,** more than one part of the fetus presents. When the presenting part does not completely occlude the pelvic inlet, a compound presentation is likely to occur. The extra space allows an arm or leg to prolapse, or slip through the opening. The most common compound presentation is an arm to prolapse alongside the head (Fig. 25–6). The incidence of compound presentation is reported to be 0.1% of deliveries (DeCherney & Pernoll, 1994).

Etiology. Prematurity and multiple gestation, in which the fetus tends to be small and the presenting part does not completely occlude the inlet, are common causes of compound presentations. An arm or leg may also prolapse alongside the presenting part if membranes rupture while the presenting part is still high and not engaged.

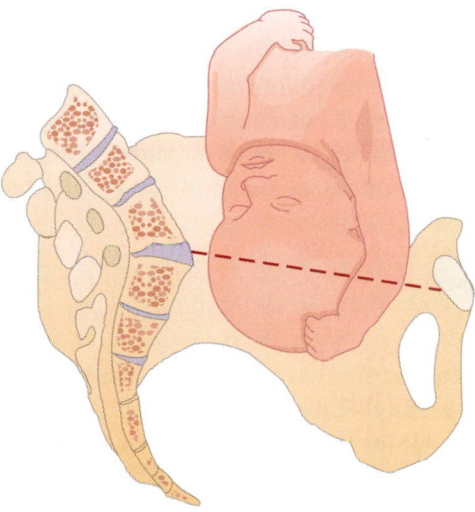

FIGURE 25–6. Compound presentation: head and hand. *(Adapted, with permission, from Oxorn, H. (Ed.). (1986). Oxorn-Foote human labor and birth (5th ed.). Norwalk, CT: Appleton & Lange, p. 278.)*

Nursing and Collaborative Management. If no complications are present, labor is permitted to continue. As the cervix dilates completely and the presenting part descends, the prolapsed arm or leg may rise out of the pelvis, allowing labor to continue normally.

The nurse should observe for an extremity in the vagina and continue to provide information to the client and her labor partner as labor progresses. Fear and anxiety, caused by seeing a prolapsed limb, may be reduced if the woman and her partner are advised of this possibility. Reassurance that labor is progressing normally may help the client to cope.

Compound presentations may be complicated by prolapse of the umbilical cord. As the presenting part moves through the pelvis with the cord beside it, the cord may become compressed, stopping the flow of oxygenated blood to the fetus. This condition is considered an obstetric emergency and requires immediate treatment to avoid fetal suffocation. (See discussion later in this chapter.)

Breech Presentation

The most common malpresentation is **breech presentation,** in which the buttocks, or breech, present. Breech deliveries occur in 3 to 4% of all single births. Breech presentations are classified as follows:

1. *Complete breech.* The buttocks is the presenting part, the fetal thighs are flexed at the hips, and the knees are flexed.
2. *Frank breech.* The buttocks is the presenting part, the fetal thighs are flexed at the hips, the legs are extended, and the feet are extended close to the face.
3. *Incomplete or footling breech.* One or two feet are the presenting part; fetal thigh(s) and knee(s) are extended.

The cause of a breech presentation is not always apparent, but prematurity, primiparity, and older maternal age have been associated with increased risk of breech birth (Rayl, Gibson, & Hickok, 1996). In addition, malpresentations are associated with great parity because of the weakened musculature of the mother. Polyhydramnios may be a factor because excessive amniotic fluid makes it easier for the fetus to change position. Hydrocephaly (enlarged head) or a low implanted placenta may also be influential, because these conditions prohibit the fetal head from entering the pelvis (Rayl, Gibson, & Hickok, 1996). Any condition that would interfere with the engagement of the fetal head could lead to a breech presentation.

Maternal Risks. Vaginal delivery of a fetus in a breech position poses several problems for the mother. Usually the labor is prolonged. The soft, irregular tissues of the breech are not as effective in dilating the cervix as are the hard bones of the fetal skull. Membranes may rupture prematurely, putting the mother at risk for developing an infection, especially if the labor is long. The head and shoulders are born last in a breech delivery and there is little or no time for molding. Manipulation and use of forceps to assist with the delivery may result in lacerations of the birth canal. Cesarean delivery of a breech fetus poses additional surgical risks to the mother because of the operative procedure involved.

Fetal Risks. Infant morbidity and mortality are thought to be increased with a breech delivery as compared with a vertex delivery. Trauma, especially to the aftercoming head, can lead to central nervous system injuries. Compression of the umbilical cord between the mother's pelvis and the aftercoming head may result in asphyxia of the fetus. Fractures of fetal bones and muscle damage are more frequent in breech than vertex presentations. Entrapment of the fetal head, prolapse of the umbilical cord, and aspiration of meconium are also directly related to a breech delivery. Several studies have demonstrated that the mode of delivery of infants in a breech presentation does not significantly affect the outcome (Albrechtsen, 1997; Erkkola, 1996; Koike, Minakami, Sasaki, Sayama, Tamada, & Sato, 1996; Robertson, Foran, Croughan-Minihane, & Kilpatrick, 1996).

Nursing and Collaborative Management. During labor, the client with a breech fetus needs to be assessed frequently for progress of labor. Labor may be long because of slow cervical dilation. The client may become exhausted as the labor continues and should be encouraged to rest between contractions. Enlisting the support of the labor partner to assist the client to rest and relax may help. Hydration must be maintained and intake and output monitored if the labor is long.

Breech presentations are associated with a prolapsed cord. The nurse should monitor the fetal heart rate (FHR) for bradycardia, which might indicate cord compression. The nurse also should visually examine the perineal area and vaginal opening for signs of the cord, which sometimes will prolapse through the cervix.

The decision between vaginal and cesarean delivery in a breech presentation is the responsibility of the physician. During labor, assessments are made of fetal size, type of presentation, and adequacy of the mother's pelvis. Whether the fetal head is flexed or extended is noted; possible congenital malformations that might interfere with the normal progress of labor are identified. If the decision is made to deliver vaginally, the delivery may be spontaneous or assisted. A spontaneous delivery requires no assistance from the attending physician or nurse-midwife. If assistance is required, it is given after the fetus has been expelled as far as the umbilicus. Forceps may be used to extract the fetal head in assisted breech deliveries (Fig. 25–7A). In rare instances, the physician may attempt to extract the total fetal body. This procedure involves manipulation to convert the frank breech to a footling breech (Fig. 25–7B). Cesarean delivery is chosen if

there is evidence that a vaginal delivery would pose a threat to either the mother or the fetus.

The vaginal delivery of a breech presentation is an area of great controversy among physicians. Some believe that normal size, term infants have the best result for vaginal deliveries. Primiparous women presenting breech are usually delivered by cesarean. With multiparous women, some physicians elect vaginal delivery; others opt for a cesarean delivery. Some physicians believe that all breech presentations should be managed by cesarean delivery regardless of the parity of the mother (Scorza, 1996). Approximately 80% of breech fetuses that are at term in the United States are delivered by cesarean (St. Saunders, 1996).

External Cephalic Version. External cephalic version (ECV) is the manipulation of the fetus through the abdominal wall to convert a breech to a vertex presentation. It is attempted in very controlled circumstances. Studies have shown that ECV after 36 weeks' gestation reduced the number of breech deliveries and cesarean deliveries (Annapoorna, Arulkumaran, Anandakumar, Chua, Montan, & Ratnam, 1997; McParland & Farine, 1996).

▶ Prolapse of the Umbilical Cord

Prolapse of the umbilical cord constitutes an obstetric emergency. Although not a common occurrence (about once in every 400 births) the condition is associated with a high fetal mortality rate. If the presenting part of the fetus is not engaged in the pelvis or if the fetus is not snug with a malpresentation, when the membranes rupture the cord can prolapse and be carried downward by the sudden gush of amniotic fluid (Fig. 25–8). Anytime the presenting part does not

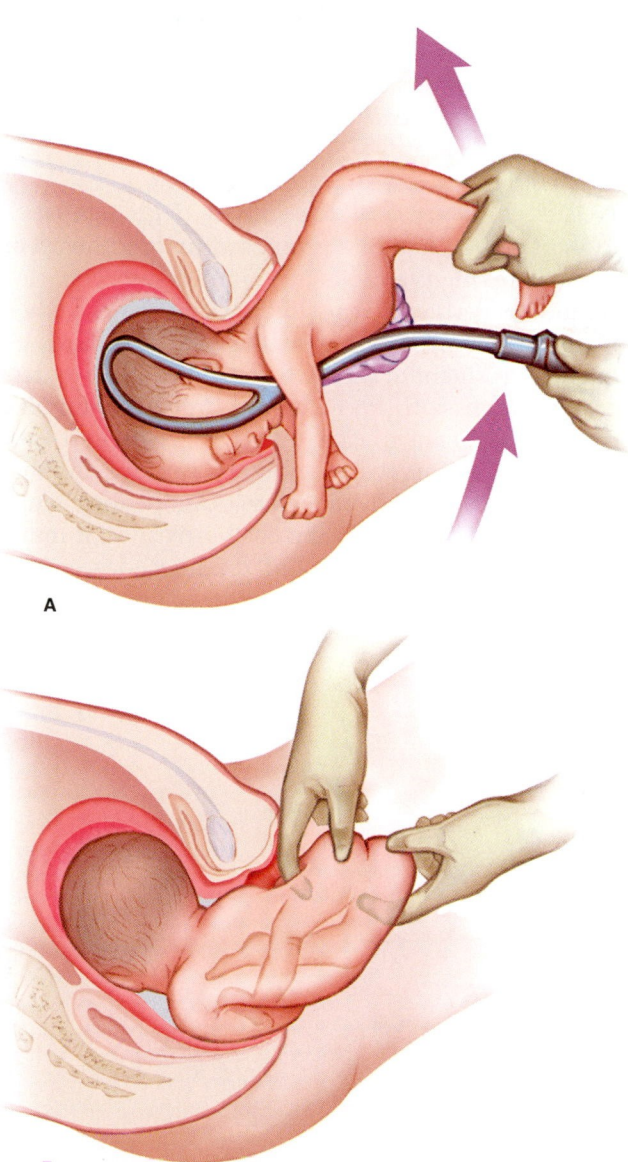

FIGURE 25–7. Delivery of breech presentation. **A.** Extraction of a complete or incomplete breech using forceps to the aftercoming head. Note the direction of movement (arrow). **B.** Extraction of a frank breech using moderate traction exerted by a finger in each groin and facilitated by generous episiotomy. *(Reproduced, with permission, from Cunningham, F.G. et al. (1997). Williams obstetrics (20th ed.). Stamford, CT: Appleton & Lange, pp. 498, 503.)*

Nursing Alert

Nursing care during external cephalic version consists of monitoring the client's vital signs, assessing the FHR for abnormal patterns, and evaluating the client's response to the procedure as it may cause discomfort. After the procedure, the nurse checks for vaginal bleeding and assesses maternal vital signs, uterine activity, and FHR.

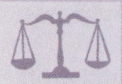

Ethical Decision Making

During the intrapartum period, complications can occur that require prompt decisions and interventions. There is controversy among health care providers about whether breech presentations should be delivered by cesarean or by vaginal delivery. Since the nurse is a key member of the interdisciplinary health care team and is a primary advocate for the client and her partner, the following issues should be considered in this situation:

1. With the current emphasis on quality care delivered in a cost-effective manner, do you think that the majority of breech presentations should be delivered vaginally or by cesarean delivery?
2. Who should make the decision about the method of delivery?
3. What factors should influence the decision-making process?
4. How would you respond if the physician disagrees with the client's choice about the method of delivery for a breech presentation?

closely adhere to the pelvis, as in fetopelvic disproportion, the potential for prolapsed cord exists. Shoulder, compound, and breech presentations are examples of malpresentations in which the cord is likely to prolapse. Risk is also increased when the fetus is small, as in prematurity and multiple gestation.

Maternal Risks. There is no direct risk to the mother with prolapsed cord. She is, however, placed at risk by attempts to save the fetus.

Fetal Risks. The mortality rate for the fetus with a prolapsed cord is high. Compression of the cord between the presenting part and the bony pelvis of the mother results in fetal hypoxia. Prolonged cord compression can lead to central nervous system damage and even death.

Nursing and Collaborative Management. Prompt recognition of a prolapsed umbilical cord and immediate interventions are important. The nurse should be alert to the possibility of a prolapse when a malpresentation is noted in the laboring client. Frequent assessment of the FHR should be done to detect cord compression, because the prolapsed umbilical cord is not always visible (occult prolapsed cord). Immediately after the membranes rupture, the nurse should check the FHR as well as examine the client for a prolapsed cord. When the cord prolapses, it may lie beside the presenting part of the inlet, descend into the vagina, or protrude outside the vagina.

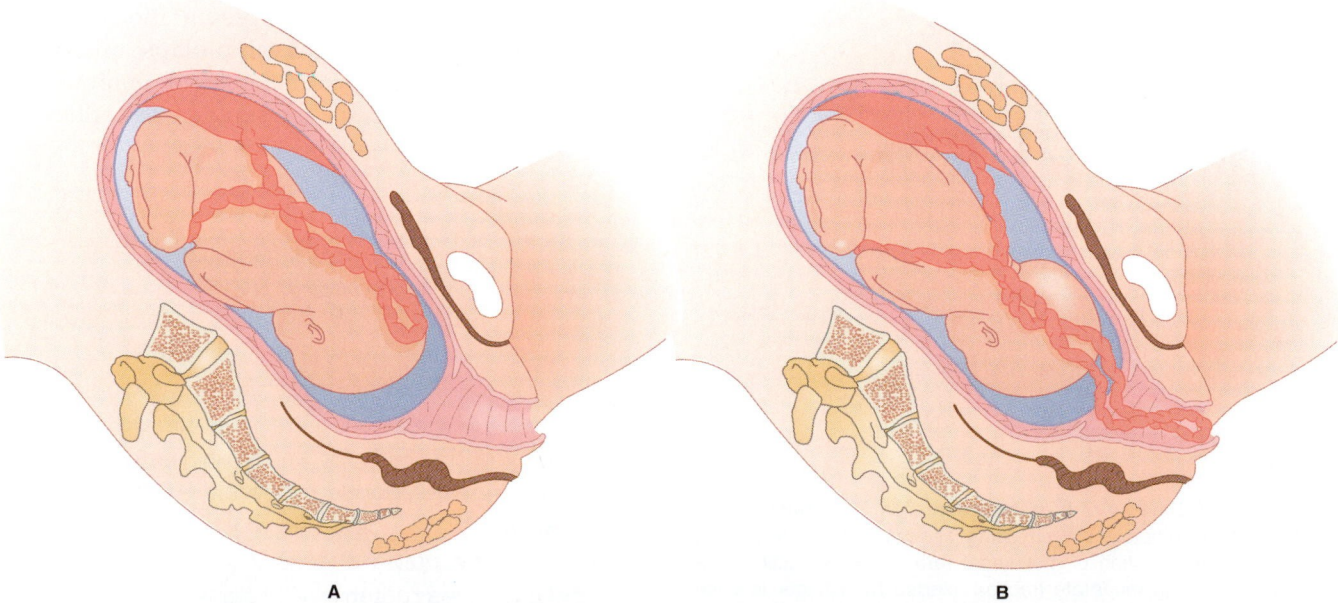

A   B

FIGURE 25–8. Prolapse of the umbilical cord. **A.** Cord prolapsed at the inlet. **B.** Cord prolapsed through the introitus. *(Adapted, with permission, from Oxorn, H. (Ed.). (1986). Oxorn-Foote human labor and birth (5th ed.). Norwalk, CT: Appleton & Lange, p. 285.)*

A prolapsed cord requires immediate action by the nurse. The client should be assisted into a position that will shift the weight of the fetus off the cord. This could be either the Trendelenburg or knee–chest position. Supplemental oxygen should be administered to the client via mask. IV fluids should be started or increased to enhance the fluid volume and circulation. The physician should be notified immediately. If the cord is protruding outside the vagina, no attempt is made to replace it or push it back in the vagina. The cord may instead be covered with sterile towels moistened with warm sterile saline to prevent it from drying and cooling.

Vaginal support of the presenting part may help relieve pressure on the cord. This is accomplished by placing a sterile gloved hand into the vagina and pushing up on the presenting part. This support may continue until a cesarean delivery is performed. Immediate cesarean delivery is recommended unless the cervix is completely dilated and a rapid vaginal delivery is possible.

When a cord prolapses, the client may be startled by the sudden rush of personnel to assist. The nurse can help the client by remaining calm despite the activity. Explanations of the procedures that are necessary can help reduce the client's anxiety and enlist her cooperation. Both the client and her labor partner may be fearful for the safety of the fetus; explaining what is being done to assist the fetus may help them cope with their fears.

► Malposition

Position of the fetus in labor refers to the relationship of the presenting part to the maternal pelvis. For identification purposes, the maternal pelvis is divided into quadrants. Left and right anterior quadrants are in the front of the pelvis near the pubic arch. Left and right posterior quadrants are in the back near the coccyx. Another reference point is the denominator, a designated point on the presenting part that is used to describe the position. In the "ideal" position, the fetal head is completely flexed on the chest and the occiput (O), which is the denominator, is in either the right or left anterior quadrant of the mother's pelvis [right occiput anterior (ROA) or left occiput anterior (LOA)].

The fetal head follows the principle of "best fit" so malpositions may occur in the presence of fetopelvic disproportion or in an abnormal pelvic inlet. The most common malpositions are the occiput posterior and occiput transverse positions.

Occiput Posterior

A fetus in an occiput posterior position is in a vertex or cephalic presentation, with the occiput (denomina-

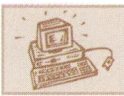

Research Abstract

Use of Critical Thinking Techniques in Intrapartal Nursing Decisions

The purpose of this descriptive, qualitative study was to determine what clinical parameters expert intrapartal nurses used to assess the severity of fetal stress. The participants in the study were 18 expert labor and delivery nurses with an average of 11.3 years of intrapartal experience.

The findings of the content analysis of clinical problem-solving indicated that the nurses' assessment of fetal stress included duration of the stress, fetal reserve status, signs of stress, and reversibility of stress. The nurses also assessed whether the pattern was short or prolonged, continuous or intermittent, and the progress of the woman's labor. Assessment of fetal reserve status included data regarding maternal pregnancy health status, gestational age of the fetus, and biophysical assessment of fetal status. Reversibility of stress was assessed by the nurses based on the responsiveness of the fetus to resuscitation.

The conclusion of this study was that clinical decision making of expert intrapartal nurses was a process with contextual features and links.

Application to Practice

This study supports the view that nurses use critical thinking techniques in assessing complications during labor and delivery. Assessment does not derive from one set of parameters, but many sets of variables. The expert labor and delivery nurse integrates knowledge in making clinical decisions that assist the client and family.

Source: Haggerty, L.A. (1996). Assessment parameters and indicators in expert intrapartal nursing decisions. Journal of Obstetric, Gynecologic, and Neonatal Nursing, 25(6), 491–499.

tor of the fetal skull) of the fetus in the left or right posterior quadrant of the mother's pelvis. Occiput posterior presentation occurs in 10 to 25% of all labors (DeCherney & Pernoll, 1994). Right occiput posterior (ROP) is five times more common than left occiput posterior (LOP). Following the "best fit" principle during labor, a fetus in a head-first position with the occiput in the posterior quadrant of the maternal pelvis enters the pelvic inlet transversely or side to side. To exit through the pelvic outlet, the fetal head must be in an anteroposterior position, that is, straight up and down. To accomplish this, rotation must take place in the midpelvis.

Rotation with the occiput in the posterior quadrant can be accomplished in one of three ways: (1) A long-arc rotation of 135° takes the fetus from a ROP position to an occiput anterior position, where the fetal head is straight up and down in an anteroposterior position; this type of rotation occurs in about 90% of occiput posterior positions. (2) Rotation of 90° moves the fetus from a ROP to a ROA position. (3) Rotation of 45° moves the fetus from a ROP to a right occiput transverse position.

Many fetuses in occiput posterior positions rotate to an anterior position spontaneously with no difficulty. Problems arise when rotation does not occur. With a persistent occiput posterior position, the fetal head does not rotate to the anterior position. Failure to rotate and cessation of descent of the fetal head indicate that labor has arrested and intervention is needed. Cephalopelvic disproportion may be a factor in occiput posterior positions. Anthropoid and android pelves, with their large posterior, sagittal diameters, lend themselves to occiput posterior positions.

Maternal Risks. Labor with a fetus in an occiput posterior position is long and difficult. Backache is common as the occiput bone presses against the mother's sacrum. If the fetus is delivered in a posterior position, perineal lacerations can occur and a large episiotomy may be needed. An episiotomy prevents tearing of the perineum, as the large back part of the head causes greater stretching during the birthing process. In the event of a cesarean delivery, the woman is at risk for surgical complications related to the operative procedure.

Fetal Risks. Molding and excessive edema of the fetal skull are common in these malpositions. Fetal asphyxia also may occur.

Nursing and Collaborative Management. A client with a fetus in an occiput posterior position may be able to help the fetus to rotate anteriorly by lying on the side opposite the fetus' back. Gravity may then assist the fetus to rotate. By squatting, kneeling, getting on hands and knees, and assuming a knee–chest position with pelvic tilting, the client may facilitate fetal rotation and descent. The nurse should assist the client in assuming these positions and give clear explanations as to why she is to do them.

Backache is a common complaint with occiput posterior positions. Sacral rubs may help. The labor partner can be encouraged to assist the client during a contraction by applying firm pressure on the sacral area. Frequent change of positions may also help.

With a persistent occiput posterior position, both the first and second stages of labor tend to be prolonged. Contractions and progress in labor should be checked and recorded at frequent intervals. FHR also should be monitored for signs of fetal distress. Hydration needs to be maintained during a long labor, usually through intravenous solutions, such as lactated Ringer's solution.

As long as labor is progressing and there is no indication of maternal or fetal distress, vaginal delivery can be anticipated. If labor becomes arrested, medical intervention is required. The fetus may be delivered vaginally using forceps provided there is no fetopelvic disproportion, the head is engaged, the cervix is fully dilated, and the membranes are ruptured. If any of these conditions are not met, vaginal delivery should not be attempted. The fetus can be delivered in the occiput posterior position or rotated with the forceps to a more anterior position for delivery. Inability to deliver vaginally or the presence of distress necessitate a cesarean delivery.

Persistent Occiput Transverse

Occiput transverse position occurs in a manner similar to that of occiput posterior as just described. The difference is that in the midpelvis, the fetal head begins to rotate to an anterior position and stops or arrests when it is transverse, with the fetal skull horizontal to the long axis of the mother. The arrest may be caused by ineffective uterine contractions or a pelvis that has a flattened anteroposterior diameter.

Maternal Risks. After a period of normal labor the client may experience a decrease in the rate and intensity of her contractions. Barring any complications from abnormal pelvic structure or fetopelvic disproportion, oxytocin may be used to stimulate the contractions. The client then is subject to any complications associated with the use of oxytocin. Delivery may be accomplished vaginally. Forceps are used to rotate the head to facilitate delivery. Lacerations of the birth canal can occur during a forceps delivery. Cesarean delivery places the mother at risk for complications related to the operative procedure.

Fetal Risks. Asphyxia may occur during a long, difficult labor. Also, if forceps are used to rotate or deliver the fetus, injury to the fetal neck or head may occur.

Nursing and Collaborative Management. Nursing care is related to the type of medical intervention selected. If oxytocin is used to augment the labor, all the activities associated with the administration of the drug must be carried out (see Chapter 24). Maternal positioning may be used to assist with rotation. The nurse needs to explain these positions and why they are being used, and to assist the client in assuming them. Throughout labor contractions, maternal vital signs and FHR are frequently assessed. Emotional support is given to both the client and her labor partner to help them cope with the dystocia.

▶ Fetal Conditions Resulting in Fetopelvic and Cephalopelvic Disproportion

In addition to malpresentation and malposition, fetal dystocia may also be caused by fetal conditions contributing to fetopelvic and cephalopelvic disproportion. Two conditions that predispose to such a situation are large fetal size and hydrocephalus.

Large Fetal Size
A fetus is termed large (or macrosomic) when he or she weighs more than 4000 g (9 pounds). This large size is often associated with maternal diabetes. Late in pregnancy, failure of the pancreas of the diabetic mother to release enough insulin to meet the increased demands results in hyperglycemia. These high levels of glucose stimulate the fetal pancreas to release insulin. The increased maternal glucose and the increased fetal insulin combine to produce excessive fetal growth (see Chapter 32). Other factors predisposing to large fetal size include delivery more than 7 days postterm, weight gain greater than 20 kg during pregnancy, multiparity, and maternal age over 35 years.

Maternal Risks. The large fetus may be delivered vaginally, provided the maternal pelvis is adequate; however, the presence of a large fetus and an average-size pelvis often results in fetopelvic disproportion. Cesarean delivery may be necessary if the fetus is too large to travel through the pelvis. A large fetus may also predispose the mother to uterine rupture and postpartum hemorrhage because of the overstretching of the myometrium.

Fetal Risks. Infant mortality related to trauma associated during the birthing process of macrosomic fetuses has been estimated at 13%, or almost 1 in 7. This compares with 4% mortality among infants of normal size (Benson & Pernoll, 1994). A large fetus whose size is underestimated may experience trauma to the head as a result of strong contractions, which force the head against the bony structures of the pelvis. Cerebral edema, neurologic damage, hypoxia, and asphyxia may result. Shoulder dystocia and fractures of the clavicle and humerus are more common with large infants (Ecker, Greenberg, Norwitz, Nadel, & Repke, 1997).

Nursing and Collaborative Management. Nursing measures are aimed at offering the mother and her labor partner support. If a vaginal delivery is planned, the second stage of labor may be prolonged and the client may need encouragement to cope. Delivery may be accomplished spontaneously, with the use of forceps, or by cesarean. The method chosen is the one that poses the least risk to mother and fetus.

Fetal Hydrocephalus
Fetal hydrocephalus is the excessive accumulation of cerebrospinal fluid in the ventricles of the brain with consequent enlargement of the cranium. Fetal hydrocephalus is often accompanied by other conditions such as spinal cord anomalies and mental retardation. It occurs in 1 in 2000 fetuses and accounts for approximately 12% of severe fetal malformations occurring at birth. In one third of the cases of fetal hydrocephalus, a breech presentation is found. Whatever the presentation, cephalopelvic disproportion is common (Cunningham et al., 1997).

Maternal Risks. Fetal hydrocephalus predisposes the laboring client to uterine rupture. In these cases, maternal mortality is very high.

Fetal Risks. The fetus with hydrocephalus is at great risk of trauma to the head. Again, high morbidity and high mortality are associated with this condition.

Nursing and Collaborative Assessment. The mother is asked to empty her bladder to facilitate abdominal and vaginal examinations. If the fetal presentation is cephalic, a broad firm mass is evident above the symphysis. The FHR is often loudest above the umbilicus, which often leads to the suspicion of a breech presentation. Vaginal examination may elicit wide suture lines and large fontanelles.

   If the presentation is breech, the condition may be more difficult to detect. Radiography or sonography may provide some confirmation of hydrocephalus.

Nursing and Collaborative Management.
For the fetus to be delivered vaginally, the size of the hydrocephalic head must be reduced. In cephalic and breech presentations, fluid is removed from the head via a needle inserted transvaginally. This procedure is called cephalocentesis. Because this procedure has a high incidence of fetal death, many hydrocephalic infants are delivered by cesarean. Even in cesarean deliveries, fluid may be removed from the fetal head. An experimental technique involving antepartal shunting of fluid from the ventricle in the head of the fetus is currently being tried.

The nurse monitors the client's vital signs and progress, if the woman has a trial of labor. Further, the nurse helps to prepare the client and her support person for any treatments or cesarean delivery. Much support is necessary for the couple coping with a difficult fetal diagnosis.

▶ Shoulder Dystocia

Shoulder dystocia occurs when the anterior shoulder of the fetus becomes impacted behind the symphysis pubis (Fig. 25–9). It is a serious complication that can result in neonatal and maternal morbidity (Piper & McDonald, 1994). Predisposing factors for shoulder dystocia include a large fetus, prolonged second stage of labor, previous delivery of an infant weighing more than 4000 g, postterm pregnancy, and a contracted pelvic outlet.

Maternal Risks. After a traumatic delivery, the mother may experience vaginal and perineal lacera-tions. These result from maneuvers to deliver the shoulders of the infant.

Fetal Risks. Shoulder dystocia increases fetal morbidity and mortality. Fetal risk is related to asphyxia resulting from prolonged cord compression when delivery is delayed and trauma to the arm and shoulder.

Nursing and Collaborative Assessment and Management. During delivery of a fetus with shoulder dystocia, the shoulders should be delivered as soon as possible after the head. Care must be taken not to exert excessive traction on the head or neck, which could stretch the neck too much or fracture the clavicle. Cesarean delivery is the method recom-mended for diabetic women with an estimated fetal weight of more than 4000 g, and should be seriously considered for those laboring women whose esti-mated fetal weight is over 4500 g and who have an abnormal labor (O'Leary, 1992).

Other methods of delivery used in the presence of shoulder dystocia are described in the literature. One approach is called the Zavanelli maneuver. After the head has been delivered and restitution has occurred, the head is returned to the prerestitutional position, maneuvers are reversed, the head is flexed and returned to the vagina, and the fetus is delivered by cesarean. Other methods include placing suprapu-bic pressure while downward traction is applied to the fetal head, delivering the posterior shoulders first, and maternal position change maneuvers (Cunning-ham et al., 1997; Piper & McDonald, 1994). One such maneuver, the McRoberts maneuver, involves sharply

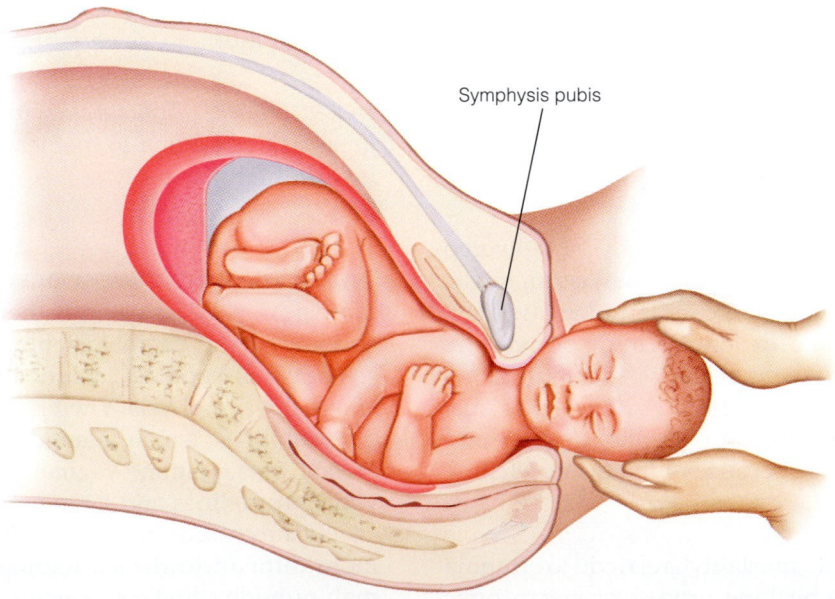

Symphysis pubis

FIGURE 25–9. Shoulder dystocia.

flexing the woman's legs upon her abdomen, causing straightening of the sacrum relative to the lumbar vertebrae with accompanying rotation of the symphysis pubis towards the head of the client, decreasing the angle of pelvic inclination (Cunningham et al., 1997).

Shoulder dystocia may be suspected when the fetus is large and the second stage of labor prolonged. If a vaginal delivery is planned, the nurse needs to prepare the client and her labor partner to expect that some difficulty may be encountered. Explanations help to reassure clients and gain their trust. Continued assessment of contractions along with the progress of labor is important. FHR should be assessed at frequent intervals and evaluated for signs of distress. During a vaginal delivery, the nurse may assist the physician by providing suprapubic pressure as it is requested.

▶ DYSTOCIA RELATED TO THE PASSAGE

Pelvic dystocia occurs when the fetus cannot enter or pass through the bony pelvis of the mother. It is due most often to contractions of the pelvis. Contractions are decreased diameters of the pelvis that are usually the result of pelvic size and shape.

Some pelves are better suited to childbirth than others. The gynecoid or female pelvis, which is considered the best, is found in about half of all women.

Factors other than pelvic size must also be considered when pelvic dystocia is suspected. A woman may have adequate pelvic measurements, but if uterine contractions are not effective, descent of the presenting part will not occur. If the fetus is too large or in a malpresentation or malposition, passage through the pelvis will be delayed or even arrested. The reverse is also true. Strong, efficient uterine contractions could move a fetus through a pelvis with borderline normal measurements. There are generally said to be three types of pelvic contractions:

1. *Inlet contraction.* Pelvic inlet contraction is present when the anteroposterior diameter of the maternal pelvis is less than 10 cm and the transverse diameter is less than 12 cm. As the presenting part first enters the pelvis through the inlet, small measurements may make engagement difficult. In an attempt to fit into the inlet, the fetal head may become malpositioned as it follows the principle of "best fit." This means the head will enter the pelvic inlet the way it is best accommodated. Difficulties may be encountered if the small moldable breech enters a pelvis with small measurements and then the aftercoming head becomes

stuck. Inlet contraction most often is caused by rickets, a vitamin D deficiency.

2. *Midpelvic contraction.* Midpelvic contraction occurs when the plane of least dimension, the midpelvic plane, is reduced. The midpelvic plane is at the level of the ischial spine. It is formed from the margin of the symphysis pubis and touches the sacrum at the junction of the fourth or fifth vertebra. An ischial spinous diameter less than 9.5 cm results in midpelvic contraction. Genetic factors responsible for the pelvic structure are the most frequent cause of this type of contraction. Midpelvic contraction often results in transverse arrest of the fetal head. The midpelvis is where internal rotation of the fetal head takes place. Contractions in this area complicate the rotation process or prevent it altogether.

3. *Outlet contraction.* With contraction of the pelvic outlet, the distance between the ischial tuberosities is less than 8 cm. This condition frequently occurs along with other contractions of the pelvis and is related to pelvic bone development.

Maternal Risks. Dystocia related to pelvic contractions prolongs labor as a result of slow dilation or fetal descent. All the problems associated with prolonged labor may occur: exhaustion, increased discomfort, and potential intrauterine infection resulting from premature rupture of membranes. Pelvic dystocia can also result in uterine rupture, as the muscles overdistend in an effort to expel the uterine contents. Forceps-assisted delivery may traumatize maternal tissues, causing profuse bleeding from the lacerations of the birth canal and perineum. Cesarean delivery may be necessary, in which case the mother is susceptible to operative complications such as hemorrhage and infection.

Fetal Risks. The fetal head is prone to injury in the event of pelvic dystocia, as it is forced against the cervix by uterine contractions. With borderline measurements, the fetal skull may have to mold excessively to pass through the pelvis. Caput succedaneum is common. Neurologic problems, as well as hemorrhage and fractures of the fetal head, can occur because of the pressing of the head against the bony pelvis.

Nursing and Collaborative Assessment. Marked deviations such as decreased pelvic diameters and abnormalities in pelvic structure may be identified during prenatal care, at which time vaginal delivery can be ruled out and cesarean delivery anticipated. Borderline measurements might indicate a trial labor. This trial of labor involves observing the woman through at least 4 hours of well-established labor for dilation or monitoring the woman in the second stage of labor for more than 2 hours for head engagement. Interventions such as maternal positioning may be attempted. Failure of the trial of labor warrants cesarean delivery. When dystocia occurs in labor and the powers and the passenger can be ruled out as the cause, pelvimetry and ultrasound should be conducted to determine pelvic measurements.

When pelvic contraction has not been identified prior to the start of labor, the nurse must monitor cervical dilation and fetal descent closely. If these fail to progress normally, pelvic contraction may be a cause.

The labor graph can be a useful tool in identifying problems. Assessment of contractions is important. With strong contractions and no fetal descent, uterine rupture is possible. Monitoring fetal heart tones is necessary to detect fetal distress. A prolapsed cord could restrict or stop the flow of oxygenated blood to the fetus. Observation of amniotic fluid is also helpful in identifying fetal distress. In the absence of a breech presentation, the presence of meconium in the amniotic fluid usually is indicative of fetal distress.

Nursing Diagnoses. After careful assessment, several nursing diagnoses may be developed concerning dystocia related to the passage or pelvis. Examples of diagnoses include:

Problem-oriented diagnoses:

- Risk for injury, related to pelvic dystocia
- Fear, related to unplanned cesarean delivery

Wellness-oriented diagnoses:

- Effective family coping, related to knowledge of diagnosis and agreement with treatment plan

Nursing and Collaborative Management. Protraction or arrest disorders that cannot be anticipated are treated by forceps-assisted or cesarean delivery; the decision depends on the location of the fetus in the pelvis and the amount of trauma each method poses to mother and fetus.

Throughout the long and difficult labor accompanying pelvic dystocia, the client and her labor partner need to be constantly informed of the interventions being done for both mother and fetus. Advising the woman of the progress in labor, such as changes in cervical dilation and fetal descent, can help to allay anxiety. Each intervention needs to be fully explained. An understanding of what is happening reduces anxiety and encourages client participation where possible. The nurse should support the client and partner in coping with unanticipated events that may occur during the labor process.

► DYSTOCIA RELATED TO THE PSYCHE

The psyche is a powerful factor during labor. Under normal conditions, the intrapartum period is one of heightened emotions and stress. When complications arise, stress increases and may develop into a crisis. The high-risk intrapartum client experiences concurrent maturational and situational crises. Nurses need to understand the psychologic aspects of labor if they are to give care and support to the client and her labor partner during crisis.

In the classic study by Lederman and coworkers (1983), a link was detected between psychosocial variables, such as the client's fears about labor; physiologic variables, such as blood levels of epinephrine and norepinephrine; and progress in labor. Thus, the client's psyche has been empirically shown to influence stress-related hormones and progress in labor. Nursing interventions related to the client's psyche are important in ensuring the normal progress of labor.

Several factors have been found to influence the psyche of the client experiencing a high-risk labor. These include the client's perception of the problem, coping strategies, available support systems, levels of fear and anxiety, image of herself, and preparation for childbirth.

► Perception of the Problem

The intensity of the woman's response is determined largely by how the problem is perceived. Several factors can alter this perception. These include emotional states, anxiety, hostility, age, and prior experience. When a complication develops during labor, the client's response can be affected by how apparent the problem is. A prolapsed cord and the possibility of fetal demise may cause a more intense response than the prospect of a prolonged labor as a result of ineffective contractions. Progress in labor also can affect the client's response. Problems that arise early in labor may be explained so that the client can understand and participate in the treatment; however, as labor progresses and the woman goes through psychologic withdrawal, her attention is focused only on the moment, and communication may be more difficult.

► Coping

To handle stress and threats to their well-being, individuals develop patterns of behavior called coping mechanisms. Clients rely on a variety of coping mechanisms to handle different levels of stress. These coping mechanisms may be constructive or destructive.

Constructive coping mechanisms lead to the resolution of a problem. Mild anxiety may be manifested in tension-releasing behaviors such as crying, sleeping, pacing, and other repetitive behaviors. These behaviors are aimed at relieving stress. The nurse should support these coping mechanisms in both the client and her labor partner if they are effective in relieving and reducing the anxiety.

As the level of anxiety increases, different behaviors will become apparent. These may include denial of the threat, projection, or repression. Although these behaviors can protect the client from feeling worthless or inadequate, they also can distort reality and interfere with interpersonal relationships. When this happens, the coping mechanisms are destructive. The nurse can help the client and her labor partner to recognize these destructive coping mechanisms and attempt to substitute more positive coping behaviors.

▶ Support Systems

The course of labor and delivery can be influenced significantly by the client's support system. A support system includes those in the environment from whom the client expects help, generally family and friends. In the labor room, the labor partner and the nurse can be a support system for the client. When a complication arises, the support system is most important. A strong support system helps the client to cope. If, however, the support system is weak or absent, the client may lose all perception of control over the situation.

▶ Fear

During labor, all women experience fear to some extent. Fear implies that the client is afraid of something that actually exists. The client may fear the process of labor or the anticipated pain. She may fear death, afraid that she may die during labor.

Three classic fears have been identified during labor: (1) fear for oneself, (2) fear for the infant, and (3) fear of the unknown. Erickson (1976), in a classic early study, identified several complications of labor that can result in the woman's fear for her infant and herself:

- Prolonged first stage of labor
- Prolonged second stage of labor
- Rotation of the fetal head
- Indicated low forceps
- Apgar scores less than 5
- Apgar scores of 5 to 7

Women's Health

The nurse needs to be alert to verbal and nonverbal cues that may indicate an excessive level of anxiety in a high-risk intrapartum client. Verbal cues may take the form of questions or statements that reflect the woman's apprehension about the well-being of her baby or the anxiety she is feeling about the situation. Nonverbal cues may be communicated through the wringing or clenching of hands, an unwillingness to change position, and discomfort that is disproportional to the stage of labor.

▶ Anxiety

With fear the client is afraid of an actual thing; with anxiety the source is not known. Fear may cause anxiety.

Anxiety is not always bad; some degree of anxiety may actually help the client deal realistically with the process of labor. But when anxiety levels reach the panic stage, the client may become immobilized and lose her ability to solve problems.

▶ Self-Image

Self-image refers to how the client feels about herself; this may be positive or negative. If the client approaches labor with realistic perceptions and goals, she maintains a positive self-image. On the other hand, perceptions and goals that are unrealistic or incongruent with labor events may lead to a negative self-image. Nurses can promote the client's positive self-image by praising her efforts during labor and explaining procedures so that the client can understand them. This is most important when complications arise in labor that interfere with the client's goal. If the client has prepared for a vaginal delivery and then must have a cesarean delivery because of a complication that arises suddenly, she may feel that she has failed and the complication is her fault. She must be helped to see that she had no control over the problem and that the ultimate goal of childbirth has been realized despite the method.

▶ Preparation for Childbirth

The labor experience is more satisfying if the client and her labor partner are prepared both physically and emotionally for the birth. Preparation for the birth can increase the client's ability to cope; decrease her stress, anxiety, and pain; and provide satisfaction with the childbearing experience. Education gives both the client and her labor partner greater opportunities to control the labor experience, resulting in a positive reaction to the birth experience.

► Nursing Diagnoses

Nursing diagnoses for dystocia related to the psyche are developed after careful assessment. Examples of diagnoses include:

Problem-oriented diagnoses:

- Powerlessness, related to slow progress in labor
- Ineffective individual coping, related to fatigue and discomfort during labor
- Altered role performance (paternal), related to unexpected course of labor

Wellness-oriented diagnoses:

- Positive interaction, related to adequate resources
- Positive maternal self-image, related to effective coping with difficult labor

► OTHER PROBLEMS

Although dystocias related to the powers, passenger, passage, or psyche are major problems occurring during the intrapartum period, other complications may arise. These complications can be associated with dystocia, or independent of it. Among these problems are abnormal fetal heart rate patterns, pregnancy-induced hypertension, heart disease, delivery of multiple fetuses, and abnormalities of the cord, amniotic fluid, and placenta.

► Abnormal Fetal Heart Rate Patterns in Labor

During a difficult labor, assessment of fetal well-being is essential. Measurement of the FHR is the chief method of fetal assessment. FHR also is an indicator of fetal distress.

Use of continuous electronic fetal monitoring in the client experiencing dystocia provides a second-by-second audio and visual FHR recording. The FHR can be monitored either externally or internally depending on whether the membranes have ruptured.

Many factors must be evaluated in determining the FHR pattern. These include baseline rate, variability, and decelerations (see Chapter 22 for an in-depth discussion of FHR patterns). Parity, progress in labor, maternal and obstetric complications, and analgesia or anesthesia must also be considered.

A FHR pattern that requires no intervention is called an innocuous or reassuring pattern. With such a pattern, there is a normal baseline FHR, accelerations with no other changes, early decelerations, mild variable decelerations, or normal variability. A nonreassuring pattern is a warning sign of possible problems. This pattern includes a decrease in variability, increase or decrease in the baseline, moderate tachycardia, or intermittent late deceleration with normal variability. An ominous pattern requires prompt intervention. This pattern includes absence of variability, marked bradycardia, persistent late deceleration with decreasing variability, and variable decelerations with absent variability. Nurses must be alert for and able to recognize these patterns during labor and notify the physician. Table 25–2 summarizes assessment of abnormal FHR patterns and nursing interventions.

The nurse should change the client's position to maximize fetal blood flow. Frequent assessment of the monitoring strip should be made for signs of decelerations and absence of variability, and the physician notified if these occur.

► Pregnancy-Induced Hypertension

Pregnancy-induced hypertension (PIH) is characterized by an elevation in blood pressure (hypertension), the presence of excess serum proteins in the urine (proteinuria), and the retention of water (edema). (See Chapter 19 for additional discussion.) It occurs only during pregnancy, labor and delivery, or soon after delivery. It is thought to be a progressive disease; if not treated aggressively, it may lead to convulsions and death.

Preeclampsia

Another name for the syndrome that includes hypertension, edema, and proteinuria is preeclampsia. A client with preeclampsia in labor must be monitored closely. Blood pressure should be taken at least every 4 hours and more frequently if it begins to rise. The blood pressure should be taken on the same arm and with the client in the same position if readings are to be accurately assessed. Intake and output should be monitored and recorded. A dipstick can be used to check for proteinuria. Edema should be assessed with particular attention to puffiness around the eyes, face, and sacrum. Placing the client in a left lateral position

▶ **TABLE 25-2**

Nursing Management of Abnormal Fetal Heart Rate Patterns

Pattern	Management
Baseline Fetal Heart Rate	
Tachycardia (161–180 beats per minute)	Observe 10 to 15 minutes; turn client to left side; hydrate to improve circulating volume; reduce stressors; report findings.
Bradycardia (<120 beats per minute)	Observe 10 to 15 minutes; turn client side to side or in knee–chest position; assess for maternal hypotension and correct; assess for prolapsed cord and correct; prepare for delivery.
Variability	
Increased (short-term variability)	Difficult to identify—assess for signs of fetal hypoxia.
Decreased (long-term variability)	Position on left side; hydrate; avoid central nervous system depressants; give oxygen by mask; assess fetal heart pattern for other signs of distress.
Decelerations	
Early	Usually does not indicate fetal distress—no treatment, differentiate from other deceleration patterns.
Late	Position on left side; assess and correct for maternal hypotension; discontinue oxytocin (if in use); administer oxygen by mask; prepare for delivery if pattern does not improve.
Variable	Check for prolapse of cord; turn on side or in knee–chest position; give oxygen by mask; hydrate; prepare for emergency delivery if pattern does not improve.

helps to improve blood flow to the uterus as well as to increase the glomerular filtration rate. Signs of central nervous system irritability such as headache, hyper-reflexia, and visual signs should be noted and reported immediately. An increase in blood pressure, proteinuria, or edema also should be reported to the physician. The FHR should be assessed closely, as placental insufficiency is associated with PIH. The client most likely will need explanations about the nursing interventions being used. The nurse can help to reduce the client's anxiety as well as encourage her participation by providing clear explanations. Supporting both the client and her labor partner helps them to cope with a situation they might not fully understand.

Severe Preeclampsia/Eclampsia

If the symptoms of preeclampsia worsen during labor, the condition becomes an obstetric emergency. Assessment of blood pressure, edema, and proteinuria is done at more frequent intervals. A Foley catheter may be placed to facilitate accurate assessment of output. The client is placed on absolute bedrest in a quiet environment to reduce central nervous system stimuli. Electronic monitoring of both mother and fetus is necessary.

Development of severe preeclampsia can lead to eclampsia, which is characterized by convulsions and increased maternal and fetal morbidity and mortality. The nurse must ensure that emergency equipment is present in the room and ready to use. This equipment includes oxygen, suction equipment, soft gag or padded tongue blades, and an airway. Emergency medications may also be included with the equipment

as well as an emergency delivery pack. The client and her labor partner will most likely become anxious with the increased activity of the personnel. The nurse should maintain a calm attitude, explain the procedures, and continue to be supportive.

Management is aimed at stabilizing the blood pressure, preventing convulsions, and delivering the fetus as soon as possible. Once the client is stabilized, delivery should proceed. Delivery is the most effective treatment for this condition.

▶ Heart Disease

Management of the pregnant woman with heart disease during labor and delivery is influenced by the functional capacity of the heart. The New York Heart Association classifies heart disease as class I, II, III, or IV, according to the physical signs exhibited by the client (class I being uncompromised and class IV very compromised). (See Chapter 19.)

In general, care of the woman with heart disease during labor focuses on prevention of cardiac decompensation, prevention of cardiac failure, relief of pain, and alleviation of apprehension. Women with class I or II disease are less at risk for cardiac complications than those with class III or IV disease (Troiano, 1992).

The woman labors in a side-lying or semirecumbent position to promote maximal oxygenation and uteroplacental perfusion and to minimize maternal exertion. Respirations are eased by the upright position. The nurse takes vital signs every 15 minutes during the first stage and every 10 minutes during the second stage of labor. A heart rate greater than 100 beats per minute and a respiratory rate greater than 24 per minute are early signs of cardiac failure necessitating intensive medical treatment. Oxygen is administered. The nurse administers and monitors the effects of other medications that may be used, such as intravenous morphine, rapidly acting digitalis, and furosemide. Electronic monitoring of uterine contractions and FHR is initiated with the onset of labor.

The nurse needs to be sensitive to the anxiety of the couple during the labor and delivery process. Continuous support by the nurse helps to allay the apprehension and fear associated with the woman's heart condition and the process of labor and delivery.

The preferred method of delivery for the woman with heart disease, regardless of functional classification, is vaginal delivery. Cesarean delivery is major surgery and much more taxing on cardiac function than vaginal delivery. Cesarean delivery is limited to such obstetric indications as fetopelvic disproportion. Signs of cardiac decompensation and failure developing after complete dilation and effacement of the cervix are indications for prompt forceps delivery unless easy spontaneous birth is expected within minutes (Cunningham et al., 1997).

Judicious use of analgesia during labor and anesthesia during delivery is required for the woman with a cardiac condition. In some women, especially nulliparas who require greater force and time to deliver the fetus, continuous epidural analgesia has been used. The major danger of conduction analgesia is maternal hypotension, which can further reduce cardiac output (Cunningham et al., 1997). Local anesthetics and pudendal blocks are preferable to general anesthetics for delivery. Oxygen may be continuously administered to the mother during the delivery process.

For women who must deliver by cesarean, a combination of thiopental, succinylcholine, nitrous oxide, and at least 30% oxygen has been used. An endotracheal tube should be in place before the anesthetic is administered (Cunningham et al., 1997).

The nurse should carefully monitor the mother during the labor and delivery process, and should assess for any signs of cardiac decompensation in the immediate puerperium. Prompt reporting and management by the interdisciplinary team is essential.

▶ Multiple Gestation

Pregnancy involving multiple fetuses is considered high risk and should be monitored closely during labor and delivery. Complications commonly found with multiple fetuses include preterm labor, uterine dystocia, abnormal fetal presentations, prolapsed umbilical cord, and premature separation of the placenta. Although pregnancies involving more than two fetuses occur, they are far less common than twin pregnancies. Therefore, this section focuses on intrapartum care of the client with twin fetuses.

Maternal Risks
The mother of twin fetuses is prone to postpartum hemorrhage, physical fatigue, and feelings of being overwhelmed with parental responsibilities. Moreover, she may experience a prolonged labor because of uterine dystocia with all its consequences.

Fetal Risks
The greatest risk to both fetuses is prematurity. There may also be a disparity in fetal size, and the first twin may benefit disproportionately from being delivered first. Hazards of twin delivery may also occur because of malpresentation. In about 40% of twins, the vertex-nonvertex presentation occurs (Boggess & Chisholm, 1997).

Nursing and Collaborative Assessment
In pregnancies involving more than one fetus, there are many positions and presentations each fetus may assume. These can be assessed in most instances by real-time sonography. During labor FHRs should be monitored frequently. External electronic monitoring is desirable until membranes rupture; then simultaneous external and internal electronic monitoring is used. The examiner may palpate multiple fetal parts and hear multiple fetal heartbeats. The nurse carefully assesses the client throughout labor and delivery for signs of complications associated with a multiple gestation, such as PIH, uterine dystocia, abnormal FHRs, and pulmonary edema. In the postpartum period, the mother is assessed for hemorrhage and infection. Infants are often placed in neonatal intensive care units for treatment and observation.

Nursing and Collaborative Management
As delivery becomes imminent, a team of health care professionals skilled in care of both the mother and the infants should be available. Whatever the type of delivery, the use of analgesia and anesthesia for the client with multiple fetuses should be judicious. Because of the possibility of fetal respiratory depression, the choice of analgesia or anesthesia is difficult.

Vaginal delivery is best accomplished if the first twin is in a cephalic presentation. If the first twin is breech, difficulties occur (e.g., prolapse of the umbilical cord) that make cesarean delivery a safer choice.

Delivery of the first twin in a cephalic presentation is the same as any delivery of a fetus in a cephalic presentation. As soon as the first twin is delivered, the second twin should be assessed for presentation, size, and relationship to the birth canal. If the vertex or the breech of the second twin is engaged, moderate fundal pressure is applied and the second set of membranes, if present, is ruptured. Labor resumes and the second twin's heart rate is closely monitored. If contractions do not resume, oxytocin in an intravenous solution may be used to stimulate labor.

If the second twin has moved down the pelvis, delivery occurs spontaneously or with minimal assistance. If the second twin does not enter the pelvic inlet, delivery becomes a problem. The choice may be to deliver the second twin by cesarean, or to manipulate the fetus to facilitate vaginal delivery.

Manipulation of the fetus can be accomplished by internal podalic version: the physician rotates the fetus in utero from a cephalic presentation to a breech presentation, so that the fetus can be extracted. The reason for turning the second twin in this manner is to avoid excess trauma to the fetal head during the more difficult second delivery.

Frequently, twins are delivered by cesarean. Pregnancies with more than two fetuses are nearly always delivered by cesarean to prevent maternal and fetal complications associated with a difficult vaginal delivery. Some practitioners advocate cesarean delivery when the second twin is in a nonvertex presentation (Boggess & Chisholm, 1997).

▶ Cord Abnormalities

Abnormalities of the umbilical cord, such as abnormalities of cord insertion and knots or loops in the cord, may affect the course of labor and delivery.

Abnormalities of Cord Insertion

Normally the umbilical cord inserts in the center of the placenta. Velamentous insertion of the cord is a condition in which the umbilical vessels of the cord separate in the membranes before reaching the placenta; thus the cord implants into the membranes rather than the placental disk. This condition occurs in approximately 1% of all placentas (DeCherney & Pernoll, 1994). The primary risk to the fetus is vasa previa during labor. In this situation, the vessels present themselves ahead of the fetus at the internal os. These vessels may rupture during labor and lead to exsanguination of the fetus.

Vaginal examination may allow the practitioner to palpate a tubular fetal vessel in the membranes over the presenting part. Confirmation may be by amnionoscopy, direct observation of the fetus and the color and amount of amniotic fluid by means of a specially designed endoscope inserted through the uterine cervix. In addition, painless vaginal bleeding, when tested, will reveal fetal hemoglobin.

If the vessels rupture during labor, there is little hope for fetal survival because of the severe blood loss. Parents require intense nursing support throughout this crisis.

Abnormalities of the Cord That May Affect Blood Flow

Knots in the Umbilical Cord. True knots of the cord occur in about 1.1% of deliveries, with a perinatal loss of 6.1%. The knots result from active movements of the fetus (DeCherney & Pernoll, 1994). As the fetus descends through the birth canal, the knot in the cord tightens, cutting off the flow of oxygenated blood to the fetus and resulting in fetal hypoxia and distress.

Loops of the Umbilical Cord. Loops are formed when the cord becomes coiled around portions of the fetus, usually the neck. One cord loop around the neck is present in 21% of deliveries (DeCherney & Pernoll, 1994).

As labor progresses, the cord may tighten during a contraction and cause deceleration of the FHR (variable or late decelerations). Fetal death or severe morbidity is a risk if the problem is not recognized.

Nursing and Collaborative Assessment. Early recognition and prompt delivery minimize the morbidity and mortality resulting from cord abnormalities that impede blood flow. Most of these abnormalities are first noted by irregularities in the FHR and pattern. During delivery, the practitioner palpates for a loop of cord around the fetal neck or arm, and removes it or clamps and cuts it.

Nursing and Collaborative Management. The nurse can indirectly assess for cord abnormalities by vigilantly monitoring the FHR, especially during contractions, when the cord may tighten or become compressed. If an abnormal fetal heart pattern is noted, the physician should be notified immediately. Again, support for the couple is vital throughout this emergency.

▶ Amniotic Fluid Abnormalities

Abnormalities of the amniotic fluid include meconium staining, polyhydramnios, and oligohydramnios.

- *Meconium-stained amniotic fluid.* Normally, meconium is not noticeably present in amniotic fluid, except in breech presentations. Fetal hypoxia, which produces a fetal defecation reflex, is the major factor contributing to meconium-stained fluid. These fetuses are considered at risk and are closely monitored.
- *Polyhydramnios.* Polyhydramnios is the presence of an excessive quantity of amniotic fluid (greater than 2000 mL) (see Chapter 19).
- *Oligiohydramnios.* Oligohydramnios is a severe deficiency of amniotic fluid—far below the normal 1000 mL, sometimes as low as a few milliliters of viscous fluid (see Chapter 19).

Maternal Risks. Meconium staining and oligohydramnios carry no maternal risks. With polyhydramnios, however, the mother may experience severe dyspnea, edema, and abdominal pain. In some cases, labor may occur prior to the 28th week of gestation.

Fetal Risks. Abnormalities of the amniotic fluid are associated with high fetal risk. Meconium staining of the amniotic fluid may indicate fetal hypoxia. Polyhydramnios may indicate such congenital conditions as fetal anencephaly, spina bifida, and esophageal atresia. Further, polyhydramnios has been associated with multiple gestation and isoimmunization.

Oligohydramnios is associated with such fetal abnormalities as pulmonary hypoplasia, obstruction of the fetal urinary tract, and severe intrauterine growth retardation. Oligohydramnios that occurs early in pregnancy can cause amniotic band syndrome, in which parts of the amnion adhere to and constrict parts of the fetus.

Nursing and Collaborative Assessment. The nurse should assess the amniotic fluid after rupture of the membranes. Any variation in color or amount of fluid may signal fetal distress or fluid abnormalities. In addition, antenatal assessments such as uterine measurements and sonography need to be reviewed.

Nursing and Collaborative Management. The FHR needs to be closely monitored for signs of fetal distress. If the cervix is fully dilated and fetal distress cannot be corrected, the mother is prepared for delivery. A cesarean delivery might be the method of choice.

If overdistension of the uterus is apparent, the mother is watched for uterine dystocia during labor and postpartum hemorrhage. The nurse is responsible for ensuring that the mother is as comfortable as possible during labor. Position change may reduce pressure on the diaphragm for the client with polyhydramnios.

▶ Placental Abnormalities

Placental abnormalities may also produce problems during labor and delivery. Included are such problems as placenta previa and abruptio placentae. (See Chapter 19 for an in-depth discussion of these placental abnormalities.) An additional problem with the placenta may occur during the third stage of labor, if there is an abnormally firm adherence of the placenta to the uterine wall. Fragments or cotyledons of the placenta may tear off and be retained as the placenta is expelled.

Further, the total placenta may adhere to the myometrium (placenta accreta), may invade the myometrium (placenta increta), or may penetrate the full thickness of the myometrium (placenta percreta) (DeCherney & Pernoll, 1994; Filardo & Nagey, 1990).

Maternal Risks. The major risk to the mother with third-stage placental adherence is postpartum hemorrhage. Further, postpartum infection is more common because of the intrauterine manipulation necessary to deliver the placenta.

Nursing and Collaborative Assessment. Inspection of the placenta is imperative to ensure that there are no retained fragments. Delayed spontaneous separation of a placenta may indicate an adherent placenta.

Nursing and Collaborative Management. The delivery of a problem placenta depends on the site of placental implantation, the depth of penetration into the myometrium, and the number of cotyledons involved. When there is minimal adherence of a few placental fragments, manual removal may be attempted. Oxytocin may be used to keep the mother's uterus contracted to prevent hemorrhage.

With total involvement and greater adherence of the placenta, attempts at manual removal will not succeed and may possibly cause severe hemorrhage. Usually, a prompt hysterectomy is done, as no other adequate management is currently available for this obstetric emergency (DeCherney & Pernoll, 1994).

Nursing management includes monitoring of maternal vital signs and maternal intake and output, observation for signs of shock and hemorrhage, and replacement of fluids, electrolytes, and blood. The nurse must provide empathetic support for the client who might or does undergo hysterectomy, and for her partner, during this crisis.

Critical Thinking in Care Planning

Care of a Client with Dystocia Related to Fetopelvic Disproportion

Lynda Turner, age 23 and pregnant with her first child, is admitted to the hospital in early labor. She is accompanied by her husband Bill. They have attended Lamaze classes together and are excited but anxious about the approaching birth. During admission, Lynda talks continually. She asks many questions and keeps wringing her hands. After the admission procedure is completed, Lynda and Bill walk around the unit. Lynda's membranes have not ruptured and walking is suggested to stimulate the contractions. As the contractions become stronger and Lynda becomes more uncomfortable, she returns to bed.

At this time, an external electronic fetal monitor is applied. Lynda is quite restless in bed. She changes position frequently, looking for one of comfort. Her facial expression indicates pain and occasionally she can be heard telling Bill that the contractions are painful. Bill and Lynda work well together. He assists her with her breathing and uses effleurage to encourage her to relax.

About 8 hours after admission, Lynda's membranes rupture spontaneously. The fluid is meconium stained. Both Lynda and Bill become upset at the sight of the greenish fluid. Lynda begins to cry and Bill demands to see the physician right away. The physician places an internal electrode on the fetal scalp which reveals a FHR of 120 with a late deceleration pattern. Contractions continue about every 2 minutes and are of strong intensity. Lynda is placed on her left side.

An hour and a half later, a vaginal examination reveals that the cervix has dilated 7 cm but that no further fetal descent has occurred. The fetus remains at station 1+ after 1½ hours of strong uterine contractions. The fetal monitor shows a FHR of 120 with late decelerations and now some decreased variability. The physician is notified. He tells Lynda and Bill that labor is not progressing normally and that the fetus is showing signs of distress. He also advises them that this lack of progress is most probably caused by fetopelvic disproportion and that, because of fetal distress, a cesarean delivery is indicated. Lynda is prepared for a cesarean delivery. She is taken to the delivery room and delivers a healthy 7½-pound male infant.

▶ Assessment

- Client talks continually and asks frequent questions
- Client wrings hands
- Client exhibits restlessness and grimacing
- Client complains of pain
- Client begins to cry; labor partner asks to see physician
- Meconium-stained amniotic fluid
- Decreasing FHR with late decelerations

Nursing Diagnosis

Anxiety, related to dystocia with first infant

Expected Client/Family Outcomes	Nursing Action/Intervention	Evaluation
Client will be able to verbalize fears and concerns during labor.	Establish a trusting relationship with client and labor partner. *Rationale:* A trusting relationship demonstrates to the client the concern of the nurse and encourages verbalization of feelings. Verbalizing feelings can reduce anxiety.	Signs of anxiety are decreased.

(continued)

Critical Thinking in Care Planning continued

Expected Client/Family Outcomes	Nursing Action/Intervention	Evaluation
	Give clear explanations of procedures. *Rationale:* Many of the client's concerns can be alleviated with explanations.	Client verbalizes understanding of procedures.
	Encourage labor partner's support of client. *Rationale:* Labor partners can often be successful in minimizing anxiety.	Client expresses less anxiety.

Nursing Diagnosis
Pain, related to intensity of labor contractions

Client will be as comfortable as possible during labor.	Reinforce breathing techniques taught at Lamaze classes. *Rationale:* Appropriate breathing techniques help client to cope with the discomfort of the contractions.	Client does not hyperventilate or hold breath and expresses minimal discomfort.
	Encourage labor partner to do effleurage. Give frequent back rubs. *Rationale:* Effleurage and back rubs stimulate the afferent nerve fibers and block pain sensation.	Client states that pain is reduced.
	Administer analgesics as necessary. *Rationale:* Analgesics provide pain relief during difficult labor.	
	Encourage client to rest between contractions. Provide calm, quiet environment. *Rationale:* Pain is exaggerated by exhaustion and fatigue.	Client rests between contractions.
	Praise and encourage client's efforts. *Rationale:* Praise enhances self-esteem and positive reinforcement promotes the continuation of breathing and relaxation techniques in a supportive environment.	Client behaves as though she is in control and states that she is.

Nursing Diagnosis
Risk for fetal injury, related to uteroplacental insufficiency

Fetus will continue to be oxygenated during labor.	Assess FHR tracing of internal monitor every 15 minutes. *Rationale:* Frequent monitoring helps identify fetal problems.	FHR pattern returns to normal.
	Place client in left lateral position. *Rationale:* Left lateral position improves blood flow to uterus by reducing pressure on vena cava.	There are no signs of uteroplacental insufficiency.

Nursing Diagnosis
Ineffective family coping: compromised, related to fear for fetus

Client and labor partner will gain control of situation as soon as possible.	Continue to inform client and labor partner of labor progress and nursing and medical interventions. *Rationale:* Keeping client and labor partner informed helps to decrease anxiety and maintain control.	Client and labor partner experience less problems with coping.

Critical Thinking in Care Planning continued

Nursing Diagnosis

Knowledge deficit, related to alteration in normal labor process

Expected Client/Family Outcomes	Nursing Action/Intervention	Evaluation
Client and labor partner will verbalize understanding of the alterations in labor.	Explain the reasons for lack of fetal descent. Explain reasons for cesarean delivery; inform couple about procedure. *Rationale:* Anxiety can be heightened by a lack of knowledge. Clear explanations can facilitate client coping.	Client and labor partner show fewer signs of anxiety. Both demonstrate an understanding of situation.

Chapter Highlights

▶ Dystocia can be classified according to factors such as the powers (uterine contractions), passenger (fetus), passage (pelvis), and the psyche.

▶ Uterine dystocia may be the result of hypotonic or hypertonic uterine contractions or precipitous labor.

▶ Dystocia may also be classified according to disorders of the preparatory, dilational, and pelvic divisions of labor.

▶ Dystocia may also result from pathologic retraction rings, of which the most common is Bandl's ring.

▶ Dystocia related to the passenger may be caused by malpresentation or malposition of the fetus, conditions contributing to fetopelvic and cephalopelvic disproportion, or shoulder dystocia.

▶ Dystocia related to the passage may be attributed to the type of pelvis, its diameters, or both.

▶ Dystocia is also associated with the state of the maternal psyche, which is influenced by the client's perception of the problem, coping strategies, available support systems, levels of fear and anxiety, self-image, and preparation for childbirth.

▶ Additional complications of labor and delivery include abnormal fetal heart rate patterns; pregnancy-induced hypertension; heart disease; delivery of multiple fetuses; and abnormalities of the cord, amniotic fluid, and placenta.

▶ The nurse is an integral member of the interdisciplinary health care team and collaborates with other professional colleagues in delivering care to intrapartum families at risk.

After reading the vignette at the beginning of this chapter, use what you have learned to answer these questions.

1. What strategies can Margaret Kiely, RN, use to help Cathleen and Bill Harris understand and cope with potential uterine dystocia?

2. What nursing interventions can the nurse implement to prevent the complications that may result from hypotonic uterine dysfunction?

3. What positive and/or negative behaviors may be exhibited by Cathleen and Bill Harris in response to a dysfunctional labor pattern?

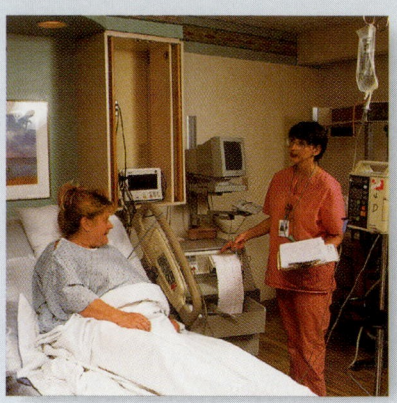

Critical Thinking Questions

▶ References

Albrechtsen, S. (1997). Evaluation of a protocol for selecting fetuses in breech presentation for vaginal or cesarean section. *American Journal of Obstetrics and Gynecology, 177*(3), 586–592.

Annapoorna, V., Arulkumaran, S., Anandakumar, C., Chua, S., Montan, S., & Ratnam, S.S. (1997). External cephalic version at term with tocolysis and vibroacoustic stimulation. *International Journal of Gynaecology and Obstetrics, 59*(1), 13–18.

Benson, R.C., & Pernoll, M.L. (1994). *Handbook of obstetrics and gynecology* (9th ed.). New York: McGraw-Hill.

Boggess, K.A., & Chisholm, C.A. (1997). Delivery of nonvertex second twin: A review of the literature. *Obstetrical and Gynecological Survey, 52*(12), 728–735.

Cunningham, F.G., MacDonald, P.C., Gant, N.F., Leveno, K.J., Gilstrap, L.C., Hankins, G.D.V., & Clark, S.L. (1997). *Williams obstetrics* (20th ed.). Stamford, CT: Appleton & Lange.

DeCherney, A.H., & Pernoll, M.L. (Eds.). (1994). *Current obstetric and gynecologic diagnosis and treatment* (8th ed.). Norwalk, CT: Appleton & Lange.

Ecker, J.L., Greenberg, J.A., Norwitz, E.R., Nadel, A.S., & Repke, J.T. (1997). Birth weight as a predictor of brachial plexus injury. *Obstetrics and Gynecology, 89*(5 Pt. 1), 643–647.

Erickson, M. (1976). The relationship between psychologic variables and specific complications of pregnancy, labor, and delivery. *Journal of Psychosomatic Research, 50,* 20–21.

Erkkola, R. (1996). Controversies: Selective vaginal delivery for breech presentation. *Journal of Perinatal Medicine, 24*(6), 553–561.

Filardo, J., & Nagey, P. (1990). An unusual presentation: Placenta percreta with uterine conservation. *Journal of Perinatology, 10,* 206–208.

Haggerty, L.A. (1996). Assessment parameters and indicators in expert intrapartal nursing decisions. *Journal of Obstetric, Gynecologic, and Neonatal Nursing, 25*(6), 491–499.

Koike, T., Minakami, H., Sasaki, M., Sayama, M., Tamada, T., & Sato, I. (1996). The problem of relating fetal outcome with breech presentation to mode of delivery. *Archives of Gynecology and Obstetrics, 258*(3), 119–123.

Lederman, R., Lederman, E., Work, B, & McCann D. (1983). Relationship of psychologic factors in pregnancy to progress in labor. In L.N. Sherwen & C.T. Weingarten (Eds.), *Analysis and application of nursing research: Parent-neonate studies.* Monterey, CA: Wadsworth.

McParland, P., & Farine, D. (1996). External cephalic version. Does it have a role in modern obstetric practice? *Canadian Family Physician, 42,* 693–698.

Notzon, F.C., Cnattingius, S., Bergsjo, P., Cole, S., Taffel, S., Irgens, L., & Daltveit, A.K. (1994). Cesarean section deliveries in the 1980s: International comparison by indication. *American Journal of Obstetrics and Gynecology, 170*(2), 495–504.

O'Leary, J.A. (1992). *Shoulder dystocia and birth.* New York: McGraw-Hill.

Piper, D.M., & McDonald, P. (1994). Management of anticipated and actual shoulder dystocia: Interpreting the literature. *Journal of Nurse-Midwifery, 39*(2 Suppl.), 91S–105S.

Rayl, J., Gibson, P.J., & Hickok, D.E. (1996). A population-based case-control study of risk factors for breech presentation. *American Journal of Obstetrics and Gynecology, 174*(1 Pt. 1), 28–32.

Robertson, P.A., Foran, C.M., Croughan-Minihane, M.S., & Kilpatrick, S.J. (1996). Head entrapment and neonatal outcome by mode of delivery in breech deliveries from 28 to 36 weeks of gestation. *American Journal of Obstetrics and Gynecology, 174*(6), 1742–1747.

St. Saunders, N.J. (1996). Controversies: The mature breech should be delivered by elective cesarean section. *Journal of Perinatal Medicine, 24*(6), 545–551.

Scorza, W.E. (1996). Intrapartum management of breech presentation. *Clinics in Perinatology, 23*(1), 31–49.

Troiano, N.H. (1992). Cardiac diseases in pregnancy. In L.K. Mandeville & N.H. Troiano (Eds.), *High-risk intrapartum nursing* (pp. 38–50). Philadelphia: J.B. Lippincott.

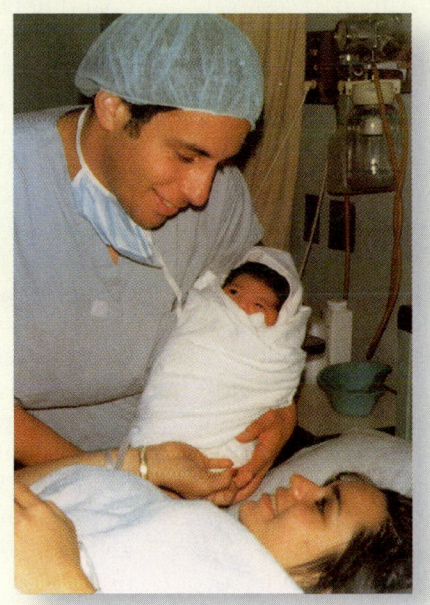

Laura and David Weiss are excited to be pregnant with their first child. Laura receives early and excellent prenatal care. The couple plans to share their baby's birth and attend childbirth education classes together. Despite her healthy pregnancy, Laura goes past her estimated date of delivery. When her pregnancy reaches 42 weeks, her obstetrician becomes concerned, and labor is induced. As her labor becomes active, Laura's pain is managed with an epidural anesthetic. Nearly 15 hours into the induction, Laura is fully dilated, but descent of the baby's head is found to have arrested. Fresh meconium is noted in the amniotic fluid and the electronic fetal monitor indicates fetal distress, which does not resolve with interventions such as changing Laura's position, administering oxygen, and shutting off the intravenous administration of oxytocin.

Laura is prepared for an emergency cesarean delivery. The surgery is uncomplicated. As soon as the baby is delivered, she is suctioned and given oxygen. When considered stable, the baby is wrapped warmly and placed into David's arms. In the recovery room, David and Laura become acquainted with Rachel. ∎

26

The Cesarean Experience

A **cesarean delivery** is a surgical procedure in which a fetus is delivered through an incision made through the abdominal wall and the uterus. Although cesarean section is a technically correct term for the operation, cesarean delivery, cesarean birth, and cesarean experience are used to highlight the importance of the birth event. As surgical and maternity clients, women who deliver in this manner present special challenges to the nurse. Cesarean clients are always considered to be high risk, because the cesarean procedure is regarded as major abdominal surgery; however, the degree of risk is related to the circumstances that led to the need for an abdominal birth. Nursing care evolves from such goals as early identification of high-risk conditions for which cesarean birth is indicated; implementation of strategies that will ensure safe, healthy delivery outcomes for mother and fetus; and the design of interventions that will promote an emotionally satisfying, family-centered birth experience.

This chapter discusses the indications, contributing factors, benefits, drawbacks, and contraindications for cesarean delivery. It also describes types of cesarean birth and explores preparation for this experience, delivery room, and postpartum care. The chapter concludes with a discussion of the qualifications and contraindications for vaginal birth after cesarean.

▶ BACKGROUND AND INCIDENCE

Cesareans are not new operations and were performed before the time of the ancient Romans. Unfortunately, survival was a major problem, and cesarean delivery was done only in desperate situations. The procedure was also performed on dead women to separate the mother and fetus. The first professional cesarean delivery in the United States took place in 1827. During the next 50 years, there were only 71 cesarean deliveries in the United States, and the mortality rate was 52%, mostly from infection and hemorrhage (Oxorn, 1986). Prior to 1882, the uterus was not usually sutured for several reasons, including the belief that sutures were unnecessary and only increased infection.

By the 1950s, the cesarean rate was about 3–4%; however, this rate continued to climb. At one time physicians had to justify why a cesarean was done. By the end of the 1970s, in a professional climate that focused on the pathologic aspects of childbirth, physicians often had to justify why a cesarean was not done (Enkin, 1977). By 1988, the cesarean rate was nearly 25% (Taffel, Placek, Moien, & Kosary, 1991) and higher in some places. While it is hard to specify what the cesarean rate should actually be, decreasing the high cesarean rate to under 15% became a national goal (Public Health Service, 1991). Due to such factors as professional and consumer concern over the high rate of cesareans and health insurance companies' reluctance to pay for routine repeat cesarean deliveries, the rate has been decreasing and was estimated to be about 20.8% in 1995 (Clarke & Taffel, 1996a, 1996b; Curtin & Kozak, 1997; U.S. Centers for Disease Control and Prevention, 1996). National rates do not reflect the variations in actual rates among communities or caregivers, however.

Unfortunately, the decrease in cesarean rates has mostly been due to an increase in vaginal birth for future delivery, rather than a decrease in the rate of first-time (primary) cesareans. Unless the primary rate decreases along with an increase in **vaginal birth after cesarean** (VBAC) (vaginal birth of an infant to a woman who has had at least one previous cesarean delivery), overall cesarean rates are likely to continue to be high (Cunningham et al., 1997; Paul & Miller, 1995; Shearer, 1996). See box entitled Examples of Strategies to Decrease the Rate of Cesarean Delivery for a description of selected activities through which this issue can be explored.

At the same time that the incidence of cesarean births has increased, perinatal and maternal mortality have decreased. Does a cause–effect relationship exist? This is a difficult question, because such factors as better prenatal and neonatal care, and not the cesarean procedure alone, might contribute to better outcomes (Cunningham et al., 1997).

The cesarean rate will probably never be zero, even with the most low-risk oriented care. Some situations are truly high risk. The complexity of the human birth experience requires that each client be evaluated on an individual basis.

▶ INDICATIONS

Cesarean delivery is performed whenever it is unlikely that a safe vaginal delivery can take place or whenever it is judged that a delay in delivery would jeopardize the well-being of mother, fetus, or both. Unfortunately, this sounds simpler than it is in clinical practice. Intrapartum complications can be complex, and it may be hard to determine whether an obstetric catastrophe will or will not take place if a cesarean is delayed. Careful client evaluation, clinical judgment, and collaboration among nurses, physicians, other health care professionals, and clients themselves are important.

► EXAMPLES OF STRATEGIES TO DECREASE THE RATE OF CESAREAN DELIVERY

- Identify rates of cesarean delivery in your setting. Remember that cesarean delivery is major abdominal surgery with a variety of high costs.
- Question high rates through appropriate channels in your setting (staff/quality assurance meetings, peer review, etc.).
- Encourage evaluation of reasons for high rates of cesarean births and identification of strategies to decrease rates if possible.
- Question routine use of technology that is associated with increased risk of cesarean delivery (epidurals, electronic fetal monitoring, etc.)
- Work with women in using alternative strategies to cope with labor. Educational efforts for medical and nursing staff can address such cesarean-related topics as the appropriate use of technology and labor dystocia.
- Work with fellow staff members (physicians, nurses) to develop attitudes and practices focusing on avoidance of cesarean delivery unless necessary.
- Encourage appropriate use of such strategies as upright position and ambulation in labor; these have been associated with lower rates of operative delivery.
- In appropriate situations, use accepted professional guidelines to decrease routine cesarean deliveries for women with history of certain infectious conditions.
- Give up the old myth, "Once a cesarean always a cesarean." Whenever appropriate, encourage and support VBAC as a safe method of future delivery.
- Work with the media in advertising the benefits of VBAC.
- Through interdisciplinary efforts, professional organizations, etc., work to address malpractice concerns related to not performing cesarean deliveries.

► CONTRIBUTING FACTORS

One or more factors can contribute to the occurrence of cesarean birth:

1. Safety of the procedure. Although a cesarean is major abdominal surgery, women can expect in nearly all cases to survive and recover. In addition, physicians practicing obstetrics or obstetric anesthesia are more skilled in this now common procedure.
2. Factors related to the health of the mother, such as severe pregnancy-induced hypertension, or preexisting conditions such as diabetes and heart disease. Certain health problems, such as uterine myomas, tend to occur in older women, and may contribute to the incidence of cesareans in older pregnant women, especially nulliparas. Obesity and excessive maternal weight gain (≥20 kg) have also been associated with an increased incidence of cesarean birth.
3. Factors related to fetal status, such as fetal distress, the most frequent reason for the increased cesarean rate, or maternal death.
4. Factors related to the interactions of maternal and fetal factors, such as uterine dystocia, failure to progress in labor, uterine rupture, placenta previa, abruptio placentae, prolapsed cord, fetal malpresentations, breech presentations (especially for primiparous women), cephalopelvic disproportion, fetal distress related to decreased placental blood flow during contractions, and certain types of prenatally diagnosed congenital abnormalities (e.g., spina bifida) in which vaginal delivery might injure the fetus.
5. Infections in the birth canal, such as active herpes lesions, because of the risk of fetal infection during the birth process. Unfortunately, professional worry over the chance of asymptomatic shedding of herpes virus in the vaginal canal at the time of delivery and of severe consequences of the virus to the newborn prompted many unnecessary routine cultures and cesareans. While the decision for a cesarean needs to be made on an individual basis, the use of guidelines issued by the American College of Obstetricians and Gynecologists (1988) has been associated with a decrease in the number of cesareans in women with a history of genital herpes (Cunningham et al., 1997; Roberts, Cox, Dax, Wendel, & Kevenko, 1995).
6. Previous cesarean or uterine surgery. The presence of a previous uterine incision remains the most common indication for cesareans in the United States, despite proven safety of VBAC for women who meet certain criteria (Harrington, Miller, McClain, & Paul, 1997).
7. Multiple fetuses. Some intrapartum problems, such as fetal malpresentations and abnormal uterine contraction patterns, occur with greater frequency in pregnancies with multiple

fetuses. In uncomplicated, progressive labors, twins may be delivered vaginally; however, cesareans are nearly always done in the United States when more than two fetuses are present.

8. Miscellaneous conditions, such as tumors in the birth canal, failed forceps delivery, and certain congenital anomalies.

9. Technologic advances, such as electronic fetal monitoring (EFM), which have led to diagnoses of fetal distress or labor arrest. Studies indicate that cesarean rates increase with continuous EFM.

10. Professional concern over potential malpractice suits. Physicians may be more willing to perform a fairly safe surgical procedure than to risk an unfavorable outcome and a malpractice suit. Concern over negative peer reactions to a poor obstetric outcome and feelings of accountability to a client and family may also influence cesarean decisions (de Costa, 1998).

11. Client request for cesarean delivery and the right of women to be actively involved in their own treatment decisions. Johnson and co-workers (1986) noted that a physician can rightfully refuse a woman's request for intervention if the risk is very large. However, they observed that although cesarean delivery is always associated with some risk, the risk is similar to that taken by the healthy woman having elective gynecologic surgery. Results of their survey of 112 obstetricians in the United States indicated that some physicians considered the client's request in itself enough reason for cesarean delivery, although this practice is controversial.

12. Evolving lack of physician experience in managing difficult deliveries. As more cesareans are done for complex births, there will theoretically be fewer physicians trained and experienced in management of problem vaginal deliveries. This factor is likely to have a large impact on the future practice of obstetrics.

13. Background of the obstetric care provider. Clients of certified nurse-midwives have been reported to have a lower rate of cesarean deliveries than women who receive obstetric care from obstetricians or family practice physicians (Lewin, 1997; Rosenblatt et al., 1997; Woolbright, 1996).

14. Positioning and activity during labor. Upright positions and ambulation during labor have been associated with lower rates of cesarean delivery (Albers et al, 1997).

15. Other nonclinical factors. Higher cesarean rates have been reported for women who have

Ethical Decision Making

Arnelle Hollis, 39 weeks' pregnant, has been diagnosed with a complete placenta previa. Her caregivers all agree that cesarean delivery is the only safe method of delivery for the baby. However, Arnelle refuses to have a cesarean and states that she "absolutely does not want to have surgery." A court order authorizing a cesarean delivery of her baby is being discussed. As a nurse caring for this client, the following questions need to be considered:

1. What issues are raised by the client's refusal of a life-saving procedure for her fetus?
2. What problems in caring for Arnelle Hollis might arise if she is forced by court order to undergo a cesarean?
3. What strategies might be used to help this client accept the cesarean?
4. How do you feel about involving the judicial system in client care decisions?

private insurance than for women who do not, and for women who deliver in for-profit proprietary hospitals, nonteaching hospitals, or hospitals with a small volume of obstetric cases (Haas, Udvarhelyi, & Epstein, 1993; Murray & Pradenas, 1997). Conversely, lower cesarean rates have been associated with attentive, high-quality nursing care (Radin, Harmon, & Hanson, 1993).

In rare instances, a cesarean delivery may be ordered by a court of law if a mother is unable or unwilling to consent (Lindgren, 1996).

Nursing Alert

Repeat cesareans, dystocia or failure to progress in labor, breech presentation, and concerns for fetal well-being are the four most frequent indications for cesarean delivery (Cunningham et al., 1997).

▶ BENEFITS

The main benefit of cesarean birth is that it is a life-saving procedure in situations of obstetric emergency and in situations in which vaginal birth is not possible. Cesarean delivery has become safe enough so that nearly all clients can expect to recover. Women who know in advance of their elective cesarean delivery also have the advantage of being able to prepare for the birth. When the delivery is scheduled in advance, couples can attend cesarean education programs and plan for a family-centered birth experience. In addition, the delivery can be timed so that the health care team and facilities necessary for the cesarean can be assembled without difficulty.

▶ DRAWBACKS

There are several drawbacks related to cesarean delivery:

1. Despite increased safety of the surgery, maternal morbidity and mortality are higher for cesarean than vaginal births. Differences among studies and difficulties in compiling data make actual comparisons difficult. As major abdominal surgery, cesarean delivery has risks, although in the United States maternal death rarely occurs. Maternal mortality rates have been estimated to range from 6.1 to 22 per 100,000 live births (Gabbe, Niebyl, & Simpson, 1996). The greatest risks for mortality are from thromboembolism, severe infection, and anesthesia. Risk of death related to aspiration pneumonia, once a major problem, has decreased due to administration of a nonparticulate antacid such as sodium citrate or citric acid solution prior to the surgery.

   Maternal morbidity for cesarean birth is considerably higher than for vaginal delivery and has been estimated to occur with a frequency of 10–80%, clearly a broad range (Zuspan & Quilligan, 1988). Infections, hemorrhage, urinary tract complications, and nonfatal thromboembolisms are major sources of morbidity (Cunningham et al., 1997). Increased maternal morbidity has also been reported when cesarean delivery is performed for high-risk conditions before 28 weeks of gestation (Evans & Combs, 1993) and when women are very obese (Perlow & Morgan, 1994).

2. The procedure itself can carry risks to the fetus. At times, miscalculation of fetal maturity has resulted in scheduling of a cesarean too early in gestation and delivery of a premature infant. This is called **iatrogenic prematurity,** because the prematurity results from inadvertent or erroneous treatment given by the physician. Strategies to evaluate fetal maturity can minimize the likelihood of this event. Another risk to the fetus is accidental injury during the uterine incision or delivery, although this does not happen often.

3. When done for medically or obstetrically high-risk clients, cesarean procedures can be complicated by preexisting conditions. For example, diabetic women whose blood sugar levels are not monitored and controlled carefully may become hyperglycemic or hypoglycemic during or after surgery. This can lead to further complications such as fluid and electrolyte imbalance.

4. There is little choice in childbirth settings for cesarean clients. As a surgical procedure, cesarean delivery is always done in an operative environment within a hospital setting. Not every hospital that encourages family-centered, "homelike" birth practices for women with vaginal deliveries creates similar experiences for cesarean clients. Women who have cesareans can find themselves with a delivery experience very different from what they may have imagined (e.g., separated from their support partner, required to have general anesthesia because of a lack of available personnel qualified to administer regional anesthesia, or recovery in a general postoperative unit where maternal–infant contact is restricted).

5. Women who have emergency cesarean deliveries must deal with an unexpected outcome of their birth plan. This is especially problematic if a woman began labor and anticipated delivery in an out-of-hospital birth environment or in a hospital birthing room. Although some women feel relief at having a cesarean terminate labor, others may have a sense of crisis and experience negative feelings such as disappointment, anger, confusion about the cesarean, and loss of self-esteem.

6. Women who deliver by cesarean have the simultaneous tasks of parenting a newborn and recovering from major abdominal surgery. Without help from family, friends, or hired assistants, this can be difficult and exhausting.

7. Cesarean birth is more expensive than vaginal birth in terms of hospital fees for the procedure and lengthened hospital stay. Out-of-hospital costs include extended child care for

children at home and the mother's needs for more assistance after discharge. In addition, the emotional cost of the cesarean to the client and her family must be considered.

8. Women who deliver by cesarean have a longer period of discomfort and restricted mobility than do women who deliver vaginally. Most cesarean clients require pharmacologic assistance with pain control. It may take about a month before a woman who delivers by cesarean can move about with complete comfort. Painful activities can include driving a car (especially with manual transmission), changing positions (e.g., from supine to sitting), or making any physical movements that require use of the abdominal muscles.

9. The presence of an abdominal scar may be upsetting to some women, especially if a vertical skin incision was used.

10. Women who undergo first-time cesarean births have a higher risk of cesarean delivery for future pregnancies.

11. Even when women attempt VBAC, delivery occurs in a setting where operative delivery is accessible. Delivery alternatives, such as the use of a free-standing birth center or home, can be restricted, because of concerns for client safety and other factors.

► CONTRAINDICATIONS

The safety level of cesarean delivery has improved so that no absolute maternal contraindications to the procedure exist. If, however, maternal blood clotting ability is greatly compromised, vaginal delivery, if possible, is preferred because it presents less risk of bleeding. Cesarean delivery is not done when the fetus is thought to be too premature to survive. This situation also raises moral and ethical questions.

► TYPES

► Definitions

A cesarean delivery may be primary (that is, a woman's first abdominal delivery) or repeat. A cesarean is called "repeat" when the woman has delivered at least once before in this manner. Both primary and repeat cesareans can be done on an elective basis or on an emergency basis. An elective cesarean is a planned abdominal delivery; the woman knows in advance that a cesarean birth will be performed. An elective cesarean may be done for a variety of reasons, including maternal diabetes, malpresentation of the fetus, placenta previa, and history of previous cesareans. Emergency cesareans are done for conditions in which prompt delivery is thought necessary to preserve the life or well-being of the mother, fetus, or both. Emergency cesareans can be performed for situations that require immediate delivery, such as abruptio placentae and acute fetal distress, or for situations in which a delay of an hour or two is unlikely to harm the mother or fetus, such as failure to progress in labor and prolonged rupture of membranes.

► Incisions

Cesarean deliveries are done using two major incisional approaches: classic and low segment. With a classic cesarean incision, a midline incision is made vertically through the skin and subcutaneous tissues and vertically into the body of the uterus. The incision extends from above the lower uterine segment to the fundus of the uterus. Advantages of this type of incision are that it:

- Provides quicker access to the fetus in an emergency
- Offers greater visibility of the pregnant uterus to the physician performing the surgery
- Allows for extension upward if more room for delivery of the fetus is needed

A classic incision is technically easier to do than a low-segment incision (described next), and therefore might be selected by an inexperienced physician handling an emergency delivery.

Several disadvantages are related to the classic cesarean incision, including:

- Greater blood loss because of the location of the incision through the uterine muscles
- Presence of a midline abdominal scar, which many women consider cosmetically undesirable
- Creation of a plane of weakness due to the scar tissue that forms vertically along the muscles in the uterus

A vertical classic incision has a greater likelihood of rupture during a future pregnancy or labor than a horizontal, low segment incision, although the chance of uterine rupture is small.

Low-segment cesarean incisions are currently the incisions most frequently performed for cesarean delivery. With this approach, a low, transverse incision is made through the skin and subcutaneous tissue at the level of the pubic hairline. This is called a

Pfannenstiel incision, after the 19th-century German gynecologist who pioneered the procedure. (The Pfannenstiel incision refers to the incision through the skin and subcutaneous tissue, but not to the type of uterine incision.) A popular term for this incision is "bikini cut," for the healed incision is most often contained within the pubic hairline, or bikini line.

Advantages of a Pfannenstiel incision include:

- Less visible abdominal scarring
- Decreased chance of wound opening or hernia development
- Lower risk of associated blood loss
- Less likelihood of the development of adhesions of abdominal organs (such as the bowel) to the healed incisional line
- Decreased risk of rupture in future pregnancy and labor

Disadvantages of the Pfannenstiel incision include less visibility of the uterus for the physician performing the surgery than with a vertical incision (especially in obese women) and difficulty in extending the incision, should the physician require more room to deliver the fetus. A greater amount of time, particularly during a repeat cesarean, is required for this incision.

Various combinations of skin and uterine incisions may be used according to the clinical situation. A horizontal, low-segment uterine incision and a vertical skin incision may be used for the very obese client, so that the skin incision does not lie directly within the deep skin folds of the obese abdomen. Occasionally, a vertical uterine incision may be accompanied by a Pfannenstiel incision. In situations such as prematurity, the lower uterine segment has not thinned as it does in late pregnancy, and this makes a horizontal incision more difficult. A vertical uterine incision may also be preferable when the fetus is in a breech position.

Skin and uterine incisions are separate. There is no way simply to look at a cesarean abdominal skin suture line or scar and identify the type of uterine incision used. This information, however, is important; it is recorded by the physician in the client's chart immediately after the procedure is completed. A client who had had a low-segment, transverse uterine incision and no other suspected recurrent risk conditions could be an excellent candidate for a future vaginal birth.

Repeat cesareans are usually performed through the same incisions, even if the previous incisions were vertical. The scar tissue, if thick, is removed. In addition to the obvious cosmetic benefit of one rather than two types of skin and uterine incisions, scar tissue of a healed incision is a plane of weakness. Minimizing the number of incision sites into the uterus is a physiologic advantage.

Cesarean hysterectomy, a surgical procedure in which the uterus as well as the fetus is removed, is performed as a last-resort measure during obstetric emergencies such as uncontrollable uterine hemorrhage, severe uterine infection, and the presence of large uterine tumors. Obviously, sterilization results from removal of the uterus and is of great consequence to women who want future pregnancies. Women who do not desire more children may also have negative feelings related to the loss of a "feminine" body organ. Cesarean hysterectomy is not a recommended method of voluntary sterilization. This procedure entails more extensive, higher-risk surgery than tubal sterilization after cesarean delivery and is truly irreversible.

The type of cesarean procedure selected depends on the clinical situation, physician's judgment, and client request. Nurses need to be able to provide information to women about cesarean procedures. Prenatally, nurses can provide teaching on this topic during prenatal visits or during prepared childbirth classes, as cesarean delivery is a potential method of delivery for all clients. Nurses can also encourage clients, as a means of participating in their own childbirth experience, to discuss this subject with their physicians or nurse-midwives prior to delivery. Although nurse-midwives do not perform cesareans, they educate clients prenatally about what to expect in case a cesarean becomes necessary. In many instances, the nurse-midwife remains with the client to provide support throughout the cesarean delivery (Varney, 1997). During the postpartum period, through interventions based on assessment of client and family responses to the cesarean, nurses can further promote client understanding of cesarean delivery.

▶ ANESTHESIA FOR CESAREAN DELIVERY

Anesthesia for cesarean delivery is discussed in Chapter 23.

▶ PREPARATION FOR CESAREAN DELIVERY

▶ Before Pregnancy

Preparation for cesarean birth actually begins prior to pregnancy. Today, cesareans are common procedures. However, as Lampman and Phelps (1997) observed in their study of male and female college students, much uncertainty about cesarean birth exists. Many couples have friends or relatives who have had cesareans; some have had previous cesarean deliveries themselves. These experiences may or may not have been positive. Television, radio, publications, and other media have also had an impact on public impressions of cesarean births. Such impressions can evolve from factually presented material or highly distorted approaches tailored to story lines.

Nurses need to be aware of how cesarean births are being portrayed by the media, as well as the nature of client perceptions of this type of childbirth. In addition, nurses should examine their own attitudes toward cesarean births. Through roles as authors, speakers, and consultants, as well as in letters to the media, nurses can affect the accuracy of information presented to the public and can promote public awareness of options available to families regarding cesarean birth.

▶ During Pregnancy

The topic of cesarean birth should be raised with all clients, regardless of risk status. Childbirth always carries an element of uncertainty; it is not possible—or wise—to promise a low-risk vaginal delivery. During prepared childbirth classes, antenatal health visits, or work with the media, the nurse is in an unique position to provide information regarding cesarean birth and options available to clients in their local hospitals. The nurse also can facilitate discussion between the pregnant couple and their physician or nurse-midwife.

Currently, a number of hospitals and organizations offer childbirth education programs specifically for the couple who will have a planned cesarean delivery. The reasons for these classes are similar to the reasons for classes for couples expecting a vaginal delivery. Physical and psychologic preparation can help couples to integrate birth, whether vaginally or abdominally, into the cycle of life events, to maintain a sense of control, and to have an emotionally satisfying, safe delivery.

Many topics are covered during cesarean birth classes. Some are also presented in standard childbirth preparation classes. Some examples follow.

- Previous cesarean experiences, plans, and goals of expectant couples attending the classes
- Attitudes toward cesarean births
- Indications for cesarean birth
- Safety and risks of cesarean birth
- Tests for fetal well-being and maturity
- Importance of good maternal health during pregnancy
- Nutrition

- Physical conditioning—exercises for relaxation, exercises to promote comfort during pregnancy and postpartum
- Cesarean prevention, VBAC
- Signs of impending labor and what to do if labor begins
- The hospital experience (tour of facility, description of admission procedures, hospital policies regarding cesarean deliveries, differences among local hospitals in policies regarding cesarean deliveries)
- Role of nurses and other health care personnel in care of the cesarean family
- Preparation for surgery, family concerns related to surgery
- Home arrangements (e.g., child care for other children, advance preparation for help at home following discharge)
- In-hospital physical preparation (e.g., blood tests, intravenous line insertion, vital signs, fetal assessment, urinary catheter, shave and scrub)
- Anesthesia options
- The cesarean procedure—what will be experienced before, during, and after the cesarean (films on cesarean birth may be shown)
- Role of the support person (what she or he will and will not be able to do, what the support person may experience)
- Appearance of the newborn and care in the delivery room
- Opportunities for parent–infant contact in delivery room and recovery area
- Recovery unit procedures and personnel; whether the client recovers in a maternity unit or in a general hospital recovery unit
- Recovery from anesthesia, pain and pain medications, relaxation exercises such as deep breathing and imagery
- Postpartum care in the recovery unit
- Postpartum care in hospital (pain management, positions and exercises to promote comfort in the first postpartum days, changing positions, ambulation, deep breathing, coughing, comfortable positions for infant care)
- Infant feeding choices, techniques, and positions
- Involution—physical and emotional changes in hospital and after discharge
- Diet and exercise
- Possibility of early discharge programs
- Managing at home after discharge (physical needs, integration of infant into family, special needs of cesarean parents)
- Emotional responses related to cesarean birth
- Value of cesarean support group

▶ Preoperative Care

Nurses in delivery room settings work with women who did not expect to have a cesarean, with women who knew in advance of their scheduled surgical birth, and with women who are planning a vaginal birth after a previous cesarean but who may undergo another cesarean if labor complications emerge. Most people have fears related to childbirth and to surgery, even if they do not initiate discussion of them. Calm, knowledgeable support can reduce the sense of crisis associated with cesarean birth. Strategies that enhance a sense of control and joy in the birth experience, such as actively encouraging the couple in the decision-making process and making the surgical birth as family-centered as possible, can foster client–staff collaboration and help ensure a positive delivery experience for the woman.

Preoperative teaching should be done for clients whether or not they have attended prepared childbirth classes and regardless of their backgrounds. This includes physicians and nurses who have cesarean births. These individuals at times have been deprived of the quality of educational preparation offered to other clients, because staff assume that they already know "all there is to know."

The importance of anticipatory guidance, teaching, and emotional support, noted earlier, remains constant throughout any nurse–client–family interactions. The actual sequence of preoperative events may vary according to the client's status and individual hospital, medical, or nursing policies.

Verification of client identification takes place as soon as the woman arrives on the unit. At this time an identification bracelet and anklet for the baby may be obtained and taped to the front of the mother's chart. This does not, however, absolve delivery room nurses from the responsibility of checking to make sure that the neonate's identification number corresponds to the mother's identification number before either leaves the delivery room.

Consent for the cesarean is obtained on admission to the unit, or at the time that the need for a cesarean is determined. Although getting consent is within the role of the physician, in many hospitals the nurse may act as a witness to the consent. For ethical and legal reasons, the nurse should not sign any consent that he or she has not directly witnessed; for the same reasons, nurses are advised not to obtain consent for the cesarean. Nursing history and physical assessment, including fetal heart rate, are done; prenatal records are reviewed; and nursing goals, intervention strategies, and expected outcomes (nursing care plan) are developed.

Preoperative testing is performed. A urine specimen is sent to the laboratory for analysis; simple testing for glucose, acetone, and protein may be done on the unit.

Blood samples are drawn for complete blood count (CBC), electrolytes, and clotting studies (when indicated). A blood sample is also sent to be typed and crossmatched with available blood bank blood in case the woman requires transfusions. In some settings, the nurse performs the venipuncture and obtains and sends the blood specimens. In other settings, technicians or house staff are available. Blood specimens must be clearly labeled and sent without delay for laboratory analysis, especially if the cesarean is being done on an emergency basis. In emergency situations, a staff member should notify the laboratory of the importance of prompt attention.

In some hospitals, scheduled elective cesarean clients may be preadmitted; that is, laboratory studies may have been done prior to their admission date. In this case, the results need to be recorded on the client's chart before the cesarean. Both physicians and nurses must know recent laboratory results for a client prior to any surgical procedure. In the interest of client well-being and in the spirit of professional collaboration, the nurse should make certain that the physician is aware of any abnormal values and that, whenever indicated, appropriate interventions have been initiated.

An intravenous line is inserted. In many labor and delivery units, this procedure is done by the nursing staff. An intravenous line is needed to provide ready intravascular access for medications, for fluid and electrolyte therapy, and for blood transfusions, if necessary. An intravenous catheter to avoid infiltration and a bore large enough for blood products should be used. Small, "butterfly" needles are not used.

Prescribed medications are administered. For example, intravenous antibiotics may be given when the woman is thought to be at risk for infection (e.g., prolonged ruptured membranes). Medications to raise gastric pH above 2.5, to promote gastric tone and emptying, and to block histamine release may be given before anesthesia. These are discussed in Chapter 23.

The abdomen is shaved and scrubbed from the xiphoid to about 2 1/2 in. below the pubic hairline. It is not necessary to shave the entire mons, although this is common practice in some hospitals.

An indwelling urinary catheter is inserted. In nonemergency cases, this can be done after establishing the regional block to avoid needless maternal discomfort. Continuous urinary drainage is established to keep the bladder decompressed during cesarean surgery and to lower the risk of surgical injury to the bladder. In women who have normal renal function and who are receiving intravenous fluid therapy, the bladder can quickly become distended during the surgery; this could also inhibit proper contraction of the uterus after delivery of the infant. Routine procedure in many hospitals calls for insertion of the catheter before the woman is brought to the delivery room. At best, this is a very uncomfortable procedure for the woman. The catheter can easily be inserted in the delivery room after the woman has been anesthetized, even when cesarean delivery is unplanned. (The nurse should be aware that diplomacy, especially in dealing with other nurses and with physicians, may be necessary in altering traditional routines.)

The father, or other support person, is assisted in preparing for the cesarean. Appropriate clothing for the delivery room is given, as well as information about what he may expect, where he will be positioned during delivery, and what his role will be. The nurse needs to provide appropriate support, as an expectant father about to see his infant born by cesarean may be experiencing feelings ranging from excitement to terror.

To promote the client's safety, side rails need to be kept raised, and the woman should not be left unattended. The labor room nurse does not leave until the client has been transferred to the cesarean delivery room and until the nurses who will attend the cesarean have directly assumed responsibility for her care. In many units, the nurses who care for the client in the labor unit also assist at the cesarean delivery. A woman who has an unplanned cesarean may have had an epidural catheter placed while she was in the labor room. During transport and transfer to the operating table, special care needs to be taken so that the epidural catheter does not become displaced or that the woman does not sustain injury as a result of impaired sensory and motor functions of her lower extremities.

The nurse also makes certain that the cesarean delivery team has been notified of the impending birth. This includes the anesthesiologist, nursery nurses, and pediatrician, as well as the obstetrician or perinatologist. When problems are expected with the newborn, a special-care nursery nurse and a neonatologist, when part of the hospital staff, may also be called to attend the birth. Throughout cesarean preparation, fetal surveillance continues.

▶ DELIVERY ROOM CARE

After the woman arrives in the cesarean delivery room, the obstetrician, medical assistants, anesthesiologist, pediatrician, and nursing staff who will assist at

the delivery assume responsibility for her and her baby. In some hospitals cesareans are performed in the general surgical suites by obstetricians or are assisted by operating room nurses who come to the maternity unit to attend the cesarean. In other hospitals, nurses who regularly work in labor and delivery may scrub and assist with the procedure. They may also circulate and assist with nonsterile functions that do not require a surgical scrub, such as aiding the anesthesia personnel, helping the scrub nurses and physicians dress in sterile attire, performing an antiseptic scrub of the operative area, verifying the initial and final sponge and instrument count with the scrub nurse, recording the time and nature of delivery room events, participating in immediate care of the neonate, and giving encouragement to the mother and her support person.

Normal maintenance of delivery rooms is in large part under nursing supervision. Rooms should be kept stocked with current equipment in good repair. Nurses attending cesarean deliveries must also know how to use the equipment properly and with ease. An actual delivery is not the time to find out that there are no more sutures, that the suction machine does not work, or that the oxytocin has expired. An operative suite equipped for cesarean delivery always needs to be ready to receive a client, even on units where cesarean deliveries are not frequently performed. In addition to the usual surgical attire of gloves, boots and gowns, all personnel assisting in cesarean deliveries need to wear goggles as well as masks to protect themselves from contamination with body fluids. Sharma and colleagues (1997) found that the masks and goggles of physicians, their assistants, and scrub nurses were often spattered with blood during cesarean deliveries.

Regional anesthesia is administered by the anesthesiologist prior to the preparation of the surgical site. This allows time for the anesthesia to take effect. If general anesthesia is to be used, the woman is completely prepared and the team is scrubbed and ready to begin the cesarean prior to the induction of anesthesia.

After the operative area has been scrubbed with an antiseptic solution, an incision is made by the physician through the skin, subcutaneous tissues, and uterus. During the procedure, retractors are used to allow for visibility of the operative field (Fig. 26–1). Suction is used to remove fluids from the operative area, and cauterization of small blood vessels is done to reduce bleeding. During the procedure, the woman's heart rate, blood pressure, respirations, and oxygen levels are monitored. The infant is delivered through the incision, and the cord is clamped and cut. A sample of cord blood is taken from the cord. Cord blood studies are based on the client's unique needs

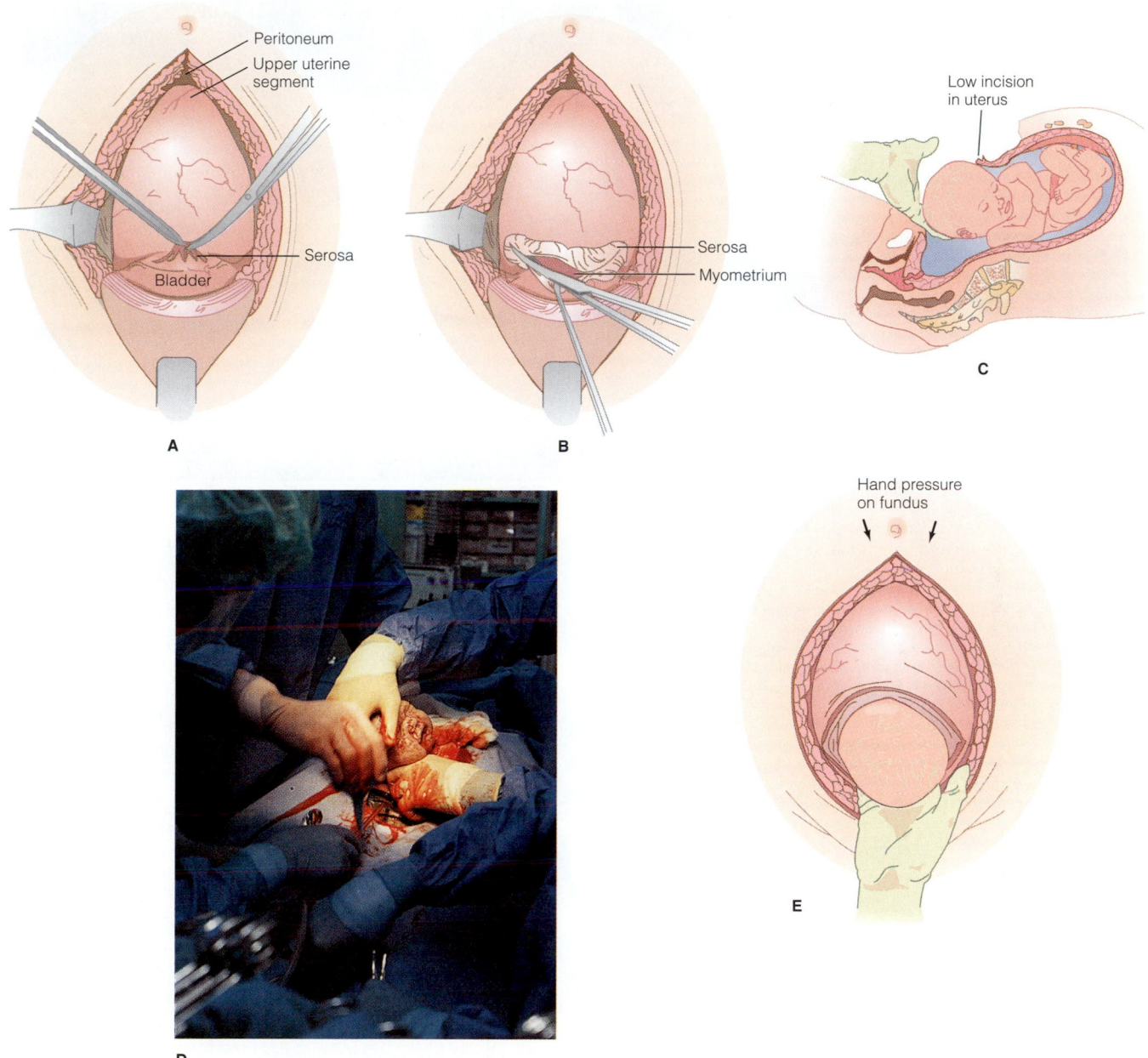

FIGURE 26–1. Cesarean delivery. **A.** The loose serosa is held in the forceps. The tip of the hemostat points to the upper margin of the bladder. The retractor is firm against the symphysis. **B.** Sterile bandage scissors are used to make the incision into the loose serosa. **C.** and **D.** After incisions are made into the uterus and fetal membranes, the physician reaches into the uterus between the symphysis pubis and the fetal head. The head is carefully lifted to bring it from beneath the symphysis forward through the uterine and abdominal incisions. **E.** As the fetal head is lifted through the incision, pressure is usually applied to the uterine fundus through the abdominal wall to help expel the fetus. *(A, B, C, and E are adapted, with permission, from Cunningham, F.G. et al. (1997). Williams obstetrics (20th ed.). Stamford, CT: Appleton & Lange, pp. 516, 519. D is courtesy of Harriette Hartigan/Artemis.)*

and hospital protocol and may include analysis of bilirubin, type, Rh factor, and pH.

After delivery of the newborn, the physician manually removes the placenta, if it has not spontaneously separated. Manual delivery of the placenta has been associated with greater blood loss and a higher incidence of postoperative endometritis than

spontaneous delivery of the placenta (Gabbe, Niebyl, & Simpson, 1996; McCurdy, Magann, McCurdy, & Saltzman, 1992). Intravenous oxytocin to stimulate uterine contraction and decrease bleeding is administered by the anesthesiologist after delivery of the fetal shoulders. The uterus is then repaired with nonremovable sutures (Fig. 26–2). In one commonly used

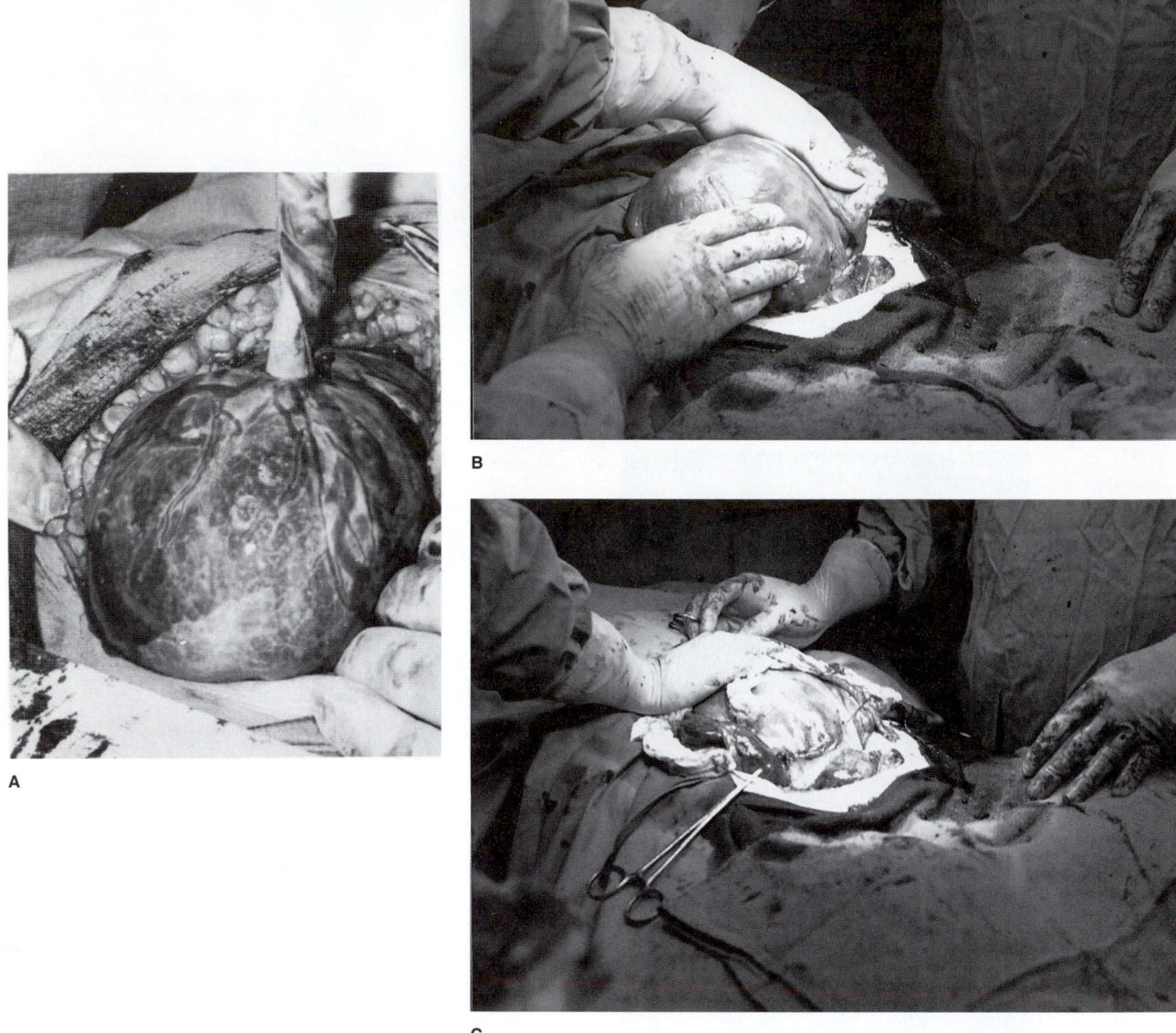

FIGURE 26–2. A. Placenta is bulging through uterine incision as uterus contracts. **B.** The uterus is replaced after repair outside the body. Ovaries, uterus, and fallopian tubes are inspected. **C.** The uterine suture line is inspected prior to closure of the subcutaneous tissues and skin. *(A is reproduced, with permission, from Cunningham, F.G. et al. (1989). Williams obstetrics (18th ed.). Norwalk, CT: Appleton & Lange, p. 451.)*

technique, the physician lifts the uterus through the abdominal incision, places it onto the sterile drapes covering the abdominal wall, and proceeds with the repair. Advantages of this include easy visualization of areas of uterine relaxation or bleeding and better visual exposure of the adnexa. Disadvantages of this technique include possible discomfort experienced by clients receiving spinal or epidural anesthesia and, occasionally, nausea and vomiting when the uterus is brought out or replaced (Cunningham et al., 1997).

While the obstetric team is involved in surgical repair, the newborn, after initial assessment, can be wrapped in a warm blanket, shown to the mother, and held by the father or support person. In this way the attachment process can be facilitated within the cesarean room. This, however, depends on the health status of the newborn and the type of anesthesia used for the mother.

After repair of the uterus, a final sponge and instrument count is taken and recorded before the abdominal wall is closed. The skin incision may be

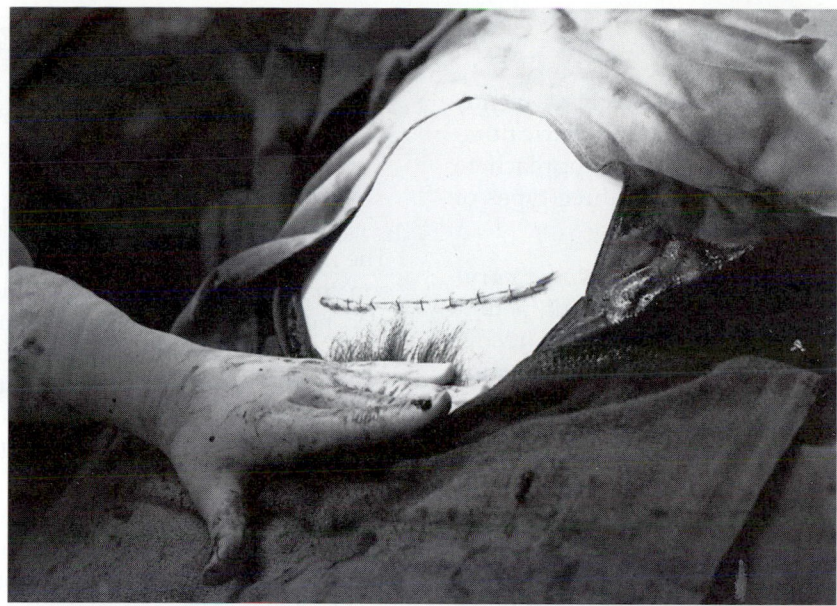

FIGURE 26–3. Repaired skin incision with staples used for closure. Note that pubic hair around the incision was removed; however, a complete pubic shave is not necessary.

closed with sutures or with staples (Fig. 26–3). A light dressing, for example three 4 × 4 sponges unfolded once and secured with tape, is applied to the skin incision. The woman is then transferred to a stretcher and brought to the recovery unit.

When a woman who received regional anesthesia for her cesarean birth is moved to an obstetric recovery unit, the support person who has attended the delivery can usually remain with her, although hospital rules vary. In certain hospitals, the newborn, if healthy, may also stay with the couple. When recovery takes place in a general postoperative recovery suite, visitor presence may be restricted. For these reasons, prior to delivery, couples need to be aware of the policy at the hospital where they plan to deliver.

▶ CARE OF NEWBORN IN DELIVERY ROOM

As a cesarean is considered a high-risk delivery, all neonates born in this manner are considered at risk and are examined carefully. Often, a member of the special-care nursery staff attends, along with a pediatrician or neonatologist. All staff responsible for the newborn need to be skilled in neonatal resuscitation techniques as well as in the immediate care of a high-risk neonate.

A heated crib with resuscitative equipment is prepared prior to the cesarean and is considered nec-

essary to any obstetric unit. The newborn is handed by the physician performing the cesarean to the nurse or pediatrician attending the newborn. The neonate is placed beneath the radiant warmer, suctioned, dried, and assessed. Apgar scores (see Chapter 30) are done at 1 and 5 minutes after birth. Identification bands with numbers corresponding to the mother's identification number are placed on the newborn's ankle and wrist, and footprints are taken. Antimicrobial eye therapy may be delayed for a short while to facilitate eye contact between the new parents and the baby. If the mother has not received general anesthesia, the baby is brought close to her, so that she may see and kiss her newborn. If all is well, the baby, wrapped warmly and wearing a hat to conserve heat, may be given to the father or support person to hold within the mother's range of vision. As the surgery is completed, the new parents may interact with their newborn. If the baby's condition is unstable, however, he or she is brought at once to the special care nursery. The parents may be extremely distressed by their newborn's uncertain status; therefore, attention needs to be focused on providing emotional support to the parents during the cesarean, as well as afterward.

Ways in which parents may be supported during the rest of cesarean delivery when neonatal outcome is poor should be discussed in staff planning meetings before crisis situations are encountered. In this way effective strategies that may be realistically used in a particular hospital setting can be developed.

► POSTPARTUM CARE

The postpartum care of the cesarean client blends principles and practices of surgical and obstetric nursing (Figs. 26–4 and 26–5). A systematic approach to the client in the recovery unit includes three types of assessment:

- *Assessment of physical and physiologic parameters.* Overall impression of the client, neurologic status, sensory and motor function (recovery from anesthesia), cardiovascular status (pulse, blood pressure, skin color), respiratory status, temperature (oral temperatures should be avoided unless the woman is completely awake), fundal height and degree of firmness, appearance of the abdominal dressing, amount and color of lochia, intravenous therapy and fluid intake, urine output and patency of catheter. Oxygen and suction are kept available for use, if needed, even when clients have received epidural or spinal anesthesia (AWHONN, 1998).
- *Assessment of pain and determination of need for analgesics as ordered.* As the effects of anesthesia wear off, the woman may be increasingly aware of pain related to the surgery. Uterine palpation to ensure that the uterus remains well contracted can be an especially uncomfortable, although necessary part of postoperative care. Intramuscular analgesics, such as meperidine, may be given when the woman is fully reactive from the anesthesia. Epidural administration of a narcotic drug, such as morphine, has provided especially effective analgesia after cesarean delivery, and is becoming an increasingly widespread alternative to intramuscular analgesics in the immediate postoperative period. (See Chapter 23 for further discussion of epidural analgesia.)
- *Assessment of psychologic parameters.* The immediate response of the woman and her partner to the cesarean delivery, the woman's desire to be with her infant, the woman's beginning acquaintance with the infant.

Nursing strategies that may promote the client's comfort in the recovery room include:

- Providing warmed blankets (these may be applied when the woman is transferred from the delivery table to the stretcher)
- Providing mouth care
- Giving a sponge bath
- Administering prescribed analgesics (unless epidural analgesia has been given)
- Assisting with positioning
- Orienting the woman and her support person to the recovery unit
- Providing reassurance that the cesarean is over
- Fostering opportunities for contact between the mother and her support person and between the couple and the newborn

The nurse needs to allow the mother and support person to express feelings about the delivery; the nurse also needs to accept these feelings as valid, whether they are positive or negative. If the newborn cannot be brought to the recovery unit, the delivery or recovery nurse, the special-care nurse, pediatrician, or neonatologist may provide information about the neonate's condition.

Several clients may be in the same recovery unit, especially if it is a general surgical recovery suite. Concern for the client's reactions to others who have just had surgery requires thoughtful placement of the client in the unit. Client privacy can be promoted by drawing drapes completely around the stretcher whenever physical assessment and care are being undertaken.

Safety is a major priority within a recovery unit. Side rails remain raised at all times. Whenever sensory or motor function has been altered, the nurse needs to take measures to protect the client against inadvertent injury. Although it is desirable to encourage early parent–newborn contact, the woman is also recovering from the effects of anesthesia and drugs that have muscle relaxant or sedative effects. The newborn may be held close to the mother by the nurse or the support person, but the baby should not be placed unsupervised on the stretcher.

► Admission to Postpartum Unit

When the woman is recovered (i.e., completely awake, and able to move independently, with blood pressure, pulse, and respirations stable, a well-contracted uterus, no excessive bleeding, and a urine output of at least 30 mL per hour), she is brought to the postpartum unit. In addition to receiving the client and her chart, the postpartum nurse takes an oral report of the woman's surgical and recovery experiences from the recovery nurse. An assessment of the client needs to be done on her admission to the postpartum floor and *before* the departure of the nurse from the recovery unit. At that time, the client's record should be reviewed to verify that all medications, fluids, physical signs, and other parameters have been documented.

Target Postdelivery LOS = 72 hours

Date of Birth: _____ Time of Birth: _____
Date of Discharge: _____ Time of Discharge: _____   Sex _____

	Prenatal by 36 weeks	Labor/ Delivery/Recovery	OR Day Postpartum	Post-OP Day 1	Post-OP Day 2	Discharge Day Post-OP Day 3	Post-OP Day 4 / Home	Post-OP Day 5
Laboratory/ Diagnostic Tests	H + H; Type and Screen; Rubella; RPR; HBSAG	CBC; MsBOS; RPR		H + H or CBC Per Order; RPR Results				
Treatments/ Assessments		Prenatal records in DR by 38 weeks; Assessment, VS	Postpartum/Post-OP Assessments; Peri care/Foley care; Oxygen PRN; Duramorph monitoring PRN	Postpartum/Post-OP Assessments; Bed bath with assist; Peri care; D/C Duramorph monitoring as indicated	Postpartum/Post-OP Assessments	Postpartum/Post-OP Assessments		Follow-up phone call by P.P nursing staff
Medications/IVs	Prenatal vitamins	Anesthesia per order	PCA pump per order; IV with pitocin per order; IM pain meds per order	D/C PCA pump; D/C IV when tolerating PO; RhoGAM PRN; Rubella PRN; PO pain meds	PO pain meds; Mylicon PRN; Stool softener PRN	D/C prescriptions		
Consultations	Social work per guideline		Social work if indicated	Lactation counselor PRN; Pediatrician; Social work PRN	Lactation counselor PRN	Lactation counseling PRN; Pediatrician; Social work PRN		
Activity		Bedrest	Bedrest; Pulmonary hygiene	OOB as tolerated; Pulmonary hygiene	Ambulation; Self-care/Peri care	Ambulation; Self-care/peri care		
Nutrition	Appropriate weight gain	NPO, ice chips	NPO, ice chips	Clear liquids	Progress to house diet	House diet		
Education/ Discharge Planning	Childbirth prep classes; Parentcraft; Breastfeeding class PRN; Tour/crit. path orientation; Contraceptive planning; Preparing for Your Baby's Birth at Jefferson; Select pediatrician; "Baby Talk" video	Relaxation technique; Orient to procedure, OR, and recovery room; Breastfeeding	Orient to PCA pump; Orient to unit; Infant feeding as indicated; Breast pump if needed	Handwashing; Baby's crib; Infant positioning, feeding; Body mechanics for OOB and ambulation; Incision care	Infant care/feeding class; D/C planning; Circumcision care as indicated; S & S of dehydration and infection	D/C instructions; Gift pack; Follow-up care; Review prescription medication	Reinforce postpartum education	
Home Care	Referral to home care		Notify home care of delivery			Home care referral	Home care visit PRN	Home care visit PRN
Variances: Order Reason Order Reason								
RN Signature:								

Target Outcome = Demonstrates parenting skills
Minimal physical discomfort

Confirmed postdelivery by obstetrician: _____   Signature _____   Date _____

FIGURE 26–4. Clinical pathway: cesarean delivery: mother. *(Courtesy of Thomas Jefferson University Hospital, Jefferson Health System, Philadelphia, PA.)*

Date of Birth: _____
Date of Discharge: _____

Time of Birth: _____
Time of Discharge: _____

Sex _____

Target LOS = 72 hours

	0–6 hours	7–12 hours	13–18 hours	19–24 hours	Day 2	Day 3	Within 2 hrs. of discharge	Home 24–48 hrs. Postdischarge
Laboratory/ Diagnostic Tests	Coombs Maternal Hep B status			Coombs results Maternal RPR status at delivery Bilirubin at age 24 hours PKU at age 24 hours	TA Bilirubin if > 5 at 24 hours	Bilirubin per protocol Bilirubin if > 5 at 24 hours		Bilirubin if > 5 or if baby jaundiced by home health nurse; report results to pediatrician
Treatments/ Procedures	Stabilization Baby ID VS as per patient standard Weight Bath	Circumcision permit and circumcision Hep B permit	Circumcision care	Circumcision care	Circumcision care	Circumcision care		
Medications/IVs	Triple dye to cord Vitamin K Erythromycin ointment to eyes	HBIG if mother is Hep B positive or status unknown Hep B vaccine						
Consultations								
Activity	Radiant warmer until stable temp	Open crib	Open crib	Open crib	Open crib	Open crib	Open crib	
Nutrition	Breast feeding/or glucose H₂O	Breast feeding/or formula at least q 4 hrs	Breast feeding/or formula at least q 4 hrs	Breast feeding/or formula at least q 4 hrs	Breast feeding/or formula at least q 4 hrs	Breast feeding/or formula at least q 4 hrs	Breast feeding/or formula at least q 4 hrs	Breast feeding/or formula at least q 4 hrs
Assessments	Apgar at 1 and 5 minutes Gestational age Nursing assessment for VS, feeding, voiding, bonding	I + O Nursing assessment for VS, feeding, voiding, bonding	I + O Assess circumcision site	Physician assessment of body systems I + O Nursing assessment for VS, feeding, voiding, bonding	I + O Nursing assessment for VS, feeding, voiding, bonding	I + O Nursing assessment for VS, feeding, voiding, bonding		HHC nurse assessment of physical environment and baby including VS, feeding, voiding, stooling, bonding, jaundice
Education/ Discharge Planning	See clinical pathway/ mother						Instructions to parents	
Home Care								
Variances:								
Order								
Reason								
Order								
Reason								

RN Signature: _____

Target discharge status = Feeding well
 Maintaining temperature
 Voiding and stooling adequately
 Bonding

Confirmed by pediatrician:

_____ _____
Signature　　　　　　　　　Date

FIGURE 26–5. Clinical pathway: cesarean delivery: infant. *(Courtesy of Thomas Jefferson University Hospital, Jefferson Health System, Philadelphia, PA.)*

▶ Stay in Postpartum Unit

Care of the postpartum cesarean woman resembles nursing care for the woman who delivers vaginally, with the following important differences.

Cesarean clients are surgical clients with all the needs of women who have had major abdominal surgery. Although cesarean women do not have the perineal discomfort experienced by women who have delivered vaginally, they may realistically have considerable incisional pain, especially on the first postpartum day, unless epidural analgesia was administered. The nurse needs to anticipate this and to *offer* analgesics and other comfort measures. Some hospitals may use client-controlled analgesics, administered by intravenous pump according to the client's own perceived needs, but with a preset safety limit for dosage. Assessment of the uterine fundus will also be painful for the cesarean client, and the nurse can organize care so that the woman receives an analgesic prior to this.

Postoperative pain limits mobility. The cesarean client will need encouragement and physical assistance, especially in changing positions, getting out of bed, and handling her newborn. Cesarean clients do need help with personal hygiene measures, such as sponge bathing hard-to-reach body areas. By the third postoperative day, showering is usually possible; however, nursing assistance may be needed. The nurse should organize the environment surrounding the client so that call bell, telephone, personal items, and other items are within easy reach. A postpartum cesarean client should not have continuous rooming-in until she is able to ambulate and hold her newborn independently.

Postanesthesia effects on respiratory function necessitate that the nurse listen for breath sounds and supervise deep breathing and coughing exercises as well as early ambulation. Assessment of respiratory status is particularly important in women who have received epidural analgesia.

The intravenous infusion may remain for 24 to 48 hours, or until the client tolerates fluids well by mouth. In addition, some postcesarean clients retain intravenous access for continued antibiotic administration.

Nearly all women have indwelling urinary catheters inserted prior to the surgery to keep the bladder decompressed and out of the surgical field. The catheter may be removed the morning after the cesarean or sooner, depending on obstetric judgment. As in caring for any catheterized client, the nurse needs to check urinary output (e.g., color, quantity), make certain that straight drainage is not impaired by "kinks" in the tubing, and minimize chance of infection through universal precautions and aseptic technique. In certain cases urine samples for urinalysis and culture may be taken before the catheter is removed; however, these tests are costly and are not routinely performed for all postcesarean clients. To prevent bladder distension and minimize the possibility of associated complications such as uterine hemorrhage and urinary tract infection, women should void spontaneously within 4 to 6 hours of removal of the catheter. Assisting the client into the bathroom, ambulation, running water in the sink, or pouring warm water over the vulva may help clients void and avert the need for reinsertion of a catheter.

On the second and third postoperative days, gas pain related to incoordinate bowel action may be a problem. Strategies such as early ambulation can be helpful. A bowel movement usually provides relief, but may need to be induced with a rectal suppository or, if ineffective, an enema, as prescribed by the physician.

The abdominal incision site needs to be inspected and any redness, swelling, oozing, or separation reported to the physician and charted. After the surgical dressing has been removed by the physician, a light dressing, without heavy tape, may be used for protection, especially if a maternity belt holding a sanitary pad would come into contact with the wound. The presence of an abdominal incision, along with the circumstances that led to the need or diagnosis of the need for the cesarean, may put the cesarean client at higher risk for infection than the woman who delivers vaginally.

Cesarean clients whose skin incisions were closed with nonabsorbable materials, such as metal skin staples, will need these removed, usually by the fourth day. Some physicians may choose to close cesarean skin incisions with absorbable sutures that do not need removal; however, suture removal from the postcesarean skin incision is fairly swift and involves minimal discomfort.

Some cesarean clients fear they will not be able to breastfeed because of the cesarean. Cesarean mothers often have their first breastfeeding experience several hours later than mothers who deliver vaginally. There is no reason, however, why a cesarean delivery alone should affect a mother's ability to breastfeed successfully. The nurse needs to identify cesarean-related fears about breastfeeding and to provide reassurance and assistance for the client who wants to breastfeed.

▶ Challenges of Early Discharge

Women with an uncomplicated postcesarean course often go home on the third postpartum day or in rare cases sooner. Over the years, the trend toward earlier discharge has reflected such factors as increasing pressures to minimize costs of hospitalization and the client's desire to go home.

Early discharge of cesarean clients presents several challenges. For example, health care providers often worry about "missing" high-risk conditions that do not emerge during shortened hospital stays. Leaving the hospital early does not mean that a woman who is only a few days beyond surgery can manage well at home with a new baby. As Brooten and col-

leagues (1996) found, women discharged early continued to have many needs at home.

Caring effectively for postcesarean clients who have early discharge requires reevaluation of traditional cesarean care. Without close to a week of traditional in-hospital care, clients need strategies that foster independence earlier, help them to manage away from direct view of health care providers, and ensure post-discharge follow-up. In order to manage well at home, clients ideally should have assistance

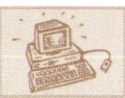 *Research Abstract*

Early Discharge and Home Care After Unplanned Cesarean Birth: Nursing Care Time

In this study of 61 women who delivered healthy infants by unplanned cesarean delivery, advanced practice nurses provided discharge planning and 8-week home follow-up with home visits, telephone calls, and daily telephone availability. The amount of time spent by the advanced practice nurses was based on the needs of the women and the judgment of the health care providers, rather than by the woman's reimbursement insurance plan. Such plans often specify and limit the amount of reimbursible time spent with clients. More than half of the subjects needed more than the two expected home visits, which averaged an hour each; all but 10 subjects needed more than the expected 10 phone calls. Forty-four percent of the women had pregnancy complications; 21% had post-discharge complications, and these clients needed extra time in discharge planning and during home visits. However, the women without complications needed extra time in telephone contact. The study highlighted the intense psychosocial needs of women who have had unplanned cesareans and the need for home visits and telephone follow-up by nurses after these clients' early discharge. With interventions by the advanced practice nurses, the women were significantly more satisfied with their care and had fewer acute care visits to hospitals or clinics; no one in the group was readmitted to the hospital. Thus, such interventions, along with the early discharge, had financial savings as well as psychosocial and physical benefits. The study concluded that the education and resource needs of such high-risk women may not be met by the one or two 1-hour home visits currently provided by health care services.

Application to Practice

Over the past two decades, length of hospital stay after cesarean delivery has decreased greatly. Women routinely are now being discharged on the third postpartum day; in some cases, women are going home sooner. What happens to these women after discharge? Unfortunately, not everyone has enough need-based, knowledgeable follow-up. This study helps to identify the amount of time women who have had unplanned cesareans need for post-discharge care. The study also underscores the importance of attending to the post-discharge needs of women who have had unplanned cesarean deliveries and highlights the cost savings, even though time-consuming interventions may be necessary. Nurses working in postpartum settings should not simply assume that going home early means that all is well for clients who have unplanned cesarean deliveries. Third party payers, nurses, and physicians need to work together to ensure that these women receive adequate and appropriate follow-up care.

Source: Brooten, D., Knapp, H., Boruki, L., Jacobsen, B., Finkler, S., Arnold, L., & Mennuti, M. (1996). Early discharge and home care after unplanned cesarean birth: Nursing care time. Journal of Obstetric, Gynecologic, and Neonatal Nursing, 25(7); 595–600.

from at least one responsible significant other, be well educated about postcesarean needs, be able to identify problems, and agree to contact their health care providers if problems arise. Early discharge does not mean the end of contact between clients and their health care providers. Such strategies as scheduled telephone calls (even to confirm wellness) and home visits can help contain costs and promote quality care.

▶ Discharge Teaching

Many aspects of discharge teaching, such as breast-feeding and sexuality, are similar for clients regardless of whether they deliver abdominally or vaginally. Teaching specific to cesarean mothers focuses on assisting the mother to continue to recover from surgery while adapting to the addition of the new-born to the family. Teaching should also include significant family members, as the client will need assistance with household responsibilities and with infant care.

Discharge teaching includes emotional reactions to the cesarean on the part of the client and her significant others. The nurse can provide reassurance and anticipatory guidance about normal reactions. The nurse can also identify clients who are having difficulty in postpartum adaptation or in coping with the cesarean delivery and then make appropriate referrals for further evaluation. Clients should be informed of support groups, which focus on the special needs of cesarean families. Nurses working with cesarean clients should be aware of such groups in their local communities, as well as the existence of national organizations.

Before discharge, the client makes an appointment for a follow-up postpartum, postcesarean examination. Clients are generally seen during the first to third week. Clients discharged before removal of staples have their staples removed at an office or home visit 3–5 days after discharge.

▶ Psychologic Responses

In the 1950s, cesarean and vaginal delivery clients were treated in a similar fashion. Childbirth was widely viewed as a pathologic event for which most people received general anesthesia and remained hospitalized for periods extending to 2 weeks. By the mid-1970s, however, prepared childbirth and family-centered, father-attended birth became widely publicized and available for women who delivered vaginally. As noted earlier, cesarean clients were denied a similar birth experience. Such negative feelings as

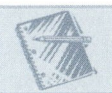

Client Teaching

Postpartum Teaching for Cesarean Clients

To help clients recover from cesarean delivery after discharge from the hospital, the nurse can suggest the following strategies:

- Rest frequently during the day.
- Restrict your activities to caring for yourself and, with help, your baby.
- To relieve pain when changing position (e.g., rising from a supine to a sitting position), roll to your side and splint the incision with one hand as you gently push yourself upward with your other hand.
- Avoid heavy lifting or other activities that can potentially strain the healing wound.
- Take the oral analgesics prescribed by your physician to relieve discomfort.
- Consult your physician before taking any over-the-counter medications.
- Be aware of danger signs of infection (redness, swelling, discharge, separation of the incision, fever, or foul-smelling vaginal discharge) and recurrent heavy bleeding. Contact your health care provider immediately if these signs occur.
- Exercise appropriately based on your situation and according to your health care provider's instructions.

anger, disappointment, loss of self-esteem, and grief were described, particularly when the woman lacked adequate information, received general anesthesia and could not be awake for her delivery, and was separated from her partner and newborn (Reichert, Baron, & Fawcett, 1993). Research from the early 1980s indicated that psychologic wounding tended to be greater in women who had valued and sought natural childbirth as a goal in itself (Sandelowski & Bustamante, 1986). These women tended to be from Caucasian middle-class backgrounds.

The great differences between the cesarean delivery and vaginal birth experiences has narrowed today, although studies on women's reactions to cesareans have had conflicting results. Most research has confirmed that women who deliver by cesarean in a family-centered atmosphere can adapt well and have satisfying birth experiences. However, studies continue to point out the importance of the supportive, as well as the technical, quality of medical and nursing care during the events surrounding the cesarean delivery (Radin et al., 1993; Reichert et al., 1993; Fawcett & Weiss, 1993). Several factors, described below, have been linked to the changing trends in women's perceptions and attitudes toward cesarean birth.

- The efforts of cesarean birth organizations, which have sought to have family-centered, culturally sensitive care, including the participation of the father or significant other in the birth, for cesarean clients.
- Inclusion of content about cesarean preparation in prepared childbirth classes, the establishment of special cesarean education programs, and greater public knowledge about cesareans, perhaps decreasing the perception of cesarean delivery as a threatening event.
- The high incidence of cesarean birth, which may make women feel less different or abnormal. Today, most women know someone who had a cesarean birth.
- Widespread media attention to cesarean birth.
- Greater acceptance of the use of technology in childbirth, and increasing emphasis on birth as more of a "high-risk" event, with cesarean birth seen as a viable method of delivery.
- Attempts of hospitals and health care providers to "normalize" the cesarean birth experience. In many places, such barriers to the childbirth experience as routine use of general anesthesia and rules against the presence of significant others in the delivery room have been lifted. Opportunities for sustained contact with the newborn are now more widely available, and women are able to go home sooner.

Much progress has been made in promoting a positive birth experience for cesarean clients. However, nurses must always be aware of the potentially wide variety of responses that clients may have toward abdominal birth, and must realize that many complex variables can affect a client's and family's responses. While working with other health care providers to decrease the cesarean rate, nurses must nevertheless identify and work to minimize potential barriers to emotionally satisfying care. Without stereotyping, nurses must be able to provide culturally sensitive care and to be aware that women from different cultures may respond differently to cesarean delivery. As the events surrounding cesarean birth change, there continues to be an ongoing need for research into perceptions and responses of women and families to cesarean birth.

▶ THE FATHER'S EXPERIENCE

Cesarean delivery presents a potential risk to the father's childbirth experience. Most hospitals currently encourage fathers to be present during the vaginal delivery of their babies. However, this policy does not automatically extend to cesarean deliveries. In some places, fathers are still regarded as intruders; sets of institutional regulations may restrict paternal participation in cesarean delivery. Ironically, the arguments that were once used to keep fathers from attending vaginal deliveries have been applied to fathers' attendance at cesarean deliveries: the infection rates may increase; the father would be in the way; the father could not "stand" to witness cesarean surgery. Neither research nor clinical reports have given evidence to substantiate barring fathers from cesarean deliveries.

Many fathers now expect to attend their partners' cesarean delivery. However, hospital policies regarding fathers' presence at cesarean deliveries vary. Most hospitals allow fathers to attend elective cesareans if they have gone to cesarean preparation classes. A few hospitals still may not permit fathers into the cesarean room under any circumstances. Some hospitals allow fathers to attend whether the cesarean is being done on an emergency or an elective basis. Attitudes of obstetricians and delivery room nurses also determine whether a father can see his infant born. In a classic study, May and Sollid (1984) observed that fathers' negative reactions did not tend to focus on the cesarean itself, but on policies that set up barriers to their participation in the birth and on physicians' and nurses' behaviors that made them feel unsupported and excluded from the birth; this happened regardless of whether they were actually present for the delivery.

Change in hospital practices has come about largely because there are so many cesareans being done and in response to consumer demand for a father-attended birth experience similar to that offered to women having vaginal deliveries. The media has done much to promote public acceptance of father-attended births, and many fathers look forward to this experience. Being ignored or denied access to the delivery can foster feelings of anger, frustration, and disappointment for fathers. At times they may blame staff or their partners. On the other hand, attendance and staff support can promote feelings of togetherness and common purpose.

Nurses can help cesarean fathers through such strategies as:

- Encouraging expectant fathers to discuss their plans, thoughts, and fears about cesarean delivery

- Providing information about options, as well as restrictions, available at local hospitals
- Developing and teaching cesarean birth classes to expectant couples
- Encouraging fathers to be present in the delivery room and to seek early contact with their infants
- Providing anticipatory guidance, even if the father has attended cesarean preparation classes
- Advising the father in aspects of the cesarean experience such as how to don surgical attire, where to stand, what to expect, and what he may do
- Providing an opportunity for fathers to discuss their feelings about the cesarean delivery
- Keeping the father informed about the progress of the cesarean
- Offering emotional support
- Inviting the father to accompany the newborn to the nursery, to observe the nursery admission procedures, and to touch and hold the newborn

At times it may not be feasible for a father to be present for the cesarean delivery, or he may choose not to be present. In such cases, the reason why the father was not present should first be identified, as interventions are affected by this reason. Fathers who decline the invitation to be present for the cesarean should be treated with respect, and staff should not attempt to "force" them to see the delivery.

▶ VAGINAL BIRTH AFTER CESAREAN DELIVERY

Vaginal birth after cesarean delivery (VBAC) is no longer a new idea and is part of routine practice in many settings. Nevertheless, whether a woman who has at one time had a cesarean birth can safely deliver vaginally in the future continues to be controversial. Early in the 20th century, Cragin's decree of "once a cesarean, always a cesarean," took hold. Despite evidence supporting VBAC for appropriate candidates, most women who have had cesareans once have cesarean deliveries again. In 1995, the VBAC rate was 35.5 per 100 women with a previous cesarean; however, this was nearly triple the 12.6% rate in 1988 (Curtin & Kozak, 1997). Trends are changing, and VBAC is occurring more often in the late 1990s and with greater support from health care providers than in the previous decades (Korte, 1998).

VBAC is usually performed within hospital settings with ready access to cesarean facilities; physi-

cians traditionally are the health care providers. However, women attempting VBAC can have family centered births within hospital birthing rooms. As Harrington and colleagues (1997) demonstrated, certified nurse-midwives can also care for these clients safely within these settings.

The argument against VBAC focuses on the possible occurrence of such major and life-threatening complications as uterine rupture. Fibrotic scar tissue from previous uterine surgery is not as strong as uncut muscle and forms a plane of weakness in the uterus. Distension of the uterus in a future pregnancy and the force of contractions during labor could theoretically exert enough pressure to split the uterus along the old incision line, although the actual incidence of this event is low. Professional fear of obstetric catastrophe has become a major reason for elective repeat cesarean birth (Cunningham et al., 1997; Miller & Sutter, 1985).

Several factors may contribute to the low incidence of VBAC. Current professional worry about potential malpractice suits supports the notion of "once a cesarean, always a cesarean." In a study of 241 women with previous cesareans, Kline and Arias (1993) found that medical indications and client personal wishes were the motivations for 77.4% of the women opting for repeat cesarean delivery. Only 6.6% of VBAC clients and 13.3% of repeat cesarean clients considered their physician's advice to be the most important factor in their decision. Hueston and Rudy (1994) found that clients with private insurance had more repeat elective cesareans. They attributed their results in part to the ability of these clients to have their desires for repeat cesareans met and to better overall compensation for health care providers.

Proponents of VBAC claim that cesareans pose greater risks than VBAC. Miller and Sutter (1985) observed that "when concrete data are examined, concerns voiced over uterine rupture seem to be exaggerated and based more on history than the current clinical environment." Morbidity rates for elective repeat cesarean deliveries have also been reported to be higher than the 3% morbidity rate associated with vaginal delivery (Hueston & Rudy, 1994). However, maternal and neonatal morbidity rates for women who attempt VBAC but require cesarean delivery are not believed to be higher than for women who have a primary cesarean after labor. Maternal and perinatal mortality rates for VBAC are not greater than those for repeat cesarean birth. In addition, repeat cesarean delivery is financially and emotionally more expensive than VBAC. With physician consultation as indicated and with readily accessible hospital services, nurse-midwives may manage and deliver clients attempting VBAC, thereby adding the benefit of choice of caregiver to VBAC.

► Qualifications and Contraindications

Vaginal birth after cesarean has been supported as a safe option to routine repeat cesarean by such groups as the Association of Women's Health, Obstetric and Neonatal Nurses (AWHONN) and the American College of Obstetricians and Gynecologists (ACOG). Third party insurers recognize VBAC as a reimbursible option. Indeed, greater scrutiny and cost-consciousness by managed care insurers, reluctant simply to pay the higher costs of routine repeat cesareans, are contributing to the increase in VBACs.

An estimated 60–80% of all clients who have a trial of labor will be able to have VBAC (Hale, 1994). About 75–80% will be able to have VBAC if the primary cesarean was done for a reason unlikely to recur, such as breech presentation. A previous vaginal delivery is a factor indicating that future VBAC can be likely. Ideally, candidates for VBAC are women who:

- Desire to avoid cesarean delivery and want to experience labor and vaginal delivery
- Have access to a hospital and staff supportive of VBAC
- Had a previous cesarean for a problem that is unlikely to recur
- Are in good physical health
- Have had a healthy pregnancy with a fetus weighing less than 4000 g
- Understand the risks and benefits of VBAC and the possibility of an emergency cesarean if labor does not progress smoothly.

Vaginal birth after cesarean would be contraindicated in any condition that of itself precludes vaginal birth (e.g., complete placenta previa), difficult fetal presentations, situations where the woman does not want to try VBAC, and in facilities where women do not have access to emergency cesarean delivery should the need arise. Women who have had more than one cesarean may have a trial of labor, although risks and benefits are not as well known as for women who have had only one previous cesarean (Cunningham et al., 1997).

Type of previous uterine incision also affects VBAC. Low transverse incisions are considered the safest for VBAC. Risk of uterine rupture from these incisions has been estimated to be 0.19–0.8% (Cowan, Kinch, Ellis, & Anderson, 1994; Flamm, Goings, Liu, & Wolde-Tsadik, 1994). However, a vertical uterine incision, extending into the upper contractile portion of

the myometrium, is believed to be a contraindication to VBAC, because of the risk of uterine rupture during labor, noted to be as high as 12% (Cunningham et al., 1997; Naef, Ray, Chaukan, Roach, Blake, & Martin, 1995). VBAC is a more controversial option for women with a vertical uterine incision that is confined to the mostly noncontractile lower uterine segment. Studies by Naef and colleagues (1995) and Adair and colleagues (1996) did not find risk of scar dehiscence to be remarkably different from risks for women laboring after low transverse uterine incisions. From their review of obstetric literature, Martin and colleagues (1997) concluded that women with one previous nonextended low-segment vertical uterine cesarean incision should be considered similar to women with a previous low segment scar and be candidates for trials of labor.

Alternative birth settings that cannot provide prompt access to facilities for cesarean delivery, if needed, are not recommended for VBAC. However, VBAC could be attempted in a hospital birthing room.

► Role of the Nurse

Nursing care of the woman attempting VBAC combines strategies for family-centered low-risk labor and delivery with strategies for care of the high-risk labor and delivery client. Ideally, the client would arrive in the labor unit with two birth plans: one for vaginal delivery and one in the event that cesarean delivery became necessary. In this situation, the client would have collaborated prenatally with her obstetric health care providers to ensure an optimal birth experience whether the birth occurred vaginally or abdominally. Support from nursing and medical staff promotes maternal confidence in attempting VBAC. During labor and delivery, careful monitoring of maternal and fetal status is essential. Actual management of the client undergoing VBAC is similar to that of a client attempting a vaginal delivery. Oxytocin and epidural anesthesia may be used (American College of Obstetricians and Gynecologists, 1995). In addition, the unit should be readied in case an emergency cesarean becomes necessary. The nurse must be able to promptly identify deviations from normal labor progression, especially indications of uterine rupture (signs of hemorrhage, shock, subjective reports of a "ripping sensation" or of sharp uterine pain, abrupt cessation of contractions, a fetus that can be palpated with excess ease) and the onset of any fetal distress. Should a threat to maternal or fetal well-being arise during the course of labor, the nurse must promptly inform the physician and prepare for the possibility of an emergency cesarean.

Women who do have VBAC may experience pride, confidence, and excitement about achieving a personal goal. Feelings may not be completely positive, if the reality of a VBAC experience is not congruent with the client's expectations.

Nurses need to provide special support to the client who attempts VBAC but requires a repeat cesarean delivery. Some clients may equate VBAC with success as a woman and are at risk for feelings of failure and disappointment if VBAC does not become possible. During prenatal preparation, nurses need to avoid equating VBAC with "success" and to make certain that clients and families understand that VBAC cannot be guaranteed. Development of a prenatal alternative birth plan can help the client and her partner retain a sense of control over their birth experience and can promote a family-centered birth.

Nurses should also anticipate negative client reactions and provide opportunity for the client and her family to express their feelings.

Nurses as well as other obstetric caregivers need to explore their own attitudes toward VBAC, to review the professional literature about VBAC, and to assist colleagues in learning about VBAC. Prenatally, clients who could potentially attempt VBAC should be taught about this option and supported so they may attempt VBAC. Clients desiring VBAC may also have to contend with negative attitudes from family members who should also be included in VBAC teaching. Through roles as authors and consultants to the media, nurses can foster public perceptions of VBAC as a safe means of delivery for many women who have had previous cesarean childbirth.

Critical Thinking in Care Planning

Care of the Client Immediately After Elective Cesarean Delivery

Jacky Vincent, G 2 P 1, 32 years old, is admitted to the delivery unit for a repeat cesarean birth. Her first child was born by emergency cesarean delivery 4 years ago as a result of failure to progress in labor and cephalopelvic disproportion.

Jacky is brought to the delivery suite at 8:00 AM. She receives spinal anesthesia and is awake for the cesarean, with her husband Jim in attendance. The Vincent's newborn son weighs 7 lbs 4 oz and has Apgar scores of 9 at 1 minute and 10 at 5 minutes. Following an uncomplicated 2-hour stay in the recovery room, Jacky is transferred to the postpartum floor. She receives 75 mg of meperidine, IM, for incisional pain. An indwelling catheter is in place and an intravenous drip of lactated Ringer's is running at 125 cc per hour.

▶ Assessment

- Blood pressure 110/70, pulse 72 and regular, respirations 17, temperature 98.2°F
- Dressing dry and intact
- Fundus firm, located at umbilicus

- Lochia rubra, moderate
- Urine clear and yellow
- Client reports incisional pain; requires assistance to turn in bed
- Client hesitant to deep breathe and cough or change position

Nursing Diagnosis

Healthy physiologic adaptation following cesarean delivery

Expected Client/Family Outcomes	Nursing Action/Intervention	Evaluation
During the postpartum period, the client will maintain normal physiologic balance.	Maintain continuous assessment (q15 min in recovery room, on admission to postpartum floor, then q4h or each shift as ordered) of:	Client's postpartum hospital stay is without complications.
	• Neurologic status and progressive recovery from anesthesia • Pulse, blood pressure, respirations • Fundal height • Lochia • Incision/dressing • Intravenous flow rate • Patency of indwelling catheter; color and amount of urinary output	
	Rationale: Assessment provides data about health status and recovery following cesarean delivery.	

Critical Thinking in Care Planning continued

Nursing Diagnosis

Pain, related to cesarean delivery

Expected Client/Family Outcomes	Nursing Action/Intervention	Evaluation
Client will report decreased discomfort related to incisional pain.	Assess incision, dressing, and nature of pain. Administer pain medications. *Rationale:* Pain in incision may indicate infection or separation, as well as normal postoperative discomfort. Analgesics relieve postoperative pain. Provide comfort measures: • Techniques of distraction, breathing, relaxation, imagery • Turn and position as indicated • Keep warm • Provide sponge bath, mouth care, back rub *Rationale:* Comfort measures will assist client to relax, improving ability to cope with postoperative incisional pain.	Client will report decreased pain related to cesarean delivery.
	Encourage husband to stay with client. Bring newborn to mother and father to see and touch after mother is made comfortable. *Rationale:* Promotes family-centered birthing experience. Promotes initial parent–infant attachment and provides alternate focus for attention.	Couple will remain together and will become acquainted with their newborn.

Nursing Diagnosis

Potential ineffective breathing pattern, related to postoperative immobility and incisional pain

Postoperatively, client will cough, deep breathe, and change position. By the end of the first postoperative day, client will be out of bed with assistance.	Assess respiration. Administer pain medication as ordered. Assist client with change of position, coughing, deep breathing, and getting out of bed. *Rationale:* Client will tolerate deep breathing, coughing, and mobility if made comfortable. Teach client importance of deep breathing, coughing, and mobility. *Rationale:* Deep breathing, coughing, and early ambulation help to prevent postoperative respiratory complications.	By the end of the first postoperative day, client is performing coughing and deep breathing and is able to get out of bed with assistance.

 *Chapter Highlights*

▶ Cesarean delivery is a surgical procedure in which delivery follows an incision through the abdominal wall and the uterus.

▶ Although the cesarean rate has decreased since the early 1990s, efforts such as client and staff education, peer review, encouragement of appropriate candidates to attempt vaginal birth for future delivery, and better understanding of electronic fetal heart rate monitoring may hopefully further decrease the incidence of cesareans.

▶ Cesarean delivery is indicated whenever it is unlikely that a safe vaginal birth can take place, or whenever it is judged that a delay in delivery would jeopardize the well-being of mother, fetus, or both.

▶ Factors that can contribute to the occurrence of cesarean birth include safety of the procedure; factors related to maternal and fetal status; infections in the birth canal; previous cesarean or uterine surgery; multiple fetuses; technologic advances in obstetric care; professional concern over potential malpractice suits; client request for cesarean delivery; lack of physician experience in managing difficult deliveries; and background of the obstetric providers.

▶ Cesarean delivery can be a life-saving procedure; however, it is major abdominal surgery with drawbacks such as a higher incidence of maternal morbidity and mortality, higher costs, longer recovery, and higher risk of future cesarean delivery.

▶ Cesarean deliveries are performed using either the classic vertical incision or low-segment incision.

▶ Preoperative, intraoperative, postoperative, and postpartum care of the cesarean client combines principles of surgical and obstetric nursing and strategies that enhance a sense of control and joy in the birth experience and foster client–staff collaboration.

▶ Postdischarge teaching that focuses on assisting the mother to recover from surgery while adapting to the addition of the newborn to the family is especially important in light of the current practice of early discharge.

▶ Cesarean delivery can result in intense emotional responses within women, including relief, depression, guilt, and crisis.

▶ Nurses can help cesarean fathers have positive experiences with these deliveries through such strategies as encouraging fathers to express their feelings about the birth, providing information about options and restrictions related to cesarean birth, and offering emotional support.

▶ Cesarean deliveries should no longer be routinely performed for women simply because they had a previous cesarean delivery; many women are appropriate candidates for a safe vaginal delivery in the future.

▶ Nursing care of women attempting vaginal birth after cesarean combines strategies for family-centered low-risk labor and delivery with strategies for care of the high-risk labor and delivery client.

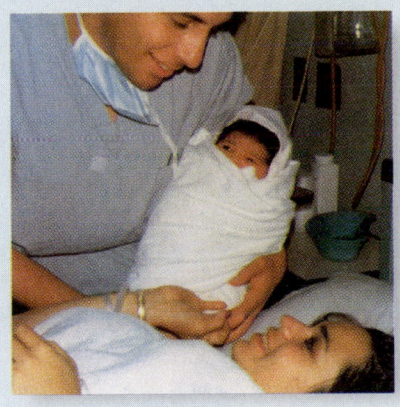

After reading the vignette at the beginning of the chapter, use what you have learned to answer these questions:

1. What reactions might David and Laura Weiss have to their unplanned cesarean delivery?

2. Which factors in this couple's experience would contribute to a positive or a negative unplanned cesarean birth?

3. What can nurses do to ensure that couples experiencing unplanned cesarean delivery have a positive experience?

Critical Thinking Questions

▶ # References

Adair, C.D., Sanchez-Ramos, I., Whitaker, D., McDyer, D.C., Farah, I., & Briones, D. (1996). Trial of labor in patients with a previous lower uterine cesarean section. *American Journal of Obstetrics and Gynecology, 174,* 966.

Albers, L.L., Anderson, D., Cragin, L., Daniels, S.M., Hunter, C., Sedler, K.D., & Teaf, D. (1997). The relationship of ambulation in labor to operative delivery. *Journal of Nurse Midwifery, 42*(1), 4–8.

American College of Obstetricians and Gynecologists. (1988). *Perinatal herpes simplex virus infections* (Technical Bulletin No. 122). Washington, DC: Author.

American College of Obstetricians and Gynecologists. (1995). *Vaginal delivery after previous cesarean birth.* Washington, DC: Author.

Association of Women's Health, Obstetric, and Neonatal Nurses. (1998). *Standards and guidelines for professional nursing practice in the care of women and newborns* (5th ed.). Washington, DC: Author.

Brooten, D., Knapp, H., Boruki, L., Jacobsen, B., Finkler, S., Arnold, L., & Mennuti. (1996). Early discharge and home care after unplanned cesarean birth: Nursing care time. *Journal of Obstetric, Gynecologic, and Neonatal Nursing, 25*(7), 595–600.

Clarke, S.C., & Taffel, S.M. (1996a). Rates of cesarean and VBAC delivery, United States, 1994. *Birth, 23*(6), 166–168.

Clarke, S.C., & Taffel, S.M. (1996b). Cesarean rates decreasing. *OB GYN News, 31,* 10.

Cowan, R.K., Kinch, R.A., Ellis, B., & Anderson, R. (1994). Trial of labor following cesarean delivery. *Obstetrics and Gynecology, 83*(6), 933–936.

Cunningham, F.G., MacDonald, P.C., Gant, N.F., Leveno, K.J., Gilstrap, L.C., Hankins, G.D.V., & Clark, S.L. (1997). *Williams obstetrics* (20th ed.). Stamford, CT: Appleton & Lange.

Curtin, S.C., & Kozak, L.J. (1997). Cesarean delivery rates in 1995 continue to decline in the United States. *Birth, 24*(3), 194–196.

de Costa, C. (1998). A sort of progress. *The Lancet, 351* (April 18), 1202–1203.

Enkin, M. (1977). Having a section is having a baby. *Birth and Family Journal, 4,* 99–104.

Evans, L.C., & Combs, C.A. (1993). Increased maternal morbidity after cesarean delivery before 28 weeks of gestation. *Internal Journal of Obstetrics and Gynecology, 40,* 227–233.

Fawcett, J., & Weiss, M.E. (1993). Cross-cultural adaptation to cesarean birth. *Western Journal of Nursing Research, 15,* 282–297.

Flamm, B.L., Goings, J.R., Liu, Y., Wolde-Tsadik, G. (1994). Elective repeat cesarean delivery versus trial of labor: A prospective multicenter study. *Obstetrics and Gynecology, 83*(6), 927–932.

Gabbe, S.G., Niebyl, J.R., & Simpson, J.L. (1996). *Obstetrics: Normal and problem pregnancies* (3rd ed.). New York: Churchill-Livingstone.

Haas, J.S., Udvarhelyi, S., & Epstein, A.M. (1993). The effect of health coverage for uninsured pregnant women on maternal health and the use of cesarean section. *Journal of the American Medical Association, 270,* 61–64.

Hale, R.W. (1994). Operative delivery. In A.H. DeCherney & M.I. Pernoll (Eds.), *Current obstetric and gynecologic diagnosis and treatment* (8th ed.) (pp. 543–573). Norwalk, CT: Appleton & Lange.

Harrington, L.C., Miller, D.A., McClain, C.J., & Paul, R.H. (1997). Vaginal birth after cesarean in a hospital-based birth center staffed by certified nurse-midwives. *Journal of Nurse-Midwifery, 42*(4), 304–307.

Hueston, W.J., & Rudy, M. (1994). Factors predicting elective repeat cesarean delivery. *Obstetrics and Gynecology, 83,* 741–744.

Johnson, S.R. (1986). Obstetric decision-making: Responses to patients who require cesarean delivery. *Obstetrics and Gynecology, 67,* 847–850.

Kline, J., & Arias, F. (1993). Analysis of factors determining the selection of repeated cesarean section or trial of labor in patients with histories of prior cesarean delivery. *Journal of Reproductive Medicine, 38,* 289–292.

Korte, D. (1998). *The expectant mother's guide to vaginal birth after cesarean.* Cambridge, MA: Harvard Common Press.

Lampman, C., & Phelps, A. (1997). College students' knowledge and attitudes about cesarean birth. *Birth, 24*(3), 159–164.

Lewin, T. (1997, April 18). Midwives deliver healthy babies with fewer interventions. *The New York Times,* p. A15.

Lindgren, K. (1996). Maternal-fetal conflict: Court-ordered cesarean section. *Journal of Obstetric, Gynecologic, and Neonatal Nursing, 25*(8), 654–656.

Martin, J.N., Jr., Perry, K.G., Jr., Robers, W.E., & Meydrech, E.F. (1997). The case for trial of labor in the patient with a prior low-segment vertical cesarean incision. *American Journal of Obstetrics and Gynecology, 177*(1), 144–148.

May, K.A., & Sollid, D.T. (1984). Unanticipated cesarean birth from the father's perspective. *Birth, 11,* 87–95.

McCurdy, C.M., Jr., Magann, E.F., McCurdy, C.J., & Saltzman, A.K. (1992). The effect of placental management at cesarean delivery on operative blood loss. *American Journal of Obstetrics and Gynecology, 167,* 1363–1367.

Miller, C.R., & Sutter, C.S. (1985). Vaginal birth after a cesarean. *Journal of Obstetric, Gynecologic, and Neonatal Nursing, 14,* 383–389.

Murray, S.F., & Pradenas, F.S. (1997). Cesarean birth trends in Chile, 1986 to 1994. *Birth, 24*(4), 258–263.

Naef, R.W. III, Ray, M.A., Chauhan, S.P., Roach, H., Blake, P.G., & Martin, J.N., Jr. (1995). Trial of labor after cesarean delivery with a lower-segment, vertical uterine incision: Is it safe? *American Journal of Obstetrics and Gynecology, 172*(6), 1666–1673.

Oxorn, H. (Ed.). (1986). *Oxorn-Foote human labor and birth* (5th ed.). Norwalk, CT: Appleton & Lange.

Paul, R.H., & Miller, D.A. (1995). Cesarean birth: How to reduce the rate. *American Journal of Obstetrics and Gynecology, 172,* 1903–1911.

Perlow, J.H., & Morgan, M.A. (1994). Massive maternal obesity and perioperative cesarean morbidity. *American Journal of Obstetrics and Gynecology, 170,* 560.

Radin, T.G., Harmon, J.S., & Hanson, D.A. (1993). Nurses' care during labor: Its effect on the cesarean birth rate of healthy, nulliparous women. *Birth, 20,* 14–21.

Reichert, J.A., Baron, M., & Fawcett, J. (1993). Changes in attitudes toward cesarean birth. *Journal of Obstetric, Gynecologic, and Neonatal Nursing, 22,* 159–167.

Roberts, S.W., Cox, S.M., Dax, J., Wenden, G.D., & Kevenko, K.J. (1995). Genital herpes during pregnancy: No lesions, no cesarean. *Obstetrics and Gynecology, 85*(2), 261–264.

Rosenblatt, R.A., Dobie, S.A., Hart, L.G., Schneeweiss, R., Gould, D., Baine, R.R., Benedetti, T.J., Pirani, M.J., & Perrin, E.D. (1997). Interspecialty differences in the obstetric care of low-risk women. *American Journal of Public Health, 87*(3), 344–350.

Sandelowski, M., Bustamante, R. (1986). Cesarean birth outside the natural childbirth culture. *Research in Nursing and Health, 9,* 81–88.

Sharma, J.B., Ekoh, S., McMillan, L., Hussain, S., & Annan, H. (1977). Blood splashes to the masks and goggles during cesarean section. *British Journal of Obstetrics and Gynecology, 104*(12), 1405–1406.

Shearer, E. (1996). Once a cesarean, always a scar. *Birth, 23*(3), 172–175.

Taffel, S.M., Placek, P.J., Moien, M., & Kosary, C.L. (1991). 1989 U.S. cesarean rate steadies—VBAC rises to nearly one in five. *Birth, 18,* 73.

U.S. Centers for Disease Control and Prevention. (1996). Births and deaths—U.S., 1995. The virtual hospital. *Morbidity and Mortality Weekly Report, 45:* 42, 9–10.

U.S. Department of Health and Human Services, Public Health Service. (1991). *Healthy people 2000: National health promotion and disease preventions objectives, full report with commentary* (DHHS Publication No. (PHS) 91-50212). Washington, DC: U.S. Government Printing Office.

Varney, H. (1997). *Varney's midwifery* (3rd ed.). Boston: Jones & Bartlett.

Woolbright, L.A. (1996). Why is the cesarean delivery rate so high in Alabama? An examination of risk factors, 1991–1993. *Birth, 23*(1), 20–25.

Zuspan, F.P., & Quilligan, E.J. (1988). *Douglas-Stromme operative obstetrics* (5th ed.). Norwalk, CT: Appleton & Lange.

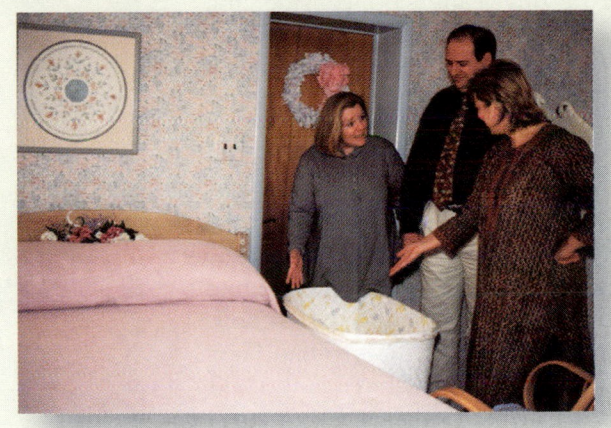

Paul and Sara Cooper are expecting their first child in 8 weeks. On the recommendation of Paul's sister, who is the mother of two children, they are visiting a birth center that is located approximately 10 miles from their house. Paul's sister gave birth to her second child at this center and, because of the positive experience that she and her family shared at this facility, she is urging Paul and Sara to consider the birth center for their delivery.

When Donna Moore, CNM, a staff member of the birth center, meets Paul and Sara and starts talking with them, she notes that, while they seem interested in learning about the care provided at the facility, they are reluctant to ask specific questions about the birthing environment and what they can expect during labor and delivery. As the nurse begins to explain the preparations involved in finalizing the birth plan and the conditions under which transfer from the birth center to an acute care hospital would be necessary, she notices that Sara is glancing nervously at Paul, who also seems uncomfortable with the information being discussed. ∎

27

Community-Based Nursing During Birth

More than twenty years ago, the ANA House of Delegates endorsed a resolution calling for a birth environment that would be physically safe, consider the psychologic well-being of the family unit, and be based on a family-centered concept of care. This resolution was, in part, an outgrowth of a prevalent trend in childbirth: that of viewing childbirth as a healthy, normal physiologic process, and not a pathologic state to be interfered with by medical intervention in a hospital environment.

The environment that best reflects this philosophy is a childbearing family's own home. Home birthing, mostly managed by nurse-midwives—both lay and certified nurse-midwives (CNMs)—had been in existence for centuries both in the United States and in Europe. However, in the early 1900s, home birth and nurse-midwives fell into disrepute due to poor care, which resulted in high maternal and infant death rates. By the mid-1930s, birth had moved into the hospital under control of the physician.

By the mid-1970s, home birth again began to be seen as one important community-based option to achieving a "natural" birth experience. While some families chose to conduct their own home birth experience, unattended by a professional, some nurse-midwives continued to do safe home deliveries. Home birth as an option, however, was threatened in the mid-1980s, when home birth practitioners were faced with the loss of insurance liability coverage for this practice. An additional problem was the lack of guidance for conduct of home births by accrediting agencies. In response, in 1989, the American College of Nurse-Midwives created the Home Birth Section of the Division of Standards and Practice to establish necessary guidelines for the conduct of home births by home birth practitioners, primarily CNMs. While insurance coverage is still a challenge for practitioners, this barrier has to some extent been resolved. Home birth still remains one community-based option for childbearing families today.

A second option for community-based birth was created by the Maternity Center Association (MCA), an organization committed to a high quality, family centered birth experience, which launched the Childbearing Center (CbC) in Manhattan in 1975. Under the guidance of Ruth Lubic, CNM, the CbC became one of the first freestanding community-based birthing centers in the country. From its inception, the CbC was developed as an alternative to hospital birth for those childbearing families who believed that the medical-hospital system of care had failed to meet their needs for personalized, health- and family-oriented services. While still not a "routine" environment for childbearing, many childbirth (also called birth) centers exist in communities today and serve a growing clientele of

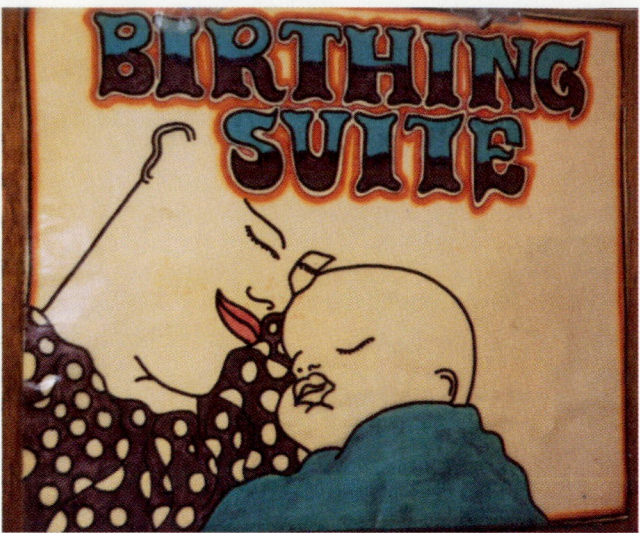

FIGURE 27–1. Entrance to a birthing suite at a childbirth center. One of the goals of the birth experience in this setting is to provide a nuturing, home-like environment for the childbearing family.

childbearing families (Fig. 27–1). Individuals managing these centers are represented by the National Association of Childbearing Centers, which assists members with standards, guidelines, continuing education, and advocacy.

This chapter discusses the historical influences on community-based birth and the issues involved in managing care in alternative birth settings. It also explores the components involved in the management of community-based birth and the safety aspects of care in both the home and in childbirth center settings. The chapter concludes with a description of the economic benefits of community-based birth settings and outlines the challenges that health care practitioners within these settings are encountering.

▶ HISTORICAL PERSPECTIVES ON COMMUNITY BIRTH

In the early 1900s, a time when virtually all births occurred in the home, the history of community-based birthing cannot be removed from the histories of public health nursing and establishment of nurse-midwifery in the United States. Of importance, the first two decades of the 20th century are also notable for the recognition of the profoundly inadequate quality of maternity care and subsequent actions taken to improve it. They are further known for the establishment of two organizations, the Children's Bureau in Washington, D.C., and the MCA in New York City. Both of these organizations have had an immense influence on the development of maternal–infant health and childbearing practices and the quality of nurse-midwifery care, both in community and hospital settings.

In 1903, Lillian Wald, a community health nurse, developed the concept of a federal Children's Bureau. President Theodore Roosevelt recommended a bill to establish such a bureau in 1909. It was not until 1912, however, that Congress passed the bill establishing the Children's Bureau. The first act of the Bureau was to conduct a study of infant deaths, which uncovered a deplorable rate of 124 infant deaths for each 1000 live births. The Bureau also noted the link between infant health and maternal health during the childbearing cycle and the importance of early and continuous prenatal care in reducing both infant and maternal mortality.

Around the same time, the New York City Health Commissioner's study of maternal and infant mortality also documented the connection between infant and maternal mortality and lack of prenatal care. From this study emerged a plan in which New York City was zoned, and a maternity center was established in each zone. The first such maternity center opened in 1917, and the MCA, a central organization of New York City maternity centers, was established in 1918. The MCA's first endeavors were development of educational materials and teaching tools for maternity practitioners and fostering the idea of prenatal care. In 1921, the concept of many regionalized maternity centers located throughout the city was dropped, and MCA became a centralized organization devoted to care of mothers and newborns in New York City throughout the childbearing cycle.

In the early 1920s the MCA and the Henry Street Visiting Nurse Association collaborated in a study that illustrated the value of specialized maternity care within a generalized public health nursing program. Subsequently, MCA began an intensive educational program in maternity care for both public and professional health personnel, especially public health nurses. Such early alliances between community nursing and maternity care foreshadowed the community-based childbearing care of today.

On the basis of their demonstration of the success in providing complete maternity care and their collaboration with the Henry Street Visiting Nurse Association, MCA concluded that nurses needed to be prepared in normal obstetrics and discussed opening a school of nurse-midwifery in the United States. Establishment of such a school was temporarily halted in the 1920s, however, due to the terrible reputation of nurse-midwives in the United States. At this time, virtually all births occurred in homes, and the primary birth practitioners were nurse-midwives (often not nurses but lay "granny" nurse-midwives). Maternal and infant deaths during birth, as demonstrated by the studies already mentioned, were a frequent occurrence. By 1930, obstetric care had moved in mass out of the home into the hospital, and laws were passed to regulate the practice of nurse-midwives. As a result of these laws, several midwifery schools were established, and formal education of nurse-midwives in the United States began. A second important factor in establishing nurse-midwifery practice as a part of the health care delivery system for childbearing families was the introduction of nurse-midwives from Europe.

▶ The Frontier Nursing Service

The first nurse-midwives to practice in community-based settings in the United States were British-trained nurse-midwives who came to this country as part of a program designed to provide health care for pregnant women and infants in rural Kentucky. At that time in Kentucky, the majority of nurse-midwifery deliveries occurred in homes located in remote communities. Nurse-midwives were brought to the United States by Mary Breckinridge, an American nurse who was also certified as a nurse-midwife in England. In 1928, the program was incorporated as the Frontier Nursing Service (FNS).

The work and record of the FNS is legendary. FNS nurse-midwives performed home births in virtually inaccessible areas of Kentucky. In 1951, statistics demonstrated that 8596 clients had been delivered by nurse-midwives since 1925, 6533 of whom were delivered in extremely primitive homes. The average maternal death rate for FNS clients during the 25 years studied was 1.2 per thousand live births, compared to a national average maternal death rate of 3.4 per thousand live births during the same period (Gabay and Wolfe, 1997). Even during these early years, it was evident that properly managed community-based birth, particularly home births, could be as safe, or safer, than hospital births.

In general, home births became a less mainstream birthing option. It was not until the mid-1970s that attention was again focused on home births. Many childbearing couples were still uncomfortable with the idea of giving birth in their home, however, but did not desire a hospital birth. Thus, the time was ripe for another alternative for giving birth in a community setting.

▶ Evolution of Childbirth Centers

The major issue that led to the development of the CbC was families' disenchantment with hospital births. A revival of interest in home birth was occurring, with some families choosing a "do-it-yourself" form of home birth. The so-called "opting-out" phenomenon, where childbearing families choose not to give birth in a hospital environment, but rather chance a potentially risky, professionally unattended birth at home, prompted MCA to develop an alternative to both hospital and home birth.

The CbC was given permanent establishment in January, 1978, by the Public Health Council of New York. It is designed as an out-of-hospital facility equipped to provide normal maternity care to carefully screened families anticipating a healthy childbearing experience. It provides a home-like environment and is minimally equipped as a hospital. However, it is not the same as a home birth. Care is provided by a team consisting of nurse-midwives, obstetricians, pediatricians, nurse-midwife assistants, public health nurses, ancillary and support personnel, and the families themselves. Full reimbursement for care is granted to clients of the CbC.

At the time of its initiation, the birth experience, including labor, delivery, and early postpartum and newborn stabilization, was managed at the CbC, with a return home in up to 12 hours. No rigid procedures were used: A mother could choose to give birth in any position she desired as long as her safety and that of the baby were ensured. Oxytocin was not used to induce or stimulate labor in the setting, nor were forceps used. The setting was most appropriate for midwifery management, but not for obstetric modalities and treatments. Risk of an obstetric emergency was an indication for transfer to the consulting or backup hospital, a necessary component of the program.

Families were encouraged to share the labor and delivery experience. Infants remained with their parents at all times. The baby was examined by a pediatrician before the family returned to their home. Home visits by nurses within 24 hours after the family left the center were usually a standard component of follow-up care. The family returned to the CbC on day 6 or 7 after delivery and during the 5th to 6th week after delivery for the postpartum check-up.

Today, many childbirth centers have their own variations of this protocol. However, the philosophy which guided the CbC remains. The CbC built its service on the following assumptions (Faison, Pisani, Douglas, Granch, & Lubic, 1979; Lubic & Ernst, 1978):

- The ultimate goal of maternity care is to provide safe, satisfying, and economic care to all childbearing families, while promoting within those families confidence in their own ability to bring forth and rear a child.
- For the majority of expectant families, childbirth is a normal physiologic experience.

- A growing segment of the American childbearing public is not content with available maternity services and is actively seeking alternatives.
- The hospital health care delivery system has failed for the most part to respond to the needs of childbearing families.
- Discontented families are ready and willing to accept the responsibilities inherent in participation in the design of their own maternity services.
- A childbirth center can serve as an alternative option acceptable to both the discontented public and concerned professionals.

On the basis of these assumptions, the CbC identified nine principles to be considered in establishing a childbirth center (Lubic & Ernst, 1978):

1. A childbirth center is an adaptation of the home, rather than a modification of the hospital.
2. A childbirth center provides safe care to healthy families anticipating a normal childbearing experience.
3. A childbirth center provides high-quality maternity care at low cost.
4. A childbirth center promotes family unity through participation of individual family members.
5. Childbirth centers are effective primary care and referral services in regionalized perinatal care programs.
6. Delineating the philosophy and nonclinical policies for a childbirth center is most effectively accomplished by a governing body responsive to the idea of birth as a normal physiologic event.
7. In order for a childbirth center to function effectively, both professionals and families must accept and respect each other's roles as members of a team.
8. Education in preparation for childbirth, infant care, parenting, and general self-help is an essential component for childbirth center operations.
9. The successful operation of a childbirth center is based upon use of CNMs, with expert physician consultation and a full range of supporting personnel and services as a backup.

Freestanding childbirth centers, while having variations and serving different populations of childbearing families, generally hold to these principles and beliefs. They constitute a major alternative to both hospital and home birth, providing, as many believe, "the best of both worlds."

► MANAGING CARE IN COMMUNITY-BASED BIRTH SETTINGS

Guidelines for managing childbearing and the birth process in both at home and in freestanding childbirth centers are similar in terms of the approach to this experience. Since almost all births in community-based settings are managed by nurse-midwives, guidelines for both settings are based on the nurse-midwifery management process. The overriding philosophy of these guidelines is that all nurse-midwives must have confidence that birth is normal and must have the ability to convey this belief to the family with reassurance and enthusiasm regardless of the setting for the birth. However, there are differences in managing childbirth in a birth center or home compared to a hospital setting. Unlike the hospital setting, which usually offers accessibility to a wide variety of procedures, equipment, resources, and personnel in the event of a sudden or acute problem, the childbirth center or home will have more limited equipment, fewer professional staff, and lack access to some specialized procedures (Jackson & Bailes, 1997). The nurse-midwife must be capable of independently stabilizing and managing clients with maternal, fetal, and newborn emergency problems and, if indicated, transporting those clients to a backup consulting hospital.

One of the most important components in managing childbearing in a community-based birth environment is the client selection process. To ensure a positive outcome, the woman and her family must not only be low risk for pregnancy, labor and delivery, postpartum, and newborn complications, but must also have other attributes that will make them good candidates for a home birth or childbirth center delivery.

► Client Criteria for Community-Based Birthing Environments

The goal of risk assessment for a community-based birth site is to select the woman and family who, by all current midwifery and medical knowledge and standards, is a low-risk client with an excellent prognosis for a normal, healthy pregnancy, delivery, and postpartum course (Jackson & Bailes, 1997). Risk assessment is an ongoing process, with a possibility of risk factors presenting during pregnancy, throughout labor, and even in the postpartum period. "Low risk" also means that the woman and family are willing to accept responsibility for self-care, have an adequate social support network for the whole childbearing cycle, have a realistic and positive expectation about natural birth, understand and agree to the criteria specific to alternative birthing (e.g., breastfeeding, preparation of participants, no medication), and have no medical or obstetric factors that would require hospitalization.

Client selection for a community-based birth setting is a complex process that includes skilled interviewing; prenatal, intrapartum, and postpartum observation and measurements; ongoing practitioner–client communication; provider judgment; and opportunities for the client to alter the risk profile by positive behaviors (Dickinson, Jackson, & Swartz, 1994). Many screening criteria used will be common to both community-based and hospital midwifery practices. There are, however, certain criteria that are unique to home and childbirth center births that assume greater significance when one of these births is considered. Specifically, in every instance, consideration should be given to the potential need for support staff and equipment that is available only in the hospital setting. Essential criteria for determining a good candidate for a community-based birthing experience include psychosocial factors, demographic factors, community practice standards, logistical factors, and medical considerations (Jackson & Bailes, 1997).

Psychosocial Factors

These factors are of paramount importance, since birth in a home or childbirth center setting occurs in an environment where the family is responsible for securing social and physical supports for pregnancy, labor, birth, and the puerperium. The woman's and family's emotional environment during the prenatal period and at the birth greatly affects labor progress, birth outcome, and postpartum health. The woman's attitude towards birth, motherhood, her body, pain, and the birth environment can all have an impact on childbearing. Similarly, the woman's partner's willingness to participate in the birth and provide support will also affect the outcome of the childbearing process.

Demographic Factors

Women and families from a great variety of socioeconomic, educational, and ethnic backgrounds seek community-based birth environments. The practitioner needs to determine whether specific demographic factors will affect the outcome of a home or childbirth center birth or the relationship between practitioner and client.

Community Practice Standards

Community practice standards may also affect eligibility for community-based birth sites. For example, there are great variations among communities, states, and regions about accepted management strategies and risk classification for conditions such as vaginal

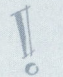

Nursing Alert

In considering candidates for the community-based birthing experience, the assessment of the family's psychosocial responses to this environment is critical. If it is determined that the woman's (or another family member's) emotional state will seriously affect either the progress and outcome of labor, communication with the labor and delivery team, or willingness to accept transfer to the consulting hospital should the need arise, then the planned birth environment should be reassessed.

birth after cesarean deliveries (VBAC), mild gestational diabetes, and prolonged rupture of membranes at term. Inclusion or exclusion of women with these conditions from a community-based birth setting depends on the individual practice guidelines of the nurse-midwives and consulting physicians, their mutual understanding or jurisdiction, and nature of their collaboration.

Logistical Factors

Specifically, for a home birth, the client and family must live within a defined service area of a hospital that has an obstetrical unit and arrangements must be made with the hospital for emergency transport in the event of complications during birth. As a standard component of its operation, a childbirth center will already have established such arrangements with a consulting hospital within an acceptable distance from the center.

Medical Considerations

In addition to the absence of medical risk factors that would classify the woman or family as a high-risk client or situation, certain other factors are routinely emphasized in determining candidacy for a community-based birth experience, such as:

- *Nutritional status.* A careful diet history of the woman at the onset of care can assist the nurse-midwife in assessing her nutritional profile. If alterations are recommended, the woman (and other family members) must demonstrate a commitment to improving the woman's diet as her pregnancy progresses.
- *Smoking.* Due to the association of smoking and complications such as low-birth-weight

infants or abruptio placentae, many nurse-midwives feel that smoking is an absolute contraindication to community-based birth environments, unless there is evidence of the woman's cessation or dramatic reduction of smoking by the second trimester.

- *Anemia.* Many midwives who practice in the home birth or childbirth center environment adhere to a standard of a specific minimum hemoglobin or hematocrit requirement that the woman must meet at term to qualify for delivery in the community setting. Adherence to a standard of 10g/dL HGB or 30% Hct can help maintain good prenatal outcomes as well as assist the woman in her postpartum recovery.
- *Medication.* Commitment to nonpharmacologic management strategies for labor pain relief is a requirement of planned home birth, and part of the philosophy for childbirth center births. The desire for pharmacologic analgesia is often considered an indication for transfer to the consulting hospital. On the other hand, the woman must be willing to accept the administration of oxytocics in the case of postpartum hemorrhage. It is usually not reasonable to wait for a transfer or even for a lengthy discussion of the benefits and need for this medication. The issue must be raised ahead of time with the woman and her family and the decision to use the oxytocic left to the judgment of the nurse-midwife.

► MANAGEMENT OF COMMUNITY-BASED BIRTHS

Community-based births—both those occurring in the home and in a childbirth center—share common management components. However, because home births occur in the family's own home, and not in an alternative facility, additional considerations are necessary. Aspects of the management program that are both common to and different in home births and childbirth center deliveries are discussed below.

► Antepartum Period

During pregnancy the woman and family are actively engaged in planning and health promotion to create the healthiest maternal and external environment in which the baby will be received and grow. Table 27–1 presents management guidelines that are observed during the antepartum period in community-based settings.

Management Guidelines for Childbirth Experiences in Community-Based Settings

Antepartum Period	Intrapartum Period	Postpartum Period	Neonatal Period
Preconception and first trimester: • Client/family exploration of birth options • Options for supporting normal pregnancy and for accessing specialized tests, care and/or resources in the event of problems (health, social, economic) • Demographics • Family history • Medical history • Nutrition, vitamin/folic acid/mineral supplementation • Accurate gestational dating • Substance use (cigarettes, alcohol, drugs, caffeine) • Infection exposure/potential and follow-up • Toxic exposure and follow-up • Pets and any necessary precautions • Domestic violence/abuse and follow-up • Genetic risks, options and follow-up • Known health risks (e.g., diabetes, hypertension) • Environmental concerns (adequate and safe housing, sanitation, heating, electricity) • Transportation options • Social supports and stresses (including economic) • Information needs (danger signs, nutrition, etc.) • Relationship expectations with providers • Maternal/fetal status • Informed consent for home or childbirth center births Second Trimester (in addition to the concerns listed above): • Client/family adaptation to pregnancy • Informational needs (premature onset of labor, fetal development, quickening, etc.) Third Trimester (in addition to the concerns listed above): • Preparation for birth and parenting • Preparation of home for birth (for home births) and parenting/infant care • Roles of woman, family members, support persons, and providers during the birth • Considerations for transfer including transportation, likely scenarios, medical and hospital back-up • Emergency provisions and action plans • Maternal/fetal status	Support normal labor and birth Monitor maternal status Monitor fetal status: • Fetal heart rate (FHR) in early labor every 30–60 minutes • FHR in active labor every 15–30 minutes and periodically listening through and for 30 seconds following a contraction • FHR in second stage of labor after each contraction or every 5 minutes Monitor emotional and relational factors that support or impede labor Assess specific problems: • Prolonged latent phase/maternal exhaustion • Fetal distress (first and second stage) • Meconium-stained amniotic fluid • Post-dates • Malpresentation of fetus • Arrest of labor or absence of progress in dilation or descent • Shoulder dystocia • Excessive bleeding during labor • Excessive bleeding after birth • Newborn distress after birth • Prolonged rupture of membranes • Signs of chorioamnionitis • Signs of pregnancy-induced hypertension • Maternal/family ambivalence about transfer to consulting hospital • Maternal/family ambivalence about staying home or in childbirth center • Effect of severe weather or natural disasters (blizzards, hurricanes, floods) on choice of birth setting • Repair of extensive or unusual lacerations Emergency provisions/action plans	Immediate monitoring of maternal status (bleeding, blood pressure, uterine involution, ability to void, etc.) Guidance about infant feeding (breastfeeding) Information needs (signs and symptoms of infections, thromboembolic phenomenon, wound care) Support systems Immediate monitoring of newborn status Maternal/paternal/sibling/infant bonding Parenting information needs Environmental hazards (second-hand smoke, etc.) Assess specific problems: • Delayed bleeding • Maternal infection • Maternal thromboembolic events • Wound breakdown • Maternal depression • Relational and social stresses • Breastfeeding problems • Impaired maternal/paternal/sibling/infant bonding Postpartum contact and follow-up for mother and baby	Normal newborn transition to extrauterine life Collection of cord blood and, if indicated, follow-up with RhoGAM administration to the mother Evaluation of breastfeeding Administration of vitamin K to the newborn Newborn eye prophylaxis Communication with the baby's long-term health care provider (family practitioner, pediatrician, pediatric nurse practitioner) Testing newborn for metabolic disorders Management of meconium-stained amniotic fluid Difficulty initiating the newborn's respirations Newborn hypoglycemia Congenital anomalies of the newborn

Source: Jackson & Bailes, 1997.

▶ Intrapartum Period

Intrapartum management in a community setting, either the home or childbirth center, requires the provider, usually the nurse-midwife, to use a wide variety of assessment and management skills that are not used as commonly in hospital settings. The nurse-midwife may be called upon to use judgment about how environments, activities, and people affect the labor's progress. He or she may determine better ways for maternal energy to be directed and may need to suggest that the mother move about in her home or the childbirth center, make changes in her behavior, and alter her interaction with others in order to achieve this objective (Fig. 27–2).

The intrapartum period poses special considerations because it is the time during which maternal or fetal status can change very quickly and require immediate, directed interventions. Consequently, for the home or childbirth center setting, the practitioner must have clear guidelines (see Table 27–1).

The most common reason for transfer from the home or childbirth center to the hospital is failure to progress in labor or maternal exhaustion. The nurse-

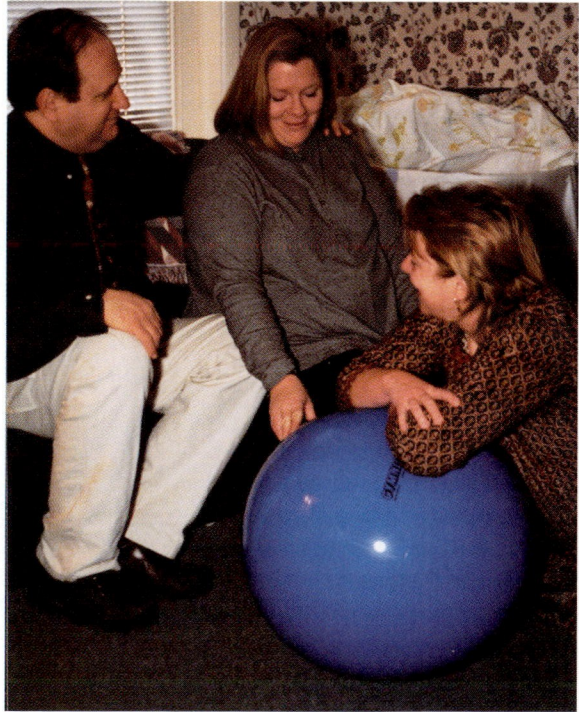

FIGURE 27–2. The staff at a childbirth center can discuss various methods, such as a birthing ball, that may help clients manage discomfort during the first stage of labor.

midwife's care during the intrapartum period may be crucial to the difference between completing a birth in a community setting or a hospital transfer.

▶ Postpartum Period

In the home or childbirth center experience, assessment and management of the postpartum period usually includes the first 3–12 hours after birth and home visits for the next few days at various intervals. Some practitioners see the woman and the new baby two or three weeks after the birth and again at six to eight weeks. Others see them only during the first few days and then at six to eight weeks. See Table 27–1 for postpartum management guidelines.

▶ Neonatal Period

Breastfeeding provides an ideal opportunity to assess the newborn's well-being. Suck and swallow reflexes, breathing patterns and general vigor can all be observed while the baby is at the breast. If the family obtains pediatric care from another provider, different guidelines apply than if the baby is followed for the first one to two months by the nurse-midwife. As in the intrapartum period, the immediate newborn period is one during which the baby's status can change quickly, and the nurse-midwife is responsible for assessment, management, and transport of the newborn if indicated (see Table 27–1).

▶ Emergency Management

Emergencies may occur during pregnancy, labor, birth, and in the immediate postpartum and neonatal periods. All nurse-midwives are taught normal birth management as well as management of certain emergency situations. In the home birth or childbirth center settings, the mother and/or neonate is transported to a hospital when it is decided that the situation requires personnel (e.g., an obstetrician or neonatologist), equipment (e.g., magnetic resonance imaging equipment), or procedures (e.g., sonogram) beyond what is available at the birthing site. The nurse-midwife will manage emergencies in different ways, depending on the interaction of many complex factors (see box entitled Factors Influencing Management of Emergencies in Community-Based Birth Settings).

► FACTORS INFLUENCING MANAGEMENT OF EMERGENCIES IN COMMUNITY-BASED BIRTH SETTINGS

SUPPORTING MEDICAL BACKUP SYSTEM

- Distance to the backup hospital
- Availability of the ambulance
- Availability of the consulting physician
- Relationship of the nurse-midwife with the consulting physician
- Prior experiences and interactions of the midwife and the consulting physician
- Attitude of the nursing and medical staff at the receiving backup hospital
- Resources available at the backup hospital
- Ability of the receiving backup hospital to perform emergency cesarean birth or other procedures

CHARACTERISTICS OF THE PARENTS

- Motivation and dedication to home or childbirth center birth
- Attitude regarding responsibility for their own health care
- Previous birth experiences
- Attitudes of other family members and social supports

- Spiritual beliefs
- Ability of the mother to push effectively and deliver
- Parity of the mother

FACTORS AFFECTING NURSE-MIDWIFERY PERFORMANCE

- Nurse-midwife's level of skill and experience with a particular emergency
- Quality of communication between parents and nurse-midwife
- Availability of supplies and backup in case of problems
- Nurse-midwife's level of fear in a particular emergency situation
- Woman's labor status
- Road conditions and weather forecast
- Mental status of the nurse-midwife (effects of conditions such as sleep deprivation and stress on performance)
- Level of competency and experience of the nurse-midwife's birth assistant

Source: Jackson & Bailes, 1997.

► Transport

Decision making about when to transport the mother or baby to the consulting backup hospital is one of the most difficult problems a nurse-midwife encounters in a community-based birth. The general rule of thumb is, if in doubt, transfer. Guidelines concerning transport include (Jackson & Bailes, 1997):

1. Maintain transport vehicle appropriately and keep the gas tank full
2. Have a well-rehearsed transport plan including map and directions to nearest hospital and consultant backup hospital if different
3. Have an extra copy of the client's chart for the hospital physician
4. Have nurse-midwife accompany the client to the hospital and stay if at all possible
5. Include on the transfer chart: time of decision to transfer; mode of transfer; time of departure from home or childbirth center; time of arrival at hospital; time interventions were implemented

► Education

In addition to the antepartal, birth, postpartum, and neonatal management program, both childbirth centers and home birth practitioners generally have a

specific educational component to their care of the family. Commonly included aspects of education offered by community-based birthing settings include (Garite, Snell, Walker, & Darrow, 1995):

- *Childbirth education.* Physical aspects of pregnancy; body care including exercises and breathing techniques (some midwives or staff at childbirth centers also offer childbirth preparation classes); and psychologic aspects of pregnancy, including such issues as feelings related to hormonal changes, psychologic preparation for birth, and new roles of family members in the postpartum period.
- *Nutrition.* Nutrition in the prenatal and postpartum periods (including home care for lactation and newborns) and general family health.
- *Parenting.* Care of newborns, sibling rivalry.

► SAFETY ISSUES INVOLVING COMMUNITY-BASED BIRTH SETTINGS

One of the main concerns relating to alternative birth settings in the community is the safety of such settings for mother and baby. Both professionals and families remember the days when birth in a community setting, especially at home, was a risky business. The safety of both home and childbirth center settings for mothers and infants has been demonstrated by numerous studies. This achievement can be attributed to the safety record of CNM deliveries, which also have been extensively documented. This section briefly reviews studies concerning both certified nurse-midwifery practice and the safety record of home and childbirth center deliveries.

► Safety of Nurse-Midwife Deliveries

Research documents that nurse-midwife-managed care for childbearing families results in similar or reduced rates of medical interventions, similar outcomes (in terms of infant and maternal mortality and morbidity), similar numbers of complications for mother and baby, and greater satisfaction with care when compared with physician-managed care (Gabay & Wolfe, 1997; Turnbull et al., 1996). Compared to physician-managed care, midwifery care is associated with a lower incidence of cesarean delivery (Butler, Abrams, Parker, Roberts & Laros, 1996), fewer operative deliveries and episiotomies, and less use of epidural anesthesia (Chambliss et al., 1992).

As early as 1986, the U.S. Congress's Office of Technology Assessment issued a report reviewing the evidence on the quality and costs of care provided by CNMs, and concluded that ". . . within their areas of competence . . . CNMs provide care whose quality is equivalent to that of care provided by physicians. Moreover . . . CNMs are more adept than physicians at providing services that depend on communication with patients and preventive actions" (U.S. Congress, Office of Technology Assessment, 1986). These findings are echoed in a study initiated in 1991 and funded by the Robert Wood Johnson Foundation, which demonstrated the major contribution by CNMs across the nation to the health care of women and infants from vulnerable populations (American College of Nurse-Midwives, 1994). While nurse-midwives still practice primarily in hospitals, approximately 20% of their births occur in a community setting (12% in childbirth centers, 8% in home births) (American College of Nurse-Midwives, 1994). It is clear that management of childbearing by CNMs, in all settings, is a safe (and even superior in some circumstances) option for giving birth.

► Safety of Home Birth Deliveries

Safety has been the focus of research on home births since 1970. Unfortunately, much research has been retrospective in nature, relying on information recorded on birth certificates. Because of the retrospective nature of the research, it has been impossible for researchers to discriminate planned home births from unplanned home births (that is, births occurring in a home setting by accident) or to determine the type of birth attendant (i.e., CNM, lay or "granny" nurse-midwife, or other person). As one would expect, given this great variability of birthing conditions, study results have been mixed. For example, some findings indicate that nurse-midwife-managed out-of-hospital births produced fewer low-birth-weight infants, better Apgar scores, while other findings indicate higher perinatal mortality rates in out-of-hospital births. In general, when such variables as congenital anomalies, unplanned home births, and birth attendants other than CNMs were excluded from the data analysis, morbidity and mortality outcomes from studies were comparable to those rates found in similar hospital populations (Jackson & Bailes, 1997). Additional studies, also controlling for these variables and comparing home births with hospital births, have also found similar or lower mortality and morbidity rates, as well as lower rates of complications and obstetrical interventions such as forceps deliveries (Durand, 1992; Mehl-Madrona & Madrona, 1997). These studies underscore the safety of home births when appropriate prenatal screening is done and higher risk pregnancies are directed to the hospital for labor and birth.

Because of the limitation of some of these studies, nurse-midwives and other professionals interested in home birth have made research in this area a priority. Several ongoing studies in this area are using better controlled designs to overcome earlier difficulties. One such study is a prospective study of CNM-attended home births originating at Columbia University School of Nursing in New York City. A second study, using both prospective and retrospective data collection techniques, is being conducted by the Midwives Alliance of North America. These studies should produce additional data concerning the safety of CNM-attended, well-managed home births (Jackson & Bailes, 1997).

► Safety of Childbearing Center Deliveries

The late 1970s saw the beginning of the alternative birthing option, the childbirth center. By 1982, an expert committee of the Institute of Medicine (IOM) and the National Research Council addressed the controversy surrounding the increase in community-based births. The committee concluded that reliable information about the safety and efficacy of different birth settings, as well as psychologic and cost issues, was lacking (Institute of Medicine and National Research Council, 1982). It recommended that high priority be given to research to document the safety and efficacy of such alternative birth settings. Acting on these recommendations, the National Association of Childbearing Centers conducted a multicenter, prospective, and descriptive study of more than 17,000 women seeking care in freestanding childbirth centers. The investigators concluded that ". . . few innovations in health service promise lower cost, greater availability, and a high degree of satisfaction with a comparable degree of safety" (Rooks, Weatherby, Ernst, Stapleton, & Rosenfeld, 1989). These results suggest that modern childbirth centers can identify women who are at low risk for obstetrical complications and can care for them in a way that provides these benefits.

Other studies have also supported the findings of the multicenter study. In a meta-analysis comparing modern childbirth centers with hospital and physician-attended births in terms of safety, rates of complications, number of invasive procedures, cost effectiveness, and client satisfaction, one investigator found that comprehensive data clearly demonstrated that childbearing centers are as safe as hospitals for low-risk births, do fewer invasive procedures and cesarean deliveries, are less expensive, and have high rates of client satisfaction. In addition, childbearing centers effectively shift control of the pregnancy from physician to mother. The investigator concluded that, for low-risk pregnancies, childbirth centers offer many advantages over conventional hospital-based births without compromising the safety of the mother or infant. The investigator also pointed to the possibilities for childbirth centers to provide excellent care to poor and minority mothers, thus helping to solve issues of access to safe care for these populations (Spitzer, 1995). While the establishment of childbirth centers was largely the result of the interest of middle-class women in a natural birth experience, several projects have already demonstrated the efficacy of childbirth centers in delivering care to poor or minority women (Dickinson et al., 1994; Garite et al., 1995). There is little doubt that freestanding childbirth centers, staffed by CNMs, provide an excellent community-based alternative to hospital births.

► COST-EFFECTIVENESS OF COMMUNITY-BASED BIRTH OPTIONS

Studies of childbirth centers often focus not only on safety, but also on cost of giving birth in such a facility as opposed to a hospital. Multiple studies over the years support claims of the economic benefits of childbirth centers. One study, conducted by Blue Cross/Blue Shield during 1976 and 1977, showed that childbirth centers provide services at about half the cost of hospitals. A survey of 46 childbirth centers in 1982 found that center charges amounted to 47.7% of the amount charged by hospitals in the same communities for comparably low-risk births. The Health Insurance Association of America found in 1989 that childbirth center care, including prenatal, delivery and postnatal care, education and home visits, cost, on average, half of the cost for prenatal care and hospital delivery (Spitzer, 1995).

Cost-effectiveness and quality of care analyses of the services provided by both childbirth centers and nurse-midwives in home birth settings are in progress. Based on the studies that have already been conducted in this area, ongoing and future analyses will continue to demonstrate the benefits of community-based birth settings for low-risk childbearing families.

► COMMUNITY-BASED BIRTH AND MANAGED CARE: CHALLENGES FOR THE FUTURE

It is still too early to know the eventual outcomes of transition from fee-for-service payment to the prepayment plans found in managed care arrangements (see Chapter 1). However, one thing is clear: In managed care and capitation arrangements, it is more profitable for providers to keep people well and use the talents of the work force efficiently. A focus on keeping childbearing families healthy has always been part of the philosophy underlying midwifery and childbirth center care. This philosophy should allow providers to focus on preventive care rather than on the more usual focus on the treatment of disease that is common in the fee-for-service model of care delivery. One of the driving forces of managed care is cost containment, combined with access to care and quality of services. Whatever changes occur, childbirth centers and midwifery care in home births will be well positioned for this change.

Several challenges remain for nurse-midwives who practice home births and in community-based childbirth centers. Although such alternatives as childbirth centers and home births may be well suited for managed care arrangements, there is the danger that they may lose those aspects that made them excellent models of care for childbearing families.

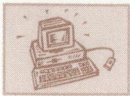

Community-Based Birth Options: An Analysis of the Cost-Effectiveness of Childbirth Centers

Freestanding community birth centers are a relatively new phenomenon. Increasingly, women are choosing fewer interventions in childbirth, such as the approach used at childbirth centers. However, there is opposition in many arenas to birth centers as an alternative to hospital care. Insurance providers claim that the childbirth center is a duplication of services already provided in the hospital, therefore increasing costs without providing economic benefits. Further, if a woman needs to be transferred out of the birth center to the hospital for any reason, there would be a further increase in costs. This study was a decision analysis of the cost-effectiveness of giving birth in a childbirth center as opposed to a hospital environment. It answered the following questions: (1) Is the birth center a cost-effective choice for delivering a baby? (2) Below what percentage of transfers to the hospital is optimal to make the birth center an economical choice with the current charges? (3) What costs would need to be accrued by admitting a woman to the birth center and then transferring her to the hospital to make the birth center an uneconomical choice?

Decision analysis is a quantitative approach that has been successfully used in medicine and nursing to reduce uncertainty in clinical management and assessing complex client problems. As a tool to assess cost-effectiveness of alternative strategies of care, decision analysis has been proven to be an objective approach for the economic evaluation of alternative health care programs. It includes the following steps: formulating the decision problem; identifying the decision alternatives; identifying the possible clinical outcomes of each decision alternative and representing the events leading to these outcomes with a series of chance and decision points; measuring the outcomes; and assigning probabilities and calculating the expected value of each decision alternative. A computer-generated, decision tree format was used to model this cost-effectiveness analysis study. Costs, defined here as the economic impact of charges to the insurer and/or client, of different alternatives for delivery of health care fall into two categories: Direct costs are the costs directly related to the care, such as cost of interventions, and indirect costs are costs not directly related, such as fixed equipment or cost of education of clinicians. Field research, in the form of interviews with such individuals as financial managers, was conducted to collect data on the costs of the alternatives. In addition, quality outcomes and utility outcomes (the appropriateness of the place of birth with regard to the clinical outcome) were also measured.

The results of this analysis suggest that a birth center is a cost-effective strategy for labor and delivery of low-risk women. The effectiveness or appropriateness of setting for the average low-risk birth was greater in the birth center than at the hospital. On the average the hospital was 38% more expensive than the birth center. The hospital further offered a less appropriate model of care for low-risk birth, thus verifying the quality of this alternative. In addition, it was not until the transfer rate became greater than 62% that the birth center stopped being the most cost-effective setting for low-risk women to give birth.

The investigators conclude that, although careful assessment with attention to possible transfer is appropriate for all women considering delivering in a birth center, the birth center should be considered a cost-effective model of care for most low-risk women. Findings of this analysis indicate that insurers and health policy decision makers should view a birth center as an economical and high-quality model of health care delivery.

Application to Practice

While this is not research in the traditional sense, this type of study, focusing on cost analysis of alternative treatment forms, will likely become a predominant form of research in the health care field. Data, such as that uncovered by this study, will be necessary to ensure high-quality, cost-effective models of care in an era of managed care. Nurses and other health care professionals need to become familiar with techniques such as decision analysis for inclusion in outcome and intervention studies.

Source: Stone, P., & Walker, P.H. (1995). Cost-effectiveness analysis: Birth center vs. hospital care. Nursing Economics, 13*(5), 299–308.*

Specifically, those responsible for childbirth centers and home births must (Dickinson et al., 1994):

- Maintain the philosophy of personalized, individualized, culturally sensitive, family-centered and safe care for mother and infant
- Maintain low staff-client ratios
- Maintain the integrity of informed consent despite algorithms or clinical pathways
- Maintain a low use of unnecessary technology, using only that which is appropriate to the needs of low-risk mothers and newborns

While managed care, with its focus on health promotion and illness prevention, is a "natural" for community-based birthing, managed care has a downside. The cost-containment aspects of managed care most often seems to be the predominant concern of care delivery under this model. Childbirth centers and home births may easily fall into the trap of putting cost containment first. Dickinson and colleagues (1994) warn that, as childbirth centers become more popular to payors because of their improved cost-efficiency, it is important for staff to maintain a philosophy of care based on the tenets detailed by Ruth Lubic and the MCA in its first endeavor, the CbC. This philosophy of family-centered care is also essential for nurse-midwives conducting home births.

Chapter Highlights

- Historically, home births and childbirth centers have evolved into important community-based options for giving birth and as alternatives to hospital births.

- Both home births and childbirth center births are most often managed by certified nurse-midwives and share a philosophy of family-centered care.

- To ensure a safe birthing experience within community-based settings, candidates should be low-risk clients with excellent prognoses for healthy pregnancy, delivery, and postpartum courses.

- Management of home and childbirth center births share many common components that are inherent in a nurse-midwife-managed birth.

- Transport to a backup or consulting hospital and/or physician is essential when risk status changes or if equipment, procedures, or personnel not present in the center or home during the birth become necessary.

- Factors that influence management of emergencies in community-based birth settings include elements of the medical backup system, characteristics of the childbearing family, and components of nurse-midwifery performance.

- Research has consistently demonstrated that, with appropriate client screening for low-risk clients and nurse-midwifery management, both home births and childbirth center births are not only as safe as hospital births, but that they also provide many advantages not offered by hospital births.

- Childbirth center births have been shown to be highly cost effective, even when considering the possibility of transfer to a consulting hospital.

- While cost-effectiveness will continue to make community-based birth options attractive in a managed care environment, it is important for practitioners to remember the philosophy that established such options as alternatives to the hospital—the philosophy of family-centered care.

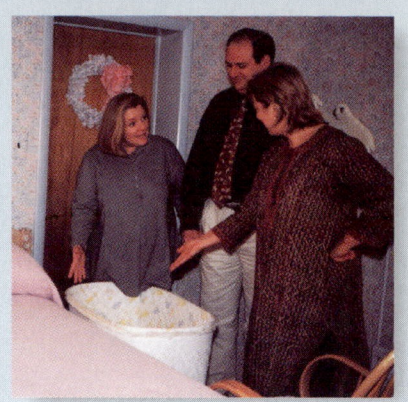

After reading the vignette at the beginning of this chapter, use what you have learned to answer these questions.

1. As the nurse responsible for managing the care of this couple, what actions would you take to promote Paul and Sara Cooper's knowledge of and comfort with their options in choosing a birthing facility?

2. How would Donna Moore's advanced preparation as a CNM enable her to anticipate the Cooper's apprehension about their choice of a birthing facility and design strategies that will resolve their concerns about this experience?

3. In what ways do the trends toward consumer involvement in childbearing care and family-centered maternity care complement one another in the situation of Paul and Sara Cooper?

Critical Thinking Questions

► References

American College of Nurse-Midwives. (1994). *Nurse-midwives: Quality care for women and newborns.* Washington, DC: Author.

Butler, J., Abrams, B., Parker, J., Roberts, J., & Laros, R. (1993). Supportive nurse-midwife care is associated with a reduced incidence of cesarean section. *American Journal of Obstetrics and Gynecology, 80,* 161–165.

Chambliss, L.R., Daly, C., Medearis, A.L., Ames, M., Kayne, M., & Paul, R. (1992). The role of selection bias in comparing cesarean birth rates between physician and midwifery management. *Obstetrics and Gynecology, 80*(2), 161–165.

Dickinson C., Jackson, D., & Swartz, W. (1994). Making the alternative mainstream: Maintaining a family-centered focus in a large freestanding birth center for low-income women. *Journal of Nurse Midwifery, 39*(2), 112–118.

Durand, M.A. (1992). The safety of homebirth: The farm study. *American Journal of Public Health, 8,* 450–453.

Faison, J., Pisani, B., Douglas, R., Granch, G., & Lubic, R. (1979). The Childbearing Center: An alternative birth setting. *Obstetrics and Gynecology, 54*(4), 527–532.

Gabay, M., & Wolfe, S. (1997). Nurse-midwifery: The beneficial alternative. *Public Health Reports, 112,* 386–394.

Garite, T., Snell, B., Walker, D., & Darrow, V. (1995). Development and experience of a university-based freestanding birth center. *Obstetrics and Gynecology, 86*(3), 411–416.

Institute of Medicine and National Research Council. (1982). *Research issues in the assessment of birth settings.* Washington, DC: National Academy Press.

Jackson M., & Bailes, A. (Eds.). (1997). *Home birth practice.* Washington, DC: American College of Nurse Midwives.

Lubic, R.W., & Ernst, E.K. (1978). The Childbearing Center: An alternative to conventional care. *Nursing Outlook, 26*(12), 754–760.

Mehl-Madrona, L., & Madrona, M.M. (1997). Physician and midwifery-attended homebirth effects of breech, twin, and post date: Outcome data on mortality rates. *Journal of Nurse-Midwifery, 42*(2), 91–103.

Rooks, J. Weatherby M., Ernst, E., Stapleton, S., & Rosenfeld A. (1989). Outcomes of care in birth centers: The National Birth Center Study. *New England Journal of Medicine, 321,* 1804–1811.

Spitzer, M. (1995). Birth Centers: Economy, safety, and empowerment. *Journal of Nurse-Midwifery, 40*(4), 371–375.

Stone, P., & Walker, P.H. (1995). Cost-effective analysis: Birth center vs. hospital care. *Nursing Economics, 13*(5), 299–308.

Turnbull, D., Holmes, A., Shields, N., Cheyne, H., Twaddle, S., Gilmour, W.H., McGinley, M., Reid, M., Johnstone, I., Geer, I., McIlwaine, G., & Lunan, C.B. (1996). Randomized, controlled trial of efficacy of midwife-managed care. *Lancet, 348,* 213–218.

U.S. Congress, Office of Technology Assessment. (1986). *Nurse practitioners, physician assistants, and certified nurse-midwives: A policy analysis* (Report No. ota-hcs-37). Washington, DC: U.S. Government Printing Office.

V

The Postpartum Period

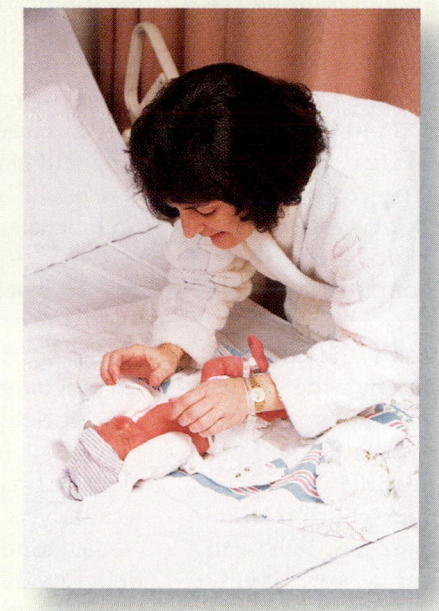

Deborah and Adam Bergman's daughter Jessica was born 6 hours ago after an uncomplicated vaginal delivery. Deborah, Adam, and their 3-year-old son Neil have been together since shortly after Jessica's birth and arranged to have Jessica stay with Deborah in her hospital room for most of their hospitalization. Adam suggests to Neil that they buy a gift for the baby, and father and son set off happily in their search.

Barbara Carson, RN, asks Deborah if she would like help with Jessica's care. Deborah smiles and states, "Thank you. I'd appreciate your being with me. I think I'm fine, but it's been 3 years since I changed a newborn's diaper." As she unwraps the blanket around Jessica, Deborah whispers softly to her daughter and strokes her arms. She states, "In some ways, she looks exactly like Neil when he was born, but in others, she's completely different. I even think she resembles my mother, especially in the shape of her mouth." ∎

28

Care of the Postpartum Family

Traditionally, the first 6 weeks following birth has been referred to as the **puerperium,** or postpartum, a time when the woman's body undergoes multiple physiologic changes in response to childbirth. Health care professionals, however, have come to believe that the period after giving birth is also a time for psychologic restoration and a time when parents develop a relationship with their infant (Ferketich & Mercer, 1995; Imle & Drayden, 1996; Mercer & Ferketich, 1990). As a result, many health care professionals view the first 6 to 8 weeks after birth as the **postpartum period;** some label the first 3 months following birth "the fourth trimester."

The postpartum period is not only the culmination of pregnancy, labor, and birth, but the beginning of the childrearing phase of the family life cycle. Structural and functional changes in the family system initiate patterns for healthy or altered family functioning, including parent–child interaction (Mercer & Ferketich, 1990; Thompson, 1997; van den Boom, 1997). The addition of a new family member may be highly stressful to the family and its members. Despite the stresses, the postpartum period is generally a time of family health and well-being.

This chapter first discusses the physiologic, psychologic, and sociocultural changes that occur within the woman and her family during the postpartum period. It then presents the assessment components that form the data base for individual clients. The chapter concludes with a description of the strategies that nurses can employ in caring for the postpartum family.

► PHYSIOLOGIC CHANGES DURING THE POSTPARTUM PERIOD

The physiologic changes that occur in the woman during the postpartum period occur in almost all of the major body systems, with the most dramatic alterations taking place during the first few days after delivery.

► Reproductive System

The return of the reproductive system to approximately its prepregnancy size and function is termed **involution.** The process takes about 6 weeks, with the exception of resumption of menses and ovulation. The most rapid changes of the reproductive system occur immediately after birth and within the first 3 to 4 days.

Uterus

Immediately after expulsion of the placenta, the uterine fundus, now firmly contracted, assumes a position approximately midway between the umbilicus and symphysis pubis. The uterine walls, now paled as a result of compression of blood vessels, are thickened and in close proximity compared with the previous pregnant state.

By 12 hours postpartum, the fundus rises to the umbilicus or slightly above. Thereafter, the uterine fundus descends 1 to 2 cm, or one fingerbreath, per day, so that by the 10th day after delivery the fundus may no longer be palpated in the abdomen. By 6 weeks postpartum, the uterus has assumed nearly its prepregnancy size and shape.

At delivery the uterus weighs approximately 2.2 pounds or 1 kg. By 6 weeks after delivery it weighs 60 to 100 g because of a reduction in uterine cell size due to autolysis of protein.

Uterine ligaments are stretched and loose after delivery, and thus their ability to support the uterus is diminished. In particular, a full bladder's ability to displace the uterus is aided by the nonsupportive uterine ligaments. As uterine involution progresses, the ligaments regain tone.

Endometrium. With the delivery of the placenta and membranes, the underlying decidua, irregular in thickness and appearance, is filled with blood. At the placental site, the tissue is raised and jagged and contains numerous thrombosed blood vessels.

During the first few days after delivery, the spongy layer of the decidua is discarded as a discharge called **lochia.** By 2 to 3 days, the basal layer of the decidua differentiates into two layers: (1) a superficial layer that, becoming necrotic, is cast off as lochia, and (2) a new basal layer adjacent to the myometrium that contains endometrial gland fundi and connective tissue, the precursors for the new endometrium. Regeneration of the endometrial tissue from the neoplacental decidua is achieved by proliferative and mitotic activity of the endometrial gland fundi and connective tissue. Within 7 to 10 days, epithelium lines the uterine cavity except at the placental site; by 3 weeks the endometrial tissue is restored (Cunningham et al., 1997).

In the initial postpartum, the uterine lochia is categorized according to color and content. During the first 2 to 3 days the lochia contains primarily decidual tissue, epithelial cells, red blood cells, white blood cells, some meconium, vernix caseosa, and lanugo; it is termed **lochia rubra** because it is red. By approximately the third day, **lochia serosa** is present, a pale serosanguinous discharge containing decidua, red blood cells, white blood cells, bacteria, and cervical mucus. Lochia serosa may continue until the 10th day after delivery and is followed by **lochia alba,** a creamy yellow discharge, which gradually ceases. Lochia alba is primarily composed of white blood cells, bacteria, some decidual cells, epithelial cells, fat, cervical mucus, and cholesterol. In general, by the time the cervix is fully closed at 2 to 3 weeks after delivery, the lochia has just about ceased. Lochia that persists past the third or fourth week following delivery warrants medical evaluation.

In the first hour postpartum, as much as 120 mL of lochia may be discharged with complete cardiovascular tolerance. Even the loss of 500 mL of blood after completion of the third stage of labor may be tolerated, although this amount was traditionally classified as postpartum hemorrhage. In general, a large peripad holds 60 to 100 mL of lochia when saturated. The primary health care provider is notified if more than one or two pads are saturated during the first hour postpartum or one pad within 15 minutes.

After the first hour postpartum, the volume of lochia discharged gradually decreases. The total discharged averages 255 mL.

A greater amount of lochia is discharged when the woman is upright after long periods in a recumbent position. Lochia tends to pool within the uterus and vagina during inactivity. Accordingly, many women note an increase in lochia in the morning, after resting during the night. Similarly, women may note the passage of small blood clots after periods of rest and concurrent pooling of blood. As long as the small clots are free of placental tissue, they are harmless. Retained placental tissue can produce large clots and hemorrhage. Persistent lochia or resumption of lochia rubra may indicate subinvolution (failure of the uterus to return to its normal size) and postpartum infection. Foul-smelling lochia may result from uterine infection. A sudden increase in physical activity in the early postpartum can increase uterine bleeding.

Placental Site. At the placental site, as necrotic tissue is sloughed off, endometrial restoration begins at the margins by extension and downward growth of tissue, as well as by proliferation of the endometrial fundi and connective tissue. This process, termed **exfoliation,** is thought to prevent the formation of scar tissue. Through exfoliation, the placental site decreases in size so that within 14 days its diameter is approximately 3 to 4 cm, and by 42 days complete involution has occurred (Cunningham et al., 1997).

Lower Uterine Segment and Cervix. After delivery, the lower uterine segment is thin and flabby and readily collapses. The muscle, however, contracts and retracts so that by 4 to 6 weeks postpartum the lower segment is identifiable as the uterine isthmus.

The cervix, also flabby, thin, and collapsed after delivery, gradually contracts so that by 2 days postpartum, it is dilated 2 to 3 cm. By the 7th day postpartum, the cervix is nearly closed and thick.

During delivery the external os is often lacerated and may be discernible later as depressions on the cervix. As the cervix involutes, the external os never regains its original oval shape, but rather is identified as a wider, transverse slit with extensions (see Fig. 6–14). Unilateral and untreated lacerations of the cervix, like those of the vagina, can be the cause of prolonged continuous bleeding in the presence of a firmly contracted uterus.

Ovulation and Menstruation. Although ovulation and menstruation may occur by 6 to 8 weeks postpartum, considerable variation exists (AWHONN/Johnson & Johnson Consumer Products, Inc., 1996). Resumption of ovulation and menstruation differs between lactating and nonlactating women, and even within these two groups of women there are variations.

In nonlactating women, menstrual flow resumes in 6 to 8 weeks for 40–45% and in 12 weeks for 65–70% (Bowes, 1996). In a study by Campbell and Gray (1993), 100% of the nonlactating women menstruated by 12 weeks. Almost all nonlactating women are menstruating by 6 months postpartum. Fifty to 60% of nonlactating women have an anovulatory menstrual flow for the first cycle. The average time for resumption of ovulation in nonlactating women is approximately 10 weeks after delivery (Resnik, 1994); however, an average of 7 weeks was reported in a small sample of nonlactating, American women (Campbell & Gray, 1993).

Lactating women often experience postpartum amenorrhea for a longer period. One plausible explanation is that the prolactin level, which is elevated during the initiation of lactation, inhibits follicular development, resulting in a failure of the ovaries to respond to gonadotropins. By 12 weeks postpartum up to 45% of lactating women may report menstruation. However, Campbell and Gray (1993) found only 20% of the lactating women menstruated by 12 weeks and, in fact, the time of their first ovulation averaged 189 days with a range of 34 to 256 days. In general, postpartum amenorrhea in lactating women ranges from 6 weeks to more than 2 years. This wide range is highly dependent on whether the woman breastfeeds continuously or breastfeeds with supplements.

Vagina and Vaginal Orifice
The vagina, vaginal outlet, and labia surrounding the outlet are stretched during delivery; rugae are

obliterated. Gradually the vagina regains shape and tone. Although rugae reappear by 3 weeks postpartum, the increase in tone and reduction in size of the vagina and vaginal outlet generally require at least 6 weeks. Once the lochia has stopped, the vagina is dry, especially in the lactating woman. Vaginal lacerations are suspected if profuse bleeding occurs despite a firmly contracted fundus. The labia become progressively less flabby, but generally do not regain the nonparous tone.

Occasionally postpartum women develop vulvar and vaginal hematomas, that is, masses that form when blood seeps into connective tissue beneath the vulvar skin and vaginal mucosa. Vulvovaginal hematomas can occur with forceps or vacuum extraction, with spontaneous vaginal delivery, and secondary to the episiotomy repair (Zahn, Hankins, & Yeomans, 1996).

During delivery of the baby, the hymen is lacerated. The lacerated edges of the hymen heal as separate tags called carunculae myrtiformes.

Perineum

The perineal body is the tissue that lies between the vaginal introitus and the anus. Because the anus is often affected by a vaginal delivery, discussion of the perineum includes content related to the anus.

During the puerperium, the perineum and anus are often uncomfortable for women who have delivered vaginally. The perineum is often edematous and ecchymotic. Perineal lacerations and episiotomies may extend into the anus and cause puerperal discomfort. The edges of the episiotomy and repaired lacerations should be approximated with sutures intact during the early postpartum. Generally, dissolvable suture is used. Within 1 to 2 weeks some women find pieces of suture on their peripad. The presence of hemorrhoids adjacent to the perineal body may heighten discomfort.

Within a week perineal and anal discomfort begins to diminish, and perineal edema and bruising may resolve. The episiotomy and lacerations usually heal within 2 to 3 weeks.

Breasts

Several changes occur in the breasts to prepare them for lactation during the postpartum period. (See Chapter 31.)

► Cardiovascular System

The cardiovascular system is greatly altered during pregnancy to meet the demands of gestation, labor, and delivery. During the postpartum, the cardiovascular system gradually resumes a nonpregnant state.

With delivery of the baby, the diaphragm is no longer pushed upward against the heart by the uterus and abdominal contents. Consequently, the heart is no longer displaced to the left and upward.

Cardiac Output, Pulse, and Blood Pressure

The increase in cardiac output, induced by pregnancy and the first and second stages of labor, begins to resolve shortly after delivery. Reflecting the diminished cardiac output, women experience bradycardia (as low as 50–70 beats per minute) for the first 6 to 10 days after delivery. Conversely, a rapid pulse rate can indicate postpartum hemorrhage, anxiety, fatigue, infection, fever, or cardiac disease.

The postpartum blood pressure should fall within the normal adult range. Increased blood pressure suggests pregnancy-induced hypertension. Decreased blood pressure suggests uterine hemorrhage, orthostatic hypotension, or a physiologic response to diminished intrapelvic pressure.

The belief that cardiovascular parameters return to prepregnant values by 6 weeks postpartum has been challenged by researchers. Capeless and Clapp (1991) found that at 12 weeks postpartum systemic vascular resistance remained decreased while stroke volume and end-diastolic volume were increased over prepregnant values. The researchers note that in previous studies baseline cardiovascular measurements were not obtained before pregnancy but rather pregnant and postpartum values were compared.

Blood Volume and Concentration

By the third week postpartum, total blood volume normally decreases from the prenatal level of 5–6 L to the nonpregnant level of 4 L (Novy, 1994). One third of the decrease takes place during delivery and soon after, and a similar amount is lost by the first week. The amount of blood lost during delivery generally determines the hemoglobin and hematocrit in the postpartum period (Novy, 1994).

During labor, erythropoiesis increases, and if accompanied by dehydration, the hemoglobin and hematocrit also increase. Erythropoietin levels may remain elevated during the first week after delivery (Novy, 1994). As fluids are replaced and fluid volume stabilizes, erythropoiesis, hematocrit, and hemoglobin decrease (Cunningham et al., 1997; Novy, 1994); by 4 days postpartum these values have stabilized (Richter, Huch, & Huch, 1995). Postpartum erythrocyte, hematocrit, and hemoglobin values much below prelabor or early-labor levels indicate that the woman has sustained a significant blood loss. Hemoglobin levels on the second postpartum day best predict hemoglobin concentration by 6 weeks postpartum. Generally, for each 450–500 mL of blood lost, the hemoglobin will decrease 1–1.5 g/dL and the hematocrit will decrease 2–4% (Grohar, 1996). Women who received intravenous solutions during labor, however, can have significantly reduced hemoglobin concentration in the first 4 days postpartum.

Leukocytes are markedly elevated in the early postpartum. Levels as high as 25,000 mm, without an infection, have been reported although the average is 14,000 to 16,000 mm (Cunningham et al., 1997; Novy, 1994). Although postpartum leukocytosis is common, an increase of more than 30% over 6 hours suggests infection (AWHONN/Johnson & Johnson Consumer Products, Inc., 1996).

Blood Loss

Blood loss during vaginal delivery of a single infant and in the first 24 hours postpartum amounts to approximately 500 to 600 mL. Approximately 930 to 1000 mL of blood are lost with the delivery of twins or in a cesarean delivery (Akins, 1994). Traditionally, a blood loss of more than 500 mL in the first 24 hours after delivery has been labeled postpartum hemorrhage; however, women can tolerate without adverse effects the loss of most of the blood added to the circulation during pregnancy (Cunningham et al., 1997). Consequently, many health care professionals now consider that an estimated blood loss greater than 500 mL is a warning that hemorrhage may be imminent; mild postpartum hemorrhage is considered a blood loss of 750 to 1250 mL. Women are at greatest risk of postpartum hemorrhage within the first 24 hours of delivery; however, late postpartum hemorrhage may occur during the 7th to 10th days after delivery when blood coagulation factors reach low levels.

Blood Coagulation

Clotting factors that increased during pregnancy tend to remain elevated during the initial postpartum period. In addition, the level of protein C, a main coagulation inhibitor, decreases slightly after delivery. By 3 to 5 days postpartum, protein C levels increase as compared with predelivery levels. Nonpregnant individuals with an inherited protein C deficiency frequently develop venous thromboembolic disorders (Sipes & Weiner, 1992). Persistent elevation in clotting factors, the low level of protein C, diminished activity, infection, and injury predispose a woman to pulmonary embolism and thromboembolism in the lower extremities.

Varicosities and Edema

Lower extremity varicosities that developed during pregnancy because of increased blood volume and dependent venous stasis are less severe shortly after delivery. Edema of the extremities, as well as of other parts of the body, diminishes. Delivery also removes the pressure of the heavy, pregnant uterus.

▶ Respiratory System

Respirations remain in the normal range during the postpartum period. As the abdominal organs resume their nonpregnant position, the respiratory diaphragm also returns to its usual position. By 2 months postpartum, total pulmonary resistance increases by 50% as compared with pregnancy. Specific airway conductance, which increased during pregnancy, returns to the nonpregnancy level by 5 to 8 weeks after delivery. The changes in airway conductance may be caused by decreased progesterone.

Generally, women who deliver vaginally do not complain of dyspnea. Women who deliver by cesarean, however, may experience abdominal pain when trying to deep breathe and cough. Any woman complaining of dyspnea, regardless of the method of delivery, should be assessed for pulmonary embolism. As with any surgical client, women who have had a cesarean need to be assessed for respiratory status, especially if they have received epidural analgesics that may affect respirations.

▶ Urinary System

In the early postpartum, the ability of the bladder to eliminate urine warrants close attention. After an uncomplicated vaginal delivery, women may get out of bed to go to the bathroom. Although some women may have the urge to void spontaneously after delivery, many do not feel the need to urinate and have difficulty with the first postpartum void. Urination is impeded by perineal lacerations, hematomas, generalized swelling and bruising of the perineum and tissues surrounding the urinary meatus, physiologic and conductive anesthesia, and diminished sensation of bladder pressure. Furthermore, using a bedpan is unpleasant and may impede urination. The postpartum woman is therefore at risk for urinary retention, bladder distension, urinary stasis, and urinary tract infection (UTI). With bladder distension the postpartum woman is also at risk for uterine atony (inability of the uterine musculature to contract), resulting in hemorrhage. Specifically, as the bladder distends, the uterus is displaced and its ability to contract lessens. When the uterus fails to contract, cut blood vessels can bleed.

Generally, within 4 to 8 hours of a vaginal delivery, women have a spontaneous urge to void. In the next 48 hours, women void frequently. Large amounts of intravenous fluids given during labor and delivery also contribute to increased urine output. Levels of endogenous oxytocin diminish after delivery. Oxytocin has an antidiuretic effect, that is, the client retains fluid. As the oxytocin level decreases, its antidiuretic effect also decreases. Fluid previously retained is therefore excreted as urine. This postpartum diuresis also causes rapid bladder filling and may contribute to bladder distension.

In the first 2 days after delivery, proteolytic enzymes promote self-digestion of protein substances from the uterine wall (autolysis). Mild proteinuria may occur as a result of this process. Pathologic conditions such as hypertensive disorders and diabetes may produce markedly elevated proteinuria and ketonuria. Urine may also test positive for acetone/ketones resulting from dehydration during a prolonged labor. Lactosuria may occur in breastfeeding women as a result of the lactation process.

Within a week of delivery, creatinine clearance, which is normally elevated during pregnancy, returns to normal. Blood urea nitrogen (BUN) increases in response to the autolytic process occurring within the uterus. By 4 to 6 weeks, kidney function is normal and the ureteral dilation of pregnancy has diminished.

▶ Musculoskeletal System

With delivery of the placenta, the influence of progesterone on the woman's general muscle tone is removed. Consequently, muscle tone is restored in the postpartum if there is a balance of rest, activity, exercise, and diet. In particular, restoration of tone in the rectus abdominis muscles, the pubococcygeal muscle, and the muscles of the lower extremities is often of concern during the postpartum period.

For most women the appearance of the postpartum abdomen causes much concern. The previously pregnant abdomen is now soft, flabby, and weak. The thick central abdominal muscles, the rectus abdominis muscles, are usually separated after the delivery, giving the abdomen the flabby appearance. Separation may be greater when there was previous muscle weakness, multiple gestation, polyhydramnios, excessive weight gain, and grand multiparity. Although muscle tone is often regained in 6 weeks, some women need more time. Some women fail to regain maximum tone, despite exercise and diet.

Childbirth is accomplished with stretching and trauma to the pubococcygeal muscle, the major pelvic sphincter. The pubococcygeal muscle usually aids in maintaining bowel and bladder function, supports the contraceptive diaphragm, and may influence vaginal responses to intercourse.

In the first 24 hours after delivery many women experience lower-extremity soreness and weakness from the muscular tension and exertion of labor and delivery. Women who received regional anesthesia may experience decreased sensation in the lower extremities (Tulman, Fawcett, Groblewiski, & Silverman, 1990).

▶ Integument

The integument undergoes overt changes during the puerperium. As estrogen and progesterone levels decrease, the deeper pigmentation that occurred during pregnancy, such as darkening areolae and nipples, facial chloasma, and linea nigra, gradually diminishes also. Striae that formed on the breasts, abdomen, and thighs during pregnancy begin to fade. They eventually appear as silver or white skin streaks. Spider angiomas and palmar erythema also begin to disappear, presumably due to diminished estrogen.

During the early postpartum the integument also aids in ridding the woman of some excess water. Specifically, during the first week after delivery, women experience diaphoresis (profuse sweating) during the night. Diaphoresis may interrupt sleep and cause chilling and discomfort.

Women may experience mild, temporary alopecia, an increase in scalp hair loss, for several weeks or months after delivery. The alopecia reduces the number of growing scalp hairs, which had increased during the last two trimesters of pregnancy due to altered androgen levels. The alopecia usually stops gradually without long-term effects. For most women, the hair loss is not noticeable to others, but merely identified by an increase in hairs lost after grooming or washing the hair.

▶ Gastrointestinal System

Immediately after a vaginal delivery many women are hungry and thirsty due to the energy spent, the nausea and vomiting that may have occurred during labor, or because they were not allowed anything by mouth during labor. This NPO policy in childbearing institutions is presently questioned (Ludka & Roberts, 1993). Healthy, low-risk women should be able to eat and drink during labor.

Whether they deliver vaginally or by cesarean, women experience sluggish bowels for several days after delivery. Decreased peristalsis occurs in response to anesthesia, surgery, diminished intraabdominal pressure, diminished muscle tone, inappropriate diet, insufficient fluid intake, or if diarrhea occurred or an enema was given during labor. In addition, pain and fear of harm from hemorrhoids, an episiotomy, or lacerations lead to a woman's decreased willingness to exert pressure on the perineum. Constipation and gas pain may result.

Many women develop hemorrhoids during pregnancy and labor and delivery. As the woman strains, internal hemorrhoids may become external and bleed. Generally hemorrhoids are painful for a couple of days after delivery. They become smaller over the next several weeks; however, many women may experience mild chronic hemorrhoidal discomfort.

▶ Endocrine System

Reproductive Hormones

With delivery of the placenta there is a rapid decline in human placental lactogen (hPL) or human chorionic somatomammotropin (hCS), human chorionic gonadotropin (hCG), estrogen, and progesterone. By 1 week postpartum, only estrogen may be discernible in plasma. In addition, levels of follicle-stimulating hormone and luteinizing hormone are very low at 10 days postpartum.

In nonlactating women, estrogen levels begin to rise to follicular levels approximately 3 weeks after delivery, followed by rising, although low, levels of progesterone. Return to prepregnancy levels of estrogen and progesterone is more variable and slower in lactating than in nonlactating women.

During pregnancy, the pituitary gland begins to secrete prolactin. As the levels of progesterone and estrogen rapidly decline after delivery, and lactation is initiated. the prolactin level rises. With increased breastfeeding, the prolactin level rises further. In nonlactating women, the prolactin level declines and reaches the nonpregnancy level by 14 days.

Thyroid Hormone

Slight nonpathologic enlargement of the thyroid gland may be caused by pregnancy-induced hyperplasia of glandular tissue, general increased vascularity, and increased iodine turnover in response to a higher glomerular filtration rate and renal iodine clearance. Additionally, during pregnancy the thyroid gland may enlarge slightly and the basal metabolic rate increases. By 6 weeks postpartum the thyroid gland should return to the prepregnant state.

A small percentage of women develop puerperal thyroiditis, an autoimmune disease characterized by increased thyroid antibody titers, painless thyroid enlargement, and either hyperthyroid or hypothyroid symptoms (Browne-Martin & Emerson, 1997). In most cases puerperal thyroiditis is self-limiting (Mestman, 1997). It may manifest as early as 3 to 4 weeks postpartum (AWHONN/Johnson & Johnson Consumer Products, Inc., 1996) and as late as 12 weeks after delivery (Mestman, 1997). Occasionally, chronic thyroid disease and recurring transient thyroid disease

with subsequent pregnancies persist (Browne-Martin & Emerson, 1997).

▶ PSYCHOLOGIC AND SOCIOCULTURAL CHANGES DURING THE POSTPARTUM PERIOD

Successful parenting is a continuous and complex interactive process that not only requires the acquisition of new skills but also the development of a loving relationship between the parent and infant and the integration of the new or expanded parent role with other existing roles. Several factors may affect the beginning of this process, and thus have the potential for long-term effects. The birthing experience (Nichols, 1993) and paternal participation in the birthing experience (Fortier, 1988; Palkovitz, 1992) have been identified as factors that may affect the parental role and early attachment behaviors of the parents. Other factors that may affect the transition to parenthood include parental expectations about parenting (Palkovitz, 1992) and their perceptions of their level of competency in performing parenting tasks (Ferketich & Mercer, 1995; Mercer & Ferketich, 1990, 1994; Pridham & Chang, 1992), their prenatal and postnatal expectations of the infant, parity (Grace, 1993), personality attributes and emotional states (Ferketich & Mercer, 1994; Mercer & Ferketich, 1994), and the support or conflict that is present in their relationship with their partner, family, and friends (Belsky & Kelly, 1994; Reece, 1993; Tiller, 1995).

▶ Transitions in Parenting

The transition to parenthood is often difficult and may be perceived as a crisis. Parents may experience difficulty in adequately communicating their needs to one another. The birth of an infant to first-time parents has also been demonstrated to result in (1) decreased affection and feelings of love for one another, (2) feelings of ambivalence toward each other, (3) greater conflict between them, and (4) diminished interest in sexual intimacy on the part of the woman (Belsky & Kelly, 1994).

Several reasons have been suggested for the nature of the difficult relationship between new parents. Being awakened at night by the infant may cause sleep deprivation. During the first few months after delivery, the infant is completely dependent on the parents, which can overwhelm them. In most societies, women have traditionally been responsible for the majority of infant care and men have been viewed as breadwinners. Despite changing attitudes and beliefs about fatherhood and the roles of women, mothers are still considered the parent responsible for the care of the young infant. The new father often feels that the mother is preoccupied with the infant and has little time for him (Belsky & Kelly, 1994). Furthermore, although modern-day fathers may be expected to participate in care of the young infant, they have not had proper role models. This problem is compounded by the fact that in the first few months after delivery, the father is often the sole breadwinner, and consequently not home most of the day. Fathers tend to continue their activities outside of the home after the birth, resulting in the mother's feeling alienated and alone. After meeting the needs of the infant all day, the new mother may be uninterested in intimacy with her partner.

By the time the infant is 6 months old, as many as 50% of new mothers are back at work, which requires that the family reorganize responsibilities. Research demonstrates that in dual-earner families, fathers adapt their roles and provide a large part of infant care (Hall, 1991). Parents who are unable to successfully reorganize responsibilities will experience role strain and marital conflict.

Often, transition to parenthood may be difficult for those parents who had not planned to have a child. Despite current contraceptive technology, many pregnancies are unplanned. Abortion, although legal, is for many an unacceptable alternative.

In addition, the change from a stable dyadic (two-person) relationship or to a series of shifting triangles places great stress on family structure and function.

► Tasks of New Parents

In addition to the difficulties of the transition to parenthood, new mothers and fathers face a variety of psychosocial tasks in assuming their role. These tasks include:

- Learning to care for their infant
- Providing a safe environment that fosters growth and development
- Attaching to the infant
- Incorporating the infant into their social sphere
- Learning to balance multiple roles and relationships
- Fostering the parental role of each parent
- Developing a sense of family
- Learning to deal effectively with problems and conflicts (Fig. 28–1)

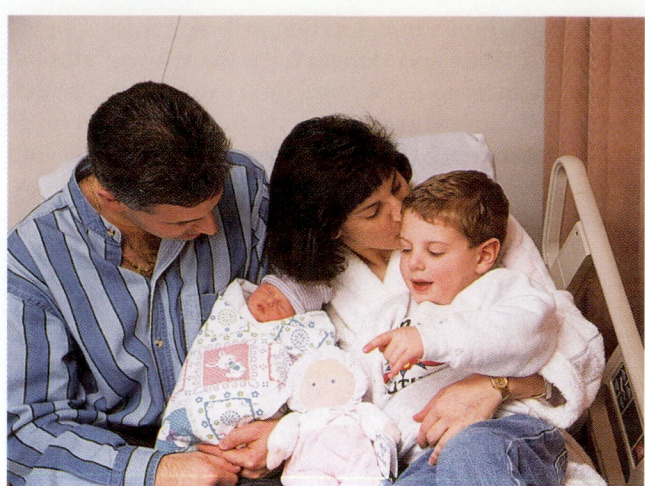

FIGURE 28–1. One of the tasks that these parents will face is incorporating the infant into the family.

The resolution of these tasks is an additional challenge for the family system that may already have its coping abilities stretched.

► Social Networks

Studies of social network ties and support systems have identified the importance of these systems in a couple's transition to parenthood. Support from their social network (friends, relatives, co-workers) promotes the couple's physical and psychologic adaptation to pregnancy and the postpartum period (Reece, 1993; Susman, 1996). In addition, Klaus and Kennell (1997) note that postpartum women who received emotional and physical support in labor from a doula, i.e., a trained lay person other than the husband or father of the baby, demonstrate greater self-esteem, less depression, a higher regard for the infant, and a greater ability to care for their infant compared to women who did not have a doula during labor.

The social network, however, is altered by the birth of a child. For example, grandparents often increase contact with new parents after the birth of the first baby. New fathers and mothers have more contact with other parents of young children. The old social networks of co-workers and friends who are not parents tend to fade, especially for mothers, after childbirth. However, when there are personal concerns or tension in the environment, helpseeking by mothers of young infants is considered appropriate and encouraged by family, friends, and professionals (Pridham, 1997). Through helpseeking, the new mother learns culturally valued practices and develops role competency (Pridham, 1997).

▶ Psychosocial Adaptation of the Mother

Maternal Role Attainment

The process of maternal role attainment begins long before the actual birth of an infant. Birth ushers in a new phase in the development of the mother–infant relationship.

Maternal role attainment is described as a process that continues over a 3- to 10-month period following the birth (Mercer, 1986). Maternal tasks during that period include attaching to the infant by identifying, claiming, and interaction (Klaus & Kennell, 1982); becoming competent in performing mothering behaviors (Mercer & Ferketich, 1990, 1994); and feeling gratification in mother–infant interactions (Mercer, 1986).

The maternal role is attained after about 1 year, at least for the first-time mother. The process is not an inevitable, step-by-step progression. Instead, peaks and valleys in behaviors indicate the course. The challenges presented by the infant's continuous and changing developmental behaviors almost invariably lead to the mother's feelings of role incompetency at different points in time (especially at the 8- to 12-month stages).

Mercer (1986) describes four phases in a mother's adaptation to her new role. They span the first year of the infant's life and include the physical recovery phase (birth to 1 month); the achievement phase (2 months to 4 or 5 months); the disruption phase (6 to 8 months); and the reorganization phase (beginning after 8 months and continuing after 12 months).

Physical Recovery Phase (Birth to 1 Month). Biologic adaptation dominates during the **physical recovery phase,** as the mother recovers from birthing and her infant makes the transition to the external world. The woman's social network often offers much-needed help.

Achievement Phase (2 Months to 4 or 5 Months). As the mother feels better, the psychologic and social levels of adaptation dominate during the **achievement phase.** The infant has settled into a predictable routine, the mother generally feels competent in care of the young infant, and the infant's socialization skills (such as the spontaneous smile) make him or her a pleasure to care for. Many mothers choose to return to work during this phase, increasing the complexity of the mothering role.

Disruption Phase (6 to 8 Months). During the **disruption phase,** the mother begins to feel stress at the social level of adaptation, as she tries to balance conflicting roles of work, mother, and wife. The

infant's developmental changes and newfound mobility challenge the mother's skills and competence, making her question herself again. A clash may develop between the infant's evolving self and the mother's need to regain a sense of herself similar to her prepregnant state.

Reorganization Phase (Beginning After 8 Months and Continuing After 12 Months). All levels of adaptation—biologic, psychologic, and social—are evident in the **reorganization phase.** Biologic changes occur as the infant continues to grow, develop, and master the environment, and as the mother begins to wean the infant. Psychologically, the mother often becomes restless with the all-consuming nature of motherhood and the burden of responsibility for her infant. Socially, she may wish to be recognized in roles other than that of mother. She individuates herself more and more from her infant as she attempts to regain some of her prepregnancy activities.

Maternal Variables. Several variables have been identified that may affect maternal role attainment. Because maternal role attainment is multidimensional and evolving, the presence of any one variable is not necessarily a sign of success in achieving the maternal role. Maternal variables are discussed in Table 28–1.

In addition to the maternal variables that can affect role attainment, the temperament and health status of the infant can also have an impact on this process. An infant who is easy to care for and demonstrates predictable behaviors increases parents' feelings of competence in their ability to deliver care. Parents, however, may perceive infant behavior differently, based on their previous experience caring for infants. Furthermore, an individual infant's temperament and patterns may be predictable, but may be in conflict with the needs, expectations, and temperament of the parent. In this latter situation, both the parents' feelings of competency and the parent–infant relationship may not be optimal. Furthermore, a premature or sick infant can affect maternal attachment process and role attainment. After delivery, a sick or premature infant may be separated from the mother. Depending upon the status of the infant at birth, the mother may not have the opportunity to hold or gaze upon her infant. Subsequently, the mother may delay attaching to the infant because of her fears that the infant may die and/or she may be unable to identify with the infant. Finally, mothers, as well as fathers, may not feel competent to deliver the more complex care required for sick or premature infants (Harrison & Magill-Evans, 1996).

▶ **TABLE 28–1**

Variables Affecting Maternal Role Attainment

Variable	Effect
Age at first birth	Greater maternal age associated with greater physical risk; more assets, education, and commitment to mothering; and more role conflict.
Perception of birth experience	Differences between expectations and actual performance in labor affects self-esteem; having a vaginal birth birth associated with a more positive self-perception after birth than when experiencing a cesarean birth.
Early mother–infant contact	Early contact associated with greater attachment behaviors.
Social support	Emotional, informational, physical, and approval support from spouse/father of the baby and extended family associated with less maternal stress and more positive self-evaluation of parenting behaviors.
	Lack of social support associated with postpartum depression.
Personality traits	Incompatibility of maternal and infant personality traits and patterns may affect maternal feelings toward infant and sense of competency.
Self-concept and competency	Positive self-concept/self-esteem predicts maternal role competency and self-evaluation of role performance.
Childrearing attitudes	Attitudes and beliefs influence mother–infant interactions, role fulfillment, and infant/child socialization.
Health status	Pain, infection, fever, fatigue, and need for recuperation associated with maternal immobilization and inability to assume care for newborn/infant; may not affect overall maternal role competence.

Role Conflict in Transition. Transition to the maternal role can result in role conflict for contemporary women. Several factors, including previous roles and relationships, may affect a woman's sense of conflict. It is not clear whether having a career in and of itself produces role conflict. Nor is it known whether the extent of role conflict differs between mothers who choose to return to work and those who must return to work. The literature indicates that new mothers lack role models for integrating roles related to work and motherhood (Hartrick, 1997; Miller 1996). In one study mothers returning to work felt that because they did not identify with any role models, they improvised and negotiated relationships to manage the practicalities of child care and career (Miller, 1996). Hartrick's (1997) phenomenologic study identified three elements by which mothers define self: (1) nonreflective doing, i.e., taking up roles that are modeled by others; (2) living in the shadows, i.e., a time when they can no longer feel secure and the foundation of their lives crumbles; and (3) reclaiming and discovery, i.e., a time in which they nurture the self and make new connections. Tulman & Fawcett (1990) found that when women perform household and social tasks and care for themselves and their infant, employed mothers function the same as nonemployed mothers. Some women may actually experience less role conflict when working due to a sense of self-fulfillment and worth, particularly if they have a supportive family and excellent child care.

The level of marital satisfaction may also contribute to a woman's transition to the maternal role. Marital satisfaction is positively related to ease of transition. Conversely, marital discord after birth may produce additional conflicts for the woman as she attempts to adapt to the maternal role.

The Maternal–Infant Dyad

Immediately after birth and for some time thereafter the mother and newborn form what is called the **maternal–infant** (or maternal–child) **dyad.** Formation of the dyad seems to be an important factor in the continued process of parent–child attachment. Historically, formation of the new family has been believed to depend to a large extent on the integrity of this dyad (Rubin, 1984). More recent literature supports that the father indirectly affects the mother's interactions with the infant and her general sensitivity, i.e, ability to appropriately respond to the infant's signals (Cowan, 1997; van IJzendoorn & De Wolff, 1997). Subsequently, when the mother is sensitive to the infant's signals, the infant experiences a successful interaction, which promotes a secure relationship (De Wolff & van IJzendoorn, 1997).

Maternal–infant bonding, as described by Klaus and Kennel (1982, 1995), is a vital component of the attachment process that occurs in the immediate postpartum period. Bonding is only one necessary component of the parent–child attachment process.

Bonding, as an isolated event, will neither doom nor ensure parent–child attachment and a healthy parent–child relationship. The attachment process is lengthy and complex, and requires positive outcomes at many levels.

Attachment begins with the embryo. The mother and fetus share a special, intense closeness and communication. After birth, the closeness between mother and newborn is akin to the relationship that existed during pregnancy.

Within the maternal–infant dyad, the behaviors of bonding occur, and the process of attachment continues to evolve during the postpartum period. About 4 to 5 months, attachment behaviors between mother and infant are joined to beginning separation or individuation behaviors (see Chapter 4). These attachment and separation or individuation behaviors continue as parallel processes throughout the first 2 years of the mother–child relationship. Ideally, the outcome of these processes will be the individuation of the child and mother into two independent, autonomous individuals—a parent and child who have a healthy, loving relationship.

Attachment Behaviors.

Various behaviors assist the bonding between a mother and her newborn in the immediate postpartum period. These behaviors are reciprocal; that is, the mother's behaviors evoke certain responses from her newborn and the newborn's behaviors elicit responses from the mother. Several maternal and infant behaviors are recognized (Table 28–2).

Identification of the Infant.

Much early thought concerning how a new mother learns to identify her infant after birth followed observations made by Rubin (1984). Although more recent research has disproven some of the early theory, much of it has yet to be tested. Rubin's ideas provide a good starting point for looking at this process.

Identification does not occur after a single contact with the infant, but with repeated contact, made most often during and after feeding (Rubin, 1984). Repeated exposures are necessary for the mother to observe characteristics of *her* infant. Rubin describes two forms of observations: tactile and visual identification.

New mothers have been observed to follow a sequence of tactile identification of their infants. Early studies found that mothers progressed from touching the infant's periphery (hands, feet) with their fingertips to touching the torso with their full palm (Rubin, 1963). Later research, however, called this sequence into question (Tulman, 1986).

Many questions remain about the process of tactile identification. More certain, however, is that a mother's touching is an important source of tenderness for her infant (Tulman, 1986) and facilitates maternal–infant attachment.

Rubin (1963) also stresses visual identification as part of a larger process called "claiming" (Fig. 28–2).

▶ **TABLE 28-2**

Maternal–Infant Bonding Behaviors

Interactions Originating in the Mother That Affect the Infant

Touch	Helps bind mother and infant together in the early part of their relationship.
Eye-to-eye contact	Well-known and frequently observed "en face position"; mutual gazing (especially about 9 to 10 in., the distance at which the neonate can best focus on objects) is a very powerful behavior for assisting maternal–infant attachment.
Mother's voice	Mother's high-pitched voice tones fit the infant's auditory perception range.
Entrainment	Rhythmic pattern of movements by which the infant responds to the mother's voice.
Reestablishment of biorhythmic cycles	Infant's intrauterine cycles (such as sleep–wake and rapid eye movement cycles) are disrupted at birth; mother's cycles and routines help the newborn to reestablish his or her daily cycles.
Breast milk and bacterial nasal flora	Both are contributed by the mother and help to protect the newborn from the new extrauterine environment.
Odor	By the fifth day, a breastfeeding newborn can distinguish the mother.
Heat	Mother provides reliable source of heat for her newborn.

Interactions Originating in the Newborn That Affect the Mother

Eye-to-eye contact	The "other half" of maternal gazing (see above, for a description of the process).
Cry	Infant's voice affects the mother; breastfeeding mothers sometimes experience the milk ejection reflex when they hear their infants cry.
Release of oxytocin and prolactin	Infant stimulates hormonal changes in the mother through suckling or other contact with the breast.
Odor	By third or fourth day, mothers have been found to recognize the odor of their own infants.
Entrainment	Infant responds to mother's voice with a "dance" or rhythmic movements.

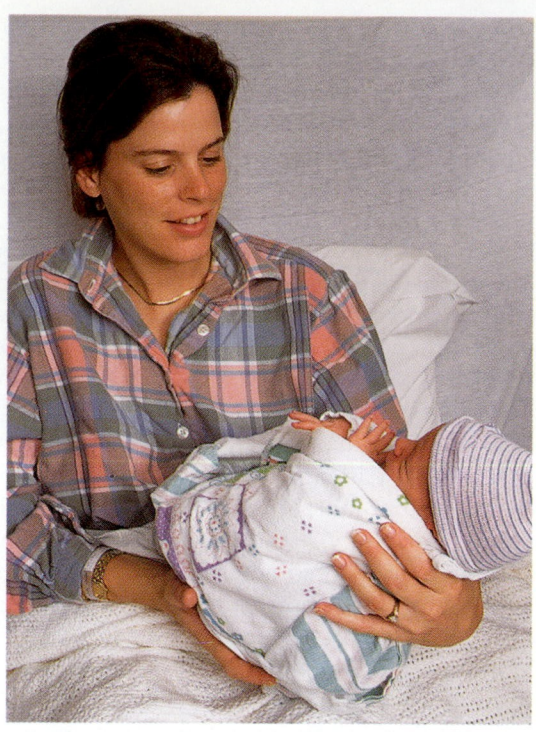

FIGURE 28–2. This new mother is engaging in visual identification of her newborn.

In this process, the mother identifies features and characteristics of the neonate that are similar to those of other family members or her own. Each aspect of the infant's appearance and behavior is linked in this way to the mother or members of the larger family system. Naming the child is an important part of the claiming process. By choosing a name, the mother and family affirm the infant's existence and belonging.

Finally, how a mother and her infant interact affects the mother's identification of her newborn. The feeding relationship is especially important in establishing harmonious maternal–infant interaction. Early feeding situations are often stressful for the mother as she attempts to prove herself a "good" mother as measured by the infant's response to feeding. A successful feeding relationship not only helps in a positive identification of the neonate, it also increases the mother's self-esteem.

Maternal Body Image

The postpartum woman often expects her body to return to normal and look like her prepregnant self. This is rarely the case.

Fawcett (1977) studied changes in perceived body space during the eighth and ninth months of pregnancy and during the first and second postpartum months. She found that women's perceived body space increased during pregnancy, decreased markedly during the first postpartum month, and then increased during the second postpartum month. By the second month, women realized that they were not as small as they would like to be.

Although the postpartum woman may feel somewhat better about her postpartum body image than about her pregnant body image, she feels more positive about her prepregnant body image than about her postpartum body image. Achieving a return to the prepregnant figure is cited by many women as their primary postpartum concern.

Along with dissatisfaction about their postpartum body image, women must also adjust to a physical separation from the fetus or infant. Some women feel a sense of nostalgia for the intimate experiences of the fetus in utero and a sense of emptiness.

Maternal Concerns

Research supports that in the initial postpartum period maternal concerns focus upon two overall issues: self-care and infant care (Birk, 1996; Imle & Drayden, 1996; Maloni, 1994; Miovech, Knapp, Borucki, Roncoli, Arnold & Brooten, 1994). Maternal concerns regarding self-care in the immediate postpartum period often relate to physical restoration and are closely related to incisional/laceration healing, diet, exercise, and fatigue. Miovech et al. (1994) reported that women who had had a cesarean delivery are initially concerned with pain, incisional problems, activity intolerance, and gastrointestinal discomfort. Similarly, Birk (1996) found that self-care of the "stitches" is concern of women after a cesarean delivery; the episiotomy is a concern of women after a vaginal delivery.

Initial postpartum concerns about integrating the infant into the family include managing multiple roles, such as housework, meeting the needs of the infant and other family members, and coping with changes in the marital or partner relationship. Based on their qualitative study of first time parents' experiences of the postpartum, Imle and Drayden (1996) report that initially postpartum women are concerned with reverting from pregnancy to normalcy and with integrating the baby into the new family unit. Men are also concerned with the integration of the family unit (Imle & Drayden, 1996).

Mothers also express concerns about infant care, specifically feedings, gastrointestinal difficulty (colic), skin irritations, and sleeping and crying problems. Maloni (1994) reported that in a sample of 33 primiparas, acquisition of knowledge about infant care and personal characteristics of their newborns was highest during postpartum hospitalization than when at home. On postpartum days 1–6, mothers learned the most about infant feeding; on days 7–13 they learned about daily infant care (Maloni, 1994). Postpartum day 1, mothers were focused on acquisition of knowledge regarding their infant's characteristics; by days 2 through 13, they focused on learning about their infant's activity (Maloni, 1994).

Although physical restoration concerns resolve in the first few postpartum weeks, psychosocial and lifestyle concerns continue. Family dynamics, return to work, and division of caregiving are areas of focus. One study of women at 8 weeks postcesarean delivery found that changes in activity, depression, family interaction, body image, child care, and work/school were major concerns (Miovech et al., 1994). Imle and Drayden's (1996) study also support that, during the late postpartum months, mothers, as well as fathers, are concerned with crying and other infant behaviors, family integration, and support for parenting.

Primiparous and multiparous women share many of the same concerns in the postpartum period; however, multiparous women voice additional concern about the strain a new child places on the rest of the family (Martell, 1996) and the new, more complex structure of the family system. Multiparous women frequently cite as major concerns meeting the needs of everyone at home and not having enough time to do so.

New mothers often experience some degree of "blues" and some may have depression after delivery (see Chapter 29).

▶ Psychosocial Adaptation of the Father

An important "discovery" of researchers and clinicians in recent years is that the neonate's experience extends beyond his or her relationship with the mother. Fathers, too, are an integral part of the neonate's life.

Paternal Role Adaptation

How the father will fulfill his new role and what his behaviors will be in that role are influenced by (1) his participation in childbirth, (2) the family role organization, (3) the father's sex role identification, (4) degree of competency in performing the role, and (5) the father's cultural background.

Participation in Childbirth. Fathers' participation in childbirth often enhances future father–infant inter-

action. Fathers who have immediate and extended contact with their newborns after birth demonstrate more subsequent behaviors such as talking to the newborn. A father's participation in the childbirth, through preparation and involvement in either vaginal or cesarean birth, seems to foster more positive feelings about birth and increases the opportunity for early contact and frequent interactions with the infant. Research supports the theory that the father's presence at the delivery and early contact with the infant can predict paternal–infant caretaking activities (Fortier, 1988). Fathers who have limited initial contact with the infant after birth, however, have successfully developed a relationship with their infant by increasing their interaction time apart from the delivery experience (Chandler & Field, 1997; Palkovitz, 1992).

Although present day childbirth settings and practices promote the presence of the father during labor and delivery, a recent qualitative study (Chandler & Field, 1997) found that fathers felt as if their presence during labor and delivery was merely tolerated by the health care providers and that they were not seen as being part of a laboring couple but rather as a support person for the laboring woman. Additionally, these fathers reported that as labor progressed they felt less confident in being able to help their wives and became more fearful about the outcome. After the delivery, the men reported that they switched their focus to their newborn and were active in baby care at 4 weeks postpartum. The childbirth experience may affect some men's self-confidence and spouse relationship more than it affects their early interaction with the infant (Nichols, 1993).

Family Structure and Sex Role Identification. Organization of the family and sex role identification affect the nature of the father's role with his newborn.

Studies indicate that in families in which both the mother and father are employed, fathers are more involved with child care (Hall, 1991). Findings, however, are not always consistent. The level of other interaction with the baby in dual-earner families may be the result of the employed mother's need to have contact with the infant, the father's need for contact, and the mother's support of the father's interaction with the infant. In families where the traditional clearly defined male and female roles are ambiguous, men may be more nurturant with their offspring and take on additional caretaking roles. In one study where 57% of the women had returned to work by 3 months, 90% of the fathers were involved in baby care and household activities (Tiller, 1995).

Degree of Competence. Research indicates that paternal role competency is a major predictor of paternal attachment to the infant (Ferketich & Mercer, 1994, 1995; Mercer & Ferketich, 1990). Paternal role competence progressively evolves from birth to 8 months postpartum for both experienced and inexperienced fathers (Ferketich & Mercer, 1994, 1995; Mercer & Ferketich, 1990). The research suggests that paternal role competence for experienced fathers is affected by the relationship between the father and his wife/partner and to the presence, if any, of paternal feelings of depression (Ferketich & Mercer, 1995). In contrast, the presence of anxiety and the degree to which the father feels he has a sense of mastery or control over his life is related to paternal role competence in inexperienced fathers (Ferketich & Mercer, 1995).

Cultural Background. The cultural background of both parents affects the father's role and behavior. Culture defines what is socially acceptable in terms of personal space, eye contact, and touch (Lipson, Dibble, & Minarik, 1996). Although participation in the birth process and early paternal–newborn physical contact may be desirable and considered to be indicative of healthy paternal behaviors, an individual's culture, background and adherence to its laws or rules may prohibit or prevent the father from demonstrating these behaviors. For example, during labor, delivery, and the postpartum period when the woman has vaginal bleeding, an Orthodox Jewish man is not permitted to touch his wife (DeSevo, 1997). He may not actively take the baby from the mother. He can, however, hold his newborn provided a person other than his wife has handed him the newborn.

Father–Infant Relationship

Studies have documented the powerful impact on the father of seeing and holding his newborn immediately after birth (Ferketich & Mercer, 1989; Nichols, 1993). Fathers react to their infants with elation, relief that the infant is healthy, pride, increased self-esteem, and feelings of closeness when the infant opens his or her eyes.

As with mothers and infants, early contact between fathers and infants increases holding and play in the early weeks of the infant's life. Research indicates that in the first 15 minutes after birth, first-time fathers spend the majority of the time gazing at the newborn, and spend less time using touch (Tomlinson, Rothenberg, & Carver, 1991). Fathers also display a progressive touch sequence with their infant over the first few days, and both fathers and mothers appear equally sensitive to the newborn's behavioral cues in the early postpartum period.

A classic study describes the father's reaction or bond to the newborn as **engrossment** (Greenburg & Morris, 1974). Engrossment is characterized by seven behaviors.

1. *Visual awareness of the newborn.* The father perceives the infant as attractive, pretty, or beautiful.
2. *Tactile awareness of the newborn.* The father has a desire to touch and hold the infant, activities that he perceives as very pleasurable (Fig. 28–3).
3. *Awareness of distinct features of the newborn.* The father feels that he can distinguish his own infant from other infants.
4. *Perception of the newborn as perfect.* In spite of some unattractiveness and awkwardness of the infant, the father sees the infant as the epitome of perfection.
5. *Strong attraction to the newborn.* The father focuses his attention on the infant.
6. *Extreme elation.* The father describes a "high" after birth of his child.
7. *Increased sense of self-esteem.* After seeing his infant for the first time, the father describes himself as feeling proud, bigger, more mature, or older.

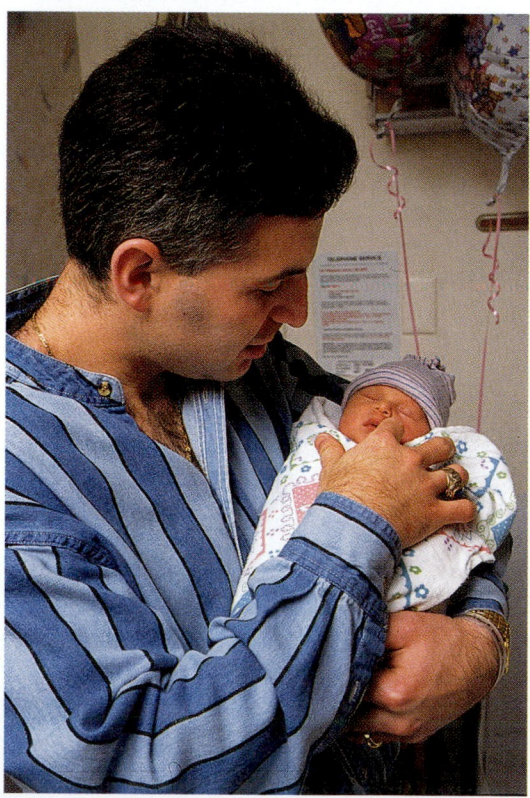

FIGURE 28–3. As part of engrossment, a father gains awareness of his daughter by stroking her cheek with his finger.

The belief that the mother is the most important figure in a child's life and that the child becomes attached to her first is not supported by research. Most infants seem to form attachments to both parents about the same time. The nature of the mother–infant relationship, however, may differ from that of the father–infant relationship. Gamble and Morse (1993) found that fathers of breastfed infants felt that the difference was due to breastfeeding. Specifically, these fathers felt inadequate and frustrated when trying to bottle-feed their infants in the absence of the mother. They compensated, however, by being involved in other infant care activities.

Parental roles are most likely the result of culture and social conventions. Hall (1991) reported that some fathers have difficulty assuming an active parental

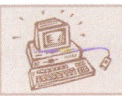 *Research Abstract*

Paternal Attitudes Toward Infant Behaviors During the First Year

This longitudinal, repeated measures study explored fathers' parenting attitudes and interactions with their infants from prebirth to one year. A nonrandomized sample, consisting of 228 first-time fathers and 65 experienced fathers, participated at the prebirth testing period. The sample size dropped to a total of 62 fathers at 3 months after the birth, and 42 fathers at 1 year. At each of the testing times, fathers completed the Adult-Adolescent Parenting Inventory (AAPI), a four-construct instrument which evaluates parental expectation of the child; the parent's ability to have empathy toward the child's needs; belief in corporal punishment; and belief in family roles. In addition, fathers completed a demographic questionnaire containing some questions on marital and family life.

Repeated one-way ANOVA was performed on mean scores of the four constructs. Because raw scores for first-time fathers did not differ from experienced fathers, analysis between test times was performed using the total sample. Scores significantly decreased between prebirth and 3 months for parental expectation of the child, and then significantly increased, returning to a level similar to preterm at 1 year. This finding demonstrated that fathers had inappropriate parental expectation of the infant at 3 months. Analysis also demonstrated that fathers had a significantly greater belief in corporal punishment at 3 months compared to either the prebirth or 1 year test periods.

At 3 months, 57% of the mothers were working; 90% of fathers helped around the house and with child care; and although all previously reported marital happiness, 48% felt their marriage was happier than at prebirth, and 4% said less happy. At 1 year 58% of the fathers reported they helped with child care as much as they did at 3 months, 37% said they helped more, and 5% said they helped less. In addition, at 1 year 75% of fathers reported their marriages were happier and 5% said less happy.

The data from this study suggest that regardless of experience, fathers undergo a transition in taking on the parental role and that the marital relationship also undergoes transition as the infant is incorporated into the family. At 3 months there is a need for fathers to develop more realistic expectations of their infants. Their heightened belief in the use of corporal punishment at 3 months may reflect stress experienced as a father and a husband.

Application to Practice

The study suggests that nurses need to provide more education to fathers or expectant fathers on infant behavior and the stress a marriage may undergo as the family adapts to new or expanded parental roles and incorporates the infant into the family. Fathers need to be taught alternatives to corporal punishment that more appropriately reflect the developmental level of their infants and which foster positive healthy parental and child behaviors.

Source: Tiller, C.M. (1995). Fathers' parenting attitudes during a child's first year. Journal of Obstetric, Gynecologic, and Neonatal Nursing, 24, *508–514.*

role because they lack a role model and are often viewed as the traditional breadwinner. In our present-day socioeconomic climate, however, parenting has become a more shared responsibility.

▶ Adjustment of Siblings

The adjustment of siblings to the newborn is often a concern of parents. Siblings create environments for each other that have the potential to affect the development of each child. In addition, parental roles evolve, in part, from complex interaction patterns with both the older child(ren) and the newborn.

The arrival of the newborn often causes siblings to feel displaced, frustrated, angry, and unloved (Sawicki, 1997). The reactions of the older child are influenced by birth or ordinal position of each child, the age difference between children, the sex of each child, and the age of the older child at the birth of the newborn. In general, children under the age of 5 years tend to be more upset than older children. In addition, the personality and temperament of the older child and the parent–child relationship may influence the child's adjustment to the newborn. A difficult, hard-to-manage child who has trouble with change reacts most negatively to the birth of a sibling. A stable, supportive parent–child relationship often fosters the child's adjustment to the newborn.

Adjustment to the birth of a half-sibling can be difficult, particularly in situations where the older child's parents are divorced or have a conflict-riddled relationship. The older child may feel that he or she does not truly belong; birth of a half-sibling may further destroy the child's hope that his or her parents will reconcile. The child's insecurities may be fostered by the biologic parents' negative and angry comments about each other.

Sibling rivalry, or the competition for love, approval, and attention from a parent, is frequently present between siblings and becomes evident with the arrival of the newborn. Manifestations of sibling rivalry include aggressive behaviors, e.g., hitting, pushing, or biting the baby; regressive behaviors, e.g., bedwetting, thumb-sucking, drinking from a bottle; attention-seeking behaviors, e.g., demanding, acting out; and independence and mastery of new skills, e.g., self-toileting (Sawicki, 1997). Siblings may also have sleep disturbances and frequent crying episodes.

While parents may expect negative behaviors, many note that older siblings demonstrate interest in the newborn (Fig. 28–4). In one study parents expected more negative behaviors in their first-born than were actually observed after the birth of their second child (Gullicks & Crase, 1993).

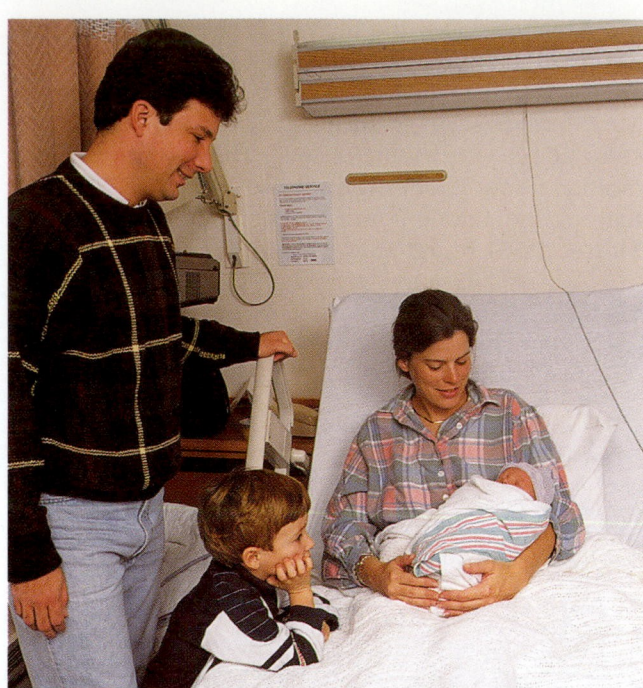

FIGURE 28–4. An older sibling shows interest and curiosity in his new brother.

Maternal Relationship to Older Children

Changes in the relationship between an older child and the mother would seem unavoidable after the birth of a new infant. The infant is totally dependent and requires much attention, attention that before had often been directed exclusively to the older child. In general, the relationship between the mother and older sibling is marked by a decrease in maternal attention and an increase in confrontation and maternal restraint. Despite expectations of negative behaviors from their older children and the emotional effects on mothers when their older children display negative behaviors, mothers elect to have their older child visit in the hospital after birth of the newborn (Mackey & Miller, 1992).

▶ Adjustment of Grandparents

Birth of a first grandchild marks the development of a multigenerational family system made up of grandparents, parents, and children (Fig. 28–5). Grandparents who are close to the new family are presented with two major themes: the "spirit of change" and "the spirit of conservation" (Taylor, 1983).

In the "spirit of change," the patterns of interaction that were used in the past are broken and new interpretations are brought to present events. A new mother may remember how her mother oriented her

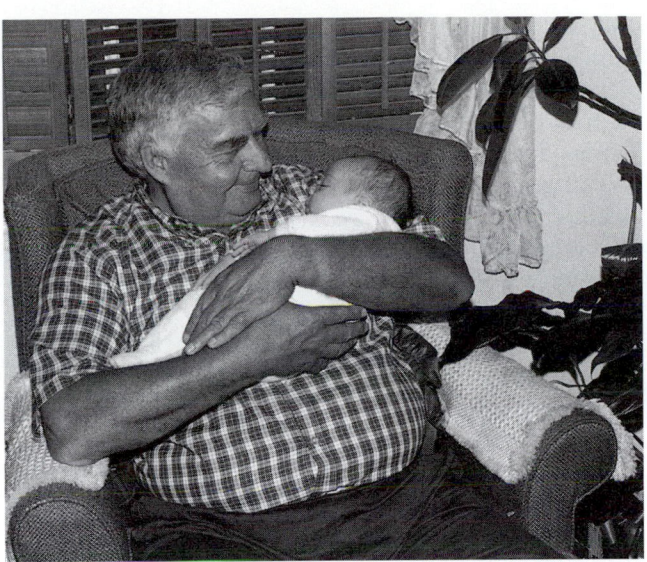

FIGURE 28–5. A grandfather with his new grandchild.

to a sex role (e.g., by teaching her to cook and clean). She may resolve to orient her new daughter (or son) in a less traditional pattern (e.g., daughters may mow lawns and sons set tables). New parents reflect on their parents' childrearing and decide to "do it differently."

The "spirit of conservation," on the other hand, maintains the continuation of family patterns from one generation to the next. These patterns of family routine and ritual form a fabric of everyday life and endure with each generation. A holiday or birthday celebration may become an enduring family ritual. Other examples include a variety of specific parenting patterns, such as reading bedtime stories to children. New parents often carry on these rituals in their own family. The spirit of conservation gives some stability to multigenerational families.

Parents and Grandparents: Role Models

The themes of change and conservation are mirrored in research concerning new parents' role models. A classic study by Mercer (1986) showed that the majority of women name their mother as their principal role model during their first year of motherhood. In addition, the majority of these new mothers rate themselves the same as their mothers in the area of child care. Other similarities include judgment and use of physical discipline. Most new mothers, however, do see themselves as more lenient or fairer than their mothers were with them. Thus, although women tend to mother as they were mothered, they may believe that they are more liberal and fairer than their mothers (Mercer, 1986).

Fathers also tend to use their own fathers as role models. Pleasant memories of being fathered or dissatisfaction with the relationship seem to motivate a new father either to repeat or successfully rework his own experiences of being parented.

After the birth of an infant, the new parents' parents remain important role models in how they care for the new child. Their proximity, support, and advice often play a vital role in the evolving parent–neonate relationship. In some cases, grandparents may have primary caretaking roles. The extent of the grandparents' role varies among cultural groups; thus the nurse will need to identify the role of grandparents in each family group. The box entitled Helpful Grandparent Behaviors presents supportive behaviors that can characterize the relationship between new parents and grandparents.

▶ Socioeconomic Influences

The socioeconomic status of the family affects the manner in which a newborn is integrated into the family. It determines the resources available to the

▶ HELPFUL GRANDPARENT BEHAVIORS

- Supporting the new mother and father in parenting activities.
- Carrying out household tasks while the mother recuperates from childbirth.
- Providing additional attention to older children.
- Supporting existing child care activities.
- Asking permission of the parents to provide care to the newborn.
- Passing on appropriate family rituals.

- Maintaining a neutral position when parents are in a conflict.
- Asking what the new parents would like to have done with regard to child care and home routines.
- Supporting the advice of the health care providers.
- Demonstrating interest in learning about current baby and postpartum care.
- Being emotionally available.
- Supporting father–infant interactions.

family to care for the newborn; it may determine the person(s) who will care for the newborn and where the child is cared for. Whether a family qualifies for local, state, or federal assistance is also determined by socioeconomic factors.

The family structure of low-income families may differ from the middle-class lifestyle of a nuclear family. The newborn may enter a family with various combinations of extended family members and friends. For example, a teenage mother may take her newborn home with her to her own mother, who lives with other children, grandchildren, aunts, uncles, or cousins. In such an instance, the grandmother may actually assume the role of mother for both her daughter and grandchild. Family structures in which several individuals fulfill the role of mother may be an adaptive means of coping with a hostile environment.

Other roles and responsibilities and circumstances may dictate that someone other than the mother take care of the newborn. For example, the new mother may need to return to work or school. Several people may need to be available to help care for the baby.

Sometimes, the newborn will not live with the mother. For example, if the newborn's parents are experiencing "hard times," they may give the newborn to a relative or close friend to raise until their economic status improves. This "informal adoption" is a way families cope in an environment of great stress such as poverty.

▶ Sociocultural Influences

Sociocultural factors influence family members' interactions with the newborn during the puerperium. The family's cultural affiliations also affect the type of care given to the newborn and the mother. For example, several cultural groups have a "nurse" come into the home to care for the newborn while the mother regains her strength.

Rituals may be another cultural influence on childrearing during the puerperium. Many religious rituals, such as baptism or bris, introduce the newborn to the religious community. Moreover, customs that family members observe may be based on their cultural background.

Other chapters focus on the African-American family, East Asian families in the United States, the Chicano (Mexican-American) family, and the Puerto Rican family to illustrate cultural influences on pregnancy and delivery. This chapter discusses the American Indian family (also referred to as Native Americans) and how it traditionally perceives childbearing

and child rearing. Nurses must be aware of the cultural orientation of a childbearing family to understand the unique needs of its members in the postpartum period. Individual differences, however, exist within any group. Although the need for individualized assessment and care cannot be overemphasized, the nurse must be alert to the importance of providing culturally sensitive care for the childbearing family.

Cultural Focus: The American Indian Family

Perhaps more than for any other minority group in the United States, it is difficult to discuss common cultural characteristics of North American Indians; they include both American Indians and natives of Alaska. There are approximately 500 Indian tribes in the United States, each with its own culture and customs (Lutz, 1997; Seideman, Jacobson, Primeaux, Burns & Weatherby, 1996). Health care professionals must learn about the culture of the community from which their clients come.

Every American Indian family should be individually assessed to determine its unique patterns and characteristics. Identification of several broad cultural patterns and characteristics, however, may help the nurse understand the responses of the client to the childbirth experience. These patterns, not the specific family structure and function, are the focus of this section.

American Indians live predominately in 26 states, mostly in the western part of the United States. States with the largest number of American Indians are Oklahoma, Arizona, California, New Mexico, and Alaska (Spector, 1996). Most major cities in the United States have populations of American Indians, Alaskan natives, or both. More than half of the American Indians and Alaskan natives do not consider reservations their principal residence.

Traditional Family Organization. Although families from different tribes have very different organizational patterns, some commonalties are observed among American Indian families. The three-generation extended family remains an ideal for many (Seideman et al., 1996). Parental activities are often delegated among grandparents, aunts, and uncles. Traditionally, cousins were considered as close as siblings, and incest taboos applied to even distant cousins. In earlier times, grandparents often had a major role in the care of infants and young children, with parents responsible for the economic matters of the family. Aunts and uncles often had particular disciplinary and teaching responsibilities, freeing the biologic parents for more pleasurable interactions with children (Seideman et al., 1996).

In that structure, which was child centered, children had ties from birth to several parental figures. They provided the security of affection and a variety of role models for the developing child. This family structure is still a highly desirable ideal, and many American Indian families strive to maintain these important ties.

Role of Women. In most American Indian nations, women are respected and influential. The woman is traditionally the most verbal family member and the member who holds the family together. Some nations are matrilineal, so children "belong" to the mother's clan. In matrilineal clans, women are often the ones to make important decisions (Kramer, 1996).

Role of Children. Children are highly prized and desired by the American Indian family. The sex of the first-born child often does not seem to matter to parents. In a matrilineal clan, however, a girl is often desired. The child's upbringing is permissive, and physical punishment rare. Children are often allowed to unfold and develop naturally, at their own pace. For example, children wean and toilet-train themselves at their own rate with little interference from adults. Although limits are set concerning proper and life-threatening behaviors toward others, the child is free to choose whether or when to engage in a wide variety of behaviors. Consequences of behaviors, rather than parental direction, teach lessons to children. Guilt is not a tool used to persuade children to conform. The children often have trouble in schools designed for children in the dominant culture (Seideman et al., 1996).

Cultural Characteristics. In the traditional American Indian culture, "present" has a different meaning from the linear concept of here and now. The American Indian's concept of present is geared to personal and seasonal rhythms. Present time orientation is flexible (Kramer, 1996) and may not be based on actual clock or calendar time. Life cycle events, such as childbearing, are rhythmic. At each stage of life, the focus is on the present, with little concern for the next or succeeding stages. Consequently, a pregnant woman may focus only on her childbearing and give little thought to care of the infant.

The American Indian desires to understand and work in harmony with natural forces. Submission, through acceptance of overwhelming natural events that cannot be controlled, is part of life for the American Indian. This attitude may lead to a high-risk pregnant mother refraining from participating in a high-tech antenatal medical regimen, which can frustrate health care professionals.

American Indians view the needs and goals of the group as more important than the needs and goals of the individual. The group may be the Indian nation, community, family, or other identifiable cluster of people. Communal sharing of essentials is important in the American Indian society. Thus, it may be difficult to convince a pregnant woman receiving benefits from the Women, Infants and Children (WIC) program to keep her milk and food for her own needs if such essentials are needed by children and other members of the extended family.

Although the group has primary importance, a person has innate, individualized potential. American Indians respect the autonomous, natural unfolding of the personality of each person, a concept called "noninterference." Generally, the American Indian speaks for him or herself except when too ill to do so (Kramer, 1996). Confrontation related to control of behavior is often limited to making sure that the other individual is aware of the consequences of behavior. Health care professionals often see this behavior as uncooperative.

The traditional American Indian believes that health is living in total harmony with nature. Each nation has its own variations in beliefs about sickness (fate, evil spirits) and health. Physical illness and genetic defects may be viewed as resulting from behaviors that are socially unacceptable, whereas mental illness may result from a loss of harmony with the environment and from breaking taboos (Kramer, 1996). Health promotion of the individual and family occurs through participation in religious ceremonies and rituals. Kramer (1996) points out that physical stamina is promoted through running and aerobic exercise performed during rituals; purification or cleansing is promoted through "sweating" rituals.

Among American Indians, the traditional healer or medicine person (shaman, spiritual leader) plays an important part in the health of the people (Kramer, 1996; Spector, 1996). This medicine person is seen as wise in the ways of nature and the relationships between humans and the environment. Medicine persons may be welcomed and necessary collaborators in health care. The traditional healer looks for the spiritual cause of a health problem. His or her cure is for the whole person.

Health Care Problems. Several specific health problems affect American Indians. Spector (1996) ranks the five primary causes of death as (1) heart disease, (2) accidents, (3) malignant neoplasms, (4) chronic liver disease and cirrhosis, and (5) cerebrovascular disease. However, according to Lutz (1997), chronic obstructive pulmonary disease and other lung diseases, heart disease, and malignant neoplasms are 20–30% less for American Indians when compared to all U.S. races. Furthermore, Lutz (1997) reports that the death rates among American Indians are 100% greater for trauma and accidents, diabetes, chronic liver disease, and cirrhosis compared to other races. Leading causes of morbidity include accidental injuries, cirrhosis, alcoholism, attempted suicide, attempted homicide, malnutrition, and deformities resulting from fetal alcohol syndrome (Spector, 1996). Gallbladder and cervical disease is also more prevalent in selected Indian populations (Lutz, 1997).

Many of the principal causes of death and illness are directly related to alcohol abuse, a widespread and severe problem in the American Indian community. Two problems facing the nurse working with mothers and infants also stem from the problems of alcohol abuse: domestic violence and fetal alcohol syndrome (Lutz, 1997).

Traditionally men and women are seen as harmonious parts of an ordered universe (Spector, 1996); however, this pattern seems threatened among American Indians, in large part due to current economic pressures. Although women can market their housekeeping skills in modern society, many men, especially in urban settings, are without work. This pattern often generates female-dominated households with poor male role models for boys. Alcohol abuse and economic pressures contribute to a woman's vulnerability to violence. Violence may occur during pregnancy. This is in conflict with the American Indian male role to protect the family and community (Kramer, 1996).

Fetal alcohol syndrome is a very difficult problem facing American Indian parents, given the high value placed upon children in this culture. Parents often deny their child's problem. Media campaigns that focus on frightening parents into sobriety seem to provide little help, and they cannot reverse the physical effects on children.

Childbearing. The birth rate for American Indians is approximately twice the national rate, with 25% being teen pregnancies and more than 50% of first-time mothers being under 25 years of age (Lutz, 1997). In the 1970s, the maternal morbidity rates for the American Indian were twice that of the white population (Lutz, 1997). By the mid-1980s, the maternal mortality rate for American Indians had dropped significantly to almost equal with all races in the United States (Lutz, 1997). Although access to health care varies depending upon whether one lives on a reservation or in an urban setting, prenatal care in the first trimester now exceeds 60% (Lutz, 1997).

In the 1960s the infant mortality rate began declining more rapidly among American Indians than among the rest of the U.S. population, and in 1982 it was slightly lower than that of the white population. The *post*-neonatal mortality rate for American Indians, however, is twice that reported for white children; low birth weight is the primary contributor. Other causes include the prevalence of diarrhea among American Indian infants and the difficult environment in which they live (Spector, 1996).

As noted earlier, the American Indian philosophy views pregnancy as part of the rhythmic, cyclic pattern of life. There is a deep respect for life, childbearing, and children (Seideman et al., 1996). Childbearing is viewed as "healthy," and mothers are encouraged to think positive thoughts. Although childbirth is approached differently among nations, several common threads are shared related to pregnancy, labor and delivery, and the puerperium (Kramer, 1996):

- Prenatal care is expected.
- Although a healer is the health care provider, the laboring woman's mother or other female kin may be a birth attendant with a normal delivery.
- The father may be expected to avoid hunting and eating meat immediately after birth until the infant's cord falls off.
- The mother and her infant recuperate indoors for 20 days or until the cord falls off.
- Pain control includes meditation and indigenous plants.

The postpartum is often highly structured by custom. For example, traditional Navajo women may deliver at home with a tribal midwife and the extended family. After the delivery, the placenta is buried (a fairly common traditional Indian practice). The postpartum Hopi woman drinks hot herbal tea, perhaps to ensure that the uterus contracts; the infant is given a herbal emetic to provoke vomiting whatever was swallowed during birth (Spector, 1996). Traditional Navajo women breastfeed their infants, but do not begin immediately. Modern Navajo women, on the other hand, may go to the Indian Health Service for delivery by a physician or midwife; breastfeeding is not as common as it is among more traditional women.

One postpartum or newborn tradition in many nations is the use of a cradle board or some variation (Fig. 28–6), which enables the infant to be easily transported with the parents as they move about. Each nation has its own rituals and ceremonies related to the cradle board, including decorations.

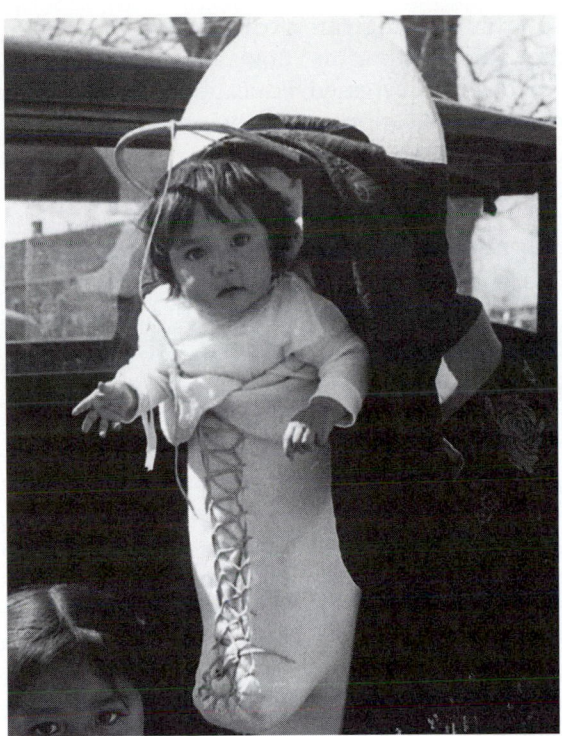

FIGURE 28–6. A Bannock infant is carried in a traditional cradle board.

atmosphere with relaxed surveillance. Postpartum assessment needs to be done to confirm wellness and identify high-risk conditions.

In the early postpartum period, the nurse plans and provides care in collaboration with certified nurse-midwives, physicians, registered dieticians, social workers, and other specialists as needed. Nurses may also refer new mothers to community resources, such as parent support groups.

In many institutions, nurses and physicians develop a list of standing orders that are effective in treating many common physiologic problems encountered in the puerperium, such as pain. The nurse then helps the woman select an appropriate treatment. If pathologic problems develop, such as hemorrhage, the nurse notifies the physician and/or nurse-midwife and a collaborative plan of care is implemented.

Because healthy women are often discharged within 24–48 hours following a normal vaginal delivery, discharge planning should ideally begin prenatally. When ongoing problems are identified, the birthing center or hospital nurse responds to the special needs of a family and may refer them to an appropriate agency for follow-up care at home. In some settings, a nurse or outreach worker may make a home visit to ensure continuity of care.

► OVERVIEW OF POSTPARTUM CARE

The postpartum is the period when a woman's physical and psychologic functioning following childbirth is restored and the foundation for relationships among the parents, newborn, and other family members are being established. Nursing care plays a critical role in the attainment of restoration and healthy family relationships.

Postpartum care is provided in a variety of settings. Traditional hospital settings provide care to women and their newborns on a postpartum unit, separate from labor and delivery. However, birthing centers and many hospitals now use the same room to provide care during labor, delivery, recovery, and postpartum in what is termed LDRP, or single room maternity care unit (SRMC). The LDRPs offer a home-like setting for childbirth within the walls of a hospital and spare the woman the transfer to another unit. In settings where LDRP is not possible, couplet care to the mother and her newborn by one nursing staff, as opposed to traditional care in which mother and newborn receive care from two separate nursing staffs, is often offered.

Postpartum assessment is the same regardless of the setting. Nurses should not confuse a relaxed

► THE DATA BASE

The initial subjective data base includes a review of systems pertinent to the puerperium. Subjective data collection also focuses on a woman's daily habits, history, changes during pregnancy, labor and delivery experience, perception of present status, and cultural and social expectations. Any current problem should have a complete symptom review, exploring onset, duration, location, quality, quantity, precipitating factors, aggravating factors, alleviating factors, time-associated factors, and previous history of a similar problem. Subjective data should also include the mother's perception of her knowledge level concerning self-care, the puerperium, infant feeding methods, infant care, and family dynamics. After the initial data base is collected, subsequent daily subjective data focus on present status and potential problems, needs, and assets.

Although most women are stable after delivery, the immediate postpartum may not be the appropriate time to obtain in-depth subjective data or to assess educational needs. The mother's need for rest, food, and fluid; her need to interact with significant others; her degree of pain and discomfort; and the effects from medications frequently determine the nature of nurse–client interactions. Further assessment is done after the mother has had an opportunity to rest.

Subjective data can be obtained prior to or along with the physical examination. As problems or needs are identified, the nurse can provide interventions at the time when the mother is physically assessed.

The objective data base includes the physical assessment data (collected through the use of inspection/observation, palpation, percussion, and auscultation) and laboratory data. Physical assessment is usually performed from the general to the specific, and in a cephalocaudal (or head-to-toe) manner. The healthy mother is given a postpartum physical examination, frequently referred to as the postpartum check. A postpartum check typically includes assessment of the mother's emotional status, blood pressure, pulse, respirations, pain/discomfort level, breasts, uterine fundus, bladder, perineum, lochia, and extremities. Temperature is assessed after delivery. During the first hour after delivery, components of the postpartum check, except for the breasts and temperature, are assessed every 15 minutes. Thereafter, in general, the postpartum check, including breasts and temperature, is once every 8 to 12 hours for healthy women who delivered vaginally. Mothers are also assessed for fatigue, hunger, and thirst. If the mother is receiving intravenous fluids, the IV site and amount of fluid infused thus far and the amount of fluid in the bag are assessed. Additional assessments are warranted for women who had a cesarean delivery, i.e., respiratory status, abdominal dressing/incision, urinary output via an indwelling catheter, and the ability to move and turn. Women who have had anesthetics need to be assessed for recovery from these agents. A description of the physical assessment of major systems is provided under the section entitled Nursing and Collaborative Assessment.

In addition to the postpartum check, the nurse collects objective data related to the mother and infant on a 24-hour basis. A postpartum flow sheet (Fig. 28–7) can be a helpful guide for postpartum assessment.

Analysis of all data identifies physical, psychosocial, and educational problems, needs, and assets from which care plans are developed. Because much of

postpartum nursing care evolves from educating the mother, the postpartum flow sheet delineating the knowledge area assessed, education given, and evaluation of the education, can be helpful in documenting this facet of care.

► NURSING AND COLLABORATIVE ASSESSMENT

► General Data and Survey

Subjective data, obtained daily, focus on the mother's own perception of her level of energy; a symptom review of discomfort and other problems; degree to which such basic needs as sleep, hunger, and cleanliness are met; ability to perform self-care; success of breastfeeding (if appropriate); emotions and feelings (about labor and delivery, the baby); knowledge of safety precautions; and identification of areas of concern or education deficits. Additionally, the mother's ongoing evaluation of the success of interventions is needed.

The objective general survey of the postpartum mother includes skin color, facial expression, grooming, posture, motor activity, gait, personal hygiene, body odor, speech, level of awareness/consciousness, mood, and affect. Data collected from the general survey, when combined with the general subjective data, often determine the focus of immediate nursing care. Complaints of extreme fatigue, lack of energy, little sleep or rest, and a high degree of discomfort coupled with a depressed mood, slouched or bent posture, and inability to provide self-care alert the nurse that the needs for physical and psychologic restoration have not been fulfilled yet. If these needs are not met, the mother may be unable to interact with and care effectively for her newborn. Subsequent nursing assessments and care are focused on the initial cues the nurse receives from the mother.

Nursing care is planned so that such assessments as vital signs and uterine, bladder, and perineal checks are coordinated. Such an approach promotes comprehensive evaluation of the client's actual status and minimizes disruptions for the client. Timing of assessments is done according to protocols for the birthing facility and as needed to ensure client well-being.

► Vital Signs

During the first hour postpartum, the mother's pulse, respirations, and blood pressure are assessed every 15 minutes. If stable, pulse, respirations, and blood pres-

Nursing Alert

A woman who has received epidural anesthesia or analgesia should not get out of bed until full sensation and movement have returned.

Client's name _____   Gravida _____   Para _____
                                    Delivery date _____

Physical assessment			
	Remarks		
Vital signs			
Blood pressure			
Pulse			
Respirations			
Temperature			
Fundus			
Condition			
Height and location			
Lochia/vaginal discharge			
Color			
Amount and condition			
Number of pads changed			
Breast			
Breast or bottle feeding			
Breast assessment			
Nipple assessment			
Incision/lacerations (REEDA)			
Perineum			
Episiotomy site			
Lacerations			
Abdominal incision			
Appearance			
Dressing change			
Wound irrigation			
Nutrition			
Diet			
Intake			
Fluids			
Type and amount			
IV solution, rate, site			
Elimination			
Voided			
Amount			
Any discomforts			
Bowel movement			
Number and type			
Constipation			
Treatments			
Comfort measures			
Rest			
Pain (type, location, intensity)			
Interventions			
Sitz bath			
Witch hazel pads			
Surgigator			
Pericare			
Analgesic perineal spray			
Analgesic (name, route, time)			
Other			

FIGURE 28–7. Postpartum flow sheet of physical and psychologic assessments and possible educational needs of the client.

Psychosocial assessment			
Remarks			
Coping 　Appearance, behavior			
Interactions 　Maternal/infant 　Paternal/infant 　Sibling visitation 　Grandparent 　Support systems			

Education			
Knowledge and skills	**Date and time**	**Present: mother, father, other supports**	**Outcome (needs reinforcement, return demonstration, assessment)**
Postpartum assessments			
Comfort measures			
Sitz bath procedure and frequency			
Pericare 　Medications			
Nutrition			
Elimination			
Exercises			
Preventive measures 　Rh (D) immune globulin 　Rubella 　Breast self-examination 　Family planning 　Reportable signs and symptoms 　Physician/midwife appointment			
Discharge planning			
Rest/sleep			
Exercises/daily activities			
Sexual activity/family planning			
Return to work			
Infant care 　　Appearance 　　Senses and reflexes 　　Temperature taking 　　Sleep/wake cycles 　　Stools 　　Feeding 　　Bathing 　　Cord care 　　Circumcision care 　　Skin 　　Handling 　　Diapering 　Community resources			
Parenting classes 　　Lactation support (consultant/group) 　　Day care 　　Car seat rental 　　Child health clinics 　　Referral			

FIGURE 28–7 *(continued).* Postpartum flow sheet of physical and psychologic assessments and possible educational needs of the client.

sure are then assessed at half-hour intervals for 1 hour, followed by vital sign checks every 4 hours for 24 hours and thereafter as needed.

A pulse rate of 50 to 70 beats per minute is quite common. High pulse rates (for example, over 100) may indicate hemorrhage, cardiac disease, infection, and anxiety. When the mother experiences tachycardia, the nurse should immediately assess for hemorrhage by focusing on the blood pressure, uterine tone, quantity of lochia, and condition of the perineum or abdominal dressing/incision.

Blood pressure should be fairly consistent with prelabor measurements. A suddenly low blood pressure alerts the nurse to hemorrhage, orthostatic hypotension, and a possible adverse reaction to regional anesthesia (if hypotension occurs shortly after administration of regional anesthesia). A blood pressure elevated well above the mother's baseline blood pressure—or an increase of 30 mm Hg in systolic pressure, 15 mm Hg in diastolic pressure, or both—suggests pregnancy-induced hypertension (PIH). The nurse needs to assess for headaches, epigastric pain, edema, and hyperreflexia. The mother should be instructed to lie on her left side, and a physician should be notified. The nurse should be prepared to place the mother on seizure precautions should the hypertension persist.

During the first 24 hours, temperature is usually normal. Slight elevations in the temperature up to 38°C (100.4°F) suggest dehydration. Higher elevations during the first 24 hours or a temperature above 38°C after 24 hours may indicate infection. Temperature is assessed at the beginning of the first hour postpartum. If the mother is afebrile, temperature is assessed at least every 8 hours during the first 24 hours, or as needed. The nurse should assess the mother for overt signs of puerperal infection (see Chapter 29).

Respirations generally are within normal limits in the puerperium. Slightly increased respirations may be present with anxiety and pain. A slightly diminished respiratory rate may be the result of analgesia and anesthesia. Women who have received certain epidural analgesics, however, need to be assessed carefully for the first 24 hours, because of the risk of respiratory depression. Respiratory depression secondary to narcotic administration is treated with a narcotic antagonist, such as naloxone (Narcan), levallorphan (Lorfan), or nalorphine (Nalline).

▶ Lungs

The nurse does not need to routinely assess the lungs of a woman who has delivered vaginally unless there are signs of respiratory infection, distress, or depression; existing PIH; cardiac disease; water intoxication; or the woman has received general or spinal anesthesia or epidural analgesia/anesthesia. The nurse, however, does need to observe the quality and rate of respirations and be alert for signs of respiratory difficulty, as some women are predisposed to embolic disease.

▶ Abdomen

General Tone

The shape, appearance, and general muscle tone of the puerperal abdomen often concern women. Postpartum women frequently express their displeasure with their flabby, still-pregnant-looking abdomens. Subjective data focus on the individual woman's perception of self, her body image; knowledge of the gradual change in the shape and appearance of her body; and knowledge of exercises.

On physical assessment the puerperal abdomen, in the first week after delivery, looks about 5 months pregnant. The abdomen is frequently flabby, unless distended with flatulence. With trapped flatus, the abdomen distends upward, as opposed to laterally, when the mother is lying down in the bed. A large, flabby abdomen indicates diminished muscle tone. Most often the rectus abdominis is separated, a condition termed *diastasis recti abdominis*. To assess for diastasis of the muscles, the mother is instructed to lie flat and then raise her head, placing her chin on her chest. A visible pouching out of the abdomen running vertically from the xiphoid process to the symphysis pubis is found on inspection. On palpation the separation of the muscles is evident and may be measured.

Bowels

The nurse takes a history of bowel elimination. Emphasis is placed on obtaining data about bowel habits, quality and timing of last bowel movement, dietary and fluid intake, how much the woman usually walks or what other exercise she achieves, presence of perineal and rectal discomfort, and use of aids to promote bowel functioning. The nurse elicits the information in terms of prepregnancy history, pregnancy history, intrapartum experience, and the postpartum.

The nurse must also take into account any analgesics and other medications given to the mother. Codeine and codeine products may promote constipation.

To assess for bowel functioning the nurse first inspects for abdominal distension as discussed previously. Then the nurse auscultates the abdomen in all four quadrants. Further assessment of the abdomen is performed through percussion and palpation. Normal bowel functioning is characterized by bowel sounds—that is, clicks and gurgles—occurring at a rate of 5 to 34 per minute; generalized tympany and areas of dullness (caused by varying amounts of fat), with a prominent tympanic gastric bubble over the stomach; and a soft abdomen. High-pitched tinkling sounds are indicative of intestinal air and fluid under tension in the bowel. Sluggish bowels, characterized by abdominal distension, infrequent bowel sounds, generalized tympany of the bowels upon percussion, and a lack of bowel movements, are common in the first few days postpartum as a result of the common occurrences of loose bowel movements or an enema during labor, lack of food ingestion while in labor, and diminished activity level after delivery. In the first few days after delivery some women do not resume their usual dietary intake. If constipation occurs, the abdomen may be distended.

As the postpartum woman's dietary intake of roughage and fluids increases, and as the effects from anesthesia and labor and delivery diminish, peristalsis increases. For many women, bowel functioning is restored without difficulty. Such conditions as episiotomies, lacerations, and hemorrhoids may be painful enough to hinder bowel movements and thereby predispose the woman to constipation.

Uterus

During the early postpartum, the mother's knowledge about uterine involution, uterine massage, and reproduction should be assessed. Additionally, the nurse collects objective and subjective data concerning characteristics of the uterus and of lochia including amount, color, odor, and changes noted, as well as data pertaining to afterpains.

Uterine Involution. With each postpartum assessment, uterine tone is evaluated by palpating the fundus. Before the procedure, the woman is asked to void, as a full bladder can push the fundus upward and to the side and prevent accurate assessment. The mother is then asked to lie with the bed flat. The nurse places one hand on the lower abdomen. The nurse moves the other hand downward, beginning a few centimeters above the umbilicus, and palpates for the fundus (Fig. 28–8).

The fundus should be contracted and firm when palpated. In addition, the fundus should be in the midline of the abdomen. Various notations are used by nurses to record fundal assessment. For example, a fundus that is firm, midline, and 1 fingerbreath below the umbilicus may be recorded as "FFU-1, midline" or "FF U/1, midline."

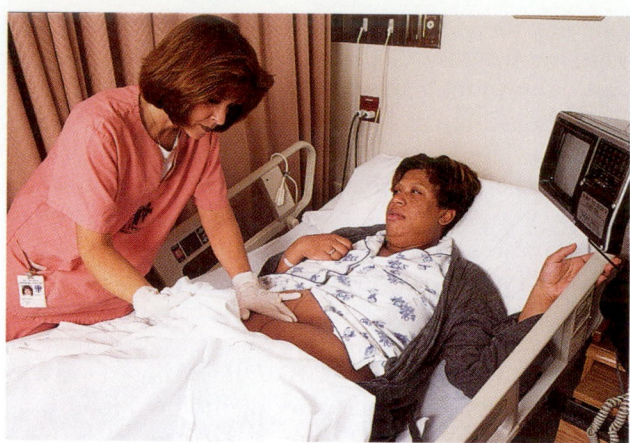

FIGURE 28–8. Nurse palpating fundus to assess uterine involution.

While palpating the uterus, the nurse should assess for excessive uterine tenderness. Abdominal guarding, facial grimacing, and subjective verbalization of extreme pain may indicate uterine tenderness and suggest an infection of the uterus. Medical follow-up and monitoring for signs and symptoms of infection are indicated.

Occasionally the nurse may find that the fundus is soft, boggy, and deviated to one side. This can be a sign of a full bladder. The woman should be asked to void and then the uterus reassessed. When the bladder is emptied, the fundus should be firm and midline. The nurse should advise the client of the need to empty the bladder frequently. External fundal massage to stimulate fundal contraction should be performed by the nurse while at the same time observing the vaginal blood flow. If the uterine atony is due to retained placental tissue, the nurse may observe that as the fundus is massaged, blood clots with tissue are expelled from the vagina. If the uterine atony is due to infection, the lochia may have a foul odor. Whenever the nurse finds a soft and boggy fundus, the amount, odor, and quality of lochia should be assessed, recorded, and reported.

The nurse should report to the physician or certified nurse-midwife if uterine atony persists after the bladder is emptied, if tissue is expelled, or if lochia is foul smelling or excessive. Lochia obtained from the uterus is collected for culture and sensitivity when an infection is suspected.

Lochia. The nurse routinely assesses the amount, consistency, color, and odor of lochia. The woman voids and cleanses her perineum before the postpartum check, and the nurse asks to see the used peripad before it is wrapped and discarded. The nurse asks how long the pad had been worn (when it was applied). Subjective data are needed regarding the amount of lochia, number of pads worn since the woman was last assessed, and passage of any blood clots. Women often express concern about the amount of lochia and seek reassurance that it is normal. Nurses should wear disposable gloves when examining the perineum or the peripads, as a precaution against transmission of any bloodborne infections.

The amount of lochia is estimated to determine whether blood loss is excessive. Immediately after delivery, lochia can be moderate and then diminishes. Usually during the first few days, lochia rubra is light to moderate, with 4–8 peripads used daily. As the lochia changes to serosa and then to alba, amounts decrease further.

Jacobson (1985) developed a standard to improve the accuracy of lochia assessment: If the stain on the peripad is less than 1 inch in size, the lochia is scant; if lochia is between 1 and 4 inches, it is light; if between 4 and 6 inches in length, it is moderate; and if the pad is saturated, lochia is heavy. In a recent study, Luegenbiehl (1997) found that nurses tend to overestimate the amount of blood loss. However, when given education regarding the specific brand of peripad and how it looked and felt with varying amounts of lochia, nurses' estimation of blood loss improved. Because brands of peripads vary in the amount of blood they can hold, Luegenbiehl (1997) recommends that each institution identify how the particular brand of peripads used looks or feels when lochia is scant (3–9 cc); light or small (14–22 cc); moderate (30–45 cc); and large or heavy (55–75 cc).

In general, saturation of one pad within 15 minutes, or saturation of more than one pad within an hour, suggests hemorrhage. If a woman reports that her pads have been saturated in a short period, the nurse should place a clean peripad, determine whether the bladder is full (see the section entitled Bladder later in this chapter), assess her vital signs, check the condition of her fundus, and monitor the amount of lochia during the next hour. A steady flow or seepage of lochia can also indicate hemorrhage (AWHONN/Johnson & Johnson Consumer Products, Inc., 1996). Suspected hemorrhage is reported to a physician or certified nurse-midwife without delay.

If a more accurate assessment of the amount of lochia is needed, the peripad can be weighed and compared to the weight of a clean, unused peripad. Linens and bed pads can also be weighed if needed. One mL of blood approximately equals 1 g.

When blood loss is considered to be significant, either intrapartum or postpartum, anemia screening is indicated. In the past, physicians routinely ordered hemoglobin and hematocrit testing on all postpartum women. This practice was based on work by Taylor and Lind (1981), which indicated that hemoglobin levels on the second postpartum day best predict hemoglobin concentration by 6 weeks postpartum. However, shortened hospital lengths of stay in various states have led to screening earlier than the second postpartum day, and treatment is often not initiated in asymptomatic postpartum women nor needed for women delivered vaginally. Nicol, Croughan-Minihane, and Kilpatrick (1997) recommend limiting anemia screening to women with a significant blood loss.

Afterpains (Postpartum Contractions). During the first few days postpartum, uterine contractions, called **afterpains,** frequently cause abdominal discomfort. More afterpains are experienced by multiparous, lactating women, and women who had a greatly distended uterus, as from multiple gestation, a large fetus, or polyhydramnios. Among multiparous women, the uterus has cycles of contracting and relaxing, whereas among primiparous women the uterus is more likely to remain contracted. Lactating women most frequently experience contractions while breastfeeding, as a result of the release of endogenous oxytocin with the milk ejection reflex. A lactating multiparous woman may experience strong contractions during infant feedings.

Bladder

To assess the urinary system and bladder functioning during the puerperium, data obtained from each woman should include her history of elimination pattern, UTI, and bladder distention or urinary retention; her current ability to void; presence of urgency, burning, or frequency; amount, color, and concentration of current voids; and whether she senses that her bladder has been emptied or that it is full. In addition, a mother's general knowledge about hygiene and how to prevent UTIs should be assessed.

Physical examination of the bladder is done when the uterus is assessed. Women at risk for difficulty in voiding are assessed frequently. The routine may be more often in some settings, for example, with bladder checks every 15 minutes for the first hour; every 30 minutes for the next 2 hours; every hour for the next 2 hours; every 4 hours for the next 24 hours; and thereafter, every 8 hours.

Prior to examination, the client is asked to void. Unless the woman has voided recently, a measured void of less than 100 mL can indicate urinary overflow from a distended bladder. With the woman supine, the nurse inspects the abdomen for bladder distention. An empty bladder will not be visible. As the bladder fills, the surfaces become convex. When the bladder contains more than 500 mL of urine, a bulge is visible in the lower abdomen. When the bladder is greatly distended, an ovoid mass well above the symphysis pubis is visible. Then the uterine fundus will be soft, boggy, and often displaced to one side. To avoid that, the client is advised to void frequently.

To percuss or palpate the bladder the nurse starts about 2 inches (5 cm) above the symphysis pubis and moves downward. Percussion of a filling or full bladder will emit a dull sound. The bladder may be palpated when it contains at least 150 mL of urine. If the bladder contains a large amount of urine, the woman will experience a sense of pressure. The palpated bladder feels soft, fluid filled, and ballottable, that is, easily pushed about.

Generally, within 4 to 8 hours of delivery women have regained their urge to void. In the next 48 hours, postpartum diuresis takes place and the woman will frequently urinate. As much as 3000 mL of urine per day, with 500 to 1000 mL of urine at one void, is possible during the 2nd to 5th postpartum days.

Because of the tendency to retain urine in the early postpartum period, there is an increased risk of developing a UTI. Women who repeatedly need to be catheterized and/or women with an indwelling catheter are also at risk for developing an urinary infection. Signs and symptoms of a puerperal UTI include: dysuria, frequency, urgency, suprapubic tenderness, and fever. When there are signs and symptoms suggestive of infection, urine is collected for culture and sensitivity and a urinalysis performed.

Strict monitoring of intake and output is necessary for postpartum women with an indwelling catheter. Less than 30 mL of urine per hour, or less than 600 mL in 24 hours, suggests a problem related to urine production. After the catheter is removed, the first few voids should be measured to establish that the voids are not merely the result of overflow.

Kidney

Kidney infection is suggested if pain is elicited when assessing the costovertebral angles (CVAs) for tenderness. The angles are formed by the 12th ribs and the vertebral column. To assess for tenderness, the nurse places the palm of the left hand over a CVA and strikes that palm with the ulnar surface of the right fist. Normally no pain is elicited; however, if it is, kidney infection is suggested.

► Back

The postpartum woman should be asked about back pain or discomfort. If an epidural or spinal anesthetic was used during delivery, the nurse checks the site for redness, swelling, or bruising. Women who received epidurals or spinals may normally report some back soreness at the site.

► Perineum

Although the perineum refers to the tissue between the vaginal introitus and anus, assessment of the perineum includes the anus as well. The comfort, or discomfort, of an episiotomy, lacerations, or hemorrhoids must be assessed. A complete symptom review is done, emphasizing the conditions that improve or worsen discomfort. In addition, the nurse must assess whether the woman can independently perform perineal care and whether the woman can identify interventions that best relieve her discomfort and at the same time promote healing.

To assess the perineum, the woman is placed in Sims' position—on the left side with right knee and thigh drawn up, and her left arm extended along her back. In this position, also called semiprone, the upper buttock is lifted so that the perineum is visible. A penlight is often needed so the perineum can be seen well.

Episiotomy and Lacerations

Postpartum women often experience much discomfort from repaired perineal lacerations and episiotomies, and the nurse assesses the area for signs of healing, trauma, and infection. Davidson (1974) identified an acronym, **REEDA,** to evaluate episiotomy healing: *Redness, Edema, Ecchymosis, Discharge,* and *Approximation.* Nurses need to describe and record the location and extent of redness, edema, and ecchymosis. Discharge, if present, should be described in terms of quality (serous, serosanguineous, bloody, or purulent) and quantity. In terms of approximation, nurses note the degree to which the episiotomy or repaired laceration is intact. The extent and depth of skin separations should be described, that is, the length of separation and the layers of skin affected.

During the first day edema and redness are common, but the edges of the episiotomy or repaired lacerations should be intact and there should be no discharge. If the perineum was traumatized during the delivery, ecchymosis may be present. Severe redness, edema, ecchymosis, and the presence of discharge inhibit healing of the perineum. In particular, moderate to severe redness and edema and the presence of discharge are indicative of infection.

Hemorrhoids

Hemorrhoidal discomfort often accompanies a vaginal delivery or a cesarean delivery after a long unsuccessful second stage of labor. Internal hemorrhoids may become external with the forces of labor. Both internal and external hemorrhoids may enlarge from the pressure exerted on the pelvic floor.

The anal area is examined for hemorrhoids. They are described in terms of number, size, presence of bleeding, and degree of tenderness.

Hematomas

Women with hematomas can be asymptomatic, but often women experience severe perineal pain or rectal pressure that may simulate a need for a bowel movement. During a physical examination, postpartum vulvovaginal hematomas are suspected when a mass which displaces the vagina and/or the rectum is found. Edema and a purplish discoloration are often present. Small hematomas may not be visible or palpable.

Hematomas may bleed and, if excessive, the woman may hemorrhage. The nurse should notify the physician or nurse-midwife of any hematomas so that prompt treatment, if needed, can be initiated. Medical treatment may involve incision and evacuation of the hematoma (see Chapter 29).

▶ Extremities

In the immediate postpartum, women who had regional analgesia or anesthesia are assessed for lower extremity sensation. Women delivered vaginally are also assessed for the ability to stand. Generally, the woman who has had an epidural for analgesia during labor has lower extremity sensation and can safely stand by the end of the first hour after delivery.

Over the next couple of days, the extremities are assessed. A history of venous disease should be determined. Swelling, skin color, signs of pain, or varicosities in the extremities should be noted. The lower extremities are routinely assessed for edema and indications of venous disease; however, the upper extremities may also be evaluated for similar signs.

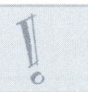 *Nursing Alert*

Bleeding caused by hematomas may not be overt. Therefore, signs of internal hemorrhage (e.g., increased pulse, decreased blood pressure, pallor, clamminess, hypovolemia, and anemia) in the postpartum woman need to be assessed carefully.

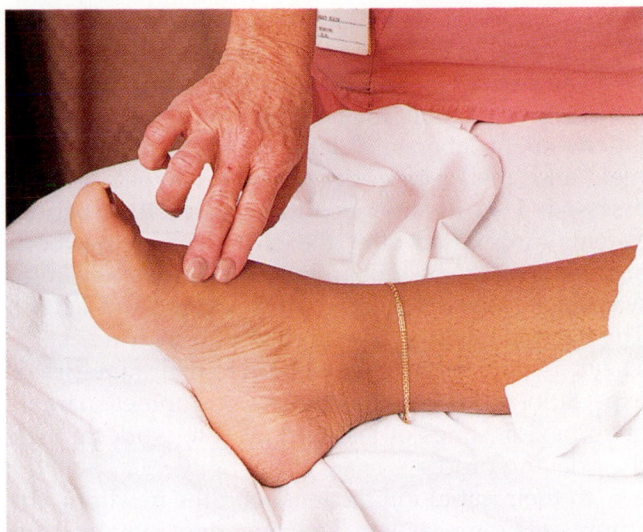

FIGURE 28–9. Nurse assessing client's foot for edema.

Edema is assessed by pressing over a bony prominence such as the dorsum of the foot and pretibial area (Fig. 28–9). If edema is present, the nurse notes if pitting occurs. The extremities are compared for temperature (by palpation). A localized area of redness, increased temperature, and tenderness over a vein suggests thrombophlebitis.

Calf pain on dorsiflexion of the foot was considered a positive Homans' sign. However, overt clinical signs and symptoms may be absent in clients with deep vein thrombosis. Therefore, Homans' sign is now considered an unreliable test for deep vein thrombosis. Nevertheless, a client's complaint of leg pain or tenderness should be reported to the nurse-midwife or physician for further investigation.

▶ Neurologic System

Reflexes are expected to be within normal limits. Women with hyperreflexia may be experiencing PIH, with the potential for a seizure. If hyperreflexia is present, the nurse should assess for other signs of PIH, such as increased blood pressure, proteinuria, and edema and inform the physician or nurse-midwife.

▶ Psychosocial Assessments

The emotional status of the mother is assessed through observations and direct verbal communication. The mother's emotional state after delivery may range from elation to exhaustion (AWHONN/Johnson & Johnson Consumer Products, Inc., 1996). By three to ten days after delivery, mothers may cry easily and relate that they have "postpartum blues."

The parents' reactions to their intrapartum experience, feelings about the baby, degree to which expectations about labor and delivery and the baby were met, and their sense of parental competency are assessed. Usually in the initial postpartum period, parents are excited after the birth of their newborn and focus on the overall appearance of their newborn, wanting to know the newborn's weight and length. The parents focus on identifying with their newborn. They compare the actual newborn to their fantasies or expectations. When expectations are unmet, parents often have feelings of loss and need to work through the grieving process.

In their initial interactions with the newborn, the parents may appear less assertive; they may wait for direction from the nurse regarding when to interact with their newborn, e.g., when to feed the baby or when to change the diaper. However, within the first day or two the parents demonstrate that they are incorporating the newborn into their family and are more autonomous in their interactions with the newborn.

To ensure that the newborn will be in a nurturing and safe environment and that appropriate newborn care will be provided, ongoing assessments are made of the parent(s)–infant interactions and extended family or significant other interactions with the newborn. In particular, the nurse assesses for signs that attachment between the parent(s) and newborn is progressing, e.g., touching, skin to skin contact, eye contact, listening to one another, positive statements by the parent regarding the newborn, acceptance of newborn's behavior, and newborn responding favorably to parents providing care and comfort.

During the early postpartum, the nurse identifies who the caretakers will be and their ability to provide care and nurture the newborn. If the caretaker is an aged grandmother who has limited mobility, follow-up in the home is indicated to assess for adaptation. Furthermore, the knowledge level and educational needs of the parents or caretakers are assessed prior to discharging the newborn from the birthing center or hospital.

▶ Socioeconomic Assessments

The socioeconomic assessment which began preconception or prenatally continues through the postpartum period. The family structure is assessed to identify resources, the support structure, the role of family members, and the ability to obtain and purchase necessary baby care items. The safety of the home environment is addressed. Women are asked where they will be living after the delivery; whether they will be returning home alone or with a support person; and whether they are homeless. At a time when confidentiality and privacy can be ensured, all mothers should be asked about domestic violence and abuse.

▶ Nursing Diagnoses

Assessment in the postpartum period provides the nurse with data about the client and her family. Diagnoses can then be developed from the subjective and objective data. These nursing diagnoses allow the nurse to plan individualized care that reflects the client's healthy and unhealthy responses.

Nursing diagnoses for the postpartum period typically focus on normal physical alterations that result from delivery, transition to parenthood, and psychosocial issues. Examples of nursing diagnoses that may apply to the client in the postpartum period include:

Problem-oriented diagnoses:

- Risk for infection, related to perineal laceration during labor and delivery
- Body image disturbance, related to changes of pregnancy in the maternal body
- Ineffective family coping: compromised, related to cultural conflicts between parents and relatives regarding newborn care

Wellness-oriented diagnoses:

- Asset in normal progress of involution, related to minimal trauma during labor and delivery and uterine contractility
- Asset in sibling coping, related to early family interaction at sibling visitation in postpartum period
- Asset in paternal–infant attachment, related to paternal engrossment behaviors
- Asset in integration of newborn in family, related to performance of cultural rituals (e.g., baptism, naming ceremonies)

▶ NURSING AND COLLABORATIVE MANAGEMENT

Working collaboratively with the postpartum woman and her family, the nurse prioritizes the plan of care. Physical restoration and relief of discomforts often are of great importance to the mother. Care needs to be directed towards meeting the woman's physical needs so that the mother can take on the tasks of motherhood. Additionally, postpartum care for the entire family focuses on helping the family members to incorporate the newborn into the family and take on new roles.

► Promoting Maternal Safety

In the immediate postpartum period, safety precautions are discussed with the mother and any family members present. The call bell should be placed within the mother's reach and she should know how to use it (Fig. 28–10). The mother's environment should be organized to allow easy access to a bedside telephone, waste baskets, and tissues. The mother is cautioned against getting out of bed unless assisted by the nurse. Assistance is necessary until she is physically stable. Because postural hypotension can occur, especially when getting out of bed for the first time after delivery, the mother is instructed to sit and dangle her feet over the side of the bed for a few minutes before standing. If she feels well, the mother can then be assisted out of bed. The nurse may carry spirits of ammonia to use if the mother becomes faint. When the mother is in the bathroom, location and use of the emergency call bell is reviewed.

► Promoting Uterine Tone and Minimizing Afterpains

Interventions are often needed to promote uterine tone. In the immediate postpartum period, the nurse

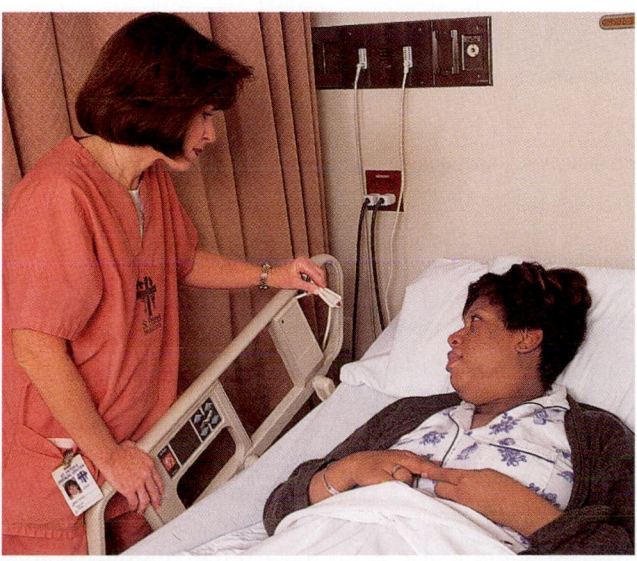

FIGURE 28–10. Nurse assessing safety measures for the new mother, such as ensuring that the call bell is in easy reach.

needs to make certain that the bladder is emptied so that uterine atony and hemorrhage are prevented. Additionally, to prevent uterine hemorrhage, fundal contraction should be stimulated with external fundal massage. Frequently women receive oxytocic agents such as methylergonovine maleate (Methergine) or oxytocin (Pitocin) to stimulate uterine contractions.

Postpartum women should receive information concerning normal uterine involution. They should be taught how to feel for the fundus and how to perform fundal message if excessive bleeding occurs. If the woman is receiving oxytocic agents to promote uterine tone, she will need information concerning their action, route of administration, expected duration of treatment, and side effects. The nurse should advise the woman that a rapid increase in activity can increase uterine bleeding. Prior to discharge from the hospital or birthing center, the woman should be counseled concerning ovulation, menstruation, sexual activity, and family planning, as discussed later in this chapter.

Interventions for uterine afterpains include suggesting that the woman do breathing and relaxation exercises or teaching her how to do them, and administering analgesics, such as ibuprofen. Lying on the abdomen or placing a warm water bag or warm heating pad against the abdomen may also promote comfort.

► Promoting Elimination Health

Establishment of healthy bowel and bladder functioning after delivery often requires nursing intervention. Postpartum women need to be informed that proper exercise and adequate diet contribute greatly to the restoration of abdominal and bowel health and promote bowel elimination and expulsion of flatus. If the women does not have a bowel movement, an enema may be indicated.

Oral stool softeners and laxatives are frequently given routinely to prevent constipation. They are the treatment of choice for women with fourth-degree lacerations, as the administration of suppositories and enemas can rupture sutures for extensive lacerations. After lacerations have healed, an enema, if needed, is permitted.

Antiflatuent medications, such as chewable simethicone (Mylicon), may be administered after meals and at bedtime to prevent the formation of gas pockets in the gastrointestinal tract. Frequent changes in position when lying in bed and early ambulation post-cesarean delivery also contribute to the release of flatus.

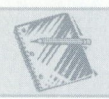

Client Teaching

Interventions to Relieve or Prevent Constipation During the Postpartum Period

The nurse can share the following strategies with the postpartum client who is either experiencing constipation or is at risk of experiencing constipation:

- Drink at least 6 to 8 glasses of nonalcoholic fluids a day to keep stool soft and promote hydration, assuming renal function is normal.
- Eat a diet that contains fresh fruits, raw vegetables, whole bran or whole grain cereals, and bread to provide fiber.
- Exercise daily to promote peristalsis.
- If unable to have a bowel movement within 2 to 3 days, take either a glycerine suppository, bisacodyl (Dulcolax) suppository, or 30 mL of milk of magnesia.

Some women are unable to void after a vaginal delivery and experience urinary distension. To stimulate voiding, several interventions may be helpful:

- Provide privacy.
- Avoid use of a bedpan if possible; have the woman get up and use the toilet.
- Run tap water.
- Pour warm water over the vulva.
- Encourage voiding in a shower or in a sitz bath followed by a shower.
- Expose the urinary meatus to fumes from peppermint spirits; 2 or 3 drops in a bedpan relaxes the meatus.
- Have the client drink a warm beverage.

If the bladder remains distended after the first void, the woman is asked to void again in 1 hour. Usually after the second void the bladder is emptied. If, however, the woman is unable to empty the bladder adequately, a straight catheterization may be advised, after which the woman is assessed frequently for bladder filling and her ability to urinate. Usually, only one straight catheterization is needed.

Because both the tendency to retain urine in the early postpartum period and the use of a catheter are associated with UTIs, interventions need to be taken to prevent these infections. Nurses should advise women to drink fluids; to ingest products rich in vitamin C; to wear cotton underwear; to carefully clean the perineum; and to urinate at least every 3 to 4 hours.

▶ Promoting Perineal Comfort

Nursing care of the perineum focuses on general pericare; Kegel exercises to strengthen the pubococcygeal muscle; interventions to reduce swelling, increase circulation, promote healing, and provide temporary relief from perineal discomfort; and ways to determine when the perineum has healed. In addition, because hemorrhoids and hematomas are in close proximity to the perineum, interventions aimed at reducing hemorrhoids and hematomas increase perineal comfort and thus are included in the discussion.

General Pericare

The postpartum woman is taught to rinse and wipe the perineum from the front toward the back after each void or defecation to prevent contamination of the vagina and urinary meatus. A plastic peribottle filled with warm water is an efficient means of rinsing the perineum. Some hospitals have surgigators in the bathroom that spray an antiseptic, water, or both, onto the perineum. A new peripad should be applied each time the woman urinates or defecates, and at least every 3 hours while the woman is awake.

Kegel Exercises

Kegel exercises in the postpartum period increase circulation to the pelvic floor and thereby promote healing of the pubococcygeal muscle, an episiotomy, and perineal laceration. (Exercise is discussed later in the chapter.)

Interventions to Reduce Swelling, Increase Circulation, Promote Healing, and Provide Temporary Pain Relief

In the first 8 to 24 hours, a cool pack should be applied to the perineum to minimize swelling through vasoconstriction. The pack may be commercially prepared or the nurse may use a rubber glove filled with ice and wrapped with a washcloth. To avoid damage to the skin, ice should not be applied directly. Some health care providers recommend a sitz bath with cool water to provide relief.

After the first 24 hours, a warm or cool sitz bath is commonly used to promote healing and comfort. Prior to using a sitz bath, the woman should cleanse the perineum with a peribottle or shower.

Sitz Bath. Most institutions provide individual plastic sitz baths that can be taken home. The plastic sitz bath consists of a basin that fits into the commode or toilet with the seat lifted away. A plastic bag with tubing, similar to an enema bag, is filled with warm or cool water and placed at a level above the basin. The tubing is then attached to the inside of the basin. The basin is filled with warm or cool water, and the tubing is clamped off. The woman is instructed to sit in the bath with her gluteal muscles relaxed so that the perineal body can receive the treatment. To freshen the water, a woman should unclamp the tube and allow water to enter the basin; excess water will flow out through the back of the basin and down into the commode or toilet. Sitz baths are effective treatments that may be used for 10 to 20 minutes, two to four times a day.

Other Treatments. For temporary pain relief, oral analgesics such as acetaminophen, ibuprofen, and oxycodone may be offered. Many women need analgesics for the first few days. Application of local anesthetic sprays and ointment and witch hazel pads to the perineum may also provide temporary relief. Placing the woman in a knee-chest position, along with Kegel exercises and buttock tucks, can promote perineal healing, minimize pain, and reduce swelling. Some health care professionals advocate sitting on a hard surface rather than a soft chair, which directs the woman's weight toward sore perineal tissues.

Care of Hemorrhoids and Hematomas

Interventions for hemorrhoids and small hematomas are similar to those used in treating an episiotomy or lacerations. In the first 24 hours after delivery, cool packs may be applied to the perineum and anus to minimize swelling. Thereafter, moist heat, as provided by a sitz bath, can help to reduce hemorrhoidal swelling and hematomas by increasing circulation. Cool witch hazel pads placed on the hemorrhoids are soothing and help to relieve and prevent itching. Women can be taught to replace the hemorrhoid into the anorectal canal with a lubricated glove or finger cot, and then assume a knee-chest position for a short period of time.

▶ Promoting Mobility

Walking in the postpartum period should be encouraged to increase circulation, prevent stasis of fluid and venous complications, and promote gastrointestinal motility. Women with edema and varicosities may be given support stockings to wear when walking. They should be encouraged to elevate their legs while lying supine and discouraged from crossing their legs or wearing tight, elastic-band knee high stockings, which impede circulation. Women should be told that as the body returns to the nonpregnant state, edema will diminish and varicosities may also lessen in severity.

▶ Immunizations

Rubella

Because of the severe birth defects that can result when a pregnant woman contracts rubella, women are screened prenatally for antibody titers. Rubella immunization, however, is deferred until the postpartum period. Consequently, during the early puerperium, the nurse identifies women who need rubella counseling and immunization (see box entitled Drug Guide: Rubella Virus Vaccine). Women who are immunized should be advised not to become pregnant for 3 months because of the potential risk to a fetus (McEvoy, 1996).

Despite the availability of the rubella vaccine, many women have not been immunized. In addition, if a girl is immunized before she is 5 years old with MMR (measles-mumps-rubella) vaccine, she may, by the time she is 20 or 30 years old, lose her immunity. Thus, rubella screening of childbearing women and immunization of appropriate postpartum women are important.

Prevention of Rh Sensitivity

The most severe hemolytic disease of the newborn results from Rho(D) isoimmunization, which occurs when the Rh-negative woman has antibodies to the Rh factor and is pregnant with an Rh-positive fetus. The antibodies destroy fetal Rh-positive red blood cells. If destruction is severe, the newborn may die.

Isoimmunization of an Rh-negative woman may be the result of a previous pregnancy if that fetus had Rh-positive blood. Although most fetal–maternal bleeding occurs during childbirth, fetal and maternal blood may come into contact at other times; for example, during antepartal bleeding, amniocentesis, or abdominal trauma. When contact occurs, an Rh-negative mother who lacks the Rh blood factor will identify the Rh-positive fetal red blood cell as an antigen. Then, unless prevented, the mother will produce antibodies to the antigen. As little as 0.1 mL of Rh-positive cells may stimulate antibody formation, although the exact number of Rh-positive cells that will provoke isoimmunization in the Rh-negative women is unknown (Pernoll, 1994).

▶ DRUG GUIDE: RUBELLA VIRUS VACCINE

ACTIONS/INDICATIONS

Rubella virus vaccine live promotes long-term immunity to rubella by inducing the production of specific antibodies in individuals over 12 months of age. Active immunity to rubella prevents intrauterine infection, which can result in miscarriage, abortion, stillbirth, and congenital measles syndrome. The combination measles, mumps, rubella virus vaccine live (MMR) is the vaccine of choice when rubella immunization is indicated and the individual is also likely to be susceptible to measles, mumps, or both.

STABILITY

In lyophilized form, vaccines containing rubella virus should be refrigerated at 2 to 8°C but may be frozen. The vials containing diluent may be stored at room temperature. After reconstitution with the diluent provided by the manufacturer, the vaccines should be refrigerated at 2 to 8°C and discarded if not used within 8 hours. Both lyophilized and reconstituted vaccines should be protected from the light.

DOSAGE

Rubella virus vaccine live is administered only by subcutaneous injection, preferably into the outer aspect of the upper arm. Vaccines containg rubella virus live are reconstituted by adding the entire amount of diluent supplied by the manufacturer to the corresponding vial of lyophilized vaccine and agitating the vial.

Reconstituted vaccine containing rubella virus live should be inspected visually for particulate matter and discoloration prior to administration. The vaccine should be reconstituted and administered using sterile syringes and needles that are free of preservatives, antiseptics, and detergents, as these substances may inactivate live viruses; a 25-gauge, 5/8-in. needle is recommended for administration of the vaccine.

The usual dose is 0.5 mL, regardless of age, administered in a single dose. Children vaccinated with MMR vaccine before age 5 may lose immunity by age 20 to 30. Children who received rubella virus vaccine live when less than 12 months of age should be revaccinated.

CONTRAINDICATIONS AND PRECAUTIONS

No allergic reactions have been reported. The vaccine is contraindicated in individuals who have had an anaphylactic reaction to topically or systemically administered neomycin because each dose contains approximately 25 mg of neomycin.

Because replication of rubella vaccine virus may be potentiated in individuals with primary immunodeficiencies (e.g., cellular immune deficiency, hypogammaglobulinemia) or with suppressed immune response resulting from leukemia, lymphoma, other malignancies affecting the bone marrow or lymphatic system, or blood dyscrasias, the rubella virus vaccine live is contraindicated. The vaccine

should not be given to an individual with a family history of congenital or hereditary immunodeficiency until the immunocompetence of the individual has been documented. The vaccine may be given to individuals with HIV infection.

Rubella virus vaccine live generally is contraindicated in individuals receiving immunosuppressive therapy (e.g., corticosteroids, corticotropin, alkylating agents, antimetabolites, radiation therapy), although the manufacturer states that the vaccine is not contraindicated in individuals receiving corticosteroids as replacement therapy. Febrile respiratory illnesses or other active febrile infections are contraindications to receiving the vaccine, whereas a simple upper respiratory infection does not preclude vaccination. Pregnancy is a contraindication to receiving rubella vaccination for 3 months after vaccination.

ADVERSE REACTIONS

Incidence increases with age of vaccine. Symptoms associated with natural rubella infections including lymphadenopathy, rash, urticaria, fever, malaise, sore throat, and headache; nausea and vomiting occur occasionally in vaccinees. Symptoms may occur 11 to 20 days after vaccination and are usually mild and transient, generally persisting 1 to 5 days. Arthralgias and rarely transient arthritis may occur.

Burning and stinging of short duration may occur at the injection site because of the slightly acidic pH of the vaccine. Induration, erythema, tenderness or pain, and wheal and flare may occur occasionally at the vaccine injection site.

The ACIP and AAP consider rubella virus vaccine live compatible with lactation, but do caution that one case of mild illness in a breastfeeding infant whose mother received the vaccine has been reported.

DRUG INTERACTIONS

- *Tuberculin.* Rubella virus vaccine live has been reported to temporarily suppress tuberculin skin sensitivity; therefore, tuberculin tests should be done before, simultaneously with, or 6 weeks after administration of the vaccine.
- *Vaccines.* Rubella virus vaccine live may be administered simultaneously with an inactivated vaccine, poliovirus vaccine live oral, measles virus vaccine live, and mumps virus vaccine live. Incidence and severity of adverse effects may be increased by concomitant administration of live virus vaccines other than measles or mumps.
- *Immunosuppressive agents.* Possible diminished response to rubella virus vaccine live and replication of virus may be potentiated. Vaccination should be deferred until the immunosuppressive agent has been discontinued for approximately 3 to 12 months. Corticosteroids for replacement are not a contraindication.
- *Immune globulins and blood products.* Vaccination should be deferred in clients who have received blood, plasma, or

► **DRUG GUIDE: RUBELLA VIRUS VACCINE** *(continued)*

more than 0.04 mL/kg immune globulin within the preceding 3 months, as these products contain antibodies that may interfere with the immune response to the vaccine. Rubella virus vaccine live should be given at least 14 days prior to or at least 6 weeks, preferably 3 months, after administration of an immune globulin.

NURSING IMPLICATIONS

- Identify women who have low or zero antibody titer against rubella.
- Advise women to avoid becoming pregnant for 3 months after immunization.

The mother with antibodies to Rh-positive blood presents a potentially dangerous situation in future pregnancies if there is maternal–fetal Rh incompatibility. Specifically, when circulating maternal antibodies cross the placenta and come in contact with the fetal antigen, the fetal red blood cell is destroyed. Hemolytic disease of the fetus and newborn results. Fortunately, Rho(D) isoimmunization can be prevented during pregnancy and the early postpartum.

On admission, maternal blood is drawn for typing. Nurses are alerted for women with Rho(D)-negative blood type. Immediately following delivery, cord blood is drawn to determine the newborn's blood type. If the newborn is Rho(D) positive, the nonsensitized mother is given 300 μg of Rho(D) immune globulin within 72 hours of delivery (see box entitled Drug Guide: Rho(D) Immune Globulin (RhoGAM, Gamulin)). Generally, the standard dose of 300 μg of Rho(D) immune globulin protects the mother against a bleed of up to 15 mL of D-positive red cells or 30 mL of fetal blood (Cunningham et al., 1997). If, however, a large fetomaternal hemorrhage occurs, a larger dose may be given. Occasionally, irritation occurs at the injection site.

► **DRUG GUIDE: RHO(D) IMMUNE GLOBULIN (RHOGAM, GAMULIN)**

ACTIONS/INDICATIONS

To suppress the active antibody response and formation of anti-Rho(D) in the Rho(D)-negative, D^u-negative individual exposed to Rh-positive blood as a result of delivery or an Rho(D)-positive or D^u-positive infant, termination of pregnancy, amniocentesis or abdominal trauma during pregnancy, or transfusion with Rho(D)-positive or D^u-positive blood. It is thought that the immune globulin binds to the antigen and prevents stimulation of the primary immune response.

DOSAGE

Administered by intramuscular injection only (to the mother and not the infant) in the deltoid muscle. *Full-term delivery:* One standard dose vial (contains enough anti-Rho(D) to suppress the immunization potential of 15 mL of Rho(D)-positive or D^u-positive packed red blood cells) in divided doses at different sites within 72 hours of delivery. *Termination of pregnancy:* Up to 12 weeks of gestation, one microdose vial (contains enough anti-Rho(D) to suppress the immunization potential of 2.5 mL of Rho(D)-positive or D^u-positive packed red blood cells) within 72 hours. At 12 or more weeks gestation, one standard dose vial is given within 72 hours.

CONTRAINDICATIONS AND PRECAUTIONS

Use with caution in clients with history of allergic reactions to preparations containing human immune globulins, and in clients with thrombocytopenia or bleeding disorders. Contraindicated in Rho(D)-positive or D^u-positive individuals or in Rho(D)-negative individuals who have been sensitized to Rho(D) or D^u antigens and have anti-Rho(D) in their serum.

ADVERSE REACTIONS

Most common: Discomfort at injection site, slight fever.
Less common: Myalgia, lethargy, splenomegaly, elevated bilirubin, allergic reactions.

NURSING IMPLICATIONS

- Assess blood group and presence of Rh factor [Rho(D)] in mother and infant.
- Explain to couple rationale for therapy.
- Inform clients who are Jehovah's Witnesses that Rho(D) immune globulin is considered a blood product.
- Administer Rho(D) immune globulin within 72 hours of delivery when mother is Rho(D) negative and infant is Rho(D) positive.
- Administer IM injection deep in muscle.

If an Rh-positive woman accidentally receives immune globulin, a generalized reaction, characterized by lysis of maternal red blood cells, can occur. Careful adherence to necessary precautions when administering medications and blood products will prevent erroneous administration.

► Sleep, Rest, and Comfort

During the normal process of labor and delivery, maternal energy expenditure is high. As a result, most women are physically exhausted. Sleep, rest, and comfort measures are needed to replenish maternal energy.

Bedrest is usually maintained during the first hour postpartum or until the woman's status has stabilized. During this initial recovery period, a quiet, warm environment should be provided for the mother, father, and their newborn. If a private room cannot be provided, the nurse should make certain that the curtains are drawn around the bed to ensure privacy. Frequently, the skin-to-skin contact between mother and newborn, using a blanket over the dyad, or both measures can provide adequate warmth. The nurse helps position the mother and her newborn to promote comfort and prevent undue stress on the tired maternal muscles. The use of supporting pillows behind the mother's head, back, and the arm that cradles the newborn minimizes the work that needs to be done by the mother's body, and thereby conserves energy.

As the initial recovery period comes to an end, the nurse helps the woman to sponge bathe or shower.

Despite the need for rest and sleep, many women are euphoric and unable to rest during the first day postpartum. The euphoria and restlessness, which usually end with the first evening after delivery, are often related to the woman's need to talk about her experience. Many women accept telephone calls and make calls to friends and relatives to talk about the birth experience.

In the hospital, nurses can plan to care for each postpartum woman so that her rest and sleep will not be disturbed. Maternal exhaustion may initially prevent a woman from providing 24-hour care for her newborn. This maternal need for physical restoration should not be viewed as a negative attachment behavior.

Once at home, physical and emotional restoration will remain a priority. Before discharge, a woman needs anticipatory guidance and education about how to get sufficient rest and sleep and how to care for her infant. Nurses help the client by providing information about resuming physical activity, described later. Nurses may also suggest to postpartum women and their partners ways that they might organize activities that are necessary in providing newborn care and self-care for mothers. Guidance is also given about how to deal with uninvited visitors at home. For example, couples are advised to tell visitors that the nurse or physician has said the mother must rest and have visitors only for a short while; or it is suggested that a note be placed on the door stating that mother and infant are sleeping; or the mother is instructed to take the telephone off the hook to prevent interruptions.

► Daily Activity and Exercise

Exercise programs and other activities should be resumed gradually.

Daily Activity

During the early postpartum, a woman is confronted with conflicting tasks: (1) physical and emotional restoration, (2) the need to assume complete responsibility for the newborn, and (3) resumption of previous activities and responsibilities. Her need to complete these tasks can create undue physical and emotional strain.

Light household chores, such as dusting furniture or preparing a meal, are appropriate physical activities for the first week postpartum. If feasible, a woman should enlist the aid of another adult to help with cleaning and laundry until she feels well enough to resume those chores. A woman who tries to resume all household tasks and responsibilities too soon may have increased uterine bleeding, with an increased risk for uterine subinvolution or hemorrhage. The woman, therefore, is taught that increased bleeding may mean she is doing too much. Lifting heavy objects is postponed until healing occurs.

Return to occupational or educational settings depends on the nature of activity that will be undertaken and the woman's unique circumstances. Generally, healthy women who deliver vaginally safely return in 4 to 6 weeks, provided the planned activities are not too strenuous. A woman who had a cesarean delivery should wait at least 6 to 8 weeks before returning to work or school. Some women return sooner.

Many women want to know when they can drive a car again. Generally, women who have delivered vaginally resume driving within a week or when they feel well enough to drive safely; however, women who delivered by cesarean should wait until driving does not cause pain.

Postpartum Exercise

Exercise for postpartum women should promote muscle tone of the pelvic floor and abdomen, and enhance circulation to the lower extremities. A postpartum program discussed with the health care provider usually begins with one exercise; each day another is added. Ideally, exercises are practiced at least twice a day. Women should be instructed that in any exercise session, each exercise (except for Kegel exercises) should be repeated four to five times for the first few days and gradually built up to repetitions of at least 10. Table 28–3 presents an example of a 9-day schedule of exercise for women who delivered vaginally. Women who have had a cesarean delivery should consult their physician before undertaking an exercise program.

More vigorous exercises, such as situps and straight leg lifts, should be postponed until approximately 3 weeks after vaginal delivery (Tulman et al.,

1990). Mothers should be cautioned not to proceed with exercise if vaginal bleeding reappears or if they do not feel well.

▶ Sexual Issues and Family Planning

Sexual Activity

Following childbirth, couples may have many questions about sexual activity; however, it is an intimate topic in many cultures, and couples may hesitate to initiate discussion. Information about sexual activity should be part of routine postpartum care and ideally should be discussed with both partners during pregnancy and prior to the client's discharge.

Traditionally, physicians advised healthy couples to refrain from intercourse until after the postpartum examination, about 6 weeks after delivery. This recommendation was based on beliefs that the perineum

---

▶ TABLE 28-3

Postpartum Exercises

DAY 1. Kegel exercises	Postpartum regeneration of the pubococcygeal muscle may be improved if, prenatally, women are taught Kegel exercises. Kegel exercises can be started soon after a vaginal delivery to strengthen the pubococcygeal muscles and promote healing of the muscle and episiotomy. Approximately 50 to 100 Kegel exercises are needed each day to be effective. To perform Kegel exercises, the woman tightens the perineal (pubococcygeal) muscle, starting at the anus and progressing toward the urinary meatus. Contraction of the perineal muscle is maintained for 5 seconds and then gradually relaxed. The woman can determine if she is doing the exercise correctly by trying the exercise while urinating. If she can stop the flow of urine, she is correctly performing Kegel exercises. They should not be routinely performed when urinating because of the potential for urinary stasis.
DAY 2. Abdominal toning exercise 1: Deep abdominal breathing	The mother, lying supine, inhales slowly and deeply to expand the abdomen. Then, exhaling slowly by either hissing or blowing through pursed lips, she tightens her abdominal muscles. Feet may alternately be moved toward the buttocks while inhaling (Fig. 28–11A).
DAY 3. Abdominal toning exercise 2: Deep breathing with chin flexion	In this modification of the deep abdominal breathing exercise, the mother slowly flexes her chin onto her chest as she inhales and lowers her head back to the floor as she exhales.
DAY 4. Abdominal toning exercise 3: Arm raises	The mother, lying supine with legs parted slightly, extends arms outward so that they are resting on the floor at right angles to the trunk of the body. The arms are gradually raised and the hands brought together. As the hands touch, the arms are gradually lowered. Mothers should be instructed to inhale as the arms are raised and exhale slowly as they are lowered (Fig. 28–11B).
DAY 5. Abdominal back toning exercise: Pelvic rocks	Lying supine with arms down at the sides, knees flexed, and feet firmly on the floor, the mother breathes in deeply and arches her back as she tightens the abdomen and buttocks. As the mother lowers her back and buttocks onto the floor, she exhales slowly (Fig. 28–11C).
DAY 6. Abdominal buttock toning exercise	Lying supine with knees and hips flexed and feet firmly on the floor, the mother tilts her pelvis inward and contracts her buttocks as she lifts her head and shoulders and reaches toward her knees. She then returns slowly to her original position and repeats the exercise, remembering to inhale at the start of the exercise (Fig. 28–11D).
DAY 7. Abdominal and thigh tighteners	Lying with legs straight, the mother raises her head and slightly raises her right knee, as her left hand reaches toward (but does not actually touch) the right knee. The mother should then slowly return to her original position and repeat the exercise using her left knee and right hand.
DAY 8. Buttock, thigh, and abdominal stretching exercise: Modified bicycling	The mother lies supine with arms at her sides and knees and hips flexed. She inhales slowly and raises one leg toward the abdomen, stretching out as if to bicycle. She returns her leg to the original position as she exhales. The exercise is then repeated for the opposite leg.
DAY 9. Buttock, thigh, and abdominal stretching exercise: Modified leg lifts	The mother lies supine with arms at sides and legs straight. One knee and hip are flexed and brought toward the abdomen. The knee is then brought slowly over the other knee (Figs. 28–11E and 28–11F). Shoulders remain flat on the floor. Slowly move leg back to beginning position.

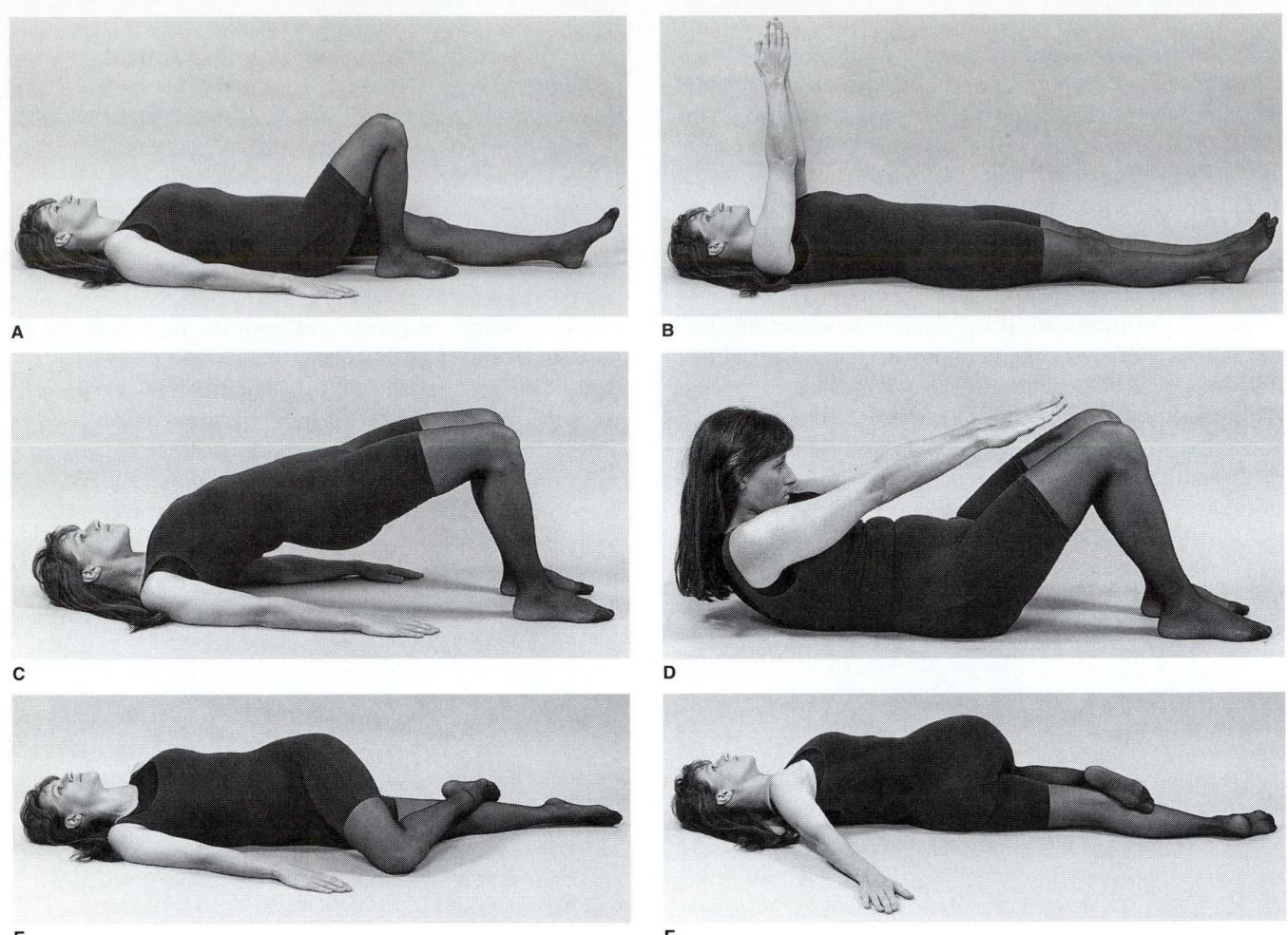

FIGURE 28–11. Postpartum exercises for women who have vaginal delivery to tone abdomen, back, and buttocks. Exercises are described in Table 28–3. **A.** Day 2. **B.** Day 4. **C.** Day 5. **D.** Day 6. **E, F.** Day 9.

needed time to heal, the woman was subject to infection, and the health care provider should confirm that healing had occurred. In reality, such a long time is not usually needed. Current recommendations vary; no specific time has been designated when intercourse should be resumed. Generally, intercourse is safe when bleeding has stopped, the client has healed, and both client and partner desire to have intercourse. For many couples, 2 to 3 weeks postpartum is appropriate (Cunningham et al., 1997; Tulman et al., 1990).

At first, couples may have difficulties with sexual activity. Reestablishment of normal prepregnancy sexual response patterns can be delayed after childbirth, and sexual interest patterns may fluctuate (see Chapter 5 for a discussion about sexuality and the childbearing couple). Discussions with the client or couple about sexual activity should explain the importance of caring, taking time with each other, and noncoital sexual options that enhance and express mutual affection (Tulman et al., 1990).

Vaginal atrophy and dryness, thought to be related to low estrogen levels, may make intercourse uncomfortable, particularly during lactation, which suppresses estrogen production (Cunningham et al., 1997). Water-soluble lubricants, such as K-Y Jelly, promote comfort. Fear of pain and being fatigued, due to the demands of infant care and the expanded family, also affect sexual activity. Moreover, some breastfeeding clients express concern about milk leaking during sexual activity. Nursing the baby prior to sexual intimacy can be helpful.

Clients may not resume intercourse because of their concern about another pregnancy. Family planning options should be discussed with every client prior to discharge.

Family Planning

Most women do not intentionally plan to become pregnant again in the early puerperium; however, some are pregnant by their 6-week postpartum

Women's Health

The use of Kegel exercises to heal the pubo-coccygeal muscle, an episiotomy, or a perineal laceration also enhances vaginal sensation and response during intercourse and can promote resumption of sexual activity during the post-partum period.

checkup. Lack of knowledge concerning resumption of ovulation and their failure to use contraception are frequently the cause.

Counseling women and their partners prior to discharge helps couples to prevent unwanted, unplanned pregnancies. Education must include information about the variations in onset of ovulation and menstruation. Nurses should stress that ovulation frequently resumes before the first menses—indeed, as early as 1 month following delivery. This early resumption occurs particularly among women who are not completely breastfeeding.

Options. Postpartum tubal ligation may be performed if a client is certain she does not want more children. Restrictions and availability, however, vary in different settings. Despite advances in reversing tubal ligations, voluntary sterilization is considered permanent and should not be selected by women who think they may want to have more children.

Condoms and contraceptive foams and gels may be prescribed until the postpartum examination. Diaphragms or cervical caps are usually not fitted until the examination, after involution of the reproductive organs. Then, accurate sizing can be done. The postpartum is not the ideal time to insert an intrauterine device (IUD). The risk of expulsion and side effects is greatest within 2 to 4 weeks postpartum; thus insertion is delayed until 4–8 weeks postpartum (Pasquale, 1996). The IUD has been used for postpartum women who may not return for a 6-week examination. One concern related to the IUD is the woman's need for access to care. Questions arise as to whether this particular method should be used by women who do not have health care readily accessible.

Oral contraceptive use is usually delayed until about 3 weeks after delivery, due to such factors as the hypercoagulable state of the postpartum client. Oral contraceptives tend to reduce milk supply and are thus not recommended for lactating women until milk

flow and breastfeeding are well established. Monitoring the baby's weight indicates adequacy of milk supply.

Medroxyprogesterone acetate (Depo-Provera) has been used for postpartum women and is effective for 3 months. It is not thought to cause such side effects as maternal thromboembolism or milk suppression but does have such side effects as amenorrhea or irregular bleeding (Cunningham et al., 1997). Other progestin-only contraceptives, such as the "minipill" or the time-release levonorgestrel implants (e.g., Norplant), are hormonal contraceptive options that have minimal effect on milk production or neonatal growth and early development (Cunningham et al., 1997).

Postpartum family planning poses a dilemma for women who will consider only natural family planning methods. They are difficult to use until a regular ovulation cycle is reestablished. Clients who will use only these methods and do not want to become pregnant may be advised to abstain from vaginal intercourse until they experience 2 or 3 regular menstrual cycles or until they can again identify changes associated with ovulation.

Breastfeeding does suppress ovulation but is not a predictable method of contraception. When other methods of family planning are either inaccessible or unacceptable, breastfeeding may prevent pregnancy better than using no method; however, suppression of ovulation tends to occur best during the first 6 months postpartum if the mother is completely and consistently breastfeeding.

Couples may elect to temporarily use, for example, condoms and contraceptive foam and then switch to a method of their choice, such as the diaphragm, when the postpartum period is complete. Health care providers must make certain that clients are discharged with plans for fertility control that are acceptable and accessible to them and that they know how to use.

▶ Pharmacotherapeutics

During the early postpartum period, pharmacologic agents may be used to promote uterine contractions and consequently minimize uterine bleeding and relieve pain and discomfort from episiotomy, lacerations, abdominal incision, abdominal flatulence, and afterpains. The nurse is responsible for monitoring the responses to pharmacologic agents.

Promotion of Uterine Contractions

Oxytocin. Synthetic oxytocin (Pitocin) is commonly used in the immediate postdelivery period to stimulate uterine contractions as a means of controlling postpartum bleeding (see box entitled Drug Guide: Oxytocin in Chapter 24). Typically the postpartum dosage of oxytocin is 10 to 40 U/1000 mL of intravenous fluid and given at a rate to control uterine atony.

Ergonovine Maleate. Ergonovine maleate (Ergotrate) is administered as a 0.2-mg oral tablet every 6 to 12 hours to promote uterine contractions postpartum. Within 6 to 15 minutes, and lasting for approximately 90 minutes, this drug produces firm tetanic contractions of the uterus. The tetanic contractions gradually change to more clonic contractions. Known side effects include hypertensive episodes, sudden allergic shock, nausea, and vomiting.

Methylergonovine Maleate. Methylergonovine maleate (see box entitled Drug Guide: Methylergonovine Maleate (Methergine)) rapidly produces a sustained tetanic contraction to minimize blood loss after delivery. This medication is used in cases of subinvolution, that is, when the uterus does not reduce in size as expected. The usual oral dose is a 0.2-mg tablet three to four times a day, up to 1 week. If intramuscular injection is desired 1 mL containing 0.2 mg of the drug is administered every 2 to 4 hours. Intravenous administration of methylergonovine maleate is discouraged for routine usage because of the increased chance of sudden hypertension or cerebrovascular accident.

Relief from Discomfort

Pharmacologic therapy for discomfort from episiotomy, lacerations, abdominal incision, or postpartum uterine contractions ranges from mild analgesics to narcotics and includes combinations of a mild analgesic and narcotic. These medications are usually available to women on an as needed (prn) basis, every 4 hours.

Analgesia. Acetaminophen and ibuprofen are effective for mild to moderate discomfort of the perineum and breasts and for uterine cramping. Acetaminophen also has antipyretic effects. In therapeutic doses acetaminophen usually does not produce side effects. In excessive amounts, acetaminophen can cause gastrointestinal irritability, nausea and vomiting, tachycardia, cyanosis, jaundice, anemia, and liver damage.

Ibuprofen (Motrin, Advil) is a nonnarcotic analgesic that also has anti-inflammatory and antipyretic properties. It blocks prostaglandin synthesis. Ibuprofen is useful in the postpartum for relief of uterine cramping and episiotomy discomfort. The usual dosage ranges from 400 to 800 mg, 3 to 4 times per day, but not to exceed 3.2 g/day. Adverse effects

---

▶ DRUG GUIDE: METHYLERGONOVINE MALEATE

ACTIONS/INDICATIONS

Directly stimulates contraction of uterine and vascular smooth muscle by interacting with receptors for biogenic amines, such as alpha-adrenergic or tryptaminergic receptors. Also produces vasoconstriction, primarily of capacitance vessels. Prevents and treats postpartum and postabortion hemorrhage caused by uterine atony or subinvolution.

DOSAGE AND ROUTE

Administered orally or IM (may be used IV if uterine bleeding is severe and it is given over more than 1 minute). *Oral:* 0.2–0.4 mg every 6 to 12 hours for 2 to 7 days. *IM or IV:* 0.2 mg every 2 to 4 hours as needed (maximum 5 doses).

CONTRAINDICATIONS AND PRECAUTIONS

Use with caution in women with cardiovascular disease or hepatic or renal dysfunction; should not be used to induce labor; hypersensitivity to phenol (injection only).

ADVERSE REACTIONS

Most common: Nausea, vomiting. *Less common:* CNS—headache, tinnitus, dizziness; CV—palpitations, arrhythmias, chest pain, hypertension (especially after rapid IV administration); GU—hematuria.

DRUG INTERACTIONS

• Regional anesthesia: Increased risk of hypertension.
• Vasoconstrictors: Increased risk of hypertension.

NURSING IMPLICATIONS

• Assess vital signs.
• Provide information regarding possible discomforts, such as cramping.

include visual disturbances, renal function changes, and increased tendency for bleeding.

Codeine. Codeine 30 to 60 mg orally is indicated for severe to moderate pain from an abdominal incision, episiotomy, lacerations, and pharmacologically induced uterine contractions. Codeine can depress respirations; decrease gastrointestinal activity, resulting in constipation and decreased mobility of the bladder; produce euphoria; and induce nausea and vomiting.

Oxycodone. Oxycodone is a derivative of morphine and related to codeine. (Percocet combines oxycodone with acetaminophen.) Side effects are the same as those for codeine and morphine.

Epidural Analgesics. Epidural analgesics are used particularly after cesarean delivery. This analgesic method is discussed in Chapter 23.

Simethicone. Simethicone (Mylicon) 40 to 80 mg is used to minimize gastrointestinal discomfort from entrapped flatus, especially after a cesarean delivery. For maximum effectiveness one tablet should be chewed after meals and at bedtime.

▶ Promoting Psychosocial Well-Being

Psychosocial nursing care of the childbearing family during the postpartum period focuses on fostering an integrated, harmonious family unit. This concept is also the basis for programs of family-centered maternity care, which promote family unity and safety. Family-centered nursing care is client oriented and is based on the family's unique needs and cultural background (Phillips, 1997).

Family-centered postpartum care is more than a system for delivering nursing care; it is a philosophy that values, respects, and focuses on the family, however the client defines her family (Phillips, 1997). Family-centered postpartum care provides a family-centered environment to foster attachment (rooming-in, flexible visitation, mother–baby dyad nursing care, and flexible visitation), planning, and discharge teaching.

Promoting Family Safety

As part of safety education in birthing centers and hospitals, parents are instructed on prevention of infant abduction. Specifically, parents are instructed

on the purpose and use of matching identification bands for parents and their newborns. Parents are cautioned to not give the newborn to anyone unless the staff member is properly identified and the parent is aware, and has validated, that the newborn is to be taken.

Attachment

During the postpartum, the nurse observes for normal family–newborn attachment and promotes attachment behaviors. Intervention and referrals to appropriate resources may be necessary if attachment seems problematic.

In observing attachment behaviors, the nurse needs to know that forms designed to measure parental (most often maternal) "bonding" must not be used rigidly. They are simply guides to help the nurse focus on appropriate behaviors. The meaning and pattern of attachment behaviors must be assessed in the context of the total family environment. The nurse should expect that different cultural groups will express attachment behaviors differently.

Promoting Maternal Attachment. Nursing strategies for promoting attachment between mother and newborn include the following:

- Provide care for the mother's dependency needs, such as bathing, rest, and food.
- Encourage the mother to discuss her labor and delivery experience. As she expresses her feelings, she begins to resolve and integrate her labor and delivery into her personal history.
- Encourage participation of the mother's significant others, for example, infant's father, friends, parents. When the mother receives nurturing from others, she can better nurture her infant.
- Encourage the mother to inspect her infant. Encourage her to take the infant out of the blanket and inspect the unclothed infant's toes, fingers, trunk, and face. Inspection fosters identification and allows the mother to replace the "fantasized" infant with the real infant. It also allows the mother to see that her baby is intact. If the infant has a visible physical handicap, the mother can observe the extent of the handicap and begin to grieve. This is an excellent chance for client teaching.
- Encourage face-to-face, eye-to-eye, and skin-to-skin contact to help establish interactions between mother and infant. This can be accomplished by teaching the mother to position the infant at an optimum gazing distance

(approximately 9 to 10 in.). The mother is also taught to interact with the infant when the infant is awake and alert. The breastfeeding mother can be encouraged to put her baby to breast.

- Allow the mother to talk about the infant. At first, the mother may express some disappointment about appearance or sex. At this time, such comments should not be confused with deficits in attachment. Talking about the infant also allows the mother to identify the infant ("Look! he has his father's ears").
- Encourage early and frequent feedings, as feeding is perceived as an act of mothering. Moreover, feeding is an opportunity for close interaction with the infant.
- Encourage the mother to talk to her infant. The infant responds to the mother's voice by moving and looking at her. This type of interaction is a positive experience for both mother and infant.
- Describe to the mother the potential responses and temperament of the infant. Parents need to understand that how the newborn interacts with them depends in part on the infant's behavioral style.
- Maximize the amount of time the mother and newborn spend together in the birthing center or hospital so that the mother may learn about her newborn and newborn care in a secure environment. This can be fostered through rooming-in and/or couplet care (see sections later in this chapter).

Promoting Paternal Attachment. Many nursing strategies that are used to promote maternal–newborn attachment are also appropriate to promote paternal–newborn attachment. Most of the described attachment behaviors are human behaviors and the same strategies work for both mother and father. Specific strategies that focus on the father include:

- Allow early, sustained contact between the father and the infant, beginning in the delivery room.
- Encourage the father to talk about the infant.
- Allow the father to inspect the infant.
- Encourage en face behavior between the father and infant.
- Encourage the father to express feelings which are often intense.

Promoting Sibling Attachment. Sibling involvement is part of family-centered care. Certain strategies can promote sibling attachment.

- Base interventions on the child's growth and developmental levels and cultural background.
- Promote sibling preparation classes, if they are not already conducted, to help siblings prepare for and adjust to the newborn.
- Educate parents about positive and negative aspects of sibling adaptation to the newborn and sibling rivalry.
- Encourage parents to show children constructive ways to express feelings.
- Praise children for positive behaviors towards the newborn.
- Encourage parents to be consistent in disciplining children.
- Allow siblings to visit their mother.
- Encourage parents to focus attention on the older child. For example, parents may present the child with a gift and play with the child alone, without the new baby present.
- Allow the child to touch or hold the infant. Some institutions have sibling rooms to promote this experience.
- Counsel parents regarding expectations of sibling attachment in relation to the child's developmental level.
- Use dolls and play equipment to help the older child express feelings about the new infant.

Promoting Grandparent Attachment. Promoting grandparent attachment is important in providing support for the family. Indeed, some grandparents will be primary caretakers for the baby. Interventions include:

- Encourage involvement with the newborn.
- Encourage visitation of the parents' parents.
- Encourage grandparents to support and help parents in the parenting roles.
- Encourage the parents to support and help the grandparents in the grandparenting role.
- Allow grandparents to discuss their feelings about the new infant and their roles.
- Institute special programs or classes for grandparents.

Rooming-In

With rooming-in, the mother and infant are in the same room for an extended period, rather than for scheduled visits (Fig. 28–12). Rooming-in provides parents and the infant the chance to be together to the extent they desire and facilitates demand feeding and the overall acquaintance process. Many birthing institutions still have a central nursery, and parents transport their infants back and forth between the nursery and room at will.

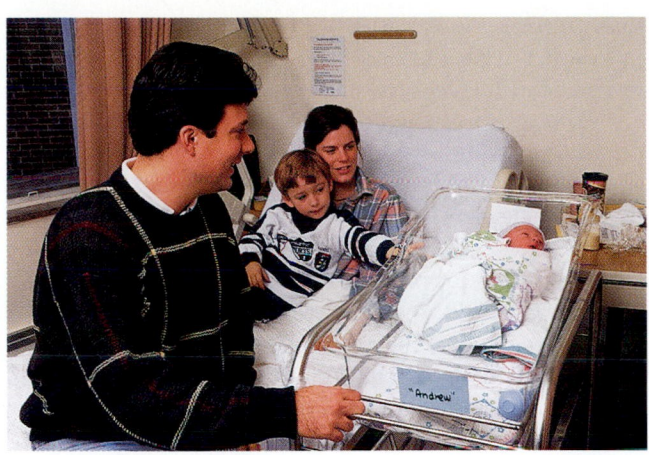

FIGURE 28–12. Rooming-in.

Caregivers should be flexible and nonjudgmental in structuring rooming-in so that each family's needs are met. Several strategies can foster a positive rooming-in experience for a family, as follows:

- Explain rooming-in. Make certain families understand that they are not being abandoned, but have an opportunity to be with their newborn.
- Be available to the family as a consultant for newborn care.
- Organize the room and supplies to facilitate family-centered care.
- Keep unpleasant stimuli, such as noise and human traffic, to a minimum.
- Plan for flexibility in parents' participation in rooming-in.

Rooming-in is not a substitute for nursing assessment and intervention. The nurse should not assume that mothers who room-in, including multiparous women, are either confident or independent. New mothers have many personal needs and require nursing care. For example, mothers who have perineal discomfort may require time to take a sitz bath. A flexible rooming-in situation permits staff to care for the infant while the mother's needs are met.

Mothers' desires for rooming-in may be affected by the method by which nursing care is delivered. Weiss and Armstrong (1991) found that mothers having dyad care preferred to have complete rooming-in, whereas nondyad mothers preferred nursery care. Mothers, regardless of parity, wanted the option of whether or not to have rooming-in or to return their newborns to the nursery at night.

Mother–Neonate Dyad Care

Mother–neonate dyad care, also known as couplet care, has become an increasingly popular postpartum delivery system. Dyad care goes beyond the rooming-in concept to encompass a family-centered philosophy (Phillips, 1997). Staff members are educated to care for both mother and newborn, who may have complete or partial rooming-in. (In traditional hospital settings, nurses tend to work only with the healthy newborn or only with the postpartum mother.) Single-room maternity care units facilitate this system and allow care for the mother and baby to be provided on a 24-hour basis in the same location. Physical care is given to both mother and newborn, client teaching is provided, and charting done. Collaboration is with obstetricians, certified nurse-midwives, pediatricians, and other health care professionals. Essentially, mother–neonate dyad care provides a safe environment for parents to learn about their newborn and for increased opportunities for education (Phillips, 1997). Numerous other benefits of dyad care have been identified: the potential to foster the mother–neonate relationship, the provision of continuity of care, less duplication of services, elimination of problems related to separate nursing staffs caring for the same client, and cost-efficiency in terms of staffing needs (Watters & Kristiansen, 1995; Weiss & Armstrong, 1991).

Actual client satisfaction with mother–neonate dyad care has had mixed reviews. Cottrell and Grubbs (1994) found that women receiving traditional care with rooming-in and those receiving dyad care were equally satisfied with the care given for themselves and their baby. However, Watters and Kristiansen (1995) found that mothers were more satisfied in terms of client education with the dyad care system than with the traditional system.

Flexible Visitation

With flexible visitation programs, fathers are not considered "visitors" and have access to the mother and newborn. Other individuals in the family—siblings, grandparents, relatives, and friends—have flexible visiting hours. (Each program is specified by the birthing institution.) Sibling visitation allows older brothers and sisters to interact with the newborn as they become acquainted.

The nurse can help ensure flexible visitation for childbearing families by educating other health care professionals concerning the benefits of flexible family visitation, instituting such policies for childbearing families in the birthing institution, and encouraging family members to establish a visiting pattern that meets their needs.

Discharge Planning

Discharge planning should take place during prenatal visits, when postpartum care plans are discussed with the client. Ideally, before delivery, women should have a clear idea of where they will receive postpartum follow-up. Care of the postpartum woman takes place in a variety of settings, including homes, birthing centers, and hospitals. Contemporary health care providers no longer view pregnancy and childbirth as illnesses, but rather as healthy phenomena. In accordance with this positive view of pregnancy and childbirth, birthing centers, both within a hospital or free standing, promote early discharge of women, often within 12 hours after a delivery. When a family elects to have an early discharge, home care follow-up is needed. However, in the late 1980s and early 1990s, in a desire to contain costs, many insurance companies revised policies and refused to pay for postpartum hospital stays much beyond 24 hours for women delivered vaginally and 48–72 hours for those delivered by cesarean. Physicians were forced to promote shortened hospital stays for all postpartum women, without taking into account the psychosocial needs of the families and regardless of the availability of postpartum home care follow-up. Because early discharge is not appropriate for all women, nor desired by all, many states have adopted laws that promote 48-hour hospital stays for the woman delivered vaginally and 72–96 hours for women delivered by cesarean.

Many facilities have instituted the use of clinical pathways. These outlines of client care promote continuity of care, minimize duplication of services, and provide a timeline that helps in setting goals and in organization of care. Clinical pathways are particularly helpful with short hospital stays, but also provide guidance and ensure that a standard of care is provided. Figure 28–13 provides an example of a clinical pathway for a woman who delivers vaginally.

Discharge Teaching

Discharge teaching is one of the most important roles of the nurse in preparing the new family to return home. In providing discharge teaching, the nurse must be aware of the socioeconomic status of a family, cultural beliefs, and defined childrearing roles so that appropriate discharge instructions are not only provided, but provided to and accepted by the appropriate people. For example, in many cases the nurse provides discharge instructions to the postpartum woman concerning her physical care; however, in a given culture or family structure, family members may be expected to assist the mother in her care. Furthermore, because many women return to work after the baby is born and in many families extended members assume childrearing roles, a variety of people, in addition to the new mother and father of the baby, may need to be taught about current baby care prac-

tices. Information that is not culturally sensitive or is in conflict with defined family roles and beliefs will not be readily accepted and used.

The resources available to care for a newborn differ among families. In providing discharge instructions concerning baby toys and equipment, the nurse needs to be sensitive to the economic status of the family. The nurse may discuss with middle-income families where appropriate toys and equipment may be purchased. However, in low-income families, the nurse may need to help the parents assess furniture or objects already in their home that might be adapted for the newborn. For example, a drawer removed from the dresser and placed on the floor might substitute for a crib, and a sink for an infant bathing tub. Families can be given information about local stores that sell second-hand infant clothes. The family's religious group might also provide supplies for the newborn. Civic or hospital auxiliary groups may be asked for donations of infant clothing or other articles much needed by impoverished families. Finally, the nurse refers to social services families meeting the state's eligibility criteria for WIC, Medicaid, and Aid to Families With Dependent Children. The nurse's creativity is needed to help financially stressed families.

Depending upon the length of stay and the potential for a home visit, the nurse prioritizes with the mother and her family topics that will be discussed before discharge. Goals of discharge planning include the client's being able to care for herself and her infant. Planning for parent education begins with assessment of the mother's and other family members' learning needs and readiness to learn. A generalized teaching checklist is then individualized for each family. The following methods may be used by the nurse:

- Small group discussion
- Individualized teaching
- Use of audiovisual aids such as diagrams and pictures and, when available, computerized programs
- Return demonstration (for example, the nurse assesses a parent bathing the newborn)
- Development of written instructions to which the family can refer at home
- Suggesting postpartum educational classes after the mother is discharged
- Referral to appropriate community services, such as a breastfeeding support group
- Providing a list of community resources to the family

Throughout the teaching-learning process, the nurse evaluates the strategies used and the family's responses.

Projected LOS: 48 hours
Actual LOS: _____

	Recovery hr.	0–24 hrs.	24–48 hrs.	Discharge (≤ 48 hrs.)	Initial PP visit (4–6 weeks)
Assessments	VS and PP checks as per policy/standard. Urine output, lochia and pain/comfort levels. Mother-infant/family-infant interaction.	Review ante- and intrapartum history and labs. Identify rubella, Rh, hepatitis status. VS, PP checks, voids, BMs, lochia, pain/comfort and family interactions per standard.	→ →	→ → →	→ Family coping/interactions
Diagnostics		CBC. RhoGAM work-up if indicated. Urine C and S if indicated.	→ → →		As indicated.
Treatment and medications	IV fluid, pitocin and analgesics prn/order. Pericare and ice to perineum.	PP kit with periaids, sitz bath (cool → warm). D/C IV as ordered. Meds: iron, vitamins, stool softener and laxatives, RhoGAM as ordered.	→ → → →	Rubella immunization if indicated. Self-care.	Vitamins
Activity	Bedrest with progression to assist to bathroom. Assisted ADL.	Progressive ADL. Up 1st time with assistance. Progress → up ad lib.	→ →	→	→
Diet	Light snacks; encourage fluids.	Regular	Regular	Regular	Regular
Psychosocial	Encourage family interaction with infant. Initiate breastfeeding if indicated.	Mother begins to provide infant care. Appropriate mother-infant/family-infant interactions. Breastfeed q 2–3 hrs. if appropriate.	Mother assumes care for infant. Alert family to signs of postpartum depression.		
Consults	Anesthesia. Social work prn. Pastoral care prn. Lactation consultant prn.	→ → →	→ → →	→ → →	→
Education	Initiate education re: pericare, infant safety, breastfeeding; current status.	Continue education: increase content of self-care, safety, physical and emotional status as per standard. Education re: infant care per nursery standard.	Reinforce education.	→	→ Identify and discuss additional education needs.
Discharge		HCC/VNA if indicated. Initiate discharge planning and instructions.	→ Discharge plan and instructions (PP).	Prescriptions given. Follow-up planned. Discharge instructions reviewed/understood and signed by client.	Plan for routine follow-up.
Outcome	Physiologically stable for transfer to PP unit. Bonding. Breastfeeding initiated.	VS stable. PP checks WNL; voiding. Client demonstrates proper pericare, understands information given.	→ → → → → →	→ → → → →	→ → → Episiotomy/laceration healed. Uterine evolution completed. Stable family-infant relationship.

FIGURE 28–13. Clinical pathway: uncomplicated vaginal delivery, postpartum. *(Courtesy of Ellen Shuzman, PhD, RN, St. Peter's Medical Center, New Brunswick, N.J.)*

► **TABLE 28-4**

Danger Signs in the Postpartum Period

Signs and Symptoms	Complication
Boggy, soft uterus that fails to contract when massaged; uterus remains at same height or rises	Subinvolution (failure of the uterus to diminish in size)
Lochia has strong, offensive odor; blood clots with white tissue; uterine pain; fever	Uterine infection
Bulging/swelling beneath skin of vulva and wall of vagina; intense perineal pain with profuse bleeding; rectal pressure	Hematoma (blood in tissue beneath skin of vulva or vaginal mucosa)
Significantly elevated blood pressure; persistent headache; dizziness; blurred vision; spots before the eyes; edema/swelling of extremities and face; epigastric pain; muscular irritability; convulsions	Pregnancy-induced hypertension
Chest pain; shortness of breath; air hunger; increased respirations; apprehension	Pulmonary embolism (blood clot in the lung)
Pain in calves; localized heat, redness, swelling, and knot-like areas on lower extremity	Thrombophlebitis (blood clot in legs)
Profuse, bright red lochia; increased pulse; large clots	Hemorrhage
Fever; pain/burning on urination; increased frequency or urination; decreased amounts of urine; spasms of urethral meatus; back pain/flank pain	Urinary tract/kidney infection

Role of the Nurse. In discharge teaching the nurse's primary role is to educate the woman and her family. The nurse teaches them how to perform pertinent assessments and what danger signs to note and report (Table 28–4). General postpartum education is also provided; additional information ideally was given in prenatal classes and will also be provided during follow-up home visits.

When delivery occurs at home or when the postpartum woman is discharged early from the hospital or birth center, a nurse may visit the family, perhaps within the first 24 hours. Additional visits and phone calls may follow (Chapter 34). In most health care systems, the postpartum woman is expected to return to the primary health care provider within 6 weeks after delivery. At that time, uterine involution, episiotomy healing, and postpartum adaptation are assessed. Regardless of the birth setting, clients need to have a source to contact for routine questions and for emergencies related to the mother or newborn.

Commonly Asked Questions

How long will my vaginal discharge (lochia) last?

Your vaginal discharge can continue for 3–4 weeks. You can expect:

- Red to reddish brown bleeding for the first 2 to 3 days after delivery.
- A pinkish discharge for several days after.
- By the 10th day after delivery the discharge is white or pale yellow.
- Rapid increases in your activity level may cause prolonged vaginal bleeding or a return of vaginal bleeding in the first few weeks postpartum.
- If you have a return of vaginal bleeding at 4–6 weeks, after a few weeks of no bleeding, you are most likely menstruating.

What should I do if I bleed heavily (saturate one pad or more in ½ hr) or pass large clots?

If you bleed heavily or pass large clots:

- Call your doctor, nurse-midwife, or nurse.
- Make certain you have emptied your bladder.
- If you delivered less than 2 weeks ago, try massaging the top of your uterus. When the uterus is massaged it contracts, becoming firm to help stop bleeding.
- Decrease activity; lie down and rest.
- Make certain you do not lift anything heavier than your newborn.
- Increase the amount of fluids you are drinking.

How should I care for my "stitches" from the episiotomy?

Your stitches are in the perineum, an area between your vagina and rectum. Care of your episiotomy and your genital area is called pericare and includes:

- Using the peri-bottle after urinating, moving your bowels, and when changing your peripad.
- Using a sitz bath 2–4 times a day until your perineum has healed.
- Using Tucks and anesthetic sprays or ointments as needed.
- Changing your peripad approximately every 3–4 hours or more frequently if needed.
- Performing pericare until your stitches are healed and your vaginal discharge has stopped.

How will I know that my perineum has healed?

You can tell that your perineum has healed when:

- You do not have any pain at the site.
- You can insert one finger, then a second finger into the vagina and you do not have any discomfort.

Do my stitches need to be removed?

No. The stitches dissolve over time, and do not need to be removed.

How will I know if I have an infection?

If you have any of the following signs or symptoms, you may have an infection:

- Fever (temperature over 101°F).
- Abdominal pain.
- Nausea, vomiting or stomach/intestinal distress.
- Burning on urination.
- Frequently having to urinate a small amount.
- Foul odor to vaginal discharge or bleeding.
- Heavy vaginal bleeding (saturating one pad in ½ hr).
- Passing large blood clots.
- Increased pain at your episiotomy site.
- If you had a cesarean delivery, incisional redness, tenderness, or discharge.
- Localized pain, swelling, or redness in one breast.

What should I do if I think I have an infection?

If you think you have an infection you should:

- Call your doctor, nurse-midwife, or nurse.
- Increase the amount of fluids you drink.
- Continue with pericare, breast care, and incisional care.

When can I resume sexual activity?

If you delivered vaginally and did not have a fourth degree tear, you can resume sexual activity:

- When your vaginal discharge has stopped.
- When your perineum has healed.
- If you do not have pain or discomfort when one finger, then two fingers, are inserted into the vagina, you can try intercourse using a lubricant such as K-Y jelly.
- If your doctor, nurse-midwife, or nurse has not advised you otherwise.

(continued)

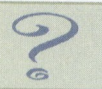 *Commonly Asked Questions* continued

- If you are aware that you may become pregnant even if you have not resumed menstruation ("period").

When will I get my period again?

Your period can return:

- As early as 4 weeks after delivery if you are not breastfeeding.

- As late as several months if you are breastfeeding.
- With or without ovulation (releasing an egg from your ovary).

Critical Thinking in Care Planning

Care of a Client Experiencing Perineal Discomfort

Linda Harris is a 24-year-old primiparous woman who delivered vaginally, with a midline episiotomy. She is presently 24 hours postpartum. On entering the room the nurse observes that Mrs. Harris is sitting awkwardly in bed, trying to breastfeed her son. As the newborn begins to suck, Mrs. Harris groans and, removing her hand from her breast and placing the hand on the bed tries to change her position. The newborn loses hold of the breast and begins to cry. Mrs. Harris looks sadly at her son and cries, "We're not doing too well, are we? I'm not helping you to feed." At this point the nurse reaches out and touches Mrs. Harris' shoulder. Mrs. Harris looks at the nurse and cries, "It hurts so much that I can't even stay in one position long enough to feed him." The nurse asks Mrs. Harris to describe where the pain is. Mrs. Harris replies that "it hurts by my stitches."

▶ Assessment

- Client states that "it hurts by my stitches"
- Pain interferes with caring for newborn
- Client unable to sit in a comfortable position
- Episiotomy red, moderate edema; approximated, no ecchymosis or discharge
- Water from peribottle provides momentary relief

- Client changes peripad every 1 to 3 hours
- Client did 100 Kegel exercises per day during third trimester; has not done Kegel exercises since before delivery
- Client does not use benzocaine spray; does not know how to use sitz bath or its purpose
- Client reports perineal discomfort while breastfeeding infant

Nursing Diagnosis

Pain, related to episiotomy repair and manifested by edema

Expected Client/Family Outcomes	Nursing Action/Intervention	Evaluation
By 1 day postpartum, client will: - State the purpose of sitz bath, benzocaine spray, witch hazel pads, assumption of side-lying position, and resumption of Kegel exercises. - Report decreased perineal discomfort with use of comfort measures.	Assess perineum and level of discomfort. Teach client proper use and purpose of sitz bath, benzocaine spray, assumption of side-lying position, and resumption of Kegel exercises. *Rationale:* Identify normal or high-risk situation. Education is needed to promote self-care; knowledge of purpose of treatment aid or comfort measure can motivate client to use those treatments, aids, and measures.	Client can state purposes of sitz bath, witch hazel pads, benzocaine spray, side-lying position, and Kegel exercises. Client begins to use perineal treatments and comfort measures. Client reports decreased discomfort.
- Demonstrate how to set up and use sitz bath.	Teach client how to set up sitz bath; have client return the demonstration. *Rationale:* Return demonstration evaluates client education.	Sitz bath is set up and used appropriately by client.

(continued)

Critical Thinking in Care Planning continued

Expected Client/Family Outcomes	Nursing Action/Intervention	Evaluation
• Use perineal aids and comfort measures.	Assess client's responses to perineal aids and comfort measures. *Rationale:* To ensure health and safety of all clients, responses to all treatments, aids, and comfort measures must be assessed.	Client uses perineal aids and comfort measures appropriately.
By the 6-week visit postpartum, client's episiotomy site will be clean, dry, intact, and without redness, ecchymosis, or edema.	Teach client self-assessment of episiotomy site. Advise client to call if problems develop. *Rationale:* Self-assessment promotes self-care, keeps client in control of her health, and allows for early interventions if problems develop.	Client reports episiotomy site is progressively healing.
	Reinforce need to continue use of peribottle, changing pads every 3 to 4 hours, after each void and bowel movement. *Rationale:* Reinforcement is a means of promoting the continuation of appropriate client actions.	Client continues to carry out pericare with peribottle, and changes pads every 3 to 4 hours.
At telephone follow-up, client will report progressive healing. At 6 weeks postpartum, client will report that she is free of perineal discomfort.	Provide telephone follow-up support for client after discharge. *Rationale:* Client needs support after discharge to assist in self-care practices.	At telephone follow-up, client reports progressive healing. At 6 weeks postpartum client is free of perineal discomfort; perineum is healed.

Nursing Diagnosis

Ineffective breastfeeding, related to maternal perineal discomfort

By the next feeding, client will obtain temporary relief of perineal pain so that she may effectively breastfeed her newborn.	Place client in side-lying position when she is lying in bed, or advise buttocks tightening prior to sitting. *Rationale:* Side-lying position and buttocks tightening reduces pressure on perineum and anus, thus providing temporary relief.	Client lies on her side in bed and uses buttocks tightening before sitting; experiences a reduction in perineal discomfort. Client is able to resume breastfeeding her newborn comfortably.
	Offer analgesic before feeding newborn if perineal discomfort is severe. *Rationale:* If needed, oral analgesics should be offered before mother interacts with newborn so that medication can have time to act, thus enabling mother to be relaxed and free of pain when with newborn.	Client reports diminished perineal discomfort.
	Teach client to use sitz bath 1/2 hour before feeding newborn. *Rationale:* Sitz bath provides moist heat, which promotes circulation and reduces edema. Sitz baths and peribottle clean perineum.	Client reports relief of perineal discomfort.
	Teach client to change peripad, apply benzocaine spray and witch hazel pads to perineum 15 minutes before feeding newborn. *Rationale:* Soiled peripads can irritate perineum and provide a medium on which microorganisms can grow. Benzocaine spray provides temporary anesthesia to perineum.	Client reports increasing comfort when breastfeeding newborn.

Chapter Highlights

▶ The postpartum period, or puerperium, is a time of physiologic changes in many of the woman's body systems, and primarily in the reproductive system within the uterus, vagina, and perineum.

▶ The addition of a new family member, the neonate, results in psychologic and sociocultural changes within the family that are reflected in transitions in parenting, mastery of new tasks, and adjustment of social networks.

▶ Psychosocial adaptation of the mother during the postpartum period consists of further refinement of the maternal role; formation of the maternal–infant dyad; adjustment to an altered body image; and attention to concerns that focus on self-care and infant care.

▶ Establishment of the mother–child relationship is accomplished through the maternal tasks of bonding with the newborn, identifying with the newborn, and developing feelings of competency in caring for the newborn.

▶ Establishment of the father–child relationship during the postpartum period is accomplished through sensitivity to the newborn's behavioral cues, use of progressive touch behaviors, and feelings of competency in the parental role.

▶ The relationship between the siblings and the newborn is influenced by the ordinal position of each child, the age differences between the children, the sex of each child, and the age of the older child at the birth of the newborn.

▶ Adjustment of grandparents to the birth of an infant is guided by the new parents' desire to either change former patterns of childrearing or continue family patterns from one generation to the next.

▶ Socioeconomic and sociocultural influences affect the way in which the newborn is integrated into the family and the nature of the interaction between each family member and the newborn.

▶ A thorough assessment of the mother and her family is the basis for developing nursing interventions in the postpartum period.

▶ Nursing assessment includes compiling subjective data and performing a general survey of the postpartum mother; monitoring vital signs; examining organs and structures such as the lungs, abdomen, uterus, back, perineum, extremities, and the neurologic system; and conducting psychosocial and socioeconomic evaluations.

▶ Nursing care of the client and family during the postpartum period includes promoting maternal safety; promoting uterine tone and minimizing uterine afterpains; promoting elimination health; promoting perineal comfort; promoting mobility; ensuring administration of necessary immunizations such as rubella immunization and Rho(D) immune globulin; promoting sleep and comfort; recommending appropriate activity and exercise programs; providing information about sexuality and family planning; administering pharmacologic agents to promote uterine contraction and relieve pain and discomfort from associated conditions resulting from labor and delivery; and promoting psychosocial well-being.

▶ Discharge planning should be initiated during prenatal visits and reinforced with the client and family during the postpartum period so that continuity of care is ensured.

▶ The role of the nurse in discharge teaching is to educate the woman and her family about how to perform necessary assessments and what danger signs to note and report during the postpartum period.

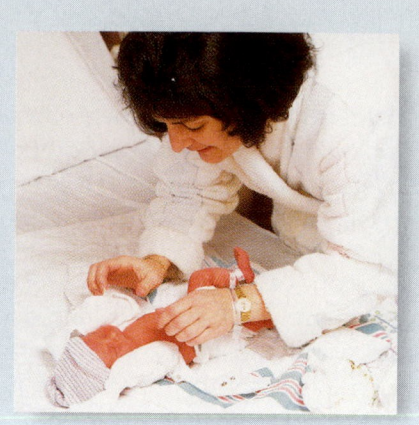

After reading the vignette at the beginning of this chapter, use what you have learned to answer these questions.

1. How can Deborah Bergman's interaction with her baby contribute to Deborah's confidence in her role as mother?

2. How can a nurse caring for a healthy hospitalized postpartum family ensure that the clients' physiologic and psychologic needs are met?

3. What aspects of Deborah Bergman's behavior are examples of attachment and maternal claiming?

Critical Thinking Questions

▶ References

Akins, S. (1994). Postpartum hemorrhage: A 90s approach to an age-old problem. *Journal of Nurse-Midwifery, 39,* 123S–134S.

AWHONN/Johnson & Johnson Consumer Products, Inc. (1996). *Compendium of postpartum care.* Philadelphia: Medical Broadcasting.

Belsky, J., & Kelly, J. (1994). *The transition to parenthood.* New York: Delacorte.

Birk, D. (1996). Postpartum education: Teaching priorities for the primipara. *Journal of Perinatal Education, 5,* 7–12.

Bowes, W.A. (1996). Postpartum care. In S.G. Gabbe, J.R. Niebyl, & J.L. Simpson (Eds.), *Obstetrics: Normal and problem pregnancies* (3rd ed.) (pp. 691–713). New York: Churchill-Livingstone.

Browne-Martin, K., & Emerson, C.H. (1997). Postpartum thyroid dysfunction. *Clinics in Obstetrics and Gynecology, 40,* 90–101.

Campbell, O.M.R., & Gray, R.H. (1993). Characteristics and determinants of postpartum ovarian function in women in the United States. *American Journal of Obstetrics and Gynecology, 169,* 55–60.

Capeless, E.L., & Clapp, J.F. (1991). When do cardiovascular parameters return to their preconception values? *American Journal of Obstetrics and Gynecology, 165,* 883–886.

Chandler, S., & Field, P.A. (1997). Becoming a father: First time fathers experience of labor and delivery. *Journal of Nurse-Midwifery, 42*(1), 17–24.

Cottrell, B.H., & Grubbs, L.M. (1994). Women's satisfaction with couplet care nursing compared to traditional postpartum care with rooming-in. *Research in Nursing and Health, 17,* 401–409.

Cowan, P.A. (1997). Beyond meta-analysis: A plea for a family systems view of attachment. *Child Development, 68,* 601–603.

Cunningham, F.G., MacDonald, P.C., Gant, N.F., Leveno, K.J., Gilstrap, L.C., Hankins, G.D.V., & Clark, S.L. (1997). *Williams obstetrics* (20th ed.). Stamford, CT: Appleton & Lange.

Davidson, N. (1974). REEDA: Evaluating postpartum healing. *Journal of Nurse-Midwifery, 19,* 6–8.

DeSevo, M.R. (1997). Keeping the faith: Jewish traditions in pregnancy and childbirth. *Lifetimes* (August), 46–49.

DeWolff, M.S. & van IJzendoorn, M.H. (1997). Sensitivity and attachment: A meta analysis of prenatal antecedents of infant attachment. *Child Development 68,* 571–591.

Fawcett, J. (1977). The relationship between identification and patterns of change in spouse's body images during and after pregnancy. *International Journal of Nursing Studies, 14,* 199–213.

Ferketich, S.L., & Mercer, R.T. (1989). Men's health status during pregnancy and early fatherhood. *Research in Nursing and Health, 12,* 137–148.

Ferketich, S.L., & Mercer, R.T. (1994). Predictors of paternal role competence by risk status. *Nursing Research, 43,* 80–85.

Ferketich, S.L., & Mercer, R.T. (1995). Predictors of role competence for experienced and inexperienced fathers. *Nursing Research, 44,* 89–95.

Fortier, J.C. (1988). The relationship of vaginal and cesarean births to father–infant attachment. *Journal of Obstetric, Gynecologic, and Neonatal Nursing, 18,* 128–134.

Gamble, D., & Morse, J.M. (1993). Fathers of breastfed infants: Postponing and types of involvement. *Journal of Obstetric, Gynecologic, and Neonatal Nursing, 22,* 358–365.

Grace, J.T. (1993). Mother's self-reports of parenthood across the first 6 months postpartum. *Research in Nursing and Health, 16,* 431–439.

Greenburg, M., & Morris, N. (1974). Engrossment: The newborn's impact upon the father. *American Journal of Orthopsychiatry, 44,* 520–531.

Grohar, J. (1996). Postpartum care. In K.R. Simpson & P.A. Creehan

(Eds.), *AWHONN's perinatal nursing* (pp. 249–270). Philadelphia: J.B. Lippincott.

Gullicks, J.N., & Crase, S.J. (1993). Sibling behavior with a newborn: Parents' expectations and observations. *Journal of Obstetric, Gynecologic, and Neonatal Nursing, 22,* 438–444.

Hall, W. (1991). The experience of fathers in dual-earner families following the births of their infants. *Journal of Advanced Nursing, 16,* 423–430.

Harrison, M.J., & Magill-Evans, J. (1996). Mother and father interactions over the first year with term and preterm infants. *Research in Nursing and Health, 19,* 451–459.

Hartrick, G.A. (1997). Women who are mothers: The experience of defining self. *Health Care for Women International, 18,* 263–277.

Imle, M.A., & Drayden, T. (1996). First time parents' perspectives of their concerns during the postpartum. *Communicating Nursing Research, WIN Assembly. Advancing Nursing Through Research, Practice, and Education, 29,* 152.

Jacobson, H. (1985). A standard for assessing lochia volume. *MCN, American Journal of Maternal-Child Nursing, 10,* 174–175.

Klaus, M.H., & Kennell, J.H. (1982). *Parent-infant bonding.* St. Louis: Mosby.

Klaus, M.H., & Kennell, J.H. (1997). The doula: An essential ingredient of childbirth rediscovered. *Acta Pediatrica, 86,* 1034–1036.

Klaus, M.H., Kennell, J.H., & Klaus, P.H. (1995). *Bonding: Building the foundations of secure attachment and independence.* Reading, MA: Addison-Wesley.

Kramer, J. (1996). American Indians. In J.G. Lipson, S.L. Dibble, & P.A. Minarik (Eds.), *Culture and nursing care: A pocket guide* (pp. 11–22). San Francisco: UCSF Nursing Press.

Lipson, J.G., Dibble, S.L., & Minarik, P.A. (1996). *Culture and nursing care: A pocket guide.* San Francisco: UCSF Nursing Press.

Ludka, L.M., & Roberts, C.C. (1993). Eating and drinking in labor. *Journal of Nurse-Midwifery, 38,* 199–207.

Luegenbiehl, D.L. (1997). Improving visual estimation of blood volume on peripads. *MCN, American Journal of Maternal Child Nursing, 22,* 294–298.

Lutz, D.J. (1997). A guest editorial: Delivery health care to native American women: The challenge continues. *Obstetrical and Gynecological Survey, 52,* 153–154.

Maloni, J.A. (1994). The content and sources of maternal knowledge about the infant. *Maternal-Child Nursing Journal, 22,* 111–120.

Mackey, M.C., & Miller, H.M. (1992). Women's views of postpartum sibling visitation. *Maternal-Child Nursing Journal, 20,* 40–49.

Martell, L.K. (1996). Is Rubin's "taking in" and "taking-hold" a useful paradigm? *Health Care for Women International, 17,* 1–13.

McEvoy, G.K. (1996). *AHFS 96 drug information.* Bethesda, MD: American Society of Health-System Pharmacists.

Mercer, R. (1985). *First time motherhood experiences form teens to forties.* New York: Springer.

Mercer, R. (1986). Predictors of maternal role attainment at one year post birth. *Western Journal of Nursing Research, 8,* 9–32.

Mercer, R.T., & Ferketich, S.L. (1990). Predictors of family functioning eight months following birth. *Nursing Research, 39,* 76–78.

Mercer, R.T., & Ferketich, S.L. (1994). Predictors of maternal role competence by risk status. *Nursing Research, 43*(1), 38–43.

Mestman, J.H. (1997). Hyperthyroidism. *Contemporary Ob/Gyn, 42,* 16, 21, 24.

Miller, S. (1996). Questioning, resisting, acquiescing, balancing: New mothers' career reentry strategies. *Health Care for Women International, 17,* 109–131.

Miovech, S.M., Knapp, H., Borucki, L., Roncoli, M., Arnold, L., & Brooten, D. (1994). Major concerns after cesarean delivery. *Journal of Obstetric, Gynecologic, and Neonatal Nursing, 23,* 53–59.

Nichols, M.R. (1993). Paternal perspectives of the childbirth experience. *Maternal-Child Nursing Journal, 21*(3), 99–108.

Nicol, B., Croughan-Minihane, M., & Kilpatrick, S.J. (1997). Lack of value of routine postpartum hematocrit determination after vaginal delivery. *Obstetrics and Gynecology, 90,* 514–518.

Novy, M.J. (1994). The normal puerperium. In A.H. DeCherney & M.L. Pernoll (Eds.), *Current obstetric and gynecologic diagnosis and treatment* (8th ed.) (pp. 240–274). Norwalk, CT: Appleton & Lange.

Palkovitz, R. (1992). Changes in father–infant bonding beliefs across couples' first transition to parenthood. *MCN, American Journal of Maternal Child Nursing, 20,* 141–154.

Pasquale, S. (1996). Clinical experience with today's IUDs. *Obstetrical and Gynecological Survey, 51,* S25–S29.

Pernoll, M.L. (1994). Late pregnancy complications. In A.H. DeCherney & M.L. Pernoll (Eds.), *Current obstetric and gynecologic diagnosis and treatment* (8th ed.) (pp. 331–343). Norwalk, CT: Appleton & Lange.

Phillips, C.R. (1997). *Mother-baby nursing.* Washington, DC: AWHONN.

Pridham, K.F. (1997). Mothers' help seeking as care initiated in a social context. *Image: Journal of Nursing Scholarship, 29,* 65–70.

Pridham, K.F., & Chang, A.S. (1992). Transition to being the mother of a new infant in the first 3 months: Maternal problem solving and self-appraisals. *Journal of Advanced Nursing, 17,* 204–216.

Reece, S.M. (1993). Social support and early maternal experience of primiparas over 35. *MCN, American Journal of Maternal Child Nursing, 21,* 91–98.

Resnik, R. (1994). The puerperium. In R. Creasy & R. Resnik (Eds.), *Maternal-fetal medicine: Principles and practice* (3rd ed.) (pp. 140–143). Philadelphia: W.B. Saunders.

Richter, C., Huch, A., & Huch, R. (1995). Erythropoiesis in the postpartum period. *Perinatal Medicine, 23,* 51–59.

Rubin, R. (1963). Maternal touch. *Nursing Outlook, 11,* 828–831.

Rubin, R. (1984). *Maternal identity and the maternal experience.* New York: Springer.

Sawicki, J.A. (1997). Sibling rivalry and the new baby: Anticipatory guidance and management strategies. *Pediatric Nursing, 23,* 298–302.

Seideman, R.Y., Jacobson, S., Primeaux, M., Burns, P., & Weatherby, F. (1996). Assessing American Indian families. *MCN, American Journal of Maternal Child Nursing, 21,* 274–279.

Sipes, S.L., & Weiner, C.D. (1992). Coagulation disorders in pregnancy. In E.A. Reece, J.C. Hobbins, M.J. Mahoney, & R.H. Petrie (Eds.), *Medicine of the fetus and mother* (pp. 1111–1138). Philadelphia: J.B. Lippincott.

Spector, R.E. (1996). *Cultural diversity in health and illness* (4th ed.). Stamford, CT: Appleton & Lange.

Susman, J.L. (1996). Postpartum depressive disorders. *Journal of Family Practice, 43,* S17–S24.

Taylor, D. (1983). Reflections on parenting: A multi-general perspectives. *Family Process, 22,* 341–346.

Taylor, D.J., & Lind, T. (1981). Puerperal haematological indices. *Journal of Obstetrics and Gynecology, 88,* 601–606.

Thompson, R.A. (1997). Sensitivity and security: New questions to ponder. *Child Development, 68,* 595–597.

Tiller, C.M. (1995). Fathers' parenting attitudes during a child's first year. *Journal of Obstetric, Gynecologic, and Neonatal Nursing, 24,* 508–514.

Tomlinson, P.S., Rothenberg, M.A., & Carver, L.D. (1991). Behavioral interaction of fathers with infants and mothers in the immediate postpartum period. *Journal of Nurse-Midwifery, 36,* 232–239.

Tulman, L. (1986). Initial handling of newborn infants by vaginally and cesarean-delivered mothers. *Nursing Research, 35,* 296–300.

Tulman, L., & Fawcett, J. (1990). Maternal employment following childbirth. *Research in Nursing and Health, 13,* 181–188.

Tulman, L., Fawcett, J., Groblewiski, L., & Silverman, L. (1990). Changes in functional status after childbirth. *Nursing Research, 39,* 70–75.

van den Boom, D.C. (1997). Sensitivity and attachment: Next steps for developmentalists. *Child Development, 64,* 592–594.

van IJzendoorn, M.H., & DeWolff, M.S. (1997). In search of the absent father—Meta-analysis of infant–father attachment: A rejoinder to our discussants. *Child Development, 68,* 604–609.

Watters, N.E., & Kristiansen, C.M. (1995). Two evaluations of combined mother-infant versus separate postnatal nursing care. *Research in Nursing and Health, 18,* 17–26.

Weiss, M.E., & Armstrong, M. (1991). Postpartum mothers' preference for nighttime care of the neonate. *Journal of Obstetric, Gynecologic, and Neonatal Nursing, 20,* 290–295.

Zahn, C.M., Hankins, D.V., & Yeomans, E.R. (1996). Vulvovaginal hematomas complicating delivery: Rationale for drainage of the hematoma cavity. *Journal of Reproductive Medicine, 41,* 569–574.

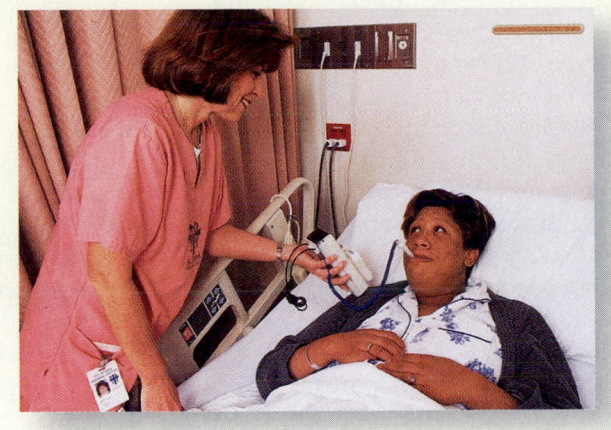

Virginia Gordon is a 28-year-old multi-gravida. She delivered 9 lb 7 oz Russell, her third child, by cesarean after a difficult labor did not progress. On the third postpartum day, Virginia tells Kim Donnelly, RN, that she "just doesn't feel well" and that she has more abdominal pain than the day before. As part of assessment, the nurse takes Virginia's temperature, which is 102°F. Virginia then worriedly states, "Russell and I are supposed to be discharged tomorrow, and I need to get home to my family. Do you think I will have to stay longer in the hospital?" ∎

29

Care of the Postpartum Family at Risk

Postpartum complications occur, even with excellent care. They may be related to problems that started before pregnancy, during pregnancy, during labor and delivery, or after the baby is born. Postpartum complications include such physiologic conditions as maternal postpartum hemorrhage, puerperal infections and thromboembolic disorders, and such psychologic conditions as postpartum blues, depression, and psychosis. High-risk postpartum conditions threaten the well-being of the mother and the family.

Many high-risk clients will not be candidates for early discharge; extended contact with the client and her family allows additional time for assessment and intervention. However, high-risk conditions can emerge suddenly during the early postpartum period in women who had previously been considered low risk. Nurses need to be experts in wellness to distinguish between variations in normal health and true complications of the puerperium. Nurses also help educate clients and families about high-risk conditions that may appear after discharge. Assessment and management by an interdisciplinary team, which includes the client and her family in decisions that affect them, are essential to the identification and treatment of high-risk postpartum conditions.

▶ POSTPARTUM HEMORRHAGE

Globally, the largest proportion of maternal deaths, directly related to obstetrics, results from hemorrhage. Most of these hemorrhages occur during the postpartum period (AbouZahr, Wardlaw, Stanton, & Hill, 1996). In addition, postpartum hemorrhage ranks as the most common cause of excessive blood loss during the childbearing cycle (Craigo & Kapernick, 1994). The life-threatening nature of hemorrhage and the perception that "pregnancy is not supposed to end this way" are frightening to clients and family members. Their fears may be compounded by worry related to such treatments as blood transfusions.

Postpartum hemorrhage may occur before, during, or after delivery of the placenta. Postpartum hemorrhage is defined by the volume of bleeding and the time when bleeding occurs.

Traditionally, postpartum hemorrhage was defined as the loss of more than 500 mL of blood after delivery of the placenta (Cunningham et al., 1997). However, about half the women who deliver vaginally lose this much blood; women who have cesarean delivery routinely lose about 1000 mL of blood. A healthy pregnant woman is estimated to have a blood volume of about 6000 mL (Gabbe, Niebyl, & Simpson, 1996). Healthy women can usu-

ally tolerate a blood loss at delivery similar to the blood volume added during pregnancy, i.e., 1000–2000 mL for an average size woman (Cunningham et al., 1997). The box entitled Classification of Postpartum Blood Loss outlines the four classes of blood loss and the physiologic effects of each type of blood loss.

Certain high-risk conditions do affect tolerance of blood loss. For example, women with severe pregnancy-induced hypertension tend to lose the hypervolemia of pregnancy and may not withstand bleeding that would usually be considered normal. In addition to prompt diagnosis, they may require such interventions as crystalloid and blood replacement (Cunningham et al., 1997). The incidence of postpartum hemorrhage serious enough to cause hypovolemic shock has been estimated to be less than 0.5 percent for women who have vaginal deliveries (Hayashi & Castillo, 1993).

Postpartum hemorrhage is further defined according to the time when it occurs. Early postpartum hemorrhage occurs within the first 24 hours of delivery. Late postpartum hemorrhage occurs at any time from 24 hours to 6 weeks postdelivery.

The term "postpartum hemorrhage" describes bleeding, but is not a diagnosis in itself. Causes of excessive bleeding need to be identified so that prompt and proper treatment can be given. Without a specific diagnosis for bleeding, unnecessary blood loss and other complications can arise (Cunningham et al., 1997).

▶ Early Postpartum Hemorrhage

Excessive bleeding from the site of implantation of the placenta, trauma to the genital tract or nearby tissues, or a combination of these factors can result in early postpartum hemorrhage (see box entitled Risk Factors and Reasons for Immediate Postpartum Hemorrhage).

Hemorrhage Related to Bleeding from the Placental Site
Hemorrhage due to uterine atony occurs when a hypotonic myometrium fails to contract effectively enough to control bleeding from the site of placental implantation. This condition has been estimated to account for about 50% of early postpartum hemorrhages (Craigo & Kapernick, 1994).

Nursing and Collaborative Assessment. Postpartum clients should be assessed for normal uterine involution with particular attention to women with risk factors. Many childbearing settings practice

▶ CLASSIFICATION OF POSTPARTUM BLOOD LOSS

CLASS 1

- Blood loss less than 900 mL
- Percent of blood volume lost: 15%
- Effects: Client rarely has signs of blood volume loss and seems otherwise well

CLASS 2

- Blood loss of 1200–1500 mL
- Percent of blood volume lost: 20–25%
- Effects: Possible increase in pulse and/or respiratory rate (possibly doubling of respiratory rate); orthostatic blood pressure changes; decreased perfusion of extremities, but not cold, clammy extremities; narrowing of pulse pressure (when pulse pressure drops to 30 mm Hg or less, the client should be evaluated for other signs of volume loss)

CLASS 3

- Blood loss of 1800–2100 mL
- Percent of blood volume lost: 30–35%

- Effects: Hypotension; cold clammy skin; increased respiratory rate (30–50 respirations/minute); tachycardia (120–160 beats/minute)

CLASS 4

- Blood loss of 2400 mL
- Percent of blood volume lost: 40% or more
- Effects: Profound shock; no discernible blood pressure; pulses absent in extremities; oliguric or anuric; circulatory collapse and cardiac arrest take place if therapy to restore volume is not started quickly
- Note: Hematocrit may not change significantly for at least 4 hours, and complete compensation usually takes about 48 hours. Therefore, hematocrit alone may not be the best indicator of hemorrhage. Vigorous fluid resuscitation may further lower hematocrit levels.

Source: Gabbe et al., 1996; Cunningham et al., 1997.

▶ RISK FACTORS AND REASONS FOR IMMEDIATE POSTPARTUM HEMORRHAGE

BLEEDING FROM PLACENTAL IMPLANTATION SITE

- Hypotonic myometrium resulting in uterine atony
- General anesthetics (e.g., halogenated hydrocarbons) that relax the uterus and increase risk of bleeding
- Poorly perfused myometrium resulting in hypotension:
  - Hemorrhage
  - Conduction analgesia
- Overdistended uterus that occurs with large fetus, multiple fetuses, or polyhydramnios; uterus may not contract firmly and a lot of blood may be lost, especially if a general anesthetic that relaxes the uterus is used
- Following prolonged labor (uterus may be hypotonic)
- Following very rapid labor (uterus that sustained an unusual workload may be hypotonic post delivery)
- Following oxytocin-induced or augmented labor (following strong labor contractions, the postdelivery uterus may be hypotonic)
- High parity
- Uterine atony in previous pregnancy
- Chorioamnionitis (infection can inhibit contractility of the myometrium, leading to excessive blood loss)

- Retained placental tissue (during the third stage of labor, constant squeezing of the contracted uterus in an attempt to separate the placenta may result in incomplete separation of the placenta, adherent pieces of placenta, uterine atony, and increased blood loss; placenta should be allowed to deliver spontaneously and manual extraction done only when necessary)
- Avulsed cotyledon
- Abnormally adherent placenta, involving one to all of the cotyledons of the placenta (placenta accreta, placenta increta, placenta percreta)

TRAUMA TO THE GENITAL TRACT

- Large episiotomy, including extension of the episiotomy
- Lacerations of the perineum, vagina, or cervix
- Ruptured uterus

COAGULATION DEFECTS

- Intensify all of the above

Source: Adapted from Cunningham et al., 1997, p. 761.

family-centered care, and significant others are encouraged to remain with the new mother, who may hold and feed her baby after delivery. During this relaxed time, however, uterine and other physical assessments should be continued, because such complications as hemorrhage might otherwise be missed. Postpartum assessment parameters are discussed in Chapter 28.

Identifying hemorrhage requires evaluating the client as a whole, rather than focusing attention on a single parameter. For example, tachycardia may indicate hypovolemia, resulting from postpartum hemorrhage; however, tachycardia also may indicate other conditions that may or may not threaten well-being. Respiratory rate alone is not a useful indicator of postpartum hemorrhage. Many such factors as anxiety, cerebral perfusion, and acidosis can change respiratory rate. Blood pressure in the postpartum period should be similar to the woman's prenatal blood pressure. A sudden drop in blood pressure, however, may indicate severe postpartum hemorrhage.

Problems can occur in using pulse and blood pressure alone as early indicators of postpartum hemorrhage since these signs may not change significantly until large amounts of blood have been lost. In early hemorrhage, systolic pressure may be normal, but diastolic pressures rises. Systolic blood pressure drops when 30% or more of the blood volume is lost. Other signs of hypovolemia related to hemorrhage include client reports of pain, fatigue, or severe thirst, low urine output, pallor, anxiety, and in extreme cases, loss of consciousness. Postpartum hemoglobin and hematocrit levels may not change for hours even after hemorrhage; however, values that drop significantly are also indicators of heavy bleeding.

Accurate estimation of actual blood loss is difficult. No clinically useful and accurate standard exists. Heavy bleeding may be missed if the blood accumulates in the uterus or other body tissues or even under the mattress of the bed or on the floor. Pools of blood may not be seen easily with certain types of break-apart labor-delivery beds (Luegenbiehl, 1997). Assessment of postpartum peripads (discussed later) remains among the most common ways to evaluate postpartum blood loss.

Uterine tone is assessed by palpating the fundus for firmness and location (see Chapter 28). A soft, boggy fundus may indicate uterine atony; a fundus that is deviated from midline may indicate atony related to a full bladder. The mother should be asked to void and the fundus reassessed after voiding. If the uterus then becomes firm and more midline, the uterine atony was probably due to a full bladder.

A fundus that is soft and boggy should be gently massaged. The expulsion of clots or tissue may indi-

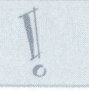

Nursing Alert

Do not expect postpartum hemorrhage only to mean blood gushing from the vagina. Bleeding may be concealed in the uterus or other tissues and may occur at a slow, steady pace. Postpartum care always requires careful assessment for bleeding.

cate uterine atony caused by retained placental fragments and should be reported to the physician or certified nurse-midwife (CNM) immediately.

If bleeding persists, despite a firmly contracted uterus, bleeding from an episiotomy or lacerations of the cervix, vagina, or uterus should be suspected.

The lochia is assessed for amount, odor, and quality each time the fundus is assessed. The amount of lochia is assessed by observing the saturation level of the peripads and the number of pads saturated within a certain time frame. Complete saturation of one pad (60–100 mL of lochia) within 15 minutes or saturation of two or more pads within 1 hour suggests hemorrhage (Jacobson, 1985). Foul-smelling lochia may indicate infection (discussed later).

Accurate assessment is crucial for nurses who rely on visual estimation of blood loss as an indication of normal or high-risk bleeding. Many nurses are not aware that different brands of peripads reveal blood in different ways, thus possibly affecting estimates of actual blood loss. In addition, without an objective and well-understood standard on which to base accurate and consistent assessments of the amount of blood on peripads, assessments may not be accurate (Luegenbiehl, 1997). Educational programs, targeted toward staff and home care nurses, that include correct estimation of blood volume on the brand of peripad used at a site may improve accuracy in estimation of blood loss.

Nursing Diagnoses. Nursing diagnoses are made after careful assessment of the woman with postpartum hemmorhage. Examples of diagnoses include:

Problem-oriented diagnoses:

- Risk for fluid volume deficit, related to excessive postpartal blood loss
- Fatigue, related to excessive blood loss
- Fear, related to diagnosis, assessment, and treatment of postpartum hemorrhage

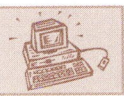

Research Abstract

Improving Visual Estimation of Blood Volume on Peripads During the Postpartum Period

Through the Association of Women's Health, Obstetric, and Neonatal Nursing (AWHONN), 387 staff members at 13 test sites (rural and urban hospitals) participated in this study, which investigated staff members' accuracy in estimating the amount of blood on peripads. Accurate estimation of blood loss is important for the detection of postpartum hemorrhage. Each site used a familiar brand of peripad. Three pads were prepared for each standard category: "scant" (3, 7, and 9 cc); "small" (14, 18, and 22 cc); "moderate" (30, 40, and 45 cc); and "large" (55, 65, and 75 cc). Subjects estimated the amount of blood on the pads (which were sealed in plastic bags and could be handled), attended a short program on accurate assessment of blood on the brand of peripad used, and then estimated the amount of blood on each peripad again.

Data were analyzed using paired *t* tests of the percent difference of estimated blood volume on the pretest and posttest pads. Among the results was the finding that the educational program could increase accuracy in estimation of blood volume lost. Students and participants with the least amount of work experience were less accurate in pretest estimations than registered nurses, although their scores improved with education. The results of the study supported previous research indicating that personnel tend to overestimate and not underestimate the amount of blood on a peripad. Although participants in the study overestimated blood loss by 102% before the educational program, this dropped to 47% overestimation (perfect estimation = 0) after the program.

Application to Practice

Assessment of blood loss is a standard part of postpartum care and is crucial to the early identification of certain types of postpartum hemorrhage. Inability to ensure accurate assessment can result in such problems as mistaken diagnoses and unnecessary interventions for bleeding. The finding that staff tend to overestimate blood loss, even after an educational program, indicates the need for further education about blood volume assessment on peripads. This study is an example of practice-based research and underscores the interest of staff members from multiple settings in improving their ability to assess this important parameter. The use of multiple and diverse sites and cooperation from such a large group of staff members support the findings and highlight the importance of in-service orientation and refresher education for all staff, including home care nurses, assessing such important parameters as blood loss. The study also highlights the importance of knowing about variation among different brands of peripads and about what different blood volumes look like on the pads used in staff members' own settings. In addition to findings that are clinically applicable, the study is an example of cooperation among a major professional organization, researchers from an educational setting, and staff in 13 different practice sites.

Source: Luegenbiehl, D.L. (1997). Improving visual estimation of blood volume on peripads. MCN, American Journal of Maternal–Child Nursing, 22(6); 294–298.

- Knowledge deficit, related to diagnosis and treatment of reasons for hemorrhage

Wellness-oriented diagnoses:

- Asset in physiologic functioning, related to good prenatal care, normal pregnancy hypervolemia, and nutrition
- Family coping: potential for growth, related to previous positive family coping strategies

- Potential for effective crisis resolution, related to physiologic assets of mother, effective treatment of the event, and appropriate resources

Nursing and Collaborative Management. Successful management depends upon prompt identification of abnormal bleeding and the reason for the bleeding, and appropriate interventions to control current bleeding and prevent future hemorrhage. All pregnant women should be assessed for the risk of postpartum hemorrhage in the prenatal and intrapartum periods. Women at risk admitted to labor units should have their blood typed and screened for antibodies. Blood should be available postdelivery if a transfusion is indicated.

After delivery, the fundus is massaged until it becomes firm. Excessive or vigorous massage should be avoided as it may interfere with normal contraction of the uterus. Oxytocics are often administered to enhance contraction of the uterus. Oxytocin (Pitocin) is usually added to a liter bottle of intravenous solution and administered to the client. A commonly used dosage is 20 units of oxytocin added to a liter of intravenous solution. Methylergonovine maleate (Methergine) 0.2 mg also may be given intramuscularly to contract the uterus. The intravenous route is rarely used for Methergine, due to the risk of such severe side effects as hypertension. In addition, the woman may be prone to intrauterine infection. Strategies to prevent infection, such as meticulous aseptic technique, are important.

When uterine atony and heavy bleeding persist, despite the use of oxytocics and manual massage of the fundus, other treatment is indicated. Examples of interventions to control bleeding include: administration of prostaglandins; bimanual compression of the uterus; exploration of the uterus and curretage; percutaneous embolization or ligation of the pelvic arteries; and hysterectomy.

Intramuscular injection of a 15-methyl derivative of prostaglandin $F_{20}c$ carboprost tromethamine may be administered to treat postpartum hemorrhage. Carboprost tromethamine has been found effective in the management of severe postpartum bleeding (Cunningham et al., 1997). The client may have side effects associated with the administration of prostaglandins, including diarrhea, hypertension, vomiting, fever, flushing, and tachycardia.

Bimanual compression of the uterus is done by the physician or nurse-midwife to control postpartum hemorrhage. One gloved hand is placed on the client's abdomen. The fundus is grasped and pushed down toward the symphysis pubis. The other gloved hand is inserted into the vagina with the closed fist pressing against the uterus. The physician or nurse-midwife maintains compression for as long as 20 to 30 minutes, while using both hands to massage the uterus, one externally and one internally (Fig. 29–1).

An intravenous solution, such as lactated Ringer's solution with oxytocin, is administered. A blood transfusion also may be ordered concurrently in severe cases of hypovolemia to replace blood loss. A Foley catheter may be inserted to prevent distension

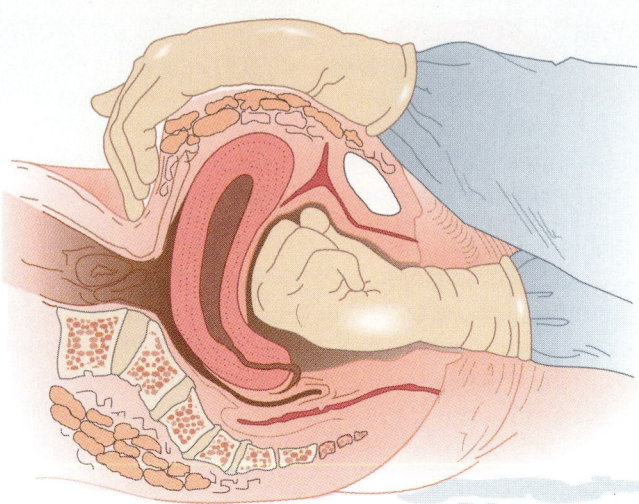

FIGURE 29–1. Bimanual compression of the uterus and massage with the abdominal hand to control hemorrhage from uterine atony. *(Reproduced, with permission, from Cunningham, F.G. et al. (1997). Williams obstetrics (20th ed.). Stamford, CT: Appleton & Lange, p. 765.)*

of the bladder and facilitate bimanual compression and massage (Craigo & Kapernick, 1994).

If the bleeding cannot be controlled by nonsurgical treatments, surgical intervention may be required. Using a vaginal approach, the uterus is explored, and any retained products of conception are removed; uterine curretage may be needed to accomplish this (Benson & Pernoll, 1994). In some cases laparotomy may be needed. During the procedure the physician may achieve immediate temporary control of the bleeding by pressure occlusion of the aorta for several minutes in an otherwise healthy woman. This gives the physician time to try to locate and control the cause of the bleeding (Craigo & Kapernick, 1994).

If heavy bleeding continues, the physician may need to ligate the uterine or hypogastric arteries. Ligation of these arteries may substantially control bleeding without cutting off the supply of blood to the uterus and pelvic structures, as the collateral circulation usually can maintain the viability of the pelvic tissue (Oxorn, 1986). If hemorrhage cannot be controlled, the physician may perform a hysterectomy (removal of the uterus) as a lifesaving measure.

The woman with postpartum hemorrhage requires intensive nursing care. Vital signs must be monitored and an accurate record of intake and output maintained. The nurse also anticipates various therapies, for example, bimanual compression and intravenous therapy, and prepares the client and her family accordingly. Simple and clear explanations are given. Mobilizing family social support is also an important function of the nurse. Family coping is enhanced by comprehensive and holistic nursing care during this crisis.

Lacerations

Lacerations and trauma are believed to account for about 20% of early postpartum hemorrhages (Craigo & Kapernick, 1994). Lacerations can occur despite attentive and skillful care. Most lacerations that require suturing are repaired at delivery and heal well (see box entitled Lacerations). However, bleeding, especially bright red bleeding, that continues although the uterus is firmly contracted suggests hemorrhage related to lacerations. As expected, large lacerations tend to present a greater danger.

Risk Factors. Risk factors for excessive bleeding from lacerations include forceps delivery, precipitous or rapid delivery, delivery of a large baby, and delivery of multiple babies. Lacerations may also occur with a normal, spontaneous delivery.

Nursing and Collaborative Assessment. The physician or nurse-midwife should carefully inspect for lacerations after delivery; staff nurses continue external assessment of the fundus, perineum, and lochia as part of routine postpartum care. Trauma to the genital tract can be associated with heavy blood loss, even if the bleeding does not outwardly appear to be excessive. For example, a laceration of the cervix may cause significant blood loss through slow, steady

▶ **LACERATIONS**

PERINEAL

- *First degree:* extends through skin
- *Second degree:* extends through muscles of perineal body
- *Third degree:* extends through perineal body to anal sphincter
- *Fourth degree:* extends through perineal body and anal sphincter and involves rectal wall

VAGINAL

- Longitudinal tears of upper vagina
- Lacerations of vulva and lower vagina
  - Superficial tears
  - Deep lacerations that may include urethra, labia minora, clitoris, and bladder

CERVICAL

- Superficial lacerations, usually at 3- and 9-o'clock positions
- Extensive lacerations of lower uterine segment

bleeding, which may be overlooked, especially if the fundus is well contracted. Uterine lacerations may also result in hemorrhage.

If external inspection does not reveal the source of heavy postpartum bleeding, a vaginal examination to visualize the cervix and upper vagina is performed by the CNM or physician. Assessment parameters for hemorrhage, related to suspected lacerations, include client's reports of discomfort, vital signs, uterine contractility, amount and nature of lochia, intake, output, pallor, and clamminess of skin.

Nursing and Collaborative Management. Lacerations that need suturing are usually repaired immediately following delivery. Occasionally, heavy postpartum bleeding requires that the client be returned for surgical repair of a laceration. To allay anxiety, the client and her significant others need to receive clear explanations and support about the procedures involved.

After surgical repair of a laceration, vital signs, fundal firmness, lochia, intake, and output are assessed and recorded. Care of a perineal laceration is similar to care of an episiotomy repair (see Chapter 28). Application of an ice pack to the perineum for the first 24 hours is believed to be helpful in minimizing swelling. After this period, sitz baths have traditionally been used to increase circulation and promote healing. Hill (1989), however, found no difference between the effects of heat and cold on perineal healing after episiotomy or laceration in the first 24 hours after delivery.

Once the client is stabilized, she may be encouraged to perform Kegel exercises to promote healing of the pubococcygeal muscle. Analgesics such as oral acetaminophen or ibuprofen and analgesic sprays applied to the perineal area may be offered to minimize perineal discomfort. The nurse should also be aware of any special herbal remedies used by the client to promote perineal comfort and healing.

Hematomas

Bleeding into the connective tissue beneath the vaginal mucosa or vulvar skin may cause the formation of vaginal and vulvar hematomas (Fig. 29–2). Hematomas develop as a result of injury to tissues with spontaneous as well as operative deliveries (e.g., forceps). Vulvar hematomas are identified as bulging masses, covered by discolored skin. Vaginal hematomas may be concealed.

Nursing and Collaborative Assessment. One of the first signs of a hematoma may be the client's report of pressure, inability to void, or pain. When bleeding occurs into tissues between the

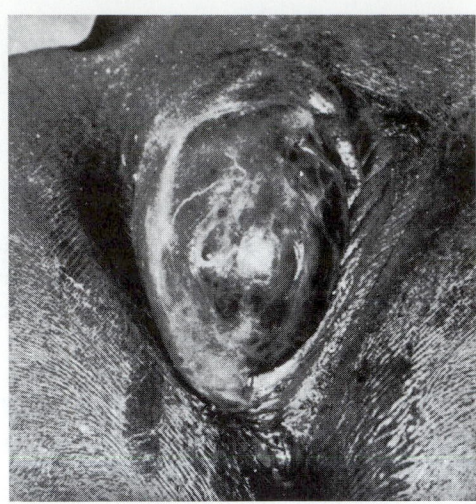

FIGURE 29–2. Vulvar hematoma bulging into the right vaginal wall. *(Reproduced, with permission, from Cunningham, F.G. et al. (1997). Williams obstetrics (20th ed.). Stamford, CT: Appleton & Lange, p. 771.)*

vagina and the rectum, the client may report feeling rectal pressure "like the need to have a bowel movement."

Vulvar hematomas can be very painful, and pain may be the first symptom of this condition. In some cases, tissues overlying the hematoma may open and produce heavy bleeding or large clots (Cunningham et al., 1997). A vulvar hematoma may present as a discolored mass that appears suddenly.

Depending upon their location and size, hematomas may either be easily seen by external examination or require vaginal examination. Most hematomas do not threaten life or long-term well-being, although bleeding into huge hematomas has been known in rare cases to cause death. In situations where continued or heavy bleeding is suspected, other assessment strategies are the same as for hemorrhage.

Nursing and Collaborative Management.
Small or moderate-sized vulvar hematomas may absorb spontaneously without operative management. Ice and heat treatments may help to reduce swelling and discomfort. When large or expanding hematomas of the vaginal walls are identified, however, incision and evacuation of the hematoma by the physician may be performed.

Hematomas may result in considerable loss of blood, which is difficult to estimate accurately. Fluid and blood replacement is therefore indicated to prevent hypovolemia in cases where blood loss is excessive. Broad-spectrum antibiotic therapy also has been useful in controlling secondary infection (Cunningham et al., 1997).

Nursing care focuses on assessment of the mother and comfort measures—for example, cold and heat treatments and analgesics—to help relieve discomfort associated with a hematoma. If surgical treatment is indicated, the nurse prepares the client and her family for the procedure and assesses the client's vital signs and perineum during and after the surgery.

▶ Late Postpartum Hemorrhage

Late postpartum hemorrhage may develop within days of delivery or later in the postpartum period, after the client is home. Prior to discharge from the health care facility, the nurse teaches the client and her partner signs and symptoms related to such problems as hemorrhage.

Late or delayed postpartum hemorrhage may be the result of **subinvolution** (delayed involution) of the uterus or, less commonly, retention of placental fragments. The exact cause of subinvolution of the uterus is unknown; however, faulty placental implantation and infection at the implantation site have been suggested as possible causes (Craigo & Kapernick, 1994).

Retention of placental fragments also may result in late postpartum hemorrhage. The retained portion of the placenta undergoes necrosis, forming fibrin deposits. These deposits form a placental polyp, which eventually detaches from the myometrium, causing hemorrhage. Retained placental tissue is also associated with placental accreta, and manual removal of the placenta (Cunningham et al., 1997).

Nursing and Collaborative Assessment
In educating the client about late postpartum hemorrhage, the nurse should:

- Explain the normal pattern of uterine involution and lochial flow
- Explain the importance of reporting any abnormalities, such as bright red bleeding, excessive clots, persistent lochia rubra, prolonged lochial discharge, foul-smelling lochia, a soft boggy fundus or pain in the perineum, rectum, abdomen, or back, to the health care provider.
- Teach the client assessment of fundal height, location, and condition.
- Teach the client fundal massage and assessment of whether the fundus becomes firm in response to the massage or remains soft and boggy.

The diagnosis of subinvolution is confirmed by bimanual pelvic examination. The uterus is found to be larger than normal for the specific postpartum stage (Cunningham et al., 1997). Retained placental tissue is diagnosed clinically, although ultrasound may be helpful in some cases.

Nursing Diagnoses

Examples of diagnoses related to delayed postpartum hemorrhage include:

Problem-oriented diagnoses:

- Altered maternal role performance, related to hospitalization for management of delayed postpartum hemorrhage
- Knowledge deficit, related to symptoms and management of delayed postpartum hemorrhage

Wellness-oriented diagnoses:

- Potential for minimal role conflicts, related to adequate family resources
- Potential for decreased anxiety concerning treatment for delayed postpartum hemorrhage, related to understanding of condition

Nursing and Collaborative Mangement

The woman with delayed postpartum hemorrhage may be hospitalized. Uncertainty about her condition and separation from the infant and other family members can increase the client's stress and anxiety. Supportive nursing actions include explaining the condition and treatment and encouraging communication among family members.

On admission, oxytocin in intravenous solution, and/or intramuscular methylergonovine maleate (Methergine) may be administered to stimulate uterine contractions. Methergine, however, is contraindicated in women who are hypertensive. If the bleeding subsides, the client is observed for several hours. Vital signs are taken, the fundus is palpated for firmness, and the lochia is assessed for quantity and quality of flow. Hemoglobin and hematocrit are obtained to assess for anemia resulting from blood loss.

If bleeding continues, uterine compression and bimanual massage (see earlier discussion) are often performed to control hemorrhage caused by subinvolution. If heavy bleeding persists, curettage may be indicated. This procedure should be carried out only when other treatment has failed because curettage may further traumatize the implantation site and cause additional bleeding. When curettage is performed, the client and her partner should be advised that hysterectomy may be necessary (Cunningham et

al., 1997). Broad-spectrum antibiotics also may be given to the client if postpartum infection is suspected.

To minimize the chance of hemorrhage related to retained placental fragments, the placenta and membranes should always be carefully inspected after delivery. If a portion of the placenta or membranes is missing, the uterus should be explored.

▶ Identifying Causes of Postpartum Hemorrhage

The degree of contractility of the uterus helps in identifying the cause of postpartum hemorrhage. If the fundus is firm and well contracted and bleeding persists, the cause is usually lacerations; if the fundus is soft and boggy, the cause is usually uterine atony. Lacerations of the cervix may produce a slow seepage of bright red blood; uterine atony may cause heavy bleeding with clots. In each case, however, serious hypovolemia may occur.

At times, bleeding may have more than one cause, for example, atony and trauma. The cervix and vagina therefore need to be inspected for lacerations even when uterine atony is present (Cunningham et al., 1997). Table 29–1 summarizes contributing risk factors and assessment findings for the client with bleeding from the placental site, trauma from lacerations, hematoma, or subinvolution.

▶ POSTPARTUM INFECTIONS

Postpartum infection is the leading reason for hospital-acquired infections and is a major cause of maternal morbidity and mortality (Clark, 1995). Postpartum infections result in such problems as disruptions in mother–infant interaction, longer hospital stays or readmission to the hospital, lactation difficulties, higher costs, and potential threats to life or long-term well-being.

Postpartum infections fall into two broad categories. The first category covers the reproductive system infections, also termed **puerperal infection** or **puerperal fever.** This refers to bacterial infections that arise in the genital tract after delivery. The second category includes non–reproductive system infections that arise in sites other than the genital tract and influence maternal morbidity during postpartum recovery. These infections, which include mastitis and urinary tract infections, are indirectly related to the reproductive cycle and physiology of pregnancy,

▶ **TABLE 29-1**

Postpartum Hemorrhage

Cause of Hemorrhage	Contributing Risk Factors	Assessment	Interventions
Bleeding from placental site	Uterine overdistension from multiple gestation or polyhydramnios Prolonged or precipitous labor Uterine infection Disseminated intravascular coagulation Bladder distension	Boggy, soft fundus Profuse, bright red lochia Blood clots Foul-smelling lochia Increase in height of uterine fundus Failure of uterus to involute	Have client empty bladder. Assess fundus for firmness. Gently massage and assess location and firmness of fundus. Take vital signs. Note amount, consistency, color, and odor of lochia. Report findings.
Lacerations	Operative delivery Vaginal birth after cesarean birth Delivery of large infant Precipitous delivery	Firm fundus (usually) Seepage of bright red blood	Observe for trickling of bright, red blood. Take vital signs. Assess fundus and lochia. Assess suture lines for REEDA.[a] Report findings.
Hematoma	Difficult delivery Operative delivery (e.g., forceps)	Complaint of pain or pressure in vagina or perineum Ecchymotic mass in perineum Inability to void	Assess vagina and perineum for mass. Take vital signs. Report findings. Place ice pack on perineum.
Subinvolution	Faulty placental implantation Infection at implantation site Retention of placental fragments	Late postpartum hemorrhage Bright red bleeding Persistent lochia rubra Prolonged lochial discharge No change or a rise in the fundal height Soft, boggy fundus	Teach couple how to assess lochia and fundus prior to discharge and contact the health care provider with abnormal findings. Assess vital signs, fundus, and lochia.

[a]REEDA = redness, edema, ecchymosis, discharge, and approximation.

labor, delivery, and lactation. Infections in the second category might also occur in nonpregnant individuals.

▶ Reproductive System Infections

The classic definition of **puerperal morbidity** resulting from infection is a temperature of 100.4°F (38.0°C) or higher on any 2 of the first 10 days postpartum exclusive of the first 24 hours, as taken orally by a standard technique at least four times a day. This definition was developed in the early 20th century, but remains the most commonly employed standard in the United States (Cunningham et al., 1997).

Although temperature is the criterion most commonly used to determine puerperal morbidity, a temperature of 100.4°F or higher in the first 10 days postpartum is also associated with benign conditions such as breast engorgement. The cause of fever in the postpartum period must therefore be investigated to allow proper treatment.

The development of better techniques for identification of causative agents and the use of antibiotics in treatment have decreased maternal deaths from bacterial infections. Despite advances in maternity care, infections still rank high in the list of complications in the postpartum period. The cost to the family is still great. The mother may be separated from her newborn and often has to spend additional days in the hospital. In addition, serious reproductive system infections may lead to sterility or problems with future childbearing. Prevention of infection is always the best possible treatment.

Bacterial Causes

A variety of bacteria are responsible for reproductive system infections. In most cases, the bacteria causing infection are those found normally in the bowel, perineum, and cervix. These bacteria, which are not usually pathogenic, may become so as a result of injury and devitalization of tissue (Cunningham et al., 1997). Anaerobic bacteria, aerobic bacteria, or a combination may be involved. Table 29–2 lists common anaerobic and aerobic bacteria responsible for reproductive system infections.

Reproductive system infections usually begin in the uterus and may spread upward to the fallopian tubes and ovaries (salpingo-oophoritis), outward to

► **TABLE 29-2**

Common Aerobic and Anaerobic Bacteria Responsible for Female Reproductive System Infections

Aerobes

Group A, B, and D streptococci
Enterococcus
Gram negative bacteria:
   E. coli
   Klebsiella
   Proteus species
Staphylococcus aureus

Anaerobes

Peptococcus species
Peptostreptococcus species
Bacteroides bivius, B. fragilis, B. disiens
Clostridium species
Fusobacterium species

Other

Mycoplasma hominis
Chlamydia trachomatis

Source: American College of Obstetricians and Gynecologists, 1988.

the parametrial cellular tissue (parametrial cellulitis), and, if more extensive, to the peritoneal cavity (peritonitis). Septic pelvic thrombophlebitis, clotting in the veins of the pelvis, may also occur (Biswas & Perloff, 1994). A severe complication of reproductive system infection is bacteremia, which can be associated with septic shock.

Risk Factors

Several risk factors associated with reproductive system infection are assessed in the antepartum and intrapartum periods (see box entitled Risk Factors Associated with Reproductive System Infections).

Many risk factors have been indirectly linked to poverty. Women in lower socioeconomic groups are at greater risk for postpartum infections, as well as other complications of pregnancy. Prevention of complications is far less costly than management of complications, both in dollars and in family functioning.

Specific Infections

Metritis. **Metritis** is a puerperal uterine infection involving the endometrium, decidua, and adjacent myometrium. This term is more specific than endometritis (infection of the endometrium) because the underlying myometrium is almost always involved in metritis.

Metritis is the most common postpartum infection (Clark, 1995). Symptoms usually begin on the third to fifth day postpartum; however, if the invading organism is a beta-hemolytic streptococcus, the onset is usually earlier (Varney, 1997). Factors contributing to the development of metritis include prolonged labor, prolonged rupture of the membranes, or introduction of pathogens from multiple vaginal examinations. The risk of metritis is greater after cesarean delivery than after vaginal delivery, and both the frequency and severity of infection are higher after abdominal birth (Blanco, 1992; Clark, 1995).

Metritis is usually caused by bacteria that invade the decidua at the placental site. The hypervascularity of the remaining decidua also makes it susceptible to the invasion of pathogens, as does injury to the cervix. The appearance of the infected decidua may vary. In some cases, the necrotic mucosa sloughs, producing an abundant, foul-smelling, bloody, and sometimes frothy discharge. In other cases, the uterine discharge may be scant and odorless (as in infection with beta-

---

► **RISK FACTORS ASSOCIATED WITH REPRODUCTIVE SYSTEM INFECTIONS**

ANTEPARTUM

- Low socioeconomic status
- Little or no prenatal care
- Premature rupture of membranes
- Silent chorioamniotic infection

INTRAPARTUM

Labor

- Introduction of pathogens from frequent vaginal examinations, especially with ruptured membranes and intrauterine fetal monitoring
- Prolonged labor
- Prolonged rupture of the membranes

Delivery and Postpartum

- Lacerations, episiotomy, tears, hematomas
- Hemorrhage, especially after excessive blood loss
- Cesarean delivery, especially after prolonged labor
- Operative delivery (e.g., forceps)
- Chorioamnionitis
- Bladder catheterization
- Retained placental fragments

HISTORY

- Acute conditions such as urinary tract infection, mastitis, pneumonia
- Chronic conditions such as diabetes, alcoholism, drug abuse, immunosuppression

hemolytic streptococcus). In either case, subinvolution of the uterus may occur (Cunningham et al., 1997).

Parametrial Cellulitis. **Parametrial cellulitis** (parametritis) is an extension of puerperal infection that begins in the uterus and spreads into the broad ligament by several means:

1. Through lymphatic transmission of bacteria from infected cervical or uterine lacerations, or uterine incision for cesarean delivery
2. By direct extension of cervical lacerations into connective tissue at the base of the broad ligaments, exposing the tissue to direct invasions by organisms
3. Secondary to pelvic thrombophlebitis, in which organisms gain access to surrounding tissue from a purulent thrombus of the venous wall

The infection involves the entire uterus and may spread to the ovaries and fallopian tubes. If parametrial cellulitis progresses, a parametrial abscess may develop and require draining to prevent its rupture into the peritoneal cavity (Varney, 1997).

Peritonitis. **Peritonitis,** an infection of the peritoneum, may spread from the uterus by way of the lymphatics to the abdominal cavity (Fig. 29–3). This serious condition may be life threatening. Purulent exudate into the abdominal cavity can cause systemic sepsis. Abscesses may form between loops of bowel. These abscesses may not respond to intravenous antibiotics and may need to be drained surgically. Pus in the peritoneal cavity leads to a paralytic ileus. An inflammatory reaction to the pus may cause adhesions to form between the loops of bowel and may ultimately result in mechanical small bowel obstruction. The cul-de-sac, subhepatic and subdiaphragmatic spaces can also be sites of abscess formation.

Septic Pelvic Thrombophlebitis. **Septic pelvic thrombophlebitis** results when an infection spreads along venous routes into the pelvis (Fig. 29–4). The placental site is the usual portal of entry of the bacteria. The bacterial infection causes thrombosis of myometrial veins, which in turn support the growth of anaerobic bacteria (Cunningham et al., 1997). The infection may spread via the pelvic veins into the right ovarian vein, which may further extend the infection to the inferior vena cava, and into the left ovarian vein, which may further extend the infection to the left renal vein. Spread of infection into the femoral vein results in femoral thrombophlebitis. Blood clots formed in these veins may embolize to the

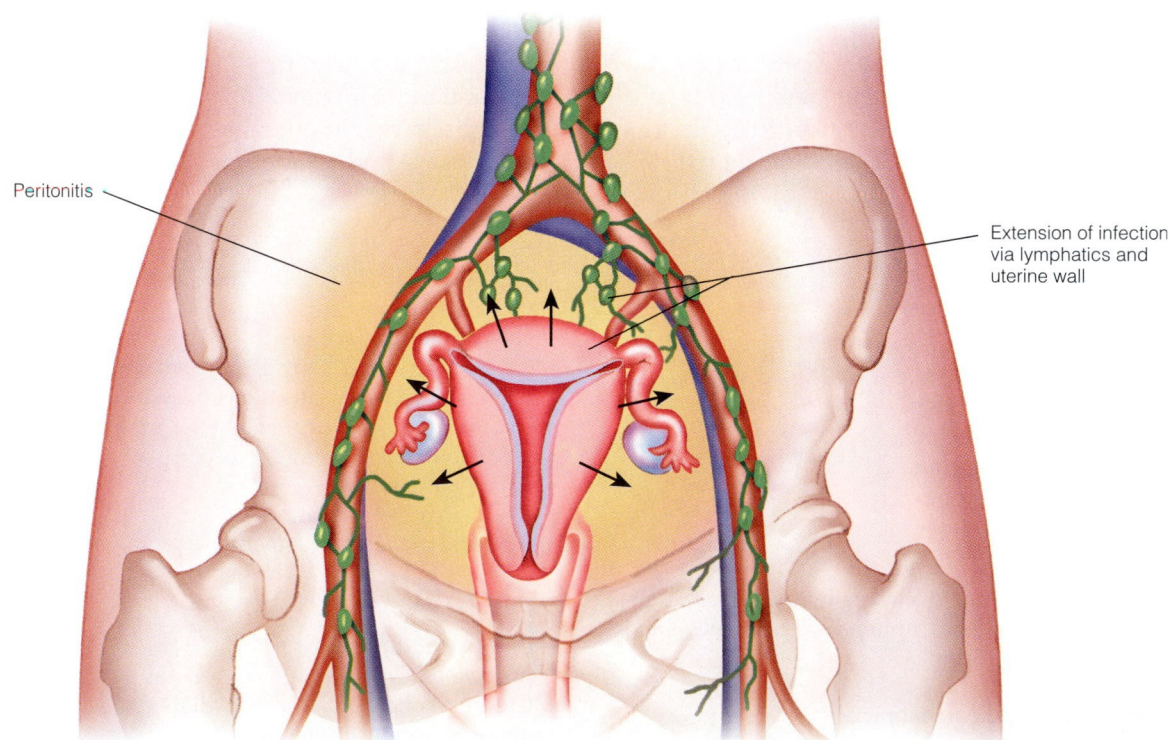

Peritonitis

Extension of infection via lymphatics and uterine wall

FIGURE 29–3. Peritonitis may develop with spread of uterine infection via lymphatics.

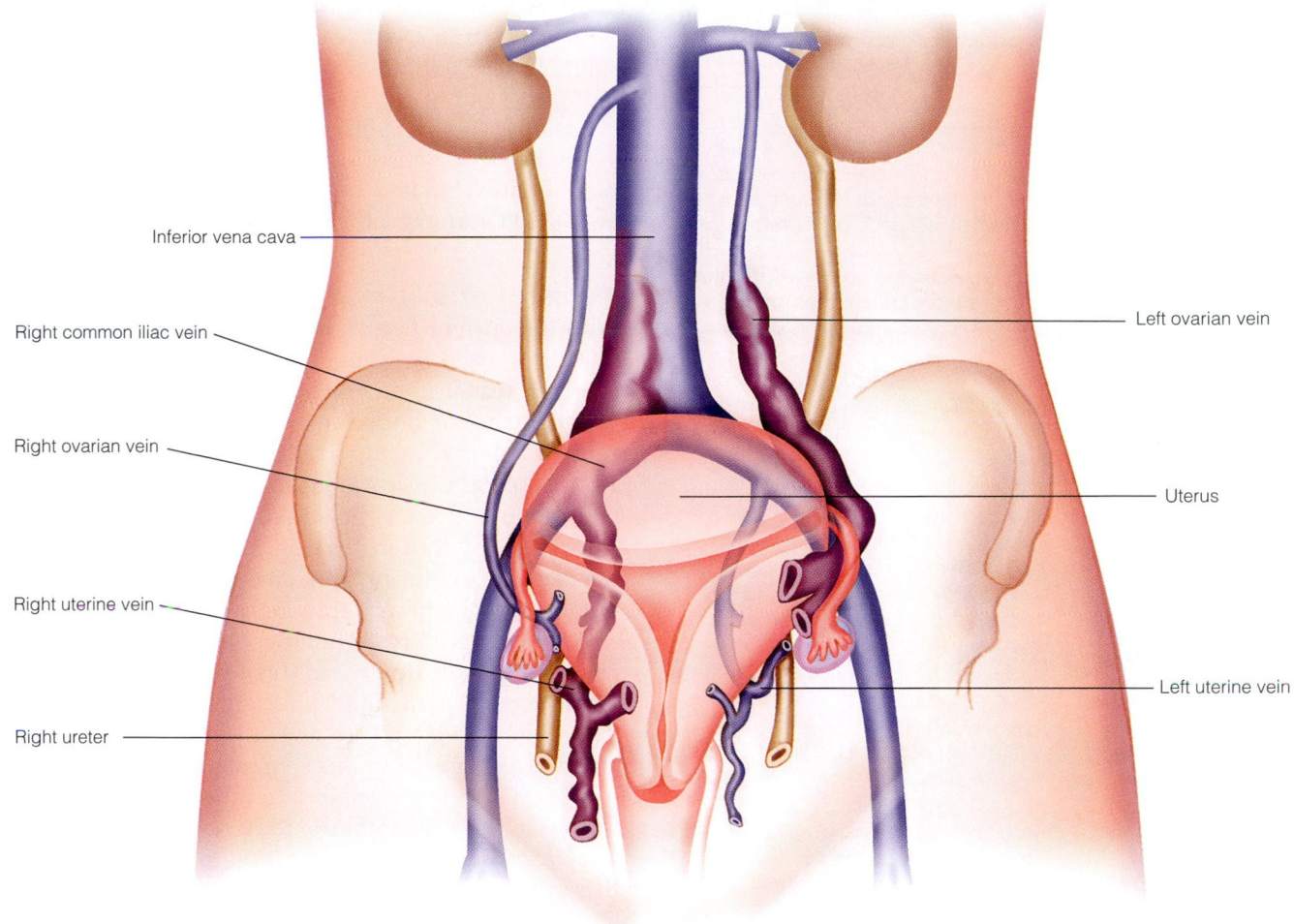

FIGURE 29–4. Septic pelvic thrombophlebitis. Any or all pelvic vessels and the inferior vena cava may be involved.

Labels on figure:
- Inferior vena cava
- Right common iliac vein
- Right ovarian vein
- Right uterine vein
- Right ureter
- Left ovarian vein
- Uterus
- Left uterine vein

lungs. Septic pelvic thrombophlebitis may present as a prolonged, spiking fever that continues despite antibiotic therapy; other physical signs may not be present, and there is no evidence of an abscess (Blanco, 1992).

Bacteremia and Septic Shock.
Bacteremia is the invasion of the blood by bacteria. The bacteria can reach the blood from the uterus through the lymphatics or veins. If the invading organism is virulent, septic shock can occur.

Nursing and Collaborative Assessment.
For each of the preceding conditions, there are both general and specific assessment parameters. Signs of infection may appear after discharge, so the client should be taught to identify problems and to call her health care provider. The range of symptoms and signs can vary with the nature and severity of infec-

tion (Clark, 1995). General parameters include elevated temperature [100.4°F (38°C) or higher], increased pulse rate, pain (local or systemic), fatigue, pallor, anorexia, nausea, vomiting, foul-smelling lochia, and subinvolution. Specific assessment parameters are summarized in Table 29–3.

Reproductive system infections in the postpartum period must be assessed for the severity of the infection and the suspected causative organism(s). A history can identify prenatal or intrapartal risk factors. A physical examination is also performed, with the examiner using a vaginal speculum to visualize the vagina, cervix, and vaginal discharge. Specimens of lochia may be taken for microscopy and culture. This is done by passing a covered swab through the vagina and uncovering the swab when the desired area (high in the vagina and uterus) is reached. The resulting specimen is then sent to the laboratory. A bimanual examination is performed to assess the

► TABLE 29-3

Summary of Specific Reproductive System Infections and Assessment Findings

Type of Infection	Assessment Findings
Metritis	Fever initially 101–102°F, (38.3–38.9°C); if infection becomes more serious, jagged temperature elevations between 101 and 104°F (38.3 and 40°C) Uterine tenderness on palpation of the fundus or on bimanual examination Grimacing, guarding, complaints of pain Prolonged or bothersome afterpains Subinvolution of uterus Bacteria revealed on culture of lochia
Parametrial cellulitis (parametritis)	Prolonged elevation of temperature to 102–104°F (38.9–40°C) with fluctuations Extension of abdominal pain laterally; possible rebound tenderness Hypotension, subinvolution, chills Decreased bowel sounds, nausea, and vomiting
Peritonitis	Elevation of temperature to as high as 105°F (40.5°C) Severe pain Paralytic ileus Abdominal rigidity Frequent vomiting with dehydration Weak and thready pulse (possible) Rapid, shallow respirations Excessive thirst, marked anxiety
Septic pelvic thrombophlebitis	Elevation of temperature to 105°F (40.5°C); dramatic fluctuations (possible) over short periods Pain in flank or lower abdomen
Bacteremia and septic shock	Rapid elevation of temperature to 103–104°F (39.4–40°C) Profuse, foul-smelling lochia Symptoms of shock Reduction in urinary output

uterus, adnexa, cellular tissues, and pelvic peritoneum for swelling and tenderness. Blood is drawn for culture if the infection is severe or if bacteremia is suspected.

Nursing Diagnoses. Examples of nursing diagnoses that can be developed for the client with a postpartum reproductive system infection include:

Problem-oriented diagnoses:

- Impaired tissue integrity, related to puerperal metritis
- Risk for infection: spread, related to uterine infection
- Hyperthermia, related to puerperal infection

- Altered parenting, related to maternal separation from newborn because of maternal infection

Wellness-oriented diagnoses:

- Positive self-concept: mothering role performance, related to relief of symptoms of infection and availability of resources

Nursing and Collaborative Management. With the current trend toward early discharge, many infections become apparent after the client is discharged. Teaching clients about signs and symptoms of infection and the importance of contacting their health care providers is an important part of postpartum care. Antimicrobial therapy is the mainstay of treatment for reproductive system infections. Other measures include rest, hydration, analgesia, teaching, and emotional support during this stressful experience. The type or combination of antibiotics used, their dosages, and route of administration depend on the suspected causative organism(s) and the degree of infection. While women with mild infections may receive oral antibiotics, moderately to severely infected women are given broad-spectrum intravenous antibiotics.

Most infections respond to broad-spectrum intravenous antibiotics within 48 to 72 hours. For the client known to be infected at the time of delivery, initial therapy consists of combination drug regimens. Table 29–4 lists information about several antibiotics commonly used to treat reproductive system infections.

If fever persists after 48 to 72 hours of antimicrobial therapy, investigation of possible other causes of infection is indicated. Antimicrobial therapy for peritonitis includes agents effective against *Peptostreptococcus, Peptococcus, Bacteroides, Clostridium,* and aerobic coliforms. As paralytic ileus may occur with peritonitis, the gastrointestinal tract is compressed by continuous nasogastric suctioning (Cunningham et al., 1997).

Septic shock is a complication of reproductive system infection and requires aggressive therapy: vigorous intravenous fluid infusion and administration of broad-spectrum antimicrobial drugs that cover suspected pathogens. Septic shock requires hemodynamic monitoring, vasoactive drugs when hypotension is not corrected by fluid treatment, and oxygen administered by mask to prevent tissue hypoxia. Nursing care for women with septic shock includes:

- Assessment of maternal vital signs (including pulse, blood pressure, and temperature)
- Careful assessment of intake and output
- Observation of lochia
- Notation of subjective complaints of the client

▶ **TABLE 29-4**

Antibiotics Commonly Used to Treat Reproductive System Infections

Antibiotic	Active Against	Dose
Ampicillin (many proprietary names)	*Escherichia coli, Proteus mirabilis, Neisseria gonorrhoeae,* enterococci, streptococci, pneumonocci	1–2 g IV every 6 hours
Cefoxitin (Mefoxin)	*E. coli, N. gonorrhoeae, Bacteroides* sp, *Clostridium* sp, *Peptococcus* sp, *Peptostreptococcus* sp, *Klebsiella* sp, *Proteus* sp	1–2 g IV every 6–8 hours
Cefotaxime (Claforan)	Similar to cefoxitin	1–2 g IV every 6–8 hours
Ceftizoxime (Cefizox)	Similar to cefoxitin	1–2 g IV every 8–12 hours
Cefotetan (Cefotan)	Similar to cefoxitin	1–2 g IV every 12 hours
Doxycycline (Vibramycin, others)	*Chlamydia trachomatis*	100 mg orally every 12 hours, or 100–200 mg IV once or twice daily
Gentamicin (many proprietary names)	Enterococci (when given with ampicillin), *E. coli, Klebsiella* sp, *Proteus* sp, *Pseudomonas*	1–2 mg/kg IV every 8 hours; adjust dose to maintain peak serum concentration of 4–8 μg/mL
Clindamycin (Cleocin)	*Bacteroides* sp, streptococci, staphylococci	600 mg IV every 6 hours or 900 mg IV every 8 hours

Monitoring hourly urine output (via indwelling catheter) is an excellent indicator of successful treatment.

Women with reproductive system infections need continuous nursing support. The client and her family may be anxious about the implications of the condition and the possible separation from the newborn. If the client is placed on a medical floor and is separated from her newborn, the nurse who cares for the newborn can coordinate communication with nurses caring for her. The client who is breastfeeding can be assured that she may continue to do so unless (1) she must be separated from the newborn, (2) she is given antibiotics that contraindicate breastfeeding, or (3) she feels too ill to breastfeed. If separation is indicated, the nurse can teach the client to maintain lactation by pumping the breasts, or to stimulate relactation once the infection has abated.

Women with serious infections may feel quite ill. They also may need to undergo additional procedures, for example, surgical drainage in the event of an abscess. Some women may be ill enough to require intensive care. In some settings, women with severe perinatal illness are admitted to a maternal–fetal intensive care unit. These units can provide critical care while meeting the complex physical and psychosocial needs associated with childbearing. Comprehensive care when infections arise usually prevents life-threatening sequelae.

Localized Infections

In addition to the reproductive system infections already mentioned, localized infections of the per-

ineum, vagina, or cesarean incision may occur in the postpartum period. Infection of the episiotomy site is relatively rare, occurring in 0.5 to 3% of women who have episiotomies. As might be expected, women with fourth degree lacerations are at greater risk for serious infection than women whose lacerations are less extensive (Cunningham et al., 1997).

Vaginal lacerations may become infected directly or by extension of infectious agents from the perineum. The abdominal incision may also become infected after cesarean delivery. These infections may be preceded by uterine infections and, in some instances, may progress to systemic infections.

Nursing and Collaborative Assessment. The classic features of infected wounds (redness, edema, ecchymosis, drainage) are present with infected episiotomy or abdominal incisions. The previously approximated edges of the incision may separate and seropurulent fluid may drain from the infection site.

The client may complain of pain and tenderness in the perineal, vaginal, or abdominal area. Temperature may rise if the incision is not opened and drained. When the wound is opened, cultures should be sent to isolate the bacteria.

Nursing and Collaborative Management. Care of localized infections focuses on establishing drainage of the infected material. An episiotomy or abdominal incision may open spontaneously. At other times, sutures are removed to allow drainage.

Sitz baths every 4 to 6 hours assist in cleansing the perineal area and provide comfort to the client with an infected perineal wound. Abdominal incision infections are treated by open drainage. The wound should be left open and packed with saline moistened gauze at least twice a day. Most of these wounds heal by secondary intention. Clean wounds with good granulation tissue may be sutured or taped closed. Analgesics can also provide some relief for discomfort related to localized infections.

▶ Non–Reproductive System Infections That Affect Postpartum Recovery

In addition to infections that directly affect the reproductive system of the postpartum client, several general infections may indirectly influence postpartum recovery. Two of the most common infections are mastitis and urinary tract infections (UTIs). Both of these can also occur in nonchildbearing women. A thorough assessment is essential to pinpoint the cause of symptoms and ensure an appropriate plan of care. Women who have chills, fever, and tenderness (common symptoms of metritis) may in fact have a UTI; women who complain of chills and fever later in the postpartum period may have mastitis.

Mastitis

Mastitis is an inflammation of the breast tissue caused by bacterial infection and found primarily in breastfeeding mothers. The bacterial organism usually enters the breast through a cracked nipple and multiplies in the milk. In some instances, infection results from stasis of milk behind a blocked duct. The causative organism is usually *Staphyloccus aureus,* which is found in the infant's nose and throat. The infant may contract the bacteria from nursery personnel, who may carry the organism, especially on the hands.

Nursing and Collaborative Assessment. Symptoms of suppurative mastitis do not appear until the second to fourth week postpartum. The client reports a painful, hardened, reddened area, usually on one breast. She may experience fever, chills, malaise, and enlarged glands in the axilla on the affected side. The breast may be engorged. Milk from the affected breast may be sent for culture and sensitivity. Results of the cultures also provide important information for surveillance about infections spread in nurseries (Cunningham et al., 1997). If not treated promptly, mastitis may progress and an abscess may form (Clark, 1995).

Nursing Diagnoses. Examples of nursing diagnoses for the woman experiencing mastitis include:

Problem-oriented diagnoses:

- Ineffective breastfeeding, related to discomfort from mastitis
- Altered maternal role performance, related to breast discomfort

Wellness-oriented diagnoses:

- Positive coping, related to knowledge of treatment for mastitis
- Positive self-concept, related to comfort secondary to treatment for mastitis

Nursing and Collaborative Management. Management focuses on treating infection and preventing stasis of milk in the breast. The woman with mastitis is managed with antibiotics, such as dicloxacillin or a cephalosporin. Continued feeding on the

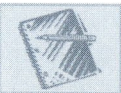

Client Teaching

Prevention of Mastitis

For the client at risk for or experiencing a recurrence of mastitis, the nurse can suggest the following strategies:

- Wash your hands before breastfeeding.
- Breastfeed frequently to prevent engorgement and stasis of milk. Avoid conditions that could foster milk stasis, e.g., constant pressure on the breast as might occur with a tight, ill-fitting brassiere, stopping the flow of milk by pressing on the areola, etc.
- Minimize the chance of cracked nipples by positioning your infant correctly on your breast, making sure that your baby latches on properly, and changing nipple pads when wet.
- If an area of your breast is distended or tender, breastfeed from the affected side first for each feeding. Remove your bra and massage the distended area as your infant nurses. Apply warm, moist heat before breastfeeding, change your baby's position on the breast, and make sure your breast is emptied after the feeding.
- Contact your health care provider if redness, fever, or pain occur in your breast(s).

affected breast is recommended, because the infant can empty the breast better than a breast pump or manual expression. Emptying of the infected breast minimizes engorgement and stasis of milk. If the woman is too uncomfortable to breastfeed on the affected side, gentle pumping until nursing can be started again is recommended (Cunningham et al., 1997). Such strategies as a well-supporting, properly fitted brassiere, analgesia, and an ice pack to the breast in between feedings or warm packs with feedings (whichever feels better) can be used (Varney, 1997). In some cases, the infant may need to be checked for bacterial colonization and, if test results are positive, treated for infection (Clark, 1995).

If the client develops a breast abscess, incision and drainage are required. Some authorities recommend discontinuation of breastfeeding on the affected breast, which is usually painful. The infant may still nurse on the opposite breast, and the client can pump the affected breast. Breastfeeding may need to be discontinued in some cases as a result of certain medications.

The woman with mastitis feels ill and may also feel discouraged about breastfeeding. The nurse can provide encouragement and ensure that the mother is given consistent, accurate information regarding the treatment for mastitis.

Urinary Tract Infections

Urinary tract infections occur in about 2 to 4% of postpartum women (Clark, 1995). *Escherichia coli* is the most frequent cause (75 to 90% of cases). Urinary tract infections can be differentiated into cystitis and pyelonephritis. **Cystitis** is inflammation of the bladder; pyelonephritis is inflammation of the renal pelves. (See Chapter 19 for discussion of UTIs during pregnancy.)

Risk Factors. Several factors place women at risk for postpartum UTIs:

- Relative hypotonicity of the lower urinary tract and bladder, which can cause stasis of urine.
- Trauma to the bladder from passage of the fetus through the pelvis.
- Catheterization. As Clark (1995) noted, 1–5% of women who have a single short-term catheterization and 50% of women who have intermittent catheterizations develop bacteruria.
- Frequent vaginal examinations during labor.

Nursing and Collaborative Assessment. In the postpartum period, distinguishing between reproductive system infections and UTIs can be difficult. Elevation in temperature may be the only presenting symptom of UTI; it should be ruled out when the postpartum woman has a temperature of 100.4°F or higher. Other signs and symptoms of UTIs are dysuria, frequency, urgency, suprapubic pain, hematuria, and pyuria. A history of urinary infections prenatally or chronic UTIs is a risk factor.

Pyelonephritis often does not become apparent until the end of the first postpartum week (Clark, 1995). The woman with pyelonephritis is usually quite ill. In addition to dysuria and frequency, signs of kidney involvement, for example, costovertebral angle tenderness, may be apparent. The woman's fever may spike as high as 104°F (40°C) and be accompanied by chills, flank pain, anorexia, and vomiting.

Relevant laboratory tests include urinalysis, complete blood count, serum creatinine and electrolyte levels, and blood and urine cultures and sensitivities. Significant bacteriuria is defined as the presence of 100,000 bacteria of the same species/mL on a clean-catch or catheterized specimen of urine. A count between 10,000 and 100,000 is ambiguous and indicates that the test should be repeated. Because of increased risk of infection, catheterization should be avoided.

Nursing Diagnoses. See Chapter 19 for examples of nursing diagnoses related to urinary tract infection.

Nursing and Collaborative Management. Management of UTIs consists of antimicrobial therapy, analgesia, and hydration. The course of treatment is usually begun before the culture and sensitivity results are obtained and adjusted if indicated by the laboratory results. High fluid intake is indicated to flush the urinary tract. Urinary anesthetics, such as phenazopyridine hydrochloride, are given for symptomatic relief of dysuria.

Management of the woman with pylonephritis includes bedrest; intravenous fluids to ensure adequate hydration and urinary output; parenteral antimicrobial therapy; and a cooling blanket (if the client has a high fever). Further tests, such as an intravenous pyelogram or ultrasound, may be done for clients with continuing problems.

Nursing care includes assessment of vital signs, intake and output, urinalysis, and urine culture and sensitivity. The postpartum client with a UTI may be relatively asymptomatic or she may be acutely ill. Although women with UTIs do not need to be separated from their infants, those who are acutely ill may find that they need someone else to provide infant care either in their room or in the nursery.

The nurse can also encourage prevention of infection by teaching the client self-care practices, for example, personal hygiene, wiping from the meatus toward the rectum to avoid bacterial contamination, and emptying the bladder frequently to avoid urinary stasis. The woman with pyelonephritis may need long-term therapy. Explanations about the condition and therapy should be provided to the client and other family members. Breastfeeding is not contraindicated, but may be delayed or interrupted if the client is acutely ill.

▶ Prevention of Infection

When the client is admitted to the birthing facility, strict asepsis should be followed. Universal precautions minimize spread of disease. Multiple vaginal examinations should be avoided. Measures also should be taken to prevent dehydration and exhaustion during labor and excessive blood loss during delivery. Operative deliveries should be minimized if possible. After delivery, the physician or CNM should inspect for and remove any retained placental tissue, as this is a focus for infection. High-risk cesarean delivery clients should receive prophylactic antibiotics in an effort to control infection.

Nurses should assist postpartum clients to void by measures such as providing privacy, helping the client to ambulate and to use a toilet instead of a bedpan, running water, and helping the client shower. These measures, although time consuming, often spare clients risk of infection, related to catheterization.

▶ THROMBOEMBOLIC DISORDERS

The prenatal, intrapartum, and postpartum phases of childbearing are high-risk periods for the development of thromboembolic disorders. These disorders include superficial venous thrombosis, limited to the superficial veins of the lower extremity, and deep venous thrombosis (DVT), involving the deep veins of the leg. Superficial venous thrombosis is associated with inflammation and may be termed "phlebitis," or superficial venous thrombophlebitis. Deep venous thrombosis is not associated with inflammation and should not be called "phlebitis."

▶ Risk Factors

The onset of thromboembolic disease is more likely in the postpartum period than in the prenatal period. Factors associated with increased risk include maternal age greater than 35, past history of thrombosis, cardiac disease, more than three previous pregnancies, cesarean delivery, obesity, varicose veins, and venous stasis caused by immobilization. The incidence of throm-

boembolic disease in the postpartum period decreased when early ambulation became widely practiced.

Stasis is probably the strongest predisposing factor to deep venous thrombosis. In addition, clotting factors generally remain elevated in the immediate postpartum period. Levels of protein C, a main coagulation inhibitor, decrease slightly after delivery and do not increase again until about 3 to 5 days postpartum. Women with such preexisting hematologic abnormalities such as sickle-cell anemia, protein C deficiency, Factor V resistance, or antithrombin III deficiency are more prone to venous thrombosis whether or not they are pregnant.

▶ Superficial Venous Thrombosis

Superficial venous thrombosis is limited to the superficial veins of the legs. The thrombus forms as a result of inflammation in the vein wall (thrombophlebitis). This type of thrombosis rarely results in serious complications, such as pulmonary embolism. If, however, thrombophlebitis extends above the knee, the woman is at higher risk for deep vein involvement.

▶ Deep Venous Thrombosis

Deep venous thrombosis in the leg may involve much of the deep venous system from the foot to the iliofemoral region. Deep venous thrombosis in the postpartum period may present with abrupt onset of pain and edema of the calf. However, the onset of DVT may not produce pain and tenderness, but only mild swelling.

Nursing and Collaborative Assessment

Through routine postpartum assessment, the nurse may be the first person to identify signs and symptoms of thromboembolic disorders. The nurse palpates the calves of the legs for heat and tenderness, and notes any subjective complaints of the mother (see Chapter 19). Diagnoses based solely on clinical signs and symptoms may be inaccurate 50% of the time (Cowchock & Merli, 1992; Weiner, 1985). For example, DVT can be present despite a negative Homans' sign. Because of the inaccuracy of the physical examination, further testing is usually necessary. Women suspected of having DVT should first be evaluated with such noninvasive tests as ultrasound or duplex scanning (see Chapter 19). Venography should only be performed when noninvasive tests are inconclusive or unavailable.

Nursing and Collaborative Management

Management for superficial venous thrombosis includes rest, elevation, the use of support hose when ambulating, analgesics for comfort and antiinflammatory agents. The nurse provides information to the client and family regarding the condition and self-care practices.

For women diagnosed with DVT, anticoagulant therapy is started with IV heparin. The initial therapy includes administration of heparin by continuous intravenous infusion. Dosages of heparin are adjusted according to coagulation studies (partial thromboplastin time 2 times control). While the client is on heparin therapy, her platelet count should be monitored because of the potential for development of heparin-induced antibodies to platelets.

Oral warfarin therapy is usually started at the time of diagnosis of DVT and continued for 3 to 6 months (see box entitled Drug Guide: Warfarin Sodium). A filter may be placed in the inferior vena cava to protect against pulmonary emboli if anticoagulation is contraindicated. The dosage of warfarin traditionally has been monitored by the prothrombin time or the protime ratio. Variations in results of this test can exist among laboratories, because of differences in the reagents used for the tests. The International Normalized Ratio (INR) is a method of standardizing prothrombin time results reported by different laboratories. With the INR system, a client's anticoagulation status can be more uniformly monitored and the likelihood of undercoagulating or overcoagulating the client may be decreased (Berkman, 1992; Jeong, 1993). Although warfarin is contraindicated in pregnancy, it may be taken postpartum. The drug is excreted into breast milk, and there is controversy over possible neonatal effects from the

---

▶ **DRUG GUIDE: WARFARIN SODIUM**

ACTION/INDICATIONS

Interferes with the synthesis of vitamin K–dependent blood coagulation factors II, VII, IX, and X. Inhibits thrombus formation when stasis is induced and may prevent extension of existing thrombi. Prophylaxis and treatment of venous thrombosis. Prophylaxis and treatment of pulmonary embolism. Treatment of atrial fibrillation with embolization. As an adjunct in treatment of coronary occlusion.

DOSAGE

Usually administered orally. *Usual initial adult dose:* 5–15 mg daily until desired INR (International Normalized Ratio) is reached. *Maintenance dose:* usually ranges from 2 to 10 mg daily, but dose is adjusted on basis of INR.

CONTRAINDICATIONS AND PRECAUTIONS

Contraindicated in active bleeding or when risk of bleeding is increased, as in hemorrhagic blood dyscrasias; ulceration of wounds of gastrointestinal, respiratory, or genitourinary tracts; cerebrovascular hemorrhage. Also in senility, alcoholism, or psychosis if client cannot be relied on to comply with therapy. Contraindicated in pregnancy. Use with caution in minor dental or surgical procedure.

ADVERSE REACTIONS

Most common: Minor bleeding episodes. *Less common:* CV—hemorrhage from any body site; necrosis, and gangrene of skin; GI—nausea, vomiting, anorexia, diarrhea, increase in liver enzymes; hematologic—leukopenia, agranulocytosis; other—dermatitis, urticaria, alopecia, fever, purple toe syndrome; fetal—congenital anomalies.

DRUG INTERACTIONS

Drugs/conditions that may potentially increase response to warfarin: acute alcohol intoxication, allopurinol, aminosalicylic acid, amiodarone, anabolic steroids, chloral hydrate, chloramphenicol, cimetidine, clofibrate, cotrimoxazole, danazol, dextrothyroxine, diazoxide, diflunisal, disulfiram, erythromycin, ethacrynic acid, fenoprofen, glucagon, ibuprofen, indomethacin, influenza virus vaccine, isoniazid, ketoprofen, meclofenamate, mefenamic acid, metronidazole, miconazole, nalidixic acid, pentoxifylline, phenylbutazone, propoxyphene, phenylketonuria, quinidine, quinine, salicylates, streptokinase, sulfinpyrazone, sulfonamides, sulindac, tetracyclines, thiazides, thyroid drugs, tricyclic antidepressants, urokinase, vitamin E.

Drugs/conditions that may potentially decrease response to warfarin: chronic alcoholism, barbiturates, carbamazepine, corticosteroids, ethchlorvynol, glutethimide, griseofulvin, mercaptopurine, methaqualone, estrogen-containing oral contraceptives, rifampin, spironolactone, vitamin K.

NURSING IMPLICATIONS

INR is determined before initiation of therapy and periodically if client is placed on maintenance dose.

- Assess for signs of bleeding.
- Teach client to wear identifying bracelet and inform other health care providers (e.g., dentists) that she is on warfarin therapy.
- Teach client to use soft toothbrush and assess for signs of hemorrhage.
- Advise breastfeeding clients that it is yet uncertain whether oral warfarin will pass into breast milk or not. They should request their physician to prescribe subcutaneous heparin, which does not have this effect.

drug. As a precaution, the breastfeeding mother should be advised to inform her health care provider so that he or she may prescribe subcutaneous heparin, which does not pass into the breast milk.

Nursing care for the woman placed on loading doses of anticoagulant therapy includes careful monitoring for signs of hemorrhage, such as epistaxis, blood in the urine and stool, and ecchymosis or petechiae. The woman who will receive protracted therapy after discharge should be taught the purpose and action of the medication and the signs of hemorrhagic complications. The woman also should wear an identification bracelet that states that she is receiving anticoagulant therapy.

▶ Pulmonary Embolism

Pulmonary embolism (PE) is a rare complication of DVT. About 35% of women who develop PE have a history of DVT. Emboli may originate in the legs or pelvic veins.

Nursing and Collaborative Assessment

Signs and symptoms of PE may include sharp chest pain or chest discomfort, dyspnea, tachypnea, and apprehension. Other symptoms include rales, air hunger, hemoptysis, cyanosis, tachycardia, and gallop rhythm over the heart when large emboli are present. However, an unexplained fever may be the only sign of a PE.

Laboratory studies include the indirect tests of serial blood gas analysis, blood coagulation studies, electrocardiogram, chest x-ray, and duplex scanning. The diagnosis of pulmonary emboli is verified by ventilation perfusion scan of the lung using radioisotopes. If this is still inconclusive, pulmonary angiography remains the most definitive way of detecting PE.

Nursing and Collaborative Mangement

The physician or nurse-midwife should be notified immediately if PE is suspected. Heparin therapy is begun (with close monitoring of partial thromboplastin time) and oxygen given (1 to 2 L/min by nasal route).

A large PE may block blood flow from the right ventricle into the lungs. This may result in right-sided cardiac failure, shock, and death. Emergency treatment may include surgical embolectomy, or use of fibrinolytic agents such as streptokinase or urokinase. However, the use of lytic agents systemically may be contraindicated in the postpartum woman.

The client with a pulmonary embolus requires intensive nursing care and crisis intervention by the interdisciplinary team. She and her family also need continuous support throughout the crisis.

▶ PSYCHOLOGIC COMPLICATIONS

During the postpartum period, many women report symptoms of increased tension, anxiety, labile moods, and negative thinking. In some women, these feelings may be symptoms of mood disorders that interfere with healthy adaptation. Psychologic conditions seen during the postpartum period include the widely experienced "postpartum blues" and the more serious conditions of postpartum depression, postpartum panic disorder, and postpartum psychosis.

▶ Postpartum Blues

Postpartum blues or **transient depression** are common terms for temporary and self-limiting depression that usually begins within the first few days after delivery. The actual causes of postpartum blues are unknown. The condition may last from a few hours or days to 2 to 3 weeks, although the exact time frame is unclear. Postpartum blues are thought to affect up to 75% of postpartum women.

Postpartum blues is the mildest form of emotional disturbance associated with childbearing (Woud, Thomas, Droppleman, & Meighan, 1997). Women with postpartum blues experience an alteration in mood, characterized by such feelings as anxiety, irritability, sadness, and tearfulness. They also have periods of happiness. These women are otherwise healthy, and their transient depression is believed to be unrelated to their own or their babies' health, obstetric problems, socioeconomic status, method of infant feeding, or hospitalization, although any of these conditions could affect the client's mood (Rosenthal, 1994). Transient depression occurs in many cultures. However, it tends to be less of a problem in cultures that encourage open expression of emotions and that surround the childbearing woman

Nursing Alert

The client on a maintenance regimen of warfarin sodium should avoid salicylates because they can cause bleeding and restrict use of alcoholic beverages since alcohol can alter response to warfarin.

with significant others to provide love, care, and support.

Postpartum blues tend to resolve spontaneously. However, postpartum blues should not be dismissed as trivial. Indeed, research has linked postpartum blues at 1 week postpartum with the development of postpartum depression at 6 and 12 weeks postpartum (Beck, Reynolds, & Rutowski, 1992). In addition, depression that persists or that is linked to a specific cause requires further assessment.

▶ Postpartum Depression

In contrast to postpartum blues, symptoms of **postpartum depression** may last for weeks. Depression may occur during pregnancy; however, postpartum depression can differ from depression during pregnancy. It may recur in future pregnancies. The onset of postpartum depression is most often seen in the fourth week after delivery and usually evolves slowly across several weeks; it can also develop at any time during the first year (Wood et al., 1997). An estimated 10–15% of women are affected by postpartum depression, which has more emotional disturbance, distorted thinking, and related problems than does postpartum blues.

The causes of postpartum depression remain unclear. A higher incidence of the syndrome has been observed in women with past personal or family psychiatric problems, interpersonal difficulties, severe postpartum blues, and life event problems (Beck et al., 1992; Rosenthal, 1994). Postpartum depression has been linked to such factors as (Beck, 1996, 1998a; Rosenthal, 1994; Wood et al., 1997):

- Prenatal anxiety/depression
- Child care stress
- Life stress
- Lack of social support
- Unstable relationships with husband and/or parents

- Personal dissatisfaction
- Perception of the infant's temperament as demanding and difficult

Postpartum depression is an emotionally painful experience for women and their families and tends to interfere with daily activities. Wood and colleagues (1997) describe this condition as a "downward spiral" of emotions that women in their study likened to "drowning," "going downhill," and "sinking deeper and deeper." Studies have further demonstrated an association between maternal depression and adverse outcomes for the child (Zuckerman & Beardslee, 1987). The box entitled Selected Characteristics of Postpartum Depression presents behavioral manifestations that may occur with this condition.

▶ Postpartum Panic Attacks and Panic Disorder

Panic attacks and panic disorder have recently been identified as psychologic problems that can occasionally occur during the postpartum period. Panic attacks are characterized by sudden terror, often associated with a feeling of impending doom; they are accompanied by such physical symptoms as shortness of breath, dizziness, nausea, palpitations, and chest pain and such psychologic symptoms as decreased cognitive functioning and fear of losing control, dying, or going crazy (Beck, 1998b). Panic disorder is identified when recurrent, unexpected panic attacks are followed by at least a month of worry about another attack or its implications or a significant behavioral change related to the attacks (American Psychological Association, 1994). Panic disorder may occur for the first time during the postpartum period or may occur prior to pregnancy or delivery. According to Zal (1990), panic disorder may be linked to genetic vulnerability and may emerge postpartum in relation to stress during pregnancy. Postpartum panic disorder complicates lives, brings about negative changes in

---

▶ SELECTED CHARACTERISTICS OF POSTPARTUM DEPRESSION

- Inability to sleep or rest
- Crying
- Changes in appetite
- Decreased energy and fatigue
- Feelings of worthlessness and despair; negative future outlook
- Sense of isolation
- Lack of concern for personal appearance

- Feelings of anxiety, irritability, loss of control
- Obsessive thoughts of being a failure
- Hostility/anger
- Problems with maternal–infant interaction; perception of infant as difficult and demanding; guilt about not being able to care adequately for the baby
- Feelings of being an inept mother, of being trapped, angry, or afraid

women's lifestyles, and affects self-esteem (Beck, 1998b). Postpartum panic disorder differs from postpartum depression, although women with postpartum panic disorder may also suffer from depression.

▶ Postpartum Psychosis

Postpartum psychosis is a severe psychiatric condition that occurs in an estimated 1 to 2% of postpartum women (Wood et al., 1997). Postpartum psychosis may be similar to nonpostpartum psychosis. Symptoms often develop from a few days to 4 to 6 weeks postpartum, although the illness may begin during the third trimester. Symptoms include restlessness, irritability, sleep disturbances, delusions, hallucinations, disorganized behavior, and withdrawn behavior. The actual cause of postpartum psychosis is unknown, and the condition may recur with future pregnancies. Women at risk for postpartum psychosis include those with previous psychiatric histories, marital and family problems, stressful life events, and lack of social support; however, postpartum psychosis can occur without these risk factors (Rosenthal, 1994).

Postpartum psychosis causes great concern, because of the risk of the mother's behavior to her infant, herself, or others. However, nonpsychotic women may also think of harming themselves or their babies and sometimes respond to such impulses (Wood et al., 1997).

▶ Nursing and Collaborative Assessment

Assessment focuses on identifying postpartum psychologic complications and contributing factors. Ideally, women at risk are identified during pregnancy, so that appropriate interventions can be started. While in the birthing facility, women are assessed for such at risk behaviors as inability to comfortably hold or feed infants (Wood et al., 1997). Data regarding the woman's postpartum adaptation include (Beck, 1998a, 1998b; Rosenthal, 1994):

1. *History.* Depression, panic disorder or other psychologic problem prior to or during pregnancy; postpartum psychologic problem with any previous pregnancy.
2. *Daily activities.* Difficulties in care of self, household, and infant; sleep; eating schedule; moods; interest in sex; energy level.
3. *Impact of childbirth events.* Frequency of thoughts about labor and delivery; feelings about the event; sense of disappointment, sadness, or ambivalence.
4. *Mother–infant interactions.* Degree of comfort while with the infant, degree of pleasure while performing infant tasks; thoughts of "something bad" happening to the infant; confused or angry feelings toward the infant; degree of comfort in being a mother; child care stress.
5. *Social activities and supports.* Perception of relationship with infant's father and significant others; time for social activities with other adults; perception of receiving emotional support; sense of isolation from other adults.
6. *Self-assessment.* Degree to which the woman rates herself as a "good person"; ability to manage her many roles; sense of physical attractiveness; predominant mood; depressive feelings, panic, or suicidal thoughts.

Assessment also is done to differentiate postpartum problems from such conditions as schizophrenia, organic brain syndromes, and substance abuse.

Nursing Diagnoses

Assessment of the client for psychologic adaptation in the postpartum period leads to the development of appropriate nursing diagnoses for postpartum depression. Examples of these diagnoses include:

Problem-oriented diagnoses:

- Impaired social interaction, related to postpartum depression
- Altered family processes, related to maternal depressive behavior
- Risk for violence: self-directed or directed at infant, related to severe postpartum depression

Wellness-oriented diagnoses:

- Positive self-concept, related to successful treatment for postpartum depression and positive social supports
- Positive social interaction with infant, related to successful management of postpartum depression

Women's Health

Certain symptoms that may indicate depression, such as exhaustion, difficulty in sleeping, and changes in appetite, may actually be manifestations of normal postpartum changes.

► Nursing and Collaborative Management

Management begins with identification of women at risk and of signs and symptoms of postpartum blues, postpartum depression, postpartum panic disorder and postpartum psychosis. Creating an environment where a client and her significant others can discuss emotional concerns is essential. Clients may feel that an emotional disorder carries a stigma or that they are alone; they may remain silent unless such topics as blues, depression, panic, and feelings of inadequacy in parenting are raised by the caregiver. Early discharge and the usual occurrence of postpartum psychologic problems after the woman is home present challenges. Assessment and management strategies for these conditions are important for such outreach as postpartum home visits, the client's routine postpartum visit(s) to the clinic or caregiver's office, and telephone follow-up programs. Strategies can include: realistic childbirth and parenting education that prepares women for real, rather than only ideal, postpartum experiences; educating women to differentiate between symptoms of postpartum blues and depression; educating about physical and psychologic components of panic attacks; and educating women and families about supportive resources and the need for intervention should psychologic symptoms occur (Beck, 1998b; Wood et al., 1997). Teaching new mothers about infant caregiving skills and appropriate responses to infant cues and helping women gain confidence in adjusting to their new roles are also necessary. In addition, appropriate referrals need to be made to community and mental health care providers and agencies.

A caring attitude is part of all nursing interventions. However, what nurses perceive as essential caring behaviors may not be perceived in the same way by mothers with postpartum depression. Beck (1995a, 1995b) studied women who had experienced postpartum depression. Through extensive, unstructured interviews, she identified the following themes the women felt were essential aspects of nurses' caring:

- Having the knowledge about postpartum depression to make a quick, accurate nursing diagnosis
- Using keen observation and intuition for an awareness that something might be wrong with the mother
- Providing hope that the mothers' living nightmares would end
- Sharing valuable time with the mother
- Making appropriate referrals
- Making an extra effort to provide continuity of care for the mother
- Understanding what the mother was experiencing

Women with postpartum blues usually recover spontaneously with support. Women with postpartum depression or panic disorder may be treated as outpatients. Medications, individual and/or group therapies may be used. Women and their significant others need to be involved. Hospitalization may be necessary for women with severe postpartum psychologic problems who are unable to manage otherwise. Regardless of diagnosis, anyone thought to be at risk to herself or others requires immediate intervention.

Critical Thinking in Care Planning

Care of the Client Experiencing Postpartum Depression

Alice and Peter Green come to the pediatrician's office for the first time with Matthew, their 2-week-old infant. This is their second son; their first child is 3 years old. The nurse practitioner takes a health history, including history of previous pregnancies and health of their first child. As the nurse is taking the history, she notes that Peter is doing all the responding and Alice is sitting in the chair with her head bent and eyes directed to the floor. Peter is holding the infant. The nurse directs her attention to Alice and asks how she is feeling. Alice replies in one or two words without raising her eyes from the floor. Alice's past history reveals previous postpartum depression. The previous postpartum depression lasted 3 weeks and was treated on an outpatient basis. Peter states that his wife's current symptoms seem more severe.

▶ Assessment

- History of postpartum depression
- Client does not make eye contact; has sad expression; does not look at or hold infant
- Client's husband does most of the responding during interview
- Client states that she wanted a girl
- Client's husband states that she needed much help in caring for first child; mother-in-law had to care for infant for first few weeks and is again helping with infant

Nursing Diagnosis

Altered family processes, related to maternal depressive behavior

Expected Client/Family Outcomes	Nursing Action/Intervention	Evaluation
Following interventions, the postpartum client will: - Communicate with the health care provider. - Communicate with her husband, infant, and other family members and demonstrate beginning social interaction with infant and others. - Demonstrate positive coping techniques.	Identify strategies used by family to cope successfully with client's postpartum depression after birth of first child. Provide support to client and partner and encourage them to verbalize concerns. Assess family's coping strategies and interactional patterns: verbal and nonverbal communication, role behavior, use of support systems. *Rationale:* Previous successful coping strategies are useful when similar crises emerge. Empathic care supports couple during a difficult time. Verbalization helps family define the crisis and coping strategies needed. Assess maternal attachment behaviors and risk for delayed attachment and abuse. *Rationale:* Postpartum depression is a painful experience for clients and families. Impaired maternal–infant attachment can increase potential for other problems. Identify family support systems and alternate caretakers for infant. *Rationale:* Social support is related to positive health care outcome.	Following interventions, client interacts with, and makes eye contact with the health care provider. Client and family discuss strategies used after birth of first child. Client demonstrates attachment behaviors with infant. Client interacts socially and communicates with infant and other family members.

Critical Thinking in Care Planning *continued*

Expected Client/Family Outcomes	Nursing Action/Intervention	Evaluation
	Encourage couple to use stress management techniques, practice relaxation techniques and get adequate rest, exercise, nutrition. *Rationale:* Stress management techniques that include positive self-help practices foster resolution of crisis in a positive manner.	Couple demonstrates and discusses stress management techniques.
	Provide referral to psychiatric clinical nurse specialist, psychologist, or psychiatrist (as necessary), specializing in postpartum depression. *Rationale:* These practitioners can provide specialized care to client and family.	Client and partner inform nurse that they have sought assistance from specialist and attended counseling sessions as necessary.
	Refer client to postpartum depression support group if appropriate. *Rationale:* Support groups can provide resources and can help clients not feel isolated as they deal with postpartum depression.	Client and partner attend support group.

Chapter Highlights

▶ Postpartum complications occur, even with excellent care, and can predate pregnancy, emerge during pregnancy, labor, or delivery, or appear only during the postpartum period.

▶ Postpartum hemorrhage is the most common cause of excessive blood loss during childbearing and attention should be given to careful postpartum physical assessment in order to identify heavy bleeding promptly and help minimize chances of unnecessary blood loss and other complications.

▶ Early postpartum hemorrhage occurs within the first 24 hours after delivery and is most often due to excessive bleeding from the site of implantation of the placenta and/or trauma to the genital tract or nearby tissues.

▶ Late postpartum hemorrhage occurs any time between 24 hours and 6 weeks postpartum and may be the result of either subinvolution or retention of placental fragments.

▶ Interventions for postpartum hemorrhage focus on early identification and treatment of the cause(s) of hemorrhage and correction of hypovolemia.

▶ Postpartum infections encompass infections that arise in the genital tract after delivery (metritis, parametrial cellulitis, peritonitis, and septic pelvic thrombophlebitis) and non–reproductive system infections (mastitis and urinary tract infections) that arise in sites other than the genital tract and influence maternal morbidity during postpartum recovery.

▶ Antimicrobial therapy, hydration, and pain relief are important components of treatment for postpartum infections.

▶ Thromboembolic disorders can also occur in the postpartum period and include such conditions as superficial venous thrombosis and deep venous thrombosis, which may lead to pulmonary emboli.

▶ Psychologic complications of the postpartum period include postpartum blues, depression, panic disorder, and psychosis.

▶ Nurses should anticipate that some women may experience psychologic difficulties during the postpartum period, provide an atmosphere that encourages discussion and identification of these problems, and be prepared to refer clients appropriately.

After reading the vignette at the beginning of this chapter, use what you have learned to answer these questions.

1. What assessment criteria might be used to determine the cause of Virginia Gordon's fever?

2. What effect might a high-risk condition such as postpartum infection have on Virginia Gordon's plans for discharge and interaction with her baby and family?

3. What nursing actions might provide physical comfort and emotional support to a client with a postpartum infection?

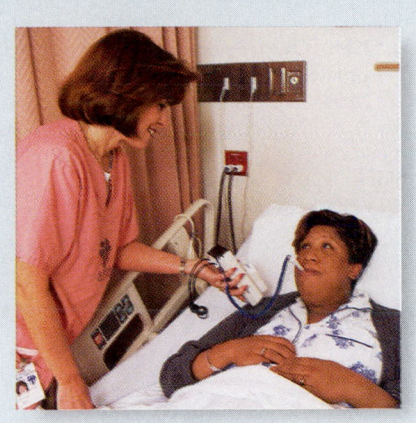

Critical Thinking Questions

▶ References

AbouZahr, C., Wardlaw, T., Stanton, C., & Hill, K. (1996). Maternal mortality. *World Health Statistics Quarterly, 49*(2), 77–87.

American College of Obstetricians and Gynecologists. (1988). *Antimicrobial therapy for obstetric patients* (Technical Bulletin No. 117). Washington, DC: Author.

American Psychological Association (1994). Diagnostic and Statistical Manual of Mental Disorders. (4th ed.) (DSM-IV). Washington DC: Author.

Beck, C.T. (1995a). Perception of nurses' caring by mothers experiencing postpartum depression. *Journal of Obstetric, Gynecologic, and Neonatal Nursing, 24*(9), 819–825.

Beck, C.T. (1995b). Effects of postpartum depression on maternal-infant interaction: A meta-analysis. *Nursing Research, 44*(5), 298–304.

Beck, C.T. (1996). A meta-analysis of the relationship between postpartum depression and infant temperament. *Nursing Research, 45*(4), 225–230.

Beck, C.T. (1998a). A checklist to identify women at risk for developing postpartum depression. *Journal of Obstetric, Gynecologic, and Neonatal Nursing, 27*(1), 39–46.

Beck, C.T. (1998b). Postpartum onset of panic disorder. *Image, 30*(2), 131–135.

Beck, C.T., Reynolds, M. A., & Rutowski, P. (1992). Maternity blues and postpartum depression. *Journal of Obstetric, Gynecologic, and Neonatal Nursing, 21,* 287–293.

Benson, R.C., & Pernoll, M.L. (1994). *Handbook of obstetrics and gynecology* (9th ed.). New York: McGraw-Hill.

Berkman, S.A. (1992). Current concepts in anticoagulation. *Hospital Practice* (February 15), 187–200.

Biswas, M.K., & Perloff, D. (1994). Cardiac, hematologic, pulmonary, renal, and urinary tract disorders in pregnancy. In A.H. DeCherney & M.L. Pernoll (Eds.), *Current obstetric and gynecologic diagnosis and treatment* (8th ed.) (pp. 428–467). Norwalk, CT: Appleton & Lange.

Blanco, J.D. (1992). Postpartum endometritis. In N. Gleicher (Ed.), *Principles and practice of medical therapy in pregnancy* (2nd ed.) (pp. 727–731). Norwalk, CT: Appleton & Lange.

Clark, R.A. (1995). Infections during the postpartum period. *Journal of Obstetric, Gynecologic, and Neonatal Nursing, 24*(6), 542–548.

Cowchock, F.A., & Merli, G.J. (1992). Pulmonary embolism and thromboembolic disorders. In N. Gleicher (Ed.), *Principles and practice of medical therapy in pregnancy* (2nd ed.) (pp. 738–743). Norwalk, CT: Appleton & Lange.

Craigo, S.D., & Kapernick, P.S. (1994). Postpartum hemorrhage and the abnormal puerperium. In A.H. DeCherney & M.L. Pernoll (Eds.), *Current obstetric and gynecologic diagnosis and treatment* (8th ed.) (pp. 574–593). Norwalk, CT: Appleton & Lange.

Cunningham, F.G., MacDonald, P.C., Gant, N.F., Leveno, K.J., Gilstrap, L.C., Hankins, G.D.V., & Clark, S.L. (1997). *Williams obstetrics* (20th ed.). Stamford, CT: Appleton & Lange.

Gabbe, S.G., Niebyl, J.R., & Simpson, J.L. (1996). *Obstetrics: Normal and problem pregnancies* (3rd ed.). New York: Churchill-Livingstone.

Hayashi, R.H., & Castillo, M.S. (1993). Bleeding in pregnancy. In R.A. Knuppel, J.E. Drukker (Eds.), *High-risk pregnancy: A team approach* (2nd ed.) (pp. 539–560). Philadelphia: W.B. Saunders.

Hill, P.S. (1989). Effects of heat and cold on the perineum after episiotomy laceration. *Journal of Obstetric, Gynecologic, and Neonatal Nursing, 18,* 124–129.

Jacobson, H. (1985). A standard for assessing lochia volume. *MCN, American Journal of Maternal-Child Nursing, 10,* 174–175.

Jeong, E. (1993). Using the international normalized ratios when monitoring protimes. *Hospital Pharmacy, 28,* 1076.

Luegenbiehl, D.L. (1997). Improving visual estimation of blood volume on peripads. *MCN, American Journal of Maternal Child Nursing, 22,* 294–298.

Oxorn, H. (Ed.). (1986). *Oxorn-Foote human labor and birth* (5th ed.). Norwalk, CT: Appleton & Lange.

Rosenthal, M.B. (1994). Psychological aspects of obstetrics and gynecology. In A.H. DeCherney & M.L. Pernoll (Eds.), *Current obstetric and gynecologic diagnosis and treatment* (8th ed.) (pp. 1087–1106). Norwalk, CT: Appleton & Lange.

Varney, H. (1997). *Varney's midwifery* (3rd ed.). Boston: Jones & Bartlett.

Weiner, C.P. (1985). Diagnosis and management of thromboembolic disease during pregnancy. *Clinics in Obstetrics and Gynecology, 28,* 107.

Wood, A.F., Thomas, S.P., Droppleman, P.G., & Meighan, M. (1997). The downspiral of postpartum depression. *MCN, American Journal of Maternal Child Nursing, 22*(6), 308–316.

Zal, H.M. (1990). *Panic Disorder: The Great Pretender.* New York: Plenum Press.

Zuckerman, B.S., & Beardslee, W.R. (1987). Maternal depression: A concern for pediatricians. *Pediatrics, 79,* 110–116.

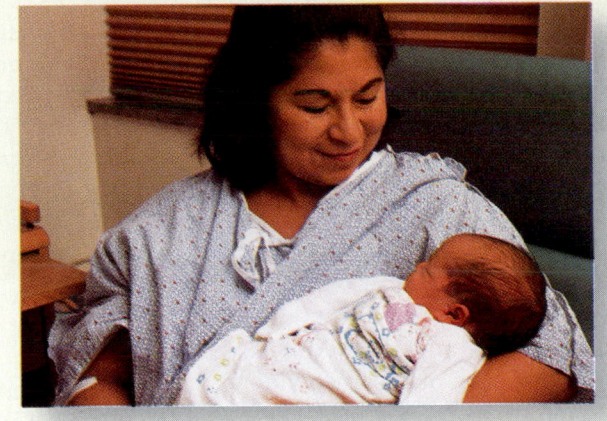

Nine-hour-old Anna Lopez is with her parents, Carmen and Emilio, in Carmen's hospital room. Anna is the couple's first child. Immediately after delivery, Anna was placed in Carmen's arms, and Carmen and Emilio were delighted to see how alert Anna was and how well she focused on their faces.

Carmen asks Gloria Rinaldi, RN, "Would you watch me as I pick Anna up? I've only done this once before and I want to be sure I'm doing it right." Carmen lifts Anna up from the crib and, cradling her against her chest, sits down in a chair. She states, "I felt much more comfortable handling Anna this time. Is there anything else we should know about caring for her?" ∎

30

Assessment and Care of the Normal Newborn

During the **neonatal period,** the first 28 days of life, family members change in response to the physiologic, psychologic, and developmental needs of the newborn. At the same time, parents and siblings have needs related to their changing roles within the family system. Coping with these roles begins in the prenatal period, when parents fantasize about their idealized infant; however, the birth of the newborn requires that family members become reality oriented as they focus attention on the care of the newborn.

The newborn has physical features that are much different from those of children and adults. The head is large in comparison to the rest of the body, the extremities are relatively short, and the abdomen is prominent. At birth, the newborn may show evidence of edema of the presenting part, or the head may be molded from the process of labor and delivery. The newborn also may have skin variations such as milia, mongolian spots, and Epstein's pearls in the mouth, which may be unfamiliar to parents. In short, the newborn's physical features may be different from those fantasized by the parents during pregnancy.

Birth requires that the newborn make several physiologic changes in adjusting to the extrauterine environment. The most critical adaptations involve the respiratory and cardiovascular systems. The newborn must also begin to regulate body temperature, an activity that was unnecessary for the fetus in utero. Several other systems also undergo major changes as the newborn moves from intrauterine to extrauterine life.

Behavioral responses of the newborn are predictable. The newborn is equipped with a repertoire of behavioral interactions that will elicit responses from caregivers. The nurse's role includes teaching parents about the normal characteristics of the newborn so that positive parent–newborn interactions can be facilitated.

Assessment of the neonate is an ongoing process during which the nurse collects physiologic and psychosocial data. Immediately after an infant's birth, the nurse determines the Apgar score, which is an assessment of the newborn's heart rate, respiratory effort, reflex irritability, muscle tone, and color. A variety of screening procedures may also be done in the early newborn period.

The health of neonates is influenced by the health of their parents, family, and environment. The data base obtained by the nurse provides relevant information about the newborn against which later comparisons can be made. Thus, it is imperative that the initial data base be comprehensive and consider all that affects the newborn.

Nursing care begins in the newborn period and focuses on preventive measures that protect the infant. Promotion of parent–newborn attachment begins at birth and continues throughout the first year. Discharge planning is important in anticipating needs of families and their newborns.

Maternity nurses coordinate care with community and pediatric nurses in an effort to provide continuity and holistic nursing services to families and their newborns. Nurses assist family members to promote the health and well-being of the neonate and infant, and educate parents about normal growth and development parameters and care of common problems that may occur during infancy.

▶ PHYSIOLOGIC ADJUSTMENT TO EXTRAUTERINE LIFE

Transition from an intrauterine to extrauterine environment is a critical period of behavioral and physiological adjustment for the newborn. To enable the newborn to adjust to the extrauterine environment, birth initiates a series of physiologic events. Respiratory adjustment (initiation of breathing), cardiovascular adjustment (circulation), hematologic adjustment (blood volume), and thermal adjustment (regulation of body temperature) are vital. Newborns who fail to make these adaptations are at serious risk for survival.

▶ Respiratory Adjustment

Respiratory effort is perhaps the most critical adjustment that the newborn must make at birth. The first breaths of air begin the following sequence of cardiopulmonary changes: (1) converting from fetal to neonatal circulation, (2) emptying the lungs of fluid, and (3) establishing the characteristics of pulmonary function.

The lungs of the fetus have developed systematically since conception. By 24 weeks of gestation, alveolar sacs in the lungs develop; by 28 weeks, the cells of the alveoli differentiate into type I and type II cells. Type I alveolar cells make gas exchange in the lungs possible. Type II cells allow for the production of surfactant. By 36 weeks of gestation, the number of type II alveolar cells has increased along with surfactant production.

During intrauterine life, exchange of oxygen and carbon dioxide occurs across the placenta from one fluid medium to another. After birth, this exchange occurs across the newborn's alveolar membrane between a gaseous medium (air in the alveoli) and a fluid medium (blood in the alveolar capillaries). One of the most crucial adaptations that the newborn must make at birth is the adjustment of respiratory function to a gaseous environment. Before the neonatal lungs can maintain respiratory function, respiratory movements must be initiated, lungs expanded, functional residual capacity established (able to retain some air in the lungs at the end of the expiration to prevent collapse of the lungs), pulmonary blood flow increased, and cardiac output redistributed.

Initiation of Respirations

Many theories address the initiation of respiration in the newborn. The theories focus on stimuli that interact to contribute to the respiratory effort. The stimuli are mechanical, chemical, and sensory. For purposes of discussion, they are presented here separately, although they influence respiratory effort simultaneously (Fig. 30–1).

Mechanical Stimuli. The fetus makes respiratory movements in utero. The lungs at birth are about half expanded with fluid secreted by the fetal lungs and the tracheal glands (Moore, 1993). The volume of this fluid is equal to almost one half of the total lung capacity. The fetal lungs also have a high vascular resistance as a result of pulmonary arterial vasoconstriction (Martin, Fanaroff, & Klaus, 1993). The transition from the uterine to the extrauterine environment requires the immediate onset of breathing, the absorption of lung fluid, its replacement with air, and a rapid increase in the blood oxygen content.

The primary mechanical stimulus that facilitates adequate neonatal respirations is the compression of the fetal chest during the delivery process. During delivery, the squeezing of the fetal thorax increases the intrathoracic pressure and expels 30 to 35 mL of fluid from the lungs. After delivery, the chest wall of the fetus recoils, creating a negative interstitial and intrapleural pressure. This recoil of the chest wall probably produces a small passive inspiration of air, forcing some of the air into the lungs and some blood into the pulmonary capillaries. An air–fluid interface is thus established within the larger airways. The aveoli would tend to collapse under these conditions were it not for the presence of surfactant.

The newborn exhales, usually with crying; this activity expands the alveolar sacs by creating a positive intrathoracic pressure. At the same time, an adequate functional residual capacity is attained to prevent collapse of the lungs. The functional residual capacity of the lungs at 10 minutes after birth is the same as that found at 5 days postdelivery. One hour after birth, the distribution of air with each breath is similar to that observed in the young adult (Martin, Fanaroff, & Klaus, 1993). The functional residual capacity of air is maintained because the surface tension of the fluid in the lungs is reduced by surfactant. This reduction in surface tension allows the aveoli to remain expanded, and some air to remain in the lungs after expiration.

Pressure changes that take place during expiration are needed for the initiation of adequate respirations. With expiration, the newborn's diaphragm descends, resulting in negative pressure. That is, pressure in the alveoli becomes considerably higher than pressure in the interstitial tissue, resulting in the flow of fluid from

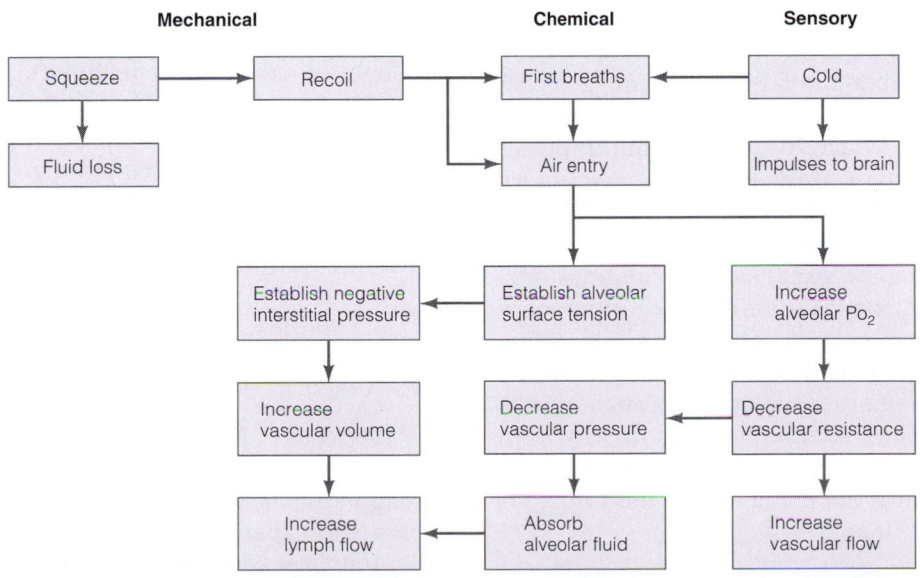

FIGURE 30–1. Stimuli influencing newborn respirations. *(Adapted, with permission, from Smith, C.A., & Nelson, N.M. (1976). Physiology of the newborn infant (4th ed.). Springfield, IL: Charles C. Thomas.)*

the alveoli to the interstitial space. From the interstitial tissue, the fluid is removed by the pulmonary capillaries and lymphatics. With each successive breath, the pulmonary vascular resistance decreases and the remainder of the fluid is absorbed. Removal of fetal lung fluid thus occurs in two stages: (1) displacement of fluid from alveolar spaces to interstitial tissue, which occurs rapidly; and (2) removal of fluid into lymph and blood vessels, which can take several hours.

Problems can occur with the onset of neonatal respirations when surfactant is deficient. The surface tension of the fluid in the lungs will not be reduced, causing the alveoli to collapse on expiration. Preterm infants may have surfactant deficiency and, as a result, serious problems with respiratory effort. Newborns delivered by cesarean may also have some difficulty with respiratory effort because they may have more fluid and less air in the lungs during the first 6 hours of life. This initial fluid retention is related to the lack of compression of the fetal chest during cesarean delivery.

Chemical Stimuli. Several chemical stimuli also contribute to the respiratory efforts of the newborn. Once the umbilical cord is cut, uteroplacental circulation stops. The placenta has acted as the "fetal lung" during pregnancy. Carbon dioxide (CO_2) readily crosses the placenta so that there is equilibrium of P_{CO_2} on both the fetal and maternal sides of the placenta. Conversely, oxygen (O_2) transport is less efficient. (Maximum P_{O_2} in the fetus is 40 mm Hg.) Yet despite the low P_{O_2}, oxygen saturation in the fetal blood is approximately 80 to 85%.

During the birth process, the uteroplacental circulation is compromised, resulting in an initial increase in the P_{CO_2} and a drop in the P_{O_2}. P_{CO_2} may rise to 80 mm Hg, and P_{O_2} may drop to 10 mm Hg (Oliver, 1987). These high carbon dioxide and low oxygen concentrations in the blood stimulate peripheral and central chemoreceptors, which in turn transmit impulses to the respiratory center of the brain. The respiratory center in the medulla then transmits impulses to stimulate the neonate's respiratory effort.

With the mechanical expansion of the lungs during the first breaths, the P_{O_2} rises, and the pulmonary vascular resistance decreases. This in turn increases pulmonary arterial blood flow that had previously bypassed the pulmonary circulation through shunts in the fetal circulation. Arterial P_{O_2} rises rapidly from less than 30 to 60 mm Hg or more in the first minutes of life, demonstrating the efficiency of the lungs for oxygen exchange (Truog, 1987).

Sensory Stimuli. The newborn is subjected to multiple sensory stimuli at birth. Combined with the mechanical and chemical stimuli, they play a role in initiation of breathing in the normal newborn.

The relative cooling effect of the environment in the delivery room stimulates sensory impulses in the trigeminal area of the face. Impulses are then transmitted to the respiratory center of the brain to initiate respirations in the newborn. Cooling is probably an intense stimulus to breathing, and the response is immediate.

Other stimuli, such as light, noise, and pain, probably also play a role in the initiation of respirations. The role of tactile stimulation is less clear and is probably of minor significance. For this reason, the slapping of the heels or buttocks of the newborn on delivery is discouraged because of the minimal effect on respiratory effort. Greater emphasis is placed on gentle physical contact.

The initiation of respirations in the newborn is thus an interaction of mechanical, chemical, and sensory stimuli. They are summarized in Table 30–1.

Newborn Respirations

The respiratory rate of the newborn is between 30 and 60 breaths per minute. Newborns have higher respiratory rates when crying, and lower rates when sleeping. The pattern of respirations is characterized by shallow, irregular breathing, sometimes interrupted by short periods of apnea. Neonatal respirations are also abdominal in nature.

▶ Cardiovascular Adjustment

Important cardiovascular changes occur when the newborn emerges from the intrauterine environment. Fetal circulation is discussed in detail in Chapter 13.

In fetal circulation, the fetal placental vessels offer little resistance to the flow of blood. The placenta has a low-resistance circuit of vessels that eventually receives blood from the fetal aorta. In contrast to the low-resistance, placental vessels in the fetus, pulmonary vascular resistance to blood flow is high. As a result, the fetal aortic blood pressure is lower than the pulmonary artery pressure, and little blood goes into the pulmonary circulation (lungs). At birth, changes occur in the pulmonary–systemic pressure relationships and in the right-to-left shunts (foramen ovale, ductus arteriosus, ductus venosus).

Conversion of Fetal to Neonatal Circulation

Change in Pulmonary–Systemic Pressure Relationships. In converting fetal to neonatal circulation two factors are important: removal of the placenta and expansion of the lungs with air. Clamping the umbilical cord at birth removes the placental circulation, the component that offers the least resistance to the flow of blood. As a result, aortic blood pressure is raised, and the return of blood from the inferior vena cava is reduced.

► **TABLE 30-1**

Mechanical, Chemical, and Sensory Stimuli that Initiate Neonatal Respirations

Stimuli	Response
Mechanical	
Squeezing of fetal chest during delivery	Increases intrathoracic pressure; expels 30–35 mL fluid from lungs.
Chest recoil	Produces small passive inspiration, forcing some of air into lungs; air–fluid interface established.
Exhalation, usually with crying (expiration)	Positive intrathoracic pressure established; adequate functional residual capacity attained; descent of the diaphragm, causing negative interstitial pressure; pressure in alveoli becomes higher than in the interstitial tissue, resulting in flow of fluid from alveoli to lymphatics.
Chemical	
Cessation of uteroplacental circulation	Initial increase in Pco_2 and drop in Po_2.
Increase in Pco_2 and decrease in Po_2	Stimulation of peripheral and central chemoreceptors, which transmit impulses to brain, stimulating respiratory effort.
Po_2 rises, pulmonary vascular resistance decreases	Increase in pulmonary arterial blood flow.
Sensory	
Cool environment in delivery room	Stimulates sensory impulses in trigeminal area of face; impulses transmitted to respiratory center of brain to initiate respirations.
Light, noise, pain	Probably stimulate respirations; exact mechanism unknown.

With the newborn's first breaths, vasodilation of pulmonary vessels occurs, producing a significant decrease in pulmonary vascular resistance and an increase in pulmonary blood flow. Neonatal lung expansion is important in stimulating pulmonary arteriolar relaxation (decreasing pulmonary artery blood pressure) and providing adequate oxygenation to the newborn. At the same time, systemic blood pressure (aortic blood pressure) increases because of the greater peripheral vascular resistance brought about by removal of the placental circulation. This reversal of pulmonary and systemic blood pressures, from fetal to neonatal circulation, affects the right-to-left shunts found in fetal circulation.

Closure of Right-to-Left Shunts. The shunts in fetal circulation (foramen ovale, ductus venosus, ductus arteriosus) are termed right-to-left shunts because they shunt blood from the right side to the left side of the heart (foramen ovale, ductus arteriosus), or from the umbilical vein to the inferior vena cava (ductus venosus). At birth, changes occur in the shunts that alter neonatal blood flow.

The foramen ovale is an opening in the interatrial septum, which shunts blood from the right atrium to the left atrium, bypassing the right ventricle and the pulmonary circulation. In fetal circulation, the pressure in the right atrium is higher than in the left. Oxygenated blood therefore flows from the right to the left atrium (area of higher pressure to lower pressure), keeping the foramen ovale open.

At birth, the decrease in pulmonary vascular resistance, combined with an increase in peripheral vascular resistance, causes an increase in the amount of blood in the left atrium. This results in an increase in left atrial pressure and a decrease in right atrial pressure, causing the foramen ovale to close within minutes of birth. Some right-to-left shunting of blood may still normally occur for a few months after birth without causing problems for the neonate.

The ductus venosus, the fetal structure that shunts blood from the umbilical vein to the inferior vena cava, closes within 3 to 7 days of birth (Fig. 30–2). After birth, umbilical venous return decreases so that very little blood flows through the ductus venosus. Although the mechanism is unknown, one possible explanation for the closure is that the ductus venosus becomes fibrotic (ligamentum venosus) from lack of circulation.

In fetal circulation, the ductus arteriosus shunts blood (right-to-left) into the descending aorta, bypassing the pulmonary circulation (Fig. 30–2). With the onset of neonatal breathing, the pulmonary vascular resistance decreases, and the systemic resistance increases, causing a reversal of the shunting of blood through the ductus (left to right).

In utero, the ductus arteriosus remains open because of the vasodilating effects of prostaglandins E_1 and E_2 found in the ductal tissue. When the oxygen tension rises after birth, constriction of the ductus occurs. This constriction, combined with the left-to-right shunting of blood, promotes closure of the ductus arteriosus beginning 4 to 12 hours postnatally; the ductus functionally closes by the time the newborn is 24 hours of age. Fibrosis of the ductus arteriosus, which closes it permanently (ligamentum arteriosus) may take as long as 3 weeks to occur.

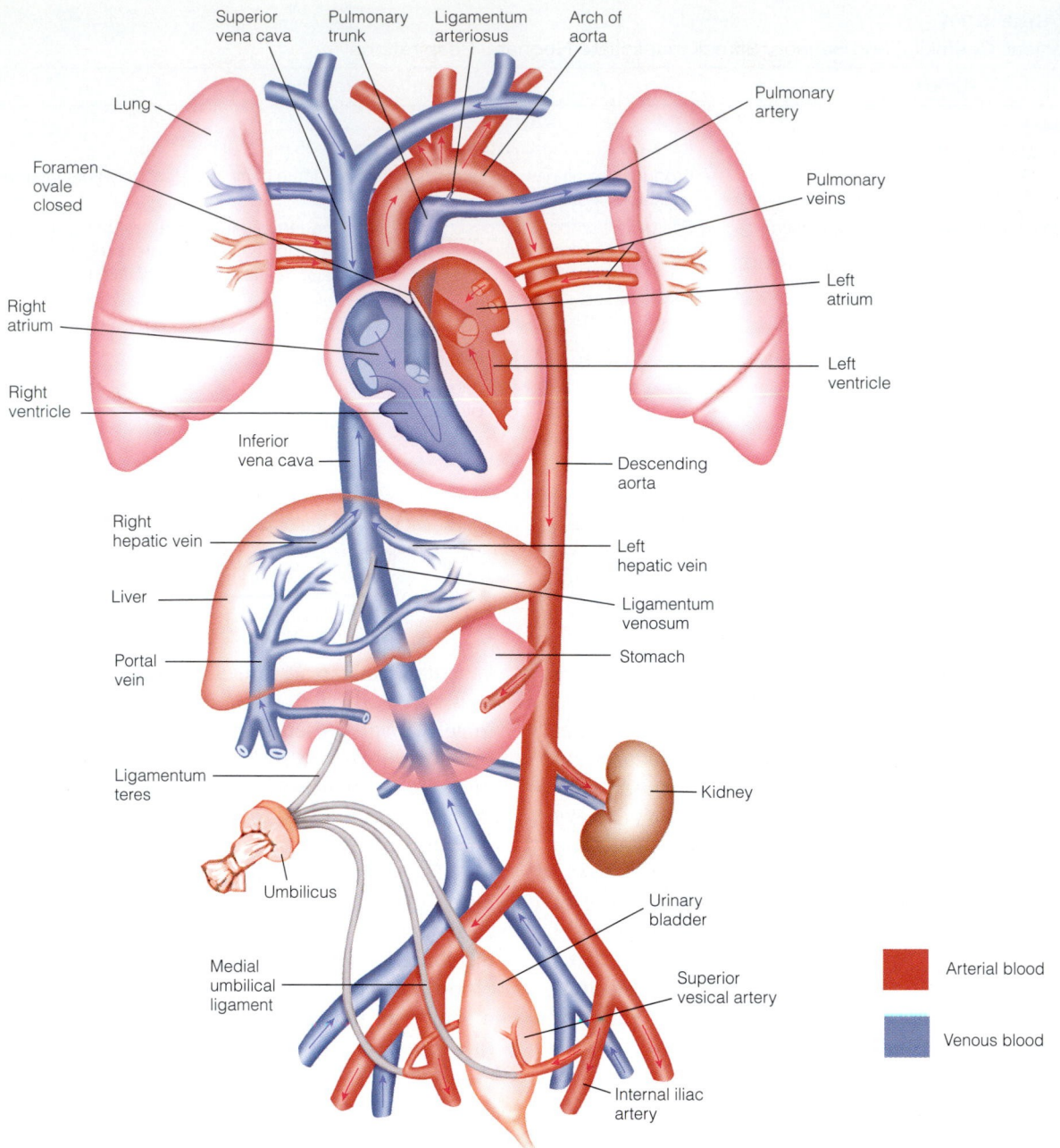

FIGURE 30–2. The newborn's circulatory system.

The interim period, before the ductus permanently closes, is termed the *transitional phase* of perinatal circulation. If, during the transitional phase, the pulmonary vascular resistance should again increase to a level higher than the systemic resistance, a reversal from neonatal to fetal circulation will occur (e.g., in a preterm newborn). During the transitional phase, left ventricular volume and pressure increase while right ventricular pressure decreases (e.g., the left ventricle pumps twice the volume load of the right ventricle). This means that the newborn has unequal volumes in the left and right ventricles during this phase, in contrast to the equal volumes of blood found in the child and adult.

Constriction of the Umbilical Arteries and Umbilical Vein. The umbilical vein carries oxygenated blood to the fetus, and the two umbilical arteries remove deoxygenated blood and waste materials from the fetal circulation. Constriction of the umbilical vein and arteries begins at birth, as a result of the increase in peripheral circulation and the removal of the placental circulation.

Neonatal Heart Rate and Blood Pressure

The heart rate of the newborn ranges between 120 and 160 beats per minute. The heart rate may increase to as much as 180 beats per minute when the newborn is crying, and may decrease to a low of 70 to 100 beats per minute when the newborn is sleeping. Transient functional cardiac murmurs may be heard in the neonatal period as a result of the changing dynamics of the cardiovascular system at birth.

During the first 12 hours of life, the mean blood pressure for a neonate weighing 3.5 kg (7.7 pounds) is 67/41. For a newborn weighing 3.6 kg (8 pounds), mean blood pressure is 80/58 during the same period. The newborn's blood pressure is highest after birth and reaches a plateau about 4 to 6 days after birth.

▶ Hematologic Adjustment

At term, the placental vasculature contains 75 to 125 mL of blood, which represents one fourth to one third of the total fetal blood volume. Blood volume in the newborn can be increased by 40 to 60% if the newborn is held below the level of the placenta and clamping of the cord is delayed. This extra blood volume provides the advantage of increased oxygen and nutrients to the newborn.

Because the fetal circulation is less efficient at oxygen exchange than the lungs, the fetus needs additional red blood cells for transport of oxygen in utero. To meet this need, the fetal bone marrow becomes hyperactive and produces increased numbers of red blood cells (erythropoiesis). The hemoglobin concentration of the newborn at birth is therefore higher than that of the child or adult. The number of reticulocytes (the precursors to mature erythrocytes) is also higher in the circulating blood of the newborn than in the child or adult. The reticulocytes at birth range from 4 to 8% of red blood cells; at 4 weeks, the range is 0 to 0.5%.

After birth, more efficient oxygen exchange takes place in the lungs of the newborn, and fewer red blood cells are required. The bone marrow of the newborn becomes hypoactive, resulting in a decrease in the concentrations of hemoglobin. The average hemoglobin concentration is 14 g/100 mL at 4 weeks and 12 g/100 mL at 8 weeks. The hemoglobin of the newborn also converts from fetal hemoglobin (hemoglobin F), which provides greater oxygen carrying capacity needed in utero, to adult hemoglobin (hemoglobin A).

The white blood cell count of the newborn at birth is usually between 15,000 and 25,000/mm³. By the 6th day postdelivery, lymphocytes predominate (37%) and persist through the first 5 years of life. The platelet count in the neonatal period averages between 150,000/ and 250,000/mm³, the same as that in the child and adult.

▶ Thermal Regulation

Children and adults are considered **homiotherms** (warm blooded) because they can maintain a constant core body temperature regardless of a wide range of environmental temperatures. Although newborns have the capabilities of homiotherms, the range of environmental temperatures to which they can adapt without being stressed is severely restricted compared with the adult.

The newborn differs from the child and adult by having a large surface area in proportion to mass, less thermal insulation (subcutaneous fat), and relatively lower vasomotor control (ability to control skin blood flow). The newborn also has greater potential for heat loss than does the adult, and differs in mechanisms of heat production (thermogenesis).

All homiotherms have a **neutral thermal environmental range,** that is, the range of environmental temperature in which an individual is able to maintain a normal internal temperature with minimal metabolism and oxygen consumption for heat production. Because the newborn differs from the adult in the proportion of surface area to mass, as well as in thermal insulation, the neutral temperature zone of the newborn is 32 to 34°C (89.6 to 93.2°F), as compared with the adult's neutral zone of 26 to 28°C (78.7 to 82.4°F). Below this range, termed the **critical temperature,** a metabolic response to cold is necessary to replace heat loss. The neutral range thus represents the thermal range of minimal stress. Table 30–2 compares factors that contribute to temperature control in the newborn and older child or adult.

Mechanisms of Heat Transfer

In utero, the internal or core temperature of the fetus is slightly higher than that of the mother. At birth, the newborn's internal temperature may drop rapidly because the delivery room is usually 25 to 30°F lower than the maternal temperature.

Heat loss in the newborn is the result of four mechanisms: (1) evaporation, (2) radiation, (3) convection, and (4) conduction (see box entitled Mechanisms of Heat Transfer). The heat transfer depends on the temperature of the environment (air and walls), air speed, and water vapor pressure or humidity.

Thermogenesis and Heat Retention

The newborn has the capability to produce and retain heat through various mechanisms. Mechanisms to produce heat include nonshivering thermogenesis, muscular activity, and positional changes. Vasomotor control is a mechanism that allows the newborn to retain heat.

▶ **TABLE 30-2**

Factors that Influence Temperature Control in the Newborn and Older Child or Adult

Newborn	Older Child or Adult
Large surface area in proportion to mass	Smaller surface area in proportion to mass
Less thermal insulation (subcutaneous fat)	Mature deposits of subcutaneous fat provide thermal insulation
Some mature vasomotor control (ability to control skin blood flow)	Mature vasomotor control
Neutral temperature zone 32 to 34°C (89.6 to 93.2°F)	Neutral temperature zone 26 to 28°C (78.7 to 82.4°F)
Nonshivering thermogenesis in response to cold stress	Shivering thermogenesis in response to cold
Six times as many sweat glands as adults, but maximum response of each gland one-third that of adult	

Nonshivering Thermogenesis. The newborn increases heat production in a cool environment mainly through **nonshivering thermogenesis,** a complex process that increases the metabolic rate and rate of oxygen consumption in the newborn. More specifically, the process includes the metabolism of brown fat for heat production when the newborn is subjected to cold stress.

Brown fat cells begin appearing in the fetus by 17 to 20 weeks of gestation (see Chapter 13). At term, brown fat accounts for 2 to 6% of the total body weight of the newborn. Brown fat is found for weeks after birth unless its stores are depleted from cold stress.

Changes in environmental temperature have the potential to disturb the core body temperature, with serious consequences to the newborn. Brown fat metabolism is activated in response to changes in environmental temperature that are perceived by the thermal sensors in the newborn's skin, even when the core temperature of the newborn is unchanged. The stability of the core body temperature is thus protected by the newborn's mechanisms of heat production.

Muscular Activity and Positional Changes. Although the newborn does not have the same capabilities as the adult to change position and increase muscular activity in response to cold, evidence suggests that these activities are important in maintaining core body temperature in cold surroundings (Hey & Scopes, 1993). When exposed to cold, the newborn may become restless and increase muscular activity. Moreover, flexion (flexing the extremities and back) helps to decrease the amount of skin surface exposed to cold and conserve heat.

Vasomotor Control. In addition to mechanisms to produce heat, the newborn's body has the ability to retain heat by controlling skin blood flow. By constricting blood vessels in the skin, heat can be retained in the tissues, thereby helping to maintain the core temperature. The newborn's thermal insulation is, however, poor compared with that of the adult; this mechanism alone is inadequate in maintaining the core temperature.

Hyperthermia

Hyperthermia develops more rapidly in the newborn than in the adult because of the larger surface-to-volume ratio of the newborn's body. Although newborn infants have six times as many sweat glands per unit area as adults, the maximum response of each gland is only one-third that of the adult. Thus, when exposed to high temperatures the newborn is unable to sweat to lower the temperature. The risk of hyperthermia to

▶ **MECHANISMS OF HEAT TRANSFER**

EVAPORATION

Water in amniotic fluid covering the newborn at birth escapes to the environment as vapor; loss depends on air speed, absolute humidity of the environment, or both

RADIATION

Heat from the newborn is transferred to cooler objects in the environment (walls of incubator or air temperature of the room)

CONVECTION

Cool air in the delivery room passes over the newborn's body and causes heat loss

CONDUCTION

Heat from the newborn is lost to cooler objects that come in contact with the body the newborn is great when the environmental temperature is above the neutral temperature zone. Heat stress will cause the newborn to increase metabolic rate and respirations in an effort to control temperature because of the inability of the sweat glands to respond.

Consequences of a Nonneutral Thermal Environment

The neutral thermal environment is the temperature range that causes minimal stress to the newborn. No single environmental temperature is best for all sizes and conditions of newborns. The environment that is appropriate for the normal newborn may be too cold for the preterm newborn. Conversely, the environmental temperature that is appropriate for the preterm newborn may be too warm for the full-term healthy newborn. Severe consequences may result when newborns are exposed to environmental temperatures above or below their neutral temperature zone.

Serious overheating of the newborn can cause cerebral damage from dehydration, heat stroke, and even death. Cold stress produces less obvious consequences, unless it is severe enough to cause neonatal cold injury. The newborn's need to increase heat production results in increased nutritional requirements, increased metabolic rate, and an increased need for oxygen. In the case of cold injury, severe cooling may result in metabolic acidosis, a decrease in the arterial oxygen blood level, and hypoglycemia. Further, fluctuations in environmental temperature can cause periods of apnea in the newborn (Klaus, Martin, & Fanaroff, 1993).

Temperature of the Newborn. The axillary temperature of the newborn averages from 36.5 to 37°C (97.6 to 98.6°F). The temperature of a full-term healthy newborn should stabilize within 10 hours of birth. An axillary temperature greater than 37.2°C (99°F) may indicate that the environment is too warm or that the newborn is suffering from either dehydration or infection. An axillary temperature below 36.1°C (97°F) may indicate a cold environment, which is subjecting the newborn to cold stress. It is important for the nurse to monitor the newborn's temperature and environment closely to prevent fluctuations in body temperature.

▶ ADJUSTMENTS IN OTHER SYSTEMS

Respiratory, cardiovascular, and hematologic system adjustments and temperature control are crucial to the health of newborns as they emerge into the extrauterine environment. Adjustment of other systems also is necessary, as outlined in the following discussion.

▶ Urinary System

The newborn's urinary system is structurally complete but physiologically immature at birth. The musculature of the bladder is underdeveloped, the epithelium of the kidney is thick, and reabsorption and filtration in the renal tubules are limited.

Due to this physiologic immaturity, the newborn is unable to concentrate urine. Maximum urine concentration is only about one-half that of the adult under conditions of thirsting. Water losses are therefore greater in the newborn than in the adult, and water requirements per kilogram of body weight are greater in the newborn period than in any other period of the life cycle. The daily fluid requirement for the healthy full-term newborn is approximately 125 mL/kg in a 24-hour period; the preterm newborn needs 150 mL/kg per day.

In the second week of life, the full-term newborn's need for water ranges from 125 to 150 mL/kg per day. Approximately one half of this is required for the formation of urine; the rest is needed to offset the insensible water loss by the lungs, skin, and other losses. The insensible water loss is directly related to the calories metabolized by the newborn (about 40 mL/100 cal) (Behrman, 1992).

The ability of the newborn to handle high-osmolarity or high-acid loads is also limited. Most newborns, however, thrive despite a high protein and osmolar intake, probably because much of this intake is used for growth and is not passed on to the kidney for excretion. The urine of the newborn may contain small amounts of proteins and excessive amounts of urates. The urates in the urine may stain the diaper pink in the first week of life.

The bladder capacity of the newborn is approximately 15 mL, and emptying of the bladder occurs frequently. The newborn usually voids at birth, but will not void again for 12 to 24 hours. After this time, the newborn may void 20 or more times a day. Voiding is a good indication that the newborn is receiving adequate fluid intake.

▶ Integument

At birth, the full-term newborn's skin demonstrates good texture and tone. During the first week postdelivery, the skin may begin peeling because of the thinness of its layers and its sensitive nature. The extrauterine environment does not provide the same protection for the skin as did the intrauterine environment. Households that are dry may cause the newborn's skin to peel and crack.

Sebaceous glands are present at birth and may be found mostly on the face and scalp. The glands that produce sweat (exocrine glands) are immature at birth so that they respond little when the newborn is overheated. The exocrine glands begin maturing within a few weeks of birth.

Newborns are born with varying amounts of hair. The hair is usually silky to the touch. During the first few months after birth, newborns may begin losing their hair. The growth of new hair usually starts on the sides of the head, with the slowest growth at the crown.

▶ Endocrine System

The endocrine system of the newborn is usually fully developed, but functionally immature. In utero, the adrenal cortex of the fetus is active in the production of maternal hormones. Because of this overactivity of the adrenals in utero, the fetal adrenal gland is extremely large during pregnancy. The adrenals rapidly involute at birth, but are still functional.

Adrenal androgen secretion is greater during the neonatal period than in later childhood. Adrenal androgens are not secreted in appreciable amounts again until puberty. The newborn also controls tissue concentrations of adrenocortical steriods by means of a hypothalamic–pituitary–adrenal homeostatic mechanism. The hypothalamus is sensitive to tissue levels of cortisol and contains an adrenocorticotropic hormone (ACTH)-releasing factor and corticotropin-releasing hormone. When cortisol levels are low, these factors stimulate the release of ACTH by the pituitary gland. Adrenocorticotropic hormone in turn stimulates cortisol biosynthesis. Increased levels of cortisol inhibit the production of ACTH (Moshang & Bongiovanni, 1993). The adrenal glands also secrete aldosterone in response to low sodium and potassium levels in the blood. This response assists the newborn in maintaining fluid and electrolyte balance.

In utero, the fetal thyroid begins functioning by 12 weeks of gestation, allowing the fetus to accumulate and concentrate iodine. At birth, the thyroid gland of the newborn is active. The amount of protein-bound iodine rises immediately after birth and remains elevated for several weeks.

Thyroid function tests are elevated in the newborn and remain elevated for the first several months of life. They are lower in premature and sick newborns than in healthy term newborns. The T_4 level of cord blood ranges from 7 to 13 $\mu g/dL$, with a mean of 10.9 $\mu g/dL$. The T_3 level of cord blood ranges from 12 to 90 ng/dL, with a mean of 48 ng/dL. Thyroid function screening is important at birth because congenital hypothyroidism may lead to serious problems in growth and development, specifically in central nervous system functioning (Moshang & Bongiovanni, 1993).

▶ Gastrointestinal System

The full-term neonate is born with the capacity to swallow, digest, metabolize, and absorb proteins and simple carbohydrates, and to emulsify lipids. With the exception of pancreatic amylase, the characteristic enzymes and digestive juices are present even in low-birth-weight neonates (Avery & Fletcher, 1993).

The motility of the gastrointestinal tract and the newborn's sphincteric control are immature. As a result, symptoms such as regurgitation, gas distension, flatus, and a wide variety of stool patterns may be found in the newborn.

Protein Digestion

The newborn efficiently digests proteins from the diet. Digestion of proteins is facilitated by rennin and then pepsin in the stomach, pancreatic proteases in the duodenum, and enteric proteases and peptidases in the intestines (Avery & Fletcher, 1993). The infant adds approximately 3.5 g protein daily to the body during the first 4 months of life.

Carbohydrate Digestion

The salivary glands do not begin functioning until 2 to 3 months of age, when drooling becomes quite evident; however, the salivary enzymes that are present are sufficient to handle simple carbohydrates in the neonatal period.

Carbohydrate digestion begins in the mouth with salivary amylase. The newborn is deficient in pancreatic amylase and thus has difficulty digesting complex carbohydrates such as starches (polysaccharides). The small intestine contains four enzymes: lactase, sucrase, maltase, and isomaltase. These enzymes convert the disaccharides lactose, sucrose, and maltose into the monosaccharides glucose, galactose, and fructose. Lactose is usually well digested by the newborn, although cases of lactose intolerance have been documented (Avery & Fletcher, 1993).

Lipid Digestion

Lipid digestion in the newborn is less efficient than in the older child and adult because of the relatively lower levels of pancreatic lipase enzyme and bile salts. The digestion of lipids begins in the stomach, stimulated by lingual lipase derived from the glands in the tongue. Hydrolysis of lipids continues in the duodenum and jejunum under the influence of pancreatic lipase, and bile salts further emulsify the lipids.

The newborn excretes 10 to 20% of the dietary intake of lipids, resulting in some steatorrhea (fatty stools). This does not produce a problem for the newborn; however, if the newborn is given fat-soluble vitamins, these may be excreted in the stool.

Stomach

The stomach of the newborn has a capacity of approximately 90 mL, with an emptying time of about 2½ to 3 hours. The pH of the stomach secretions is high (5 to 6) at birth, but falls to normal adult values within a few hours.

Stools

Meconium, the first stool of the newborn, is usually passed within 12 to 36 hours of birth. This first stool appears sticky and greenish black.

By the third day postdelivery, the newborn passes **transitional stools,** which appear watery or loose and greenish brown to yellowish brown. The change in stool color (and consistency) is a result of the newborn's ingestion of formula or breast milk. By the fourth day, the typical **milk stools** are observed. Milk stools are yellow; they are pasty or watery, varying according to the feeding method and the individual newborn (see Chapter 31).

▶ Hepatic Regulation

The liver of the newborn is immature, but has several important functions, among them the conjugation of bilirubin and a role in blood coagulation.

Conjugation of Bilirubin

One of the functions of the liver is the conjugation of bilirubin. As red blood cells die, heme, a component of hemoglobin found in red blood cells (and other proteins), is liberated. Heme is metabolized to unconjugated bilirubin (indirect bilirubin). The bilirubin is carried to the liver by albumin and other blood proteins. Within the liver cells, bilirubin is transported by ligandin (Y protein) to a site where conjugation occurs. The enzyme glucuronyl transferase is needed for the conjugation process. The conjugated bilirubin is transported into the bile, which then enters the intestinal tract. Bacteria in the small intestine convert bilirubin into stercobilinogen, which is excreted from the body in the feces, and urobilinogen, which is excreted in the urine.

If the feces are not expelled, unconjugated bilirubin levels may again rise. As a result of factors such as the enzyme beta-glucuronidase, the conjugated bilirubin may be hydrolyzed to unconjugated bilirubin within the bowel lumen and reabsorbed, thereby again increasing overall unconjugated bilirubin levels and the potential for neonatal jaundice.

Neonatal Physiologic Jaundice (Icterus Neonatorum). Neonatal **physiologic jaundice** is defined as an unconjugated bilirubin concentration that peaks at less than 12.9 mg/dL, with a rise in bilirubin levels of less than 5 mg/dL per day. Conjugated bilirubin levels remain less than 1.5 mg/dL. Bilirubin levels return to normal around 10 days after birth. Physiologic jaundice may result from an increased load of bilirubin on the liver cells or decreased bilirubin clearance from the plasma (Maisels, 1993). Physiologic jaundice is a common occurrence in healthy newborns.

An increased load of bilirubin on the liver is related to bilirubin production and enterohepatic circulation. It is estimated that the newborn produces 8 to 10 mg/kg of bilirubin per day. This production is related to the newborn's high circulating red cell volume (per kilogram), the shorter mean red cell life span, and an early bilirubin peak in the blood. The production of bilirubin decreases with increasing postnatal age, but is still twice the adult production at 2 weeks of life. The newborn also absorbs larger quantities of unconjugated bilirubin (indirect) from the enterohepatic circulation (intestines, liver) than does the adult. Moreover, newborns have fewer bacteria in the small intestines and greater activity of the deconjugating enzyme beta-glucuronidase. As a result, conjugated bilirubin is hydrolyzed to unconjugated bilirubin, and the larger quantities of unconjugated bilirubin place additional stress on the newborn's immature liver, contributing to neonatal jaundice (Maisels, 1993).

The decreased ability of the liver to clear bilirubin from the plasma is associated with decreased transport of bilirubin by ligandin in the liver cells and decreased conjugation. Uptake of bilirubin from the plasma takes place when the bilirubin binds to the proteins in the liver. The predominant bilirubin-binding protein ligandin is relatively deficient in the newborn liver for about the first 5 days after birth (Maisels, 1993).

Conjugation of bilirubin also is impaired in the newborn. There is less glucuronyl transferase produced by the liver. At the same time, the newborn is breaking down red blood cells. The result is an increase in blood levels of unconjugated bilirubin. This, accompanied by the newborn's reabsorption of larger quantities of unconjugated bilirubin from the bowel, contributes to physiologic jaundice beyond the first 24 hours after birth.

In normal circumstances, the neonatal liver is capable of excreting bilirubin that has been conjugated (direct bilirubin). Thus, serum levels of conjugated bilirubin usually are not elevated in physiologic jaundice; however, the ability of the neonatal liver to secrete conjugated bilirubin is more limited than that of the adult. If there are significant increases in bilirubin levels, as in hemolytic disease, the ability to excrete conjugated bilirubin will be impaired. Elevated serum levels of conjugated bilirubin are thus indicative of nonphysiologic jaundice (Maisels, 1993).

Chilling, decreased fluid and calorie intake, and weight loss also may contribute to jaundice in the newborn. Chilling can cause the newborn's core temperature to decline, bringing on metabolic acidosis. The state of acidosis, in turn, can reduce the capacity of bilirubin to bind to albumin, thereby causing an increase in the serum level of unconjugated bilirubin.

Decreased fluid and caloric intake and weight loss have been associated with elevated bilirubin levels in the neonate. Early and frequent feedings reduce weight loss and promote adequate fluid and caloric intake. Such feedings also promote more frequent stools and a decrease in the enterohepatic circulation (Maisels, 1993).

Breastfeeding Jaundice. Breastfed newborns sometimes have increased serum bilirubin concentrations. The bilirubin rises progressively from the fourth day of life, reaching a maximum level of unconjugated bilirubin of 10 to 30 mg/dL by 10 to 15 days of life. This condition, referred to as **breast milk jaundice syndrome,** is a relatively benign condition.

Breastfeeding jaundice is thought to be multifactorial. Some cases are linked to a hormonally induced delay in bilirubin conjugation (Cashoro, 1993). In one study, serum bilirubin levels of breastfed newborns were also associated with the frequency of feeding in the first 3 days of life. Researchers found that newborns who nursed 8 or more times a day had significantly lower bilirubin levels than those who nursed fewer than 8 times in 24 hours (De Carvalho, Klaus, & Merkatz, 1982). Mothers should thus be encouraged to breastfeed early and frequently during this period. Feeding the newborn on demand will usually accomplish this goal.

Some investigators believe that a double standard should be used in the classification of hyperbilirubinemia for bottle-fed and breastfed infants. In a large study (2416 infants), it was found that the upper limit for bilirubin concentration for formula-fed infants was 11.4 mg/100 mL, and that for breastfed infants it was 14.5 mg/100 mL. The investigators suggest that a diagnosis of jaundice, requiring further testing, may not be indicated unless the serum bilirubin exceeds 15 mg/dL in the breastfed infant or 12 mg/dL in the formula-fed infant (Maisels & Gifford, 1986).

Role of the Liver in Coagulation

The liver plays an important role in blood coagulation as a source of coagulation factors II, VII, IX, and X. These coagulation factors, as well as prothrombin, are dependent on the synthesis of vitamin K. For the first few days of life, however, the newborn lacks the bacterial flora in the gastrointestinal tract necessary for vitamin K synthesis. Thus, during this period, the newborn may be deficient in prothrombin and other coagulation factors.

Bacterial colonization of the intestines occurs with the intake of formula or breast milk. Newborns are at risk for vitamin K deficiency when their mothers have taken anticonvulsant medications (e.g., phenobarbital, dilantin) prenatally.

Since 1961, it has been common practice to administer a prophylactic injection of vitamin K_1 at birth to prevent hemorrhagic disease of the newborn (see the section entitled Preventing Hemorrhage later in the chapter).

▶ Immunologic System

Newborns, especially full-term newborns, are born with the capability to combat some infections as a result of placental transmission of maternal antibodies. The newborn also has the potential for both cell-mediated and antibody-mediated immune responses.

Cell-mediated immunity depends on the T lymphocytes, which develop from stem cells in the embryonic mesenchyme and appear in the embryonic yolk sac. These T lymphocytes migrate to the fetal liver and then from the liver to the thymus where they differentiate into functional types. T lymphocytes are mediated by antigens, dividing and increasing their numbers at the site of an antigen reaction. They also play an indirect role in stimulating circulating antibodies.

B lymphocytes also originate in the embryonic mesenchyme and mature in the fetal liver. B lymphocytes are differentiated into plasma cells in the bone marrow, lymph nodes, and spleen. They also differentiate into plasma cells in the presence of helper T lymphocytes. The function of the B cells is also antigen mediated, stimulating the production of antibodies. By 15 weeks of gestation, circulating B lymphocytes are found in the same numbers as they are found in the adult.

Antibody-mediated immunity depends on B lymphocytes producing specific antibodies called immunoglobulins. The principal groups of immunoglobulins are immunoglobins G, M, and A.

Immunoglobulin G (IgG) readily crosses the placenta from the maternal to the fetal circulation. Placental transfer of IgG begins during the 3rd month of gestation, but markedly increases in the 3rd trimester. The short-lasting immunity that the newborn receives from the IgG is called **passive immunity.**

Over the first 3 months of life, maternal IgG levels are depleted in the infant; however, the infant synthesizes IgG during the same period, partially making up for this depletion. The newborn receives passive immunity to diseases for which the mother has developed specific antibodies. Among the diseases are diphtheria, tetanus, poliomyelitis, measles, mumps, and gram-positive cocci such as pneumococcus. The schedule of immunizations for infants is based on the premise that the infant receives only passive immunity from the mother and needs to develop his or her own antibodies for protection from some of the common childhood diseases.

As IgG is transferred in increased amounts during the last trimester, the premature newborn is at a deficit in combating infections. Moreover, all newborns, whether full term or premature, are not protected from gram-negative bacterial infections by maternal IgG.

Immunoglobulin M (IgM) is the immunoglobulin that contains antibodies to gram-negative bacteria as well as to blood group antigens and some viruses. Maternal IgM does not cross the placenta, although by 30 weeks of gestation, the fetus can produce IgM in response to exposure to infection. At birth, the normal serum IgM concentration is usually below 20 mg/dL, so that the newborn has increased susceptibility to infection with gram-negative bacteria such as *Escherichia coli*. The level of IgM increases rapidly during the first month of life, and is approximately one-half that found in the adult by 6 months of age.

Immunoglobulin A (IgA) does not cross the placenta, and there is no evidence that the fetus synthesizes this immunoglobulin. It is found in two forms, circulating IgA and secretory IgA. Secretory IgA is found over secreting surfaces of the body, such as the intestinal and respiratory mucosa, the eyes, and the epithelium of the urinary tract. It resists destruction by pH and enzymatic sources. Secretory IgA helps protect the newborn from infection on secretory surfaces. Breast milk, especially colostrum, contains a significant amount of secretory IgA, thereby providing the newborn with some passive immunity. IgA begins to be produced by the first month of life.

The full-term newborn is usually able to combat minor infections; however, the neonatal immune response is deficient. For example, the absence of IgM contributes to the increased susceptibility of the newborn to gram-negative bacterial infections. Newborns also have difficulty in localizing infections because they cannot clear bacteria from the blood as quickly as adults. Moreover, antibody production is dependent on exposure to antigens, which usually does not occur until after birth. The development of immunocompetence to such bacteria as *Haemophilus* does not occur until after the neonatal period. Premature newborns, especially those less than 34 weeks of gestation, are especially prone to infections because of their immature immune response.

▶ Neurologic System

The normal full-term newborn has an intact, although immature, nervous system. The development of the nervous system occurs in stages in utero. In the first stage, completed by midpregnancy, the fetus develops the actual number of nerve cells that will exist for the remainder of the life span. During the second stage, rapid growth of neurons occurs. In the third stage, beginning in the latter part of gestation and continuing through the 4th year of life, the number of glial cells and dendrites increases. Myelination of neurons begins at about the fourth month of gestation and continues through the 4th year.

Neurologic development follows cephalocaudal and proximodistal patterns. Myelin, which increases the speed and accuracy of nerve impulses, develops earliest in the transmitters of sensory impulses and the nerves of the brain stem. The newborn, therefore, has an acute sense of hearing, smell, and taste. The newborn also is able to survive by breathing and maintaining acid-base balance because of this early myelination.

Motor Behavior and Reflexes

Gross motor behavior begins with movements in the upper part of the body. The newborn is able to move the eyes and fixate on human faces. Newborns are also able to control their heads and make movements with their mouths. Fine motor behavior begins with purposeless flailing of the arms and progresses to purposeful movements during infancy, such as reaching for objects. As the infant grows and develops, sensorimotor coordination further develops, as shown by the ability to walk by 12 to 18 months of age.

Primitive reflexes also are found in the newborn. These reflexes assist the newborn's survival and safety. Among the primitive reflexes found in the newborn are the Moro, palmar and plantar grasp, tonic neck, sucking and rooting, swallowing, Babinski, stepping, Galant, crossed extension, magnet, traction, arm recoil, crawling, and glabellar reflexes (see section entitled Neonatal Reflexes later in the chapter). As the infant develops, these primitive reflexes give way to righting reflexes (e.g., righting of the neck and head) and protective reactions.

The Senses

The newborn is capable of responding to a variety of stimuli through the senses. The behaviors are related to the newborn's level of arousal and orienting response.

Visual Responses. At birth, the newborn can process complex visual information and track an object in space (Fig. 30–3). Newborns also respond to unpleasant visual stimuli, such as a bright light, by blinking and withdrawing their heads. If stimulation is repeated, newborns can shut out the stimulus which enables them to better meet other physiologic demands (Brazelton, 1993).

Newborns prefer complex visual stimuli, and are fascinated by geometric shapes, large circles, dots, and squares. They focus their attention on patterned objects rather than plain ones and prefer black-and-white contrast.

Research also indicates that newborns prefer a human face to other objects and will follow a drawing that resembles a human face 90 to 180 degrees (Rantz,

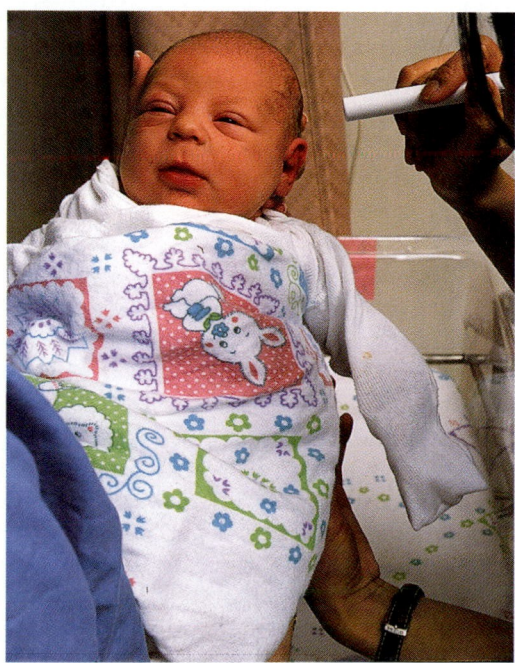

FIGURE 30–3. The tracking response of a newborn is elicited by moving an object or a penlight 9 to 12 inches away from the newborn's line of vision.

1965). They also have the ability to scan the environment to focus on preferred stimuli.

A newborn's visual acuity is difficult to measure; however, it appears to range from 20/100 to 20/400. Newborns, however, can define the edges of 1/8- and 1/16-inch strips at 9 and 12 inches, and can fixate on objects for 4 to 10 seconds. They can also refixate every 1.0 to 1.5 seconds.

Brazelton (1993) describes the optimal response to visual stimulation as an initial alerting, attention that increases, a gradual decrease in interest, and a final turning away from a monotonous stimuli.

Hearing. The anatomic structures of the ear are well developed at birth. The newborn's eustachian tube is shorter and wider than that of the adult. The newborn also has specific and well-organized auditory responses.

Brazelton (1993) notes that when the newborn is presented with an interesting stimulus, such as a rattle, he or she will become alert, breathing will become irregular, eyes will open, and the newborn will scan the environment, turning toward the sound. As with visual responses, repeated auditory stimuli cause the newborn to shut out the stimuli.

Newborns are able to discriminate between sounds, and seem especially responsive to the human voice in the range of 500 to 900 Hz (Eisenberg, 1970). Low-frequency stimuli (25 to 40 dB) soothe the newborn; high-frequency stimuli (about 4000 Hz) produce an immediate response but may cause distress (Brazelton, 1993). Research has shown that newborns as young as 3 days old can discriminate between their mother's voice and the voice of another woman (De Casper & Fifer, 1980).

Olfactory Response. Newborns have a highly developed sense of smell. They prefer sweet odors. Evidence has shown that a 5-day-old newborn can distinguish his or her own mother's breast pad from those of other mothers (MacFarlane, 1975).

Taste. Newborns also have a discriminating sense of taste. They prefer sweet fluids to unsweetened or salty fluids. When newborns are given a sweet fluid (e.g., 15% sucrose), they suck more frequently and initially take shorter rest periods; however, they suck more slowly with increasing concentrations of sucrose.

When the newborn is fed cow's milk formula, she or he will suck continuously, pausing irregularly. If breast milk is then substituted, the newborn recognizes the change in taste, sucking in bursts with frequent pauses. The pauses are thought to be related to the taste of the breast milk, and the burst–pause pattern of the sucking is related to accommodation to a different stimulus (Brazelton, 1993).

Response to Tactile Stimuli.

Research indicates that newborns respond to touch in a variety of ways. When newborns are upset, they appear to be quieted by gentle, soothing patting or stroking. On the other hand, when newborns are quiet, a disturbing tactile stimulus quickly brings them to an alert state and may cause distress. Stroking a newborn's cheek elicits the rooting and sucking reflexes, which aid feeding.

Periods of Reactivity in the Newborn

Within the first 24 hours of birth, newborns demonstrate predictable periods of reactivity: a first period of reactivity, a period of sleep or inactivity, and a second period of reactivity. These periods are characterized by physiologic adjustments and behavioral states of the newborn. The sleep–wake patterns and physiologic adjustments of newborns during the periods of reactivity are influenced by the difficulty of the labor and delivery and any medications that the mother may have received during the labor and delivery process.

First Period of Reactivity.

The first period of reactivity occurs during the 30 minutes immediately after birth. In the initial phase of this period, newborns are in a state of quiet alertness. Their eyes are open and bright. They can focus attention on their parents' faces and attend to voices, especially those of their mothers. This phase lasts approximately 15 minutes and is followed by a phase of active alertness.

In the phase of active alertness, neonates have frequent bursts of movements, which may be accompanied by crying. They have a strong sucking reflex and appear hungry. This phase also lasts approximately 15 minutes.

The first period of reactivity is characterized by physiologic as well as behavioral responses. Rapid, shallow respirations may be accompanied by transient flaring of the nares, grunting, and retractions of the chest. The heart rate is rapid and irregular. Bowel sounds are absent and stools are present, although passage of meconium may or may not occur during this period.

Period of Sleep or Inactivity.

After the first 30 minutes, newborns become drowsy and fall asleep. During the sleep state, newborns are relatively unresponsive and difficult to awaken. Respiratory and heart rates slow and become more regular. The temperature of the newborn may drop. Posture appears relaxed and bowel sounds are present. Because of the relative inactivity of the newborn, it is difficult to ini-

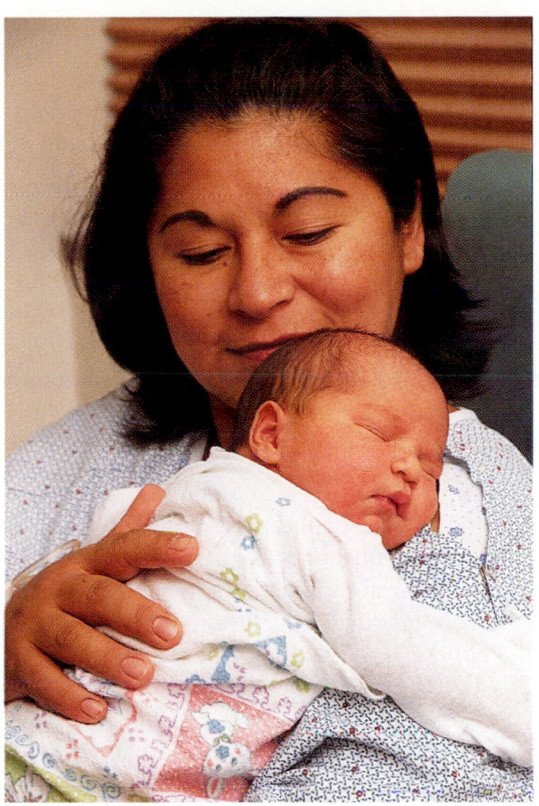

FIGURE 30–4. Period of inactivity.

tiate feeding. This period of inactivity may last from 2 to 4 hours (Fig. 30–4).

Second Period of Reactivity.

After the period of sleep or inactivity, newborns enter the second period of reactivity. This period may last from 4 to 6 hours in the normal newborn. The newborn is awake and alert during this period and may demonstrate alternate states of quiet alertness, active alertness, and crying.

The newborn's physiologic responses also may vary during this period. Respiratory and heart rates may change rapidly. Newborns should be observed for tachypnea and apnea during this period. Newborns produce gastric and respiratory mucus, which may cause them to regurgitate and gag. They also may demonstrate changes in color, with transient phases of mild cyanosis. Bowel sounds increase during this period, and the newborn may pass the first meconium stool. The first voiding also may occur.

During this period, the nurse can provide the parents opportunities to begin attachment behaviors. Feeding also may be begun if it was not initiated during the first period of reactivity. The neonate sucks, roots, and swallows, and becomes interested in feeding.

► BEHAVIOR

Newborns respond interactively and reciprocally with their caregivers. Newborns also demonstrate several other characteristic behavioral responses.

► Behavioral State

Brazelton's classic research in 1973 on newborn behavior and neurologic responses was described as the newborn's state of consciousness. The newborn's behavioral state can be categorized into six levels of arousal:

1. *Deep sleep.* The newborn's face appears relaxed; the eyelids are closed with no movement. Breathing is regular and deep. Little or no motor activity occurs, with the exception of an occasional startle or fine mouth movements.
2. *Light sleep.* The newborn's eyes are closed and rapid eye movements (REMs) occur. Occasional body activity, ranging from minor twitches to stretching of the extremities, can be noted. Breathing is irregular and more rapid than in deep sleep.
3. *Drowsiness or semidozing.* The newborn's eyes may be open or closed. If open, the eyes appear glazed and do not focus. Some motor activity may occur, with an occasional startle. Respirations are fairly regular, but faster than in sleep states.
4. *Quiet alert.* Newborns' eyes are open, bright, and alert. They focus on and follow appealing objects, such as a red ball. Newborns also attend to auditory stimuli, such as their mothers' voices.
5. *Active alert.* Newborns experience frequent bursts of movement of the extremities. Their eyes are open, scanning the environment. This state is apparent prior to feeding or when the infant is fussing.
6. *Intense crying.* Newborns have periods of motor activity, accompanied by continuous bursts of crying. This state helps newborns to shut out disturbing stimuli and alerts the caregiver to hunger and discomfort of the newborn.

► Sleep–Wake Cycle

Newborns appear to have individualized sleep–wake patterns. In general, sleep cycles (light REM sleep and deep sleep) at term occur in intervals of 45 to 50 min-utes, with premature babies having shorter intervals. Rapid eye movement sleep, which occurs in the deep sleep state as well as the light sleep state, contributes to the growth and maintenance of neural structures (Brazelton, 1993).

The newborn's sleep–wake cycles become patterned so that eventually diurnal patterns of daytime wakefulness and night sleeping occur. These diurnal patterns are influenced by appropriate feeding patterns, sufficient nurturing activities, and a fussing period prior to a long sleep (Brazelton, 1993). Weight also influences diurnal patterns. When newborns weigh approximately 12 pounds, they begin stretching their feeding times, and eliminating nighttime feedings.

► Behavioral Responses

Newborns demonstrate several predictable responses when interacting with caregivers and when responding to environmental stimuli. Brazelton's (1973) early research demonstrates that newborns can be assessed for these responses, which vary depending on their behavioral state. For example, when newborns are in the deep sleep state, they respond only slightly to a moderately loud rattle. In the active alert state, on the other hand, newborns respond to the rattle by becoming quiet, alerting, and then turning to the rattle as if searching for it. Brazelton also found that newborns can be assessed for orienting response, habituation, consolability and self-quieting, cuddliness, and motor organization.

Orienting Response

The response of newborns to stimuli is called the orienting response. Research indicates that newborns become more alert when they sense a new stimulus, and less responsive when orienting to a repetitive stimulus (Als & Brazelton, 1981). This ability to respond less to repetitive stimuli is termed the response decrement. This phenomenon allows neonates to control their behavioral state. Overresponsive newborns are said to lack response decrement. They are easily aroused and tend to respond to many stimuli by crying. Unresponsive newborns are relatively inactive and difficult to arouse. Quiet alert newborns respond to stimuli with a normal response decrement.

Habituation

Habituation is the process whereby newborns shut out disturbing or overwhelming stimuli. This process allows the newborn to respond less to a repeated stimulus. Stimuli such as light or noise will first alert the newborn to the stimulus. With repeated applications of the stimulus, however, the response of the newborn will decrease. Parents need to understand this concept. As one parent stated, "I was so worried that my baby could not hear. He seemed to startle and awaken when our dog barked when we first took him home. Now, he sleeps even when the dog is barking."

Along with habituation, newborns appear to have clear preferences for certain stimuli. They prefer female voices over male voices and human faces over other objects (Brazelton, 1993).

Consolability and Self-Quieting Behavior

The consolability of the newborn, either by intervention of the caregiver or by self-consolation, is important to the success of parent–newborn interactions. Consolability refers to the way in which newborns are able to change from the crying to the active alert, quiet alert, drowsy, or sleep state. Parents who are successful in consoling their newborns experience a sense of satisfaction. As one mother proudly noted, "When my baby is crying, it seems that only my husband or myself can quiet her." On the other hand, the inability to console may be very distressing to the parents.

Newborns also have the ability to console themselves. This is referred to as self-quieting behavior. Self-quieting or self-consoling behaviors include hand-to-mouth movements, sucking, alerting to external stimuli such as voices or faces, and motor activity.

Nurses can assist parents in identifying self-quieting behaviors of their newborn so that they will not feel they have to pick up the newborn as soon as she or he starts to cry. Nurses also should assist the parents in identifying behaviors that will help console the newborn, such as rocking, holding, and patting.

Cuddliness

Cuddliness is the newborn's response to being held by the caregiver; specifically, it is the degree to which a newborn nestles into the contours of the caregiver's body. Many newborns cuddle; some resist being held. Nurses can foster cuddling by assisting parents to assume comfortable positions, and explaining that newborns differ in this response.

Motor Organization

Motor organization refers to those activities that enable the newborn to control and coordinate movement. When stimulated, newborns with good motor organization demonstrate movements that are rhythmic and spontaneous. For example, when roused from sleep, they may initially startle and then attempt to bring their hands to their mouths. To bring the hand to the mouth, the newborn may turn the head to one side, thus displaying control of one side of the

body. The newborn then extends and flexes the arm to enable the hand to reach the mouth. As the hand reaches the mouth, the newborn's body relaxes and the face softens as he or she attempts to insert the clenched fist. When these efforts are successful, the newborn maintains a quiet state of semi-alertness. Such motor behavior is a good indication of central nervous system organization in newborns (Brazelton, 1993).

▶ Attachment/Bonding

The newborn's behavioral state also affects the attachment behaviors of parents and infants. Understanding newborn behavior helps parents be sensitive to the cues of their newborn. Over time, parents and infants get to know each other well and modify their behaviors accordingly.

▶ NURSING AND COLLABORATIVE ASSESSMENT

Several methods of assessment are used for the newborn. Findings from each assessment are compared with previous observations to ensure that the newborn continues to develop normally or to promptly identify any high-risk conditions. Information is gathered from a variety of sources: interviews with the parents, maternal and paternal records, prenatal and delivery room records, various assessment tools, and observation and physical examination of the neonate as an individual and as a member of a family unit.

One of the first assessments is assignment of an Apgar score. The score is a widely used measurement of the neonate's physiologic status. After the initial evaluation is completed, screening procedures, a health history, complete physical examination, and assessment of gestational age are carried out.

▶ Apgar Score

The **Apgar score** was developed in 1953 by Virginia Apgar, M.D., to assess the neonate's condition at birth. Five parameters are assessed 1 minute and 5 minutes after birth: heart rate, respiratory effort, reflex irritability, muscle tone, and color.

Heart Rate

The heart rate of the neonate is counted for a full minute by means of auscultation or palpation. A score of 2 is given if the heart rate is more than 100/min; a score of 1 is given if the heart rate is less than

100/min; a score of 0 is given if the heart rate is absent.

Respiratory Effort

Respiratory rate is assessed by counting the respirations for 1 full minute. Respirations may be assessed by means of observation or auscultation. A score of 2 indicates regular respirations or crying; a score of 1 indicates slow, irregular respirations; and a score of 0 indicates absent respirations (apnea).

Reflex Irritability

Reflex irritability is assessed by observing the neonate's response to a stimulus, such as rubbing the back or gently flicking the soles of the feet. A score of 2 is given when the neonate responds to the stimulus by crying; a score of 1 is given when the neonate responds by grimacing or frowning; and a score of 0 is given when the neonate has no response.

Muscle Tone

Muscle tone is assessed by observing the neonate's activity level, the level of resistance when the examiner extends the neonate's extremities, and how fast the extremities return to a state of flexion. A score of 2 is given when the neonate demonstrates good muscle tone, activity, and spontaneous flexion of the extremities; a score of 1 is given when there is some activity, some flexion of the extremities, and some resistance to extension; and a score of 0 is given when the neonate is limp or completely flaccid.

Color

The color of the neonate also is assessed at 1 and 5 minutes after birth. Most neonates are somewhat cyanotic at birth. With the onset of respirations, the skin becomes pink, but the extremities may remain cyanotic. A score of 2 for color is given when the neonate is completely pink; a score of 1 is given when the extremities are blue or pale and the body is pink; and a score of 0 is given when the newborn is blue or pale.

Summarizing Results

Table 30–3 summarizes the Apgar score. The score helps caregivers determine how much, if any, resuscitation the neonate will need. A total score of 7 to 10 indicates that the neonate is in good condition and will need only possible suctioning of the mouth and nose and observation. A score of 3 to 6 indicates a moderately depressed neonate who will need some resuscitation and close observation. A score of 0, 1, or 2 indicates a severely depressed neonate who will need resuscitation, possible ventilatory assistance, and intensive observation and care.

Neonates who are at term or close to term when delivered are more likely to have higher Apgar scores than those who are premature. Of the five categories of assessment, heart rate is the least affected by gestational age; muscle tone, reflex irritability, and respiratory effort increase with advancing gestational age. Color is the most unreliable parameter at any given gestational age.

► Screening Procedures

Screening procedures for the neonate may include determinations of cord blood type, blood group, and Coombs' reaction; testing for metabolic diseases such as phenylketonuria (PKU), hypothyroidism, and galactosemia; tests for sickle-cell disease and syphilis; and an initial hearing screening.

Cord Blood Type, Group, and Coombs' Reaction

A sample of cord blood is collected in the delivery room and sent to the laboratory. The cord blood is tested for blood type and group. A Coombs' test should also be performed for neonates, especially for those whose mothers have type O or Rh-negative blood or for neonates who become significantly jaundiced. The direct Coombs' test will determine if antibodies are present in the neonate's blood. (See Chapter 32.)

► **TABLE 30–3**

The Apgar Score

Sign	0	1	2
Heart rate	Absent	Less than 100/min	Greater than 100/min
Respiratory effort	Absent	Slow, irregular	Regular or crying
Reflex irritability	No response	Grimace, frown	Cry, cough
Muscle tone	Limp	Some motion, some flexion of extremities, some resistance to extension of extremities	Active, spontaneous flexion, good tone
Color	Cyanotic or pale	Body pink, extremities cyanotic	Completely pink

Test for Phenylketonuria

To test for PKU, a blood sample is taken from the heel after the neonate has ingested sufficient quantities of milk (24 to 36 hours of milk ingestion). Phenylketonuria is an autosomal recessive disease of protein synthesis in which the blood level of the amino acid phenylalanine becomes very high; the disorder results in mental retardation. The incidence of PKU is 1 in 15,000. Retardation can be prevented through dietary control.

Test for Galactosemia

The blood sample taken from the neonate's heel to test for PKU is also used to test for galactosemia. Galactosemia is another autosomal recessive disease in which the inborn error of metabolism involves the body's inability to convert galactose to glucose. The surplus of galactose in the body causes liver and brain damage. Infections and cataracts are seen in infancy. The incidence of galactosemia is 1 in 40,000. If found early, it may be treated with a galactose-free diet.

Test for Hypothyroidism

Mass neonatal screening for hypothyroidism is a cost-effective measure for preventing mental retardation caused by thyroid dysfunction in neonates. A sample of the neonate's blood is taken and usually sent to an outside laboratory. The incidence of hypothyroidism (1 in 4000) and the effectiveness of early replacement therapy in preventing mental retardation make this an appropriate screening test for neonates (Di George, 1992).

Test for Sickle-Cell Disease

Sickle-cell disease can be detected in the newborn period using the same blood sample obtained for other newborn screenings. Sickle-cell disease is an autosomal recessive disorder occurring in certain ethnic groups, most commonly African-Americans. Other groups known to be affected include people of Mediterranean, Carribean, Arabian, East Indian, and South and Central American ethnic origins.

Sickle-cell disease is marked by crescent-shaped red blood cells caused by defective hemoglobin. Severe, life-threatening health problems may result. Early detection of sickle-cell disease can reduce morbidity and mortality.

Among the variations of sickle-cell disease the most common form occurs in African-Americans and has an incidence of 1 in 375. Because of the variations noted in the disease, it is recommended that all babies be screened, because screening programs targeting a specific ethnic group may not identify all affected infants (Sickle Cell Disease Guideline Panel, 1993).

Test for Syphilis

Because the incidence of syphilis has increased among neonates, many institutions routinely test for the condition. The Venereal Disease Research Labs (VDRL) test or the rapid plasma reagent (RPR) test is used.

Initial Hearing Screening

Hearing can initially be assessed when a neonate is in the quiet alert state. A hand clap or ringing bell near the ear will usually cause a startle or blink response. If the neonate does not respond to the sound initially, a retest for hearing should be done.

▶ Health History

Interviewing parents is an important step in data gathering. The time spent also promotes development of a trusting relationship between parents and nurse.

The health history includes prenatal and postnatal histories; family history; a family profile, which includes developmental, psychologic, sociocultural, and environmental factors; and information on adaptation of the neonate (Fig. 30–5). The information will vary with the age of the neonate. The form used may also vary from agency to agency depending on policies and procedures, but the information is generally standardized. The nurse should not feel limited to the questions included in the form, but should pursue and include relevant, important information if indicated. The nurse may also construct a health history form that is tailored to a particular setting.

▶ Physical Examination

Throughout the immediate postnatal period, the neonate continues to adapt to extrauterine life and to demonstrate several physical and physiologic changes. For that reason, appraisals of the neonate should be dated and timed.

Timing of Evaluation

The first physical examination is performed at delivery regardless of the setting. Coupled with the Apgar score, it confirms the general condition of the neonate. A more comprehensive examination is done within the first 24 hours after birth. Another should be performed before the neonate is discharged and again at 2 and 4 weeks of age.

The Setting

If possible, the neonate's parents are present during the examination. Parents often worry about small

Neonatal assessment data

Date _____

	At birth	Today
Name _____	weight _____	weight _____
Birthdate _____	Length _____	Length _____
Birthtime _____	H.C. _____	H.C. _____
Race _____	Chest _____	Chest _____
Sex _____	Blood type _____	
	APGAR 1 _____ 5 _____	

Biographic data

	Mother	Father	Siblings
Name	_____	_____	_____
Age	_____	_____	_____
Occupation	_____	_____	_____
Religion	_____	_____	_____
Insurance	_____	_____	_____

Family medical history

Heart disease _____   Diabetes _____   Allergies _____
Hypertension _____   Arthritis _____   Migraines _____
Blood disorders _____   Obesity _____   Other _____
Renal disease _____   Mental illness _____
Cancer _____   Seizure disorder _____

Genogram

Mother's prenatal history   G _____   P _____   A _____   SB _____

Date prenatal care started _____   Blood type _____

Medications _____   Vitamins _____   Nutritional status: *good* _____
    fair _____

Alcohol ingestion _____   Other substances _____   *poor* _____
Smoking _____   Exposure to radiation _____
Sexually active until _____ month gestation
Weight gain _____ pounds

Health problems:
    hypertension _____   bleeding _____   infection _____
    diabetes _____   control: *diet* _____ *insulin* _____
    accidents _____   other _____

Childbirth preparation classes: _____   who attended _____

FIGURE 30–5. Sample neonatal assessment tool.

Mother's prenatal history (con't)

Delivery: *vaginal* _____   *forceps* _____   *vacuum extraction* _____
            C/S _____   indication _____
            anesthesia _____   medications _____
            complications _____
Support system during L&D _____
Attachment experience immediately postdelivery _____

Postnatal history

Physical abnormalities _____
Health problems_____
Discharged with mother _____

Nutritional status

Breast _____   *Bottle* _____
Feeding: *well* _____   *fair* _____   *poor* _____
Tolerated: *well* _____   *fair* _____   *poor* _____
Breast: _____ min/breast   frequency _____ hours
   P.C. supplement: what_____   how often _____   how much_____
Formula: type _____   amount_____ oz   frequency _____ hours
Vitamins: _____
Bowel movements: color_____   consistency_____   frequency_____ /day
            problems_____
Urination: frequency_____ /day   problems _____

Developmental status

Regards face _____   smiles responsively_____
Lifts head when prone _____

Sociocultural status

Primary caretakers _____
Grandparents: Maternal   Paternal
   supportive?   _____   _____
   available?   _____   _____
Significant others
   relationship _____
   available   _____

Environment/safety

Safety seat _____ use: *front*_____   *rear* _____   *both*_____
Smoke detectors _____
Smokers in home _____
Pets/animals in home _____
Number of residents in home _____
Water supply: city/fluoride treated _____   well _____
Other:

FIGURE 30–5. *Continued*

Physical assessment

T. _____ H.R. _____ R.R. _____ B/P _____

General appearance:

flexed _____ extended _____ symmetric_____

if not, describe _____

muscle tone: WNL _____ hypotonic _____ hypertonic _____

state of arousal: deep sleep _____ light sleep _____

drowsy _____ quiet alert _____

active alert _____ crying _____

strong/lusty _____

high pitch/shrill _____

weak _____

tremors _____

Other:

Skin: pink _____   meconium staining _____   turgor/tenting   Y _____   N _____

dusky _____   petechiae _____   location _____

cyanotic _____   rash _____ pustules _____ vesicles _____

acrocyanosis _____   ecchymosis _____

pale _____

jaundice _____

beefy red _____

Other:

Head: fontanelles _____

soft/flat _____

depressed _____

bulging _____

sutures _____

WNL _____

open/wide space _____

closed _____

hair

silky smooth _____   wooly _____

distribution WNL _____   *if not, describe* _____

Face: symmetric/proportional _____   *if not, describe* _____

Eyes: iris color   sclera color   R   L

dark blue/gray _____   white _____   blink reflex _____   _____

brown _____   jaundice _____   pupillary reflex _____   _____

true blue _____   red reflex _____   _____

pink _____

conjunctiva: pink _____   erythema _____   discharge _____   hemorrhages _____

tears: present _____   not present _____   excessive _____

Other:

Ears: position WNL _____   low set _____

pinnae developed/firm _____   shapeless/floppy _____

TMs color _____   bony landmarks _____   intact _____   mobile _____

acoustic blink or startle reflex + _____ – _____

Other:

FIGURE 30–5. *Continued*

Nose: mucus: none _____ small amt. _____ mod. amt. _____ copious _____
          appearance WNL _____ *if not, describe* _____
          nasal flaring: Y_____ N _____

Mouth and throat: symmetric _____ *if not, describe* _____
          buccal mucosa/gingiva: pink _____ moist _____ lesions _____
                   other _____
          soft/hard palate: intact _____ jaundice _____
                 Epstein's pearls _____ other _____
          mucus: none _____ small amt. _____ mod. amt. _____ copious _____
          tongue: midline _____ symmetric _____
              frenulum WNL _____ *if not, describe* _____
              macroglossia _____ protruding _____ other _____
          Other:

Neck: muscle tone WNL _____ *if not, describe* _____
          full range of motion _____ *if not, describe* _____
          rigid _____ torticollis _____ webbing _____
          masses _____ *if so, describe* _____

Chest: symmetric _____ *if not, describe* _____
          clavicles intact _____
          nipples WNL _____ *if not, describe* _____
          breath sounds _____ bilateral _____
          expiratory grunting _____
          inspiratory wheeze _____
          retractions _____ *if so, describe* _____
          gasping _____ apnea > 15 sec _____
          Other:

Heart: location of PMI _____

pulses	Full	Symmetric
apical	_____	_____
femoral	_____	_____
dorsalis pedis	_____	_____
brachial	_____	_____

          murmurs _____ *if so, describe* _____
          Other:

Abdomen: symmetric _____ *if not, describe* _____
          soft _____ tense _____ concave _____ distended _____
          umbilical cord: on _____ off _____
            number of vessels _____ arteries _____ vein
            drying WNL _____ bleeding _____ discharge _____ other _____
          bowel sounds regular _____ increased _____ decreased _____ absent _____
          masses or organomegaly _____ *if so, describe* _____
          liver edge felt _____ *if so, where* _____

Genitalia: WNL _____ *if not, describe* _____
          male: circumcised _____ uncircumcised _____
              meatal opening: tip of glans _____
                   hypospadias _____ *if so, describe* _____
                   epispadias _____ *if so, describe* _____
             testes descended _____
               hydrocele _____
          age of 1st voiding _____ hrs _____
            urinary stream: adequate _____ dribbles _____
          Other:

Anus and rectum: patent _____ + wink reflex _____ fissures _____
          other _____
          age when meconium first passed _____

FIGURE 30–5. *Continued*

Extremities: symmetric _____ *if not, describe* _____

full ROM _____ *if not, describe* _____

muscle tone: good _____ hypotonic _____ hypertonic _____

hip　　　　　　　　　　　R　　　　　　　　L

　Ortalani _____　_____

　leg length _____　_____

　creases _____　_____

　knee height _____　_____

Other:

Spine:　appears WNL _____ *if not, describe* _____

Reflexes:	Present	Abnormal		Present	Abnormal
Moro	_____	_____	placing	_____	_____
palmar	_____	_____	crossed extension	_____	_____
grasp	_____	_____	magnet	_____	_____
tonic neck	_____	_____	traction	_____	_____
sucking	_____	_____	arm recoil	_____	_____
rooting	_____	_____	crawling	_____	_____
swallowing	_____	_____	Galant's	_____	_____
Babinski	_____	_____	glabellar	_____	_____
stepping	_____	_____			

Assessment summary

FIGURE 30–5. *Continued*

"imperfections" that health care providers regard as normal. Performing the examination with the parents in attendance allows the nurse to discuss normal findings and normal variations. The nurse can also answer any questions or allay any fears that parents might have. At the same time, the nurse can demonstrate techniques for handling the neonate as well as assess the parental responses to these interventions.

The physical examination should be performed with the neonate lying unclothed in a warm, well-lighted area. Radiant warmers often are used in the nursery for the initial examination. Careful hand-washing and cleansing of the stethoscope and the other instruments used should precede the examination. In addition, the nurse should use universal precautions, especially as the newborn may still have some dried blood on the body or hair. The nurse should also obtain baseline data for comparison with observations made at a later date. These data include vital signs; weight; length; and head, chest, and abdominal circumferences. The data may be determined before or during the examination.

Baseline Data

Vital Signs. Temperature, heart rate, and respiratory rate are always measured. Blood pressure may not be routinely assessed unless specifically indicated, for example, if a cardiac problem is suspected. Table 30–4 summarizes neonatal vital signs.

Temperature generally is measured by the axillary route (Fig. 30–6). Electronic thermometers are quicker than standard mercury thermometers and afford a reading within 1 minute. At times, an electronic thermometer may indicate a low temperature. The nurse must check the equipment to make sure this reading is accurate and not due to rundown batteries, positioning of the probe, or other mechanical problems. Standard mercury thermometers should be held in place for 3 minutes. Previously, the initial temperature was taken rectally to rule out imperforate anus; however, now it is generally accepted that the passage of meconium is sufficient to validate a patent anus.

The normal neonatal heart rate can average between 120 and 160 beats per minute, ranging from

▶ **TABLE 30–4**

Summary of Neonatal Assessment: Usual Findings, Acceptable Variations, and Abnormal Findings

Area Assessed	Usual Findings	Acceptable Variations	Abnormal Findings
Temperature	Axillary route preferable Averages between 36.5 and 37°C (97.6 and 98.6°F) Stabilized by 10 hours of age	Ranges from 36.1 to 37.2°C (97 to 99°F)	>37.2°C (99°F) (may indicate excessively warm environment, dehydration, infection/sepsis, brain damage) <36.1°C (97°F) (may indicate cold environment, infection)
Heart rate	Average apical pulse at rest 120–160 beats per minute Heart rate regular Increases with crying and movement Decreases with quieting and sleep	70–100 beats per minute sleeping; 180 beats per minute crying Irregular heart rate for brief periods or after crying	Tachycardia: >160 beats per minute awake and at rest Bradycardia: <120 beats per minute awake and at rest Irregular heart rate
Respirations	Average 40 respirations per minute Abdominal breathing Quiet and shallow Irregular, periodic breathing	35–60 respirations per minute Cheyne–Stokes–type breathing without evidence of respiratory distress Transient tachypnea, especially in the newborn period Apnea lasting 5–15 seconds	Tachypnea: >60 respirations per minute Bradypnea: <30 respirations per minute Apnea lasting longer than 15 seconds

Blood pressure	At birth
	  Systolic 60–90 mm Hg
	  Diastolic 40–60 mm Hg
	0–6 months:
	  Systolic 80–110 mm Hg
	  Diastolic 45–60 mm Hg
		Change in activity level will cause variations in readings	Hypotension (may indicate hypovolemia or shock)
			Hypertension (may be sign of coarctation of aorta, especially if there is a difference in blood pressure readings between the upper and lower extremities)

Weight	Full term (gestation 38–42 weeks), birth weight >2500 g Full term, average weight 3400 g (7 pounds 8 oz) Preterm (gestation <37 weeks), birth weight <2500 g	Birth weight 2500–4000 g (5 pounds 8 oz to 8 pounds 13 oz) Approximately 10% weight loss after birth Will regain birth weight by 10–14 days of age	Weight loss > 10–15% Weight inappropriate for gestational age
Length	Average length 50 cm (20 in.)	45–55 cm (18–22 in.)	<45 cm (18 in.) (may indicate congenital dwarf)
Head circumference	Average head circumference 33–35 cm (13–14 in.)	32.5–37.5 cm (12.5–14.5 in.)	Microcephaly <32.5 cm >37.5 cm (hydrocephalus should be considered)
General appearance	Normal resting position: flexion Good muscle tone Body size proportional Umbilicus center of body Body movement symmetric Strong, lusty cry	Jerky movements Tremors of arms, legs, and body with vigorous crying or at rest during the first 48 to 72 hours of life	Hypotonia Hypertonia Tremors Associated with hypoglycemia or hypocalcemia At rest at 4 days of age (may indicate CNS disease) Birth defects High-pitched or shrill cry (may indicate neurologic impairment) Weak or absent cry (indicates severe illness or mental retardation) Asymmetric body movement (may indicate central or peripheral neurologic deficits, birth injuries, or congenital anomalies)

Skin	Pink color (varies according to racial background)
	Nailbeds pink
	Familial and racial features
	Milia
	Good skin turgor, no tenting
		Desquamation
		Acrocyanosis
		Mottling
		Harlequin color change
		Petechiae over presenting part
		Erythema toxicum
			Jaundice after 24 hours of life
			Physiologic jaundice
			  Formula: >12–13 mg/dL
			  Breast: >15 mg/dL
			Cyanosis/duskiness
			Beefy red (may be associated with polycythemia)

(continued)

▶ **TABLE 30–4** *(continued)*

Summary of Neonatal Assessment: Usual Findings, Acceptable Variations, and Abnormal Findings

Area Assessed	Usual Findings	Acceptable Variations	Abnormal Findings

Skin *(continued)*	Lanugo
	Vernix caseosa
		Capillary hemangiomas (telangiectatic nevi)
		Ecchymosis
		Mongolian spotting
		Physiologic jaundice
		  Formula: <12–13 mg/dL
		  Breast: <15 mg/dL
		Nevus flammeus
		Nevus vascularis
		Cavernous hemangiomas
			Petechiae on nontraumatized body areas
			Tenting (may indicate poor hydration)
			Generalized pallor (may indicate anoxia or anemia)
			Pustules, vesicles, rashes
			Meconium staining (indicates fetal stress)

Head	Anterior fontanelle
	  Diamond shape at junction of coronal/sagittal sutures
	  Soft/flat
	Posterior fontanelle: triangular shape at junction of sagittal/lambdoidal sutures
	Silky smooth hair distributed evenly over scalp
		Molding
		Fontanelle size
		Caput succedaneum
		Cephalhematoma
		Scalp abrasions, lacerations, punctures from forceps, vacuum extractor, scalp pH determinations, internal monitor probe, or delivery trauma
			Widely spaced suture lines (may indicate hydrocephalus)
			Closed suture lines (indicates synostosis)
			Very large anterior fontanelle (may indicate hypothyroidsm)
			Bulging fontanelle (may indicate increased intracranial pressure)
			Depressed fontanelle (may be a sign of dehydration)
			"Wooly," fine hair found on premature neonates
			Unusual hair lines (may be associated with chromosomal disorders)

Face	Symmetric facial features well positioned and proportional Facial movement equal bilaterally Eyebrows, eyelashes, hairline present Receding chin	Small degree of asymmetry (may be the result of intrauterine positioning)	Facial palsy when neonate grimaces or cries (may be caused by intrauterine positioning, forceps, or birth trauma) Distorted facies (may be seen in newborns with chromosomal disorders)

Eyes	Symmetric in shape, movement, and placement
	Iris color
	  Dark blue (Caucasians)
	  Brown (dark-skinned infants)
	Positive blink reflex
	Tears may not be observed
	Conjunctiva pale pink
	Pupillary size and shape equal bilaterally
	Positive pupillary reflex bilaterally
	Sclera white with slight bluish tint
	Movement of eyeballs random and uneven
	Fixates momentarily
	May follow to midline
	Pseudostrabismus
	Doll's-eye phenomenon
	Positive red reflex
		Transient lid edema (may be caused by maternal hormones or eye prophylaxis)
		Subconjunctival hemorrhages
		Transient strabismus or nystagmus
		Brushfield's spots (may also be found in newborns with Down syndrome or other conditions associated with mental retardation)
		Epicanthal folds in newborn of Asian descent (may also be present in newborns with chromosomal disorders)
			Dacryostenosis
			Dacryocystitis
			Eye discharge related to bacterial infection or chemical conjunctivitis related to eye prophylaxis
			Sclerae yellowish (indicative of jaundice)
			Corneal opacities
			Ptosis
			Gross nystagmus
			Constant strabismus
			Coloboma
			Pink iris (albinism)
			True blue sclera (osteogenesis imperfecta)

Ears	Top of ear in alignment with inner and outer canthi of eyes
	Well formed with firm cartilage
	Patent ear canals
	Tympanic membranes
	  Pearly gray
	  Intact
	  Translucent and bony middle ear landmarks visible
		Crumpled and flattened against side of head (as a result of intrauterine positioning)
		Vernix caseosa in ear canals
		Floppy if premature
			Unilateral or bilateral preauricular skin tags
			Low-set ears (may indicate chromosomal aberrations)
			Malformations of the ear (may be associated with renal problems)
			Floppy if full term

▶ **TABLE 30–4** *(continued)*

Summary of Neonatal Assessment: Usual Findings, Acceptable Variations, and Abnormal Findings

Area Assessed	Usual Findings	Acceptable Variations	Abnormal Findings
Ears *(continued)*	Mobile Positive acoustic blink or startle reflex		
Nose	Placement should be midline on face Nostrils patent Sneezing to clear nostrils Pink, moist, mucous membranes	Small amount of mucus Misshapened nose (may result from intrauterine positioning)	Copious mucus Flaring nostrils (indicates respiratory distress) Malformed or misshapened (may occur in chromosomal problems) Choanal atresia Deviated septum
Mouth and throat	Lips and lip movement symmetric Lips pink and moist Tubercle on upper lip from sucking Buccal mucosa and gingiva pink and moist Edentulous Hard and soft palates intact Uvula midline Tongue freely moveable and symmetric in shape and movement Sucking pads No tonsilar tissue	Short frenulum without tongue tie Cysts in floor of mouth near frenulum Epstein's pearls	Precocious teeth Cleft lip, cleft palate, or both Protruding tongue (may be a sign of chromosomal problems) Macroglossia (may be early sign of hypothyroidism or may be caused by hemangioma) Micrognathia (associated with Pierre Robin or other syndromes) Short frenulum (tongue tie) Yellowish palate (indication of jaundice) Excessive saliva (may indicate tracheoesophageal fistula or atresia) Oral thrush Continuous inspiratory and expiratory stridor (may indicate small larynx or tracheomalacia)
Neck	Short, straight with many skin folds Trachea midline Full range of motion Adequate muscle strength Thyroid not palpable	Palpable cervical lymph nodes < 5mm	Masses Rigidity/torticollis Webbing or abnormally short neck (may be associated with chromosomal disorders)

Chest	Symmetric in size, shape, and movement
	Cylindrical shape
	Circumference equal to or less than head circumference
	Nipples symmetric and developed
	Breath sounds clear and equal bilaterally
		Xyphoid process may be prominent
		Ribs may be noted on deep inspiration
		Breast engorgement (caused by maternal hormones)
		"Witch's milk"
		Supernumerary nipples
		Transmitted upper airway sounds, should clear on crying
			Asymmetric in shape and movement
			Funnel-shaped (pectus excavatum)
			Fractured clavicles
			Signs of respiratory distress
			  Unequal chest expansion
			  Decreased breath sounds
			  Rales or adventitious sounds
			  Expiratory grunting
			  Retractions
			  Nasal flaring
			  Gasping
			Inspiratory wheeze
			Decreased, increased, or abnormal breath sounds

Heart	Point of maximal impulse lateral to midclavicular line in third or fourth left intercostal space Femoral, dorsalis pedis, brachial pulses full and symmetric S_1 and S_2 clearly heard throughout the precordium S_2 splitting	Point of maximal impulse visible Functional heart murmur	Arrhythmias Asymmetric femoral and apical pulse (may indicate cardiac anomaly) Heart sounds heard prominently on right instead of left side of chest with dextrocardia Murmurs associated with congenital defects

(continued)

▶ **TABLE 30-4** *(continued)*

Summary of Neonatal Assessment: Usual Findings, Acceptable Variations, and Abnormal Findings

Area Assessed	Usual Findings	Acceptable Variations	Abnormal Findings

Abdomen	Cylindrical in shape, protrudes slightly
	Superficial abdominal veins
	Umbilical cord
	  Two arteries and one vein
	  Shrivels and blackens second or third day of life
	Bowel sounds present in all four quadrants
	Stomach percussion tympanic
	Liver and spleen percussion dull
	Liver
	  Span 5.6–5.9 cm
	  Palpated 1–2 cm below right costal margin
	Edge feels soft
	Spleen tip palpated under left costal margin
	Kidneys
	  Palpated adjacent to vertebral column approximately 1–2 cm above umbilicus
	Lower half of right kidney and tip of left kidney palpable
	Meconium passed within 24 hours of delivery
	First voiding within 24 hours of delivery
		Umbilical hernia reducible
		Irregular bowel sounds
			Concave (may indicate diaphragmatic hernia)
			Distended or tense
			Increased, decreased, or absent bowel sounds
			Umbilical cord
			  Single artery
			  Granuloma
			  Bleeding
			  Infection
			  Discharge
			Omphalocele
			Abdominal masses
			Organomegaly
			Inguinal hernias, male > female

Genitalia	Female
	  Edematous clitoris and labia majora
	  Increased pigmentation of external structures (as a result of hormonal influences)
	  Whitish mucoid or pseudomenstruation (as a result of hormonal influences)
	  Smegma under labia
	Male
	  Foreskin not retractable if not circumcised
	  Smegma under foreskin if not circumcised
	  Meatal opening is a centrally located slit on tip of glans
	  Strong, arching, urinary stream
	  Penile erection when stimulated or with urination
	  Scrotum: pink or dark brown depending on complexion, rugae (full term), both testes descended, positive cremasteric reflex
	Male and female
	  Uric acid crystals in urine
		Female
		  Vaginal/hymenal tags
		  Fusion of labia minora
		Male
		  Testes at junction of external inguinal rings
		  Hydroceles
			Female
			  Ambiguous, hypertrophied, or underdeveloped genitalia
			Male
			  Ambiguous, hypertrophied, or underdeveloped genitalia
			  Hypospadias or epispadias
			  Cryptorchidism
			  Phimosis (usually not evident until infant is older)

Anus and rectum	Anus patent Good sphincter tone Positive wink reflex Passage of meconium within 24 hours	Meconium passage within 48 hours	Meconium present in other genital orifices Imperforate anus Anal fissures

► **TABLE 30–4** *(continued)*

Summary of Neonatal Assessment: Usual Findings, Acceptable Variations, and Abnormal Findings

Area Assessed	Usual Findings	Acceptable Variations	Abnormal Findings

Extremities	Symmetric and equal in size and movement
	Full range of motion
	Flexed position
	Good tone
	Nails present on fingers and toes
	Plantar creases over anterior half of sole of foot
	Fat pads on feet give flat-footed appearance
		Extended knees with breech presentation
		Misaligned position as a result of intrauterine positioning
		Absent plantar creases as a result of prematurity
			Developmental dysplagia of the hip
			  Positive Ortolani movement
			  Unequal leg length
			  Unequal thigh creases and gluteal folds
			Polydactyly
			Syndactyly
			Simian line (may indicate chromosome abnormality such as Down syndrome)
			Erb-Duchenne palsy
			Talipes equinus (clubfoot)
			Metatarsus varus

Spine	Appears straight but can easily be flexed Can lift head and turn side to side when prone	Pilonidal dimple without tuft of hair or discharge	Pilonidal dimples with tuft of hair (may be associated with spina bifida occulta) Pilonidal cyst Myelomeningocele or meningocele Masses

as low as 70 to 90 while sleeping to as high as 180 while crying. The rate should be counted for a full minute to recognize normal fluctuations and to detect abnormalities.

Respiratory rates vary between 35 and 60 breaths per minute. Respirations are abdominal and can easily be counted by observing the rise and fall of the abdomen. The neonate's respiratory pattern is characterized by shallow, irregular breaths, often interrupted by short periods of apnea lasting 5 to 15 seconds. Respiratory function is evaluated by observing the breathing pattern for 1 full minute.

Recent data suggest that both heart and respiratory rates are affected by age. Full-term neonates will demonstrate a decrease in respiratory rate, with a mean of 38.5 at 4 weeks of age compared with a mean of 45.1 at birth. Heart rate shows an increase from a mean of 116.3 at birth to 141.3 at 15 days, and then decreases to 136.2 at 4 weeks of age.

Blood pressure is evaluated using the Doppler method of electronic monitoring or auscultated with a stethoscope. A 1-inch cuff is used with the stethoscope placed over the brachial artery. Neonatal blood pressure is highest immediately after birth, but falls to a minimum within 3 hours. It then begins to rise steadily and reaches a plateau about 4 to 6 days after birth. This measurement is usually equal to the blood pressure immediately after birth. The average blood pressure in a neonate weighing more than 4 kg is 72/55 but the reading will vary with activity (Behrman, 1992).

Parameters of Physical Growth. Parameters of physical growth must be carefully assessed. Because a neonate's progress is validated by these parameters, it is important to measure and record them accurately. Serial measurements are used to determine growth patterns. Recordings can be made on growth charts and compared with the previous readings.

The following measurements are made during each routine assessment. Table 30–4 summarizes physical assessment findings.

Weight. Neonates are usually weighed on admission to the nursery. They are placed unclothed in the

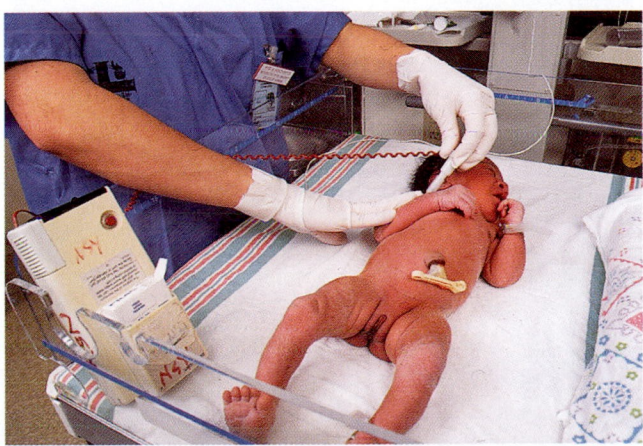

FIGURE 30–6. A neonate's axillary temperature is measured using an electronic thermometer.

center of a properly balanced scale. The examiner places one hand lightly over the neonate to prevent her or him from falling off the scale. While in the hospital, the neonate is usually weighed at the same time every day. The weight is recorded in grams or kilograms but converted to pounds for the benefit of the parents.

The average birth weight is 3400 g, or 7 pounds 8 ounces. Weight ranges from 2500 to 4000 g (5 pounds 8 ounces to 8 pounds 13 ounces). Neonates lose weight after birth, generally 10% of the birth weight or less, but regain their birth weight by 10 to 14 days of age.

Length. The average length of the newborn is 20 inches (50 cm), with a range of 18 to 22 inches (45 to 55 cm). This measurement is often difficult to obtain because of the position of flexion that the neonate assumes. The neonate should be flat on the back and the knees held in an extended position. The soles of the feet should be perpendicular to the surface. The examiner then measures using an accurate tape measure from the top of the head to the soles of the feet (Fig. 30–7).

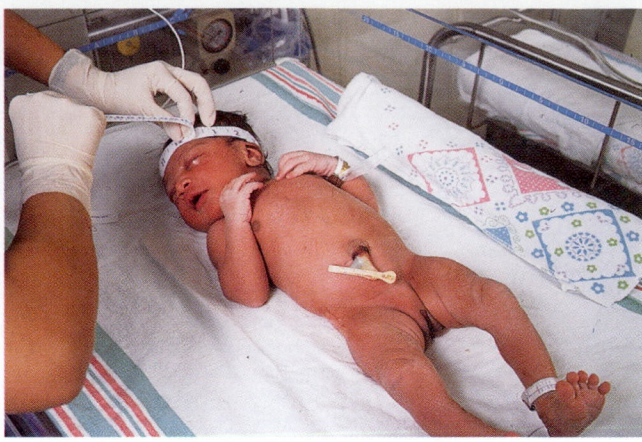
FIGURE 30–8. Measuring a newborn's head circumference. (The range is 33 to 35 cm.)

Head circumference is measured at the widest diameter, which is the occipitofrontal diameter (Fig. 30–8). The head may initially be misshapened as a result of molding, and therefore should be measured until it regains its original shape, within several days of birth. The average head circumference is 33 to 35 cm (13 to 14 inches).

The chest circumference is obtained by placing the tape around the chest at the nipple line (Fig. 30–9). The chest circumference may be equal to the head circumference but should not exceed it. Generally, it is about an inch less.

Abdominal circumference is measured by placing the tape around the abdomen at the level of the umbilicus. Abdominal measurements are usually

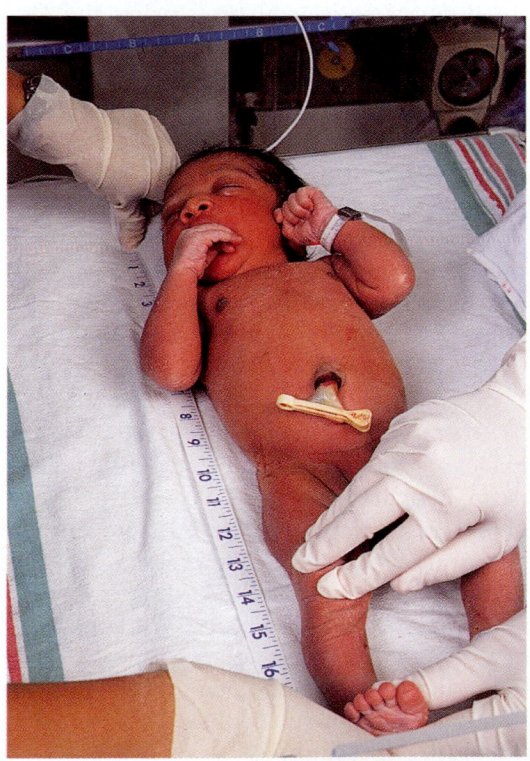
FIGURE 30–7. Measuring the length of a neonate. Often it is helpful if two staff members work together to ensure the accuracy of the procedure.

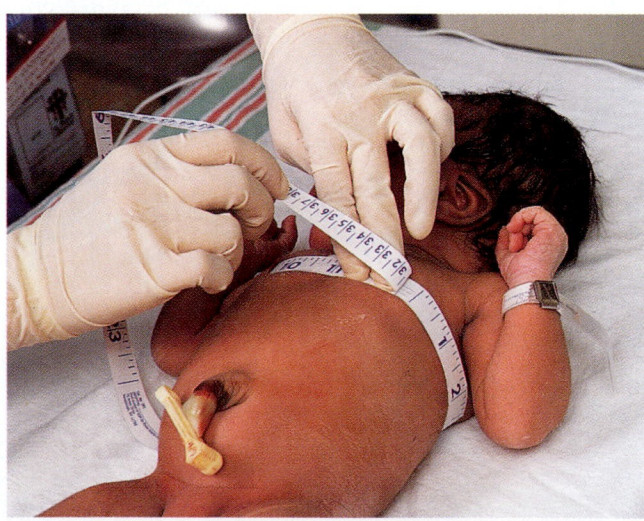
FIGURE 30–9. Measuring chest circumference. (Measurement is about that of the head circumference, but should not exceed it.)

made when there is a suspicion of pathology that causes abdominal distension.

General Appearance

The normal resting position of the neonate is flexion. Both the arms and legs are adducted and flexed. The head is large in proportion to body length, averaging about one fourth of the total. The umbilicus is the center of the neonate's body. The neck is short and the abdomen is prominent.

The nurse begins by noting the neonate's state of arousal and orienting response (see earlier section entitled Behavioral State). The examination is easiest to accomplish with the neonate in the quiet state. The characteristics of color, flexion, muscle tone, symmetry, obvious birth defects, respiratory patterns, and body movements can then be noted. The neonate should have a strong, lusty cry that is neither high pitched nor shrill. The latter may indicate neurologic impairment.

Skin

The neonate's skin is observed for color and color changes during activity, familial and racial features, rashes, milia, anomalies or deformities, birthmarks, jaundice, petechiae, forceps marks (Fig. 30–10), tone, and hydration status. These characteristics should be recorded.

Color varies according to racial background, pigmentation, and physiologic changes. The neonate is generally pink. **Acrocyanosis,** characterized by bluish discoloration of the hands and feet, is normal immediately after birth or if the neonate is exposed to a cold environment (Charlton & Phibbs, 1996) (Fig. 30–11). It is believed to be caused by a normal newborn condition of vasomotor instability and poor peripheral circulation. Acrocyanosis caused by vasomotor instability can be differentiated from true

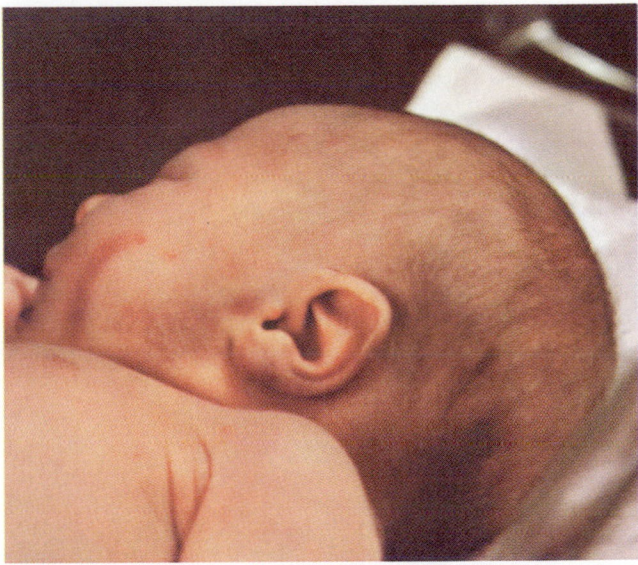

FIGURE 30–10. Forceps marks on the newborn. Pressure marks from forceps used during delivery are usually located on the cheek and jaw. They usually disappear within a day. *(Reproduced, with permission, of Mead Johnson & Company, Evansville, Indiana.)*

cyanosis by vigorously rubbing the sole of the foot, which will turn pink if the acrocyanosis is due to vasomotor instability.

Mottling (blotches of discoloration) may occur in response to temperature changes. However, pale, mottled skin may be a sign of such serious conditions as sepsis (Charlton & Phibbs, 1996). Occasionally a neonate may experience a **harlequin color change** whereby one side of the body develops a deep red color. It is a response to a normal vasomotor disturbance causing the blood vessels on one side of the body to constrict while those on the other side dilate. The condition may last for a few seconds or minutes and may occur again. This change should be recorded

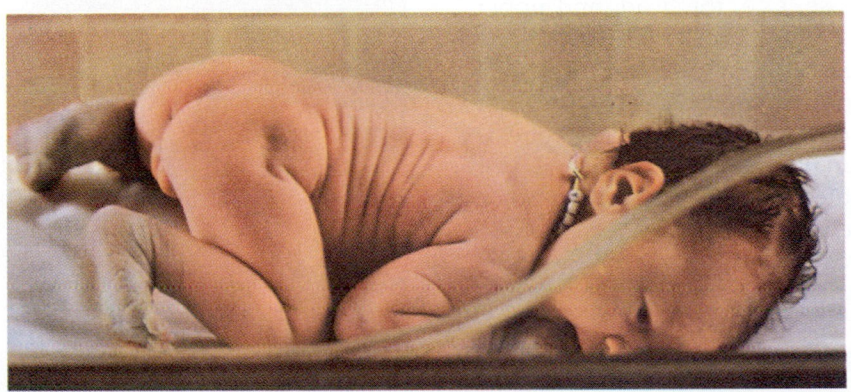

FIGURE 30–11. Acrocyanosis in the newborn. *(Reproduced, with permission, of Mead Johnson & Company, Evansville, Indiana.)*

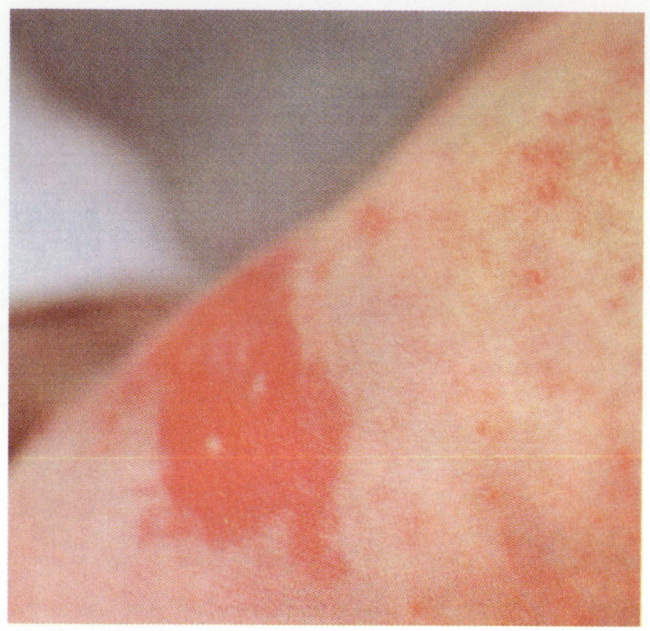

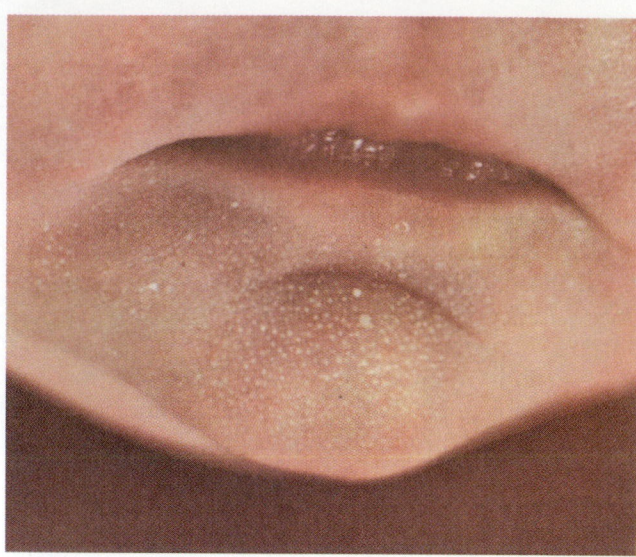

FIGURE 30–13. Milia. The spots usually disappear spontaneously within a few weeks. *(Reproduced, with permission, of Mead Johnson & Company, Evansville, Indiana.)*

FIGURE 30–12. A newborn with erythema toxicum. This condition is noted during the newborn's first 24 hours and may remain for about a week, most commonly on the trunk and diaper area. *(Reproduced, with permission, of Mead Johnson & Company, Evansville, Indiana.)*

and reported, although it is of unknown pathologic origin (Charlton & Phibbs, 1996).

Other normal variations include **petechiae,** which are tiny hemorrhagic spots found over the presenting part; **erythema toxicum** (Fig. 30–12), a transient newborn rash characterized by white vesicles with a red macular base; and capillary hemangiomas **(telangiectatic nevi),** commonly called **"stork bites,"** which are often on the nape of the neck, bridge of the nose, forehead, and eyelids. Stork bites on the face commonly disappear by several months of age; those on the neck remain longer. **Milia** are small (1-mm diameter) white papules caused by plugged sebaceous glands on the nose, face, forehead, and upper torso (Fig. 30–13).

Ecchymoses may result from birth trauma, use of forceps, or both. **Mongolian spotting,** large irregular darkly pigmented areas on the posterior lumbar region, is common among African-American, Asian, or American Indian neonates (Fig. 30–14). It may also be found among white neonates who have a dark complexion. The spotting may not disappear for 2 years.

At birth, the skin is covered by vernix caseosa. Lanugo may also be present in varying degrees, but is most prevalent on the back, shoulders, pinnae, and forehead.

Physiologic jaundice, a yellow discoloration of the skin that is caused by bilirubin metabolism, may

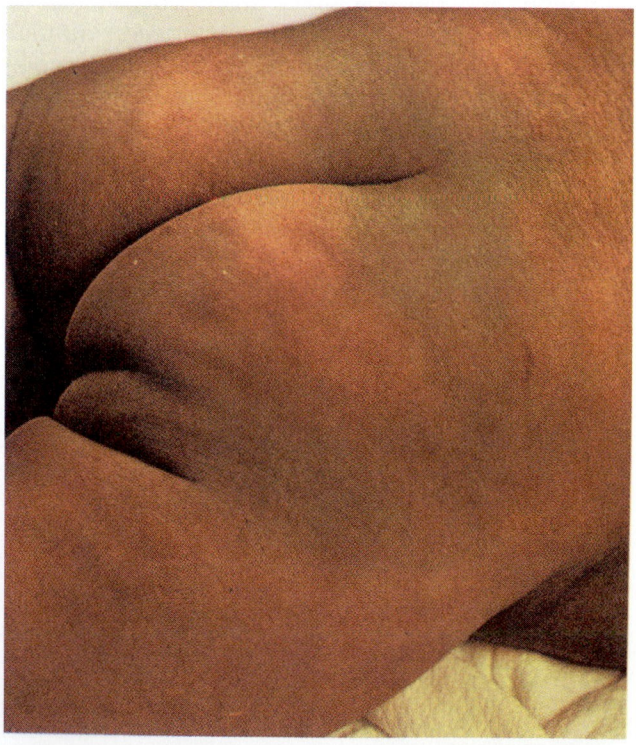

FIGURE 30–14. Mongolian spotting. *(Reproduced, with permission, of Mead Johnson & Company, Evansville, Indiana.)*

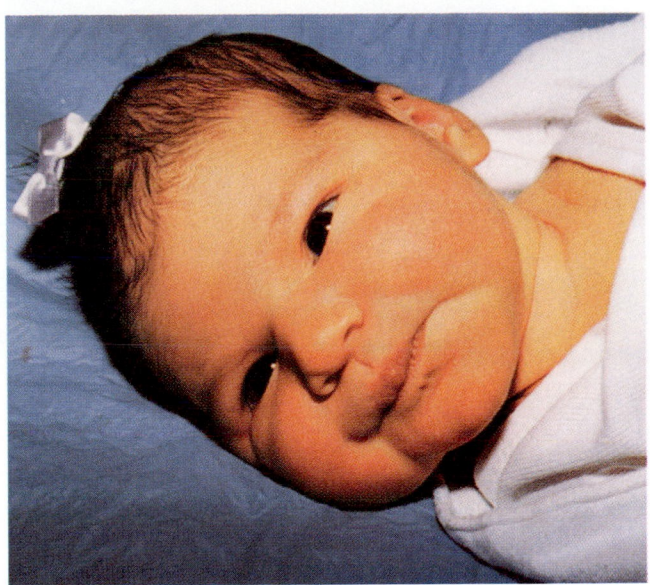

FIGURE 30–15. Physiologic jaundice in a newborn.

appear after the first 24 hours of life (Fig. 30–15). It can easily be identified by using a finger to press on the infant's skin (e.g., over the bridge of the nose) and observing whether a yellow color is present in the area that was pressed. Jaundice that occurs before 24 hours of age is considered pathologic.

The skin is also inspected for birthmarks, and their location, color, size, characteristics, and distribution are noted. Hemangiomas, or vascular tumors, include **nevus flammeus,** or **port-wine stain;** nevus vascularis, or strawberry marks (Fig. 30–16); and cav-

ernous hemangiomas. Nevus vascularis and cavernous hemangiomas usually begin to disappear several weeks after birth, but may not completely fade until the child is 7 years old. Nevus flammeus does not disappear with time.

The skin is palpated for texture and tone. A neonate's skin is very sensitive. It commonly desquamates during the first or second week of life. Skin turgor is checked by gently pinching the neonate's skin and noting the return to normal.

Head

The shape and symmetry of the neonate's head are greatly affected by the forces of delivery, a process known as molding (Fig. 30–17). Head circumference is noted. The nurse should palpate the head, feeling for the fontanelles and suture lines. In a vaginal delivery, the suture lines may be overriding, a condition caused by the shifting of the bony plates of the skull. This will usually correct itself after birth.

The condition of the suture lines should be noted. They should be palpable. Widely spaced suture lines may indicate hydrocephalus, an excessive accumulation of cerebrospinal fluid in the ventricles of the brain. Closed sutures indicate synostosis, a premature closing of the skull that can prevent normal brain growth and development.

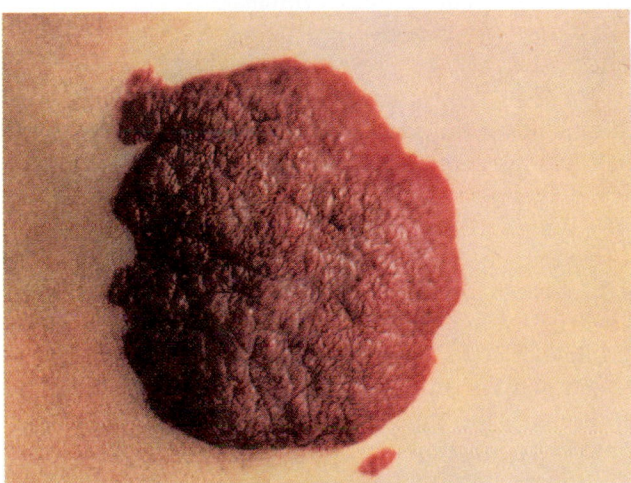

FIGURE 30–16. Strawberry mark (nevus vascularis). The typical lesion is raised, sharply demarcated, and resembles a ripe strawberry. (Reproduced, with permission, of Mead Johnson & Company, Evansville, Indiana.)

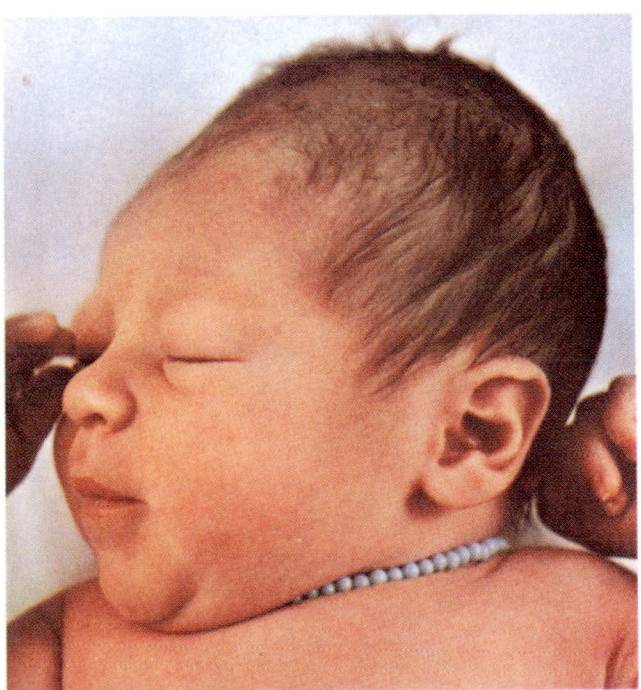

FIGURE 30–17. Molding. The asymmetry that results from compression during delivery usually disappears by the end of the first week. (Reproduced, with permission, of Mead Johnson & Company, Evansville, Indiana.)

The fontanelles are palpated and measured. The anterior fontanelle is located at the junction of the sagittal and coronal sutures and is diamond-shaped. The fontanelle usually feels soft and pulsations may be noted. The posterior fontanelle, a triangular depression, is located at the junction of the lambdoidal and sagittal sutures, and is usually palpable (Fig. 30–18).

Fontanelles will vary in size. On average, the anterior fontanelle is 3 to 4 cm long by 2 to 3 cm wide and should be soft and flat. The posterior fontanelle is between 0.5 and 1.0 cm long; it may be just palpably open or open only fingertip size.

Hypothyroidism may be suspected in neonates whose anterior fontanelles are very large. A tense or bulging fontanelle may indicate increased intracranial pressure. A fontanelle that is severely depressed indicates dehydration.

The scalp is also palpated for **caput succedaneum,** a soft tissue edema that occurs from the pressure of delivery. It crosses the suture lines, which distinguishes it from **cephalhematoma,** a subperiosteal hemorrhage that is limited to one side of the scalp (Fig. 30–19). This condition may take several weeks to recede. Occasionally a neonate may have bilateral cephalhematomas, or cephalhematoma and caput succedaneum.

The scalp is also inspected for abrasions or lacerations that may occur as a result of forceps use; blistering or a circular hematoma at the site of a vacuum extractor; or puncture wounds related to fetal monitor electrodes or fetal blood gas sampling.

The texture and distribution of hair are noted. The amount and color will vary and are dependent on

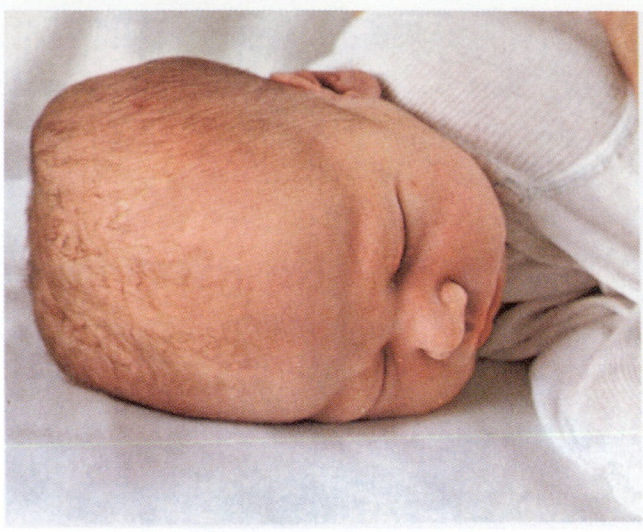

FIGURE 30–19. Cephalhematoma. *(Reproduced, with permission, of Mead Johnson & Company, Evansville, Indiana.)*

genetic factors. The neonate's hair is usually silky and smooth. Unusual distribution or texture should be noted.

Face

The overall appearance of the neonate's face is noted. It should be symmetric, with features well positioned and proportionate. Eyebrows, eyelashes, and hairline should be present. The chin appears to recede. Facial movements should be equal bilaterally. The neonate may have a small degree of asymmetry as a result of intrauterine positioning. Facial palsy, resulting from use of forceps or intrauterine positioning, is evident when the neonate cries or grimaces.

Eyes

The neonate's eyes are observed for symmetry and placement on the face. The examiner needs to check that eyes are present by gently parting the newborn's closed lids. Babies can be born without one or both eyes. With eyelids present, they may simply appear to have their eyes closed. They are normally dark blue, or in dark-skinned neonates, brown. Eyelids should move easily and have eyelashes on both the upper and lower lids. The blink reflex should be evident when a light is directed to the eyes. Tears may not be observed, as the tear ducts and lacrimal glands are not completely functional for at least 1 month after birth.

Silver nitrate, if applied prophylactically, may cause some transient lid edema. Neonates who have had silver nitrate administered may also experience some eye discharge or chemical conjunctivitis. To avert this, many hospitals now use an erythromycin

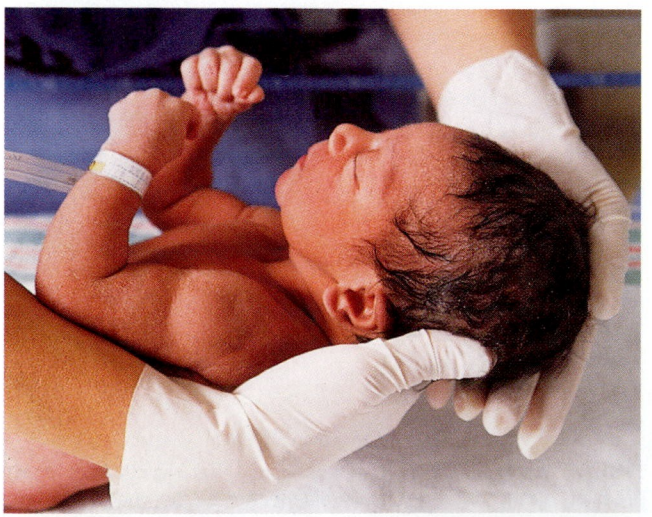

FIGURE 30–18. Nurse palpates a newborn's posterior fontanelle.

ointment or drops. Dacryocystitis, blocked tear ducts, can also cause eye discharge.

The conjunctiva should be pale pink. The size and shape of the pupils are noted. The pupillary reflex is elicited by shining a bright light into the eyes; whether the pupils constrict equally is observed.

The sclerae usually have a slight bluish tint; a definite blue is abnormal and may indicate osteogenesis imperfecta. A yellowish hue is indicative of jaundice. Occasionally, the nurse may note subconjunctival hemorrhages on the sclerae caused by the birth process. They usually disappear within a few weeks.

Movement of the eyeballs is also noted. The neonate can focus momentarily and may follow to midline, but eye movements are characterized as random and uneven. The examiner may note some transient strabismus or nystagmus due to immature neuromuscular control. This may last up to 4 months. When the neonate's head is rotated from side to side, the eyes do not follow the movement but instead move in the opposite direction (doll's-eye phenomenon). The movement usually persists about 10 days after birth. The "setting sun" sign may also be observed. Although the sign, in which a downward gaze allows visualization of the sclera above the pupil, may be seen briefly in some normal newborns, it often indicates hydrocephalus.

The neonate's corneas are observed for opacity. The light from an ophthalmoscope falling on the retina will elicit the red reflex. This procedure is performed most easily if the neonate is held upright or semi-upright, as the eyes will open spontaneously.

Brushfield's spots, black and white specks around the periphery of the irises, may be seen in normal neonates, but more often in a newborn with Down syndrome. Coloboma, the absence of part of an iris, may also be noted.

Neonates of Asian descent normally have epicanthal folds, which are vertical folds of skin covering the inner canthus of the eye. In infants who are not Asian, these folds may indicate a chromosomal disorder.

Ears

The neonate's ears are examined, noting their size, shape, and position on the head. The top of the ear should be in alignment with the inner and outer canthi of the eyes (Fig. 30–20). The ears may appear crumpled and flattened against the side of the head, but should be well formed with firm cartilage. Occasionally, preauricular skin tags are present, either unilaterally or bilaterally.

Low-set ears may indicate a variety of syndromes and chromosomal aberrations. Malformations of the ear may also be associated with renal problems.

The ear canal should be inspected for patency. Vernix caseosa may be present in the canals for several days after birth, making visualization of the tympanic membranes difficult. To facilitate visualization of the inner ear, the neonate should be prone. The examiner stabilizes the neonate's head and pulls the pinna down and back. The otoscope is then inserted using the other hand. The tympanic membrane is observed for color, translucency, and landmarks. The neonate's head is then turned to inspect the other ear.

Nose

The neonate's nose is examined for size, shape, patency of the nostrils, mucous membrane integrity, and discharge. The nose should be on the midline of the face. Neonates are nose breathers; sneezing clears partially obstructed nares. The mucous membranes are pink and moist and may have a small amount of mucus but no heavy drainage. Flaring of the nostrils

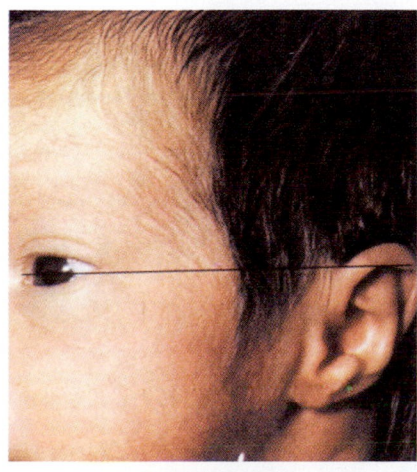
Normal position

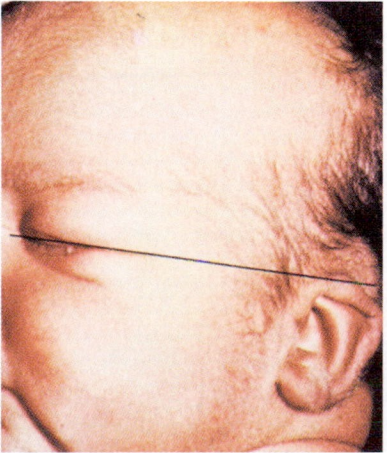
Twisted or pseudo low-set

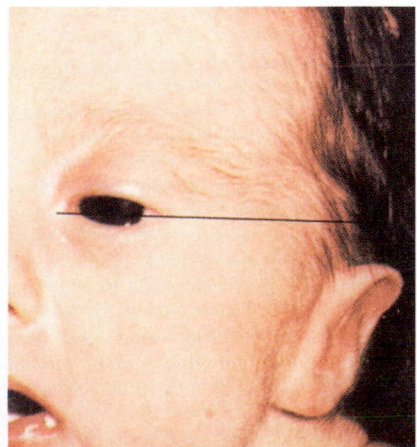
True low-set

FIGURE 30–20. External ear positions. *(Reproduced, with permission, of Mead Johnson & Company, Evansville, Indiana.)*

indicates obstruction of the nares as well as respiratory distress. A malformed or misshapened nose may occur in certain chromosomal abnormalities. The inability to pass a small catheter through each nostril may indicate choanal atresia.

Mouth and Throat

The mouth is inspected and palpated. Symmetry of the lips and lip movement and the internal structures of the mouth is noted. The lips are pink and moist. Most neonates develop a tubercle in the middle of the upper lip from sucking.

The buccal mucosa and gingiva should be pink and moist. Some neonates are born with precocious teeth. They are usually pulled if they are loose, as they are hazardous to the neonate. Both the hard and soft palates are inspected for the presence of cleft palate. The shape of the palate is noted. The uvula should be midline.

The size and placement of the tongue are noted. The tongue should move freely; its shape and movement should be symmetric. The characteristics of the frenulum should be checked. Occasionally, a neonate may have a shortened fibrous frenulum (tongue tie), but if the tongue can extend to the alveolar ridge, intervention is not indicated.

Epstein's pearls, small white epithelial cysts on the hard palate and gums, may be present (Fig. 30–21). Sucking pads may be palpated inside the cheeks. To elicit the sucking reflex, the examiner places a gloved finger inside the neonate's mouth.

The posterior pharynx should be visualized. It is easiest to see when the neonate is crying. Saliva is usually scant, because the salivary glands are immature. The presence of excessive saliva in a neonate should alert the nurse to the possibility of tracheoesophageal fistula or atresia.

Neck

The neck of the neonate is short and straight with many skin folds. To inspect the neck, the examiner holds the neonate's shoulders and head in one hand and gently extends the neck. The neck should be held in the midline and moved symmetrically from side to side.

The position of the trachea is palpated. The thyroid is usually not palpable in the neonate. The nurse also feels for masses. Palpable cervical lymph nodes are usually small, less than 5 mm in diameter. Muscle strength can be assessed by palpation.

Chest

Assessment of the neonate's chest requires inspection, palpation, and auscultation. Percussion is of limited value because the chest is small. The chest is observed for symmetry, size, shape, and respiratory movements. It is cylindrical, with the circumference equal to or less than the head circumference. The xyphoid process is frequently seen under the skin because of the thinness of the chest wall. The ribs may also be noted on deep inspiration.

The breasts in both male and female neonates may be engorged because of the influence of maternal hormones. This condition usually regresses by the end of the second week of life. Occasionally, a whitish secretion is noted from the nipples. This discharge, known as "witch's milk," is also the result of maternal hormones. The nipples should be symmetric on the

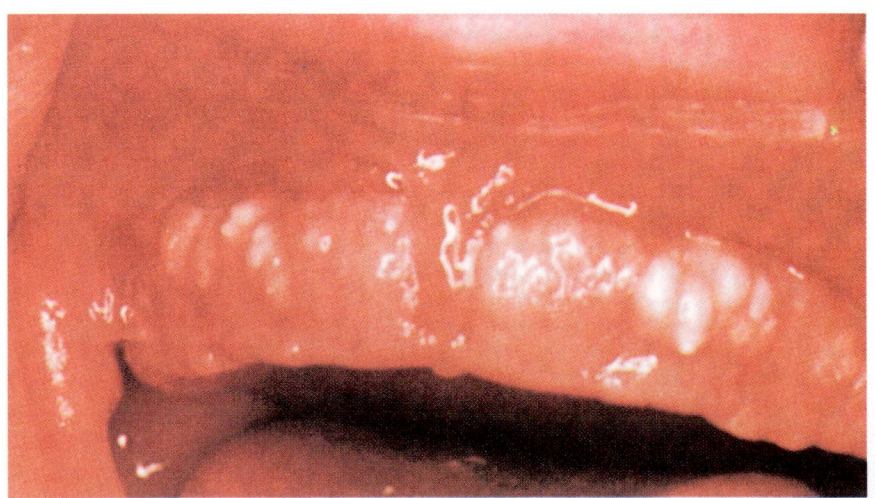

FIGURE 30–21. Epstein's pearls. These cysts usually disappear spontaneously within a few weeks. (*Reproduced, with permission, of Mead Johnson & Company, Evansville, Indiana.*)

chest. Some neonates may also have supernumerary nipples, located below the true nipples along the nipple line. These do not contain breast tissue.

The examiner should palpate the clavicles for any fractures. They can occur during delivery and impair the neonate's arm motion.

Both axilla should be palpated for nodes. Small nodes may be present in a small percentage of well neonates; however, nodes are normally not felt. Neonates with perinatal human immunodeficiency virus (HIV) exposure and infection may exhibit some degree of axillary lymphadenopathy.

The character of the respiratory cycle is noted. In the neonate, respiratory movements are abdominal in nature. The rate and rhythm of respirations as well as the quality are noted. The movement of the chest should be equal throughout the cycle.

Breath sounds are auscultated in both the anterior and the posterior lung fields. The neonate's breath sounds are normally bronchial in nature, because the chest cavity is short and the chest wall is thin. Occasionally, transmitted upper airway sounds are heard, but these generally clear with crying.

The nurse also notes signs of respiratory compromise: unequal chest expansion, decreased breath sounds, rales or any adventitious sounds, grunting, retractions, and nasal flaring. Intercostal retractions may frequently be seen during crying; however, the presence of subcostal or supraclavicular retractions indicates a severely compromised neonate.

Heart

The neonate's circulatory system is dependent on the normal structure and function of the heart and major blood vessels. Initial inspection of the neonate includes the color of the skin, mucous membranes, lips, and nailbeds, which should be pink. Apical pulsation, or the point of maximal impulse (PMI), may be visible, usually lateral to the midclavicular line in the third or fourth interspace.

The PMI should be palpated and noted. The neonate's other pulses (femoral, dorsalis pedis, and brachial) should also be palpated. Because the pedal pulses may not always be palpable, their absence is not necessarily abnormal. Absence of the femoral pulses is abnormal and indicates decreased aortic blood flow caused by coarctation of the aorta. It is best to palpate with the index fingers and simultaneously feel the bilateral pulses to assess their equality and fullness.

Auscultation of the heart involves the use of both the bell and the diaphragm of the stethoscope (Fig. 30–22). Careful listening is needed to distinguish between breath sounds and heart sounds. The heart should be auscultated at all four areas—aortic, pul-

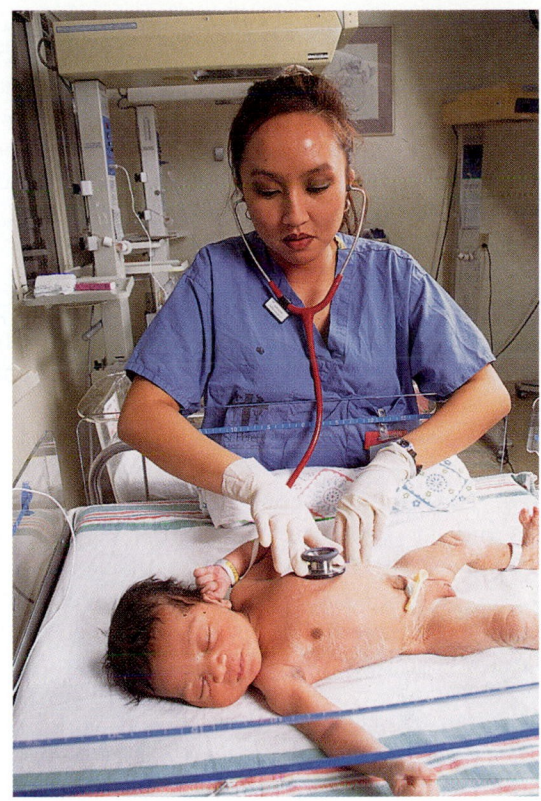

FIGURE 30–22. Auscultation of the heart.

monic, tricuspid, and mitral—and below the left axilla and posteriorly below the left scapula. Both S_1 and S_2 heart sounds should be clearly heard. S_1 is the first heart sound, and is caused by closure of the mitral and tricuspid valves. It is loudest at the apex. S_2, the second heart sound, is best heard at the upper sternal border. It is caused by closure of the aortic and pulmonic valves. S_2 splitting, a normal finding, may be difficult to distinguish due to the neonate's rapid heart rate.

It is important to note on which side of the chest the heart sounds are heard. If the neonate's heart is abnormally positioned on the right side of the chest (dextrocardia), the sounds will be heard on that side.

Nursing Alert

Signs of a congenital heart defect include heart sounds greatest over the right upper chest, cyanosis, murmur, and tachypnea and diaphoresis with feeding.

Heart murmurs are reported; some may be functional, resulting from the changing hemodynamics of birth. Other murmurs may be caused by congenital defects. The location, quality, timing, and loudness of murmurs should be noted. In addition, their appearance or disappearance over time is important in identifying their significance.

Abdomen

The neonate's abdomen appears cylindrical and protrudes slightly. Shape, contour, respiratory pattern, and defects should be noted. Superficial abdominal veins are normal.

The presence of the umbilical cord is noted, and in the early neonatal period, the vessels should be counted. The umbilical cord normally contains two arteries and one vein. The cord begins to dry several hours after birth, and shrivels and blackens by the second or third day of life. The umbilicus should be inspected frequently for signs of infection (foul odor, redness, and/or purulent drainage), granuloma (small, red, raw polyp where the umbilical cord separates), bleeding, and discharge. The cord normally falls off by 2 weeks after birth. By the time the neonate is 1 month old, the umbilicus should be healed.

Umbilical hernias are a common problem and are easily visualized when the neonate is crying. The size and characteristics of hernias should be noted and reported. They are caused by a persistent separation of the rectus muscles (diastasis recti), and may resolve without treatment by the age of 1 year (Taeusch, 1991).

The abdomen should be observed for signs of distension or gross bulging, which may be due to obstruction, infection, or a solid mass. Visible peristaltic waves and upper left quadrant distension suggest pyloric or duodenal obstruction, especially if accompanied by vomiting. Serial abdominal circumference measurements are used to document the progress of abdominal distension.

Auscultation of the abdomen should be performed before palpation and percussion. The nurse listens for peristaltic sounds in all four quadrants. The sounds are usually heard within 1 to 2 hours after birth, and may be irregular.

The abdomen is percussed over the stomach, liver, and spleen. Liver and spleen percussion produces a dull sound; stomach percussion results in a tympanic sound.

Light and deep techniques are used to palpate the abdomen. The neonate's knees are flexed to relax the abdominal muscles. The liver of the average neonate spans 5.6 to 5.9 cm, and can be felt 1 to 2 cm below the right costal margin (Charlton & Phibbs, 1996). Normally, the liver edge feels soft. The spleen tip can be felt just under the left costal margin.

The kidneys are best palpated within the first 6 hours after birth before the abdomen becomes distended with air and feedings. The kidneys can be felt adjacent to the vertebral column, approximately 1 to 2 cm above the umbilicus. Normally, the lower half of the right kidney and the lower tip of the left kidney are felt. The examiner should place one finger under the neonate's flank and press upward. The other hand then presses downward. The kidney should be felt as a firm oval structure.

The passage of meconium is noted. The neonate's bowels can occasionally be palpated. The cecum, in the lower right quadrant, and the sigmoid, in the lower left quadrant, are easiest to feel.

The bladder may be percussed just above the symphysis pubis. The presence of urine will produce a tympanic sound. The time of the first voiding should be noted.

The examiner lightly strokes each of the four quadrants around the umbilicus to assess superficial abdominal reflexes. Using the index finger, diagonal strokes are made in the form of a diamond. The abdominal muscles and umbilicus should move in the direction of the quadrant that is assessed.

Masses in the lower abdominal area should be noted. Inguinal hernias are common in neonates, more prevalent among males. Palpable inguinal nodes are a common benign finding in the neonatal period.

Genitalia

Assessment of the genitalia involves both inspection and palpation. The color, size, shape, and position of the various structures of both the male and female organs are noted.

The female neonate usually has an edematous clitoris and labia majora. The clitoris appears large and may be sensitive to touch. Often, increased pigmentation of the external structures, resulting from hormonal influences, is evident. The labia majora are drawn slightly apart to inspect the labia minora. The vaginal opening is observed. Variations in the appearance of the hymen are common and normal. Vaginal or hymenal tags (short appendages) may be observed. They often disappear within a few weeks of birth. The nurse may also note a whitish mucoid or blood-tinged vaginal discharge resulting from the withdrawal of maternal hormones. The bloody discharge is known as pseudomenstruation. A white cheeselike substance called smegma may be found under the labia. The internal structures of the female genitalia are not routinely assessed.

In the male neonate, the nurse examines both the penis and the scrotum. The penis, about 3–4 cm long, should be intact with no additional orifices on the ventral surface (hypospadias) or dorsal surface (epispadias). Penile length less than 2.5 cm is not considered normal; endocrine evaluation is indicated (Charlton & Phibbs, 1996). The foreskin of an uncircumcised neonate may not be retractable and should not be forcibly retracted. Circumcision removes the foreskin and exposes the glans penis. The meatal opening should be seen as a slit centrally located on the tip of the glans. The nurse should note the adequacy of the urinary stream. The penis may become erect when stimulated or just before urination.

The color of the scrotum may vary from pink in light-skinned neonates to dark brown in darker-complexioned neonates. Rugae, or wrinkle formations, are noted on the surface of the scrotum in full-term neonates. The testicles should be compared. In many neonates, they are not fully descended and can be felt just at the junction of the external inguinal ring. The thumb and forefinger are used to assess testicular size. Using the first two fingers of the other hand, gentle pressure can be exerted on the inguinal canal in a downward position to keep the testicles from retracting. **Hydroceles,** caused by an accumulation of fluid around the testes, are a common finding. They can easily be transilluminated with a light and usually decrease in size. The examiner should assess for an inguinal hernia when a hydrocele is persistent.

The cremasteric reflex can be elicited by stroking the inner thigh; bilateral retraction of the testes will occur.

Occasionally, abnormalities in genital development are evident at birth. Organs may appear hypertrophied, underdeveloped, or ambiguous. If the true gender of the neonate is questionable, gender is not assigned. A diagnosis is made through buccal smear for karyotype and blood tests for ketosteroids. The testing is usually done within the first 3 days of life.

Another common finding among neonates is rust-colored stains on the diaper. As discussed earlier, they are caused by uric acid crystals in the urine and may resemble blood spots.

Anus and Rectum

The position of the anus in relation to the genitalia is noted. The passage of meconium from the rectum should be recorded, as it assures the patency of the anus. Meconium found in other genital orifices is abnormal and should be recorded. The anus should have good sphincter tone as noted by observation. The wink reflex, or contraction of the anal sphincter, can be elicited by gently stroking the perianal area.

Extremities and Spine

The extremities and spine may be assessed during the neurologic examination, although the two examinations are presented separately here.

The extremities are inspected for symmetry, equality, muscle tone, and range of motion. The neonate is examined for gross abnormalities. Movement of the extremities should be symmetric and subject to full range of motion.

The hands and arms are inspected. Arm lengths should be equal. Nails should be present. Extra digits **(polydactyly)** are sometimes found on the hands or feet. Fingers or toes may be fused **(syndactyly).** The palms are inspected for creases. The simian line, a single palmar crease, is often found in Down syndrome (Fig. 30–23).

Arm movement should be assessed. Occasionally, trauma to the brachial plexus during a difficult delivery will result in brachial palsy. The most common type of palsy involves the fifth and sixth cervical nerve roots **(Erb–Duchenne paralysis).** In this condition, the affected arm is held in a position of tight adduction and internal rotation at the shoulder. Although the grasp reflex on the affected side may be intact, the Moro reflex (described in the following section) cannot be elicited. Restoration of function is dependent on the degree of injury. With treatment, most neonates have complete recovery.

Leg length is assessed by extending both legs at the same time. They should be equal with symmetric skin folds. The legs should be inspected in both the prone and supine positions. A neonate who is delivered in a breech presentation may have extended knees. Hip integrity is assessed by using the Ortolani and Barlow maneuvers. The nurse exerts downward pressure on the hips while the neonate's knees are flexed. The hips are abducted at least 70 degrees and then adducted (Fig. 30–24). The motion should be smooth; no unusual clicks felt. A click, unequal movement, or presence of extra skin folds is a positive response, indicating that the hip is dislocated. The neonate should be referred for further assessment.

The legs are assessed for evidence of clubfoot (talipes equinus) or other anomalies. Both feet are put through range of motion; misaligned feet may result from intrauterine positioning.

The soles of the feet are inspected for creases; premature newborns have none, or a few in the anterior portion of the foot. The fat pads of the feet give the neonate the appearance of being flat-footed.

The neonate's spine is examined for obvious defects. The spine appears straight but can easily be flexed. A prone neonate should be able to lift the head and turn from side to side. The nurse may also palpate the vertebrae for abnormalities. The presence of a pilonidal dimple should be noted. Dimples containing a tuft of hair are often associated with spina bifida occulta.

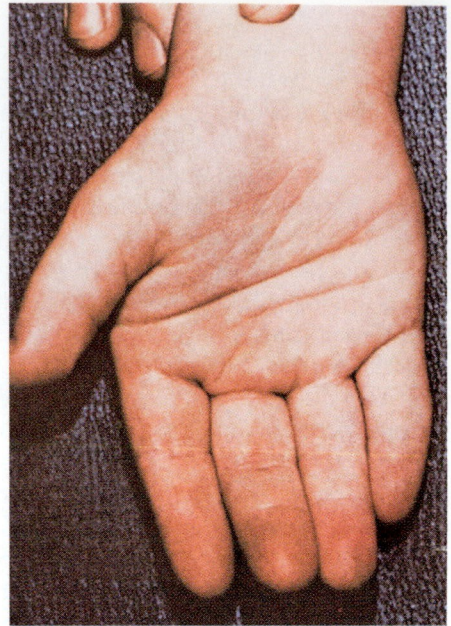 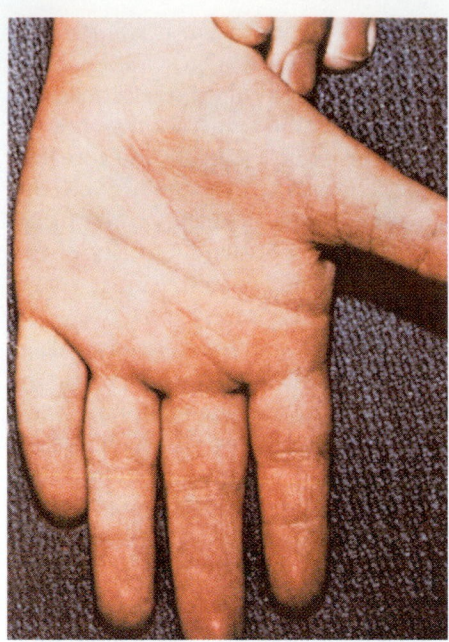

FIGURE 30–23. Palmar creases in Down syndrome. *(Reproduced, with permission, of Mead Johnson & Company, Evansville, Indiana.)*

Neonatal Reflexes

The neurologic system of the neonate is examined by determining the presence of reflexes and assessing neuromuscular movement. Specific reflexes are identified and tested. Throughout the examination, the neonate is observed for movement and symmetry. Many reflexes are present at birth and remain as the neonate matures; others disappear within the first weeks to the first year of life. These reflex behaviors are necessary for the neonate's survival and safety. Their absence may indicate central nervous system

(CNS) damage. Reflexes that persist beyond the time they normally disappear may also indicate CNS problems.

Moro Reflex. The **Moro reflex** is elicited by holding the neonate in a semisitting position and allowing the head and trunk to fall backward a few centimeters. It may also be elicited by striking a flat surface adjacent to where the neonate is lying supine. The neonate abducts and extends the arms symmetrically. The fingers will fan out, with the thumb and forefin-

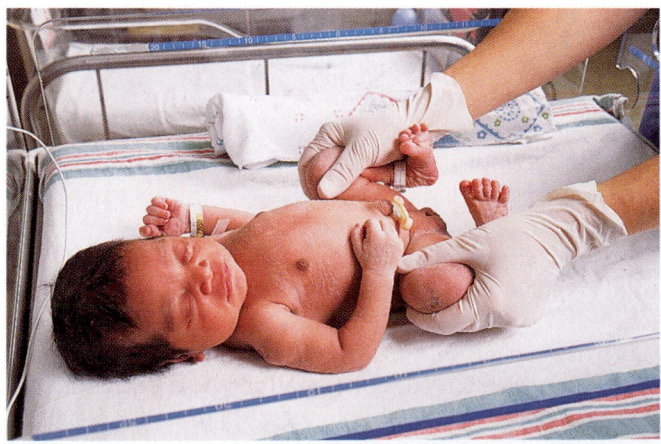 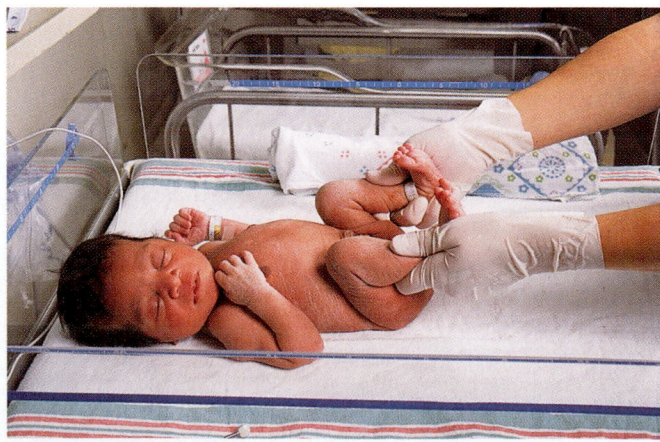

FIGURE 30–24. Hip integrity is assessed in a newborn by observing and feeling the smoothness of movement in the joint.

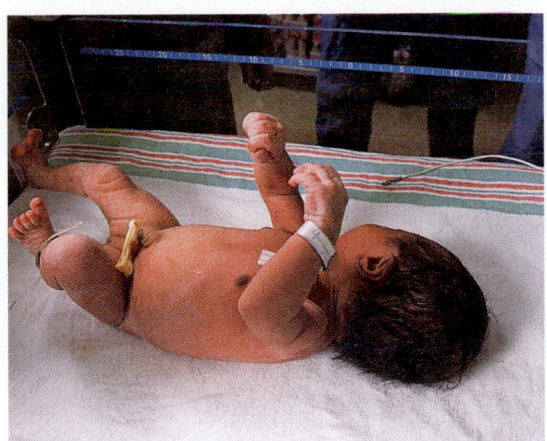

FIGURE 30–25. Newborn exhibiting Moro reflex.

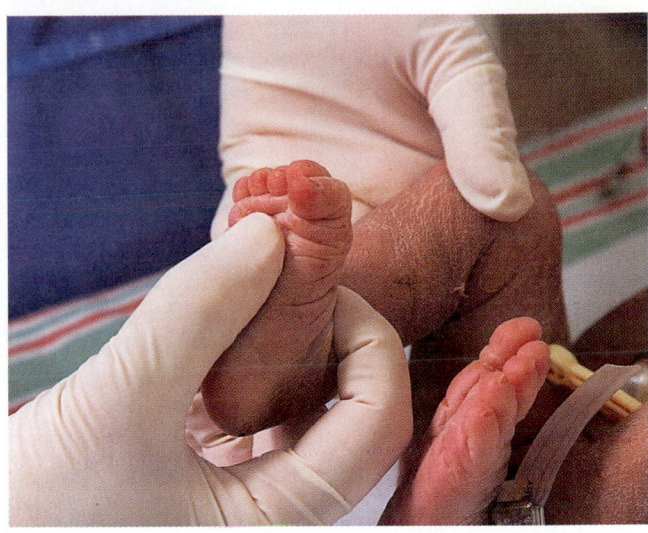

FIGURE 30–27. Newborn exhibiting plantar grasp reflex.

ger forming a "C" (Fig. 30–25). The arms then adduct in an embracing movement and return to their relaxed position. The legs may follow in a similar motion. The Moro reflex should be present at birth and usually disappears by 3 to 4 months of age. Persistence of the reflex beyond 6 months of age warrants further assessment.

Palmar and Plantar Grasp Reflexes. To elicit the **palmar grasp reflex,** the examiner places a finger in the neonate's palm approaching from the ulnar side (Fig. 30–26). The neonate's fingers will curl around the examiner's finger with a firm grasp that enables the neonate to be raised from the supporting surface. This reflex disappears by 2 to 4 months of age.

The **plantar grasp reflex** is elicited by placing the thumb at the base of the neonate's toes. The toes curl downward in response (Fig. 30–27). This reflex diminishes by 8 months of age.

Tonic Neck Reflex. The **tonic neck reflex (or fencing position)** is elicited by quickly turning the neonate's head to one side while she or he is lying on the back. The extremities on that same side extend and those on the opposite side flex, giving the neonate the appearance of a "fencer" (Fig. 30–28). The reflex usually fades by 3 to 4 months, although some children may assume this position during sleep as late as 2 to 3 years. Persistence of this reflex in an alert infant beyond 4 months of age may indicate cerebral palsy.

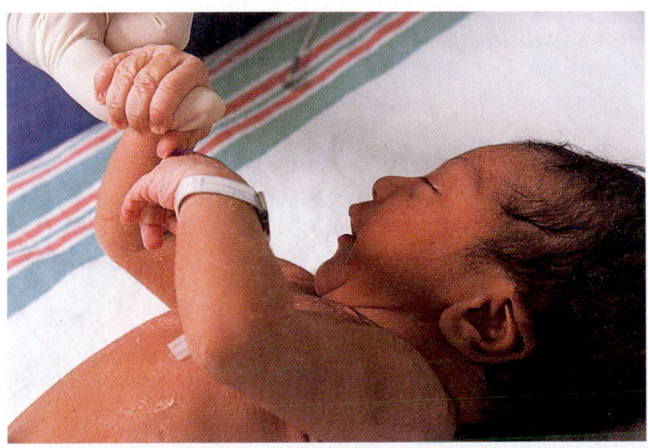

FIGURE 30–26. Newborn exhibiting palmar grasp reflex.

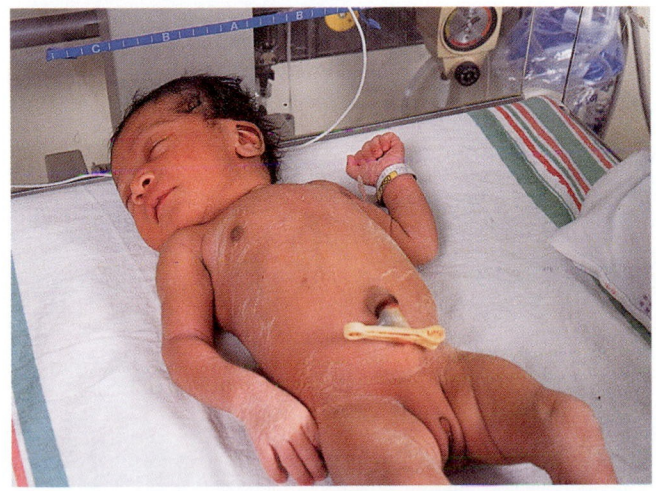

FIGURE 30–28. Newborn exhibiting the tonic neck reflex.

Sucking and Rooting Reflexes. The **sucking reflex** and **rooting reflex** are elicited by touching the neonate's cheek, lip, or corner of the mouth with a nipple or other stimulus. The neonate responds by turning in the direction of the stimulus, opening the mouth, and beginning to suck. These reflexes usually disappear by 7 months of age.

Swallowing Reflex. The **swallowing reflex** can be observed during feeding. Fluid should be ingested easily without gagging, coughing, or vomiting. Swallowing may be poorly developed in a premature newborn or in a newborn with a neurologic defect.

Babinski Reflex. To elicit the **Babinski reflex,** the lateral aspect of the sole is stroked upward across the ball of the foot with an object. The neonate responds by hyperextending the toes and dorsiflexing the great toe (Fig. 30–29). The Babinski reflex disappears after 1 year of age.

Stepping and Placing Reflexes. The **stepping reflex** is elicited by holding the neonate in an upright position and allowing one foot to touch a flat surface (Fig. 30–30). Alternate stepping movements that simulate walking are observed. To elicit the **placing reflex,** the neonate is positioned upright, with the dorsal surface of the feet placed against the edge of the table. The neonate responds by flexing the knees and hips and moving the legs up to the table surface. These reflexes usually disappear by 4 months of age.

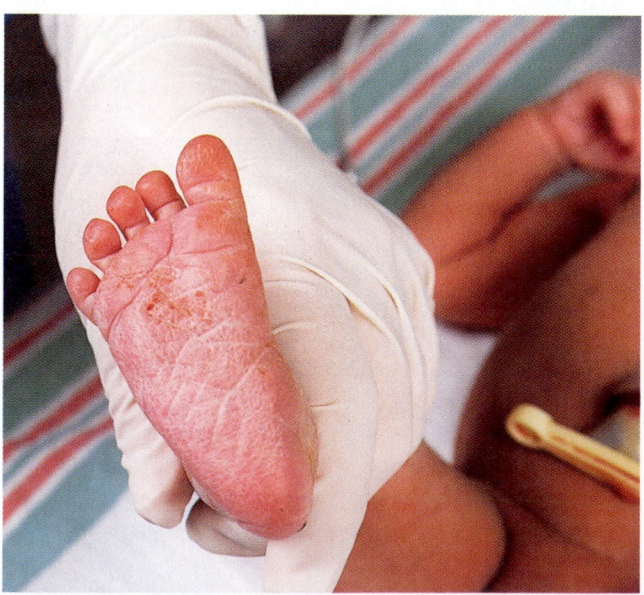

FIGURE 30–29. The Babinski reflex. The newborn's toes hyperextend and the great toe dorsiflexes.

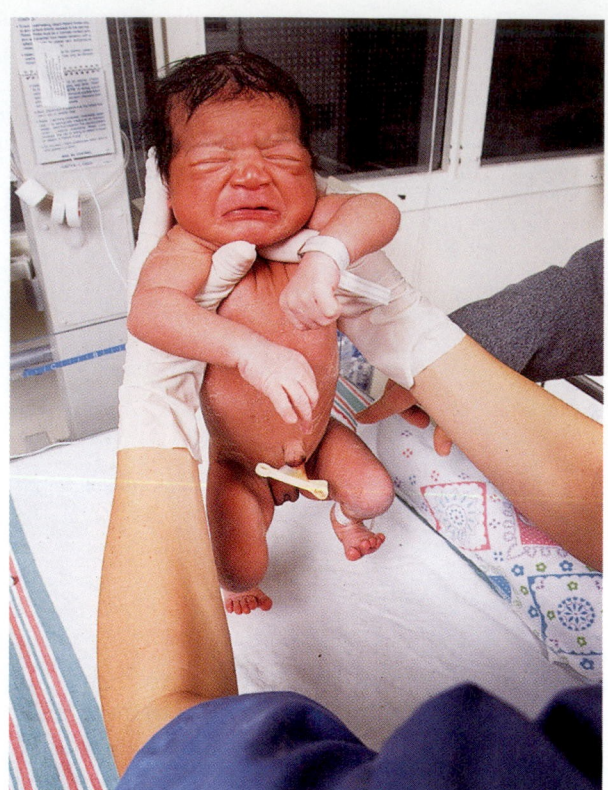

FIGURE 30–30. Newborn exhibits the stepping reflex. Alternate foot movements simulate walking.

Galant's Reflex. **Galant's reflex (trunk incurvation)** is elicited by placing the neonate in a prone position. The newborn's back is firmly stroked about 5 cm (2 inches) from the spine in a downward motion. The neonate responds by curving the body to the side of the stimulus. The opposite side is then checked. This response diminishes by 2 to 3 months of life.

Crossed Extension. With the neonate lying on the back, the examiner extends one leg, pressing the knee down to the surface of the examining table. The foot of the extended leg is stimulated. The opposite leg responds by flexing, adducting, and extending.

Magnet Reflex. The neonate is placed on the back. The examiner partially flexes both legs, applying gentle pressure to the soles of the feet. The neonate responds by extending both legs against the source of pressure.

Traction Reflex. The examiner pulls the neonate up by the wrists from a supine position. Head lag is noted first; the neonate then responds by lifting the head and holding it upright before allowing the head to fall forward on the chest. The amount of head lag noted depends on the maturity and muscle tone of the neonate.

Arm Recoil. Both arms are extended together by pulling them down by the wrists. Brisk flexion of the elbows is noted when the arms are quickly released.

Crawling Reflex. The neonate should make crawling movements when placed in a prone position. This usually disappears by 6 weeks of age.

Glabellar Reflex. With the neonate's eyes open, the examiner taps lightly over the forehead or bridge of the nose. The neonate responds by blinking for the first four or five taps. Continued blinking with repeated taps may indicate an extrapyramidal disorder.

▶ Gestational Age Assessment

Assigning gestational age on the basis of the maternal menstrual cycle and expected date of delivery is inadequate for assessing neonatal outcome. The combination of neonatal size and weight may also confuse the examiner about expected behavioral patterns and physical appearance.

Neonates can be identified according to birth weight as being small-for-gestational-age (SGA), average-for-gestational-age (AGA), or large-for-gestational-age (LGA) (Fig. 30–31). This classification is valid whether the neonate is preterm (before 38 weeks), term (between 38 and 42 weeks), or postterm (after 42 weeks) (Battaglia & Lubchenco, 1967).

Gestational age assessment is based on the work of Dubowitz and coworkers (1970). It is used to determine the appropriate gestational age of the neonate regardless of birth weight. Research focusing on the characteristics and neurologic development of neonates began about 1950. Synthesizing the findings of earlier investigators, Dubowitz and his colleagues developed a reliable method of assessment. Ballard and colleagues modified the original Dubowitz tool in 1979. More recently, the tool has been refined and expanded to assess neonates from 20 to 44 weeks of gestation (Ballard, Khoury, Wedig, Wang, Eilers-Walsman, & Lipp, 1991). The New Ballard Score (NBS) includes criteria for extremely premature infants and allows for a more accurate assessment of more mature infants (Fig. 30–32).

Gestational age of the newborn using the NBS is based on neurologic signs, including posture and primitive reflexes, which vary with gestational age; and both external and superficial characteristics of the newborn, which change with gestational maturity.

This assessment is reliable immediately after birth and within the first 24 hours. According to the authors, it may be used up to 3 to 5 days after birth, but then becomes unreliable because of the maturational changes that occur. For infants less than 26 weeks of gestation, the tool is most valid within the first 12 hours of life. The tool contains 12 parameters of assessment (6 neuromuscular and 6 physical maturity criteria). The method was designed for those who care directly for the neonate. As nurses care for neonates around the clock, the tool is an easy and accurate way for them to assess gestational age and identify potential problems on the basis of their findings.

The neuromuscular criteria are determined by assessing complete body posture; square window flexion of the wrist (Fig. 30–33), arm recoil, popliteal angle, scarf sign of the arm and shoulder (Fig. 30–34), and heel-to-ear placement. The physical maturity criteria are determined by inspecting the neonate for quality of skin texture and appearance, presence of lanugo on the back, plantar surface appearance, breast size, ear and eye development, and genital development. The scores for each category are added. The total score may range between –10 and 50, indicating gestational ages between 20 and 44 weeks.

▶ Behavioral Assessment

Several tools have been used to assess the neonate's behavioral responses and predict maternal–neonate interactions. These include the Neonatal Perception Inventory developed by Broussard and Hartner (1971) and the Brazelton Neonatal Behavioral Assessment Scale devised by Brazelton (1984).

Neonatal Perception Inventory
The Neonatal Perception Inventory (NPI) is used to assess maternal perception of certain neonatal behaviors, and may predict the behavioral interaction between mother and newborn. The inventory consists of two similar instruments administered on the first or second postpartum day and repeated when the neonate is 1 month old. Crying, feeding, spitting up, sleeping, elimination, and predictable patterns of eating and sleeping are addressed. The mother is asked to compare her concept of the "average" newborn with her perceptions of her own newborn at two different points in time. In optimal situations, a mother rates her own baby as better than average. This inventory, along with other observations and history, assists the nurse to identify potential problems in the interaction between mother and neonate.

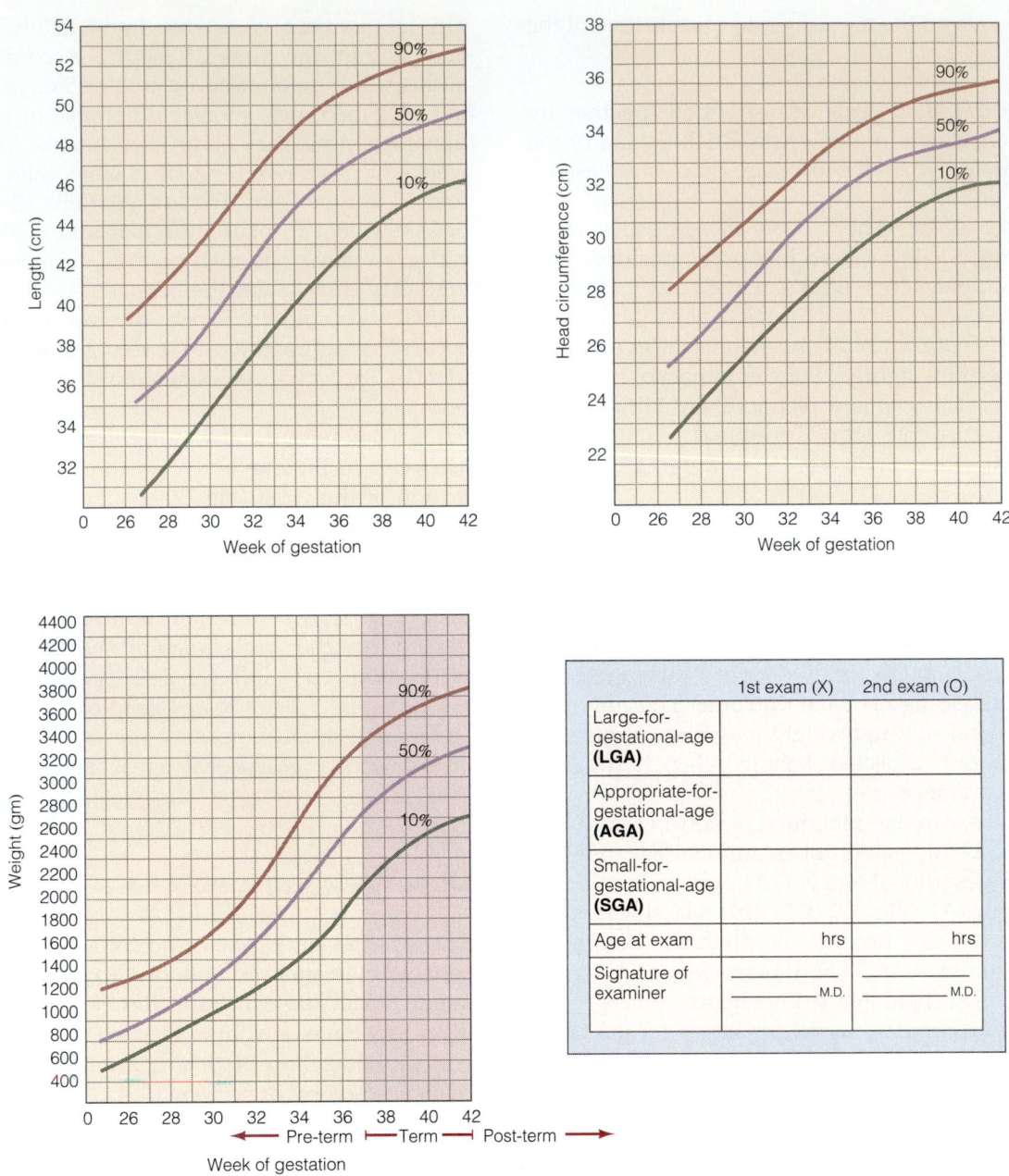

FIGURE 30–31. Gestational age assessment tool. *(Reproduced, with permission, from Battaglia, C., & Lubchenco, L.O. (1967). A practical classification of newborn infants by weight and gestational age.* Journal of Pediatrics *71:159–163.)*

Brazelton Neonatal Behavioral Assessment Scale

The Brazelton Neonatal Behavioral Assessment Scale (BNBAS) assesses newborn behavior and neurologic integrity. Neonates have many behaviors and neurologic responses that allow them to control their responses to the environment. The BNBAS evaluates the neonate's state and response to stimulation by assessing interaction with the environment, motor processes, defensive reactions, and organizational processes. The neonate's consciousness is important when interpreting the reactions to stimuli, as reactions will depend on the neonate's state at the time of testing.

Brazelton's research was based on the descriptions of the neonate's states of consciousness (see earlier section entitled Behavioral State). The neonate

Name _____ **Date/time of birth** _____ **Sex** _____

Hospital no. _____ **Date/time of exam** _____ **Birth weight** _____

Race _____ **Age when examined** _____ **Length** _____

APGAR score: 1 minute _____ 5 minutes _____ 10 minutes _____ **Head circ.** _____

Examiner _____

Neuromuscular maturity

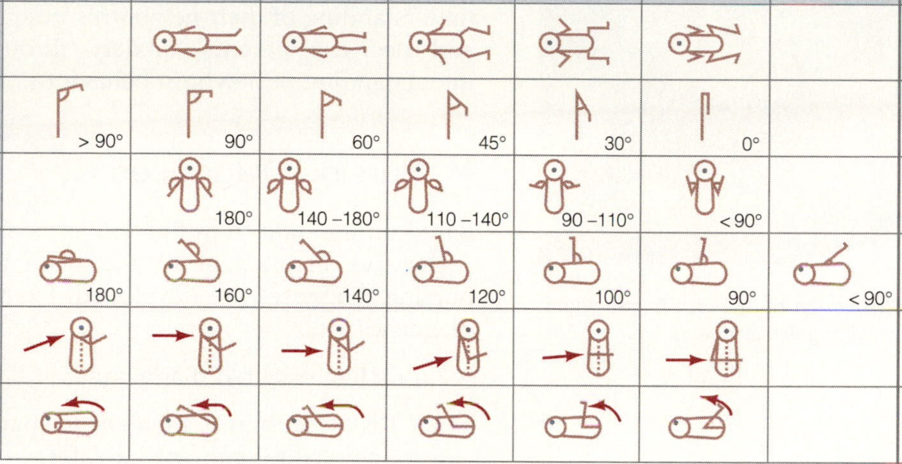

Neuromuscular maturity sign	Score							Record score here
	−1	0	1	2	3	4	5	
Posture								
Square window (wrist)	> 90°	90°	60°	45°	30°	0°		
Arm recoil		180°	140–180°	110–140°	90–110°	< 90°		
Popliteal angle	180°	160°	140°	120°	100°	90°	< 90°	
Scarf sign								
Heel to ear								

Total neuromuscular maturity score

Physical maturity

Physical maturity sign	Score							Record score here
	−1	0	1	2	3	4	5	
Skin	sticky friable transparent	gelatinous red translucent	smooth pink visible veins	superficial peeling and/or rash, few veins	cracking pale areas rare veins	parchment deep cracking no vessels	leathery cracked wrinkled	
Lanugo	none	sparse	abundant	thinning	bald areas	mostly bald		
Plantar surface	heel-toe 40–50 mm: −1 < 40 mm: −2	> 50 mm no crease	faint red marks	anterior transverse crease only	creases anterior two-thirds	creases over entire sole		
Breast	imperceptible	barely perceptible	flat areola no bud	stippled areola 1-2 mm bud	raised areola 3-4 mm bud	full areola 5-10 mm bud		
Eye/ear	lids fused loosely: −1 tightly: −2	lids open pinna flat stays folded	sl. curved pinna; soft; slow recoil	well-curved pinna; soft; but ready recoil	formed and firm, instant recoil	thick cartilage ear stiff		
Genitals (male)	scrotum flat, smooth	scrotum empty faint rugae	testes in upper canal rare rugae	testes descending few rugae	testes down good rugae	testes pendulous deep rugae		
Genitals (female)	clitoris prominent and labia flat	prominent clitoris and small labia minora	prominent clitoris and enlarging minora	majora and minora equally prominent	majora large minora small	majora cover clitoris and minora		

Total physical maturity score

Score

Neuromuscular _____

Physical _____

Total _____

Maturity rating

Score	Weeks
−10	20
−5	22
0	24
5	26
10	28
15	30
20	32
25	34
30	36
35	38
40	40
45	42
50	44

Gestational age (weeks)

By dates _____

By ultrasound _____

By exam _____

FIGURE 30–32. Ballard tool for gestational assessment. (*Reproduced, with permission, from Ballard, J.L. et al. (1991). New Ballard score, expanded to include extremely premature infants*. Journal of Pediatrics. *119:417–423*)

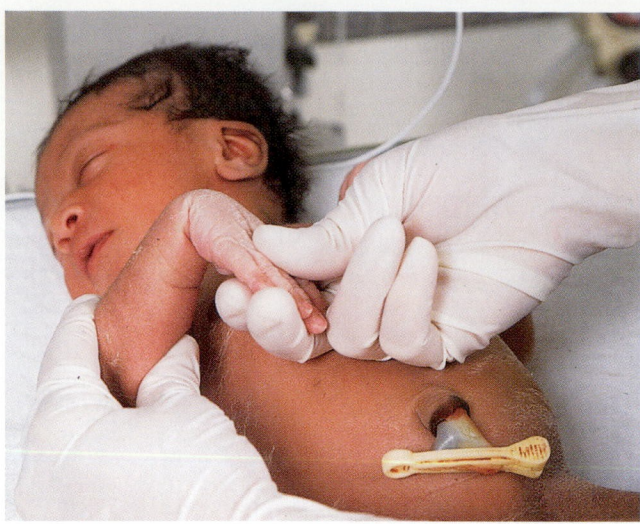

FIGURE 30–33. Square window flexion of the wrist is one neuromuscular criterion used in assessing gestational age.

is assessed on 28 behavioral items that are scored on a 9-point scale. In addition, the examiner elicits 18 neurologic responses that are scored on a 3-point scale. The criteria are tested as the neonate proceeds from one state to the next in a sequential order. The midpoint of most of the scales is considered the norm. As labor, delivery, and medication use influence neonatal reactions, the behavior on the third day of life is considered the expected mean. The neonate is scored on the best, not average, behavior.

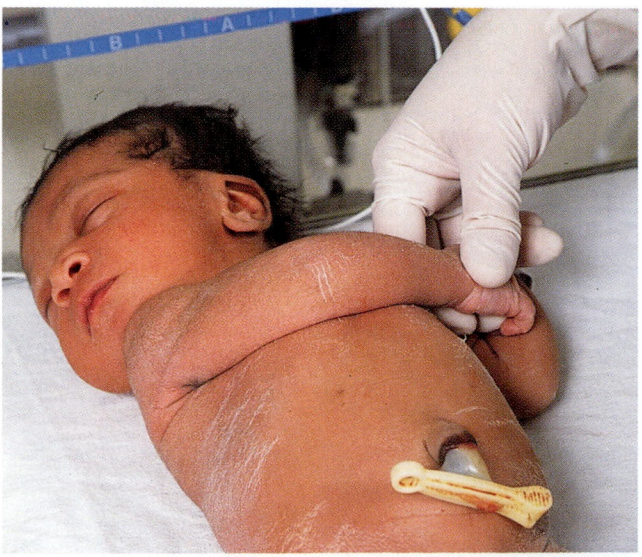

FIGURE 30–34. The scarf sign is an indicator in gestational age assessment.

The assessment is conducted in a quiet, dimly lit environment to avoid distractors. It takes approximately 30 minutes to complete. At present, special training is needed to use the BNBAS with a high degree of reliability and test validity; however, the information obtained has several benefits. It can assist the nurse in developing a more comprehensive care plan for the neonate and family, promote parents' understanding of their newborn's unique capabilities, and decrease parents' anxiety through improved understanding of newborn behavior.

▶ Nursing Diagnoses

Based on the data from the delivery record and comprehensive assessment of the neonate after birth, nursing diagnoses are developed. Examples of these diagnoses are:

Problem-oriented diagnoses:

- Risk for injury, related to parents' lack of knowledge of infant car safety

Wellness-oriented diagnoses:

- Effective breastfeeding, related to good sucking and rooting reflexes
- Effective infant feeding pattern, related to appropriate intake of nutrients and fluid
- Positive parenting, related to maternal–neonate eye-to-eye contact, maternal enfolding, touching behaviors

▶ NURSING AND COLLABORATIVE MANAGEMENT

The immediate neonatal period is usually a time of joy and relief for parents. They may also worry about the well-being of their newborn and their new roles as parents. Nursing care in the immediate neonatal period focuses on helping the newborn to adjust to his or her environment and helping family members to adjust to their new roles. Several goals guide nursing care of the newborn in this period, including maintaining a patent airway, promoting thermoregulation, preventing hemorrhage, preventing infection, promoting initial parent–newborn attachment, identifying the newborn, promoting nutritional well-being, and meeting the educational needs of parents. Through discharge planning, the nurse ensures follow-up care for the newborn and family after they leave the health care facility. Discharge planning is very important because today mothers and their newborns are going home earlier than they did previously.

► Maintaining a Patent Airway

Immediately after delivery, the newborn may need suctioning to remove fluid from the mouth and nares. Suctioning should be done gently with a bulb syringe or other neonatal suction, removing fluid first from the newborn's mouth and then from the nares. If the nares are suctioned first, the newborn may be stimulated to develop an inspiratory gasp, which may cause aspiration of fluid into the lungs.

The newborn with good respiratory effort and heart rate needs little suctioning beyond that done after delivery with the bulb syringe. Excessive suctioning may produce trauma, with mucosal swelling and partial occlusion of the airways (Nelson, 1993). Drainage can be facilitated by placing the newborn in a side-lying position. A bulb syringe should be placed by the crib in the event that further suctioning is necessary.

The nature of respiratory efforts is determined by observation and auscultation of breath sounds and heart rate. If the pulse rate is over 100 beats per minute, respiratory movements are observed to be unlabored, and the respiratory rate is at 30–60 breaths per minute or if the newborn is crying, the transition from intrauterine to extrauterine life is assumed to be progressing normally. Close observation of the newborn, however, is still essential during the first days of life.

► Promoting Thermoregulation

As stated earlier, newborns lose heat through radiation, evaporation, conduction, and convection when exposed to cold. Initial nursing care includes maintenance of a neutral thermal environment for the newborn. The goal of temperature control is thermoneutrality.

Drying the Newborn's Body

The decrease in core and skin temperatures is most rapid immediately after birth. A large amount of heat is lost through evaporation from the wet body of the newborn. Newborns who remain wet in a delivery room have a mean decline in rectal temperature of 2.1°C (3.8°F) and a mean decline in skin temperature of 4.6°C (8.3°F) within 30 minutes of birth. In contrast, newborns who are dried and placed under a radiant heater experience a decline in core temperature of only 0.7°C (1.3°F) and a decrease in skin temperature of 0.8°C (1.5°F).

Simply drying and wrapping the newborn in a warm blanket also decreases heat loss considerably. The importance of drying the newborn cannot be overemphasized. A family-centered approach to care includes drying and wrapping newborns and giving them to their mother and father to cuddle.

Incubators

Incubators are one of the most commonly used devices for warming the newborn. In an incubator, the newborn is heated by convection; however, because temperature of the walls of the incubator cannot be controlled, the newborn may lose heat through radiation. In an effort to prevent radiant heat loss in incubators, some incubators are equipped with clear cylindrical plastic heat shields. Radiant losses are diminished by the use of the shield because the warm incubator air heats the shield to the same temperature as the air within the incubator. The newborn radiates heat only to the plastic shield instead of to the cooler walls of the incubator.

Radiant Heaters

Radiant heaters (Fig. 30–35) are warming panels that are placed above the newborn in an effort to prevent heat loss through radiation. These devices provide heat from infrared energy. Under the radiant heater, radiant losses are reduced; however, convective and evaporative losses are markedly increased because of the increased insensible water loss. Special heat

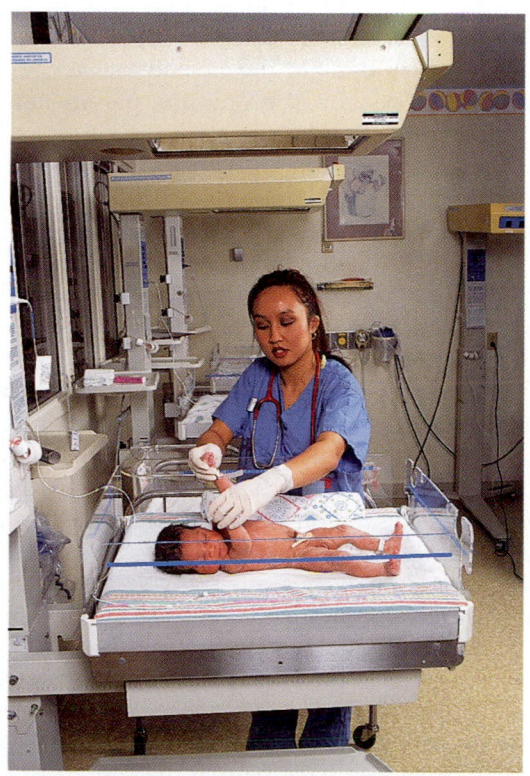

FIGURE 30–35. Nurse assessing newborn who is placed under a radiant warmer.

shields have been used in an effort to prevent this evaporative water loss. Although radiant heaters are generally more convenient in intensive-care situations, well-humidified incubators may provide a more stable thermal environment (Hey & Scopes, 1993).

In traditional hospital settings, radiant heaters are commonly used in the delivery room and for an initial period in the newborn nursery. The thermostat of the radiant heater is controlled by a sensing thermistor taped to the newborn's abdomen or leg; this helps to adjust the temperature of the radiant heater to the temperature of the newborn. An alarm alerts staff to changes in temperature of the neonate's skin or to the sensor's losing contact with the skin.

In general, within 4 hours the newborn's temperature stabilizes and the dressed newborn can be placed in an open crib. Many institutions will place a hat on the newborn's head to prevent heat loss from the head and to help control the thermal environment.

Parent–Newborn Contact

Early parent–newborn contact is a principle of a family-centered approach to care. Research has shown that contact with one or both parents in the delivery room is a method for controlling the newborn's temperature. Hill and Shronk (1983) found that when newborns were properly dried and wrapped and given to one or both of their parents, their temperatures were similar to those of newborns who were immediately placed in a heated transporter. This inexpensive way to regulate the newborn's temperature has the added benefit of promoting parent–newborn attachment in the delivery room.

▶ Preventing Hemorrhage

Newborns have a deficiency of vitamin K-dependent factors, which places them at risk for bleeding. An injection of vitamin K (phytonadione) is therefore indicated for prevention and treatment of hypothrombinemia and treatment of neonatal hemorrhagic disease. Phytonadione's activity is the same as naturally occurring vitamin K, which is required in the synthesis of blood coagulation factors II (prothrombin), VII, IX, and X in the liver.

Phytonadione is most often given once intramuscularly immediately after delivery (0.5 to 1.0 mg). It may be repeated after 6 to 8 hours if necessary. The injection is given in the lateral aspect of the newborn's thigh. The nurse periodically observes the injection site for hematoma, redness, and nodule formation. The infant may also have pain at the site.

Alternatively, 1 to 2 mg may be given orally immediately after delivery and repeated after 12 to 48 hours if necessary.

Nursing Alert

When phytonadione is given intramuscularly or orally to prevent hemorrhage in the newborn, it is relatively nontoxic. However, adverse reactions to phytonadione may include signs of gastric distress or a rash, urticaria, erythema, hemolytic anemia, kernicterus, or allergic reaction.

Phytonadione is administered intravenously to a newborn only in emergency situations, as an anaphylactic-type reaction may occur. The newborn may exhibit cardiac irregularities, chest pain, cyanosis, convulsive movements, dulled consciousness, flushing face, circulatory collapse, bronchospasm, rapid and weak pulse, shock, and death.

Vitamin K antagonizes the anticoagulant activity of warfarin if the two drugs are both administered. Phytonadione is stored in a light-resistant container because light will destroy the vitamin.

▶ Preventing Infection

Scrupulous handwashing by health care workers is probably the single most important factor in preventing infections in the nursery. Some birthing institutions require that health care workers perform a 3 to 5 minute scrub of the hands and arms before entering the nursery at the beginning of the shift. At the least, health care workers should wash their hands with soap and water before caring for each newborn. In addition, health care workers who have infections should not care for newborns.

In the United States many birthing institutions also have specific regulations aimed at preventing infections in the nursery. Health care workers use universal precautions to protect against spread of HIV and other blood-borne or body fluid–borne infections. Newborns have their own equipment and cribs in an effort to prevent infection. Other measures implemented to prevent infection in the newborn include neonatal eye care and cord care.

Eye Care

Prenatal care should routinely include culturing maternal cervical secretions for gonococci and treatment of women who are infected. Even when this is done, the routine use of a prophylactic agent in the newborn's eyes is recommended to prevent infection with *Neisseria gonorrhoeae* (ophthalmia neonatorum, which can cause neonatal blindness).

Prophylactic agents that are currently recommended for instillation into the newborn's eyes to prevent gonococcal ophthalmia include erythromycin, 0.5% ophthalmic ointment or drops in single-dose tubes or ampules; tetracycline, 1% ophthalmic ointment or drops in single-dose tubes or ampules; and 1% silver nitrate solution in single-dose ampules. One of these agents is instilled into the eyes of the newborn within 1 hour after delivery. It is recommended that the agent not be flushed from the eyes after the application (Charlton & Phibbs, 1996).

The nurse instills the medication by pulling down on the lower eyelid and instilling drops or ointment into the lower conjunctival sac. The eyes are then closed so that the medication can permeate the eyes. The medications, especially silver nitrate, can cause mild conjunctivitis, which may interfere with the quiet alert state of the newborn. For this reason, eye prophylaxis is often delayed up to an hour to facilitate initial interactions between parents and their newborns.

Chlamydial ophthalmia, caused by *Chlamydia trachomatis*, is believed to be more prevalent than gonococcal ophthalmia. Because no topical treatment currently is effective in preventing chlamydial ophthalmia, preventive measures are aimed at detecting and treating chlamydial infection in the mother. If the newborn becomes infected, the treatment of choice is erythromycin administered orally, 50 mg/kg per day, in three or four divided doses for 10 to 14 days. Topical therapy of the newborn's eyes has been associated with a 60 to 80% failure rate (Hammerschlag, 1989), as compared to a 10 to 20% failure rate for systemically administered erythromycin.

Cord Care

The cord is clamped in the delivery room and the clamp remains in place at least 24 hours. Some nurseries apply an aseptic solution, such as triple-dye, erythromycin solution, or alcohol, to the cord to prevent infection. Triple-dye causes the cord to turn dark blue. The nurse explains this procedure to parents, and assures them that this is a normal reaction.

The nurse observes the cord for signs of hemorrhage or infection. If bleeding is noted, a second clamp is applied and the physician notified.

▶ Promoting Initial Parent–Newborn Attachment

The nurse can help to promote initial parent–newborn attachment by enabling the parents to hold and touch their newborn in the delivery room. During the first and second periods of reactivity, the nurse can promote attachment behaviors between newborns and parents. Because the newborn demonstrates good sucking reflexes during the first period of reactivity, if the mother wishes to breastfeed she can be encouraged to put the newborn to breast at this time.

▶ Identification of Newborn

Identification of the newborn usually is done using ankle and wrist bracelets for the newborn and a wrist bracelet for the mother. The same information is placed on each bracelet and includes mother's name, sex of newborn, hospital number, and date and time of delivery. The nurse prepares and places the identification bracelets on the mother and newborn before they leave the delivery room. Some states require footprints of the newborn, although that is probably not a reliable method of identification (a perfect print of the great toe would reliably identify the newborn). Problems in identification arise as staff may lack skill in producing adequate footprints.

▶ Promoting Nutritional Well-Being

One of the first acts of parenting is feeding the newborn. Parents, especially mothers, tend to judge their parenting skills by how well the newborn feeds on the breast or bottle and how much weight the newborn is gaining. If problems occur with the feeding experience, parents often become frustrated and their confidence as caretakers may be affected. (See Chapter 31 for a complete discussion of newborn nutrition.)

Initial Feeding

The breastfed newborn may be put to breast immediately after delivery or during the first period of reactivity if the mother so desires. Breastfeeding of newborns soon after birth promotes mother–newborn interaction. During the first period of reactivity, the newborn is awake and alert and tends to latch onto the breast. The mother will have a sense of accomplishment if the newborn nurses even for a short period of time. An additional benefit of early breastfeeding is stimulation of lactation.

Newborns who are bottle fed may also be given sterile water. An initial feeding of a few milliliters of sterile water allows the nurse to assess the newborn's sucking, swallowing, and gag reflexes. Sterile water is used instead of glucose water or formula because if the newborn should aspirate the feeding the sterile water will be absorbed easily by the lungs.

During the initial feeding the nurse assesses the newborn for such symptoms as regurgitation and cyanosis, which may point to complications. These symptoms may indicate the presence of tracheoesophageal fistula (an abnormality in which the esophagus is connected to the trachea by an opening) or esophageal atresia. In this latter condition, the esophagus ends in a blind pouch instead of in the stomach. As the pouch fills with fluid from the feeding, regurgitation of the fluid results. If there is a question as to the patency of the esophagus or to the possibility of tracheoesophageal fistula, assessment of the gastrointestinal tract is performed.

The first formula feeding for the bottle fed newborn may occur after the newborn has ingested sterile water for one to two feedings, usually according to the protocol of the birthing institution. Newborns will usually consume one-half to one ounce during this feeding.

▶ Meeting Educational Needs of Parents

Parents have many educational needs that can be met prior to discharge from the birthing institution. Common parental concerns in the neonatal period focus on handling and positioning the neonate, nasal and oral suctioning, circumcision care, cord care, bathing and skin care, elimination patterns, and clothing and wrapping the neonate. Other aspects of newborn care such as promoting normal growth and development, preventing communicable diseases and accidents, promoting normal sleep patterns, and providing support for working parents are also discussed prior to discharge. These concerns can be priorities of the nurse during discharge planning from the birthing facility.

Handling and Positioning

Parents should be taught various positions in which to hold the neonate, including the cradle hold, the football hold, and the upright position. The parents and the neonate should feel comfortable in whatever position is chosen. It is important to teach parents to support the neonate's head and neck in all the positions.

In the cradle hold, the parent cradles the neonate in the arm against the chest. This position is often used for feeding. The advantages of this hold is that the parent may use the other hand, the neonate feels secure, and the parent can look at the neonate when feeding.

In the football hold, the parent holds the neonate's head in the palm of the hand, and the remainder of the body straddles the forearm. This position allows the parent to hold the neonate while keeping the other hand free to wash the neonate's hair, hold a bannister while walking up steps, hold another child's hand, and so forth.

The neonate may be held upright, using both hands so that the neonate's head rests on the parent's shoulder. This position is often used for burping the neonate.

Parents should also be taught to position a newborn on the back or side. A rolled towel or small baby blanket may be used to support the infant's back in a side-lying position. Newborns should not be placed on their abdomens because of the possible relationship of this position to sudden infant death syndrome (SIDS).

When picking the neonate up from a crib, the parent is taught to place one hand under the neck and shoulders and the other hand under the buttocks. With a slow, smooth motion, the neonate is then lifted from the crib. Another technique is to swaddle the neonate in a blanket before picking up the neonate, with both hands.

The nurse demonstrates different positions for handling and holding the neonate to the parents and the parents should return the demonstration. Parents should feel comfortable in handling and holding the neonate by discharge.

Nasal and Oral Suctioning

Neonates are compensatory nose breathers and at times may sound as if they are nasally congested when in fact they are not. The neonate may sneeze to clear the nasal passage; this does not indicate an upper respiratory infection. At times, however, excess mucus or regurgitated milk may need to be cleared from the oral and nasal passages. The nurse should therefore teach the parents to use a bulb syringe.

Parents are taught to place the neonate in a football hold, leaving one hand free to manipulate the bulb syringe. The bulb of the syringe is compressed and then the tip is placed in the neonate's mouth. The bulb should be compressed before placing in the mouth and not while in the infant's mouth or nose. (Placing the syringe in the mouth first prevents an inspiratory gasp that might occur if the syringe were placed in the nasal passage, instead.) The tip of the syringe is aimed at the side of the mouth and the parents slowly release the compression of the bulb to draw in the secretions; the tip of the syringe is then removed from the mouth and the secretions released into a tissue. This procedure is repeated in the nares. After use, the bulb syringe should be washed with soap and water and stored near the neonate. The bulb syringe should be used only when necessary.

Circumcision Care

Circumcision is the surgical removal of the foreskin, exposing the glans penis. Opinions of health care providers concerning circumcision have varied greatly over the years. In 1975, the American Academy of Pediatrics changed a long-standing position recommending circumcision for male infants. At that time, the Academy stated that routine circumcision was not medically indicated. In 1989, however, the Academy again changed its position, advising that circumcision may have medical benefits as well as risks. Benefits of circumcision, according to the Academy, include possible prevention of such diseases as urinary tract infection and cancer of the penis. Risks, on the other hand, include potential postprocedure bleeding and infection (American Academy of Pediatrics, 1989). Routine circumcision is likely to remain controversial. Some parents may choose to have their male newborns circumcised for religious or cultural reasons.

Neonatal circumcisions are usually performed by physicians, or in the Jewish tradition, by specially trained individuals known as mohels. In some states, certified nurse-midwives perform newborn male circumcisions. Circumcisions are the only male procedures routinely performed by obstetricians.

Circumcision is done in the birthing facility or, in the Jewish culture, in a home or synagogue. In the birthing facility, an informed consent is obtained from the parent or parents. The neonate is restrained on a circumcision board, draped with sterile towels, and the penis is cleansed. A topical or regional anesthetic is also recommended. Sterile technique is used to remove the foreskin.

Equipment for the procedure may include a scalpel and Gomco clamp. The clamp is used to minimize bleeding during and after the procedure. When the Gomco clamp is used, the prepuce is first separated from the glans penis with a sterile probe and stretched over a metal cone. The Gomco clamp is applied and after 4 to 5 minutes the prepuce above the clamp is removed with a scalpel. The Gomco clamp is removed immediately after the procedure.

After the procedure, the nurse observes the neonate for normal voiding and for bleeding at the circumcision site. A dressing of petroleum gauze may be placed loosely around the penis at the time the procedure is completed. Vitamin A and D ointment or white petroleum may be used to prevent friction from the diaper; in one technique, the A and D ointment or white petroleum is placed on the diaper area that will cover the circumcision site. The diaper is then placed loosely around the neonate. The neonate should be given to the mother or parents as soon after the procedure as possible to allay their anxiety and for his comfort. The neonate should be kept off his abdomen for 12 hours after the circumcision to prevent irritation of the wound by friction.

No special care of the circumcision is required at home. The nurse teaches the parents to observe the penis for signs of bleeding and normal healing. A small yellow exudate may be seen on the second day after circumcision. This is part of the healing process and should not be removed by the parents. Tub baths should be avoided until the circumcision is healed. As circumcisions may be done after the neonate has left the birthing institution as part of religious rituals, these parents will also need information related to circumcision care prior to discharge.

Cord Care

Parents should be advised that the cord will dry and fall off in approximately 5 to 10 days. The application of antiseptic solutions such as triple-dye to the cord should also be discussed with parents. Parents are taught signs of infection (that is, redness, swelling, and drainage) that should be reported to the physician. Cord care is also taught to the parents. This may include applying alcohol to the cord, including its base, with each diaper change to help it dry. Parents are taught to diaper the neonate with the diaper folded down away from the cord to prevent rubbing and to expose the cord to the air. Sponge bathing is recommended until the cord falls off. Parents may ask the nurse about the use of bellybands. In some cultures the use of bellybands is thought to prevent umbilical hernias. The nurse should explain to the parents that bellybands do not prevent umbilical hernias and in fact may delay drying of the cord.

Bathing

The newborn is given an initial bath if the vital signs are stable. Current research indicates that healthy full-term newborns with rectal temperatures higher than 36.5°C can be bathed after the initial assessment, and that the traditional delay in bathing is not needed. This procedure decreases chances of staff exposure to potentially infected birth fluids covering the baby (Penny-MacGillivrary, 1996). Sponge baths are given until the cord drops off. The nurse uses mild soap and water and observes the newborn throughout the bathing procedure for signs of physiologic and behavioral adaptations. The purpose of the initial bath is to remove blood and birth fluids. Gloves should be worn by the nurse during the first bath and whenever the nurse may come in contact with urine, feces, and body fluids. Care must be taken to keep the newborn warm during the bath, as well as during any assessments.

A bath demonstration by the nurse teaches the parents techniques of bathing the neonate. The parents can return the demonstration to ensure their comfort with bathing. Both sponge bathing and tub bathing are taught to parents.

Before the bath begins, all necessary equipment is gathered, including towels, washcloths, mild soap, mild shampoo, baby lotion, vitamin A and D ointment or white petroleum jelly, diapers, clothing, and blankets. The water should be a safe temperature, approximately 98°F (37°C), or warm to the touch. If a parent does not have a thermometer at home to test the water, he or she may insert an elbow into the water. The water should feel warm, not hot. The room where the bath will be given should also be warm and free from drafts. The neonate should be washed from head to toe, leaving the diaper area last because it is most soiled. Bathing time should be enjoyable for both neonate and parents and parents can time baths to best meet the needs of their newborn and their family. There is no set time that a bath must be done.

The bath is a time when parents can inspect their newborn. The nurse should point out characteristics and common variations among newborns, such as molding, to reassure parents of the newborn's normalcy.

Sponge Bath.   The part of the neonate being bathed is exposed while the rest of the body is covered. Bathing begins with the eyes, which are washed with a cotton ball or washcloth and clear water. Each eye is wiped from the inner to the outer corner. A new cotton ball or portion of the washcloth is used for each eye to prevent cross-contamination. Any crusted material is wiped from the nose with the washcloth or a tissue. The ears are then washed by twisting the washcloth

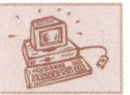

Research Abstract

Effect of Early Admission Bathing on Thermoregulation in Newborns

Blood and blood-stained amniotic fluid present a risk of serious infection to health care workers. Although universal precautions are recommended by the Centers for Disease Control, a perception of minimal risk or anticipated maternal objection have been shown to lessen health care workers' strict compliance with the precautions when caring for newborns. In an effort to decrease health care workers' exposure to blood-borne pathogens early bathing of newborns has been recommended. The current practice in the setting of the investigator was to delay admission bathing until normal body temperature is achieved and maintained. However, the investigator noted that the exact timing of the completion of thermoregulation of the newborn was not completely known and no evidence existed to support delaying admission bathing until body temperature is sustained. The purpose of the study was to determine the effects of early admission bathing on thermoregulation in newborns.

The sample consisted of 100 healthy full-term newborns. Through random assignment 49 newborns were bathed in the experimental group after the admission examination to the nursery was completed, the average age being 61.15 minutes old. Fifty-one newborns in the control group were bathed at 4 hours of age. Vital signs including rectal temperature, apical heart rate and respiratory rate, and air temperature were recorded on admission to the nursery, before and after bathing, one hour and two hours after bathing. The results of the data collected demonstrated that newborns who were bathed after the admission assessment to the nursery showed no significant difference in rectal temperatures compared to those who were bathed at the traditional four hours of age.

Application to Practice

This study adds to our knowledge of newborn thermoregulation and thereby directly affects clinical practice. The findings indicate that healthy full-term newborns can be bathed soon after one hour of life, thus decreasing health care professionals' risk of contact with blood-borne pathogens. The investigator challenged the "traditional practice" with scientific reasoning and added to the ever-growing body of nursing research.

Source: Penny-MacGillivrary, T. (1996). A newborn's first bath: When? Journal of Obstetric, Gynecologic, and Neonatal Nursing, *25, 481–487.*

around the finger and washing around the pinna and in the area behind the ears. Cotton-tipped swabs should not be inserted into the nares or ear canals. They can cause injury to the nasal mucosa and tympanic membrane. The parents should be taught that the eventual development of cerumen (earwax) in the external ear canal is normal. Swabs should not be placed in the ear canal to remove cerumen, as they can cause the cerumen to become packed in the ear canal, resulting in discomfort to the neonate. After washing the ears, the rest of the face is washed with warm water.

While the neonate is still dressed the hair may be cleansed with water or shampooed with a mild shampoo. To shampoo the hair the neonate is placed in a football hold over a basin of water. The scalp is wiped or lathered and rinsed with warm water. Parents sometimes worry that they will injure the "soft spot" when washing the hair. They should be reassured that the head may be washed over the fontanelle without causing any injury. The hair is then towel dried and brushed with a soft brush.

The neonate's shirt is then removed and the folds of the neck, the arms, axillae, chest, back, and abdomen are washed with a mild soap and rinsed with a wet washcloth. The cord is kept dry during the bath. The skin is then thoroughly dried and the upper part of the body wrapped with a blanket to prevent chilling. The neonate's legs and feet are then unwrapped and washed with mild soap and water and dried thoroughly.

The genitalia and buttocks are washed last with mild soap and water. Cleansing of the female genitalia is done from the front to back to avoid contamination of the urethra and vagina with fecal material. The scrotum and the penis in the male are also washed with mild soap and water. Uncircumcised males should not have the foreskin retracted for cleansing. Forcibly retracting the foreskin may cause edema and constriction of blood vessels. The penis of the circumcised male is also washed gently with soap and water and dried. The buttocks and anal area are then washed thoroughly with soap and water. The genitalia, buttocks, and anal area should also be washed after each diaper change to prevent skin irritation.

Lubricants such as unscented lotions, vitamin A and D ointment, and white petroleum jelly, are effective for skin care. Powders and oils are not recommended for the neonate's skin. Oils may clog the pores, and the small particles of powders may be inhaled by the neonate, causing respiratory difficulty.

Tub Baths. After the cord falls off, tub bathing of the neonate is possible. Parents do not need to buy an expensive infant tub. The kitchen sink is a satisfactory infant tub; however, certain safety precautions are necessary for parents who bathe the neonate in the sink. The sink should be cleaned before the neonate is bathed. A folded towel can be placed in the bottom of the sink to help prevent sliding. Cold water should be run through the faucet before the neonate is placed in the bath and the faucet should be turned away from the neonate to prevent accidental burns.

As with the sponge bath, parents should have all the equipment for the bath prepared and available before beginning the bath. Two or three inches of water should be placed in the tub or sink and the water temperature tested for comfort.

The neonate's eyes, nose, ears, and face are washed as in the sponge bath. The head is washed in the same manner. The neonate is then placed in the tub. While the parent supports the head and neck, the body is washed. The neonate may also be lathered sparsely with soap and then placed in the tub or sink for rinsing. Parents may wish to place a towel on their arm and then cradle the neonate in the towel when placing the neonate in the tub. This provides additional traction to help prevent slipping in the tub.

Neonates do not have to be completely bathed every day, although the diaper area is cleansed at each changing. The parents or other caretakers should schedule the bath at a time that is convenient for them.

Care of Nails. Parents are often concerned about how to cut the neonate's nails. The best time to cut the nails is when the neonate is sleeping. The parent may use an infant scissor and cut the nails straight across if the nails are long and the neonate is scratching himself or herself. An emery board may also be used and may prevent injury to the infant's skin. The fingernails and toenails may sometimes grow inward and adhere to the skin. Parents should be reassured that this is normal and should not attempt to cut the nails in this case, to avoid cutting the skin.

Infant Sucking Needs

Neonates may have sucking needs beyond those for feeding. For breastfed infants, artificial nipples should be discouraged during the first few weeks, because they can cause nipple confusion. Nurses should assess the parents' likes and dislikes regarding the use of pacifiers. For the neonate who needs additional sucking, pacifiers may be used if the parents wish. Neonates who thumb suck usually did so in utero. Thumb sucking may continue into the preschool years.

Elimination Patterns

Parents need to be aware that urates in the urine may stain the diaper pink during the first week of life and that this is a normal occurrence. Parents are often concerned about the elimination pattern of their neonate. After the initial meconium and transitional stools, breastfed neonates will have stools that are loose and yellow. They may pass stools up to 10 times a day, or go several days without a stool. Formula-fed infants, on the other hand, have stools that are firmer and yellow brown. Soy-based formulas produce stools that are greenish brown and pasty. A neonate may void 20 or more times a day.

Diapering. Parents and other caretakers should be informed about the types of diapers that are available and shown how to diaper an infant. Diapers are disposable or made of cloth. To accommodate urethral anatomy, some disposable diapers are constructed differently for girls and boys: girls' diapers have extra padding toward the back; boys' diapers have extra padding in the front. Disposable diapers offer a variety of features ranging from colors and prints to contoured shapes. These features often add to the cost of these items. Clients who need to be cost conscious and who wish to use disposable diapers can do well with "no frills," house-brand types.

Disposable diapers are costly and are often not biodegradable, yet many parents choose to use them. If stools are firm enough, they should be emptied from the diaper into a toilet before the diaper is thrown away.

Cloth diapers should be folded with consideration to absorbency; that is, they should be folded with additional thickness toward the back for girls and toward the front for boys.

Clothing and Wrapping

The neonate should be dressed for appropriate warmth and comfort. In general, neonates should wear a T-shirt, diaper, and light- to medium-weight sleeper that covers the neonate from neck to toe. Clothing should not be too warm in warm temperatures or too light in cold. To avoid chilling in air conditioning, a blanket may be used over the newborn's clothing.

The neonate's head should be covered with a hat when outdoors in the sun or when the temperature is cool. The neonate should not be placed directly in the sun, as the skin is sensitive and will burn easily. Sunscreen products made specifically for a neonate's sensitive skin may be used.

Parents are taught to launder the newborn's clothing and cloth diapers separately from other family clothing. A mild soap should be used and the clothing and diapers rinsed thoroughly to avoid any residue that might cause irritation. Fabric softeners may also irritate the skin.

The nurse should also teach parents how to wrap their newborn (Fig. 30–36). The baby blanket is placed on a flat surface. The neonate's head is placed at one corner, and one side of the blanket is wrapped over the infant and under the opposite side. The bottom corner of the blanket is then folded upward over the feet toward the chest, and the other side of the blanket is wrapped over the neonate. The newborn feels secure when wrapped in this manner, and parents are able to cradle the infant with more confidence.

Promoting Growth and Development

Growth is a product of the continuous and complex interaction of heredity and environment. Why growth occurs is not known; however, it is known that although growth rate may vary, the patterns remain stable. Growth is quantitative; that is, it can easily be observed and objectively measured. An important part of infant assessment is measurement of height, weight, and head and chest circumference. The infant's growth is charted during health care visits to identify and monitor the progress and pattern of growth.

Development is an interaction of the processes of physical growth, learning, and heredity. Development

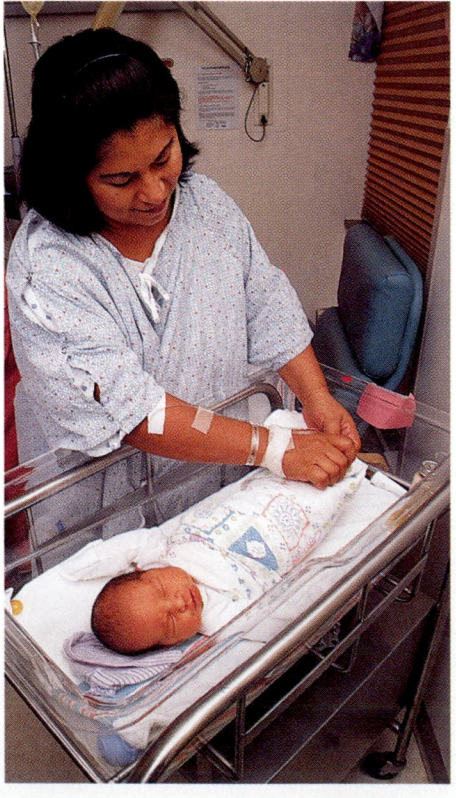

FIGURE 30–36. Wrapping the newborn facilitates the parents' cradling of the infant.

Commonly Asked Questions

Can my baby see?

Newborns can see several inches in front of them and prefer to look at faces more than anything else.

How often should I clean the umbilical cord area?

The umbilical cord can be cleaned with rubbing alcohol every time the diaper is changed. Be sure to clean the base of the cord at the level of the skin.

Is it normal for my newborn girl to have swollen "private parts"?

Yes, it is very normal. The genital area is swollen due to the maternal hormones she was exposed to when in the womb. It is also normal to have a small amount of bleeding from the vagina due to maternal hormones as well.

How often should I bathe my newborn?

A newborn does not need to be bathed every day. Every other day should be enough. A sponge bath is performed until the cord falls off. The baby can then be tub bathed. The diaper area should be cleaned well with every diaper change. Urine and stool can cause the skin to become irritated or to break down.

How will I know my newborn has a fever?

Taking your newborn's temperature either under the arm or in the rectum will let you know. Call your healthcare provider if the baby's temperature is 99.4°F when taken under the arm and 100.4°F when taken in the rectum.

What should I do if my newborn has a fever?

A newborn with a rectal temperature of 100.4°F or more needs to be seen by a primary care provider, an emergency department, or a clinic as soon as possible.

How do I know if my newborn is constipated?

Constipation is seen when your newborn passes hard, rock-like stool. Grunting, getting red in the face, and squirming are normal for newborns when they are passing stool. This does not mean they are constipated. Newborns can even go several days without stooling and still be normal.

What is jaundice and why is my newborn yellow?

Jaundice occurs where there are high amounts of bilirubin in the body that cause your newborn's skin and eyes to look yellow. When a red blood cell is no longer needed by the body, it breaks down into different parts; one of these parts is called bilirubin. Our bodies normally get rid of bilirubin through the liver and stool. But a newborn's liver is not fully mature and needs extra time to get rid of the bilirubin. You can do several things to help clear the bilirubin and the yellowness of your infant. First feed your infant frequently; one effect of feedings is causing the infant to stool and pass bilirubin from the body. Placing your infant near a closed window in the sunlight will also help clear bilirubin from the body.

---

is a qualitative continuous process that begins at conception. Developmental changes evolve from a complex interaction of such factors as maturation and experience. Development of locomotion skills and cognition is the result of an interaction between maturation and learning. Regardless of how much practice is provided, an infant cannot walk until myelination occurs and a certain level of maturity is reached. The cognitive, sensory, and motor development contributes to the child's eventually walking.

Although the processes underlying growth and development are complex, general principles indicate how development proceeds:

1. Growth and development are orderly and usually do not vary. Throughout infancy definite patterns in motor, physical, cognitive, and psychosocial growth can be observed. Although the time at which these occur may vary, there are definite periods when behaviors are expected to emerge. All early physical and motor development is "directional." Development is **cephalocaudal** (head-to-tail). The maturation process of the central nervous system is similar; the cervical area of the spinal cord matures earlier than the lumbar and sacral areas. Thus, infants are able to lift their heads

before they can lift the chest area, and they can sit before they stand. Development also has a **proximodistal** dimension. Development proceeds from the center of the body and moves outward toward the extremities. Infants use their fingers as a unit before they are able to control finger movements, and they gaze at items before they can reach out and grasp them.

2. Behavior becomes more versatile as development proceeds. Fine motor, social, and cognitive behaviors develop as the baby gets older. For example, infants communicate their needs through crying. Communication progresses to cooing, babbling, and single words in infancy to the ability to express complex thoughts and feelings during late childhood and adolescence. Behavior is influenced by genetics and environment. The time at which behaviors occur can vary within limits and under a variety of environmental conditions.

3. Development is patterned and continuous, but it may be stable at one time and change often at another. Development may accelerate in one area, and lag in another. For example, an infant's motor ability may progress rapidly while speech progresses more slowly.

4. Continuing interaction occurs between a changing individual and a changing environment. Responses of the infant to the environment produce changes in the infant so that later responses to similar or other events in the environment differ from earlier behaviors. For example, infant sucking patterns become modified with practice, and the infant is able to distinguish between nutritive and nonnutritive sucking and modify modes of sucking.

Although development is patterned and predictable, it cannot proceed without appropriate stimulation. Kaye (1982) and other investigators observed that infants have learning abilities as early as the first days of life; they conclude that the infant's abilities are more sophisticated and organized than was formerly believed. In providing teaching, the nurse must understand infant growth and development, psychosocial theory, psychosexual development, cognitive growth, and separation–individuation.

One of the most important factors in infant development is the quality of caretaking. All infants must establish a trusting relationship with at least one caretaker who will meet his or her needs. The mutual interaction that occurs contributes to the infant's gratification and growing sense of confidence that specific

behaviors will get positive responses from caretakers. Nurturing helps stimulate the development of language, social skills, and learning that are the foundation for further achievement.

Language, cognitive, social, and motor skills can be developed if the primary caretakers respond to the appropriate infant cues at the appropriate time. For example, the best method for teaching language is to talk to the infant and respond to his or her crying, cooing, and babbling.

Table 30–5 outlines language, cognitive, social, and motor development in the first 12 months of life.

Development occurs as a natural process in all infants according to their potential as long as they have a variety of experiences in which they actively participate. The quality and quantity of development are influenced by such factors as temperament, readiness, mastery of previously developed skills, and environment.

Preventing Communicable Diseases

Immunization against communicable disease is an important aspect of disease prevention and health promotion throughout childhood. Communicable diseases among infants and children are some of the oldest known public health problems. Public concern and scientific discovery have resulted in development of many effective and powerful immunizing agents that are readily available to children.

The American Academy of Pediatrics' Committee on Infectious Disease recommends that immunizations be started when an infant is 2 months of age, with the exception of the hepatitis B vaccine, the first dose of which can be given at birth (American Academy of Pediatrics, 1997). Some antibodies are transferred via the maternal–fetal circulation in utero, and that provides passive immunity for the infant. For approximately 6 months to 1 year, the infant is protected against diseases for which the mother has antibodies.

Active immunity is given through the introduction of a vaccine that stimulates the body to produce antitoxins or antibodies. The vaccine can be given in the form of a toxoid, live attenuated virus, or killed inactivated virus. The box entitled Vaccine Profile discusses the uses of the hepatitis B and polio vaccines in preventing these diseases in infants. Table 30–6 presents a recommended schedule for the hepatitis B vaccine.

The immunization schedule (Table 30–7) is flexible; immunity is achieved whether the interval between doses is short or long. What is important is that the correct dose be administered. Immunizations are contraindicated when there is an acute illness

▶ **TABLE 30–5**

Developmental Milestones

Behavior Progression	Approximate Age Behavior Develops
Language	
Responds to stress by crying	Birth
Coos and babbles; "talks" when spoken to; squeals with pleasure	3 months
Babbles; makes sounds to inanimate objects	6 months
Imitates sounds	9 months
Vocalizes some words, e.g., Mama, Dada	1 year
Cognitive	
Exhibits inborn primitive reflexes; becomes efficient at sucking	Birth
Repeats reflexes spontaneously, e.g., moves hands to mouth	1 month
Exhibits coordination between motor skills and vision	4 months
Exhibits object permanence; distinguishes self from others	8 months
Social	
Follows objects with eyes; responds by crying	Birth
Smiles socially	1 month
Laughs aloud; may show preference for usual caretakers	6 months
Cries and becomes tense in strange situations and with strangers	9 months
Responds to "no"; understands names of objects	1 year
Motor	
Lifts head while lying on abdomen; holds hands in fixed position	Birth
Lifts head 90 degrees; supports weight on forearms; clasps and unclasps hands voluntarily; turns head toward moving objects	3 months
Turns over	5 months
Transfers objects from hand to hand; sits with support	6 months
Sits without support; crawls; pulls self to standing position; uses pincer grasp	9 months
May begin to walk	1 year

accompanied by fever and severe reactions to a previous vaccine (e.g., convulsions and high fever). The common cold and upper respiratory infections usually are not contraindications; however, this guideline can be confusing and may cause parents to delay further immunizations until respiratory symptoms disappear.

The nurse involved in health care of infants must be an effective teacher who can provide, interpret, and reinforce information given to parents. In addition, the nurse must know about new immunizations and changes in recommendations for well-known ones (e.g., varicella and polio vaccine) and the infectious process and understand antigen–antibody relationships and immunization schedules and procedures.

The nurse should discuss the benefits and risks of immunizations with parents and ask them to sign an informed consent prior to the administration of immunizations to the infant. An immunization record is then given to the parents and updated as additional immunizations are provided.

Preventing Accidents

Home safety and accident prevention are essential components of health maintenance. Accidents are one of the top ten leading causes of death in the first year of life. Most accidents are preventable. Parents must be made aware of the extent of accidental death and injury and can be helped to form an effective accident prevention plan.

Both the stage of development and maternal (or primary caretaker) factors influence infant accident rates. Mothers whose infants are at the highest risk for accidental death tend to be young and poorly educated women who have more than one child. Limited access to health care and poverty are variables that are associated with poor education and teenage pregnancy; the infants of these young women are at a particularly high risk for accidental injury and death.

The infant is totally dependent on caregiver supervision for the prevention of accidents. One can easily understand how the overextended mother with several children, the young mother who has developmental needs of her own, and the poorly educated

HEPATITIS B VACCINE

The hepatitis B vaccine protects against infection by the hepatitis B virus. The hepatitis B virus is in the viral class *Hepadnaviridae* and is the most common viral illness in the world. Infection with hepatitis B causes acute and chronic hepatitis, cirrhosis, and primary hepatocellular carcinoma.

The virus is transmitted from person to person via parenteral or mucosal exposure. The largest amount of virus is found in the blood and serous fluids; lower amounts are in saliva and semen. Due to the large amount of blood and serous fluid present at birth, a hepatitis B–positive mother can very effectively transmit the virus to her newborn.

The hepatitis B vaccine is recommended for all infants and consists of a series of 3 injections to confer immunity. The first injection can be given within the first 24 to 48 hours of life. The schedule for the hepatitis B vaccine can be found in Table 30–6.

Infants born to mothers who are carriers of hepatitis B virus must receive both hepatitis B vaccine and hepatitis B immune globulin (HBIG) at birth. The HBIG is given to offer passive immunity and prevent an infection by the virus. Table 30–6 summarizes the hepatitis B vaccine schedule for an infant born to a hepatitis B positive mother.

POLIO VACCINE

The oral poliovirus vaccine (OPV) and the inactivated poliovirus vaccine (IPV) are the vaccines which are used to promote immunity to three types of polio viruses. OPV is a live attenuated vaccine and IPV is an inactivated form of the three polio viruses developed into a vaccine. The only side effect to receiving the OPV is the possibility of contracting vaccine-associated paralytic polio; the overall risk is 1 in 2.4 million.

An infection by the poliovirus can manifest itself in a variety of ways; 95% of poliovirus infections are subclinical and without symptoms. About 2% of infections lead to paralytic poliomyelitis, characterized by permanent paralysis and in some cases death (American Academy of Pediatrics, 1997). The poliovirus is transmitted by the oral-fecal route.

Poliomyelitis has become rare in the United States. There have been no reported cases of poliomyelitis caused by the wild virus since 1980 in the U.S. and no cases of this type of poliovirus in the Western hemisphere since 1991 (American Academy of Pediatrics, 1997).

The only reported cases of poliomyelitis have been those caused by giving the OPV. Since 1980, approximately 8 to 9 cases of vaccine-associated paralytic polio (VAPP) have been reported yearly (American Academy of Pediatrics, 1997). For this reason, the U.S. Centers for Disease Control and Prevention's (CDC) Advisory Committee for Immunization Practices as well as the American Academy of Pediatrics have recommended a change in the schedule for polio vaccine. See Table 30–7 for a summary of the polio vaccine schedule and all the recommended childhood immunizations. By using the sequential schedule, IPV at 2 months of age and 4 months of age and OPV at 12 to 18 months and 4 years of age, the incidence of VAPP is expected to decline by 50 to 75% (American Academy of Pediatrics, 1997).

It is the nurse's role to educate parents and reinforce the need for timely vaccinations. The nurse must be informed of the changes in vaccination schedules and be able to explain these changes to parents and families. For more information regarding vaccines, contact the CDC, 1600 Clifton Rd., Atlanta, Georgia 30333.

▶ **TABLE 30-6**

Recommended Schedule of Hepatitis B Immunoprophylaxis to Prevent Perinatal Transmission[1]

Vaccine Dose and HBIG	Age
Infant Born to Mother Known To Be HBsAg Positive	
First	Birth (within 12 hr.)
HBIG[2]	Birth (within 12 hr.)
Second	1–2 mo
Third	6 mo
Infant Born to Mother Not Screened for HBsAg	
First[3]	Birth (within 12 hr.)
HBIG[2]	If mother is HBsAg-positive, give 0.5 mL as soon as possible, not later than 1 wk after birth
Second	1–2 mo
Third	6–18 mo[4]

[1]HBsAG indicates hepatitis B surface antigen; HBIG, hepatitis B immune globulin.
[2]HBIG (0.5 mL) given intramuscularly at a site different from that used for vaccine.
[3]First dose is same as that for infant of HBsAg-positive mother. Subsequent doses and schedules are determined by maternal HBsAg status.
[4]Infants of HBsAg-positive mothers should be vaccinated at 6 months of age.

Source: Reprinted, with permission, from American Academy of Pediatrics. (1997). 1997 Red book: Report of the committee on infectious diseases *(24th ed.). Elk Grove Village, IL: Author, p. 258.*

▶ **TABLE 30-7**

Recommended Childhood Immunization Schedule United States, January–December 1998[a]

Age ▶ / Vaccine ▼	Birth	1 mo	2 mos	4 mos	6 mos	12 mos	15 mos	18 mos	4–6 yrs	11–12 yrs	14–16 yrs
Hepatitis B[2,3]	Hep B-1									Hep B[3]	
		Hep B-2			Hep B-3						
Diphtheria, Tetanus, Pertussis[4]		DTaP or DTP	DTaP or DTP	DTaP or DTP		DTaP or DTP[4]			DTaP or DTP	Td	
H. influenzae type b[5]		Hib	Hib	Hib[5]	Hib[5]						
Polio[6]		Polio[6]	Polio		Polio[6]			Polio			
Measles, Mumps, Rubella[7]						MMR			MMR[7]	MMR[7]	
Varicella[8]						Var				Var[8]	

[a]Vaccines[1] are listed under the routinely recommended ages. Bars indicate range of acceptable ages for vaccination. Shaded bars indicate *catch-up vaccination:* at 11–12 years of age, hepatitis B vaccine should be administered to children not previously vaccinated, and Varicella vaccine should be administered to children not previously vaccinated who lack a reliable history of chickenpox.

[1]This schedule indicates the recommended age for routine administration of currently licensed childhood vaccines. Some combination vaccines are available and may be used whenever administration of all components of the vaccine is indicated. Providers should consult the manufacturers' package inserts for detailed recommendations.

[2]Infants born to HBsAg-negative mothers should receive 2.5 µg of Merck vaccine (Recombivax HB) or 10 µg of SmithKline Beecham (SB) vaccine (Engerix-B). The 2nd dose should be administered ≥ 1 mo after the 1st dose. The third dose should be given at least 2 mos after the second, but not before 6 mos of age. Infants born to HBsAg-positive mothers should receive 0.5 mL hepatitis B immune globulin (HBIG) within 12 hrs of birth, and either 5 µg of Merck vaccine (Recombivax HB) or 10 µg of SB vaccine (Engerix-B) at a separate site. The 2nd dose is recommended at 1–2 mos of age and the 3rd dose at 6 mos of age. Infants born to mothers whose HBsAg status is unknown should receive either 5 µg of Merck vaccine (Recombivax HB) or 10 µg of SB vaccine (Engerix-B) within 12 hrs of birth. The 2nd dose of vaccine is recommended at 1 mo of age and the 3rd dose at 6 mos of age. Blood should be drawn at the time of delivery to determine the mother's HBsAg status; if it is positive, the infant should receive HBIG as soon as possible (no later than 1 wk of age). The dosage and timing of subsequent vaccine doses should be based upon the mother's HBsAg status.

[3]Children and adolescents who have not been vaccinated against hepatitis B in infancy may begin the series during any childhood visit. Those who have not previously received 3 doses of hepatitis B vaccine should initiate or complete the series during the 11–12 year-old visit and unvaccinated older children should be vaccinated whenever possible. The 2nd dose should be administered at least 1 mo after the 1st dose, and the 3rd dose should be administered at least 4 mos after the 1st dose and at least 2 mos after the 2nd dose.

[4]DTaP (diphtheria and tetanus toxoids and acellular pertussis vaccine) is the preferred vaccine for all doses in the vaccination series, including completion of the series in children who have received ≥1 dose of whole-cell DTP vaccine. Whole-cell DTP is an acceptable alternative to DTaP. The 4th dose DTaP may be administered as early as 12 months of age, provided 6 months have elapsed since the 3rd dose, and if the child is considered unlikely to return at 15–18 mos of age. Td (tetanus and diphtheria toxoids, absorbed, for adult use) is recommended at 11–12 years of age if at least 5 years have elapsed since the last dose of DTP, DTaP, or DT. Subsequent routine Td boosters are recommended every 10 years.

[5]Three H. influenzae type b (Hib) conjugate vaccines are licensed for infant use. If PRP-OMP (PedvaxHIB [Merck]) is administered at 2 and 4 mos of age, a dose at 6 mos is not required. After completing the primary series, any Hib conjugate vaccine may be used as a booster.

[6]Two poliovirus vaccines are currently licensed in the US: inactivated poliovirus vaccine (IPV) and oral poliovirus vaccine (OPV). The following schedules are all acceptable by the ACIP, the AAP, and the AAFP, and parents and providers may choose among them:

  1. IPV at 2 and 4 mos; OPV at 12–18 mos and 4–6 yr
  2. IPV at 2, 4, 12–18 mos, and 4–6 yr
  3. OPV at 2, 4, 6–18 mos, and 4–6 yr

The ACIP routinely recommends schedule 1. IPV is the only poliovirus vaccine recommended for immunocompromised persons and their household contacts.

[7]The 2nd dose of MMR is routinely recommended at 4–6 yrs of age or at 11–12 yrs of age, but may be administered during any visit, provided at least 1 month has elapsed since receipt of the 1st dose and that both doses are administered at or after 12 months of age.

[8]Susceptible children may receive Varicella vaccine (Var) at any visit after the first birthday, and those who lack a reliable history of chickenpox should be immunized during the 11–12 year-old visit. Children ≥ 13 years of age should receive 2 doses, at least 1 mo apart.

Source: Reprinted, with permission, from American Academy of Pediatrics. (1997). 1997 Red book: Report of the committee on infectious diseases (24th ed.). Elk Grove Village, IL: Author, pp.18–19.

mother who has limited problem-solving skills or little knowledge of infant development, could easily overlook or fail to recognize the safety needs of her infant.

An effective accident prevention plan must take into consideration the needs and development of both infants and caretakers. It is not too early to begin discussing newborn safety during the prenatal period, with reinforcement sessions at each well-child and postpartum visit. Nurses who work with infants and caretakers, whether it be in hospitals, clinics, physicians' offices, or home visiting agencies, are in a position to play an active role in accident prevention. The U.S. Consumer Product Safety Commission, Washington, DC 20207, is an excellent source of information and teaching materials that may be shared with parents and primary caretakers.

Knowledge about infant abilities at specific ages and developmental stages is the basis of every accident prevention plan. Health care providers are encouraged to share pamphlets in the caretaker's language and articles concerning normal infant development along with any accident prevention information that may be disseminated. And, as with all educational efforts, the needs, abilities, and environment of the learner cannot be overlooked.

Accident prevention information (Table 30–8) is most useful when taught with developmental activities and abilities that place the infant at risk for a particular accident.

Parents and primary caretakers must understand the importance of accident prevention. Simply mentioning accident prevention is not sufficient. For example, despite public awareness campaigns about car safety seats, infants and children are still seen unrestrained in cars. Parent education can help address this problem.

Numerous films and teaching materials are available in a variety of languages for use in prenatal

▶ **TABLE 30–8**

Accident Prevention During the First Two Months

Developmental Ability	Preventive Action
Weak gastroesophageal sphincter; vomits and regurgitates easily.	**Aspiration** Hold infant 15 to 30 minutes after feeding to prevent vomiting.
Only beginning head and neck control.	Do not offer solid foods.

Engages in movement that may propel or project the infant:
  Kicks legs.
  Rolls from side to supine.
  Lifts head momentarily.
  Rotates and extends head.
  Has grasp reflex.
  Moves arms and hands.
	Pacifiers should be of one-piece construction with a large shield to prevent entry into mouth.
	
	Suffocation
	Never leave infant alone in any amount of water.
	Avoid sleeping with infant.
	Avoid the use of plastic of any sort; discard plastic bags immediately.
	Crib slats should not be more the 2⅜ inches apart.
	Cover crib slats with bumpers.
	Remove unnecessary pillows, blankets, and stuffed toys from crib.
	
	Strangulation
	Avoid use of necklaces, straps, ties, or cords around neck or near crib.
	Do not hang pacifier around infant's neck.
	Remove bibs for naps.
	Be cautious of any toys with straps or cords.
	
	Falls
	Never leave infant unattended on high surfaces (place infant on floor if need be).
	Supervise toddlers and young children around infant.
	Avoid placing infant in high chairs or grocery carts until the infant can sit well.
	Use security straps in infant seats and strollers.
	
	Motor Vehicles
	Always use an infant seat, even with premature infants.
	At this age place infant seat facing rear of car.
	Never leave infant unattended in carriages or strollers.
	Never leave infant unattended in cars.
	Car seat placement—*All* infant car seats should be in the center of the back seat, rear facing. *None* should be in the front seat regardless of the presence of an air bag.
	
	Burns
	Check surface temperature of car seats and belts.
	Avoid smoking around infant.
	Expose to direct sunlight only for brief periods.
	Cover infant's head when in sun; head is largest body surface of infant.
	Check bath and formula temperatures carefully.
	Avoid drinking or pouring hot liquids while holding infant.
	Keep infant away from hot objects.
	Avoid use of hot-mist vaporizers.
	
	Bodily Injury
	Always close safety pins.
	Avoid sharp objects or toys.
	Be careful with sharp jewelry or clasp pins for jewelry.

classes and clinics, well-child clinics, physicians' offices, day care centers, and other facilities in which parents, infants, and primary caretakers may be encountered. Parents and primary caretakers must become active participants in recognizing the dangers in their own automobiles and homes and the methods by which those dangers can be removed.

Promoting Normal Sleep Patterns

Sleeping patterns vary among infants and change with maturation. Generally speaking, infants between 2 and 6 weeks of age show a great variation in sleep patterns but gradually phase into a diurnal cycle (Edelman & Mandle, 1994). In the first 2 weeks of life, most newborns sleep the same number of hours during the day as they do during the night. By 5 weeks of age, 66% of infants begin to sleep longer at night, and by 3 months of age, 98% of infants sleep longer at night. The pattern that is established by 4 to 5 months of age is usually one of 2- to 4-hour naps after feedings and 6 to 7 hours of sleep through the night. Around 6 months of age, nap periods shorten to a morning and afternoon nap after meals and sleeping through the night. Infants may wake during the night at about 7 months of age, when they begin to experience separation anxiety. By 1 year of age, some infants give up the morning nap, sleep longer in the afternoon, and sleep through the night, although there is variability in infant sleep patterns.

Sleep problems, particularly not sleeping through the night, may cause great stress to families and create problems of sleep deprivation, exhaustion, and irritability for caretakers. Awakening in the night itself is not considered a problem; rather, awakening and then crying and not returning to sleep is what is defined as a problem by parents. New, young, inexperienced parents, or parents lacking an experienced and knowledgeable support system, may have more difficulty than experienced parents. Problems may arise when parents do not understand normal infant sleep behaviors and view the sleepless, crying infant as a sign of their incompetence as parents, or view the sleepless crying as an attempt by the infant to manipulate the parent. More commonly, parents have difficulty with the night awakening because they are exhausted the next day and find it hard to meet the demands and obligations of managing a home, job, and personal and professional relationships.

The age of the infant when sleep problems are reported influences the management of the problem. There is so much variation among infant sleeping patterns in the first 6 weeks of life that parents must be educated to the fact that a "normal" infant sleeping pattern does not exist. Parents may require instruction as well as emotional support during this period. To gather accurate information about the infant's sleeping, waking, and crying times, parents are instructed to keep a record during two or three 24-hour periods. Most young infants sleep 15.4 hours in 24 hours (although how those 15.4 hours are spread throughout the 24-hour period may vary), and cry 1½ to 3½ hours per day. Parents may just need to understand

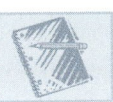

Client Teaching

The nurse can suggest the following strategies to help parents address their specific concerns regarding care of their newborn:

- Never leave your newborn alone on a changing table, a couch, or bed. The baby can easily roll off the surface and fall to the floor, causing serious injury.

- To prevent suffocation, your newborn should be placed on their side or back when being put to sleep. Roll a small receiving blanket and place it against your baby's back to maintain the side position. No stuffed animals or pillows should be in your newborn's sleeping area as they may cause suffocation.

- All infants and children up to 40 pounds must be placed in an approved car safety seat whenever they are in a vehicle (cars, trucks, vans). Your newborn's infant car seat should be secured in the center of the back seat, facing out the rear window and in the semi-reclined position. Be sure to read the instructions for your specific type of car seat so that it is properly belted into a vehicle.

- Remember to gather all your equipment for the bath first. Choose a quiet time of the day when you can pay full attention to your infant while he or she is in the bath water. Also choose an area of your home free from drafts. When giving a sponge bath, leave your infant covered with an undershirt or towel until you get to that body part to prevent chilling. In bathing, start with the cleanest area and move to the dirtiest; for example, clean your infant's eyes first, then face, neck, arms, hands, legs, and feet. Save the diaper area until last.

that their infant is behaving normally. Nurses should not overlook the fact that when parents are complaining of a sleep problem in their young infant, they may actually be having difficulty with the infant's crying and not his or her awake state. Education of the parent as to individual temperamental traits and interventions for excessive crying (discussed later under Colic) may help the parent cope with this early period (Edelman & Mandle, 1994).

Supporting Working Parents

The number of families in which both parents work outside of the home continues to grow. As a result, concern has increased about the effect of parental absence on an infant. Questions today center on when a mother should return to work and the infant's response to maternal absence, paternal absence, or both. Another important issue of concern to working parents is obtaining affordable, appropriate child care. Unfortunately, many working parents do not have wonderful, inexpensive care available. Media attention to cases of an infant's abuse while in the care of a "nanny" has further added to parental worry about returning to work. In addition, not all employers or jobs are helpful to parents of young children. Attention must be directed toward a better understanding of how two-income and single-parent families provide child care for their infants.

The characteristics of a caretaker could have implications for the psychologic well-being of parents and their children. Most children in day care spend more than 30 hours per week with their caretakers, who have responsibility for all aspects of the infant's care during the parents' absence; the caregivers provide for the infant's social, emotional, and cognitive development, as well as more basic needs.

Owen and colleagues (1984) studied the parent–child relationships in 59 dual-income families and their infants. The quality of the mother–infant attachment did not decrease when the mother returned to work. Whether the mother returned to work when the child was an infant or toddler did not seem to affect the stability or quality of development.

► Discharge Planning

Discharge planning should include teaching related to infant care, parental concerns, and management of the infant at home. The nurse makes certain that prior to discharge parents have identified a care provider who will continue care for the infant. The nurse can also assist parents with making well-baby appointments.

Parents need to have the chance to discuss child care concerns at their well-baby visits. Advice should

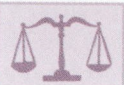

Ethical Decision Making

Given the fact that noted child authorities like Brazelton have suggested that the primary caregiving parent remain at home during the first 4 months to get to know the infant and thus establish a greater level of attachment and intimacy, parents may ask the nurse his or her opinion about staying home with the child instead of returning to work. If you were the nurse caring for a family in this situation, consider the following issues:

1. Whose rights, the parent's to be able to return to work for career or economic needs or the infant's to have a parent at home, should take precedence in this situation?
2. What other approaches can be used to enhance attachment between the infant and the primary caregiver who is employed full-time that would benefit both the infant and the parent?
3. Should employers provide alternative employment options that include parental leave to help families cope with this problem?

be based on an understanding of the family's needs and services available in the community. Such topics as age of siblings asked to babysit and how to evaluate a potential child care situation can be addressed.

► SELECTED NEONATAL AND INFANT STRESSORS

The neonate and infant possess unique physiologic capabilities to adapt to stress, both internal and external. Occasionally, however, interventions are necessary to ensure or ease a return to wellness. Many stressors identified during the neonatal and infant periods can be managed through nursing interventions or through joint protocols developed with medical and other health care professional colleagues. The following sections discuss nursing care of physiologic jaundice, obstructed lacrimal ducts, skin problems, thrush, regurgitation, colic, and fever.

▶ Physiologic Jaundice

Physiologic jaundice is a common condition during the early neonatal period, occurring in approximately 50% of term infants during the first week of life, usually on the second or third day. (See discussion earlier in this chapter about Hepatic Regulation.) The condition most often occurs when the neonate's immature liver is unable to handle the breakdown of protein, resulting in hyperbilirubinemia, an excess of bilirubin in the blood.

Jaundice present at birth or within the first 24 hours is considered pathologic. See Chapter 32 for discussion of the criteria that differentiates pathologic jaundice from physiologic jaundice.

A serum bilirubin level of 2.0 mg/dL or greater is a common finding in neonates during the first week of life. Usually jaundice is not visible until the serum concentration exceeds 7.0 mg/dL. Traditionally, the peak level for physiologic jaundice in normal neonates is 12.9 mg/dL.

Breastfed neonates may normally have a higher bilirubin than bottle-fed newborns. However, neonates need to be evaluated on an individual basis.

Assessment for jaundice is discussed earlier in the chapter in the section entitled Skin. Neonates of dark-skinned or olive-complexioned parents may appear to be jaundiced when in actuality they are not.

Although serum bilirubin levels have been the traditional method used to screen for hyperbilirubinemia, many institutions now employ noninvasive, transcutaneous bilirubinometry methods. One method uses an icterometer, an inexpensive Plexiglas strip on which are painted five yellow transverse stripes that are precisely colored. The Plexiglas strip is pressed against the neonate's skin and the color of the skin is compared with the color on the stripes. A jaundice score is then assigned. Another method uses a jaundice meter that measures the intensity of the yellow color in the skin through spectrophotometry. The jaundice meter is placed against either the neonate's forehead or sternum. Both methods are considered appropriate in screening for jaundice (Schumacher, Thornberg, & Gutcher, 1985), and decrease the number of serum samples that must be taken for analysis. If bilirubin levels exceed acceptable levels, phototherapy will be instituted (see Chapter 32). (Acceptable levels may vary from institution to institution.)

Nursing care of the newborn with physiologic jaundice centers on providing clear and appropriate explanations to the parents. Too often a newborn is taken for a blood test with the explanation that a "bilirubin level" is needed. Even the most knowledgeable of parents may have little understanding of the meaning of such a test. Clear explanations of the physiology and purpose of testing will allay parents' anxieties.

Protocols for treatment of breastfeeding jaundice vary. If the mother continues to nurse, elevated levels of bilirubin may persist, reaching normal values by 3 to 12 weeks of age. If breastfeeding is interrupted, serum bilirubin levels decline within 48 hours and bilirubin levels rise only about 1 to 3 mg/dL after nursing is resumed. Some investigators conclude that when the serum bilirubin concentration approaches 17 mg/dL, breastfeeding should be interrupted for 48 hours, at which time it can be resumed (Maisels, 1993). If this protocol is chosen, the nurse needs to support the mother and allay any fears she may have that there is something wrong with her milk or that she is doing harm to the newborn by breastfeeding. The nurse should also assist the mother to maintain lactation through the use of manual expression and breast pumps.

Other practitioners have attempted to supplement breastfed newborns with glucose water. This practice does not reduce the serum bilirubin level. In fact, using glucose water may increase the level of bilirubin (Maisels, 1993). Supplementing with plain water is thought to have no effect on the bilirubin concentration (De Carvalho, Hall, & Harvey, 1981).

One study of bottle- and breastfed infants found a greater excretion of bilirubin in those who had a greater stool output. Bottle-fed infants were found to have more frequent stools, whereas breastfed infants experienced a greater weight loss in the immediate neonatal period. It was suggested that hyperbilirubinemia in breastfed infants could be minimized by earlier stimulation of intestinal motility (De Carvalho, Robertson, & Klaus, 1985). Nurses can support this by explaining the benefits of early rooming-in, and frequent nursing to reestablish hydration as well as promoting the early onset of milk supply. If the mother does not desire to have the newborn room-in, every effort should be made to bring the newborn to her when hungry, instead of imposing a routine schedule.

▶ Obstructed Lacrimal Ducts

New mothers may be concerned about constant tearing and a mucoid discharge from either one or both of the neonate's eyes. Lacrimal outlet obstruction, or dacryostenosis, occurs in more than 50% of neonates in the first week of life. Usually the nasolacrimal ducts spontaneously open by 3 months of age. Parents can be taught to massage the ducts to promote mucous drainage. Massage is accomplished by firm pressure in a small circular motion along the side of the nose toward the eye and the opening of the lacrimal duct at the inner canthus. The drainage is then cleared away with a cotton ball and warm water, wiping from the inner to the outer canthus. This process is repeated three to four times a day in the affected eye.

Rarely does acute infection (dacryocystitis) occur. This is characterized by purulent discharge, swelling in the inner canthal region, and tenderness and redness over the area. Topical and systemic antibiotics are usually indicated for dacryocystitis. Eye hygiene is the same as for dacryostenosis.

▶ Skin Problems

Numerous skin problems may be noted in infancy. Fortunately, the most common are also usually the most benign. The common skin problems of infants include cradle cap, which is a form of seborrheic dermatitis, and diaper dermatitis, which includes contact, ammoniacal, and fungal diaper rash.

Cradle Cap

Cradle cap is a form of seborrheic dermatitis that results from a buildup of sebaceous matter on the scalp, usually over the anterior fontanelle. It differs from more severe and chronic forms of seborrheic dermatitis because it is easily treated with proper washing of the scalp. Infants with cradle cap have the characteristic yellow, crusty, waxy patches restricted to the anterior scalp. Infants with other, more severe forms of seborrheic dermatitis have lesions on the eyebrows, eyelids, chest, cheeks, neck, and axilla, as well as the scalp and behind the ears.

Shampooing should be demonstrated to the mother or caretaker, who often is surprised that the scalp can be thoroughly washed without causing damage. Baby oil may be massaged into the scalp 15 to 30 minutes prior to shampooing; then with gentle but firm rubbing with a dry washcloth or combing with a fine-tooth comb, some of the crusty patches can be lifted from the scalp. The scalp and hair may then be washed with a mild shampoo and rinsed well with tepid water. The parent is instructed to repeat this procedure daily until the cradle cap is removed.

In more severe cases of cradle cap, an antiseborrheic shampoo may be indicated. It should also be noted that secondary infections can develop on the scalp that may require antimicrobial treatment.

Diaper Dermatitis

Diaper dermatitis, or contact dermatitis, is a general term for numerous and distinct skin irritations and inflammations that occur in the diaper area. The specific causes vary and require different treatments. Determining the cause is a primary focus of care.

The diagnosis of the type of diaper dermatitis is based on the erythema and thickening of the skin. In primary irritant contact dermatitis, the skin may look red and scalded. It occurs when the infant's diaper area is repeatedly subjected to moisture from frequent urination and friction from the diaper itself. Diaper dermatitis attributed to *Candida albicans* can result from invasion secondary to a preexisting skin irritation; in some cases, *C. albicans* can be a primary invader (Leyden, 1986). The lesions of *Candida* diaper dermatitis are well circumscribed. They are characteristically vivid "fire-engine" red and appear pustulovesicular. Satellite lesions may appear on thighs and abdomen.

The goal of treatment is to keep the diaper area clean, dry, and aerated without causing additional trauma or irritation. The nurse should provide reassurance to the parent or primary caretaker as she or he often feels ashamed and at fault for the problem. Further information can be given to parents during discharge planning in an effort to promote health and prevent the problem. The nurse can provide written instructions and demonstrations of skin care if needed, including the following points:

1. Check and change both cloth and disposable diapers frequently so that urine and feces are not in prolonged contact with the skin.
2. Avoid the use of baby wipes that may not adequately cleanse the skin.
3. Rinse the diaper area with tepid water after each voiding and use a mild soap and tepid water rinse after each bowel movement. Gently dry the skin thoroughly.
4. Expose the skin to air for approximately 10 minutes before reapplying diaper.
5. Avoid plastic and rubber pants, as they permit excessive moisture buildup. Use a thick two- to three-layer diaper and place the infant on a covered changing mat to avoid constant wetting of bed linen.
6. When disposable diaper intolerance is suspected, try cloth diapers. Some infants may simply be sensitive to the elastic or plastic used on some disposable diapers and a simple change in the type or brand of diaper may be all that is needed.
7. Wash cloth diapers with a mild soap and rinse twice, using one-half cup of either vinegar or bleach in the last rinse. Clothes softeners usually contain perfumes and chemicals that may be irritating to infant skin; currently, unscented fabric softeners are available.

Machine-drying cotton diapers at a high temperature destroys organisms and softens cotton without the use of a softener. If a commercial diaper service is used, parents should inquire about their methods of diaper washing.

8. For infants with a diarrhea-induced rash, apply a small amount of A&D ointment, Desitin, *or* zinc oxide to the cleaned, irritated skin to provide a protective barrier against the diarrhea. Gently cleanse the skin with a mild soap and tepid water after each bowel movement, gently pat dry, and reapply the ointment. Desitin or zinc oxide are removed more easily with mineral oil than with soap and water.

9. Treat severe irritant dermatitis with 1% hydrocortisone as prescribed.

10. Avoid the use of powders or lotions when the skin is inflamed or broken.

11. Nystatin (Mycostatin) cream should be used as prescribed with each diaper change to treat diaper dermatitis caused by *Candida albicans*.

▶ Thrush

Thrush is an oral infection by the fungus *Candida albicans*. The infection may result from contact with an infected vaginal canal during delivery. Other sources of contamination include hands, bottles, or nipples.

The peak incidence is usually around the second week of life, long after the neonate has been discharged from the hospital. Thrush may also occur after antibiotic therapy, as the medication destroys the normal flora and allows opportunistic organisms to flourish.

The infection appears in the mouth as white patches, which the mother may at first interpret as milk curds. The lesions can be on the buccal mucosa, the gums, the tongue, and the hard and soft palate. Some neonates may experience sucking difficulties if the involvement is extensive.

Oral thrush can easily be treated with a topical fungicide, such as nystatin suspension. The medication is administered four times a day for 1 week. The mother can be taught to instill a dropperful of medication into the side of each cheek, and then "paint" the lesions with a cotton-tipped applicator.

Everything that comes in contact with the neonate's mouth must be clean. This precaution must be stressed to parents. Bottle nipples and pacifiers should be boiled after use. Handwashing is very important.

▶ Regurgitation

Regurgitation, or "spitting up," is the effortless bringing up of a small amount of formula (usually one or two mouthfuls) and does not lead to nutritional deficiency.

Excessive air swallowing (or aerophagy) may increase the incidence of regurgitation. Prolonged crying, as is seen in underfeeding and delayed feeding, improper size of nipple hole, or sucking on an empty bottle, results in air swallowing.

Improper positioning of the infant may also cause regurgitation. Parents should be instructed to avoid added pressure on the infant's stomach. For example, they should not allow the infant to double over at the waist while sitting, double up the infant's legs when changing diapers, use tight diapers or clothing, position the infant too high on the caretaker's shoulder so that there is pressure directly on the stomach, or lay the infant down too soon after a feeding. Caretakers can also be advised to use a cloth diaper or small towel to protect their own clothing when feeding.

The infant may be positioned in an infant seat that is angled at 50° to 60° for ½ to 1 hour after each feeding. The infant seat should be made comfortable so that the infant may nap or play without difficulty.

If advised by the health care provider, feedings may be thickened with infant cereal (1 tablespoon of cereal to 4 ounces of formula) to help the formula remain in the stomach. The nurse should reassure parents that the condition is due to an immature lower esophageal sphincter and that the problem is usually corrected by 6 months of age and, at the latest, by walking age.

▶ Colic

Colic and paroxysmal fussiness are terms used for unexplained crying. The infant cries suddenly, loudly, and continuously for no apparent reason; sometimes the crying lasts hours. Other signs that may be observed include a flushed face; distended, tense abdomen; legs drawn to the abdomen; cold feet; and clenched fists.

Colic, seen in approximately 10% of all infants, has no proven organic basis. The crying episodes begin early, often in the first weeks of life, and continue until approximately 3 months of age. Infants with sensitive or vigorous temperaments and infants who seem to need less sleep than the norm tend to be colicky. The crying also tends to occur at the same time each day, usually late in the afternoon or early evening or during the busiest time of the day (Behrman, 1992).

Although the exact cause of colic is unknown, overfeeding, primary caretaker anxiety, milk allergy, excessive air swallowing, formulas with a high carbohydrate content, intestinal allergy, immaturity of the digestive system, and tension in the household may all contribute to crying episodes (Crawshaw, 1985).

The goal of management is to determine, if possible, the factors that contribute to an episode of colic in the individual infant, to provide support for the parents, and to provide relief for the infant. No one method of treatment seems to consistently provide relief. Parents are taught numerous possible interventions to allay the infant's crying and discomfort.

Infants should not be overfed or offered food every time they cry. The nurse should review overfeeding, calorie and ounce requirements, formula preparation, and feeding techniques with the primary caretaker.

Prior to an anticipated episode, the infant should be dressed warmly and comfortably, with socks or booties. Some infants respond to being wrapped snugly in a blanket. The infant should be engaged in a rhythmic, soothing activity, as can be achieved in an automatic swing, a back or chest carrier, vibrating mat or chair, a rocking cradle or chair, a ride in the stroller or car, or by a gentle massage. Some infants are soothed by a pacifier or by thumb sucking.

Some infants respond to warmth, as provided by a warm bath or placement on a well-covered, partially filled hot-water bottle or heating pad at the lowest setting. Extreme caution should be exercised to avoid burning or overheating the infant. Lying prone on a hard surface such as a parent's knees or a firm mattress may provide relief.

A reduction in activities, tension, and noise during the time that the crying episode occurs may also soothe the infant. Soft, continuous or monotonous music or sound helps some infants. Two ounces of sweetened, noncaffeinated peppermint tea has been found useful by some parents.

Parents should avoid becoming fatigued or exhausted. The nurse should explore possible options with the parents. If all else fails, the parents should ensure that the infant is safe, fed, and dry; position the infant in the crib or rocking cradle in a different room; and let the infant cry until he or she falls asleep. Some parents play music as distraction from the crying. If this suggestion sounds particularly unkind, the reality of an infant who cries for periods of 2 hours or longer should be considered. The nurse should encourage the parents to be loving, kind, and supportive with the infant. The infant does not have control over the discomfort.

▶ Fever

A fever is a body temperature elevated above normal. Fever is the most common reason that parents seek medical attention for their infants and children. Parents often lack knowledge not only about fever, but about the measurement and management of fever as well. It is a problem that must be addressed at all educational and socioeconomic levels.

To be reliable partners with health care providers, parents must know normal and elevated temperature values, know how to take a temperature and reduce a fever, be able to follow treatment orders and administer medications safely, and know when to seek further assistance from health care personnel. In the neonatal period, fever above 99°F axillary or 100.4°F rectally is cause for parents to seek advice from the health care provider. Fever is often the first sign that the newborn has a bacterial infection in the blood (septicemia), the urine (urinary tract infection), lung (pneumonia), or meninges (meningitis) (Behrman, 1992). Newborns with a fever need prompt attention. In teaching parents about fever, the nurse can reinforce this important point. The nurse should validate that parents know how to correctly take an axillary or rectal temperature and read a thermometer.

Critical Thinking in Care Planning

Care of a Newborn During Assessment

Melissa Lee is a 2-day-old newborn of Chinese-American parents, Steven and Kimberly Lee. Steven is 26 years old and is a manager of a bookstore. Kimberly is 24 years old and is a student at a nearby community college. They have been married for 3 years and are renting a two-bedroom apartment. Melissa is their first child. The health history reveals no parental or family health problems. Steven smokes cigarettes in the home and car.

Melissa was delivered vaginally with low forceps after approximately 9½ hours of labor without complication. Mother had an epidural block but no other medications were used during labor or delivery. Father was present during labor and delivery. Parents and Melissa spent approximately one-half hour together in the delivery room afterwards.

Melissa had no problems at birth and had Apgar scores of 9 at 1 minute and 9 at 5 minutes. Her birth weight was 7 pounds 2 oz and her blood type O+. Melissa has been breastfed since birth. She is now 2 days old and weighs 6 pounds 8 oz. Melissa is rooming-in with her mother. The parents are concerned about Melissa's weight loss, the color and consistency of her stools, and "bruising" on her back.

The results of a physical examination are as follows:
Age: 2 days
Weight: 6 pounds 8 oz (25th percentile)
Length: 19 in. (25th percentile)
Head: 34 cm (25th percentile)
Chest: 33.5 cm
VS: 98.2°F, HR: 130, RR: 40
General appearance: Neonate is a content, alert, responsive female who appears in no acute distress.
Skin: Pink; mongolian spot at posterior lumbar region approximate 2 × 3-cm area; milia on nose; good turgor; no rashes, petechiae, or lesions; nails pink with rapid capillary refill.
Head: Round, anterior and posterior fontanelles soft and flat; anterior fontanelle 1 × 1 cm; posterior fontanelle ½ cm; suture lines palpable within nor-

mal limits; no caput succedaneum or cephalhematoma; no abrasions, lacerations, or lesions; full head of black silky hair.
Face: Symmetric with Asian features; movement equal bilaterally.
Eyes: Sclera clear; conjunctiva clear and pink; bilateral epicanthal folds, no ptosis, lid lag, or deformity; eye movements random without pseudostrabismus; positive blink reflex; cornea and lens clear; positive red reflexes bilaterally; irises dark gray/black; no coloboma or Brushfield's spots.
Ears: Pinnae well formed and firm with instant recoil; normal alignment with eyes; no preauricular skin tags; auditory canals patent bilaterally; tympanic membranes translucent, mobile with normal light reflex; responds to bell.
Nose: Symmetric, patent without septal deviation, mucosa pink without discharge; no flaring of nostrils.
Mouth and Throat: Lips symmetric and pink without lesions; gums and mucosa pink, moist without lesions; tongue midline, symmetric; Epstein's pearls noted midline on hard palate; soft and hard palate intact without lesions; saliva within normal limits; uvula midline.
Neck: Supple with full range of motion; trachea midline; no masses or lymphadenopathy.
Chest: Symmetric without masses or tenderness; nipples symmetric without supernumerary nipples; clavicles within normal limits; breath sounds clear and equal bilaterally without rales, rhonchi, or wheezing; no retractions or grunting.
Heart: Pulse regular; PMI, left fourth intercostal space at midclavicular line, diameter 1 cm; femoral, dorsalis pedis, and brachial pulses full and equal throughout; S_1 and S_2; no murmur, gallop, or extra sounds.
Abdomen: Symmetric, rounded, soft, nontender without masses or organomegaly; umbilical cord attached with application of triple-dye stain, umbilicus healing without signs of infection, or bleeding, discharge; no umbilical or inguinal hernia; bowel

(continued)

Critical Thinking in Care Planning continued

sounds active in all four quadrants; superficial abdominal reflexes within normal limits.

Genitalia: External female genitalia within normal limits without erythema, rash, or discharge.

Anus and rectum: Anus midline, patent; adequate sphincter tone with positive wink reflex; no fissures, bleeding, or rashes.

Extremities and spine: Extremities symmetric in movement and appearance; muscle tone within normal limits; full range of motion throughout; hips abduct equally with negative Ortolani movement; no polydactyly or syndactyly; creases within normal limits; spine straight, flexible without deformities; no pilonidal dimple.

Neonatal reflexes: Primitive reflexes within normal limits; positive Moro, palmar and plantar, tonic neck, sucking, swallowing, rooting, Babinski, stepping and placing, Galant's, crossed extension, magnet, traction, arm recoil, crawling, and glabellar reflexes.

▶ Assessment

- Well 2-day-old Asian female neonate
- Weight loss in normal range
- Stools of breastfed infant
- Mongolian spot present

- Parents are concerned about neonate having lost weight, about "diarrhea," and about "bruising" on her back
- Father smokes cigarettes in the home and car

Nursing Diagnosis

Knowledge deficit (parental), related to normal newborn characteristics and variations

Expected Client/Family Outcomes	Nursing Action/Intervention	Evaluation
By the 3rd postpartum day, parents will verbally express understanding of selected normal newborn characteristics, including: - Weight loss - Bowel and bladder elimination - Skin variations	Encourage parents to be present at physical examination so that newborn characteristics can be demonstrated and explained, including voiding and stool patterns for breastfed neonates and skin features. Teach parents physiologic reasons for weight loss and normal patterns of weight gain in neonates. Give parents written literature about newborn characteristics to reinforce verbal explanations. Provide anticipatory guidance to parents about resources for concerns and questions. *Rationale:* Uncertainty increases anxiety. Increased knowledge tends to decrease anxiety. Anticipation of parents' concerns will help decrease fears of the unknown.	When asked, parents describe characteristics and patterns of weight gain in the neonate.

Critical Thinking in Care Planning continued

Nursing Diagnosis

Risk for injury, related to father's smoking in the home and car

Expected Client/Family Outcomes	Nursing Action/Intervention	Evaluation
By the first well-child visit, neonate's environment will be smoke free.	Provide parents with information about passive smoking and increased risk for respiratory disease when exposed to cigarette smoke. *Rationale:* Passive smoke inhalation increases the risk of respiratory disease. Assist parents in developing a plan to maintain a "smoke-free" environment for neonate both at home and in car. Refer father to smoking cessation program. Specialized strategies and support may be necessary to eliminate smoking habit. Provide anticipatory guidance about fire safety in home: • Smoke detectors • Fire extinguishers • Plan for escape from home • Home fire drills • Easy access to phone numbers for fire department • Tot-finder labels for windows and doors	At first well-child visit, parents describe measures instituted to provide smoke-free environment for neonate. At the first well-child visit, parents describe safety features that have been instituted in the home.

Chapter Highlights

▶ Critical events of transition from intrauterine to extrauterine life include respiratory adjustment, cardiovascular adjustment, hematologic adjustment, and thermal regulation.

▶ Other neonatal body systems that adjust at birth include the urinary, integumentary, endocrine, gastrointestinal, hepatic, immunologic, and neurologic systems.

▶ Neonates have characteristic behavioral states and responses that can be categorized into six levels of arousal: deep sleep, light sleep, drowsiness or semidozing, quiet alert, active alert, and intense crying.

▶ Newborns behave in predictable ways, such as the orienting response, habituation, consolability, cuddliness, and motor organization, and parents need to know about these behaviors so they can be sensitive to the newborn's cues.

▶ The immediate nursing assessment of the newborn includes assignment of an Apgar score and screening procedures for phenylketonuria, galactosemia, hypothyroidism, sickle-cell disease, syphilis, and hearing.

▶ The newborn's first physical examination upon admission to the nursery includes vital signs, growth parameters (weight and length), physical assessment, assessment of gestational age, and behavioral assessment.

▶ Nursing care of the neonate focuses on maintaining a patent airway; promoting thermoregulation; preventing hemorrhage; preventing infection; promoting parent–newborn attachment; identifying the newborn; promoting nutritional well-being; and assessing the educational needs of parents.

▶ Major concerns of parents of the newborn include handling and positioning; nasal and oral suctioning; circumcision care; cord care; bathing and skin care; elimination patterns; clothing and wrapping; promoting growth and development; preventing communicable diseases; preventing accidents; normal sleep patterns; and consequences of being a working parent.

▶ Several stressors that may affect the neonate are physiologic jaundice, obstruction of the lacrimal ducts, skin problems, thrush, colic, and fever.

▶ Nursing care through discharge planning includes parent teaching and coordinating follow-up with community-based nurses and the primary care provider.

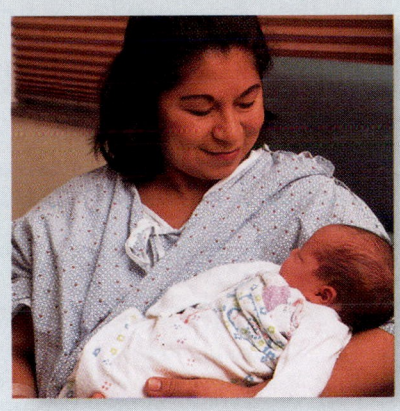

After reading the vignette at the beginning of this chapter, use what you have learned to answer these questions.

1. What advice can the nurse give this couple about infant safety?

2. What strategies can Gloria Rinaldi, RN, use to promote Carmen and Emilio Lopez's confidence in caring for their baby?

3. What should new parents be taught about the care of the healthy newborn?

Critical Thinking Questions

▶ # References

Als H., & Brazelton, T.B. (1981). A new model of assessing behavioral organization in preterm and full-term infants. *Journal of the American Academy of Child Psychiatry, 20,* 239.

American Academy of Pediatrics. (1989). Report of the task force on circumcision. *Pediatrics, 84,* 388–391.

American Academy of Pediatrics. (1997). *1997 red book: Report of the Committee on Infectious Diseases* (24th ed.). Elk Grove Village, IL: Author.

Avery, G.B., & Fletcher, A.B. (1993). Nutrition. In G. Avery (Ed.), *Neonatology: Pathophysiology and management of the newborn* (4th ed.) (pp. 330–356). Philadelphia: J.B. Lippincott.

Ballard, J.L., Khoury, J.C., Wedig, K., Wang, L., Eilers-Walsman, B.L., & Lipp, R. (1991). New Ballard Score, expanded to include extremely premature infants. *Journal of Pediatrics, 119,* 417–423.

Battaglia, F.C., & Lubchenco, L.O. (1967). A practical classification of newborn infants by weight and gestational age. *Journal of Pediatrics, 71,* 159–163.

Behrman, R.E. (1992). *Nelson textbook of pediatrics* (14th ed.). Philadelphia: W.B. Saunders.

Brazelton, T.B. (1973). *The neonatal behavioral assessment scale* (National Spastics Foundation No. 50). London: William Heinemann.

Brazelton, T.B. (1984). *Neonatal behavioral assessment scale* (2nd ed.). Philadelphia: J.B. Lippincott.

Brazelton, T.B. (1993). Behavioral competence of the newborn infant. In G. Avery (Ed.), *Neonatology: Pathophysiology and management of the newborn* (4th ed.) (pp. 289–300). Philadelphia: J.B. Lippincott.

Broussard, E.R., & Hartner, M.S. (1971). Further considerations regarding maternal perception of the first born. In J. Hellmuth (Ed.), *Exceptional infant: Studies in abnormalities* (vol. 2) (pp. 432–439). New York: Brunner/Mazel.

Cashoro, W.J. (1993). Hyperbilirubinemia. In J.J. Pomerance & C.J. Richardson (Eds.), *Neonatology* (pp. 231–241). Norwalk, CT: Appleton & Lange.

Charlton, V.E., & Phibbs, R.H. (1996). Examination of the newborn. In A.M. Rudolph (Ed.), *Rudolph's pediatrics* (pp. 208–218). Norwalk, CT: Appleton & Lange.

Crawshaw, J.P. (1985). The fussy infant: Dealing with colic. *Patient Care, 19,* 93.

De Carvalho, M., Hall, M., & Harvey, D. (1981). Effects of water supplementation in physiologic jaundice in breast-fed babies. *Archives of Disease in Childhood, 56,* 568–569.

De Carvalho, M., Klaus, M.H., & Merkatz, R.B. (1982). Frequency of breast-feeding and serum bilirubin concentration. *American Journal of Diseases of Childhood, 136,* 737–738.

De Carvalho, M., Robertson, S., & Klaus, M. (1985). Fecal bilirubin excretion and serum bilirubin concentrations in breast-fed and bottle-fed infants. *Journal of Pediatrics, 107,* 786–790.

De Casper, A., & Fifer, W. (1980). Of human bonding: Newborns prefer their mother's voices. *Science, 208,* 1174–1176.

Di George, A.M. (1992). Disorders of the thyroid gland. In R.E. Behrman (Ed.), *Nelson Textbook of Pediatrics* (pp. 1414–1421) Philadelphia: W.B. Saunders Company.

Dubowitz, L.M., Dubowitz, V., Goldberg, C. (1970). Clinical assessment of gestational age in the newborn infant. *Journal of Pediatrics, 77,* 1–10.

Edelman, C., & Mandle, C. (1994). *Health promotion throughout the lifespan* (3rd ed.). St. Louis: Mosby.

Eisenberg, R.B. (1970). The development of hearing in man: An assessment of current status. *Journal of the American Speech and Hearing Association, 12,* 119–123.

Hammerschlag, M.R. (1989). Medical progress: Chlamydial infections. *Journal of Pediatrics, 114,* 727–734.

Hey, E., & Scopes, J.W. (1993). Thermoregulation in the newborn. In G. Avery (Ed.), *Neonatology: Pathophysiology and management of the newborn* (4th ed.) (pp. 357–365). Philadelphia: J.B. Lippincott.

Hill, S.T., & Shronk, L.K. (1983). The effect of early parent-infant contact on newborn body temperature. In L.N. Sherwen & C.T. Weingarten (Eds.), *Analysis and application of nursing research: Parent-neonate studies* (pp. 239–247). Belmont, CA: Wadsworth.

Kaye, K. (1982). *The mental and social life of babies.* Chicago: University of Chicago Press.

Klaus, M.H., Martin, R.J., & Fanaroff, A.A. (1993). The physical environment. In M.H. Klaus & A.A. Fanaroff (Eds.), *Care of the high-risk neonate* (4th ed.) (pp. 114–129). Philadelphia: W. B. Saunders.

Leyden, J.J. (1986). Diaper dermatitis. *Pediatric Dermatology, 4,* 23–28.

MacFarlane, A. (1975). Olfaction in the development of social preferences in the human neonate. In *Parent-infant evaluation* (Ciba Foundation Symposium vol. 33). New York: American Elsevier.

Maisels, M.J. (1993). Jaundice. In G. Avery (Ed.), *Neonatology: Pathophysiology and management of the newborn* (4th ed.) (pp. 630–725). Philadelphia: J.B. Lippincott.

Maisels, M.J., & Gifford, K. (1986). Normal serum bilirubin levels in the newborn and the effect of breastfeeding. *Pediatrics, 78,* 743.

Martin, R.J., Fanaroff, A.A., & Klaus, M.H. (1993). Respiratory problems. In M.H. Klaus & A.A. Fanaroff (Eds.), *Care of the high-risk neonate* (4th ed.) (pp. 228–259). Philadelphia: W.B. Saunders.

Moore, K.L. (1993). *The developing human: Clinically oriented embryology* (5th ed.). Philadelphia: W.B. Saunders.

Moshang, T., & Bongiovanni, A.M. (1993). Endocrine disorders of the newborn. In G. Avery (Ed.), *Neonatology: Pathophysiology and management of the newborn* (4th ed.) (pp. 764–791). Philadelphia: J.B. Lippincott.

Nelson, N.M. (1993). In G. Avery (Ed.), *Neonatology: Pathophysiology and management of the newborn* (4th ed.) (pp. 223–247). Philadelphia: J.B. Lippincott.

Oliver, T.K. (1987). The newborn. In V.C. Kelley (Ed.), *Practice of pediatrics* (vol. 2) (pp. 1–16). Philadelphia: Harper & Row.

Owen, M.T., Easterbrooks, M.A., Chase-Lansdale, L., & Goldberg, W.A. (1984). The relation between maternal employment status and the stability of attachments to mother and father. *Child Development, 55,* 1894–1901.

Penny-MacGillivray, T. (1996). A newborn's first bath: When? *Journal of Obstetric, Gynecologic, and Neonatal Nursing, 25*(6), 481–487.

Rantz, R.L. (1965). Visual perception from birth as shown by pattern selectivity. *Annals of the New York Academy of Sciences, 118,* 793.

Schumacher, R.E., Thornbery, J.M., & Gutcher, G.R. (1985). Transcutaneous bilirubinometry: A comparison of old and new methods. *Pediatrics, 76,* 10–14.

Sickle Cell Disease Guideline Panel. (1993). *Sickle cell disease: Screening, diagnosis, management, and counseling in newborns and infants. Clinical practice guideline no. 6* (AHCPR Pub. No. 93-0562). Rockville, MD: Agency for Health Care Policy and Research, Public Health Service, U. S. Department of Health and Human Services.

Taeusch, H.W. (1991). Initial evaluation: History and physical examination of the newborn. In H.W. Taeusch, R.A. Ballard, & M.E. Avery (Eds.), *Schaffer and Avery's diseases of the newborn* (6th ed.) (pp. 207–224). Philadelphia: W.B. Saunders.

Truog, W.E. (1987). Care of the newborn in the delivery room. In V.C. Kelley (Ed.), *Practice of pediatrics* (vol. 2) (pp. 1–7). Philadelphia: Harper & Row.

U.S. Centers for Disease Control and Prevention. (1996). Hepatitis B. In W. Atkinson, L. Furphy, M. Gantt, M. Mayfield, & G. Thyne (Eds.), *Epidemiology and prevention of vaccine-preventable diseases* (3rd ed.) (pp. 125–144). Washington, DC: U.S. Department of Health and Human Services.

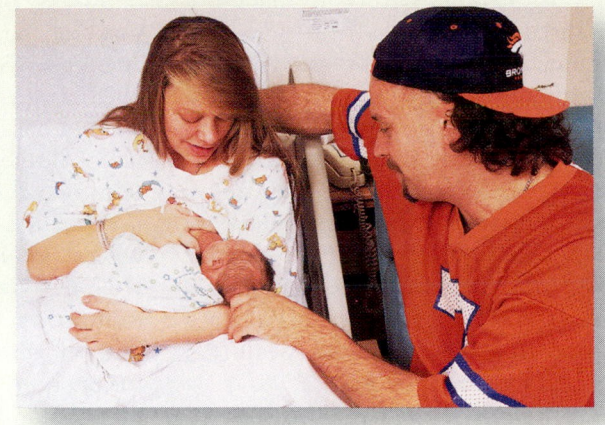

Allison and George Mahoney decided early in Allison's pregnancy that they wanted to breastfeed their baby. Immediately after their daughter Lisa was born, Allison breastfed her for the first time. Since that initial feeding, Allison has been eager to learn about breastfeeding techniques and feels confident about being able to provide for her baby's needs.

The family is visiting together and Allison is breastfeeding Lisa. As Lucy Salas, RN, checks on their progress, George, who has his arm around his wife and baby, states, "I'm really glad that Allison is doing so well with breastfeeding. I only wish that I could be a little more involved with feeding Lisa. What can I do that would help with her care?" ∎

31
Postpartum and Newborn Nutrition

Nutrition is integral in promoting a healthy recovery for the new mother. Postpartum women have unique nutrient needs which must be met in order for them to meet the demands of motherhood. If a woman chooses to breastfeed her infant, then the role of her diet takes on an even greater significance in promoting overall wellness. Meeting the specific needs of infants is critical in promoting the rapid growth and development that normally occurs during the first year of life. Breast milk or infant formula should be provided until the infant reaches one year of age. Solid foods can be introduced into the infant's diet based on the developmentally appropriate time. Nurses have a key role as client educators in promoting healthy nutrition for new mothers and their babies.

▶ POSTPARTUM NUTRITION

▶ Restoration of Nutritional Status

The nutrient needs of a postpartum woman are related to her decision to breastfeed, the demands of replacing nutrient stores, and the desire to return to prepregnancy weight. Each of these conditions creates unique nutrient needs for the postpartum mother and influences dietary recommendations. Many factors place postpartum mothers at nutritional risk. Stores of calcium, folic acid, and vitamin B6 may decrease during gestation (Mitchell, 1997). Mothers who had poor gestational weight gain, multiple births, and low body weight may be at nutritional risk. Fatigue, weight loss, and changes in appetite are areas of special concern that need to be addressed during dietary counseling. Women who are identified as having poor diets should supplement their food intake with a prenatal vitamin and mineral supplement.

▶ Postpartum Body Weight

After birth of their infant, most postpartum mothers have a strong desire to return to their normal prepregnancy weight. More than two-thirds of the weight gained during pregnancy is due to an increase in maternal tissue and water. The additional weight is derived from increases in plasma volume and red blood cell mass. Maternal fat deposition during pregnancy serves as an adaptation that provides adequate energy for the last trimester and helps to support the energy needs of lactation. The immediate weight loss after delivery is approximately 10–12 pounds. It includes 1.5 pounds for the placenta, 2 pounds of blood and amniotic fluid, and the weight of the baby.

Within the next 2–4 days, diuresis results in the loss of an additional 5 pounds. With complete involution, about 1.8 pounds will be lost. Additional weight is lost for several weeks as a result of circulatory changes (Greene, Smiciklas-Wright, Scholl, & Karp, 1988). If gestational weight gain is excessive, then the mother has an increased risk for pregnancy-associated weight retention and postpartum overweight and obesity (Scholl, Hediger, Schall, Ances, & Smith, 1995).

Several strategies can be advised for mothers whose goal is to return to normal prepregnancy weight. For the breastfeeding mother, a significant reduction in kcal should be avoided, as this may interfere with normal lactation. Dietary recommendations for postpartum women promote a healthy eating plan that contains a variety of foods with adequate portion sizes such as illustrated by the USDA Food Guide Pyramid. Quick weight loss plans should be avoided, as they may prevent nutrient restoration and contribute to the mother's fatigue. An aerobic exercise program can be advised to facilitate weight loss of stored body fat.

▶ Nutritional Needs of Breastfeeding Mothers

To provide enough nutritionally adequate breast milk, a lactating mother needs a diet higher in calories and fluids than that of a nonpregnant, nonlactating woman. Lactating women on average require an additional 640 kcal/day during the first six months of breastfeeding and an additional 510 kcal for the second six-month period. Kcal needs thereafter are determined by the frequency of feeding and thus the average daily milk production. As fat storage during pregnancy provides between 100 and 150 kcal/day for the first six postpartum months, an increase of 500 kcal/day over nonpregnant intake is required for lactation. The total daily energy requirements vary among women but, in general, 2700 kcal/day is recommended. Caloric intake frequently needs to be further adjusted when the mother breastfeeds the infant more than 3 months, when there is more than one infant, and when the mother is below her ideal weight (National Research Council, 1989).

Lactating women need approximately 2500 to 3000 mL of fluid each day to produce enough breast milk. The breastfeeding woman should therefore be encouraged to consume up to 8 glasses of fluids per day. Excessive maternal sweating and thirst during hot weather and strenuous activity are indications that fluid intake needs to be increased. Additionally, the infant may demand more breast milk during growth spurts and in hot weather, requiring that the mother in turn increase her fluid intake.

The increased calories and fluids should provide the nutrients required for breast milk production and nutritionally adequate breast milk. Table 31–1 provides the Recommended Daily Allowances for lactating women. Several nutrients are needed in greater amounts during lactation. A total daily protein intake of 62 to 65 g per day is required to support the energy and nutritional needs of lactation. Lactating women are advised to continue to consume at least 1200 mg of calcium per day. Phosphorus, which is also needed for infant skeletal development, should be increased by 400 mg over the nonpregnant level. If too much phosphorus is ingested, calcium absorption will be decreased; if not enough calcium is ingested and absorbed, calcium deposited in maternal bones will be depleted. Requirements for water soluble vitamins are also increased to aid in energy production by the body. Increased amounts of vitamins A, C, and E are needed to promote functional and structural properties of cells. Trace mineral requirements are also increased to meet the losses that occur during lactation.

▶ TABLE 31–1

Recommended Dietary Allowances for Lactation

Nutrient	Nonlactating Women (25–50 y)	Lactating Women 0–6 mo	Lactating Women 6–12 mo
Energy (kcal)	2200	2700	2700
Protein (g)	50	65	62
Vitamin A (RE)	800	1300	1200
Vitamin C (mg)	60	95	90
Vitamin D (µg)	5	10	10
Vitamin E (mg)	8	12	11
Vitamin K (µg)	65	65	65
Thiamin (mg)	1.1	1.6	1.6
Riboflavin (mg)	1.3	1.8	1.7
Niacin (mg)	15	20	20
Vitamin B_6 (mg)	1.6	2.1	2.1
Vitamin B_{12} (µg)	2.0	2.6	2.6
Folate (µg)	180	280	260
Calcium (mg)	800	1200	1200
Phosphorus (mg)	800	1200	1200
Magnesium (mg)	280	355	340
Iron (mg)	15	15	15
Iodine (µg)	150	200	200
Zinc (mg)	12	19	16
Selenium (µg)	55	75	75

Source: National Research Council, Food and Nutrition Board, 1989.

A healthy diet during lactation is just as important as it was during pregnancy. Table 31–2 provides a daily food guide for lactating women. Breastfeeding women should receive dietary counseling to assist them in making healthy food choices. Because of the increased need for nutrients, lactating women also are sometimes advised to take a vitamin and mineral supplement.

Caffeine and alcohol consumption by the lactating mother may have negative effects on the infant. Large amounts of caffeine-containing beverages can cause irritability and wakefulness in infants. Alcohol, when consumed by the nursing mother, is secreted in the breast milk. Among other serious effects on the infant, alcohol can cause a decrease in infant consumption of milk and can interfere with the milk letdown reflex (Mennella & Beauchamp, 1991). Breastfeeding mothers should therefore be advised to avoid alcohol and large amounts of caffeine in their diet.

▶ PROMOTING NUTRITIONAL WELL-BEING IN INFANTS

The interaction that occurs between the mother and newborn during the act of feeding is vital for both the physical and psychologic development of the baby. Knowledge about the nutritional needs of infants, lactation, formula feeding, feeding patterns, feeding recommendations, and feeding problems is important in ensuring the nutritional and emotional health of the infant and family.

▶ Nutritional Needs of the Newborn/Infant

The Food and Nutrition Board bases its recommended dietary allowances for infants during the first 6 months of life on the nutrients in human milk and the amount of that milk ingested by healthy infants of well-nourished mothers (National Research Council Food and Nutrition Board, 1989). The American Academy of Pediatrics recommends that all infants be breastfed until they are at least 1 year old (American Academy of Pediatrics, 1997). The Recommended Dietary Allowances (RDAs) are used as a guide in predicting the nutritional requirements for each infant and are presented in Table 31–3.

Infants need the same nutrients as older children and adults; however, a larger quantity of each nutrient is needed per unit of infant body weight. For example, the infant needs 115 kcal/kg body weight

▶ **TABLE 31–2**

Daily Food Guide for Lactating Women

Food Group	One Serving Equals		Recommended Minimum Servings
Protein Foods Provide protein, iron, zinc, and B vitamins for growth of muscles, bone, blood, and nerves. Vegetable protein provides fiber to prevent constipation.	**Animal Protein** 1 oz cooked chicken or turkey 1 oz cooked lean beef, lamb, or pork 1 oz or 1/4 c fish or other seafood 1 egg 2 fish sticks or hot dogs 2 slices luncheon meat	**Vegetable Protein** ½ c cooked dry beans, lentils, or split peas 3 oz tofu 1 oz or ¼ c peanuts, pumpkin, or sunflower seeds 1½ oz or ½ c other nuts 2 tbsp peanut butter	7 One serving of vegetable protein daily
Milk Products Provide protein and calcium to build strong bones, teeth, healthy nerves and muscles, and to promote normal blood clotting.	8 oz milk 8 oz yogurt 1 c milk shake 1½ c cream soup (made with milk) 1½ oz or ⅓ c grated cheese (like cheddar, monterey, mozzarella, or swiss)	1½-2 slices presliced American cheese 4 tbsp parmesan cheese 2 c cottage cheese 1 c pudding 1 c custard or flan 1½ c ice milk, ice cream, or frozen yogurt	3
Breads, Cereals, Grains Provide carbohydrates and B vitamins for energy and healthy nerves. Also provide iron for healthy blood. Whole grains provide fiber to prevent constipation.	1 slice bread 1 dinner roll ½ bun or bagel ½ English muffin or pita 1 small tortilla ¾ c dry cereal ½ c granola ½ c cooked cereal	½ c rice ½ c noodles or spaghetti ¼ c wheat germ 1 4-inch pancake or waffle 1 small muffin 8 medium crackers 4 graham cracker squares 3 c popcorn	7
Vitamin C–Rich Fruits and Vegetables Provide vitamin C to prevent infection and to promote healing and iron absorption. Also provide fiber to prevent constipation.	6 oz orange, grapefruit, or fruit juice enriched with vitamin C 6 oz tomato juice or vegetable juice cocktail 1 orange, kiwi, mango ½ grapefruit, cantaloupe ½ c papaya 2 tangerines	½ c strawberries ½ c cooked or 1 c raw cabbage ½ c broccoli, Brussels sprouts, or cauliflower ½ c snow peas, sweet peppers, or tomato puree 2 tomatoes	1
Vitamin A–Rich Fruits and Vegetables Provide beta-carotene and vitamin A to prevent infection and to promote wound healing and night vision. Also provide fiber to prevent constipation.	6 oz apricot nectar or vegetable juice cocktail 3 raw or ¼ c dried apricots ¼ cantaloupe or mango 1 small or ½ c sliced carrots 2 tomatoes	½ c cooked or 1 c raw spinach ½ c cooked greens (beet, chard, collards, dandelion, kale, mustard) ½ c pumpkin, sweet potato, winter squash, or yams	1
Other Fruits and Vegetables Provide carbohydrates for energy and fiber to prevent constipation.	6 oz fruit juice (if not listed above) 1 medium or ½ c sliced fruit (apple, banana, peach, pear) ½ c berries (other than strawberries) ½ c cherries or grapes ½ c pineapple ½ c watermelon	¼ c dried fruit ½ c sliced vegetable (asparagus, beets, green beans, celery, corn, eggplant, mushrooms, onion, peas, potato, summer squash, zucchini) ½ artichoke 1 c lettuce	3
Unsaturated Fats Provide vitamin E to protect tissue.	⅓ medium avocado 1 tsp margarine 1 tsp mayonnaise 1 tsp vegetable oil	2 tsp salad dressing (mayonnaise-based) 1 tbsp salad dressing (oil-based)	3

Source: Reproduced, with permission, from Mitchell, M.K. (1997). Nutrition across the life span. Philadelphia: W.B. Saunders.

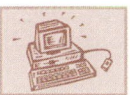

Research Abstract

Nutritional Inadequacies in the Diets of Low-Income Breastfeeding Women

The American Academy of Pediatricians (1997) recommends breastfeeding for all newborn infants (with a few execptions) for at least the first 12 months of infancy. In 1995, 59.7% of U.S. newborns were breastfed (American Academy of Pediatrics, 1997). Breastfeeding mothers have increased energy and nutrient needs to meet the demands of lactation. Despite the evidence for breastfeeding promotion and the increased nutrient needs for lactation, there is limited research in the area of actual nutrient intake of American women who choose to breastfeed their infants.

This study investigated the energy and nutrient intakes of 183 low-income breastfeeding women at 3 months postpartum. The subjects were participants of the Canadian health promotion program "Better Beginnings, Better Futures." Participants were interviewed by trained research assistants who collected sociodemographic information, breastfeeding information, and a 24-hour dietary recall. The mean age of the participants was 29 years of age, and 55% had completed some education beyond high school despite their low-income financial status. The researchers noted that the breastfeeding mothers were more highly educated than the other mothers who chose to participate in the Better Beginnings, Better Futures projects and suggested that they may be experiencing recent poverty rather than chronic poverty.

Both the mean and median intakes of energy were lower than the Recommended Dietary Allowances (RDAs) for lactating women (2190 kcal versus 2700 kcal). Median intake of folate, calcium, thiamin, iron, zinc, and vitamin A were also below the recommended intake. Protein intakes met the RDAs. The average kcal distribution of the energy nutrients were as follows: protein, 16.2%; carbohydrate, 54.3%; and lipid, 30.4%. Dietary deficiencies can cause depletion of nutrient maternal stores and tissue levels. If lactating women are malnourished, the fatty acid and vitamin content of the milk may also be altered.

Twenty-five percent of the subjects reported taking supplements. The nutrient intake from supplementation was not incorporated into the dietary intake analysis. The researchers did not find an association between level of poverty and energy and nutrient intake. They attributed this lack of correlation to the high educational level of the participants.

Application to Practice

Breastfeeding promotion interventions should include strategies to encourage a healthy diet for the lactating mother. Particular attention should be given to promoting an adequate energy intake, including foods concentrated in calcium, folate, zinc, and iron. Low-income breastfeeding mothers should be referred to the Women, Infants, and Children Supplemental Food Program (WIC). Eligible participants of WIC can receive individual nutritional counseling and vouchers to purchase healthy foods.

Source: Doran, L., & Evers, S. (1997). Energy and nutrient inadequacies in the diets of low-income women who breastfeed. Journal of the American Dietetic Association, 97(11); 1283–1287.

per day during the first 6 months of life as compared with the adult female, who needs 36 kcal/kg body weight. The infant's kilocalorie need per unit of weight is therefore more than three times that of the adult.

Energy Needs
The energy needs of a newborn are determined by the basal metabolic rate, physical activity, growth and maintenance, urinary and fecal losses, and the thermic effect of food. The RDA for energy is 115 kcal/kg per day (52 kcal/pound) during the first 6 months and 105 kcal/kg per day (47 kcal/pound) during the second 6 months (National Research Council Food and Nutrition Board, 1989).

To assess if an infant's energy intake is sufficient, height and weight measurements should be monitored regularly. Increases in height and weight growth

► **TABLE 31-3**

Recommended Dietary Allowances for Normal Infants During the First Year

	0–6 Months	6–12 Months
Weight		
kg	6	9
pounds	13	20
Height		
cm	60	71
inches	24	28
Nutrient	**RDA**	**RDA**
Protein, g	13	14
Vitamin A, µg RE[a]	375	375
Vitamin D, µg[b]	7.5	10
Vitamin E, mg TE[c]	3	4
Vitamin K, mg	5	10
Ascorbic acid, mg	30	35
Thiamine, mg	0.3	0.4
Riboflavin, mg	0.4	0.5
Niacin, mg NE[d]	5	6
Vitamin B_6, mg	0.3	0.6
Vitamin B_{12}, µg	0.3	0.5
Folacin, µg	25	35
Calcium, mg	400	600
Phosphorus, mg	300	500
Magnesium, mg	40	60
Iodine, µg	40	50
Iron, mg	6	10
Zinc, mg	5	5
Selenium, µg	10	15

[a]Retinol equivalents. 1 retinol equivalent = 1 µg retinol or 6 µg beta-carotene.
[b]As cholecalciferol, 10 µg cholecalciferol = 400 IU of vitamin D.
[c]Alpha-tocopherol equivalents. 1 mg d-alpha-tocopherol = 1 alpha-TE.
[d]1 NE (niacin equivalent) is equal to 1 mg of niacin or 60 mg of dietary tryptophan.
Source: National Research Council, Food and Nutrition Board, 1989.

should progress at approximately the same rate. If an infant loses weight, does not gain weight, or reduces his or her rate of growth, then the kcal and nutrient intake of the diet should be closely examined. If growth in height slows or stops, the diet should also be evaluated. If weight gain greatly exceeds the growth in height, the energy intake of the infant should also be evaluated (Pipes, 1996).

Protein

Protein is required for growth and maintenance of tissue. Human milk provides the infant with about 2.2 g protein/kg per day during the first month of life. By the sixth month, protein in breast milk has fallen to 1.5 g/kg per day. The RDA for protein for the first 6 months is 13 g/day, and during the second 6 months, 14 g/day.

Carbohydrates

Lactose accounts for about 40% of the calories in human milk. The lactose content of human milk is higher than that of cow's milk. For this reason, lactose or other simple carbohydrates are added to commercial formulas. The Food and Nutrition Board does not include a recommended daily carbohydrate allowance for infants, but carbohydrates should provide 30–60% of the total kcal (Pipes, 1996).

Lipids

Lipids are needed during infancy to meet the high energy requirements of growth and development. Approximately 45 to 50% of the calories in human milk and most formulas are provided by fat. The fat linoleate supplies 6 to 9% of the calories in human milk. Formulas that furnish 3% of the calories as linoleic acid will meet the infant's needs.

Vitamins

Human milk and commercially prepared formulas furnish most of the RDAs for vitamins. Human milk and cow's milk contain adequate amounts of A and B-complex vitamins; however, although human milk also meets the ascorbic acid (vitamin C) needs of the infant, cow's milk does not. Thus, most commercial formulas are fortified with ascorbic acid. If the formula is not fortified with ascorbic acid, a supplement should be given. The RDA allowance for ascorbic acid is 30 mg/day for the first 6 months of life, and 35 mg/day for the second 6 months.

The RDA for vitamin D is 10 µg (400 IU) per day during the first year of life. Commercial formulas are fortified with vitamin D. Breastfed infants can obtain the required vitamin D through exposure to sunlight, a good source of the vitamin.

The synthesis of vitamin K is delayed for several days after birth because the newborn lacks the necessary intestinal bacterial flora. An intramuscular injection of 0.5 to 1.0 mg of vitamin K (vitamin K_1) is therefore recommended at birth to prevent neonatal hemorrhage.

Minerals

Human milk and commercially prepared formulas fulfill most of the RDAs for minerals. Ensuring adequate iron intake probably requires the most attention in infancy. The iron stores of a healthy infant of a well-nourished mother are adequate for the first 4 to 6 months of postnatal life. The average need of the infant for iron is 1.5 mg/kg per day. The RDA for iron is 6 mg daily for the first 6 months of life and 10 mg daily for the next 6 months.

Although the iron content of breast milk is low, about one half of the iron present in breast milk is absorbed by the infant. Only an estimated 10% of iron is absorbed from formulas. The American Academy of Pediatrics advises the use of iron-fortified formula for formula-fed infants from birth to one year of age (American Academy of Pediatrics, 1993).

Breastfed infants obtain 60 mg calcium per kilogram body weight. The RDA for this mineral is 60 mg/kg per day. Breastfed infants retain about two-thirds of their total calcium intake. Bottle-fed infants retain less than 50% of the total calcium intake from cow's milk formula; however, as formulas contain a higher proportion of calcium than breast milk, the net retention is the same (Mitchell, 1997).

The RDAs for magnesium and zinc are met by both breast milk and formulas. Fluoride is important in preventing tooth decay. However, controversy exists regarding fluoride supplementation in infants. The American Academy of Pediatrics advises fluoride supplements (0.25 mg/day) only in infants to children three years of age whose water fluoride content is less than 0.3 ppm (American Academy of Pediatrics, 1995). Excess fluoride can cause dental fluorisis, a mottling of the enamel of the teeth (Touger–Decker, 1996).

Water

An infant requires more water in relation to body weight than an adult, because the infant's kidneys are unable to concentrate waste efficiently. An infant therefore excretes more water to carry off wastes than an adult. Daily water excretion of the infant is high, about 15% of the body weight. The National Research Council recommends an intake of 1.5 mL/kcal/day of water (National Research Council Food and Nutrition Board, 1989). Breast milk and most commercially prepared infant formulas contain this kcal-to-water content ratio. Supplemental water is usually not required until infants are fed solid foods, with the possible exception of formula-fed infants during hot weather and infants suffering from vomiting and diarrhea.

▶ Differences Between Human Milk and Cow's Milk

The most balanced food available for the human infant is human milk; it is species specific. The nutrients found in human milk are more easily digestible than those contained in cow's milk or artificial formulas. The high lactose content of breast milk facilitates calcium absorption.

Sixty percent of the protein in human milk consists of lactalbumin, which has an amino acid composition very similar to that of human body tissues. In contrast, only 15% of the protein in cow's milk is lactalbumin. The higher percentage of lactalbumin in human milk makes it more easily digestible than cow's milk or artificial formulas. The remaining protein in both human and cow's milk is primarily casein. As whey is easier to digest, the increased whey-to-casein protein ratio in human milk also makes the absorption and utilization of human milk higher than that of cow's milk or artificial formulas. Fifty percent of the kcal content of human milk is derived from lipids. The first milk secreted (called the fore milk) is low in fat but as the breastfeeding session continues, there is a gradual increase in fat content of the milk. Therefore, it is important that infants are breastfed for an adequate time period to obtain more high-fat hind milk.

Although human milk and cow's milk are both low in iron, the iron in human milk is absorbed better than the iron in cow's milk (Lawrence, 1997). Cow's milk contains higher levels of calcium, phosphorus, sodium, and potassium than human milk; however, more calcium is retained from human milk than from cow's milk. Also, the balance of minerals in human milk is sufficient to meet the newborn's needs.

Human milk furnishes the ascorbic acid needs of the infant, whereas cow's milk does not. There is also more vitamin A in human milk than in cow's milk. Both milks are deficient in vitamin D. Additional components present in human milk include folate and thyroid hormone. These are important for DNA synthesis and growth.

▶ Lactation

Establishing and maintaining lactation are highly integrated psychophysiologic processes that occur within the mother–infant dyad. Although in reality the processes are indivisible, the following discussion is divided into three components—anatomic, physiologic, and psychologic—for conceptual ease.

Anatomy of the Breast

The mature human female breast is composed of glandular epithelial tissue embedded in adipose tissue and supported by fibrous connective tissue. Externally, in the center of each mature female breast is the areola, distinguished as the circular pigmented skin area that surrounds the nipple. Montgomery tubercles, small sebaceous glands of the areola, lubricate the nipples.

Each breast, known as a mammary gland, is organized into approximately 15 to 20 lobes. Each lobe, in turn, is divided into lobules. The lobules contain connective tissue that houses alveoli, the secretory cells of the mammary gland. Alveoli are clustered around ductules. These ductules unite to form a single excretory lactiferous (mammary) duct in each lobe. The lactiferous ducts enlarge slightly to form sinuses, or ampullae, behind the nipple and underlying the areola. Each sinus terminates in a small opening on the surface of the nipple, called the mammary papilla. The nipple is well supplied with nerve endings that are particularly sensitive to touch. Each nipple contains bundles of smooth muscle fibers that stiffen to allow for better grasp by the breastfeeding infant.

Physiology of Lactation

Lactation involves the synthesis of human milk by the alveolar cells, the release of milk into the alveolar lumen (secretion stage of lactation), and the ejection of milk through the ductal system (ejection stage of lactation). To prepare for lactation the human mammary gland undergoes physiologic changes during pregnancy and the early postpartum. The changes are accompanied by anatomic changes in breast tissue (see Fig. 6–19). Prenatally, estrogen stimulates proliferation and differentiation of the ductal system within the breast. Progesterone increases the lobes, lobules, and alveoli. By the end of pregnancy, the anterior pituitary gland secretes increasing levels of prolactin, resulting in additional proliferation of epithelial cells in the mammary glands and in the production of a new group of enzymes involved with carbohydrate metabolism. In addition, hPL stimulates the alveolar cells to begin lactogenesis, or milk production, so that by the third trimester the breasts may secrete colostrum, a yellow, premilk substance. Colostrum is high in protein and contains antibodies, particularly immunoglobulins G and A (IgG and IgA). The antibody-rich colostrum may act protectively in the newborn's gastrointestinal system. Colostrum production gradually diminishes after delivery. In some primiparous women, colostrum production may persist for a couple of weeks.

As the production of true breast milk begins, the breasts become larger, firmer, heavier, and more tender. The breast veins distend and become more prominent. By 3 to 5 days after delivery, bluish white milk is produced. In some multiparous women breast milk production begins before 3 days postpartum. The bluish white milk is slightly lower in protein than colostrum.

Secretion Stage. Prolactin is the hormone primarily responsible for stimulating the synthesis of milk and its release into the alveolar lumen. With delivery of the placenta, levels of progesterone and estrogen decrease, thereby diminishing their probable inhibitory effect on prolactin production. In addition, the hypothalamus no longer produces a prolactin-inhibitory factor following delivery. Consequently, with the removal of prolactin-inhibitory agents, the anterior pituitary gland's secretion of the hormone increases soon after delivery. Prolactin acts on the alveolar cells. Within those cells, lactose, fat, casein, and some proteins are synthesized and combined with other proteins, vitamins, minerals, and water from maternal plasma. In a few days, true human milk is produced. It is secreted into the alveolar lumen and remains there, awaiting ejection stimuli.

Although prolactin is directly responsible for milk secretion, other factors indirectly influence the process. For example, enough growth hormone and adrenal corticosteroids are needed to begin lactation. More important, the frequency and the length of time the infant suckles influence the amount of milk secreted. In the first few weeks, the mother usually produces more milk than is required for her infant. Gradually, however, the amount of milk produced is reduced to meet the amount demanded by the infant. In essence, the mother's supply of breast milk becomes synchronized with the infant's need and demand. As the infant grows and demands more milk, the breasts produce more. Generally, the more frequent the feedings, the more milk is secreted. Inadequate emptying of the breasts usually results in less milk secretion (Kearney, Cronenwett, & Barrett, 1990).

Ejection Stage. The movement of milk through the ductal system is accomplished through a neurohormonal reflex known as the **milk ejection reflex,** previously called the **let-down reflex** (Shrago & Bocar, 1990). Primarily in response to the infant's sucking on the breast, the posterior pituitary gland secretes oxytocin. Influenced by the oxytocin, myoepithelial cells surrounding the alveoli contract and propel milk through the ductal system to the infant.

The milk ejection reflex may take several days or weeks to establish. Some women are not physically aware of the reflex, but instead note their infant's behavior. For example, at the beginning of a feeding, the infant in search of milk takes quick, almost frantic, sucks. Then the mother feels a tingling sensation within her breasts as milk is propelled through the ducts. Subsequently the mother observes the infant taking longer, more relaxed sucks.

Psychologic Aspects of Lactation

Inseparable from the physiology of lactation is the psychology of lactation. Successful lactation occurs when the physiologic and psychologic aspects of mother and infant are in synchrony. Although most women are physiologically and anatomically capable of lactation, psychologic conditions may inhibit lactation (Hill & Humenick, 1989). In some cases, the physiologic mechanism of lactation may stimulate sexual arousal, with psychologic implications for some women.

One of the most important factors contributing to the success of breastfeeding is the mother's willingness to breastfeed. Women who have a strong desire to breastfeed tend to continue longer than women who have negative or ambivalent feelings toward breastfeeding. Women who have a strong desire to breastfeed often demonstrate more tolerance for breast discomforts, such as cracked or sore nipples or leakage of milk and are more accepting of the need for more frequent feedings with infant growth spurts.

Not all women who decide to breastfeed are eager to. Many women do not feel comfortable exposing their breasts and in many cultures breastfeeding in public is not approved. Some women believe that breastfeeding interferes with their home and work routines, but decide to breastfeed out of guilt. Other women may have had a negative experience with breastfeeding in the past or simply lack the social support. These women are often frustrated and anxious while breastfeeding.

Women who have negative or ambivalent feelings toward breastfeeding, as well as those who lack encouragement from significant others, tend to wean the infant whenever a problem arises, whether it is directly related to breastfeeding (cracked nipples) or to a variety of other factors (infant crying). These women tend to have more difficulty handling the normal growth spurts common in infants at 10 days, 3 weeks, and 3 months of age. Frequently, women with negative or ambivalent feelings believe that they cannot produce a sufficient quantity or quality of breast milk. A mother's misconceptions are often reinforced by well-meaning but erroneous advice from significant others who are not knowledgeable about breastfeeding. If interventions are not instituted, the woman's beliefs become reality in a cycle of events. The woman, for example, may become anxious, diminishing or even totally inhibiting the milk ejection reflex; the infant in turn becomes frustrated and increases the demand for milk (Kearney et al., 1990). If this cycle is not interrupted with effective interventions, the mother will eventually give up breastfeeding.

Psychologic Stimulation of Milk Ejection.
Although the primary stimulus for initiating the milk ejection reflex is the infant's sucking on the breast, several psychologic factors can also stimulate the reflex. A lactating mother may suddenly experience leakage of breast milk when she hears an infant cry, when she thinks about her infant, or when she anticipates a feeding. As the mother and infant become synchronized for feedings, the mother's milk may leak at the precise moment the baby awakes for a feeding, even if the mother and infant are not in the same area.

Sexual Arousal and Sexual Activity.
The physiologic responses of breastfeeding are closely tied to responses from sexual arousal (Lawrence, 1989) (see Chapter 5 for a discussion about sexuality and the childbearing couple).

Desire for sexual activity may be affected by lactation. Lactating women may experience less sexual desire. In addition, cultural beliefs may prohibit sexual intercourse for lactating mothers, which could decrease the couple's desire for sexual relations. However, many couples do experience an increased desire for sexual intercourse, because of such factors as frequent nipple stimulation, ease with normal body changes, increased comfort since the end of late pregnancy, or a belief that the chances of conception are diminished during lactation.

Breast Evaluation and Interventions
Subjective data from the mother are needed regarding the method of infant feeding; the mother's knowledge of breast care, lactation, and suppression of lactation; previous experience with breastfeeding; a history of breast disease, problems, or lactation risks; and whether or not the mother practices breast self-examination. The nurse should ask the breastfeeding mother about progress in breastfeeding and status/condition of the breasts. The bottlefeeding mother should also be asked about the status of her breasts and suppression of lactation.

Physical examination of each breast should begin with inspection. The nurse should first note if the mother is wearing a brassiere. Both breastfeeding and bottlefeeding mothers may be more comfortable with support provided by a well-fitting brassiere or breast binder. During the examination the brassiere should be removed. The breasts are inspected for shape, contour, general symmetry, direction of nipples, degree of nipple prominence, condition of nipples and areolae, areas of redness, venous distension, fullness, and leakage. The breasts may then be palpated to determine temperature and degree to which the breasts are filling with milk. (A routine postpartum breast assessment differs from a clinical breast examination in which all areas of the breasts are thoroughly palpated to identify breast lumps.) As the nurse palpates the breasts, the mother is asked whether she is experiencing any discomfort or tenderness. Nipple function may be assessed by asking the client to compress the areola between thumb and forefinger. The nipple will respond normally by protracting or abnormally by retracting or inverting (Fig. 31–1) (Riordan & Auerbach, 1993).

During the physical examination of the breasts, the nurse can reinforce general breast care. The nurse also has the opportunity to teach or reinforce breast self-examination, although due to breast changes the postpartum period is not an ideal time to teach the procedure. Many women, however, have contact with health care providers only during childbearing, and this time may be the only opportunity for a woman to learn this potentially life-saving self-care procedure.

Engorgement. **Primary breast engorgement,** also called **physiologic breast engorgement,** is swelling of the breasts that results from an increase in the blood and lymph supply to the breasts and the beginning of full milk production. With primary engorgement, the breasts are full, heavy, and tender. The tissue is compressible, milk flow is present, and the infant can nurse.

Secondary engorgement, sometimes called **pathologic engorgement,** can result when the breasts are not sufficiently drained, for example, because of the infant's incorrect positioning and sucking or because the baby's access to the breast is restricted (Chute, 1992). Milk then accumulates in the ducts and alveoli, the breast alveoli become distended, and milk-secreting cells are flattened and drawn out and may rupture. With this condition, the breasts become hard, shiny, and painful. The areola flattens and

hardens, making it difficult for the infant to latch onto the breast. As a result, milk flow decreases. Lactation may be suppressed if the pressure of engorgement continues and the breasts are not emptied.

Applying cabbage leaves to the breast has been reported to reduce engorgement, although the scientific basis or actual effectiveness of this natural remedy is not established. With one technique, the mother places cool, raw cabbage leaves that have been washed and dried, on the affected breast or breasts; holes are cut in the leaves for the nipples to keep them dry. The leaves are changed every 2 hours or when they wilt. Breastfeeding mothers remove the leaves during nursing and reapply them after the infant has fed. Nikodem and colleagues studied the effects of cabbage leaves on mothers' perceptions of breast engorgement and how breastfeeding practices were influenced at 72 hours and 6 weeks postpartum (Nikodem, Danziger, Gebka, Gulmezoglu, & Hofmeyr, 1993). The mothers who used the cabbage leaves tended to report less breast engorgement than mothers who had routine care, although the trend was not statistically significant. At 6 weeks, the women who used the cabbage leaves were more likely to be breastfeeding exclusively and had greater breastfeeding success. Citing a need for further investigation, the researchers questioned whether their results reflected the effects of the cabbage leaves or the extra attention and reassurance, which may have supported the confidence and self-esteem in subjects who used the leaves.

Engorgement may also occur in mothers who do not breastfeed. Other treatments discussed later for

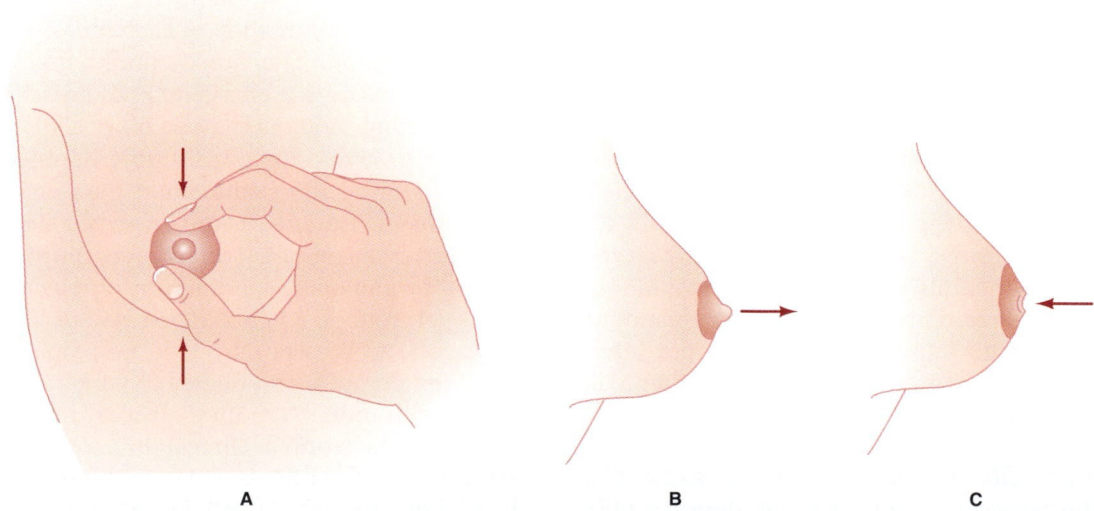

FIGURE 31–1. Nipple assessment includes a pinch test **(A).** Normal response is nipple protraction **(B);** abnormal response is inversion **(C).**

engorgement depend on whether the mother has chosen to bottlefeed or breastfeed her infant.

Interventions for the Breastfeeding Mother.
The mother may be more comfortable wearing a well-fitting, supportive brassiere during the early puerperium or until discomfort from breast fullness passes. The mother may be able to remove the brassiere at night, during sleep hours, if she so desires. The supportive brassiere minimizes the heavy feeling in the breasts that occurs and also provides support for the breasts and back.

To minimize discomfort and help resolve engorgement, the breasts need to be emptied frequently (about 10 feedings per 24-hour period); feeding times need not be restricted (Brown, 1992; Chute, 1992). The mother can assist emptying the breast during the feeding by massaging the breast, especially the tail and upper, outer quadrant. As the milk drains from the alveolar lumina and arrives at the lactiferous sinuses, the infant's sucking will slow and become more rhythmic to withdraw the milk. If the infant does not drain the breasts, the mother can relieve engorgement by manual or mechanical expression of milk.

With engorgement, the breast swells with added blood, lymph, and milk. The nipple and areola may be too firm to allow the infant to grasp on for feeding. The mother may experience acute pain as the infant tries to grasp the nipple; in this situation a mild analgesic, administered before the feeding, is appropriate. Additionally, prior to the feeding the areola and nipple can be softened by releasing some milk. A warm shower or application of warm compresses to the breast may provide enough stimulation to release some milk from the breasts. If not, the manual expression of some of the milk is indicated.

The breastfeeding mother who is experiencing extreme discomfort from engorgement can try applying cool packs to the breasts. As the infant is still stimulating the breast when feeding, the use of cool packs does not often result in an inadequate milk supply.

Interventions for a Mother Who Is Bottlefeeding.
Lactation must be suppressed to resolve engorgement in mothers who are bottlefeeding. Medications (hormonal and nonhormonal) were at one time widely used to inhibit lactation; however, each had drawbacks and risks and overall did not greatly reduce breast engorgement. Currently, many health care providers recommend simple mechanical inhibition, such as avoiding breast stimulation, wearing a support bra or compression binder continuously (but not while showering) as soon as possible after delivery, and applying cool packs to the breasts and axillae.

These measures relieve the discomfort of engorgement as well as help suppress lactation. Analgesics also reduce discomfort.

Usually discomfort subsides in 5 to 7 days; however, small amounts of milk may remain for a month or longer.

Some mothers may choose to relieve the discomfort associated with engorgement by expressing some colostrum or milk.

Sore Nipples.
Mothers may experience nipple tenderness during the first few days of breastfeeding. Normally, sensations of mild tenderness subside after the first few minutes of breastfeeding and resolve spontaneously in a few days. Painful soreness, however, related to trauma differs from tenderness. Research indicates that nipple tenderness or soreness is not related to frequency or duration of feedings, prenatal preparation, or skin color (Riordan & Auerbach, 1993; Zeimer & Pigeon, 1993).

A nurse should question the mother about nipple discomfort and, as part of breast assessment, inspect the nipples for signs of irritation. Periodic observation of the infant at the breast is necessary to identify improper techniques that lead to nipple trauma. Soreness may evolve into cracking and bleeding, which can worsen if the infant is improperly positioned at, does not correctly latch onto, or is improperly removed from the breast. If the nipples bleed, small amounts of blood may be found in the infant's mouth or in regurgitated milk. Women may continue to breastfeed, but should be aware of potential infection.

The mother should experience a slight pulling sensation as the baby nurses. Painfully sore nipples, however, can indicate a problem in breastfeeding technique.

Several measures may be suggested for a woman to use in treating her sore nipples.

- If nipples are painful, take a mild analgesic before feeding.
- Manually express some milk before feeding to enable the infant to latch onto the nipple more easily.
- Make certain that the infant is positioned appropriately and latches on well with a wide open mouth.
- Offer the breast that is less sore first, to minimize the most vigorous infant sucking on the nipple with more discomfort.
- When the infant is finished nursing, express a small amount of hind milk and massage the milk onto the nipple and areola. The antibodies and leukocyte content are thought to help minimize the possibility of infection.

- Air dry nipples after feeding.
- Moist compresses applied to the nipples may relieve some discomfort. In her study of 65 breastfeeding women with sore nipples, Lavergne (1997) found that clean breast pads or tea bags, moistened with warm water and applied to the sore nipples at least four times daily, provided better relief than no treatment. Study subjects also kept their bras open under their clothes for 15 minutes following each treatment.
- To promote hygiene, always wash hands before feeding. During daily bath or shower, wash nipples with plain water.
- Avoid the use of plastic-lined bras.
- Inform the health care provider of skin breakdown or severe discomfort.

Candida infection may be present if nipples are bright red and severely sore, if shooting pain occurs after breastfeeding has been established, or following antibiotic therapy. The baby may or may not have evidence of oral *Candida* infection. *Candida* may be transferred back and forth between infant and mother and require antifungal treatment for the mother's nipples and baby's mouth.

Guidance. Breastfeeding guidance should be given during the initial feedings and should continue until the mother can breastfeed independently (Fig. 31–2). Staff and clients need to understand this can take a great deal of time and patience. Mothers often believe that they are expected to know how to breastfeed or that it should be easy. Consequently, they are reluctant to ask for help or give up breastfeeding because they think it is too hard or that they are unable to succeed. The nurse needs to encourage a mother to express her concerns.

Inverted Nipples. Some mothers have **inverted nipples.** True inverted nipples remain flat or retract inward when stimulated, making it difficult for an infant to latch on. Nipples that appear inverted may be drawn out manually or with a breast pump before feeding. A nipple shell worn between feedings may also help draw the nipple out (Fig. 31–3).

Effects of Drugs and Other Substances on Breast Milk

Drugs pass into breast milk via mechanisms similar to those used by substances moving across the placenta (Blackburn & Loper, 1992). Drugs, environmental pollutants, alcohol, and nicotine are examples of substances that can be found in human milk and that may harm breastfeeding infants. For example, mothers should be advised to avoid alcoholic beverages (beer, wine, whiskey) as no safe level has been established. Nurses can also discuss reducing environmental exposure to pollutants; for example, mothers should be counseled to wash fruits and vegetables well because of insecticidal residue and to avoid places recently sprayed with insecticides.

Mothers are advised to consult their health care provider before taking drugs of any kind and to inform their health care providers, including their dentists, that they are breastfeeding. Appendix A lists drugs that may pass through breast milk and their effects on the infant.

Special Considerations Related to Breastfeeding

HIV Infection. The human immunovirus can be transmitted in breast milk from a mother to her newborn. Consequently, women who carry HIV are advised not to breastfeed.

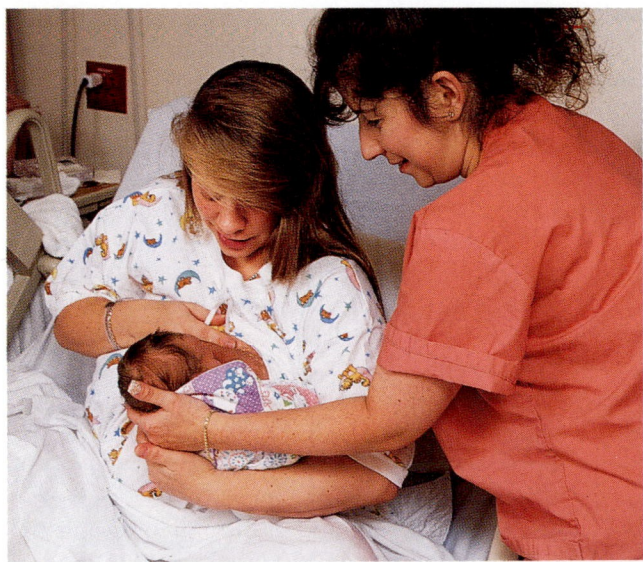

FIGURE 31–2. Nurse providing guidance about breastfeeding to a new mother.

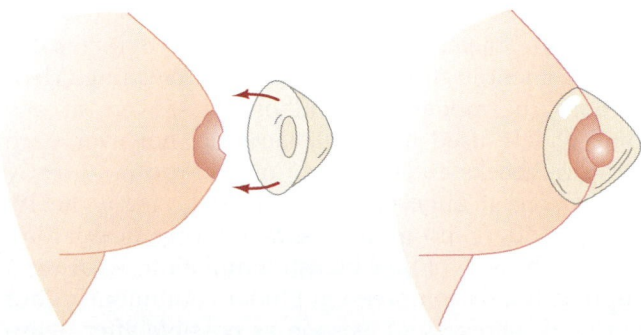

FIGURE 31–3. Breast shell for inverted nipples.

Breast Surgery, Breast Cancer, or Functional Loss of a Breast. Breast surgery, treatment for breast cancer that conserves the breast (lumpectomy, radiation), and such conditions as severe, chronic mastitis, are risks to lactation (Hughes & Owen, 1993; Robbins, 1992). Surgical and oncologic lactation risks are becoming increasingly common as women bear children at older ages and as cosmetic breast surgery becomes more available. Breast surgery, especially periareolar incisions, may sever milk ducts and affect nerve innervation in the breast. Radiation therapy may cause diffuse damage with atrophied lobules, preventing normal prenatal and lactation changes.

Many women who have had breast surgery, such as reduction or augmentation, will be able to breastfeed (Hughes & Owen, 1993). They may, however, experience difficulties and will benefit from teaching, based on their specific needs. The nurse's ability to identify the amount of surgical disruption to the ducts and nerves in the breasts can help develop realistic expectations for lactation.

Interventions for women with previous surgery depend on the reason for surgery and the type and extent of surgery. Intervention may include the following steps:

- Supporting the mother's decision to try breastfeeding.
- Presenting strategies for successful lactation (discussed earlier in this chapter).
- Encouraging the use of a breast pump after feedings, if appropriate, to foster milk production in the surgically altered breast.
- Suggesting use of a supplementary feeding method if needed.
- Encouraging the mother to express her feelings related to previous surgery and breastfeeding.
- Referring the woman to a lactation consultant for ongoing, one-on-one assistance.

Women with breast implants may have pronounced postpartum breast engorgement (Neifert, 1991). Breast pain, diffuse swelling, excess milk pressure, and inadequate infant latch-on may hinder milk flow and result in involution of mammary glandular tissue. In such cases, useful strategies include applying warm packs to the breast before feedings, gentle breast massage, cool packs between feedings, and regular use of a piston electric breast pump to remove residual milk after feedings.

Women who have had a double mastectomy are unable to breastfeed because both breasts have been removed. Reconstructive surgery does not make a difference to breastfeeding.

With education and encouragement, women with one functional breast can often breastfeed successfully.

Identifying lactation risks is part of postpartum assessment. Breast examination can reveal reasons for problematic breastfeeding. At times, full breastfeeding may not be possible; however, partial breastfeeding can provide the benefits of breast milk to the infant and a satisfying experience for the mother.

Breastfeeding More Than One Infant. Women can successfully breastfeed two or more infants (Biancuzzo, 1994; Gromada, 1991; Robbins, 1992), even when the mother is separated from them. Breastfeeding one infant can be difficult for a new mother; breastfeeding more than one adds complexity to the process. Teaching must be tailored to those complexities (see box entitled Strategies to Help Mothers Breastfeed More Than One Infant). A mother may be encouraged by her own confidence, prior breastfeeding success, and support from health care providers, family, and other women who have had positive experiences breastfeeding following a multiple birth. However, problems related to organization, social support, and mistaken beliefs that women with more than one neonate cannot breastfeed, prevent many women from even trying to breastfeed.

The advantages of breastfeeding more than one infant include frequent mother–baby interaction with each infant, even if two feed at the same time; identification of breastfeeding as an easier, cheaper, and more efficient method, once lactation and babies' routines are developed (between 4 and 8 weeks); nutritional and immunologic benefits of breast milk; and opportunities to sit and rest.

Difficulties include the demands of frequent feeding, garnering support from skeptical family and friends, and the organization required to feed more than one infant.

Figure 31–4 illustrates the positions for breastfeeding two infants.

Breastfeeding During Pregnancy. In the American culture, most women do not continue to breastfeed an older sibling when they become pregnant, although in other countries it is widely practiced. Some women will not volunteer information about continuing to breastfeed, for fear of disapproval from health care providers. Generally, breastfeeding does not pose physical risk to a healthy woman with an uncomplicated pregnancy. Increased nausea during the first trimester and nipple or breast tenderness have been reported with breastfeeding. A woman's diet needs to be carefully evaluated to ensure that she is receiving adequate nutrition. Most children wean themselves during pregnancy, possibly as a result of changes in the milk or in their own growth and development.

▶ **STRATEGIES TO HELP MOTHERS BREASTFEED MORE THAN ONE INFANT**

- Unless breastfeeding is contraindicated, which is rare, encourage it as an appropriate choice for mothers of multiples; breastfeeding can be complete or partial. Include significant others in education about breastfeeding.
- Prepare a woman prenatally for breastfeeding more than one infant; begin during the second trimester or earlier, due to the higher incidence of preterm birth of multiples.
- Identify maternal/fetal/neonatal lactation risk factors and develop appropriate strategies to promote lactation (for example, mother and infants may be separated).
- Make sure that the client receives lactation assistance if necessary (lactation consultant, skilled in working with mothers of multiples, support groups for breastfeeding mothers of multiples, printed literature, videos).
- Promote early lactation. Assist stable women to begin breast pumping within 6 hours of birth if the babies cannot breastfeed. Encourage suckling, rather than pumping, if the infants are able.
- Promote strategies that foster a mother's physical and emotional resources (e.g., creation of a "breastfeeding station" at home, where finger foods, beverages, and how-to literature are easily accessible during breastfeeding; teaching the importance of help from significant others at home).
- Assist the mother with learning to differentiate between her infants and devising realistic care, based on their individual needs.

- Suggest strategies to help the mother organize for breastfeeding (keeping simple checklists to chart times of each baby's feedings, bowel movements, and so forth, can help).
- Teach feeding positions for one or two babies at a time. If the mother has more than two infants, help devise feeding patterns (e.g., alternating infants and breasts at each feeding; alternating infants and breasts every 24 hours, or for even-numbered multiple sets; or assigning a specific breast to each infant).
- Avoid strategies that do not promote establishment of successful breastfeeding (supplementing every feed, alternating breastfeeding sessions with bottlefeeding sessions). Supplementing is usually not a problem for milk production if feeding on each breast occurs 8 to 12 times per day. If possible, supplementing should be avoided until lactation is well established.
- Avoid strategies that can interfere with the mother–infant relationship (e.g., exclusively breastfeeding one healthy infant and exclusively bottle feeding the other healthy infant).
- Educate staff about ways to support breastfeeding mothers of multiples.

Source: Gromada, 1991; Robbins, 1992.

Tandem Breastfeeding. Tandem breastfeeding refers to breastfeeding one child throughout a subsequent pregnancy and then continuing to breastfeed that older sibling and the newborn. Due largely to cultural norms, this is not widely practiced in the United States, although it is in other cultures.

Colostrum is produced despite the older sibling's breastfeeding throughout the pregnancy (Gromada, 1991). Transient changes in the composition of the feed can be manifested by looser stools of the sibling during the early postpartum. Despite the feeding pattern of the older sibling, the newborn has the same needs as any breastfed newborn and should have unrestricted, demand feedings 8 to 12 times per 24 hours. Assigning a child to a particular breast is unnecessary; it has the same advantages and disadvantages as when feeding infants from a multiple birth. Temporary breast assignment, however, may be practiced if one of the triad develops an infection, such as *Candida* (Gromada, 1991). Both children must be assessed for adequate nutritional intake.

Organizing tandem breastfeeding sessions depends upon such factors as the age of the older sibling

and the mother's physical and emotional comfort. Tandem feeds may be given separately or simultaneously, with the newborn usually positioned first and the older child often capable of self-positioning.

Educational Preparation for Breastfeeding

The Decision to Breastfeed. Many women decide to breastfeed early in pregnancy, or even before they become pregnant. In 1995, 59.4% of women in the United States were breastfeeding either exclusively or with formula feeding supplementation when discharged from the hospital (Chute, 1992; Ryan, 1997). Breastfeeding rates are highest among higher income, college-educated women older than 30 years of age (Ryan, 1997). Prenatal factors, such as maternal confidence, social learning and behavioral beliefs about breastfeeding (convenience, healthfulness, embarrassment), and support networks (social and professional) influence the duration of breastfeeding (Janke, 1994; O'Campo, Faden, Gielen, & Wang, 1992). For these reasons, preparation for breastfeeding should be part of prenatal education. Ideally, breastfeeding should be presented as early as possible.

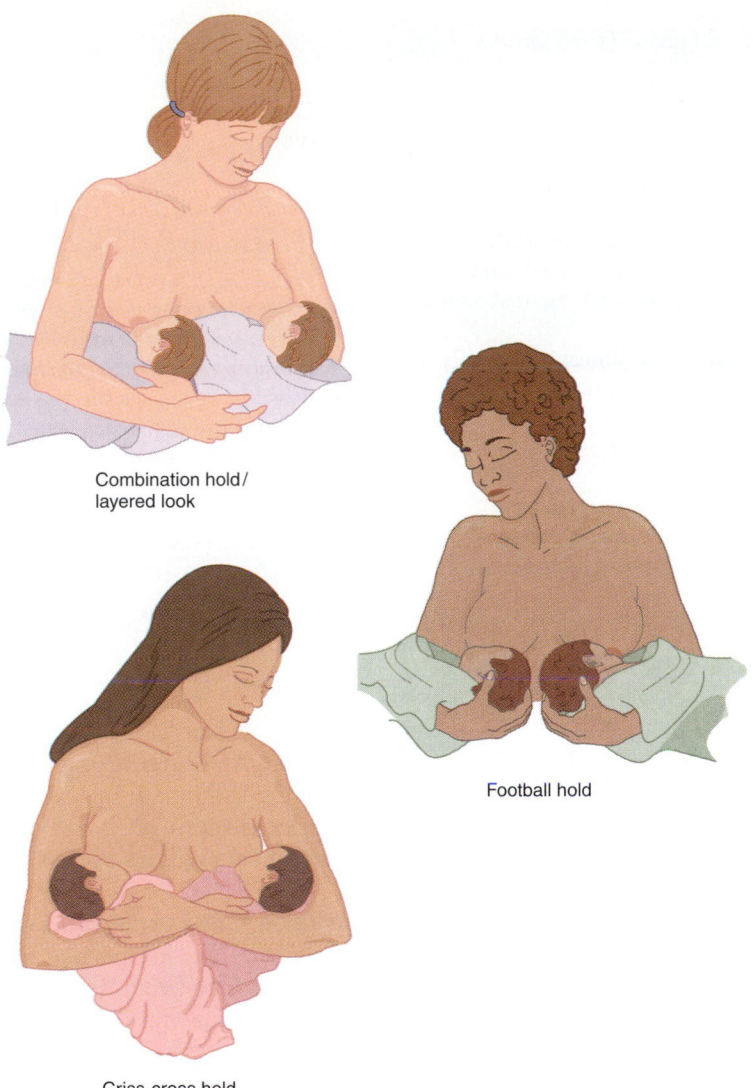

Combination hold/
layered look

Football hold

Criss-cross hold

FIGURE 31–4. Positions for breastfeeding two infants. *(Reproduced, with permission, from Spangler, A. (1992). Breastfeeding: A parent's guide. PO Box 501046, Atlanta, GA 31150-1046: Amy Spangler, p. 40.)*

According to Chute (1992), breastfeeding topics should be part of health and reproduction classes for elementary and secondary school students so that adolescents and young adults can come to accept breastfeeding as the norm.

Breastfeeding is more than a feeding method; it involves complex relationships and communication between a lactating woman and her infant. The decision to breastfeed is affected by such factors as the woman's cultural background, socioeconomic status, presence of breastfeeding role models and support people, media images of breastfeeding, previous experiences with breastfeeding, and hospital policies related to infant feeding.

Breastfeeding, rather than bottle feeding, has been supported as the ideal method of infant feeding by major health care organizations, such as the Association for Women's Health, Obstetric and Neonatal Nurses (AWOHNN), the American Academy of Pediatrics (AAP), and the American College of Obstetricians and Gynecologists (ACOG). The United States' National Health Promotion and Disease Prevention Objectives have targeted the year 2000 for increasing to at least 75% the proportion of mothers who breastfeed their babies in the early postpartum, and to at least 50% the proportion who continue breastfeeding until their babies are 5 to 6 months old. This objective is based on the 1988 estimate that 54% of women breastfed when

► ADVANTAGES OF BREASTFEEDING

BENEFITS OF BREASTFEEDING FOR THE INFANT

- Contains suitable nutrient composition for infant growth and development
- Is maintained at the correct temperature for feeding
- Contains living leukocytes, certain antibodies, and other antimicrobial factors that may protect against certain infections
- Decreases incidence of food-borne illness, especially in geographic/economic areas where storage of formula is difficult
- Decreases incidence of otitis media, possibly due to the nature of the infant's suckling
- Decreases incidence of necrotizing enterocolitis
- Decreases incidence of lower respiratory infections
- May decrease incidence and severity of allergies

- Easy to digest and decreases the incidence and severity of diarrhea

BENEFITS OF BREASTFEEDING FOR THE MOTHER

- Encourages a sense of empowerment
- Promotes a one-to-one physical interaction with the baby
- Decreases postpartum bleeding
- Promotes more rapid uterine involution
- Possibly decreases the risk of such diseases such as ovarian and premenstrual breast cancer
- Is highly accessible (no shopping or additional costs)

Source: American Academy of Pediatrics, 1997; Chua, Arulkumaran, Lim, Selamat, & Ratnam, 1994.

---

discharged from their birth sites and only 21% continued to breastfeed at 5 to 6 months (U.S. Department of Health and Human Services, 1991). See box entitled Advantages of Breastfeeding for discussion of the benefits of breastfeeding for infants and mothers.

Breastfeeding should be initiated shortly after birth, optimally within the first hour (American Academy of Pediatrics, 1997). The availability of continuous rooming-in helps to facilitate breastfeeding. Despite breast milk's providing ideal infant nutrition and despite such benefits as close physical contact, many healthy women do not initiate breastfeeding or do not continue to breastfeed much beyond discharge from the birthing facility. They may be influenced by numerous obstacles such as negative attitudes of significant others, lack of education and guidance for breastfeeding, and difficulties integrating breastfeeding into their lifestyles.

Many women mistakenly believe they should naturally "know how" to breastfeed. Many published sources give that impression. Although nearly every confident woman with perseverance and good support can breastfeed, it takes time and commitment. The most challenging period is the early postpartum, when the milk supply is being established and when the mother and infant are becoming acquainted and learning to work together with breastfeeding.

Nurses can provide crucial support that may make a difference between success or discontinuation of breastfeeding. Nurses should examine policies and practices in the maternity unit to identify obstacles to breastfeeding. Such practices as supplemental feedings and required nursery stays are still being implemented in some units, despite research indicating their ineffectiveness. Nurses should assume that all postpartum clients will have questions and need assistance.

Infant Characteristics That Aid in Feeding. At birth, an infant has several characteristics and reflexes that promote breastfeeding. The less prominent lower jaw and fat pads in the cheeks aid in sucking. The sucking and gag reflexes help control fluid intake, and the rooting reflex helps orient an infant to the breast. To use the rooting reflex, the mother should stroke the infant's lips with her nipple and wait for the baby's mouth to open wide.

Positioning Infant and Mother. Proper positioning of the mother and infant enables the infant to latch onto the nipple and areola effectively and fosters the mother's comfort during feeding (Chute, 1992; Riordan & Auerbach, 1993). The infant's nose must be at the level of the nipple, and the ear, shoulder, and hip should be aligned and the baby well supported. Prior to feeding, the mother may massage her breast to move the milk toward the nipple; a small amount of milk may be expressed. To place the infant onto the breast, the mother holds her breast with her thumb on top and fingers underneath. Keeping the fingers away from the areola allows the infant to grasp as much of the areola as necessary for a good latch on. Figure 31–5 illustrates three comfortable positions for breastfeeding.

The mother may stroke the infant's mouth with her nipple until the infant opens the mouth wide. The

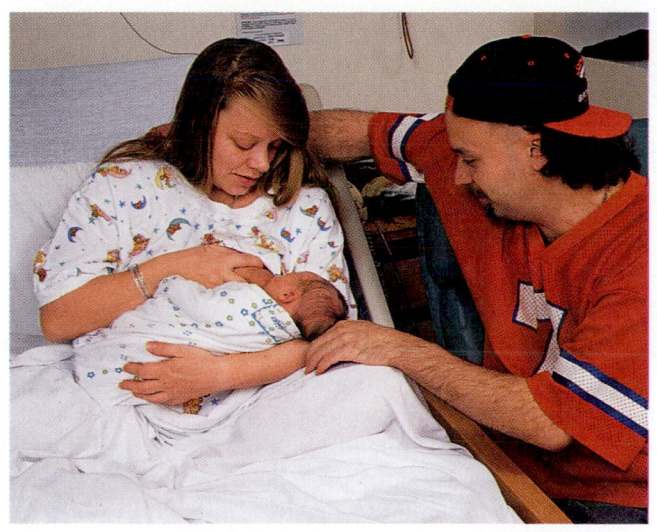

A

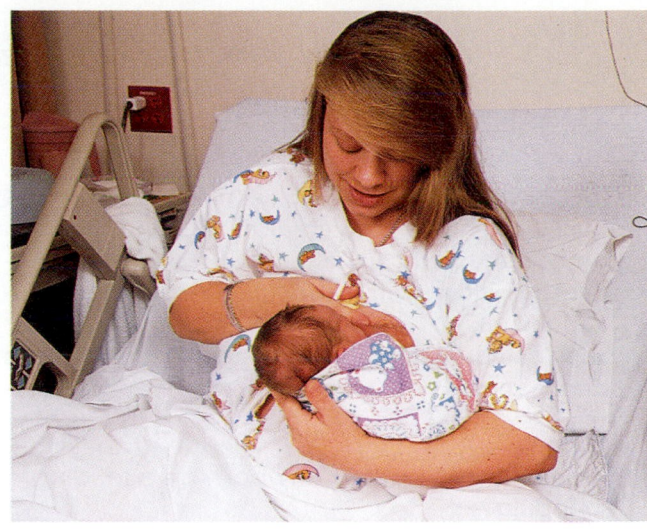

B

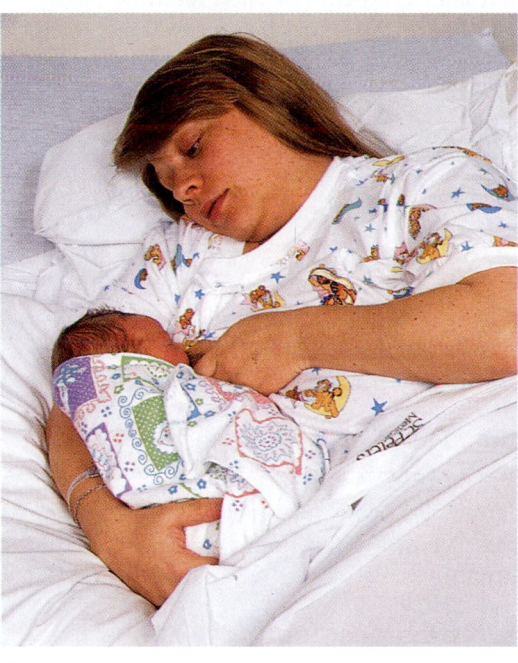

C

FIGURE 31–5. Three positions that are often used for breastfeeding are the cradle hold **(A)**, the football hold **(B)**, and the side-lying position **(C).**

mother then quickly brings the infant to the breast and points the nipple toward the upper part of the infant's mouth. The infant's lips should be flanged outward, and the chin pressed into the breast tissue. The tongue should be over the lower jaw and seen if the lower lip is gently lowered. With proper latch on, the mother experiences a gently pulling sensation. If the mother is uncomfortable, she can first remove the infant from the breast by placing her finger in the infant's mouth between the upper and lower jaws to break the suction. She may then go through the procedure again to adjust the infant's positioning.

Nurses should assume that new mothers need help in finding a comfortable position to breastfeed.

Mothers who have abdominal or perineal discomfort may be more comfortable lying on their sides with pillows for support. The infant is then placed in a side-lying position supported along the back by a pillow or rolled blanket. The infant's mouth is parallel to the nipple and the feet toward the mother's waist. The infant's side-lying position can be altered so that the feet are toward the mother's head.

Many mothers prefer to sit in a chair or on a bed while breastfeeding. Support for the mother's back and arms provides comfort and reduces strain. A pillow under the mother's knees if she is in bed or a stool on which to rest her flexed legs if she is sitting in a chair provides additional support.

Commonly Asked Questions

How soon can I breastfeed after delivery?

The newborn may be put to the mother's breast immediately after delivery if mother and newborn are healthy. Early initiation of breastfeeding provides the infant with nourishing colostrum, stimulates the infant's digestive tract, promotes lactation, helps build maternal confidence, and stimulates uterine contractions, which help to control postpartum bleeding.

Should I try to put my newborn on a feeding schedule?

No. Successful lactation is fostered by feeding soon after delivery and then feeding when the newborn is ready to nurse. The neonate tends to nurse about 10 times per 24 hours. Frequent breastfeedings have been associated with adequate milk volume and decreased serum bilirubin levels. As the mother's milk supply becomes synchronized with the infant's demand for milk, the infant may begin to increase the interval between feedings, so that feedings are closer to every 3 hours and at times even less frequent.

My baby was sleepy and refused the breast when I first tried to feed her. Can I be successful in breastfeeding?

Yes. A newborn's initial or intermittent refusal to breastfeed does not doom a woman's ability to breastfeed and is not an indication simply to switch to formula feeds. Feedings need to be tailored to the baby's needs, rather than a hospital's schedules. An infant's refusal of the breast tends to be more likely when hospital routines dictate a rigid "every 4 hour" feeding schedule.

Are there some women and infants who are unable to breastfeed?

There are some instances in which maternal or infant factors, or a combination of both, can result in an infant's receiving insufficient milk. However, nearly all women can have a satisfying breastfeeding experience with confidence and proper support. A women who needs to use formula supplements can also put her baby to her breast and need not be denied the breastfeeding experience.

Should I restrict my baby's feedings to a certain amount of time for each breast?

No. Restricting feeding times may prevent adequate nipple stimulation and emptying of the breasts. However, newborns may only nurse for a short time at the initial feedings.

Is it a must for infants to nurse for the same amount of time on both breasts at every feeding?

No, though common practice has been to advise women to offer both breasts at a feeding, possibly to help relieve discomfort related to breast fullness. Some infants only nurse at one breast for a feeding and some nurse at both breasts. In order to keep both breasts stimulated to produce milk and to promote comfort, mothers can be advised to alternate the breast that is offered first at each feeding. However, one study found no difference in infant behavior or mothers' satisfaction in women who fed their neonates on one breast or both during each feeding.

Are there times when a growing infant will again feed more frequently?

Yes. During growth spurts, such as around 10 days, 3 weeks, and 3 months after birth, infants require more milk. They may breastfeed more frequently for a day or two or until the milk supply is once again synchronized with the baby's needs.

Are the breasts ever completely empty?

No. The term "empty" is commonly used to refer to the breasts after a thorough breastfeeding session. However, milk is continually being produced in the lactating woman.

Is supplementing breast feedings with formula or glucose water all right?

Supplementing breast feedings with formula or glucose water is not advised for the woman establishing a normal breastfeeding pattern and can interfere with establishment of successful lactation. Mothers can pump their breasts to provide breast milk, which may be fed to the infant in a bottle when breastfeeding is not possible (for example, when the mother is working). In rare instances supplementation may be advised to prevent neonatal dehydration.

How will I know if my baby is getting enough milk?

Indications that the baby is receiving enough milk include the infant's overall appearance of wellness

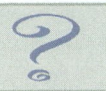

Commonly Asked Questions *continued*

and production of at least 6 voids per day of straw-colored urine. Placing a facial tissue in the diaper can help indicate wetness when super absorbent diapers are used. Infants who are not wetting diapers as expected, who seem lethargic, or otherwise unwell should be seen by their health care provider. Bowel movements are also indicative of adequate intake of breast milk. Many breastfed newborns will have a loose bowel movement with each feeding. At least 4 stools per 24 hours are expected after the first week and during the first 2 months. Appro-

priate weight gain indicates the infant is getting enough milk. However, a newborn normally may lose up to 10% of the birth weight, so weight gain is not among the earliest signs.

Should I have a glass of beer or wine to relax before I breastfeed?

No. Breastfeeding women should not drink alcoholic beverages, because alcohol passes into breast milk and can be potentially harmful to the newborn.

A mother may find that placing the infant on a pillow on her abdomen helps to reduce strain. When sitting, the mother usually cradles the infant; however, she may place the baby in a football hold.

Signs of Successful Lactation. A major concern of breastfeeding mothers is knowing whether the infant is receiving enough milk. In the first days after birth, colostrum provides enough nourishment to meet the infant's nutritional needs. Mothers should be reassured that newborns do not require a large intake during this period. Only a small percentage of mothers are actually unable to provide sufficient nutrition through breastfeeding.

Documentation. Traditionally, nurses have evaluated and documented a breastfeeding session as "good," "fair," or "poor." In relation to breastfeeding, however, these terms have no widely accepted, standard definition; the interpretation can vary with each nurse. In addition, this type of documentation neither effectively identifies breastfeeding problems nor encourages communication among staff members about the problems. There is a real need for a simple, reliable tool to evaluate breastfeedings and predict problems (Riordan & Koehn, 1997). A few rating scales have been developed to help staff score or evaluate breastfeeding, but their reliability and validity have been questioned. Further refinement and research are needed before clinical decisions are based on findings from such tools. Checklists or narrative documentation about breastfeeding may include considerations described in the box entitled Documentation of Breastfeeding: Factors to Be Considered.

Lactation and Responsibilities Out of the Home. Many women decide to continue breastfeeding as they resume their roles outside the home. If a mother is to return to full or part time work soon after birth, she will require teaching and support to help her continue breastfeeding. Ideally, planning for blending breastfeeding and out-of-home responsibilities begins before or during pregnancy. When feasible, talking with employers in advance may help in devising plans to support breastfeeding after the woman returns to work (National Healthy Mothers, Healthy Babies Coalition, n.d.).

Three main alternatives are available to the mother returning to out-of-home activities. The alternative she chooses will be influenced by her responsibilities outside the home, the degree to which she can maintain lactation while separated from her infant, and her physiologic and psychologic responses to assuming multiple roles.

As a first alternative, mothers who have flexible schedules and environments may have the infant with them or brought to them for feedings. This option usually requires that the infant be on a feeding schedule to enable the mother to plan for feedings. Wearing two-piece outfits or clothes that button in front make breastfeeding or pumping easier (National Healthy Mothers, Healthy Babies Coalition, n.d.).

As a second alternative, mothers may decide to have their infant fed breast milk when they are not available for the feeding. To provide a supply of breast milk for bottlefeedings, the mother should pump her breasts when she misses a feeding and express any milk left at the end of each feeding. The mother will need information on the expression and proper storage of the milk.

► DOCUMENTATION OF BREASTFEEDING: FACTORS TO BE CONSIDERED

- Baby's state and behavior at the time of feeds. Is the baby alert, sleepy, fussy, etc.? How does the mother respond to the behaviors?
- Positioning of infant's mouth on the breast. Are lips flanged so that about 1½ inches of areola beyond the everted part of the nipple is within the baby's mouth?
- Infant's sucking pattern. Are the infant's cheeks rounded during sucking? Can jaw movement be seen as far back as the infant's ears? If the cheeks are sucked inward and not rounded, the infant's latch onto the breast is incorrect. Is the baby sucking well on his or her own in bursts of 5–7 sucks with a short rest period, followed by another phase of sucking? The baby who spontaneously sucks for 5–10 minutes on a breast is likely to have latched on well.
- Signs of milk transfer. Is a change in the infant's sucking pattern noted? Does the mother have signs of the milk ejection reflex? Uterine cramping is a sign of oxytocin release and an indicator that the milk ejection reflex has been stimulated. Does the baby have audible swallowing? Does the baby burp or pass stool after feeding?
- The baby's general appearance. Despite voiding or stooling, is the baby's weight appropriate or is excess weight being lost?
- Mother's need for help. What type of help does the mother need (positioning, latch on, etc.)? Is she independent in breastfeeding? What background factors (family support for breastfeeding, previous experiences, etc.) need to be considered?
- Mother's own evaluation of her breastfeeding. Does she report feeling confident, unsure, etc.?
- Response to breastfeeding of significant others.

Source: Riordan & Koehn, 1997.

The amount of milk pumped is generally less than that obtained by an infant's suckling. The mother needs to anticipate that her milk may diminish at first; however, her supply can be maintained by continuing to pump her breasts and by frequent nursing when she is with the infant. The mother may also find that the infant may independently wean from specific feedings; for example, some 2- to 3-month-old infants no longer require a late evening feeding. The mother can express and store milk from those feedings that the infant no longer requires. This alternative for maintaining a supply of breast milk for bottle feeding can be very successful.

Some women feel guilty if they are too physically or psychologically exhausted to maintain a sufficient supply of stored milk. Indeed, juggling breastfeeding and out-of-home responsibilities can at times be very stressful. Nurses can help those mothers anticipate possible problems in maintaining an adequate milk supply, identify ways to handle the stress of other responsibilities, and select appropriate alternatives.

As a third alternative, formula can be provided when the mother misses a feeding. Essentially, the infant is weaned off breast milk for a given feeding. This alternative works well for mothers who are unable to pump their breasts regularly. Initially, the mother may experience breast fullness and leaking of milk when she misses a feeding. Wearing breast pads may help manage leakage. To relieve breast discomfort that results from missed feedings, the mother can express some milk. Without sufficient stimulation, lactation eventually ceases for those feedings from which the infant is weaned.

Manual and Mechanical Expression of Milk.

All breastfeeding women should be taught how to express milk from their breasts and the proper method of storage. Breast milk may be expressed to relieve breast engorgement, to maintain lactogenesis when the mother and infant are separated, and to provide human milk for the infant when conditions prevent the infant from breastfeeding.

Both manual and mechanical expression of milk begins with bringing the milk from the alveolar lumina through the ductal system toward the areola. Application of moist heat to the breasts in the form of a shower or compresses, followed by breast massage, promotes the initial release of milk through the ductal system. Breast massage may be accomplished by encircling the periphery of the breast and applying gentle traction toward the nipple. Breast massage may also be performed by supporting the breast with one hand and, with either the flat surface or fist of the other hand, firmly, repeatedly stroking the breast from the periphery toward the center until the entire breast is massaged (Figs. 31–6A and 31–6B). After breast massage, the milk is ready to be expressed. If the milk is to be saved and used later, a sterile container should be used to collect the milk.

To express milk manually, the thumb is placed on the upper outer edge of the areola while the fingers are placed on the lower edge. The thumb and fingers exert pressure back toward the chest wall and then are

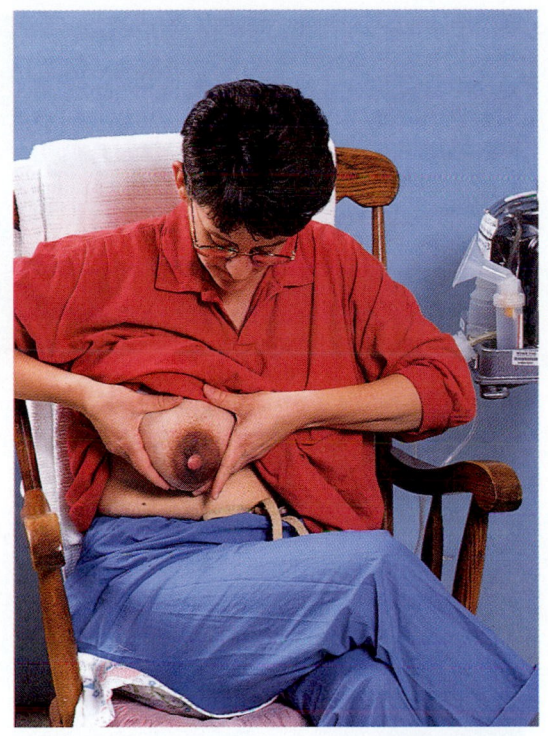

A

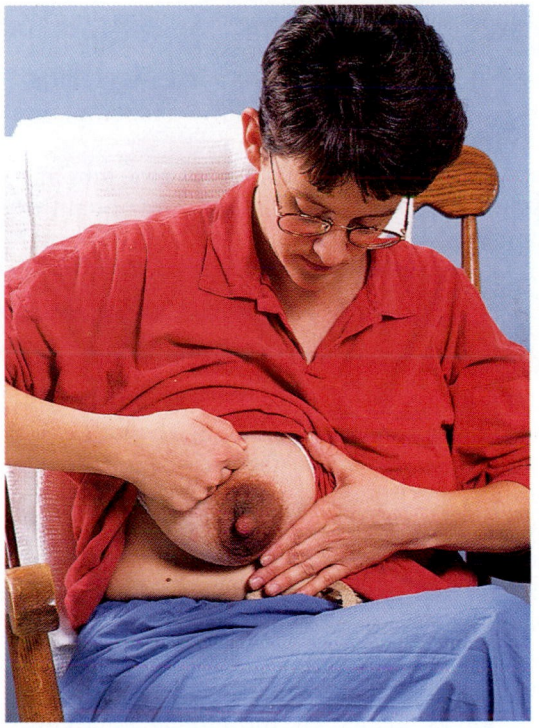

B

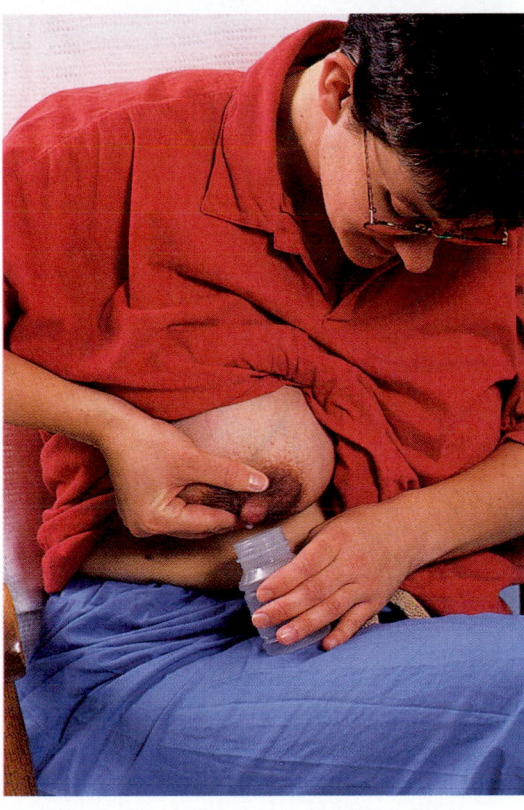

C

FIGURE 31–6. Manual expression of milk from the breast. **A.** and **B.** Breast massage stimulates release of milk from the ducts. **C.** Initially only a small amount of milk is secreted.

compressed together. Initially a small amount of milk is expressed (Fig. 31–6C). After a while, the mother experiences the milk ejection reflex; however, if the manual expression immediately follows a feeding, the milk ejection reflex may not be elicited.

The mother should be informed that the amount of milk expressed by hand usually does not equal the amount of milk the baby obtains by sucking. Whereas an infant may obtain at least 3 oz of milk from a breast, the mother may only be able to express an ounce or two from a full breast.

If a mother wishes to use a breast pump, the nurse can help her decide which type of pump will meet her needs and those of the infant. The La Leche League, a support group for breastfeeding mothers, as well as lactation consultants, can also provide information about breast pumps.

Breast pumps consist of a glass or plastic funnel attached to a glass or plastic receptacle. Until recently, manual breast pumps (e.g., Lloyd B pump) created suction by squeezing either a bulb or a handle attached to a funnel. With the Kaneson or Ross pump, however, suction is created by the mother's moving an inner cylinder funnel back and forth within an outer cylinder. A variety of battery-operated pumps are also available. Pumps are appropriate for mothers who want to maintain lactogenesis when temporarily separated from their infant.

Mothers who collect milk for premature infants or for infants who cannot suck because of a health problem may want to rent an electric pump (Fig. 31–7). When the infant cannot suck for an extended period, an electric pump can best stimulate lactogenesis and empty the breasts completely. The mother should pump each breast for about 15 minutes on each side.

Breast pumps should be thoroughly cleaned after each use.

To store breast milk, a clear container is recommended. At home, some mothers prefer to store milk in sterile plastic disposable bottle inserts. All milk stored in the hospital needs to be labeled with the mother's name, date, time, and amount. At home, milk should be labeled with the date, time, and amount. Breast milk can be safely stored for 72 hours in a refrigerator and up to 3 months in the main storage area of the freezer of a two-door refrigerator/freezer unit.

Frozen milk can be defrosted by placing it under warm tap water or placing it in the refrigerator for a few hours. The bottle is then placed under warm tap water. As stored breast milk often separates, the bottle needs to be shaken. Frozen milk should not be defrosted in a microwave oven.

Supplementary Feedings. Hospitals often provide dextrose and water or plain water bottles for

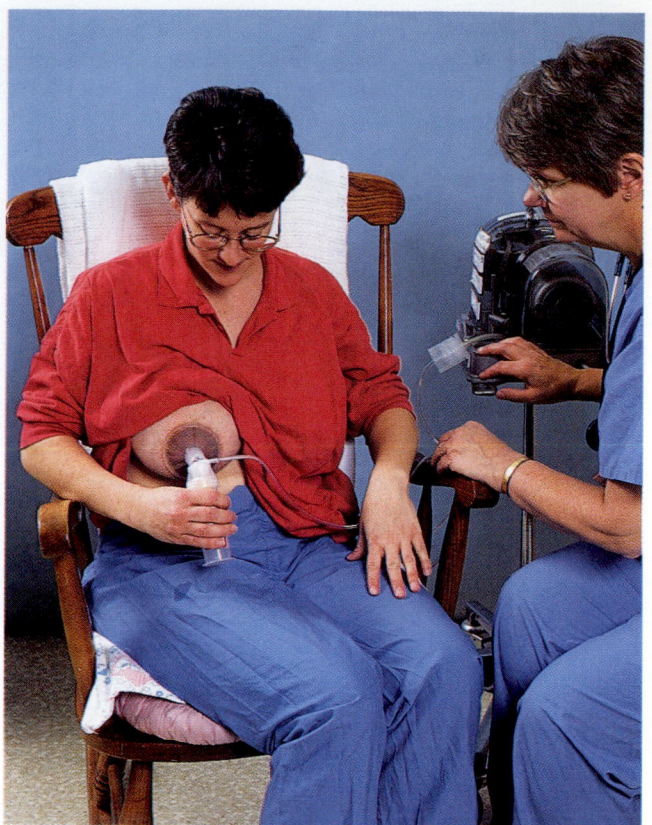

FIGURE 31–7. Nurse helps mother use an electric breast pump.

breastfeeding infants. In a normal term infant, however, such feedings are not needed; indeed, they may impede breastfeeding. Many lactating women, fearing that their infants are not receiving enough nourishment, are tempted to give them supplementary bottles. In the early puerperium, frequent bottle supplements may confuse some breastfed infants. The sucking mechanism of breastfeeding differs from that needed with bottle feeding in terms of effort exerted, use of muscles, amount of air taken in, and direction in which the tongue is thrust.

In breastfeeding, the infant must suck vigorously to stimulate the milk ejection reflex. Aided by facial muscles, the infant thrusts the tongue up and forward to grasp and draw the human nipple into the mouth and against the hard palate. The areola is compressed by the gums, limiting the amount of air swallowed. Many breastfed infants do not need to be burped frequently.

With bottle feeding, the facial muscles are relaxed as the tongue is thrust forward to control the flow of milk from the rubber nipple. Closure of the infant's mouth around the rubber nipple is incomplete, resulting in the ingestion of air and the need for frequent burping.

If the breastfed infant receives a supplementary bottle frequently in the first few weeks of life, the infant may refuse the breast when breast milk does not flow immediately as does formula. In general, supplementary bottles should be avoided until lactation is well established.

If the mother chooses to miss a feeding she will need to express her milk instead so she will be comfortable. The baby can be fed milk with a bottle, cup, or spoon.

▶ Formula Feeding

The Decision to Formula Feed

Some women choose to formula feed their infants or discontinue breastfeeding soon after discharge. Personal factors, the environment in which a women lives, the infant's "personality," ease in breastfeeding, and personal definitions of health that extend beyond nutritional qualities are examples of influences on their decision (Gigliotti, 1995). Nevertheless, with the current nursing emphasis on the benefits of breastfeeding, bottlefeeding mothers have at times been made to feel "less than" good mothers or have felt they had to defend their decisions to bottlefeed to disapproving staff, friends, and family.

Formula feeding is a safe choice for families who can obtain, properly prepare, and store infant formula. Indeed, infants who have been formula fed do grow into healthy children from loving families. Nurses need to be careful to support the decision of clients to formula feed or breastfeed their infants. In helping families to be satisfied and independent in feeding their babies, nurses need first to examine their own values and biases related to infant feeding.

Commercially Prepared Formulas

Commercially prepared formulas (e.g., Enfamil, Similac, SMA) are patterned on the nutrient content of human milk, although none of the formulas is identical to human milk. Many of the commercially prepared formulas are based on cow's milk, using nonfat dry milk. Several adaptations are available.

- Protein content is decreased; protein is treated to produce a fine, flocculent, easily digested curd.
- Butterfat is removed, and vegetable oils, such as corn oil, are substituted to increase the linoleic acid content.
- Cholesterol content is reduced.
- Lactose or other carbohydrates are added.
- Levels of calcium, phosphorus, and other minerals are reduced by dilution.
- Vitamin A, C (ascorbic acid), D, and E are added.

- Iron may be added because of the infant's need for iron in the first year of life.

Other formulas such as soy-based formulas are available instead of milk-based formulas for infants who have an intolerance to milk-based formulas. Soy-based formulas also are fortified with iron. Table 31–4 compares the constituents of several commercial formulas.

Commercially prepared formulas are available as liquid concentrates or powders or in ready-to-use forms. Parents should be taught about the different types of formulas and the appropriate method of preparation for each.

Safety of Formulas

The American Academy of Pediatrics, in 1976, proposed minimum levels for essential nutrients in infant formulas (American Academy of Pediatrics Committee on Nutrition, 1976). In 1980, the Infant Formula Act was passed by the federal government, requiring that the Food and Drug Administration (FDA) regulate the composition of all infant formulas to ensure safety and wholesomeness. Manufacturers of formula must keep accurate records, and notify the FDA about any proposed change in composition of their products.

Safety also can be taught to parents with regard to formula preparation. Labels should be carefully read so that infants are not inadvertently given concentrated formula for ready-to-feed formula. Parents also should be taught sterilization techniques if these are deemed necessary (see later discussion).

▶ Volume and Frequency of Feeding

Healthy newborns, whether breast or bottle fed, should be fed on a demand basis. They will regulate their feedings to their needs.

To calculate the amount of breast milk or formula needed by the infant, the following guide can be used:

Based on a kilocalorie need of 115 kcal/kg body weight, a 7 pound (3.18 kg) newborn should receive 115 kcal × 3.18 kg, or 365.6 kcal, daily. As breast milk and formulas contain 20 kcal/oz, the newborn requires 365.7 kcal divided by 20 kcal, or 18.28 oz of breast milk or formula.

Breastfed neonates will nurse between 8 and 12 times a day. It may be assumed that they are receiving an adequate supply of milk if they seem satisfied after nursing, urinate at least 6 times per day, and gain weight after the initial weight loss.

Formula-fed neonates may feed 6 to 8 times per day. They can usually go longer between feedings because formula is digested more slowly than breast

▶ **TABLE 31-4**

Constituents of Several Commercial Formulas[a]

	Infant Formulas				Whole Cow's Milk	Soy Protein Formulas			
	Human Milk	SMA[b]	Similac w/FE[b]	Enfamil w/Fe[b]		Nursoy[b]	Isomil	Prosobee	I-Soyalac
Protein (W/V)[c]	1.2%	1.5%	1.5%	1.5%	3.4%	2.1%	1.8%	2.0%	2.1%
Casein	40%	40%	82%	40%	82%	—	—	—	—
Whey protein	60%	60%	18%	60%	18%	—	—	—	—
Fat (W/V)[c]	3.6%	3.6%	3.6%	3.8%	3.4%	3.6%	3.7%	3.6%	3.7%
% Polyunsaturated	14.2	14.5	41.2	31.8	4.0	14.5	37.1	28.9	60.5
% Monounsaturated	41.6	41.2	14.7	16.9	30.5	41.2	17.1	15.4	23.9
% Saturated	44.2	44.2	44.1	51.2	65.5	44.2	45.7	55.6	15.6
Vitamin E IU/L	3.4	9.5	20	21	1.3	9.5	20	21	16
Minerals (mg/100 mL[mEq/L])									
Total (ash)	210	250	330	300	740	350	380	400	400
Na	15 (7)	15 (7)	22 (10)	18 (8)	51 (22)	20 (8.7)	32 (14)	29 (13)	28.5 (12)
K	55 (14)	56 (14)	81 (21)	72 (18)	157 (40.2)	70 (18)	95 (24)	78 (20)	79 (20)
Ca	34 (17)	42 (21)	51 (25)	46 (23)	123 (61.2)	60 (30)	71 (35)	63 (32)	69 (35)
P	14 (9)	28 (18)	39 (25)	32 (21)	96 (61.9)	42 (27)	51 (33)	50 (32)	48 (31)
C1	37 (11)	37.5 (11)	51 (15)	42 (12)	96 (27.1)	37.5 (11)	44 (12)	55 (16)	53 (15)
Iron (per L)	0.8 mg	12 mg[d]	12 mg[d]	12 mg[d]	0.5 mg	11.5 mg	12 mg	12.7 mg	13 mg
Carbohydrate (W/V)[c]	7.2% (lactose)	7.2% (lactose)	7.2% (lactose)	6.9% (lactose)	4.8% (lactose)	6.9% (sucrose)	6.8% (corn syrup solids, surcrose)	6.8% (corn syrup solids)	6.8% (sucrose, tapioca dextrins)

[a]All data for competitive products derived from product labels, *Physicians Desk Reference,* or analyses.
[b]Concentrate with iron (standard dilution).
[c]W/V = weight per volume.
[d]SMA lo-iron. Enfamil and Similac contain 1.4 mg iron per quart. Infants fed these formulas should receive supplemental dietary iron from an outside source to meet daily requirements.

Courtesy of Wyeth Labs, Philadelphia. © 1986.

milk, thereby causing the neonate to feel satisfied longer. Formula-fed infants can be assessed for adequate intake by noting the number of bottles, and the amount of formula in each bottle consumed in a 24-hour period. Assessing the newborn's weight gain and the number of wet diapers also indicates nutritional status.

▶ Feeding Patterns

Feeding the neonate is one of the first acts of parenting. The nurse should support the parents' decision about whether to breastfeed or bottlefeed. Healthy newborns should be fed on a demand basis. The parents are taught that neonates and infants also experience growth spurts during which they need to be fed more frequently. Growth spurts occur at about 10 days, 3 weeks, and 3 months after birth. Parents should feed the neonate or infant on demand during these times. Growth spurts last for several days and are self-limiting. Anticipatory guidance by the nurse will help parents deal effectively with their neonate's

or infant's demands during these times. Parents should be reassured that during growth spurts the infant's needs can be met by either the breast or bottle without supplementary feeding.

During the first year of life infants have changing needs related to breastfeeding or bottle feeding. Table 31–5 is a guide related to the frequency and ounces per feeding in the first year. Breastfed infants usually

▶ **TABLE 31-5**

Schedule For Milk Feedings During The First Year

Age	Number of Feedings Per 24 Hours	Amount Per Feeding (oz)	Total Amount Per 24 Hours (oz)
1 week	6	2–3	12–18
2–4 weeks	6	3–5	18–30
2–3 months	5	4–6	20–30
4–5 months	5	5–7	25–35
6–7 months	4	7–8	28–32
8–12 months	3	8	24

Reproduced, with permission, from Lewis, C.M. (1984). Nutrition and nutritional therapy in nursing. Norwalk, CT: Appleton-Century-Crofts.

nurse more frequently than bottlefed infants because breast milk is more easily digested than formula. Parents are also taught that the infant will usually sleep through the night when he or she has reached 12 pounds or in about 8 weeks, although this is highly individualized for each infant.

Patterns of Breastfeeding

Parents should be informed that the mother's milk supply will become synchronized with the neonate's demand for milk. In general, neonates should nurse for 10 to 20 minutes on each breast every 2 to 3 hours. Mothers are also taught that they can keep the baby on each breast during a feeding for as long as the baby seems to want to nurse. The mother's nipples will not get sore as long as the infant's grasp on the nipple is correct. Improper infant positioning, grasp, or latch on to the nipple has been linked to nipple soreness (Riordan & Auerbach, 1993). The box entitled Teaching Guide for Breastfeeding Positioning and Schedule describes guidelines related to breastfeeding patterns and positions.

Patterns of Formula Feeding

Parents are taught that formula-fed neonates will take about 2 to 3 oz per feeding or 12 to 15 oz per day in the first week of life. Neonates will increase their consumption of formula at each feeding as their stomach capacities increase. Another rule of thumb that can be taught to parents is that neonates will initially consume 2½ oz per pound of body weight in the first

weeks of life. If, for example, the neonate weighs 8 pounds, he or she will consume 20 oz in a 24-hour period. If the 20 oz is consumed in eight feedings, the neonate will take 2.5 oz per feeding; if taken in 6 feedings, the neonate will take 3.3 oz per feeding.

Techniques for Bottle Feeding and Formula Preparation

Parents and other caretakers should be taught to hold the neonate in a comfortable position when bottle-feeding. The bottle should be held upright so that milk and no air is in the nipple and neck of the bottle. This prevents the neonate from swallowing air that may cause discomfort from gas. Several different types of bottles and nipples are sold. The opening in the nipple should allow a steady flow of formula but should not be too large as it will cause the neonate to swallow too much liquid and regurgitate the formula.

Commercial formulas are sold in concentrated liquids, powders, ready-to-feed, and prepackaged ready-to-feed formula in bottles. The concentrated liquids and powders require mixing with water and should be prepared exactly according to their package directions. The concentrated formulas and powders are less expensive than the ready-to-feed formulas.

Parents should be taught to carefully read the labels on commercially prepared formulas. Use of concentrated formula without dilution can cause metabolic problems and dehydration in the neonate. Formulas should be prepared for a 24-hour period if concentrated liquid is used. Once prepared, they

---

► **TEACHING GUIDE FOR BREASTFEEDING POSITIONING AND SCHEDULE**

POSITIONING MOTHER

Assist mother to find the most comfortable position. The *least* comfortable position is leaning back in the bed. For the beginning feedings, seat mother in a comfortable chair, arrange pillows on mother's lap, behind her back, and under arm and shoulder on the side in which the baby is to nurse; if mother has had an epidural, mother may lie on her side with pillows between her knees and at her back. For the initial feeding in the delivery room, place mother on her side with pillows to support her back.

POSITIONING INFANT

Instruct mother to position the infant's head so that it is rotated toward her and the nose is at the level of the mother's nipple; teach the mother to support her breast in a "C-hold" (thumb above the areola and the rest of the

fingers under the breast); when infant opens mouth in response to brushing nipple against baby's lower lip, signal the mother to slip the nipple and top of areola into infant's mouth.

SCHEDULE

Feed infant on demand; in the beginning both breasts should be offered at each feed to stimulate response; if infant does not nurse on both breasts, single alternating breast feedings of whatever duration should be offered frequently. *There is no need to restrict nursing time.* Infant may feed in "bunches," that is, frequent feedings whenever he or she wants. Most newborns require 20 to 40 minutes to complete a feeding; allow the baby to nurse from the first breast until he or she spontaneously pulls away so that the baby gets the benefit of the fatty hind milk as well as the low-fat fore milk.

should be stored in the refrigerator for no longer than 48 hours. The bottle may be taken out of the refrigerator one-half hour before use or run under warm water to take the chill out of the formula. Formula feeds should not be heated in microwave ovens. Powders and ready-to-feed formulas may be prepared for each feeding. Once the can of ready-to-feed formula is opened, it should be refrigerated and discarded if not used within 48 hours. The can of powdered formula may be stored at room temperature, once opened, for a period of 3 weeks or for the length of time advised by the manufacturer.

Parents are cautioned to avoid propping the bottle. The neonate may regurgitate and aspirate the formula when the bottle is propped. Neonates who nurse from propped bottles are also prone to nursing bottle mouth syndrome (see later discussion).

Bottle Sterilization

Parents and other caretakers are taught that the bottles and nipples should be washed with soap and water. The dishwasher may be used effectively to wash the bottles. If the water supply is not purified or if there is a question about the cleanliness of the water supply, sterilization procedures are taught to parents.

When bottle sterilization is indicated, two methods may be used: the terminal method and the aseptic method. For either method, the first step is to wash the bottles (other than bottles that use liners to hold the milk), nipples, and bottle caps in soapy, warm water. An inexpensive bottle brush is helpful in removing residue.

Terminal Method. After the equipment is washed, the formula is prepared according to the directions on the can. The bottles are filled with the formula and the nipples are inverted into the bottles with the caps loosely applied. The bottles are placed in a large kettle in 2 or 3 inches of water or, alternately, in a bottle sterilizer. The kettle or sterilizer is covered and the bottles are boiled for 25 minutes. The bottles remain in the sterilizer until cool. They are then removed, the lids are tightened, and the bottles stored in the refrigerator.

Aseptic Method. After the equipment is washed, it is placed in a large kettle or sterilizer and boiled for 5 minutes. The amount of water needed to mix concentrated formula is boiled separately for 5 minutes. The bottles, caps, and nipples are removed with tongs from the sterilizer or kettle. A sterilized measuring pitcher is used to measure the appropriate amount of water and formula into each bottle. Bottles are refrigerated until needed.

Burping

Neonates and infants should burp (eruct) at least twice during a feeding (Fig. 31–8). Parents are taught to rec-

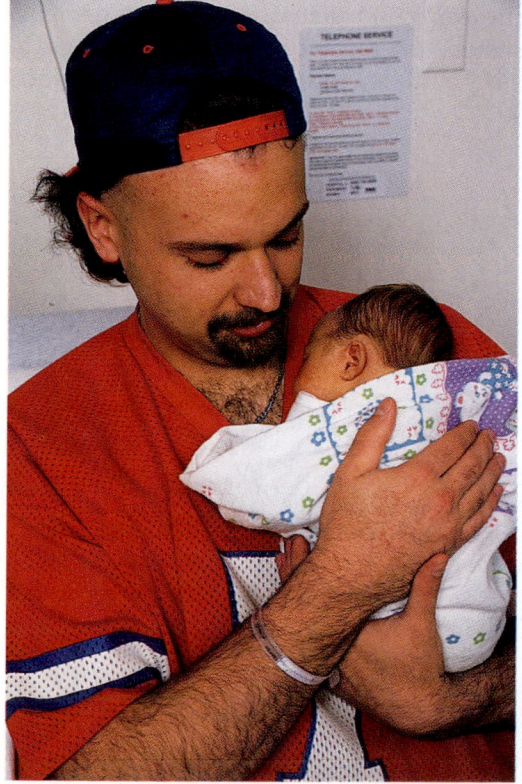
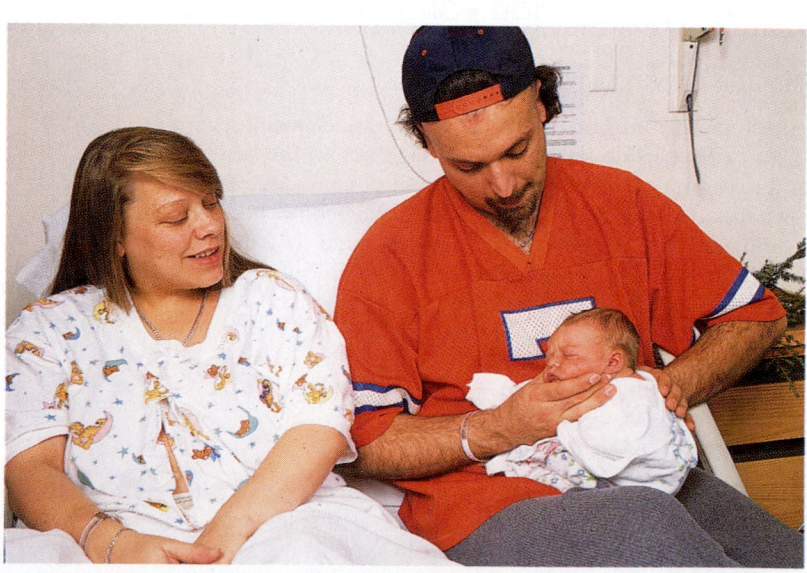

A
B

FIGURE 31–8. Upright **(A)** and sitting **(B)** positions in which a neonate may be burped.

ognize their neonate's signals related to burping: the neonate will stop sucking when he or she needs to be burped; if the neonate does not burp after several minutes, he or she probably does not need to burp. The neonate may be burped upright on the parent's shoulder. The infant's back is patted gently. Alternately, the neonate may be placed in a sitting position with one hand holding the chin for head support and the other hand gently patting the back. This position allows the parent to watch the neonate during burping.

▶ Infant Feeding Recommendations

Adequate nutrition is considered the single most important factor affecting infant physical growth and development. The first 4 to 6 months constitute the most rapid period of growth for the infant. Because requirements for nutrition are most critical during this period, nutritional deficiencies can have long-term effects on growth and development (Mitchell, 1997).

Food in an infant's diet must be adequate in energy, vitamins, and minerals. It also must meet the needs of the developing digestive tract and renal capacity while supporting the rapid growth rate of the first year of life. Infants double their birth weight by the 5th month and triple it by the 12th month. In addition, length usually increases by 50%. These large increments require a consistent and adequate food supply. An inadequate diet during the first year cannot support optimal growth and nutrient storage.

Solid foods are introduced into the diet as a supplement to the breast milk or infant formula. It is important that solids (sometimes called beikost) be provided at the developmentally appropriate time. Human milk or infant formula alone provides the best nutrition for infants in the first 4 to 6 months of life. The full-term infant has iron stores in the body that are estimated to be adequate until 4 to 6 months. After this time, exogenous iron should be added to the diet of breastfed babies to decrease the risk of development of iron-deficiency anemia. Iron-fortified dry infant cereal is an excellent low-cost source of iron for infants. The American Academy of Pediatrics (1993) recommends the use of iron-fortified formulas for bottle-fed babies.

Individual custom, beliefs, and practices may dictate when parents decide to introduce solid foods into the infant's diet. Solid foods should not be introduced before 4 to 6 months of age for several reasons (Mitchell, 1997). By 16 weeks of age infants have developed a more mature sucking pattern; they can move the tongue back and forth and hold the head more erect and in the midline. Hand–eye coordination is also developing; by 24 weeks the infant can grasp

an object in sight and place it in the mouth. Chewing movements begin between the 24th and 28th weeks. All of these developmental achievements indicate that infants are ready to feed finger foods to themselves. Physiologically, the gastrointestinal tract has matured and is producing the digestive enzymes necessary for absorption and metabolism of fats, protein, and starches. The excretory capacity of the kidneys also has adapted to larger osmolar loads. Early introduction of supplementary foods (before 4 months) may interfere with lactation by causing satiety and therefore decrease the infant's desire to nurse. Early introduction of solid food may also stimulate an allergic reaction to the food (Rolfes, DeBruyne, & Whitney, 1990).

Parents should be taught to introduce solid foods slowly. A single-grain, ready-to-serve, iron-fortified dry cereal is usually the first solid food offered to the infant. Rice is the least allergenic of the cereals and is recommended as the first cereal to be introduced. Cereal is followed by fruits and juices and pureed yellow and green vegetables. Pureed meats do not need to be added until 9 months of age. Foods should be introduced one at a time and fed to the infant for 3–5 days before a new food is given. In this way if food intolerance or allergy develops, the allergen can be readily identified. Once a variety of foods have been introduced, foods can be combined and new textures and flavors introduced. As food intake increases, milk intake should decrease; however, breast or formula feedings are still important to supply nutrients needed by the infant. Infant foods can be selected from commercial baby food manufacturers or prepared at home. Special safe food handling practices should be used for home-made baby food to prevent any food-borne illnesses.

The transition to solid foods offers an excellent opportunity for parents or other caretakers to set the stage for healthy eating habits. Acquired tastes for salts, sugars, and empty caloric foods may be established at this time. Effective teaching techniques and a sound knowledge base in nutrition and infant growth and development can serve as effective tools for the nurse in providing anticipatory guidance about infant nutrition.

Weaning and Introduction of Solid Food

Weaning usually occurs between 6 months and 1 year of age and should be done gradually. One study of breastfeeding mothers investigated patterns of weaning that could be chosen by mothers. Three patterns were found: gradual weaning, minimal breastfeeding, and sudden severance. The mothers who chose gradual weaning replaced total breastfeeding with cow's milk or formula and/or solid foods over a period of 1 to 8 weeks. Mothers who chose minimal breastfeeding gradually reduced the number of feedings until the infant was breastfeeding only twice a day; thus, when the mother wished to terminate breastfeeding completely, only two feedings needed to be eliminated. In the third pattern, sudden severance, the breastfeedings were totally eliminated in one day (Williams & Morse, 1989). The investigators concluded that gradual weaning was preferable.

The transitions from breast to bottle, from breast to cup, or from liquids to solids all describe weaning. Improved hand–eye coordination, attempts to hold the bottle, decreased interest in breastfeeding or bottle feeding, and an interest in chewing are signs that the infant is ready to respond to feeding changes. Many parents and health care professionals feel that this is an appropriate time to introduce solids. At the same time, the amount of milk and the number of feedings should be reduced.

Weaning to the cup should be attempted when the infant is ready. The infant's age, signs of readiness, number of milk feedings per day, ability to use a cup, and way in which sucking needs are met should be assessed prior to counseling parents.

▶ Feeding Problems

The most common feeding problems encountered in the first year of life are underfeeding, overfeeding, regurgitation, and colic (Behrman, 1992). Regurgitation and colic are discussed in Chapter 30. Feeding and food consumption in infancy have far greater implications than the obvious provision of nutrients for energy, maintenance, and growth. Feeding is usually the first and perhaps the most important sharing behavior that is experienced between the infant and the primary caretaker. It is a function necessary for sustaining physical life that has far-reaching effects on the psychosocial well-being of both infant and parent.

Underfeeding

The underfed infant usually eats all the food, formula, or breast milk that is offered, but has a history of inadequate weight gain, irritability, and fussing between feedings. On occasion, underfeeding may result when the infant refuses feedings that are offered (Hambridge, 1997).

The underfed infant is not an infant with organic or systemic disease. Rather, the problem is one of the infant not being offered adequate nutrition or there being some mechanical or feeding technique problem that prohibits the adequate intake of nutrition. There may be a psychologic component such as a problem with mother–infant attachment, but more commonly there is a lack of knowledge on the part of the mother or primary caretaker (Hambridge, 1997). Some mothers may be inexperienced and lack an effective support system in the home; other mothers may be concerned with obesity, overfeeding, or spoiling the child by feeding on request. Due to lack of money and ability to obtain formula or lack of understanding, some mothers may "water down" the infant's formula. Still other mothers may be responding to pressures in the home from family members who have their own ideas about infant feeding. Finally, in conjunction with other indicators, underfeeding may signal child neglect or abuse. The health care provider is cautioned to assess for other signs before drawing this conclusion on the basis of underfeeding alone.

A complete and thorough feeding history must be obtained. The mother or primary caretaker must be instructed in every aspect of infant feeding, including calorie and ounce requirements, formula preparation, proper holding of the infant, effective breastfeeding and bottlefeeding techniques, and adequate eructation (or burping) of the infant. Bottles and nipples should be examined for air leaks and appropriate nipple hole size.

The mother's attitude, expectations, ideas, and desires about infant feeding as well as those of other significant family members are also explored. Any conflict or stress that may be affecting the feeding of the infant must be addressed and settled. Lastly, the mother or primary caretaker and significant others may be made active members in the solution of the underfeeding problem. Growth charts and desired outcome goals may be shared with these individuals as the infant is followed closely to ensure adequate weight gain. In some cases, after a careful assessment, referral to social or legal agencies may be appropriate.

Overfeeding

Most authorities agree that it is seldom the breastfed infant who has a problem with overfeeding and subsequent problems such as regurgitation, vomiting, and obesity (Behrman, 1992). The feeding practices most frequently associated with overfeeding are bottlefeeding, excessive amounts of formula, overly concentrated formula, and the early introduction of nonmilk solids (Lawrence, 1985).

Bottlefed infants tend to be overfed because parents expect the infant to empty the bottle at each feeding and persist until the infant does so, and because the bottle may be offered by some parents whenever the infant makes any demand of his or her environment. The parent misreads the infant's need for play, stimulation, attention, affection, or some other discomfort as a need for food. Parents may also use the bottle simply to keep the infant quiet.

Overly concentrated formulas are usually the result of errors in preparation rather than the makeup of the formula itself. For this reason, formula preparation cannot be taken for granted, either during discharge planning or at well-infant visits, and should be reviewed with all mothers who use formula and in particular when diarrhea or loose stools are noted in the neonate or excessive weight gain is noted in the older infant. (See earlier discussion of techniques for bottlefeeding and formula preparation.)

Nursing management focuses on the following recommendations.

1. Encourage breastfeeding until at least 6 months of age if possible, as breastfeeding infants seldom have problems with overfeeding.
2. Instruct parents to avoid feeding their infants sweeteners, sugar, and solids. Semisolid foods may be introduced at 4 to 6 months of age.
3. Use growth charts to help parents understand normal growth in height and weight.
4. Review calorie and ounce requirements of the infant at each health visit and discourage parents from forcing infants to empty every bottle.
5. Review the correct mixing and concentration of formulas when the infant is bottlefed.
6. Review with parents the cues that infants use to indicate hunger and satiety.
7. Encourage parents to read solid food labels and avoid those high in carbohydrates.
8. Instruct parents that when solid foods are started, they should avoid mixed dinners and use plain vegetables and meats, as these contain fewer additives and carbohydrates.
9. Present information so that the parents can make informed decisions and choices. Remember that some cultures value "plump" babies.

► Tooth Decay

In the first year of life the oral cavity is routinely examined during visits to the well-child clinic. To avoid the high incidence of dental problems that continue to plague children in our society, early teaching of parents concerning proper dental care should be instituted at the first well-child visit. The primary teeth usually do not begin to erupt until approximately 5 months of age, but dental care initiated prior to this time will establish healthy dental habits for the child later in life.

Most children are not able to manage a toothbrush before 18 months of age, but an infant's caretaker can cleanse the gums and developing teeth by wrapping a thin layer of fine mesh gauze around the little finger and gently "sweeping" the gums and teeth to remove milk and food residue.

To prevent the development of "nursing bottle mouth syndrome," parents should be discouraged from giving the infant and young child a bottle at bedtime or naptime. The continuous bathing of the teeth with carbohydrate liquids such as milk, juices, and sugar water, for prolonged periods, is the primary cause of the syndrome. Although this condition is not seen until 18 months or later, the habit of sleeping with a bottle is established in early infancy.

Critical Thinking in Care Planning

Care of an Infant Experiencing Feeding Problems

Amy Hirschburg and her son Jason, 6 months old, visit the clinic for a six-month checkup. Amy reports that Jason has been very irritable lately and has not been sleeping through the night. She also reports that she has been "watering down" the formula lately to "make it last." Her husband Stephen has recently lost his new job as a city bus driver and they have had difficulty in paying their bills and having enough money to buy food for the family. Jason's weight is 13.5 pounds and his height is 24.5 inches. This places him in the 10th percentile for weight and the 15th percentile for height. Income screening reveals that the family is eligible for WIC.

▶ Assessment

- 6-month-old male infant experiencing growth failure
- Weight: 13.5 lbs (10th percentile)
- Height: 24.5 in. (15th percentile)

- Mother reports "watering down" infant formula to "make it last"
- Mother reports lack of money for food or formula purchases
- Family is income eligible for WIC

Nursing Diagnosis

Altered nutrition, less than body requirements, related to infant's inadequate formula intake

Expected Client/Family Outcomes	Nursing Action/Intervention	Evaluation
By the end of the visit, the client will: • Identify how improper feeding can lead to infant growth failure.	Explain importance of preparing infant formula according to package directions. *Rationale:* Growth failure is due to insufficient kcal and nutrient intake.	Client provides return demonstration on correct preparation of formula and describes the effects of feeding diluted formula.
• Make appointment for enrollment in WIC.	Contact local WIC program for client referral. *Rationale:* Referral to WIC provides a means of obtaining necessary food in order to prevent further weight loss in infant.	Client reports that she has contacted WIC and is receiving benefits.
• Receive WIC vouchers for infant formula, infant cereal, and infant juice.	Review how WIC foods/formula can be integrated into meal plan. *Rationale:* Enrollment in WIC provides sufficient formula and infant food.	
• Work with the nurse in developing a healthy menu plan for the infant.	Develop a healthy meal schedule for infant. *Rationale:* Client and family benefits from a specific plan to follow.	Client describes menu plan and family's adherence to it.

Chapter Highlights

► Nutrition during the postpartum period is important in promoting restoration of nutrient stores in the mother and providing adequate energy for the demands of caring for a newborn.

► The process of lactation creates significant demands on the mother's body which must be met by an increase in energy and nutrient intake.

► Infants need the same nutrients as older children and adults; however, a larger quantity of each nutrient (protein, carbohydrates, lipids, vitamins, minerals, and water) is needed per unit of infant body weight.

► Lactation involves synthesis of human milk by the alveolar cells in the breast, secretion of milk into the alveolar lumen, and ejection of milk through the ductal system.

► Psychologic conditions may facilitate or hinder lactation and one of the most important factors contributing to the success of breastfeeding is the mother's willingness to breastfeed.

► Breast evaluation consists of the physical examination of each breast and recommendations for interventions relating to comfort measures, engorgement, sore nipples, and inverted nipples.

► The decision to breastfeed is influenced by many factors and nurses can provide the support necessary that may make a difference between success or discontinuation of breastfeeding.

► Women may choose to formula feed their infants for many reasons and nurses must support the decisions of their clients in the choice of a feeding method.

► Infants should either be breastfed or formula fed until one year of age with the introduction of solid foods at approximately 4–6 months of age.

► The most common feeding problems encountered in the first year of life are underfeeding and overfeeding and can be managed by providing client education in all aspects of infant feeding.

After reading the vignette at the beginning of this chapter, use what you have learned to answer these questions.

1. What strategies can Lucy Salas, RN, suggest to help George Mahoney participate in his baby's care?

2. What information concerning maternal and newborn nutritional requirements should Lucy Salas, RN, provide to the Mahoney family?

3. What behaviors would indicate the family's successful adaptation to breastfeeding?

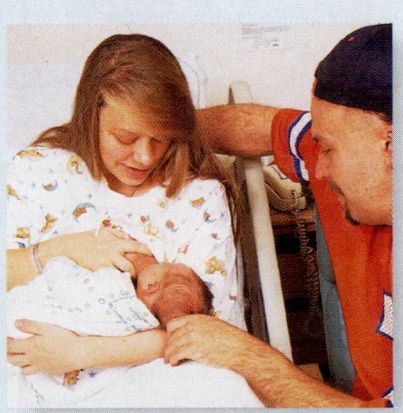

Critical Thinking Questions

► References

American Academy of Pediatrics, Committee on Nutrition. (1976). Commentary on breast feeding and infant formulas, including proposed standards for formulas. *Nutrition Review, 34,* 248–256.

American Academy of Pediatrics, Committee on Nutrition. (1995). Fluoride supplementation for children: Interim policy recommendation. *Pediatrics, 95*(5), 777.

American Academy of Pediatrics. (1997). Workgroup on breastfeeding: Policy statement. *Pediatrics, 100*(6), 1035–1039.

Behrman, R.E. (1992). *Nelson textbook of pediatrics* (14th ed.). Philadelphia: W.B. Saunders.

Biancuzzo, M. (1994). Breastfeeding preterm twins: A case report. *Birth, 21*(2), 96–100.

Blackburn, S.T., & Loper, D.L. (1992). *Maternal, fetal, and neonatal physiology: A clinical perspective.* Philadelphia: W.B. Saunders.

Brown, L.P. (1992). Breastfeeding and jaundice: Cause for concern? *Clinical Issues in Perinatal Women's Health Nursing, 3,* 613–619.

Chua, S., Arulkumaran, S., Lim, I., Selamat, N., & Ratnam, S.S. (1994). Influence of breastfeeding and nipple stimulation on postpartum uterine activity. *British Journal of Obstetrics and Gynecology, 101*(9), 804–805.

Chute, G.E. (1992). Promoting breastfeeding success: An overview of basic management. *Clinical Issues in Perinatal Women's Health Nursing, 3,* 570–582.

Doran, L., & Evers, S. (1997). Energy and nutrient inadequacies in the diets of low-income women who breastfeed. *Journal of the American Dietetic Association, 97*(11), 1283–1287.

Gigliotti, E. (1995). When women decide *not* to breastfeed. *MCN, American Journal of Maternal-Child Nursing, 20*(6), 315–321.

Gromada, K.K. (1991). Breastfeeding more than one: Multiples and tandem breastfeeding. *Clinical Issues in Perinatal Women's Health Nursing, 3,* 656–666.

Greene, G.W., Smiciklas-Wright, H., Scholl, T.O., & Karp, R.J. (1988). Postpartum weight change: How much of the weight gained during pregnancy will be lost after delivery? *Obstetrics and Gynecology, 71*(5), 701–707.

Hambridge, M. (1997). Nutrition and feeding. In G.E. Merenstein (Ed.), *Handbook of pediatrics* (18th ed.) (pp. 50–84). Norwalk, CT: Appleton & Lange.

Hill, P.D., Humenick, S.S. (1989). Insufficient milk supply. *Image, 21,* 145–148.

Hughes, V., & Owen, J. (1993). Is breast-feeding possible after breast surgery? *MCN, American Journal of Maternal-Child Nursing, 18*(4), 213–217.

Janke, J.R. (1994). Development of the breast-feeding attrition prediction tool. *Nursing Research, 43,* 100–104.

Kearney, M.H., Cronenwett, L.R., & Barrett, J.A. (1990). Breast-feeding problems in the first week postpartum. *Nursing Research, 39*(2), 90–95.

Lavergne, N.A. (1997). Does application of tea bags to sore nipples while breastfeeding provide effective relief? *Journal of Obstetric, Gynecologic, and Neonatal Nursing, 26*(1), 53–58.

Lawrence, R.A. (1985). Approach to breastfeeding. In W.A. Walker & J.B. Watkins (Eds.), *Nutrition in pediatrics: Basic science and clinical application.* Boston: Little, Brown.

Lawrence, R.A. (1989). *Breastfeeding: A guide for the medical profession* (3rd ed.). St. Louis: Mosby.

Lawrence, R.A. (1997). *A review of the medical benefits and contraindications to breastfeeding in the United States.* Arlington, VA: National Center for Education in Maternal and Child Health.

Mennella, J.A., & Beauchamp, G.K. (1991). The transfer of alcohol to human milk: Effects in flavor and the infant's behavior. *New England Journal of Medicine, 325*(4), 981.

Mitchell, M.K. (1997). *Nutrition across the life span.* Philadelphia: W.B. Saunders.

National Healthy Mothers, Healthy Babies Coalition. (n.d.). *Working and breastfeeding* [Booklet]. Washington, DC: Author.

National Research Council Food and Nutrition Board (1989). *Recommended dietary allowances* (10th ed.). Washington, DC: National Academy Press.

Neifert, M. (1991). Breastfeeding after breast surgical procedure or breast cancer. *Clinical Issues in Perinatal Women's Health Nursing, 3,* 673–682.

Nikodem, V.C., Danziger, D., Gebka, N., Gulmezoglu, A.M., & Hofmeyr, G.J. (1993). Do cabbage leaves prevent breast engorgement? A randomized controlled study. *Birth, 20*(2), 61–64.

O'Campo, P, Faden, R.R., Gielen, A.C., & Wang, M,C. (1992). Prenatal factors associated with breastfeeding duration: Recommendations for prenatal interventions. *Birth, 19,* 195–201.

Pipes, P. (1996). Nutrition in infancy. In L.K. Mahon & S. Escott-Stump (Eds.), *Food, nutrition, and diet therapy* (9th ed.) (pp. 213–256). Philadelphia: W.B. Saunders.

Riordan, J., & Auerbach, K.G. (1993). *Breastfeeding and human lactation.* Boston: Jones & Bartlett.

Riordan, J.M., & Koehn, M. (1997). Reliability and validity testing of three breastfeeding assessment tools. *Journal of Obstetric, Gynecologic, and Neonatal Nursing, 26*(2), 181–187.

Robbins, M.J. (1992). Breastfeeding in the face of adversity. *MCN, American Journal of Maternal-Child Nursing, 17*(5), 242–245.

Rolfes, S.R., DeBruyne, L.K., & Whitney, E.N. (1990). *Lifespan nutrition: Conception through life.* St. Paul, MN: West.

Ryan, A.S. (1997). The resurgence of breastfeeding in the United States. *Pediatrics 99*(4), E12.

Scholl, T.O., Hediger, M.L., Schall, J.I., Ances, I.G., & Smith, W.K. (1995). Gestational weight gain, pregnancy outcome, and postpartum weight retention. *Obstetrics and Gynecology, 86*(3), 423–427.

Shrago, L., & Bocar, D. (1990). The infant's contribution to breast-feeding. *Journal of Obstetric, Gynecologic, and Neonatal Nursing, 19,* 209–215.

Touger-Decker, R. (1996). Nutrition in dental health. In L.K. Mahon & S. Escott-Stump (Eds.), *Food, nutrition, and diet therapy* (9th ed.) (pp. 581–593). Philadelphia: W.B. Saunders.

U.S. Department of Health and Human Services, Public Health Service. (1991). *Healthy people 2000: National health promotion and disease preventions objectives, full report with commentary* (DHHS Publication No. (PHS) 91-50212). Washington, DC: U.S. Government Printing Office.

Williams, K.M., & Morse, J.M. (1989). Weaning patterns of first-time mothers. *MCN, American Journal of Maternal-Child Nursing, 14*(3), 188–192.

Ziemer, M.M., & Pigeon, J.G. (1993). Skin change and pain in the nipple during the 1st week of lactation. *Journal of Obstetric, Gynecologic, and Neonatal Nursing, 22*(3), 247–256.

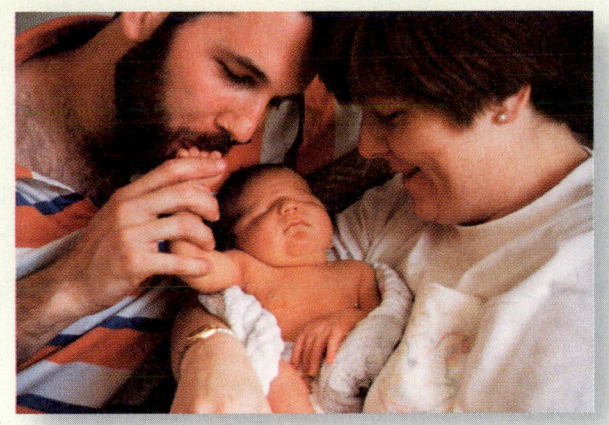

Six-pound Ryan Blair is born anophthalmic, because early in gestation, his eyes never formed. He is an otherwise healthy term infant. His condition is recognized in the nursery when his fused eyelids cannot be separated for the standard eye ointment given to newborns. Neither Ryan's parents, Megan and Ray Blair, nor their health care providers had any prior idea that the baby would be totally blind or that he would have a congenital anomaly. His two-year-old sister Suzanne is healthy and sighted. Unlike other organs, eyes have not been transplanted; Ryan will be blind throughout his life. ∎

32

Assessment and Care of the Newborn at Risk

Major technologic and therapeutic advances have produced significant and often parallel changes in perinatal and neonatal nursing care. Mortality and morbidity rates for pregnant women have improved and currently more infants survive the immediate birth experience than at any other time in history. Despite these advances, the first month of life, the neonatal period, is a risky time for many infants. Although more neonates are surviving the birth experience, some require complex care to adapt to or to survive the early months of life. These neonates are at risk for physical, developmental, and psychosocial problems that may have long-term effects.

The neonatal nurse plays an extremely important role in identifying risk factors or problems that can complicate the neonate's transition to extrauterine life. The nurse is a key member of the interdisciplinary team that works to support the neonate through this transition by providing an environment that promotes optimal growth and development.

▶ THE HIGH-RISK NEONATE

A neonate is described as high risk when physical or social factors affecting the prenatal course, labor and delivery, the transition to extrauterine life, or the newborn period threaten life or well-being. Maternal risk factors, such as lack of prenatal care, poor nutrition, and substance abuse, create a difficult prenatal environment for the fetus and may alter fetal development. Neonates of mothers with medical conditions such as diabetes may also have difficulty in adjusting to extrauterine life.

Premature birth poses special challenges for the neonate. The premature neonate often requires maximum physiologic and environmental support from specially skilled interdisciplinary teams (see Chapter 33). Other neonates may develop special problems in the first hours or days of life that also make the transition to extrauterine life difficult. Such conditions as anemia, inborn errors of metabolism, and congenital heart disease may not have been suspected during pregnancy. These disorders are identified after birth when abnormal signs and symptoms are assessed and further evaluated.

Nurses working in normal newborn nurseries have a special challenge. They must be able to distinguish normal neonatal behavior and physiologic functioning from abnormal signs and symptoms. They must do this by observing and interpreting subtle changes in the neonate. The interdisciplinary health care team, recognizing high-risk problems, may opt to transfer the neonate to a special care or intensive care nursery in the same or another hospital. An interdisciplinary team usually includes nurses, physicians, and respiratory therapists, who carefully coordinate the neonate's care during the transport between hospitals when this is necessary. Early identification of high-risk problems and neonatal transport to level III regional centers have resulted in a decline in neonatal mortality (see Chapter 2).

Transition to parenthood is a process of change and stress even in the best of circumstances. The birth of a seriously ill newborn intensifies the stress and can create a crisis for the family. No physical abnormality or complication can be treated without addressing the emotional concerns of the family (see Chapter 12).

Many assessment and management strategies require procedures that can be restrictive, unpleasant, or painful for the high-risk neonate. Nurses are challenged to integrate soothing and emotionally supportive strategies into their physical care of the newborn. Organizing care to avoid constant or inappropriate stimulation of the neonate, controlling environmental noise and lighting, fostering parent–newborn interaction, and ensuring that the neonate is treated with dignity, touched gently, and cuddled if possible, help to ease the high-risk experience for tiny clients too young and too sick to be advocates for themselves.

▶ NEONATAL PROBLEMS RELATED TO ALTERATIONS IN MATERNAL FUNCTIONING DURING PREGNANCY

▶ The Neonate of a Substance-Abusing Mother

Any prenatal substance abuse can have lifelong adverse consequences for the neonate. The pregnancy of a substance-abusing woman is associated with higher morbidity and mortality for the mother and the neonate. These pregnancies may be complicated by inadequate prenatal care, poor nutrition, sexually transmitted and other infectious diseases, pregnancy-induced hypertension, premature rupture of membranes and the delivery of preterm and small-for-gestational age neonates (Behrman & Kliegman, 1996). Multiple substances may be used; the mother and/or father may have fragile or poor parenting skills. Drug-dependent mothers often lack knowledge about child development and may themselves have experienced physical, sexual, or verbal abuse and/or multiple social, family, and interpersonal losses. For example, mothers of cocaine-addicted infants may have high levels of anxiety and depression (Ludwig, Marecki,

Wooldridge, & Sherman, 1996). At the time of delivery or during the postpartum, the parents may continue to be involved with drugs.

The most commonly abused substances include alcohol, marijuana, cocaine, and opiates (heroin and methadone). Periodic episodes of cerebral anoxia, caused by repetitive in utero withdrawal of the abused substance, can cause permanent brain damage in the fetus. Withdrawal from the addicting agents can also occur after birth, causing multiple physiologic problems for the neonate. In addition, the neonate may demonstrate a number of behavioral and attachment problems and often has difficulty adjusting to environmental stimuli such as noises and bright lights.

Drug Abuse

Nursing and Collaborative Assessment.
Assessment of the pregnant woman must include a maternal history of drug use during pregnancy. Unfortunately, this information is difficult to obtain with accuracy because the mother may be reluctant to share any details or may be an unreliable historian. Identification of drugs used immediately prior to delivery is of utmost importance too. Drugs crossing the placenta may seriously compromise the neonate's ability to adjust to extrauterine life immediately after birth.

Recognition of the most common signs of drug withdrawal in the neonate, sometimes called neonatal abstinence syndrome, is an important part of ongoing nursing assessment. Neonates exhibit central nervous system, gastrointestinal, respiratory, and vasomotor symptoms as a result of drug withdrawal. Table 32–1 lists some of the most common symptoms observed in neonates suffering from drug withdrawal. Most neonates exhibit signs of withdrawal in the first 24 to 72 hours of life. Many nurseries have special checklists on which withdrawal symptoms can be quickly docu-

mented throughout the neonate's hospital stay. Figure 32–1 gives an example of a withdrawal symptom checklist.

Nursing and Collaborative Management.
Early identification of drug abuse in pregnant women is important for the prompt delivery of appropriate treatment for the neonate. The main treatment goal is to support the neonate's physical needs while maintaining an environment that promotes adequate adjustment to extrauterine life. Specific nursing interventions include the following:

- Identifying the neonate at risk for drug withdrawal
- Decreasing environmental stimuli to reduce irritability, conserve energy, and promote sleep and rest; limiting loud noises and bright lights; swaddling the neonate; and approaching the neonate calmly
- Balancing small, frequent feedings with frequent rest periods to conserve energy and promote nutrition and growth
- When possible, feeding the neonate "on demand" rather than according to a predetermined feeding schedule
- Supporting the neonate's self-comforting measures, such as making the pacifier easily available
- Promoting the neonate's skin integrity by changing the neonate's position and by frequently cleaning and drying the skin, in particular the diaper area
- Providing support and education to the parents in a nonjudgmental, nonpunishing manner. Indeed, these clients present major challenges. In their study of neonatal nurses' knowledge of and attitudes toward caring for cocaine-

▶ **TABLE 32–1**

Signs of Neonatal Narcotic Withdrawal

W	=	wakefulness
I	=	irritability
T	=	tremulousness, temperature variation, tachypnea
H	=	hyperactivity, high-pitched cry, hyperacusis, hyperreflexia, hypertonus, hiccups
D	=	diarrhea, diaphoresis, disorganized suck
R	=	rub marks (excoriations on knees and face), regurgitation (vomiting)
A	=	apneic spells, autonomic dysfunction
W	=	weight loss (or failure to gain weight)
A	=	alkalosis (respiratory)
L	=	lacrimation
S	=	stuffy nose, sneezing, seizures

Source: Reproduced, with permission, from Rudolph, A.M., Hoffman, J.I.E., & Rudolph, C.D. (Eds.). (1996). Rudolph's pediatrics (20th ed.). Stamford, CT: Appleton & Lange, p. 840.

System	Signs and Symptoms	Score	AM				PM					Comments
Neonatal abstinence syndrome assessment scoresheet						Name: _____						
						Date: _____						
Central nervous system disturbances	Excessive high pitched (or other) cry	2										Daily weight:
	Continuous high pitched (or other) cry	3										
	Sleeps < 1 hour after feeding	3										
	Sleeps > 2 hours after feeding	2										
	Sleeps < 3 hours after feeding	1										
	Hyperactive moro reflex	2										
	Markedly hyperactive moro reflex	3										
	Mild tremors, disturbed	1										
	Moderate-severe tremors, disturbed	2										
	Mild tremors, undisturbed	3										
	Moderate-severe tremors, undisturbed	4										
	Increased muscle tone	2										
	Excoriation (specify area): _____	1										
	Myoclonic jerks	3										
	Generalized convulsions	5										
Metabolic/vasomotor/respiratory disturbances	Sweating	1										
	Fever (< 101° F; 99–100.8° F; 37.2–38.2° C)	1										
	Fever (38.4°C and higher)	2										
	Frequent yawning (> 3–4 times/interval)	1										
	Mottling or webbing	1										
	Nasal stuffiness	2										
	Sneezing (> 3–4 times/interval)	1										
	Nasal flaring	2										
	Respiratory rate > 60/minute	1										
	Respiratory rate > 60/minute with retractions	2										
Gastrointestinal disturbances	Excessive sucking more than 5 minutes after feeding	1										
	Poor feeding, poorly coordinated sucking and swallowing reflex	2										
	Regurgitation	2										
	Projectile vomiting	3										
	Loose stools	2										
	Watery stools	3										
Total score												
Initials of scorer												

FIGURE 32–1. Neonatal abstinence syndrome assessment scoresheet. *(Courtesy of Thomas Jefferson University, Philadelphia, PA.)*

exposed infants and their mothers, Ludwig and colleagues (1996) found that nurses lacked knowledge about caring for these clients. The nurses' attitudes toward the mothers were generally negative and/or judgmental. The nurses who had more experience with this population and who worked in higher acuity settings tended to have more positive attitudes toward the babies but not toward their mothers.

• Promoting parent–infant bonding, whenever feasible. The substance-abusing parent requires support, but also supervision. In some cases, the parent may be too affected by drug use to hold and care for the newborn safely. Grandparents or other relatives may be primary caretakers for the infant and therefore need support and education to help in building their confidence and their relationship with the baby.

• Maintaining an interdisciplinary approach, so that interventions for the family as well as the newborn can be started or continued.

Medications and other therapies may be required for these neonates. Medications for neonatal withdrawal are based on the type of drug or drugs affecting the neonate and the severity of withdrawal symp-

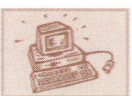

Research Abstract

Neonatal Nurses' Knowledge of and Attitudes Toward Caring for Cocaine-Exposed Infants and Their Mothers

A questionnaire survey was used to identify the knowledge, attitudes, and backgrounds of 215 nurses who worked in Level I, II, or III nurseries of 6 hospitals in northwestern New York State. The sample represented 35% of questionnaires; considering this was an anonymous survey that offered no special compensation or follow-up for nonrespondents, the researchers were pleased with the return. They were careful to identify potentials for sampling biases, related to the return rate, location, etc. The level of nurses' knowledge about cocaine abuse and its implications for nursing cocaine-addicted infants and their mothers was found to be low; the nurses' attitudes toward the mothers, but not toward their infants, were found overall to be negative and/or judgmental. Greater experience with caring for cocaine-addicted infants and higher acuity of the neonatal unit in which the nurse worked correlated with more positive attitudes toward the infants, but not their mothers. Weak correlations were found between knowledge and attitude and formal education, inservice education and self-education; nurses who had more educational experiences tended to have more positive attitudes, although the researchers questioned whether nurses with more positive attitudes sought more education about cocaine-addicted infants.

Application to Practice

A basic belief of professional nursing is that care should be delivered in a nonjudgmental manner. But what happens when the clients have high-risk lifestyles, such as prenatal cocaine use, that go against what is socially acceptable and result in harm to their infants? This study indicates that nurses do harbor negative, judgmental attitudes toward such clients. In addition, such attitudes were accompanied by overall lack of knowledge about prenatal cocaine use and its effects on babies. While the study did not specifically identify how the care the nurses delivered was actually affected, it seems as if respondents had a lot of their own feelings to overcome before they could provide support and therapeutic care to these high-risk mothers. Nevertheless, women who use cocaine are still mothers, although they are considered high risk; cocaine-exposed infants do go home to their families. The study challenges nurses in practice to identify their own attitudes, to assess how staff care for cocaine-addicted clients and babies in their own settings, and to seek, design, or implement the kind of educational programs that will help staff to work with such clients in a caring and professional manner.

Source: Ludwig, M.A., Marecki, M., Wooldridge, P.J., & Sherman, L.M. (1996). Neonatal nurses' knowledge of and attitudes toward caring for cocaine-exposed infants and their mothers. Journal of Perinatal and Neonatal Nursing, 9(4); 81–95.

toms. Severe irritability that disrupts normal sleeping or feeding patterns, poor weight gain, diarrhea, and seizures are signs that indicate treatment.

Heroin and methadone withdrawal have been treated successfully with various combinations of narcotics, sedatives, and hypnotics. The doses and duration of treatment are ordered and adjusted to control symptoms. For example, phenobarbital has been used to decrease irritability and prevent seizures. Weaning the infant from the drug is individualized and based on the baby's progress. Babies with severe autonomic symptoms may be treated with medications such as paregoric.

Prenatal Alcohol Use

Alcohol easily crosses the placenta and produces fetal blood levels similar to those of the pregnant woman. The fetal liver is immature, and the developing fetus is therefore exposed to the harmful effects of alcohol for a longer time period (Gardner, 1997). Alcohol exposure can damage the fetus and cause birth defects, including mental retardation and neurodevelopmental deficits. The type of birth defects and long-term problems, related to fetal alcohol exposure, vary and depend upon such factors as the gestational age of the fetus and the level of alcohol exposure (Gardner, 1997). For example, exposure to alcohol during the first trimester places a fetus at risk for organ and musculoskeletal anomalies; exposure during the second and third trimesters increases the risk of such problems as intrauterine growth retardation and preterm delivery. The most important factor in alcohol-related anomalies is believed to be the peak blood alcohol level. Binge drinking therefore poses an especially great risk to fetal development (Gardner, 1997).

In addition to alcohol, some women use other drugs, like cocaine and heroin. Such polydrug use jeopardizes fetal as well as maternal health and safety.

No safe level has been identified for alcohol intake during pregnancy. Therefore, to prevent alcohol related harm to the fetus, women who desire to become pregnant or who are pregnant should be advised not to consume any alcohol (Cunningham et al., 1997).

Assessment of maternal alcohol consumption and the mother's knowledge of its effects on an unborn child must ideally occur before conception. Alcohol education, including facts about the consequences of alcohol consumption during pregnancy, should be provided to women of childbearing age. Preconceptional as well as prenatal health visits should include the topic of alcohol. The American Academy of Pediatrics (1993) advocates that alcohol educational programs be integrated in elementary, junior high, senior high, and postsecondary education settings.

Nursing and Collaborative Assessment.

Assessment of pregnant women includes maternal history of alcohol use before and during pregnancy. A nonjudgmental, conversational calm approach is the best method for obtaining an accurate history. Certain questions may be useful in identifying the alcohol-using mothers.

- Have you had any beer, wine, wine coolers, or any other alcoholic beverage since you became pregnant or began trying to get pregnant?
- When was the last time you drank beer, wine, or wine coolers or any other alcoholic drink? Do you recall how much you had to drink at that time? Was this what you usually drink? Please describe.
- How often do you think you drink too much? How often have you had alcoholic beverages since you became pregnant?
- Please describe any other drugs used along with alcoholic beverages.
- Do you feel you have or ever had a drinking problem? If so, in what ways have you tried to deal with your drinking?
- Does anyone in your family have a drinking problem? Please describe.

- Are you aware that alcoholic drinks can affect an unborn baby?
- Are you currently receiving help for a drinking problem? If not, would you like help?

Some clients may not be aware of the effects that alcohol can have on their unborn child. Clients falling into the high-risk group of heavy alcohol consumption require additional information, intervention, and support directed by a multidisciplinary team. Nurses must reinforce the importance of continued prenatal care. When appropriate, nurses can refer these clients to programs specializing in care of pregnant, substance-abusing women. Maintaining contact throughout the pregnancy is important to ensure proper follow-up care.

Assessment of the neonate begins with identification of maternal alcohol use. At times, however, identification is not possible prior to delivery of the neonate.

Fetal alcohol syndrome (FAS) is the term given to a group of abnormalities found in neonates who are exposed to unsafe levels of alcohol during pregnancy. Estimates indicate that FAS occurs in 1 to 3 of 1000 live births; however, the incidence is believed to be higher among certain populations, for example, among some Native American communities and underreported in the general population (Gardner, 1997). Unfortunately, FAS often goes undiagnosed and unreported for several reasons. For instance, physicians may not diagnose FAS, particularly among clients whose social standing is similar to theirs; health care providers may be reluctant to make a diagnosis that would give a negative label to a woman and infant; and women who drink heavily also may not accurately reveal the amount of their drinking.

About one third of infants of alcoholic women demonstrate FAS. The major characteristics are (Gardner, 1997):

- Prenatal and postnatal growth retardation (failure to thrive, low birth weight, microcephaly)
- Mental impairment (delayed development; hyperactivity; learning or attention disorders; poor motor coordination; mental retardation)
- Craniofacial abnormalities (Fig. 32–2) (small palpebral fissures [eye openings]; flat maxillary area, thin upper lip; flat or absent philtrum; short, upturned nose).

About 50% of affected infants have poor coordination, hypotonia, attention deficit disorders with hyperactivity, and decreased adipose tissue in early childhood (American Academy of Pediatrics, 1993). Other problems associated with FAS include cardiac anomalies, hemangiomas, eye and ear anomalies, and weak sucking ability. About two thirds of infants born

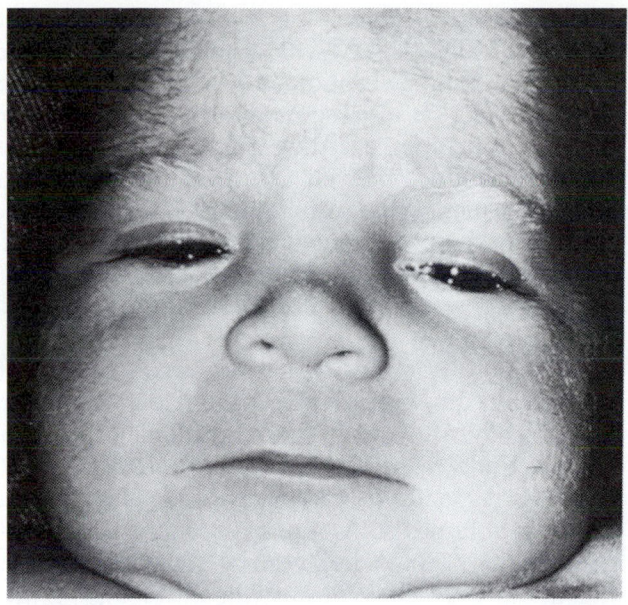 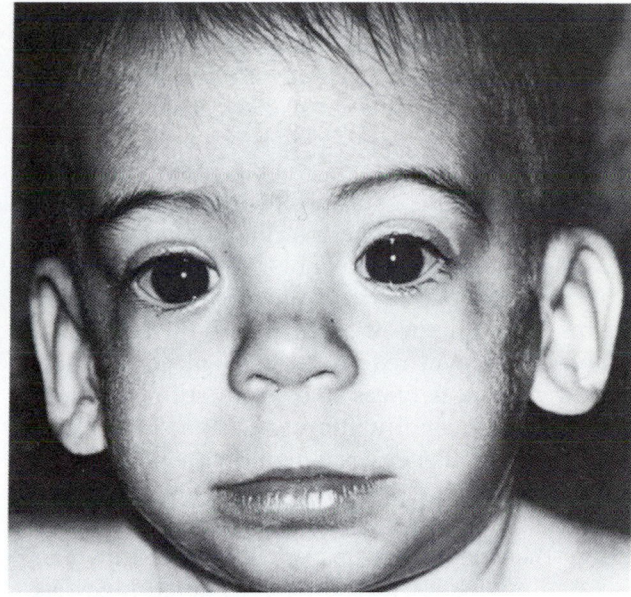

A   B

FIGURE 32–2. Facial features of a child with fetal alcohol syndrome at **(A)** 1 week and **(B)** 1 year of age. Note the narrow palpebral fissures at one week, short nose with broad low bridge, and absent philtrum with narrow lip. *(Reproduced, with permission, from Rudolph, A.M., Hoffman, J.I.E., & Rudolph, C.D. (Eds.). (1996).* Rudolph's pediatrics *(20th ed.). Stamford, CT: Appleton & Lange, p. 420.)*

to alcoholic women develop alcohol related birth defects (ARBD) and have some of FAS' physical anomalies or alcohol-related neurodevelopmental disorder (ARND) and show some of the neurodevelopmental anomalies of FAS. These children have a variety of problems and are prone to attention deficit disorders with hyperactivity, fine-motor impairment, clumsiness, and delays in speech development (American Academy of Pediatrics, 1993).

Nursing Diagnoses. Nursing diagnoses for the neonate with FAS are based on a comprehensive assessment. Examples of nursing diagnoses include:

Problem-oriented diagnoses:

- Altered growth and development, related to teratogenic effects of alcohol on fetus
- Altered nutrition: less than body requirements, related to weak neonatal sucking ability
- Altered family processes, related to alcohol-impaired interactions

Wellness-oriented diagnoses:

- Potential for enhanced neonatal development, related to participation in infant development program
- Potential for progressive family coping, related to parental participation in treatment and in support groups

Nursing and Collaborative Management. Care of the neonate with FAS focuses on providing supportive and palliative interventions. Special attention should be taken to avoid overstimulating the neonate. Keeping lights low, minimizing noise, swaddling the baby with blankets, and offering a pacifier are particularly helpful in soothing and quieting the neonate. Ongoing assessment of neurologic function should include observation of the neonate's alertness, body position, muscle tone, movement, and reflexes. Seizures are treated with anticonvulsant medications. (See the section on Neonatal Seizures near the end of the chapter.) Enteral or parenteral feedings may be necessary if the neonate's ability to suck is too weak to meet nutritional and hydration needs.

Infants with FAS/ARND need interventions that monitor developmental progress, health, and home environment. Parents and family members need ongoing support. They must be given accurate information about how the neonate will respond to stimuli and strategies that can be used to console the neonate when at home. Prior to discharge, parents should be given opportunities to feed the neonate; the nurse can use this time to offer suggestions that will assist parents in providing the neonate with adequate nutrition, as discussed earlier. Referral services for parents and infants are needed. These infants can be difficult to care for and parents frequently need ongoing help with parenting skills.

The effects of FAS do not disappear as the infant grows older. The problems associated with FAS and ARND described earlier can persist throughout the life of the affected individual (American Academy of Pediatrics, 1993). Parents and family members must be aware that support and management strategies introduced in the neonatal period must continue in varying degrees throughout the child's life.

Women who abuse alcohol may also use other drugs. Combinations of drugs increase risk of severe problems for the fetus. Women who have additional substance abuse will require further support, education, and referral services. Neonates suffering from both drug and alcohol withdrawal have special care needs, such as a quiet environment, frequent feedings, and ongoing medical follow-up. Mothers who have abused drugs and alcohol during pregnancy to such an extent that the neonate suffers from withdrawal or has related anomalies should be considered high-risk clients for parenting disorders. Drug abuse impairs parental judgment and the ability to care for a neonate, especially a neonate who is difficult to feed and comfort.

Evaluation of the mother's social situation and the family's home environment is important to ensure safety and security of the neonate. Interdisciplinary collaboration, including nurses, physicians, and social workers, is essential in identifying the neonate's special needs. Inclusion of other family members in planning for care (such as the neonate's grandparents), is essential because these individuals may become the primary care providers at home. At times the home environment may be so unstable that foster care becomes necessary. Social workers will be able to identify appropriate community agencies and resources for the neonate, mother, and family to assist with this difficult process. In addition, such strategies as residential treatment centers for substance-using mothers and neonates to facilitate parenting abilities may also be needed.

▶ The Neonate of a Diabetic Mother

Diabetes mellitus is a major high-risk condition of pregnancy (see Chapter 19). A woman may be diabetic before pregnancy or diabetes may emerge during pregnancy. Maternal diabetes is associated with a higher than normal rate of such problems as congenital anomalies and fetal death. In addition, the children of women who had uncontrolled or poorly controlled diabetic pregnancies may be at risk for developing insulin resistance, or Type II, non-insulin dependent diabetes mellitus (Doshier, 1995).

Reducing risk for the neonate of a diabetic mother ideally begins with establishment of good control prior to conception and then careful prenatal care, focusing on glucose monitoring, metabolic control, and teaching regarding diet and medication so that plasma glucose levels are safely maintained during pregnancy (Blackburn & Loper, 1992; Doshier, 1995). The goals are to monitor the pregnancy closely so that the neonate can be born at term with minimal complications and to treat actual and potential problems of the newborn.

Alterations in glucose metabolism in the diabetic mother can dramatically affect the fetus in utero and immediately after birth. Hyperglycemia in the diabetic mother causes fetal hyperglycemia. The fetal pancreas responds to this hyperglycemia by producing large volumes of insulin, a condition called hyperinsulinemia. The hyperglycemia and hyperinsulinemia in the fetus affect intrauterine physiologic growth and development. The fetus is at risk for developing problems in many body systems, for example, congenital heart defects.

The birth of the neonate of the diabetic mother may be complicated by a preterm delivery or a difficult term delivery. The neonate may develop problems after birth because the neonate's pancreas continues to produce larger volumes of insulin resulting in a drop in the glucose level. If untreated, the neonate can develop hypoglycemia and other serious complications.

Nursing and Collaborative Assessment

Appearance. The infant of a diabetic mother often has a large body (macrosomia; Fig. 32–3). The neonate appears plump, plethoric (beefy red), and puffy. The macrosomia is believed to result from an increase in cell number and size, due to the effects of circulating insulin (Suevo, 1997). The neonate may become floppy and lethargic and suck poorly or may become jittery and irritable. Neonates of diabetic mothers also may be small for gestational age as a result of placental insufficiency in utero.

Assessment of the neonate both at rest and during activities such as feeding is important. Accurate measurements of height, weight, and head and chest circumferences should be plotted on the neonate's growth chart.

Intrauterine Growth. Hyperglycemia and hyperinsulinemia affect the intrauterine growth of neonates of diabetic mothers. Intrauterine growth can be accelerated, causing some neonates of diabetic mothers to be large for gestational age (LGA) (Samson,

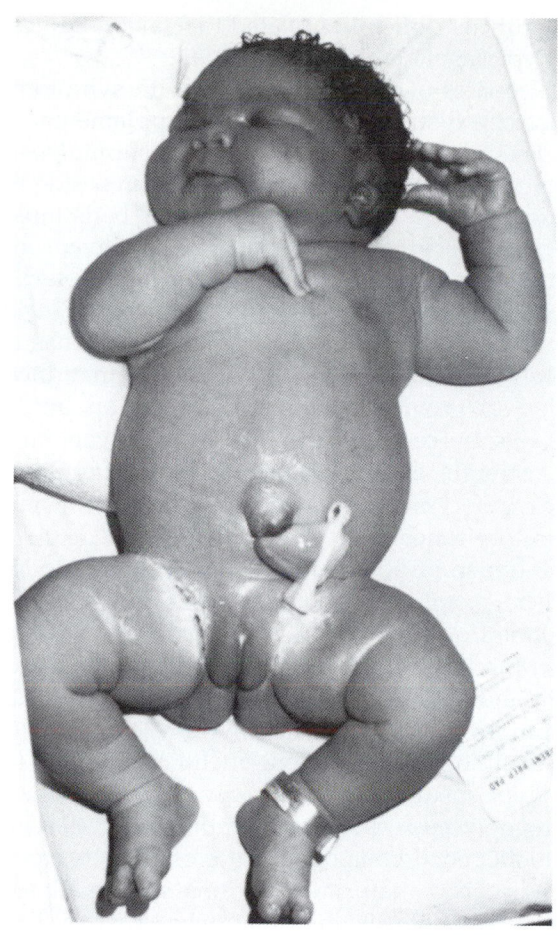

FIGURE 32–3. This macrosomic infant weighing 6050 g was born to a woman with gestational diabetes.

1992; Suevo, 1997). When intrauterine growth is accelerated, most body organs except the brain are prone to be larger. Unlike other LGA neonates, LGA neonates of diabetic mothers characteristically have subcutaneous fat deposits rather than increased length and head size (Fig. 32–3). Large-for-gestational-age neonates are at greater risk for injuries during delivery. Cesarean delivery may be warranted to prevent traumatic birth injuries such as shoulder dystocia, clavicular fractures, depressed skull fractures, brachial plexus palsy, and facial paralysis.

Conversely, some neonates of diabetic mothers may be low birth weight and/or small for gestational age, particularly if they are delivered prematurely or if there is maternal vascular disease associated with the diabetes (Behrman & Kliegman, 1996). These neonates require special attention related to their low-birth-weight and potentially compromised metabolic state.

Respiratory Distress. The neonate of a diabetic mother is at risk for developing respiratory distress and hyaline membrane disease after birth. Surfactant is the phospholipoprotein required for adequate respiration in the newborn. Surfactant production is altered by the hyperinsulinemia in the fetus. As a result, the neonate of a diabetic mother may not produce enough surfactant before birth. The neonate may develop signs and symptoms of respiratory distress. A high respiratory rate (greater than 60 breaths per minute when sleeping or quiet) may be observed. The neonate may have an expiratory grunt with each breath, exhibit retractions or nasal flaring, and require supplemental oxygen. The nurse should assess the color of the neonate's skin, mucous membranes, and nail beds. Pale, dusky, or blue color changes indicate increasing respiratory distress requiring immediate intervention.

Congenital Anomalies. The neonate of a poorly controlled or uncontrolled diabetic mother is at risk for congenital anomalies. Preconceptional and early first trimester hyperglycemia have been associated with such congenital malformations as cardiac defects (Doshier, 1995). Cardiovascular anomalies associated with infants of diabetic mothers include transposition of the great vessels, coarctation of the aorta, atrial and ventricular septal defects, and cardiomegaly (Samson, 1992; Suevo, 1997). Skeletal and central nervous system malformations include neural tube defects and caudal regression syndrome. Ear anomalies and renal and gastrointestinal malformations have also been associated with infants of diabetic mothers.

Assessment of the neonate with suspected cardiac anomalies includes attention to heart rate, blood pressure, peripheral pulses, color, and activity level. A neonate who has sustained tachycardia, weak peripheral pulses, and a pale or dusky coloring, and who tires quickly with feedings or activity should be assessed further. Abnormalities of the spine may be apparent at birth and are managed according to the anomaly. The nurse assesses the neonate's musculoskeletal system, noting the presence of obvious abnormalities and the neonate's ability to move all extremities equally well.

Metabolic Disturbances. The neonate of a diabetic mother is at risk for numerous alterations in metabolic functioning. These neonates often develop hypoglycemia (low blood glucose level) as a result of the presence of high levels of insulin in the absence of the maternal source of glucose (see Alterations in Metabolic Functioning later in the chapter). Insulin levels are initially high at birth because the fetal pancreas attempts to respond to high glucose levels in utero. Adjustment to normal limits usually occurs in the first few days of life. Polycythemia may result from dehydration related to intrauterine hyperglycemia or chronic fetal stress (Suevo, 1997). Respiratory distress, related to decreased alveolar gas exchange from this condition, may occur.

These neonates are also at risk for hyperbilirubinemia related to delayed transition from fetal to adult hemoglobin or from normal red blood cell breakdown in the polycythemic infant (Suevo, 1997) (see Alterations in Hematologic Functioning later in the chapter). Hypocalcemia may also be found during the neonatal assessment. Hypocalcemia may be related to abnormalities in maternal calcium levels, prematurity, or a difficult delivery. Glucagon production in the liver may decrease in response to the low glucose levels found in the neonate of the diabetic mother after delivery. Nursing assessment of the neonate of a diabetic mother includes the assessment of signs and symptoms of metabolic disturbances as well as the monitoring of laboratory test results.

Nursing Diagnoses

Nursing diagnoses for the neonate of a diabetic mother are developed on the basis of a comprehensive assessment. Examples of nursing diagnoses for a macrosomic neonate include:

Problem-oriented diagnoses:

- Risk for trauma to the neonate during labor and delivery, related to large size
- Altered nutrition: less than body requirements, related to hypoglycemia in the newborn period

Wellness-oriented diagnoses:

- Effective family coping, related to understanding physiologic bases of neonatal macrosomia
- Potential for normal neonatal growth and development, related to maternal glycemic control during pregnancy

Nursing and Collaborative Management

Care of the neonate of a diabetic mother must address the actual and potential complications of delivering a macrosomic and LGA newborn. The initial and ongoing newborn assessments include inspection for traumatic birth injuries. Management is determined by the type and severity of the actual injuries sustained by the neonate. Small-for-gestational age neonates are less likely to sustain traumatic birth injuries. They do, however, face high-risk deliveries because of maternal complications related to severe diabetes, low birth weight, and in many cases prematurity (see Chapter 33). They also are at great risk, after delivery, of devel-

oping further difficulties related to fetal hypoglycemia and hyperinsulinemia.

Neonates of diabetic mothers with symptoms of respiratory distress may require supplemental oxygen. The infant should be placed in a supine position with the head of the bed elevated, or in a side-lying position. Side rails of cribs or warmer beds must be raised and secured in that position to prevent infant falls, especially when the head of the bed is elevated.

Respiratory distress can progress to hyaline membrane disease if surfactant production has been severely altered. Mechanical ventilation may then be needed to provide adequate oxygenation until the lung disease resolves and the neonate can breathe well enough without assistance. Continuous cardiorespiratory monitoring and ongoing assessment of respiratory function are therefore essential.

If hyperbilirubinemia is expected, bilirubin levels must be monitored. Phototherapy is the most common treatment for mild to moderate hyperbilirubinemia. Muscle irritability may be related to hypocalcemia and should be confirmed by obtaining serum calcium levels. Supplementation of calcium via intravenous fluid is the treatment of choice.

Hyperinsulinemia is directly related to the risk for hypoglycemia, the most common alteration in the metabolic functioning of neonates of diabetic mothers. Hypoglycemia may have obvious signs and symptoms or it may be asymptomatic. In either case, early identification and management can prevent further high-risk complications for the neonate. Neonatal hypoglycemia is addressed in more detail in the later section, Alterations in Metabolic Functioning.

Neonates of diabetic mothers require close observation, because problems involving many organ systems may emerge soon after delivery. The length of a neonate's stay in an intensive care nursery will be determined by how quickly the infant is able to make successful transition to extrauterine life and by how quickly the blood glucose level stabilizes. Parents require ongoing support and information from the interdisciplinary team in caring for the neonate.

▶ The Neonate of an Infected Mother

Infections in the neonate are the result of preconceptional, prenatal, intrapartal, or postpartal exposure to harmful microorganisms. Infections acquired before conception, such as human immunodeficiency virus, can affect the neonate. Some infections can pose a potential threat during pregnancy. One such group of infections, called the TORCH infections, is discussed in Chapter 19. Intrapartal infections occur when the neonate is exposed to organisms such as *Chlamydia trachomatis* or herpes simplex virus, which can be found in the mother's genital tract. This exposure can occur after membranes rupture or during passage through the birth canal. Postnatal infections can be caused by contact with these same organisms; however, many postnatal infections have been found to be nosocomial (hospital-acquired) infections. These infections are caused by normal human flora or pathogens that are transmitted from neonate to neonate on the hands of nursery staff (Cunningham et al., 1997).

Each newborn is at risk of being infected. Unfortunately, neonatal intensive care nurseries pose many risk factors for infections. Consistent use of universal precautions, and, particularly, good hand washing techniques, is essential for staff working in any setting, and especially in working with such vulnerable populations as newborns. Use of universal precautions prevents and limits spread of infections to other infants and to health care providers as well.

Neonatal Sepsis

The term *sepsis* currently refers to a systemic inflammatory response syndrome (SIRS), resulting from infection (Jacobs & Darville, 1996). Infection is often due to bacteria, although such microorganisms as viruses and fungi may cause sepsis (Tangredi, 1998). In sepsis, infection provokes a cascade of metabolic,

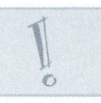

Nursing Alert

The most common means of transmitting bacterial infection is through either direct contact, for example, in the birth canal or from caregivers' hands, or indirect contact, for example, via a contaminated object like a thermometer or droplets from coughing or sneezing (Askin, 1995).

immune, and clinical changes. Without successful treatment, sepsis can produce shock and result in multiple organ dysfunction and death. Table 32–2 presents definitions of sepsis and septic shock. The box entitled Group B Streptococcal Infection in the Newborn describes Group B streptococcus (GBS), the leading bacterial infection causing illness or death in newborns (Mitchell, Stefferson, Hogan, & Brooks, 1997).

Early onset of congenital neonatal sepsis usually emerges within the first 24 hours to 4 days after birth and tends to progress faster than late onset sepsis (Askin, 1995). Such microorganisms from the normal

---

▶ **TABLE 32-2**

Definitions of Sepsis and Septic Shock

Systemic Inflammatory Response Syndrome (SIRS): A characteristic clinical response manifested by two or more of the following conditions:

Hyper- or hypothermia	Temperature ≥38.4°C or <36°C
Tachycardia	Infant heart rate >160 bpm
	Child heart rate >150 bpm
Tachypnea	Infant respiratory rate >60 bpm
	Child respiratory rate >50 bpm
Pathologic white blood cell count	>15,000 cells/µL, <5000 cells/µL, or >10% immature (band) forms

Sepsis: The systemic inflammatory response due to infection

Severe SIRS: SIRS or sepsis associated with one of the following manifestations of organ hypoperfusion:

Lactic acidosis	
Oliguria	Urine output <0.5 mL/kg/h for 2 hrs.
Altered mental status	
Inadequate oxygenation	A-a gradient >40 mm Hg, Pao_2 <70 on room air or Sao_2 <92% on room air

Severe sepsis: All of the above plus clinical evidence of infection

Shock due to SIRS: Meet the criteria for SIRS plus one of the following:

Hypoperfusion requiring >40 mL/kg isotonic fluid (crystalloid or colloid) and/or inotropic support

Hypotension

More than one manifestation of organ hypoperfusion

Septic shock: The above criteria plus clinical evidence of infection

Source: Reproduced, with permission, from Rudolph, A.M., Hoffman, J.I.E., & Rudolph, C. D. (Eds.). (1996). Rudolph's pediatrics (20th ed.). Stamford, CT: Appleton & Lange, p. 532.

▶ GROUP B STREPTOCOCCAL INFECTION IN THE NEWBORN

Group B beta-hemolytic streptococcus (GBS) or *Streptococcus agalactiae*, a gram-positive aerobic coccobaccilus, is responsible for the leading bacterial infection causing illness or death in newborns. Of the estimated 4 million births each year in the United States, up to 8000 cases of GBS occur, with about 300 resulting neonatal deaths; survivors may suffer long-term problems (Glantz & Kedley, 1998; Mitchell et al., 1997). An average of 20% of pregnant women are believed to carry GBS in the rectum or lower genital tract during pregnancy, as the gastrointestinal tract is the most common reservoir for GBS (Glantz & Kedley, 1998). GBS is not the same organism as group A streptococcus or *Streptococcus pyogenes*, which is the cause of the common "strep throat" infections. GBS infections may be early or late onset. Mothers are often asymptomatic.

EARLY ONSET GBS:

- Most common type of GBS infection
- Acquired from the mother (vertical transmission) during pregnancy or birth
- Occurs within 7 days of birth (average age of infant is 20 hours)
- Most infants are full term, but an estimated 30–50% are premature
- Other risk factors include a maternal history of premature ruptured membranes, maternal fever in labor and chorioamnionitis
- Associated with higher morbidity and mortality than late onset GBS (Askin, 1995; Mitchell et al., 1997). An estimated 40–70% of infants of mothers who are colonized at delivery become colonized with the identical group B streptococcal serotype by 3–5 days after delivery; however, only about 1% develop invasive disease (Friedland & McCracken, 1996). Group B streptoccal serotypes I, II, and III equally result in early onset sepsis

Signs and Symptoms

Because GBS may masquerade as other conditions often seen in the newborn, early detection may be difficult. First signs of early onset GBS sepsis may be respiratory distress (most common sign), lethargy, poor muscle tone and feeding behaviors, hypoglycemia, inability to maintain body temperature, tachycardia, jaundice, and pallor. Onset may also be sudden and accompanied by severe symptoms. The primary focus may be the lungs, although meningitis may sometimes be present. Septic shock may occur. Indications of poor perfusion, which is seen in this condition, are mottled skin, weak pulses, capillary refill longer than 2 seconds (seen best in the big toe), oliguria, metabolic acidosis, and hypotension. Respiratory distress due to GBS is hard to distinguish from respiratory distress due to other causes.

Assessment

Early identification of signs of GBS; cultures on blood and cerebrospinal fluid (CSF); CBC with differential shows neutropenia and thrombocytopenia; tests for GBS antigen, e.g., latex agglutination testing of urine; countercurrent immu-noelectrophoresis (CIE) on urine, blood, or CSF; cultures on tracheal or gastric aspirates can indicate exposure to GBS but do not identify tissue invasion without positive blood cultures; monitoring of intake and output, blood glucose levels, electrolytes, acid-base balance.

Management

Includes such antibiotics as penicillin G (often the drug of choice), ampicillin, or aminoglycosides (especially gentamicin) alone or in combination; NICU care; supportive therapy to avoid or minimize complications and to ensure adequate fluids, nutrition, ventilation, oxygenation, and tissue perfusion; interventions to manage seizures and increased intracranial pressure for infants with meningitis.

LATE ONSET GBS

- Affects infants from 8 days to 3 months old, but occurs most often at 2–4 weeks of age
- Maternal acquisition is the most common cause
- Infants become colonized during birth, but why some infants progress to active infection and others do not is unknown
- Staff who are themselves colonized can transmit GBS
- Without strict use of universal precautions by staff and all those caring for the infant, GBS can be spread from infected to well infants

Signs and Symptoms

Poor feeding and fever may be the first symptoms; many of these infants have had a respiratory infection. The following may occur:

- Meningitis: signs include fever, irritability, high pitched cry, poor feeding, seizures and tachypnea (Mitchell et al., 1997). Streptococcal group B III accounts for 90% of meningitis caused by these microbes; about half the survivors of neonatal group B streptococcal meningitis have some degree of neurologic impairment (Friedland & McCracken, 1996). Confirmed by lumbar puncture.
- Bacteremia (signs include poor feeding, irritability, fever, "acute" illness)

Management

Similar to interventions for an infant with early onset GBS disease; focuses on hydration, oxygenation, ventilation, tissue perfusion, and intravenous antibiotics. Infants may recover completely.

Around 20% of GBS infections cannot be categorized as early or late syndromes; they involve many different organ systems and spread over a broad clinical spectrum. Examples of these "miscellaneous syndromes" include cellulitis, scalp abscess, conjunctivitis, and peritonitis (Friedland & McCracken, 1996).

The social, financial, and emotional cost of GBS is so high that the American Academy of Pediatrics (1997), the U.S. Centers for Disease Control and Prevention (1996), and the American College of Obstetricians and Gynecologists (1996) have developed prevention guidelines which focus

► **GROUP B STREPTOCOCCAL INFECTION IN THE NEWBORN** *(continued)*

on screening of all pregnant women, either by rectovaginal cultures or through analysis of their risk factors for GBS. Despite some variations, the protocols help to decrease transmission of GBS disease from mother to infant. Women testing positive for GBS or who are at risk may receive intrapartum antibiotic prophylaxis (IAP) treatment during labor to prevent their transmitting GBS to their infants (Mitchell

et al., 1997). With IAP, infants without symptoms may not routinely need a full sepsis workup and antibiotics. Limited testing, for example complete blood count and blood culture, may be recommended if IAP was received less than 4 hours before delivery. Because of the risk of missing GBS infection, infants of mothers with positive cervical cultures may be treated.

vaginal flora as group B beta-hemolytic streptococcus, *H. influenzae,* listeria monocytogenes, *E. coli,* and *S. pneumoniae* are believed to cause early onset sepsis.

Late onset or acquired sepsis presents after 4 days (Askin, 1995). This condition progresses more slowly and has less related mortality than early onset sepsis, but does have greater morbidity. A variety of microorganisms can be responsible for late onset sepsis, which may be acquired from the birth canal or the external environment. Examples of these microorganisms include *S. aureus, S. epidermidis,* group B beta-hemolytic streptococcus, and pseudomonas. Unfortunately, the neonatal intensive care unit presents a risk factor for neonatal sepsis, particularly for the youngest and smallest infants, who may have more than one episode of sepsis while in these units (Baley & Goldfarb, 1993).

Nursing and Collaborative Assessment. Nurses are often the first health care providers to recognize signs of neonatal sepsis, because of their ongoing contact with the infants. Table 32–2 summarizes signs that define sepsis and septic shock. In addition, the septic infant may be pale or cyanotic, jaundiced, and/or lethargic. He or she may feed poorly, have a high-pitched cry, or seizures. Neonates respond globally; infection primarily in one site, such as the meninges, can cause alterations in other systems throughout the body. Signs and symptoms of neonatal sepsis are often subtle and appear gradually; therefore, when a neonate does not seem "healthy," careful assessment for signs of sepsis should be made.

Assessment focuses on maternal, fetal, and neonatal history; the neonate's activity and behaviors (alertness, feeding, crying); ability to establish and maintain temperature; heart rate, respirations, and blood pressure; presence of seizures; and onset and degree of jaundice. Diagnostic tests for neonatal sepsis include cultures of blood, urine, and spinal fluid. In addition, cultures are taken from any areas with suspicious drainage, such as the eyes or umbilical stump.

Other diagnostic tests include complete blood count with differential, serum electrolytes, and glucose; blood gas analysis; urinalysis; and chest x-ray. These series of tests are often called a "sepsis workup" and are performed when specific clinical indications are present. The results of these tests guide decisions for further evaluation and treatment. However, the manner in which blood specimens are collected and analyzed can affect results; therefore, correlation of history and clinical findings with laboratory results is essential (Polinski, 1996). Knowledge of results of a maternal cervical culture is also helpful in identifying sources of infection.

Nursing and Collaborative Management. Antimicrobial therapy and supportive care form the bases of management for neonatal sepsis (Cavaliere, 1995). The goals of management are to identify the type and source of infection, to initiate treatment that cures the infection and minimizes or prevents related complications, and to support the neonate's parents through this difficult period.

The neonate is housed in a nursery, equipped for administration of antibiotics and treatment of neonatal sepsis. After cultures are taken, antibiotic therapy is begun. During treatment, peak and trough antibiotic levels are obtained to ensure that therapeutic levels of antibiotics are maintained. Other physiologic interventions will be related to the nature of organ system involvement. Management includes strategies to ensure hydration, oxygenation, ventilation, adequate nutrition, and tissue perfusion. For example, a ventilator may be needed for respiratory support, and a radiant warmer may be used to stabilize body temperature. Management also includes strategies for care of other co-existing problems, such as prematurity and hyperbilirubinemia.

The nurse needs to provide ongoing support and education for the parents of a septic neonate. This is especially important if the mother is separated from her baby due to her own illness or if the infant is transported to a neonatal intensive care unit at another hospital. (See Chapter 12 for a discussion of psychosocial needs of parents of infants who are in or are transported to a neonatal intensive care unit.)

As a preventive strategy for management of neonatal sepsis, *all* staff members need to practice universal precautions. Nosocomial infections and prevention of spread of infections in the nursery should be topics for orientation and ongoing inservice education programs.

Human Immunodeficiency Virus (HIV) Infection

Human immunodeficiency virus (HIV) is a retrovirus that attacks the T lymphocytes in the human immune system. HIV was first identified in 1981 in adults; the first pediatric case of acquired immune deficiency syndrome (AIDS) was identified in November, 1982 (Mofenson, 1997a). Women of childbearing age are one of the fastest growing groups with AIDS; in 1984 they accounted for only 6% of AIDS cases, reported to the Centers for Disease Control and Prevention, but by 1995 they accounted for 19% of AIDS cases (Rogers, 1997). This does not even account for the number of unreported or undiagnosed HIV infected women of childbearing age. An estimated 15,000 perinatally infected children were born in the United States from 1978 to 1993; an estimated 1 million children have been infected globally; as many as 5–10 million are forecast to be infected by the year 2000 (Mofenson, 1997b). Although impossible to know for certain the exact number of infected women and neonates, it is clear that perinatal HIV is a major and growing public health concern. Prevention of transmission of HIV is a public health priority.

Women who are infected with HIV have an estimated 15 to 25% chance of passing the virus to their fetuses during the childbearing process (U.S. Centers for Disease Control and Prevention, 1998). Maternal and newborn treatment with the antiretroviral agent zidovudine (AZT or ZDV) has been shown to decrease perinatal transmission substantially (Connor et al., 1994; Mofenson, 1997b). Transmission from an HIV infected mother may occur prenatally, during the birth process, or through breastfeeding.

Nursing and Collaborative Assessment. Assessment begins with identifying mothers and neonates in high-risk groups. Maternal blood tests for the presence of HIV antibodies may be performed with clients' permission. Because of issues regarding confidentiality and the emotional and social impact of making the diagnosis of HIV infection, many agencies have developed special protocols for obtaining consent for blood tests from clients identified in high-risk

groups. Routinely, counseling accompanies testing for HIV. Health care professionals should also provide information and support to individuals who are in high-risk groups or who test positive (or negative) for HIV antibodies.

Mothers who have been infected with HIV and who have positive HIV antibodies in their blood may be asymptomatic; however, their HIV antibodies cross the placenta and are found in the neonate's blood. Neonates of mothers who are HIV positive will also test positive at birth, because of the presence of maternal antibodies. Not all neonates testing positive at birth will actually be infected. The neonate of an HIV-infected mother must be closely followed.

Diagnosis of true HIV infection in babies by available tests such as ELISA or Western blot tests is delayed until the infant is about 15 months of age, when maternal antibodies are no longer present in the infant's circulatory system. With these tests, identification of antibodies in the newborn indicates the mother is infected. However, these tests do not give information about whether or not the child actually has the virus, too. Currently, several new techniques have been used to diagnose children less than 1 year old. Such tests as the polymerase chain reaction and the HIV culture test for DNA components of the virus, or for the virus itself, can identify true infection in the infant. However, these tests require expert interpretation, tend to be expensive, and are not widely available (Sherwen, 1995).

Some neonates found to have HIV antibodies and who develop the HIV infection may demonstrate symptoms at birth. About one third of vertically infected infants develop early AIDS within the first year after birth; the remainder develop AIDS more slowly, and some can be asymptomatic for several years (De Rossi, Ometto, Masiero, Zanchetta, & Chieco-Bianchi, 1997). A sign of HIV infection in the neonate is sepsis or repeated opportunistic infections with, for example, the following organisms: *Pneumocystis carinii, Cytomegalovirus, Mycobacterium avium-intracellulare,* herpes simplex virus, *Candida albicans, cryptococcus neoformans,* and *Toxoplasma gondii.*

Other signs of HIV infection include failure to thrive, diarrhea, anemia, thrombocytopenia, respiratory distress, generalized lymphadenopathy, neurologic dysfunction, developmental delays, and hepatosplenomegaly (Klaus & Fanaroff, 1993).

Nursing and Collaborative Management. HIV infection cannot be cured. Interventions to decrease transmission focus on reducing maternal viral load, enhancing maternal and infant HIV–specific immune response, pharmacologic prophylaxis for the newborn, and attempts to decrease peripartum and postpartum exposure to the virus. A variety of therapeutic protocols exist. Even if these interventions do not completely prevent transmission, they may be able to slow the progress of HIV disease among babies who do become infected (Mofenson, 1997a).

Zidovudine controls the replication of the virus and slows progression of symptoms in children (as well as adults). Management for neonates and children also focuses on treating secondary infections and symptoms related to immunosuppression.

Special attention to nutritional support is required, because of the many gastrointestinal problems associated with infection. This may include the use of tube feedings or total parenteral nutrition. Attempts may be made to prevent infection through use of prophylactic antibiotics or gamma globulin. Treatment of persistent infections may include long-term administration of antibiotics. The neonate often becomes weak and requires supplemental oxygen. Skin care becomes essential in the presence of recurrent diarrhea and skin rashes caused by *Candida albicans*. The neonate or infant with diagnosed HIV infection or disease requires ongoing care after discharge that must include close supervision, meticulous hygiene, special feeding techniques, medication administration, and ongoing medical follow-up. These neonates frequently require lengthy and repeated hospitalizations.

The emotional and social implications of HIV infection are significant for both the neonate and the family. Collaborative interdisciplinary approaches to the management of the neonate with HIV infection and his or her family are therefore imperative. Parents of neonates diagnosed with HIV infection are high-risk clients. Concurrent family problems, including the illness of one or both parents, drug use, lack of support systems, poverty, and the social stigma attached to HIV, further complicate the care of the neonate with HIV infection. Evaluation of the family's social situation and home environment is important for the future safety and special needs of the neonate with HIV infection.

Parents preparing for the discharge of their neonate require much support and education from the interdisciplinary health care team. Preparation may be complicated by the fact that an HIV-positive mother may be a single parent, solely responsible for the care of the infant. These parents may be learning about their own illness in addition to their neonate's; they will be afraid and worried. Support groups and community agencies can be identified to assist the parents with the neonate's home care, the impact of the diagnosis of HIV infection, and the financial resources available to them. Parents should be familiar with the many health care professionals, nurses, physicians, and social workers who will follow the neonate on an ongoing basis. They should be encouraged to ask questions, and all information and answers must be offered in a nonthreatening, nonjudgmental manner.

Because of illness or social circumstances, the biologic parents may be unable to provide necessary care to the neonate. Extended family members or foster families require thorough education regarding the neonate's current and future special care needs. They too can be referred to the appropriate community agencies and support networks for additional help.

▶ SPECIFIC PROBLEMS CAUSING ALTERATIONS IN NEONATAL FUNCTIONING

▶ Alterations in Hematologic Functioning

Jaundice

Jaundice, a yellow discoloration of the skin, sclera, and mucous membranes, results from hyperbilirubinemia or high levels of unconjugated bilirubin (Ruchala, Seibold, & Stremsterfer, 1996). Neonatal jaundice is observed during the first week of life in 60% of term and 80% of preterm neonates (Bucuvalas & Balistreri, 1996). Jaundice is usually seen when the total serum bilirubin level is greater than 7 mg/dL (Poland & Ostrea, 1993). The degree of yellow discoloration is not a direct indication of increases or decreases in the serum bilirubin level. The yellow discoloration is, however, the result of an accumulation of unconjugated or indirect bilirubin, which is lipid soluble and diffuses most freely into body tissues and organs. The presence of jaundice in the neonate should be considered a risk factor directly related to hyperbilirubinemia.

Hyperbilirubinemia is an abnormally high level of bilirubin in the blood. This occurs when normal pathways of bilirubin metabolism and excretion in the newborn are altered. Total serum bilirubin levels greater than 12 mg/dL in the term formula-fed newborn, 14 mg/dL in the breastfed newborn, and 15 mg/dL in the preterm newborn usually indicate hyperbilirubinemia. Hyperbilirubinemia is often considered a common neonatal condition with physical symptoms exhibited within the first 36 to 72 hours after birth. Most preterm newborns show symptoms after 48 hours of age (Bucuvalas & Balistreri, 1996). Ethnic and geographic variables may influence the incidence of hyperbilirubinemia. For example, East Asian and American Indian neonates have average serum bilirubin levels that are higher than the rest of the population. Neonatal jaundice also tends to run in families (Maisels, 1994).

Kernicterus, or bilirubin encephalopathy, is a neurologic syndrome resulting from deposits of unconjugated bilirubin in brain cells (Behrman & Kliegman, 1996). The exact level at which indirect-reacting bilirubin becomes toxic to the baby is unclear; however, in healthy term infants, without another cause for hemolysis, kernicterus is rare if the serum bilirubin level is under 25 mg/dL. However, preterm and low-birth-weight newborns may be more susceptible to potential toxicity at lower serum bilirubin levels than term newborns (Behrman & Kliegman, 1996). At toxic levels, unconjugated or indirect bilirubin diffuses freely into brain tissue, causing neurologic damage. The severity of the symptoms is related to the degree of toxicity.

Neonates with kernicterus become lethargic with poor tendon reflexes and hypotonia. The Moro reflex disappears. The neonate develops difficulty feeding as a result of vomiting and the inability to suck strongly enough to draw milk from a nipple effectively. Extraocular muscles are paralyzed, and the neonate gazes downward (the "setting sun" sign). Although floppy and weak at the onset of the syndrome, the neonate later becomes irritable, hypertonic, and may develop seizures. Death may also occur (Poland & Ostrea, 1993). Unfortunately, the symptoms of kernicterus are not reversible. The long-term effects include a wide range of sensory, perceptual, and motor defects; mental retardation; and seizures. Management focuses on prevention of bilirubin toxicity through prompt identification and treatment of hyperbilirubinemia.

Physiologic Jaundice. Hyperbilirubinemia that occurs as the result of normal newborn metabolism during the first week of life is called **physiologic jaundice** (see Chapter 30). This type of jaundice is different from the more serious alteration in functioning known as pathologic jaundice, described later. Jaundice and hyperbilirubinemia in a neonate warrant immediate evaluation to identify any actual danger to the neonate and treatment needed.

Understanding the metabolism of bilirubin is essential to the effective management of a neonate with jaundice and hyperbilirubinemia (see Fig. 32–4 and discussion in Chapter 30).

The red blood cell volume of the neonate is significant because bilirubin is a product of red blood cell catabolism, or breakdown. Neonates are prone to **polycythemia,** a condition in which there is a surplus of red blood cells. Polycythemia is diagnosed when venous hemoglobin is greater than 22 g/dL and venous hematocrit is greater than 65% (Phibbs, 1996a). There are numerous potential causes of polycythemia in the newborn period (Table 32–3).

Although the neonate has a larger volume of circulating red blood cells (RBCs), the life span of fetal RBCs is only 90 days, in contrast to the 120-day life span of adult RBCs. The increased volume of RBCs with a comparatively shorter life span gives rise to a state of active RBC breakdown. This increased rate of RBC breakdown, along with an immature liver, place the neonate at risk for increased bilirubin production. In addition to polycythemia, other conditions causing red blood cell breakdown, such as blood incompatibilities, can lead to abnormally high bilirubin production.

Pathologic Jaundice. **Pathologic jaundice** is suspected when the yellow discoloration of the skin, sclera, and mucous membranes is visible before 24 hours of life in a term infant and before 48 hours in a preterm infant; total serum bilrubin levels exceed 12 mg/dL in the term newborn and 15 mg/dL in the preterm newborn; and the total serum bilirubin level increases by more than 5 mg/dL in 24 hours. Pathologic jaundice within the first 36 hours after birth is usually due to excessive bilirubin production, since slow clearance rarely causes very high levels at this age (Poland & Ostrea, 1993).

Various conditions can cause pathologic jaundice:

- Enclosed hemorrhage or a hematoma such as a cephalhematoma, which may contribute to the increased volume of hemolyzed RBCs, causing an increase in the level of serum bilirubin.
- Neonatal hepatitis and congenital atresia of the bile ducts, which alter the ability of the liver to conjugate and excrete bilirubin in the neonatal period.
- Metabolic factors such as sepsis, hypoxia, respiratory distress, and lack of carbohydrate intake, which may contribute to altered bilirubin metabolism and excretion.
- Other factors, such as RBC or enzyme abnormalities or drug-induced hemolysis, which increase bilirubin levels.
- Hemolytic diseases of the newborn; the most common of these are Rh incompatibility and ABO incompatibility, in which maternal antibodies are actively sensitized against the RBCs of the neonate. Sensitized maternal antibodies cross the placenta and lead to overwhelming destruction of fetal RBCs.

Hemolytic Diseases of the Newborn

As discussed earlier, the major and most serious causes of pathologic jaundice are **hemolytic diseases of the newborn.** Maternity clients whose fetuses are at risk for the development of hemolytic disease in the

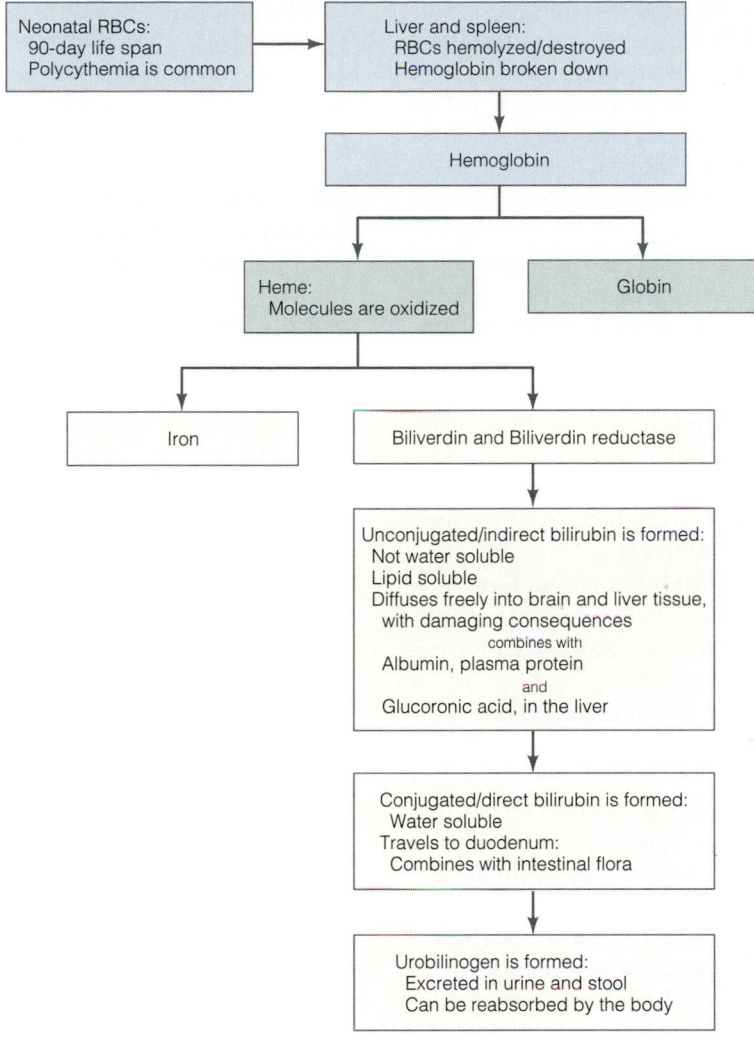

FIGURE 32–4. Bilirubin metabolism.

▶ **TABLE 32-3**

Potential Causes of Neonatal Polycythemia

Maternal–fetal transfusion	Occurs when blood is shunted from the maternal circulation to the fetal circulation.
Placental–fetal transfusion	Occurs when there is a delay in clamping the umbilical cord, or when the cord is manipulated, causing blood from the placenta to enter the fetal circulation.
Twin-to-twin transfusion	Occurs when blood is shunted from one twin to the other twin in utero or during delivery.
Chronic fetal hypoxia	Causes an increase in fetal red blood cell production.
Maternal metabolic or endocrine alterations (e.g., maternal diabetes)	Cause an increase in the viscosity of the blood.

neonatal period can usually be identified in the prenatal period. Questions that the nurse may ask the mother to help identify prenatal risk factors include the following:

- How many times have you been pregnant?
- How many of your children were born alive? Include details regarding the delivery and postnatal course of each infant.
- Have you ever delivered a stillborn infant? Include details regarding the delivery of each infant.
- How many spontaneous abortions (miscarriages) have you had?
- How many induced abortions (planned abortions) have you had?
- What is your blood type? (to be confirmed by laboratory analysis)

- What is the blood type of the father of this fetus? What is the blood type of the father of other pregnancies if it is known to be different?
- Have you ever received a medication called RhoGAM during pregnancy or after delivering an infant or after an abortion?
- Can you tell me why you received this medication?
- Have any of your other children been diagnosed with hyperbilirubinemia or "yellow jaundice"?
- Have any of your other children been diagnosed with a hemolytic disease, or were you told they have a different blood type from yours?
- Did any of your children have to stay longer in the hospital when they were born because they had to lie under special lights?
- Did any of your children have to receive a blood transfusion?
- Why did the infant have to receive phototherapy or a blood transfusion?
- Have you received regular prenatal care?
- Did you have any problems during your pregnancy?
- Did you have to have any special tests done while you were pregnant? If so, what tests were done, and do you know why they were done?

Information about ABO blood types and Rh blood groups must be obtained. Blood types include A, B, AB, and O. The blood type of the fetus is genetically determined, based on the blood types of the parents. In addition to blood types, blood group must also be identified. There are two blood groups, Rh+ and Rh−. The Rh blood group is determined by the presence of certain antigens. The combination of antigens that exists determines whether the Rh factor is present (Rh+) or absent (Rh−). For example, if the Rh factor is present in an individual with type O blood, that individual will have type O, group Rh+ blood, or O+ blood. The most common and strongest Rh+ antigen is the D antigen. It is the antigen that is involved in the hemolytic process of Rh incompatibility. (See Chapter 19 for further discussion of Rh isoimmunization.)

Pregnant women should have serum antibody testing early in pregnancy as part of routine prenatal care. The anti-D titer indicates the extent to which the mother is producing antibodies against the D antigens of the Rh+ red blood cells of the fetus. A measurable antibody titer at the beginning of pregnancy, a rapidly rising titer, or a titer of 1:64 or higher is significant. If the mother has an anti-D titer of 1:16 or higher at any time during a future pregnancy, the extent of disease in the fetus should be assessed with such tests as

amniocentesis, percutaneous umbilical blood sampling (PUBS), and ultrasound. Women who have had a previously affected infant or stillbirth can be carrying a fetus who is equally or more severely affected (Behrman & Kliegman, 1996).

ABO Incompatibility. **ABO incompatibility** is a hemolytic condition that occurs when the major blood group of the mother is incompatible with that of the fetus. Maternal antibodies may be formed against the cells of the fetus' blood type. The most common incompatibility occurs when the mother is type O and the fetus is type A or type B. It can also occur when the mother is type A and the fetus is B, or if the mother is type B and the fetus is type A. About one third of type A or B infants of O mothers have identifiable maternal antibodies on their red cells. This condition occurs more often in type B than A infants and is more likely in black than white infants whether they are A or B. However, only a small number of these infants develops clinical disease (Phibbs, 1996b). Maternal antibodies causing ABO incompatibility can affect the first as well as subsequent pregnancies.

The action of maternal antibodies against the fetus' cells causes agglutination, or clumping of the cells. These clumps of cells get caught in small peripheral blood vessels where they hemolyze, producing large quantities of bilirubin. Severe hyperbilirubinemia is a complication of this form of ABO incompatibility. Damage related to the blocked peripheral blood vessels is observed in rare instances. For example, renal failure may result from blockage of small blood vessels in the kidney. Effects of ABO incompatibility on the neonate, however, are usually mild.

Assessment shows signs of neonatal jaundice in the first 24 hours of life. A weak to moderate positive direct Coombs' test and hyperbilirubinemia are generally the main clinical indicators. The direct Coombs' test detects the presence of maternal antibodies in the neonate's blood. The presence of these antibodies indicates that a reaction causing clumping or destruction of RBCs is likely to occur or is occurring. Although most neonates progress well without specific treatment, phototherapy is usually indicated if the bilirubin continues to rise toward toxic levels. An exchange transfusion may be indicated in the presence of severe hemolytic disease and severe hyperbilirubinemia, but this is uncommon. Future pregnancies should be monitored to identify the presence of an ABO incompatibility; however, no treatment is available to prevent the possible future recurrence of ABO incompatibility.

Rh Incompatibility. Rh incompatibility causes a hemolytic disease in the fetus and newborn. The perinatal mortality of neonates with Rh incompatibility is 17.5%, with 14% of these deaths occurring as still-births.

Rh incompatibility occurs when an Rh– mother is pregnant with an Rh+ fetus (see Chapter 19). In the most common situation, the fetal red blood cells (RBCs) contain D antigens, which are lacking on the RBCs of the mother. Conditions such as fetal–maternal bleeding in a current or prior pregnancy (for example, mixing of fetal and maternal blood during delivery in a previous pregnancy), previous failure to receive RhoGAM or an inadequate amount of RhoGAM following pregnancy or abortion, and a previous blood transfusion may result in maternal isoimmunization or sensitization and the initial formation of maternal antibodies to the D antigen. It is rare, however, that the fetus in the first pregnancy in which sensitization occurs will become affected by the antibodies.

During the current pregnancy in a mother who has been exposed to the D antigen, antigens from the Rh+ fetus stimulate additional maternal production of antibodies against D antigens. These anti-D antibodies return to the fetal circulation, where they attach to and destroy the fetal RBCs. (Maternal sensitization can also occur in response to other irregular fetal Rh blood group antigens.) The condition characterized by fetal or neonatal hemolytic anemia resulting from incompatibility between the maternal and fetal blood groups is termed erythroblastosis fetalis (Dunn, Bhutani, Weiner, & Ludomirski, 1988). As RBCs are destroyed, the fetus responds by increasing erythropoietic activity in the liver, spleen, and bone marrow. The severity of erythroblastosis fetalis is therefore related to the amount of fetal RBC destruction and how well the fetus can produce new RBCs in response to the anemia.

Severe fetal RBC destruction in utero may lead to a condition termed hydrops fetalis. In this condition, the fetus' ability to produce enough new RBCs is exhausted. This can lead to multisystem failure in which, for example, the cardiovascular, respiratory, and hepatic (liver) systems cannot function properly. Hydrops fetalis is also characterized by massive edema, pleural effusions, and ascites, and may progress to death in utero. If hydrops fetalis is present at birth, cardiovascular and respiratory collapse is likely. Aggressive resuscitation is necessary; however, progressive failure of the neonate may occur (Avery, Fletcher, & MacDonald, 1994).

Nursing and Collaborative Assessment.
Assessment of the neonate with jaundice or suspected jaundice begins with identification of known risk factors. Neonates with prenatal risks such as Rh incom-

patibility, intrapartum risks such as cephalhematoma, or postpartum risks such as prematurity or sepsis, must be monitored carefully. Infants without identifiable risks yet with yellow discoloration of the skin, sclera, or mucous membranes in the first days to weeks of life must be evaluated. Because the observed degree of yellow discoloration is not a direct indication of the severity of jaundice, serum bilirubin levels are necessary to validate clinical findings. Serial serum bilirubin levels can determine the severity of progressing jaundice. The levels of bilirubin indicate what treatment should be considered.

The age of the neonate in hours or days at the onset of jaundice is essential to the diagnosis of an underlying clinical cause. The assessment must also include evaluation of feeding techniques, oral intake, and bowel and bladder activity.

When Rh incompatibility is known or anticipated, thorough and ongoing assessment of the neonate is imperative. Attention should be paid to the amniotic fluid at birth. High levels of bilirubin pigments, produced as a result of fetal RBC destruction, can produce a yellow discoloration of the amniotic fluid, umbilical cord, and the vernix caseosa. The severity of hemolytic disease depends upon the nature of the infant's immune response and may range from mild to severe and life threatening. When the ability of the hematopoietic system to handle the hemolysis is exceeded, severe anemia results in pallor and signs of cardiac decompensation (cardiomegaly, respiratory distress, generalized swelling, and circulatory collapse). This clinical picture, hydrops fetalis, often results in fetal death or death of the newborn shortly after birth. Hydrops fetalis can also be caused by such non-immune conditions as certain infections, tumors, metabolic problems, and chromosomal syndromes (Behrman & Kliegman, 1996). Jaundice is not present at birth, as the excessive amounts of bilirubin produced in utero are eliminated through the placenta and maternal circulation. Jaundice will become obvious during the first day of life, and the bilirubin level will continue to rise rapidly (Behrman & Kliegman, 1996).

Hemolytic diseases of the neonate such as ABO and Rh incompatibilities can prove to be life threatening. Quick and accurate assessment by nurses is essential to identification of the presence of these alterations. Table 32–4 reviews key elements of both ABO and Rh incompatibilities.

Nursing and Collaborative Management.
Management of the neonate with Rh incompatibility is aimed at prevention. Rho(D) immune globulin (RhoGAM) is an anti-Rh immunoglobulin that is administered to women after the delivery or abortion

▶ **TABLE 32-4**

Comparison of ABO Incompatibility and Rh Incompatibility

	ABO Incompatibility	Rh Incompatibility
Definition	Incompatibility between the major blood types (A, B, AB, O) of the mother and the fetus. When fetal blood mixes with the maternal blood a reaction occurs causing the fetal RBCs to be destroyed.	Incompatibility between the Rh blood groups of the mother and fetus. Occurs when an Rh– mother is pregnant with an Rh+ fetus. When maternal and fetal blood mix a reaction is caused. The mother's body produces antibodies against the fetal RBCs that carry the Rh+ antigen (D). This causes the fetal RBCs to be destroyed through a process called immunization or sensitization. If a mixture of maternal and fetal blood cells occurs during labor, subsequent pregnancies with an Rh+ infant will be affected.
Incidence	Occurs in 20 to 25% of all pregnancies; in 10% of these cases, the newborn develops hemolytic disease.	Occurs in 9% of all pregnancies; 1 in 15 newborns of these pregnancies develops hemolytic disease.
Signs and symptoms	After 24 hours of life, may develop during first pregnancy.	Often begins in utero; sensitization occurs during a first pregnancy, abortion, or blood transfusion; signs and symptoms generally appear in a subsequent pregnancy.
Common signs and symptoms	Jaundice related to hyperbilirubinemia.	Yellow amniotic fluid, umbilical cord, and vernix caseosa. Jaundice related to hyperbilirubinemia. Anemia. Enlarged liver and spleen. Petechiae and purpura. Possible cardiorespiratory collapse.
Laboratory tests	Weak to moderately positive Coombs' test. Bilirubin greater than 12 mg/dL in term newborn and greater than 15 mg/dL in preterm newborn.	Positive Coombs' test. Bilirubin greater than 12 mg/dL in term newborn and greater than 15 mg/dL in preterm newborn. Hemoglobin less than 13 g/dL or hematocrit less than 40%. Increased reticulocyte count.
Management	Phototherapy. Exchange transfusion in severe circumstances.	Phototherapy. Exchange transfusion. Administration of Rho(D) immune globulin to an Rh– mother at 28 weeks' gestation and after every pregnancy with an Rh+ fetus, whether the pregnancy reaches term or terminates in abortion.

of an Rh+ newborn or fetus. The anti-Rh immunoglobulin helps destroy the Rh+ cells that were transferred to the mother from the fetus. The destruction of these cells prevents further maternal production of anti-Rh antibodies. Thus, anti-Rh antibodies will not be present in the mother's circulation at the time of another pregnancy. An Rh– client who delivers an Rh+ infant, has an abortion, or who undergoes a procedure in which fetal and maternal blood may be mixed should receive prophylactic treatment. An Rh– client who is still unsensitized may also receive RhoGAM during the 24th week of pregnancy. Prevention of Rh sensitization is 90% effective with the administration of Rho(D) immune globulin after delivery (Phibbs, 1996b).

If the hemolytic process is detected while the fetus is still in utero, management is aimed at preventing intrauterine death. Induction of an early delivery may be necessary to prevent progression of the life-threatening condition. Intrauterine transfusions may also be used for the severely compromised fetus.

The birth of a neonate with known or suspected Rh incompatibility poses a tremendous challenge to the delivery room and nursery teams. The immediate goal is to assess the newborn swiftly and begin resuscitative measures if necessary. Complete blood count with differential, blood type, reticulocyte count, platelet count, blood gas, Coombs' test, and direct and total bilirubin levels may be performed on cord blood samples (Dunn et al., 1988); however, any intrauterine transfusions may affect results of blood type and Coombs' tests.

Results of serial laboratory tests must be examined. The main goals of management then become treatment of anemia and prevention of severe hyperbilirubinemia, which could cause neurologic damage (see earlier discussion of kernicterus). Phototherapy is the method of treatment used when mild to moderate hyperbilirubinemia is identified. In critical situations, an exchange transfusion is performed.

Phototherapy. Phototherapy is used to decrease serum bilirubin in neonates with hyperbilirubinemia as a result of conditions accompanied by mild to moderate jaundice. Settings for phototherapy include the normal newborn nursery, the intensive care nursery, the mother's hospital room, or the home.

Phototherapy exposes the neonate to a special high-intensity fluorescent light source, which oxidizes the unconjugated bilirubin in the skin. The unconjugated bilirubin then becomes water soluble and is excreted in both the bile and the urine without going through the usual conjugation process in the liver.

Several types of light sources are used to provide phototherapy, such as daylight, white fluorescent light, special blue fluorescent light, green fluorescent light, and quartz halogen light. Although blue light sources are effective, they have been reported to irritate the eyes of health care providers. Skin color changes can be difficult to see under colored lights and therefore may be missed if the neonate is not observed carefully.

Some centers still use the traditional phototherapy lights, although more and more have made the transition to the biliblanket system, described later. With the traditional system, the number and type of light sources used to provide treatment are based on the severity of the hyperbilirubinemia. For example, the neonate may receive single phototherapy, using one light source, or double phototherapy, using two light sources. The amount of energy delivered from the light source that results in the maximum elimination of bilirubin is 420 to 475 nanometers (nm) (Wilkerson, 1989). The nurse checks the intensity of light each time the neonate is placed in phototherapy. A hand-held meter, called an irradiance meter, can be used to check the output of the fluorescent light source. The light meter is held at the level of the neonate and in the area of greatest illumination. The light output is measured in units of microwatts per square centimeters per nanometer. A range of 7 to 10 µW/cm per nm is appropriate when a single light source is being used, and a level of 15 µW/cm per nm is desirable when double light sources are used.

The neonate receiving traditional phototherapy will have his or her eyes covered by a shield or mask to prevent potential retinal damage caused by the fluorescent lights. The nurse should observe the neonate to ensure that the eyepatches stay properly positioned. Eyepatches should be removed at least every 6 hours in order to assess the eyes for the presence of irritation (Wilkerson, 1989). Removing the eyepatches during feedings and parental visits will also provide the neonate with necessary visual stimulation. It is also recommended that the neonate's genital area be shielded as well. Surgical masks tied like a bikini or diapers can be secured around the neonate's groin to provide this protection.

With traditional phototherapy, maximum exposure is achieved by placing the neonate unclothed in the path of the light source. The use of an isolette or radiant warming bed allows the neonate to remain unclothed while providing the appropriate thermal environment. Phototherapy lights and the thermal environment can cause insensible water loss in the neonate. In addition, neonates receiving phototherapy often have frequent loose green stools. The nurse should assess the skin and mucous membranes for signs of dehydration. The neonate's intake and output should be strictly maintained. Urine specific gravity may be monitored to indicate dehydration as well. Small frequent feedings of formula or breast milk are recommended to maintain adequate fluid intake.

The neonate receiving phototherapy is at risk for alterations in skin integrity. The intensity of the light source can cause redness or burns if not properly maintained and positioned at least 12 inches away from the neonate (Wilkerson, 1989). The application of eyepatches can cause irritation on the face. Frequent stools and the use of coverings other than a diaper over the genitals can lead to excoriation. Careful and frequent cleansing of the neonate's skin is essential. The use of ointments or lotions is not recommended because they could cause further skin irritation or burning during phototherapy.

The sight of a neonate in an isolette, eyes covered with a mask and lying under a bright light, can frighten parents. They need to know why the neonate requires phototherapy, the expected length of treatment, and if the jaundice will recur. Scheduling phototherapy treatments around parents' visits will provide special stimulation and interaction for both.

Sunlight provides natural phototherapy for mild hyperbilirubinemia. After discharge, the pediatrician may recommend that parents expose the neonate to indirect sunlight coming through the window for short periods; for example, for 15 to 20 minutes four times daily. To avoid skin burning, however, the neonate should not be placed unprotected in bright outdoor sunlight; to avoid cold stress, the neonate should not be left exposed to cool room temperatures. The neonate requiring treatment for hyperbilirubinemia should be followed by a health care provider after discharge as indicated by the neonate's condition.

A newer and now more commonly used method for delivering phototherapy directly to the skin of the jaundiced neonate consists of a fiberoptic biliblanket and halogen light source (Fig. 32–5). The biliblanket is attached to the light source with a coupler device. The light source is placed on the infant's bed or on a nearby table. The biliblanket is placed under the axilla and wrapped around the trunk of the neonate. A baby shirt is placed over the biliblanket and the neonate is covered with a blanket. The light source stays on at all times. This method does not require that the neonate's eyes be patched and also allows easier observation of the infant's color. Unlike the traditional phototherapy system, the infant is not at risk for loss of fluid. The neonate and this portable phototherapy system can be moved into the mother's hospital room. The neonate can be held, changed, and fed with the system in use. In addition, this method can be useful for home care of the neonate requiring phototherapy.

The effectiveness of inpatient phototherapy is evaluated by serial serum bilirubin tests performed at least every 8 to 12 hours during the therapy. Serum bilirubin levels are monitored daily for infants receiving home phototherapy. Once serum bilirubin levels return to normal, phototherapy is discontinued. Additional serum bilirubin tests will then be performed to ensure that the levels do not begin to rise again. Parents should be aware of the serial blood tests that the neonate will receive and be given the option to remain with the neonate during the tests if they desire.

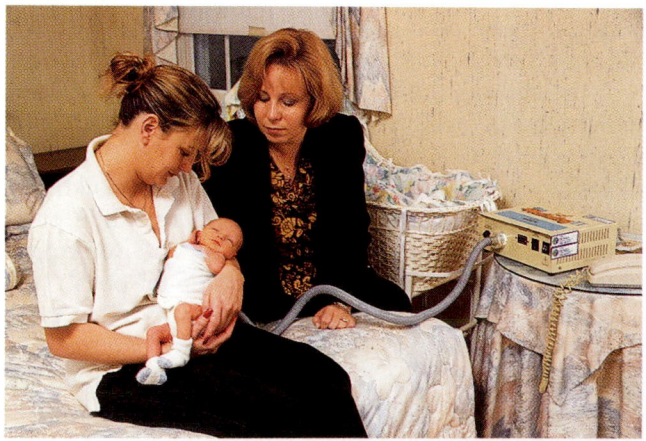

FIGURE 32–5. A newborn receiving phototherapy in the home.

Exchange Transfusion. In an exchange transfusion, blood is withdrawn from the neonate and replaced with compatible adult blood. Exchange transfusions are completed in neonatal or pediatric intensive care units. Exchange transfusions are done in critical circumstances, as in the following situations:

- Anemia and hyperbilirubinemia appear to be progressing to dangerous levels.
- Neonate's hemoglobin is less than 10 mg/dL.
- Cord bilirubin level is greater than 5 mg/dL.
- Reticulocyte count is greater than 15%.
- Neonate is further compromised by prematurity.
- Family history reveals that siblings experienced life-threatening hemolytic processes (Behrman & Kliegman, 1996).
- Severe sepsis and acidosis are unresponsive to other measures.

The goals of an exchange transfusion are removal of unconjugated bilirubin from the neonate, removal of sensitized maternal RBCs from the neonate, removal of circulating immune antibodies from the neonate, replacement of nonsensitized compatible RBCs, restoration of blood volume, and correction of anemia (Phibbs, 1996b).

Rh– whole blood compatible with the sera of the neonate is used for the actual exchange transfusion. The blood and the baby's identification must be verified prior to administration of the blood and according to the policy of the institution where the baby is being treated. Blood is withdrawn in small aliquots, usually 5 to 10 mL, through the umbilical vein. An equal volume of donor blood is then administered. The donor blood is usually warmed, using a blood warmer and coil set specifically designed to warm blood to the appropriate temperature.

The process of withdrawing and replacing equal volumes of blood continues until the neonate has received two times her or his blood volume. Normal blood volume equals 85 mL/kg (Behrman & Kliegman, 1996; Poland & Ostrea, 1993).

The following safety measures are necessary during the exchange transfusion:

- The neonate must be placed on a cardiorespiratory monitor.
- The neonate's blood pressure must be monitored continuously.
- The neonate should have stomach contents aspirated prior to the start of the procedure.
- The neonate must have a peripheral intravenous line in place to receive maintenance intravenous fluids during the procedure.

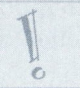

Nursing Alert

Blood should never be warmed in a hot water bath or in the microwave.

- The neonate's temperature must be monitored and maintained during the procedure; a radiant warming bed is usually used.
- Resuscitation equipment must be readily available.
- Blood glucose level should be assessed pre- and post-exchange to minimize risk of hypoglycemia.

During the procedure the nurse is responsible for monitoring and documenting the neonate's vital signs every 15 minutes. Laboratory tests, such as calcium and glucose levels, are done during the exchange transfusion. According to unit protocols, in many places hemoglobin and hematocrit, electrolytes, and bilirubin are checked immediately after the transfusion is completed and then serially every 4 to 8 hours afterward.

Exchange transfusions can have numerous complications during and after the procedure, including embolism, thrombosis, volume overload, electrolyte imbalances, hypothermia, and infection from the intravenous line (Poland & Ostrea, 1993). In addition there is an increased risk for necrotizing enterocolitis occurring post-exchange via umbilical venous catheter. For this reason, assessment should include measurement of abdominal girth and assessment of stool for presence of blood. The neonate with a hemolytic disease such as Rh incompatibility must therefore receive careful and ongoing assessment. Laboratory data in addition to the physical examination will confirm that the hemolytic process has subsided, the anemia is resolving, and the bilirubin level is maintained below a dangerous level. Parents require continuous support throughout the neonate's hospitalization.

Anemia

Anemia exists in the neonate when the hemoglobin level is less than 13.5 g/dL or the hematocrit is less than 45%. During the weeks after birth, the hemoglobin undergoes typical physiologic changes, resulting in values that are falsely indicative of anemia. True (pathologic) anemia can result from several different pathophysiologic processes in the neonate. To differentiate physiologic from pathologic anemia, a thorough history and definitive laboratory studies are required. This ensures that the appropriate corrective therapy is promptly initiated.

Anemia may result from blood loss related to prenatal pathophysiology, often abruptio placentae and placenta previa. Intrapartum blood loss, for example, from an accidental tear in the umbilical cord, also accounts for some cases of anemia in the neonate. Postnatal blood loss may be attributed to an intravascular hemorrhage, accidental rupture of internal organs, hemolytic diseases of the newborn such as Rh or ABO incompatibility, or birth injuries such as cephalhematoma. Sick or preterm newborns may undergo frequent blood samplings for laboratory analysis, which could result in iatrogenic, or hospital-acquired, anemia.

The most commonly observed anemia is physiologic anemia. Although the healthy newborn has higher hemoglobin and hematocrit levels than older children or adults, a decline begins the first week. The term neonate reaches the lowest hemoglobin level, 9–12 g/dL, between 8 and 12 weeks of age. The preterm neonate reaches the lowest hemoglobin level, around 7–9 g/dL, by 3–6 weeks; the levels can be even lower in very small, preterm babies. This anemia stimulates the production of erythropoietin and red blood cells. Iron stores are also used in the production of these RBCs, and both term and preterm neonates may need iron supplements.

Nursing and Collaborative Assessment. Assessment of the neonate with anemia or suspected anemia begins with identification of known risk factors that would predispose to the condition. Any neonate found to have experienced a prenatal, intrapartum, or postnatal condition that is related to anemia must be carefully monitored. Neonates with anemia may demonstrate the following signs: poor feeding, lethargy, pale color, apnea, weak cry, and tachycardia. As in many abnormal neonatal conditions, the signs are nonspecific. Monitoring of neonatal activity, physical assessment, and laboratory tests, such as hemoglobin, hematocrit, reticulocyte count, and platelets, are essential. Serial hemoglobin hematocrit levels should be monitored closely for changes.

Nursing and Collaborative Management. Management begins with the identification of the cause of the anemia. If physiologic anemia is identified, ongoing monitoring of the hemoglobin and hematocrit levels may be the only interventions warranted. The process may, however, become more complicated in the case of Rh incompatibility. The smaller number of RBCs present in anemia limits the oxygen-carrying capability of the neonate. Sick or preterm neonates with other problems that affect adequate oxygenation, such as hyaline membrane disease, are further compromised. The neonate may require supplemental oxygen until the oxygen-carrying capacity can be increased and maintained. These neonates also may require a transfusion of packed RBCs. The volume of the transfusion is always carefully calculated. Transfusion volumes of only a few milliliters may be used for the very-low-birth-weight neonate.

Careful management of blood sampling may reduce the number of transfusions required. A cumulative record of all blood withdrawn should be maintained for all neonates. Replacement is done with packed red blood cells when 5 to 10% of the neonate's blood volume has been lost. Up-to-date laboratory equipment and sampling techniques are essential to ensure that the minimum amount of blood is drawn from these neonates. Additional treatments such as iron supplementation and routine monitoring of hemoglobin and hematocrit may also be necessary. Special treatments may be necessary to manage the underlying cause of the anemia.

▶ Alterations in Metabolic Functioning

In utero, the placenta regulates the metabolism of the fetus. The transition to extrauterine life demands that the neonate's own metabolism immediately take over this essential function. Even in the healthy term neonate, the new energy needs and physiologic adjustments at birth can make this transition process difficult. Neonates who have experienced altered metabolic regulation in utero (e.g., the neonate of a mother with diabetes or a neonate who experienced intrauterine malnutrition) have greater metabolic demands during and after birth. Also, neonates who are preterm or who are experiencing other physiologic stresses, such as respiratory distress or sepsis, have additional difficulty in regulating their own metabolic needs. Common alterations affect the metabolism of calcium, magnesium, and glucose.

Hypocalcemia and Hypercalcemia

Calcium is a key element of normal metabolic functioning. Calcium freely crosses the placenta to meet the growth needs of the fetus. Between 28 and 38 weeks, fetal calcium needs increase dramatically. At birth, the endocrine system makes many adjustments to continue to supply the amount of calcium needed by the neonate.

If calcium needs are high and calcium reserves are low, the neonate is in danger of developing hypocalcemia (low serum calcium level). Alterations in calcium levels in the neonate include the following:

- *Early neonatal hypocalcemia,* which includes preterm newborns, newborns suffering from birth asphyxia, and newborns of insulin-dependent diabetic mothers; this usually occurs at 24–48 hours after birth (Koo & Tsang, 1994).
- *Late neonatal hypocalcemia,* which is related to hypomagnesemia and intestinal malabsorption of calcium; this may be seen late in the first week after birth and often presents with neonatal tetany (Koo & Tsang, 1994).
- *Hypoparathyroidism,* which occurs as a result of maternal hyperparathyroidism in utero (Kliegman, 1993).

Hypocalcemia usually manifests 24 to 48 hours after birth. A serum calcium level less than 7 mg/dL indicates hypocalcemia. Signs related to hypocalcemia include muscle twitching, irritability, increased muscle tone, jitters, high-pitched cry, cyanosis, vomiting, refusal to feed, and seizures. Many of these signs could be related to different neonatal illnesses such as sepsis. In addition, some neonates with hypocalcemia may be asymptomatic. Laboratory analysis of serum calcium levels is necessary to confirm the medical diagnosis. Calcium levels are not routinely drawn for normal term newborns; however, calcium assessment would be indicated for any newborn with the preceding signs.

Management of hypocalcemia begins with identification of the potential cause. Calcium supplements may be added to intravenous solutions. A dose of 24 to 35 mg/kg per 24 hours is commonly used (Kliegman, 1993). If the neonate has seizures, which may become life threatening, intravenous calcium may be given in a bolus dose. A bolus dose refers to the administration of a specific amount of medication at one time rather than via a continuous infusion. Extreme caution must be used with the administration of intravenous calcium in this manner as rapid administration may cause bradycardia or asystole

Nursing Alert

Calcium cannot be administered in an intravenous solution containing sodium bicarbonate because a precipitate will form.

(Koo & Tsang, 1994). Assessment and documentation of continued clinical symptoms of hypocalcemia are essential. Intravenous sites must be assessed and monitored carefully for infiltration. Additional treatments are included if the hypocalcemia is related to a cause other than the stress of extrauterine transition.

Hypercalcemia occurs infrequently in the neonatal period. Serum calcium levels greater than 11 mg/dL or ionized calcium greater than 5 mg/dL indicate hypercalcemia (Blackburn & Loper, 1992). The causes of hypercalcemia can include congenital primary hyperparathyroidism, hypervitaminosis, or underlying genetic and metabolic diseases. The neonate with hypercalcemia can demonstrate poor feeding, vomiting, polyuria, hypotonia, lethargy, hypertension, and seizures.

Management of hypercalcemia is directed at the identified underlying cause. Laboratory tests such as total and ionized calcium levels, phosphate levels, and vitamin D levels will be monitored. Treatment includes reducing calcium intake. In some cases, beginning enteral feedings can improve the absorption and excretion of calcium by the gastrointestinal tract. When hypercalcemia is severe, diuretics such as furosemide (Lasix) can be used to reduce serum calcium levels. Fluid and electrolytes must be closely monitored whenever diuretics are used.

Hypomagnesemia and Hypermagnesemia

Magnesium is actively exchanged between the mother and the fetus in utero and plays a key role in overall metabolic functioning (Kliegman, 1993). Magnesium is important for the proper functioning of the parathyroid gland. If the magnesium level is abnormal, parathyroid functioning, such as the release of hormones, is affected. If that occurs, the serum calcium level will be altered, and overall metabolic balance disrupted.

The magnesium level is significantly affected by both intrauterine and postnatal factors, including poor maternal diet; maternal diabetes; placental insufficiency; administration of certain medications, for example, magnesium sulfate; decreased intestinal absorption; and loss of magnesium during an exchange transfusion (Behrman & Kliegman, 1996).

Alterations in magnesium metabolism can result in either hypomagnesemia or hypermagnesemia. Hypomagnesemia is an abnormally low serum magnesium level (less than 1.5 mg/dL). Symptoms similar to those seen with hypocalcemia occur with serum magnesium levels less than 1.2 mg/dL. Often, the only way to distinguish which metabolic alteration is present is by the results of serum laboratory analysis (Behrman & Kliegman, 1996). Management of hypomagnesemia includes the administration of 50% magnesium sulfate, 0.2 mL/kg via an intramuscular injection daily in the presence of severe symptoms. In less severe circumstances, oral magnesium supplements can be given with feedings. Oral doses of magnesium range from 20 to 40 mg/kg per day. Accompanying hypocalcemia often corrects itself as hypomagnesemia resolves.

Hypermagnesemia is an abnormally high serum magnesium level (greater than 2.8 mg/dL); serious symptoms occur with levels above 5 mg/dL. The symptoms of hypermagnesemia include central nervous system depression, which can result in respiratory depression, apnea, hypotension, lethargy, and depressed reflexes. Calcium gluconate may be administered to an infant who is hypermagnesemic as a result of the mother's receiving high doses of magnesium sulfate during labor. Interventions are required when symptoms are severe.

Hypoglycemia and Hyperglycemia

Glucose is an essential element in all body functioning. Glucose metabolism is the first level of defense in the stress response and in the response to an increase in physiologic energy needs. The fetus relies on glucose metabolism in utero, especially during periods of rapid growth. The many physiologic changes that occur at birth demand large amounts of energy. As maternal glucose supplies are no longer present, the neonate must immediately respond to these physiologic demands. Alterations in glucose metabolism occurring in utero or after birth have the potential to compromise the neonate. Some of the major causes of altered glucose metabolism are maternal diabetes; diminished production of glucose in the liver; multiple physiologic stresses, such as transition to extrauterine life, acidosis, hypothermia, congenital heart disease, and sepsis; low birth weight; poor oral intake; and intravenous glucose infusions. Glucose metabolism may be altered causing either hyperglycemia, the presence of a serum glucose level greater than 125 mg/dL, or hypoglycemia, the presence of a serum glucose level less than 40 mg/dL.

Hypoglycemia. Hypoglycemia is a condition in which the blood glucose level is abnormally low. Hypoglycemia is defined as a serum glucose level less than 40 mg/dL in a term or preterm infant (Brooks, 1997). Variations in definitions of hypoglycemia exist; for this reason, it is difficult to specify the precise incidence of this condition.

Neonates are vulnerable to hypoglycemia in the first days of life. During the birth process, the neonate expends large amounts of energy. One important source is the metabolism of glucose. After birth, the neonate can no longer rely on maternal glucose. This change in metabolic functioning can cause hypoglycemia. Hypoglycemia is seen most commonly in infants of diabetic mothers. An estimated one fourth to one half of infants of diabetic mothers develop hypoglycemia within the first 24 hours, particularly if they are macrosomic (Ogata, 1996). Neonates whose growth was retarded before birth are prone to hypoglycemia if they experienced intrauterine malnutrition. The preterm neonate is also at risk for hypoglycemia, because of insufficient stores of glycogen and immature hepatic enzymes. Other conditions that place the infant at risk for hypoglycemia include sepsis, shock, asphyxia, and hypothermia. Hypoglycemia may occur after an exchange transfusion (because blood only has the dextrose equivalent of 5% dextrose solution) and after abrupt discontinuation of intravenous fluids, after malposition of umbilical catheters, and with the administration of certain medications.

Neonatal hypoglycemia often manifests in subtle ways. Physical signs include refusal to eat, vomiting, cyanosis, hypothermia, respiratory distress, lethargy, and jitteriness, tremors, or seizures (Brooks, 1997; Ogata, 1996). Hypoglycemia can also be confused with such conditions as hypocalcemia and hypomagnesemia, because such signs as poor feeding, tremors, and jitteriness are similar (Suevo, 1997). Evaluation of serum calcium and magnesium levels is therefore indicated.

Some hypoglycemic neonates have severe signs and symptoms; others are asymptomatic. Most infants initially demonstrate subtle symptoms; the nurse therefore must closely monitor for onset and/or progression of symptoms in any neonate with risk factors for hypoglycemia.

Hypoglycemia is often difficult to identify by symptoms alone and is confirmed by serum glucose levels. Capillary blood glucose monitoring is a quick method of glucose assessment, which requires only a drop of blood. Abnormal results must be confirmed by laboratory analysis. A neonate with symptoms of hypoglycemia, risk factors for developing hypoglycemia, or capillary blood glucose levels less than 40 mg/dL warrants assessment. Assessment also includes further evaluation when other conditions associated with hypoglycemia, such as sepsis and respiratory distress, are suspected.

Management begins with accurate monitoring of the glucose of the newborn. Nurseries have specific screening glucose protocols. In many nurseries, neonates at risk for hypoglycemia have glucose levels assessed in the first hour of life, then every 2 hours for the first 8 hours of life. Glucose testing is then done every 4 to 6 hours until the neonate is 24 hours old.

Neonates who are able to feed orally should be given a 5% dextrose solution, 20 kcal/oz formula, or breast milk within 2 hours of birth (Brooks, 1997). In some settings, infants at risk are tested for hypoglycemia within the first 30 minutes after birth. Those with capillary glucose results of 40 mg/dL or less are then gavage fed with formula. Feedings are then continued according to protocols for each unit. For example, preterm infants may be fed every 2 to 3 hours; breastfed babies are fed on demand; bottlefed babies may be fed every 3 to 4 hours. Nurses must make sure that feedings occur on time. Parents require support and teaching regarding specific feeding.

Neonates who feed poorly may be started on orogastric feedings. If the infant is too ill to tolerate enteric feedings, intravenous therapy is indicated. For example, to manage symptomatic hypoglycemia, a 2–4 mL/kg infusion of D10W may be administered over 2 minutes; a continuous infusion of D10W (approximately 8 mg/kg per minute of glucose) is then often ordered (Brooks, 1997; Suevo, 1997). However, glucose infusions more than 12 mg/kg per minute may place the infant at risk for further insulin release and rebound hypoglycemia (Cordero & Landon, 1993). Intravenous sites should be checked at least every hour, as the glucose solution may cause problems with neonatal tissue burning and sloughing. A central line may be used to decrease the risk of tissue extravasation in neonates who require dextrose solutions greater than 12.5% (Brooks, 1997).

Once intravenous therapy is started, the neonate's condition and peripheral glucose levels must be monitored carefully until hypoglycemia resolves and the neonate establishes normal glucose levels with feeding. Care must be taken to minimize stresses that can add to problems related to hypoglycemia. For example, a neutral thermal environment should be maintained, because cold stress increases the neonate's glucose metabolism (Suevo, 1997).

Parents continue to need support and teaching about the neonate's condition. They also need instruction regarding expression and storage of breast milk and support as they begin to feed their baby. Parents must be given enough opportunity to feed their infant

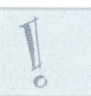

Nursing Alert

Faulty techniques in blood glucose sampling can lead to misdiagnosis and improper treatment. Staff who do blood sampling should be carefully trained in the specific method used in their own settings (Brooks, 1997).

and discuss home feeding schedules before the infant is discharged.

Hyperglycemia. Hyperglycemia is usually related to extreme prematurity and intravenous glucose infusions. It often occurs when the neonate is stressed by multiple physiologic problems simultaneously. The symptoms include glucosuria (glucose in the urine) and changes in fluid and electrolyte balances. Risk for intraventricular hemorrhage is increased with hyperglycemia. It occurs when fluid balance in the brain is altered, causing bleeding to occur. Management focuses on prevention of glucose imbalances, especially in the preterm newborn. A glucose infusion must be carefully monitored. Intermittent serum glucose tests are important in confirming that glucose levels are within an acceptable range. In severe circumstances, regular insulin may be given, with the dose carefully calculated on the basis of the serum glucose level.

Inborn Errors of Metabolism

Inborn errors of metabolism is the term used to describe a large number of genetically determined diseases that cause alterations in metabolic functioning (Rezvani & Rosenblatt, 1996). The altered metabolic functioning is usually the result of deficient enzyme activity in the body, leading to disorders of amino acid metabolism, uric acid cycle defects, and organic acidemias, among others. The most common amino acid disorder is **phenylketonuria (PKU).** (See the box entitled Phenylketonuria). Other inborn errors in metabolism include galactosemia and maple syrup urine disease. Table 32–5 lists common inborn errors of metabolism identified in the neonatal period. Most inborn errors of metabolism are inherited as autosomal recessive traits (Rezvani & Rosenblatt, 1996). Mothers with the autosomal recessive trait often have only 50% of normal metabolic function themselves. This level is usually adequate to make up for their own altered enzyme activity. The maternal metabolism is also able to substitute for the enzyme activity lacking in the fetus, thereby preventing the toxic buildup of the products of fetal metabolism in utero. After birth, the deficient enzyme activity continues to alter normal metabolic functioning (Mamunes, 1980). In mild disorders, these conditions may remain undetected for the individual's entire life. More severe cases demonstrate symptoms soon after birth and may prove to be life threatening (American Academy of Pediatrics, 1992; Klaus & Fanaroff, 1993).

When left untreated, inborn errors of metabolism cause irreversible brain damage. This brain damage can be minimized with the early identification of the abnormality and the initiation of an aggressive treatment plan. The importance of precise and early diagnosis of metabolic disease cannot be overemphasized because of the need to individualize treatment plans and minimize brain damage (American Academy of Pediatrics, 1992).

Nursing and Collaborative Assessment. Inborn errors of metabolism, identified in the neonatal period, are usually severe and require careful assessment. The first step in assessment is a thorough family history. Important points to note are the death of another child in the neonatal period, especially if the cause of death was not truly identified; the presence of a sibling with similar signs and symptoms; the presence of a similar metabolic disorder in the family of either parent; and the presence of consanguinity of the parents, where the parents are relatives such as first cousins. Absence of a family history of the preceding factors does not rule out the presence of an inherited metabolic disease.

Signs and symptoms of neonates with inborn metabolic disorders include lethargy, apnea, or tachypnea, poor feeding and vomiting, poor muscle tone, seizures, hepatosplenomegaly (enlarged liver and spleen), hypoglycemia, jaundice, enlarged tongue, diarrhea, and unusual odor of the neonate's body or excretions (Rezvani & Rosenblatt, 1996).

Inborn errors of metabolism can cause abnormal amounts of metabolites (products of metabolism) to accumulate in the neonate's body. For example, in amino acid disorders, ingested protein is not fully metabolized. The symptoms of disorders are caused by the accumulated metabolites. The identification of organic acidemias is often preceded by severe metabolic acidosis, which may cause tachypnea.

Although alterations in metabolism are quite complex, the symptoms are nonspecific, mirroring those of other neonatal illnesses or diseases, for example, congenital heart disease or sepsis. Neonates with metabolic disorders can quickly become debilitated and are prone to developing infections. A neonate who becomes severely ill without obvious cause or is suspected of being septic should be assessed for the presence of metabolic disorders (Rezvani & Rosenblatt, 1996).

The medical diagnosis of inborn errors of metabolism is suggested by an analysis of the signs and symptoms and is confirmed by laboratory analysis (see Table 32–5). Laboratory analysis for inborn errors of metabolism includes a broad range of serum and urine tests. Most tests identify the presence of abnormal levels of certain metabolites. The findings indicate where the abnormality occurs in the neonate's metabolism.

► PHENYLKETONURIA

Phenylketonuria (PKU) is an inborn error of metabolism that occurs in 1 of 10,000 to 20,000 persons (Nyhan, 1996). It is transmitted as an autosomal recessive trait and is the most common amino acid disorder. Phenylalanine is an essential amino acid that is converted into tyrosine by the liver enzyme, phenylalanine hydroxylase. The basic defect in PKU is absence of phenylalanine hydroxylase. Consequently, phenylalanine accumulates in the body; high levels disrupt normal metabolism and cause brain damage (Rezvani, 1996). In addition to classic PKU, described here, varieties of conditions related to abnormal phenylalanine metabolism exist.

SIGNS AND SYMPTOMS

The affected neonate is normal at birth; however, after ingestion of breast milk or formula that contains protein, phenylalanine begins to build in the neonate's blood. Mental retardation may evolve gradually and not be apparent for a few months (Rezvani, 1996). If the condition is not diagnosed in the infant's first 3–6 weeks of life, toxic levels can cause brain damage (Burton, 1987). Symptoms that may be observed include vomiting, irritability, seborrheic skin rash, unusual musty odor, and hyperactive reflexes. In addition, 90% of neonates with PKU are fair haired, fair skinned, and have blue eyes (Nyhan, 1996).

Older infants and children may have the following additional symptoms: seizures, purposeless movements, microcephaly, and growth retardation.

ASSESSMENT

PKU is confirmed by high levels of phenylalanine in the body. Blood tests are recommended at 48–72 hours after birth and after the infant has time normally to ingest breast milk or formula which contains proteins. Early discharge presents problems of false negative results, due to inadequate time for feedings. Although many hospitals require testing before discharge, parents of infants discharged early need to be counseled to bring the baby back for repeat testing. PKU testing after discharge may be done during a home visit.

In collecting specimens for PKU testing, drops of blood need to completely fill disks marked on special filter paper. The specimen and relevant data about the neonate are mailed to a screening laboratory. When the Guthrie test is used for PKU assessment during the first 3–4 days after birth, a phenylalanine level of 4–6 mg/dL may indicate a neonate is at risk. Phenylalanine and tyrosine plasma concentrations are then assessed. Criteria for diagnosis of PKU include:

- Plasma phenylalanine levels persistently higher than 20 mg/dL
- Normal plasma tyrosine levels
- Increased phenylalanine metabolites in the urine
- Infant inability to tolerate an oral challenge of phenylalanine
- Abnormal serum concentrations of cofactor tetrahydrabiopterin

MANAGEMENT

Management begins with prevention; attention is given to mass screening tests for PKU in every neonate. The goal of management is to reduce serum phenylalanine levels, thereby minimizing brain damage. A diet low in phenylalanine is begun as soon after birth as possible; a special formula is recommended (American Academy of Pediatrics, 1992). Frequent determinations of serum phenylalanine levels should be done. A recommended optimal serum level is between 3 mg/dL and 15 mg/dL. Care must be taken to prevent too low levels of phenylalanine, a condition that causes symptoms similar to those of PKU. Dietary restrictions may be somewhat reduced between the ages of 6 and 8 years; however, when to relax restrictions is controversial, and some form of restriction of dietary phenylalanine is needed indefinitely (Rezvani, 1996). Neonates and parents require additional support and care for special needs related not only to maintaining a difficult diet, but also to any occurrence of brain damage.

Girls treated successfully for PKU have now grown up and have become pregnant. By adulthood, these women tend to be off the special diets that they followed as children. However, they can have high phenylalanine levels that create a metabolic environment that harms fetal development. Maternal PKU syndrome occurs in infants of these women, although most of the infants do not have PKU themselves. Pregnant women with PKU who are not controlled on a low phenylalanine diet have higher risks of spontaneous abortions. Their infants have high rates of mental retardation, microcephaly, congenital heart disease, and altered facial features. To minimize or prevent problems, a low phenylalanine diet, started before pregnancy, is recommended so that phenylalanine levels can be kept below 10 mg/dL during pregnancy (Burton, 1994).

► **TABLE 32-5**

Inborn Errors of Metabolism Frequently Identified in the Neonatal Period

	Failure to thrive, poor feeding	Vomiting	Diarrhea	Lethargy/coma	Hypo/hypertonicity	Seizures	Respiratory distress, apnea	Jaundice	Hepatosplenomegaly	Coarse facial features	Abnormal odor	Dysmorphic features	Abnormal eye findings	Abnormal hair	Macroglossia	Laboratory Findings	Metabolic acidosis	Hypoglycemia	Hyperammonemia	Elevated transaminase	Non-glucose-reducing substances	Ketonuria	(+) Ferric chloride in the urine	Neutropenia	Thrombocytopenia	Anemia	Vacuolated lymphocytes
Disorders of Carbohydrate Metabolism																											
Galactosemia	X	X	X		X	X		X	X				X				X	X			X	X					X
Glycogen storage disease type I	X		X		X	X			X								X	X									
Pyruvate dehydrogenase deficiency	X				X	X											X										
Pyruvate carboxylase deficiency	X			X	X	X											X	X			X						
Disorders of Amino Acid Metabolism																											
Organic acidemias																											
Methylmalonic acidemia	X	X		X	X	X	X										X	X	X			X		X	X	X	
Propionic acidemia	X	X		X	X	X											X		X			X		X	X		
Isovaleric acidemia	X	X		X	X	X	X										X		X						X	X	
Multiple carboxylase deficiency	X	X		X	X	X											X		X			X					
Glutaric acidemia type II	X	X				X					X						X	X									
Urea cycle defects																											
Carbamyl phosphate synthetase deficiency	X			X	X	X	X												X						X		
Ornithine transcarbamylase deficiency	X			X	X	X	X		X										X	X							
Citrullinemia	X	X		X	X	X	X												X								
Argininosuccinic aciduria	X			X	X	X	X		X					X					X	X							
Other disorders of amino acid metabolism																											
Maple syrup urine disease	X		X	X	X	X											X	X						X	X		
Nonketotic hyperglycinemia	X			X	X	X	X					X													X		
Phenylketonuria	X	X				X						X												X			
Hereditary tyrosinemia	X	X	X					X				X								X		X	X	X	X	X	
Lysomal storage disorders																											
Gangliosidosis type I	X						X		X	X		X	X		X												X
Cell disease	X								X	X		X	X		X												
Sialidosis type II	X								X	X		X	X		X												X
Other inborn errors of metabolism																											
Congenital adrenal hypoplasia	X	X			X																						
Cystic fibrosis	X		X																								
Hypophosphatasia	X				X																						
Alpha-antitrypsin deficiency	X						X	X	X											X							
Fatty acyl coenzyme A dehydrogenase deficiency	X	X		X	X	X												X	X	X							
Zellweger syndrome	X			X	X				X				X														
Neonatal adrenoleukodystrophy	X			X	X							X	X														

Recognition of symptoms is an essential part of the daily nursing assessment and care of the neonate. Suspected abnormalities should be reported to the physician to aid in the further assessment of the neonate. The nurse also plays a key role in obtaining specimens for laboratory analysis. Often specimens must be obtained before or after feedings; thus, the neonate's feeding schedule must be closely monitored. When obtaining urine specimens, the nurse must avoid contamination with stool or lotions applied to the diaper area. In blood tests obtained by nurses, such as the test for phenylketonuria, specific spots on a test card must be completely covered by the neonate's blood. Patience and accuracy are essential in obtaining a specimen appropriate for the particular test.

Great strides have been made in recent years in identifying and managing inborn errors of metabolism. One important reason is the early identification of metabolic abnormalities through the use of neonatal screening tests. Screening tests are usually done before the neonate's discharge from the hospital when health care providers have access to the neonate and before the negative effects of the condition progress. The most common mass neonatal screening test is for PKU; however, many states routinely screen for other inborn errors of metabolism or hormonal disorders such as hypothyroidism.

Nurses must be aware of the neonatal screening tests performed in their state. The nurse can ensure that necessary screening tests are completed prior to the neonate's discharge. The nurse must be aware of special factors that affect the accuracy of the test. For example, newborns should have at least 24 hours of protein feeding before a specimen is taken for a PKU test, because adequate feeding is needed to raise levels in infants with this problem (Forsberg, 1997). Infants who are discharged early may have testing or repeat testing done after discharge. Neonates who require lengthy hospitalizations, transfers between newborn nursery and the intensive care nursery, or transfers between hospitals require meticulous attention to ensure that the necessary screening tests are completed and the results obtained in a timely manner.

Parents may question the necessity of screening tests or may request information about the disorders for which the neonate is being tested. Basic information should be shared with parents without unnecessarily alarming them. Parents can be directed to contact their primary health care provider to obtain the results of the screening tests.

Nursing and Collaborative Management.

As soon as an inborn error of metabolism is confirmed, referral should be made to physicians specializing in the care of infants and children with metabolic diseases. Long-term management and family support are essential in the ongoing treatment of these neonates. As these metabolic diseases are genetically transmitted, a genetic evaluation of the family should be included in the treatment plan as well.

Management then is directed at minimizing the alteration in the metabolism. Because of the complexity of each of the inborn errors of metabolism, specific treatment regimens are necessary. Many inborn errors of metabolism are successfully managed with strict dietary regimens or vitamin or hormonal supplements. Consistent and ongoing implementation of these treatments is essential for the future well-being of the child.

Neonates with severe metabolic diseases, especially those who are not diagnosed in the first weeks of life, may sustain irreversible brain damage. The brain damage may range from mild retardation to profound and severe mental retardation. Infants may not demonstrate signs of brain damage until they are several months old. Careful developmental assessment is essential in their ongoing care. Families require support and education from the interdisciplinary health care team. They often can benefit from referrals to community agencies in their local area.

▶ Alterations in Nutrition and Gastrointestinal Functioning

Neonates have special nutritional needs. Nutritional management focuses on maintaining cellular functioning, promoting growth and development, and replacing fluids and nutrients lost in urine, feces, or sweat. High-risk, immature, or undernourished neonates pose even greater nutritional challenges to members of the interdisciplinary team.

Nursing and Collaborative Assessment

Assessment of the high-risk neonate's nutritional needs includes the following factors (Klaus & Fanaroff, 1993):

1. *Gestational age and weight.* Preterm neonates have limited fat and glycogen stores, and low albumen, iron, and calcium levels, which must be carefully considered in planning nutritional intake. Reflexes essential to oral feeding (e.g., the gag reflex) are not present until 32 weeks of gestation.
2. *Gastrointestinal functioning.* The neonate's stomach empties slowly in the first few weeks of life. Esophageal sphincters may also have

poor tone and cause the stomach contents to reflux into the esophagus or trachea. Congenital anomalies of the gastrointestinal tract can further complicate the neonate's ability to feed orally.

3. *Metabolic functioning.* Preterm or malnourished neonates may require a different combination of nutrients because of a changing metabolism. For example, low-birth-weight neonates may require some amino acids that are not essential to the healthy term neonate.

4. *Temperature stability.* Neonates with unstable temperatures should be fed in the regulated environment of a radiant warmer or an incubator. However, these thermal environments raise the neonate's fluid requirements.

5. *Respiratory functioning.* A neonate experiencing respiratory distress is not able to bottlefeed or breastfeed. A neonate who requires oxygen may have higher oxygen needs during activities such as feeding. The neonate who has a weak cry or changes color with crying may not be able to safely nipple feed.

6. *Coordination of sucking and swallowing.* Sucking and swallowing activities begin before birth but are not fully developed until after birth. Sucking begins before swallowing is seen. Swallowing, which allows food to enter the stomach and not the trachea, develops at 32 to 34 weeks of gestation. Sucking and swallowing may not be coordinated at birth and must be assessed before oral feedings begin.

Assessment of intake begins with growth. Adequate growth is assessed on the basis of weight, length, total body fat, and head circumference. The indicators are plotted in percentiles on a growth chart. The goal is to maintain growth within or above the birth percentiles (Klaus & Fanaroff, 1993). The long-term goal of supporting adequate growth of a neonate focuses on ongoing, progressive nutritional management.

Nursing and Collaborative Management

Nutritional management of high-risk neonates must be highly individualized. It is aimed at providing the necessary combination of nutrients in the safest, most effective method for each neonate. Nutrients can be provided parenterally (through intravenous lines) or enterally (via the gastrointestinal system). In each case, the contents of the feeding are specially calculated in response to the neonate's nutritional needs. The high-risk neonate's response to the feedings and the methods by which the feedings are administered are always assessed.

Parenteral Feedings. Parenteral (or intravenous) fluids are usually administered through a peripheral vein in the extremity or scalp. Initially, intravenous fluids contain glucose, sodium, and potassium. Magnesium and calcium may also be given. If the neonate requires intravenous nutrition for longer than several days, total parenteral nutrition (TPN) is begun. Total parenteral nutrition is an intravenous solution containing essential and nonessential amino acids and nonprotein calories, usually in the form of glucose. Vitamins, minerals, and electrolytes may also be added. Depending on the concentration, TPN solutions can be administered either through peripheral veins or through deep or central venous routes. While potential complications related to metabolic imbalances, alterations in liver functioning, and infection of the intravenous access site may accompany the use of TPN, they do not prevent its use. Meticulous management of peripheral intravenous lines is required when TPN is infused peripherally to prevent infiltration and sloughing of skin or subcutaneous tissue. X-ray confirmation for placement of central catheters must be done before any infusion takes place through them.

Intralipids may also be administered intravenously. Intralipids are fat emulsion solutions that are high in calories. These solutions allow high caloric intake while limiting volume and are usually infused over a 24-hour period. Intralipid solutions do not require central venous access and are often given simultaneously with TPN. Intralipids prevent the essential fatty acid deficiency associated with prolonged use of other parenteral methods. Intralipids must be used cautiously in neonates who have difficulty excreting free fatty acids. Those at risk include preterm and small-for-gestational-age neonates. Intralipids may also interfere with serum bilirubin measurements. In addition, administration of intralipids in infants with respiratory distress syndrome may further worsen the condition by interfering with oxygen transfer by the red blood cells.

Accurate and safe administration of parenteral nutrition requires collaboration between health care providers so that proper solutions and rates of infusion are calculated and administered. The neonate's weight must be monitored and documented daily. Intravenous lines and sites should be meticulously cared for and observed for signs of infiltration and infection.

The neonate's parenteral and enteral intake and urinary and gastrointestinal output must be carefully documented hourly. Monitoring of intermittent glucose levels and other laboratory studies are necessary in calculation of the neonate's future nutritional needs.

Enteral Feedings. Nutritional feedings, administered through the gastrointestinal tract, are called enteral feedings. The patent gastrointestinal tract is able to digest enteral feedings and provide the neonate with the necessary nutritional intake. Enteral feedings include oral feedings, such as breastfeedings and bottle feedings, in which the neonate feeds from a nipple, as well as tube feedings. Enteral feedings of breast milk or formula are the only way a healthy neonate needs to be fed. For preterm or sick neonates, oral enteral feeding may be the last of many steps in a long process.

Tube Feedings. The transition from parenteral feedings to enteral feedings may require the temporary use of tube feedings to provide adequate nutrition. A tube is passed through the nose or mouth into the stomach. Once the tube is inserted, placement is confirmed by aspiration of stomach contents or auscultation of a bolus of air injected into the stomach. The tube is taped in position to prevent it from dislodging during the feeding (see box entitled Placement of a Tube for Gavage Feeding).

Before administering the feeding, any residue from the previous feeding is identified by gentle aspiration of the stomach contents. The volume, color, and consistency of the residue are noted, and it is then refed to the neonate. Parameters may be set regarding an acceptable residual volume for each neonate. Nurses should notify physicians when the residual volume exceeds designated parameters, as it may indicate intolerance of the feedings.

Tube feedings may be gavage (bolus) feedings, in which a specific volume is administered over a limited period. In many cases, the tube is inserted immediately before the gavage feedings and removed afterward. High-risk neonates may also receive continuous tube feedings, in which the nasogastric tube is taped in place and the prescribed feeding is delivered usually by a pump at a continuous rate. The method of tube feeding and the type of feeding pump used depend on the neonate's condition and special needs (Ferraro-McDuffie, Huddleston, Smith, Karotkin, & Gardner, 1994).

Careful handling and positioning of the neonate during and after the feeding are necessary to reduce the likelihood of regurgitation and to prevent aspiration of the feeding. If the neonate's condition allows, parents may be encouraged to hold the neonate with the head elevated during tube feedings. If the neonate is not being held, the right lateral position is preferred, with the head of the bed elevated. This position promotes stomach emptying and reduces the risk of regurgitation. Immediately after the feeding, the neonate should be placed in the proper position.

Offering a pacifier to an infant (after 34 weeks' gestation) during tube feedings may help stimulate sucking and swallowing reflexes in preparation for future oral feedings.

Transition to Oral Feedings. The transition from tube feedings to oral feedings is often a gradual process. Initially, nipple feeding is attempted once a day, then gradually increased to every third, then every other feeding. The nurse should be prepared to spend at least 20 minutes with the neonate who is nipple feeding. For small or sick neonates, eating is an activity that requires a large amount of energy; therefore, frequent rest periods are often needed. The neonate may suck vigorously in short bursts and then swallow, indicating immature sucking/swallowing coordination. The neonate may require support under the chin and on the cheeks to facilitate successful feeding. The nurse should burp the neonate after at least every 15 mL of the feeding. If the neonate is not able to ingest enough nutrition through oral feedings, alternative strategies must be identified. For example, if the neonate is only able to nipple- or breastfeed half the necessary volume of formula, the remainder of the feeding may be administered by tube.

Communication between nurses and physicians is essential to identify the best strategy for each neonate. Parents are often anxious to nipple feed their neonates. During the beginning stages of nipple feeding in the high-risk neonate, parents require encouragement and support through what can prove to be a very frustrating process.

Breast milk can be the ideal nutritional product for the high-risk term neonate. It is easily digested and contains several important protective antibodies; however, high-risk term neonates are not always able to begin nursing when their mothers' milk supply begins. Nursing staff should be prepared to offer information and support to the woman who may need to pump her breasts regularly until her infant is able to be put to breast. Expressed breast milk may be given in tube feedings or bottle feedings until the neonate is able to be put to breast.

Studies indicate that unless very weak or ill, even a small preterm neonate can eventually successfully breastfeed. Breastfeeding readiness is indicated when the neonate experiences short wakeful periods, exhibits a sucking reflex, tolerates gavage feedings, and no longer requires oxygen therapy or ventilatory support.

Breast milk of the preterm mother differs in composition from the term mother's milk (Beckholt, 1990). For example, preterm breast milk contains more protein, nitrogen, calcium, sodium, and chloride, and lower levels of lactose, than term milk. After the first

► PLACEMENT OF A TUBE FOR GAVAGE FEEDING

OBJECTIVE

To insert accurately and safely an orogastric or nasogastric tube

To administer accurately and safely a tube feeding to the neonate who, because of gestational age or illness, cannot bottlefeed or breastfeed

EQUIPMENT

- Appropriate-size feeding tube (5 or 8 French)
- Tape
- Sterile water
- Appropriate-size syringe (5 to 20 cc)
- Formula or breast milk in the appropriate volume
- Stethoscope
- Pacifier

PROCEDURE

1. Orogastric feedings are usually preferred, as newborns are nose breathers and a nasogastric tube may partially occlude the airway; however, oral tubes can cause excessive gagging in some neonates, making use of the nasal route necessary. To determine how far the tube should be inserted: measure the distance from the nose to the ear to the xiphoid process. Mark the tube with tape to indicate how far it should be inserted.

2. Safely position the baby. Use a mummy-type of blanket restraint to prevent the baby from moving during the procedure.

3. Lubricate the tip of the feeding tube with water, insert it into the back of the throat, and gradually ease it down until the marker is at the neonate's lips (if an orogastric tube) or at the tip of the nose (if a nasogastric tube). If resistance is met and the tube cannot be advanced, remove it, allow the neonate to rest, and begin again. Caution should be used as some neonates may experience a vagal response, including bradycardia, when the tube is inserted.

4. Remove the tube immediately if the infant coughs excessively, chokes, becomes cyanotic, or cannot vocalize or cry.

5. Check for proper placement by aspirating for stomach contents and gently pushing 1 to 5 cc of air into the stomach while listening over the upper left quadrant of the abdomen with the stethoscope. If stomach contents cannot be aspirated and air is not auscultated entering the stomach, remove the tube. Once placement has been confirmed, aspirate the air in the stomach before begin-

ning the feeding. Amount, color, and consistency of aspirate should be recorded. Feeding volumes may be altered or feedings withheld based on this information and the particular situation.

6. Secure the tube to the infant's cheek using tape or a transparent dressing. Avoid taping the tube to the forehead to prevent irritation to the nostril.

7. If possible, the neonate should be dressed and held during the feeding. This is often a good time to involve the parents. If the neonate cannot be held, he or she should be positioned on the right side with the head of the bed elevated slightly to facilitate gastric emptying.

8. Attach the syringe without the plunger and fill it with the amount of formula or breast milk to be given. If the syringe cannot hold the total volume of the feeding, slowly add the remaining formula before the syringe empties to prevent excess air from entering the stomach. Gentle pressure may be applied with the plunger to initiate gravity drainage. Feedings should not be pushed or forced. The amount of the feeding should be based on the neonate's fluid and caloric requirements, which are calculated according to the weight in kilograms.

9. An orogastric tube may stimulate the sucking reflex. Offer the neonate a pacifier during tube feedings as nonnutritive sucking is a valuable form of stimulation.

10. When the feeding is completed, pinch the tube and gently remove it. In some instances, a nasogastric tube is left in place between feedings.

11. Place the neonate on the right side, with the head of the bed slightly elevated.

12. Record the data, including confirmation of tube placement; amount and quality of stomach aspirate; type and amount of feeding; tolerance of the feeding, as indicated by the presence of vomiting or diarrhea; ability or interest in sucking during the feeding; and overall readiness to begin nipple feedings.

13. If the feedings are to be continuous, the tube is left in place and secured with tape. Care should be taken to tape the tube in a position that will not place pressure on the nares and cause irritation. Feedings may be given as continuous or bolus, using a pump. Continuous feedings should be administered by an infusion pump at a constant rate. Syringe, tubing, and feeding tube changes are done according to unit policy.

Adapted, with permission, from Willett, M.J., Patterson, M., & Steinbock, B. (1986). *Manual of neonatal intensive care nursing*. Boston: Little, Brown, pp. 67–68.

month, the nutrient levels of preterm milk are similar to term milk. For this reason, preterm breast milk may not be nutritionally adequate for the preterm neonate, especially after the first month of lactation. Fortifying or supplementing breast milk may allow breastfeeding to continue and meet the special needs of the preterm neonate.

Attempting to provide breast milk for a sick or preterm neonate may be very difficult for a mother and requires a commitment by both the mother and the nursing staff who will support her. Realistic goals regarding the neonate's readiness to breastfeed must be communicated to the parents. Identification of the role that the father desires to have in feeding the neonate or questions and concerns he may have about breastfeeding must be explored as well. Encouraging parents to participate in other feeding activities, such as holding the neonate or offering the pacifier, can be very satisfying as they look forward to the time when the neonate will be able to breastfeed. When the neonate is ready to breastfeed for the first time, parents need additional support and education.

Congenital Abnormalities

Maintaining adequate nutrition for the high-risk neonate may be further complicated by congenital anomalies in the gastrointestinal tract. The most frequent anomalies are categorized as follows:

- *Atresia.* **Atresia** is a congenital absence of an opening in a structure or system of the body. In esophageal atresia, the esophagus ends in a blind pouch. The neonate gags and vomits frequently when trying to feed, because the feeding cannot continue beyond the blind pouch. Aspiration pneumonia can occur. Neonates with esophageal atresia often have an opening between the area of the esophagus below the blind pouch and the trachea. This is called a tracheoesophageal fistula; it must be repaired surgically. Many of these infants are unable to handle their own secretions and may seem "bubbly" during the first day of life. The nurse may identify this anomaly when unable to pass a suction catheter or feeding tube into the neonate's stomach.
- *Stenosis.* This narrowing in the lumen of some part of the gastrointestinal tract may be caused by a web of tissue or it can involve the entire thickness of the bowel wall. A common site of stenosis is the pyloric sphincter, where the stomach empties into the duodenum. Neonates with pyloric stenosis often progress to projectile vomiting within the first 4 to 6 weeks of life. The neonate acts hungry, loses weight, and becomes dehydrated. Waves of peristalsis, movement of the intestinal muscles, are visible across the abdomen. An ultrasound or barium study is used to confirm the diagnosis. Surgical repair of the stenosis is the treatment required. Oral feedings of 5% glucose can usually be started 4 to 6 hours after surgery. Feedings are gradually increased in volume and strength. The neonate is usually feeding well with no further complications 48 hours after the surgical procedure.
- *Duplications.* These congenital cystlike projections or tubular structures can form anywhere along the gastrointestinal tract. These structures can be blind tubelike extensions of an area of the intestine that open into the lumen of the intestine. Duplications can cause obstructions. Duplications that open into the lumen of the intestine produce acid secretions that irritate the bowel lining and can cause perforation. A duplication can simply be a palpable mass. Surgical repair is indicated based on the type of structure and the complications it causes.

Learning that their neonate has an abnormality of the gastrointestinal tract can be frightening for parents. They will have many questions about the causes of the abnormality and its management. Some abnormalities require only one surgical intervention, which allows the neonate to return to oral feedings quickly. Other abnormalities require more complicated surgical procedures, in which oral feedings are the last of many steps in the neonate's recovery. Until the abnormality is corrected, the neonate requires careful attention to nutritional needs and may require intravenous fluids such as total parenteral nutrition. In addition, the neonate may require special feeding procedures, such as tube feedings, at home until he or she is able to eat normally. Parents require the support of the interdisciplinary health care team as they move through the necessary steps of the treatment. Parents must be aware of the importance of the special follow-up care required after the neonate is discharged.

▶ Alterations in Cardiac Functioning

Alterations in cardiac functioning place the neonate at particular risk during the transition to extrauterine life. At birth, dramatic cardiac and hemodynamic changes take place (see Chapter 30). Alterations in cardiac functioning in the neonate may be the result of acute disease processes, such as persistent pulmonary hypertension, or of congenital heart diseases caused by defects in the heart and cardiac blood vessels. Many abnormalities in the heart pose acute and chronic life-threatening risks for the neonate and growing infant. Careful assessment is essential to swift and accurate identification of the disorder and the implementation of an effective treatment plan.

Persistent Pulmonary Hypertension

The adjustment from fetal to neonatal circulation that occurs at birth is essential to the neonate's survival in the environment outside the uterus. At birth, the lungs of the healthy neonate expand with air, blood vessels in the lungs dilate, pulmonary vascular resistance decreases quickly, shunts close, and the right ventricle of the heart sends blood to the lungs for gas exchange (Hansen, 1996). The heart, now exerting greater "pressure," is able to pump blood to the vessels of the lungs, which have become areas of lower "pressure" and do not "resist" the blood's entry. After birth, blood is thus oxygenated in the lungs, and the left side of the heart becomes and remains a higher pressure system than it was during fetal development, when the lungs were not the source of oxygenation of the blood (DeBoer & Stephens, 1997).

Once the fetus has been delivered and the cord clamped, he or she can never truly go back to "fetal circulation," because the newborn is no longer attached to the placenta. However, in certain neonates, a modified fetal circulation pattern continues, to some degree, as follows (Hansen, 1996):

- Blood vessels in the lungs do not dilate well when the baby breathes air after birth; they remain constricted. Unlike in normal transitions of the fetus to neonate, the pulmonary vascular resistance remains high.
- Due to this high pulmonary vascular resistance, blood entering the right side of the heart does not flow to the lungs to become oxygenated, but instead is shunted right-to-left across the ductus arteriosus to the descending aorta. As pressure in the right ventricle and right atrium rises, blood is shunted from the right atrium across the foramen ovale to the left atrium. These right-to-left shunts cause hypoxemia. The result of this situation is that blood returns to the systemic circulation without going to the lungs for oxygenation.

The full or postterm neonate with perinatal hypoxia is at risk for developing a persistent fetal circulation, which is more accurately called persistent pulmonary hypertension (PPHN). The neonate with PPHN may have a history of meconium staining, fetal distress, or other risk factors for sepsis or pneumonia. The box entitled Causes of Persistent Pulmonary Hypertension of the Newborn summarizes causes of PPHN, which may be transient or persist. The infant with PPHN may seem healthy at birth; however, progressive cyanosis develops over the next 12 hours. Other signs include tachypnea, respiratory grunting, and retractions; resuscitation may be needed. A systolic murmur is heard, but systemic blood pressure and cardiac output can be normal at first, unless severe asphyxia or sepsis is present (Hansen, 1996). If these signs are observed, the neonate must be assessed aggressively to confirm the presence of an alteration in cardiac functioning and its possible causes.

► CAUSES OF PERSISTENT PULMONARY HYPERTENSION OF THE NEWBORN

TRANSIENT

- Hypoxemia with or without acidosis
- Hypothermia
- Hypoglycemia
- Hyperviscosity

PERSISTENT

- Active vasoconstriction
  - Sepsis/pneumonia
  - Meconium or amniotic fluid aspiration
- Anatomic abnormalities of pulmonary vessels

- Underdevelopment of the lung
  - Diaphragmatic hernia
  - Potter syndrome
  - Other causes of oligohydramnios
- Maldevelopment of pulmonary vessels
  - Chronic intrauterine hypoxemia
  - Aspiration syndromes
  - Intrauterine closure of ductus arteriosus
  - Idiopathic

Source: Reproduced, with permission, from Rudolph, A.M., Hoffman, J.I.E., & Rudolph, C.D. (Eds.). (1996). *Rudolph's pediatrics* (20th ed.). Stamford, CT: Appleton & Lange, p. 1609.

The primary goal of management is to maintain adequate oxygenation. PPHN requires complex and intensive care which can include supplemental oxygen and mechanical ventilation; avoiding cold stress; treating such reversible causes of PPHN as hypoxia, hypoglycemia, and hypothermia; sedation; volume replacement to support the systemic circulation; vasopressors to improve cardiac contractility; increase cardiac output and raise systemic pressure; and medications to improve pulmonary blood flow. New, promising therapies include surfactant replacement, high-frequency ventilation and extracorporeal membrane oxygenation (ECMO). With ECMO, the infant is placed on a type of lung bypass; an external membrane oxygenator maintains oxygenation for the infant (DeBoer & Stephens, 1997; Hansen, 1996).

Prompt interventions may prevent problems related to PPHN from worsening. Considered a disorder of transition from fetal to extrauterine life, PPHN with treatment is usually a self-limiting disease, resolving within 3 to 5 days. Unfortunately, PPHN can be life threatening, and the mortality rate depends upon the underlying cause. Some infants who survive have such long-term problems as hearing difficulty, neurologic impairment, and chronic lung disease (Hansen, 1996).

Congenital Abnormalities

Congenital heart diseases occur in at least 1% of live-born infants; the incidence is higher in preterm infants and in fetuses who are born dead or who die before birth (Hoffman, 1996). The exact cause of a congenital heart disease is often difficult to identify. Factors may include genetic abnormalities such as Down syndrome and trisomy 18; environmental factors such as viral infections (e.g., rubella); or exposure to teratogens such as alcohol or drugs (e.g., the anticonvulsant phenytoin, dextroamphetamines, and lithium chloride). However, no clear-cut cause can be identified for most congenital heart diseases.

Congenital heart defects in the neonate cause a wide range of hemodynamic alterations (Fig. 32–6). Congenital heart defects are separated into two categories, based on the presence of cyanosis, which results from the altered hemodynamic states. Alterations that cause cyanosis are called **cyanotic heart defects,** and alterations that do not cause cyanosis are called **acyanotic heart defects.** Cyanotic heart diseases include tetralogy of Fallot and transposition of the great vessels. Acyanotic heart diseases include ventricular septal defects, atrial septal defects/atrioventricular canal defects, pulmonary stenosis, patent ductus arteriosus, aortic stenosis, and, coarctation of the aorta.

Nursing and Collaborative Assessment. Assessment of the neonate's cardiac and circulatory status is essential in determining whether alterations in cardiac functioning are caused by congenital heart defects. Assessment of the neonate must include the following components:

1. Questioning the mother about prenatal history and noting maternal risk factors that are related to cardiac abnormalities.
2. Careful monitoring of vital signs, including temperature, apical heart rate, respiratory rate, and blood pressure; for neonates found to have a murmur or suspected to have a cardiac disease, blood pressures must be taken on each extremity with the appropriate-size blood pressure cuff.
3. Assessing heart sounds to identify the presence of abnormal sounds including murmurs.
4. Assessing the quality of pulses in all four extremities; assessing bilateral femoral pulses.
5. Assessing respiratory status, including the neonate's skin color, respiratory effort, breath sounds, presence of respiratory distress, and the need for supplemental oxygen and ventilatory support.
6. Assessing the neonate's activity level, including the length and quality of activities and the presence of color changes during activities (crying and feeding are both important activities to be noted).
7. Assessing strict intake and output including measurements of the specific gravity of the urine.
8. Assessing the neonate's weight at least once a day.

In addition to physical assessment of the neonate, diagnostic tests may include arterial blood gases, glucose and calcium levels, and hemoglobin and hematocrit; invasive diagnostic tests, including cardiac catheterization; and noninvasive diagnostic tests, including chest x-rays, electrocardiograms, and echocardiograms. Abnormal assessment findings in the neonate suspected to have an alteration in cardiac functioning must be documented. The information obtained in the physical assessment is often the key to identifying a particular alteration or defect. The clinical presentation of a neonate with severe cardiac disease usually includes one or more of the following: cyanosis, respiratory distress, congestive heart failure, diminished cardiac output, abnormal cardiac rhythm, cardiac murmurs.

Nursing Diagnoses. Nursing diagnoses are developed for the neonate with altered cardiac functioning

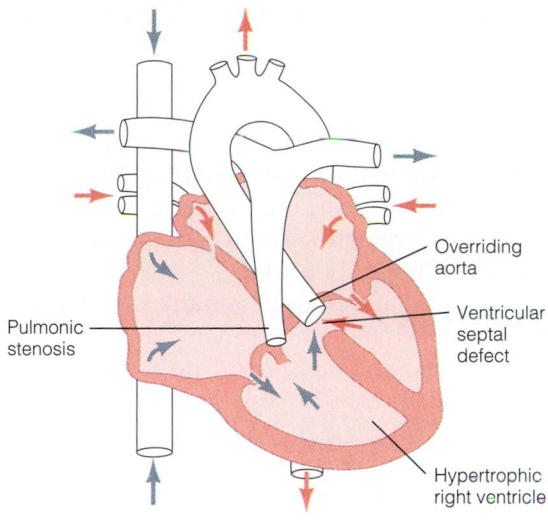

Tetralogy of Fallot

Tetralogy of Fallot is characterized by the combination of four defects: (1) pulmonic stenosis (2) ventricular septal defect (3) overriding aorta (4) hypertrophy of right ventricle. It is the most common defect causing cyanosis in clients surviving beyond two years of age. The severity of symptoms depends on the degree of pulmonary artery stenosis, size of the ventricular septal defect, and degree to which the aorta overrides the septal defect.

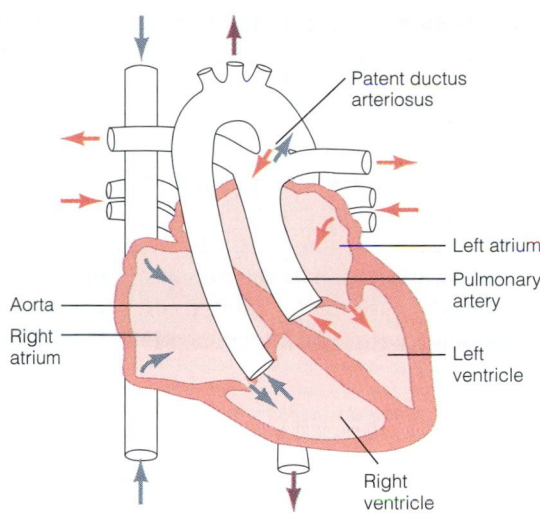

Transposition of great vessels

This anomaly is an embryologic defect caused by a straight division of the bulbar trunk without normal spiraling. As a result, the aorta originates from the right ventricle, and the pulmonary artery from the left ventricle. An abnormal communication between the two circulations must be present to sustain life.

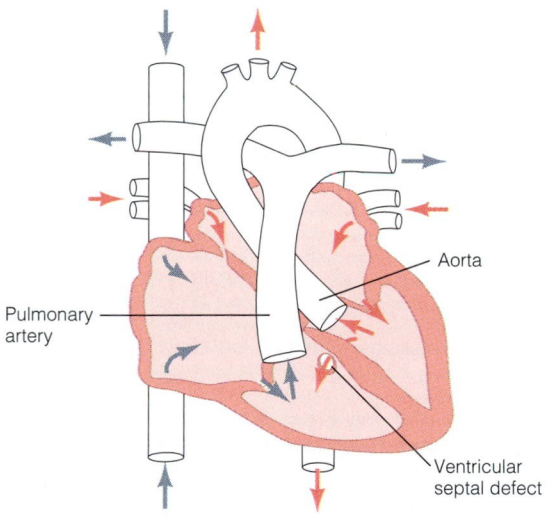

Ventricular septal defects

A ventricular septal defect is an abnormal opening between the right and left ventricle. Ventricular septal defects vary in size and may occur in either the membranous or muscular portion of the ventricular septum. Because higher pressure is in the left ventricle, blood is shunted from the left to the right ventricle during systole. If pulmonary vascular resistance produces pulmonary hypertension, the shunt of blood is then reversed from the right to the left ventricle and cyanosis results.

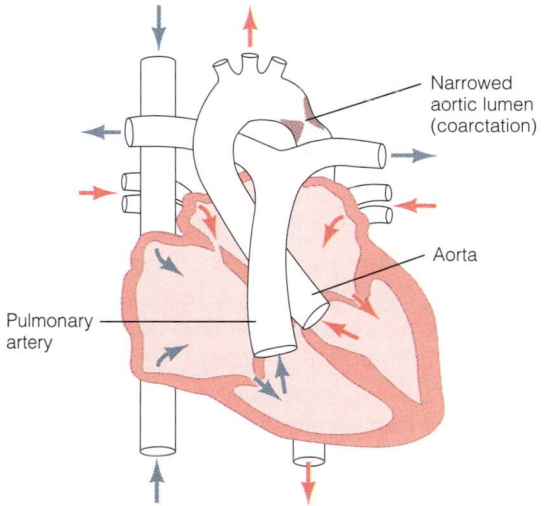

Coarctation of the aorta

Coarctation of the aorta is characterized by a narrowed aortic lumen. Coarctations vary greatly in anatomic features. The lesion produces an obstruction to the flow of blood through the aorta causing an increased left ventricular pressure and workload.

FIGURE 32–6. Congenital abnormalities of the heart. *Cyanotic defects:* tetralogy of Fallot and transposition of the great vessels. *Acyanotic heart defects:* ventricular septal defect and coarctation of the aorta. *(Reproduced, with permission, from Congenital Heart Abnormalities: Clinical Education Aid no. 7. Columbus, OH: Ross Laboratories, n.d.)*

after comprehensive assessment. Examples of diagnoses related to neonatal cardiac functioning include:

Problem-oriented diagnoses:

- Altered cardiopulmonary tissue perfusion, related to persistent pulmonary hypertension in the neonatal period
- Decreased cardiac output, related to patent ductus arteriosus in the neonatal period
- Altered parenting, related to transport of neonate with cardiac condition to intensive care unit

Wellness-oriented diagnoses:

- Asset in physiologic adaptation, related to spontaneous closure of patent ductus arteriosus

Nursing and Collaborative Management.

Neonates with cardiac disease require care from the interdisciplinary team in a specialized nursery environment equipped for care of such infants. The neonate may need to be transferred to a hospital with an intensive care nursery, usually a level III facility. It is a frightening, stressful time for parents. Nurses can support and console them as they cope with the neonate's condition and transfer (see Chapter 12).

Interventions are initiated once the neonate's needs are clearly identified. For example, large amounts of energy are required for the sucking, swallowing, and breathing activities needed during feedings. The neonate may require tube feedings for all or some feedings to conserve energy; may require oxygen during activities such as bottle feedings or breastfeedings; may be fluid restricted and permitted a limited number of nipple feedings each day; and may require clustering of care as well as ongoing diagnostic studies. If the neonate develops serious life-threatening complications, such as congestive heart failure, aggressive treatment may be indicated. The neonate may require cardiovascular medications, such as digoxin, to regulate and strengthen the heartbeat, or diuretics, such as furosemide (Lasix), to eliminate or prevent fluid overload. If a congenital heart defect is identified, the neonate may require surgical repair of the defect soon after birth or years later.

Discharge Planning.

The discharge of a neonate with altered cardiac functioning often includes ongoing interventions begun in the hospital. For example, some parents must learn how to care for their neonate receiving oxygen at home. Teaching will include safety information as well as the skills needed to bathe and feed the neonate receiving oxygen. Parents must demonstrate understanding of the medication(s) they will be administering, the purpose(s) and side effects of the medications; in addition, they must be able to measure the correct dose of the medication(s) and administer it according to schedule, and know when to notify the physician. For some neonates, fluid intake may be restricted at home as well. Parents must demonstrate competency in preparing the correct amount of formula for every feeding. Nurses can further assist parents learning to care for these neonates by offering strategies about coordinating feeding schedules with family activities.

Many cardiac disorders require long-term collaborative management among members of the interdisciplinary team such as nurses, physicians, surgeons, and social workers. Parents must be aware of the importance of regular follow-up care for their neonate, and become familiar with the health care professionals who will manage the care. Parents will have many questions about the neonate's cardiac disease and what to expect in the future. They require consistent support and education about the changes that will occur in the neonate's condition or treatment plan. Identifying community support groups or financial resources prior to the neonate's discharge can further assist parents.

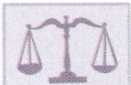

Ethical Decision Making

Suzette Stevens is assessed to be 39 weeks' gestation and weighs 5 lbs 8 oz. Born with Down syndrome and cardiac anomalies, she becomes cyanotic with activity, feeds poorly, and tires easily. Without cardiac surgery, which could correct her heart problem, she is not expected to survive. Suzette's parents, Peter and Michelle Stevens, are devastated at having a child with Down syndrome and express their fears about trying to raise a child with lifelong special needs. They will soon have to face the decision to sign consent for surgery or to make Suzette as comfortable as possible and let her die without surgery. If you were the nurse caring for this family, consider the following questions:

1. What ethical dilemmas are raised by the situation that Peter and Michelle Stevens face?
2. Would these dilemmas exist if their infant did not have Down syndrome?
3. Should the nature of congenital anomalies or genetic disorders affect the care a baby receives?

► Alterations in Neurologic Functioning

The central nervous system of the fetus and neonate is vulnerable to factors that may temporarily or permanently affect neurologic functioning. These factors may be the result of congenital malformations or may be induced by the prenatal or postnatal environments. Early identification of risk factors of physiologic abnormalities is essential in limiting or preventing long-term neurologic impairment.

Congenital Abnormalities

One group of congenital malformations in the central nervous system comprises anomalies that occur during fetal development of the nervous system. Some abnormalities result from the failure of the neural tube to develop and close correctly. The neural tube is the embryonic structure that eventually develops into the brain and spinal cord. Failure of the neural tube to develop properly leads to three main defects (Cohen, 1987):

1. **Anencephaly.** The skull and the cerebral hemispheres are absent; only the brainstem may be visible at the base of the skull. The head looks very small and abnormally shaped (Fig. 32–7).
2. **Spina bifida.** There are three abnormalities related to spina bifida. In **spina bifida occulta,** the vertebral laminae do not fuse in an isolated area of the spine; in **meningocele,**

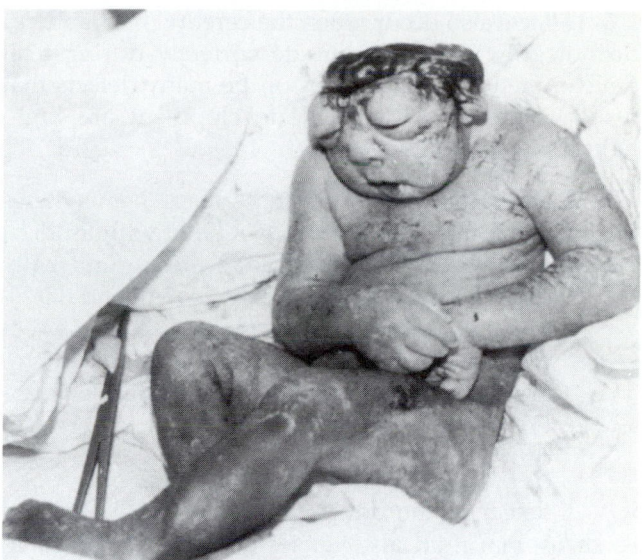

FIGURE 32–7. Anencephalic infant. *(Reproduced, with permission, from Cunningham, F.G. et al. (1997). Williams obstetrics (20th ed.). Stamford, CT: Appleton & Lange, p. 907.)*

meninges protrude from the spinal canal but the spinal cord is in correct position; in **meningomyelocele** both the meninges and the spinal cord protrude through the spinal canal (Fig. 32–8).

3. **Encephalocele.** Brain tissue and meninges protrude in a sac through a defect in the skull.

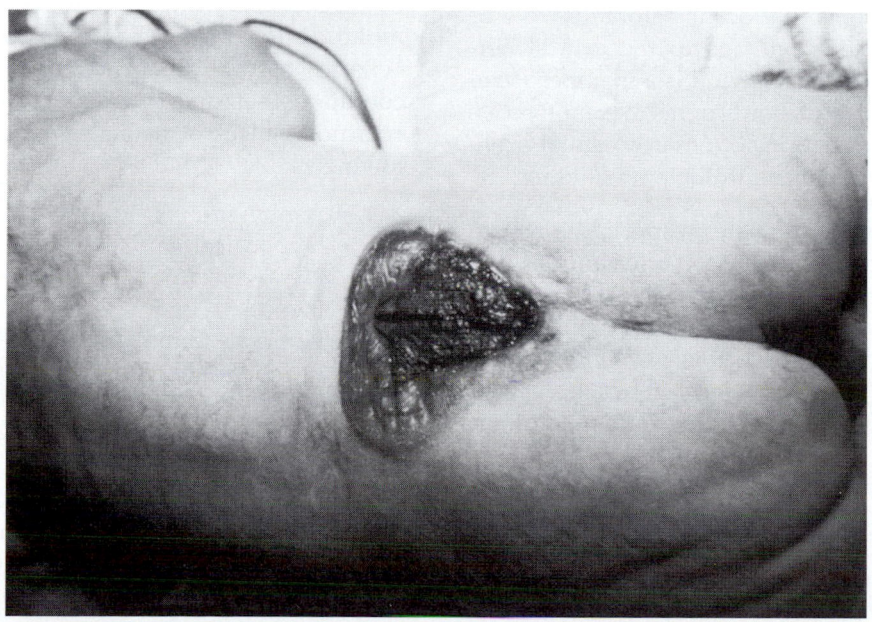

FIGURE 32–8. Large lumbar meningomyelocele. *(Courtesy of Dr. Victor Klein from Cunningham, F.G. et al. (1997). Williams obstetrics (20th ed.). Stamford, CT: Appleton & Lange, p. 908.)*

Defects also occur when the cerebral hemispheres do not grow and differentiate correctly during fetal development. Two examples of the many defects that result from such abnormal development are highlighted here:

1. **Hydranencephaly.** The cerebral hemispheres are absent and the space is filled with fluid.
2. **Microcephaly.** The head appears unusually small because of the limited growth and development of the brain. The brain is only 15% of the size of the normal neonatal brain. Microcephaly is also caused by intrauterine infections, anoxia, malnutrition, and other syndromes.

A defect in the development and circulation of cerebrospinal fluid also causes congenital malformations. A major neurologic alteration that occurs with this defect is **hydrocephalus.** In this condition, the head appears abnormally large. There is an abnormality in the circulation of cerebrospinal fluid. Circulating hydrocephalus is caused by an abnormality in the ventricles in the brain that prevents the cerebrospinal fluid from emptying properly. Communicating hydrocephalus occurs when the cerebrospinal fluid is not absorbed effectively. These abnormalities cause an increase in the amount of cerebro spinal fluid present in the brain, which causes the ventricles in the brain to dilate. This enlargement causes so much swelling that the sutures of the skull and the fontanelles spread, causing the neonate's head to become enlarged (Behrman & Kliegman, 1996).

The second group of abnormalities is the result of environmental problems that occur before delivery or in the postnatal period. Damage to the central nervous system in the perinatal period is a major cause of intellectual handicap and nonprogressive motor disorders. Three main categories of environmental problems may seriously impair neurologic functioning:

1. *Cerebral anoxia.* Neonates, especially preterm neonates, are more likely to suffer injuries as a result of anoxia. Anoxic damage leads to a disease process called periventricular leukomalacia in which decreased flow of blood to areas of the brain near the lateral ventricles causes infarction. This leads to long-term neurologic damage.
2. *Meningeal infection.* The infection damages the brain cells. The most common are rubella, cytomegalovirus, herpes virus, coxsackievirus, and *toxoplasma* infections.
3. *Metabolic alterations.* Altered metabolic states that remain uncontrolled, such as diabetes and hyperbilirubinemia, can damage brain tissue and prevent further normal development.

Neonates who suffered from an injury to the brain tissue before, during, or after birth can demonstrate a wide range of symptoms. Although symptoms of the initial insult may begin to subside, long-term residual effects may not be truly realized until years later. This produces a difficult situation for both the parents and the nurses and physicians caring for the neonate. The neonate may look healthy, and the natural tendency is for the parents to be reassured by the neonate's appearance. Nurses need to reinforce to the parents the importance of follow-up care.

Growth and development must be monitored closely throughout infancy for the presence of abnormalities that would require further medical and other treatment. These infants may develop seizures. Later, problems with cognitive functioning may be identified. In addition to ongoing neurologic assessment, developmental assessments must be included. The developmental assessment determines the infant's ability to reach developmental milestones, such as sitting alone, crawling, and making verbal sounds, at the appropriate point in her or his growth and development. As the infant gets older, developmental assessments may assist in identifying special learning needs as well.

Neonatal Seizures

Seizures are one of the most common abnormal neurologic findings in the neonatal period (Blackburn & Loper, 1992). They are chain reactions of repetitive abnormal electrical signals occurring in the cerebral neurons. Neonatal seizures differ from seizures of the older child or adult because generalized, tonic-clonic convulsions do not tend to take place in the first month after birth (Behrman & Kliegman, 1996). Seizures may be a sign of many different abnormal conditions; seizures themselves are not diseases. Some common causes of neonatal seizures include the following:

- Asphyxia
- Hypocalcemia
- Hypoglycemia
- Hyponatremia
- Hypernatremia
- Intracranial hemorrhage
- Infections
- Congenital central nervous system malformations
- Familial (autosomal dominant) characteristics
- Inborn errors of metabolism
- Withdrawal from drugs (including anesthetics)

In an estimated 25% of infants, no cause for seizures will be found (Nordli, Pedley, & De Vivo, 1996). Because neonates have an immature neurologic system, seizures may be difficult to identify. Any type of unusual behavior in the neonate may indicate seizure activity; therefore, careful assessment of the neonate is essential.

Nursing and Collaborative Assessment.

Table 32–6 describes five types of seizures that may be seen in the neonate. Behaviors such as grimacing, chewing, repetitive swallowing and yawning, tongue thrusting, staring, involuntary muscle contractions, and alterations in respiratory rhythm may be evident. Different types of seizures cause different abnormal movements. In observing unusual behaviors in the neonate, the nurse must:

- Establish that a seizure is taking place; expert knowledge of normal variations in newborn behavior is required.
- Make sure that the neonate is in a safe environment where behavior can be closely observed; for example, if the neonate begins to seize during a feeding or while being held, he or she

should be placed in a side-lying position in the crib. Equipment in the crib should be removed for safety.

- Note the exact time the seizure began and how long it lasted.
- Note the different types of behaviors and movements that occur as part of the seizure.
- Note which body parts are involved in seizure activity; note if one or both sides of the body are affected.
- Monitor vital signs including apical heart rate, respiratory rate, and blood pressure.
- Make sure that suction emergency equipment is readily available.
- Note medication and dose administered, the time given, and the neonate's response.
- Assess neurologic status and vital signs at the end of the seizure.
- Continue to monitor the neonate, noting when normal activity level resumes.

▶ **TABLE 32-6**

Types of Seizure Activity

Type of Seizure	Description/Neonatal Behaviors	Type of Seizure	Description/Neonatal Behaviors
Subtle seizures	Subtle seizures are commonly associated with severe central nervous system insults in both the preterm and term neonate. Behaviors observed include repetitive sucking, a fixed posture, pedaling movements of the legs and paddling movements of the arms, blinking or a fixed gaze, and apnea.	Multifocal clonic seizures	Multifocal clonic seizures are also often the result of generalized cerebral disturbances and are usually seen in the term neonate. Behaviors include rhythmic jerking movements that start in one area of the body, such as the right arm, and spread to other areas of the body. The spread of the jerking movements is usually nonorderly and can progress to the point where the entire body is found to have generalized clonic movements.
Tonic seizures	The tonic seizure is the most common seizure seen in preterm neonates with intraventricular hemorrhages. Behaviors include decerebrate posturing in which there is rigid extension of the arms and legs, with the palms of the hands and the soles of the feet facing downward. The neck is hyperextended, and the neonate may arch the back. This position may be held consistently until the seizure is over. It may also be seen intermittently during the seizure.	Myoclonic seizures	When seen in the term neonate, myoclonic seizures are often related to metabolic disturbances. Behaviors include synchronized, rapid, isolated jerking of both the upper and lower extremities. A myoclonic seizure looks similar to the Moro reflex. Extreme caution must be used in differentiating the Moro reflex, which occurs as a response to a loud noise or a jolt of the crib, and the myoclonic seizure, which is spontaneous and cannot be provoked.
Focal clonic seizures	Focal clonic seizures may be seen in the neonate as a result of generalized cerebral disturbances, such as asphyxia or metabolic disturbances. It is most common in the term neonate. Behaviors include rhythmic jerking of muscle groups. Focal clonic seizures are seen when only one part of the body develops rhythmic jerking, for example, the right arm.		

Several diagnostic tests are recommended, in addition to observation, to determine the underlying cause of the seizure. For example, blood glucose levels are assessed for hypoglycemia, and serum bilirubin levels for hyperbilirubinemia. A lumbar puncture is done to obtain samples of cerebrospinal fluid. The fluid is cultured to identify infection causing meningitis. Cerebrospinal fluid may also indicate bleeding or hemorrhage if large amounts of red blood cells are found. An electroencephalogram (EEG) is done to pinpoint the area in the brain where the seizure is occurring. Computerized tomographic (CT) scanning and ultrasound tests can also identify areas of bleeding in the brain or other brain abnormalities.

Other indications of neurologic problems should be identified. Intracranial pressure can increase as a result of increases in brain volume, of the cerebral blood volume, and the cerebrospinal fluid volume. The pressure increase may be caused by bleeding, obstruction, edema, or an abnormal structure such as a tumor. Critical changes, such as apnea and bradycardia, will occur in the neonate's vital signs. Cranial sutures may separate and the fontanelles begin to bulge. Increased intracranial pressure also causes changes in the neonate's neurologic status; for example, lethargy and abnormal posturing may be seen.

Nursing and Collaborative Management.
Management of a neonate with seizures can be complicated. Normal newborn behavior such as rapid eye movement in light sleep and Moro reflexes have, at times, been mistakenly identified as seizures. Every seizure workup entails not only a financial, but an emotional cost to the parents. Neonates may be transferred to an intensive care nursery in the hospital where they were born or to another hospital that specializes in the care of sick newborns. Nursing and medical expertise in caring for normal neonates is needed to differentiate abnormalities from normal behavior (Weingarten, 1988).

Efforts to identify the cause or source of a seizure are essential. Sometimes, however, the cause is never revealed. Some conditions that cause seizures in the neonate such as electrolyte imbalances, may have no long-term effect and do not require long-term treatment. On the other hand, conditions such as hypoxic brain damage and intraventricular hemorrhage are serious. Neonates with these conditions require aggressive follow-up care to prevent further neurologic damage and identify potential growth and development problems.

Acute management begins with treatment of the seizure with anticonvulsants and antiepileptics. Medications are probably the most effective means to control seizures. Phenobarbital is the anticonvulsant drug often used for neonates. Doses are calculated on the basis of the neonate's needs and range between 8 and 10 mg/kg per day. Serum levels of phenobarbital are monitored to ensure that the correct amount of medication is given to prevent the seizures. Often, the neonate must continue to take the medication after discharge. Discharge teaching should be provided to parents in a supportive manner. To assess retention of the discharge teaching, the nurse should ask parents to explain why the neonate is receiving the medication, list the side effects of the medication, administer the medication correctly, and describe when the physician should be notified.

The discharge of a neonate with alterations in neurologic functioning usually initiates a long process of follow-up and collaborative services. These neonates may exhibit behaviors such as irritability and short attention spans that make caring for them difficult. Nurses need to encourage parent–infant contact to promote attachment and recognition of the neonate's strengths. The possibility that their child has a brain disorder frightens most parents. Parents need realistic yet supportive advice and explanations. They should be encouraged to ask questions and discuss their concerns openly with the nurses and physicians caring for the neonate. They need support in dealing with the uncertainties of their child's future and in clearly understanding the role they play in the neonate's ongoing care. Nurses should make early referrals for available support services in the family's local community in preparation for discharge.

Critical Thinking in Care Planning

Care of the Neonate of a Diabetic Mother

Baby Margie Myers was born by spontaneous vaginal delivery at 38 weeks of gestation to an insulin-dependent diabetic mother. Mrs. Myers experienced difficulty in controlling her serum glucose levels throughout her pregnancy. Baby Myers weighed 9 pounds 10 oz at birth. She was puffy and had a capillary glucose of 40 at 15 minutes of age. Her respirations were initially labored at a rate of 40 breaths per minute. Her head was molded and she moved all four extremities independently and symmetrically when stimulated and crying. Baby Myers was given formula via feeding tube in the delivery room.

▶ Assessment

- Capillary blood glucose at delivery 40, confirmed by laboratory analysis
- Capillary blood glucose following feeding 75
- Respiratory rate 40
- No retractions, flaring, grunting
- Color pink in room air
- No supplemental oxygen given

- Moving all four extremities independently and symmetrically
- Facial movements are present and symmetrical
- Head is molded and symmetric without depression; no signs of bruising
- Cord bilirubin 1.5; no yellow discoloration of skin, sclera, or mucous membranes

Nursing Diagnosis

Alteration in metabolism, secondary to maternal diabetes

Expected Client/Family Outcomes	Nursing Action/Intervention	Evaluation
Neonate will be free of signs and symptoms of hypoglycemia after birth.	Observe for signs and symptoms of hypoglycemia (weak cry, apnea, cyanosis, hypothermia, lethargy, feeding problems, tremors, or seizures). *Rationale:* Early identification of signs and symptoms can lead to prompt treatment preventing serious harm to neonate.	Neonate is pink in color, has a strong cry, and is feeding well.
Neonate will have normal glucose level while tolerating feedings every 3 hours for at least 24 hours before planned discharge.	Gavage feed with formula after birth for glucose of 40 or less. Check capillary glucose before feedings. *Rationale:* Offering an early feeding will provide glucose to treat hypoglycemia.	Capillary glucose 75 following early feeding. Glucose values range between 90 and 100 after 8 hours of life.

(continued)

Critical Thinking in Care Planning continued

Nursing Diagnosis

Potential for ineffective breathing pattern, related to possible inadequate surfactant production in utero

Expected Client/Family Outcomes	Nursing Action/Intervention	Evaluation
Neonate will maintain adequate respiratory status in room air.	Ongoing assessment for signs of respiratory distress, increased respiratory rate, presence of retractions, nasal flaring, grunting, cyanosis. *Rationale:* Early identification of respiratory distress will lead to prompt treatment and prevention of serious harm to neonate.	Neonate remains pink, breathing easily at a rate of 40.

Nursing Diagnosis

Potential for musculoskeletal trauma during birth, related to macrosomia and large size

Neonate will demonstrate independent symmetric movement of all four extremities following labor and delivery.	Assess for presence of paralysis, asymmetric movement of extremities or face, bruising, etc. *Rationale:* Identification of traumatic injuries will lead to prompt treatment.	Neonate able to independently and symmetrically move all four extremities.
Neonate will demonstrate symmetric facial movements following labor and delivery.		Facial movements are equal and symmetric. No bruising is present.
Any evidence of trauma (bruising, impaired movement, etc.) will be promptly identified.	Document color, temperature, tone, movement, and presence and quality of pulses in extremities. *Rationale:* A traumatic injury may result in compromise of neurologic or cardiovascular functioning requiring intervention. Consistent documentation will demonstrate clinical changes over time.	Neonate's extremities remain pink and warm, with strong palpable pulses present. Neonate moves extremities independently and with tactile stimulation.

Nursing Diagnosis

Risk for alteration in metabolism, related to potential hyperbilirubinemia

Neonate will maintain bilirubin level within normal limits.	Assess for presence of yellow discoloration of skin, sclera, or mucous membrane. *Rationale:* Yellow discoloration can be a sign of jaundice and must be documented and further evaluated.	Any yellow discoloration is promptly identified.
	Monitor intake (volume and frequency of oral feedings) and output (volume and frequency of urine and stool). *Rationale:* Bilirubin is excreted in urine and stool; adequate intake and output will promote excretion of bilirubin.	Neonate breastfeeds well; has at least 6 wet diapers in 24 hours and 4 stools in 24 hours.
	Monitor serum bilirubin. *Rationale:* Serum bilirubin values are accurate indicators of the presence of abnormal levels of bilirubin requiring additional therapy.	Serum bilirubin level remains within normal limits.

Chapter Highlights

▶ A neonate is considered high risk when any physical or social factors affecting the prenatal course, labor and delivery, transition to extrauterine life, or newborn period threaten life or well-being.

▶ Maternal prenatal substance abuse can harm the developing fetus and newborn and presents special challenges for care of the newborn.

▶ The nature of the problems of a neonate of a substance-abusing mother depends on such factors as the drug or drugs used, the duration, and dosage.

▶ Maternal diabetes poses risks to the fetus and newborn ranging from metabolic disturbances to congenital defects and fetal death.

▶ Infections in the neonate result from preconceptional, prenatal, intrapartal, or postpartal exposure to harmful microorganisms.

▶ Good handwashing and use of universal precautions help decrease spread of infections from staff and other caretakers to infants.

▶ Jaundice may normally occur in newborns for physiologic reasons or be caused by such pathologic conditions as hemolytic diseases of the newborn.

▶ Interventions for high bilirubin levels depend on the cause of the disorder and include phototherapy and exchange transfusion (in severe circumstances).

▶ Several alterations in metabolic function can occur in newborns, such as hypocalcemia, hypercalcemia, hypomagnesemia, hypermagnesemia, hypoglycemia, and hyperglycemia.

▶ Inborn errors of metabolism is a term describing a large number of genetically determined diseases that cause alterations in metabolic functioning.

▶ Many physical conditions that place an infant at risk are accompanied by feeding problems; nutritional assessment and intervention need to consider such factors as gestational age and weight, respiratory status, gastrointestinal and metabolic functioning, temperature stability, coordination of sucking, and swallowing.

▶ Alterations in cardiac functioning in the neonate may be the result of acute disease processes, such as persistent pulmonary hypertension, or of congenital heart diseases, caused by defects in the heart and cardiac blood vessels.

▶ Neonatal seizures are among the most common abnormal neurologic findings in the neonatal period; care focuses on identification of the cause of seizures and their treatment.

After reading the vignette at the beginning of this chapter, use what you have learned to answer these questions.

1. What are the implications of caring for a baby who is blind from birth?

2. What difficulties might Megan and Ray Blair have in telling relatives and friends about Ryan?

3. What can a nurse say and do to help this family cope with this rare and severe congenital anomaly?

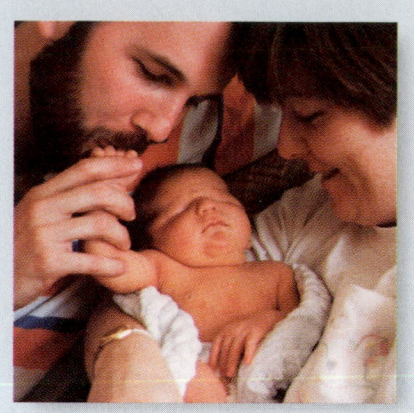

Critical Thinking Questions

► References

American Academy of Pediatrics, Committee on Genetics. (1992). New issues in newborn screening for phenylketonuria and congenital hypothyroidism. *Pediatrics, 69,* 104–106.

American Academy of Pediatrics, Committee on Substance Abuse and Committee on Children with Disabilities: Fetal alcohol syndrome and fetal alcohol effects. (1993). *Pediatrics, 91,* 1004–1066.

American Academy of Pediatrics, Committee on Infectious Diseases and Committee on Fetus and Newborn. (1997). Revised guidelines for prevention of group B streptococcal (GBS) infection. *Pediatrics, 99,* 489–496.

American College of Obstetricians and Gynecologists, Committee on Obstetric Practice. (1996). *Prevention of early onset group B streptococcal disease in newborns* (Committee Opinion No. 173). Washington, DC: Author.

Askin, D.F. (1995). Bacterial and fungal infections in the neonate. *Journal of Obstetric, Gynecologic, and Neonatal Nursing, 24*(7), 635–643.

Avery, G.B., Fletcher, M.A., & MacDonald, M.G. (1994). *Neonatology: Pathophysiology and management of the newborn* (4th ed.). Philadelphia: Lippincott-Raven.

Baley & Goldfarb. (1993). Neonatal infections. In M.H. Klaus & A.A. Fanaroff (Eds.), *Care of the high-risk neonate* (4th ed.) (pp. 323–344). Philadelphia: W.B. Saunders.

Beckholt, A.P. (1990). Breast milk for infants who cannot breastfeed. *Journal of Obstetric, Gynecologic, and Neonatal Nursing, 13,* 216–220.

Behrman, R.E., & Kliegman, R.M. (1996). *Nelson textbook of pediatrics* (15th ed.). Philadelphia: W.B. Saunders.

Blackburn, S.T., & Loper, D.L. (1992). *Maternal, fetal, and neonatal physiology: A clinical perspective.* Philadelphia: W.B. Saunders.

Brooks, C. (1997). Neonatal hypoglycemia. *Neonatal Network, 16*(2), 15–21.

Bucuvalas, J.C., & Balistreri, W.F. (1996). The liver and bile ducts. In A.M. Rudolph, J.I.E. Hoffman, & C.D. Rudolph (Eds.), *Rudolph's pediatrics* (20th ed.) (pp. 1134–1137). Stamford, CT: Appleton & Lange.

Burton, B. (1987). Inborn errors of metabolism: The clinical diagnosis in early infancy. *Pediatrics, 79,* 359–368.

Burton, B. (1994). Inherited metabolic disease. In G.B. Avery, M.A. Fletcher, & M.G. MacDonald (Eds.), *Neonatology: Pathophysiology and management of the newborn* (4th ed.) (pp. 726–743). Philadelphia: Lippincott-Raven.

Cavaliere, T.A. (1995). Pharmacologic treatment of neonatal sepsis: Antimicrobial agents and immunotherapy. *Journal of Obstetric, Gynecologic, and Neonatal Nursing, 24*(7), 647–658.

Cohen, F. (1987). Neural tube defects: Epidemiology, detection and prevention. *Journal of Obstetric, Gynecologic, and Neonatal Nursing, 16*(2), 105–115.

Connor, E.M., Sperling, R., Gelber, R., Kiselev, P., Scott, G., O'Sullivan, M.J., VanDyke, R., Bey, M., Shearer, W., Jacobson, R.L., et al. (1994). Reduction of maternal–infant transmission of human immunodeficiency virus type 1 with zidovudine treatment. Pediatric AIDS Clinical Trials Group Protocol 076 Study Group. *New England Journal of Medicine, 331*, 1173–1180.

Cordero, L., & Landon, M.B. (1993). Infant of the diabetic mother. *Clinics in Perinatology, 20*(3), 635–648.

Cunningham, F.G., MacDonald, P.C., Gant, N.F., Leveno, K.J., Gilstrap, L.C., Hankins, G.D.V., & Clark, S.L. (1997). *Williams obstetrics* (20th ed.). Stamford, CT: Appleton & Lange.

DeBoer, S.L., & Stephens, D. (1997). Persistent pulmonary hypertension of the newborn: Case study and pathophysiology review. *Neonatal Network, 16*(1), 7–13.

De Rossi, A., Ometto, L., Masiero, S., Zanchetta, M., Chieco-Bianchi, L. (1997). Viral phenotype in mother-to-child HIV-1 transmission and disease progression of vertically acquired HIV-1 infection. *Acta Paediatrica Supplement, 421*, 22–28.

Doshier, S. (1995). What happens to the offspring of diabetic pregnancies. *MCN, American Journal of Maternal-Child Nursing, 20*(1), 25–28.

Dunn, P.A., Bhutani, V., Weiner, S., Ludomirski, A. (1988). Care of the infant with erythroblastosis fetalis. *Journal of Obstetric, Gynecologic, and Neonatal Nursing, 17*, 382–386.

Ferraro-McDuffie, A., Huddleston, K., Smith, M., Karotkin, E., & Gardner, K. (1994). How well do enteral feeding pumps perform? *MCN, American Journal of Maternal-Child Nursing, 19*, 144–147.

Forsberg, S.A. (1997). Infant metabolic screening: a total quality management approach. *Journal of Obstetric, Gynecologic, and Neonatal Nursing, 26*(3), 257–261.

Friedland, I.R., & McCracken, G.H. (1996). Neonatal sepsis and meningitis. In A.M. Rudolph, J.I.E. Hoffman, & C.D. Rudolph (Eds.), *Rudolph's pediatrics* (20th ed.) (pp. 536–544). Stamford, CT: Appleton & Lange.

Gardner, J. (1997). Fetal alcohol syndrome: Recognition and intervention. *MCN, American Journal of Maternal-Child Nursing, 22*(6), 318–322.

Glantz, J.C., & Kedley, K.E. (1998). Concepts and controversies in the management of group B streptococcus during pregnancy. *Birth, 25*(1), 45–53.

Hansen, T.N. (1996). Persistent pulmonary hypertension of the newborn. In A.M. Rudolph, J.I.E. Hoffman, & C.D. Rudolph (Eds.), *Rudolph's pediatrics* (20th ed.) (pp. 1608–1611). Stamford, CT: Appleton & Lange.

Hoffman, J.I.E. (1996). Congenital heart diseases. In A.M. Rudolph, J.I.E. Hoffman, & C.D. Rudolph (Eds.), *Rudolph's pediatrics* (20th ed.) (pp. 1457–1458). Stamford, CT: Appleton & Lange.

Jacobs, R.F., & Darville, T. (1996). Bacteremia, sepsis and shock. In A.M. Rudolph, J.I.E. Hoffman, & C.D. Rudolph (Eds.), *Rudolph's pediatrics* (20th ed.) (pp. 530–536). Stamford, CT: Appleton & Lange.

Klaus, M., & Fanaroff, A. (1993). *Care of the high-risk neonate* (4th ed.). Philadelphia: W.B. Saunders.

Kliegman, R.M. (1993). Problems in metabolic adaptation: Glucose, calcium and magnesium. In M.H. Klaus & A.A. Fanaroff (Eds.), *Care of the high-risk neonate* (4th ed.) (pp. 282–301). Philadelphia: W.B. Saunders.

Koo, W.W.K., & Tsang, R.C. (1994). Calcium and magnesium homeostasis. In G.B. Avery, M.A. Fletcher, & M.G. MacDonald (Eds.), *Neonatology: Pathophysiology and management of the newborn* (4th ed.) (pp. 585–604). Philadelphia: Lippincott-Raven.

Ludwig, M.A., Marecki, M., Wooldridge, P.J., & Sherman, L.M.

(1996). Neonatal nurses' knowledge of and attitudes toward caring for cocaine-exposed infants and their mothers. *Journal of Perinatal and Neonatal Nursing, 9*(4), 81–95.

Maisels, J. (1994). Jaundice. In G.B. Avery, M.A. Fletcher, & M.G. MacDonald (Eds.), *Neonatology: Pathophysiology and management of the newborn* (4th ed.) (pp. 630–725). Philadelphia: Lippincott-Raven.

Mamunes, P. (1980). Neonatal screening tests. *Pediatric Clinics of North America, 27*, 733–749.

Mitchell, A., Steffenson, N., Hogan, H., & Brooks, S. (1997). Neonatal group B streptococcal disease. *MCN, American Journal of Maternal-Child Nursing, 22*, 249–253.

Mofensen, L.M. (1997a). Interaction between timing of perinatal human immunodeficiency virus infection and the design of preventive and therapeutic interventions. *Acta Paediatrica Supplement, 421*, 1–9.

Mofensen, L.M. (1997b). Reducing the risk of perinatal HIC-1 transmission with zidovudine: Results and implications of AIDS Clinical Trials Group Protocol 076. *Acta Paediatrica Supplement, 421*, 89–96.

Nordli, D.R., Pedley, T.A., & De Vivo, D.C. (1996). Seizure disorders in infants and children. In A.M. Rudolph, J.I.E. Hoffman, & C.D. Rudolph (Eds.), *Rudolph's pediatrics* (20th ed.) (pp. 1941–1967). Stamford, CT: Appleton & Lange.

Nyhan, W.L. (1996). Disorders of amino acid metabolism. In A.M. Rudolph, J.I.E. Hoffman, & C.D. Rudolph (Eds.), *Rudolph's pediatrics* (20th ed.) (pp. 306–322). Stamford, CT: Appleton & Lange.

Ogata, E.S. (1996). The infant of the diabetic mother. In A.M. Rudolph, J.I.E. Hoffman, & C.D. Rudolph (Eds.), *Rudolph's pediatrics* (20th ed.) (pp. 248–252). Stamford, CT: Appleton & Lange.

Phibbs, R.H. (1996a). Neonatal polycythemia. In A.M. Rudolph, J.I.E. Hoffman, & C.D. Rudolph (Eds.), *Rudolph's pediatrics* (20th ed.) (pp. 252–255). Stamford, CT: Appleton & Lange.

Phibbs, R.H. (1996b). Hemolytic anemias. In A.M. Rudolph, J.I.E. Hoffman, & C.D. Rudolph (Eds.), *Rudolph's pediatrics* (20th ed.) (pp. 1193–1203). Stamford, CT: Appleton & Lange.

Poland, R.L., & Ostrea, E.M. (1993). Neonatal hyperbilirubinemia. In M. Klaus & A. Fanaroff (Eds.), *Care of the high-risk neonate* (4th ed.) (pp. 302–322). Philadelphia: W.B. Saunders.

Polinski, C. (1996). The value of the white blood cell count and differential in the prediction of neonatal sepsis. *Neonatal Network, 15*(7), 13–23.

Rezvani, I. (1996). Defects in metabolism of amino acids. In R.E. Behrman & R.M. Kliegman (Eds.), *Nelson textbook of pediatrics* (15th ed.) (pp. 329–333). Philadelphia: W.B. Saunders.

Rezvani, I., & Rosenblatt, D.S. (1996). An approach to inborn errors of metabolism. In R.E. Behrman & R.M. Kliegman (Eds.), *Nelson textbook of pediatrics* (15th ed.) (pp. 328–329). Philadelphia: W.B. Saunders.

Rogers, M.F. (1997). Epidemiology of HIV/AIDS in women and children in the USA. *Acta Paediatrica Supplement, 421*, 15–16.

Ruchala, P.L., Seibold, L., & Stremsterfer, K. (1996). Validating assessment of neonatal jaundice with transcutaneous bilirubin measurement. *Neonatal Network, 15*(4), 33–37.

Samson, L.F. (1992). Infants of diabetic mothers: Current perspectives. *Journal of Perinatal and Neonatal Nursing, 6*, 61–70.

Sherwen, L.N. (1995). Human immunodeficiency virus infection during the perinatal period: A review of literature concerning pregnant women and neonates. *Journal of Perinatology, 15*(1), 54–66.

Suevo, D.M. (1997). The infant of the diabetic mother. *Neonatal Network, 16*(5), 25–33.

Tangredi, M. (1998). Clinical snapshot: Septic shock. *American Journal of Nursing, 98*(3), 46–47.

U.S. Centers for Disease Control and Prevention. (1996). Prevention of perinatal group B streptococcal disease: A public health perspective. *Morbidity and Mortality Weekly Report, 45*(RR-7), 1–24.

U.S. Centers for Disease Control and Prevention. (1998). 1998 guidelines for treatment of sexually transmitted diseases. *Morbidity and Mortality Weekly Report, 47*(RR-1), 1–111.

Weingarten, C.T. (1988). Caring for parents of a newborn transferred to a regional intensive care nursery: A challenge for low-risk obstetric specialists. *Journal of Perinatology, 8,* 271–275.

Wilkerson, N. (1989). Treating hyperbilirubinemia. *MCN, American Journal of Maternal-Child Nursing, 14,* 32–36.

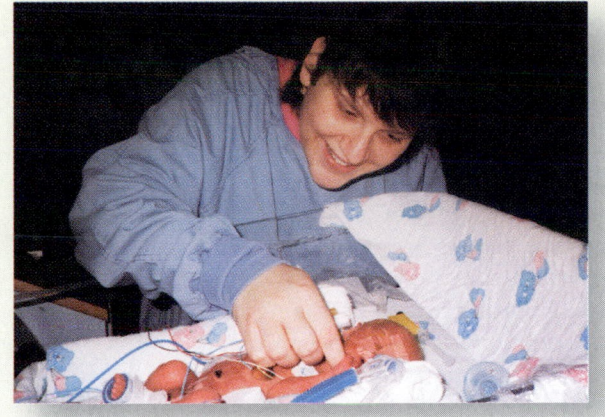

Luke Farrell was born prematurely at 31 weeks' gestation and weighed 2400 g. On Luke's fourth day in the NICU, he seems fatigued and Eileen Taylor, RN, notes the following signs: abdominal distension and blood in the stool. Diagnostic tests reveal that Luke is experiencing necrotizing enterocolitis.

Although Luke's parents, Gail and Rob Farrell, are very anxious about the effects of this disorder on Luke's health, they are determined to be involved in his care. The nurse encourages them to speak to Luke and touch him. As Gail bends over Luke, she gently strokes his chest with her finger and whispers softly to him. She smiles and states, "I always feel better when I'm close to Luke. It's almost as if, despite all the tubes and monitors he's connected to, he knows I'm here with him." ∎

33

Risk Related to Gestational Age and Birth Weight

Historically, birth weight was considered to be the most important indicator of a neonate's well-being; however, with advances in neonatology has come the realization that birth weight alone is not an accurate indicator of risk factors facing the newborn. The assessment of both gestational age and birth weight provides a more complete perspective on neonatal functioning. By focusing on gestational age and birth weight, health care providers can prevent the intrauterine growth retarded, full-term infant from being identified inaccurately as premature or the macrosomic or large premature neonate from being identified as full term. By appropriately assessing gestational age and size, health care providers can make important decisions about neonatal maturation and functioning and identify special risk factors that may affect the neonate.

▶ ASSESSMENT OF GESTATIONAL AGE AND SIZE

A newborn's weight, intrauterine growth, and gestational age are important indicators of maturity. These data can assist nurses and physicians in predicting potential gestational age and size problems that the newborn may face in the neonatal period. No one method of estimating gestational age or development is sufficient. Prenatal, delivery, and postnatal data and assessments together provide the most reliable prediction of gestational development and intrauterine growth.

▶ Gestational Age

Neonatal assessments for gestational age are based on examination of the neonate for certain physical and neuromuscular signs. A commonly used gestational age assessment tool was devised by Dubowitz and colleagues (1970). This tool uses 21 criteria to assess gestational age, regardless of birth weight. The Dubowitz Gestational Age Tool is most valid when used for neonates between 28 and 43 weeks' gestation. Ballard's (1991) adaptation of the Dubowitz tool and the Brazelton Neonatal Behavioral Assessment Scale (1984) are two other tools available to assess gestational age after birth (see Chapter 30).

▶ Intrauterine Growth

Once the neonate's birth weight is obtained and the gestational age assessed, intrauterine growth is determined. The birth weight, length, head circumference, and gestational age are plotted on standard intrauterine growth charts. Based on where the neonate falls on the chart, he or she is classified as small-for-gestational-age (SGA), appropriate-for-gestational-age (AGA), or large-for-gestational-age (LGA).

▶ Small-for-Gestational-Age Neonate

Neonates identified as **small-for-gestational-age** have experienced intrauterine growth retardation. These neonates usually have a birth weight below the 10th percentile for their gestational age (Behrman & Shiono, 1997). The SGA neonate can be premature, term, or postterm.

Fetal growth retardation may occur early or late in gestation. Fetal cellular growth occurs in two phases. In the first phase, virtually all growth is due to increases in the number of cells in the fetal body. Interference with growth of the fetus during this phase results in the fetus' production of fewer than the normal number of cells. This type of growth impairment is called symmetric growth retardation, because all parts of the body are equally small as a result of in utero malnutrition which has persisted long enough to slow all growth and because of the overall lower number of body cells. The fetus is not able to make more cells and can only continue to grow and develop with that number of cells (Nagey & Viscardi, 1993).

Asymmetric intrauterine growth retardation is another type of fetal growth retardation. The fetus may have an appropriate-size head and an appropriate length, but the overall body weight and organ size are diminished (Fig. 33–1). The fetus physiologically appears to respond to in utero malnutrition by using stored hepatic glycogen for energy needs unmet by the mother. Shrinkage of the fetal liver and abdomen results. Thus, initially, most fetal body parts seem to grow normally, while the abdomen actually shrinks. By shunting blood to the heart and brain, the malnourished fetus increases the chance to survive at the expense of normal growth of less essential body parts (Nagey & Viscardi, 1993).

Several factors contribute to impaired growth in the fetus:

* Uteroplacental dysfunction (related to maternal hypertension or pregnancy-induced hypertension, severe maternal diabetes, multiple gestations, maternal renal disease, placental infarcts or abruptions, altitude, etc.)—asymmetric type
* Genetic causes (congenital and chromosomal abnormalities)—symmetric type

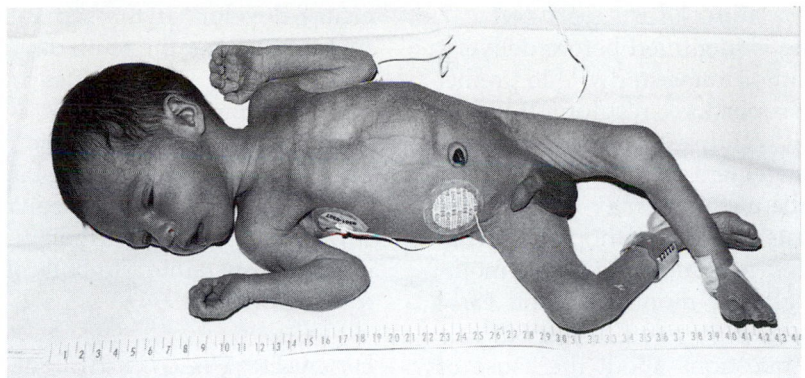

FIGURE 33–1. Neonate at 37 weeks of gestation with asymmetric intrauterine growth retardation. *(Reproduced, with permission, from Rudolph, A.M., Hoffman, J.I.E., & Rudolph, C.D. (Eds.). (1996).* Rudolph's pediatrics *(20th ed.). Stamford, CT: Appleton & Lange, p. 246.)*

- Infections (syphilis, rubella, toxoplasmosis, etc.)—symmetric type
- Inborn errors of metabolism—symmetric type
- Environmental factors (smoking and drugs such as heroin, alcohol [symmetric]); drugs and alcohol are also related to combined types of in utero growth retardation
- Placental unit insufficiency (placental infarcts or abruptions, multiple gestations)—combined types

The SGA neonate appears thin and wasted at birth. The skin is often loose, dry, and scaling. SGA neonates lack subcutaneous fat stores and often appear to have muscle wasting. The umbilical cord may be thin from a lack of Wharton's jelly. These neonates are usually alert and active and seem hungry, although they may go 24 hours or longer without voiding if fluids are not provided early and in sufficient quantity.

The SGA neonate is at risk for several clinical alterations, including respiratory distress; asphyxia; hypoglycemia; infections, especially those related to intrauterine infections; polycythemia; and hypothermia.

Nursing and Collaborative Management

Management of the SGA neonate ideally begins with the identification of prenatal risks for intrauterine growth retardation. If possible, steps can be taken to limit or to prevent growth retardation before birth. Specific treatments are directed toward alteration in functioning of the SGA neonate. For example, frequent glucose tests and a strict feeding schedule may be implemented for the neonate with hypoglycemia, antibiotics will be initiated for the neonate with an infection, and the hypothermic neonate will be placed in a thermally controlled isolette.

Overall management includes assessment of the SGA neonate's growth progress. Serial height and weight measurements are documented during the hospitalization. Parents should be aware of any special treatment needs the neonate may require at home. In addition, parents must be aware of the goal weight that the neonate must reach before discharge. Parents are anxious to learn of any weight gains and often ask for that information on a daily basis. Including parents in the care and feeding of the SGA neonate helps promote attachment, especially if the neonate's discharge is delayed. The nurse can observe the parent–neonate interaction and offer suggestions and support as parents master the care of their neonates.

▶ Large-for-Gestational-Age Neonate

Large-for-gestational-age neonates have birth weights that exceed the 90th percentile for their gestational age (Behrman & Shiono, 1997). The very large or macrosomic neonate is often born to a diabetic mother (see Chapter 32). Other conditions, such as Wiedemann-Beckwith syndrome (an autosomal dominant congenital syndrome) can cause the newborn to be macrosomic (Wiedemann, Kunze, & Grosse, 1997). Large parents can have large neonates who do not have any special problems. Also, some cultural groups, such as American Indian tribes, are more likely to have LGA neonates. The incidence of diabetes is also high among these groups. The LGA neonate may be premature, term, or postterm.

Nursing and Collaborative Management

Ideally the LGA neonate is identified before delivery. This allows the physician or nurse-midwife to predict potential fetopelvic disproportions, resulting from the neonate's large size, that could result in birth trauma.

After delivery, management includes treatment of any injuries related to the birth and may include consultations with specialists, such as orthopedic physicians. Large neonates and neonates of diabetic mothers may require serial glucose monitoring and early feedings or intravenous therapy (see Chapter 32).

Parents may have questions about the cause of the neonate's macrosomia and often ask about the neonate's future expected growth rate. Discharge instructions should include appropriate feeding guidelines to prevent concerned parents from potentially overfeeding or underfeeding the LGA neonate at home.

► Appropriate-for-Gestational-Age Neonate

The premature, term, or postmature neonate may also be **appropriate-for-gestational-age** in size and development. This indicates that the neonate has been able to grow and develop in utero at the appropriate rate; however, being appropriate-for-gestational-age does not eliminate problems associated with prematurity or postmaturity. The term neonate who is appropriate-for-gestational-age may also face risk factors that complicate the delivery and postnatal period, such as asphyxia and persistent pulmonary hypertension.

► Multiple Gestation

In multiple gestations, more than one fetus is present in the uterus. Two types of multiple gestation can occur. In a monovular pregnancy, one ovum separates into two or more embryos (monozygotic twins). In a binovular pregnancy, more than one ovum is fertilized (dizygotic twins).

Twins are the most common type of multiple gestation. The greater the number of fetuses, the greater the morbidity and mortality.

Monovular Pregnancy

In a monovular pregnancy, the embryos are monozygous or identical. Monozygous neonates are the same sex. They have the same general appearance, including eye and hair coloring. These neonates even have identical or very similar fingerprints.

If separation of the single embryo occurs early in the pregnancy, before the fifth day, two separate pla-

centas develop. If the separation occurs later in the pregnancy, after the tenth day, the embryos may share one placenta. The neonates may be conjoined if the embryo separates after the tenth day of pregnancy. When conjoining occurs, the neonates are connected by a common bridge of skin or even share entire organs or limbs. These neonates may be able to be surgically separated if the nature of their attachment is not life sustaining to both of them (Avery, Fletcher, & MacDonald, 1994).

Binovular Pregnancy

In a binovular pregnancy, separate placentas and embryos develop from each fertilized ovum. This produces dizygous, nonidentical, or fraternal neonates. Dizygous neonates can be the same sex but are often different sexes. These neonates exhibit similarities as would ordinary brothers and sisters that are the products of single pregnancies. Binovular pregnancies are more common with a positive familial history of multiple births, if the mother is over 35 years of age, has had infertility treatment, and has had other pregnancies.

Special Problems Related to Gestational Age and Size in Twins

Intrauterine growth is similar in twins and singletons until 30 weeks, when intrauterine growth diminishes in both monozygous and dizygous twins. At birth, twins are usually smaller than a singleton neonate of the same gestational age. The main deficit in the intrauterine growth of twins occurs in the last 8 to 10 weeks of gestation. Twins are usually not the same weight at birth. Birth weights may be close or differ substantially (Fig. 33–2). Multiple gestations account for 17% of intrauterine growth retardation, with monochorionic twins showing greater degrees of variation in birth weight than dichorionic twins (Avery, Fletcher, & MacDonald, 1994). Twins may also be large-for-gestational-age, although this is not as common as small for gestational age.

Fetal growth retardation, causing one or both twins to be small-for-gestational-age, results from special problems (discussed next) often experienced by a mother with a multiple gestation. Poor nutrition, anemia, and iron and folic acid deficiencies can contribute to fetal growth retardation. Fetal growth retardation in twins can also be related to a twin transfusion syndrome, in which one twin loses blood to the other twin through a common placental blood vessel (Avery, Fletcher, & MacDonald, 1994). Although the fetuses may have normal growth potential, altered placental functioning may not allow them to receive the necessary nutrients to sustain appropriate growth for their gestational age. Vascular abnor-

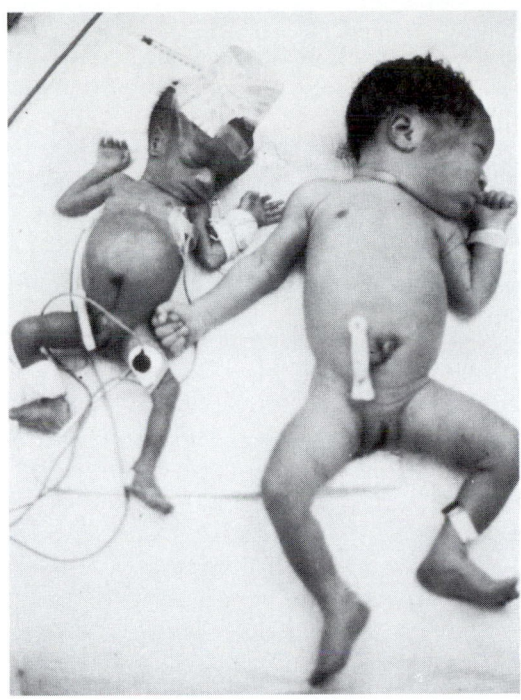

FIGURE 33–2. Marked birth weight disparity in dizygotic twins. The larger twin weighed 2300 g, appropriate for gestational age. The markedly growth-retarded smaller twin weighed only 785 g. *(Reproduced, with permission, from Cunningham, F.G. et al. (1997). Williams obstetrics (20th ed.). Stamford, CT: Appleton & Lange, p. 872.)*

malities of the placenta or premature separation of the placenta also can cause the fetuses to develop chronic fetal distress with the growth retardation.

Nursing and Collaborative Management. In most cases, confirmation of more than one fetus occurs before 33 weeks of gestation. However, multiple gestations are at times diagnosed late in pregnancy or at birth, especially if the woman has not received consistent prenatal care. During pregnancy, the uterus is found to be larger than expected for the length of time since the mother's last menstrual period. Multiple gestation is usually confirmed by ultrasound.

The mother expecting twins must be assessed closely for signs and symptoms of alterations that would place the twins at risk for preterm birth or intrauterine growth retardation. Serial ultrasound tests are done to monitor intrauterine growth and development.

Management of twins begins with the mother with a multiple gestation and must include careful prenatal assessment. The mother is at risk for special problems, among them hyperemesis; discomfort related to increased abdominal pressure, such as gas-

trointestinal discomfort and shortness of breath; anemia and iron and folic acid deficiencies; pregnancy-induced hypertension; antenatal and intrapartum hemorrhage; polyhydramnios; premature labor or premature rupture of membranes; and obstructed labor caused by fetal malpresentations (Revenis & Johnson, 1994).

Prematurity is the most frequent cause of mortality in multiple gestations, especially if the neonates are born before 33 weeks of gestation. Efforts to prevent a premature delivery are therefore essential. The mother requires additional rest, especially after 24 weeks of gestation. She may also require restricted activity between 26 and 36 weeks of gestation. Tests to assess fetal maturity are routinely done at 34 weeks. It can, however, be difficult to accurately interpret laboratory tests such as the lecithin to sphingomyelin ratio, which helps to identify fetal lung maturity, as there is more than one fetus to consider. Ultrasound becomes an important tool in predicting fetal size, gestational age, and readiness for delivery.

Parents require consistent support as they anticipate the birth of multiples. They must be aware of potential complications as the pregnancy continues and the importance of adhering to special instructions such as dietary and activity restrictions.

▶ THE PREMATURE NEONATE

The **premature neonate** is defined as a baby born before the end of 37 weeks' gestation, i.e., less than 259 days after the date of the mother's last menstrual period (Behrman & Shiono, 1997). Prematurity accounts for at least 75% of neonatal deaths that do not result from congenital malformations (Simpson, 1997); in the United States, the prematurity rate (about 10%) has remained remarkably constant. Prematurity and low birth weight often occur together. Indeed, any very premature infant will have a low birth weight (see discussion later in this chapter). Being SGA adds complications related to intrauterine growth retardation.

Premature neonates must be assessed for appropriate intrauterine growth. These neonates may be small for gestational age, appropriate for gestational age, or large for gestational age. A premature LGA neonate may look like a term neonate. Conversely, the term neonate that is SGA may appear to be premature. Accurate identification of the neonate's gestational age, weight, and intrauterine growth is essential because each situation poses very different problems for the neonate (see box entitled Factors Associated With Prematurity and Low Birth Weight).

> ► FACTORS ASSOCIATED WITH PREMATURITY AND LOW BIRTH WEIGHT

DEMOGRAPHIC FACTORS

- Age (younger than 18; older than 35)
- Low socioeconomic status
- Unmarried
- African American

RISK FACTORS EXISTING BEFORE PREGNANCY

- High parity (more than 4)
- Low weight for height
- Chronic hypertension
- Lack of immunity to such diseases as rubella
- Poor obstetric history (previous low-birth-weight infant)
- Maternal genetic factors
- Other chronic health conditions

RISK FACTORS DURING PREGNANCY

- Multiple fetuses
- Short pregnancy interval
- Pregnancy-induced hypertension
- Infections

- Bleeding
- Placental problems
- Fetal anomalies
- Incompetent cervix
- Premature rupture of membranes
- Uterine irritability
- Other maternal illnesses
- Trauma

LIFESTYLE FACTORS

- Smoking
- Alcohol and other drug use

OTHER IMPORTANT FACTORS

- Inadequate or no prenatal care
- Stress
- Iatrogenic prematurity

Source: Behrman & Shiono, 1997.

The general appearance of the premature neonate will vary dramatically with the gestational age and with how sick the neonate becomes after the delivery. Table 33–1 presents an overview of some common characteristics of the premature neonate.

The premature neonate is likely to develop certain problems related to immaturity of various organ systems. Some common problems are respiratory distress syndrome, periodic breathing and apnea, retinopathy of prematurity, anemia, intracranial hemorrhages, temperature instability, feeding problems, necrotizing enterocolitis, and hyperbilirubinemia (Behrman & Shiono, 1997). Many of these complications are not exclusive to prematurity and can be noted in the term and postterm neonate as well. The following discussion highlights some of the major alterations related to prematurity.

► Alterations in Respiratory Functioning

Respiratory Distress Syndrome (RDS)

Respiratory distress syndrome (RDS) or **hyaline membrane disease** (HMD) is a pulmonary disorder that occurs in neonates born with immature lung development. RDS remains a major clinical problem in preterm infants; however, some term neonates may also develop RDS. Precipitating factors for RDS

> ► **TABLE 33-1**
> Common Characteristics of the Premature Neonate

Position	At 28 weeks of gestation, the neonate is floppy and hypotonic; at 32 weeks, the neonate flexes the lower extremities; and at 36 weeks, the neonate flexes all four extremities.
Skin	The premature neonate's skin is almost transparent and is ruddy in color. The neonate is covered with fine downy hair called lanugo. Vernix caseosa, the cheesy covering on the skin of the neonate, is minimal at 28 weeks of gestation and increases with gestational age.
Head	The premature neonate has wide, soft fontanelles with overriding sutures. The head appears large for the size of the body.
Ears	The 28- to 35-week gestation neonate has thin, pliable, inelastic ears, as cartilage does not begin to develop until after 35 weeks of gestation.
Chest	The overall chest appears small and malleable. The breast tissue is usually not palpable before 35 weeks of gestation. The neonate's cry is weak and poorly sustained.
Abdomen	The premature neonate's abdomen often appears distended because of poor muscle tone and the transparent skin.
Genitalia	The premature male neonate has a poorly developed scrotum with few skin folds and undescended testicles. The labia minora and the clitoris appear large in the premature female neonate as the labia majora are not fully developed.

Reproduced, with permission, from Avery, G.B., Fletcher, M.A., & MacDonald, M.G. (1994). Neonatology: Pathophysiology and management of the newborn (4th ed.). Philadelphia: Lippincott-Raven.

include prematurity, especially less than 35 weeks' gestation; asphyxia at birth; maternal diabetes, especially if less than 38 weeks' gestation; cesarean section without labor; acute antepartum hemorrhage; second-born twin; and male sex (Beachy & Deacon, 1993).

RDS occurs when the neonate's lungs lack the pulmonary surfactant required for respiration. Without pulmonary surfactant, the alveoli collapse and each successive breath becomes more difficult for the neonate. The collapsed (or atelectatic) alveoli cannot allow for the exchange of oxygen and carbon dioxide, and hypoxia (defined as an arterial oxygen tension of 50 mm Hg or less) may quickly occur. Hypoxia leads to vasoconstriction of the pulmonary vessels, making it more difficult for blood to flow to the lungs. Blood is then redirected through other routes such as the foramen ovale and the ductus arteriosus. (See Chapter 30 for a discussion of conversion of fetal to neonatal circulation.) The extra work demanded for the increasing respiratory distress can quickly deplete the neonate's available energy.

Nursing and Collaborative Assessment.

Assessment begins prior to delivery with identification of fetuses likely to develop RDS. Delay of delivery until fetal lungs are mature is the ideal solution. If that is not possible, arrangements should be made to deliver the neonate in a hospital with specialized facilities and staff to care for the potentially ill newborn.

The neonate who develops RDS has increasing respiratory difficulty in the first 3 to 6 hours of life. Tachypnea (a respiratory rate above 60 breaths per minute); retractions (Fig. 33–3): grunting; nasal flaring; and cyanosis (a blue discoloration noted in the nailbeds, lips, mouth, extremities, face, and trunk) are noted. Apneic episodes may occur. The infant's oxygen requirements increase and lung compliance decreases. Diagnostic x-ray findings are seen. Signs and symptoms can be modified in many low-birth-weight infants as a result of early assisted ventilation and surfactant therapy (Martin & Fanaroff, 1997).

The neonate with RDS will also have altered gas exchange, demonstrated by abnormal arterial blood gas values. Specifically, there will be hypoxemia, an abnormally low oxygen level and hypercarbia, a high carbon dioxide level, if gas exchange is severely impaired. Acidosis may develop. Oxygen levels may also be assessed in a noninvasive manner. A transcutaneous monitor or pulse oximeter are two devices that are applied to the neonate's skin. They detect oxygen levels in the peripheral blood supply. The chest x-ray of an infant with RDS often shows a diffuse reticulogranular (ground glass) pattern in both lung fields.

Neonates who are identified to be at high risk for developing RDS or who have symptoms of RDS must be closely monitored in the first hours and days of life. Careful and ongoing assessment is necessary to help prevent life-threatening complications such as

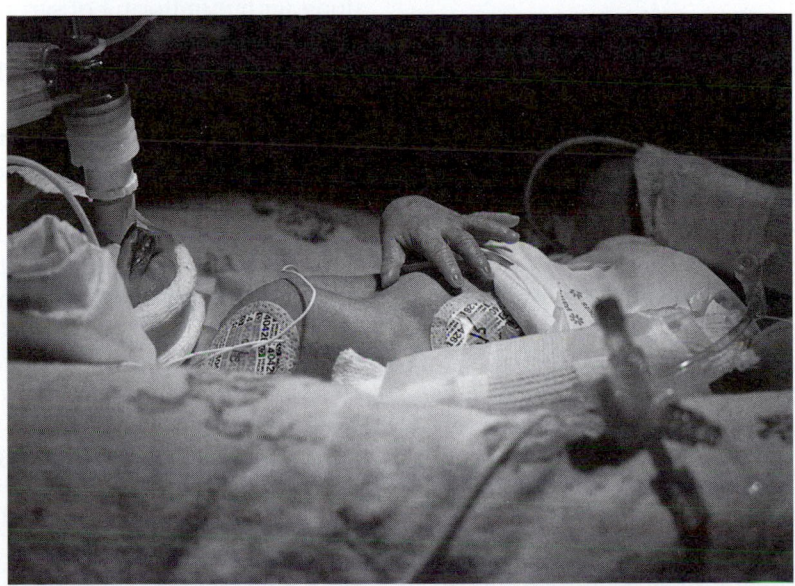

FIGURE 33–3. Neonate in respiratory distress. Note retractions in the chest of the newborn.

apnea, the absence of respirations, which can result from severe respiratory distress.

Nursing Diagnoses.

On the basis of the comprehensive assessment, nursing diagnoses for the preterm neonate with respiratory distress syndrome are developed. Examples of diagnoses include:

Problem-oriented diagnoses:

- Ineffective breathing pattern, related to deficient surfactant
- Ineffective airway clearance, related to excess secretions
- Impaired gas exchange, related to immaturity of newborn's lungs and decreased surfactant

Wellness-oriented diagnoses:

- Potential asset in resolution of RDS, related to neonatal weight greater than 1500 g

Nursing and Collaborative Management.

Management of the neonate with RDS focuses on resolution of the severe respiratory distress and the resulting hypoxia, retention of carbon dioxide, and acidosis. Supplemental warmed, humidified oxygen is administered to maintain PaO_2 levels between 50 and 80 mm Hg, and $PaCO_2$ levels at 40–50 mm Hg (Martin & Fanaroff, 1997). Oxygen may be administered via oxyhood or by continuous positive airway pressure (CPAP) via nasal prongs or an endotracheal tube. CPAP provides a certain amount of consistent positive pressure in the lungs to prevent collapse (atelectasis) of alveoli or bronchioles, the smaller extensions of the main pulmonary airways. If the neonate requires additional support, intubation and assisted ventilation can be instituted. Assisted ventilation to aid the infant's breathing uses mechanical support, or a ventilator.

If the neonate requires intubation, the nurse assesses:

- Respiratory status including color, breath sounds, number and quality of spontaneous respirations, presence of signs of respiratory distress, oxygen saturation, and/or transcutaneous monitoring, and results of arterial blood gas tests.
- Placement of an endotracheal tube. (This includes being careful when suctioning or positioning the neonate to prevent the tube from accidentally dislodging. An accidental or unplanned extubation can lead to an emergency in trying to provide the neonate with adequate ventilation in the absence of a tube in the trachea. The physician must be notified immediately if an accidental extubation occurs.)
- Patency of the endotracheal tube. (This includes as-needed suctioning and noting the amount, color, and consistency of secretions.)
- Ventilator settings, to ensure that they are appropriately maintained.

The nurse must notify the physician immediately of any changes in the neonate's status, and be prepared to provide such information as the infant's vital signs and results of pertinent laboratory tests.

An intubated infant who seems to be "fighting the respirator" may actually be indicating that something is wrong (Wung, 1993). For example, the endotracheal tube may need repositioning or it may be blocked by secretions that need to be suctioned, a pneumothorax may have occurred, respirator settings may be incorrect, the respirator may be malfunctioning, or the infant may need comforting. Sedation may be used for infants who are agitated for no definable reason. Prior to pharmacologic intervention, however, the causes of infant agitation should be identified and appropriate actions taken.

Neonates with respiratory distress who require intubation will have difficulty clearing secretions from their lungs. Chest vibration may be performed gently if needed to prevent atelectasis and build-up of secretions. In chest vibration, a vibrator is used over the lung fields to loosen secretions from the smaller airways.

As RDS worsens, the pulmonary blood vessels constrict in response to acidosis, allowing fetal circulatory structures, such as the ductus arteriosus, to remain open. Careful fluid management is needed, along with monitoring of serum electrolytes and body weight. Diuretics, such as furosemide (Lasix), may be given if signs of congestive heart failure are seen. Additional management may include specific treatment of a patent ductus arteriosus, using indomethacin or surgical repair. (See discussion of patent ductus arteriosus later in this chapter.)

Surfactant deficiency is the primary cause of RDS; consequently, surfactant replacement therapy has become an acceptable form of therapy. The development and use of exogenous surfactant in neonates with immature lungs is believed to decrease complications of RDS, minimize the severity of the syndrome, and decrease mortality related to the condition (Martin & Fanaroff, 1997). Exogenous surfactant therapy has been studied with various therapeutic protocols and drug preparations. Currently, it is recommended for prophylactic or preventive treatment and for rescue treatment for established RDS (Martin & Fanaroff, 1997). Three types of exogenous surfactant preparations may be used: natural surfactant, artificial surfactant, and synthetic surfactant (Boeckling, 1992). They are given to the neonate via an endotracheal tube, which allows the exogenous surfactant to be dispersed throughout the lung. The goal of surfactant replacement therapy is for infants to need less ventilatory support and oxygen, and thus be weaned sooner from assisted ventilation.

Liquid ventilation is a new and highly specialized therapy that has been used in treatment of infants who do not respond to conventional therapy for RDS or respiratory failure. With this type of therapy, special inert perfluoro-chemical liquids that have high solubility for respiratory gases are introduced into the lungs. The infused liquid spreads throughout the lungs and eliminates surface tension–related forces, thereby allowing oxygen and carbon dioxide to be exchanged more freely. Several modified approaches have also been used. For example, liquid ventilation has been combined with gas ventilation.

Management of the neonate with RDS must also include careful consideration of nutritional needs. The neonate experiencing severe respiratory distress is not able to take oral feedings. Intravenous fluids are indicated. If the neonate requires prolonged intravenous therapy, total parenteral nutrition may be started (see Chapter 32). As the neonate recovers, enteral feedings may be started. These neonates often begin with nasogastric or orogastric feedings before nipple feedings are attempted. Calories and fluid requirements are specially calculated, based on the weight and energy and nutritional needs of the neonate.

Neonates with severe respiratory distress can become debilitated quickly. Universal precautions and ongoing assessments for signs of potential infections are essential. The nurse should monitor the neonate's temperature as well as laboratory results. The intubated neonate is at special risk for lung infections. Meticulous care should be taken during suctioning procedures. Neonates who develop infections are treated with antibiotics.

Neonates with respiratory distress expend large amounts of energy because of the increased work of breathing. This additional energy expenditure can place them at risk for an unstable temperature. Hypothermia not only requires greater energy production to raise the neonate's temperature, but can increase oxygen demands significantly and contribute to acidosis. Through the use of radiant warmers and isolettes, it is possible to maintain a neutral thermal environment. This decreases the potential stress on the neonate's energy stores and promotes improved oxygen use.

Complications of RDS may occur spontaneously or result from therapeutic interventions. Major complications are associated with mechanical ventilation, oxygen administration, endotracheal tubes, and arterial catheter placement (Fanaroff & Merkatz, 1993). They include pulmonary air leaks, particularly pneumothorax and pulmonary interstitial emphysema; bronchopulmonary dysplasia; retinopathy of prematurity; hypotension; patent ductus arteriosus; infection; and intraventricular hemorrhage. Careful medical management and astute nursing assessment and intervention are essential to prevent complications.

RDS may peak in severity by day 2 to 3. Without further complications, improvement from RDS is generally seen by 72 hours after birth. Surfactant therapy may shorten this period (Martin & Fanaroff, 1997). Respiratory rate and retractions decrease and oxygenation and ventilation improve, thus allowing weaning from respiratory support. In very-low-birth-weight infants, recovery may be prolonged, and continued oxygen and respiratory support may be needed.

Bronchopulmonary Dysplasia (BPD)

Bronchopulmonary dysplasia (BPD) is a chronic obstructive pulmonary disorder of premature infants who have required mechanical ventilation and/or high levels of oxygen in the first weeks of life. The most significant risk factor for development of BPD is the degree of prematurity and low birth weight. An estimated 5000 to 10,000 new cases occur each year (Bland & Tooley, 1996). BPD is thought to develop as follows:

1. Neonatal lungs are exposed to damaging stimuli (barotrauma, oxygen toxicity).
2. Direct damage occurs to lung tissue.
3. Lungs become inflamed and edematous.
4. An influx of mononuclear cells and proliferation of fibroblasts occurs with subsequent pulmonary fibrosis.
5. Airway changes develop with abnormal growth and inflammation followed by smooth-muscle hypertrophy (Razycki & Kirkpatrick, 1993).

Three definitions are used to confirm the diagnosis of BPD.

1. A clinical scoring system of radiographic sequence, with stage I the least severe and stage IV indicating chronic disease.
2. Oxygen dependence for more than 28 days with persistent x-ray changes.
3. Oxygen dependence beyond 36 weeks corrected postnatal gestational age (Fanaroff & Merkatz, 1993).

Nursing and Collaborative Assessment. The infant with BPD demonstrates persistent signs of respiratory distress, including an increase in ventilatory requirements or inability to wean from the ventilator, hypoxia, hypercapnia, acidosis, rales, rhonchi, wheezing, retractions, bronchospasm, and fluid intolerance (Beachy & Deacon, 1993). The infant may also have intermittent episodes called "BPD spells." During BPD spells the infant becomes irritable, agitated, and dusky and demonstrates signs of acute respiratory distress, including retractions, nasal flaring, tachypnea, and cyanosis. Bronchopulmonary dysplasia spells may resolve spontaneously or may require specific interventions. Interventions may include the use of increased supplemental oxygen, chest vibration and suctioning, and administration of aerosolized bronchodilators, medications that help resolve constriction and spasm of the small airways in the neonate's lungs.

Nursing and Collaborative Management. Management of the infant with BPD includes supportive care similar to that required by the neonate with RDS. The following are management priorities:

1. Provision of supplemental oxygen and ventilatory support.
2. Provision of diuretics to control fluid retention and subsequent pulmonary edema.
3. Administration of bronchodilators, medications such as theophylline, to relieve and prevent bronchospasms. (Bronchodilators may also be administered via aerosolized breathing treatments.)
4. Restriction of fluid to help reduce pulmonary edema.
5. Provision of optimal nutrition to promote growth and healing of the lungs and to compensate for increased work of breathing.
6. Provision of chest physiotherapy and suctioning.
7. Provision of a neutral thermal environment.
8. Provision of developmental care. (See this section later in this chapter.) Clustering of care to ensure periods of rest and sleep. (Infants with BPD often require such frequent contact that they may be unable to obtain adequate rest. The development of a daily schedule in coordination with the care plan is an ideal way to allow for needed periods of rest. Controlling noise, light, and other environmental stimuli also promotes rest.)
9. Provision of auditory, visual, and tactile stimulation according to the infant's tolerance and developmental care plan. (Black-and-white pictures of geometric shapes, pictures of parents, mobiles, and a mirror are ways to provide stimulation for the neonate without demanding great energy expenditure. Tape recorders are also stimulating. Parents should be involved early in their infant's care and taught to provide appropriate sensory interventions that enhance development.)
10. Prevention of infections, especially respiratory infections that could further aggravate bronchospasms.
11. Use of steroids to assist with lung compliance and ability to wean from ventilatory support.

Most infants with BPD show gradual improvement during their hospitalization and eventually recover from their chronic lung disease to be well enough to go home. Their needs upon discharge often include supplemental oxygen, a cardiorespiratory monitor, chest physiotherapy, medications, and extensive follow-up services. Discharge planning, coordination of home care, and follow-up services are essential, as these infants require constant treatment and monitoring after discharge.

Parents of an infant with BPD face a great challenge in caring for a chronically ill child at home. Prior to discharge they must demonstrate the ability to provide such care as feeding, oxygen support, suctioning, giving medications, and monitoring. Hospitalizations, financial burdens, complex daily medications, and treatment schedules at home can stress the family. Parents must be able to assess changes in the infant's status and notify health care providers appropriately. They need to rely on consistent nursing support as their infant's complex requirements change.

Growth delays, recurrent pulmonary infections, and pulmonary sequelae are commonly seen in infants with BPD (Rozycki & Kirkpatrick, 1993). Growth delays may be due to poor nutrition, related to increased caloric needs. The infant's caloric needs are higher due to the increased work of breathing and chronic hypoxia. Supplemental oxygen should be provided to maintain oxygen saturation greater than or equal to 88 to 90%. Recurrent pulmonary infections also affect growth. Infants with BPD have an increased incidence of upper and lower respiratory infections requiring prompt treatment. Recent reports indicate that children with BPD have abnormal lungs and abnormal pulmonary function (airway obstruction, airway hyperactivity and hyperinflation.) These children are at an increased risk for readmission to the hospital during early childhood because of infection or reactive airway disease.

Periodic Breathing and Apnea

Premature neonates are at special risk for developing irregular breathing patterns, called **periodic breathing.** In periodic breathing, the neonate has periods of 5 to 10 seconds in which he or she does not take a breath, followed by periods of 10 to 15 seconds in which breathing proceeds at a rate of 50 to 60 breaths per minute. This recurring, irregular pattern is so common that it is considered normal in preterm infants (Miller, Fanaroff, & Martin, 1997a). During periodic breathing, there is no change in the neonate's color, heart rate, or temperature. Periodic breathing is more common in preterm neonates less than 36 weeks' gestation.

Apneic episodes are periods in which respiration stops for at least 10–15 seconds. They can be complicated by cyanosis, pallor, hypotonia, or bradycardia. Tiny infants are at greater risk for these responses than more mature infants, even when the apnea does not last as long. The apneic infant may also have frequent swallowing-like movements in the pharynx during the apnea (Miller, Fanaroff, & Martin, 1997a). Prolonged or repeated apnea can lead to neurologic injury if untreated.

Apnea of prematurity is usually related to the immaturity of the respiratory regulatory system in the central nervous system (Avery, Fletcher, & MacDonald, 1994). Other potential causes of apnea include the following.

- *Neurologic disorders.* Seizures, asphyxia, intraventricular hemorrhage
- *Metabolic abnormalities.* Hypoglycemia, hyperglycemia, hypocalcemia, hyponatremia, hyperbilirubinemia, and acidosis
- *Respiratory disorders.* Pulmonary obstruction, RDS, aspiration, pneumonia, acidosis
- *Infection.* Septicemia, pneumonia, meningitis
- *Temperature instability.* Hypothermia, hyperthermia
- *Impaired oxygenation.* Patent ductus arteriosus, hypotension, congestive heart failure, pulmonary edema, anemia
- *Malnutrition.* Abdominal distension, necrotizing enterocolitis, abdominal obstruction, gastroesophageal reflux
- *Drugs.* Maternal (narcotics, analgesics), neonatal (anticonvulsants, narcotics/analgesics)

Nursing and Collaborative Assessment. The diagnosis of apnea of prematurity is made by the exclusion of other causes of apnea and bradycardia. The infant is evaluated for a possible underlying cause. After metabolic, hematologic, neurologic, and infectious causes of apnea have been ruled out, recurrent apnea in a preterm infant is classified as apnea of prematurity. The evaluation of the infant with apnea includes a physical exam; review of documented apneic episodes; concurrent use of a pulse oximeter to identify whether desaturation occurs at the same time; such laboratory studies as complete blood count and differential, blood glucose, electrolytes, calcium, phosphate, and magnesium to rule out metabolic problems, infection, and respiratory alterations; pneumocardiogram and chest x-ray; and possible EEG, cranial ultrasound, barium swallow, and pneumogram (Beachy & Deacon, 1993).

Nursing and Collaborative Management. Periodic breathing and apneic episodes are frequent findings in the premature neonate. Therefore, these neonates are placed on continuous cardiorespiratory monitors until normal breathing patterns are observed. Monitor alarms must be set for the correct parameters of heart rate and respiratory rate and must always remain in the "on" position with alarm volumes audible. Alarms must be answered immediately to prevent a life-threatening emergency.

Nursing interventions that may reduce and prevent occurrence of apnea include the maintenance of a neutral thermal environment; avoidance of triggering reflexes, such as vigorous suctioning; and placing a neck roll under the infant's neck and shoulders (Beachy & Deacon, 1993; Grisemer, 1993). The nurse witnessing an apneic episode should use gentle tactile stimulation to arouse the neonate. This stimulation can include tapping the feet, stroking the back, or changing the neonate's position. If the neonate does not begin to breathe, positive pressure ventilation with 100% oxygen via bag and mask is given. If the neonate does not begin to breathe spontaneously, intubation and mechanical ventilation will be required.

The neonate found to have periodic breathing or recurrent apneic episodes must be assessed to identify the underlying cause. Nasal CPAP at low pressures may be used to decrease the incidence of apnea (Grisemer, 1993). If the frequency of apneic episodes increases to several per hour or if cyanosis develops, treatment with a methylxanthine drug (aminophylline, theophylline, or caffeine) may be prescribed to be administered intravenously or orally to the neonate (Avery, Fletcher, & MacDonald, 1994). These medications act as stimulants to the neonate's central nervous system and work to eliminate the irregular breathing patterns.

Most apnea of prematurity resolves by the time the infant reaches a postconceptional age of 34 to 36 weeks; occasionally, apnea can persist for several weeks postterm (Grisemer, 1993). Home apnea monitoring and medication may be necessary after discharge. Parents must receive special discharge teaching regarding the safe use of the monitor and how to respond if the monitor signals an alarm. Instruction also includes training in infant cardiopulmonary resuscitation (CPR) for parents and adults who will be caring for the baby. In addition, parents must demonstrate knowledge of the correct administration of medication.

Identification of an irregular breathing pattern in the neonate can be frightening to parents. In addition to concerns about the neonate's prematurity, parents face caring for the neonate at home with medications and an apnea monitor. A referral for home monitoring should be made early, as well as arrangements for home care follow-up. The nurse should allow parents ample time to familiarize themselves with the neonate's usual daily care, such as bathing and feeding, before teaching about the monitor. This allows the parents to gain comfort and confidence in caring for the neonate before adding more complicated skills, such as monitor training and CPR, to their discharge plan.

Parents must have ready access to a phone and must know how to notify the emergency rescue system in their community if the neonate does stop breathing. In addition, they need to let the electric company know that they must maintain electricity at all times. They also need emergency numbers in case of power outage. Parents are instructed to notify the physician if the monitor alarms frequently while the neonate is sleeping or if they observe an apneic episode. Regular follow-up visits are important to assess the neonate's progress, as well as to reinforce discharge teaching. Follow-up visits also allow planning for further evaluation to assess the infant's breathing pattern as he or she gets older. The apnea monitor and medications are continued until the infant is found to have a regular breathing pattern. See the box entitled Nursing Strategies: Preparation for Home Apnea Monitoring.

The nurse is advised to assess the family's home environment and situation prior to discharge. In one example, a community health nurse making a home visit found that a single mother was not using the apnea monitor. On further evaluation, it was discovered that the dwelling had one functional electrical outlet into which a space heater was plugged. When faced with a choice of heat for the family or use of the monitor, the mother met the most basic need first—warmth.

Retinopathy of Prematurity (ROP)

Retinopathy of prematurity (ROP) is a disease process that occurs in the blood vessels in the retina of the eyes; it affects preterm infants because the retinal blood vessels are immature. Normal development of the preterm infant's retinal vessels initially can be stopped or harmfully altered by such factors as hyperoxia, shock, asphyxia, hypothermia, vitamin E deficiency, and light exposure (Perlstein, 1997; Phelps, 1997). It is unclear why the retinal vessels of some babies can withstand such problems and continue to develop in a normal fashion and why the retinal ves-

---

▶ **NURSING STRATEGIES: PREPARATION FOR HOME APNEA MONITORING**

- Assess the family's needs, level of education, available supports among friends and family, overall health, financial level, particular demands of job, home, and family, and current level of understanding of neonate's condition.
- Educate family about apnea; fill in gaps in knowledge.
- Review all home care therapies (including medication administration, side effects, and so on).
- Help family to locate appropriate and available family and community resources (e.g., Visiting Nurses Association).
- Help family locate home monitoring company.
- Refer family to social services if financial arrangements must be negotiated (e.g., obtaining a telephone).
- Help family to design a practical and safe placement of monitor in the home.
- Make sure family has a telephone or access to one for possible emergencies.

- Assist family in notifying local emergency services of potential need for services (e.g., police, fire, electric company).
- Demonstrate, then observe family as they practice with the machine.
- Carefully explain CPR techniques. (Allow time for demonstration; provide written materials for quick referral.)
- Make sure that safety precautions are understood and that troubleshooting for potential mechanical problems is clearly understood.
- Demonstrate how to maintain a log of apneic episodes.
- Prepare and support the family regarding lifestyle changes. (Include other children and relatives as necessary.)

Adapted with permission, from Norris-Berkemeyer, S., & Hutchins, K. (1986). Home apnea monitoring. *Pediatric Nursing, 12*, 259–262.

sels of other babies follow a pathologic course. Indeed, ROP can result in outcomes ranging from normal vision to blindness. An estimated 400 babies each year are blinded and 4300 are left with retinal scars from ROP (Phelps, 1997). Both the incidence and severity of ROP are greater with decreasing gestational age and birth weight. For example, ROP is rare in infants over 1500 g; most significant disease is seen in infants who weigh less than 1250 g at birth (Phibbs, 1996).

ROP was originally attributed only to the effects on the retinal vessels of high concentrations of oxygen, used as part of respiratory therapy for preterm infants. However, ROP is now believed to be multifactorial in origin. The current increase in ROP seems to be related to the increased survival of infants so immature at birth that cautious use of oxygen is not a major factor (Phelps, 1997).

The retina of the eye is not fully developed until 40 to 44 weeks' gestation. At 32 weeks' gestation, the blood vessels in the temporal peripheral area of the retina remain immature. This temporal peripheral area of the retinal blood vessels becomes most vulnerable to damage.

With ROP, the retinal arterioles, the small branches of arteries in the retina, constrict or narrow. This constriction decreases the volume of blood that flows to the retina of the eye. If the constriction is not resolved, the affected retinal blood vessels may be destroyed. When this occurs, the growth of undamaged retinal blood vessels will increase to try to reestablish the damaged retinal circulation. These new blood vessels grow very rapidly and tend to be weak or abnormal. The weakened blood vessels can allow blood and fluid to leak into the vitreous of the eye. Over time, this can result in the development of scar tissue that places tension on the retina. This damage to the retina can cause severe impairment in vision or even blindness. Retinopathy of prematurity has been described in four stages or five grades, based on the abnormalities that develop in the retina and retinal blood vessels (Table 33–2).

Nursing and Collaborative Assessment and Management. Management of ROP begins with identifying neonates who are at risk and prompt diagnosis. The premature low-birth-weight neonate is at special risk for this condition because of the immaturity of retinal blood vessels. Management includes careful attention to the neonate's oxygen needs, which can fluctuate even in infants who are fairly stable. Prompt weaning from oxygen should be initiated as soon as it is safe for the neonate. Some units administer the antioxidant vitamin E. Cryotherapy and laser photocoagulation are therapies that have had favorable results (Phelps, 1997).

▶ **TABLE 33-2**
Classifications of Retinopathy of Prematurity

Classification by International Proliferative-Phase Fundus Changes

Stage I	Demarcation line seen between vascularized and avascularized retina
Stage II	Demarcation line is elevated to a ridge
Stage III	Ridge has increased growth of extraretinal blood vessels
Stage IV	Retinal detachment

Classification by Cicatrical-Phase Fundus Changes

Grade I	Small areas of retinal pigment irregularities are seen
Grade II	The disc is distorted
Grade III	The retinal fold is seen
Grade IV	Incomplete retrolental mass, partial retinal detachment
Grade V	Complete retrolental mass, total retinal detachment

Serial ocular examinations should be performed by an ophthalmologist who is experienced with ROP. In many units, examinations are performed for premature infants and for all infants who received oxygen therapy. Follow-up exams are based on the condition of each infant.

Before the ophthalmologic examination, a series of drops will need to be placed in the neonate's eyes to dilate the pupils. The drops are often administered according to a special time schedule ordered by the physician performing the examination. Once the neonate's pupils are dilated, the neonate may be sensitive to the bright lights of the nursery. Care should be taken to lower the lights over the neonate's bed or shade the bed if possible. The nurse may also be asked to assist in the examination by holding the neonate's head in the necessary position.

Parents will be anxious to know the outcome of the ophthalmologic examination and whether the neonate will have a vision impairment. Parents require continued support as information about long-term vision is often obtained only after serial examinations as the infant grows. Parents must be aware of the importance of follow-up visits with the ophthalmologist for continued assessment and management.

▶ **Alterations in Cardiovascular Functioning**

Patent Ductus Arteriosus

As discussed in Chapter 30, in the fetus the ductus arteriosus is a functional cardiac structure; it connects the left pulmonary artery and the aorta and shunts blood away from the lungs in fetal circulation. The ductus arteriosus constricts after birth. Closure is influenced by such factors as the muscular development of the ductus, blood oxygen levels, and prostaglandin levels. Functional closure takes place within the first 12 hours in the mature infant, although permanent closure may take several weeks.

Patent ductus arteriosus (PDA) is a condition in which the ductus remains open after birth. The incidence of patent ductus arteriosus increases in premature infants, although the exact mechanism is unclear (Heymann et al., 1993). Several conditions can maintain a patent ductus or stimulate the ductus to reopen. For example, premature neonates are more likely than term neonates to experience respiratory complications that compromise their arterial oxygen levels. Without adequate oxygen levels, the smooth muscle of the ductus will not constrict and the ductus will stay open. Also, the ductus arteriosus in the premature neonate is less muscular than the ductus in the term neonate. Thus, conditions such as acidosis and the presence of prostaglandin E_2, which in fetal life helps the smooth muscle of the ductus remain relaxed, more quickly affect the ductus in the premature neonate to prevent closure (Avery, Fletcher, & MacDonald, 1994).

Hypoxia, acidosis, and the presence of prostaglandin E_2 also affect the closure of the ductus in the term neonate. Even if closed, the ductus can reopen in the presence of these conditions. In neonates with cyanotic heart disease, such as transposition of the great vessels, the presence of a PDA is beneficial, as the PDA can provide for the necessary mixing of oxygenated and unoxygenated blood (Avery, Fletcher, & MacDonald, 1994; Heymann et al., 1993).

Nursing and Collaborative Assessment. The term or premature neonate with a small PDA is likely to be asymptomatic. The larger the patent ductus, however, the more hemodynamic complications that arise. When the ductus remains open, there is shunting of the blood from the left side of the heart to the pulmonary system. Blood from the aorta is shunted into the pulmonary artery, increasing the blood flow to the lungs. In the large PDA, this blood is shunted with higher pressure because it is coming from the aorta and the systemic circulation. This increased blood flow to the lungs can cause congestive heart failure. This in turn can cause congestion in the lungs that interferes with necessary gas exchange and may cause hypoxia. Signs and symptoms of PDA include (1) a continuous murmur, called a Gibson murmur, which is a crescendo systolic murmur with clicks heard at the base of the heart; (2) in a large PDA, bounding peripheral pulses and a wide pulse pressure in the blood pressure; and (3) persistent respiratory distress and hypoxia (Avery, Fletcher, & Mac-

Donald, 1994; Heymann et al., 1993). Signs of congestive failure include edema, poor weight gain, recurrent pulmonary infections, and persistent respiratory distress and hypoxia.

Patent ductus arteriosus is confirmed through diagnostic testing. A chest x-ray will show an enlarged heart, pulmonary congestion, and a prominent pulmonary artery and left atrial enlargement. An electrocardiogram will show abnormalities that indicate left ventricular hypertrophy. An echocardiogram will demonstrate the ductus arteriosus, its size, and direction of flow across the defect.

Nursing and Collaborative Management. Initial management is directed at relieving the symptoms related to respiratory distress and congestive heart failure. Supplemental oxygen and ventilatory support are administered, based on the results of arterial blood gas tests. The neonate's fluid status must be carefully calculated to prevent both fluid overload and dehydration. The neonate's intake and output and daily weight are strictly monitored. The administration of diuretics, such as furosemide (Lasix), helps to eliminate and prevent fluid overload. Calorie needs are carefully calculated to ensure that sufficient calories are provided for the neonate's energy needs. Nutrition can be provided in enteral or parenteral feedings.

Once fluid and calorie needs have been addressed, management of the PDA itself is considered. In some cases, indomethacin, a prostaglandin inhibitor, is administered to promote closure of the ductus. If indomethacin is ineffective in producing closure or if indomethacin is contraindicated, surgical ligation of the ductus may be done.

Parents must receive careful explanation of the presence of a PDA and its effects on the neonate's condition. The parents of a critically ill newborn can easily become overwhelmed when approached with yet another "problem." Parents must also be informed about the use of indomethacin and the results obtained and advised if the persistence of a PDA will require surgical repair. Pictures or diagrams can be extremely useful in explaining PDA, its effects on the neonate, and the surgical repair procedure.

▶ **Alterations in Neurologic Functioning**

Intracranial Hemorrhage

Intracranial hemorrhage can be a major problem, especially for the premature, very-low-birth-weight neonate, although this condition can occur in near term or term neonates. An intracranial hemorrhage occurs when blood leaks into the cranial cavity from the vascular system in the brain. Bleeding can range from a small amount of oozing to a massive hemorrhage. Bleeding usually originates from the rich supply of small blood vessels in the germinal layer of the brain in the periventricular area. The fragile walls of the small arteries, capillaries, and veins in the neonate can easily be damaged, causing bleeding to occur. The most common type of intracranial hemorrhage in very-low-birth-weight premature neonates is periventricular, intraventricular hemorrhage (PIVH) (Reed & Blumer, 1997).

The actual incidence of PIVH is unknown, due to a lack of epidemiologic data. However, frequency reports range from 20 to 50%, with discrepancies in the rates reflecting such factors as differences in the newborn populations reported (Papile & Brann, 1993). PIVH increases as gestational age and birth weight decrease.

PIVH can be graded according to the site of hemorrhage and the presence or absence of ventricular dilatation (Table 33–3) (Rozmus, 1992). Grades I and II are graded as "mild," Grade III is "moderate," and Grade IV is graded "severe." An isolated subependymal hemorrhage takes place in about 40% of infants with PIVH; about 60% of infants with PIVH sustain intraventricular hemorrhages.

There are many potential causes of PIVH, the origin is often multifactorial, and infants with PIVH may have different combinations of factors. Factors involved in the development of PIVH include very-low-birth-weight, hypoxia, respiratory failure requiring mechanical ventilation, fluctuations in cerebral blood flow and pressure, alterations in platelet function and coagulopathy, ischemia, pneumothorax, PDA, hypothermia, and rapid administration of volume expanders.

Consequences associated with PIVH include dilation of the ventricles of the brain, posthemorrhagic hydrocephalus, and parenchymal hemorrhage. Associated brain lesions, such as ischemic injuries to the white matter of the brain, can also occur. PIVH can cause long-term neurologic impairment or death; however, it is often difficult to predict whether and to what extent a surviving newborn will be affected later in life. Prognosis also depends on other complications the neonate may have as a result of prematurity.

Nursing and Collaborative Assessment. The majority of intraventricular hemorrhages manifest during the first 2 days and nearly all PIVH occur within the first week after birth (Sims et al., 1993). An estimated 25–70% of PIVH occurs in the first 6 hours after birth (Reed & Blumer, 1997). Presentation ranges from unnoticeable to dramatic. Symptoms may include a sudden change in respiratory status, such as episodes of apnea; hypotension; a dropping hematocrit level that fails to rise after blood transfusions; a full and bulging fontanelle; and a change in activity such as an unwillingness to suck, myoclonic movements, lethargy, seizures, and decreased muscle tone.

In addition to the identification of symptoms, intracranial hemorrhage is confirmed by ultrasound examination of the neonate's head. Because 50% of premature neonates with intracranial hemorrhage may be asymptomatic, ultrasound of the head is often done to screen for the presence of an intracranial hemorrhage in these neonates. CT brain scanning or magnetic resonance imaging may also be used in assessment (Sims et al., 1993).

Nursing and Collaborative Management. Collaborative management of the neonate with an intracranial hemorrhage, such as PIVH, includes prevention, short-term management, and long-term management (Avery, Fletcher, & MacDonald, 1994).

Prevention of premature, very-low-birth-weight birth would have a major impact on eliminating the incidence of intracranial bleeding; however, upon birth of a premature neonate, prevention is directed at maintaining adequate ventilation and maintaining the perfusion in the vulnerable germinal matrix of the brain. This includes preventing sudden or wide fluctuations in systemic blood pressure. Any intrusive procedures can increase systemic blood pressure. Sudden increases in blood pressure have been noted in premature neonates during motor activity, diagnostic procedures, handling, seizures, and mechanical ventilation. For this reason care of the newborn should be clustered so there is minimal handling of susceptible infants. Caution must be used when caring for the premature neonate who requires treatments and activities; health care providers should be prepared to intervene swiftly when problems arise (Avery, Fletcher, & MacDonald, 1994).

▶ **TABLE 33-3**

Classification of Periventricular, Intraventricular Hemorrhage (PIVH)

Mild
Grade I: Isolated germinal matrix hemorrhage
Grade II: Intraventricular hemorrhage with normal ventricular size

Moderate
Grade III: Intraventricular hemorrhage with acute ventricular dilation

Severe
Grade IV: Parenchymal hemorrhage

Source: Pomerance & Richardson, 1993, p. 426.

Acute management begins with the identification of the symptoms related to an intracranial hemorrhage. An ultrasound of the neonate's head must be quickly obtained. Further management is then focused on treatment of the particular abnormality identified. For example, a severe hemorrhage could cause multisystem abnormalities that require aggressive intervention. Seizures would be treated with medications such as phenobarbital; apnea, with oxygen and mechanical ventilation.

PIVH can be a serious type of intracranial hemorrhage. The ventricles in the brain can become dilated with excessive amounts of cerebrospinal fluid. This is called posthemorrhagic ventricular dilation. This ventricular dilation can cause an inappropriate increase in head circumference, demonstrated by full and bulging fontanelles. Ventricular size is monitored by serial ultrasound examinations of the head and serial accurate head measurements.

If the ventricular dilation does not stop spontaneously, intervention is necessary. Serial lumbar punctures (spinal taps) can help to decrease excessive accumulations of cerebrospinal fluid. If the accumulation continues and causes an increase in intracranial pressure, neurosurgical intervention is required. This would include surgical placement of a ventricular peritoneal shunt. In this procedure a shunt is placed in the ventricles of the brain to drain the excessive amounts of cerebrospinal fluid into the peritoneal cavity.

Nursing care of the premature neonate with PIVH includes careful and ongoing assessment for key symptoms. Once the neonate has been diagnosed with PIVH, both the neonate and the parents require aggressive support. In addition to learning about the many interventions needed to manage the neonate's changing condition, parents will be extremely concerned with the severity and the extent of the damage caused by the hemorrhage and the possible long-term consequences.

Neurologic abnormalities appear more often with large severe hemorrhages; however, the best indicators of long-term deficits related to PIVH are regular developmental and neurologic assessments of the neonate's growth and development over time. If the older infant or child demonstrates neurologic or developmental delays, the parents will be referred to the community programs that best meet that child's special needs. Management strategies then focus on parental education and the long-term care related to the child's problems.

Thermoregulation

After birth, the neonate expends large amounts of energy to regulate his or her own body temperature in a different environment. Heat losses after delivery can

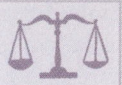

Ethical Decision Making

Baby Kobi was born at an estimated 25 weeks' gestation and weighed 600 g. Shortly after birth, he sustained a severe PIVH. Three days after birth, he continues to be unstable and is being maintained through life-supporting technology.

If you were the nurse caring for Baby Kobi, consider the following questions:

1. How would you feel about vigorous and expensive interventions to maintain life?
2. Do you feel that technology should or should not be used to support life for extremely low-birth-weight infants whose course is uncertain? Should any limits be set?
3. What strategies would you use to help Baby Kobi's parents?

be great and occur as a result of evaporation, convection, conduction, and radiation (see Chapter 30).

The premature neonate cannot immediately compensate for these heat losses. These neonates are at greater risk than the term neonate because of their greater body surface area. Brown fat tissue is an important mechanism for producing heat for the neonate. The premature neonate, however, cannot fully rely on this mechanism, as brown fat cells do not begin to appear until 26 or 30 weeks of gestation.

Infants get cold when their heat loss is greater than their heat production (Perlstein, 1997). Premature neonates are at great risk for **cold stress,** especially if their body temperatures fall below 35°C (95°F) (Nagey & Viscardi, 1993). During cold stress, metabolic needs increase dramatically.

The premature or sick neonate is less likely to adapt to those greater oxygen needs related to environmental temperature changes. The premature neonate who has lung disease, such as RDS, is likely to become severely compromised if temperature instability further increases oxygen needs. This would place the premature neonate at risk for developing hypoxia, metabolic acidosis, and further temperature instability.

In addition to cold stress, the premature neonate is also sensitive to increases in environmental temperatures. These neonates may develop an abnormally high body temperature, higher than 37°C (98.6°F), if wrapped in multiple blankets in a warm environment

(Nagey & Viscardi, 1993). Temperature increases that would be expected in the presence of infection are often only low-grade increases of normal temperatures in the neonate, because of the immaturity of their temperature regulation mechanisms.

Nursing and Collaborative Assessment.
Common signs of inadequate temperature regulation in the neonate are central nervous system depression, including lethargy, fatigue, and poor feeding behaviors; cardiac arrhythmias, especially bradycardia; cardiovascular instability, including an unstable blood pressure; depressed respirations and periods of apnea; and metabolic abnormalities (Avery, Fletcher, & MacDonald, 1994).

Nursing Diagnoses.
Nursing diagnoses are developed after comprehensive assessment of the neonate. Examples of diagnoses related to thermoregulation in the preterm neonate include:

Problem-oriented diagnoses:

- Ineffective thermoregulation, related to immature central nervous system and decreased brown fat
- Risk for altered body temperature, related to inability to maintain a neutral thermal environment
- Hypothermia, related to immature thermoregulating mechanism and cold environment
- Hyperthermia, related to immature thermoregulating mechanism and hot environment

Wellness-oriented diagnoses:

- Potential asset for maintaining a neutral thermal environment, related to controlled temperature in radiant warmer or isolette

Nursing and Collaborative Management.
To assist in thermoregulation, the preterm neonate should be dried thoroughly in the delivery room, and the wet linens should be immediately removed. After delivery, the premature neonate will require an artificially warmed environment, such as an isolette or a radiant warming bed. The neutral thermal temperature must be carefully calculated for each neonate, based on the gestational age and weight. A smaller neonate usually requires a warmer environmental temperature than a larger neonate to maintain body temperature properly.

Initially, the isolette or the radiant warmer is used in the servo mode. The servo mode allows a temperature probe to be taped to the neonate's skin. As the neonate's temperature needs increase and decrease, the environmental temperature is automatically adjusted within a preset range (Nagey & Viscardi,

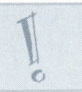

Nursing Alert

Radiant warmers increase an infant's insensible fluid loss. This is considered when fluid needs are calculated and may be a factor in choice of a radiant warmer or isolette for an infant.

1993). Caution must be used to ensure that temperature alarms are set in the *on* position and are functioning properly. This prevents problems and ensures that the radiant temperature is safely maintained. Neonates in radiant warmers should be dressed only with a diaper, so that their temperature can be properly maintained in the servo mode and overheating can be prevented. The nurse also should monitor the neonate's temperature regularly with a thermometer to ensure proper functioning of the isolette or radiant warmer, as well as to assess the neonate's temperature stability.

Once the neonate is able to regulate his or her own temperature, weaning from the warmed environment of the isolette or radiant warmer to an open crib can begin. The neonate is dressed with a shirt, hat, and double or triple blankets while in the crib. The neonate's temperature must be monitored every 30 minutes to 1 hour until temperature stability is confirmed (Avery, Fletcher, & MacDonald, 1994). The neonate's temperature can be monitored every 3 to 4 hours thereafter (Nagey & Viscardi, 1993).

Parents of premature neonates who require an isolette or radiant warmer can feel isolated from their child. Parents should be encouraged to touch the neonate in the warmer bed or through the portholes of the isolette. The neonate, if properly wrapped and dressed, can tolerate visits with parents outside of the isolette before being fully weaned to an open-air crib. Including parents in the weaning process can be an important step in facilitating parent–infant attachment prior to discharge. In addition, kangaroo care is appropriate for many preterm infants and is a way to promote the parent–infant relationship (see Chapter 12).

▶ Alterations in Gastrointestinal Functioning

Preterm infants can have major nutritional problems associated with gestational age and weight, metabolic and gastrointestinal functioning, temperature instability, respiratory status, and coordination of immature feeding reflexes, such as sucking and swallowing.

Care of the preterm neonate must therefore include nutritional considerations. In addition, alterations in gastrointestinal functioning can be related to life-threatening conditions such as necrotizing enterocolitis.

Necrotizing Enterocolitis (NEC)

Necrotizing enterocolitis (NEC) is a potentially life-threatening gastrointestinal disease seen in the sick newborn. It is the most common acquired intestinal emergency in the NICU (Crissinger, 1997). Necrotizing enterocolitis occurs in 1 to 10% of infants hospitalized in neonatal intensive care units, with 90% of the cases occurring in premature infants (Avery, Fletcher, & MacDonald, 1994; Crissinger, 1997). With increased survival of low-birth-weight infants, the incidence of NEC may increase (Andrews & Krowchuk, 1997).

The cause of NEC is multifactorial and not fully known (Kitterman, 1996). It occurs in the setting of a stressed gut with immature protective mechanisms (Crissinger, 1997). It has been observed to occur in clusters of neonates at one time; however, a single causative factor cannot be linked among the cases. Some sources better describe the disease process as a syndrome with many associated factors. Risk factors commonly associated with NEC include the following:

- Hypoxemia
- Bowel immaturity
- Perinatal asphyxia
- Bowel ischemia
- Hypertonic substances introduced into the gut
- Overgrowth of enteric bacteria
- Polycythemia
- Very low birth weight
- Acidosis
- Indwelling enteric feeding tubes
- Sepsis
- Placement of umbilical catheters

Feeding might also increase the risk of intestinal tissue hypoxia due to increased intestinal oxygen demands during absorption of nutrients. The increased metabolic demands may lead to tissue hypoxia and then injury to the mucosa, bacterial invasion, and NEC (Crissinger, 1997). For this reason, beginning feedings may be delayed in the very-low-birth-weight infant and in infants who are hypoxic.

Nursing and Collaborative Assessment. The clinical signs and symptoms of NEC are usually seen between 3 and 10 days after birth but have been found as late as 3 months of age. Symptoms and signs may occur gradually or suddenly and include (Kitterman, 1996):

- Apneic periods
- Abdominal distension (the most common finding; usually the presenting sign); progression to visible loops of bowel
- Feeding intolerance with increased residuals (increasing volumes or bile staining are serious signs)
- Blood in the stool (may be occult)
- Erythema of the abdominal wall (may indicate peritonitis; can be visible in babies who at first do not seem very ill, especially very premature infants with thin abdominal walls)
- Lethargy (often an early sign)
- Carbohydrate intolerance (reducing substances in the stool)
- Sepsis (infection is usually a late sign)

Abdominal x-ray can reveal the following: pneumatosis intestinalis (small gas bubbles in the bowel wall are a definitive diagnosis); fixed, dilated bowel loop indicating lack of peristalsis and possible bowel necrosis; and free intraperitoneal gas, indicating intestinal perforation (a severe sign). Laboratory findings may show thrombocytopenia, which may indicate necrotic bowel, metabolic acidosis, and signs of coagulopathy (Kitterman, 1996).

A recent study (Andrews & Krowchuck, 1997) identified differences in stool patterns between infants with NEC and infants who did not develop NEC. Infants with NEC passed the first stool around 14 hours after their first feedings, tended to have a higher number of stools, and had stools described more often as seedy than infants who did not have NEC. Despite sample sizes of 34 infants in each group, the study suggests the importance of including assessment of stool patterns in identification of NEC.

The signs of NEC can be severe and life threatening for the premature neonate who is already ill with conditions such as RDS and infection. If a perforated intestine occurs, signs of cardiovascular and respiratory collapse will be seen as shock develops.

Nursing and Collaborative Management. NEC requires swift medical and nursing intervention. Often, the first signs are observed by the nurse. The physician is notified without delay. The neonate should be placed on a cardiorespiratory monitor for continuous assessment and can be placed on a radiant warmer bed to provide the necessary thermal environment and allow easy observation of any changes in condition (Fig. 33–4).

Management begins with the immediate discontinuation of all enteral feedings. An orogastric tube is placed into the neonate's stomach to decompress the

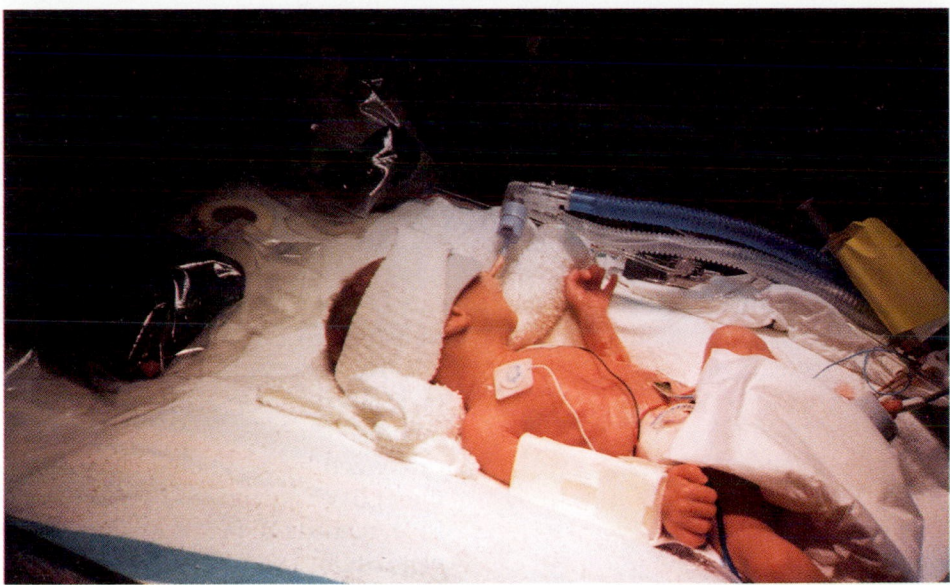

FIGURE 33–4. A premature newborn with necrotizing entercolitis requires intensive care.

GI tract. Position of the tube is checked by radiograph, rather than by instilling air in the catheter and listening to the stomach. Abdominal girth is measured at the same place on the abdomen once a shift to check for increasing distension. A surgical pen can be used to mark the abdomen for placement of the measuring tape. In addition, the abdomen is assessed for the presence of visible loops of bowel. Bowel sounds should be assessed in all four quadrants.

The amount, color, and consistency of the drainage from the orogastric tube should be closely monitored and documented. The gastric drainage should also be tested for the presence of occult blood. All stools are also tested for the presence of occult blood. Testing for occult blood may be done by using a standard Gastrocott and Hemoccult kit, or specimens may be sent to the laboratory for testing.

Feedings are withheld for a minimum of 7 to 10 days or until the disease process resolves. During that time the neonate requires total intravenous nutritional support and careful fluid and electrolyte management. This includes the calculation and administration of total parenteral nutrition (see Chapter 32) (Avery, Fletcher, & MacDonald, 1994).

Because of the risk of sepsis and potential for peritonitis with the presence of bacteria in the neonate's intestine, intravenous antibiotics are administered. Antibiotic susceptibilities of the organisms commonly encountered in the nursery affect the choice of antibiotics. Intravenous sites must be assessed regularly for signs of redness or swelling that may indicate infiltration or infection.

Surgical resection of the bowel is indicated only if perforation occurs. A colostomy or ileostomy may be required in the presence of extensive intestinal damage. Removal of large segments of damaged intestine could leave the neonate with a short bowel. This may result in long-term nutritional and absorption problems for the infant. Additional management includes cardiovascular support if signs of shock develop and respiratory support since the infant is a "belly breather"; he will guard a painful abdomen and attempt to breathe much more shallowly.

Attention should be given to pain management. Analgesics such as morphine may be used; however, intubation and mechanical ventilation should be available if apnea is sustained.

The neonate's recovery from NEC may be complicated and require prolonged hospitalization. The gradual return to enteral feedings may be further delayed by malabsorption of the food ingested or recurrent diarrhea. Neonates who have a short bowel from surgical resection could require parenteral nutrition for years. Recurrent intestinal obstructions may result from scar tissue narrowing the intestinal lumen as the damaged bowel heals. Additional complications related to the neonate's prematurity, such as RDS, may further delay full recovery and discharge home.

Parents require extensive support and education through this very stressful time. Parents will have questions about when the neonate can resume feedings and often become frustrated when setbacks further delay the neonate's discharge. It is extremely stressful for anyone to learn to care for a neonate with an ostomy. Parents need to identify one other adult who can assist them in sharing caretaking activities for the neonate. Parents must understand the importance of attending routine follow-up visits with the physician and must be familiar with symptoms that require immediate medical attention.

▶ Very-Low-Birth-Weight and Extremely-Low-Birth-Weight Neonates

Advances in neonatology have resulted in survival of smaller and sicker neonates. The decrease in neonatal mortality since the early 1960s has been related to such factors as technology, regionalization of perinatal/neonatal care with transports to tertiary care centers, and most recently, the widespread use of exogenous surfactant in NICUs (Bennett, 1997). Special categories have been developed to describe the tiniest neonates (Behrman & Shiono, 1997):

- **Low-birth-weight (LBW)**—a neonate weighing less than 2500 g at birth
- **Moderately-low-birth-weight**—a neonate who weighs between 1500 and 2499 g at birth.
- **Very-low-birth-weight (VLBW)**—a neonate who weighs less than 1500 g at birth.
- **Extremely-low-birth-weight (ELBW)**—a neonate who weighs less than 1000 g at birth.

The most significant cause of low birth weight is prematurity. Premature neonates with low birth weights can also be described as SGA, AGA, or LGA.

Birth weight is an important indicator of neonatal outcome. Any neonate with a birth weight under 2500 g is at risk for special problems in the postnatal period. Neonates who are VLBW and ELBW have multiple problems that can have long-term effects or that can cause death. For example, a relatively high rate of disabilities has been noted in the population of infants weighing less than 750 g at birth; although these infants once were considered too small to live, their survival now is probable (Als, 1997; Hack, 1997). The health of a LBW infant is related directly to his or her gestational age; the younger the baby, the greater the risks. It is often not possible to forecast whether and to what extent an infant will have long-term problems, even with the best care.

The most common problems experienced by VLBW or ELBW neonates are related to prematurity; however, these neonates are at special risk because, in addition to their prematurity, they have minimal energy stores to battle the complications of prematurity resulting from their small birth weight. This combination of risk factors can pose a tremendous challenge to the interdisciplinary neonatal team that will work together to help the neonate survive the premature birth with as few long-term complications as possible (Stevenson, Petersen, Yates, Benitz, & Gale, 1988).

The care and treatment of the premature VLBW or ELBW neonate can extend over many weeks and months. The neonate's hospital stay is often further prolonged by additional complications. For example, the ELBW neonate is at increased risk for developing BPD related to the need for prolonged mechanical ventilation. The lengthy hospitalization of a VLBW or ELBW neonate results in tremendous financial obligations for both parents and/or their third-party payers.

The parents of a VLBW or ELBW neonate can quickly become overwhelmed by the many problems that can complicate the neonate's hospital course. Although it is important to keep the parents informed about any changes in the neonate's status, positive advances must be discussed along with the setbacks. Parents need to be presented with the neonate's prognosis in the immediate and long-term future. They may be faced with difficult decisions about initiating or continuing certain treatments for the VLBW or ELBW neonate who is experiencing life-threatening complications. Parents confronted with hard decisions are under great stress and require thorough explanations with opportunities to ask questions. Parents often find strength in ongoing and consistent support by the physicians, nurses, and other health care providers caring for their neonate (see Chapter 12).

▶ THE POSTMATURE NEONATE

The neonate born after the end of 42 weeks of gestation is termed **postmature** or **postdate.** Three to twelve percent of all pregnancies extend more than 2 weeks beyond the estimated date of confinement. The postmature neonate is more likely to experience fetal distress during labor and suffer ill effects from prolonged pregnancy (Avery, Fletcher, & MacDonald, 1994). The effects of postmaturity on the fetus are referred to as postmaturity syndrome.

Postmaturity syndrome results from physiologic changes related to the neonate's prolonged gestation. A major problem in the development of postmaturity syndrome is the inability of the placenta to continue to nourish the fetus adequately. This occurs because the aging placenta gradually loses its ability for gas and nutrient exchange.

The postmature neonate has normal length and head circumference at birth. Often the neonate weighs more than 4000 g; however, this neonate may also show signs of intrauterine weight loss, such as loss of subcutaneous fat and muscle mass. Characteristically, the postmature neonate will have peeling skin, long fingernails, and a wide-eyed gaze. The amniotic fluid, umbilical cord, and skin are often meconium stained. Oligohydramnios also may be observed.

Problems related to postmaturity syndrome are linked to the length of the gestation and the amount of stress that the fetus has suffered as a result of the prolonged pregnancy. Large neonates are at risk for birth injuries and may need to be delivered by cesarean because of cephalopelvic disproportion (Avery, Fletcher, & MacDonald, 1994). Placental insufficiency can place the neonate at risk for altered gas exchange that can result in life-threatening problems such as asphyxia and meconium aspiration syndrome (see later discussion).

Management of the postmature neonate is linked to the stress placed on the fetus as a result of prolonged pregnancy. Serial ultrasounds are often done if a pregnancy is suspected to be postdate. This assists in eliminating questions regarding the correct calculation of the estimated data of confinement. In addition, a biophysical profile may be done to assess the status of the fetus in utero.

Immediate assessment of the neonate and the amniotic fluid after delivery assists the delivery room team in responding appropriately to potential problems. Many postmature neonates tolerate labor and delivery well and progress without difficulty. Other neonates suffer serious consequences of complications related to postmaturity. Problems such as severe or recurrent asphyxia and meconium aspiration syndrome can be life threatening and must be aggressively managed. Postmature neonates found to be at risk for alterations after delivery are best observed in an intensive care nursery where expert care can be initiated immediately should problems arise.

► Asphyxia

Asphyxia, a potentially life-threatening condition, is a state of altered gas exchange in which there is a decrease in oxygenation and an increase in carbon dioxide in the body (Avery, Fletcher, & MacDonald, 1998). When asphyxia occurs, sufficient oxygen does not enter the fetal circulation and carbon dioxide is not removed from the blood. The tissues of the fetus'

body continue to use what little oxygen is available. This results in a lack of available oxygen, and hypoxia, an arterial oxygen level less than 50 mm Hg, occurs (Heymann et al., 1993). For the sick neonate, an arterial oxygen level between 60 and 80 mm Hg is desirable. When hypoxia occurs, anaerobic metabolism becomes active. This results in the production of large amounts of metabolic acids in the body. If not resolved immediately, asphyxia can result in death or severe physiologic damage (Avery, Fletcher, & MacDonald, 1994).

There are many potential causes of asphyxia in the fetus. Some of the most common causes are listed here:

- Interruption of umbilical blood flow such as would occur if the umbilical cord is compressed during labor
- Interruption of placental blood flow related to placental separation, abruption, or infarct
- Inadequate perfusion on the maternal side of the placenta, related to maternal hypotension
- Anemia in the fetus that makes it difficult for that fetus to tolerate the mild transient hypoxia that can occur normally during labor
- Failure of the neonate's lungs to inflate after delivery, related to an obstructed airway and possibly meconium aspiration (Avery, Fletcher, & MacDonald, 1994)

Asphyxia can occur suddenly and, in severe episodes, can be lethal in less than 10 minutes. Repeated episodes of mild asphyxia that are resolved can eventually produce a cumulative effect similar to that of a severe episode of asphyxia. Asphyxia should be anticipated in prematurity, postmaturity, multiple gestation, maternal diabetes, maternal hypertension and placental abruption, maternal and fetal anemia, breech presentation and delivery, and prolapse or compression of the umbilical cord (Avery, Fletcher, & MacDonald, 1994).

Nursing and Collaborative Assessment. The asphyxiated neonate has cyanosis, demonstrated by a blue coloring of the face, extremities, lips, and trunk. The neonate is limp and unresponsive to stimulation, and may demonstrate weak, gasping breaths or may not be breathing at all. Asphyxia is a medical emergency and must be treated immediately.

Nursing and Collaborative Management. Immediate assessment of the asphyxiated neonate is essential to identify the care required. If the neonate has been severely asphyxiated, resuscitation is necessary (see the box entitled Resuscitation of the Neonate).

► RESUSCITATION OF THE NEONATE

1. Establish unresponsiveness of the neonate and need for resuscitation.
2. Place the neonate on the radiant warmer bed. Quickly, dry thoroughly and remove wet linens. This assists in maintaining the neonate's temperature, and allows easy visibility and access to the neonate.
3. Assess the neonate's heart rate and respiratory rate and place the neonate on a cardiorespiratory monitor.
4. Provide positive pressure ventilation (PPV) with 100% oxygen by bag and mask if the infant is apneic, gasping, or has a heart rate less than 100 beats/minute.
5. Initiate cardiac compressions if heart rate is less than 60 or between 60 and 80 beats/minute and not increasing after 30 seconds of PPV with 100% O_2 (Fig. 33–5).
6. Establish intravenous access through peripheral IV or umbilical venous catheter.
7. Administer medications as ordered.
8. Assess the neonate's fluid and metabolic balances and initiate intravenous fluids as ordered.

The resuscitation process can be fast paced and filled with tension for all of the staff involved. The nurse must be familiar with the resuscitation process and his or her role, the correct use and calculation of medications, and the correct technique for bag and mask ventilation and cardiac compressions (Fig. 33–5).

The neonate who has experienced asphyxia but does not require resuscitation at birth will also require special care and observation. Continued assessment of the neonate's respiratory functioning may indicate the need for additional oxygen and ventilatory support. If hypoxia persists, additional problems such as persistent pulmonary hypertension should be suspected.

The central nervous system can be severely affected by asphyxia. The lack of oxygen to the brain can lead to brain damage and seizures. The neonate with brain damage related to asphyxia initially is found to be hypertonic with a poor sucking response. The neonate becomes progressively hypotonic at about 8 to 10 hours of age. Seizures will occur in the first 24 hours of life. Seizures may be in the form of tonic-clonic jerking movements or may look like lip smacking, chewing, or eye blinking. (See Chapter 32 for discussion of neonatal seizures.) The neonate with seizures requires careful observation, as well as medications to stop the seizures and to prevent their recurrence.

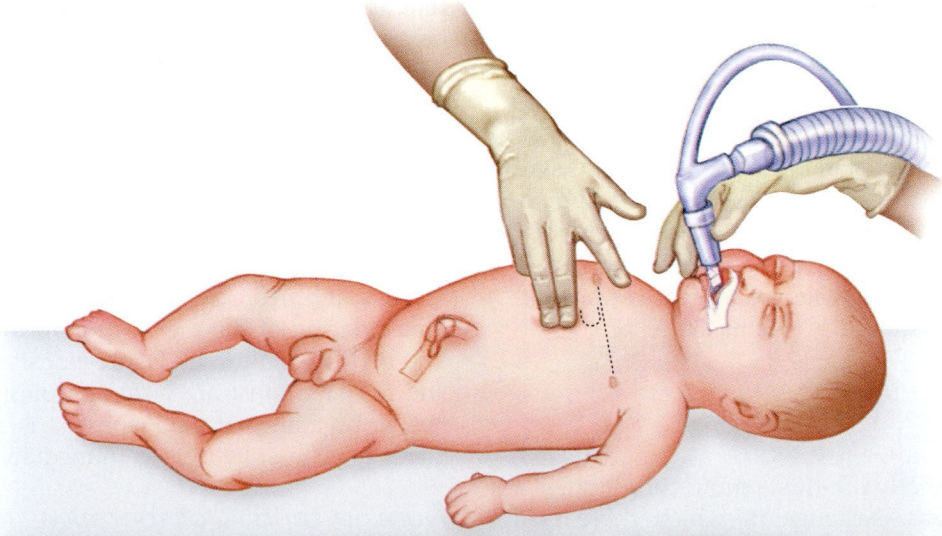

FIGURE 33–5. One technique for closed chest cardiac compression of the neonate. The infant lies on a firm surface. The third and fourth fingers of one hand are placed at neonate's nipple line, with the index finger raised from the surface of the body. Chest compression can also be done using the pads of both thumbs. *(Adapted, with permission, from the American Heart Association. (1997). Basic life support. Dallas, TX: American Heart Association. Copyright American Heart Association.)*

Additional sequelae of asphyxia can be seen in all major organ systems. The severity of the alterations depends on the severity of the asphyxia. When asphyxia occurs, blood is shunted away from the gastrointestinal system and sent to the major organs, such as the heart and the brain. This shunting of blood can damage the intestines, resulting in such problems as poor feeding and even necrotizing enterocolitis. Blood is also shunted away from the kidneys and may result in acute renal failure with low or no urine output.

The neonate who has experienced asphyxia requires intensive care for a prolonged period. This neonate is at high risk for developing numerous complications throughout the hospital stay. Parents of the asphyxiated neonate require enormous support from the interdisciplinary neonatal team. These parents need consistent, honest updates on the neonate's progress and compassionate support if the neonate's death is likely. The parents may be faced with the news that their neonate will survive but with significant problems related to damage caused by the lack of oxygen. (See Chapter 12 for discussion of psychosocial implications of the high-risk childbearing family.)

▶ Meconium Aspiration Syndrome

Meconium aspiration syndrome is a serious condition in which the fetus aspirates or breathes meconium (fetal stool) found in the amniotic fluid into the trachea or lungs. In response to physiologic stress, such as hypoxia and asphyxiation, peristalsis increases in the fetus and the anal sphincter relaxes, allowing the meconium to pass into the amniotic fluid. Although meconium is seen in the amniotic fluid of some preterm neonates, it is more likely to occur after 34 weeks of gestation and especially in the mature fetus (Miller, Fanaroff, & Martin, 1997b). Presence of meconium in the amniotic fluid in any presentation but breech is an abnormal finding (Avery, Fletcher, & MacDonald, 1994). The quantity of meconium passed affects the appearance and viscosity of the amniotic fluid. Meconium-stained amniotic fluid can range in appearance from a greenish-tinged fluid to a thick pea soup consistency.

Under normal conditions, the fetus has breathing movements in utero. In the presence of asphyxia and fetal distress, the fetus has gasping-type movements. During these gasping movements in utero, meconium can be easily aspirated into the trachea. Whenever meconium has been aspirated into the trachea, there is significant risk that the meconium can be aspirated into the lungs. Meconium can then be aspirated further into the lungs when the newborn takes the first breath at the time of delivery (Miller, Fanaroff, & Martin, 1997b).

Aspiration of meconium into the smaller airways in the lungs can result in significant morbidity and mortality in the neonate. Meconium is often thick and sticky and can partially or completely obstruct the airway. This obstruction prevents oxygen from entering the lungs and also traps air in the smaller airways distal to the obstruction. This air trapping can lead to a pneumothorax, a collapse in part or all of one or both of the lungs. It can also result in atelectasis, or collapse of the alveoli, the small air sacs in the lungs where gas exchange occurs. These alterations in the lungs cause increased hypoxia and further alter gas exchange.

Nursing and Collaborative Assessment. The neonate who has aspirated meconium demonstrates signs of respiratory distress. The distress may occur immediately at delivery or within the first hours of life. The signs of respiratory distress include tachypnea, cyanosis, grunting, nasal flaring, and retractions. The neonate's chest can appear overinflated. Breath sounds will be coarse and wet on auscultation. The neonate may be cyanotic, with a blushing coloring of the face, lips, trunk, and extremities. Arterial blood gas tests will reveal an abnormally low arterial oxygen level and an abnormally high carbon dioxide level. Additional laboratory studies may also demonstrate acidosis. The chest x-ray will show coarse irregular pulmonary densities with areas of atelectasis. The lungs can also be hyperinflated, and the diaphragm may be flattened. The infant may also show signs of classic postmaturity with evidence of weight loss and yellowish staining of nails, skin, and cord (Miller, Fanaroff, & Martin, 1997b). About 80% of term infants born with meconium aspiration have signs of undernutrition; only about 2% show signs of infection. However, about 80% of *preterm* infants with meconium aspiration have signs of infection (Gregory, 1996).

Nursing and Collaborative Management. Management of the neonate at risk for meconium aspiration syndrome begins with the removal of meconium that is in the neonate's airways before the first breath is taken. As the head is delivered, upper airway suctioning is performed by the obstetrician. Both the nose and the pharynx are suctioned to clean any remaining meconium. After the neonate's delivery, and ideally before the first breath, the trachea is suctioned under direct visualization. In direct visualization of the trachea, the physician uses a laryngoscope to examine the neonate's airway. With the laryngoscope, the vocal cords can be seen and any meconium found can be suctioned out. After suctioning, the neonate will require 100% oxygen administered with bag and mask ventilation.

Agressive suctioning prior to delivery and by endotracheal intubation will not always prevent meconium aspiration syndrome (Hageman et al., 1988). If, despite interventions in the delivery room, the neonate develops meconium aspiration syndrome, transfer to a neonatal intensive care nursery is necessary. Management of the neonate's respiratory distress is aimed at eliminating hypoxia, hypercarbia (high levels of carbon dioxide in the blood), and acidosis. Many of these neonates require intubation and mechanical ventilation. Because of the sticky and viscous nature of meconium, it may be difficult to provide adequate ventilation through the clogged airways. To prevent pushing meconium into smaller airways, positive-pressure resuscitation should not be performed until adequate laryngotracheal toilet has been done (Miller, Fanaroff, & Martin, 1997b).

The presence of meconium in the smaller air passages and the increased pressures needed to deliver the breaths can place the neonate at risk for a pneumothorax, which occurs when air enters the pleural space. The air leak may result when alveoli rupture in the presence of high ventilatory pressures. Signs of a pneumothorax include sudden cyanosis; respiratory distress including tachypnea, grunting, and flaring; unequal breath sounds; unequal chest expansion; a shift in where the apical heartbeat is auscultated; bradycardia; sudden decrease in the arterial oxygen level; sudden increase in the arterial carbon dioxide level; and hypotension. Sometimes a pneumothorax is seen on the x-ray, although the neonate is asymptomatic. This neonate must be observed closely for future signs of respiratory distress.

The neonate who develops severe symptoms related to a pneumothorax must be treated swiftly. Management includes the placement of a chest tube, which can be done at the bedside. A chest tube is a catheter that is placed into the pleural space under sterile conditions. After placement, the catheter is connected to low continuous suction via a special canister. The placement of the chest tube and the administration of additional oxygen usually resolve the pneumothorax in 24 to 72 hours (Martin & Fanaroff, 1993). Important nursing interventions include continual assessment of the neonate's respiratory status and monitoring of the chest tube and chest drainage system to ensure that it remains functional. Any alteration in the neonate's condition should be reported to the physician immediately.

Because meconium is a foreign substance in the lungs, it can be extremely irritating to the lung tissue. The inflammation that results can be treated with steroids. The irritation that develops in the lungs can also place the neonate at risk for developing sec-

ondary respiratory infections, which are treated with antibiotics (Avery, Fletcher, & MacDonald, 1994). Meconium may inhibit the function of surfactant, and exogenous surfactant therapy may be used (Miller, Fanaroff, & Martin, 1997b).

Meconium aspiration will result in asphyxiation, if the neonate's airways remain blocked by the sticky substance and adequate ventilation cannot be initiated. This is a medical emergency, demanding immediate resuscitation efforts. Infants with meconium aspiration syndrome may be candidates for extracorporeal membrane oxygenation (ECMO) therapy (Cornish, 1993). ECMO is used for infants who are in respiratory failure and who do not respond to conventional pulmonary interventions. ECMO involves the use of a complex machine that allows blood to be oxygenated while bypassing the infant's lungs; it gains time while healing occurs. While on ECMO, infants require anticoagulation; this necessary therapy can increase the risk of hemorrhage elsewhere in the infant's body, especially the brain. For this reason, the benefits are weighed against the risks for small or premature infants. ECMO therapy is generally given from 3 to 10 days and is delivered in a special intensive care setting. It differs from the heart-lung bypass used in the operating room.

Parents of the neonate who develops meconium aspiration syndrome will have questions in the delivery room as they see the neonate being whisked away to be suctioned. If meconium aspiration is a potential risk for a neonate, the parents should be made aware of the necessary treatments to expect after delivery. Parents will need additional support and information if the neonate develops severe respiratory distress and requires transfer to an intensive care nursery.

▶ PAIN

At one time it was believed that neonates, particularly premature neonates, were not neurologically developed enough to experience pain. This belief and concern about the effects of analgesics and anesthetics led to invasive procedures being performed without attention to pain management for the newborn. Premature and term neonates, however, do experience pain, and physiologic responses indicate distress (Stevens, Johnston, & Grunau, 1995). Such physiologic responses include release of catecholamines and cortisol; changes in heart and respiratory rates, which can increase oxygen consumption; increased glucose consumption and metabolic rate, which results in greater energy demands; and elevated blood pressure, which contributes to increased intracranial pressure. Even a routine procedure, such as a heel stick to obtain a blood sample, elicits physiologic responses (Stevens & Johnston, 1994).

Pain is an additional burden to already stressed neonates and contributes to the risk of such complications as hypoxia and PIVH (Blackburn & Lopez, 1992). Long-term effects of neonatal pain on personality and psychological development are unknown, although the structures for long-term memory are well developed in the newborn period (Stevens, Johnston, & Grunau, 1995).

► Management

Health care providers must identify pain as a priority in the care of newborns, especially premature, sick neonates. First, the staff needs to identify potential sources of pain, such as necrotizing enterocolitis, invasive procedures, such as surgical insertion of an intravenous line, and even certain ways of handling an infant.

The staff must be alert to responses in the neonate that may indicate pain (Blackburn & Lopez, 1992).

- Motor responses (generalized motor activity, changes in motor tone, pulling away, thrashing, wiggling, etc.)
- Facial expressions (grimace, cry face, wincing, etc.)
- Vocalizations (cry, whimper)
- Sleep–wake activity disturbance (agitation, lethargy, restlessness, changes in activity, inability to sustain state)
- Autonomic responses (changes in heart or respiratory rate, decreased oxygen saturation, apnea, increased ventilatory needs, changes in

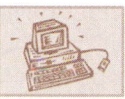 *Research Abstract*

Physiological Responses of Premature Infants to Pain

The goal of this study was to describe the physiologic responses (heart rate, oxygen saturation, and intracranial pressure) of premature infants to an acute tissue-damaging stimulus (a routine heel stick procedure). A convenience sample of 124 premature infants between 32 and 34 weeks' gestational age were studied during four phases of the procedure, i.e., a baseline observation, warming of the heel, heel stick, and heel squeezing. The effects of the infants' behavioral states and severity of illness were also considered. Results indicated that preterm infants of 32 to 34 weeks' gestation did have physiologic responses to heel-lancing. Several physiologic responses changed significantly during sticking and squeezing, which were the most invasive phases. Among their findings, the researchers observed that infants in a quiet sleep state at the time of the procedure evidenced significant differences in all physiologic variables between the baseline and warming phases of the procedure. The researchers suggested that in premature infants, even as small a procedure as heel-warming or handling may be invasive enough to initiate the sympathetic stress response. They also suggested that behavioral state is an important factor to consider when evaluating the premature infant's physiologic response to tissue-damaging stimuli.

Application to Practice

Neonatal intensive care is an invasive environment for premature infants. Heel sticks are only one example of stressful procedures that are done in the provision of daily care. Unlike adults or older children, premature infants cannot voice their responses to noxious stimuli. Recently, attention has focused on premature infants' physiologic and behavioral responses to painful stimuli. This study has many implications for nursing practice. Nurses need to be alert for physiologic responses that may further compromise fragile infants, to consider ways to minimize unpleasant handling of premature infants, and to devise strategies that promote comfort and soothe premature infants during and after procedures. The study focuses attention on the need for additional research on such topics as premature infants' responses to daily care and pain management in the intensive care nursery.

Source: Stevens, B.J., & Johnston, C.C. (1994). Physiological responses of premature infants to a painful stimulus. Nursing Research, 43, 226–231.

carbon dioxide level, increased blood pressure, hyperglycemia, increased intracranial pressure, increased serum cortisol, etc.)

Pain management evolves from an understanding of each neonate's unique situation. Care is organized to minimize pain during procedures, and an infant is handled gently. Procedures are coordinated with the infant state when possible so that a sleeping infant is not startled awake, for example, with a needle stick.

Anesthesia and analgesia are used judiciously. Nonpharmacologic interventions may enhance the therapeutic effects of pharmacologic agents and help manage mild to moderate pain. Such interventions may include providing a pacifier, swaddling, reducing environmental stimulation, and holding and comforting the infant.

▶ DEVELOPMENTAL CARE FOR PRETERM INFANTS

The NICU is a stressful environment for the preterm infant. The baby-unfriendly NICU world of lights, noise, frequent procedures, and handling in an intensive care setting that knows no day or night are believed to have negative effects on the development of these neonates (Als, Lawhon, Duffy, McAnulty, Gibes-Grossman, & Blickman, 1994; Brown & Heerman, 1997). A well known initiative, the Neonatal Individualized Developmental Care and Assessment Program (NIDCAP), was devised by Als and colleagues (1986) to alter the neonatal environment to better meet the unique developmental needs of each infant. NIDCAP interventions are developed to decrease the infant's unnecessary exposure to light and noise; regulate the amount of medical and nursing handling; promote the use of special positioning techniques that improve cerebral venous return and provide boundaries to improve motor, autonomic, and state stability; encourage parental participation and educate parents so they can provide interventions that minimize stress and maximize the quality

of interactions. Specific interventions include reorganizing the infant's immediate environment so that rest and sleep can occur; clustering care so the infant is not constantly being interrupted; educating parents about the benefits of snuggling with the infant through "kangaroo care"; and involving parents in caretaking activities for their babies. Specialized training is available for a program such as NIDCAP. Brown and Heermann (1997) found that implementing developmental care for preterm infants, when only part of the staff was trained, was associated with such positive outcomes as decreased incidence of intraventricular hemorrhage, fewer days of ventilatory support, shorter hospitalization, and greater weight gain among the premature infants studied. (See Research Abstract.)

Nurses can implement the principles of developmental care in their own settings (Brown & Heermann, 1997). For example, positioning and gravity are believed to have negative impact on neuromuscular development of VLBW infants. Short and colleagues (1996) studied the effects of swaddling (a technique of wrapping an infant in a blanket to keep upper and lower extremities in flexion with hands positioned near the mouth) versus standard positioning (routine nursery prone, lateral and supine positions, supported by blanket rolls when needed) upon VLBW infants. Their results indicated that swaddling as a positioning technique may enhance neuromuscular development of the VLBW infant.

By assessing their own NICU environment, identifying special needs and risk factors of each preterm infant client, and recognizing ways in which the NICU's practices and environment support or hinder the newborn's experience, nurses can better meet the developmental needs of preterm infants. In addition to environmental changes, developmental care includes observational skills, accurate interpretation of observations, and ability to tailor developmentally supportive care to the needs of each infant. Attending educational programs and networking with colleagues who successfully implement developmentally centered care can help staff evolve strategies for an infant-centered initiative in their own NICUs.

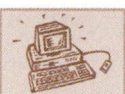

Research Abstract

The Effect of Developmental Care on Preterm Infant Outcome

Developmental care has been linked to positive outcomes for premature infants housed within the stressful environment of the NICU. The Neonatal Individualized Developmental Care and Assessment Program (NIDCAP) provides a model to address NICU stresses and improve outcomes for these infants. However, the training for NIDCAP can be costly in time and money. This study analyzed the effects on neonatal outcome if only 10% of the staff received training. The study used a retrospective, comparative design; outcome measures were collected through a chart review. The sample consisted of 25 preterm infants less than 1500 g who were cared for during the NIDCAP implementation and training period. They were matched for gestational age and birth weight with infants in the NICU before the study. The nurses who received the training provided inservice education for other interested staff. Results of the study indicated that NIDCAP infants had significantly fewer and less severe intraventricular hemorrhages, fewer days of ventilatory support, shorter hospitalizations and a higher rate of weight gain than the infants in the NICU before NIDCAP.

Application to Practice

Through the development of the technology that allowed preterm babies to survive, the role of stressful factors, related to the NICU itself, and the importance of meeting the unique developmental needs of each tiny baby have been overlooked. Developmental care is a very practical and logical way to care for infants. The researchers demonstrate how an actual established program can be modified for a different clinical setting. The study also highlights the importance of evaluating modifications through research. The authors do identify limitations related to a small study size. However, their practice-based research has cost saving implications for developmentally based care approaches in NICUs.

Source: Brown, L.D., & Heermann, J.A. (1997). The effect of developmental care on preterm infant outcome. Applied Nursing Research, 10(4), 190–197.

Critical Thinking in Care Planning

Care of the Preterm Infant

Following spontaneous rupture of her membranes at 32 weeks of gestation, Wendy Harris, age 27, G1P1, delivered a live male neonate weighing 1500 g (3 pounds 5 oz). The neonate's physical appearance and behaviors were appropriate for gestational age. No maternal or paternal history of infection, drug use, or other risk factors for preterm delivery could be identified. Since birth 3 days ago, Baby Robert has been cared for in the neonatal intensive care unit because of his prematurity. Although he has been progressing well, he has required 35% supplemental oxygen via an oxyhood. His pulse oximetry reading is 94%. His heart rate is 140 to 150; his respiratory rate is 40 to 50 with no signs of respiratory distress. His temperature is maintained at 98.0°F on a radiant warmer. Wendy and her husband, Steve, want the neonate to be breastfed and spend most of each day or evening at his bedside.

▶ Assessment

- Birth weight 1500 g
- Respiratory assessment: neonate born at 32 weeks of gestation; receiving 35% warmed, humidified oxygen in oxyhood; neonate on radiant warmer
- Respirations 40 to 50; heart rate 140 to 150
- No retractions, nasal flaring, or grunting
- Pink skin color without any cyanosis
- Pulse oximetry reading: 94%
- Neonate unable to feed via nipple because of oxygen therapy and immature sucking reflex at 32 weeks of gestation; IV therapy in progress; gavage fed

- Temperature 98°F
- Bilirubin levels of neonate of 32 weeks of gestation: cord bili 1.5, bilirubin 4.0 on second day
- Skin assessment: thin skin with some adipose tissue; no areas of skin breakdown
- Mother expresses desire to breastfeed neonate
- Mother visits neonate often and spends most of each day and evening with neonate

Nursing Diagnosis

Alteration in respiration, related to birth at 32 weeks of gestation

Expected Client/Family Outcomes	Nursing Action/Intervention	Evaluation
Neonate will maintain respiratory status with progression to room air before discharge.	Monitor respiratory effort. Report and record respiratory rate, presence of retractions, grunting, flaring, cyanosis. Auscultate breath sounds every 2 hours as needed. *Rationale:* Assessment of respiratory status allows for prompt identification of respiratory distress, treatments to be modified or maintained, and progress to be shared among health care providers.	Neonate's respiratory status continues to improve. Neonate no longer requires oxygen supplementation and oxyhood to maintain normal respiratory status.

Critical Thinking in Care Planning continued

Nursing Diagnosis

Altered nutrition, related to oxygen therapy and prematurity

Expected Client/Family Outcomes	Nursing Action/Intervention	Evaluation
After initial weight loss (≥10%), neonate will demonstrate appropriate weight gain after initiation of gavage feeding.	Check daily weights on same scale with neonate completely undressed. Record results and report weight changes. *Rationale:* Weight changes reflect nutritional status and progress.	After initial weight loss of 10% of body weight, neonate gains weight appropriately; normal nutritional status is maintained.
	Monitor intake and output; weigh diapers; assess specific gravity, skin turgor, mucous membranes, and fontanelles. *Rationale:* Hydration status is monitored so adequate hydration can be prescribed.	Normal hydration status is maintained.
	Continue IV therapy using an infusion pump. *Rationale:* Infusion pumps allow for safe administration of fluids.	IV therapy via infusion pump maintains hydration status.
	Initiate gavage feedings using breast milk pumped by mother and fortified prior to feeding. *Rationale:* Fortified breast milk is well suited to preterm neonate's nutritional needs. Fortifiers are especially useful for neonates under 1500 g.	Neonate tolerates breast milk gavage feeding.
	Check abdominal girth, tube placement, and gastric residuals; hold feedings for residual. *Rationale:* Checking placement, abdominal girth, and residuals allows for safe administration of feeding. Presence of large residual feedings and enlarged abdominal girth may indicate inability to tolerate feedings.	Abdominal girth appropriate; feeding tube placement appropriate and functioning.

Nursing Diagnosis

Ineffective thermoregulation, related to prematurity

Neonate will maintain a normal body temperature of 36.2–37°C in open crib and during kangaroo care prior to discharge.	Check neonate's axillary temperature every 4 hours. *Rationale:* Preterm neonates are at risk for temperature instability. Normal body temperature on radiant warmer reflects proper functioning of equipment.	Neonate maintains normal body temperature while on radiant warmer progressing to open air crib, and during kangaroo care.
	Skin temperature control set on appropriate level to maintain temperature in normal range. *Rationale:* Radiant warmer is used to provide heat safely. Radiant warmer allows for observation and access to neonate on respiratory support.	

(continued)

Critical Thinking in Care Planning *continued*

Expected Client/Family Outcomes	Nursing Action/Intervention	Evaluation
	When appropriate, wean neonate to open air crib by introducing time periods in open air crib, wrapping neonate well and applying hat, and checking temperature and gradually increasing time out of radiant warmer until neonate maintains temperature independently; implement kangaroo care as tolerated. *Rationale:* Weaning process prevents complications associated with sudden body temperature drop for preterm neonates. Kangaroo care provides skin-to-skin contact and fosters parent–infant relationship while maintaining infant's temperature.	

Nursing Diagnosis

Alteration in bilirubin metabolism, related to prematurity

Neonate's bilirubin levels will remain within normal limits.	Observe neonate for presence of jaundice. *Rationale:* Yellowing of skin and sclera indicate increasing bilirubin levels.	Bilirubin levels remain within normal limits.
	Check bilirubin levels every 12 hours; report and record results. *Rationale:* Prompt identification of abnormally high bilirubin levels allows for treatment to prevent complications related to bilirubin toxicity (e.g., neurologic impairment).	
	If bilirubin levels continue to increase, begin phototherapy as ordered. *Rationale:* Phototherapy lowers serum bilirubin levels.	

Nursing Diagnosis

Risk for impaired skin integrity, related to prematurity and neonatal intensive care unit procedures

Neonate will not develop skin breakdown during hospital stay.	Examine neonate's skin for signs of breakdown, especially areas in contact with equipment such as restraints. Document findings; report abnormal findings. *Rationale:* Prompt identification and treatment prevents further skin breakdown. Written records document observations of normality or problems. Maintaining skin integrity is a health team effort.	Neonate's skin remains intact throughout hospitalization.
	Change neonate's position at least every 2 hours. *Rationale:* Position changes minimize skin breakdown related to prolonged pressure.	
	Use minimal tape; avoid tight restraints. *Rationale:* Materials such as tape and pressure from equipment can promote skin breakdown.	
	Use pectin barrier under tape or other protective material as per unit protocol. *Rationale:* Such barriers can reduce chance of skin tears.	

Critical Thinking in Care Planning *continued*

Nursing Diagnosis
Delayed breastfeeding, related to prematurity

Expected Client/Family Outcomes	Nursing Action/Intervention	Evaluation
Mother will maintain lactation prior to initiation of breastfeeding.	Encourage mother's desire to breastfeed. *Rationale:* Mothers of preterm neonates need support to build confidence in decision to breastfeed. Pumping breasts helps establish and maintain lactation while baby is unable to breastfeed.	Mother maintains lactation.
Mother will independently pump and store breast milk for neonate during hospital stay.	Assess mother's knowledge of breast pumping. As needed, provide instruction in use of breast pumps. Provide privacy for pumping when mother visits neonate. Facilitate access to electric breast pumps in hospital. *Rationale:* Breast pumping is necessary to build milk supply in a mother whose neonate is initially unable to breastfeed.	Mother pumps breast milk and stores milk, which is then fed to neonate.
	As prescribed, use mother's breast milk in gavage feedings. Add fortifiers as prescribed. *Rationale:* Breast milk provides excellent nutrition for 32-week preterm neonate if fortified.	Mother expresses satisfaction from providing breast milk and breastfeeding; neonate's nutritional needs are met.
Mother will independently breastfeed neonate by discharge.	Provide support and supervision as mother begins breastfeeding neonate. *Rationale:* Effectively breastfeeding a preterm neonate can be difficult. Mothers need expert assistance to learn breastfeeding technique and support to relieve anxiety and build confidence.	By discharge, mother is able to breastfeed neonate independently.

Chapter Highlights

▶ A newborn's gestational age, intrauterine growth, and weight are important indicators of maturity since these data assist health care professionals in predicting potential problems, related to gestational age and size, that the newborn may face.

▶ A premature neonate can be small (less than the 10th percentile), appropriate, or large (greater than the 10th percentile) for gestational age, and birth weight can further be divided into low, moderately low, very low, and extremely low.

▶ With multiple gestations, gestational age and size need to be assessed for each neonate.

▶ An infant born before the end of the 37th week of gestation is considered premature; such factors as technology, regionalization of perinatal and neonatal care, and exogenous surfactant therapy have allowed younger and sicker babies to survive.

▶ The specific nature of problems for premature infants relates to such factors as reasons for prematurity or low birth weight, immaturity of organ systems, and complications arising during NICU care.

▶ Prematurity affects the entire neonate; for example, immature respiratory, cardiovascular, neurologic, and gastrointestinal functioning present unique problems.

▶ The postmature neonate is born after the end of the 42nd week of gestation and is more likely to experience fetal distress during labor and suffer ill effects from prolonged pregnancy.

▶ Pharmacologic and nonpharmacologic interventions to relieve pain and discomfort experienced by the newborn can promote well-being and reduce complications for infants.

▶ Developmental care provides an approach that focuses on reducing environmental stressors for infants, accurately indentifying and interpreting infant cues and behaviors, supporting optimal parent–newborn interaction, and designing care uniquely tailored to the needs of each infant.

After reading the vignette at the beginning of this chapter, use what you have learned to answer these questions.

1. What nursing interventions can be used to care for a premature newborn with necrotizing enterocolitis?

2. What strategies can Eileen Taylor, RN, suggest to promote Gail and Rob Farrell's involvement in their baby's care within the NICU?

3. How can principles of developmental care be applied to care of premature and sick newborns like Luke Farrell?

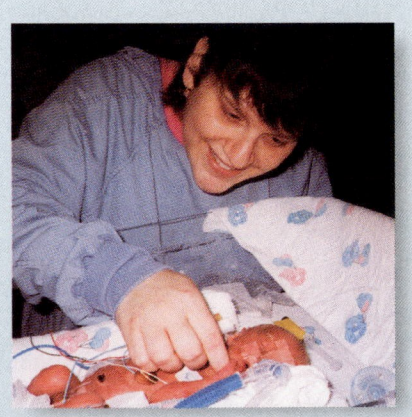

Critical Thinking Questions

► References

Als, H. (1997). Neurobehavioral development of the preterm infant. In A.A. Fanaroff & R.J. Martin (Eds.), *Perinatal-neonatal medicine* (6th ed.) (pp. 964–989). St. Louis: Mosby.

Als, H., Lawhon, G., Brown, G., Gibes, R., Duffy, F.H., McAnulty, G., & Blickman, J.G. (1986). Individualized behavioral and environmental care for the very low birth weight preterm infant at high risk for bronchopulmonary dysplasia: Neonatal intensive care unit and developmental outcome. *Pediatrics, 78,* 1123–1132.

Als, H., Lawhon, G., Duffy, F.H., McAnulty, G.B., Gibes-Grossman, R., & Blickman, J.G. (1994). Individualized developmental care for the very low-birth-weight preterm infant. Medical and neurofunctional effects. *Journal of the American Medical Association, 272,* 853–858.

Andrews, J.D., & Krowchuk, H.V. (1997). Stool patterns of infants diagnosed with necrotizing enterocolitis. *Neonatal Network, 16*(6), 51–57.

Avery, G.B., Fletcher, M.A., & MacDonald, M.G. (1994). *Neonatology: Pathophysiology and management of the newborn* (4th ed.). Philadelphia: Lippincott-Raven.

Ballard, J.L., Khoury, J.C., Wedig, K., Wang, L., Eilers-Walsman, B.L., & Lipp, R. (1991). New Ballard Score, expanded to include extremely premature infants. *Journal of Pediatrics, 119,* 417–423.

Beachy, P., & Deacon, J. (Eds.). (1993). *Core curriculum for neonatal intensive care nursing.* Philadelphia: W.B. Saunders.

Behrman, R.E., & Shiono, P.H. (1997). Neonatal risk factors. In A.A. Fanaroff & R.J. Martin (Eds.), *Perinatal-neonatal medicine* (6th ed.) (pp. 3–12). St. Louis: Mosby.

Bennett, F.C. (1997). The low birth weight, premature infant. In R.T. Gross, D. Spiker, & C.W. Haynes (Eds.), *Helping low birthweight premature babies: The Infant Health Development Program.* Stanford, CA: Stanford University Press.

Blackburn, S.T., & Loper, D.L. (1992). *Maternal, fetal, and neonatal physiology: A clinical perspective.* Philadelphia: W.B. Saunders.

Bland, R.D., & Tooley, W.H. (1996). Persistent respiratory distress syndromes. In A.M. Rudolph, J.I.E. Hoffman, & C.D. Rudolph (Eds.), *Rudolph's pediatrics* (20th ed.) (pp. 1619–1625). Stamford, CT: Appleton & Lange.

Boeckling, A.C. (1992). Exogenous surfactant therapy for premature infants. *Journal of Perinatal and Neonatal Nursing, 6,* 59–66.

Brazelton, T.B. (1984). *Neonatal behavioral assessment scale* (2nd ed.). Philadelphia: J.B. Lippincott.

Brown, L.D., & Heermann, J.A. (1997). The effect of developmental care on preterm infant outcome. *Applied Nursing Research, 10*(4), 190–197.

Cornish, J.D. (1993). Extracorporeal membrane oxygenation for severe cardiorespiratory failure. In J.J. Pomerance & C.J. Richardson (Eds.), *Neonatology for the clinician* (pp. 325–338). Norwalk, CT: Appleton & Lange.

Crissinger, K.D. (1997). Necrotizing enterocolitis. In A.A. Fanaroff & R.J. Martin (Eds.), *Perinatal-neonatal medicine* (6th ed.) (pp. 1333–1337). St. Louis: Mosby.

Cunningham, F.G., MacDonald, P.C., Gant, N.F., Leveno, K.J., Gilstrap, L.C., Hankins, G.D.V., & Clark, S.L. (1997). *Williams obstetrics* (20th ed.). Stamford, CT: Appleton & Lange.

Dubowitz, L.M., Dubowitz, V., & Goldberg, C. (1970). Clinical assessment of gestational age in the newborn infant. *Journal of Pediatrics, 77,* 1–10.

Fanaroff, A.A., & Merkatz, I.R. (1993). Antepartum and intrapartum care of the high risk infant. In M. Klaus & A.A. Fanaroff (Eds.), *Care of the high-risk neonate* (4th ed.) (pp. 1–37). Philadelphia: W.B. Saunders.

Gregory, G.A. (1996). Meconium aspiration. In A.M. Rudolph, J.I.E.

Hoffman, & C.D. Rudolph (Eds.), *Rudolph's pediatrics* (20th ed.) (p. 1605). Stamford, CT: Appleton & Lange.

Grisemer, A.N. (1990). Apnea of prematurity: Current management and nursing implications. *Pediatric Nursing, 16,* 606–611.

Hack, M. (1997). Follow up for high risk neonates. In A.A. Fanaroff & R.J. Martin (Eds.), *Perinatal-neonatal medicine* (6th ed.) (pp. 952–957). St. Louis: Mosby.

Hageman, J.R., Conley, M., Francis, K., Stenske, J., Wolf, I., Santi, V., & Farrell, E.E. (1988). Delivery room management of meconium staining of the amniotic fluid and the development of meconium aspiration syndrome. *Journal of Perinatology, 8,* 127–131.

Heymann, M.A., Teitel, D.F., & Leibman, J. et al. (1993). The heart. In M. Klaus & A.A. Fanaroff (Eds.), *Care of the high-risk neonate* (4th ed.) (pp. 345–373). Philadelphia: W.B. Saunders.

Kitterman, J.A. (1996). Necrotizing enterocolitis. In A.M. Rudolph, J.I.E. Hoffman, & C.D. Rudolph (Eds.), *Rudolph's pediatrics* (20th ed.) (pp. 257–260). Stamford, CT: Appleton & Lange.

Martin, R.J., & Fanaroff, A.A. (1997). The respiratory distress syndrome and its management. In A.A. Fanaroff & R.J. Martin (Eds.), *Perinatal-neonatal medicine* (6th ed.) (pp. 1018–1028). St. Louis: Mosby.

Martin, R.J., Fanaroff, A.A., & Klaus, M.H. (1993). Respiratory problems. In M. Klaus & A.A. Fanaroff (Eds.), *Care of the high-risk neonate* (4th ed.) (pp. 228–259). Philadelphia: W.B. Saunders.

Miller, M.J., Fanaroff, A.A., & Martin, R.J. (1997a). Respiratory disorders in term and preterm infants. In A.A. Fanaroff & R.J. Martin (Eds.), *Perinatal-neonatal medicine* (6th ed.) (pp. 1040–1065). St. Louis: Mosby.

Miller, M.J., Fanaroff, A.A., & Martin, R.J. (1997b). Meconium aspiration syndrome. In A.A. Fanaroff & R.J. Martin (Eds.), *Perinatal-neonatal medicine* (6th ed.). St. Louis: Mosby.

Nagey, D.A., & Viscardi, R.M. (1993). Retarded intrauterine growth. In J.J. Pomerance & C.J. Richardson (Eds.), *Neonatology for the clinician* (pp. 83–92). Norwalk, CT: Appleton & Lange.

Papile, L., & Brann, B. (1993). Intracranial hemorrhage: Periventricular, intraventricular hemorrhage. In J.J. Pomerance & C.J. Richardson (Eds.), *Neonatology for the clinician* (pp. 425–435). Norwalk, CT: Appleton & Lange.

Perlstein, P.H. (1997). Physical environment. In A.A. Fanaroff & R.J. Martin (Eds.), *Perinatal-neonatal medicine* (6th ed.) (pp. 481–497). St. Louis: Mosby.

Phelps, D.L. (1997). Retinopathy of prematurity. In A.A. Fanaroff & R.J. Martin (Eds.), *Perinatal-neonatal medicine* (6th ed.) (pp. 1701–1706). St. Louis: Mosby.

Phibbs, R.H. (1996). Supportive care of the premature and sick newborn. In A.M. Rudolph, J.I.E. Hoffman, & C.D. Rudolph (Eds.), *Rudolph's pediatrics* (20th ed.) (pp. 229–237). Stamford, CT: Appleton & Lange.

Pomerance, J.J., & Richardson, C.J. (1993). *Neonatology for the clinician.* Norwalk, CT: Appleton & Lange.

Reed, M.D., & Blumer, J.L. (1997). Pharmacologic treatment of the fetus. In A.A. Fanaroff & R.J. Martin (Eds.), *Perinatal-neonatal medicine* (6th ed.) (pp. 157–187). St. Louis: Mosby.

Revenis, M.E., & Johnson, L.A. (1994). Multiple gestations. In G.B. Avery, M.A. Fletcher, & M.G. MacDonald (Eds.), *Neonatology: Pathophysiology and management of the newborn* (4th ed.) (pp. 417–426). Philadelphia: Lippincott-Raven.

Rozmus, C. (1992). Periventricular-intraventricular hemorrhage in the newborn. *MCN, American Journal of Maternal-Child Nursing, 17,* 74–81.

Rozycki, H.J., & Kirkpatrick, B.V. (1993). New developments in bronchopulmonary dysplasia. *Pediatric Annals, 22,* 532–538.

Short, M.A., Brooks-Brunn, J.A., Reeves, D.S., Yeager, J., & Thorpe, J.A. (1996). The effects of swaddling versus standard positioning on neuromuscular development in very low birth weight infants. *Neonatal Network, 15*(4), 25–31.

Simpson, K.F. (1997). Preterm birth in the United States: Current issues and future perspectives. *Journal of Perinatal and Neonatal Nursing, 10*(4), 11–15.

Sims, L.M., Verdeyen-Douglass, J., & Pomerance, J. (1993). Diseases mimicking infection in the newborn. In J.J. Pomerance & C.J. Richardson (Eds.), *Neonatology for the clinician* (pp. 211–229). Norwalk, CT: Appleton & Lange.

Stevens, B.J., & Johnston, C.C. (1994). Physiological responses of premature infants to a painful stimulus. *Nursing Research, 43,* 226–231.

Stevens, B.J., Johnston, C.C., & Grunau, R.V.E. (1995). Issues of assessment of pain and discomfort in neonates. *Journal of Obstetric, Gynecologic, and Neonatal Nursing, 24*(9), 849–855.

Stevenson, D.K., Petersen, K.R., Yates, B.L., Benitz, W.E., & Gale, R. (1988). Outcome of neonates with birth weights of less than 801 grams. *Journal of Perinatology, 8,* 82–87.

Weidemann, H.-R., Kunze, J., & Grosse, F.-R. (1997). *Clinical syndromes* (3rd ed.). St. Louis: Mosby-Year Book.

Wung, J. (1993). Mechanical ventilation using conventional infant respirators. In J.J. Pomerance & C.J. Richardson (Eds.), *Neonatology for the clinician* (pp. 279–309). Norwalk, CT: Appleton & Lange.

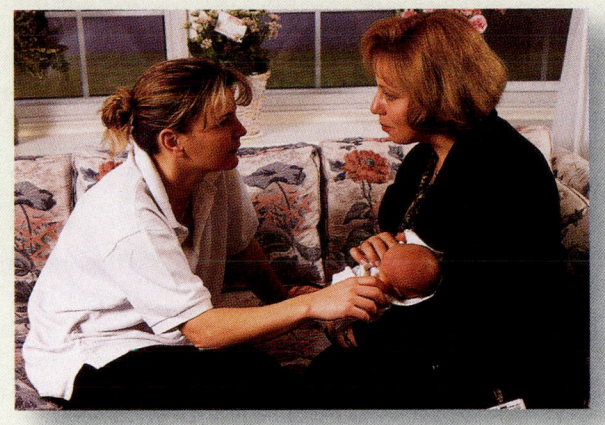

Claire Watson, NP, MSN, is conducting a home care visit with Brenda Dillon and her 1-week-old daughter Meredith. Meredith was diagnosed with hyperbilirubinemia 36 hours after her birth and received phototherapy in the newborn nursery. When she was discharged, Brenda and her husband Michael were instructed on the use of a home phototherapy unit for Meredith. The nurse has been visiting the Dillons daily to check on both Brenda and Meredith and to obtain a blood sample from the baby for serum bilirubin level testing.

Holding the baby in her arms, the nurse tells Brenda that Meredith's bilirubin level is returning to normal and asks her if she has any questions. Brenda, while stroking Meredith's cheek, looks at the nurse and states, "I'm so relieved that she's getting better. It's really been helpful having you visit these past few days. I hope that we'll be able to manage any other problems Meredith may have as well as this one." ■

34

Community-Based Nursing During the Postpartum Period

Childbirth is one of the most common causes of hospital admission in the United States (Germano & Bernstein, 1997). Increased focus on health care cost containment in the early 1990s led to programs designed to shorten typical postdelivery hospitalizations (Brooten et al., 1996; Germano & Bernstein, 1997). As the length of the hospital stay for the postpartum woman and newborn has been reduced, community-based nursing services have moved to the forefront as a key component in postdelivery care. These changes in postpartum care have necessitated the refinement of the practice standards used by maternal–child home care nurses.

▶ GOALS OF COMMUNITY-BASED CARE DURING THE POSTPARTUM PERIOD

Postpartum community-based nursing care focuses on the identification and treatment of postpartum complications, client and family education, and health promotion for both mother and baby (Williams & Cooper, 1996). The direct clinical nursing postpartum and newborn assessments and interventions must meet established standards of care whether they be completed in the hospital or at home. The home nursing visit, like in-hospital postpartum nursing care, includes maternal and newborn physical assessments, planned interventions and detailed education (see box

entitled Components of the Home Visit for the Postpartum Family). Therefore, the nurse providing the postpartum home care visit must demonstrate competency in the care of both the mother and newborn. (see box entitled Key Components of a Home Nursing Assessment).

▶ THE SETTING

The postpartum community-based care visit is completed in a location most convenient for the woman and her family. Most women return to their own home following discharge while others stay with extended family members. Once the nurse confirms the mother's address and arrives at the home, she must identify an area in the home conducive to privacy for the completion of the assessment and teaching. For example, the nurse may recommend that the living room sofa be the best place for the assessment of a postpartum woman with a cesarean section to avoid unnecessary trips upstairs. The nurse may need to take additional steps to close the curtains, lock the door, and obtain a sheet to assure the woman's privacy during the exam. When examining the newborn, the nurse may choose to use the area in the home where the parents change and dress the infant. This provides the nurse the opportunity to demonstrate strategies to keep the infant safe, such as keeping her hand on the infant at all times and, to

▶ COMPONENTS OF THE HOME VISIT FOR THE POSTPARTUM FAMILY

- Inform the family about the purpose of the nursing visit.
- Establish a time to schedule the visit at the family's convenience.
- Obtain written consent for the skilled nursing services to be provided.
- Obtain a physician's order for procedures or treatments such as blood tests.
- Obtain a complete health history for both mother and neonate.
- Perform complete physical assessment for the mother including vital signs, breast exam, fundal height, lochia, and episiotomy or abdominal incision if present.
- Perform complete physical assessment for the neonate including vital signs, weight, hydration, bowel and bladder functions, and color.
- Give treatments or perform procedures, such as a PKU blood test, ordered for the neonate.

- Assess the safety of the home environment including the presence of adequate utility services, food, and accommodations, such as a crib.
- Assess home equipment such as a breast pump for safety and proper usage.
- Identify medications prescribed for mother and neonate and assess client's knowledge and ability to follow the physician's directions.
- Assess client's ability to provide appropriate routine and emergency care.
- Identify client's knowledge base and continue teaching plan begun in hospital.
- Develop plans for subsequent visits if authorized.
- Evaluate for other family concerns and dynamics.
- Provide the family with a list of community resources and telephone numbers.

► KEY COMPONENTS OF A HOME NURSING ASSESSMENT

MATERNAL

Physical Assessment
- Temperature
- Heart rate
- Respiratory rate
- Blood pressure

Abdominal Assessment
- Fundal height
- Incisions

Perineal Assessment
- Lochia
- Episiotomy
- Hemorrhoids

Breast Assessment

Nutritional Assessment
- Hydration

Breastfeeding Assessment
- Technique
- Positioning
- Support

Psychosocial Assessment
- Mother–infant attachment
- Mother–father relationship
- Family support

Environmental Assessment
- Home safety

NEWBORN

Physical Assessment
- Axillary temperature
- Weight
- Length
- Apical heart rate
- Respiratory rate
- Head circumference
- Chest circumference

Respiratory Assessment

Neurologic Assessment

Nutritional Assessment
- Breastfed
- Bottlefed
- Feeding patterns
- Hydration

Skin Assessment
- Birthmarks
- Rashes
- Color
- Jaundice

Genitourinary Assessment
- Vaginal discharge
- Circumcision

Psychosocial Assessment
- Parental–newborn attachment
- Family support

Environmental Assessment
- Home safety

maintain good hygiene, washing her hands after diaper changes.

► CLIENT GROUP

The postpartum home care visit focuses on the well-being of the mother and newborn. However, since the visit is in the home, the nurse often has access to the woman's immediate family, extended family, and other friends and supporters. It is imperative that the nurse's initial assessment of the family includes determining who her visit and teaching should include. Religious, cultural, and social differences affect how

the mother and family members deal with the postpartum period and therefore how each participate in the home care visit (Narayan, 1997).

► THE ENVIRONMENT

One of the most important skills of the community-based nurse is the ability to assess the environment (Narayan & Tennant, 1997). After hospital discharge, clients realize that their home may not be as comfortable or as easy as they remember (Narayan & Tennant, 1997). The postpartum woman's physical discomforts place new demands on her when she is in her own home.

The home care nurse must assess the environment to be sure that the home environment:

1. Meets the client's needs
2. Keeps the client safe
3. Promotes a sense of well-being in the client.

The Joint Commission on Accreditation of Healthcare Organizations (JCAHO) requires home care organizations to demonstrate assessments of safety in the home for every home care client (Joint Commission on Accreditation of Healthcare Organizations, 1997). Minimally this includes fire resource, electrical safety, environmental and mobility safety, bathroom safety, and medication safety.

The community-based nurse is always a guest in the client's home and therefore must demonstrate respect for the client's home while providing necessary input about the environment. The home care nurse often begins this assessment by observing the environment to see if it meets the client's basic survival needs (Narayan & Tennant, 1997) (see box entitled Key Components of a Home Care Environmental Assessment).

The maternal–child home care nurse must assess the environment for both mother and baby. For example, consider the maternal–child nurse who arrived at the home of the postpartum woman discharged home 3 days following a cesarean section. The woman was alone all day until her husband returned from work. The house had one bathroom on the second floor. The kitchen and living room are on the first floor. This woman was overwhelmed with trying to go up and down the stairs to use the bathroom every few hours. She did not want to stay upstairs since she had few support persons to assist her in meal preparation and bringing liquids to drink.

The nurse used the opportunity to teach the woman about postpartum activity, nutrition, and hydration as a way to recommend alternatives to the woman's current routine at home. Since the woman strongly preferred to stay downstairs during the day, the nurse was able to recommend the use of a portable commode while on the first floor. The woman was able to ask her sister to stop in for short visits during the day to empty her commode. Her husband assisted with the commode when he returned from work. While perhaps an unusual solution to this postpartum woman's environmental challenges, this example illustrates the important role of the community-based nurse in considering the safety of the environment in the care of the client.

► PATERNAL ROLES IN POSTPARTUM COMMUNITY-BASED NURSING VISITS

Shortened postpartum hospital stays can limit true opportunities to provide teaching and guidance to fathers. Anderson (1996) used a qualitative research approach to ask new fathers open-ended questions

---

► KEY COMPONENTS OF A HOME CARE ENVIRONMENTAL ASSESSMENT

PHYSIOLOGIC AND SURVIVAL NEEDS

- Food
- Fluids
- Eating
- Elimination and toileting
- Hygiene, bathing, and grooming
- Clothing and dressing
- Rest and sleep
- Medications
- Shelter

SAFETY AND SECURITY

- Mobility and fall prevention
- Fire and burn prevention
- Crime and injury prevention

LOVE AND BELONGING

- Caregiver
- Communication
- Family, friends, and pets

SELF-ESTEEM, SELF-ACTUALIZATION

- Enjoyable and meaningful activities

Source: Narayan & Tennant, 1997.

about their relationships with their newborn. The study found that fathers need reassurance that their relationship with their infants may evolve more slowly than the mother–infant relationship, and that fathers need direction, opportunity, and support to develop their relationship with the infant. Postpartum home nursing visits provide a valuable opportunity for nurses to interact with fathers.

The postpartum community-based nursing visit is ideally scheduled at a time when both mother and father are available. This means that they may occur in the evening or on the weekend. During the visit, the nurse must welcome the father in all aspects of the assessment of the mother, infant, and associated teaching. Again, culture and social differences in families will predict the role of both the father and mother and how they will each best interact with the home care nurse.

Strategies such as asking the father to hold the infant as the nurse takes vital signs or requesting the father's help in redressing the infant after the assessment provide the nurse opportunities to ask and answer questions about the care of the infant.

▶ POSTPARTUM AND INFANT CARE TEACHING STRATEGIES IN THE HOME CARE SETTING

Postpartum women have many concerns and questions about their own recovery and about their newborn. These questions can begin in the prenatal period, continue through the postpartum hospital stay, and follow into discharge to home. The community-based nursing care visit provides an opportunity to identify and meet these educational needs.

Moran, Holt, and Martin (1997) surveyed primipara and multipara women about their perceived need for more self-care and baby care information. The study found that first-time mothers wanted information on self-care topics such as exercise, diet, nutrition, feelings of fatigue, and resuming normal activities. Multiparas wanted information about getting along with their other children, exercise, diet, nutrition, and feelings of fatigue. The most common baby care topics asked for by both groups included recognizing illness in the baby, learning about the baby's schedule, and calming the baby. First-time mothers wanted more information about baby care topics while multiparas wanted more information about self-care topics. Younger first-time mothers asked more self-care questions whereas younger multipara mothers asked more baby care questions.

The home care nurse must carefully assess the types of concerns that the mother identifies during the home care visit (see boxes entitled Client Education in the Home Setting: Maternal Concerns and Client Education in the Home Setting: Newborn Concerns). Providing direct information for specific questions is important. Nurses in the home can observe and offer guidance as the mother interprets the infant's behaviors and responds successfully. For example, if the mother says, "I know that cry—I am sure he is hungry," the nurse can respond, "You really recognize the differences in his cry." This type of feedback is essential as new mothers master problem solving techniques with their infants (Sullivan, 1997). The home care nurse can refer the mother to printed resources and handouts the hospital staff provided her. Finally, if the mother has additional questions that cannot reasonably be answered during the home care visit, the home care nurse should refer the woman to her physician or the baby's pediatrician for ongoing support.

▶ CLIENT EDUCATION IN THE HOME SETTING: MATERNAL CONCERNS

- Personal care
- Bathing
- Perineal care
- Breast care
- Incisional care
- Nutrition and hydration
- Elimination and bowel movements
- Rest and activity
- Pain relief

- Signs and symptoms of infection
- Lochia
- Postpartum musculoskeletal changes
- Postpartum emotional changes
- Exercise
- Family relationships
- Resumption of sexual activities
- Birth control
- Physician follow-up

▶ CLIENT EDUCATION IN THE HOME SETTING: NEWBORN CONCERNS

- Daily newborn care
- Bathing
- Dressing
- Diapering
- Nutrition
- Breastfeeding
- Formula preparation
- Elimination patterns
- Cord care
- Circumcision care
- Infant sleep and activity

- Newborn safety
- Positioning
- Calming the baby
- Use of bulb syringe and thermometer
- Signs and symptoms of infection
- Signs and symptoms of dehydration
- Normal growth and development
- Physician follow-up
- Immunizations
- PKU test

▶ SPECIALIZED HOME CARE FOR HIGH-RISK INFANTS

The goal of high-risk perinatal care is to prevent premature births and have a positive impact on infant mortality and morbidity. Unfortunately, even the best efforts can fail to prevent the birth of a sick or premature infant. These infants suffer a variety of rather predictable medical problems as a result of prematurity and medical complications (see Chapter 33). Once stabilized in the neonatal intensive care setting, these babies are deemed ready for discharge. This "readiness" is relative for each child and family.

High-risk infants can include any newborn that the interdisciplinary team identifies as requiring

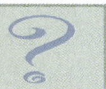

Commonly Asked Questions

Will a nurse come to my home to check on me and my baby after delivery?

Many women receive a home nursing visit as part of the maternity benefits offered by insurance companies. You can contact the Member Services Department at your health insurance company to learn more about maternity and postpartum benefits.

Will I have to pay for the home care visit if it is part of my health insurance benefits?

All insurance plans are different. It is best to call member services to obtain specific information about copayments or deductible requirements that may apply to a home care visit.

I have two other children. Do I have to accept the postpartum home care visit offered by my insurance company?

Clients always have the right to accept or decline care. However, the postpartum home care visit is designed to help support the mother, baby, and family during the transition to home. The home nursing transition visit can provide you a one-on-one opportunity to ask questions and to receive an examination to assure you and your baby are progressing well.

Can I still receive a postpartum home care visit if my insurance company does not offer one?

Postpartum home care visits are usually provided by a local home care agency. You can contact the home care agency directly to inquire about costs of postpartum home care services.

I do not have health insurance. Can someone still come to my home to check on me and the baby?

The social worker may have additional information about postpartum home care programs available for individuals who do not have insurance. Let me call the social worker to come and speak with you.

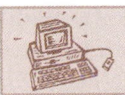

Research Abstract

Enhancing Early Discharge with Home Follow-Up

Early discharge decreases costs of hospital stays, but also decreases the chance for women to learn about mothering from health care providers. A new mother may not have contact with health care providers from the time of discharge until the scheduled newborn or postpartum visit several weeks later. In this pilot project, staff nurses, who usually worked on a hospital's maternity unit, made home follow-up visits to low-risk postpartum women–infant dyads; for reasons of safety and expertise, two nurses (a maternity and a newborn nurse) visited. An assessment interview was done by telephone 24 hours after discharge, and two nurses then made a home visit within 72 hours of the mother's hospital discharge. Mothers received a second follow-up phone call a week later and a second home visit during the third postpartum week. Assessment, teaching, and appropriate referrals were made. The project director, a faculty member from the college of nursing at a health science center, telephoned the project's mothers 6–8 weeks postpartum to assess such factors as satisfaction with hospital stay and follow-up program, adherence to follow-up care, and the need for unscheduled health visits. Of 41 mothers recruited, 29 (71%) of the mother–infant dyads completed the project. An additional 29 mother–infant dyads were randomly selected from the hospital's delivery log, received the usual standard of care, and served as the control group.

The investigators concluded that knowledge deficit related to infant or self-care was an appropriate diagnosis for 97% of the women in the project. Age, educational level, and parity did not seem to affect questions asked or information sought. The project's nurses observed that the older mothers seemed to need the project more than younger mothers, because they had fewer resources available. The control group spent more than 10 times as much for nonroutine health care than the project group. The authors felt that women who were educated about illness in themselves or their infants and who were comfortable contacting a nurse for advice were less likely to have unscheduled health care visits for minor concerns. The investigators also identified such benefits of the home visits as the chance to identify problems and begin interventions. Other outcomes related to the study included very positive responses of the staff nurses who participated in the project, a high level of client satisfaction, and desire expressed by clients to refer others to the hospital because of this service.

Application to Practice

Although a pilot study, this project has important implications for practice. The investigators identify major knowledge deficits in low-risk postpartum women after earlier discharge and the study highlights the need for health assessment and intervention in the home setting during the early postpartum period. In addition to psychosocial benefits, the study documents financial savings and advantages of such a program of well-planned home follow-up. With two nurses at each home visit, staff in other settings might claim that such a program is probably beyond their resources. However, the positive outcomes described in the study, staff and consumer satisfaction, and potential for further income-generating referrals to the sponsoring hospital helps to make the program cost-effective. It could possibly be a model for other such programs.

This study also is an example of successful collaboration between staff at a university hospital and the college of nursing at a health science center. Blending talents of individuals from education and practice backgrounds led to the development of a pilot study and program with many positive outcomes. Such collaboration makes possible research and programs that could not otherwise exist.

Source: Brown, S.G., & Johnston, B.T. (1998). Enhancing early discharge with home follow-up: A pilot project. Journal of Obstetric, Gynecologic, and Neonatal Nursing, 27 (1), 33–38.

specialized care or treatment to assure the infant's well-being. High-risk infants may have a wide range of physical illnesses or familial or social challenges.

High-risk infants have often endured extended stays in intensive care or transitional care units. There is limited ability for parents to get to know their infants with isolettes, intravenous lines, cardiac monitors, and ventilators standing between them. The family will be primarily responsible for care of the infant at home. Therefore, parent visits focus on mastering the clinical skills required to care for the infant at home as outlined in the discharge plan. One technique for educating families prior to the discharge of their high-risk infant is using a **care-by-parent program.** In this program one or both parents live in the hospital for 24 to 48 hours in an area separate from the nursery to simulate a homelike environment. During this time, parents are responsible for the complete care of the infant. Professional nursing staff serve as consultants to the parents should questions arise.

Many high-risk infants and their families require additional care and support at home after discharge. Madigan (1997) describes five categories of infants that benefit from home care services:

1. Technology-dependent infants, which include infants whose regular care and well-being requires the use of technology such as ventilators, tube feedings, or total parenteral nutrition.
2. Infants whose condition makes leaving the home burdensome; e.g., a child whose clothes or dressings make sitting safely in a car seat difficult or impossible.
3. Family comprehension of necessary teaching is questionable; e.g., a young adolescent postpartum mother who would benefit from additional education about the infant's care in the home environment where other family members could best support her.
4. Family follow-up for the infant's care is questionable; e.g., a mother who did not receive any prenatal care prior to delivery and has not identified a pediatrician for the infant's follow-up care prior to discharge. Families who require additional referrals to social services agencies can be included in this group.
5. Families living in outlying areas, far from a tertiary care center, caring for a child with an unusual illness or condition. These infants require regular assessment to identify complications early so travel to the tertiary care center can begin before a crisis occurs (Madigan, 1997).

Community-based nursing services for the high-risk newborn can fall into two categories. First, newborns can receive home nursing visits which are typically one hour long and can be completed one or more times a day (Madigan, 1997). These visits are often used when the infant is receiving intermittent therapy such as IV antibiotics or home phototherapy for hyperbilirubinemia. Second, infants can receive "continuous care" services, which are typically nursing shifts ranging from 4 to 24 hours per day (Madigan, 1997). Continuous home care shifts are used when the infant is receiving complex or multiple therapies such as continuous oxygen therapy, ventilator and tracheostomy care, tube feedings, or IV total parenteral nutrition via a central line.

Home care services are a supportive supplement to a level of care already provided safely by the family. Therefore, involvement of the home care nurse in the child's discharge planning sets the stage for a trusting relationship among the nurse and family members. This provides a framework for the health care team to work with the family to define the skills they must master prior to the infant's discharge. Parents must then receive complete discharge training including return demonstration of critical tasks such as flushing the IV line or suctioning the tracheostomy tube prior to the infant's actual discharge with home care services.

It can be difficult for parents to assume the medical-nursing caregiving role along with their new role as parents (May, 1997). Fatigue, variable schedules, learning new and often technical skills, and interaction with multiple staff members in their home causes added stress for the client.

It is not unusual for parents faced with the complex care of their infant at home to feel overwhelmed. These parents crave normalcy (May, 1997). Families give up privacy when continuous home nursing care begins. While nurses arrive for the designated shifts, parents still worry if the dishes were done, the toys were picked up, or the laundry was folded. Home nursing caregivers may not be consistent day to day, thereby disrupting family life. Usual routines are changed. For example, consider the parents receiving night shift home nursing care for an infant on an apnea monitor. Although a nurse is just a few rooms away, parents may still jump out of bed at the sound of the monitor alarm. Parents may choose to wear clothes to bed rather than pajamas so that they are readily available to the nurse should the alarm go off. This change in routine may affect the parent's personal comfort or sleep patterns, causing additional stress.

Family members change the way they communicate with each other when continuous home care occurs. It is not unusual for day-to-day conversations to consistently include some aspects of the child's care. Parents worry about confronting the nurses about problems with care for fear that the nurse would later not give the child the best care. Disagreements and arguments between parents can be guarded when occurring in front of the home nursing staff. Parents worry about the opinions other nursing staff have about them.

Previous family dynamics can be disrupted by the discharge of a high-risk infant receiving home care. Extended family members struggle with feelings of worry. Siblings of the high-risk infant may feel "lost" in the activity and focus on the infant's complex needs. Parents can feel a loss of control in juggling these family demands along with providing the specialized care their infant needs.

Home care nurses must recognize that even the most talented caregiving parent needs support in learning to develop traditional parenting skills. Nurses should watch for cues when parents seek information or assistance. By providing education and support in regular and consistent ways, parents gain confidence in both their caregiver and parent roles. In a descriptive study, May (1997) studied the process that mothers use to seek help when giving care to low-birth-weight infants at home. The study identified that mothers who perceived themselves as having more resources expressed less sense of burden in caring for their infant at home.

Home care nurses must continue to work to align parents with resources, information, and support to maximize the parents' role as the parent and caregiver. Community health nurses must be knowledgeable about community resources, specialty groups, and funding sources applicable to families with high-risk infants. Families must be educated about state and federal programs from which they and their baby could benefit. Finally, community-based nurses must serve as public advocates for families with high-risk infants by working on legislation and public policy.

▶ HEALTH MAINTENANCE OF THE HIGH-RISK INFANT

One of the major problems facing families is finding a professional to deliver primary pediatric care for their high-risk infant. The hospital or community nurse may help the family locate a community-based pediatrician who can provide the necessary specialized care for the high-risk infant.

Another problem that faces families is establishing an immunization schedule for the infant. The nor-

mal, designated schedule may be altered because of the long hospitalization or repeated minor illnesses. Parents need to be informed that immunizations can be given on an altered schedule. Health care is the major concern of mothers of premature infants after taking the infant home (Brooten et al., 1996). Parents must know what they can safely handle at home, how to handle it, and when to call for professional help.

Safety for the infant in the home is a concern to families of high-risk infants. The community-based nurse must assess the home environment and the infant's state to help parents maintain a safe environment without being overprotective of their child. This assessment includes evaluation of the physical home environment, the parents' ability to competently meet the infant's physiologic needs, and the integrity of the family system in support of the care of the child (Narayan & Tennant, 1997).

Finally, the nurse who visits the home is also in a good position to assess the manner in which the infant is being integrated into the family system. The parent–infant (and sibling–infant) attachment process may be strained because of the burden of care on the family.

As infants with multiple problems receive services from many professionals, coordination of services is essential. Nurses participating in discharge planning and practicing in the community are often the persons who can most effectively coordinate services and who are in the best position to help the family locate and use community resources (Brooten et al., 1996).

▶ ROLE OF THE NURSE DELIVERING CARE IN THE COMMUNITY

Community-based care for childbearing families requires that the nurse be skilled in maternal–child health nursing practices as well as community practice (Williams & Cooper, 1996). The professional nurse who delivers care in the community has a vital role in assuring quality care for mothers and infants in both low-risk and high-risk situations. These nurses support clients in adapting care practices begun in the hospital to the home environment using creative techniques. The nursing role incorporates health promotion, direct care, epidemiology, counseling, and political involvement. The nurse should be conversant with systems theory. This will support the nurse's assessment of both the community and the family.

The nurse should understand the ethnic, political, and demographic makeup of community that his or her agency serves. Community resources (financial, support, therapeutic, and informational) should be identified for the family by the nurse.

The nurse acts as a client advocate in using the political system to influence health care policy. For example, nurses who care for childbearing families may contact legislators to influence health policy for preventive childbearing services as well as high-risk services.

The community nurse must become experienced with establishing a role on the interdisciplinary health care team. The nurse may coordinate care with occupational therapists, physical therapists, nutritionists, and home health care aides.

The home health care aide is one team member who has had an increasing role with pregnant and postpartum women, neonates, and their families. Programs have been developed to prepare already skilled homemaker–home health aides to work specifically with parents and high-risk infants.

Home health aides perform homemaker tasks such as meal preparation for pregnant clients with activity restrictions or medical complications. Home health aides can also ease the postpartum transition for well mothers and well infants. These home health aides perform homemaker tasks as well as assisting with the personal care needs of both mother and infant.

The role of the community nurse and other professionals who work with the family during the infant's transition from newborn nursery or neonatal intensive care to home is frequently to offer practical and emotional support. Helping the family to develop effective crisis management and coping strategies can affect positive long-term care of the low- and high-risk infant. Specific nursing activities include (1) providing information, (2) fostering decision making, (3) helping to identify financial resources and child care support, (4) helping families activate a support system, (5) identifying high-risk respite care programs, and (6) making referrals (such as siblings to therapeutic play programs or day care) (May, 1997). Families who feel prepared with more resources will continue to gain confidence in the care of their at-risk infant and to minimize feeling burdened by the complexity of the care.

▶ WORKING FOR CHANGE

Community-based care for childbearing families has become a priority for the health care system. Nurses are the primary care providers who assume responsibility for home care of mothers, infants, and families. Many low- and high-risk care activities, especially health promotion for healthy childbearing families, should be available in the home. Without, however, a payment system directed toward preventive services and direct reimbursement to nurses for delivery of care in the home, the needs of many childbearing families will go unmet (Madigan, 1997). The nurse must take an active role in changing health policy (Germano & Bernstein, 1997).

Home health care includes the low- and high-risk postpartum family. A nursing discharge plan from the birthing institution helps the nurse who practices in the community provide comprehensive care to the family. In doing so, the nurse uses the components of the nursing process.

Community-based care delivered to low-risk postpartum families includes teaching traditionally done during the stay in the birthing institution. Thus, this care can fill any gap engendered by early discharge of mothers and neonates.

One major change in the home setting is the presence of sick, high-risk, or premature infants, making homes into "mini-NICUs." Prematurity and other newborn conditions can result in a variety of short- and long-term physiologic conditions requiring care of the infant in the home. Nurses must have the specific technical skills needed to care for infants with conditions resulting from prematurity and other problems, including respiratory disorders, cardiovascular disorders, apnea, and neurologic and gastrointestinal disorders. Nurses also require skills to teach parents to deliver care. Specialized nursing skills that are required to care for the infant in the home include managing an infant on an apnea monitor, caring for an infant requiring oxygen therapy or mechanical ventilation, caring for an infant with a tracheostomy, and supervising infant stimulation programs. The nurse has the task of teaching parents these skills, as they will be responsible for the infant's ongoing care.

The family of a high-risk infant must deal with several issues on a day-to-day basis, including financial support, availability of community resources, and treatment strategies. The nurse in the home care setting must be adept at providing direct care while supporting families as they master the complex care of the infant and the use of resources themselves.

Chapter Highlights

▶ Home nursing services are a key component in postdelivery care.

▶ The home nursing visit includes maternal and newborn physical assessments, planned interventions, and detailed education.

▶ Home nursing visits provide a valuable opportunity for the nurse to interact with and provide support and education to fathers and extended family members.

▶ The home nursing visit must address the postpartum woman's questions about both self-care and baby care topics.

▶ High-risk or premature newborns require specialized care and treatment after discharge to ensure the infant's well-being.

▶ Specialized home care for high-risk infants are a supportive supplement to a level of care already provided safely by the family.

▶ Parents caring for high-risk infants who perceive themselves as having more resources feel less burdened by their caregiver role.

▶ The role of the home care nurse incorporates health promotion, direct care, epidemiology, counseling, and political involvement in her professional role and responsibilities.

After reading the vignette at the beginning of this chapter, use what you have learned to answer these questions.

1. What information can Claire Watson, NP, MSN, provide to help Brenda and Michael Dillon care for their baby?

2. What are the benefits of delivering community-based care to the Dillon family?

3. In what ways can the community-based nurse offer emotional support to a family caring for a high-risk newborn?

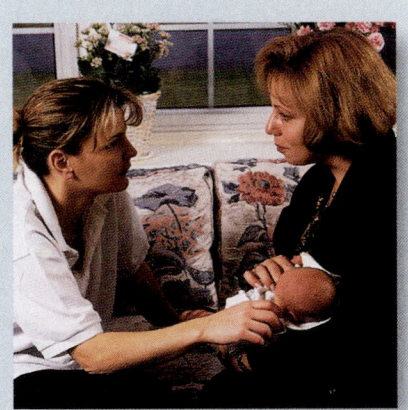

Critical Thinking Questions

► References

Anderson, A.M. (1996). The father–infant relationship: Becoming connected. *Journal of the Society of Pediatric Nursing, 1*(2), 83–91.

Brooten, D., Knapp, H., Boruki, L., Jacobsen, B., Finkler, S., Arnold, L., & Mennuti. (1996). Early discharge and home care after unplanned cesarean birth: Nursing care time. *Journal of Obstetric, Gynecologic, and Neonatal Nursing, 25*(7), 595–600.

Brown, S.G., & Johnston, B.T. (1998). Enhancing early discharge with home follow-up: A pilot project. *Journal of Obstetric, Gynecologic, and Neonatal Nursing, 27*(1), 33–38.

Germano, E., & Bernstein, J. (1997). Home birth and short-stay delivery. Lessons in health care financing for providers of health care for women. *Journal of Nurse-Midwifery, 42*(6), 489–498.

Joint Commission on Accreditation of Healthcare Organizations. (1997). *Comprehensive accreditation manual for home care.* Oak Brook, IL: Author.

Madigan, E.A. (1997). An introduction to pediatric home health care. *Journal of the Society of Pediatric Nursing, 2*(4), 172–178.

May, K.M. (1997). Searching for normalcy: Mothers' caregiving for low birth weight infants. *Pediatric Nursing, 23*(1), 17–20.

Moran, C.F., Holt, V.L., & Martin, D.P. (1997). What do women want to know after childbirth? *Birth, 24*(1), 27–34.

Narayan, M.C. (1997). Cultural assessment in home healthcare. *Home Healthcare Nurse, 15*(10), 663–670.

Narayan, M.C., & Tennant, J. (1997). Environmental assessment. *Home Healthcare Nurse, 15*(11), 798–805.

Sullivan, J. (1997). Learning the baby: A maternal thinking and problem solving process. *Journal of the Society of Pediatric Nursing, 2*(1), 21–28.

Williams, L.R., & Cooper, M.K. (1996). A new paradigm for postpartum care. *Journal of Obstetric, Gynecologic, and Neonatal Nursing, 25*(9), 745–749.

Appendix A

Transfer of Drugs and Other Chemicals into Human Milk

The following group of tables are reproduced here with the permission of *Pediatrics*. The data, which appeared in the January 1994 issue of the journal (pp. 137–146), were obtained by a search of the medical literature. An extensive reference list is published with the journal article. The compilation is a statement of the American Academy of Pediatrics Committee on Drugs.

As with any drug administration, the possibility of individual variation must be taken into account. As a statement that accompanied the tables emphasizes, "The fact that a pharmacologic or chemical agent does not appear on the lists is not meant to imply that it is not transferred into human milk or that it does not have an effect on the infant; it only indicates that there were no reports found in the literature."

▶ TABLE A–1

Drugs that are Contraindicated During Breastfeeding

Drug	Reason for Concern, Reported Sign or Symptom in Infant, or Effect on Lactation
Bromocriptine	Suppresses lactation; may be hazardous to the mother
Cocaine	Cocaine intoxication
Cyclophosphamide	Possible immune suppression; unknown effect on growth or association with carcinogenesis; neutropenia
Cyclosporine	Possible immune suppression; unknown effect on growth or association with carcinogenesis
Doxorubicin[a]	Possible immune suppression; unknown effect on growth or association with carcinogenesis
Ergotamine	Vomiting, diarrhea, convulsions (doses used in migraine medications)
Lithium	One-third to one-half therapeutic blood concentration in infants
Methotrexate	Possible immune suppression; unknown effect on growth or association with carcinogenesis; neutropenia
Phencyclidine (PCP)	Potent hallucinogen
Phenindione	Anticoagulant; increased prothrombin and partial thromboplastin times in one infant; not used in United States

[a]Drug is concentrated in human milk.

▶ **TABLE A-2**

Drugs of Abuse: Contraindicated During Breastfeeding[a]

Drug Reference	Reported Effect or Reasons for Concern
Amphetamine[b]	Irritability, poor sleeping pattern
Cocaine	Cocaine intoxication
Heroin	Tremors, restlessness, vomiting, poor feeding
Marijuana	Only one report in literature; no effect mentioned
Nicotine (smoking)	Shock, vomiting, diarrhea, rapid heart rate, restlessness, decreased milk production
Phencyclidine (PCP)	Potent hallucinogen

[a]The Committee on Drugs strongly believes that nursing mothers should not ingest any compounds listed. Not only are they hazardous to the nursing infant but they are also detrimental to the physical and emotional health of the mother. This list is obviously not complete: no drug of abuse should be ingested by nursing mothers even though adverse reports are not in the literature.
[b]Drug is concentrated in human milk.

▶ **TABLE A-3**

Radioactive Compounds that Require Temporary Cessation of Breastfeeding[a]

Drug	Recommended Time for Cessation of Breastfeeding
Copper 64 (^{64}Cu)	Radioactivity in milk present at 50 hr
Gallium 67 (^{67}Ga)	Radioactivity in milk present for 2 wk
Indium 111 (^{111}In)	Very small amount present at 20 hr
Iodine 123 (^{123}I)	Radioactivity in milk present up to 36 hr
Iodine 125 (^{125}I)	Radioactivity in milk present for 12 days
Iodine 131 (^{131}I)	Radioactivity in milk present 2–14 days, depending on study
Radioactive sodium	Radioactivity in milk present 96 hr
Technetium-99m (^{99}Tc), ^{99m}Tc macroaggregates, ^{99m}Tc O4	Radioactivity in milk present 15 hr to 3 days

[a]Consult nuclear medicine physician before performing diagnostic study so that radionuclide that has shortest excretion time in breast milk can be used. Before study, the mother should pump her breasts and store enough milk in freezer for feeding the infant; after study, the mother should pump her breasts to maintain milk production but discard all milk pumped for the required time that radioactivity is present in milk. Milk samples can be screened by radiology departments for radioactivity before resumption of nursing.

▶ **TABLE A-4**

Drugs Whose Effect on Nursing Infants Is Unknown but May Be of Concern[a]

Drug	Reported or Possible Effect
Antianxiety	
Diazepam	None
Lorazepam	None
Midazolam	—
Perphenazine	None
Prazepam[b]	None
Quazepam	None
Temazepam	—
Antidepressant	
Amitriptyline	None
Amoxapine	None
Desipramine	None
Dothiepin	None
Doxepin	None
Fluoxetine	—
Fluvoxamine	—
Imipramine	None
Trazodone	None
Antipsychotic	
Chlorpromazine	Galactorrhea in adult; drowsiness and lethargy in infant
Chlorprothixene	None

▶ **TABLE A–4** *(continued)*

Drug	Reported or Possible Effect
Antipsychotic *(con't.)*	
Haloperidol	None
Mesoridazine	None
Chloramphenicol	Possible idiosyncratic bone marrow suppression
Metoclopramide[b]	None described; dopaminergic blocking agent
Metronidazole	In vitro mutagen; may discontinue breastfeeding 12–24 hr to allow excretion of dose when single-dose therapy given to mother
Tinidazole	*See* Metronidazole

[a]Psychotropic drugs, the compounds listed under antianxiety, antidepressant, and antipsychotic categories, are of special concern when given to nursing mothers for long periods. Although there are no case reports of adverse effects in breastfeeding infants, these drugs do appear in human milk and thus could conceivably alter short-term and long-term central nervous system function.
[b]Drug is concentrated in human milk.

▶ **TABLE A–5**

Drugs that Have Been Associated with Significant Effects on Some Nursing Infants and Should Be Given to Nursing Mothers with Caution[a]

Drug	Reported Effect
5-Aminosalicylic acid	Diarrhea (1 case)
Aspirin (salicylates)	Metabolic acidosis (1 case)
Clemastine	Drowsiness, irritability, refusal to feed, high-pitched cry, neck stiffness (1 case)
Phenobarbital	Sedation; infantile spasms after weaning from milk containing phenobarbital; methemoglobinemia (1 case)
Primidone	Sedation, feeding problems
Sulfasalazine (salicylazosulfapyridine)	Bloody diarrhea (1 case)

[a]Measure blood concentration in the infant when possible.

▶ **TABLE A–6**

Maternal Medication Usually Compatible with Breastfeeding[a]

Drug	Reported Sign or Symptom in Infant or Effect on Lactation	Drug	Reported Sign or Symptom in Infant or Effect on Lactation
Acebutolol	None	B₆ (pyridoxine)	None
Acetaminophen	None	B₁₂	None
Acetazolamide	None	Baclofen	None
Acitretin	—	Barbiturate	*See* Table A-5
Acyclovir[b]	None	Bendroflumethiazide	Suppresses lactation
Alcohol (ethanol)	With large amounts, drowsiness, diaphoresis, deep sleep, weakness, decrease in linear growth, abnormal weight gain; maternal ingestion of 1 g/kg daily decreases milk ejection reflex	Bishydroxycoumarin (dicumarol)	None
		Bromide	Rash, weakness, absence of cry with maternal intake of 5.4 g/d
Allopurinol	—	Butorphanol	None
Amoxicillin	None	Caffeine	Irritability; poor sleeping pattern; excreted slowly; no effect with usual amount of caffeine beverages
Antimony	—		
Atenolol	None	Captopril	None
Atropine	None	Carbamazepine	None
Azapropazone (apazone)	—	Carbimazole	Goiter
Aztreonam	None	Cascara	None
B₁ (thiamine)	None	Cefadroxil	None
		Cefazolin	None

(continued)

▶ **TABLE A–6** *(continued)*

Drug	Reported Sign or Symptom in Infant or Effect on Lactation	Drug	Reported Sign or Symptom in Infant or Effect on Lactation
Cefotaxime	None	Hydroxychloroquine[b]	None
Cefoxitin	None	Ibuprofen	None
Cefprozil	—	Indomethacin	Seizure (1 case)
Ceftazidime	None	Iodides	May affect thyroid activity
Ceftriaxone	None	Iodine (povidone–iodine/ vaginal douche)	Elevated iodine levels in breast milk, odor of iodine on infant's skin
Chloral hydrate	Sleepiness		
Chloroform	None	Iodine	Goiter
Chloroquine	None	Iopanoic acid	None
Chlorothiazide	None	Isoniazid	None; acetyl metabolite also secreted; ? hepatotoxic
Chlorthalidone	Excreted slowly		
Cimetidine[b]	None	K₁ (vitamin)	None
Cisapride	None	Kanamycin	None
Cisplatin	Not found in milk	Ketorolac	—
Clindamycin	None	Labetalol	None
Clogestone	None	Levonorgestrel	—
Clomipramine	—	Lidocaine	None
Codeine	None	Loperamide	—
Colchicine	—	Magnesium sulfate	None
Contraceptive pill with estrogen/progesterone	Rare breast enlargement; decrease in milk production and protein content (not confirmed in several studies)	Medroxyprogesterone	None
		Mefenamic acid	None
		Methadone	None if mother receiving ≤20 mg/24 h
Cycloserine	None	Methimazole (active metabolite of carbimazole)	None
D (Vitamin)	None; follow up infant's serum calcium level if mother receives pharmacologic doses		
		Methocarbamol	None
Danthron	Increased bowel activity	Methyldopa	None
Dapsone	None; sulfonamide detected in infant's urine	Methyprylon	Drowsiness
		Metoprolol[b]	None
Dexbrompheniramine maleate with d-isoephedrine	Crying, poor sleeping patterns, irritability	Metrizamide	None
		Mexiletine	None
		Minoxidil	None
Digoxin	None	Morphine	None: infant may have significant blood concentration
Diltiazem	None		
Dipyrone	None	Moxalactam	None
Disopyramide	None	Nadolol[b]	None
Domperidone	None	Nalidixic acid	Hemolysis in infant with glucose-6-phosphate dehydrogenase (G6PD) deficiency
Dyphylline[b]	None		
Enalapril	—		
Erythromycin[b]	None	Naproxen	—
Estradiol	Withdrawal, vaginal bleeding	Nefopam	None
Ethambutol	None	Nifedipine	—
Ethanol (cf. alcohol)	—	Nitrofurantoin	Hemolysis in infant with G6PD deficiency
Ethosuximide	None; drug appears in infant serum		
Fentanyl	—	Norethynodrel	None
Flecainide	—	Norsteroids	None
Flufenamic acid	None	Noscapine	None
Fluroescein	—	Oxprenolol	None
Folic acid	None	Phenylbutazone	None
Gold salts	None	Phenytoin	Methemoglobinemia (1 case)
Halothane	None	Piroxicam	None
Hydralazine	None	Prednisone	None
Hydrochlorothiazide	—	Procainamide	None

► **TABLE A–6** *(continued)*

Drug	Reported Sign or Symptom in Infant or Effect on Lactation	Drug	Reported Sign or Symptom in Infant or Effect on Lactation
Progesterone	None	Sulfisoxazole	Caution in infant with jaundice or G6PD deficiency, and ill, stressed, or premature infant; appears in milk
Propoxyphene	None		
Propranolol	None		
Propylthiouracil	None	Suprofen	None
Pseudoephedrine[b]	None	Terbutaline	None
Pyridostigmine	None	Tetracycline	None; negligible absorption by infant
Pyrimethamine	None	Theophylline	Irritability
Quinidine	None	Thiopental	None
Quinine	None	Thiouracil	None mentioned; drug not used in United States
Riboflavin	None		
Rifampin	None	Ticarcillin	None
Scopolamine	—	Timolol	None
Secobarbital	None	Tolbutamide	Possible jaundice
Senna	None	Tolmetin	None
Sotalol	—	Trimethoprim/ sulfamethoxazole	None
Spironolactone	None		
Streptomycin	None	Triprolidine	None
Sulbactam	None	Valproic acid	None
Sulfapyridine	Caution in infant with jaundice or G6PD deficiency, and ill, stressed, or premature infant; appears in milk	Verapamil	None
		Warfarin	None
		Zolpidem	None

[a]Drugs listed have been reported in the literature as having the effects listed or no effect. The word *none* means that no observable change was seen in the nursing infant while the mother was ingesting the compound. It is emphasized that most of the literature citations concern single case reports or small series of infants.
[b]Drug is concentrated in human milk.

► **TABLE A–7**

Food and Environmental Agents: Effect on Breastfeeding

Agent	Reported Sign or Symptom in Infant or Effect on Lactation
Aflatoxin	None
Aspartame	Caution if mother or infant has phenylketonuria
Bromide (photographic laboratory)	Potential absorption and bromide transfer into milk; *see* Table A-6
Cadmium	None reported
Chlordane	None reported
Chocolate (theobromine)	Irritability or increased bowel activity if excess amounts (16 oz/d) consumed by mother
DDT, benzenehexachlorides, dieldrin, aldrin, hepatachlorepoxide	None
Fava beans	Hemolysis in client with glucose-6-phosphate dehydrogenase deficiency
Fluorides	None
Hexachlorobenzene	Skin rash, diarrhea, vomiting, dark urine, neurotoxicity, death
Hexachlorophene	None; possible contamination of milk from nipple washing
Lead	Possible neurotoxicity
Methyl mercury, mercury	May affect neurodevelopment
Monosodium glutamate	None
Polychlorinated biphenyls and polybrominated biphenyls	Lack of endurance, hypotonia, sullen expressionless facies
Tetrachlorethylene cleaning fluid (perchloroethylene)	Obstructive jaundice, dark urine
Vegetarian diet	Signs of B_{12} deficiency

Standard Laboratory Values for the Childbearing Woman

	Nonpregnant	Pregnant
Hematology (Peripheral Blood Values)		
Red blood cells (mL/mm^3)	4.2–5.4	4.2–5.4; red cell mass increases
Hemoglobin (g/dL)	12–16	11–12
Hematocrit (%)[a]	37–47	32–36
MCV (mean corpuscular volume) (μm^3)	80–98	80–95
MCH (mean corpuscular hemoglobin) (pg)	27–31	27–31
MCHC (mean corpuscular hematocrit) (%)	32–36	32–36
White blood cells (μL)	5000–12,000	5000–16,000
Differential		
Neutrophils (%)	50–60	50–70
Lymphocytes (%)	25–35	25–44
Eosinophils (%)	1–4	1–4
Monocytes (%)	2–6	2–6
Platelets (mm^3)	150,000–450,000	150,000–450,000
Prothrombin time (s)	11–15	11–15
Partial thromboplastin time (s)	60–70	Slightly shortened
Activated partial prothrombin time	25–45	Slightly shortened
Fibrinogen (mg/dL)	150–400	400–500
Bleeding time (min)	1–6 (Ivy)	1–6 (Ivy)
	1–3 (Duke)	1–3 (Duke)
Blood Chemistries		
Total bilirubin (mg/dL)	0.2–0.9	Slightly increased
Creatinine (mg/dL)	0.5–1.0	0.3–0.6
Folate (folic acid) (mg/L)	4–16	4–14
Blood sugar		
Fasting (mg/dL)	70–100	65–100
Postprandial (mg/dL)	< 120(2 hrs, blood)	< 140 (2 hrs, blood)
Iron (μg/dL)	50–150	50–120
Iron-binding capacity (mg/dL)	250–450	300–500

(continued)

▶ **APPENDIX B**

Standard Laboratory Values for the Childbearing Woman *(continued)*

	Findings During Pregnancy

Hormones

Human chorionic gonadotropin (hCG)

Urine	Positive
If quantified	> 1000 IU/24 hr
Serum	Positive
If quantified	Steady rise, by 45 days 50,000 IU; by 60 days as high as 600,000 IU; then drops to stable level of approximately 20,000 IU by 100th day

Human placental lactogen (hPL)

Weeks of Gestation	ng/mL
24–28	2.0–5.5
29–32	2.5–7.5
33–36	3.5–9.5
37–40	4.0–10.0

Urinalysis

Color	Pale straw
Appearance	Clear
Specific gravity	1.015–1.024
pH	4.5–8 (6 is average)
Protein	Negative–trace
Glucose	Negative–trace
Ketones	Negative
Microscopic red blood cells	1–2 per lower-power field
White blood cells	3–4
Casts	Occasional hyaline

Antibody Screen

Indirect Coombs' test	Negative

HTLV-III Screen[b]

ELISA[b]	Negative
Western blot	Negative

Serology

FTA-ABS[b]	Negative; nonreactive
VDRL test[b]	Negative
Rubella titer (hemagglutination-inhibition test)	> 1:8 immune

[a]At sea level. Values of 32 to 35% indicate physiologic anemia.
[b]HTLV-III, human T-cell leukemia/lymphoma virus; ELISA, enzyme-linked immunosorbent assay; FTA-ABS, fluorescent treponeal antibody-absorption test for syphilis; VDRL, Venereal Disease Research Laboratory.

Appendix C

Resources: Selected Maternal-Child Health Internet Sites

▶ Abortion

Academic Press Dictionary of Science and Technology
http://www.apnet.com/inscight/04231997/spontan1.htm
Comprehensive CD-rom access to numerous abortion sites.

Alan Guttmacher Institute
http://www.hhpcc.com/abordeth.htm
Link to the Alan Guttmacher Institute and numerous abortion statistics.

Congressional Research Service
http://www.clark.net/pub/pennyhill/abortion.html
Information about abortions in the military.

Health Answers
http://www.healthanswers.com/database/ami/converted/000907.h
Site contains statistics pertaining to spontaneous abortion. Links to other sites.

Library of Congress
http://www.oclc.org:5046/~vizine/concept/testcase-1A.100/oca
Access to Library of Congress abortion statistics.

Merck Manual
http://www.merck.com/!!v8SY71tWp/pubs/mmanual/html
Connects to the 16th Edition of the Merck Manual which contains current data on abortion.

University of Michigan
http://www.umd.umich.edu/HyperNews/get/marcyb/106w97/relatio
Links to the Michigan University Medical School. Contains a research module on abortion.

University of Tulane
http://www.mcl.tulane.edu/classware/pathology/medical_pathol
Links to the University of Tulane. Contains information on ectopic pregnancy.

▶ Breastfeeding

Breastfeeding Advocacy Page
http://clark.net/pub/activist/bfpage.html
Informative articles available.

Breastfeeding Information
http://www.bright.net~ghalley/wc_breastfeeding_links.html
Many links to different breastfeeding sites.

Breastfeeding and the Law
http://www.lalecheleague.org/LawMain.html
Links to the La Leche League. Explains women's rights about breastfeeding.

Breastfeeding and Parenting
http://www.prairienet.org/community/health/laleche/other.htm
Collection of links to web pages which features breastfeeding, lactation, and nutritional information.

Breastfeeding in Public
http://www.sheppnews.com.au/issues/messages/119.html
Articles about views on breastfeeding in public.

Medela
http://www.medela.com/header.htm
Links to Medela's board certified lactation consultants. Includes information about breastfeeding products.

▶ Childbirth

Changing Childbirth
http://www.cant.ac.uk/depts/acad/nursing/12-3-24.htm
Evaluates local and national initiatives and implementation of the Changing Childbirth Report.

Childbirth Choices—The Natural Procedure
http://babyzone.com/natural.htm
Links to the BabyZone midwife site.

Family Childbirth Center
http://www.familyinternet.com/pregcom/04010305.htm
Links to information about childbirth center rooms and hospital-based childbirth center rooms.

Family and Childbirth Education Support
http://www.macomb.lib.il.us/community/clubs/faces/index.html
High-risk pregnancy helpline. Includes information on problem pregnancies, postpartum period, and cesarean support.

Natural Childbirth and Family Clinic
http://katu.citysearch.com/E/V/PDXOR/0004/48/46/cs1.html
Links to a clinic in Portland, Oregon which seek to promote a better way to welcome children into the world.

National Childbirth Trust
http://www.netlink.co.uk/users/bilan/society/groups/nct.html
Links to non-profit organization which offer a large variety of services to help parents choose an approach to pregnancy, birth, and feeding best suited to them.

Pregnancy & Childbirth Information
http://www.childbirth.org/
Links to prenatal care, nutrition, birth, and labor sites. Includes weekly interactive tool updates.

► Community-Based Nursing

Community Health Nursing Education
http://www.nln.org/press-061697.htm
Links college nursing departments and nursing homes.

Home Nursing Agency
http://www.hhdev.psu.edu/nurs/hna.htm
Link to the Pennsylvania State University System. Discusses the home nursing agency's mission. Also links to the Rural Nursing Center Project.

Lee Community Nursing Service
http://www.citipage.com/lee/comnurse.html
Addresses every aspect of home care from preventing the hospital stay to care required following hospital discharge. Non-profit organization.

National League of Nurses
http://www.nln.org/abstracts/evenabs44.htm
Discusses concepts for community education. Links to other sites.

NLN Student Affairs Committee
http://www.org/info-survey.htm
Link to the NLN Student Affairs Community-Based Health Care Curriculum.

Teaching in the Community
http://www.nln.org/books/147262.htm
Discusses what nursing students must do to prepare to practice in the new community-based health care system.

UBC School of Nursing
http://www.nursing.ubc.ca/docs/bios/CCanam.html
Links to the University of British Columbia School of Nursing with research in numerous community workshops and presentations.

Widener University School of Nursing
http://www.widener.edu/nursing/art2.html
Links to Widener University site which discuss the need for family nurse practitioners to work in community health care environments.

► Gestational Diabetes

Children's Hospital of British Columbia
http://www.childhosp.bc.ca/childrens/GestD/Homepag.htm
Links to the gestational diabetes screening test information. Links to many other sites.

Diabetes Organization Council
http://www.diabetes.org/councils/pregnancy/particles.html
Explains medical diagnosis of gestational diabetes with treatments.

Gestational Diabetes Site
http://www.grin.net/~holden94/diabetes/gestational.htm
Site describes relationship between blood glucose level in the mother and high insulin levels in the fetus. Describes macrosomia.

Health Education Update
http://webadv.chron.com/nonprof/house/business/nonprof/speci
Describes risk factors for women who develop gestational diabetes and their newborns.

Indiana University
http://medicine.indiana.iupui.edu/diabetes.htm
Connects to the Indiana University Medical School.

Jefferson Health Network
http://www.jeffersonhealth.org/diseases/diabetes/gdcomps.htm
Links to the Jefferson Health Network. Discusses complications for the newborn.

Medical Link
http://www.medicallink.se/medlink/press/DIABETOLOGNYTT/updat
Site explains relationship between gestational diabetes and difficult labor and delivery. Links to other sites.

Methodist Health Network
http://www.methodisthealth.com/diabetes/gesta.htm
Links to the Methodist Health Network. Discusses developing factors of gestational diabetes.

Methodist Health Network
http://www.methodisthealth.com/diabetes/gdcomps.htm
Links to the Methodist Health Network. Discusses complications during childbirth and postdelivery.

NICHD—Understanding Gestational Diabetes
http://www.nih.gov/health/chip/nichd/ugd/affect.html
Link to many sites about gestational diabetes.

► High-Risk Pregnancies

Coalition for Positive Outcomes in Pregnancy
http://www.storknet.org/CPOP/bfbcard.htm
Internet message board for high-risk pregnant mothers.

Innerbody
http://www.innerbody.com/text/birth11.html
Discusses risk factors for high-risk pregnancy. Explains role of family practitioner.

Loyola University Medical Center
http://www.lumc.edu/lumc/media/newsrel/apr97/gian.htm
Connects to Loyola University Medical Center site. Contains links to other sites.

Marquette General Hospital
http://www.mgh.org/ob/obdept.html
Links to the high-risk services site of Marquette General Hospital.

Maternal Fetal Medicine and Genetic Center
http://www.stvincent.org/healthservices/womenandchildrens/mf
Describes full range of antepartal testing services, including non-stress tests.

Phoenix Perinatal Associates
http://www.perinatal.com/index.html
Links to the Phoenix Perinatal Associates site. Contains information about high-risk pregnancy.

Saint Margaret Mercy—Perinatal Center
http://www.smmh.com/health/index.html
Links to Saint Margaret Mercy Health Care Center. Contains information about high-risk pregnancies, including statistics and nutrition.

Sidelines
http://wwwthebabynet.com/babyboard/messages/5814.html
Non-profit organization which offers support for high-risk pregnancies.

University of Northern Minnesota
http://som.unm.edu/clerkship/obgyn/obgyn108.html
Links to the University of Northern Minnesota high-risk pregnancy site.

University of Pennsylvania
http://www.med.upenn.edu/health/hi_files/phw/serv_prog/hi_ri
Connects to Children's Hospital of Philadelphia.

▶ Nutrition

American Diabetic Association
http://www.eatright.org
Offers a variety of nutrition information on current issues in nutrition. Links to other resources.

American Heart Association
http://207.211.141.25/
Links to the American Heart Association site. Provides a variety of information on preventing cardiovascular disease.

Center for Science in the Public Interest
http://cspinet.org
Non-profit consumer advocacy organization for nutrition issues.

Tufts University Nutrition Navigator
http://www.navigator.tufts.edu
Links to Tufts University. Also links to a wide variety of nutrition websites.

USDA Nutrient Values
http://www.rahul.net/cgi-bin/fatfree/usda/usda.cgi
Part of the USDA website. Provides nutrient analysis on a variety of foods.

WIC Program
http://www.usda.gov/
Provides information on the Women's, Infants, and Children's (WIC) Supplemental Food Program.

▶ Perinatal Health

U.S. Centers for Disease Control
http://www.cdc.gov/genetics/temp/screening.htm
Centers for Disease Control.

Health Center
http://www.health-center.com/english/family/newborn/equipmen
Links to the Health Center. Describes and explains different materials that are safe for babies, such as plastic.

Merck Manual
http://www.merck.com/!!v8fBt07xOv8fBt07xO/pubs/mmamual/html
Describes health management in normal neonates, infants, and children.

OSDH Medical Journal
http://cajunnet2.cajunnet.com/~abdk/index.html
Links to OSDH journal articles.

Sympatico Health Links
http://www1.sympatico.ca/healthyway/REV_HTML/R6311.html
Links to the Sympatico Health System. Rates content and depth of different articles regarding newborn health.

▶ Pregnancy

BabyZone
http://babyzone.com
Links to the BabyZone. Features checklists and charts to monitor pregnancy.

Health During Pregnancy
http://pregnancy.minigco.com/msubhealth.htm
Links to bulletin boards and feedback guides regarding pregnancy.

Pregnancy
http://www.publich.asu.edu/~ide4bubu/sexlinks/preg.html
Links to the childbirth services pregnancy page.

Pregnancy and Childbirth
http://www.suite101.com/links/page.cfm/496
Links to the unassisted childbirth page. Includes information about unassisted childbirth.

Pregnancy Journals
http://www.thelaboroflove.com/websearch/links/Pregnancy/Jour
Links to journal search engine with many articles relating to pregnancy.

Pregnancy and Parenting
http://www.thelaboroflove.com/websearch/links/Pregnancy/Supp
Links to Pregnancy Today. Also includes pregnancy support groups.

Yahoo! Health
http://www.yahoo.com/Health/Reproductive_Health/Pregnancy_an
Links to pregnancy and birth indices. Includes pregnancy and parenting search engine.

▶ Pregnancy Education

BBC Education
http://ftp.bbc.co.uk/education/health/parenting/index.shtml
Links to the BBC Healthsite. Includes information about parenthood.

Dartmouth-Hitchcock Medical Center
http://pegasus.cc.ucf.edu/~feecwg/teen.html
Links to Florida Education information. Includes self-help information.

Pregnancy and Birth
http://www.yt.sympatico.ca/Contents/Health/LISTS/B9-C02-02-0
Links to articles and frequently asked questions about health and pregnancy.

Pregnancy and Parenting
http://www.thelaboroflove.com/websearch/links/Education/Reso
Links to many search engines regarding pregnancy education.

Sexuality Education and Teen Pregnancy
http://www.fpcai.org/wpasexed.htm
Links to educational sites regarding unintended pregnancies in adolescents.

Teen Pregnancy
http://www.aclin.org/other/health/cinch/profiles/00400.htm
Links to a directory of services regarding teen and adolescent pregnancy. Issues include counseling and parent education.

Women's Health
http://www.yt.sympatico.ca/Contents/Health/LISTS/B9-C02-02_a
Health links to many sites about women's health education and pregnancy.

▶ Pregnancy-Induced Hypertension (PIH)

Biomedics
http://www.biomed.lib.umn.edu/hmed/980116_preg.html
Links to Biomedics site in which different tests are explained to diagnose PIH.

Canadian Hypertension Society
http://osler.med.und.nodak.edu/clinical/pregnancyHypertension
Links to the Canadian Hypertension Society.

CCS Publishing
http://www.ccspublishing.com/journals2/pregnancy%20complicat
Links to journals which help describe different complications of pregnancy, including hypertension.

Pregnancy-Induced Hypertension
http://www.andrews.edu/IPA/education/adolescent_health/Nutri
Explains and defines PIH. Links to other sites.

► **Premature Infants**

Babies Planet
http://www.thebabiesplanet.com/1bpremat.htm
Contains information about premature delivery. Links to other sites.

Kids Health Organization
http://kidshealth.org/parent/healthy/preemies.html
Links to the Kids Health Organization. Lists statistics of premature babies.

Premature Baby Diary
http://ats.com.au/prem/index.html
Links to a mother's diary of her premature baby from delivery at 25 weeks to 40 weeks.

Premature Child Family Support
http://www.comeunity.com/preemie/index.html
Links to Internet resources regarding family support in families with premature children.

Glossary

ABO incompatibility   Disease that occurs when the fetus and mother have different blood groups. Mixing of fetal and maternal blood leads to hemolysis of fetal red blood cells and an increase in bilirubin levels in the neonate.

abortion   Termination of pregnancy before the fetus is viable outside the uterus (usually before 20 to 24 weeks of gestation or weighing less than 500 g).

complete a.   Abortion in which all products of conception have been expelled, including fetus, placenta, and decidua.

elective a.   Interruption of pregnancy before viability at the decision and request of the woman which is not based on maternal or fetal disease.

habitual a.   Spontaneous abortion occurring in three or more consecutive pregnancies.

incomplete a.   Pregnancy termination resulting in retention of parts of the products of conception.

induced a.   Intentional abortion that is artificially initiated by the use of medications or mechanical means for therapeutic or personal reasons.

inevitable a.   Imminent abortion characterized by cervical dilation, bleeding, and pain.

missed a.   Condition in which the fetus dies in utero and the products of conception are retained in the uterus.

spontaneous a.   Spontaneous expulsion of the products of conception occurring naturally and without external cause.

threatened a.   Condition in which there are signs and symptoms of impending loss of the pregnancy, such as bleeding, uterine cramping, and backache. It may progress to an inevitable abortion or it may be averted through medical treatment.

abortus   Fetus or embryo that is spontaneously delivered at less than 20 weeks of gestational age, or weighs less than 500 g or measures less than 25 cm.

abruptio placentae   Partial or complete separation of a normally implanted placenta from the uterine wall prior to the delivery of the infant.

absent variability   A persistently flat baseline fetal heart rate; a sign of potential fetal distress in labor.

acceleration phase   Phase of labor characterized by an intense increase in the rate of cervical dilation from approximately 3 to 5 cm.

accessory glands   Glands of the male reproductive system consisting of the seminal vesicles, the prostate gland, and the bulbourethral glands.

achievement phase   Period between 2 and 5 months postpartum during which mother begins psychologic and social role adaptation and infant develops a predictable routine.

acrocyanosis   Blue discoloration of the extremities present in most infants at birth; may persist for 7 to 10 days; caused by vasomotor instability and poor peripheral circulation during transition to extrauterine life.

acrosome   Membrane covering the head of the spermatozoon; contains enzymes that help sperm enter the ovum.

acrosome reaction   Sequence of events in which the acrosome of the sperm undergoes structural changes in its outer membrane and releases enzymes that dissolve the membranes of the ovum.

active immunity   Development of acquired resistance as a result of an illness or immunization.

active phase   Phase of labor that begins when the cervix is dilated to 3 cm and ends with the full dilation of the cervix.

acyanotic heart defect   Heart defect that does not cause cyanosis, for example, pulmonary stenosis and a patent ductus arteriosus.

adolescence   Period in human development between childhood and adulthood.

afterpains   Pain resulting from uterine contractions that occur after birth of an infant; tend to last 2 to 3 days and are more severe during breastfeeding and in multiparous women.

alpha-fetoprotein   Glycoprotein that is synthesized in the embryonic yolk sac, developing gastrointestinal tract, and fetal liver; crosses the placenta and can be found in the maternal blood.

amenorrhea   Absence of menses.

amniocentesis   Transabdominal withdrawal of fluid from the amniotic sac via insertion of a needle into the uterus through the abdominal wall; used to assess fetal health and maturity.

amnion   Membrane that lines the amniotic cavity and contains the embryo/fetus and amniotic fluid.

amniotic fluid index (AFI)   Method of approximating the volume of amniotic fluid in the uterus through the measurement of the deepest vertical pockets of amniotic fluid in each quadrant of the uterus.

analgesia   Reduction of pain without loss of consciousness.

androgynous   Term used to describe the incorporation of both male and female characteristics.

android pelvis   Pelvis characterized by a heart-shaped outline; also called male pelvis.

anemia   Decrease in both the circulating red blood cell mass and the cells' capacity to carry oxygen to vital organs of the mother and the fetus.

anencephaly   Absence of the cerebrum, cerebellum, and flat bones of the skull as a result of a congenital deformity. The head is small and abnormally shaped.

anesthesia   Partial or complete loss of sensation with or without loss of consciousness.

    epidural a.   Pharmacologic therapy administered by injection of a local anesthetic agent into the epidural space; also called an epidural block.

    general a.   Complete loss of sensation and consciousness as a result of pharmacologic therapy; used for cesarean or operative vaginal deliveries.

    regional a.   Pharmacologic therapy causing loss of sensation along nerve pathways of a particular organ and surrounding tissues.

    spinal a.   Pharmacologic therapy administered by an injection into the spinal subarachnoid space that causes loss of sensation in affected tissues; also called a spinal block or subarachnoid block.

anorexia nervosa   Eating disorder characterized by extreme weight loss greater than 15% of ideal body weight related to inadequate intake of nutrients.

anteflexion   Displacement of the uterus in which the uterus bends forward onto itself.

anthropoid pelvis   Pelvis characterized by the anteroposterior diameter being equal to or greater than the transverse diameter.

anthropometry   Measurement of physical characteristics of the body.

Apgar score   Numerical scoring system used to assess a newborn's heart rate, respiratory effort, reflex irritability, muscle tone, and color at 1 and 5 minutes after birth.

apneic episodes   Absence of respirations for at least 10 to 15 seconds or a pause in respirations that causes bradycardia or cyanosis.

appropriate-for-gestational-age (AGA)   Birth weight that is appropriate for the length of gestation.

areola   Darkened pigmented ring surrounding the nipple.

asphyxia   Life-threatening condition caused by lack of oxygen and accumulation of carbon dioxide in the body.

assessment   First phase of the nursing process that consists of the collection of data to determine a client's present and past health and functional status and to evaluate the client's coping patterns and responses to therapeutic interventions.

atresia   Congenital absence or pathologic closure of a normal body opening.

attachment relationship   Affectional ties among mother, father, and infant that develop over the first year of life based on response patterns that ensure that the infant will be cared for during his years of dependency.

attitude   Relationship of the fetal parts to each other.

augmentation   Stimulation of labor once natural labor has begun. Medications such as oxytocin or activities such as breast stimulation may be used to stimulate labor.

autosome   Any of the 22 pairs of identical chromosomes in males and females.

Babinski reflex   Hyperextension of the toes with dorsiflexion of the great toe in response to stroking the lateral aspect of the sole upward across the ball of the foot.

bacteremia Presence of bacteria in the blood.

balanced translocation carrier Individual with a chromosomal abnormality who demonstrates no missing or extra chromosomes, but in whom genetic material is arranged abnormally.

ballottement Diagnostic technique used to detect a floating object in the body. In pregnancy, the fetus, when tapped, moves away and then returns to touch the examiner's fingers.

Bandl's ring Type of pathologic retraction ring that can impede labor. The upper segment of the uterus overretracts while the lower segment overdistends; parts of the fetus may be trapped above and below the ring.

Barr body Represents the genetically inactive, late-replicating X chromosome.

Bartholin's glands Two small mucus-secreting glands located on either side of the vaginal orifice.

baseline fetal heart rate Average fetal heart rate between contractions. Normally the rate is 120 to 160 beats per minute.

bicornate uterus Uterus being completely or partially Y-shaped; also called a septate uterus.

bilateral tubal ligation Method of female sterilization accomplished by a surgical procedure in which the fallopian tubes are intentionally obstructed with rings or bands or are intentionally severed.

binuclear family Family that consists of two parents who have terminated the spousal relationship, live in two separate households, and cooperate in the responsibilities of parenting.

biparietal diameter (BPD) Transverse diameter of the fetal parietal bones, which is the widest diameter of the fetal skull; used as a determinant of fetal growth and gestational age.

birth center Free-standing center that provides homelike birthing experiences outside of the hospital setting.

birth plan Plan in which the expectant couple identifies a list of options preferred for their labor and delivery experience.

birth rate Annual number of live births per 1000 people.

bisexual Person who has erotic attractions for and may have had sexual experiences with individuals of both sexes.

blastocyst Term used to describe the morula about 3 days after fertilization when it develops two layers of cells with fluid-filled spaces.

bloody show Blood-tinged mucous vaginal discharge that occurs as the cervix begins to dilate.

body boundary Barrier that keeps the fetus inside the woman's protective container of a body.

body mass index Measure of a person's weight in relation to height; determined by dividing the weight (in kilograms) by the square of the height (in meters):

$$BMI = \frac{weight\ (kg)}{height\ (m)^2}$$

bonding Rapid process occurring immediately after birth that reflects mother-to-infant attachment (not the infant's attachment to the mother).

bony pelvis Bony ring formed by the sacrum, coccyx, and two innominate (hip) bones.

brachystasis Process in which a muscle does not relax to its former length following contraction.

Braun von Fernwald's sign Unilateral softening and enlargement of the uterus at the site of implantation.

Braxton Hicks contractions Irregular painless uterine contractions without cervical dilation that occur during pregnancy but are not associated with true labor.

bregma Anterior fontanelle.

broad ligaments Ligaments that extend from each side of the uterus to the pelvic wall; serve to stabilize the uterus in a midline position.

bronchopulmonary dysplasia (BPD) Chronic pulmonary disease that occurs in infants who have required mechanical ventilation and high levels of oxygen in the first weeks of life.

brow Located between the anterior and posterior fontanelles and bounded laterally by the parietal bones.

brown fat Fat deposits present in the fetus and neonate that are found around the adrenals, kidneys, in the neck, between the scapulas, and behind the sternum.

bulbourethral glands Glands located on the floor of the pelvic cavity on either side of the membranous urethra in the male; also called Cowper's glands. They secrete a mucinous substance that coats the surface of the urethra.

bulimia nervosa Eating disorder characterized by binge eating followed by purging by self-induced vomiting.

calendar method Pregnancy prevention method in which intercourse is avoided in the presence of an ovum; focuses on the timing of ovulation, the life span of sperm, and the life span of the ovum.

capacitation Enzymatic process that results in the removal of the plasma protein over the acrosome of the sperm.

caput succedaneum Edema of the presenting part of the fetal head that occurs during labor and delivery.

cardinal movements of labor Simultaneous accommodation of the fetal anatomy to the maternal pelvis and the birth canal, and passage of the fetus from the abdominal site to the external world.

care-by-parent program Component of the hospital care of high-risk newborns whereby one or both parents live in the hospital for a set period before the infant's discharge and are responsible for the infant's complete care.

carpal tunnel syndrome Compression of the median nerve in the carpal tunnel of the wrist, causing pain, edema, and altered sensation; may be caused by increased fluid retention during pregnancy.

cephalhematoma Collection of blood beneath the periosteum of the neonate's skull caused by ruptured blood vessels during labor and delivery; also called cephalohematoma.

cephalic index Ratio of the biparietal diameter to the occipitofrontal diameter of the fetal skull; indicator of fetal growth and development.

cephalocaudal Long axis of the body; head to tail.

cerclage Procedure in which a suture is used to encircle the cervix to keep it closed; treatment of choice for an incompetent cervix occurring between 14 and 20 weeks of gestation.

cervical cap Small cap-shaped contraceptive that is individually sized to fit over the cervix; provides a barrier to sperm during intercourse.

cervical ripening Process by which the cervix softens and begins to thin out.

cervix "Neck" of the uterus, which lies between the body of the uterus and the external os. The lower portion of the cervix extends into the vagina.

cesarean delivery Delivery of a fetus through an incision made in the abdominal wall and uterus.

Chadwick's sign Bluish discoloration of the mucous membranes of the vulva, vagina, and cervix observed around the fourth week of pregnancy that is caused by vasocongestion.

chloasma Irregular areas of deeper pigmentation on the forehead, nose, and cheeks observed during pregnancy ("mask of pregnancy") or in women taking oral contraceptives; also called melasma.

chorioamnionitis Infection of the chorion, amnion, amniotic fluid, and the fetus caused by organisms in the amniotic fluid, which then becomes infiltrated by polymorphonuclear leukocytes.

chorion Cellular membrane that is formed from the trophoblast.

chorionic villi Thin, hairlike projections from the chorion.

chorionic villus sampling Procedure performed during the first trimester to obtain fetal cells for diagnosis of chromosomal and congenital disorders.

circumcision Surgical removal of the foreskin, exposing the glans penis.

cleavage Rapid division of the zygote, producing blastomeres; occurs between 1 and 3 days after fertilization.

climacteric Gradual decrease (5-10 year period) in ovarian hormone production prior to menopause.

clinical reasoning Decision making process used by nurses when caring for clients in a variety of clinical situations.

clitoris Small oval body of erectile tissue located at the anterior junction of the female vulva; comparable to the male penis.

coitus interruptus Pregnancy prevention method in which, during intercourse, the man withdraws his penis from the woman's vagina and ejaculates outside of the vagina.

cold stress Excessive body heat loss that results in compensatory mechanisms such as nonshivering thermogenesis to maintain the core body temperature.

colic Acute paroxysmal episodes of pain, crying, and irritability in an infant; often caused by swallowing air, overfeeding, intestinal allergy, or emotional factors.

colostrum Precursor of milk composed mainly of serum and white blood cells that is usually secreted from the breasts after the 16th week of pregnancy. Colostrum is high in protein and provides immune properties.

communal family Group of unrelated adults and children dedicated to a common purpose.

conception Union of male sperm and female ovum resulting in fertilization.

condom Male or female birth control device; helps protect against the transmission of some sexually transmitted diseases, including HIV infection.

male c. Thin sheath worn over the erect penis during intercourse to prevent sperm from entering the vagina. Latex is thought to decrease the transmission of some STDs.

female c. Polyurethane sheath that fits into the vagina to block sperm. A ring is fitted at either end of the sheath. One ring remains outside the vagina; the other fits over the symphysis in the same manner as a diaphragm.

constriction ring Type of pathologic uterine retraction ring resulting from tetanic contractions; may trap the fetus and prevent descent.

contraction stress test (CST) Method used to evaluate the fetal response to spontaneous or induced uterine contractions; performed during the third trimester.

corpus Body of the uterus.

couvade syndrome Psychophysiologic response in the male partners of pregnant women in which the men experience physical symptoms, such as nausea and vomiting. In some cases, the syndrome is manifested by an individual who is not the father, for example, a friend.

Couvelaire uterus Condition that occurs in severe abruptio placentae when blood extravasates into the uterine musculature, the connective tissue of the broad ligaments, and the peritoneal cavity.

Cowper's glands *See* bulbourethral glands.

cradle cap Seborrheic dermatitis in the newborn characterized by an oily, yellow, crusty buildup on the scalp and face.

Cri du chat syndrome Chromosomal structural abnormality caused by a deletion; characterized by catlike cry, microcephaly, low birth weight, wide-set eyes, and mental and physical retardation.

crisis Impact of an event that challenges the assumed state of an individual and forces that individual to change his or her view of, or readapt to, the world, to himself or herself, or to both.

accidental c. *See* crisis, situational.

developmental c. Considered a normal part of growth and development; generally viewed as a period of marked physical, psychologic, and social change characterized by disturbances in life patterns; also called maturational crisis.

maturational c. *See* crisis, developmental.

situational c. Unexpected, stressful external event that may or may not coincide with a developmental crisis; also called accidental crisis.

critical temperature Temperature range that necessitates a metabolic response to cold in order to replace heat loss.

critical thinking Inherent cognitive activity in the clinical reasoning process and is an approach to inquiry in which nurses examine clinical and professional issues and search for effective answers.

culdocentesis Use of a needle or incision to aspirate fluid from the cul-de-sac of Douglas through the vagina; used to confirm an ectopic pregnancy.

cyanotic heart defect Congenital cardiac defect that causes blood to shunt from the right side to the left side of the heart, producing cyanosis. An example is tetralogy of Fallot.

cystitis Inflammation and infection of the urinary bladder.

deceleration phase Phase of labor characterized by cervical dilation from 8 to 10 cm in which effacement is nearly complete; transition phase.

decidua Mucous membrane lining of the uterus (endometrium) that surrounds the ovum and is shed after delivery.

d. basalis Portion of the decidua directly beneath the site of implantation from which the maternal portion of the placenta develops.

d. capsularis Portion of the decidua that surrounds the developing ovum and separates it from the rest of the uterine cavity.

d. vera Nonplacental decidual lining of the uterus.

deep venous thrombosis Thrombosis formation in a deep vein without the presence of inflammation.

denominators Landmarks of the fetal skull used to describe the relationship of the fetal presenting part to the maternal pelvis during delivery.

descent Movement downward; movement of the presenting part of the fetus into the birth canal that begins at the onset of labor and continues as the cervix effaces and dilates.

diagnostic-related groups (DRGs) Legislated prospective payment system whereby hospitals receive payment for expected services rendered to clients based on their diagnosis.

diagonal conjugate Measurement from the sacral promontory to the lower posterior border of the symphysis pubis.

diaper dermatitis Inflammation of the neonate's skin in the perineal area.

diaphragm Flexible disk that is inserted vaginally to cover the cervix; used to prevent pregnancy.

diastasis recti Separation of the rectus muscles along the midline of the abdomen occurring during pregnancy as a result of stretching of the abdominal wall.

dilation Widening of the external os of the cervix from a few millimeters to 10 cm to provide for passage of the fetus.

dilation and curettage Method of pregnancy termination in which the cervix is dilated enough to allow passage of a curet into the uterus. The curet is used to scrape away the endometrium to empty the uterine contents or to obtain tissue for further examination.

dilation and evacuation Method of pregnancy termination in which the cervix is dilated and the uterine walls are scraped to remove the contents.

direct maternal death Death of the mother resulting from reproductive complications of pregnancy, labor, postpartum, or interventions.

disruption phase Period between 5 and 8 months postpartum during which the mother begins to feel conflict in balancing multiple roles as the infant's newfound mobility and activity level challenge her feelings of competence.

disseminated intravascular coagulation (DIC) Complex disorder of the clotting mechanism in the blood that can lead to overwhelming hemorrhage; may be caused by abruptio placentae, sepsis, or fetal demise.

dizygotic twins Fetuses that originate from two separate zygotes; also called fraternal twins; more common than monozygotic twins.

dominant Gene that is expressed by the individual.

douching Cleansing of the vagina that is usually done to cleanse or apply medication; not advised as a method of postcoital birth control.

Down syndrome *See* trisomy 21.

ductus deferens Duct that arises from the wall of the testis, joins with the spermatic cord, and continues to the posterior wall of the bladder. The enlarged portion of the ductus deferens (the ampulla) stores sperm; also called vas deferens.

dysmenorrhea Pain during menstruation.

dystocia Difficult labor as a result of mechanical factors such as size of the fetus, pelvic diameter, and uterine activity.

eclampsia Condition in which preeclamptic signs are accompanied by grand mal seizures, coma, and/or shock; occurs during pregnancy (usually after 20 weeks) or postpartum.

ectoderm The outermost layer of cells of the three primary germ layers of the embryo.

ectopic pregnancy Pregnancy that occurs when the fertilized ovum implants in tissue other than the lining of the uterus.

effacement Process in which the uterine cervix thins, shortens, and flattens during late pregnancy, labor, or both.

effleurage Massage technique that employs light, gentle stroking; often used on the abdomen during labor.

ejaculatory duct Duct formed by the union of the seminal vesicle and the ductus deferens; extends through the prostate gland and ends at the prostatic urethra.

embryoblast The inner layer of cells of the developing blastocyst.

embryonic disc Embryonic layer of cells that develops from the blastocyst and forms the two layers that will become the amnion and yolk sac.

embryonic period Period that begins the second week after fertilization and continues until approximately the eighth week.

emergency contraception Contraceptive methods that can be used as back-up, emergency measures to prevent pregnancy after unprotected intercourse.

encephalocele Protrusion of the brain through an opening in the skull caused by a congenital abnormality or trauma.

endoderm The innermost layer of cells of the three primary germ layers of the embryo.

endometrial cycle Cycle of changes in the uterus that is stimulated by hormones during the ovarian cycle; consists of proliferative, secretory, and menstrual phases; also called uterine cycle.

endometriosis Condition in which endometrial tissue grows outside of the uterine cavity; frequently associated with infertility.

endometrium Innermost mucous layer of the uterus made up of a single layer of ciliated columnar epithelium, glands, and stroma.

engagement Point at which the widest diameter of the presenting part of the fetus has passed through the inlet of the maternal pelvis.

engorgement Distension or vascular congestion of the breast.

   primary e. (physiologic breast e.) Swelling of breast resulting from increased blood and lymph supply to breast and beginning of full milk production.

   secondary e. (pathologic e.) Accumulation of milk in ducts and alveoli; may result when breasts are not adequately drained. Breast alveoli distend and milk-secreting cells flatten, are drawn out, and rupture. Breasts become hard, shiny, and painful.

engrossment Parent's (usually, the father's) intense interest in or preoccupation with an infant.

epididymis Coiled portion of the excretory duct of the testis through which sperm travels.

epidural block *See* anesthesia, epidural.

episiotomy Surgical incision of the perineum performed in the second stage of labor to provide a wider vaginal opening of the perineal tissue as the fetus is delivered.

Epstein's pearls Small white cysts seen along the edge of the gum where the hard and soft palates meet; a normal condition in the neonate.

Erb-Duchenne paralysis Paralysis of the deltoid, biceps, anterior brachial, and long supinator muscles caused by traumatic injury to the brachial plexus; related to forcible traction during delivery. The neonate holds the affected arm tightly adducted and internally rotated.

erythema toxicum Benign pink papular rash with superimposed vesicles identified in the first 48 hours of life; resolves spontaneously within a few days.

ethical decision making Problem-solving process with specific emphasis on the careful examination of alternatives and thoughtful justification of the choice of actions required.

eutocia Normal labor.

evaluation Last phase of the nursing process and is a review of the changes experienced by the client as a result of the actions of the nurse.

exfoliation Scaling or flaking of the horny layer of the skin; separation of tissue into thin layers; occurs at the placental site as necrotic tissue is sloughed off and endometrial restoration begins in the postpartum period.

extended family Any family or individual who has a relationship with a nuclear family and to whom the nuclear family looks for consultation and support.

external os Portion of the cervix that opens into the vagina.

external rotation Normal mechanism of labor whereby the fetal head rotates outward as the shoulders rotate inward.

extremely-low-birth-weight (ELBW) A neonate who weighs less than 1000 g at birth.

fallopian tubes Slender, tubelike structures that extend laterally from each side of the uterus toward the ovary; also called oviducts. They serve as a canal through which the ovum passes after release from the ovary and through which sperm travel and as a site for fertilization.

false pelvis Bony area above the true pelvis and linea terminalis; bounded posteriorly by the lumbar vertebrae, laterally by the iliac fossae, and anteriorly by the anterior abdominal wall.

family Small social system made up of individuals related to each other by reason of strong reciprocal ties and constituting a permanent household (or cluster of households) that persists over years. *See also* extended family and nuclear family.

family developmental tasks Basic family tasks that are specific to a given stage of development in the family life cycle.

fecundability Chance of becoming pregnant per month of exposure.

fecundity Ability to participate in the production of a child.

female pelvis *See* gynecoid pelvis.

femininity Culturally prescribed, reinforced characteristics of the female sex, independent of gender.

fencing position *See* tonic neck reflex.

ferning Fernlike pattern of the cervical mucus seen under microscopic examination; peaks at midcycle in response to high estrogen levels.

fertilization Process in which sperm penetrates the outer layer of the ovum and begins a chain of events resulting in development of the human embryo.

fetal alcohol syndrome Group of congenital malformations observed in infants of mothers with excessive alcohol intake during pregnancy. The syndrome is characterized by anomalies such as intrauterine growth retardation, facial abnormalities, cardiac defects, abnormalities of the limbs and joints, mental retardation, developmental delays, and small-for-gestational-age weights.

fetal biophysical profile Fetal diagnostic technique that combines nonstress testing with ultrasonic evaluation of several parameters, such as fetal heart rate reactivity, fetal breathing movements, fetal body movements, fetal tone, and amniotic fluid volume.

fetal dystocia Labor complicated by malpresentation or malposition.

fetal period Period that begins at the eighth week and continues to birth.

fimbriae Fringe or fingerlike structures, for example, the fingerlike opening of the fallopian tubes.

flexion Fetal position in which the head bends forward so that the chin approaches the chest; occurs as the fetus moves through the pelvic inlet and reaches the pelvic floor.

folk health care system Provision of health care by people who are not formally educated but who help people in their communities based on local beliefs and values.

fontanelle Membrane-filled area or soft spot on the fetal skull; located between the cranial bones.

anterior f. Membrane-filled space located at the anterior junction of the sagittal and coronal sutures; bregma.

posterior f. Membrane-filled space located at the posterior junction of lambdoidal and sagittal sutures; lambda.

Friedman curve Graphic representation of the latent and active phases in labor.

Galant's reflex Normal reflex in which the neonate, placed in the prone position, curves the body toward the side of the stimulus when the back is stroked in a downward motion; also called trunk incurvation.

gamete intrafallopian transfer (GIFT) procedure Direct transfer of ova and washed sperm into fallopian tubes; used in the treatment of infertility.

gametogenesis Process by which the sperm and ovum are produced.

gender Biologic concept that refers to an individual's sex, male or female.

genotype Hereditary makeup of an individual resulting from combinations of genes.

Goodell's sign Softening of the cervix; a probable sign of pregnancy.

gravidity State of being pregnant.

gynecoid pelvis Pelvis in which the inlet is slightly oval and the anteroposterior diameter of the inlet is slightly less than the transverse diameter; also called female pelvis.

habituation Process whereby newborns shut out disturbing or overwhelming stimuli.

harlequin color change Neonatal vasomotor disturbance characterized by dilation of blood vessels on one side of the neonate's body causing a deep red color; a normal finding that resolves spontaneously.

health maintenance organization (HMO) System of health care provision in which a provider is paid in advance a set amount of money per person, regardless of the health care services actually used by the client.

Hegar's sign Widening of the isthmus of the uterus to the point where the isthmus can be compressed on bimanual examination; probable sign of pregnancy.

hemoglobin C disease Hemoglobinopathy in which lysine replaces glutamine at position 6 on the beta chain of the hemoglobin molecule. This reduces the amount of normal hemoglobin in the blood.

hemoglobinopathy Hereditary disorder characterized by an abnormal form of hemoglobin.

hemolytic diseases of the newborn Conditions in which maternal antibodies are actively sensitized against the fetal red blood cells. These sensitized maternal antibodies cross the placenta and destroy fetal or neonatal red blood cells. ABO incompatibility and Rh incompatibility are examples.

heterozygous Having one dominant and one recessive gene for a trait.

high-risk client Person whose physical, emotional, or social situation presents some threat to his or her health, well-being, or development.

high-risk perinatal nursing Practice of nursing of childbearing families who have an increased probability of either psychosocial or physical illness, disability, or death.

homoiotherms Person or animal able to maintain a constant core body temperature regardless of a wide range of environmental temperatures.

homozygous Having two identical genes for a trait.

hospital birthing room Hospital room in which the woman labors, delivers, and recovers; characterized by a family-centered homelike birth experience.

human response patterns Patterns that reflect the pattern and organization of individuals as they interact with the environment.

hyaline membrane disease *See* respiratory distress syndrome.

hydramnios *See* polyhydramnios.

hydranencephaly Condition in which the cerebral hemispheres are absent and the space is filled with fluid.

hydrocele Condition caused by an accumulation of fluid around the testes.

hydrocephalus Excessive fluid collection in the cerebral ventricles of the fetus, causing dilation of the ventricles, thinning of brain tissue, and a markedly enlarged head.

hymen Membranous partition that partially or wholly blocks the orifice of the vagina.

hyperbilirubinemia Presence of an abnormally high level of bilirubin in the blood.

hyperemesis gravidarum Severe and prolonged vomiting during pregnancy usually beginning in the first trimester; also called pernicious vomiting of pregnancy.

hysterosalpingogram Diagnostic procedure performed in the early proliferative phase of the ovulatory cycle in which a radiopaque dye is injected into the uterus and fallopian tubes to determine their patency.

hysterotomy Removal of the products of conception through an incision in the uterine and abdominal walls.

iatrogenic prematurity Planned delivery of a fetus prior to term.

icterus neonatorum *See* physiologic jaundice.

implantation Attachment of the blastocyst to the endometrium; occurs 7 to 9 days after fertilization.

implementation Fourth phase of the nursing process that comprises the start and completion of actions necessary to accomplish previously defined goals.

impotence Inability to achieve an erection.

inborn errors of metabolism Genetically determined diseases that cause alterations in metabolic functioning.

incompetent cervix Anatomic defect of the cervix that results in painless dilation of the cervix without uterine contractions, usually during the second or early third trimester of pregnancy.

indirect maternal death Death of a mother not directly related to the childbearing cycle but resulting from a previously existing disease or a disease not related to reproduction that developed during the childbearing cycle and was aggravated by the pregnancy.

induction Artificial initiation of labor by the use of medications, primarily oxytocin, or surgical rupture of the membranes.

infant mortality rate Number of deaths of infants under 12 months of age per 1000 live births.

infertility Diminished or absent ability to conceive or produce a viable offspring.

internalization Unconscious process by which attributes, attitudes, or standards are taken within oneself.

internal os Portion of the cervix that opens into the uterus; divides the uterine cavity and the cervical canal.

internal rotation Movement of the fetus during labor in which the anteroposterior diameter of the fetal head rotates to align with the anteroposterior diameter of the maternal pelvis.

intrauterine device Small metal or plastic form that is placed in the uterus to prevent implantation of a fertilized ovum.

introitus Entrance or opening of the vagina.

inverted nipples Nipples that remain flat or retract into the areola when stimulated.

in vitro fertilization-embryo transfer (IVF-ET) Technique used in the management of infertile couples that encompasses removal of a mature ovum from a woman's ovary, fertilization of the ovum with sperm in a petri dish, and reimplantation of the embryo into the woman's uterine cavity.

involution   Return of the female reproductive system to its prepregnancy size and function.

isochromosome   Structural abnormality of the sex chromosome caused by injury to the X chromosome during meiosis.

isthmus   Portion of the uterus located between the corpus and the cervix.

jaundice   Yellow discoloration of the skin, sclera, and mucous membranes caused by serum bilirubin levels greater than 5 to 7 mg/dL.

breast milk j. syndrome   A relatively benign condition of increased serum bilirubin concentrations in the breastfed newborn. Bilirubin rises progressively from the fourth day of life, reading a maximum level of unconjugated bilirubin of 10–30 mg/dL by 10 to 15 days of life.

pathologic j.   Jaundice that occurs before 24 hours of life in a term infant and 48 hours in a preterm infant and is related to hyperbilirubinemia. Causes include hemolytic diseases of the newborn, injuries in which an increased volume of red blood cells are hemolyzed, hepatitis, and sepsis.

physiologic j.   An unconjugated bilirubin concentration that peaks at less than 12.9 mg/dL, with a rise in bilirubin levels of less than 5 mg/dL per day. Conjugated bilirubin levels remain less than 1.5 mg/dL. Bilirubin levels return to normal around 10 days after birth. Also called icterus neonatorum.

kangaroo care   Skin-to-skin contact between infants and parents.

karotype   Arrangement of a set of chromosomes by numerical order; used to assess actual or potential genetic alterations.

kernicterus   Neurologic syndrome that results from bilirubin toxicity. The deposition of unconjugated bilirubin in the brain can result in death or impaired function.

labia majora   Two folds or lips of the female external genital organs that arise just below the mons pubis and surround the vulva.

labia minora   Two narrow longitudinal folds enclosed in the cleft of the labia majora.

labor   Involuntary process by which the fetus and placenta are propelled from the uterus of the mother to the external environment.

first stage of l.   Process of dilation whereby the cervix opens from 0 to 10 cm or to a diameter wide enough to accommodate passage of the fetus. The first stage begins with the onset of true labor and ends when dilation is accomplished.

second stage of l.   Process that begins with the complete dilation and effacement of the cervix and ends with birth of the baby.

third stage of l.   Process that begins with the birth of the baby and ends with the expulsion of the placenta and membranes.

fourth stage of l.   Process that begins with the delivery of the placenta and membranes and ends with the initial physiologic adjustment and stabilization of the mother's body system (1 to 4 hours).

lactiferous ducts   Ducts within the female breast that convey milk to the nipple.

Ladin's sign   Softening of the anterior part of the uterus at the midline, where the uterus and cervix join; occurs at about 6 weeks of gestation; probable sign of pregnancy.

Lamaze technique   Psychoprophylactic method of childbirth preparation.

lambda   Posterior fontanelle.

lanugo   Fine, downy hair that develops on the fetus during the fourth month of gestation.

laparoscopy   Procedure performed in the early follicular phase of the menstrual cycle in which a laparoscope is inserted through the abdominal wall to the abdomen and pelvis.

large-for-gestational-age (LGA)   Birth weight that exceeds the 90th percentile for gestational age.

latent phase   Phase of labor that begins with the onset of true labor and ends when the cervix dilates to 3 cm.

lecithin:sphingomyelin ratio (L:S ratio)   Ratio of lecithin to sphingomyelin in the amniotic fluid; used to assess fetal maturity. An L:S ratio equal to or greater than 2:1 indicates fetal lung maturity.

Leopold's maneuvers   Series of four maneuvers used to determine fetal lie, presentation, position, and engagement.

lesbian   Woman whose primary erotic attractions and affectional desires are for women.

let-down reflex   *See* milk ejection reflex.

leukorrhea   Whitish or yellowish mucous discharge from the cervix or vagina.

lie   Relationship of the long axis of the fetus to the long axis of the mother; can be longitudinal, transverse, or oblique.

lightening   Descent of the presenting part of the fetus into the pelvis; occurs especially in primigravidas.

linea nigra   Line of darker pigmentation extending from the symphysis pubis to the top of the fundus; seen in some women during pregnancy.

linea terminalis   Bony line that divides the false pelvis from the true pelvis.

live birth   Birth of an infant who demonstrates signs of life such as breathing, heartbeat, and voluntary muscle movements.

lochia   Spongy layer of the decidua that is discarded as vaginal discharge during the first few days after delivery.

l. alba   Creamy yellow vaginal discharge that follows lochia serosa on about the 10th postpartum day and continues to about 3 weeks postpartum; composed of white blood cells, bacteria, decidual cells, epithelial cells, fat, cervical mucus, and cholesterol.

l. rubra   Red, blood-tinged vaginal discharge that occurs following delivery and in the first 2 to 3 days postpartum; contains primarily decidual tissue, epithelial cells, and red and white blood cells.

l. serosa   Pale, serosanguineous vaginal discharge that follows lochia rubra on about the third day after delivery and continues to about the 10th postpartum day; contains decidua, red blood cells, white blood cells, bacteria, and cervical mucus.

long-term variability   Rhythmic fluctuation in the fetal heart rate; appears as waves on the fetal heart monitor tracing.

low-birth-weight (LBW)   Neonate weighing less than 2500 g at birth.

magnetic resonance imaging (MRI)   Assessment technique that provides a computer-derived image based on the detection of energy in the nuclei of atoms within the body.

male pelvis   *See* android pelvis.

malpresentation   Abnormal presentation; occurs when the presenting part entering the inlet is other than the completely flexed head of the fetus.

mammary gland   Accessory gland of the female reproductive system that is the site of lactation during pregnancy; breast.

mammography   X-ray imaging of the breasts commonly used to screen for breast abnormalities.

masculinity   Culturally prescribed, reinforced characteristics of the male sex, independent of gender.

mastitis   Inflammation of breast tissue caused by a bacterial infection; occurs primarily in breastfeeding mothers.

maternal–infant dyad   Term used to describe the mother and neonate immediately after birth.

maternal mortality rate   Number of maternal deaths resulting from the reproductive process per 100,000 live births.

maternal sensitive period   Period immediately following birth in which complex interactions occur between mother and infant that help to bind them together.

maternal transport   Transfer of a pregnant woman from one health care facility to another for the purpose of providing her and her fetus with specialized intensive care.

maternity care   Health care provided to the childbearing family; involves physiologic, psychosocial, and cultural aspects of care.

mature gravida   Woman who gives birth after age 35.

McDonald's sign   Ability of the uterus to be easily flexed at the site where the uterus and cervix join; probable sign of pregnancy.

meconium   Fetal material that contains amniotic fluid, blood, mucus, and bile pigments that is found in the first stool of the neonate.

meconium aspiration syndrome   Condition in which the fetus aspirates or breathes fetal stool found in the amniotic fluid into the lungs or trachea, resulting in respiratory distress after delivery.

meiosis   Process during which the parent cell with 46 paired chromosomes forms four daughter cells, each with 23 unpaired chromosomes.

melasma   *See* chloasma.

menarche   First menstrual period at puberty.

Mendelian inheritance   *See* single-gene inheritance.

meningocele   Condition in which the meninges protrude from the spinal cord but the spinal cord is in correct position.

meningomyelocele   Condition in which both the meninges and the spinal cord protrude through the spinal canal.

menopause Permanent cessation of ovarian function and is defined retrospectively after there have been no menstrual periods for 12 consecutive months.

menstrual cycle Cyclic process occurring in the sexually mature female during the reproductive years that includes the ovarian cycle and the endometrial cycle.

menstrual extraction Method of pregnancy termination in which a plastic cannula is inserted into the endometrial cavity and uterine contents are removed with suction.

menstruation Shedding of the uterine lining at the end of the menstrual cycle; normal physiologic process during the reproductive years.

mentum Chin; the guiding point for face presentations, which occur when the head is in complete extension.

mesoderm Intermediate germ layer of cells found at the bottom of the primitive streak; gives rise to muscle and connective tissues and other essential organs.

metritis Puerperal uterine infection involving the endometrium, decidua, and adjacent myometrium.

microcephaly Condition in which the head and brain are abnormally small in relation to the body.

midpelvis Area between the pelvic inlet and pelvic outlet; also called the pelvic cavity.

midwife Provider of care to childbearing women; derived from *mid* meaning "with" and *wif* meaning "wife" or "women."

  certified nurse-m. Professional nurse who has completed a formal program in care of the childbearing family and who has successfully passed a certification examination.

  lay m. Person who helps women with childbirth; may have formal training or no training in childbirth practices.

midwifery Practice of assisting in childbirth.

milk ejection reflex Neurohormonal reflex that causes the ejection of breast milk through the ductal system; previously called the let-down reflex.

milia Small, white papules caused by plugging of the sebaceous glands on the nose, face, forehead, and upper torso of the neonate; a normal condition that disappears within a few weeks.

milk stools Yellow and pasty or watery stools that appear by the fourth day postdelivery.

mimicry Copying of behaviors, practices, or customs of another.

minipill Oral contraceptive pill containing only progestin.

mitosis Replicative division in which a parent cell having 46 chromosomes forms two daughter cells, each with the same number of chromosomes as the parent cell.

mittelschmerz Ovulatory pain occurring at the time of ovulation in the lower quadrant of the abdomen; a sign of ovulation.

moderately-low-birth-weight A neonate weighing between 1500 and 2499 g at birth.

molding Fetal skull changes that occur during labor and delivery; caused by accommodation of the fetal head to the maternal pelvis.

mongolian spot Irregular dark pigmented area on the posterior lumbar region; may persist until age 2. These areas have no clinical significance.

monosomy Chromosomal abnormality in which one chromosome is missing so that the human body cells contain one less than the normal complement of 46 chromosomes.

monozygotic twins Twins that originate from one zygote; also called identical twins.

mons veneris Pubic mound; pad of fatty tissue over the symphysis pubis in the female.

Montgomery glands Modified sebaceous glands on the surface of the areola that enlarge during pregnancy and lactation.

morning sickness Nausea and vomiting that occur in 50 to 80% of pregnant women; usually begins shortly after the first missed menses and ends by the 12th week of gestation. Symptoms can occur at any time of day.

Moro reflex Normal reflex in which the neonate responds to a sudden stimulus by first abducting and extending the arms symmetrically and then adducting them in an embracing movement prior to returning to a relaxed position.

morula Development stage of the ovum that occurs about the third day after fertilization; a mulberrylike mass of cells consisting of about 12 to 16 blastomeres.

mosaicism Genetic mutation that results in an unequal number of chromosomes in the cells. Some cells are normal whereas others are not.

mucous plug Mucus that blocks the cervical canal during pregnancy, acting as a barrier to protect the fetus from some infections.

multifactorial pattern of inheritance Pattern of inheritance in which the presence of multiple genes and environmental influences determines a certain genetic trait; also called non-Mendelian inheritance.

multigravid Having been pregnant more than one time.

multiparous Having had two or more pregnancies that terminated at a stage at which the fetuses were viable.

myometrium Middle layer of the uterine corpus, which is continuous with the muscular layer of the fallopian tubes and the vagina.

myotonia Muscle tension that increases throughout the body during sexual stimulation.

Nägele's rule Most common method of determining a delivery date; obtained by subtracting 3 months from the first day of the last normal menstrual period and then adding 1 year and 7 days to that date.

natural childbirth Method of childbirth in which neither analgesics nor anesthetics are used.

necrotizing entercolitis (NEC) Acute, potentially life-threatening gastrointestinal disorder in the sick newborn.

neonatal mortality rate Number of infant deaths occurring in the first 28 days of life per 1000 live births.

neonatal period First 28 days of life.

neonatal transport Transfer of a neonate from one health care facility to another, usually for the purpose of providing intensive or specialized care.

neural tube defect Group of central nervous system malformations that occur when the embryonic neural tube does not develop normally. The brain, spinal cord, and overlying tissues may be affected.

neutral thermal environmental range A range of environmental temperatures at which an individual is able to maintain a normal internal temperature with minimal metabolism and oxygen consumption for heat production.

nevus flammeus Congenital red discoloration of the skin caused by an overgrowth of the cutaneous capillaries; also called port-wine stain.

nondisjunction Failure of homologous pairs of chromosomes to separate, or the failure of two chromatids of a chromosome to split; results in an abnormal number of chromosomes in the daughter cell..

nonshivering thermogenesis A heat-generating process that increases the metabolic rate and rate of oxygen consumption in the neonate.

nonstress test (NST) Assessment technique performed in the third trimester to monitor response of the fetal heart rate to movement.

nucal translucency Opaque thickness in the neck of the fetus <3 mm.

nuclear family Family grouping generally including one or two parents and their children.

nulligravid Never having been pregnant.

nulliparous Not having delivered a child that reached viability.

nursing diagnosis Nursing judgment or conclusion referring to a potential or actual problem or strength of a client that falls within the scope of nursing intervention.

nursing process Systematic method of delivering nursing care; a problem-solving process.

obstetric conjugate True anteroposterior diameter of the pelvic inlet; usually about 11 cm.

obstetrics Branch of medicine that deals with the phenomena and management of pregnancy, labor, and the postpartum period.

occiput Region in the back of the head, behind and inferior to the posterior fontanelle.

oligohydramnios Lower-than-normal volume of amniotic fluid.

oogenesis Process of ovum cell formation.

oral contraceptive Pill taken orally to prevent pregnancy; currently among the most effective methods of reversible pregnancy prevention.

organogenesis Period of embryonic development between 4 and 8 weeks during which all major organ systems are formed.

osteoporosis Disease in which deterioration of the microarchitecture of the bone leads to a decrease in bone mass.

outcome criteria Preset client goals that are evaluated in the final step of the nursing process.

ovarian cycle Part of the menstrual cycle that consists of the follicular phase, ovulation, luteal phase, and premenstrual phase.

ovary One of two almond-shaped organs located in the upper pelvic cavity near the ends of the fallopian tubes.

oviduct *See* fallopian tubes.

ovulation Periodic release of a mature, unfertilized ovum from the ovary.

palmar erythema Redness of the palms of the hands that may occur during pregnancy because of high estrogen levels; disappears after pregnancy.

palmar grasp reflex Normal reflex in which the neonate's fingers curl around an object (such as a finger) that is pressed against the palm.

paracervical block Type of regional anesthesia in which a local anesthetic agent is injected directly into the cervix. This relieves (or "blocks") discomfort from uterine contractions and cervical dilation during labor.

parametrial cellulitis Puerperal infection that begins in the uterus and spreads into the broad ligament; may spread to the ovaries and fallopian tubes; also called parametritis.

parametritis *See* parametrial cellulitis.

paraurethral glands *See* Skene's gland.

parity Number of past pregnancies that have reached viability.

passive immunity Short-lasting immunity provided by the transfer of maternal antibodies (IgG) to the fetus in utero.

patent ductus arteriosus (PDA) Neonatal condition in which the ductus arteriosus does not close spontaneously in the first weeks of life.

patterns Sequences of behavior over time, rather than isolated instances.

pelvic cavity *See* midpelvis.

pelvic inlet Upper entrance to the true pelvis; also called the superior strait.

pelvic outlet Lower aperture of the pelvic canal; the lower border of the true pelvis.

pelvimetry Measurement of diameters or distances between the bony structures of the pelvis.

penis Male organ of copulation; deposits sperm into the vagina during sexual intercourse; also conducts urine.

percutaneous umbilical blood sampling (PUBS) Technique that provides direct access to the fetal circulation via insertion of a needle through the abdominal wall of the mother into the umbilical cord to obtain fetal blood samples.

perimenopause Period of time which includes the climacteric, menopause, and the first few years after menopause.

perimetrium Outermost serous layer of the uterus.

perinatal death Type of loss related to pregnancy and fertility, including spontaneous abortion, missed abortion, fetal death, and neonatal death.

perinatal mortality rate Number of stillbirths plus number of neonatal deaths per 1000 live births.

perinatal nursing Practice of professional nursing in response to the needs of the high-risk or low-risk family through the prenatal, intrapartum, postpartum, and neonatal periods.

perinatal period Period extending from the 20th week of gestation through the 28th day of neonatal life.

perinatal transmission Transmission of an infection from the mother to the fetus during pregnancy.

perineum Area between the vagina and the anus.

periodic breathing Breathing pattern in which the neonate has 5- to 10-second periods of apnea, followed by periods of 10 to 15 seconds in which the respiratory rate is 50 to 60 breaths per minute; commonly seen in preterm neonates.

peritonitis Inflammation of the peritoneum.

pernicious vomiting of pregnancy *See* hyperemesis gravidarum.

petechiae Tiny hemorrhagic spots on the skin that result from increased intravascular pressure in the capillaries during delivery.

phase of maximum slope Greatest increase in the rate of cervical dilation in which dilation averages 3 cm an hour.

phenotype Characteristics or appearance of an individual that results from interaction of a genotype and environmental factors.

phenylketonuria (PKU) Inborn error of metabolism transmitted by an autosomal recessive trait that causes excess phenylalanine to build up in the body. If not treated, PKU can result in brain damage and mental retardation.

physical recovery phase Period from birth to 1 month during which biologic adaptation dominates as the mother recovers from birthing and the neonate makes the transition to the external world.

physiologic retraction ring   Area of constriction that develops in normal labor between the upper active segment of the uterus and the lower more passive segment of the uterus.

pica   Unusual craving for nonfood or nonnutritive substances that may occur as a result of emotional disturbances, malnutrition, or pregnancy.

Piskacek's sign   Uterine asymmetry in the cornual area of uterus occurring early in pregnancy.

placental membrane   Multiple-layer membrane of fetal tissue composing the chorionic villi.

placenta previa   Implantation of the placenta over or very near the cervical os.

placing reflex   Normal reflex action in which the neonate flexes the knees and hips and moves the legs upward when positioned upright with the dorsal surface of the feet placed against the edge of the table.

planning   Third phase of the nursing process that involves setting goals, prioritizing, and designing methods to resolve problems and reach goals.

plantar grasp reflex   Normal reflex in which the neonate's toes curl downward in response to pressure at the base of the toes.

platypelloid pelvis   Pelvis characterized by the inlet being oval with a wide transverse diameter and a short anteroposterior diameter.

point of viability   Point at which the fetus can reasonably survive outside of the uterus; usually considered to be 20 weeks of gestation.

polycythemia   Condition in which there is a surplus of red blood cells in the circulation.

polydactyly   Presence of extra digits on the hands or feet.

polyhydramnios   Excessive quantity of amniotic fluid, usually greater than 2000 mL; also called hydramnios.

port-wine stain   *See* nevus flammeus.

position   Relationship of landmarks (denominators) of the fetal presenting part to the sides, front, or back of the maternal pelvis.

postcoital test   Diagnostic procedure in which the cervical mucus is examined 6 hours after intercourse during the period of ovulation to determine the integrity of the mucus and assess for the presence of sperm; also called Sims–Huhner test.

postdate neonate   *See* postmature neonate.

postmature neonate   Baby born after the end of 42 weeks of gestation; also called postdate neonate.

postovulation method   Method of pregnancy prevention in which a couple abstains from intercourse after the occurrence of ovulation has been determined.

postpartum blues (transient depression)   Temporary and self-limiting depression usually beginning 3 to 10 days after delivery. The cause(s) is unknown. The time frame is unclear; it may last a few hours to 2 to 3 weeks. It is characterized by altered mood, anxiety, and tearfulness and is usually unrelated to actual circumstances.

postpartum depression   Depressive state that may occur during pregnancy but more often occurs in weeks or months following delivery. Considered a nonpsychotic depressive syndrome, it is characterized by mood instability, fatigue, appetite and sleep disturbances, feelings of isolation and hopelessness, difficulties in interpersonal relationships, and negative emotions while with the infant.

postpartum hemorrhage   Hemorrhage occurring from birth canal after third stage of labor in vaginal delivery. Early postpartum hemorrhage occurs within 24 hours of delivery; late postpartum hemorrhage occurs from 24 hours to 6 weeks after delivery.

postpartum period   First 6 to 8 weeks after birth during which the woman undergoes physiologic changes and psychologic restoration and the parents develop a relationship with their infant.

postpartum psychosis   Severe psychiatric condition that occurs in the puerperium, but may begin in the third trimester, and is characterized by delusions, hallucinations, and disorganized or withdrawn behavior.

postterm pregnancy   Pregnancy that continues past the estimated date of delivery (beyond 42 weeks of gestation).

preeclampsia   Progressive form of pregnancy-induced hypertension characterized by proteinuria and/or generalized edema that occurs initially after 20 weeks of gestation; also called toxemia of pregnancy. Mild forms of the disorder can quickly become severe and critical.

preembryonic period   First 14 days after conception; characterized by rapid cellular multiplication and differentiation, establishment of embryonic membranes, and development of primary germ layers.

pregnancy-induced hypertension Conditions characterized by an abnormal rise in blood pressure during pregnancy or postpartum; may be accompanied by edema, proteinuria, and hyperreflexia; may progress to eclampsia.

premature ejaculation Untimely ejaculation.

premature neonate Neonate born before the end of 37 weeks of gestation.

premenstrual syndrome (PMS) Syndrome of physical, emotional, and behavioral symptoms that can occur during the luteal phase of the menstrual cycle and can decrease or disappear at the start, or shortly after the start, of menstruation.

prenatal attachment Maternal behaviors related to the developing relationship with the fetus; includes calling the fetus by name, imagining what the fetus looks like, imagining the role of mother, and choosing names.

presentation Denotes the part of the fetus that is closest to the pelvic inlet of the mother.

brow p. Presentation in which the fetal head is partially extended and the presenting part is the brow.

complete breech p. Presentation in which the fetus presents buttocks first with flexion at both hips and knees.

compound p. Presentation in which more than one part of the fetus presents, for example, the head and an arm.

face p. Presentation in which the fetal head is completely extended with the widest part of the face presenting for delivery.

footling breech p. Presentation in which the presenting part is one or both feet with extension at both hips and knees; also called incomplete presentation.

frank breech p. Presentation in which the buttocks present with the thighs flexed and the legs extended over the anterior surface of the fetal body.

shoulder p. Presentation in which the long axis of the fetus is perpendicular to the long axis of the mother; also called transverse lie.

vertex p. Most efficient type of fetal presentation. The head is flexed and the occiput is the presenting part.

preterm birth Delivery of a neonate after the age of viability but before the completion of 37 weeks of gestation.

preterm labor Any true labor experienced between 20 and 38 weeks of gestation.

primary infertility Inability to conceive with no previous history of pregnancy.

primigravid Pregnant for the first time.

primiparous Having one pregnancy that terminated at the stage when the child was viable.

primitive reflexes Those reflexes that assist a newborn's safety and survival; for example, sucking and rooting.

primitive streak Groove that appears on the ectoderm of the embryonic disc at the end of the second week of development.

professional health care system Provision of health care by a group of health care professionals who have been educated through formal programs of professional education.

prostaglandin instillation Method of terminating a pregnancy around 15 weeks of gestation in which prostaglandins are administered intravaginally or intraabdominally, causing uterine contractions to empty the uterus.

prostate gland Gland located beneath the bladder in the male that secretes the milky fluid that is added to semen.

proteinuria Presence of 300 mg or more of serum protein in the urine.

proximodistal Proceeding from the central axis of the body and moving outward toward the extremities.

psychoprophylaxis Training of mind and body to cope with stressful stimuli; a childbirth preparation technique.

ptyalism Excessive salivation; often occurs during the first trimester.

puberty Developmental phase in males and females that results in physical maturity and the capacity to reproduce.

pudendal block Type of regional anesthesia in which a local anesthetic is injected in the area of the pudendal nerves. This relieves (or "blocks") sensations around the vagina.

puerperal fever *See* puerperal infection.

puerperal infection Bacterial infection that arises in the genital tract after delivery; also called puerperal fever.

puerperal morbidity Infection as demonstrated by a temperature of 100.4° (38°C) or higher on any 2 of the first 10 days postpartum (exclusive of the first 24 hours).

puerperium First 6 weeks after delivery during which the woman's body undergoes multiple physiologic changes in response to childbirth.

quickening Mother's first perception of fetal movements; usually occurs between 17 and 20 weeks of gestation.

recessive Gene that is present but not expressed by the individual.

reconstituted family Family that consists of remarried adults with children from the husband's and/or the wife's previous marriage.

REEDA An acronym created to evaluate episiotomy healing: Redness, Edema, Ecchymosis, Discharge, and Approximation.

regionalization Method of organizing services within a geographic area or health delivery network so that maternal and perinatal health care is maximally used in the safest and most cost-effective way.

reorganization phase Period that begins around 8 months postpartum and continues beyond 12 months during which maternal biologic, psychologic, and social adaptation is evident. The mother individuates and returns to prepregnancy activities. The infant continues to grow, develop, and master the environment.

respiratory distress syndrome (RDS) Pulmonary disorder in which the lungs lack the pulmonary surfactants required for respiration; occurs most often in preterm neonates; also called hyaline membrane disease.

restitution Turning of the fetal head after it emerges from the birth canal back to the position it assumed when it first entered the pelvis; restores anatomic alignment of the neck and shoulders.

retinopathy of prematurity (ROP) Disease process that occurs in the blood vessels in the retina of the eyes and can lead to significant vision impairment.

retrocession Displacement of the uterus in which both the cervix and corpus bend backward toward the sacrum.

retroflexion Displacement of the uterus in which the corpus bends back toward the cervix, resulting in a sharp angle.

retrograde ejaculation Condition in which the sperm flows backward into the bladder instead of out of the penis.

retroversion Displacement of the uterus in which the uterus tips backward so that the uterine fundus is lying in the pouch of Douglas instead of anteriorly on the bladder.

Rh isoimmunization Hemolytic disease arising from incompatibility of Rh factors of maternal and fetal blood which causes an antigen–antibody reaction.

rooting reflex Normal reflex in which stroking the neonate's cheek, lip, or mouth causes the neonate to turn his or her head in the direction of the stimulus.

round ligaments Ligaments found on either side of the fundus that are continuous with the ovarian ligaments and extend into the broad ligament.

rupture of membranes Tearing of the amniotic membranes prior to or during labor; may be spontaneous or artificial.

    artificial r.o.m. Intentional rupture of the amniotic membranes during labor through the use of an instrument such as an amnihook. Also called amniotomy.

    premature r.o.m. Spontaneous rupture of the amniotic membranes before the onset of active labor and contractions.

    spontaneous r.o.m. Natural tearing of the amniotic membranes.

saline termination Method of terminating a pregnancy after 16 weeks of gestation in which saline solution is injected into the amniotic sac, causing uterine contractions that expel the products of conception.

same-sex family Family that consists of two adults of the same sex with or without children.

scrotum Pouchlike structure divided in the middle by a septum, forming two sacs, each containing one testis, one epididymis, and part of the spermatic cord.

secondary infertility Inability to conceive after one or more successful pregnancies.

semen Fluid ejaculated from the erect penis that contains sperm and secretions of the accessory glands and epididymis.

seminal vesicle Pouchlike structure that joins the end of each ductus deferens to become the ejaculatory ducts.

seminiferous tubule Tubule of the testes that carries sperm.

separation–individuation Process by which the infant separates psychologically from the mother to become an autonomous individual.

septate uterus *See* bicornate uterus.

septic pelvic thrombophlebitis Puerperal infection that originates in the uterus and spreads along the venous route into the pelvis; causes thrombosis within the veins, which fosters growth of bacteria.

sex role behaviors Behaviors assigned to men and women on the basis of gender.

sexuality Part of life that has to do with being male or female.

sexually transmitted disease (STD) Category of disease transmitted through sexual intercourse and intimate sexual contact with the genitals, mouth, or rectum.

short-term variability Normal variation between successive cardiac cycles; the change in fetal heart monitoring from one beat to the next.

shoulder dystocia Difficult labor that occurs when the anterior shoulder of the fetus becomes impacted behind the symphysis pubis.

sickle-cell anemia Genetically transmitted hemoglobinopathy in which valine is substituted for glutamine at position 6 on the beta chain of the hemoglobin molecule. This causes the hemoglobin molecules to assume a sickle shape and results in blood flow impairment that can lead to organ failure.

Sims-Huhner test *See* postcoital test.

single-gene inheritance Pattern of inheritance in which the presence of one gene can cause the expression of a certain trait; also called Mendelian inheritance. There are four types of single-gene inheritance: autosomal dominant, autosomal recessive, X-linked dominant, and X-linked recessive.

single-parent family Family that consists of one parent raising children as a result of separation, divorce, death, or being unmarried.

Skene's gland Paraurethral gland; one of numerous mucous glands in the wall of the female urethra.

small-for-gestational-age (SGA) Birth weight below the tenth percentile for gestational age.

spermatic cord Structure that contains the vas deferens, blood vessels, nerves, and muscle fibers and supports the testes within the scrotum.

spermatogenesis Process by which spermatogonia, fetal sperm cells, are transformed into spermatozoa, or mature sperm.

spermicidal agent Chemical substance that destroys sperm; used as a contraceptive method.

spina bifida occulta Condition in which the vertebral laminae do not fuse in an isolated area of the spine.

spinal block *See* anesthesia, spinal.

spinal headache Severe headache often associated with neck stiffness when the woman is upright. A potential side effect of spinal anesthesia.

spinnbarkeit Elasticity of the cervical mucus present at ovulation.

squamocolumnar junction Location in the cervical canal where squamous epithelium cells meet columnar epithelium cells. The exact location will vary according to a woman's age and number of deliveries.

station Relationship of the presenting part of the fetus to an imaginary line drawn between the pelvic ischial spines.

stepping reflex Normal steplike movements of the feet and legs elicited by holding the neonate in an upright position and allowing one foot to touch a flat surface.

sterility Absolute inability to conceive; state of being free of living microorganisms.

stillbirth An infant past the point of viability who is born dead.

stork bites *See* telangiectatic nevi.

striae gravidarum Reddish or purple streaks that develop in the skin over the maternal abdomen, breasts, thighs, and hips; also called stretch marks.

subinvolution Delay or failure of the uterus to return to normal size in the postpartum period.

sucking reflex Normal reflex present in a term neonate that is stimulated by hunger or the rooting reflex.

superficial thrombophlebitis Inflammatory process involving clot formation within a superficial vein.

superior strait *See* pelvic inlet.

supine hypotensive syndrome Decrease in venous return from the lower portion of the body caused by a heavy uterus pressing on the inferior vena cava and abdominal aorta, resulting in arterial hypotension; also called vena caval syndrome.

surfactant Phospholipid that maintains alveolar patency and lowers surface tension in the lungs.

sutures Connection of adjoining bones of the skull. In the fetus, these are membrane-filled spaces.

> **coronal s.** Membrane-occupied space found between the parietal and frontal bones, extending transversely on both sides of the anterior fontanelle.

> **frontal s.** Membrane-occupied space between the two frontal bones.

> **lambdoidal s.** Membrane-occupied space between the occipital bone and the two parietal bones, extending transversely on either side of the posterior fontanelle.

> **sagittal s.** Membrane-occupied space between the parietal bones that follows the anteroposterior direction of the skull.

swallowing reflex Normal reflex present in the newborn that involves the transfer of oral feedings from the mouth to the esophagus.

symptothermal method Pregnancy prevention method in which basal body temperature is taken daily and cervical mucus is assessed daily to predict ovulation.

syncytial membrane Thin membrane that results from changes in the placental membrane; lies in close proximity to fetal circulatory network.

syndactyly Malformation in which fingers or toes are webbed or fused together.

telangiectasis Small dilated end-arterioles thought to be related to increased estrogen production during pregnancy; also called vascular spiders.

telangiectatic nevi Capillary hemangiomas found on a newborn's neck, eyelids, forehead, and nose; also called stork bites.

testes Two oval-shaped organs located in the scrotum in which testosterone and sperm are produced.

thalassemia Form of anemia that results from an alteration in the gene normally controlling the rate of polypeptide chain synthesis; a hypochromic microcytic anemia.

therapeutic decision making Component of clinical reasoning used by nurses when they plan and implement nursing care.

thrush Fungal infection caused by *Candida albicans* and characterized by small white patches on the tongue and buccal membranes.

tonic neck reflex Normal reflex elicited by turning the neonate's head to one side. The extremities on the same side extend and the extremities on the opposite side flex; also called fencing position.

total abstinence Complete avoidance of intercourse to prevent pregnancy.

toxemia of pregnancy *See* preeclampsia.

toxic shock syndrome Acute illness caused by a toxin produced by a strain of the *Staphylococcus aureus* bacterium.

transcultural nursing Nursing care that recognizes and respects the way in which different cultures perceive, know, and practice health care.

transitional stools Watery or loose, greenish brown to yellow brown stools that appear by the third day postdelivery.

transverse lie *See* shoulder presentation.

trisomy Chromosomal abnormality in which three homologous chromosomes are present rather than the normal two.

trisomy 21 Most common numerical autosomal abnormality in which there are three number 21 chromosomes instead of two; also called Down syndrome. The affected infant is characterized by mental retardation and mongoloid features.

trophoblast Outer layer of cells of the developing blastocyst that will establish the nutrient relationship with the uterine endometrium.

true conjugate Measurement from the upper margin of the symphysis pubis to the sacral promontory.

true pelvis Area of the pelvis located below the linea terminalis. The upper portion is bounded by the sacral promontory, linea terminalis, and upper margins of the pubic bones; the lower part is bounded by the margins of the ischial tuberosities and the end of the coccyx.

trunk incurvation *See* Galant's reflex.

Turner's syndrome Genetic abnormality in which a female has only one X chromosome. Nondisjunction during spermatogenesis results in the absence of the paternal X chromosome.

ultrasound Technique that involves the use of high-frequency (greater than 20,000 Hz) sound waves.

urethra Tubular passageway for urine in the female and for urine and sperm in the male.

urethral meatus External opening of the urethra.

uterine cycle *See* endometrial cycle.

uteroplacental apoplexy *See* Couvelaire uterus.

uterosacral ligaments Ligaments extending from the supravaginal portion of the cervix to the sacrum. They support the corpus and cervix, keeping the uterus in the anterior position.

uterus   Pear-shaped muscular organ that, in the nonpregnant woman, is located between the urinary bladder and the rectum.

vaccum aspiration   Method of terminating a pregnancy of less than 12 to 13 weeks in which a cannula is inserted into the uterus and the uterine contents are withdrawn using suction.

vagina   Musculomembranous tube extending from the uterus to the vulva and measuring 10 cm in length. It is located between the rectum and bladder.

vaginal birth after cesarean (VBAC)   Vaginal birth of an infant to a woman who has had at least one previous cesarean delivery.

vascular spiders   *See* telangiectasis.

vas deferens   *See* ductus deferens.

vasectomy   Method of male sterilization accomplished with a surgical procedure during which both vasa are isolated, cut, and tied.

vasocongestion   Pooling of blood causing enlargement of a body area.

vernix caseosa   Fatty secretion from fetal sebaceous glands and epidermal cells that covers the fetus, protecting the skin from abrasions or damage in utero.

vertex   Area of the head between the anterior and posterior fontanelles and bounded laterally by the parietal bones.

very-low-birth-weight (VLBW)   Neonate weighing less than 1500 g at birth.

vulva   External female genitalia, including the mons veneris, labia majora, labia minora, clitoris, and vestibule.

Wharton's jelly   Connective tissue rich in mucopolysaccharides surrounding and protecting the blood vessels in the umbilical cord.

yolk sac   Structure that transfers nutrients to the embryo while the uteroplacental circulation is being established and provides blood cells until embryonic/fetal hemopoiesis begins.

zygote   One-celled animal formed by the union of the sperm and ovum.

zygote intrafallopian transfer (ZIFT)   Combination of IVF and GIFT in which the ova are fertilized in the laboratory and then transported to the fallopian tube for development and transport to the uterus.

index

Page numbers in *italics* denote figures; those followed by "t" denote tables.

Temperature Equivalents

CELSIUS (C°)	FAHRENHEIT (F°)	CELSIUS (C°)	FAHRENHEIT (F°)
34.0	93.2	38.6	101.4
34.2	93.6	38.8	101.8
34.4	93.9	39.0	102.2
34.6	94.3	39.2	102.5
34.8	94.6	39.4	102.9
35.0	95.0	39.6	103.2
35.2	95.4	39.8	103.6
35.4	95.7	40.0	104.0
35.6	96.1	40.2	104.3
35.8	96.4	40.4	104.7
36.0	96.8	40.6	105.1
36.2	97.1	40.8	105.4
36.4	97.5	41.0	105.8
36.6	97.8	41.2	106.1
36.8	98.2	41.4	106.5
37.0	**98.6**	41.6	106.8
37.2	98.9	41.8	107.2
37.4	99.3	42.0	107.6
37.6	99.6	42.2	108.0
37.8	100.0	42.4	108.3
38.0	100.4	42.6	108.7
38.2	100.7	42.8	109.0
38.4	101.0	43.0	109.4

Conversion of Celsius (Centigrade) to Fahrenheit: (9/5 × temperature) + 32
Conversion of Fahrenheit to Celsius (Centigrade): (Temperature − 32) × 5/9

Weight Equivalents (Conversion of Pounds and Ounces to Grams)

							OUNCES									
POUNDS	0	1	2	3	4	5	6	7	8	9	10	11	12	13	14	15
0	—	28	57	85	113	142	170	198	227	255	283	312	340	369	397	425
1	454	482	510	539	567	595	624	652	680	709	737	765	794	822	850	879
2	907	936	964	992	1021	1049	1077	1106	1134	1162	1191	1219	1247	1276	1304	1332
3	1361	1389	1417	1446	1474	1503	1531	1559	1588	1616	1644	1673	1701	1729	1758	1786
4	1814	1843	1871	1899	1928	1956	1984	2013	2041	2070	2098	2126	2155	2183	2211	2240
5	2268	2296	2325	2353	2381	2410	2438	2466	2495	2523	2551	2580	2608	2637	2665	2693
6	2722	2750	2778	2807	2835	2863	2892	2920	2948	2977	3005	3033	3062	3090	3118	3147
7	3175	3203	3232	3260	3289	3317	3345	3374	3402	3430	3459	3487	3515	3544	3572	3600
8	3629	3657	3685	3714	3742	3770	3799	3827	3856	3884	3912	3941	3969	3997	4026	4054
9	4082	4111	4139	4167	4196	4224	4252	4281	4309	4337	4366	4394	4423	4451	4479	4508
10	4536	4564	4593	4621	4649	4678	4706	4734	4763	4791	4819	4848	4876	4904	4933	4961
11	4990	5018	5046	5075	5103	5131	5160	5188	5216	5245	5273	5301	5330	5358	5386	5415
12	5443	5471	5500	5528	5557	5585	5613	5642	5670	5698	5727	5755	5783	5812	5840	5868
13	5897	5925	5953	5982	6010	6038	6067	6095	6123	6152	6180	6209	6237	6265	6294	6322
14	6350	6379	6407	6435	6464	6492	6520	6549	6577	6605	6634	6662	6690	6719	6747	6776
15	6804	6832	6860	6889	6917	6945	6973	7002	7030	7059	7087	7115	7144	7172	7201	7228
16	7257	7286	7313	7342	7371	7399	7427	7456	7484	7512	7541	7569	7597	7626	7654	7682
17	7711	7739	7768	7796	7824	7853	7881	7909	7938	7966	7994	8023	8051	8079	8108	8136
18	8165	8192	8221	8249	8278	8306	8335	8363	8391	8420	8448	8476	8504	8533	8561	8590
19	8618	8646	8675	8703	8731	8760	8788	8816	8845	8873	8902	8930	8958	8987	9015	9043
20	9072	9100	9128	9157	9185	9213	9242	9270	9298	9327	9355	9383	9412	9440	9469	9497
21	9525	9554	9582	9610	9639	9667	9695	9724	9752	9780	9809	9837	9865	9894	9922	9950
22	9979	10007	10036	10064	10092	10120	10149	10177	10206	10234	10262	10291	10319	10347	10376	10404

Conversion of pounds and ounces to grams: (Pounds × 453.6) + (ounces × 28.35)
Conversion of grams into ounces (16 oz = 1 lb): Grams + 28.35